CONTENTS

Critical Care Nursing

Diagnosis and Management 8th edition

Linda D. Urden, DNSc, RN, CNS, NE-BC, FAAN

Professor and Director
Master's, Healthcare Informatics and International Nursing Programs
Hahn School of Nursing and Health Science
Beyster Institute for Nursing Research, Advanced Practice and Simulation
University of San Diego
San Diego, California

Kathleen M. Stacy, PhD, RN, CNS, CCRN, PCCN, CCNS

Critical Care Clinical Nurse Specialist
Clinical Associate Professor
Hahn School of Nursing and Health Science
Beyster Institute for Nursing Research, Advanced Practice and Simulation
University of San Diego
San Diego, California

Mary E. Lough, PhD, RN, CCRN, CNRN, CCNS, FCCM

Critical Care Clinical Nurse Specialist
Stanford Health Care
Clinical Assistant Professor
Stanford University
Stanford, California

ELSEVIER

ELSEVIER

3251 Riverport Lane
Maryland Heights, Missouri 63043

Notices

ISBN: 978-0-323-44752-2

Executive Content Strategist: Lee Henderson
Content Development Manager: Lisa Newton
Content Development Specialist: Melissa Rawe
Publishing Services Manager: Jeff Patterson
Project Manager: Anne Konopka
Designer: Amy Buxton

Printed in Canada.

Last digit is the print number: 9   8   7   6   5   4   3   2   1

Working together
to grow libraries in
developing countries

www.elsevier.com • www.bookaid.org

To future and current critical care nurses—may you always focus on caring and integration of evidence principles in your practice!

LDU

To my Dad with love!
Thank you for encouraging me to do my best!

KMS

Thank you to my family—Jim, Madeleine, and Michael—for all your support and love in a wildly tumultuous year.

MEL

Linda D. Urden, DNSc, RN, CNS, NE-BC, FAAN

Linda Urden received her diploma in nursing from Barnes Hospital School of Nursing, St. Louis, Missouri; her BSN from Pepperdine University, Malibu, California; her MN, Cardiovascular Clinical Nurse Specialist, from UCLA; and her DNSc from the University of San Diego. She is doubly credentialed as a clinical nurse specialist and in Executive Nursing by the American Nurses Credentialing Center and is a Fellow in the American Academy of Nursing. Linda has held a variety of clinical and administrative positions, with accountabilities for quality, evidence-based practice, research, education, and advanced practice. In her various positions, she has striven to create cultures that are sensitive to differentiated practice and ensure healthy work environments supporting excellence in nursing practice. In addition to this text, Linda coauthored *Priorities in Critical Care Nursing*. Other publications are in the areas of heart failure, ethics, research, outcomes measurement, management and care delivery redesign, executive decision support databases, collaborative practice models, clinical nurse specialist outcomes, and Magnet environments. Her research integrates clinical, fiscal, quality, and behavioral outcomes of care delivery and services. In addition, she is a member of editorial boards and is a peer reviewer for several nursing journals.

Kathleen M. Stacy, PhD, RN, CNS, CCRN, PCCN, CCNS

Kathleen Stacy has been a nurse for 38 years, the majority of which she has spent working in critical care. She graduated in 1978 with a BS in nursing from the State University of New York at Plattsburgh, in 1989 with an MS in critical care nursing from San Diego State University, and in 2010 with a PhD in nursing from University of San Diego. She has held a variety of positions, including staff nurse, clinical educator, outcomes manager, nurse manager, and clinical nurse specialist. Currently Kathleen is a clinical associate professor at the Hahn School of Nursing and Health Science at University of San Diego. Her research focus is on quality, patient safety, and palliative care. In addition to this text, Kathleen coauthored *Priorities in Critical Care Nursing*.

Mary E. Lough, PhD, RN, CCRN, CNRN, CCNS, FCCM

Mary Lough is a critical care nurse with more than 30 years of experience as a staff nurse, educator, and clinical nurse specialist. Mary received her BSN from the University of Manchester in England and her MS and PhD from the University of California, San Francisco (UCSF). Mary is the clinical nurse specialist for the medical/surgical/neuroscience/trauma ICU at Stanford Health Care in Palo Alto, California. She holds a clinical faculty position in the Medical School at Stanford University. She is also a clinical professor in the Department of Physiological Nursing at her alma mater, UCSF. Mary is very active with the American Association of Critical Care Nurses (AACN) and is a fellow of the Society of Critical Care Medicine (SCCM).

Mary has been involved with all eight editions of *Critical Care Nursing: Diagnosis and Management*, and she has published many other articles and research abstracts. As a clinician, Mary appreciates the benefits of a clinically grounded textbook because when she began her career as a critical care nurse so little information was available.

Deanne A. Blach, MSN, RN
Nurse Educator, Conference Chair, and Primary Nurse Planner
DB Productions of NW AR, Inc.
Green Forest, Arkansas
Concept Map Illustrator

Darlene M. Burke, PhD, MS, MA, RN
Lecturer, School of Nursing
San Diego State University
San Diego, California;
Associate Professor, Nursing & Allied Health
MiraCosta College
Oceanside, California
*Chapter 22, Neurologic Clinical Assessment and Diagnostic
Procedures*

Beverly Carlson, PhD, RN, CNS, CCRN-K, FAHA
Assistant Professor
School of Nursing
San Diego State University
San Diego, California
*Chapter 34, Shock, Sepsis, and Multiple Organ Dysfunction
Syndrome*

Jacqueline F. Close, PhD, APRN
Clinical Associate Professor
University of San Diego
San Diego, California
*Chapter 28, Gastrointestinal Clinical Assessment and Diagnostic
Procedures*
*Chapter 29, Gastrointestinal Disorders and Therapeutic
Management*

Kelly K. Dineen, RN, JD, PhD
Assistant Professor
Saint Louis University School of Law & Center for
Health Care Ethics
St. Louis, Missouri
Chapter 2, Ethical Issues
Chapter 3, Legal Issues

Joni L. Dirks, MS, RN-BC, CCRN
Manager Clinical Educators and ICU Educator
Providence Urban Hospitals
Spokane, Washington
Chapter 15, Cardiovascular Therapeutic Management

Caroline Etland, PhD, RN, CNS, AOCN, ACHPN
Director of Education, Research, and Professional Practice
Department of Nursing
Bioethics Consultant
Sharp Chula Vista Medical Center
Chula Vista, California
Chapter 10, End-of-Life Care

Lorraine Fitzsimmons, PhD, APRN, FNP, ANP-BC
Chair, Advanced Practice Nursing of Adults and Elderly
Director, Adult-Gerontology NP Program
San Diego State University School of Nursing
San Diego, California
*Chapter 34, Shock, Sepsis, and Multiple Organ Dysfunction
Syndrome*

Céline Gélinas, PhD, RN
Associate Professor
Ingram School of Nursing
McGill University;
Researcher
Centre for Nursing Research and Lady Davis Institute for
Medical Research
Jewish General Hospital
Montreal, Quebec, Canada
Chapter 8, Pain and Pain Management

Inna Goldvarg-Abud, FNP-C, MSN
Liver Transplant and Liver Clinic Nurse Practitioner
Ochsner Multi-Organ Transplant Institute
New Orleans, Louisiana
Chapter 36, Organ Donation and Transplantation

Margaret Jordan Halter, PhD, APRN
Editor, *Foundations of Psychiatric Mental Health Nursing*;
Adjunct Faculty
College of Nursing
Ohio State University
Columbus, Ohio,
Clinical Nurse Specialist
Cleveland Clinic Akron General
Akron, Ohio
Chapter 6, Psychosocial Alternations and Management

Christine Hartley, MS, RN, ACNP-BC
Nurse Practitioner
Critical Care Services
Stanford Health Care
Stanford, California
Chapter 36, Organ Donation and Transplantation

Annette Haynes, MS, RN, CNS, CCRN
Cardiology Clinical Nurse Specialist
Stanford Health Care
Stanford, California
Chapter 14, Cardiovascular Disorders

Susie Hutchins, DNP, RN, CNE
Associate Professor
MEPN Coordinator of Simulation
University of San Diego
Hahn School of Nursing and Health Science
San Diego, California
Chapter 38, The Obstetric Patient

Lourdes Januszewicz, MSN, RN, CNS, CCRN
Clinical Nurse Specialist
District Stroke Program Coordinator
Palomar Health
Escondido, California
Chapter 23, Neurologic Disorders and Therapeutic Management

Misty Jenkins, MSN, APRN, ACNP-BC, CCRN
Acute Care Nurse Practitioner, Pulmonary Critical Care
Ochsner Medical Center, New Orleans
New Orleans, Louisiana
Chapter 40, The Older Adult Patient

Cynthia A. Lewis, RN, MS, CNS, CPN
Pediatric Clinical Nurse Specialist
Medical and Pulmonary Units
Rady Children's Hospital San Diego
San Diego, California
Chapter 39, The Pediatric Patient

Mary E. Lough, PhD, RN, CCRN, CNRN, CCNS, FCCM
Critical Care Clinical Nurse Specialist
Stanford Health Care
Clinical Assistant Professor
Stanford University
Stanford, California;
Clinical Professor
Department of Physiological Nursing
University of California, San Francisco (UCSF)
San Francisco, California
Chapter 4, Genetic Issues
Chapter 9, Sedation, Agitation, and Delirium Management
Chapter 11, Cardiovascular Anatomy and Physiology
Chapter 12, Cardiovascular Clinical Assessment
Chapter 13, Cardiovascular Diagnostic Procedures
Chapter 24, Kidney Anatomy and Physiology
*Chapter 25, Kidney Clinical Assessment and Diagnostic
    Procedures*
Chapter 26, Kidney Disorders and Therapeutic Management
Chapter 30, Endocrine Anatomy and Physiology
*Chapter 31, Endocrine Clinical Assessment and Diagnostic
    Procedures*
Chapter 32, Endocrine Disorders and Therapeutic Management
Chapter 36, Organ Donation and Transplantation

Jeanne M. Maiden, PhD, RN, CNS-BC
Associate Dean and Professor
Director Graduate Program of Nursing
School of Nursing
Point Loma Nazarene University
San Diego, California
Chapter 18, Pulmonary Diagnostic Procedures

Kasuen Mauldin, PhD, RD
Assistant Professor
Nutrition, Food Science, and Packaging
San Jose State University
San Jose, California
Chapter 7, Nutrition Alterations and Management

Barbara Mayer, PhD, MS, RN, CNS
Director of Nursing Quality
Stanford Health Care
Stanford, California
Chapter 5, Patient and Family Education

Eugene E. Mondor, RN, BScN, MN, CNCC(C)
Clinical Nurse Educator–Adult Critical Care
Royal Alexandra Hospital
Edmonton, Alberta, Canada
Chapter 33, Trauma

Robyn Myers, RN, CPNP, WCC
Pediatric Nurse Practitioner
Washington University
St. Louis Children's Hospital
St. Louis, Missouri
Chapter 35, Burns

Denise O'Brien, DNP, RN, ACNS-BC, CPAN, CAPA, FAAN
Perianesthesia Clinical Nurse Specialist
Department of Operating Rooms/PACU
University of Michigan Hospitals & Health Centers
Adjunct Clinical Instructor
University of Michigan School of Nursing
Ann Arbor, Michigan
Chapter 41, The Perianesthesia Patient

Carrie J. Scotto, PhD, RN
Associate Professor
School of Nursing
University of Akron
Arkon, Ohio
Chapter 6, Psychosocial Alternations and Management

Jennifer Seigel, RN, CPNP, CWCN
Pediatric Nurse Practitioner
Washington University
St. Louis Children's Hospital
St. Louis, Missouri
Chapter 35, Burns

Teresa J. Shafer, RN, MSN, CPTC
President, Texas Transplantation Society;
Associate Editor, *Progress in Transplantation*;
Expert Reviewer, Transplant Library, Center for Evidence in
    Transplantation, Royal College of Surgeons of England
Fort Worth, Texas
Chapter 36, Organ Donation and Transplantation

Kathleen M. Stacy, PhD, RN, CNS, CCRN, PCCN, CCNS
Critical Care Clinical Nurse Specialist
Clinical Associate Professor
Hahn School of Nursing and Health Science
Beyster Institute for Nursing Research, Advanced Practice and
    Simulation
University of San Diego
San Diego, California
Chapter 16, Pulmonary Anatomy and Physiology
Chapter 17, Pulmonary Clinical Assessment
Chapter 19, Pulmonary Disorders
Chapter 20, Pulmonary Therapeutic Management
Chapter 21, Neurologic Anatomy and Physiology
Chapter 27, Gastrointestinal Anatomy and Physiology

Carol A. Suarez, MSN, RN, CNS, PHN, FNP
Clinical Nurse Specialist
Pulmonary Progressive Care Unit & Medical Acute Care Unit
Palomar Pomerado Health
Escondido, California
Chapter 37, Hematologic Disorders and Oncologic Emergencies

Linda D. Urden, DNSc, RN, CNS, NE-BC, FAAN
Professor and Director
Master's, Healthcare Informatics and International Nursing
    Programs
Hahn School of Nursing and Health Science
Beyster Institute for Nursing Research, Advanced Practice and
    Simulation
University of San Diego
San Diego, California
Chapter 1, Critical Care Nursing Practice

Julie M. Waters, MS, RN, CCRN
Clinical Nurse Educator for CICU
Sacred Heart Medical Center
Spokane, Washington
Chapter 15, Cardiovascular Therapeutic Management

Schawnté Williams-Taylor, BSN, RN, CCRN, CPTC
Managing Director
Life Gift
Lubbock, Texas
Chapter 36, Organ Donation and Transplantation

Carrie M. Wilson, MSN, RN, CPNP-PC, CPNP-AC, WCC
Pediatric Nurse Practitioner
Pediatric General Surgery
Washington University
St. Louis Children's Hospital
St. Louis, Missouri
Chapter 35, Burns

Fiona Winterbottom, MSN, RN, APRN, ACNS-BC, CCRN
Clinical Nurse Specialist for Critical Care
Ochsner Medical Center—New Orleans
New Orleans, Louisiana
Chapter 40, The Older Adult Patient

REVIEWERS

Marcia Bixby, RN, MS, CCRN, APRN-BC
Critical Care Clinical Nurse Specialist
Consultant
Randolph, Massachusetts

James Graves, PharmD
Staff Pharmacist, Certified Immunizer
St. Mary's Health Center
Jefferson City, Missouri

Rosemary K. Lee, DNP, ARNP-BC, CCNS, CCRN
Clinical Nurse Specialist
Critical Care Department, Homestead Hospital
Homestead, Florida

Judith Young, DNP, CNE
Clinical Assistant Professor
Department of Community and Health Systems
Indiana University School of Nursing
Indianapolis, Indiana

We are most grateful to the many students and nurses who made the previous editions of this book successful. This success has validated our commitments to proclaiming the outstanding contributions of critical care nurses and to promoting evidence-based nursing practice in the complex critical care environment. We actively solicited feedback from users of the previous editions and eagerly incorporated their comments and suggestions regarding format, content, and organization. And so, with this eighth edition, we again present to you a book that is thorough in all that is most pertinent to critical care nurses in a format that is organized for clarity and comprehension.

ORGANIZATION

The book's nine units and two appendices are organized around alterations in dimensions of human functioning that span biopsychosocial realms.

The content of Unit I, "Foundations of Critical Care Nursing," forms the basis of practice, regardless of the physiologic alterations of the critically ill patient. Although chapters in the book may be studied in any sequence, we recommend that Chapter 1, "Critical Care Nursing Practice," be studied first because it clarifies the major assumptions on which the entirety of the book is based. Chapter 2, "Ethical Issues," delineates theories and strategies for dealing with the ethical dilemmas that arise on a daily basis in critical care. Chapter 3, "Legal Issues," provides a base of information to help the critical care nurse be cognizant of practice issues that may have legal implications.

Chapter 4, "Genetic Issues Critical Care," provides information on the biologic basis of genetics; descriptions of the different types of *genetic* and *genomic* studies are included, plus examples of genetic diseases and pharmacogenetic syndromes encountered in critical care. The genomic arena mandates a new range of clinical and ethical competencies for nursing practice, and this list is included in the chapter.

Teaching and learning theory and strategies to best meet the learning needs of critical care patients are delineated in Chapter 5, "Patient and Family Education." Chapter 6, "Psychosocial Alterations and Management," examines the theoretic basis and nursing process for alterations in self-concept, spiritual practices, and coping. Chapter 7, "Nutrition Alterations and Management," examines the nutrition needs of critically ill patients and provides specific recommendations for different disorders. The concepts of pain and pain management in critically ill patients are discussed in Chapter 8, "Pain and Pain Management." Sedation, agitation, and delirium are described in Chapter 9, "Sedation, Agitation, and Delirium Management." Chapter 10, "End-of-Life Issues," delineates special needs for dealing with end-of-life and palliative care.

Unit II, "Cardiovascular Alterations," and Unit III, "Pulmonary Alterations," are each structured with the following chapters:
- Anatomy and Physiology
- Clinical Assessment
- Diagnostic Procedures
- Disorders
- Therapeutic Management

This organization permits easy retrieval of information for students and clinicians and provides flexibility for the instructor to individualize teaching methods by assigning chapters that best suit student needs. Unit IV, "Neurologic Alterations"; Unit V, "Kidney Alterations"; Unit VI, "Gastrointestinal Alterations"; and Unit VII, "Endocrine Alterations," are organized similarly. However, in these units, the assessment parameters including clinical and diagnostic procedures are discussed in one chapter. Also, disorders and therapeutic management are combined into one chapter.

Unit VIII, "Multisystem Alterations," covers disorders that affect multiple body systems and necessitate discussion as a separate category. Unit VIII consists of five chapters: "Trauma"; "Shock, Sepsis, and Multiple Organ Dysfunction Syndrome"; "Burns"; "Organ Donation and Transplantation"; and "Hematologic Disorders and Oncologic Emergencies."

Unit IX, "Special Populations," addresses the needs of critically ill obstetric, pediatric, and older adult patients in the critical care unit and the management of the recovery of perianesthesia patients in Chapters 38 through 41.

Appendix A, "Nursing Management Plans of Care," contains management plans organized alphabetically by nursing diagnosis for easy access by students and practitioners.

Finally, Appendix B, "Physiologic Formulas for Critical Care," features commonly encountered hemodynamic, pulmonary, and other calculations presented in easily understood formulas. Recommendations for nutrition supplements also are included.

NURSING DIAGNOSIS AND MANAGEMENT

A dominant theme of the book continues to be nursing diagnosis and management, reflecting the strength of critical care nursing practice. Wherever possible, evidence-based critical care practice is incorporated into nursing interventions. To foster critical thinking and decision making, a boxed "menu" of nursing diagnoses complete with specific etiologic or related factors accompanies each medical disorder and major medical treatment discussion and directs the learner to Appendix A, where appropriate nursing management is detailed. To facilitate student learning, the nursing management plans of care incorporate nursing diagnosis definition, etiologic or related factors, clinical manifestations, and interventions with rationale. The nursing management plans are liberally cross-referenced throughout the book for easy retrieval by the reader.

INCLUDED IN THIS EDITION

- **QSEN boxes**—a variety of additional QSEN boxes have been added to this addition. These boxes highlight quality and safety issues that are key to the care of critically ill patients. Boxes devoted to this material are identified with the QSEN icon and address the following issues:
  - Patient-Centered Care
  - Teamwork and Collaboration
  - Evidence-Based Practice (EBP)
  - Quality Improvement (QI)
  - Safety
  - Informatics

Special Features

- **Concept Maps** appear in the disorders chapters. There are 17 concept maps portraying the nursing care and treatment for complex medical conditions. The map design has been updated from the last edition. The maps portray the *outcome* approach to nursing care, depicting how the nursing interventions will alter a nursing diagnosis once they are implemented. The diagnosis is substantiated by the pathophysiology, by the things that are known to exist within the patient. The illustrations provide an additional learning tool for users to understand the complexity of the various conditions.
- **Case Studies** promote student learning and critical thinking by illustrating the clinical course of a patient experiencing the history, clinical assessment, diagnostic procedures, and diagnoses discussed in the related unit or chapter. All Case Studies include critical thinking questions to facilitate discussion. Answers to the questions are available on the Evolve website as a special resource for instructors.
- **Evidence-Based Practice** special feature highlights important research-based articles on key topics in critical care and critical care nursing.
- **Pharmacologic Management** tables are found in the therapeutic management chapters and outline common medications, along with any special considerations, used in treatment of the different disorders presented in the text.
- **Patient Education** boxes are placed in the disorders chapters and list the special topics that should be taught to the patient and family to prepare them for discharge.
- **Data Collection** boxes are located in the clinical assessment chapters and contain information that should be included as part of the patient's history.
- **Nursing Diagnoses** boxes display the diagnoses associated with particular disorders in a summary format with references to the corresponding nursing management plans in Appendix A.

EVOLVE RESOURCES FOR *CRITICAL CARE NURSING*

We are pleased to offer additional new and updated resources for students and instructors on our companion site, Evolve Resources for *Critical Care Nursing*.

Student Resources

Student resources are available at http://evolve.elsevier.com/Urden/criticalcare/ and include the following:
- Self-assessment opportunities including:
  - NCLEX® Examination Review Questions
  - CCRN Review Questions
  - PCCN Review Questions
- A selection of assessment animations and video clips for specific chapters

Instructor Resources

Instructor resources, available at http://evolve.elsevier.com/Urden/criticalcare/, provide a variety of aids to enhance classroom instruction. Instructors have access to all the above-listed Student Resources as well as the following:
- TEACH for Nurses—a new feature that replaces the Instructor Manual. TEACH for Nurses consists of detailed lesson plans that offer:
  - Lists of all student and instructor chapter resources found on Evolve
  - Teaching Strategies that present a chapter outline, content highlights, and learning activities
  - Answers to the textbook Case Studies provided for select chapters
  - Test Bank of approximately 1200 questions
  - PowerPoint presentation by chapter, consisting of approximately 1500 lecture slides, including two or three audience response questions for each chapter and a progressive Case Study in three therapeutic management chapters.
- Image Collection containing all the images from the text

Critical Care Nursing: Diagnosis and Management, 8th edition, represents our continued commitment to bringing you the finest in all things a textbook can offer: the best and brightest contributing and consulting authors, the latest scientific research befitting the current state of health care and nursing, an organizational format that exercises diagnostic reasoning skills and is logical and consistent, and outstanding artwork and illustrations that enhance student learning. We pledge our continued commitment to excellence in critical care education.

Linda D. Urden
Kathleen M. Stacy
Mary E. Lough

ACKNOWLEDGMENTS

A project of this book's magnitude is never merely the work of its authors. The concerted talent, hard work, and inspiration of a multitude of people have produced *Critical Care Nursing: Diagnosis and Management,* 8th edition, and have helped to make it the state-of-the-science text we affirm it to be. A "tradition of publishing excellence" has been evident throughout our partnership with Elsevier. We deeply appreciate the assistance of Lee Henderson, Executive Content Strategist, and Melissa Rawe, Content Development Specialist, who have helped us document and refine our ideas and transform our book into a reality. Their creativity, expertise, availability, and generosity of time and resources have been invaluable to us throughout this endeavor. We are also grateful to Anne Konopka, Senior Project Manager, for her scrupulous attention to detail.

Finally, we wish to thank the authors who contributed work to the first six editions of this book. Without the foundation they provided, an 8th edition would not have been born. We continue to be proud of our partnership with Elsevier, the teamwork and mutual respect among the three co-editors, and the final published book.

Linda D. Urden
Kathleen M. Stacy
Mary E. Lough

CONTENTS

1

Critical Care Nursing Practice

Linda D. Urden

OVERVIEW

Health care is undergoing dramatic change at a speed that makes it almost impossible to remain current and be proactive. The chaos and many challenges facing health care providers and consumers are evident in critical care, in which new treatment modalities and technology interface with the continuing effort to strive for quality care and positive outcomes. Efficiency and cost-effectiveness in relation to health care services are frequently discussed and are emphasized to all health care providers. To some, it appears that quality patient care has taken a back seat to the emphasis on cost containment and that quality and cost-effectiveness are not congruent. It is incumbent on all critical care health care providers to face these challenges from the scope of practice of their individual discipline and collectively from collaborative and interdisciplinary approaches.

The ever-changing health care environment creates many challenges for providers and consumers of care. Sensitivity to the appropriate time to eliminate or modify practices and adopt innovations is key to maintaining quality, cost-effective care delivery. Willingness to step outside of traditional structures and roles is the first step in making necessary changes. Change is constant. Flexibility and adaptation to change are essential to maintaining personal and organizational balance and to surviving in today's health care environment.

This chapter provides an overview of the evolution of critical care and describes the trends and current issues affecting critical care nurses and interdisciplinary teams. The information in this chapter serves as the framework for the remainder of the book in the areas of professional nurse decision making, holistic care, interdisciplinary collaboration, evidence-based practice (EBP), quality, and safety.

HISTORY OF CRITICAL CARE

Critical care evolved from the recognition that the needs of patients with acute, life-threatening illness or injury could be better met if the patients were organized in distinct areas of the hospital. In the 1800s, Florence Nightingale described the advantages of placing patients recovering from surgery in a separate area of the hospital. A three-bed postoperative neurosurgical intensive care unit (ICU) was opened in the early 1900s at

Johns Hopkins Hospital in Baltimore. This was soon followed by a premature infant unit in Chicago.[1]

Major societal issues have affected the development of intensive care as a specialty. During World War II, shock wards were established to care for critically injured patients. The nursing shortage after the war forced the grouping of postoperative patients into designated recovery areas so that appropriate monitoring and care could be provided. The technologies and combat experiences of health care providers during the wars of the 20th century also provided an impetus for specialized medical and nursing care in the civilian setting. The 1950s brought the new technology of mechanical ventilation and the need to group patients receiving this new therapy in one location.

CRITICAL CARE NURSING

Critical care nursing was organized as a specialty less than 70 years ago; before that time, critical care nursing was practiced wherever there were critically ill patients. The development of new medical interventions and technology prompted recognition that nursing was important in the monitoring and observation of critically ill patients. Physicians depended on nurses to watch for critical changes in the condition of patients in the physicians' absence, and they sometimes depended on the nurses to initiate emergency medical treatment.

As sophisticated technology began to support more elaborate medical interventions, hospitals began to organize separate units to make more efficient use of equipment and specially trained staff. Postoperative care, once provided by private duty nurses on general nursing wards throughout the hospital, was moved into recovery rooms where nurses with specialized knowledge regarding anesthesia recovery provided the patient care. Medical and surgical ICUs segregated the most critically ill patients in locations where they could be cared for by nurses with specialized knowledge in those areas of care. By the 1960s, nurses had begun to consolidate their knowledge and practice into focused areas such as coronary care, nephrology, and intensive care. In the hospital units established for patients needing such specialized care, nurses assumed many functions and responsibilities formerly reserved for physicians, and they assumed a new authority by virtue of their knowledge and expertise.

1

CONTEMPORARY CRITICAL CARE

Modern critical care is provided to patients by a multidisciplinary team of health care professionals who have in-depth education in the specialty field of critical care. The team consists of physician intensivists, specialty physicians, nurses, advanced practice nurses (APNs) and other specialty nurse clinicians, pharmacists, respiratory therapy practitioners, other specialized therapists and clinicians, social workers, and clergy. Critical care is provided in specialized units or departments, and importance is placed on the continuum of care, with an efficient transition of care from one setting to another.

Critical care patients are at high risk for actual or potential life-threatening health problems. Patients who are more critically ill require more intensive and vigilant nursing care. There are more than 500,000 nurses in the United States who care for critically ill patients.

These nurses practice in various settings: adult, pediatric, and neonatal critical care units; step-down, telemetry, progressive, or transitional care units; interventional radiology departments; and postoperative recovery units.[2] Nurses are now considered to be knowledge workers because they are highly vigilant and use their intelligence and cognition to go past tasks and quickly pull together multiple data to make decisions regarding subtle or deteriorating conditions. Nurses work technically with theoretical knowledge.[3]

A growing trend in acute care settings is the designation of progressive care units, considered to be part of the continuum of critical care. In past years, patients who were placed on these units would have been exclusively in critical care units. However, with the use of additional technology and monitoring capabilities, newer care delivery models, and additional nurse education, these units are considered the best environment. The patients are less complex, are more stable, have a decreased need for physiologic monitoring, and have more self-care capabilities. They can serve as a bridge between critical care units and medical-surgical units, while providing high-quality and cost-effective care at the same time.[4] Additionally, these progressive units can be found throughout the acute care setting, leaving critical care unit beds for patients who need the highest level of care and monitoring.[5]

CRITICAL CARE NURSING ROLES

Nurses provide and contribute to the care of critically ill patients in a variety of roles. The most prevalent role for the professional registered nurse (RN) is that of direct care provider. The American Association of Critical-Care Nurses (AACN) has delineated role responsibilities important for acute care and critical care nurses (Box 1.1).[6]

Expanded-Role Nursing Positions

Nurses in expanded-role nursing positions interact with critical care patients, families, and the health care team. Nurse case managers work closely with the care providers to ensure appropriate, timely care and services and to promote continuity of care from one setting to another. Other nurse clinicians, such as patient educators, cardiac rehabilitation specialists, physician office nurses, and infection control specialists, also contribute to care. The specific types of expanded-role nursing positions are determined by patient needs and individual organizational resources.

Advanced Practice Nurses

APNs have met educational and clinical requirements beyond the basic nursing educational requirements for all nurses. The

most commonly seen APNs in critical care areas are the clinical nurse specialist (CNS) and the nurse practitioner (NP) or acute care nurse practitioner (ACNP). APNs have a broad depth of knowledge and expertise in their specialty area and manage complex clinical and systems issues. The organizational system and existing resources of an institution determine what roles may be needed and how the roles function.

CNSs serve in specialty roles that use their clinical, teaching, research, leadership, and consultative abilities. They work in direct clinical roles and systems or administrative roles and in various other settings in the health care system. CNSs work closely with all members of the health care team, mentor staff, lead quality teams, and consult on complex patients. They are instrumental in ensuring that care is evidence based and that safety programs are in place. They may be organized by specialty, such as cardiovascular care, or by function, such as cardiac rehabilitation. CNSs also may be designated as case managers for specific patient populations.

NPs and ACNPs manage direct clinical care of a group of patients and have various levels of prescriptive authority, depending on the state and practice area in which they work. They also provide care consistency; interact with families; plan for patient discharge; and provide teaching to patients, families, and other members of the health care team.[2]

CRITICAL CARE PROFESSIONAL ACCOUNTABILITY

Professional organizations support critical care practitioners by providing numerous resources and networks. The Society of Critical Care Medicine (SCCM) is a multidisciplinary, multispecialty, international organization. The mission of SCCM is to secure the highest quality, cost-efficient care for all critically ill patients.[1] Numerous publications and educational opportunities provide cutting-edge critical care information to critical care practitioners.

The organization most closely associated with critical care nurses is AACN. Created in 1969, it is the world's largest specialty nursing organization. AACN is focused on "creating a healthcare system driven by the needs of patients and their families, where acute and critical care nurses make their optimal contribution."[7] The top priority of the organization is education of critical care nurses. AACN publishes numerous materials, EBP summaries, and practice alerts related to the specialty and is at the forefront of setting professional standards of care.

AACN serves its members through a national organization and many local chapters. The AACN Certification Corporation, a separate company, develops and administers many critical care specialty certification examinations for RNs. The examinations are provided in specialties such as neonatal care, pediatric care, critical care, progressive care, "virtual" ICU, and remote monitoring (e-ICU). Certification is considered one method to maintain high quality of care and to protect consumers of care and services. Research has demonstrated more positive outcomes when care is delivered by health care providers who are certified in their specialty.[8] AACN also recognizes critical care and acute care units that achieve a high level of excellence through its Beacon Award for Excellence. A unit that receives this award has demonstrated exceptional care through improved outcomes and greater overall satisfaction. It reflects on a unit with a supportive overall environment with teamwork and collaboration that is distinguished by lower turnover and higher morale.[9]

EVIDENCE-BASED NURSING PRACTICE

Much of early medical and nursing practice was based on non-scientific traditions and intuition. These traditions and rituals, which were based on folklore, gut instinct, trial and error, and personal preference, were often passed down from one generation of practitioner to the next. Some examples of critical care nursing practice based on nonscientific traditions include Trendelenburg positioning for hypotension, use of rectal tubes to manage fecal incontinence, gastric residual volume and aspiration risk, accuracy of assessment of body temperature, and suctioning artificial airways every 2 hours. To deliver the highest quality of care, EBP is essential and must be embraced by all nurses.[10] Munro and Savel[11] described courageous care as consisting of both quality and research, with knowledge as the basis. They stated that it takes courage to search for new evidence, create care guidelines, and make changes with health care providers. Bridges et al[12] reported that research studies are driving change in critical care and that future studies will focus on problematic practice issues.

The dramatic and multiple changes in health care and the ever-increasing presence of managed care in all geographic regions have placed greater emphasis on demonstrating the effectiveness of treatments and practices on outcomes. Emphasis is on greater efficiency, cost-effectiveness, quality of life, and patient satisfaction ratings. It has become essential for nurses to use the best data available to make patient care decisions and carry out appropriate nursing interventions.[10,13] By using an approach employing a scientific basis, with its ability to explain and predict, nurses are able to provide research-based interventions with consistent, positive outcomes. The content of this book is research-based, with the most current, cutting-edge research abstracted and placed throughout the chapters as appropriate to topical discussions.

The increasingly complex and changing health care system presents many challenges to creating an EBP. Appropriate research studies must be designed to answer clinical questions, and research findings must be used to make necessary changes for implementation in practice. Multiple EBP and research utilization models exist to guide practitioners in the use of existing research findings. One such model is the Iowa Model of Evidence-Based Practice to Promote Quality Care, which incorporates evidence and research as the basis for practice.[14]

QSEN   BOX 1.2   QSEN: Evidence-Based Practice

AACN Practice Alerts

- Family Presence During Resuscitation and Invasive Procedures (February 2016)
- Family Presence: Visitation in the Adult ICU (February 2016)
- Initial and Ongoing Verification of Feeding Tube Placement in Adults (February 2016)
- Prevention of Aspiration in Adults (February 2016)

Cullen and Adams describe a framework with four key phases to implement EBP: (1) create awareness and interest, (2) build knowledge and commitment, (3) promote action and adoption, and (4) pursue integration and sustained use. Each step has multiple strategies that facilitate successful progression to the next phase. The authors indicate that this model is particularly suited to complex static organizations.[13]

Just as there has been such an exponential growth of EBP literature, reports, publications, and acceptance, others are posing the question, "But at what cost?" Newhouse[15] described this as a complex issue to address and stated that economists would go beyond the costs of human labor and materials in their analysis. Another way to evaluate this is to examine "whose" cost is being considered. More recently, a published article reported estimates of costs per event for several health-acquired conditions. The estimated cost of care for one catheter-associated urinary tract infection was $758, a patient fall was estimated to cost $4,233 per fall, and a surgical "never event" cost $62,000 per event. These are most likely underestimated, but it is easy to realize the tremendous impact of situations that should not occur because there is sufficient evidence to prevent such outcomes.[16] Thus, inquisitive practitioners who strive for best practices using valid and reliable data demonstrate quality outcomes-driven care and practices.

Evidence-based nursing practice considers the best research evidence on the care topic, clinical expertise of the nurse, and patient preferences. For example, when determining the frequency of vital sign measurement, the nurse would use available research and nursing judgment (stability, complexity, predictability, vulnerability, and resilience of the patient),[17] along with the patient's preference for decreased interruptions and the ability to sleep for longer periods of time. At other times, the nurse would implement an evidence-based protocol or procedure that is based on evidence including research. An example of an evidence-based protocol is one in which the prevalence of indwelling catheterization and incidence of hospital-acquired catheter-associated urinary tract infections in the critical care unit can be decreased.[18]

AACN has promulgated several EBP summaries in the form of a "Practice Alert." These alerts are short directives that can be used as a quick reference for practice areas (eg, oral care, noninvasive blood pressure monitoring, ST segment monitoring). They are succinct, supported by evidence, and address both nursing and multidisciplinary activities. Each alert includes clinical information followed by references that support the practice.[19] Some published Practice Alerts are listed in Box 1.2.

HOLISTIC CRITICAL CARE NURSING

Caring

The high technology–driven critical care environment is fast paced and directed toward monitoring and treating life-threatening changes in patients' conditions. For this reason, attention is often focused on the technology and treatments necessary for maintaining stability in the physiologic functioning of the patient. Great emphasis is placed on technical skills and professional competence and responsiveness to critical emergencies. In this fast-paced, highly technologic health care environment, there is concern that diminished emphasis on the caring component of nursing may occur. Nowhere is this more evident than in areas in which critical care nursing is practiced. Keeping the *care* in nursing care is one of our biggest challenges. The critical care nurse must be able to deliver high-quality care skillfully, using all appropriate technologies, while incorporating psychosocial and other holistic approaches as appropriate to the patient and his or her condition.

The caring aspect between nurses and patients is most fundamental to the relationship and to the health care experience. The literature demonstrates that nurse clinicians focus on psychosocial aspects of caring, whereas patients place more emphasis on the technical skills and professional competence.[20] Noncaring is indicated by physical and emotional absence, inhumane and belittling interactions, and lack of recognition of the patient's uniqueness. Holistic care focuses on human integrity and stresses that the body, the mind, and the spirit are interdependent and inseparable. All aspects need to be considered in planning and delivering care.

Individualized Care

The differences between nurses' and patients' perceptions of caring point to the importance of establishing individualized care that recognizes the uniqueness of each patient's preferences, condition, and physiologic and psychosocial status. It is clearly understood by care providers that a patient's physical condition progresses in predictable stages, depending on the presence or absence of comorbid conditions. What is not understood as distinctly is the effect of psychosocial issues on the healing process. For this reason, special consideration must be given to determining the unique interventions that can positively affect each person and help the patient progress toward the desired outcomes.

An important aspect in the care delivery to and recovery of critically ill patients is the personal support of family members and significant others. The value of patient-centered and family-centered care should not be underestimated. It is important for families to be included in care decisions and to be encouraged to participate in the care of the patient as appropriate to the patient's personal level of ability and needs.

Cultural Care

Cultural diversity in health care is not a new topic, but it is gaining emphasis and importance as the world becomes more accessible to all as the result of increasing technologies and interfaces with places and peoples. Diversity includes not only ethnic sensitivity but also sensitivity and openness to differences in lifestyles, opinions, values, and beliefs. Significant differences exist among the cultural beliefs and practices of racial and ethnic minority groups and the level of their acculturation into the mainstream American culture.

Unless cultural differences are taken into account, optimal health care cannot be provided. More attention has been directed more recently at determining the physiologic differences and differences of disease development and progression among various ethnic groups. An increased sensitivity to

the health care needs and vulnerabilities of all groups must be developed by care providers.

Cultural competence is one way to ensure that individual differences related to culture are incorporated into the plan of care.[21,22] Nurses must possess knowledge about biocultural, psychosocial, and linguistic differences in diverse populations to make accurate assessments. Interventions must be tailored to the uniqueness of each patient and family.

COMPLEMENTARY AND ALTERNATIVE THERAPIES

Consumer activism has increased, and consumers are advocating for quality health care that is cost-effective and humane. They are asking whether options other than traditional Western medical care exist for treating various diseases and disorders. The possibilities of using centuries-old practices that are considered alternative or complementary to current Western medicine have increased in demand. These types of therapies can be seen in all health care settings including the critical care unit. Complementary therapies offer patients, families, and health care providers additional options to assist with healing and recovery.

The two terms *alternative* and *complementary* have been in the mainstream for several years. *Alternative* denotes that a specific therapy is an option or alternative to what is considered conventional treatment of a condition or state. The term *complementary* was proposed to describe therapies that can be used to complement or support conventional treatments.[23] This section includes a brief discussion about nontraditional complementary therapies that have been used in critical care areas.

Guided Imagery

One of the most well-studied complementary therapies is guided imagery, a mind-body strategy that is frequently used to decrease stress, pain, and anxiety.[24] Additional benefits of guided imagery are (1) decreased side effects, (2) decreased length of stay, (3) reduced hospital costs, (4) enhanced sleep, and (5) increased patient satisfaction.[24] Guided imagery is a low-cost intervention that is relatively simple to implement. The patient's involvement in the process offers a sense of empowerment and accomplishment and motivates self-care.

Massage

Back massage, previously practiced as part of routine care of patients, has been eliminated for various reasons, including time constraints, greater use of technology, and increasing complexity of care requirements. However, there is a scientific basis for concluding that massage offers positive effects on physiologic and psychological outcomes.

A comprehensive review of the literature revealed that the most common effect of massage was reduction in anxiety, with additional reports of a significant decrease in tension. There was also a positive physiologic response to massage in the areas of decreased respiratory and heart rates and decreased pain. The effects on sleep were inconclusive. The study authors concluded that massage was an effective complementary therapy for promoting relaxation and reducing pain, and they thought it should be incorporated into nursing practice.[25]

Animal-Assisted Therapy

The use of animals has increased as an adjunct to healing in the care of patients of all ages in various settings. Pet visitation programs have been created in various health care delivery settings,[26] including acute care, long-term care, and hospice. In the acute care setting, animals are brought in to provide additional solace and comfort for patients who are critically or terminally ill. Fish aquariums are used in patient areas and family areas because they humanize the surroundings. Scientific evidence indicates that animal-assisted therapy results in positive patient outcomes in the areas of attention, mobility, and orientation. Other reports have shown improved communication and mood in patients.[27]

TECHNOLOGY IN CRITICAL CARE

Growth in technologies has been seen throughout health care, especially in critical care settings. All providers are challenged to learn new equipment, monitoring devices, and related therapies that contribute to care and services. An example is the evolving electronic health record (EHR) that was originally designed to capture data for clinical decision making and to increase the efficiency of health care providers. There are complexities inherent in providing a "user-friendly" EHR. Thus, one that meets the needs and reflects the thought processes and actual work flow of diverse clinicians has been greatly lacking. Add to that the fact that staff-created "work-arounds" to some of the software and procedures have not significantly reduced errors or increased productivity. There is a tremendous amount of data, but those data are not translated into meaningful information with which to make decisions.[28] For this reason, it is important that critical care nurses are involved in the selection, trial, education, and evaluation of any health care informatics technologies that are being considered for their practice areas. Nurse informaticians, CNSs, educators, and managers are also essential in the selection processes so that all aspects are considered.[29] Another area for involvement of critical care nurses is in assessing new products that come into the system. There are often numerous "avenues" through which products enter such as product fairs, individual physicians, vendors, and supply departments. It is important that all proposed new products are overseen by a central committee or group who establishes criteria by which to select, pilot, evaluate, adopt, and communicate about the new product. Criteria that can be used in the initial assessment include (1) clinical relevance, (2) clinical void, (3) cost, (4) extra costs, and (5) safety.[30] This type of process ensures consistency and the same standards regarding product selection across the organization.

A more recent opportunity for critical care nurses is working in a role that encompasses the tele-ICU. Telemedicine was initially employed in outpatient areas, remote rural geographic locations, and areas where there was a dearth of medical providers. At the present time, tele-ICUs are in areas where there are limited resources on site. However, experts (critical care nurses, intensivists) are located in a central distant site. Technologies relay continuous surveillance with monitoring information and communication among care providers. Each tele-ICU varies in size and location; the key component is the availability of back-up experts. Goran describes competencies for critical care nurses who practice in a tele-ICU.[31]

INTERPROFESSIONAL COLLABORATIVE PRACTICE

The growing managed care environment has placed emphasis on examining methods of care delivery and processes of care by all health care professionals. Collaboration and partnerships have been shown to increase quality of care and services, while

BOX 1.3 QSEN: Teamwork and Collaboration

Core Competencies for Interprofessional Collaborative Practice

Values/Ethics for Interprofessional Practice
- Work with individuals of other professions to maintain a climate of mutual respect and shared values.

Roles/Responsibilities for Collaborative Practice
- Use the knowledge of one's own role and the role of other professions to appropriately assess and address the health care needs of patients and populations served.

Interprofessional Communication
- Communicate with patients, families, communities, and other health professionals in a responsive and responsible manner that supports a team approach to maintaining health and treatment of disease.

Interprofessional Teamwork and Team-Based Care
- Apply relationship-building values and principles of team dynamics to perform effectively in different team roles to plan and deliver patient/population-centered care that is safe, timely, efficient, effective, and equitable.

containing or decreasing costs.[32–37] It is more important than ever to create and enhance partnerships because the resulting interdependence and collaboration among disciplines is essential to achieving positive patient outcomes.[38] Tschannen et al[39] reported study findings in which physician-nurse relationships improved collaboration after physicians and nurses met together to create a method to change the unit culture. The physicians and nurses met together to examine collaboratively what the issues were and create strategies to resolve them. There were higher scores on openness of communication within groups, between groups, accuracy between groups, and overall collaboration.[39] Despins[40] described a study in which implementation of Crew Resource Management Training led to increased participation of all health care providers, resulting in better patient outcomes. In a study by Boev and Xia,[41] nurse-physician collaboration was again cited as evidence that hospital-acquired infections were statistically decreased.[41]

The Interprofessional Education Collaborative (IEC) published *Core Competencies for Interprofessional Collaborative Practice* in 2011. The IEC sponsors included associations of nursing, dentistry, medicine, osteopathy, public health, and pharmacy. Their goal was to establish a set of competencies to serve as a framework for professional socialization of health care professionals. They also intended to assess the relevance of the competencies and develop an action plan for implementation.[42] These competencies are especially important at the present time as we move forward with health care reform and explore innovative care delivery models using the skill sets of all health care providers in the most effective and efficient manner. Box 1.3 delineates the four core competencies.

INTERDISCIPLINARY CARE MANAGEMENT MODELS AND TOOLS

Several models of care delivery and care management are used in health care. An overview of the various terms and models is presented in this chapter, but readers are encouraged to seek additional resources and consultation for a more in-depth explanation of the models.

Care Management

Care management is a system of integrated processes designed to enable, support, and coordinate patient care throughout the continuum of health care services. Care management takes place in many different settings; care is delivered by various professional health care team members and nonlicensed providers, as appropriate.

Coordination of care and services may be done by the health care staff or the insurance or payer staff. Care management must be patient focused, continuum driven, and results oriented, and it must employ a team approach. Another term associated with this model of care is *disease state management*, which connotes the process of managing a population's health over a lifetime. However, in disease state management, there is a focus on managing complex and chronic disease states such as diabetes or heart failure over the entire continuum.

Case Management

Case management is the process of overseeing the care of patients and organizing services in collaboration with the patient's physician or primary health care provider. The case manager may be a nurse, allied health care provider, or primary care provider. Case managers are usually assigned to a specific population group and facilitate effective coordination of care services as patients move in and out of different settings. Ideally, the case manager oversees the care of the patient across the continuum of care.

Care Management Tools

Many quality improvement tools are available to providers for care management. The three evidence-based tools addressed in this chapter are clinical algorithm, practice guideline, and protocol.[43] All these tools may be embedded in the EHR.

Algorithm

An *algorithm* is a stepwise decision-making flowchart for a specific care process or processes. Algorithms guide the clinician through the "if, then" decision-making process, addressing patient responses to particular treatments. Well-known examples of algorithms are the advanced cardiac life support algorithms published by the American Heart Association. Weaning, medication selection, medication titration, individual practitioner variance, and appropriate patient placement algorithms have been developed to give practitioners additional standardized decision-making abilities.

Practice Guideline

A *practice guideline* is usually created by an expert panel and developed by a professional organization (eg, AACN, SCCM, American College of Cardiology, government agencies such as the Agency for Health Care Research and Quality). Practice guidelines are generally written in text prose style rather than in the flowchart format of algorithms.

Protocol

A *protocol* is a common tool in research studies. Protocols are more directive and rigid than guidelines, and providers are not supposed to vary from a protocol. Patients are screened carefully for specific entry criteria before being started on a protocol. There are many national research protocols, such as for cancer and chemotherapy studies. Protocols are helpful when built-in *alerts* signal the provider to potentially serious problems. Computerization of protocols assists providers in being more proactive regarding dangerous medication interactions, abnormal laboratory values, and other untoward effects that are preprogrammed into the computer.

Order Set

An *order set* consists of preprinted provider orders that are used to expedite the order process after a standard has been validated through analytic review of practice and research. Order sets complement and increase compliance with existing practice standards. They can also be used to represent an algorithm or protocol in order format.

Managing and Tracking Variances

All variances must be addressed and managed in a timely manner by the health care team members. All the previously described tools provide methods to track variances. Whether variance coding is included in the EHR or is tracked by another quality improvement method, the individual and aggregate data must be assessed and analyzed. Except for protocols, which are more rigid and research based, algorithms and guidelines can be used according to the practitioner's discretion. Tracking variances from the expected standard is one method to determine the utility of the tools in particular settings and patient populations. There must be a link between the care management system and the quality improvement program so that changes, as appropriate, can be made to positively affect the outcomes of care and services.

QUALITY, SAFETY, AND REGULATORY ISSUES IN CRITICAL CARE

Quality and Safety Issues

Patient safety has become a major focus of attention by health care consumers, providers of care, and administrators of health care institutions. The Institute of Medicine (IOM) publication *Crossing the Quality Chasm: A New Health System for the 21st Century* was the impetus for debate and actions to improve the safety of health care environments. In this seminal report, information and details were given indicating that health care harms patients too frequently and routinely fails to deliver its potential benefits.[44] The definitions of medical errors and approaches to resolving patient safety issues often differ among nurses, physicians, administrators, and other health care providers.[45] Subsequently through its use of expert panels, the IOM has published numerous other important reports related to quality, safety, and the nursing environment.

Patient safety has been described as an ethical imperative and one that is inherent in the actions and interpersonal processes of health care professionals.[46] In critical care units, where there is little room for error and safety is essential, errors may occur because of the hectic, complex environment.[46,47] In this environment, patients are particularly vulnerable because of their compromised physiologic status, multiple technologic and pharmacologic interventions, and multiple care providers who frequently work at a fast pace. It is essential that care delivery processes that minimize the opportunity for errors are designed and that a "safety culture" rather than a "blame culture" is created.[48] One author discussed results of a research study in which nurses were hesitant to report medication errors or unsafe practices so that they would not be ridiculed or "talked about" by their peer nurses. This uncivil behavior was thought to continue to contribute to an unsafe environment and one in which true error or unsafe practices and systems were greatly unreported.[49]

Medication administration is one of the most error-prone nursing interventions for critical care nurses.[50] The hectic, fast-paced environment where unplanned events are the norm can lead to medication errors.[51–53] Many medication errors are related to system failures, with distraction as a major factor. Various interventions have been created in an attempt to decrease medication errors. One article reported establishing a "no interruption zone" for medication safety in a critical care unit. In this pilot study, there was a 40% decrease in interruptions from the baseline measurement. Although researchers questioned the feasibility of sustaining this decrease in interruptions in the future,[54] this is an example of an approach that could be used to increase medication safety in the critical care unit.

When an injury or inappropriate care occurs, it is crucial that health care professionals promptly give an explanation of how the injury or mistake occurred and the short-term or long-term effects on the patient and family. The patient and family should be informed that the factors involved in the injury will be investigated so that steps can be taken to reduce or prevent the likelihood of similar injury to other patients.

It has been shown that intimidating and disruptive clinician behaviors can lead to errors and preventable adverse patient outcomes. This category includes verbal outbursts, physical threats, and more passive behaviors such as refusing to carry out a task or procedure. These types of behaviors are not rare in health care organizations. If these behaviors go unaddressed, it can lead to extreme dissatisfaction, depression, and turnover. There also may be systems issues that lead to or perpetuate these situations, such as push for increased productivity, financial constraints, fear of litigation, and embedded hierarchies in the organization.[48]

Technologies are both a solution to error-prone procedures and functions and another potential cause for error. Consider bar-code medication administration procedures, multiple bedside testing devices, computerized medical records, bedside monitoring, computerized physician order entry, and many other technologies now in development. Each in itself can be a great assistance to the clinician, but each must be monitored for effectiveness and accuracy to ensure the best in outcomes as intended for specific use.[50]

Quality and Safety Regulations

There are numerous regulations governing health care, including local, state, national, Medicare/Medicaid, and payer requirements. In this chapter, key regulations and accreditation standards impacting most critical care areas are discussed.

The Joint Commission (TJC) is an independent, not-for-profit organization that certifies more than 19,000 health care organizations in the United States. Its goal is to evaluate these health care entities using their preestablished standards of performance to ensure that high levels of care are provided in these entities. It establishes National Patient Safety Goals (NPSGs) annually[55] that are to be implemented in health care organizations (Box 1.4). TJC has also mandated a "Do Not Use" List. This list consists of abbreviations that may be confused with other similar ones. For example, do not use "U" or "u" for unit; instead, write out "unit." Another example is do not use "IU"; instead write out "international unit." Refer to TJC for a complete "Do Not Use" List.[56]

QSEN BOX 1.4   QSEN: Safety

2016 Hospital National Patient Safety Goals

- Identify patients correctly
- Improve staff communication
- Use medications safely
- Use alarms safely
- Prevent infection
- Identify patient safety risks
- Prevent mistakes in surgery

From The Joint Commission. National Patient Safety Goals Effective January 1, 2016. Hospital Accreditation Program. Oak Brook Terrace, IL: The Joint Commission; 2016.

The Safe Medical Devices Act requires that hospitals report serious or potentially serious device-related injuries or illness of patients or employees to the manufacturer of the device and to the US Food and Drug Administration (FDA) if a death has occurred. In addition, implantable devices must be documented and tracked.[57] This reporting serves as an early warning system so that the FDA can obtain information on device problems. Failure to comply with the Act results in civil action.

The FDA requires that a drug company place a boxed warning on the labeling of a prescription drug or in literature describing it. This boxed warning (also known as a "black box warning") signifies that medical studies indicate that the drug carries a significant risk of serious or life-threatening adverse effects.[58] Examples include warfarin, celecoxib (Celebrex), rosiglitazone (Avandia), and ciprofloxacin (Cipro). Alerts are published as soon as a drug is found to meet the criteria. Providers are to use caution when prescribing the medications and to consider alternative medications that have less adverse effects.

Quality and Safety Resources

The Institute for Safe Medication Practices is a not-for-profit organization dedicated to medication error prevention and safe medication use. It has numerous tools to assist care providers including newsletters, education programs, safety alerts, consulting, patient education materials, and error reporting systems. One newsletter is devoted specifically to nurses. It offers a very comprehensive array of tools.[59]

The Institute for Healthcare Improvement (IHI) is an interdisciplinary organization focused on quality that also offers many tools and resources including educational materials, conferences, case studies, publications, white papers, and quality measure tools. IHI developed the "bundle" concept, which consists of EBPs on specific high-risk quality issues as determined by a multidisciplinary group. There are many bundles published by IHI such as central line, ventilator, and sepsis bundles.[60] The National Quality Forum is another not-for-profit organization that facilitates consensus building with multiple partners to establish national priorities and goals for performance improvement. They also establish common definitions and consistent measurement. In addition, their goal is that all health care providers and stakeholders are educated regarding quality, priorities, and outcomes.[61]

The Healthcare Information and Management Systems Society is an interdisciplinary organization focused on patient safety and quality of care. This organization specifically focuses on integration of patient safety tools and practices to enhance communication, quality, efficiency, productivity, and clinical

QSEN BOX 1.5   QSEN Competencies

Patient-Centered Care

- Recognize the patient or designee as the source of control and full partner in providing compassionate and coordinated care based on respect for patient's preferences, values, and needs.

Teamwork and Collaboration

- Function effectively within nursing and interprofessional teams, fostering open communication, mutual respect, and shared decision making to achieve quality patient care.

Evidence-Based Practice

- Integrate best current evidence with clinical expertise and patient/family preferences and values for delivery of optimal health care.

Quality Improvement

- Use data to monitor the outcomes of care processes and use improvement methods to design and test changes to continuously improve the quality and safety of health care systems.

Safety

- Minimizes risk of harm to patients and providers through both system effectiveness and individual performance.

Informatics

- Use information and technology to communicate, manage knowledge, mitigate error, and support decision making.

From Cronenwett L, et al. Quality and safety education for nurses. *Nursing Outlook.* 2007;55(3):122.

QSEN BOX 1.6   QSEN: Informatics

Internet Resources

American Association of Critical-Care Nurses (AACN): http://www.aacn.org

Healthcare Information and Management Systems Society (HIMSS): http://www.himss.org

Institute for Healthcare Improvement (IHI): http://www.ihi.org

Institute of Medicine (IOM): http://www.iom.gov

Institute for Safe Medicine Practices (ISMP): http://www.ismp.org

The Joint Commission (TJC): http://www.jointcommission.org

National Database of Nursing Quality Indicators (NDNQI): http://www.nursingquality.org

National Quality Forum (NQF): http://www.nqf.org

Quality and Safety Education for Nurses (QSEN): http://www.qsen.org

Society of Critical Care Medicine (SCCM): http://www.sccm.org

Multicultural Resources

- Ethnomed: www.ethnomed.org
- Refugee Health Information Network: http://www.rhin.org
- Culture Clues: http://depts.washington.edu/pfes/CultureClues.htm
- Medline Plus: Health Information in Multiple Languages: http://www.nlm.nih.gov/medlineplus/languages/languages.htlm
- Patient information resources in Asian languages: htpp://spiral.tufts.edu
- Patient information resources in Spanish languages: http://www.nlm.nih.gov/medlineplus/spanish

support systems.[62] The National Database of Nursing Quality Indicators (NDNQI) is a national quality database devoted entirely to nursing. The database provides ongoing nurse-sensitive indicator consultation and research-based expertise. The mission of the NDNQI is to aid the RN in patient safety and quality improvement efforts. It is the only nursing national quality measurement program that provides hospitals with unit-level quality performance comparison reports.[63]

The Quality and Safety Education for Nurses (QSEN) project established standards for educating RNs at the baccalaureate and master's levels of academic education. In this model, knowledge, skills, and attitudes were created so that nurses would be able to continuously improve the quality and safety of the health care systems for which they work. There are six major categories that delineate knowledge, skills, and attitudes for each section (Box 1.5).[64] Boxes that address one of the QSEN competencies are presented throughout the book; the QSEN icon **QSEN** appears in these boxes. Box 1.6, QSEN: Informatics, lists the website addresses of all the quality, safety, and regulatory resources mentioned in this chapter.

Privacy and Confidentiality

A landmark law was passed to provide consumers with greater access to health care insurance, promote more standardization and efficiency in the health care industry, and protect the privacy of health care data.[65] The Health Insurance Portability and Accountability Act of 1996 (HIPAA) has created additional challenges for health care organizations and providers because of the stringent requirements and additional resources needed to meet the requirements of the law. Most specific to critical care clinicians is the privacy and confidentiality requirement

related to protection of health care data. This requirement has implications when interacting with family members and others and in regard to the often very close work environment, tight working spaces, and emergency situations. Clinicians are referred to their organizational policies and procedures for specific procedures for their organizations.

Communication Among Health Care Providers

The transfer of appropriate and accurate information from one care provider to another is an essential component of communication in health care. This point of information exchange is most commonly termed "handoff." It occurs at shift change; handover to a new clinician on the case; transfer to another unit, level of care, or procedure department; and discharge. Clinical environments are dynamic and complex, presenting multiple challenges for communication among care providers. Specialized care units, shortened hospital stays, complex conditions, and treatment plans requiring multiple specialist clinicians also add to the potential for unclear and missing communication. Halm[66] described many potential barriers for effective communication including time, staffing, equipment, education, human factors, culture, patient-related factors, and environmental factors. During an effective handoff, critical information is relayed, and continuity of care and treatment is maintained. Ineffective handoffs lead to adverse events and patient safety risks. For nursing, the greatest number of handoffs occur daily during the exchange of patient information at change of shift.[67] Many procedures, guidelines, and communication tools have been developed that facilitate an effective handoff.[68] One widely used communication tool is the SBAR tool created by AACN (Box 1.7).

HEALTHY WORK ENVIRONMENT

The health care environment is stressful; increasing challenges in the areas of financial constraints, regulatory requirements,

QSEN BOX 1.7 QSEN: Teamwork and Collaboration

SBAR Communication Tool

Critical information needs to be transmitted quickly and action taken.

S—Situation: Identify yourself and position, and give patient's name and the current situation. Give a clear, concise overview of pertinent issues.

B—Background: State the relevant history and physical assessment pertinent to the problem, treatment/clinical course summary, and any pertinent changes.

A—Assessment: Offer your conclusion about the present situation. Summarize facts and give your best assessment. What is going on? Use your best judgment.

R—Recommendation: Explain what you think needs to be done and when.

Follow-up action: What are the next steps? Who is responsible for follow-up? Verify any critical information received, seek clarification, ask questions, and read back critical test results. SBAR does not replace verbal communication whether over the phone or in person.

From American Association of Critical-Care Nurses. www.aacn.org/wd/hwe/docs/sbardcard.pdf; accessed 7-17-2016.

BOX 1.8 Healthy Work Environment Standards

Standard I: Skilled Communication
Nurses must be as proficient in communication skills as they are in clinical skills.

Standard II: True Collaboration
Nurses must be relentless in pursuing and fostering true collaboration.

Standard III: Effective Decision Making
Nurses must be valued and committed partners in making policy, directing and evaluating clinical care, and leading organizational operations.

Standard IV: Appropriate Staffing
Staffing must ensure the effective match between patient needs and nurse competencies.

Standard V: Meaningful Recognition
Nurses must be recognized and must recognize others for the value each brings to the work of the organization.

Standard VI: Authentic Leadership
Nurse leaders must fully embrace the imperative of a healthy work environment, authentically live it, and engage others in its achievement.

From American Association of Critical-Care Nurses (AACN). *Standards for Establishing and Sustaining Healthy Work Environments. A Journey to Excellence.* 2nd ed. Aliso Viejo, CA: AACN; 2016.

consumer scrutiny, quickly changing technologies and treatment regimens, and workforce diversity contribute to conflicts and difficulties on a daily basis. In this environment, it is essential to offer support for health care providers that can mitigate these challenges and ensure a healthy place to work.

There is an increasing amount of evidence that unhealthy work environments lead to medical errors, suboptimal safety monitoring, ineffective communication among health care providers, and increased conflict and stress among care providers. Synthesis of research in the area of work environment has demonstrated that a combination of leadership styles and characteristics contributes to the development and sustainability of healthy work environments (HWEs).[69]

AACN has formulated standards for establishing and sustaining HWEs.[70] The intent of the standards is to promote creation of environments that have a positive impact on nursing and patient outcomes. Evidence-based and relationship-centered principles were used to create the standards of professional performance. A summary of the six standards is provided in Box 1.8. Fig. 1.1 illustrates the interdependence of each standard and the ultimate impact on optimal patient outcomes and clinical excellence.

Everyone has a role in creating and sustaining the HWE. Although the manager has a major role in establishing the culture, the staff members greatly impact the culture by mentoring new staff members, role modeling behaviors, and leading interdisciplinary teams. This peer pressure has the most impact on all other staff.[71,72] Bylone[73] discussed her experience of talking with many staff members about how they think that they can influence the work unit culture. She recommends asking them how they influence each of the HWE standards, making it a personal experience and journey in achieving the HWE. Kupperschmidt et al[74] proposed a five-factor model for becoming a skilled communicator: (1) becoming aware of self-deception, (2) becoming authentic, (3) becoming candid, (4) becoming mindful, and (5) becoming reflective. All these factors lead to being a skilled communicator, creating the HWE. An additional approach for implementing the HWE model was offered by Blake,[75] who suggested five steps: (1) rallying the team, (2) surveying the team, (3) establishing work groups, (4) setting goals and developing action steps, and (5) celebrating successes along the way. The approach taken depends on the passion and commitment of the team. Blake et al[76] reported research findings that demonstrated a greater staff nurse intent to remain in their current pediatric ICU positions after the HWE was created.

SUMMARY

- Sensitivity to appropriate times to eliminate or modify practices and adopt innovations is key to maintaining quality, cost-effective care delivery.
- It is essential for nurses to use the best data available to make patient care decisions and to carry out the appropriate interventions.
- The critical care nurse must be able to deliver high-quality care skillfully, using all appropriate technologies, while incorporating psychosocial and other holistic approaches as appropriate to the time and condition of the patient.
- Nurses must possess knowledge about biocultural, psychosocial, and linguistic differences in diverse populations to make accurate assessments and plan interventions.
- Although nursing has independent and dependent nursing actions, it is essential that an interdependence with all health care providers is actualized.
- Multiple quality indicators have been developed for critical care; nurses are pivotal in quality monitoring and improvement.

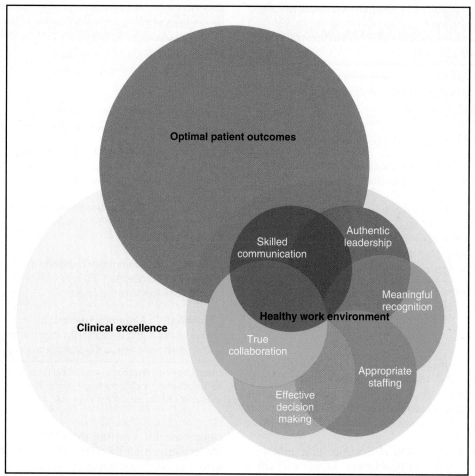

FIG. 1.1 Interdependence of Healthy Work Environment, Clinical Excellence, and Optimal Patient Outcomes. (From American Association of Critical-Care Nurses [AACN]. *Standards for Establishing and Sustaining Healthy Work Environments.* 2nd ed. Aliso Viejo, CA: AACN; 2016.)

- AACN Practice Alerts are succinct, evidence-based directives for critical care nurses and other health care providers to ensure that the most current evidence is used to provide safe care.
- HWEs are essential for establishing collaborative, trusting, and safe environments for the delivery of patient care.
- ⓔ Visit the Evolve site for additional study materials.

REFERENCES

1. Society of Critical Care Medicine. About SCCM: History of critical care. http://www.sccm.org. Accessed March 28, 2016.
2. American Association of Critical-Care Nurses. About critical care nursing. http://www.aacn.org. Accessed March 28, 2016.
3. Jost SG, et al. Integrated primary nursing: a care delivery model for the 21st-century knowledge worker. *Nurs Admin Q.* 2010;34(3):208.
4. Stacy KM. Progressive care units: different but the same. *Crit Care Nurse.* 2011;31(3):77.
5. American Association of Critical-Care Nurses. Progressive care unit fact sheet. http://www.aacn.org. Accessed April 1, 2016.
6. American Association of Critical-Care Nurses. AACN Scope and Standards for Acute and Critical Care Nursing Practice. http://www.aacn.org. Accessed April 1, 2016.
7. American Association of Critical-Care Nurses. AACN Fact Sheet. http://www.aacn.org. Accessed March 28, 2016.
8. American Association of Critical-Care Nurses. Value of certification resource center. http://www.aacn.org. Accessed March 28, 2016.
9. American Association of Critical-Care Nurses. Welcome to the Beacon Award for Excellence. http://www.aacn.org. Accessed March 28, 2016.
10. Makic MB, et al. Evidence-based practice habits: putting more sacred cows out to pasture. *Crit Care Nurse.* 2011;31(2):38.
11. Munro CL, Savel RH. Our view of courageous care. *Am J Crit Care.* 2015;24(5):372.
12. Bridges E, McNeill M, Munro N. Research in review: driving critical care practice change. *Am J Crit Care.* 2016;25(1):76.
13. Cullen L, Adams SL. Planning for implementation of evidence-based practice. *J Nurs Adm.* 2012;42(4):222.
14. Titler MG, et al. The Iowa model of evidence-based practice to promote quality care. *Crit Care Nurs Clin North Am.* 2001;13(4):497.
15. Newhouse R. Do we know how much the evidence-based intervention cost? *J Nurs Adm.* 2010;40(7/8):296.
16. Schifalacqua MM, et al. Does evidence-based nursing increase ROI? *Am Nurse Today.* 2012;7(1):32.
17. Schulman CS, Staul L. Standards for frequency of measurement and documentation of vital signs and physical assessments. *Crit Care Nurse.* 2010;30(3):74.
18. Gray M. Reducing catheter-associated urinary tract infection in the critical care unit. *AACN Adv Crit Care.* 2010;21(3):247.
19. American Association of Critical-Care Nurses. Practice alert. http://www.aacn.org. Accessed March 28, 2016.
20. Patistea E, Siamanta H. A literature review of patients compared with nurses' perceptions of caring: implications for practice and research. *J Prof Nurs.* 1999;15(5):302.
21. Gonzales R, et al. Eliminating racial and ethnic disparities in health care. *Am J Nurs.* 2000;100(3):56.

22. Leonard B, Plotnikoff GA. Awareness: the heart of cultural competence. *AACN Clin Issues.* 2000;11(1):51.

23. Kreitzer MJ, Jensen D. Healing practices: trends, challenges, and opportunities for nurses in critical care. *AACN Clin Issues.* 2000;11(1):7.

24. Tusek DL, Cwynar RE. Strategies for implementing guided imagery program to enhance patient experience. *AACN Clin Issues.* 2000;11(1):68.

25. Richards KC, et al. Effects of massage in acute and critical care. *AACN Clin Issues.* 2000;11(1):77.

26. McKenney C, Johnson R. Unleash the healing power of pet therapy. *Am Nurse Today.* 2008;3(5):29.

27. Cole K, Fawlinski A. Animal-assisted therapy: the human-animal bond. *AACN Clin Issues.* 2000;11(1):139.

28. Harrington L, Kennerly D, Johnson C. Safety issues related to the electronic medical record (EMR): synthesis of the literature from the last decade, 2000-2009. *J Healthc Manag.* 2011;56(1):31.

29. McLane S, Turley JP. Informaticians: how they may benefit your healthcare organization. *J Nurs Adm.* 2011;41(1):29.

30. Tottle J. Applying a systematic approach to new-product assessment. *Am Nurse Today.* 2008;3(9).

31. Goran SF. A new view: tele-intensive care unit competencies. *Crit Care Nurse.* 2011;31(5):17.

32. Wheelan SA, et al. The link between teamwork and patients' outcomes in intensive care units. *Am J Crit Care.* 2003;12(6):527.

33. Boyle DK, Kochinda C. Enhancing collaborative communication of nurse and physician leadership in two intensive care units. *J Nurs Adm.* 2004;34(2):60.

34. Falise JP. True collaboration: interdisciplinary rounds in nonteaching hospitals—it can be done!. *AACN Adv Crit Care.* 2007;18(4):346.

35. Golanowski M, et al. Interdisciplinary shared decision-making—taking shared governance to the next level. *Nurs Admin Q.* 2007;31(4):341.

36. Reina ML, et al. Trust: the foundation for team collaboration and healthy work environments. *AACN Adv Crit Care.* 2007;18(2):103.

37. Manojlovich M, Antonakos C. Satisfaction of intensive care unit nurses with nurse-physician communication. *J Nurs Adm.* 2008;38(5):237.

38. Lavoie-Tremblay M, et al. Effective strategies to spread redesigning care processes among healthcare teams. *J Nurs Scholarship.* 2015;47(4):328.

39. Tschannen D, et al. Implications of nurse-physician relations: report of a successful intervention. *Nurs Econ.* 2011;29(3):127.

40. Despins LA. Patient safety and collaboration of intensive care unit team. *Crit Care Nurs.* 2009;29(2):85.

41. Boev C, Xia Y. Nurse-physician collaboration and hospital-acquired infections in critical care. *Crit Care Nurs.* 2015;35(2):66.

42. Interprofessional Education Collaborative Expert Panel. *Core competencies for interprofessional collaborative practice: Report of an expert panel.* Washington, DC: Interprofessional Education Collaborative; 2011.

43. D'Arcy Y. Practice guidelines, standards, consensus statements, position papers: what they are, how they differ. *Am Nurse Today.* 2007;2(10):23.

44. Institute of Medicine. *Crossing the Quality Chasm: A New Health System for the 21st Century.* Washington, DC: National Academy Press; 2001.

45. Cook A, et al. An error by any other name. *Am J Nurs.* 2004;104(6):32.

46. White GB. Patient safety: an ethical imperative. *Nurs Econ.* 2002;20(4):195.

47. Henneman EA, et al. Strategies used by critical care nurses to identify, interrupt, and correct medical errors. *Am J Crit Care.* 2010;19(6):500.

48. The Joint Commission. Behaviors that undermine a culture of safety. *Sentinel Event Alert.* 2008. http://www.jointcommission.org/sentinel_event.aspx. Accessed March 28, 2016.

49. Covell CL. Can civility in nursing work environments improve medication safety? *J Nurs Adm.* 2010;40(7/8):300.

50. Henneman EA. Patient safety and technology. *AACN Adv Crit Care.* 2009;20(2):128.

51. Henneman E. Unreported errors in the intensive care unit: a case study in the way we work. *Crit Care Nurs.* 2007;27(5):27.

52. Flynn L, et al. Nurses' practice environments, error interception practices, and inpatient medication errors. *J Nurs Scholarsh.* 2012;44(2):180.

53. Flannery AH, Parli SE. Medication errors in cardiopulmonary arrest and code-related situations. *Am J Crit Care.* 2016;25(1):12.

54. Anthony K, et al. No interruptions please: impact of a no interruption zone on medication safety in intensive care units. *Crit Care Nurse.* 2010;30(3):21.

55. The Joint Commission. 2012 Hospital National Patient Safety Goals. http://www.jointcommission.org. Accessed March 28, 2016.

56. The Joint Commission. Facts about the official "Do Not Use" List. http://www.jointcommission.org. Accessed March 28, 2016.

57. Medical Device Reporting (MDR). http://www.fda.gov/MedicalDevices/Safety/ReportaProblem/default.htm. Accessed March 28, 2016.

58. *US Department of Health and Human Services, Food and Drug Administration: Warnings for Industry: Warnings and precautions, contraindications, and boxed warning sections of labeling for human prescriptive drug and biological products-content and format;* October 2011.

59. Institute for Safe Medication Practices. About ISMP. http://www.ISMP.org. Accessed March 28, 2016.

60. Institute for Healthcare Improvement. Using bundles to improve health care quality. http://www.ihi.org. Accessed March 28, 2016.

61. National Quality Forum. About NQF. http://www.NQF.org. Accessed March 28, 2016.

62. Healthcare Information and Management Systems Society. Patient safety and quality outcomes. http://www.HIMSS.org. Accessed March 28, 2016.

63. American Nurses Association (ANA). National Database Nursing Quality Indicators (NDNQI). http://www.nursingquality.org. Accessed March 28, 2016.

64. Quality Safety Education for Nurses. http://www.QSEN.org. Accessed April 1, 2016.

65. Centers for Medicare and Medicaid Services. The HIPAA law and related information. http://www.cms.gov/Regulations-and-Guidance/HIPAA-Administrative-Simplification. Accessed March 28, 2016.

66. Halm MA. Nursing handoffs: ensuring safe passage for patients. *Am J Crit Care.* 2013;22:158.

67. Gregory S, et al. Bedside shift reports: what does the evidence say? *J Nurs Adm.* 2014;44(10):541.

68. Friesen MA, White SV, Byers JF. Handoffs: implications for nurses. In: Patient Safety and Quality: An Evidence-Based Handbook for Nurses. vol 2. http://www.NCbi.NLM.NIH.gov/books. Accessed March 28, 2016.

69. Pearson A, et al. Comprehensive systematic review of evidence on developing and sustaining nursing leadership that fosters a healthy work environment in healthcare. *Int J Evid Based Healthc.* 2007;5:208.

70. American Association of Critical-Care Nurses. AACN standards for establishing and sustaining healthy work environments. A Journey to Excellence. 2nd ed. http://www.aacn.org. Accessed March 28, 2016.

71. Bylone M. Healthy work environments: whose job is it anyway? *AACN Adv Crit Care.* 2009;20(4):325.

72. Bylone M. I think they are talking about me!!. *AACN Adv Crit Care.* 2009;20(2):137.

73. Bylone M. Health work environment 101. *AACN Adv Crit Care.* 2011;22(1):19.

74. Kupperschmidt B, et al. A healthy work environment: it begins with you. *The Online Journal of Issues in Nursing.* 2010;15(1). manuscript 3. http://nursingworld.org/mainmenucategories/ANAMarketplace/ANAPeriodicals/OJIN. Accessed February 17, 2010.

75. Blake N. Practical steps for implementing healthy work environments. *AACN Adv Crit Care.* 2012;23(1):14.

76. Blake N, et al. Healthy work environments and staff nurse retention. *Nurs Admin Q.* 2013;37(4):356.

2

Ethical Issues

Kelly K. Dineen

It is essential that critical care nurses have an understanding of professional nursing ethics and ethical principles and that they are able to use a decision-making model to guide nursing actions. This chapter provides an overview of ethical principles and professional nursing ethics. An ethical decision-making model is described and illustrated, and recommendations are given concerning methods to use when confronting ethical issues in the critical care setting.

DIFFERENCES BETWEEN MORALS AND ETHICS

Morals are traditions of belief about right or wrong human behavior. Informed by individual and group values, morality consists of standards of conduct that include moral principles, rules, virtues, rights, and responsibilities. Moral norms form the basis for right action and provide a framework for the evaluation of behavior through a system of ethics.[1-3]

Ethics is a generic term for the reasoned inquiry and understanding of a moral life—in other words, a systematic examination of right and wrong behavior. Different theories or systems of ethics identify which moral norms (or rules) should be used and prioritized to evaluate whether conduct is ethical.[1,2] Applied ethics, of which health care ethics is a branch, is the attempt to use moral norms to evaluate conduct and to resolve particular ethical problems in context.[1] The extreme situations at the end of life or beginning of life garner most of the attention around health care ethics; however, day-to-day nursing decisions and actions implicate ethics. Day-to-day decisions fall within the realm of ethics if they (1) pertain to things within the nurse's control and (2) will show respect or fail to show respect for patients (or their loved ones).[4] Therefore most nursing decisions and interactions with patients fall within the realm of ethics. Most of the time, there is a right thing to do, and it can be done without conflict or resulting harm.

Ethical problems (also called ethical or moral dilemmas) occur only when there is some conflict surrounding an ethical decision.[4] An ethical problem exists if a person is morally obligated or appears to be obligated to two or more conflicting potential courses of action. The result is that both something right and something wrong will occur.[1,5] There are three kinds of ethical problems: cognitive, social, and volitional. In the nursing context, cognitive problems occur when the nurse is truly uncertain about the right thing to do. Social problems occur when there is disagreement among members of the health care team, family members, or other stakeholders about the right thing to do. Volitional problems occur when a nurse knows the right thing to do but does not know if he or she will

do it or can do it, usually because of power imbalances or organizational pressures. Volitional problems are often associated with moral distress.[4]

Nurses, Moral Distress, and Moral Courage

Nurses work in a system in constant flux. Health care is a highly regulated, complicated industry. Health care organizations are complex systems with varying authority structures and power dynamics. Nurses must navigate the complexities while managing frontline patient care, including emergency situations; increasingly innovative and highly technical care delivery; financial and staffing constraints; emotional and behavioral responses from patients and families, coworkers, and themselves in what is a naturally high-stakes, high-stress environment; and the reality that nurses are the most constant health professional presence at the bedside in critical care. These direct care, organizational, and structural pressures lead to an increasingly complex moral environment and frequent ethical dilemmas.[6] These factors as well as feelings of powerlessness and lack of control can contribute to detachment from the ethical impact of day-to-day decisions and contribute to professional "burnout."[6,7]

Moral distress has recently been widely discussed in the literature as a serious problem for nurses.[6-9] Moral distress often occurs with volitional ethical problems: The nurse knows the ethically appropriate action but feels unable to act consistent with that course or acts inconsistently—and therefore unethically—because of one or more barriers.[4,10] These barriers can include the medical plan of care, workplace dynamics, organizational rules, imbalanced power dynamics, interpersonal conflict, or individual psychosocial processes.

The pressure to act unethically can result in nursing behavior that is contrary to personal and professional values. Significant emotional and physical stress and resulting feelings of loss of personal integrity and professional dissatisfaction are common. Relationships with coworkers and patients and the quality of care are negatively impacted. Personal relationships and family life may also be negatively affected; nurses experiencing moral distress may resign their position or even leave the profession.[8] Tools to address and resolve moral distress are critical. Box 2.1 provides a position statement on moral distress, promulgated by the American Association of Critical-Care Nurses (AACN).[10] This evidence-based document provides additional references for the reader and suggested actions for direct care staff nurses and employers.

The AACN has also created a framework—"The 4 A's to Rise Above Moral Distress"—to support nurses who are experiencing moral distress (Fig. 2.1).[11] *Ask*, the first stage, is directed

BOX 2.1   American Association of Critical-Care Nurses Position Statement: Moral Distress

Issue

Moral distress is a serious problem in nursing. It results in significant physical and emotional stress, which contributes to nurses' feelings of loss of integrity and dissatisfaction with their work environment. Studies demonstrate that moral distress is a major contributor to nurses leaving the work setting and profession. It affects relationships with patients and others and can affect the quality, quantity, and cost of nursing care.

Definition

Moral distress occurs when

- You know the ethically appropriate action to take, but are unable to act upon it.
- You act in a manner contrary to your personal and professional values, which undermines your integrity and authenticity.

Evidence

Compelling evidence indicates that moral distress has a negative impact on the health care work environment. In one study, one in three nurses experienced moral distress.[1] In another, nearly half the nurses studied left their units or nursing altogether because of moral distress.[2]

Additional studies have shown

- Among 760 nurses, nearly 50% had acted against their consciences in providing care to terminally ill patients.[3]
- Nurses lose their capacity for caring, avoid patient contact, and fail to give good physical care as a result of moral distress.[1]
- Nurses experience physical and psychological problems as a result of moral distress.[4-10]
- Nurses physically withdraw from the bedside, barely meeting the patient's basic physical needs, or they leave the profession altogether.[1,2,4,5,11,12]

Summary

Moral distress is a key issue affecting the workplace environment. Research demonstrates that moral distress is a significant cause of emotional suffering among nurses and contributes to loss of nurses from the workforce. Further, it threatens the quality of patient care. In recognition of these harmful effects, the provision of education and tools to address and manage moral distress in the work environment is imperative and will lead to essential improvements in patient care and outcomes.

American Association of Critical-Care Nurses Policy Position

Moral distress is a critical, frequently ignored, problem in health care work environments. Unaddressed, it restricts nurses' ability to provide optimal patient care and to find job satisfaction. The American Association of Critical-Care Nurses (AACN) asserts that every nurse and every employer is responsible for implementing programs to address and mitigate the harmful effects of moral distress in the pursuit of creating a healthy work environment.

American Association of Critical-Care Nurses Calls to Action

For Nurses

Every nurse must

- Recognize and name the experience of moral distress (moral sensitivity).
- Affirm the professional obligation to act and commit to addressing moral distress.
- Be knowledgeable about and use professional and institutional resources to address moral distress, such as
  - American Nurses Association *Code of Ethics for Nurses*
  - International Council of Nurses *Code of Ethics for Nurses*
  - AACN *4 A's to Rise Above Moral Distress Handbook*
  - AACN *4 A's to Rise Above Moral Distress Facilitators Toolkit*
- Actively participate in professional activities to expand knowledge and understanding of the impact of moral distress.
- Develop skill, through the use of mentoring and resources, to decrease moral distress.
- Implement strategies to accomplish desired changes in the work environment, while preserving personal integrity and authenticity.

For Employers

Every organization must

- Implement interdisciplinary strategies to recognize and name the experience of moral distress.
- Establish mechanisms to monitor the clinical and organizational climate to identify recurring situations that result in moral distress.
- Develop a systematic process for reviewing and analyzing the system issues enabling situations that cause moral distress to occur and for taking corrective action.
- Create support systems that include
  - Employee assistance programs
  - Protocols for end-of-life care
  - Ethics committees
  - Critical stress debriefings
  - Grief counseling
- Create interdisciplinary forums to discuss patient goals of care and divergent opinions in an open, respectful environment.
- Develop policies that support unobstructed access to resources such as the ethics committees.
- Ensure nurses' representation on institutional ethics committees with full participation in all decision making.
- Provide education and tools to manage and decrease moral distress in the work environment.

References

1. Redman B, Fry ST: Nurses' ethical conflicts: what is really known about them? *Nurs Ethics* 7(4):360, 2000.
2. Millette BE: Using Gilligan's framework to analyze nurses' stories of moral choices, *West J Nurs Res* 16(6):660, 1994.
3. Solomon M, et al.: Decisions near the end of life: professional views on life sustaining treatments, *Am J Public Health* 83:14, 1993.
4. Kelly B: Preserving moral integrity: a follow-up study with new graduate nurses, *J Adv Nurs* 28:1134, 1998.
5. Wilkinson JM: Moral distress in nursing practice: experience and effect, *Nurs Forum* 23(1):16, 1987-1988.
6. Perkin RM, et al.: Stress and distress in pediatric nurses: lessons from Baby K, *Am J Crit Care* 6:225, 1997.
7. Fenton M: Moral distress in clinical practice: implications for the nurse administrator, *Can J Nurs Adm* 1:8, 1988.
8. Davies B, et al.: Caring for dying children: nurses' experiences, *Pediatr Nurs* 22:500, 1996.
9. Krishnasamy M: Nursing, morality, and emotions: phase I and phase II clinical trials and patients with cancer, *Cancer Nurs* 22:251, 1999.
10. Anderson SL: Patient advocacy and whistle-blowing in nursing: help for the helpers, *Nurs Forum* 25:513, 1990.
11. Heffernan P, Heilig S: Giving "moral distress" a voice: ethical concerns among neonatal intensive care unit personnel, *Cambridge Q Healthc Ethics* 8:173, 1999.
12. Corley MC: Moral distress of critical care nurses, *Am J Crit Care* 4:280, 1995.

Bibliography

Corley MC, et al.: Development and evaluation of a moral distress scale, *J Adv Nurs* 33(2):250, 2001.
Corley MC, Minick P: Moral distress or moral comfort, *Bioethics Forum* 18(1-2):7, 2002.
Cronqvist A, et al.: Caring about–caring for: moral obligations and work responsibilities in intensive care nursing, *Nurs Ethics* 11(1):63, 2004.

Continued

BOX 2.1   American Association of Critical-Care Nurses Position Statement: Moral Distress—cont'd

Erlen JA, Sereika SM: Critical care nurses, ethical decision making and stress, *J Adv Nurs* 26:953, 1997.

Jameton A: Dilemmas of moral distress: moral responsibility and nursing practice, *Clin Issues Perinat Womens Health Nurs* 4:542, 1993.

Jameton A: *Nursing Practice: The Ethical Issues*, Englewood Cliffs, NJ, 1984, Prentice-Hall.

Kalvemark S, et al.: Living with conflicts: ethical dilemmas and moral distress in the health care system, *Soc Sci Med* 58(6):1075, 2004.

Liaschenko J: Artificial personhood: nursing ethics in a medical world, *Nurs Ethics* 2:185, 1995.

Penticuff JH, Waldren M: Influence of practice environment and nurse characteristics on perinatal nurses' responses to ethical dilemmas, *Nurs Res* 49(2):64, 2000.

Raines ML: Ethical decision making in nurses: relationships among moral reasoning, coping style, and ethics stress, *JONAS Healthc Law Ethics Regul* 2(1):29, 2000.

Rushton CH: The Baby K case: ethical challenges of preserving professional integrity, *Pediatr Nurs* 21:367, 1995.

Storch JL, et al.: Listening to nurses' moral voices: building a quality health care environment, *Can J Nurs Leadersh* 15(4):7, 2002.

Sundin-Huard D, Fahy K: Moral distress, advocacy and burnout: theorizing the relationships, *Int J Nurs Pract* 5(1):8, 1999.

U.S. General Accounting Office. Nursing *Workforce: Emerging Nurse Shortages Due to Multiple Factors* [Report to the Chairman, Subcommittee on Health, Committee on Ways and Means, House of Representatives]. Washington, DC: US General Accounting Office.

From American Association of Critical-Care Nurses. *Position Statement: Moral Distress.* Aliso Viejo, CA: American Association of Critical-Care Nurses; 2008.

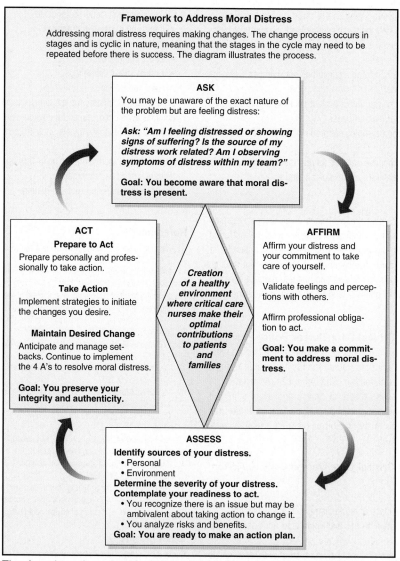

FIG. 2.1 The American Association of Critical-Care Nurses "4 A's to Rise Above Moral Distress." (From American Association of Critical-Care Nurses. Position Statement: Moral Distress. Aliso Viejo, CA: AACN; July 8, 2004.)

at self-awareness and reflection on the existence and impact of moral distress. *Affirm*, the second stage, includes a commitment to self-care. *Assess*, stage three, includes an assessment of the timing, context, and severity of distress as well as the readiness to act. *Act*, the final stage, consists of preparation, action, and maintenance of the desired change. Although the model was created by AACN, the framework can be used in diverse settings and by various health care professionals.[11,12] McCue[12] reported using the AACN framework in resolving an issue between a chief nurse executive and chief executive officer; the outcome had an impact at the organizational level.

Moral courage is defined by Lachman et al[13] as "the willingness to stand up for and act according to one's ethical beliefs when moral principles are threatened, regardless of the perceived or actual risks (such as stress, anxiety, isolation from colleagues, or threats to employment)." Moral courage is compromised by situations in which nurses are not free to advocate for themselves, for their patients, and for practices and policies that serve the ends of caregiving. Organizations have an ethical obligation to support a culture of moral courage through policies and practices that allow for a diversity of opinions, foster peer support, foster education, and support continued inquiry. Other authors have reported that moral courage is needed in everyday practice and that one must act ethically even in the presence of risk.[9,14] Courage is often described as a virtue; the American Nurses Association (ANA) defines courage as "the virtue that strengthens one's response in difficult or threatening circumstances or situations."[15]

Virtues

Virtues are habits of character or learned behaviors that predispose individuals to behave ethically.[15] In addition to courage, the virtues commonly expected of nurses include knowledge, wisdom, patience, compassion, and honesty. In contrast to personality traits or actions, virtues focus on the nurse's character or ways of being as a moral person.[16]

An often overlooked but critical virtue for all health care professionals is humility. The virtue of humility encompasses several other practices, including self-knowledge, reflection and perspective taking, and intellectual honesty (admitting what you do not know and seeking help).[17] The virtue of caring may be of particular importance for nursing; some have distinguished between caring about the patient and caring for the patient as two kinds of embodied virtues in nursing.[18] Practicing these virtues can better prepare nurses to act in an ethically appropriate and professional manner.

ETHICAL PRINCIPLES

As mentioned before, moral norms (or rules) form the basis of ethics. In health care, certain principles—descriptive and prescriptive rules that provide a basis for ethical reasoning and actions—are commonly appealed to norms.[15] These norms create nurses' obligations and corresponding patients' rights; they also form the basis of the most prevalent ethical framework of principlism. Under principlism, four principles are most commonly appealed to: (1) respect for persons/autonomy, (2) beneficence, (3) nonmaleficence, and (4) justice. These principles are used in this chapter and explained in Box 2-2.

If an action comports with one or more principles and does not conflict with any other principles, there is no ethical problem. For example, providing comfort through positioning or massage to a patient corresponds to beneficence. As long as that is done with the patient's permission and there is no risk associated with the actions, there is no conflict.

In addition, providers make daily decisions in which underlying principles conflict, but there is no ethical problem because everyone is in agreement with the right action and that action can be taken. In these instances, a principle is adhered to while others are overridden, but a conscious analysis is not always undertaken. Nonetheless, the justification and specification is occurring on some level.[1] For example, drawing arterial blood gases (ABGs) carries risks and does harm to the patient through puncturing the skin and causing pain; therefore the action is contrary to the principle of nonmaleficence. However, the action is taken based on a desire to benefit the patient's respiratory status by allowing interventions tailored to the patient's current ventilation and oxygenation status. Thus the principle of nonmaleficence is overridden by the principle of beneficence, and that action is justified because the information (ABG results) will allow for adjustments to respiratory care for the patient.

Respect for Persons/Autonomy

The principle of respect for persons requires nurses to respect the patient's inherent dignity and capacity for rational choice; this includes the obligation to honor the patient's right to autonomy, which is the right to determine what is done to or for them without coercion or undue interference from others.[18] Autonomy is also the foundation of the legal and ethical requirement of informed consent and includes the right of patients with decision-making capacity to refuse some or all treatments.[1] Decision-making capacity requires that the patient possesses a

---

BOX 2.2   Ethical Principles in Critical Care

Principle	Definition	Example Nursing Obligations	Patient Rights
Respect for persons/autonomy	Respect for the inherent and unconditional dignity of persons and to freely exercise choice about what happens to them	Truth-telling; provision of complete, accurate, and understandable information; timely communication; maintaining privacy and confidentiality; self-reflection to minimize bias	Self-determination; privacy; confidentiality
Beneficence	Promoting and maximizing benefit	Competent practice; advocacy for patient safety; acting for best interest of the patient	Appropriate, evidence-based care; effective care
Nonmaleficence	Avoiding and minimizing harm	Careful practice; self-reflection to minimize errors	Safe care and treatment
Justice	Equitable distribution of benefits and burdens and scare resources	Advocacy for equitable public policy in health care; self-reflection and advocacy to minimize disparities in care	Access to care; equitable care

set of values and goals, is able to understand the nature of the illness or injury, is able to reason through available treatment options and consequences of each (including doing nothing), and can communicate choice. Decision-making capacity is a fluid concept and can fluctuate based on health status.

Promoting autonomous decision making is a crucial and sometimes difficult responsibility of critical care nurses. Patients in critical care may lack decision-making capacity because of their illness or injury. Capacity may also fluctuate during treatment. When a patient lacks capacity, decisions are made by surrogate decision makers—typically family, friends, or others who have been named as the preferred decision maker by the patient or as designated by state laws. One exception to the need for informed consent is in emergency situations when treatment needs are emergent. The emergency treatment exception is limited, and every effort should be made by the critical care nurse to keep the surrogate decision maker informed as soon as possible.

Surrogate decision makers are required by law to make the decision that the patient would have made if he or she were able to; this is called the substituted judgment standard. This means surrogates should not choose based on their own personal preferences but instead based on their knowledge of the patient's values and preferences. Patients and families must have all the relevant information and the ability to understand and weigh options before they can make a decision that is consistent with the patient's values. Only when that is not possible should surrogates make decisions based on the patient's best interest.[16] In this situation, the nurse is a crucial member of the health care team—as patient advocate, the nurse provides and clarifies information, encourages reflection, and provides support during the decision-making process. Nurses frequently advocate for the patient, and by extension the surrogate decision maker, with other members of the health care team.

Confidentiality of patient information and privacy in patient interactions must be protected and honored by health care providers out of respect for persons and nonmaleficence. Confidentiality relates to information or data, whereas privacy relates to the person (eg, privacy is what a patient expects in a clinical encounter; confidentiality is how the information from the clinical encounter is treated). Confidentiality requires that patient information may be shared only with individuals involved in the care of the patient. Exceptions to this occur only if maintaining confidentiality seriously jeopardizes the welfare of others. These exceptions are usually reflected in state or federal laws, such as mandatory reporting laws. Privacy is closely aligned with confidentiality of patient information but relates to the person. Nurses must minimize violations of patient privacy by ensuring that doors and curtains are closed during interactions and taking extra steps to keep the patient covered during procedures. The 2015 ANA Position Statement on Privacy and Confidentiality is provided in Box 2.3.

BOX 2.3 American Nurses Association Position Statement on Privacy and Confidentiality

Purpose
Ongoing advances in technology, including computerized medical databases, telehealth, social media, and other Internet-based technologies, have increased the likelihood of potential and unintentional breaches of private/confidential health information. The purpose of this position statement is to speak to the role of nurses in protecting privacy and confidentiality and provide recommendations to avoid a breach.

Statement of American Nurses Association Position
The American Nurses Association (ANA) believes that protection of privacy and confidentiality is essential to maintaining the trusting relationship between health care providers and patients and integral to professional practice[15]. ANA supports legislation, policies, and standards that protect individually identifiable health information.

Recommendations
In keeping with the profession's commitment to patient advocacy and the trust that is essential to the preservation of the high quality of care that patients expect from registered nurses, ANA supports the following recommendations with respect to patient privacy and confidentiality:

- The patient's right to privacy of individually identifiable health information, including genetic information, is established statutorily with specific exceptions. Individuals retain the right to decide to whom, and under what circumstances, their individually identifiable health information will be disclosed. Confidentiality protections should extend not only to health records, but also to other individually identifiable health information, including clinical research records, oral reporting, images, and mental health therapy notes. This protection should be maintained in the treatment setting and in all other venues.
- Patients should receive accurate information regarding federal legislation (Health Insurance Portability and Accountability Act [HIPAA] and Genetic Information Nondiscrimination Act [GINA]) addressing individually identifiable health information and any limitations or exceptions to that legislation.

- A patient has the right to access personal health information and to supplement that information with what is necessary to make informed health care decisions, to correct erroneous information, and to address discrepancies that they perceive.
- Patients should receive written, clear notification of how their health records are used and when their individually identifiable health information is disclosed to third parties.
- The use or disclosure of individually identifiable health information without an individual's informed consent is prohibited. Exceptions should be permitted only if a person's life is endangered, if there is a threat to the public, or if there is an existing legal requirement. In the case of such exceptions, information should be limited to the minimum necessary for the situation. Individuals should be notified in writing of what information will be released, who is releasing the information, who will be receiving the information, and the purpose of revealing the information, with the signature of the disclosing provider.
- Organizations must develop appropriate administrative, physical, and technical safeguards required to protect the confidentiality, integrity, and availability of individually identifiable health information.
- Legislative or regulatory protections on individually identifiable health information should not unnecessarily impede public health efforts or clinical, medical, nursing, or quality of care research.
- Strong and enforceable remedies for violations of privacy protections should be established, and health care professionals who report violations should be protected from retaliation.

Background
Continuous developments in technology have changed the delivery of health care and the systems used to record, retrieve, and share patient information. Health professionals, insurers, and others routinely employ computers, phones, faxes, and other technologies to record and transfer information. This information, which may include diagnoses, prescriptions, or insurance information, is readily

BOX 2.3 American Nurses Association Position Statement on Privacy and Confidentiality—cont'd

available to anyone within proximity of the technology used to record, transfer, or share the data. This lack of privacy can undermine patients' relationships with providers and may adversely affect the quality of care if patients are reluctant to share personal health information. Despite the existence of laws and organizational policies intended to provide protection, patients may also worry that the exposure of personal health information, including genetic tests, may result in the loss or denial of health insurance, job discrimination, or personal embarrassment.

Summary

Quality patient care requires the communication of relevant information between health care professionals and/or health systems. The rapid evolution of communication, recording, and retrieval technologies poses challenges to maintaining the privacy, confidentiality, and security of this information. Breaches of health information can have serious personal and reputational consequences for both patients and providers in addition to a financial and organizational impact. Ensuring the integrity of the health information protection process is a shared responsibility of all health care providers and is vital to the fiduciary relationship with patients. Nurses and other health care professionals should contribute to the development and implementation of legislation, policies, and standards that protect patient privacy and the confidentiality of patient information.

Supportive Material

Code of Ethics for Nurses with Interpretive Statements[15]: Provision 3, interpretive statement 3.1, titled "Protection of the Rights of Privacy and Confidentiality" affirms the nurse's role in this process." Nurses safeguard the right to privacy for individuals, families, and communities. The nurse advocates for an environment that provides sufficient physical privacy, including privacy for discussions of a personal nature. Nurses also participate in the development and maintenance of policies and practices that protect both personal and clinical information at institutional and societal levels …. The nurse has a duty to maintain confidentiality of all patient information, both personal and clinical, in the work setting and off duty in all venues, including social media or any other means of communication (p. 9) …. When using electronic communications or working with electronic health records, nurses should make every effort to maintain data security "(p. 10).

Nursing: Scope and Standards of Practice (2015): Standard 1, Assessment, states, "The registered nurse collects pertinent data and information relative to the healthcare consumer's health or the situation" (p. 4). This standard further states that the nurse "[a]pplies ethical, legal, and privacy guidelines and policies to the collection, maintenance, use, and dissemination of data and information" (p. 54). Standard 7, Ethics, states, "The registered nurse practices ethically" and details the need further: "Safeguards the privacy and confidentiality of healthcare consumers, others, and their data and information within ethical, legal and regulatory parameters" (p. 67).

American Nurses Association. Essentials of Genetic and Genomic Nursing: Competencies, Curricula Guidelines, and Outcome Indicator (2008): This document defines essential genetic and genomic competencies for all registered nurses and identifies areas of knowledge and clinical performance indicators associated with protection of privacy and confidentiality.

The United States Department of Health and Human Services (DHHS) Privacy Rule and Security Rule: The Standards for Privacy of Individually Identifiable Health Information (Privacy Rule) went into effect in 2003 to implement the requirement of HIPAA with the goal "to assure that individuals' health information is properly protected while allowing the flow of health information needed to provide and promote high quality health care and to protect the public's health and well-being" (HHS, 2003, p. 1). The Security Rule operationalizes the protections contained in the Privacy Rule by addressing required technical and nontechnical safeguards that secure individuals' electronic protected health information.

The Joint Commission: The Joint Commission provides several accreditation programs based on the type of health organization or facility. Each accreditation program has a specific set of standards, one of which is information management (IM). The IM standard emphasizes the importance of protecting the privacy of individually identifiable health information and monitoring access to that information.

The Genetic Information Nondiscrimination Act: As noted in the International Society of Nurses in Genetics Position Statement, Privacy and Confidentiality of Genetic Information: The Role of the Nurse (2010), "Assuring privacy and confidentiality of genetic information demands continued vigilance on the part of all nurses as genetic technologies and discoveries are translated into clinical application and practice" (p. 1). This vigilance includes an awareness of the provisions in GINA. Signed into law in 2008, GINA has two parts: Title 1 prohibits health insurance providers from using genetic information to make decisions about an individual's eligibility or coverage. Title 2 prohibits employers from using genetic information to make decisions about hiring, promotion, or other terms of employment. There are limited exceptions to both Title 1 and Title 2.

American Nurses Association: Principles for Social Networking and the Nurse (2011): This document provides guidance on using social networking media in a manner that protects patients' privacy and confidentiality and maintains the standards of professional nursing practice. The six essential principles are relevant to all registered nurses and nursing students across all roles and settings.

References

American Nurses Association: *Code of Ethics for Nurses With Interpretative Statements*, Silver Spring, MD. www.Nursesbooks.org, 2015.

American Nurses Association: *Nursing: scope and Standards of Practice*, ed 3, Silver Spring, MD. www.Nursesbooks.org, 2015.

American Nurses Association: *ANA's Principles for Social Networking and the Nurse: guidance for the Registered Nurse*, Silver Spring, MD. www.Nursesbooks.org, 2011.

American Nurses Association: Essentials of Genetic and Genomic Nursing: competencies, Curricula Guidelines, and Outcome Indicators. http://www.nursingworld.org/MainMenuCategories/EthicsStandards/Genetics-1/EssentialNursingCompetenciesandCurriculaGuidelinesforGeneticsandGenomics.pdf, 2008.

International Society of Nurses in Genetics: Position statement: privacy and confidentiality of genetic information: the role of the nurse. http://www.isong.org/pdfs2013/PS_Privacy_Confidentiality.pdf, 2013.

Jackson J, Fraser R, Ash P: Social media and nurses: insights for promoting health for individual and professional use, *OJIN* 19(3), 2014. Manuscript 2. http://nursingworld.org/MainMenuCategories/ANAMarketplace/ANAPeriodicals/OJIN/TableofContents/Vol-19-2014/No3-Sept-2014/Insights-for-Promoting-Health.html.

Kiel J: An analysis of the management and leadership roles of nurses relative to the Health Insurance Portability and Accountability Act, *Health Care Manag (Frederick)* 34(1):76, 2015.

McGowan C: Patients' confidentiality, *Crit Care Nurse* 32(5):61, 2012.

Spector N, Kappel D: Guidelines for using electronic and social media: the regulatory perspective, *OJIN* 17(3), 2012. Manuscript 1. http://www.nursingworld.org/MainMenuCategories/ANAMarketplace/ANAPeriodicals/OJIN/TableofContents/Vol-17-2012/No3-Sept-2012/Guidelines-for-Electronic-and-Social-Media.html.

Taitsman J, Grimm C, Agrawal S: Protecting patient privacy and data security, *N Engl J Med* 368(11):977, 2013.

The Office of the National Coordinator for Health Information Technology: Guide to privacy and security of electronic health information. http://www.healthit.gov/sites/default/files/pdf/privacy/privacy-and-security-guide.pdf, 2015.

The Joint Commission: Information about our standards. http://www.jointcommission.org/standards_information/standards.aspx.

United States Department of Health and Human Services: Genetic information. http://www.hhs.gov/ocr/privacy/hipaa/understanding/special/genetic/.

United States Department of Health and Human Services: OCR privacy brief: summary of the HIPAA privacy rule. http://www.hhs.gov/ocr/privacy/hipaa/understanding/summary/privacysummary.pdf, 2003.

From American Nurses Association. Position Statement on Privacy and Confidentiality. Approved June 2015. http://www.nursingworld.org/DocumentVault/Position-Statements/Ethics-and-Human-Rights/Position-Statement-Privacy-and-Confidentiality.pdf. Accessed March 1, 2016.

Beneficence and Nonmaleficence

The ethical principles of beneficence and nonmaleficence require actions that maximize good and minimize harm to the patient, often in a delicate balance. The principle of beneficence presupposes compassion and requires the promotion of others' well-being through positive action and the desire to do good.[1] In contrast, nonmaleficence dictates that nurses prevent and minimize harm and correct harmful situations. Benefits must be maximized, and harms must be minimized. In critical care practice, every decision to act or not to act carries the serious potential for harm even though the intent is to benefit the patient. Thoughtfulness and care are necessary in defining and balancing benefit and harm in terms of both immediate and long-term goals for the patient.

Justice

The principle of justice means that there is an equitable distribution of limited resources. The most common example of the principle of justice is the allocation of organs for transplant. Another is access to health care, which is an issue of social justice, although it is not a constitutional right in the United States. Countless studies have demonstrated the negative impact of the system of care delivery on the health status of US residents. The Affordable Care Act has attempted to improve the just distribution of health care access by increasing the availability of health insurance for many Americans. At the same time, escalating health care costs, expanded technologies, an aging population, and a scarcity of health care personnel in some settings make the issue of health care allocation more complex.

CONFLICTING PRINCIPLES, PATERNALISM, AND MEDICAL FUTILITY

Conflict between principles is common and usually does not lead to an ethical problem. For example, suppose a patient is unconscious and needs emergency surgery for suspected peritonitis secondary to appendicitis and rupture. Surgery does harm to the patient and carries the potential for further harm to the patient in terms of risks; however, the benefits of surgery outweigh the need to avoid harm because of the known general clinical effectiveness of the intervention and the lack of reasonable, less harmful alternatives. In addition, the potential for further harm in the absence of surgical intervention is very high in terms of sepsis and possible death. Therefore on balance, surgery honors beneficence. Because the patient is unconscious and cannot consent, autonomy is overridden. However, this is justified because time is of the essence, and delay would increase the likelihood of harm in this particular situation. It is justifiable to override autonomy in this situation because of the competing reality of death in a patient with a treatable condition. Two common examples of the unethical resolution of conflicting principles are paternalism and medical futility.

Paternalism is an example of an unethical resolution of conflicting principles of beneficence and autonomy. Paternalism exists when the nurse or physician makes a decision for the patient without consulting the patient or by disregarding the patient's preferences. Until the 1970s, health care was almost entirely paternalistic, relying on the control of providers under a "doctor knows best" approach. Active involvement by various organizations, agencies, and consumer groups, as well as legal decisions, have changed the standards in health care to deference to the patients' values and preferences. However, fast-paced and high-pressure health care environments may lead less than thoughtful providers to impose their recommendations on patients.

Nurses must guard against their own paternalism in critical care and practice the virtues of humility through careful self-reflection. Postoperative care, which is designed to assist the patient with achieving a quick recovery, is a good example. Encouraging the patient to turn, cough, and deep breathe and increasing the patient's activity in the form of dangling, sitting in a chair, and ambulating all promote beneficence and nonmaleficence. However, forcing this activity over the patient's objection is paternalistic. Nurses are obligated to address underlying reasons for refusal such as pain and sleep deprivation and offer the patient options. Open and effective communication can usually lead to a resolution that both benefits the patient and is not paternalistic.

The concept of *medical futility* is difficult to define, and disputes have resulted in various discussions and proposed criteria to predict outcomes of care.[19-23] Futile care generally means there would be no useful results of health care interventions. Medical futility has been defined in countless ways; many prefer the terms *medically ineffective* or *nonbeneficial care*.[19] In general, futility means that the treatments—especially aggressive critical care—do not meet the underlying goals of care (eg, the treatment is harming the patient in some way without countervailing justification, such as benefit for the patient's overall condition). This usually occurs when there is a conflict between beneficence, nonmaleficence, and sometimes autonomy.

Some authors divide futility into categories such as physiologic or scientific futility, meaning the intervention cannot treat the problem.[2,19] The classic example of physiologic futility is administering antibiotics for a viral infection. A closely related concept is quantitative or probabilistic futility, which refers to, based on statistical evidence, "any effort to achieve a result that is possible but that reasoning or experience suggests is highly improbable and that cannot be systematically reproduced."[20] However, there is a lack of generalizable research as well as conflicting thresholds for treatments to be considered futile.[19]

Ethical futility is treatment that would not serve the underlying interests, values, and preferences of the patient.[2] Perhaps a useful way to think about futility in the context of critical care is as an unethical balance of the principles of beneficence and nonmaleficence (doing harm with no balancing or overriding benefit) or as paternalism (imposing the provider's idea of benefit contrary to the values and preferences of the patient). It can also occur when providers continue nonbeneficial care because a patient's surrogate wants "everything done" (eg, deference to autonomy despite no benefit and continued harm).

In critical care, futility is most often discussed in the context of end-of-life interventions. This is a pervasive ethical problem in the United States. According to Hofmann and Schneiderman,[24] "death is not necessarily a medical failure; a bad death is not only a medical failure, but also an ethical breakdown." Too many people in the United States experience a bad death. In general, providers fail to discuss death with patients, fail to refer to programs such as hospice or even palliative care appropriately, and persist in aggressively treating patients in high-tech settings far past the appropriate time. Moral distress is extremely common among nurses who feel compelled to provide continued, painful, invasive care that will not benefit the patient or is contrary to the patient's wishes.[22,23] Critical care nurses are on the forefront of this reality and can educate patients and families about options, clarify the realities associated with coding patients, and work with health care colleagues to foster thoughtfulness about the goals of care. Communication and problem-solving skills are essential to preventing conflicting goals and the provision of nonbeneficial care at the end of life.

PROFESSIONAL NURSING ETHICS AND THE NURSING CODE OF ETHICS

A professional ethic forms the framework for any profession[25] and is based on three elements: (1) the professional code of ethics, (2) the purpose of the profession, and (3) the standards of practice of the professional. The code of ethics developed by the profession is the delineation of its values and relationships with and among members of the profession and society. The need for the profession and its inherent promise to provide certain duties form a contract between nursing and society. The professional standards describe specifics of practice in various settings and subspecialties. Nursing professionals must stay consistent with their values and ethics and ensure that the ethical environment is maintained wherever nursing care and services are performed.[26-28] Each element is dynamic, and ongoing evaluations are necessary as societal expectations change, technologies increase, and the profession evolves.

The nursing code of ethics contains statements and directives for ethical nursing behavior.[28] The ANA Code of Ethics for Nurses, updated in 2015,[16] provides the major source of ethical guidance for the nursing profession. The nine statements of the code are presented in Box 2.4. Further delineation of each of the provisions along with in-depth discussion and examples of application can be found on the ANA website, www.nursingworld.org.

SITUATIONAL AND ORGANIZATIONAL ETHICAL DECISION MAKING IN CRITICAL CARE

As discussed earlier, the critical care nurse encounters ethical issues on a daily basis. Pavlish et al[29] studied nurses involved in ethical problems, their early indicators and risk factors, nurse actions, and outcomes. From this study, they derived risk factors for patients, families, health care providers, and health care organizations. Additionally, they delineated several early indicators for ethical dilemmas (Box 2.5). Research has indicated that screening critically ill patients periodically may help identify ethical conflicts earlier.[30] Specific actions for nursing leaders to address ethically complex situations and facilitate resolution include fostering open and early communication, providing robust ethics education, and promoting interdisciplinary collaboration.[31]

Health care organizations and authors have emphasized that responding to individual ethical issues is not enough; there must be a proactive program with a systematic approach to address ethical situations.[32,33] Preventive programs should identify, prioritize, and address concerns about ethics at an organizational level. Over time, measurable outcomes should demonstrate reduced disparities between current practices and ideal practices.[34]

Neglect of ethical problems or inadequate process or resolution at the individual or systems level results in harm to more than patients; this often results in poor staff morale, moral distress, increased operational and legal costs, negative public relations, and loss of trust in the profession. Because nurses are on the frontline of health care ethics, especially in the critical care setting, they have a unique and essential role in the resolution of ethical problems. Box 2.6 lists resources related to ethics.

Framework for Resolving Ethical Problems

Ethical problems are ubiquitous in critical care and often related to conflicts surrounding the use of technology, including the withdrawal of technology. As mentioned earlier, ethical problems in critical care occur when there is (1) conflict between the right action and the ability to take it, (2) uncertainty about the right action, or (3) conflict about which of several right actions is most ethical.[4] Dealing with an

---

BOX 2.4 American Nurses Association Code of Ethics for Nurses

1. The nurse practices with compassion and respect for the inherent dignity, worth, and unique attributes of every person.
2. The nurse's primary commitment is to the patient, whether an individual, family, group, community, or population.
3. The nurse promotes, advocates for, and protects the rights, health, and safety of the patient.
4. The nurse has authority, accountability, and responsibility for nursing practice; makes decisions; and takes action consistent with the obligations to promote health and provide optimal care.
5. The nurse owes the same duties to self as to others, including the responsibility to promote health and safety, preserve wholeness of character and integrity, maintain competence, and continue personal and professional growth.
6. The nurse, through individual and collective effort, establishes, maintains, and improves the ethical environment of the work setting and conditions of employment that are conducive to safe, quality health care.
7. The nurse, in all roles and settings, advances the profession through research and scholarly inquiry, professional standards development, and the policy generation of both nursing and health policy.
8. The nurse collaborates with other health professionals and the public to protect human rights, promote health diplomacy, and reduce health disparities.
9. The profession of nursing, collectively through its professional organizations, must articulate nursing values, maintain the integrity of the profession, and integrate principles of social justice into nursing and health policy.

From American Nurses Association. *Code of Ethics for Nurses*. Washington, DC: ANA; 2015.

BOX 2.5 Early Indicators for Ethical Dilemmas

- Signs of patient suffering (prolonged, unrelieved pain)
- Signs of unrealistic expectations (unwavering belief in patient recovery)
- Signs of nurses' moral distress (believe treatment not helpful, causes suffering)
- Signs of conflict (disagreement, different opinions)
- Signs of poor communication (avoidance of end of life and other difficult topics)
- Signs of ethics violations (disrespect for autonomy, disregard of right to information)

From Pavlish CL, et al. Screening situations for risk of ethical conflicts: a pilot study. *Am J Crit Care*. 2015;24:13.

QSEN BOX 2.6   QSEN: Informatics

Internet Resources

Ethics Resources

American Association of Critical-Care Nurses (AACN): www.aacn.org
    Joint Position Statement on ICU Overflow Patients
    Acute and Critical Care Choices—Guide to Advanced Directives
    Clinical Practice Guidelines for Quality Palliative Care
    Clinical Practice Guideline on Shared Decision Making in the Appropriate Initiation of Withdrawal From Dialysis
    Last Acts: Precepts of Palliative Care
    Pain Assessment in Nonverbal Patients
American Journal of Bioethics: www.bioethics.net
    Bioethics news and blog
American Nurses Association (ANA): www.nursingworld.org
    Multiple position statements on ethical issues in nursing
    Nursing Care and Do Not Resuscitate (DNR) and Allow Natural Death Decisions
    Reduction of Patient Restraint and Seclusion in Health Care Settings
    Forgoing Nutrition and Hydration
    Registered Nurse's Roles and Responsibilities in Providing Expert Care and Counseling at End of Life
    The Nurse's Role in Ethics and Human Rights: Protecting and Promoting Individual Worth, Dignity, and Human Rights in Practice Settings
    Active Euthanasia
American Society for Bioethics and the Humanities (ASBH): www.asbh.org
    Not-for-profit organization committed to education and research in clinical ethics

    Core Competencies for Clinical Ethics Consultants
    Code of Ethics for Clinical Ethicists
    Nursing ethics interest group (affinity group)
Catholic Health Care Association of the United States: http://www.chausa.org/ethics/overview
    Catholic health care facilities are the largest group of nonprofit health care facilities in the United States and require consideration of additional ethical norms, the Ethical and Religious Directives for Catholic Health Care, in delivering care and resolving problems
The Hastings Center: www.thehastingscenter.org
    Independent, nonpartisan, nonprofit bioethics research institute
    Provides educational resources and conferences, publications, and ethics consultation
International Council of Nurses (ICN): www.icn.org
    International Code of Ethics for Nurses
Presidential Commission for the Study of Bioethical Issues: http://www.bioethics.gov/
    Advisory panel of US leaders in health care, science, law, and ethics that seeks to develop policies to foster socially and ethically responsible delivery of health care and technology development
United States Department of Veterans Affairs: www.ethics.va.gov
    Created ISSUES preventive ethics model
    Preventive ethics tools, educational resources, and toolkit for implementing the model
    Integrated ethics program materials available

BOX 2.7   Ethics and the Nursing Process

Initial Steps: Clarify and Define Nature of the Problem
- What is the crisis (or dilemma) requiring a decision?

Assessment: Identify Key Facts and Values That Are Applicable
- What are the crucial facts of the case?
- What moral principles are at issue here?
- What decision-making procedure is appropriate?

Planning: Explore Available and Best Means to Reach Our Goal
- What is the primary aim or good for which we are acting?
- What objectives, benefits, and moral goals are achievable?
- What previous cases or contingencies should we take into account?

Implementation: Take Decisive and Effective Action to Implement Plan
- How do we begin, continue, and finish the process of intervention?

- How do we assess costs/benefits of the intervention?
- How do we monitor success/failure in the overall process?

Evaluation: Evaluate Progress and Outcomes With Planned Objectives
- What means have we set up for debriefing and feedback?
- Have we used the "right" means to a "good" end?
- How do we review the pros/cons for the action taken?

Final Steps: In Retrospect, Apply the Following Tests
- Could I/we provide a reasonable ethical justification for the course of action taken?
- Can I/we identify what we have learned from applying this model to decision making?
- How do we integrate this learning into the next decision-making cycle?

From Thompson IE, et al. *Nursing Ethics*. 5th ed. London: Churchill Livingston; 2006.

---

ethical problem effectively requires the individuals involved to pause, expand group consciousness about the issue, validate assumptions, look for patterns of thoughts or behaviors, and facilitate reflection and inquiry before making any decision.[35]

To facilitate the ethical decision-making process, a model or framework should be used to organize the relevant concerns, examine the issues, and generate possible solutions. There are numerous ethical decision-making models in the literature.[1,4,19,36,37] Some have modeled consideration of ethical issues as mapped onto the nursing process. Box 2.7 lists this framework. The SFNO model is provided here because it is easy to remember and useful both for individual patient dilemmas and for examining organizational dilemmas.

SFNO MODEL FOR DELIBERATION OF ETHICAL PROBLEMS

SFNO is an easily memorized acronym that stands for (1) Stakeholders, (2) Facts, (3) Norms, and (4) Options.[4] Using

QSEN BOX 2.8 QSEN: Patient-Centered Care

SFNO Approach to Case Analysis

"So Far No Objections"

Stakeholders
- Who has a stake in the decision being made? Why?
- Who will be significantly affected by the decision made? Why? Please be specific.
- Are there reasons to give priority to one stakeholder over another?

Facts
- What additional facts are necessary to inform your decision-making process?
- What factual issues might generate disagreement?
- What facts are relevant to a solution?

Norms
- What ethical principles, norms, or values are at stake?
- Which do you think are relevant, and which might appear to conflict or generate disagreement?

Options
- Consider a wide variety of alternatives. Resist the urge to quickly reach a recommendation.
  - What actions or policies deserve serious consideration?
  - Explore the values behind the alternatives (cognitive dissonance and perspective taking foster ethical and professional development).

- Explore the processes and strategies that can improve decision making. Compensatory strategies for professional decision making include seeking help, managing emotions, anticipating consequences (including short-term and long-term consequences), recognizing rules and context, and testing your assumptions and motives (SMART Strategies[a]).
- Narrow the options to arrive at a few ethically acceptable options.
  - If the ethical ideal is not possible, what compromise solutions are most attractive?
- Justification criteria may be helpful in explaining your reasons for selecting one or two options as superior.
  - *Necessity:* Is it necessary to infringe on the values or norms under consideration to achieve the intended goal?
  - *Effectiveness:* Will the action be effective in achieving the desired goal?
  - *Proportionality:* Is the desired goal important enough to justify overriding another principle or value?
  - *Least infringement:* Is the policy or action designed to minimize the infringement of the principle or value that conflicts with it?
  - *Proper process:* Has the decision been made using proper processes?

[a]SMART strategies are explained in DuBois JM, et al. Professional decision-making in research (*PDR*): the validity of a new measure. *Science and Engineering Ethics.* 2016 Apr 22(2); 391-416. adapted from DuBois JM. Solving ethical problems: analyzing ethics cases and justifying decision. In: *Ethics in Mental Health Research.* Oxford: Oxford University Press; 2008; and Volpe RL, et al, editors. Guidance for facilitators and facilitation guide. In: *Exploring Integrity in Medicine: The Bander Center for Medical Business Ethics Casebook.* St. Louis: Saint Louis University; 2014.

this model, the nurse should first identify the ethical question; for example, should the ventilator be withdrawn from a patient. Thereafter, the nurse should use SFNO model as an organizing device that allows the nurse (and health care team) to ensure that important considerations are identified and that group deliberation is facilitated by use of a framework. Box 2.8 provides a useful guide to use of the SFNO model.

To illustrate the use of this model, consider the following straightforward example. An elderly woman with chronic obstructive pulmonary disease (COPD) is on a ventilator, receiving artificial nutrition through a gastric tube, intravenous fluids, and antibiotics for pneumonia. The patient does not have capacity and does not have an advance directive. The patient's only child, an adult daughter, approaches the team and says the patient would not want to remain on the ventilator and requests that it be withdrawn. The treating physician believes that after the pneumonia is treated, it may be possible to wean the patient from the ventilator. The initial question is whether withdrawing the ventilator is ethically appropriate.

Stakeholders: The patient, the patient's adult daughter, and extended family all are stakeholders. The nurses, other health care team members, and the health system are also stakeholders. Other similarly situated patients are more remote stakeholders.

Facts: Many facts are not immediately available. These include, but are not limited to, whether there are other relevant stakeholders in terms of family members or loved ones; the underlying severity of the COPD; the degree to which the patient

has previously expressed her wishes to her daughter and in what context; information about the patient that reveals her likes, dislikes, and values; the patient's prognosis if the pneumonia is treated; the degree to which the patient is in pain or is suffering; the likelihood of suffering both with continued ventilation and if the ventilation is withdrawn; the time in which evidence of improvement from the pneumonia is expected; the anticipated likelihood of successfully weaning the patient from the ventilator; the underlying cognitive status of the patient; and the likelihood that the patient will be able to engage in activities that are consistent with her values if treatment is continued.

Norms: Respect for persons means that the patient's autonomous decisions should be honored. However, we do not yet know to what extent the request is an expression of the wishes of the patient or of the daughter. Beneficence requires the caregivers to maximize benefit, whereas nonmaleficence requires the caregivers to minimize harm. The extent to which the current treatments honor these norms depends on the specific answers to the above-listed facts. Conversely, if information becomes available that the patient clearly expresses a wish to not be on a ventilator under any circumstance, respect for persons may trump beneficence.

Options: The team could do nothing (eg, maintain the ventilation). The team could also begin weaning the ventilator but continue the other treatments. For example, if improvement from the pneumonia is expected after a few additional days of intravenous antibiotics, the team could work with the daughter to reach agreement to postpone removal for a few days and reassess the situation in light of the facts at that time. Mediating options are always worth exploring and often offer additional time to collect the information identified as necessary in the facts session. The team could also explore withdrawal of all but comfort care measures if that is consistent with the patient's previously expressed wishes or the patient's values.

STRATEGIES FOR PROMOTION OF ETHICAL DECISION MAKING

The complexity of health care and ethical dilemmas encountered frequently in clinical practice demand the establishment of expertise in clinical ethics and mechanisms and processes for resolution. The field of clinical ethics (also known as health care ethics or bioethics) arose directly from dilemmas in critical care situations such as the availability of artificial cardiopulmonary support, dialysis, and organ transplantation in the last 40 years. Clinical ethics is now an established, interdisciplinary profession, and hospitals almost always have resources available to assist with mitigation and resolution of ethical problems.

Institutional Ethicists, Ethics Committees, and Ethics Consultation Services

Almost every hospital has an institutional ethics committee (IEC), and many have ethics consultation services or individual professional ethicists assigned to hospitals. IECs arose as a response to ethical and legal dilemmas in the 1960s and 1970s. In some states, law requires them, and they are strongly encouraged as part of accreditation by The Joint Commission.

IECs were originally envisioned to provide education and foster ethical approaches to systemic and organizational issues. IECs still function this way at some facilities when individual ethicists or consultation services exist to assist providers and families at the bedside with ethical dilemmas. At others, IECs serve primarily as consultation services to assist with individual ethical problems. Many facilities have specialized or subdivided IECs based on clinical service. Regardless of the person, service, or committee involved, every hospital should have one or more ways to assist with ethical problems at the bedside (ethics consultations). Ethics consultations can provide the various stakeholders involved with an informed "outside" perspective and use professional expertise to assist with resolution. Recommendations issued in response to ethics consultations are generally guidance rather than mandates.

Ethics Rounds and Conferences

At hospitals with individual ethicists or consultation services, ethicists often round with other providers on each patient in critical care. In the absence of this more structured approach, nurses may consider developing a regular method of conducting ethics rounds with the assistance of their facility's ethicist or a member of the IEC. Ethics rounds can increase early identification of risk factors for emerging ethical problems and allow for proactive resolution. An individual patient ethics conference may be scheduled to include appropriate stakeholders or multidisciplinary group to discuss unit issues.[35,38]

IPCP   CASE STUDY 2.1   Patient With Ethical Dilemma

Brief Patient History

Mr. X is a 67-year-old obese man. He has a 2-year history of emphysema (100 packs/year history of tobacco abuse in the past) with two recent hospitalizations for pneumonia that required ventilatory support. Mr. X states that he does not want to be placed on a ventilator again but does not want to suffer either. He was involved in a motor vehicle accident and sustained blunt trauma to the trunk and lower extremities, with bilateral femur fractures. Although his condition is critical, he is expected to recover. Mr. X received morphine 5 mg by intravenous push in the emergency department, with minimal pain relief; however, he has experienced new-onset confusion. Mr. X's spouse and children express concern about the risk of respiratory depression from pain medication. They state that they would rather Mr. X experience pain than have him placed on the ventilator again.

Clinical Assessment

Mr. X is admitted to the critical care unit from the emergency department with blood transfusions in progress. Buck's traction (5 lb) has been applied to both lower extremities. He is awake, alert, and oriented to person, time, place, and situation. Mr. X is breathing through his mouth, taking shallow breaths. He complains of right upper quadrant abdominal pain when taking a deep breath. His skin is warm and dry. Mr. X is able to move his toes on command, and lower extremity sensation to touch is intact; however, he is complaining of severe bilateral lower extremity pain with restlessness.

Diagnostic Procedures

Arterial blood gas values are as follows: Pao_2, 55 mm Hg; $Paco_2$, 28 mm Hg; pH, 7.35; HCO_3^-, 24 mEq/L; O_2 saturation, 88%. Hematocrit is 24%, and hemoglobin is 8 g/dL. Patient reports pain as a 10 on the Baker-Wong Faces Scale. Riker Sedation-Agitation Scale score is 5.

Medical Diagnosis

Mr. X is diagnosed with a hepatic hematoma and bilateral femur fractures from a motor vehicle accident.

Questions

1. What major outcomes do you expect to achieve for this patient? What problems or risks must be managed to achieve these outcomes?
2. What interventions could be initiated to monitor, prevent, manage, or eliminate the problems and risks identified?
3. Assuming the patient consents, what interventions could be initiated to promote optimal functioning, safety, and well-being of the patient?
4. What possible learning needs would you anticipate for this patient?
5. What cultural and age-related factors might have a bearing on the patient's plan of care?
6. What were the circumstances of his previous need for mechanical ventilation? Was he adequately sedated? What is the basis for not wanting ventilation—fear of suffering, fear of never coming off the ventilator, something else? What goals of the patient should be prioritized?
7. Does he have an advance directive that further explains his wishes? Has he previously appointed a surrogate decision maker in the event of his incapacity?
8. Who are the stakeholders involved?
9. What ethical principles are in conflict here? Are other relevant legal norms involved?
10. What are the options? How do they play out in the short-term and long-term?
11. How would you resolve this problem?

SUMMARY

- Day-to-day decisions in critical care fall within the realm of ethics; each act can show or fail to show respect for the person or patient. The daily practice of critical care nursing involves ethical decision making and frequently involves ethical problems.
- Ethical problems occur when there are alternative potential actions for a patient and those actions are in conflict; individuals may be uncertain about the right thing to do, or there may be disagreement among team members about the right thing to do.
- Moral distress occurs when a nurse feels unable to act in an ethical manner because of the medical plan of care, organizational restraints, workplace dynamics, or other barriers. The AACN framework to address moral distress provides insight and guidelines for critical care nurses who experience moral distress.
- Ethical principles help guide practice, but often one action simultaneously honors one principle while overriding another. Overriding a principle must be justified in the context of the situation.
- By using an ethical decision-making framework, nurses and other stakeholders can arrive at a decision that considers and honors the patient's values and preferences and is consistent with ethical principles and the nurse's professional code of nursing ethics.
- The practice of nursing is built on a foundation of moral and ethical caring; the critical care nurse is pivotal in identifying patient situations with an ethical component and can participate in the decision-making process to address the issues.
- All facilities have professional ethics resources available to nurses and providers; these include IECs, individual clinical ethicists, and clinical ethics consultation services.
- ⓔ visit the Evolve site for additional study materials.

REFERENCES

1. Beachump TL, Childress JF: *Principles of Biomedical Ethics*, ed 5, Oxford, 2001, Oxford University Press.
2. Furrow B, et al.: *Bioethics: Health care law and ethics*, ed 7, Eagan MN, 2013, West Publishing.
3. Thompson IE, Melia KM, Boyd KM, Horsburgh D: *Nursing Ethics*, ed 4, London, 2006, Churchill Livingston.
4. DuBois JA: *Framework for Analyzing Ethics Cases, Ethics in Mental Health Research*, New York, 2008, Oxford Press (accessed February 15, 2016). https://sites.google.com/a/narrativebioethics.com/emhr/home.
5. Purtilo RB, Doherty RF: *Ethical Decisions in the Health Professions*, ed 5, St. Louis, 2011, Saunders.
6. LaSala CA, Biarnason D: Creating workplace environments that support moral courage, *OJIN* 15(3), 2010.
7. Cummings CL: *Nurse Leader*, 2010. Moral distress and the nursing experience, 8(6):37–39, November–December, 2010.
8. Epstein EG, Delgado S: Understanding and addressing moral distress, *OJIN* 15(3), 2010. Manuscript 1.
9. Gallagher A: Moral distress and moral courage in everyday nursing practice, *OJIN* 16(2), 2010.
10. AACN: Position statement: moral distress. http://www.aacn.org. Accessed March 1, 2016.
11. AACN: The 4A's to rise above moral distress. http://www.aacn.org. Accessed March 1, 2016.
12. McCue C: Using the AACN framework to alleviate moral distress, *OJIN* 16(1), 2010.
13. Lachman VD, et al.: Doing the right thing: pathways to moral courage, *American Nurse Today* 7(5):24, 2012.
14. Murray JS: Moral courage in healthcare: acting ethically even in the presence of risk, *OJIN* 15(3), 2010. Manuscript 2.
15. American Nurses Association: Silver Springs MD Glossary. In *Code of Ethics for Nurses With Interpretative Statements*, 2015, p 42. Glossary.
16. American Nurses Association: *Code of Ethics for Nurses With Interpretative Statements*, 2015, p 11.
17. Dineen KK: Addressing prescription opioid abuse concerns in context: synchronizing policy solutions to multiple complex public health problems, *Law Psychol Rev. Pending*, 2016.
18. Benjamin M, Curtis J: *Ethics in Nursing: Cases, Principles, and Reasoning*, ed 4, New York, 2010, Oxford.
19. Jonsen A, et al.: *Clinical Ethics: a Practical Approach to Ethical Decisions in Clinical Medicine*, ed 6, 2006.
20. Schneiderman LJ, et al.: Medical futility: its meaning and ethical implications, *Ann Intern Med* 112(12):949, 1990.
21. Bernat JL: Medical futility: definition, determination, and disputed in critical care, *Neurocrit Care* 2(2):198, 2005.
22. Jox RJ, et al.: Medical futility at the end of life: perspectives of intensive care and palliative care clinicians, *J Med Ethics*, 2012.
23. Schwarzkopf D, et al.: Making it safe speak up about futile care: a multi-perspective survey on leadership, psychological safety and perceived futile care in the ICU, *Crit Care* 19(Supp 1):P567, 2015.
24. Hofmann PB, Schneiderman LJ: Physicians should not always pursue a good clinical outcome, *Hastings Cent Rep*, 2007. May-June, 37(3), inside back cover.
25. Lachman VD: Practical use of the nursing code of ethics: part I, *Medsurg Nurs* 18(1):55, 2009.
26. Curtin L: Ethics for nurses in everyday practice, *American Nurse Today* 5(2), 2010.
27. Murray JS: Creating ethical environments in nursing, *Am Nurse Today* 2(10):48, 2007.
28. Winland-Brown J, et al.: The New Code of Ethics for Nurses with Interpretative Statements (2015): practical Clinical Application, Part 1, *Medsurg Nurs* 24(4):268, 2015.
29. Pavlish C, et al.: Early indicators and risk factors for ethical issues in clinical practice, *Image J Nurs Sch* 43(1):13, 2011.
30. Pavlish CL, et al.: Screening situations for risk of ethical conflicts: a pilot study, *Am J Crit Care* 24(3), 2015.
31. Pavlish CL, et al.: Avenues of action in ethically complex situations, *J Nurs Adm* 45(6), 2015.
32. United States Department of Veterans Affairs: Preventative ethics. http://www.ethics.va.gov. Accessed March 15, 2015.
33. Epstein EG: Preventative ethics in the intensive care unit, *AACN Adv Crit Care* 23(2):217, 2012.
34. Rushton CH: Ethical discernment and action: the art of pause, *AACN Adv Crit Care* 20(1):108, 2009.
35. Robichaux C: Developing ethical skills: from sensitivity to action, *Crit Care Nurse* 32(2):65, 2012.
36. Rushton CH, Penticuff JH: A framework for analysis of ethical dilemmas in critical care nursing, *AACN Adv Crit Care* 18(3):323, 2007.
37. Clark AP: A model for ethical decision making in cases of patient futility, *Clin Nurse Spec* 24(4):189, 2010.
38. Pavlish CL, et al.: Nursing priorities, actions, and regrets for ethical situations in clinical practice, *Image J Nurs Sch* 43(4):385, 2011.

3

Legal Issues

Kelly K. Dineen

OVERVIEW

The law routinely influences and intersects with the practice of nursing and with health care in general. This influence extends far beyond the common notion of malpractice and the trial system. Legal systems operate at the local, state, and federal levels and range from matters handled through the courts to matters handled through administrative agencies to agreements between private individuals or organizations. Regardless of the setting, the law in general is concerned with minimum standards rather than best practices or even ethical practice. In other words, practice that meets legal criteria is often far less than what meets ethical criteria or criteria for best practices. Nursing licensure is one example; licensure indicates only that a nurse has demonstrated the basic competencies to safely practice as an entry-level nurse. Licensure does not set best practice.

Effective nursing is about more than minimal competencies. The National Council of State Boards of Nursing (NCSBN), an organization that works to develop policy and consistent standards throughout the state licensing boards, defines nursing as (1) a scientific process founded on a professional body of knowledge, (2) a learned profession based on an understanding of the human condition across the life span and the relationship of a client with others and within the environment, and (3) an art dedicated to caring for others.[1] The NCSBN further describes nursing as a "dynamic discipline that increasingly involves more sophisticated knowledge, technologies, and client care activities." As nurses practice in this increasingly complex and rapidly evolving health care system, it is critical to understand some basic principles of law, the differences between legal thresholds and quality and scope of practice, as well as the ways laws impact practice and the ability of nurses to impact health law and policy.

This chapter highlights some of the laws and legal systems that figure prominently in nursing practice, including (1) administrative law (illustrated by the regulation of the profession by state boards of nursing [BONs]), (2) tort law (lawsuits brought by patients for the actions or inactions of nurses), (3) constitutional law (illustrated through a discussion of the legal rights of patients to make decisions to accept or refuse treatment), and (4) federal and state health care statutory laws (illustrated through self-determination laws and select federal laws).

ADMINISTRATIVE LAW: PROFESSIONAL REGULATION

For most nurses, the first professional interaction with a legal system is through the process of licensure. The ability to practice as a licensed professional nurse is a privilege granted by the state and is a function of each state's authority to promote and protect the health and welfare of its citizens. State BONs are administrative bodies created by—and that operate under—state nursing practice acts (NPAs). NPAs are state laws (statutes) that are written with more general standards by state lawmakers, passed by state legislatures, and signed by the governor. The BONs develop more specific rules (or regulations) for interpreting and enforcing the NPAs.

This process is consistent throughout every administrative system, whether federal or state. Administrative bodies are created and granted power under statutes written and passed by legislatures and signed by the governor (in the case of state law) or the president (in the case of federal law). Administrative agencies develop, propose, and enforce specific regulations in their areas. These regulations can be changed by the administrative agencies through a process of rule making that allows the agencies to adapt to changes in their relative areas without requiring the action of the legislature. For example, NPAs are state statutes that establish the scope of practice in each state. More specific standards are created as rules or regulations through a rule-making process by BONs, state administrative agencies, to further define the scope of practice and delineate standards of practice and criteria for licensure. In other words, BONs are responsible for "the interpretation and enforcement of the provisions" of NPAs.[2] The work of the BONs is just one tangible example of an administrative system but is perhaps the most important to nurses because BONs control the ability to practice.

Functions of Boards of Nursing

The regulation of nursing practice is intended to protect the health and safety of state citizens by (1) regulating the conditions of licensure, (2) regulating the scope of practice, (3) establishing a framework of standards of nursing practice, (4) removing incompetent or unsafe practitioners through disciplinary actions, and (5) prohibiting unlicensed persons from providing services reserved for licensed individuals. In addition, the regulation of nursing can enhance the professional status and the public's trust of nurses.

Scope of Practice

BONs maintain expectations for and limits of nursing practice in each state through the licensure of nurses and through challenges to non-nurses engaged in professional activities that intrude on the nursing scope of practice. The scope of practice generally refers to the broad range of activities that nurses perform and manage in the delivery of care that "require education and training consistent with professional standards …

commensurate with the RN's education, demonstrated competencies, and experience."[3] Scope of practice is framed broadly not only to account for the many professional nursing settings and roles but also to account for activities that are reserved for professional nurses and activities that may be delegated with appropriate supervision. Scope of practice provisions are also intended to prevent unlicensed professionals from providing services that are reserved to licensed professionals.

The absolute outside limits of the scope of practice are sometimes difficult to define and sometimes the subject of disciplinary actions by BONs or other professional licensure boards and legal challenges through the court system. In some cases, these challenges arise from other professional licensing boards, such as state medical boards, in response to circumstances within their state. The importance of the scope of practice has been demonstrated by several important legal cases. In *Sermchief v Gonzales*,[4] the Supreme Court of Missouri heard a case involving two nurses who worked with several physicians in rural Missouri to provide women's health care services. The nurses engaged in health counseling, routine pelvic examinations, and testing such as Pap smears, as well as community education under standing orders from physicians. Quality of care was not at issue: All the parties agreed that the nurses provided excellent care and that the patients were satisfied. The issue was strictly whether they were practicing within the scope of nursing practice or if they were infringing on the scope of medical practice (practicing medicine without a license). The court held in favor of the nurses because their work was within the boundaries of the NPA in existence at the time and within the limits of the physicians' orders.

The field of obstetrics has commonly served as an example for scope of practice issues. A case in Ohio, *Marion Ob/Gyn v State Med. Bd.*,[5] established that delivering infants was beyond the scope of physician assistant practice in Ohio but not beyond the *nursing* scope of practice because the NPA allowed licensed nurses to practice midwifery. In Kansas, lay midwives can deliver infants without infringing on the scope of nursing or medical practice. In *State Board of Nursing v Ruebke*,[6] the Kansas Supreme Court held that midwives working under the supervision of a physician are not engaged in the unauthorized practice of medicine.

Standards of Practice

NPAs establish the scope of nursing practice, whereas BONs usually develop standards of practice at the state level through administrative rule making. The NCSBN publish Model Rules for BONs to use as an example of appropriate standards.[7] These standards of practice communicate the expectations of safe and effective nursing practice within the scope of practice. State standards of practice also assist BONs in evaluating the ongoing practice of nursing. "The NPA may require safe practice, whereas the rules may specify a plan for safe practice."[8] Thus, to fully understand the expectations for and limitations of nursing in a particular state, it is necessary to review both the NPA and the rules or regulations of the BON.

The Model Nursing Act (Model Act) and Model Administrative Rules (Model Rules) developed by the NCSBN are example NPAs and regulations, respectively, for individual states in regulating nursing practice.[9] Actual state laws governing professional nursing practice vary from state to state in the degree to which they have adopted all or part of the current or previous model acts and rules. Nonetheless, the Model Act scope of practice provisions (Box 3.1) and the Model Rules for

---

BOX 3.1 Scope of Practice (Activities of Professional Nurses)

Model Nursing Act (Model Statutory Law)

The practice of registered nursing shall include
1. Providing comprehensive nursing assessment of the health status of patients.
2. Collaborating with health care team to develop and coordinate an integrated patient-centered health care plan.
3. Developing the comprehensive patient-centered health care plan, including (a) establishing nursing diagnoses, (b) setting goals to meet identified health care needs, and (c) prescribing nursing interventions.
4. Implementing nursing care through the execution of independent nursing strategies and the provision of regimens requested, ordered, or prescribed by authorized health care providers.
5. Evaluating responses to interventions and the effectiveness of the plan of care.
6. Designing and implementing teaching plans based on patient needs.
7. Delegating and assigning nursing interventions to implement the plan of care.
8. Providing for the maintenance of safe and effective nursing care rendered directly or indirectly.
9. Advocating the best interest of patients.
10. Communicating and collaborating with other health care providers in the management of health care and the implementation of the total health care regimen within and across care settings.
11. Managing, supervising, and evaluating the practice of nursing.
12. Teaching the theory and practice of nursing.
13. Participating in development of health care policies, procedures, and systems.
14. Wearing identification that clearly identifies the nurse as an RN when providing direct patient care, unless wearing identification creates a safety or health risk for either the nurse or the patient.
15. Other acts that require education and training consistent with professional standards as prescribed by the BON and commensurate with the RN's education, demonstrated competencies, and experience.

BON, state board of nursing.
Modified from National Council of the State Boards of Nursing (NCSBN). NCSBN Model Act. Chicago, IL: NCSBN; 2012, updated 2014.

---

standards of practice (Box 3.2) are useful in illustrating the differences between scope and standards. For example, the ninth activity listed within the scope of practice is "advocating the best interest of clients." Within the standards of practice in Box 3.2, the standards related to advocating for the patient include seven detailed expectations and actions for nurses in meeting their obligation to advocate for clients.

In addition to standards developed by BONs, many specialty nursing organizations have developed standards of practice. The BON standards establish broad expectations of safety and efficacy, whereas specialty standards are more targeted and aimed at fostering excellence in the specialized field. An example of specialty standards are those developed by the American Association of Critical-Care Nurses (AACN).[10] The AACN standards are presented in Box 3.3. These specialty standards are helpful in establishing and measuring quality care and often reflect a consensus opinion of experts in the particular specialty of appropriate nursing care.

The extent to which specialty standards are introduced in a legal context varies widely from state to state. It is critical to understand that the legal term of art, *standard of care*, is not

BOX 3.2   Standards of Practice[a]

Model Nursing Administrative Rules, Standards of Nursing Practice (Model Regulations or Administrative Rules)

1. Standards Related to RN Professional Accountability

The RN

a. Practices within the legal boundaries for nursing through the scope of practice authorized in the Nurse Practice Act and rules governing nursing.

b. Demonstrates honesty and integrity in nursing practice.

c. Bases nursing decisions on nursing knowledge and skills, the needs of patients, and registered nursing standards.

d. Accepts responsibility for judgments, individual nursing actions, competence, decisions, and behavior in the course of nursing practice.

e. Maintains competence through ongoing learning and application of knowledge in registered nursing practice.

f. Reports violations of the act or rules by self or other licensees.

2. Standards Related to RN Scope of Practice

The RN

a. Conducts a comprehensive nursing assessment.

b. Applies nursing knowledge based on the biologic, psychological, and social aspects of the patient's condition.

c. Detects faulty or missing patient information.

d. Plans nursing care and nursing interventions consistent with the patient's overall health care plan.

e. Uses decision making, critical thinking, and clinical judgment to make independent nursing decisions and nursing diagnoses.

f. Seeks clarification of orders when needed.

g. Implements treatment and therapy, including medication administration and delegated medical and independent nursing functions.

h. Obtains orientation/training for competence when encountering new equipment and technology or unfamiliar care situations.

i. Demonstrates attentiveness and provides patient surveillance and monitoring.

j. Identifies changes in patient's health status and comprehends clinical implications of patient's signs, symptoms, and changes as part of expected and unexpected patient course or emergent situations.

k. Evaluates the patient's response to nursing care and other therapy, including (1) patient's response to interventions; (2) need for alternative interventions; (3) need to communicate and consult with other health team members; (4) need to revise the plan of care.

l. Communicates and consults with other health team members, including (1) patient concerns and special needs; (2) patient status and progress; (3) patient response or lack of response to interventions; (4) significant changes in patient condition.

m. Documents nursing care.

n. Revises care plan as needed.

o. Takes preventive measures to protect patient, others, and self.

p. Provides comprehensive nursing and health care education in which the RN (1) assesses and analyzes educational needs of learners; (2) plans educational programs based on learning needs and teaching-learning principles; (3) ensures implementation of an educational plan either directly or by delegating selected aspects of education to other qualified persons; (4) evaluates education to meet the identified goals.

3. Standards Related to the RN's Responsibility to Advocate for the Patient

The RN

a. Respects the patient's rights, concerns, decisions, and dignity.

b. Identifies patient's needs.

c. Attends to patient's concerns or requests.

d. Promotes safe patient environment.

e. Communicates patient's choices, concerns, and special needs with other health team members regarding (1) patient's status and progress; (2) patient's response or lack of response to therapies; (3) significant changes in patient's condition.

f. Maintains appropriate professional boundaries.

g. Assumes responsibility for nurse's own decisions and actions.

4. Standards Related to RN's Responsibility to Organize, Manage, and Supervise the Practice of Nursing

The RN

a. Assigns to another only nursing measures that fall within that nurse's scope of practice, education, experience, and competence or unlicensed person's role description, including (1) assigning nursing care within the RN scope of practice to other RNs; (2) assigning nursing care to an LPN within the LPN scope of practice based on the RN's assessment of the patient and the LPN's ability; (3) supervising, monitoring, and evaluating the care assigned to an LPN.

b. Delegates to another only nursing measures for which that person has the necessary skills and competence to accomplish safely. In maintaining accountability for the delegation, an RN shall ensure that the (1) UAP has the education, legal authority, and demonstrated competency to perform the delegated task; (2) tasks delegated are consistent with the UAP's job description and can be safely performed according to clear, exact, and unchanging directions; (3) results of the task are reasonably predictable; (4) task does not require assessment, interpretation, or independent decision making during its performance or at completion; (5) selected patient and circumstances of the delegation are such that delegation of the task poses minimal risk to the patient and the consequences of performing the task improperly are not life-threatening; (6) RN provides clear directions and guidelines regarding the delegated task or, for routine tasks on stable patients, verifies that the UAP follows each written facility policy or procedure when performing the delegated task; (7) RN provides supervision and feedback to the UAP; (8) RN observes and communicates the outcomes of the delegated task.

c. Matches patient needs with personnel qualifications, available resources, and appropriate supervision.

d. Communicates directions and expectations for completion of the delegated activity.

e. Supervises others to whom nursing activities are delegated or assigned by monitoring performance, progress, and outcomes and ensures documentation of the activity.

f. Provides follow-up on problems and intervenes when needed.

g. Evaluates the effectiveness of the delegation or assignment.

h. Intervenes when problems are identified and revises plan of care as needed.

i. Retains professional accountability for nursing care as provided.

j. Promotes a safe and therapeutic environment by (1) providing appropriate monitoring and surveillance of the care environment; (2) identifying unsafe care situations; (3) correcting problems or referring problems to appropriate management level when needed.

k. Teaches and counsels patient and families regarding their health care regimen, which may include, but is not limited to, general information about health and medical condition, specific procedures, and wellness and prevention.

[a]Methods by which nurses safely and effectively deliver care within the scope of practice.

LPN, licensed practical nurse; *UAP*, unlicensed assistive personnel.

Modified from National Council of the State Boards of Nursing (NCSBN). *NCSBN Model Rules*. Chicago, IL: NCSBN; 2012, updated 2014.

BOX 3.3 Standards of Care for Acute and Critical Care Nursing

Standard 1: Assessment

The nurse caring for the acutely and critically ill patient collects comprehensive data pertinent to the patient's health or situation.

Assessment Competencies:

1. Collects data from the patient, family, other health care providers, and the community, as appropriate, to develop a holistic picture of patient's needs
2. Prioritizes data collection based on patient's characteristics related to the immediate condition and anticipated needs
3. Uses valid evidence-based assessment techniques, instruments, and tools
4. Documents relevant data in a clear and retrievable format

Standard 2: Diagnosis

The nurse caring for the acutely and critically ill patient analyzes and synthesizes data from the assessment in determining nursing diagnoses or conditions relevant to care.

Diagnosis Competencies:

1. Derives diagnoses or relevant conditions from the assessment data
2. Validates diagnoses with the patient, family, and other health care providers
3. Documents diagnoses and relevant issues in a clear and retrievable format

Standard 3: Outcomes Identification

The nurse caring for the acutely and critically ill patient identifies expected outcomes for the patient.

Outcomes Identification Competencies:

1. Identifies outcomes from assessments and diagnoses
2. Respects patient and family perspectives and values in formulating culturally appropriate outcomes in collaboration with the patient and family and with the interprofessional team
3. Considers associated risks, benefits, current evidence, clinical expertise, and cost when formulating expected outcomes
4. Modifies expected outcomes based on changes in patient's condition or situation
5. Documents outcomes as measurable goals in a clear and retrievable format

Standard 4: Planning

The nurse caring for the acutely and critically ill patient develops a plan that prescribes strategies and alternatives to attain outcomes.

Planning Competencies:

1. Employs critical thinking and judgment in developing an individualized plan using best evidence
2. Collaborates with the patient, family, and interprofessional team to develop the plan
3. Establishes priorities and continuity of care within the plan
4. Includes strategies for health promotion and prevention of further illness or injury within the plan
5. Considers associated risks, benefits, current evidence, clinical expertise, resources, and cost when developing the plan
6. Documents the plan in a clear and retrievable manner

Standard 5: Implementation

The nurse caring for the acutely and critically ill patient implements the plan.

Implementation Competencies:

1. Employs strategies to promote and maintain safe environment
2. Coordinates implementation of the plan with the patient, family, and interprofessional team
3. Intervenes to prevent and minimize complications and alleviate suffering
4. Facilitates learning for patients, families, and the community
5. Documents implementation in a clear and retrievable format
6. Provides age-appropriate and developmentally appropriate care in a culturally and ethnically sensitive manner

Standard 6: Evaluation

The nurse caring for the acutely and critically ill patient evaluates processes and outcomes.

Evaluation Competencies:

1. Conducts systematic and ongoing evaluations using evidence-based techniques, tools, and instruments
2. Collaborates with the patient, family, and interprofessional team in the evaluation process
3. Revises the assessment, diagnoses, outcomes, and interventions based on the information gained during the evaluation process
4. Documents the results of evaluation in a clear and retrievable format

Modified from American Association of Critical-Care Nurses. *AACN Scope and Standards for Acute and Critical Care Nursing Practice*. Aliso Viejo, CA: AACN; May 2015.

the same as the standards of practice. In some cases, specialty standards of practice or care have been introduced in court to help establish a legal standard of care, but not all courts will consider these. The legal standard of care and the use of specialty standards are discussed further in the following section on tort law.

TORT LAW: NEGLIGENCE AND PROFESSIONAL MALPRACTICE, INTENTIONAL TORTS

Many civil lawsuits for injuries fall under the legal heading of torts. Anyone can find themselves as a party in such a lawsuit. Torts are civil lawsuits based on unintentional acts (failure to act or negligence that results in harm) or intentional acts, such as assault, battery, or defamation. For the lay public, the standard for behavior for negligence is based on reasonableness, or what a reasonably prudent person would do in the same situation. This is also known as ordinary negligence.

In a professional capacity, individuals are judged based on their professional standard of care. Nurses caring for acutely and critically ill patients may be alleged to have acted in a manner that is inconsistent with the professional standard of care as part of a lawsuit that focuses in whole or in part on the alleged failure. This is professional malpractice or negligence law applied to professional behavior.

There are many types of cases based in tort law, but this chapter focuses on negligence and professional malpractice, intentional torts of assault and battery, and some cases based on specific clinical circumstances. These include respiratory management of acutely and critically ill patients as well as liability associated with blood transfusions, infection control, and informed consent.

Ordinary Negligence

Generally, the standard for negligence is failing to act as a reasonably prudent person would under similar circumstances. There are four criteria or elements for all negligence cases: (1) duty to another person, (2) breach of that duty, (3) harm that would not have occurred in the absence of the breach (causation), and (4) damages that have a monetary value. All four elements must be satisfied for a case to go forward. For example, suppose a grocery store employee mops the floor but fails to block off the area or put up a "wet floor" sign, and a customer walks in the area, falls and breaks a hip, and is left with hospital bills and lost wages. The grocery store has a duty to its customers to provide a reasonably safe environment and warn customers of areas of danger. Warning customers by blocking off the wet area or using a sign is what a reasonably prudent grocery store would do. Failing to warn customers is a breach of that duty. Because the customer had no warning, she walked on the wet floor, fell, and suffered the harm of a broken hip. The customer would not have suffered the broken hip if the area had been blocked off. Finally, there are monetary damages in the form of hospital bills and lost wages. This is an example of ordinary negligence in which any person could make a determination of what is reasonable in a given circumstance. A juror need not hear from a professional to determine what is a reasonably prudent practice for the grocery store (standard for nonnegligent behavior) in this case. Negligence in the professional health care context differs in that expert testimony is needed to establish the standard of care. These cases are referred to as professional negligence or professional malpractice.

Professional Malpractice

Although negligence claims may apply to anyone, malpractice requires the alleged wrongdoer to have special standing as a professional. In civil cases alleging wrongdoing by health care professionals, the terms *malpractice* and *negligence* (meaning professional negligence) are used interchangeably. Malpractice is a negligence action applied to a professional, as the court in *Candler General Hospital Inc. v McNorrill* explained.[11]

If a nurse caring for acutely and critically ill patients is accused of failing to act in a manner consistent with the standard of care, that nurse (and usually his or her employer) is subject to liability for professional negligence. Just as in ordinary negligence, the person bringing the lawsuit must prove the elements of negligence. In the health care context, the patient-plaintiffs (person[s] bringing the lawsuit) must prove (1) that the nurse had a duty to care for the patient, (2) that the nurse breached that duty by deviating from the standard of care, (3) that the breach caused harm that would not have occurred in the absence of negligence, and (4) that the plaintiff should be compensated for the resulting damages.

The legal standard of care for nurses is established by expert testimony and is generally "the care that an ordinarily prudent *nurse* would perform under the same circumstances."[12] The standard of care determination focuses more on accepted practice of competent nurses rather than best practice of excellent nurses (which may be reflected in some specialty standards of practice). In addition to expert testimony, courts may rely on multiple types of evidence to establish the standard of care.

In *Gould v NY City Health and Hospital*,[13] the court looked more closely at the standard of care and identified three basic measures for the nursing standard of care. The nurse should (1) possess the requisite knowledge and skill possessed by an average member of the profession, (2) exercise reasonable and ordinary care in the application of professional knowledge and skill, and (3) use best judgment in the application of professional knowledge and skill.

Duty

Duty to the injured party is the first element of a malpractice case and is premised on the existence of a nurse-patient relationship. Nurses assume a duty to the patient to provide care that is consistent with the standard of care when the nurse-patient relationship is established. Cases from many states recognize the nurse-patient relationship as a separate and distinct relationship[14] and as a prerequisite for determining whether a nurse owes the patient a duty to provide care in accordance with the requisite standard of care. If a nurse shows that he or she (1) was not assigned to that particular patient on the date that the negligence allegedly occurred or (2) was not working on the day or at the time the negligence allegedly occurred, there was no relationship and therefore no duty. Because no duty is imposed on the nurse, negligence allegations will fail.[15]

If the patient establishes that a specific nurse actually rendered care, the nurse will be found to have assumed a duty to provide reasonable care for the patient. This duty cannot be waived or overridden by the instructions of a physician or hospital administrator. *Lunsford v Board of Nurse Examiners*[16] illustrates this principle. In this case, Donald Floyd arrived at an emergency department (ED) in Texas complaining of chest pain and pressure that radiated down his left arm. Mr. Floyd was accompanied by Ms. Farrell, who asked a physician who was sitting at the nurses' station to examine Mr. Floyd. The physician told Ms. Farrell that Nurse Lunsford would interview Mr. Floyd before he would see a physician. The physician then instructed Nurse Lunsford to transfer Mr. Floyd to a neighboring hospital located 24 miles away because the equipment that would likely be needed to treat Mr. Floyd was already in use by another patient.

Nurse Lunsford then interviewed Mr. Floyd and suspected cardiac involvement. Because of the transfer instruction that she received from the physician, Lunsford instructed Ms. Farrell to drive Mr. Floyd to the neighboring hospital and to speed and drive with her flashers on. Reportedly, Lunsford also asked Ms. Farrell if she knew cardiopulmonary resuscitation and suggested that she might need to perform cardiopulmonary resuscitation at some point on the way. Within approximately 5 miles of the Harlingen ED, Mr. Floyd died as a result of cardiac arrest in Ms. Farrell's car.

An administrative complaint was subsequently filed with the Texas Board of Nurse Examiners alleging negligence and challenging Lunsford's nursing licensure. After a hearing on the matter, the Texas Board of Nurse Examiners suspended the license of Lunsford for 1 year. Lunsford appealed the decision and the court determined that Lunsford as well as other nurses who are similarly situated have a duty to (1) evaluate the status of persons who are ill and seeking professional help and (2) implement care needed to stabilize a patient's condition and to prevent complications. According to the Texas Court of Appeals, Lunsford failed to act reasonably and breached her duty to Mr. Floyd when she failed to (1) assess him, (2) inform the physician of the life-threatening nature of his condition, and (3) take appropriate action to stabilize him and prevent his death. The court also pointed out that hospital policy or physician orders do not relieve a nurse of his or her duty to a patient.

Breach

Breach is the failure to act consistently within applicable standards of care. For a nurse to be found negligent, the patient-plaintiff must establish that the nurse had a duty to provide care and that the nurse failed to provide care consistent with those standards. Moreover, the nurse's failure, or breach, must have caused the damages about which the patient-plaintiff seeks redress. A breach of duty does not exist if the standard of care is met.

In *Sparks v St. Luke's Regional Medical Center*,[17] the family of Thomas Sparks sued St. Luke's Regional Medical Center and treating physicians, alleging that their negligence resulted in Thomas Sparks sustaining brain damage after he was extubated. The case reached the Idaho Supreme Court. The court concluded that although Mr. Sparks suffered severe harm, no breach of duty existed and the evidence established that the standard of care for extubation and subsequent hospital care was met.

The *Sparks* case demonstrated that courts often consider many sources of evidence in determining the standard of care. These may include applicable NPAs; specialty practice standards; job descriptions; and organizational policies, procedures, protocols, and pathways, together with other reference sources including case law, journal articles, textbooks, and other manuscripts.

Actions that are consistent with professional practice standards may be used as evidence that the nurse did not breach his or her duty to patients. Even if not used as evidence for the standard of care, these standards provide guidance on quality nursing care. Nurses caring for acutely and critically ill patients should practice in accordance with the practice specialty standards issued by the AACN (see Box 3.3). These standards provide guidance for nurses, and they increasingly provide definitive guidance in courtrooms.

For example, in *Newsom v Lake Charles Memorial Hospital*,[18] the court used AACN standards along with expert testimony to evaluate the action of critical care nurses caring for a patient who died shortly after the removal of an intraaortic balloon pump. Viewing the totality of the circumstances, the court determined the hospital, through its nurses, was negligent in failing to properly alert the patient's physician of a 60-point drop in systolic blood pressure and failure to closely monitor the patient for bleeding.

Documents or policies specific to the nurse's employer or practice setting may also be used to inform the appropriate standard of care. For example, a nurse's job description or employment contract may contain provisions that require a nurse to act or to refrain from acting in a specific manner and within a specific period of time. Failure to adhere to those provisions could give rise to negligence causes of action wherein the patient-plaintiff asserts that the nurse failed to act in accordance with his or her job description or employment contract. Accordingly, job descriptions and employment contracts should reflect the standard of care and articulate reasonable expectations of behavior. Nurses caring for acutely and critically ill patients are required to act in a manner that is consistent with organizational policies, procedures, protocols, and clinical pathways. Failure to do so may result in liability if a patient is harmed because of the failure. For example, in *Teffeteller v University of Minnesota*,[19] a nurse's failure to follow an institutional protocol resulted in liability after a critically ill pediatric patient died of narcotic toxicity.

Harm Caused by the Breach

Patient-plaintiffs must prove that the nurse breached his or her duty to the patient and that the breach caused the patient to sustain injuries or damages for which he or she seeks monetary remuneration. Causation of the harm is a pivotal element in civil cases filed against nurses. If patient-plaintiffs fail to establish that some act or omission directly resulted in the harm or if something else can be shown to have caused the harm, recovery will be denied.

McMullen v Ohio State University Hospitals[20] dealt with the causation issue and was ultimately decided by the Ohio Supreme Court. In *McMullen*, an intubated patient on mechanical ventilation experienced oxygen desaturation and hypotension and exhibited cyanosis and dyspnea. The nurse also reported an audible squeak, thought to be a cuff leak on the endotracheal tube. The nurse believed that the patient was dying and paged the on-call physicians "stat." However, before the physicians arrived, the nurse removed the patient's endotracheal tube. Thereafter, it took more than 20 minutes to successfully reintubate the patient; the patient never regained consciousness and died 7 days later. The patient's estate brought a wrongful death cause of action against the Ohio State University Hospitals based on the nurse's negligence in removing the endotracheal tube (and thereby causing the loss of an airway). After appeals to the Ohio Supreme Court, the court held the nurse's actions caused the harm because the removal of the patient's endotracheal tube in an uncontrolled environment was negligent and set into motion a chain of events that directly caused the patient to die of anoxic brain injury.

Damages

The fourth element of negligence is damages. Damages are the monetary value or cost of the injury suffered. For liability to be imposed against a nurse caring for an acutely or critically ill patient, that patient must prove that something the nurse did or failed to do was inconsistent with the standard of care and that the inconsistency caused harm or injury that has a monetary value. Patient-plaintiffs in a malpractice case can usually point to additional medical bills associated with their injuries to satisfy this element.

The number of nurses being named defendants in these cases is increasing, and this is especially true for advanced practice nurses. Nurses caring for acutely and critically ill patients need to carefully consider whether to purchase professional liability insurance and, if so, the amount and type of coverage that is needed. Most institutions will provide some level of malpractice insurance coverage for nurses, but the amount and circumstances under which each nurse is covered are important considerations.

Professional Malpractice and the Nursing Process

Malpractice claims may be premised on care delivered at any point from the moment a nurse-patient relationship is established to patient discharge. What constitutes reasonable care has been the focus of many cases filed against health care professionals and the hospitals in which they practice. For nurses, there seems to be an emerging trend. If the nurse reasonably executes every component of the nursing process by assessing, planning, implementing, and evaluating the care in accordance with the requisite standard of care, reasonable care will have been provided. However, if the nurse fails with regard to a single component of the nursing process, care provided to an acutely or critically ill patient may be deemed insufficient, unreasonable, and negligent. The following cases are examples of malpractice resulting from failures in particular stages of the nursing process.

Assessment failure: failure to assess and analyze the level of care needed by the patient. Nurses caring for acutely and critically ill patients have a duty to assess and analyze the level of care needed by their patients. Where a nurse allegedly fails to fulfill this responsibility, liability for negligence may be threatened. *Brandon HMA, Inc. v Bradshaw*[21] demonstrates how courts handle failure to assess and analyze the level of care needed by acutely and critically ill patients.

In *Brandon*, Dawn Bradshaw sustained permanent injuries because of negligence on the part of the nursing staff during her hospitalization at Rankin Medical Center for bacterial pneumonia. After a chest tube was inserted, nurses failed to assess or take vital signs on Ms. Bradshaw for 4 hours and 30 minutes. When the patient was finally assessed, she was nauseated, disoriented, sweating profusely, and unable to follow verbal commands. Approximately 10 minutes later, she experienced cardiac arrest. Although the patient was resuscitated, she sustained brain injury from anoxia and was discharged to a rehabilitation facility specializing in the treatment of brain injury. The case was tried before a jury, and the jury agreed that Ms. Bradshaw sustained permanent, severe brain damage related to oxygen deprivation because of the negligence of the nursing staff. The nurse's failure to assess Ms. Bradshaw made it impossible to intervene earlier to prevent the cardiac arrest and therefore her oxygen deprivation. The jury awarded Ms. Bradshaw $9 million in damages.

To withstand allegations of failure to assess and analyze, it is important for nurses not only to assess and analyze the level of care needed by patients but also to document their assessment findings as well as all actions taken to properly care for patients. Failure to assess and analyze the situation and to document the assessment findings, the interventions, and the patient's response to those interventions exposes the nurse and, as in the *Brandon* case, the hospital to liability for negligence.

Assessment failure: failure to assess and clarify patient's condition. Nurses are responsible for obtaining appropriate and complete information on a patient's condition on assuming care, adequately assessing the patient, and clarifying and reporting any discrepancies. A case from Alabama illustrates these responsibilities. In *Brookwood Health Services v Borden*,[22] Mr. Borden developed severe back and leg pain and new-onset numbness in his legs at home a few days after a lumbar laminectomy. After phone consultation with his surgeon, Mr. Borden was taken to the ED, where he exhibited some motor deficits to his toes and ankles; he could lift his legs off of the bed and was continent. A computed tomography scan revealed a small hematoma. Mr. Borden was admitted to the hospital around midnight under his surgeon's care with orders that included neurovascular checks every 2 hours and an order to "call admitting physician for any questions, problems, change of status, or for further orders."

The nurse receiving Mr. Borden on the unit, Nurse Tolbert, assessed him at 12:15 am and documented that he was wet from incontinence, that he could not move his legs at all, and that his pedal pulses were weak. Nurse Tolbert did not notify the physician or check his ED records. At trial, Nurse Tolbert said she had received an oral report from an ED nurse and that his condition was consistent with that report. However, she did not document that report. The day nurse received a report from Tolbert and documented an assessment at 7:00 am that was consistent with Tolbert's. Mr. Borden's physician discovered the change in condition a few hours later and ordered an emergency computed tomography scan that revealed a large hematoma compressing the cauda equina that required emergency surgery. Mr. Borden was left permanently disabled with chronic pain, incontinence, significant mobility problems, and impotence.

Based on the nurse's failure to adequately assess Mr. Borden; consider his present status in light of his clinical history (eg, he was walking and continent less than 8 hours earlier); and clarify Mr. Borden's status via discussion with Mr. Borden, the ED record, or the physician, Mr. Borden sued the hospital for negligence that resulted in his permanent disability that may have been prevented with earlier intervention and emergency surgery. The jury awarded him $5 million in damages. The Alabama Supreme Court ultimately changed that award based on the failure of Mr. Borden's attorney to present adequate expert testimony of the nursing standard of care; however, the facts of the case serve as an example of how nursing vigilance or lack thereof can severely impact a patient's life and lead to liability.

Planning failure: failure to appropriately diagnose. Nurses caring for acutely and critically ill patients must plan effective courses of treatment. Such a course of treatment depends on a proper diagnosis. Historically, cases of failure to diagnose have been filed against physicians, rather than nurses. However, nurses who diagnose patient conditions may find themselves the target of a failure to diagnose a case and need to be aware that liability may be imposed if the plan of care is based on an erroneous diagnosis.

Implementation failure: failure to communicate patient findings in a timely manner. Nurses spend more time with patients than any other health care professionals do, and this is especially true for nurses caring for acutely and critically ill patients. As a result, these nurses are in the best position to promptly detect changes in a patient's condition. However, detection is only the first step. Nurses caring for acutely and critically ill patients must promptly communicate troublesome patient findings. Failure to properly communicate patient findings can be devastating for patients and can be the reason that patients file malpractice causes of action. *Denesia v St. Elizabeth Community Health Center*[23] exemplifies how courts handle these kinds of cases. In *Denesia*, it was alleged that the death of patient Lucille Denesia was the result of failure of the nursing staff to appropriately notify the physician in a timely manner of an alarmingly high partial thromboplastin time (PTT) and change in patient status indicative of neurologic compromise. Ms. Denesia was admitted to the hospital with suspected embolic stroke secondary to her history of atrial fibrillation. To prevent further emboli, anticoagulation therapy including heparin injection, a heparin drip, and oral warfarin (Coumadin) was ordered, along with a PTT level 4 hours after initiation. The PTT level was obtained at 4:00 pm, and at 5:30 pm the laboratory notified the nurse that the level was 200 seconds (far beyond the therapeutic range). The nurse reported placing a call to the physician's answering service, but she did not follow up.

Shortly after 6:30 pm, the nurse noted a 6-second arrhythmia and noted the patient was vomiting with headache pain. The nurse called Ms. Denesia's cardiologist but did not document her conversation and could not recall the details; the cardiologist contended that she reported only the arrhythmia and not the PTT level or status change. Approximately 75 minutes later, the nurse spoke with the primary treating physician; again, she did not document the conversation and could not remember what she told him. The primary treating physician testified that he was not informed of the PTT result but that he ordered the intravenous infusion of heparin to be reduced.

Over the next several hours, Ms. Denesia had multiple vomiting episodes despite repeated administration of antinausea medication. She slept for a few hours but awoke with vomiting followed by lethargy, motor weakness, and other symptoms of neurologic compromise. The primary physician was notified; he discontinued the heparin and transferred the patient to the critical care unit, where Ms. Denesia lapsed into a coma and died of a massive cerebral hemorrhage.

The case was appealed to the Supreme Court of Nebraska, where the justices ordered that the case be retried, but the parties likely settled before a retrial; the outcome is not available. Nonetheless, the case provides a cautionary tale on the importance of monitoring patient status, communicating changes, and documenting those communications. For nurses caring for acutely and critically ill patients, it is imperative that interactions with physicians, whether in person or over the telephone, be documented, as well as the information conveyed during those interactions. Had the nurse taken the time to document what she told the cardiologist and the primary treating physician, this litigation might have been avoided.

Implementation failure: failure to take appropriate action. Cases from across the United States continue to affirm that it is the nurse's responsibility to take affirmative action when action is indicated. *Garcia v United States*[24] is one such case. In *Garcia*, Candido Garcia was admitted to a Veterans Administration Medical Center for removal of chronic subdural hematomas with insertion of Jackson-Pratt drains and revision of a ventriculoperitoneal shunt. He arrived to the unit around 6:25 pm. His nurse briefly assessed him and went to lunch. Around 7:00 pm, his daughter reported that her father was making strange hand movements and snorting noises and emitting white bubbles from his mouth. Mr. Garcia's wife also noted the changes and reported the occurrence to another nurse on the ward, who dismissed her concerns. At around 7:30 pm, Mr. Garcia's nurse returned from lunch and found him unconscious and red blood in his surgical drains. The nurse did not document actions taken in alerting Mr. Garcia's physicians, and his physicians reported they received a routine page shortly before 8:00 pm and therefore did not see Mr. Garcia until 8:15 pm. Although he underwent emergency craniotomy for bleeding, the delay in obtaining proper medical assistance resulted in more severe long-term disability; he was a quadriplegic, required a tracheostomy, and had cognitive impairments. The hospital was liable for negligence based on the inaction of the nurses, and Mr. Garcia was awarded more than $2.3 million in damages. In reaching its decision, the court found that the nursing staff should have recognized the emergency nature of the situation and taken proper steps to notify the attending physician.

Failure to take appropriate action in cases involving acutely and critically ill patients has included not only issues regarding physician notification but also failure to follow physician orders,[25,26] failure to properly treat,[27] and failure to appropriately administer medication.[27–29] To avoid allegations of failure to take appropriate action, nurses caring for acutely and critically ill patients need to recognize signs and symptoms of complications and patient compromise. Nurses must also ensure that those signs and symptoms are communicated to the physician in a timely manner and take other affirmative action that is authorized and appropriate. Patient findings, interventions, and actions taken, and patient responses to interventions must be documented.

Implementation failure: failure to document. Nurses caring for acutely and critically ill patients are required not only to take appropriate action but also to accurately document their findings, interventions performed, and patients' response to interventions. Failure to thoroughly and accurately document any aspect of care gives rise to negligence causes of action.

Haney v Alexander,[30] a case from North Carolina, demonstrates how courts and juries deal with a nurse's failure to properly document. In *Haney*, a nurse caring for a patient who was experiencing atrial fibrillation failed to take, record, and communicate all the patient's vital signs and failed to properly document medication orders and administration, leading to a double dose. Shortly after the second dose of medication, the patient was found dead. The court of appeals concluded that the nurse was negligent in several respects, including failure to document vital signs, medication orders, and administration, and that the nurse's negligence contributed to the patient's death. The *Haney* case, along with many of the other cases discussed so far illustrate the consequences of inadequate documentation of care delivered, communications with other team members, interventions and actions taken, and the response of the patient to interventions and actions. Failure to thoroughly document prevents nurses from defending their actions in professional malpractice.

Implementation failure: failure to preserve patient privacy. Nurses have a legal duty to preserve patient privacy and confidentiality. State and federal statutes and case law affirm this duty. For example, in *Randi A.J. v Long Island Surgical Center*,[31] the patient was awarded more than $300,000 in damages after a nurse disclosed her confidential information to the patient's mother; furthermore, the patient had given the surgical center specific instructions not to call her home, as she wished to keep her information private. The nurse's failure to preserve the patient's privacy coupled with the facility's lack of a procedure or policy for preserving privacy led to their liability.

In addition, the actions of nurses could expose their employers to severe penalties from the federal government for violations of federal laws, such as the Health Insurance Portability and Accountability Act.[32] Nurses can ensure that the privacy of acutely and critically ill patients is protected by following patient directives as well as institutional policies and procedures, which should comply with state privacy laws and federal laws. Nurses must also avoid any discussions about specific patients with anyone except other health care professionals involved in the patient's care in nonpublic settings. Discussions about specific patients are never appropriate in public areas, such as elevators, cafeterias, gift shops, and parking lots.

Evaluation failure: failure to act as a patient advocate. From admission to discharge, nurses have a duty to act as a patient advocate. For nurses caring for acutely and critically ill patients, this duty imposes the responsibility to evaluate the care that is being given to patients. The landmark failure to advocate case was *Darling v Charleston Community Memorial Hospital*,[33] a case decided by the Illinois Supreme Court in 1965. Dorrence Darling II was an 18-year-old athlete treated at Charleston Community Memorial Hospital after a leg fracture. Dorrence was placed in traction, and his broken leg was placed in a plaster cast. Shortly after the cast was applied, he began to complain of new severe pain in the casted leg, and his toes protruding from the cast became swollen and discolored; later, the toes were cold and insensitive to tactile stimulation. The following day, his physician cut small notches in the cast around the toes. The following day, he cut 3 inches off the cast from the foot. On the third day, the physician used a saw to split the sides of the cast and in the process cut both sides of Dorrence's broken leg. By this time, the nursing staff noted blood, drainage, and a terrible odor. At no point did the nurses advocate for more aggressive treatment, a second opinion, or notify the hospital administration. Dorrence was transferred to another hospital 14 days after his admission to Charleston Community Memorial Hospital, and he eventually required a below-the-knee amputation because of the severe necrotic tissue secondary to circulatory compromise from improper casting.

A jury found the hospital liable for Mr. Darling's injuries through the negligent actions of the nursing staff and the physician. The case was appealed to the Illinois Supreme Court, which upheld the verdict, stating that the nursing staff failed to properly assess circulation, failed to promptly recognize that circulatory compromise was occurring, and therefore failed to prevent the irreversible effects of prolonged inadequate circulation. Had they recognized the significance of the symptoms they were seeing, the nursing staff could have exercised their duty to inform hospital authorities so that appropriate action could be taken. Because they failed to act as a patient advocate, Dorrence lost his leg, and the hospital was liable for their failure.

Although the *Darling* case was decided in 1965, courts continue to hold that all nurses, including nurses caring for acutely and critically ill patients, have a nondelegable duty to act as patient advocate. Failure to act as patient advocate exposes the nurse to substantial liability and, more importantly, exposes patients to life-altering and life-ending complications that could have been avoided. Advocating for the patient means taking concerns up the chain of command. Documenting concerns is insufficient to protect the nurse from liability.

For example, in *Rowe v Sisters of Pallottine*,[34] Mr. Rowe was seen in an ED after a motorcycle accident with pain in his left knee, numbness, and an absent pulse in his left foot. The ED physician discharged Mr. Rowe with instructions to return if his symptoms worsened. The nurse caring for Mr. Rowe repeatedly assessed Mr. Rowe; questioned the physician's decision to discharge Mr. Rowe; and extensively documented her concerns in the nursing notes, especially regarding the lack of a pulse. She also instructed Mr. Rowe's parents, who were with him, that there was no pulse in the foot. At trial, she explained her documentation as an effort to "cover herself." Nonetheless, the jury awarded Mr. Rowe nearly $1 million, in part, based on negligence of the nurses in failing to properly advocate for the patient. The nurses had breached the standard of care by not adequately advocating for the patient when he was discharged with unexplained and unaddressed symptoms. The court explained that nurses were obligated to take their concerns up the chain of command.

Wrongful Death

Wrongful death cases are a variation of negligence action in which the harm is the death of the individual. Similar to ordinary negligence, wrongful death claims can also be brought against nonprofessionals. However, in the professional health care context, these claims are identical to professional negligence cases except that the harm caused by the professionals is the death of the patient and the plaintiff is the survivor of the patient, such as a spouse or adult child.

For families and health care professionals, wrongful death cases are among the most traumatic. In these cases, the life-and-death nature of the health care experience is exposed. In reviewing these kinds of cases, one learns that what is at issue is rarely the use, misuse, or malfunction of sophisticated, cutting-edge technology or the miscalculation of a complex formula. On the contrary, a review of wrongful death cases suggests that the alleged failures at issue are typically foundational matters of patient care and critical thinking. For instance, failure to thoroughly assess a patient, to take vital signs, to properly administer medication, or to administer portable oxygen to a patient with respiratory compromise has been the focus of most of the wrongful death cases discussed in this chapter. To avoid wrongful death liability, it is imperative that nurses caring for acutely and critically ill patients remain vigilant, recognize the signs and symptoms of complications and compromise, and take affirmative action to advocate for the best interest of the patient.

Assault and Battery

Assault and battery are examples of intentional torts that are frequently brought against health care providers. Although they are often used together, they are actually two separate torts. Assault is any intentional act that creates reasonable apprehension of immediate harmful or offensive contact with the plaintiff. With assault, no actual contact is necessary. Battery is any intentional act that brings about actual harmful or offensive contact with the plaintiff.

In health care cases, patient consent is a defense to these claims. Assault occurs if a patient fears harmful or offensive touching. Assault may be alleged if a patient was aware that he or she was going to be touched in a manner not authorized by informed consent. For example, the act of telling a patient that he or she will be restrained may be assault. Battery occurs if the health care professional touches the patient in an unauthorized manner. The act of restraining a patient without consent is battery. Another defense to assault and battery is an emergency situation. Thus, cutting a patient's throat to create an emergency tracheostomy to create an airway may be justified, whereas cutting a patient's neck on the wrong side in opposition to the informed consent may be battery.

Special Clinical Circumstances and Professional Malpractice

This section addresses specific areas of care that result in legal action. These issues include respiratory management, liability associated with blood transfusions, and infection control issues.

Respiratory Management

The management of the respiratory status of an acutely or critically ill patient gives rise to more litigation than the management of any other physiologic system. Respiratory management involves issues ranging from appropriate use of supplemental oxygen to care of patients with artificial airways.

In *Manning v Twin Falls Clinic & Hospital*,[35] a nurse was liable for failing to keep an oxygen-dependent patient attached to a portable oxygen supply during a transfer. The patient, Mr. Manning, had end-stage chronic obstructive pulmonary disease with associated hypoxemia and hypercapnia. He was dependent on continuous supplemental oxygen by a nasal cannula. On his admission to the hospital, Mr. Manning was classified as a "no code" after discussions between his physician and family members that he likely only had days to live. In preparing to transfer the patient to a private room, his nurse disconnected the oxygen supply despite an order for continuous oxygen and over the voiced objections and explanations of his dependence on it from family members. After the bed had been moved approximately 15 feet, Mr. Manning experienced a respiratory arrest and died.

Dixon v Taylor[36] is a case of inappropriate extubation and inadequate preparation for emergencies. Willie L. Dixon, a patient in critical care for pneumonia, experienced a respiratory arrest and then cardiac arrest from which she was successfully resuscitated. She was intubated during the code and remained on mechanical ventilation. Less than 24 hours after her respiratory arrest, her physician directed her nurse and a respiratory therapist to extubate Ms. Dixon. However, they extubated her without a fully stocked crash cart and without even an oxygen mask. She initially received oxygen via nasal prongs, but this was insufficient. The patient was left unmonitored while the respiratory therapist went to another unit to obtain an oxygen mask. When he returned, Ms. Dixon was not breathing.

The nurse and respiratory therapist immediately attempted to reintubate Ms. Dixon, but the crash cart was not stocked, and the appropriate equipment for intubation was missing. During the delay, Ms. Dixon progressed to cardiac arrest. She was successfully reintubated and resuscitated minutes later, but she sustained catastrophic neurologic damage from anoxia and died 10 months later. Her survivors sued for wrongful death, and a jury awarded them nearly $1 million for negligence of the respiratory therapist in failing to voice concerns about her readiness for extubation to the physician before extubation, failing to stock the crash cart, and failing to properly prepare for Ms. Dixon's extubation and possible reintubation.

Moon v St. Thomas Hospital[37] is an example of the need to protect an intubated patient's airway. Mr. Moon underwent coronary artery bypass graft surgery and remained intubated postoperatively. His nurse documented two separate times in less than 2 hours that he was restless and was biting down on his endotracheal tube but did not notify the physician, order a bite block, or reposition the tube. Mr. Moon then transected the tube by biting through it, and a portion of the tube had to be removed from his airway. During attempts at reintubation, Mr. Moon suffered a fatal myocardial infarction. The family of Mr. Moon alleged that permitting him to bite on the endotracheal tube to the extent that it was transected was negligent and that a physician should have been notified, a bite block inserted, or the endotracheal tube repositioned to avoid the transection.

In *Owensboro Mercy Health System v Payne*,[38] a jury awarded $2,270,000 in damages for the negligent transfer of Mr. Payne from the operating room to the critical care unit. Mr. Payne had undergone 8 hours of surgery for extensive trauma. After the surgery, the health care providers transferred him from the operating room to the critical care unit without monitoring equipment or supplemental oxygen, and his respiratory demise went undetected, resulting in permanent brain injury.

In *Miller v Marymount Medical Center*,[39] Mrs. Miller, a 31-year-old pregnant woman, was admitted to Marymount Medical Center to give birth. She gave birth 2 days later via cesarean section to a healthy girl. After the cesarean section, the patient began having respiratory problems. A chest radiograph obtained on the morning after the cesarean section revealed that Mrs. Miller had pneumonia. A blood gas analysis done that same morning indicated that her Po_2 was 64.4 mEq/L. Antibiotic therapy was started, and a nasal cannula was applied to improve

oxygenation. Mrs. Miller was also treated for pain and stress with meperidine (Demerol) and hydroxyzine (Vistaril) injections. Throughout the day, her respiratory distress continued.

At 9:45 pm that same night, her physician told the Miller family that a pulmonologist was going to be called. The nurse administered Demerol and Vistaril injections 5 minutes later. Mrs. Miller's physician returned to her room 10 minutes after the injections to find Mrs. Miller unresponsive and in respiratory arrest. Five minutes later, Mrs. Miller was intubated, placed on an oxygen bag delivering 100% oxygen, and transferred to the critical care unit. Mrs. Miller was breathing without assistance 12 minutes after she was intubated and transferred to the critical care unit, but she never regained consciousness. She was eventually transferred to a nursing home in a permanent vegetative state.

Mrs. Miller's family filed a malpractice action that included allegations that the nursing staff failed to furnish treating physicians with up-to-date information, failed to obtain repeat blood gas analyses as ordered, and failed to question and proceeded to administer Demerol despite the fact that Demerol can accelerate the progression of acute respiratory distress syndrome, which is the condition the experts retained by the family concluded that Mrs. Miller had on the morning the chest radiograph was obtained. The family settled with the physicians but went to trial on the negligence claims against the hospital. The trial lasted 7 days, and the jury returned a defense verdict because they were unable to definitively determine that negligence of the nursing staff was the proximate cause of Mrs. Miller's injuries.

In a case from Philadelphia, *Small v Temple Univ. Hospital*,[40] a patient in the critical care unit died after his endotracheal tube became obstructed by a mucous plug and the nurses failed to suction the tube or act based on patient and family reports. Hours before he died, the patient wrote a note to his daughters saying he could not breathe. The daughters informed the nurses, who failed to communicate this information to the physicians. Later, when the man's breathing struggles worsened, he became agitated and tried to remove the tube. The physician, thinking he was suffering from critical care unit psychosis, gave him sedatives and had him restrained. The jury awarded his family $1.7 million in damages against the hospital for the negligent acts of the nurses.

These cases serve as a stark reminder of the life-altering and life-ending implications associated with management of the respiratory status of an acutely or critically ill patient. Consequently, nurses caring for patients with respiratory compromise must diligently assess, plan, and implement care and evaluate these patients with vigilance. These cases also highlight the importance of listening to patient and family concerns and of the physical assessment of patients. The life of an acutely or critically ill patient depends on it.

Blood Transfusions and Infection Control

Tobin v Providence Hospital[41] serves as a reminder that blood transfusions are associated with considerable risks. Rollin Tobin underwent hip replacement surgery but died of sepsis and disseminated intravascular coagulation. Mr. Tobin's wife asserted that he died because blood contaminated with *Yersinia* bacteria was administered to him during surgery.

Before surgery, Mr. Tobin donated 3 units of his own blood, and those 3 units were transfused in the operating room as well as an additional allogeneic unit. After Mr. Tobin's death, the

American Red Cross and the Centers for Disease Control and Prevention investigated the situation and determined that the fourth unit administered to Mr. Tobin was contaminated with *Yersinia* bacteria.

Mr. Tobin's family filed a wrongful death cause of action, contending that failure to monitor or record his temperature before, during, and after the operation caused his death. This case went to trial, and the jury returned a verdict of more than $6 million in favor of the estate of Mr. Tobin. However, because there was an absence of testimony on the standard of care in monitoring or recording the patient's temperature before, during, and after the operation and because of other evidentiary errors, the Michigan Court of Appeals ordered a new trial.

Similar to managing a patient's respiratory status, the administration of blood and blood products, although routine in critical care settings, is a high-risk intervention that can prove to be deadly. Often, seemingly simple measures, such as monitoring and documenting temperatures and taking appropriate action, help avoid prolonged legal battles. To avoid liability associated with administration of blood and blood products, nurses must carefully follow organizational procedures and protocols that govern these interventions. They must then take the time to thoroughly document the care that was given to protect the patient.

Several additional infection control cases demonstrate the value of nursing actions in shaping hospital policy and procedure, including taking action to correct dangerous situations. In *Carroll v Sisters of St. Frances Health Services*,[42] Bessie Mae Carroll was visiting her sister, a patient in the critical care unit. After washing her hands, she attempted to remove a paper towel from the container located adjacent to the sink. She thought the container was a paper towel dispenser and inserted her right hand into the opening at the top of the container, which was actually a sharps container. She had needle sticks in three fingers. After she told a nurse that she hurt her fingers on the paper towel dispenser, the nurse told Ms. Carroll that the container was a receptacle for contaminated needles.

Ms. Carroll developed a fear of contracting acquired immunodeficiency syndrome (AIDS) and filed this negligence-based cause of action against the hospital, contending that the container had been placed too close to the wash basin and that a warning should have been placed on the container indicating its purpose and contents. The claim was ultimately dismissed by the Court of Appeals. Nonetheless, thoughtful decisions about adequate environmental design and warnings could have avoided the injury in the first instance as well as the years and expense of litigation in this case.

CONSTITUTIONAL LAW: PATIENT DECISION MAKING

Patient autonomy or self-determination is a patient right guaranteed by state law and the US Constitution under the 14th Amendment. The right of competent adult patients to refuse treatment is well established. This right has evolved from the laws of informed consent, the laws of assault and battery (the right to be free from fear of harm and unwanted touching), and historic legal rights granted to individuals to say what is done with their own bodies. The US Supreme Court described this as the right to "possession and control of his own person, free from all restraint or interference of others, unless by clear and unquestionable authority of law."[43]

Patients With Decision-Making Capacity

Decision-making capacity means a person has the ability to (1) take in and understand information, (2) process the information in accordance with his or her own personal values and goals, (3) make a decision based on the information, and (4) communicate the decision. A person does not lack decision-making capacity merely because the decision is at odds with what others would decide or even if it seems foolish.[44] A person with decision-making capacity is often described as having capacity or as competent.

In the health care setting, a *competent adult* patient has the right to refuse even life-sustaining treatment for any reason, without regard for that individual's motivations. *Bouvia v Superior Court*[45] is representative of this principle. In *Bouvia*, a young woman with significant mobility disabilities refused to eat, and the facility in which she resided placed a nasogastric tube in Ms. Bouvia against her will out of concern that she was starving to death. The facility also subjected her to countless competency and psychiatric evaluations, all of which indicated she was fully competent (or had decision-making capacity). Ms. Bouvia sued the facility, asking the court to issue an order preventing them from treating her against her will. The facility countered by arguing that Ms. Bouvia should not be allowed to accept their treatment of her in some respects (basic skin care, mobility, wound care, and pain medications) and refuse it in others (force feedings). The court strongly disagreed with the facility and held that because she was a competent adult who understood the consequences of her decisions, she was free to consent to some but not all treatments and that she could not be compelled to accept food.

It is now well settled that competent adult patients may refuse treatment (in all or in part) for any reason or no reason at all. US law values individual autonomy to such a degree that a competent patient's wishes can almost never be legally overruled. However, no constitutional right is absolute, and there are legal frameworks for determining when a competing state interest may outweigh an individual right. For example, the right to refuse treatment or restrictions on movement can, in extreme situations, be overcome by state's interest in the health and safety of citizens. Mandatory quarantine after exposure to lethal infections, such as Ebola, is one such example. In the typical health care setting, there is little legal justification to override the wishes of a competent patient to *refuse* medical treatment. The reverse is not true: Patients have no constitutional right to demand treatment.

Critical care nurses are involved in many instances of refusal of treatment or the decision to withdraw or withhold possible treatment. This situation is difficult whether or not the patient has decision-making capacity, and it is important for nurses to keep in mind that there are times when the legal rights of patients and what feels like the "right thing to do" will match and times when these will seem at odds. Health care decisions become most complex when patients lose the capacity to make their own decisions personally. These decisions can also be difficult in patients who were never competent to make their own decisions. Navigating the law surrounding the right to refuse treatment in patients who do not have decision-making capacity is much more legally complicated than in patients with decision-making capacity.

Patients Without Decision-Making Capacity

Patients without decision-making capacity include individuals who were previously competent (individuals who reached adulthood but lost competence because of illness or injury), individuals who were never competent (individuals born with severe to profound cognitive disabilities), individuals who are not yet competent (primarily children younger than 18 years old), and individuals with fluctuating competence (eg, individuals with cyclic disorders, such as the manic phase of bipolar disorder, that can seriously impair decision making). The law allows for others to stand in their place as surrogate decision makers. The law also imposes standards of judgment for surrogate decision makers to guide and evaluate decisions.

Numerous legal mechanisms exist that can simplify at least the legal issues surrounding decision making for patients without decision-making capacity (the ethical and emotional issues are much more nuanced). These mechanisms include state probate laws that may allow courts to appoint guardians for all or some decisions. There are also various state law–based procedures for individuals with decision-making capacity to direct their future care through advance directives (statements of wishes in future situations or the appointment of a future decision maker in the event they should lose capacity). These include, but are not limited to, living wills, individual directives, durable powers of attorney, and physician orders for lifesaving treatment. The legal requirements and analyses are more stringent for decisions that may directly impact life, including decisions to forgo or withdraw treatment at the end of life.

Never and Not Yet Competent Patients

Competent adults can refuse treatment for any reason, even if others believe it is in opposition to their best interests. However, for patients who are not yet competent (ie, children) and the patients who were never competent, the law imposes a best interest standard. The standard is self-explanatory; parents and legal guardians of children have a legal obligation to make informed decisions based on the best interests of the patient. As a child matures, there are increased legal obligations to involve the patient in health care decision making based on what is developmentally appropriate in each particular situation.

It is inevitable that occasionally the judgment of a parent or guardian will clash with that of the provider or the maturing child. Every effort should be made by the nurse and the extended health care team to facilitate discussion, understanding, and resolution without resorting to the courts. However, there are procedures in every state to petition the court on an emergent basis to evaluate and rule on what is in the best interest of the patient. A common example in critical care is involving courts to request an override of parents' refusal of blood administration to their children based on religious objections. Courts should take the totality of the situation into account in making such a determination. Factors such as the likelihood of success in ordering such an intervention, the degree of invasion involved, and prognosis of the patient, as well as any expressed wishes of the child are all considered.

Previously Competent Patients

Most legal authority surrounds cases that involve a decision to withdraw or forgo life-sustaining treatment in patients without decisional capacity and who have not specified their wishes at an earlier time when they had capacity. The rapid advancement of medical care coupled with the emergence of critical care units and associated technologies, such as mechanical ventilation, vasopressive and inotropic agents, and resuscitation techniques, in the second half of the 20th century brought new challenges. For the first time, hospitals were keeping patients alive with technology but without a legal framework for discontinuation.

The courts began hearing these challenges in the late 1960s; several highly publicized cases beginning in the 1970s concerned the withdrawal of treatment in young women who were previously competent. In each of these cases, the patient had sustained devastating neurologic injury, and a legal challenge was presented to their families' ability to decide to refuse continued treatment, including nutrition and hydration.[46–48] In each case, the same family members were entrusted for years to make medical decisions for complex and life-threatening procedures on behalf of the patients, but the request to withdraw care was met with years of struggle in the legal system. This was, in part, because of a state's right to establish high standards for evidence of what the patient would have wanted.

In addition to affirming the states' ability to set high evidence standards in favor of preserving life, these cases established that in the absence of specific directions from the patient, surrogate decision makers should make a substituted judgment standard. This means that decision makers must base their decisions on the patient's known preferences and values before they lost capacity and best estimation of what the patient would have decided. The surrogate decision maker's own judgment about what should be done may differ from what they determine the patient would have wanted. He or she must abandon personal values and preferences and instead assume the preferences and values of the patient in making the decision. This is an enormous responsibility as well as a difficult task. To the extent patients can make their wishes known in advance, the agony already associated with these difficult decisions can by lessened.

These decisions, beginning with *In re Quinlan* in 1976, initiated the slow process of state-by-state legislation to provide competent adults with a way to legally direct their care in the event of future incapacity. Today, there are a wide variety of state law–based procedures for individuals with decision-making capacity to direct their future care through documents and the appointment of surrogate decision makers in the event they should lose capacity. Each state has resources on the available options for residents.

Advance Directives

Patients themselves can provide clear direction by preparing statements (usually required to be in writing) in advance that specify their wishes. *Advance directive* is a generic term meaning all statements of future health care wishes in the event of incapacity. These statements include the living will and the durable power of attorney for health care. The *living will* specifies that if certain circumstances occur, such as terminal illness, the patient will decline specific treatments, such as cardiopulmonary resuscitation and mechanical ventilation. It has proven to be of limited value because it does not cover all treatments; for example, in some states, nutritional support may not be declined through a living will. Advance directives vary by state but are generally legally binding documents that allow individuals to specify a variety of preferences, particular treatments they want to avoid, and circumstances in which they wish to avoid them. These directives also can be of limited value because it may be difficult to impossible to anticipate each situation and possible intervention in advance. The *durable power of attorney for health care* is a directive through which a patient designates an "agent," someone who will make decisions for the patient if the patient becomes unable to do so. The agent is obligated to use the patient's values and preferences to make the decision the patient would make if he or she were able to do so. This is perhaps the most useful tool if the agent is selected carefully and understands his or her responsibilities. This is not an easy task, and individuals are urged to carefully consider their choice of agent. Each state has requirements for advance directives and the form they must take to be valid and legally enforceable. Once a patient creates an advance directive in his or her own state, other states will honor it under the full faith and credit doctrine. Nurses may care for critically ill patients in one state who have executed an advance directive in another. The fact that it was drafted in another state does not negate its validity.

The Patient Self-Determination Act of 1990[49] is an example of a federal statute that impacts practice. The Act was a response to medicine's ability to keep people alive with advanced technology and the decision-making difficulties that arose in response. It was designed to encourage competent patients to consider what they would want in the event of serious illness and to encourage them to complete advance directives. The Act requires most health care institutions to provide patients at the time of admission written information of their rights under state law to make medical decisions, including the right to refuse treatment and the right to formulate advance directives. The Act also makes it illegal for a facility to require advance directives or discriminate against patients based on their advance directive or lack thereof.

Providers must have written policies and procedures (1) to inform all adult patients at initiation of treatment of their right to execute an advance directive and of the provider's policies on the implementation of that right, (2) to document in the medical record whether an individual has executed an advance directive, (3) *not* to condition care and treatment or otherwise discriminate on the basis of whether a patient has executed an advance directive, (4) to comply with state laws on advance directives, and (5) to provide information and education to staff and the community on advance directives.

Futile (or Nonbeneficial) Treatment and Orders Not to Resuscitate

Especially in critical care, nurses face situations in which continued aggressive treatment is extremely unlikely to benefit the patient. This may mean that supportive care and comfort are the best actions for the patient's well-being. All critical care nurses will observe and deliver care at some point that feels useless, unnecessary, and even harmful and painful to the patient. Nurses play an incredibly valuable role in the health care team by advocating for the best interest of the patient in a holistic way. Nurses may be responsible for reminding the team of the "big picture" and the need to provide quality of life and compassionate care to the patient.

Many providers have reported feeling obligated to continue treating patients in the absence of any reasonable chance of improvement. There is no legal obligation to provide care that is not, in the provider's judgment, reasonably calculated to improve the patient's condition or symptoms. Nurses sometimes face situations in which the patient (or the patient's family or surrogate decision maker) wants to stop treatment, but the treating physician is opposed. At other times, the entire health care team believes that aggressive treatment is no longer appropriate, but the family resists. Although patients have a legal right to refuse treatment, there is no corresponding right to receive treatment.

To deal with these situations, most institutions have futility policies for discontinuing nonbeneficial care. Some states have state laws to deal with these situations designed to facilitate communication between the providers and patients with procedures for resolution. A section of the Texas Advance Directives Act, often deemed the Texas Futile Care Law,[50] creates a specific process for providers withdrawing or refusing to provide futile care, even over the objections of the patient.

Do not resuscitate (DNR) orders are perhaps the oldest form of effectuating patient's wishes to refuse future medical treatment. However, they historically were the purview of the physician alone rather than an order communicating the shared decisions of the patient and providers. As part of some institutional futility policies, unilateral DNR orders (meaning ordered by the physician without the agreement of the patient) are permitted but should be rarely used. Institutional DNR policies should be well established and tested after decades of implementation. Policies that address orders to withhold or withdraw treatment should exist in all critical care units, and nurses should be familiar with those policies. The policies should include the patient's diagnosis, prognosis, and consent if competent or the surrogate decision maker's consent if not competent. Any conflict with advance directives or family member opinion should also be documented. DNR orders often require a second practitioner's concurrence and should require periodic review. Most importantly, they should be specific and clear. Nurses caring for patients with DNR orders should understand exactly what that means in terms of appropriate intervention.

Other orders to withhold or withdraw treatment may involve any intervention, including mechanical ventilation, oxygen, intravenous vasoactive agents or other medications, serial laboratory tests, imaging tests, pulmonary artery catheters, and other invasive monitoring. The legal and ethical implications of these orders for each patient must be carefully considered. Hospital policies should exist to guide the withdrawal of care in light of state and federal legal constraints. In addition, hospital ethicists and ethics committees can play a valuable role to providers negotiating the complexities of these decisions.

Brain Death

Since 2013, new legal issues surrounding brain death have emerged that have relevance for critical care nurses. Patients are legally dead by the *irreversible cessation* of either (1) the cardiopulmonary system or (2) the entire brain, including the brainstem. Death is pronounced in accordance with acceptable medical standards.[51] Typically, the determination of death by neurologic criteria is done in accordance with hospital policy and follows the guidelines set out by the American Academy of Neurology.[52] It is crucial that critical care nurses understand the difference between catastrophic neurologic injury and brain death, which means that examinations have been conducted in accordance with guidelines and the patient has no function of the brain or brainstem. Nurses are responsible for correctly using this terminology, especially when communicating with family members of the patient. Once testing consistent with brain death is confirmed, the patient is declared dead and either prepared for the allocation of organs or all mechanical support is removed because they are *legally dead*. This is not the same thing as withdrawal of care for terminally ill, but still alive, patients.

The states of California and New York allow for a short delay in removing equipment to accommodate family concerns, typically interpreted as 24 hours. The state of New Jersey allows for families to refuse a declaration of brain death based on religious objections.

However, increasingly, local judges have granted orders on behalf of patient families to temporarily prevent hospitals from removing mechanical ventilation and other supporting interventions. These orders typically allow for second opinions and additional testing to confirm death by irreversible cessation of total brain function, including the brainstem. In some cases, they have turned into protracted legal battles, as in the case of Jahi McMath,[53] a legally dead girl who has been on mechanical ventilation for 2 years as of this writing.

In addition, recent research suggests that not all institutional policies are consistent with following evidence-based guidelines in making a determination of death.[54] Critical care nurses are essential in these efforts, and they must understand the physical condition the patient must be in for testing to commence and serve as an advocate with the physician in ensuring testing is conducted appropriately. For example, the patient's partial pressure of carbon dioxide levels and temperature must be normalized, and certain drugs must be absent or at low levels before testing.

LEGAL ISSUES LOOKING FORWARD

This chapter could not begin to cover the labyrinth of legal issues affecting nursing practice. Each year brings new developments in legislation, case law, and administrative law that can change nursing practice. Most recently, the Patient Protection and Affordable Care Act of 2010 (ACA),[55] upheld by the United States Supreme Court in 2012,[56] instituted sweeping changes in areas ranging from eligibility for health care coverage to funding of medical and nursing research to numerous workplace programs that are intended to enhance to supply of advanced practice nurses. Of particular interest to nurses, many aspects of the ACA enhance the value and reimbursement of advanced practice registered nurses

CASE STUDY 3.1 Patient With Legal Issues

Brief Patient History

Mr. A is an 87-year-old man. He has a history of aortic stenosis; however, he has been relatively healthy until recent episodes of syncope. Mr. A lives in an assisted living facility because of forgetfulness but was independent in activities of daily living before this hospitalization.

Clinical Assessment

Mr. A was admitted to the critical care unit yesterday, after undergoing aortic valvuloplasty. Mr. A has not received any opioids or benzodiazepines since the interventional procedure yesterday. The night nurse reported that Mr. A was confused to place when awakened during the night but commented that this is normal for an 87-year-old. This morning, Mr. A was oriented to person, time, place, and situation. He is easily aroused but dozes off and on when unstimulated. Although Mr. A is able to follow simple commands, he requires repeated instructions. The nurse failed to document or report the patient's mental status change or abnormal serum electrolyte findings to the physician.

Diagnostic Procedures

Mr. A's baseline vital signs were as follows: blood pressure of 110/62 mm Hg, heart rate of 82 beats/min (sinus rhythm), respiratory rate of 18 breaths/min, and temperature of 98.4°F. The chest radiograph is normal; oxygen saturation (pulse oximetry) is 96% on room air. Results from serum electrolyte analysis include the following: sodium of 120 mmol/L, potassium of 4.1 mmol/L, chloride of 95 mmol/L, carbon dioxide of 25 mEq/L, blood urea nitrogen of 60 mg/dL, and creatinine of 2 mg/dL.

Medical Diagnosis

Mr. A is diagnosed with delirium secondary to hyponatremia.

Questions

1. What major outcomes do you expect to achieve for this patient?
2. What problems or risks must be managed to achieve these outcomes?
3. What interventions must be initiated to monitor, prevent, manage, or eliminate the problems and risks identified?
4. What interventions should be initiated to promote optimal functioning, safety, and well-being of the patient?
5. What possible learning needs would you anticipate for this patient?
6. What cultural and age-related factors might have a bearing on the patient's plan of care?

SUMMARY

- Nursing is (1) a scientific process founded on a professional body of knowledge, (2) a learned profession based on an understanding of the human condition across the life span and the relationship of a patient with others and within the environment, and (3) an art dedicated to caring for others.
- The ability to practice professional nursing is a privilege granted by state law and under the direction of BONs, state administrative agencies charged with protecting the health and welfare of state citizens by limiting nursing practice to qualified individuals who have demonstrated at least minimal competencies.
- Nursing scope of practice is defined by state NPAs. Standards of practice are delineated by BONs and are used as a basic measure of safe and effective nursing practice.
- Standards of practice and standards of professional performance, such as those promulgated by the AACN, further delineate expectations of nurses in providing quality nursing care and may help inform the standard of care in the legal context.
- Common legal theories based on civil litigation include professional negligence, wrongful death, and assault and battery. Nurses have a duty to their patients to provide care that is consistent with what a reasonably prudent nurse in the same situation would provide. This is the legal standard of care.
- Taking affirmative action that is responsive to the patient's condition and documenting those actions can diminish the risk of liability.
- Thorough documentation regarding actions taken to protect the patient is essential.
- Nurses can minimize the risk of liability by remaining true to the professional obligations to advocate for the best interests of the patients, attending to the patient's status, including carefully listening to and acting on patient reports or changes in status, documenting all of these issues, and

taking unresolved or unexplained concerns up the chain of command.

- A competent patient has a constitutional right to refuse treatment, including lifesaving treatment.
- States may require additional procedural protections when a decision maker wishes to withdraw care from patients who are not competent.
- Judicial intervention in decision making is an option but should be seen as a last step. Interdisciplinary cooperation, discussion, and collaboration between providers and decision makers should be fully explored first.
- Providers of health care must comply with requirements relating to patient advance directives.
- Any orders to withdraw or withhold treatment, including DNR orders, should be entered into the patient's medical record with full documentation by the responsible physician about the patient's prognosis and the patient's agreement or, alternatively, the family's consensus. These should be done in compliance with institutional policy.
- Brain death has a very specific clinical and legal meaning. Declaration of death by neurologic criteria requires examination in accordance with evidence-based medical standards, and hospital policies should comport with these standards. Critical care nurses should be familiar with these standards.

ⓔ Visit the Evolve Site for additional study materials.

REFERENCES

1. National Council of the State Boards of Nursing (NCSBN). NCSBN Model Nursing Practice Act and Model Nursing Administrative Rules. Chicago, IL: NCSBN; 2011.
2. National Council of the State Boards of Nursing (NCSBN). NCSBN Model Act. Chicago, IL: NCSBN; 2012, updated 2014.
3. National Council of the State Boards of Nursing (NCSBN). NCSBN Model Act. Chicago, IL: NCSBN; 2012, updated 2014, p. 2.
4. *Sermchief v Gonzales*, 660 SW2d 683 (Mo 1983).
5. *Marion Ob/Gyn v State Med. Bd.*, 137 Ohio App. 3d 522 (Ohio Ct. App., Franklin County 2000).
6. *State Bd. of Nursing v Ruebke*, 259 Kan. 599 (Kan. 1996).
7. National Council of the State Boards of Nursing (NCSBN). NCSBN Model Act. Chicago, IL: NCSBN; 2012, updated 2014.
8. Russell KA. Nurse Practice Acts guide and govern practice. J Nurs Regul. 2012: 36-40, 38.
9. National Council of the State Boards of Nursing (NCSBN). NCSBN Model Act. Chicago, IL: NCSBN; 2012, updated 2014. National Council of the State Boards of Nursing (NCSBN). NCSBN Model Rules. Chicago, IL: NCSBN; 2012, updated 2014.
10. American Association of Critical-Care Nurses (AACN). AACN Scope and Standards for Acute and Critical Care Nursing Practice. Aliso Viejo, CA: AACN; 2015.
11. *Candler General Hospital Inc. v McNorrill*, 354 SE2d 872 (Ga. 1987).
12. Painter L, et al. The nurse's role in the causation of compensable injury. J Nurs Care Qual. 2011;26(4):311–319.
13. *Gould v New York City Health and Hospital Corp.*, 490 NYS.2d 87 (1985).
14. For example, California: *Ybarra v Spangard*, 154 P.2d 687 (Cal. 1944); Colorado: *Wood v Rowland*, 592 P.2d 1332 (Colo. 1978); Delaware: *Larrimore v Homeopathic Hospital Association*, 176 A.2d 362 (Del. 1962); Minnesota: *Plutshack v University of Minnesota Hospital*, 316 NW2d 1 (Minn. 1982); Montana: *Hunsaker v Bozeman Deaconess Foundation*, 588 P.2d 493 (Mont. 1978); Pennsylvania: *Baur v Mesta Machine Co.*, 176 A.2d 684 (Pa. 1962); Texas: *Childs v Greenville Hospital Authority*, 479 S.W.2d 399 (Tx. 1972); and Washington: *Stone v Sisters of Charity of the House of Providence*, 469 P.2d 229 (Wash. 1970).
15. *Clough v Lively*, 387 SE2d 573 (Ga. 1989).
16. *Lunsford v Board of Nurse Examiners*, 648 SW2d 391 (Tx. App. 1983).
17. *Sparks v St. Luke's Regional Medical Center*, 768 P.2d 768 (Idaho 1989).
18. *Newsome v Lake Charles Hospital*, 954 So. 2d 380 (La Ct. App. 2007).
19. *Teffeteller v University of Minnesota*, 645 NW2d 420 (Minn. 2002).
20. *McMullen v Ohio State University Hospitals*, 725 NE2d 1117 (Ohio 2002).
21. *Brandon HMA, Inc. v Bradshaw*, 809 So.2d 611 (Miss. 2001).
22. *Brookwood Health Services v Borden*, Sup. Ct. Alabama (2015) (slip opinion).
23. *Denesia v St. Elizabeth Community Health Center*, 454 NW2d 294 (Neb. 1990).
24. *Garcia v United States*, 697 F.Supp. 1570 (Colo. 1988).
25. *Keyser v Garner*, 922 P.2d 409 (Idaho 1996).
26. *Long v Methodist Hospital of Indiana*, 699 NE2d 1164 (Ind. 1998).
27. *Richardson v Miller*, 44 SW3d 1 (Tenn. 2000).
28. *Ginsberg v St. Michaels Hospital*, 678 A.2d 271 (N.J. 1996).
29. *G.S. v Dep't of Human Servs.*, Div. of Youth & Family Servs., 723 A.2d 612 (N.J. 1999).
30. *Haney v Alexander*, 323 SE2d 430 (1984).
31. *Randi A. J. v Long Island Health Care*, 842 N.Y.S.2d 558 (N.Y. App. 2007).
32. The Health Insurance Portability and Accountability Act of 1996 (HIPAA), Public Law 104–191, enacted on August 21, 1996.
33. *Darling v Charleston Comm. Mem. Hosp.*, 211 NE2d 614 (Ill. 1965).
34. *Rowe v Sisters of Saint Pallottine Missionary Society*, 560 S.E.2d 491 (2007).
35. *Manning v Twin Falls Clinic & Hospital*, 830 P.2d 1185 (Id. 1992).
36. *Dixon v Taylor*, 431 SE2d 778 (N.C. 1993).
37. *Moon v St. Thomas Hospital*, 983 SW2d 225 (Tenn. 1998).
38. *Owensboro Mercy Health System v Payne*, 24 SW3d 675 (Ky. 1999).
39. *Miller v Marymount Medical Center*, 125 SW3d 274 (Ky. 2004).
40. *Small v Temple Univ. Hosp.*, 2008 Phila. Ct. Com. Pl. LEXIS 258 (Pa. C.P. 2008).
41. *Tobin v Providence Hospital*, 624 NW2d 548 (Mich. 2001).
42. *Carroll v Sisters of St. Francis*, 868 SW2d 585 (Tenn. 1993).
43. *Cruzan v Director*, Missouri Department of Mental Health, 497 U.S. 261 (1990).
44. Berg JW, et al. Constructing competence: formulating standards of legal competence to make medical decisions. Rutgers L Rev 1996;48:345.
45. *Bouvia v Superior Court*, 179 Cal. App. 3d 1127, 225 Cal. Rptr. 297, 1986 Cal. App. LEXIS 1467 (Cal. App. 2d Dist. 1986).
46. *In re Quinlan*, 70 N.J. 10 (N.J. 1976).
47. *Cruzan v Director*, Missouri Department of Mental Health, 497 U.S. 261 (1990).
48. *In re Schiavo*, 851 So.2d 182 (Fla. Ct. App. 2003).
49. *Patient Self Determination Act, Omnibus Budget Reconciliation Act of 1990*, Pub.L. 101-508 (1990).
50. For example, the *Texas Advance Directives Act*, Texas Health and Safety Code, Section 166 (1999).
51. Uniform Determination of Death Act (1981).
52. Wijdicks EFM, et al. Evidence-based guideline update: determining brain death in adults, report of the Quality Standards Subcommittee of the American Academy of Neurology. Neurology 2010;74:1912.
53. For example, Onishi N. A brain is dead, a heart beats on, New York Times (January 3, 2014); Lyons K. Jahi McMath's family takes brain-death lawsuit to federal court, SF Gate (December 24, 2015).
54. Greer DM, et al. Variability of brain death policies in the United States. JAMA Neurol 2016;73(2):213–218.
55. Patient Protection and Affordable Care Act and Reconciliation Act (2010).
56. *National Federation of Independent Business v Sebelius*, U.S. (2012).

4

Genetic Issues

Mary E. Lough

The field of genetics and genomics continues to expand and affect crucial aspects of health care. Genetic testing does not yet have a large role in critical care, but given the exponential growth of knowledge in this field and the decreasing costs of genomic sequencing, the day when personalized health care will include a genetic screen to tailor treatment to individual biology is on the horizon.[1] This is described as *precision medicine* and is supported by the National Institutes of Health Precision Medicine Initiative Cohort Program launched in 2015.[2-5] This chapter includes an overview of the biologic basis of genomics; a description of the different types of genetic and genomic studies; some examples of genetic diseases and pharmacogenetic syndromes; social, ethical, and legal concerns; and discussion of genetic and genomic competencies for nurses. A list of genetic and genomic terms is provided at the end of the chapter.

GENETICS AND GENOMICS

Genetics is the study of heredity, particularly as it relates to the ability of individual genes to transfer heritable physical characteristics. *Genes* are specific sequences of deoxyribonucleic acid (DNA) located on chromosomes within the nucleus of each cell (Fig. 4.1). Genes contain the blueprint for protein production that results in the physical characteristics of each individual. The pioneering work in human genetics has focused on single-gene variants that are rare in the population but have a large impact for the affected individual and follow classic inheritance patterns. Approximately 6000 rare disorders have been identified, and although single-gene conditions are relatively rare in the population, cumulatively they affect approximately 25 million people.[6] Single-gene disorders include Huntington disease, Tourette syndrome, cystic fibrosis, and Duchenne muscular dystrophy.[6] In single-gene variant disorders, the influence of genetics is strong, and the environmental effect is very weak.[7]

Genomics refers to the study of all of the genetic material within the cell and encompasses the environmental interaction and impact on biologic and physical characteristics. Thus, genomics is a much larger and more complex area of study. The *genome* is the complete set of DNA in an organism. Each human nucleated somatic cell contains a copy of the complete genome. The exceptions are reproductive cells (oocytes and sperm), which contain only one half of the paired chromosomes, and red blood cells because they do not have a nucleus. The human genome contains 20,000 to 25,000 protein-coding genes, which represent less than 2% of the total genome.[8]

Many disease conditions that are commonly seen in the modern world result from a confluence of environmental and genomic influences. These are described as *complex traits* or *polygenic* conditions. Furthermore, environmental conditions can alter the expression of different genes and consequently enhance the signs and symptoms associated with a disease. This represents a relatively new field of research known as *epigenetics*. Coronary artery disease is an example of a widespread disease that has both a strong environmental component (diet, obesity, diabetes, smoking) and a genomic effect that alters the risk of developing the condition.[9] Whole genome sequencing methods and genome-wide association studies (GWAS) are employed to examine multiple genes simultaneously. As the cost of genomic sequencing decreases, this is an increasingly viable clinical option.[10] Nowhere is the genomic influence more evident than in pharmacogenomics, or the unique individual response to medications (environmental impact) based on gene expression (genomic impact).[11,12]

GENETIC AND GENOMIC STRUCTURE AND FUNCTION

Chromosomes

The nucleus inside each human cell contains each person's full genetic blueprint of 23 pairs of chromosomes—22 pairs of autosomes and 1 pair of sex chromosomes—making a total of 46.[9] A number system is used to identify each chromosome. The chromosomes are traditionally arranged in order of size, starting with the largest (chromosome 1) to the smallest (chromosome 22), with the sex chromosomes placed last or to the side. A schematic of this chromosome arrangement to show the variation in size is shown in Fig. 4.2A; the chromosomes are not arranged this way inside the cell. A *karyotype* is the arrangement of human chromosomes from largest to smallest, as shown in the sequence in Fig. 4.2B.

Each chromosome consists of an unbroken strand of DNA. To fit all this genetic material inside the cell nucleus, the DNA is tightly coiled inside the chromosomes in a hierarchical order of compact structures. A specialized class of proteins called *histones* organizes the double-stranded DNA into what looks like a tightly coiled telephone cord (see Fig. 4.1).

Each somatic chromosome, also called an *autosome*, is made of two strands, called *chromatids*, which are joined near the center (see Fig. 4.1). This central region is called the *centromere*, and the ends of the chromatids are called *telomeres*. The segments of the chromosome separated by the centromere are called *arms*. The shorter arm of each chromosome is called *p* (for *petit*, or small), and the longer arm is called *q*. Differential staining of chromosomes produces alternating dark and light transverse *bands*. The bands are labeled p1, p2, p3, and so forth on the p arm and q1, q2, q3, and so forth on the q arm, counted from the centromere toward the telomeres.

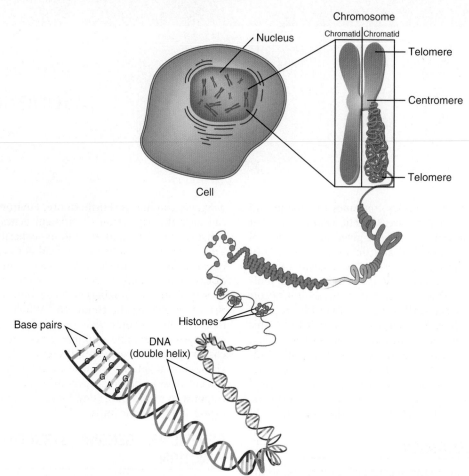

FIG. 4.1 Chromosomes are tightly packed with DNA and reside in the nucleus of the cell.

The p and q labels and bands are used to specify the location of specific DNA sections on the chromosome. There are also subbands within the major bands. This series of letters and numbers is the equivalent of an address for the location of a gene on a chromosome. For example, the cystic fibrosis gene *CFTR* (cystic fibrosis transmembrane conductance regulator) is located at 7q31.2, which indicates it is on chromosome 7, q arm, band 3, subband 1, and sub-subband 2.[13]

DNA and the Double Helix

DNA is foundational to genetics. Within the nucleus of the cell within each chromosome, DNA is arranged like a ladder, with two long strands of subunits twisted around each other to form the double-stranded three-dimensional helix.

DNA Base Pairs

The subunits within each DNA strand are called *nucleotides* or *bases*, and they are combined in pairs to form the rungs of the DNA ladder. Four nucleotide bases—adenine (A), thymine (T), guanine (G), and cytosine (C)—comprise the "letters" in the genetic DNA "alphabet." Each nucleotide base is attached to a phosphorylated molecule of the five-carbon sugar deoxyribose that forms the backbone of the DNA chain and can be visualized as the two sides of a ladder that have been twisted around (Fig. 4.3). The bases in the double helix are paired T with A and G with C. The nucleotide bases are designed so that only G can pair with C and only T can pair with A to achieve a consistent distance across the width of the DNA strand. The TA and GC

combinations are known as *base pairs* (see Fig. 4.3). There are approximately 3 billion bases in the human genome, based on findings from the Human Genome Project.[8]

The two DNA strands are orientated in opposite directions. Each DNA strand has a specific direction that is labeled as the 3′ end or the 5′ end (pronounced 3 prime, and 5 prime) (see Fig. 4.3). Because the DNA strands face in opposite directions, the 3′ end of one strand is always matched to the 5′ end of the other strand. This fact becomes important for replication (discussed next). The 3′ end is described as the *leading strand* because new nucleotides can be added only at the 3′ end.

DNA Replication

Before a cell divides, it needs to make a second copy of the entire DNA content within the cell. This process is called *DNA replication*. Sections of the DNA double helix separate longitudinally, creating openings between base pairs, known as *replication bubbles*, and mirror-image copies are made from the original strands. Stated another way, the original DNA strands provide a template that will be copied. The original is called the *parent strands*, and the mirror-image copies are described as the *daughter strands*. In Fig. 4.4, the parent strand is illustrated by the color blue with the 5′ and 3′ ends of each parent strand labeled. The daughter strands are colored red. The replication process is facilitated by DNA polymerase, an enzyme that lengthens the DNA strand by the addition of new nucleotide bases at the 3′ end of the daughter strand (see Fig. 4.4). After DNA replication is accomplished, the cell uses a

A   Autosomes   Sex chromosomes

B

FIG. 4.2 (A) Schematic of standard chromosomal arrangement used for classification of chromosomes by number, arranged from the largest (chromosome 1) to the smallest (chromosome 22). Chromosomes 1 to 22 are known as autosomes. Autosomal chromosomes are present in two identical copies, which are the same in males and females. The sex chromosomes are X (female) and Y (male). (B) This is a male karyotype because the sex chromosome arrangement is XY. The striped bands that appear on the chromosomes are achieved by use of specialized staining techniques.

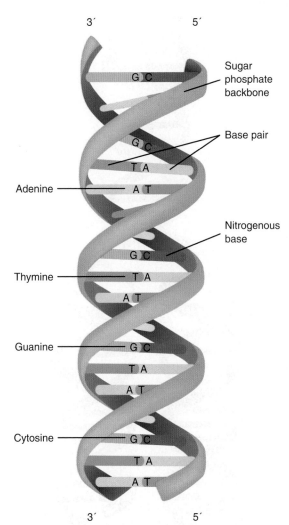

FIG. 4.3 Deoxyribonucleic Acid (DNA) Double Helix.

sophisticated mechanism for identifying and fixing errors in the replicated strand.[14] Following this procedure, the cell is ready to divide, and each new cell will contain a copy of the original DNA code.

DNA Alphabet

The nucleotides A, T, C, and G can be thought of as "letters" of a genetic alphabet that are combined into three-letter "words" that are transcribed (written) by the intermediary of ribonucleic acid (RNA). RNA translates the three-letter words into the amino acids used to make the polypeptide chains that constitute proteins. This process may be written as DNA → RNA → protein.[9,15]

Transcription

The process of making an RNA strand from a DNA strand is known as *transcription*. The strand with the genetic code that is to be transcribed is labeled as the *sense* strand or sometimes as the *coding strand*. The other strand, which is the RNA mirror image, is called the antisense or noncoding strand (Fig. 4.5). The reason there are two strands oriented in opposite directions is to facilitate replication of a DNA strand during cell division (see Fig. 4.4) or when proteins are needed (see Fig. 4.5) without compromising the original genetic material. To visualize how the process of transcription works, it may be helpful to study

Translation

The next step is to translate the RNA bases into three-letter words (eg, AUC, UGA) called *codons* that can be used to specify an amino acid. The three-base RNA codons are designed to code for 1 of 20 amino acids. Some codons signal to stop the sequence; these termination sequences are UAA, UAG, and UGA. The three-letter codons are not unique; for example, both UAU and UUC code for the amino acid phenylalanine. Most amino acids can be made from more than one codon. This can be appreciated by an examination of the list of three-letter codons, the corresponding three-letter amino acid abbreviation, the single-letter abbreviation, and the name of the amino acid in Table 4.1. The process by which proteins are made from instructions encoded in DNA is called *gene expression.*

Only a brief review of how DNA contributes to the genetic code is possible in this chapter. The volume of information that underpins genetics and genomics reflects the work of many scientists who performed research to advance this knowledge, and it may take some individual study or additional classes to master the content. An excellent free online tutorial called "DNA From the Beginning" is available through the Cold Spring Harbor Laboratory website.[15] The 41 modules use animation, video interviews, and text to present an interesting and informative introduction to the history and science of genetics.[15]

Telomeres

Telomeres are the biologic structures that protect the ends of the DNA strands from unraveling.[16] Telomeres are often likened to the plastic caps placed on the ends of shoelaces to stop the laces unraveling (Fig. 4.1).

Genetic Variation, Mutation, and Polymorphism
Variation

Genetic variation is common to all species. It means that individuals do not have the same nucleotides (A, C, T, G) in exactly the same position on the DNA strand. Some nucleotide differences result in the expression of different proteins and physical traits. Many nucleotide changes produce no visible external alteration, although those that have health-related consequences are of great interest to clinicians, patients, and researchers. Genetic variation can result from a variety of changes. It can be a single-letter substitution of one nucleotide base for another that can produce an inappropriate stop codon or produce a codon for a different amino acid. The amino acid codes are shown in Table 4.1. An example of a single-letter switch that results in an increased risk for disease is the G-to-A substitution at nucleotide 1691 in the coagulation factor V gene. This is also an example of a relatively rare single-gene variant that alters the protein product and increases the incidence of deep vein thrombosis (DVT), as described in Box 4.1.[17]

Genetic material in the chromosome can also be deleted (Fig. 4.6A), new information from another chromosome can be inserted (Fig. 4.6B), or a tandem repeat (multiple repeats of the same sequence) may produce duplicate genetic material within the chromosome (Fig. 4.6C). *Translocation* of genetic material describes a process in which chromosomes break and genetic material is moved from one chromosome to another. For example, the Philadelphia chromosome, or Philadelphia translocation, is a specific chromosomal abnormality associated with chronic myelogenous leukemia. It results from a reciprocal translocation between chromosomes 9 and 22, in which parts

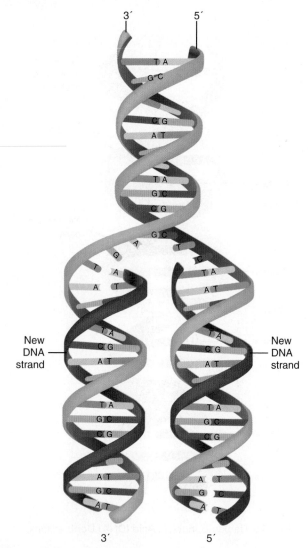

FIG. 4.4 DNA Replication Occurs Before Cell Divides. The template is provided by the original DNA strand (colored blue). The mirror-image DNA strand (colored red) is adding nucleotides to elongate the new DNA strand.

Fig. 4.5 and locate the names of the different strands; the DNA strand is colored blue, and the RNA strand is colored green to make the distinction clear.

Transcription occurs under the guidance of the enzyme RNA polymerase; sections of the DNA double helix unfold and separate into two single strands within the length of the double helix (see Fig. 4.5). The mirror-image DNA strand (shown in red in Fig. 4.4) serves as a template for the synthesis of a complementary, mirror-image strand of RNA (shown in green in Fig. 4.5). The purpose of transcription is to have the RNA mirror strand replicate the genetic code in the original DNA sense strand.

When RNA transcribes DNA nucleotides, one significant change occurs. The adenosine (A) DNA base is paired with a uracil (U) base in the RNA transcript (see Fig. 4.5). Each RNA strand also has a 3′ end (can be conceptualized as a head) and a 5′ end (conceptualized as a tail), and the growing RNA strand adds bases only at the 3′ leading end. The RNA strand, called *messenger RNA*, then leaves the nucleus of the cell, and the next action takes place in the cytoplasm.

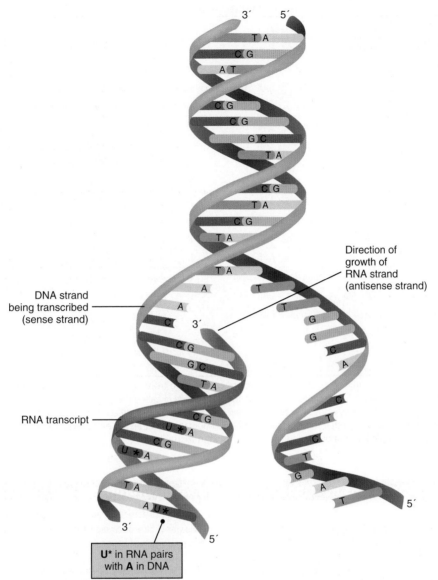

FIG. 4.5 DNA Transcription and Production of Complementary RNA Strand. The template DNA strand is colored blue. The RNA nucleotide uracil (U) pairs with the DNA nucleotide adenine (A) in the growing RNA strand (colored green).

of these two chromosomes switch places, producing the oncogenic Philadelphia chromosome and development of dysregulated tyrosine kinase.[18,19]

Mutation

The term *genetic mutation* refers to a change in the DNA genetic sequence that can be inherited. The term *mutation* typically is used to describe alterations that occur in less than 1% of a population. This use of the word *mutation* does not have the negative connotation of being more deadly than other genetic changes. It just means the incidence is rare.

Single Nucleotide Polymorphisms

When a genetic variant occurs frequently and is present in 1% or more of the population, it is described as a *genetic polymorphism*. The most common change is the substitution of one single-nucleotide base. A single-letter switch is known as a *single nucleotide polymorphism* (SNP; pronounced "snip") (Fig. 4.7). This is significant when the SNP occurs in a region of

DNA that codes for an amino acid. If the SNP change alters the amino acid product that is produced, it is called a *nonsynonymous SNP*, or *missense SNP*.[20] If a nonsynonymous SNP occurs in a coding region, it may affect protein structure and lead to alterations in phenotype (disease manifestation). An example is the G-to-A coding SNP at the 1691 site of the factor V gene associated with blood coagulation.[17] This polymorphism leads to the substitution of an arginine (A) by glutamine (G) at amino acid position 506, which alters one of the cleavage sites for activated protein C. Factor Va inactivation is slowed down because the cleavage site is atypical. This change in one amino acid reduces the anticoagulant activity of factor V, induces a hypercoagulable state, and consequently increases risk of DVT (see Box 4.1).

Approximately 5% of the population carries one copy of the factor V allele (heterozygous), which increases their lifetime risk of venous thrombosis threefold to fivefold compared with noncarriers.[20] A person with two copies of the factor V allele has a 10-fold increased lifetime risk of venous thrombosis

TABLE 4.1 The Genetic Code: Amino Acids[a]

First nucleotide in codon	Second nucleotide in codon — U	A	C	G	Third nucleotide
U	UUU Phe F *Phenylalanine*	CUC Ser S *Serine*	UAU Tyr Y *Tyrosine*	UGU Cys C *Cysteine*	U
	UUC Phe F *Phenylalanine*	UUC Ser S *Serine*	UAC Tyr Y *Tyrosine*	UGC Cys C *Cysteine*	C
	UUA Leu L *Leucine*	UCA Ser S *Serine*	UAA Termination	UGA Termination	A
	UUG Leu L *Leucine*	UCG Ser S *Serine*	UAG Termination	UGG Trp W *Tryptophan*	G
C	CUU Leu L *Leucine*	CCU Pro P *Proline*	CAU His H *Histidine*	CGU Arg R *Arginine*	U
	CUC Leu L *Leucine*	CCC Pro P *Proline*	CAU His H *Histidine*	CGC Arg R *Arginine*	C
	CUA Leu L *Leucine*	CCA Pro P *Proline*	CAA Gln Q *Glutamine*	CGA Arg R *Arginine*	A
	CUG Leu L *Leucine*	CCG Pro P *Proline*	CAG Gln Q *Glutamine*	CGG Arg R *Arginine*	G
A	AUU Ile I *Isoleucine*	ACU Thr T *Threonine*	AAU Asn N *Asparagine*	AGU ser S *Serine*	U
	AUC Ile I *Isoleucine*	ACC Thr T *Threonine*	AAC Asn N *Asparagine*	AGC ser S *Serine*	C
	AUA Ile I *Isoleucine*	ACA Thr T *Threonine*	AAA Lys K *Lysine*	AGA Arg R *Arginine*	A
	AUG Met M *Methionine*	ACG Thr T *Threonine*	AAG Lys K *Lysine*	AGG Arg R *Arginine*	G
G	GUU Val V *Valine*	GCU Ala A *Alanine*	CAU Asp D *Aspartic acid*	GGU Gly G *Glycine*	U
	GUC Val V *Valine*	GCC Ala A *Alanine*	GAC Asp D *Aspartic acid*	GGC Gly G *Glycine*	C
	GUA Val V *Valine*	GCA Ala A *Alanine*	GAA Gl u E *Glutamic acid*	GGA Gly G *Glycine*	A
	GUG Val V *Valine*	GCG Ala A *Alanine*	GAG Gl u E *Glutamic acid*	GGG Gly G *Glycine*	G

[a]Amino acids are the building blocks of proteins. The 20 amino acids are constructed from information contained in the DNA blueprint that is translated and transcribed by RNA. This transfer of information from DNA to amino acids is called the genetic code. Triple sets of bases (codons) are transcribed into the 20 amino acids. There are 64 possible combinations of codons, and several codons code for the same amino acids. The amino acids are connected in long polypeptide chains that form proteins. Three combinations signal the end of a protein chain: UAA, UAG, and UGA. Each three-letter codon also has a single-letter abbreviation, which is shown in the table.

BOX 4.1 Genetic Conditions in Critical Care: Deep Vein Thrombosis and Factor V Leiden

Clinical Presentation
Carriers of the coagulation factor V Leiden polymorphism are at increased risk for venous thromboembolism, identified by DVT or pulmonary embolism. The phenotype (clinical signs and symptoms) is defined by an increased incidence of DVT. Factor V Leiden thrombophilia is suspected in individuals with a history of DVT or pulmonary embolism and in people with first-degree family members who have experienced recurrent thromboemboli. Assessment is warranted for women who experience DVT during pregnancy or DVT while on oral contraceptives or hormone replacement therapy (HRT).[17] Factor V Leiden is found in up to 25% of patients with venous thromboembolism and in 50% of patients with familial thrombophilia.[17]

Genetic Evidence
The factor V (*F5*) gene is located on chromosome 1 on the long arm at position 23 (1q23). Factor V Leiden polymorphism refers to the specific G-to-A substitution at nucleotide 1691 in the coagulation factor V gene (genotype). This causes a single amino acid replacement at position 506 from arginine to glutamine. The resultant nonfunctional gene protein is called factor V Leiden.[17]

Normal factor V circulates in plasma as an inactive cofactor. Activation by thrombin results in the formation of factor Va, which serves as a cofactor in the conversion of prothrombin to thrombin. To express its anticoagulant function, normal factor Va must be cleaved by activated protein C (APC) at arginine in the 506 position and then at other sites within the factor Va molecule. Factor Va Leiden cannot be cleaved by APC because there is a glutamine at the 506 position. Therefore, factor Va Leiden is inactivated more slowly than normal factor Va. This leaves more factor Va available within the prothrombin complex, which increases coagulation because of ongoing generation of thrombin.

The term *Leiden* in the name refers to the town in The Netherlands where the gene was initially discovered. Factor V Leiden is also the most common cause of APC resistance, which may additively increase the risk of thrombosis.

Gene-Environment Interactions
The standard risk factors for DVT also apply to patients with factor V Leiden. The risk for DVT is increased by smoking, obesity, immobility, and trauma. Several additional genetic defects in the factor V gene have been identified as possible risk factors for thrombosis. One study identified seven other SNPs associated with DVT occurrence. Individuals with two or more genetic risk factors (gene-gene interactions) are at much higher risk for DVT.[17] Studies to evaluate this risk more clearly are ongoing.

Inheritance
The factor V Leiden allele is inherited in an autosomal dominant pattern.[17] This means a person needs only one copy (allele) of the factor V Leiden gene (heterozygous) to have a threefold to eightfold increased risk for DVT.[17] People who are homozygous have two copies of the variant gene (one from each parent) and have a 10-fold to 80-fold increased risk of DVT.[17]

Who Should Undergo Genetic Testing?
Genetic testing is reserved for individuals in high-risk groups who have experienced a first DVT before age 60 years; individuals who have experienced a first, unprovoked (no environmental stimuli) DVT at any age; and individuals with a history of recurrent DVT. There is no recommendation to test asymptomatic family members unless they have additional risk factors.[17]

To test for factor V Leiden, the first step is to do an APC resistance assay. If the blood test shows APC resistance, it is likely the individual carries the factor V Leiden variant, and genetic testing is undertaken as a secondary analysis.[17]

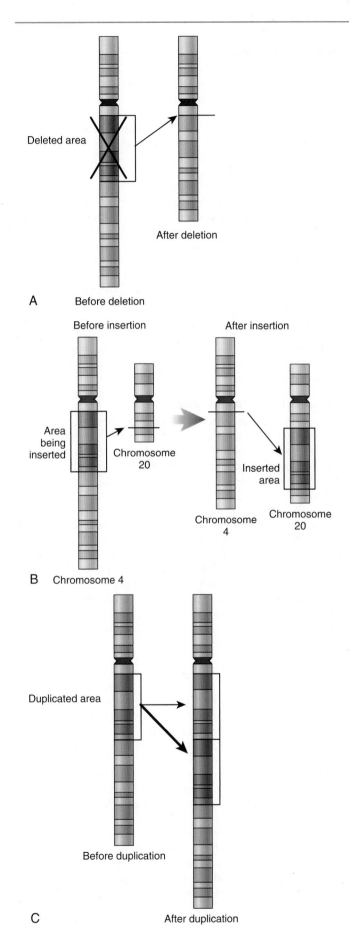

A   Before deletion

B   Chromosome 4

C   After duplication

FIG. 4.6 (A) Deletion of chromosomal genetic material. (B) Insertion of genetic material from one chromosome to another. (C) Duplication of chromosomal genetic material.

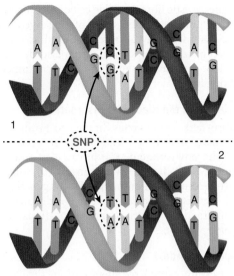

FIG. 4.7 Single nucleotide polymorphism (SNP) where one nucleotide base letter is replaced by a different base letter.

compared with noncarriers.[20] Factor V thrombophilia is one of several genetically inherited conditions that increase the risk of venous thrombosis.[20,21]

Alleles

Another name for a variant of a gene that occurs at a single locus is an *allele*. Allele symbols consist of the gene symbol, an asterisk, and the italicized allele designation. For example, the apolipoprotein E gene (*APOE*) has three major alleles (*APOE2, APOE3, APOE4*), and each allele codes for a different isoform of the ApoE protein.[22] *APOE4* expression is associated with late-onset Alzheimer disease (LOAD). In practical terms, a person with one *APOE4* allele has a risk of developing LOAD 5 years earlier; a person with two copies of the *APOE4* allele has a risk of developing LOAD 10 years earlier. Conversely, the average onset of Alzheimer disease is delayed by 5 years if a person has one copy of the *APOE2* allele.[22]

Not all changes in the DNA sequence have deleterious effects. Most SNPs have no effect because they are *synonymous SNPs*, variants that code for the same amino acid (see Table 4.1), or because they are located in noncoding genomic regions.

GENETIC INHERITANCE

Genetic Disorders

All genetic and genomic disorders do not have the same cause. The categories of disorders are chromosome disorders, single-gene disorders, complex gene and multifactorial disorders, and mitochondrial disorders.

Chromosome Disorders

In chromosome disorders, the entire chromosome or very large segments of the chromosome are damaged, missing, duplicated, or otherwise altered. Down syndrome (trisomy 21), in which there is an extra copy of chromosome 21, is an example of a chromosome disorder.

Single-Gene Disorders

In single-gene disorders, a single gene is altered. Single-gene disorders can result from inheritance of one dominant gene or two recessive genes. Cystic fibrosis, sickle cell disease, hemophilia A, and Marfan syndrome are examples of single-gene disorders. Single-gene disorders may also be described as monogenetic or Mendelian gene disorders. Single-gene disorders are rare in the population but have a significant physical impact on the affected individual.[9]

Complex Gene and Multifactorial Disorders

In some disorders, many genes interact to produce the condition, or there must be an interaction between vulnerable genes and the environment. Cardiovascular atherosclerotic diseases and type 2 diabetes are examples of complex gene disorders that result from an interaction of genetic and environmental factors.[9] Pharmacogenetic syndromes, resulting from the interactions of genes and medications, are also in this category.[1]

Mitochondrial Disorders

Some diseases are caused by alterations in the DNA of the mitochondria, which are intracellular organelles found in the cytoplasm. Mitochondrial DNA is totally different and separate from the double-helix DNA found in the nucleus. Mitochondrial DNA is transferred to offspring by maternal transmission only because mitochondria are preserved in oocytes but are destroyed in sperm during fertilization. Most mitochondrial genetic diseases are associated with disorders of enzyme function that disrupts mitochondrial energy production. Tissues and organs that have high-energy requirements such as skeletal muscles, the heart, and the central nervous system are most often affected.[23-25]

Genotype and Phenotype

The *genotype* refers to the genetic makeup at a particular locus or location on a specific chromosome within the genome; this is conceptually similar to a unique street address. The *phenotype* refers to the signs and symptoms that are clinically associated with a particular genetic condition; this is conceptually similar to describing the defining characteristics of the house, apartment, boat, dorm room, or castle at this particular address.

Genetic History and Family Pedigree

One of the tools used to determine whether a disease has a genetic component is construction of a family pedigree.[26] For clinicians, it is important to develop the skills to ask questions to elucidate which family members are affected and which are unaffected and then to identify the individuals who may carry the gene in question but do not have symptoms (carriers).[9] Standardized symbols are used in the construction of a pedigree.[26] The use of a legend to explain what the symbols mean prevents misinterpretation. The *proband* or *consultand* is the name given to the first person diagnosed in the family pedigree.[26] Examples of three simple pedigrees that illustrate the single-gene inheritance patterns and the symbols used to construct a pedigree are shown in Fig. 4.8 with examples described subsequently.

Homozygous Versus Heterozygous

Each individual inherits genetic material from his or her father and mother. If an individual inherits the same gene at a specific locus (genetic address) from both parents, the person is described as homozygous for that gene. If the genes donated by the parents differ at that locus, the person is described as heterozygous for that gene.[27]

Modes of Inheritance

One of the keys to understanding genetics is to understand the vocabulary. All humans have 23 pairs of chromosomes. One pair is sex linked: XX for a woman and XY for a man. The other 22 chromosomes are called *autosomes*; the term *autosomal inheritance* is derived from this word. The differences between some of the major forms of autosomal inheritance are described in the following sections.

Autosomal Dominant Inheritance

Autosomal dominant inheritance is described as a dominant pattern because only one copy of an affected gene is required to transmit the condition. The person has inherited one affected gene from one parent and one healthy gene from the other parent and is described as heterozygous for that gene. Typically, the disease appears in every generation. Each child of an affected parent has a 50% chance of inheriting the condition, depending on whether or not a parent has transmitted the affected gene. Male and female offspring are equally likely to inherit and transmit the condition (see Fig. 4.8A). Examples of conditions with autosomal dominant inheritance patterns include familial hypercholesterolemia, Marfan syndrome, and hypertrophic cardiomyopathy.[9]

Autosomal Recessive Inheritance

With an autosomal recessive pattern of inheritance, the disease or condition manifests only if the person has received an affected gene from both parents. The parents are carriers of the gene but are not themselves affected. The parents are heterozygous because they have one copy of a normal gene and one copy of an affected gene. Any of their children has a 25% chance to inherit in the following combinations: one normal and one affected gene (heterozygous carrier), two normal genes (unaffected), or two affected genes (homozygous affected). Persons who are homozygous for the gene associated with the disease always are affected, which means they demonstrate the phenotype of the disease (see Fig. 4.8B). In autosomal recessive inheritance, the phenotype associated with the condition is seen more often in siblings (sibships) than in the parents. Conditions associated with autosomal recessive inheritance include cystic fibrosis and sickle cell disease.

Sex-Linked Inheritance

Traits controlled by genes located on the sex chromosomes are sex-linked. Red-green color blindness and hemophilia are examples of X-linked conditions.[9] Women always have two X chromosomes (XX), one from the mother and one from the father. Even if the mother carried an affected *F8* gene, the gene on the unaffected X chromosome from the father confers the ability to make the coagulation factor, and female offspring avoid hemophilia. However, male (XY) offspring inherit one X chromosome from their mother and one Y chromosome from their father. If the mother's X chromosome carries the affected *F8* gene, the male offspring is unable to make sufficient factor VIII and manifests the bleeding disorder known as hemophilia A. The same inheritance pattern occurs with an affected *F9* gene that cannot produce coagulation factor IX resulting in hemophilia B. Both conditions can result in life-threatening bleeding.

In an X-linked disorder, each son has a 50% chance of being hemophiliac, and each daughter has a 50% chance of being a carrier. In a family pedigree, the absence of direct male-to-male

AUTOSOMAL DOMINANT INHERITANCE
Three-Generation Family Pedigree

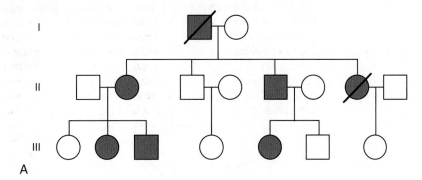

A

AUTOSOMAL RECESSIVE INHERITANCE
Four-Generation Family Pedigree

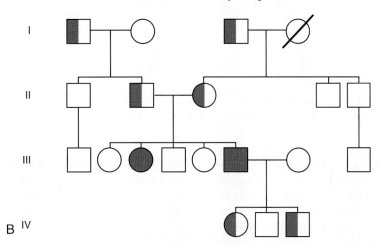

B

X-LINKED INHERITANCE
Four-Generation Family Pedigree

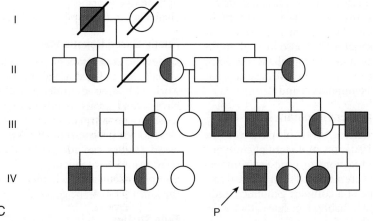

C

P

FIG. 4.8 (A) Pedigree of a dominant mode of inheritance. (B) Pedigree of a recessive mode of inheritance. (C) Pedigree of an X-linked mode of inheritance. See text for further information. (D) Symbols used to construct a pedigree.

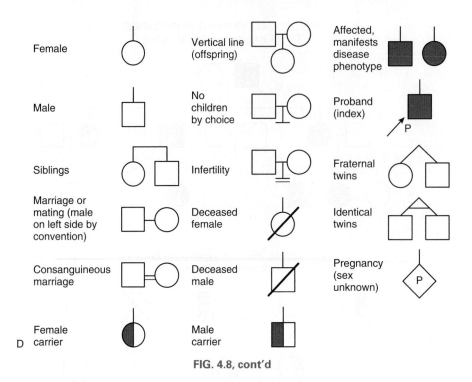

FIG. 4.8, cont'd

transmission makes this condition identifiable as an X-linked disorder. Hemophilia A is an example of a single-gene disorder. Fig. 4.8C illustrates an X-linked family pedigree for hemophilia A; a man who is affected (generation I) may pass the X-linked *F8* gene only to his daughters (generation II), who may pass the gene to sons who will be affected or to daughters who will be carriers (generation III). A girl will be affected only if she receives an affected X-linked gene from both her father and her mother as occurs in generation IV.

Hemophilia A and Hemophilia B. Hemophilia is an example of a single-gene X-linked pattern. The *F8* gene, which codes for the protein that makes coagulation factor VIII, is located on the X chromosome and is associated with hemophilia A.[28] Hemophilia B is also sex-linked because the *F9* gene, which codes for the protein that makes coagulation factor IX, is also located on the X chromosome.[28] At the present time, hemophilia is treated by replacement clotting factors. Researchers are investigating gene therapy as a potential cure for hemophilia A and B.

Complex Gene-Gene and Gene-Environment Disorders

Many genomic disorders are complex, and multiple factors are thought to contribute to manifestation of disease phenotypes. They result from gene-gene interactions or gene-environment interactions. Many patients who are admitted to the critical care unit may exhibit the phenotype of a complex genomic condition if they are obese, have type 2 diabetes, or have atherosclerotic disease.

OBTAINING INFORMATION ABOUT GENETICS AND GENOMICS

Genetic information can be collected in many ways. Often, when a gene is selected, all the methods described here may be used to link the phenotype, genotype, and environmental effects.

Genetic Epidemiology and Phenotypes

Genetic epidemiology represents the fusion of epidemiologic studies and genetic and genomic research methods. Before a gene can be mapped (genotyped), it is essential to have a reliable phenotype that can be consistently measured.[29] One of the challenges in applying genetics to the critical care environment is that the genotype is stable, but the phenotype is dynamic. Phenotypes are different at different stages of a disease and are influenced by medications, environmental factors, and gene-gene interactions.[29] It is helpful to discuss the methods used outside of the critical care unit as a way of understanding the challenges in the application of genomics in this arena.

Family-Based Genetic Studies

In genetic epidemiologic research of a rare disease, it can be a challenge to find enough people to study. One method is to work with large, extended families, known as *kinships*, which have several family members affected with the disease. Genetic testing is done to construct a genetic linkage map of the area close to the polymorphic gene found in that family.[30] Family-based studies can identify a significant phenotype-genotype relationship. Subsequently, it is important to do studies of other groups to determine whether the original finding is unique to the kinship or can be generalized to people outside the family.

Twin Studies

Studies of identical twins offer a unique opportunity to investigate the association of genetics, environment, and health. Identical twins are monozygotic and share an identical genome. Twin studies to compare the effects of genetics versus environment have been conducted by studying identical twins separated at birth. This situation occurs much less frequently today because tremendous efforts are made to keep siblings together when they are adopted.

Genetic Association Studies

Genetic association studies are usually conducted in large, unrelated groups based on demonstration of a phenotype (disease trait or symptoms) and associated genotype. In genetic association studies, it is important to recruit a diverse group of individuals to determine whether a trait is universal or found only in selected groups. Genetic studies can be conducted in isolated populations, in which population stratification is expected, or in highly mixed groups. It is important to collect information about ancestral and racial heritage to enable linkage of phenotypic and genotypic data. Diverse populations are sometimes called *admixed populations*, indicating that many different heritage groups have been included in the mix of people. The purpose of these different kinds of studies is to make a clear phenotype-genotype match and to identify which genetic conditions are associated with specific racial or ethnic groups and which genetic conditions are universal.

Case-Control Studies

In case-control studies, individuals are identified with the phenotypic and genotypic traits of a disease (cases). These cases are then matched to nonrelated control subjects by age, race, sex, and sometimes other associated disease factors.

Candidate Gene Studies

Candidate gene studies usually are exploratory studies in which a gene is suspected as a contributor to a phenotype or disease. Unrelated individuals with the phenotype are then tested for presence of the gene. These studies are usually smaller, and there is a strong biologic rationale for investigating the association between genotype and phenotype.

Genome-Wide Association Studies

GWAS examine the breadth of the human genome and typically use very large samples. The intent is to use genetic microarray technology and statistical computational power to find SNPs associated with a disease. Some GWAS are conducted with the intent of finding additional genes. However, one of the strengths of the GWAS model is that it does not have to begin with a biologic model in mind as long as the disease of interest is sufficiently common in the population; by testing thousands of SNPs, the researchers may find associations that have not been detected by other methods. A classic example is a GWAS of 14,000 individuals (cases) with 3000 shared controls genotyped to find SNPs associated with seven common diseases.[31] Significant new SNPs were found for five of seven diseases: type 1 diabetes, type 2 diabetes, rheumatoid arthritis, Crohn disease, and coronary artery disease.[31] New GWAS are published every month, and the National Human Genome Research Institute maintains an online catalog of published studies that can be searched by disease trait, chromosomal region, gene, or SNP.[32,33]

Genome Mapping Projects
Human Genome Project

The Human Genome Project was a huge, internationally collaborative project that began in 1990 with the goal of making a map of all the human genes (the genome). The final genome sequence was published in 2003. Big discoveries came out of the Human Genome Project, including a map of the human genome and a wealth of new clinical and computational tools that could be used for future studies.

The human genome map was created from the DNA of only a few people.[34] One of the surprising discoveries was that the number of genes possessed by humans was not as large as expected. The number of protein-coding genes in the chromosome is estimated to be between 20,000 and 25,000.[8] Although researchers were initially surprised that the gene number was not higher, it has become apparent than many posttranscriptional alterations occur to actively change the protein product. The ongoing research agenda is to understand all of these additional sequence elements as described in the following sections.

ENCODE Project

The *ENC*yclopedia *Of DNA E*lements (ENCODE) pilot project involved a detailed analysis of 1% of the human genome using cell lines.[35] The goal was to elucidate all the functional elements that enable relatively few human genes to produce such a wide variety of biologic products (eg, proteins). The second phase of the ENCODE project examined the entire genome in 147 different cell types. The focus was on the regulatory role of RNAs as either direct modulators of cellular functions or indirect modulators by encoding other active molecules.[35,36] Across coding and noncoding areas, 80% of the human genome is involved in at least one biochemical RNA or chromatin-associated event in the cell types examined.[36]

HapMap Project

The International HapMap Project database[37] contains greater than 4 million SNPs from 270 individuals representing four populations: African (Yoruba, Nigeria), European American (Utah), Japanese (Tokyo), and Han Chinese. HapMap displays short linear sections of genetic loci on the same chromosome known as *haplotypes* or *haplotype blocks.* Loci are grouped as a haplotype if they are close to each other on a chromosome and are inherited as a linear group. Genetic epidemiologists call this grouped pattern *linkage disequilibrium.*[30] In other words, the loci are linked by shared ancestry; genetic information is inherited in genetic "chunks" or "blocks" rather than as individual genes. The mixing of sections of different chromosomes that are inherited from each parent is called *recombination.*[30] The resultant linked genetic loci are called *haplotypes.* The edges of the haplotypes are conceptualized as *recombination hotspots* where little ancestral relationship remains. In the human genome, thousands of hotspots representing recombination and change over time have been identified. A theoretic expected haplotype change over 150,000 years from African ancestral chromosomes to modern chromosomes is shown in Fig. 4.9. The biologic rationale for recombination is to increase genetic diversity.

1000 Genomes Project

The 1000 Genomes Project builds on the information gained in the HapMap project because it greatly increases the number of included genomes. Scientific goals of the 1000 Genomes Project were to produce a catalog of human genomes identifying genetic variants that occur at 1% or greater frequency in the human population across most of the genome and at 0.5% frequency or lower within genes.[38] The 1000 Genomes Project did not collect any health-related phenotypic information.

Exome Sequencing Project

Exons are the sections of DNA that code for proteins. The Exome Sequencing Project searches for more information

FIG. 4.9 Effect of recombination on ancestral chromosomes. A gene is labeled *A* on the red ancestral chromosome. It is an example of a gene that has been conserved in modern chromosomes in one-third of cases. The gene (*A*) is associated with a specific phenotype or trait (shown as a checkmark). Because of recombination of chromosomes over thousands of generations, two-thirds of modern chromosomes no longer carry this gene.

about single-gene disorders, sometimes called *Mendelian gene disorders*, or *monogenetic disorders*, such as sickle cell disease and cystic fibrosis.[39] The use of next-generation whole exome sequencing increases the detection of disease-causing mutations because 85% of known mutations are within the exon regions.[40]

Human Proteome Project

The goal of the Human Proteome Project is to catalog all protein-coding genes. An initial draft of the proteome has been developed from analysis of 30 normal human tissue samples and cell types using mass spectrometry.[41-43] The process of protein manufacture is diagrammed as follows: DNA (exon or protein coding gene) → messenger RNA → transfer RNA → 3 nucleotide amino acid (codon) → chain of amino acids → protein.

Initial findings display the specificity of many protein-coding genes, including genes that function during one phase of life (in utero) and are silenced after birth.[41] The *Human Protein Atlas* documents the proteome.[44] The study of protein coding genes is a further step toward understanding genetic influence on human tissues in health and disease states.

Human Microbiome Project

In the healthy human body, microbial cells vastly outnumber human cells, sometimes being described as our second genome.[45] The human body is host to many microbial communities (human microbiome) located on the skin and in the nose,

mouth, and gastrointestinal and urogenital tracts. The spectrum of these microbial communities was previously almost entirely unknown. The Human Microbiome Project is designed to identify the core human microbiome and to determine whether changes in the human microbiome can be correlated with changes in human health.[45] The human microbiome project is highly relevant to critical care because so many patients experience antibiotic-associated disruption of the gastrointestinal tract and diarrhea from infection with *Clostridium difficile*.[46] The interaction of host bacteria, pathologic bacteria, the critical care environment, and pharmacogenetics has the potential to bring novel insights to current understanding of critical illness.

Genetic Diversity

The oldest human genetic lineages originate from the continent of Africa. The migration of a subset of humans out of Africa toward northern latitudes resulted in loss of genetic diversity because the genetic pool was smaller. Numerous studies have shown higher levels of nucleotide and haplotype diversity of nuclear and mitochondrial genomes in Africans compared with non-Africans.[47]

Copy Number Variation

Copy number variation (CNV) adds another level of variation to the human genome. CNV describes structural changes of DNA, larger than 1 kilobase, that include insertions, deletions, and inversions. The impact of CNVs on frequently seen diseases appears to be negligible,[48] but when rare DNA loci associated with a disease state are inserted, the "dose" of affected DNA can alter disease expression. Examples include familial Parkinson disease[49] and schizophrenia.[50] CNVs either can be associated with a Mendelian gene inheritance or can appear de novo, as a new variant, in the genome.

Individual Genome Sequences

It used to be stratospherically expensive to sequence the genome of an individual. However, the price has decreased dramatically, and the goal of a $1000 individual genome may soon be a reality. One of the many challenges is how to use all the data provided by genome analysis.[51] Another issue is personal privacy. These issues require serious legal and ethical discussion at individual and societal levels.[52]

GENETICS IN CRITICAL CARE

The next step in the genomics revolution will be to connect the growing amounts of research data to clinical interventions that may help patients.[53] The areas of clinical practice that have received the most genetic attention are cancer,[54] cardiovascular disease,[55] and pharmacogenomics.[12]

Gene Editing—CRISPR-Cas9 Technology

Gene editing, once the realm of science fiction, is now feasible for any sequenced genome. The technology, known as *CRISPR-Cas9*, which stands for "clustered regularly interspaced short palindromic repeat" (Cas9), has revolutionized the field of gene editing in the biologic sciences.[56] The Cas9 enzyme creates breaks at a target site of double-stranded DNA. The gene can then be disabled, or a new gene with a different function can be inserted at the site. This technology has the potential to offer a cure for diseases caused by a single gene, such as Huntington disease and hemophilia. This research is already progressing in animal models. The balance of ethical issues and benefit versus risk for individual patients will need to be carefully assessed.[57]

Cancer Genetics

Somatic Mutations

The word *somatic* means "related to the body." Somatic mutations are changes within a specific group of body tissues that are not heritable. Somatic changes often are related to changes in genetic markers associated with cancer or cardiovascular disease.

The Cancer Genome Atlas

There is strong evidence that many forms of cancer are caused by epigenetic alterations; one mechanism is the addition of methyl groups to specific genes to block their effect, a process sometimes referred to as *gene silencing*. Epigenetic changes can disrupt the normal balance in cell proliferation, cell survival, and cell differentiation. The Cancer Genome Atlas (TCGA) project was established to accelerate understanding of the molecular basis of human cancers.[58] The large-scale genome sequencing techniques, first developed in the Human Genome Project, are used to sequence genes associated with lethal and common cancers.[58] The goal is to document all cancer genetic changes from chromosomal rearrangements to DNA mutations to epigenetic changes (chemical modifications of DNA that can turn genes on or off without altering the DNA sequence). TCGA is an international pan-cancer research initiative that has demonstrated it may be more important to identify and target specialized biologic pathways in many lethal cancers than single genes.

Cardiovascular Genetics

Genetic markers are now included in many cardiovascular research studies to improve understanding of the genomic and environmental factors that underpin cardiovascular disease.

Long QT Syndrome

Long QT syndrome (LQTS) is a hereditary cardiac channelopathy with many different genotypes (LQTS 1 through 13)[59] and a phenotype that manifests as a prolongation of the corrected Q–T interval (Q–Tc) on the electrocardiogram (ECG). More than 90% of cases of LQTS are caused by three gene mutations.[59] Affected individuals have an increased risk of sudden cardiac death (SCD) (Box 4.2).[60-65] Not all patients who have the LQTS genotype are aware of their condition, and not all have a prolonged Q–Tc at rest. In the critical care unit, these patients are at high risk of gene-environment or gene-medication interactions that can lengthen the Q–Tc interval and entrain polymorphic ventricular tachycardia, also known as *torsade de pointes*[60]; see discussion of torsade de pointes in Chapter 12.

Cardiomyopathy

There is a very wide spectrum of cardiomyopathy genotypes and phenotypes. Some are single-gene disorders (inherited), and some are complex trait disorders with a strong environmental component in which cardiomyopathy has resulted

---

BOX 4.2 Genetic Conditions in Critical Care: Long QT Syndrome

Clinical Presentation

LQTS is a cardiac genetic disorder identified by prolongation of the Q–T interval. This is defined as a corrected Q–T interval (Q–Tc) longer than 500 msec on a resting ECG. LQTS is estimated to affect 1 in 5000 individuals and is one of the primary causes of SCD. In children, it is often called congenital LQTS.

Patients are frequently identified following a syncopal episode, a life-threatening dysrhythmia such as torsades de pointes, or an aborted SCD.[61-63] Treatment regimens include beta-blockers.[63,64] For patients with LQTS who are at high risk of cardiac arrest, insertion of a pacemaker/internal cardioverter defibrillator is warranted.[63,64]

Critically ill patients with undiagnosed LQTS are vulnerable to additional prolongation of the Q–T interval from various medications. The American Heart Association recommends monitoring of the Q–Tc interval.[60]

Genetic Evidence

Several genes have been identified for LQTS 1–10, and the three most common are listed here. All encode protein components of the cardiac ion channels and modulate ionic flow. Sometimes these disorders are described as "channelopathies."[64]

- LQTS1 is caused by a mutation in the *KCNQ1* gene (also known as the *KvLQT1* gene), which encodes a potassium channel protein active in phase 3 of the cardiac action potential (I_{ks} current). It is seen in 35%–50% of LQTS cases.
- LQTS2 is caused by a mutation in the *KCNH2* gene (also known as the *HERG* gene), which encodes a potassium channel protein that normally terminates the cardiac action potential (I_{kr} current). It is seen in 25%–30% of cases.
- LQTS3 is caused by a mutation in the *SCN5A* gene, which encodes a sodium channel protein in phase 0 of the cardiac action potential (NaV15 current). It is seen in 5%–10% of cases.

Gene-Environment Interactions

Gene-environment interactions are significant for patients with LQTS and vary by genotype and by individual:

- Patients with LQTS1 have a higher incidence of ventricular dysrhythmias and SCD events during exercise, especially swimming (physical exertion trigger).
- Patients with LQTS2 have a higher incidence of ventricular dysrhythmias and SCD events during sleep and are very sensitive to sudden loud noises that cause a startle reflex (auditory trigger).
- Patients with LQTS3 have a higher incidence of ventricular dysrhythmias and SCD events during sleep and rest.

Inheritance

Both autosomal dominant and autosomal recessive patterns of inheritance occur. LQTS1, LQTS2, and LQTS3 all have an autosomal dominant pattern of inheritance.[65] Not all individuals have the same phenotype even with the same genotype.[65] This is thought to be due to the influence of additional genes acting in concert with the primary gene to alter the cardiac action potential, to cause Q–Tc prolongation.

Who Should Undergo Genetic Testing?

Clinical genetic testing is available for LQTS. Genetic testing is very helpful in families of patients with LQTS. If the family member has a prolonged Q–Tc interval, the reasonable assumption during the cardiac and genetic work-up is that they have the mutation. It is also important to test family members with a normal Q–Tc interval, as up to 50% have "concealed" LQTS, meaning that they have a positive genotype and negative phenotype (normal Q–Tc interval on resting ECG).[64] This is because of a genetic concept termed *penetrance*, in which the same gene does not have the same phenotypic effect on everyone who is affected. If a person carries the genetic mutation but has a normal Q–Tc interval at rest, he or she may still be vulnerable during exercise or physiologic stress.

from ischemic or valvular heart disease (see cardiomyopathy in Chapter 13).

Hypertrophic cardiomyopathy. Hypertrophic cardiomyopathy is the most frequently encountered inherited cardiomyopathy.[66] It is both genetically and phenotypically heterogeneous with documented mutations in more than 11 genes that encode for cardiac sarcomere proteins.[66] Most mutations are missense SNPs in which the normal nucleotide is replaced; this alters the resultant protein. The risk of SCD is high for patients who manifest the phenotype of a hypertrophied ventricle or hypertrophied ventricular septum. To identify other members of the family who may be affected, it is recommended to construct a three-generation pedigree and perform genetic testing.[66]

Dilated cardiomyopathy. Familial dilated cardiomyopathy is associated with mutations in more than 30 genes,[67] most with an autosomal dominant mode of inheritance.[67] The phenotype is left ventricular enlargement with systolic dysfunction, often with affected family members. Phenotype presentation is variable even in patients with a known causative gene.[67] In patients older than age 40 years, a diagnosis of idiopathic dilated cardiomyopathy can be made based on the phenotype when other structural causes have been ruled out. Genetic testing is rarely performed in older adults, although the declining costs of genomic sequencing may make this feasible in the future.[68]

Restrictive cardiomyopathy. Familial restrictive cardiomyopathy is the least common inherited cardiomyopathy. The condition is usually not identified until the patient is symptomatic and the restrictive disease is at an advanced stage.[69]

Pharmacogenetics

Pharmacogenetics is the study of gene-medication interactions. Pharmacogenetics is likely to be the most visible impact of genetics encountered in the adult critical care unit particularly in relation to the cytochrome P450 (CYP450) family of enzymes involved in medication metabolism.

Cytochrome P450 Family and Medication Metabolism

The CYP450 enzymes are a superfamily of heme-containing enzymes that are vital for medication metabolism. The CYP450 family contains 57 functional genes that code for enzymes involved in medication metabolism. The isoenzymes CYP3A4 and CYP3A5 metabolize approximately 50% of medications, and they constitute approximately 60% of the total hepatic CYP450 enzyme content.[70] The metabolism of more than 90% of the most clinically important medications can be accounted for by seven CYP isoenzymes: 3A4, 3A5, 1A2, 2C9, 2C19, 2D6, and 2E1.[70] CYP3A4 can be used to understand what the abbreviations represent. *CYP* represents the symbol for all cytochrome P450 proteins, *3* denotes the gene family, *A* designates the subfamily, and *4* represents the individual gene.[70] The US Food and Drug Administration requires that new medications undergo testing for interactions with the CYP450 pathway before release.

Warfarin

Warfarin (Coumadin) is a frequently prescribed anticoagulant for patients with atrial fibrillation, mechanical cardiac valves, or thrombotic disorders. Variants in the CYP450 enzyme *CYP2C9* gene and in the vitamin K epoxide reductase complex subunit 1 gene (*VKORC1*) contribute to the considerable dose variation seen with this anticoagulant.[71] The vitamin K epoxide reductase (VKOR) enzyme activates the vitamin K–dependent clotting factors (II, VII, IX, X). Warfarin is used to inhibit the VKOR complex to prevent clot formation.

Warfarin dose variability between patients to achieve a therapeutic international normalized ratio (INR) ranges from 10% to 45% depending on *CYP2C9* and *VKORC1* polymorphisms.[72] Genetic testing is not currently recommended for everyone who takes warfarin. Laboratory tests to detect the *CYP2C9* and *VKORC1* variants are available at specialized reference laboratories.[73] The Food and Drug Administration added a warning label on the package to alert clinicians about *CYP2C9* and *VKORC1* polymorphism interactions and their effects on warfarin dosing.

Malignant Hyperthermia

Malignant hyperthermia is a rare inherited genetic disorder that negatively affects skeletal muscle on exposure to volatile anesthetics and depolarizing muscle relaxants. It may be unexpectedly discovered during general anesthesia. In malignant hyperthermia, calcium is released from the muscle sarcoplasmic reticulum and induces life-threatening muscle contracture with skeletal muscle rigidity, acidosis, and elevated temperature. The first gene to be identified was the ryanodine receptor 1 gene (*RYR1*) associated with calcium release in the sarcoplasmic reticulum.[74] Malignant hyperthermia is described in more detail in Box 4.3.[74]

GENETICS, GENOMICS, AND NURSING

As genetics and genomics exert more influence in clinical practice, there will be implications for the knowledge base of nurses and other professionals in health care. The learning curve may be steep. The addition of genetics also introduces new ethical and legal dilemmas into health care discussions. Genetics and genomics will have a big impact on how health and illness are conceptualized in the future. Genetics and genomics are already required content for baccalaureate nursing education, and this knowledge is now recommended for nurses with graduate degrees.[75] Essential competencies for nursing practice have been developed by the American Nurses Association, and examples are listed in Table 4.2.[76] It is always demanding to embrace a new model of health care delivery, and that is the challenge for all health care professionals in the coming decades. The tsunami of genetic information that is now flowing into research journals will rapidly make its way into clinical practice, including into critical care. This flood of new and relevant information will mandate that nurses understand genetic terms, incorporate genetic pedigree information into the history and physical examination, and have knowledge about pharmacogenetic interventions. Genetics and genomics constitute a complex area of study, made more so by the rapid evolution of scientific knowledge. One way to begin is to look at some of the free, Internet-based, interactive educational tutorials listed in Box 4.4 at the end of this chapter and to become familiar with the genetic and genomic vocabulary in the key terms list at the end of the chapter.

Ethical and Legal Issues in Genetics and Genomics

A paramount concern in the genomic era is to protect the privacy of individuals' unique genetic information. Many countries have established biobanks as repositories of genetic material, and many tissue samples are stored in medical center tissue banks. Because all of the individual's genome is contained

BOX 4.3   Genetic Conditions in Critical Care: Malignant Hyperthermia

Clinical Presentation

Malignant hyperthermia is a pharmacogenetic syndrome. It is a disorder of skeletal muscle calcium regulation. On exposure to volatile anesthetics and depolarizing muscle relaxants, susceptible patients experience life-threatening symptoms including sustained muscle contracture with skeletal muscle rigidity, which causes metabolic acidosis, tachycardia, and fever. The symptoms result from an abnormally high release of intracellular calcium in skeletal muscle.[74]

Genetic Evidence

Genetic linkage studies associated the malignant hyperthermia phenotype with the ryanodine receptor 1 gene (RYR1) at chromosome 19q13.1 in affected families.[74] Calcium transport from muscle sarcoplasmic reticulum through the ryanodine receptor into the sarcoplasm occurs during muscular excitation and contraction. The RYR1 gene is highly polymorphic with more than 400 variants, of which 31 mutations are known to cause the condition.[74] The presence of any of these mutations is diagnostic for malignant hyperthermia susceptibility. Genetic testing is available for causative RYR1 gene mutations.[74]

Gene-Environment Interactions

Malignant hyperthermia is an example of a gene-environment interaction. It is not an allergy, and it occurs under the specific environmental condition of general anesthesia with inhalation anesthetics (eg, chloroform, desflurane, enflurane, halothane, isoflurane, methoxyflurane, sevoflurane, trichloroethylene) and depolarizing muscle relaxants (eg, succinylcholine).

Inheritance

Malignant hyperthermia is inherited in an autosomal dominant pattern. This means that only one affected allele is needed to have the condition and that children of an affected person have a 50% chance of inheriting the mutated RYR1 gene.

Who Should Undergo Genetic Testing?

Malignant hyperthermia crisis under general anesthesia is rare. The genetic test for RYR1 is not recommended as a general screening test. Genetic testing is recommended only for individuals who have experienced an MH crisis, individuals who are first-degree relatives of a person with known MH, or individuals who have had a positive result from a muscle biopsy. The value of the genetic test is that when a mutation is discovered, family members with the same mutation are considered susceptible to MH and can avoid a diagnostic muscle biopsy. The major advantage of being aware of the diagnosis is that high-risk anesthetics can be avoided for general anesthesia in individuals susceptible to MH.

Online Resources

European Malignant Hyperthermia Group: http://www.emhg.org

Malignant Hyperthermia Association of the United States: http://www.mhaus.org

Online Mendelian Inheritance in Man (OMIM), ryanodine receptor 1 gene (RYR1): http://omim.org/entry/180901

Direct-to-Consumer Tests

A new frontier in genomics testing is the ability of any individual to voluntarily undergo genetic testing. Several private companies advertise this service on the Internet. Patients send a sample of their DNA, usually a swab from the inside of the cheek (buccal swab), to check for selected genetic risks. Other websites offer paternity testing from buccal swabs of the child and father. Many countries are now enacting laws to ensure individuals' genomic information is protected. Genetic counselors caution that the results may be hard to understand or misleading for some individuals, but clearly this information is of great interest to many people.[78]

Genetic Information Nondiscrimination Act

The Genetic Information Nondiscrimination Act (GINA) of 2008 is an essential piece of legislation designed to prevent abuse of genetic information in employment and health insurance decisions in the United States.[79] The purpose of GINA is to protect individuals who may have the gene for a disorder—but do not manifest the phenotype—from being penalized. Some people who may be at risk for a genetic disorder may not undergo testing because they fear that a positive result would affect their employability. GINA also mandates that genetic information about individuals and their families have the same protections as health information. It is important that clinicians understand that the GINA legislation does not cover all categories of insurance. It offers no protection against discrimination for life insurance, disability insurance, or long-term care insurance. The GINA legislation does not cover members of the military, individuals covered by the US Department of Veterans Affairs, or individuals covered by the Indian Health Service.[80]

HUMAN GENETICS KEY TERMS

Allele: One of several alternative gene variants that can exist at a single locus (location) on a chromosome. The term *allele* may also be used when referring to SNP variants. The most frequently found allele in a population is called the *wild-type allele*.

Candidate gene: A gene that is believed to cause or contribute to a disease. This term is typically used when the gene will be included in a research study.

Chromosomes: Structures made of DNA and proteins and located in the nuclei of cells. Chromosomes come in pairs, and a normal human cell contains 46 chromosomes: 22 pairs of autosomes and a pair of sex chromosomes. Chromosomes are composed of genes, regulatory sequences, and noncoding DNA segments.

Codon: Three-sequence nucleotide bases that code for an amino acid.

DNA: Deoxyribonucleic acid is made up of four nucleotide bases: adenine (A), guanine (G), cytosine (C), and thymine (T). DNA is heritable genetic information that resides in chromosomes inside each cell nucleus.

Epigenetic: Chemical modifications of DNA that can turn genes on or off without altering the DNA sequence. Epigenetic changes are not heritable.

Gene: A unit of inheritance; a working subunit of DNA. Each of the 20,000 to 25,000 genes in the body contains the code for a specific product, typically a protein such as an enzyme, and other specific tissue cells.

Gene expression: The process by which the coded information of a gene is translated into the structures present and operating in the cell such as proteins or RNA.

within the cell, genomic identity or susceptibility to diseases can easily be determined from a small sample. It is essential to ensure that ethical and legal protections keep pace with technical innovation. Key issues are who *owns* the genetic material and *consent* as to who has access to the genetic information. Debate about these issues is expected to continue as new advances push the technical limits of what can be discovered from a few drops of blood, a muscle biopsy sample, or a cheek swab.[77]

TABLE 4.2   Essential Genetics and Genomics Competencies for Nurses

Domain	Competencies of the Registered Nurse
Professional Responsibilities	
Competent nursing incorporating genetic and genomic knowledge and skills	Recognizes when one's own attitudes and values related to genetic and genomic science may affect care provided to patients
	Advocates for patients' access to desired genetic or genomic services and resources, including support groups
	Examines competency of practice on a regular basis, identifying areas of strength and areas in which professional development related to genetics and genomics would be beneficial
	Incorporates genetic and genomic technologies and information into registered nurse practice
	Demonstrates in practice the importance of tailoring genetic and genomic information and services to patients based on their culture, religion, knowledge level, literacy, and preferred language
	Advocates for the rights of all patients for autonomous, informed genetic and genomic related decision making and voluntary action
Professional Practice and Assessment	
Application and integration of knowledge	Demonstrates an understanding of the relationship of genetics or genomics to health, prevention, screening, diagnostics, prognostics, selection of treatment, and monitoring of treatment effectiveness
	Demonstrates an ability to elicit a minimum of three generations of family health history information
	Constructs a pedigree from collected family history information using standardized symbols and terminology
	Collects personal, health, and developmental histories that consider genetic, environmental, and genomic influences and risks
	Conducts comprehensive health and physical assessments that incorporate knowledge about genetic, environmental, and genomic influences and risk factors
	Critically analyzes the history and physical assessment findings for genetic, environmental, and genomic influences and risk factors
	Assesses patients' knowledge, perceptions, and responses to genetic and genomic information
	Develops plan of care that incorporates genetic and genomic assessment information
Identification of needed information	Identifies patients who may benefit from specific genetic and genomic information or services based on assessment data
	Identifies credible, accurate, appropriate, and current genetic and genomic information, resources, services, and technologies specific to given patients
	Identifies ethical, ethnic or ancestral, cultural, religious, legal, fiscal, and societal issues related to genetic and genomic information and technologies
	Defines issues that undermine the rights of all patients for autonomous, informed genetic and genomic related decision making and voluntary action
Assistance with referrals	Facilitates referrals for specialized genetic and genomic services for patients, as needed
Provision of education, care, and support	Provides patients with interpretation of selective genetic and genomic information or services
	Provides patients with credible, accurate, appropriate, and current genetic and genomic information, resources, services, and technologies that facilitate decision making
	Uses health promotion and disease prevention practices that consider genetic and genomic influences on risk with personal and environmental risk factors
	Incorporates knowledge of genetic or genomic risk factors (eg, patient with a genetic predisposition for high cholesterol levels who can benefit from a change in lifestyle to decrease the likelihood that the genotype will be expressed)
	Uses genetic- and genomic-based interventions and information to improve patients' outcomes
	Collaborates with health care providers in providing genetic and genomic health care
	Collaborates with insurance providers or payers to facilitate reimbursement for genetic and genomic health care services
	Performs interventions and treatments appropriate to patients' genetic and genomic health care needs
	Evaluates impact and effectiveness of genetic and genomic technology, information, interventions, and treatments on patients' outcome

From Consensus Panel on Genetic/Genomic Nursing Competencies. *Essentials of Genetic and Genomic Nursing: Competencies, Curricula Guidelines, and Outcome Indicators.* 3rd ed. Silver Spring, MD: American Nurses Association; 2009.

Gene map: A description of the relative positions of genes on a chromosome and the distance between them.

Genetic linkage maps: DNA maps that assign relative chromosomal locations to genetic locations—either genes for known traits or distinctive sequences of DNA on the basis of how frequently they are inherited together.

Genetics: The scientific study of heredity, which is how particular qualities or traits are transmitted from parents to offspring. Traditionally, the focus has been on individual genes and their impact on uncommon single-gene disorders. At the present time, the study of genetics also involves multigene disorders and gene-environment interactions.

Genomics: The expansive study of all the genes in the human genome, including gene-gene interactions, gene interactions with the environment, and the influence of other psychosocial and cultural factors.

Genotype: The genetic code sequence carried by an individual.

Haplotype: Closely linked loci on a chromosome. Haplotype blocks denote chromosomal regions where SNPs are in strong linkage disequilibrium, and they are mapped in the HapMap Project database.

HapMap Project: A map of haplotype blocks that researchers use when searching for candidate genes. Haplotypes are cataloged according to racial and ethnic group in the HapMap database.

Heterozygous: Possessing two different sequences (alleles) of a particular gene, with one inherited from each parent.

Homozygous: Possessing two identical sequences of a particular gene, with one inherited from each parent.

Linkage: The association of genes or markers that lie very near each other on a chromosome. Linked genes and markers tend to be inherited together.

Linkage analysis: A gene-mapping technique that finds patterns of heredity in large, high-risk families to locate a disease-causing gene mutation by identifying traits that are coinherited with the gene.

Linkage disequilibrium: The nonrandom association between alleles at different loci. These alleles at loci occur together on the same section of a chromosome more often than would be predicted by chance alone. This technique has been used to determine which genes are linked and inherited together.

Locus, loci: The place on a chromosome where a specific gene is located, similar in concept to a street address for the gene. The singular term is *locus*, and the plural is *loci*.

Mendelian diseases: Single-gene disorders that appear in families in dominant or recessive inheritance patterns.

Mutation: A change, deletion, or rearrangement in an individual's DNA sequence that may lead to the synthesis of an altered protein or the inability to produce the protein. The term *mutation* is used when the variant occurs in less than 1% of the population.

Nucleotide: A building block of DNA or RNA that consists of one nitrogenous base, one phosphate molecule, and one glucose molecule.

Pedigree: A graphic multigenerational family health history that uses standardized symbols.

Pharmacogenomics: The study of genetically determined responses to medications, genetic variation in medication metabolizing enzymes, and consequent alteration in medication effectiveness across the genome.

Phenotype: The observable manifestation of a genetic trait that results from a specific genotype or gene-environment interaction. These are physical characteristics, such as the signs and symptoms associated with a disease.

Polymorphism: A common variation in the sequence of DNA that occurs in more than 1% of the population. The most frequent sequence is referred to as the *wild type*, and less common variants are called *polymorphisms.*

Proband: The first person diagnosed with a condition in a family pedigree. An arrow in the family pedigree identifies the proband.

Single nucleotide polymorphism (SNP): A change in the DNA nucleotide sequence caused by replacement of a single nucleotide base. If the change of nucleotide results in a

different protein product, it is called a *nonsynonymous SNP*. If the protein product is not changed, it is called a *synonymous SNP*.

Somatic cells: All body cells except the reproductive cells.

Transcription: The process used by DNA to code for messenger RNA.

Translation: The process used by RNA to code for a protein.

Whole exome sequencing: Sequencing of protein-coding regions of DNA.

QSEN   BOX 4.4   QSEN: Informatics

Internet Resources

Genomic Databases and Reference

GeneReviews, University of Washington, Seattle, WA: http://www.genetests.org/

Online Mendelian Inheritance in Man (OMIM), Johns Hopkins University: http://www.ncbi.nlm.nih.gov/omim/

Genome-wide association studies (GWAS) catalog maintained by NHGRI: http://www.genome.gov/gwastudies/

The Cancer Genome Atlas (TCGA): http://cancergenome.nih.gov/

The International HapMap Project: http://www.hapmap.org/

The 1000 Genomes Project: http://www.1000genomes.org/

Encyclopedia of DNA Elements (ENCODE): http://genome.ucsc.edu/ENCODE/

Personal Genome Project: http://www.personalgenomes.org

Organizations

International Society of Nurses in Genetics (ISONG): http://www.isong.org/

National Coalition of Health Professional Education in Genetics (NCHPEG): http://www.nchpeg.org/

Tutorials and Education

Learn Genetics, The University of Utah: http://gslc.genetics.utah.edu/

Educational materials about genetics and genomics from NHGRI: http://www.genome.gov/Education/

Current Topics in Genome Analysis 2012, NHGRI: http://www.genome.gov/12514288

DNA Learning Center, Cold Spring Harbor Laboratory: http://www.dnalc.org/home.html

NHGRI, National Human Genome Resource Institute.

SUMMARY

- DNA is arranged inside the nucleus of the cell. DNA resembles a ladder with two long strands twisted around each other to form a double-stranded helix made up of nucleotide base pairs. There are 20,000 to 25,000 genes in the human genome.
- Coagulation-related conditions that may have a genetic component include factor V Leiden thrombosis and hemophilia A and B.
- Pharmacogenetic syndromes represent medication-gene interactions; examples include malignant hyperthermia secondary to *RYR1* polymorphisms and warfarin dosage affected by *CYP2C9* and *VKORC1* polymorphisms.
- Cardiac conditions that have a genetic component include hypertrophic cardiomyopathy and LQTS.
- The GINA legislation in the United States is designed to prevent the use of an individual's genetic risk profile in employment and insurance decisions.
- Genetic and genomic competency is recommended for all RNs.
- ⊝ Visit the Evolve site for additional study materials.

REFERENCES

1. Fox CS, et al. Future translational applications from the contemporary genomics era: a scientific statement from the American Heart Association. *Circulation*. 2015;131(19):1715-1736.
2. Precision Medicine Initiative Cohort Program. https://www.nih.gov/precision-medicine-initiative-cohort-program. Accessed January 1, 2016.
3. Collins FS, Varmus H. A new initiative on precision medicine. *N Engl J Med*. 2015;372(9):793-795.
4. Aronson SJ, Rehm HL. Building the foundation for genomics in precision medicine. *Nature*. 2015;526(7573):336-342.
5. Williams JK, et al. Advanced nursing practice and research contributions to precision medicine. *Nurs Outlook*. 2015;64(2):117-123.
6. Rare Diseases Act of 2002. *Public Law*. November 6, 2002:107-280. https://history.nih.gov/research/downloads/PL107-280.pdf. Accessed March 12, 2016.
7. Marian AJ. Clinical applications of molecular genetic discoveries. *Transl Res*. 2016;168:6-14.
8. International Human Genome Sequencing Consortium: Finishing the euchromatic sequence of the human genome. *Nature*. 2004;431(7011): 931-945.
9. Musunuru K, et al. Basic concepts and potential applications of genetics and genomics for cardiovascular and stroke clinicians: a scientific statement from the American Heart Association. *Circ Cardiovasc Genet*. 2015;8(1):216-242.
10. Ashley EA, et al. Clinical assessment incorporating a personal genome. *Lancet*. 2010;375(9725):1525-1535.
11. Chan SL, et al. Progress in understanding the genomic basis for adverse drug reactions: a comprehensive review and focus on the role of ethnicity. *Pharmacogenomics*. 2015;16(10):1161-1178.
12. Chang MT, McCarthy JJ, Shin J. Clinical application of pharmacogenetics: focusing on practical issues. *Pharmacogenomics*. 2015;16(15):1733-1741.
13. Brennan ML, Schrijver I. Cystic fibrosis: a review of associated phenotypes, use of molecular diagnostic approaches, genetic characteristics, progress, and dilemmas. *J Mol Diagn*. 2016;18(1):3-14.
14. Odell ID, Wallace SS, Pederson DS. Rules of engagement for base excision repair in chromatin. *J Cell Physiol*. 2013;228(2):258-266.
15. DNA from the Beginning. http://www.dnaftb.org. Accessed January 1, 2016.
16. Sarek G, et al. Molecular basis of telomere dysfunction in human genetic diseases. *Nat Struct Mol Biol*. 2015;22(11):867-874.
17. Kujovich JL. Factor V Leiden thrombophilia. *Genet Med*. 2011;13(1):1-16.
18. Bennour A, Saad A, Sennana H. Chronic myeloid leukemia: relevance of cytogenetic and molecular assays. *Crit Rev Oncol Hematol*. 2016;97:263-274.
19. Tefferi A. Myeloproliferative neoplasms: a decade of discoveries and treatment advances. *Am J Hematol*. 2016;91(1):50-58.
20. MacCallum P, Bowles L, Keeling D. Diagnosis and management of heritable thrombophilias. *BMJ*. 2014;349:g4387.
21. Morange PE, Suchon P, Tregouet DA. Genetics of venous thrombosis: update in 2015. *Thromb Haemost*. 2015;114(5):910-919.
22. Yu JT, Tan L, Hardy J. Apolipoprotein E in Alzheimer's disease: an update. *Annu Rev Neurosci*. 2014;37:79-100.
23. Schapira AH. Mitochondrial diseases. *Lancet*. 2012;379(9828):1825-1834.
24. Ng YS, Turnbull DM. Mitochondrial disease: genetics and management. *J Neurol*. 2016;263(1):179-191.
25. Wahbi K, et al. Long-term cardiac prognosis and risk stratification in 260 adults presenting with mitochondrial diseases. *Eur Heart J*. 2015;36(42):2886-2893.
26. Bennett RL, et al. Standardized human pedigree nomenclature: update and assessment of the recommendations of the National Society of Genetic Counselors. *J Genet Couns*. 2008;17(5):424-433.
27. Shendure J, Akey JM. The origins, determinants, and consequences of human mutations. *Science*. 2015;349(6255):1478-1483.
28. Jayandharan GR, Srivastava A. Role of molecular genetics in hemophilia: from diagnosis to therapy. *Semin Thromb Hemost*. 2012;38(1):64-78.
29. Wojczynski MK, Tiwari HK. Definition of phenotype. *Adv Genet*. 2008;60:75-105.
30. Ott J, Wang J, Leal SM. Genetic linkage analysis in the age of whole-genome sequencing. *Nat Rev Genet*. 2015;16(5):275-284.
31. Wellcome Trust Case Control Consortium: Genome-wide association study of 14,000 cases of seven common diseases and 3,000 shared controls. *Nature*. 2007;447(7145):661-678.
32. Welter D, et al. The NHGRI GWAS Catalog, a curated resource of SNP-trait associations. *Nucleic Acids Res*. 2014;42(Database issue):D1001-D1006.
33. GWAS Central. http://www.gwascentral.org. Accessed January 1, 2016.
34. Collins A, Tapper WJ. Genome variation: a review of Web resources. *Methods Mol Biol*. 2011;713:129-139.
35. The ENCODE Project Consortium: Identification and analysis of functional elements in 1% of the human genome by the ENCODE pilot project. *Nature*. 2007;447(7146):799-816.
36. The ENCODE Project Consortium: A user's guide to the encyclopedia of DNA elements (ENCODE). *PLoS Biol*. 2011;9(4):e1001046.
37. The International HapMap Consortium: A second generation human haplotype map of over 3.1 million SNPs. *Nature*. 2007;449(7164):851-861.
38. 1000 Genomes Project Consortium, et al. A map of human genome variation from population-scale sequencing. *Nature*. 2010;467(7319):1061-1073.
39. Bamshad MJ, et al. Exome sequencing as a tool for Mendelian disease gene discovery. *Nat Rev Genet*. 2011;12(11):745-755.
40. Rabbani B, Tekin M, Mahdieh N. The promise of whole-exome sequencing in medical genetics. *J Hum Genet*. 2014;59(1):5-15.
41. Kim MS, et al. A draft map of the human proteome. *Nature*. 2014;509(7502): 575-581.
42. Wilhelm M, et al. Mass-spectrometry-based draft of the human proteome. *Nature*. 2014;509(7502):582-587.
43. Uhlen M, et al. Proteomics. Tissue-based map of the human proteome. *Science*. 2015;347(6220):1260419.
44. The Human Protein Atlas. http://www.proteinatlas.org/humanproteome. Accessed January 1, 2016.
45. Jones ML, et al. Emerging science of the human microbiome. *Gut Microbes*. 2014;5(4):446-457.
46. Schubert AM, et al. Microbiome data distinguish patients with Clostridium difficile infection and non-C. difficile-associated diarrhea from healthy controls. *MBio*. 2014;5(3):e01021-01014.
47. Gomez F, Hirbo J, Tishkoff SA. Genetic variation and adaptation in Africa: implications for human evolution and disease. *Cold Spring Harb Perspect Biol*. 2014;6(7):a008524.
48. The Wellcome Trust Case Control Consortium: Genome-wide association study of copy number variation in 16,000 cases of eight common diseases and 3,000 shared controls. *Nature*. 2010;464(7289):713-720.
49. Pankratz N, et al. Copy number variation in familial Parkinson disease. *PLoS One*. 2011;6(8):e20988.
50. Sakai M, et al. Assessment of copy number variations in the brain genome of schizophrenia patients. *Mol Cytogenet*. 2015;8:46.
51. Johansson AC, Feuk L. Characterizing and interpreting genetic variation from personal genome sequencing. *Methods Mol Biol*. 2012;838:343-367.
52. Dondorp WJ, de Wert GM. The "thousand-dollar genome": an ethical exploration. *Eur J Hum Genet*. 2013;21(suppl 1):S6-S26.
53. Zhang X, Kuivenhoven JA, Groen AK. Forward individualized medicine from personal genomes to interactomes. *Front Physiol*. 2015;6:364.
54. Robson ME, et al. American Society of Clinical Oncology policy statement update: genetic and genomic testing for cancer susceptibility. *J Clin Oncol*. 2015;33(31):3660-3667.
55. Ashley EA, et al. Genetics and cardiovascular disease: a policy statement from the American Heart Association. *Circulation*. 2012;126(1):142-157.
56. Doudna JA, Charpentier E. Genome editing. The new frontier of genome engineering with CRISPR-Cas9. *Science*. 2014;346(6213):1258096.
57. Lander ES. Brave new genome. *N Engl J Med*. 2015;373(1):5-8.
58. The Cancer Genome Atlas. http://cancergenome.nih.gov. Accessed January 1, 2016.
59. Schwartz PJ, Crotti L, Insolia R. Long-QT syndrome: from genetics to management. *Circ Arrhythm Electrophysiol*. 2012;5(4):868-877.
60. Drew BJ, et al. Prevention of torsades de pointes in hospital settings: a scientific statement from the American Heart Association and the American College of Cardiology Foundation. *Circulation*. 2010;121(8):1047-1060.
61. Mullally J, et al. Risk of life-threatening cardiac events among patients with long QT syndrome and multiple mutations. *Heart Rhythm*. 2013;10(3): 378-382.

62. Bezzina CR, Lahrouchi N, Priori SG. Genetics of sudden cardiac death. *Circ Res*. 2015;116(12):1919-1936.

63. Goldenberg I, et al. Beta-blocker efficacy in high-risk patients with the congenital long-QT syndrome types 1 and 2: implications for patient management. *J Cardiovasc Electrophysiol*. 2010;21(8):893-901.

64. Goldenberg I, Moss AJ. Long QT syndrome. *J Am Coll Cardiol*. 2008;51(24):2291-2300.

65. Nannenberg EA, et al. Mortality of inherited arrhythmia syndromes: insight into their natural history. *Circ Cardiovasc Genet*. 2012;5(2):183-189.

66. Maron BJ, Maron MS, Semsarian C. Genetics of hypertrophic cardiomyopathy after 20 years: clinical perspectives. *J Am Coll Cardiol*. 2012;60(8):705-715.

67. Hershberger RE, Hedges DJ, Morales A. Dilated cardiomyopathy: the complexity of a diverse genetic architecture. *Nat Rev Cardiol*. 2013;10(9):531-547.

68. Morales A, Hershberger RE. The rationale and timing of molecular genetic testing for dilated cardiomyopathy. *Can J Cardiol*. 2015;31(11):1309-1312.

69. Daneshvar DA, et al. Familial restrictive cardiomyopathy with 12 affected family members. *Am J Cardiol*. 2012;109(3):445-447.

70. Mann HJ. Drug-associated disease: cytochrome P450 interactions. *Crit Care Clin*. 2006;22(2):329-345.

71. Johnson JA, et al. Clinical pharmacogenetics implementation consortium guidelines for CYP2C9 and VKORC1 genotypes and warfarin dosing. *Clin Pharmacol Ther*. 2011;90(4):625-629.

72. Johnson JA, Cavallari LH. Warfarin pharmacogenetics. *Trends Cardiovasc Med*. 2015;25(1):33-41.

73. Johnson M, et al. Warfarin dosing in a patient with CYP2C9*3*3 and VKORC1-1639 AA genotypes. *Case Rep Genet*. 2014;2014:413743.

74. Rosenberg H, et al. Malignant hyperthermia: a review. *Orphanet J Rare Dis*. 2015;10:93.

75. Greco KE, Tinley S, Seibert D. *Essential Genetic and Genomic Competencies for Nurses with Graduate Degrees*. Silver Spring, MD: American Nurses Association and International Society of Nurses in Genetics; 2011.

76. Jenkins J. *American Nurses Association: Essentials of Genetic and Genomic Nursing Competencies, Curricula Guidelines and Outcome Indicators*. 2nd ed. Silver Spring, MD: American Nurses Association; 2009.

77. Lough ME, Seidel GD. Legal and clinical issues in genetics and genomics. *Clin Nurse Spec*. 2015;29(2):68-70.

78. Goldsmith L, et al. Direct-to-consumer genomic testing: systematic review of the literature on user perspectives. *Eur J Hum Genet*. 2012;20(8):811-816.

79. Health law—genetics—Congress restricts use of genetic information by insurers and employers. Genetic Information Nondiscrimination Act of 2008, Pub. L. No. 110-233, 122 Stat. 881 (to be codified in scattered sections of 26, 29, and 42 U.S.C.). *Harv Law Rev*. 2009;122(3):1038-1045.

80. Laedtke AL, et al. Family physicians' awareness and knowledge of the Genetic Information Non-Discrimination Act (GINA). *J Genet Couns*. 2012;21(2):345-352.

5

Patient and Family Education

Barbara Mayer

CHALLENGES OF PATIENT AND FAMILY EDUCATION

At no other point in history has information within the general population been so readily available. Televisions are in practically every home, computers with wireless access to the Internet are available for use almost anywhere at any time, and young and old people carry cell phones. It seems as adults in the 21st century cannot tolerate a lack of information. The ease of access to the world's library of information meets a compulsive need to satisfy a desire for immediate gratification. Gathering information in bits and pieces from various sources allows people to collect information at their own pace and to gather as much or as little information as they desire. These "knowledge bites" are sorted and stored on an individual's "cerebral hard drive." The "file" is retrieved and "opened" whenever the situation warrants.

When alterations in health arise in daily life, people use all available resources to discover information to help them cope and adapt to the new experience. This type of consumerism has developed a populace that is more educated in health matters than ever before. It is our duty as health professionals to assist patients and families with information gathering and self-care management skills so that they can lead lives of the best quality possible. According to The Joint Commission, patients must receive "sufficient information to make decisions and to take responsibility for self-management activities related to their needs."[1] The goals of patient and family education are to improve health outcomes by promoting healthy behavior and involvement in care and care decisions.[1]

Admission to a critical care unit usually is an unexpected event in anyone's life. The seriousness of the situation and unfamiliarity of the hospital or unit environment evoke a stress response in patients and their families. Nursing care is focused on improving the patient's physiologic stability and promoting end-organ tissue perfusion. Promoting the most basic human physiologic survival need for cellular oxygenation is the priority. Alterations in normal functioning related to progression of the disease process, sedation, assist devices, or mechanical ventilation contribute to the possibility of mental alterations in the patient. Sleep deprivation and sensory overload add to the complexity of the issues that affect the patient's ability to receive and understand medical information. Mental alterations may limit the effectiveness of the teaching-learning encounter. These physical and cognitive limitations prevent patients from receiving or understanding information related to their care and impair their ability to make an informed decision.[2] At these times, critical life-or-death care decisions are transferred to a proxy, usually an immediate family member. The designated proxy has the responsibility to make informed treatment decisions for the patient. These types of situations present the nurse with special challenges in the education of patients and families.

Critical illness disrupts the normal patterns of daily life. Stress and crisis can develop within the family unit and stretch its members' coping resources.[3] These many emotional factors build barriers to the teaching-learning process and can become frustrating for the learner and the nurse. Amid the chaos, how do bedside nurses effectively provide patient and family education that can optimize outcomes and deliver quality, cost-effective care? It is the nurse's responsibility to educate himself or herself about concepts that provide insight into the framework for patient and family education. Adult educational concepts, such as adult learning principles, types of educational needs, barriers to learning, stress and coping strategies, and evidence-based interventions, must be used to develop an individualized education plan to meet the identified learning needs of the patient and family.

EDUCATION

Definition

Patient education is a process that includes the purposeful delivery of health-related information to promote changes in behavior that will optimize health practices and assist the individual in attaining new skills for living.[4,5] This concept can be overwhelming in the fast-paced, technology-rich setting of the critical care environment. The bedside nurse must incorporate the abundant educational needs of the patient or family into the education plan and be aware of the requirements of regulatory agencies and the legalities of documenting the teaching-learning encounter.

Benefits

Studies have documented that quality education shortens hospital length of stay, reduces readmission rates, and improves self-care management skills.[4-6] Complications associated with the physiologic stress response may be prevented if the patient or family perceives the education encounter as positive. Positive encounters decrease the stress response, relieve anxiety, promote individual growth and development, and increase patient and family satisfaction.[4-6] Examples of positive outcomes associated with a structured teaching-learning process include the following:[7,8]

- Clarification of patients' understanding and perceptions of their chronic illness and care decisions
- Improved health outcomes relative to self-management techniques, such as symptom management

- Promotion of informed decision making and control over the situation
- Diminished emotional stress associated with an unfamiliar environment and unknown prognosis
- Improved adaptation to stressful situations
- Improved satisfaction with the care received
- Improved relationship with the health care team
- Promotion of self-concept

Education Process

The education process follows the same framework as the nursing process: assessment, diagnosis, goals or outcomes, interventions, and evaluation.[4] Although this chapter discusses these steps individually, they may occur simultaneously and repetitively in practice. The teaching-learning process is a dynamic, continuous activity that occurs throughout the entire hospitalization and may continue after the patient has been discharged. This process is often envisioned by the nurse as a time-consuming task that requires knowledge and skills to accomplish. Although knowledge and skills can be obtained, time in the critical care unit is a scarce commodity. Many nurses believe they cannot educate unless formal blocks of education time are planned during the shift. Although this type of education encounter is optimal, it is unrealistic for contemporary nursing. The nurse must recognize that teaching occurs during every moment of a nurse-patient encounter.[9] Instructions for how to use the call bell or explanations of events and sensations to expect during a bed bath can be considered an education session. It is the nurse's role to recognize that education, no matter how brief or extensive, affects the daily lives of each person with whom he or she comes in contact. By following the nursing process, the physical assessment and education assessment can occur simultaneously.

STEP 1: ASSESSMENT

According to The Joint Commission, education provided should be appropriate to the patient's condition and should address the patient's identified learning needs.[1] The assessment is an important first step to providing need-targeted patient and family education. It begins on admission and continues until the patient is discharged. A formal, comprehensive, initial education assessment produces valuable information; however, it can take the nurse hours to complete. The nurse must focus the initial and subsequent education assessments on identifying gaps in knowledge related to the patient's current health-altering situation.

Learning needs can be defined as gaps between what the learner knows and what the learner needs to know, such as survival skills, coping skills, and ability to make a care decision. Identification of actual and perceived learning needs directs the health care team to provide need-targeted education. Need-targeted or need-to-know education is directed at helping the learner to become familiar with the current situation. Educational needs of the patient and family can be categorized as (1) information only (environment, visitation hours, get questions answered); (2) informed decision making (treatment plan, informed consent); or (3) self-management (recognition of problems and how to respond).[5,10] Patient education to be included in the education plan should address the plan of care, health practices and safety, safe and effective use of medications, nutrition interventions, safe and effective use of medical equipment or supplies, pain, and habilitation or rehabilitation needs.[1]

Learning needs may change from day to day, shift to shift, or minute to minute. Educational needs are influenced by how the patient or the family perceives or interprets the critical illness.[11] Perceptions of experiences vary from person to person, even if two people are involved in the same event. This intense internal feeling affects the desire to learn and understanding of the current situation. Satisfaction with the learning encounter is often judged to be positive if the nurse meets the expected learning needs of the patient and family. Congruency between nurse-identified needs and patient-identified needs brings about more positive learning experiences and encourages the learner to seek further information. The nurse must actively listen, maintain eye contact, seek clarification, and pay attention to verbal and nonverbal cues from the patient and the family to gather relevant information concerning perceived learning needs. The nurse should seek to first understand the learning need from the patient's point of view and then seek to be understood.

Strategic questioning provides an avenue for the nurse to determine whether the patient or family has any misconceptions about the environment, the patient's illness, self-management skills, or the medication schedule. Health care providers use the term *noncompliant* to describe a patient or family members who do not modify behaviors to the meet the demands of the prescribed treatment regimen, such as following the rules of a low-fat diet or medication dosing. However, the problem behind noncompliance may not be a conscious desire to defy the treatment plan but instead may be a misunderstanding of the importance of the treatment or how to follow the treatment plan. The technique of asking open-ended questions ("Can you tell me what you know about your medication?") can elicit more information about the patient's knowledge base than asking closed-ended questions ("You know this is your water pill, right?"). Open-ended questions provide the nurse an opportunity to assess actual knowledge gaps, rather than assuming knowledge by obtaining a yes-or-no response. These types of questions also assist the patient and family to tell their story of the illness and communicate their perceptions of the experience,[5] allowing the adult learner to feel respected and involved in the treatment process. Questions that elicit a yes-or-no response close off communication and do not provide an interactive teaching-learning session. Box 5.1 contains sample questions the nurse can use in an assessment to obtain needed information. Generally, with practice and effort, it can be determined what educational information is needed in a brief period without much disruption in the routine care of the patient. Patients and families are multidimensional. Even with good questioning skills, the nurse cannot assess many aspects of the learner during the initial contact or even during the hospital stay.

Learner Identification

Identifying learner characteristics benefits the nurse and results in optimal communication and the patient's understanding of information. Certain factors can affect the education process. Culture or ethnicity, age, and adult learning principles influence the manner in which information is presented and concepts are understood.[5,12]

Family

A family can be defined as a group of individuals who are bonded by biologic, legal, and social relationships.[3] The modern

---

BOX 5.1   Assessment Questions

- Why have you come to the hospital today?
- What problem are you having?
- How can we help you today?
- When did these problems start?
- Have you had these problems before?
- Have you been hospitalized for these problems before?
- Who is your doctor for this problem? Who is your family doctor?
- What medications are you taking?
- Can you tell me why you take each medication?
- How do you care for yourself at home? Do you have help?
- Are any family or friends with you today?
- Are these people your main support system?
- Are there any special needs, religious or otherwise, that we need to be aware of while you are in the hospital?
- What is your goal for coming to the hospital today?
- How can we help you reach this goal?
- Is there any information that I can give you right now that would help you understand more about why you are here or about your plan of care?
- What information have you received from other members of the health care team today?

---

family is diverse in ethnic backgrounds, sexual orientation, age, gender, work experience, physical or mental challenges, communication skills, educational backgrounds, work experience, geographic location, lived experiences, and religious beliefs.[13-15] A picture of the modern family would resemble that of a large patchwork quilt. Patches of different sizes, ethnicities, religions, cultures, attitudes, stages of development, and lived experiences would overlap and occupy their own individual spaces within the quilt framework. Bedside practitioners are expected to provide culturally competent care to each individual in the critical care setting. Culturally competent care is the delivery of sensitive, meaningful care to patients and families from diverse backgrounds.[15] This implies that the practitioner must value diversity and become knowledgeable concerning the cultural strengths and abilities of the people for whom they care.[16] Communication and understanding impact the education process. Provision of language-appropriate literature and translation services and recognition of cultural or religious differences in the perception of illness and treatment influence the education encounter.[15]

Age-Specific Considerations

The critical care patient population differs culturally and by age and stages of human development. Older adult patients may have more difficulty reading patient educational materials or the label on the bottle of prescription medication than younger adults. Printed materials with larger fonts may be needed for these patients. Older adults were not exposed to technology during their youth and may find it difficult to navigate the fragmented maze of modern health care. Because of advanced age, this population of adults may have prescriptions for multiple drug therapies. Education to prevent adverse drug reactions may be required because of the prevalence of multiple drug therapies.[17] Older adults may also be coping with end-of-life issues and need information to make informed decisions. Young adults may struggle with the issue of how to incorporate intimacy into their lives without feeling isolated from the mainstream social scene. The need for privacy and peer support may

be required to assist the young adult in coping with the current situation. The practitioner must recognize these age-specific issues and incorporate them into the education plan.[1]

Adult Learners

Adults learn in large part through lived experiences. The motivation to learn is internal and problem-oriented, focusing on life events. Malcolm Knowles described these principles of adult learning in a model known as *andragogy*. Adult learning theory stresses concepts of individualism, self-assessment, self-direction, motivation, experience, and autonomy. Adults tend to have a strong sense of self-concept, are goal-oriented learners, and like to make their own decisions.[18] They take responsibility and accountability for their own learning and want to be respected as individuals as well as recognized for accomplished life experiences. Adults have individualized learning styles and often lack confidence in their ability to learn. Education is resisted when the information given is perceived to be in conflict with the individual's self-image.

The learning process generally involves altering some part of current behavior to produce changes in lifestyle, incorporating the new or chronic illness into daily living. Coping mechanisms such as anger, disbelief, and denial affect the willingness of the patient or family to learn. The unwillingness to change behavior to manage health needs adds to the complexity of the critical care teaching-learning encounter. The nurse must provide need-to-know information in easy, understandable terms and in short bursts. Positive feedback and repetition of information may also be required before health education is incorporated into the patient's or family's bank of experiences.[18] Adults are sensitive about making mistakes and tend to view mistakes as failures. Learning situations that the patient and family interpret as belittling or embarrassing or that are perceived as insurmountable will be avoided or disregarded. The nurse should act more as a coach or facilitator of information instead of a didactic instructor.[12] The teacher can only show the learner to the door; the learner must decide to walk through that door. Learning is an active process that occurs internally over time and cannot be forced. Bedside nurses are obliged to be proactive and to have a good understanding of adult learning theory and to incorporate its concepts into the assessment of learning needs, development of an education plan, implementation of the plan, and evaluation of the outcomes of the education encounter.

Factors Affecting the Learning Process

Information must also be gathered on factors that affect the education process and impair the ability of the patient or family to respond, including (1) desire and motivation, (2) physical or cognitive limitations, (3) cultural and religious views of illness or health, (4) emotional barriers, and (5) barriers to effective communication.[1]

Readiness, Willingness, Ability

For teaching to be successful and learning to be achieved, the patient or family must be ready, willing, and able to learn. The ability to learn is the capacity of the learner to understand, pay attention, and comprehend the material being taught. Willingness to learn describes the learner's openness to new ideas and concepts. Readiness to learn is the motivation to try out new concepts and behaviors.[5] Even if the inventive teaching methods, well-considered education materials, and amounts of time are unlimited, learning cannot take place if the patient or family is not ready, willing, and able to learn.[19] Several factors affect the ability, willingness, and readiness to learn as well as the ability to cope and adapt to the current situation. These factors include physiologic, psychological, sociocultural, financial, and environmental aspects.[5,12]

Physiologic Factors

The need for oxygen and survival predominates over all other human needs. This need is described by a theory known as Maslow's hierarchy of human needs. It is a concept in which lower level, physiologic needs must be satisfied before an individual can move on to higher level, self-esteem–building issues. The motivation to meet the need to survive and to feel safe and secure predominates over the need to learn a lifestyle change such as smoking cessation. Only when lower level needs are met can the patient be open to learning new concepts and skills. There is an instinctive need to decrease the effects of stressors and reestablish a normal daily routine. A physical assessment can supply the nurse with information concerning the patient's response to the stressors.

Physiologic alterations in heart rate and blood pressure can be measured and taken into consideration during the teaching-learning encounter.[3] Sources of physiologic stress in a critically ill patient include medications, pain, hypoxia, decreased cerebral and peripheral perfusion, hypotension, fluid and electrolyte imbalances, infection, sensory alterations, fever, and neurologic deficits.[12] Experiencing one or more of these stressors may completely consume all the patient's available energy and thoughts, affecting his or her ability to interact, comprehend, and respond to teaching.

Health Literacy

Patients and families may be ready and willing to learn but lack the ability to comprehend and act on the information presented to them. In its report *Health Literacy: A Prescription to End Confusion*, the Institute of Medicine states that nearly half of adult Americans struggle to understand and follow the health information they are provided. The Institute of Medicine defines health literacy as "the degree to which individuals have the capacity to obtain, process, and understand basic health information and services needed to make appropriate health decisions." However, health literacy goes beyond the individual. Practitioners must develop the ability to present information and instructions in a way that patients and families can best understand.[20]

Assessing health literacy is not an easy task, but knowing what to look for can make it easier. Several tools are available to assist health care professionals to screen for low literacy skills. Generally, these tools fall into four categories: (1) word recognition, (2) reading comprehension, (3) functional health literacy, and (4) informal methods.[21,22] Each tool has positive and negative aspects to its use.

Word recognition tests consist of lists of health care terms that patients are asked to read. The patient is given a time limit, and scoring is based on how many words the patient can correctly pronounce. Examples of word recognition tests include the Rapid Estimate of Adult Literacy in Medicine (REALM), Wide Range Achievement Test-Revised (WRAT-R), Short Assessment of Health Literacy for Spanish Adults (SAHLSA-50), and Medical Terminology Achievement Test (MART). These tests can often be administered in 5 to 10 minutes; however, they test only the reading abilities of the individual, not comprehension or interpretation.

Reading comprehension tests assess understanding of health care information presented but do not demonstrate the individual's ability to apply this information. Reading comprehension tests are extremely time-consuming and are not often used in the clinical setting.

Functional health literacy tests assess the individual's level of comprehension and ability to put into action what they have learned. Examples of these tests include the Test of Functional Health Literacy in Adults (TOFHLA)[4] and the Newest Vital Sign (NVS).[21-22] The TOFHLA requires the individual to complete missing sections of written statements to assess the ability to read and comprehend directions for taking medications, monitoring blood glucose, and keeping appointments.[23] The tool takes 20 to 30 minutes to administer and score, making it undesirable for use in the critical care setting. An abbreviated version, the S-TOFHLA, is now available. It takes approximately 10 to 12 minutes to complete and score. Fig. 5.1 shows the NVS tool and scoring sheet.

Informal methods include identifying socioeconomic characteristics, observation of behaviors, and direct questioning. A common misconception among health care providers is that reading and comprehension levels are directly related to wealth and level of education; the implication is that someone with a graduate-level education has a higher reading level than someone who completed only grade school. This is not true; wealth and education levels do not necessarily correlate with the ability to read and comprehend health care information.

Shame has been cited as one of the most common emotions associated with low health literacy.[24] Behaviors such as handing a form to a family member to complete, claiming to be too tired, or "forgetting" their glasses are a few behaviors that may be used by individuals to hide their limitations. Other behaviors that may also provide clues to a patient's health literacy are listed in Box 5.2.

In some cases, asking a direct question can elicit an individual's level of health literacy. For example, how the individual answers questions such as "How comfortable are you in reading medicine labels?" or "How well do you understand your disease process?" may help the practitioner gain insight into the level of health literacy and plan appropriate educational interventions.

Sociocultural Factors

Variables such as culture, ethnicity, values, beliefs, lifestyle, and family role influence the way an individual perceives illness, pain, and healing.[15] Culturally sensitive educational strategies should be developed to communicate specific needs to other members of the health care team and achieve optimal learning outcomes.[1]

Financial Factors

Patients and families often worry about financial issues related to the hospitalization and the possibility of long-term disability. Examples of financial concerns are (1) fear of income loss related to time away from work or possible long-term disability, (2) how health care expenses will be paid, and (3) complex insurance coverage issues. Patients may be more concerned with the amount of out-of-pocket expenses they will have to pay for the illness rather than receiving information on symptom management strategies. The nurse must recognize these issues as patient concerns and mobilize resources to calm financial anxiety. Practitioners in other disciplines, especially social work, are available to assist patients and families to obtain community resources to help cover expenses such as medication costs.

Score Sheet for the Newest Vital Sign
Questions and Answers

READ TO SUBJECT:
This information is on the back of a container of a pint of ice cream.

	ANSWER CORRECT?	
	yes	no

1. If you eat the entire container, how many calories will you eat?
   Answer: 1,000 is the only correct answer

2. If you are allowed to eat 60 grams of carbohydrates as a snack, how much ice cream could you have?
   Answer: Any of the following is correct: 1 cup (or any amount up to 1 cup), half the container. Note: If patient answers "two servings," ask "How much ice cream would that be if you were to measure it into a bowl?"

3. Your doctor advises you to reduce the amount of saturated fat in your diet. You usually have 42 g of saturated fat each day, which includes one serving of ice cream. If you stop eating ice cream, how many grams of saturated fat would you be consuming each day?
   Answer: 33 is the only correct answer

4. If you usually eat 2,500 calories in a day, what percentage of your daily value of calories will you be eating if you eat one serving?
   Answer: 10% is the only correct answer

READ TO SUBJECT:
Pretend that you are allergic to the following substances : penicillin, peanuts, latex gloves, and bee stings.

5. Is it safe for you to eat this ice cream?
   Answer: No

6. (Ask only if the patient responds "no" to question 5): Why not?
   Answer: Because it has peanut oil.

   Number of correct answers: _____

Interpretation

Score of 0–1 suggests high likelihood (50% or more) of limited literacy.
Score of 2–3 indicates the possibility of limited literacy.
Score of 4–6 almost always indicates adequate literacy.

Pfizer Working together for a healthier world™

February 2011

Nutrition Facts

Serving Size	½ cup
Servings per container	4

Amount per serving

Calories	250	Fat Cal	120

	%DV
Total Fat 13g	20%
Sat Fat 9g	40%
Cholesterol 28mg	12%
Sodium 55mg	2%
Total Carbohydrate 30g	12%
Dietary Fiber 2g	
Sugars 23g	
Protein 4g	8%

*Percentage Daily Values (DV) are based on a 2,000 calorie diet. Your daily values may be higher or lower depending on your calorie needs.

Ingredients: Cream, Skim Milk, Liquid Sugar, Water, Egg Yolks, Brown Sugar, Milkfat, Peanut Oil, Sugar, Butter, Salt, Carrageenan, Vanilla Extract.

FIG. 5.1 The Newest Vital Sign (NVS) Health Literacy Test Tool and Scoring Sheet. (Courtesy Pfizer, New York, NY.)

BOX 5.2   Behavioral Cues Indicating Low Health Literacy

- Requests family to always be present
- Opens a medication bottle to identify a medicine
- Makes excuses:
  "I forgot my glasses."
  "I want my son to read it first."
  "I'll take it home with me."
- Refers to medications by shape or color rather than name
- Cannot teach-back
- Frequently misses appointments
- Postpones decision making
- Watches or mimics behavior or responses of others
- Pretends to read material—eyes wander over page, slow to read
- Does not complete forms or asks staff or family to complete

Psychological factors

When confronted with a life-altering situation such as admission to a critical care unit, patients and families may experience anxiety and emotional stress. Anxiety and fear disrupt the normalcy of daily life. Sources of emotional stress include fear of death, uncertain prognosis, role change, self-image change, social isolation, disruption in daily routine, financial concerns, and unfamiliar critical care environment.[3,20] These intense emotions can lead to a crisis situation and alter the ability of the patient and family to cope.[25,26] During the critical illness, an individual's ability to process or retain information and ability to participate in the treatment plan could be altered.[2] If the disease process or physiologic stressors impair the patient's ability to make decisions, the burden of decision making will transfer to the family. Gender differences affect a patient's reaction to stress. For example, women who have experienced a myocardial infarction report higher anxiety levels than men at all

TABLE 5.1 Teaching-Learning Process in Adaptation to Illness

Stage of Adaptation	Characteristic Patient Response	Implications for Teaching-Learning Process
Disbelief	Denial	Orient teaching to present.
		Teach during other nursing activities.
		Reassure patient about safety.
		Explain all procedures and activities clearly and concisely.
Developing awareness	Anger	Continue to orient teaching to present.
		Avoid long lists of facts.
		Continue to foster development of trust and rapport through good physical care.
Reorganization	Acceptance of sick role	Orient teaching to meet patient.
		Teach whatever patient wants to learn.
		Provide necessary self-care information; reinforce with written material.
Resolution	Identification with others with same problem; recognition of loss	Use group instruction.
		Use patient support groups and visits by recovered patients with same problem.
Identifying change	Definition of self as one who has undergone change and is now different	Answer the patient's questions as they arise.
		Recognize that as basic needs are met, more mature needs will arise.

points during the hospital stay.[27] Physiologic alterations caused by anxiety have a negative impact on the recovery process and the long-term prognosis.[27] In critical situations, the nurse may find it necessary to repeat information or limit teaching sessions to short bursts rather than one long encounter. Medical jargon should be limited and replaced by terms that are easy to understand. Provision of honest and accurate information about the disease state may decrease the effects of stressors and alleviate anxiety and fear.

Coping

Coping refers to the way a person manages stressful events that are straining or exceeding personal resources.[5,28] The stressful event is appraised according to the level of threat to the individual and is managed by focusing on the problem at hand or the emotions felt at the moment.[29] Critical illness disrupts the normalcy of daily routines. Coping strategies are used by the patient and family to help maintain control over the situation and encourage hope and stability in life. Disbelief and denial may be present any time during the hospitalization. Phrases such as "Why me" and "I can't believe this is happening" are common in the critical care setting. Other coping mechanisms, such as denial and anger, hamper the ability of the patient or family to problem solve and cope with the situation. All are barriers to the ability of the patient to receive information and incorporate it into the self-concept. Adults must be physically ready and emotionally willing to learn. Therefore teaching new skills or self-management techniques to the adult learner presents a special challenge to the nurse in critical care. For example, until the patient accepts the diagnosis of heart failure as part of who he or she is, he or she will not make appropriate changes in lifestyle to avoid an exacerbation of the disease.

Adaptation

A stressor can be any condition, situation, or perception that requires an individual to adapt.[30] All situations in a critical care facility may well be considered stressful. The capacity of an individual to adapt is paramount in breaking down emotional barriers that affect willingness and readiness for learning.

Culture, beliefs, attitudes, and ability to mobilize resources affect a person's ability to respond to a crisis situation.[28] General characteristics of the stages of adaptation to illness are outlined in Table 5.1 with corresponding applications for the teaching-learning process. Patients and families move through these stages on an individual timeline and at a variable pace. A person may move back and forth between stages and may skip a stage altogether. The patient and each member of the family may be experiencing different stages in the adaptation process at the same time. The education encounter may need to be modified to meet the needs of the patient and family.

Environmental Factors

The critical care environment can be considered a source of stress to the learner. Although sounds, people, and state-of-the-art equipment are familiar and mundane for the nurse, this environment may appear foreign and intimidating to the patient and family. Prior exposure to a critical care unit is a double-edged sword. Depending on whether the outcome of the experience was positive or negative, it may help alleviate or heighten anxiety. The nurse must pay attention to the perceptions of the environment by the patient and family and alter the teaching-learning encounter accordingly. Sleep cycle alterations caused by sleep deprivation or sensory overload related to continuous noise from machines or people affect the patient's ability to concentrate and comprehend information. Allowing frequent uninterrupted rest periods assists the patient in obtaining structured sleep.[30]

For patients and families to value education, they must believe the information source is reliable. The bedside nurse is the most available source of information in the critical care unit. It is important for him or her to develop a rapport and establish a sense of trust within the nurse-patient relationship. These positive characteristics are recommended for a supportive learning environment. Assignment of multiple caregivers may negatively affect the ability of the patient and family to form a trusting relationship with the nursing staff. Arranging consistency in the assigned caregivers can help promote rapport and trust, decrease anxiety, and enhance comfort level with the environment.[5,28]

STEP 2: EDUCATION PLAN DEVELOPMENT

Education must be ongoing, interactive, and consistent with the patient's plan of care and education level.[1] The nurse must analyze information gathered from the assessment to prioritize the educational needs of the patient and family. The nursing diagnosis for deficient knowledge and accompanying interventions can be applied to any situation. The nurse must also consider the patient's physical and emotional status when setting education priorities. Ability, willingness, and readiness to learn are factors that can impair acceptance of new information and add to the complexity of the teaching-learning encounter. These factors should be recognized by the nurse before implementation of teaching. The written teaching plan should identify the learning need, goals, or expected outcome of the teaching-learning encounter; interventions to meet that outcome; and appropriate teaching strategies.

Research and accepted national guidelines or standards can be used to assist the practitioner in developing an evidence-based plan for education. Examples of organizations that offer education standards are the American Association of Critical-Care Nurses, the American Heart Association Guidelines for Practice, and the Society of Critical Care Medicine. A database for nursing interventions and outcomes has been developed from research that began in the 1980s. This research is known as the IOWA Project. It can be used in daily practice and can be found in two books: *Nursing Interventions Classification (NIC)* and *Nursing Outcomes Classification (NOC)*. These evidence-based interventions and outcomes assist the nurse in providing consistent outcomes and interventions from nurse to nurse, shift to shift, and discipline to discipline.

Determining What to Teach

It can be difficult to prioritize the multitude of learning needs that practitioners are required to address during a period in critical care. Learning needs in the critical care unit, the progressive care setting, or the telemetry setting can be separated into four different categories to help set teaching priorities in each phase of the hospitalization (Table 5.2). Learning needs during the initial contact or first hours of hospitalization can be

TABLE 5.2 Categories of Educational Needs in Critical Care	
Phase	**Educational Needs**
Initial contact or first visit, with focus on immediate needs	Preparation for the visit: patient representatives or nurses can prepare the family and patient for the first visit
	What to expect in the environment
	How long the visit will last
	What the patient may look like (eg, tubes, IV lines)
	Orientation to the unit or environment: call light, bed controls, waiting rooms, unit contact numbers
	Orientation to unit policies and hospital policies
	HIPAA, advanced directives, visitation policies
	Equipment orientation: monitors, IV pumps, pulse oximetry, pacemakers, ventilators
	Medications: rationale, effects, side effects
	What to do during the visit: talk to the patient, hold the patient's hand, monitor length of visits (if applicable)
	Patient status: stable or unstable and what that terminology means
	What treatments and interventions are being done for the patient
	Upcoming procedures
	When the physician visited or is expected to visit
	Disciplines involved in care and the services they provide
	Immediate plan of care (next 24 h)
	Mobilization of resources for crisis intervention
Continuous care	Day-to-day routine: meals, laboratory visits, physician visits, frequency of monitoring (VS), nursing assessments, daily weights, and shift routines
	Explanation of any procedures: expected sensations or discomforts (eg, chest tube removal, arterial sheath removal)
	Plan of care: treatments, progress, patient accomplishments (eg, extubation)
	Medications: name, why the patient is receiving them, side effects to report to the nurse or health care team
	Disease process: what it is and how it will affect life, symptoms to report to health care team
	How to mobilize resources to assist the patient and family in coping with stress and crisis: pastoral care, social workers, case managers, victim assistance, domestic violence counseling
	Gifts: When a loved one is ill, it is traditional to send flowers, balloons, or cards; if your unit has restrictions on gifts, make the family aware
	Begin teaching self-management skills, and discuss aftercare information
Transfer to different level of care	**Sending Unit**
	Acknowledge positive move out of critical care
	When the transfer will occur
	Why the transfer is occurring
	What to expect in the different unit
	Name of the new caregiver
	Availability of care provider
	Visiting hours

TABLE 5.2 Categories of Educational Needs in Critical Care—cont'd

Phase	Educational Needs
Planning for aftercare, discharge planning	Directions for how to get there; the new room number and phone number
	Receiving Unit
	Orientation to environment, visitation policies, visitors
	Unit routine, meals, shift changes, physician visits
	Expectations about patient self-care; ADLs
	Medication and diagnostic testing routine times
	Self-care management: symptom management, medication administration, diet, activity, durable medical equipment, tasks or procedures
	What to do for an emergency
	What constitutes an emergency or when to call the physician
	How to care for incisions or procedure sites
Completed throughout hospital stay	Return appointment: name of physician practice, practice phone numbers and contacts
	Obtaining medications: prescriptions, pharmacy, special medication ordering information
	Required lifestyle changes: mobility and safety issues for paraplegic patient or patient with stroke, ADLs issues relative to medications or symptoms
	Potential risk modifications: smoking cessation, diet modifications, exercise
	Resources: cardiac rehabilitation, support groups, home care agencies
End-of-life care	End-of-life care: participation in care, services available, mobilizing resources
	Palliative care
	Hospice

ADLs, activities of daily living; *HIPAA,* Health Insurance Portability and Accountability Act; *IV,* intravenous; *VS,* vital signs.

predicted. Education during this time frame should be directed toward the reduction of immediate stress, anxiety, and fear rather than future lifestyle alterations or rehabilitation needs. Interventions are targeted to promote comfort and familiarity with the environment and surroundings.[31] The plan should focus on survival skills, orientation to the environment and equipment, communication of prognosis, procedure explanations, and the immediate plan of care.

Three learning domains are considered when developing an individualized education plan: knowledge, attitude, and skills. The knowledge domain is centered on the acquisition of information or facts by the patient about a given topic, such as listing the signs and symptoms of hypoglycemia and knowing what to do if he or she becomes symptomatic. A patient who has had diabetes for years has life experiences with his or her disease process that are different from those of the newly diagnosed patient. Even though two patients have the same diagnosis, educational needs differ. The attitude domain includes the incorporation of new values, beliefs, or attitudes into patients' behavior, such as believing smoking is bad for them and then exerting a conscious effort to stop. The skills domain is involved with the acquisition of skills that enable a person to perform a new technique, such as endotracheal suctioning or dressing changes. The nurse may incorporate one or more of these domains into the education plan.

Patients and their families are attempting to cope with the seriousness of the current situation and need information continually to adapt their behavior accordingly. Leske and Molter's hallmark research in the area of needs of the families of critically ill patients has provided nursing with a scientific body of knowledge for identification of the learning needs of this population. Results of these studies found that families of critically ill patients needed to have their questions answered honestly and to have a feeling of hope.[32] The outcomes of this research can be used in developing interventions for the initial phase in

BOX 5.3   QSEN: Patient-Centered Care

Interventions for Identified Patient and Family Needs

- Answer questions openly and honestly.
- Give as much or as little realistic information as the patient and family members need to understand about the situation or the patient's physiologic condition.
- Provide specific facts about the patient's daily or hourly progress.
- Provide information in simple terms that are understandable.
- Use short sentences, and incorporate only a couple of pieces of information at one time.
- Provide emotional comfort to reduce anxiety and facilitate the feeling of hope.
- Prepare the patient and family for their first visit to the unit.
- Explain the possible appearance of the patient, purpose of the equipment, the family's role in visitation, and the unit environment.
- Keep the family informed and involved in the daily plan of care.
- Explain what procedures will be done, why they are being done, and what information is hoped to be gained from each procedure.

the hospitalization process. Box 5.3 includes a sample listing of interventions that can be used to help meet the needs of the family. During this time of elevated stress, the nurse may have to refocus the patient and family to help concentrate efforts on coping with the present instead of dwelling on possibilities of the future. Not addressing these immediate concerns can result in further anxiety, affect the ability to cope, and prevent open and honest communication.[3]

As the hospital length of stay increases, patients and families begin to adapt to the situation, and learning needs change. The patient and family develop positive feelings of relief and happiness in the fact that survival has been achieved. Because lower level, physiologic needs are met, the patient's efforts can be concentrated on modifying behavior to meet higher level needs, such as self-concept and self-actualization. Teaching during the continuous phase of nursing care is aimed at answering the patient's or family members' questions about the treatment plan or how the critical illness will impact their daily lives. Education on lifestyle modification and self-management skills should be presented during this phase of nursing care.

Discharge planning is also part of the education process and should start with admission to the hospital. Instructions for home care, also known as aftercare, should be accomplished before the day of discharge to avoid decreased retention of education that occurs with information overload.

Patient Education boxes are placed in each Disorders chapter. Special topics that should be taught to patients and families in preparation for discharge are listed.

Writing Goals or Outcomes

An outcomes statement helps clarify to the teacher and the learner what is to be taught, what is to be learned, what is to be evaluated, and what is to be documented. When goals or expected outcomes of the education encounter are clearly stated, the teacher and the learner understand the expectations and will do their best to achieve them. These statements differ from interventions in that they reflect what the learner is to accomplish, not what the nurse is to teach.[33] Identifying and writing outcomes may be the most difficult aspect in the development of the education plan of care. The written outcomes provide direction for the teaching-learning process and should be straightforward, should be attainable, and should include one task or learning domain.[33]

The three components in the outcomes statement are (1) the individual who will meet the objective, (2) a measurable or observable verb, and (3) the content to be evaluated or learned. Examples of measurable verbs include define, list, identify, perform, prepare, and demonstrate, whereas nonmeasurable, higher level verbs include believe, value, and understand. Remember the "KISS" rule: *Keep It Simple, Simon.* Outcomes should include behavioral lifestyle changes for self-management, psychomotor skill acquisition, and acquisition of knowledge. The following is an example of a clearly stated outcome: "The patient and family will list the signs and symptoms of postoperative infection."

Developing Interventions

Interventions describe how a nurse will become involved in providing education to the patient or the family. Determining education interventions is part of clinical decision making.[34] Nurse-initiated interventions are based on clinical knowledge and judgment and have a direct impact on the outcome of the teaching encounter.[34] Although physiologic problems occupy most of the nursing plan of care, it is essential to incorporate teaching interventions into the daily plan to create positive patient outcomes. Nurses just entering the profession readily refer to education plans developed by experienced nurses to guide them in their new role of patient educator.[35] Carefully planned and developed interventions support nurses, patients, and families focused on achievable outcomes. Education interventions are targeted toward information to be taught, such as how to care and use oxygen or how to recognize signs and symptoms of an infection. The following is an example of a

clearly stated research-based intervention: "Instruct the patient and family on proper name of prescribed diet."[34]

Standardized Education Plans

Standardized education plans provide the health care team with consistent outcomes and interventions. Although standardized plans are easy to implement, they must be individualized to meet the specific needs of the patient or family.[7] Examples of standardized plans of care include patient pathways and traditional nursing care plans for Deficient Knowledge. Examples of nursing management plans for Deficient Knowledge are included in Appendix A.

STEP 3: IMPLEMENTATION

After the assessment is completed and the education plan is developed, need-targeted education can commence. Beginning practitioners differ from experienced practitioners in their skills of implementing the education plan of care. Experienced practitioners use their intuition and knowledge base to anticipate learning needs and form a mental list of interventions and possible outcomes.[35] Practitioners just starting in the profession need the concrete education plan that has been developed to guide the teaching-learning encounter.[35]

Setting up the Environment

The optimal environment for learning is one that is nonthreatening, comfortable, open, and honest. Many factors concerning the critical care environment can be threatening or anxiety producing. The practitioner must assess for these distractions and control them as much as possible. Providing the family with open visitation and access to the patient and health care providers can help decrease their anxiety level and improve satisfaction with care.[3] Current Health Insurance Portability and Accountability Act requirements for patient confidentiality necessitate a need for privacy during the teaching-learning encounter. The attention of the bedside practitioner to this detail in open environments, such as critical care units, waiting rooms, and emergency departments, is important in creating an environment of trust and reassurance. Supportive education promotes behaviors that facilitate motivation to learn and adherence to lifestyle changes.[36] The following is a list of strategies the practitioner can implement to facilitate learning[36]:

- Show empathy and concern. Actively listen to the learner and acknowledge lived experiences and ideas.
- Use language and nonverbal communication to enhance choice and promote problem solving.
- Reduce language that is controlling, criticizing, guilt provoking, judgmental, or punishing.
- Provide rationale for self-management behaviors: the importance of changing lifestyle to manage symptoms.

One example of the difference between supportive education and nonsupportive education is demonstrated by a patient with a diagnosis of chronic heart failure who is experiencing an exacerbation of symptoms related to dietary salt intake. Suppose the patient states that he or she is doing "okay" at adhering to the low-salt diet, but family members complain that he or she eats too many processed foods and too much take-out fast food. This is an example of a nonsupportive teaching phrase: "You know salt isn't good for you."[36] This phrase is judgmental, critical, and guilt provoking and makes an assumption of the patient's level of knowledge. By revising the wording in the phrase, the meaning of the information is changed. This is an example: "I know it is difficult not to eat all your favorite foods. Adding salt is up to you. Do you understand that salt will affect your heart condition?"[36] This supportive statement transfers accountability of performing the self-management skill from the nurse to the patient and motivates the patient to make the conscious decision to limit salt intake.

Teaching Strategies

The nurse may be the first health care provider to initiate patient teaching. Bedside nurses are in a unique position to facilitate, mentor, and coach patients through the endless maze of information presented in the critical care arena. Information overload often occurs, and the information taught can easily be forgotten. Nurses may become frustrated when family members and patients ask the same questions repeatedly. Patience with repeated questioning is essential because information taught may be lost within minutes after its presentation. Although health care providers would like patients and families to retain 100% of information given, in reality, learning does not take place in one session or may not occur at all. An individual may be able to remember only two or three pieces of information in one education session.

Nurses are continuously interacting with patients and discussing their progress, updating them on treatment plans, and describing procedures. With that in mind, every patient contact can be thought of as a brief teaching-learning encounter. The Ask Tell Ask method of determining the patient's or family's understanding of their care is one technique that can be used during any care encounter. For example, the nurse first asks the patient what he or she understands of the plan of care, then clarifies what the patient did not understand, then asks for verification of understanding.[37] The nurse must use every teachable moment and take advantage of the patient's readiness and willingness to learn. When educating adults, a combination of teaching strategies should be used to facilitate giving and receiving information. Each individual has a different learning style: visual, auditory, or tactile. Common strategies include discussion, demonstration, and use of media.

Discussion

Informal discussion can take place anywhere and at any time. This strategy allows for interaction between the teacher and the learner. Discussion occurs one-on-one or in groups. Education sessions need to be adapted quickly, as they are occurring, to meet the ever-evolving needs of the patient and family. Although teaching through discussion is informal, the information given should promote the goals of the education plan. Focus on what the patient or family wants or *needs* to know at that moment, rather than on what might be *nice* to know. Obtaining and maintaining the learner's attention during the discussion may be challenging. The nurse must use different teaching strategies and techniques and modify them frequently according to the situation and the response of the patient or family to the education.

Several strategies are used to maintain a positive teaching-learning encounter:
- Addressing the patient and family members by name
- Clearly stating the purpose of the education encounter
- Getting and keeping the patient and family involved in the learning process
- Maintaining eye contact during the encounter

- Keeping the encounter brief and to the point
- Giving positive reinforcement
- Communicating with professionals in other disciplines about the progress and additional learning needs of the patient and family[4,5]

Demonstration and Practice

Demonstration and practice are the best strategies for teaching technical skills. Adults learn best when they are able to participate in the learning process. Involving the learner, providing consistent step-by-step instructions, and presenting a visual demonstration of the skill being performed are important strategies to achieve successful task acquisition. By allowing the patient or family to practice the skill in a simulated or real situation, the outcome of the teaching encounter can be evaluated. This strategy allows the nurse to offer positive reinforcement and constructive feedback during the learning encounter, building learner confidence in performing the newly acquired skill. Many demonstration sessions and repetitive practice may be required for the patient or family to acquire and feel comfortable with the new skill.

Use of Media

Video-assisted instruction. For decades, videos have provided a simple and convenient method of presenting patient education. Presentation format can make a tremendous difference in how successful the learning experience is. Traditional videos using spoken or graphic representation are convenient and efficient in providing information but have been shown to be less effective when behavior modification is the objective.[38] To effect behavior modification, two techniques can be used to improve the effectiveness of educational videos: (1) showing real people representing the behavior to be changed and (2) presenting information in gain-framed messaging rather than loss-framed messaging, for example, "patients who do not smoke experience fewer heart attacks" rather than "patients who smoke are more likely to have a heart attack."[39]

Videos supply the learner with a large amount of information in a relatively short period and enable different nurses to distribute information that remains consistent from patient to patient and family to family. Videos can be used to educate patients on various topics, including medications, disease processes, procedures, symptom management, weight monitoring, laboratory tests, diet, surgery, and health maintenance issues. Interactive video technology offers on-demand educational and health information video programs delivered to the patient through television. Patients and families are able to access education videos anytime during their hospital stay. The digital video system allows multiple TVs to show the same video at the same time. Bedside call systems are linked to a computer server, which allows patient selection of videos from the bedside. These systems can be customized to meet the needs of specialty patient populations (eg, cardiac, obstetrics). Reports can be generated to list all educational films viewed during the patient's stay. Evaluation of learning can be achieved through the system by administration of a pretest or posttest available on the system.

However, viewing a video does not ensure retention of information or knowledge acquisition. Patient education videos should not be used in place of interaction with the patient and family. After the patient watches the video, the nurse must review the content and reiterate key points of information.

This postvideo encounter is also used to evaluate the outcome of the teaching-learning encounter. To review the content with the patient or family, the nurse must also watch the video and choose key points to discuss with the learner in the postvideo discussion. Video presentation should be used to assist the learner in meeting identified educational needs.

Written materials. Written media, such as brochures, pamphlets, patient pathways, and booklets, are common in outpatient and inpatient areas of health care. They usually are inexpensive and offer opportunities for a wide range of education: education about the disease process, information on risk factor modification, procedure education, medication education, and education about use of medical equipment in the home setting. Written materials address multiple learning styles and offer learner-centered teaching with concrete, basic information that can be placed at the learner's fingertips for immediate review as well as future review anytime the learner desires. The practitioner must ensure that written materials are appropriate for the patient population as a whole and for a particular individual patient or family. Several factors should be considered when choosing printed materials for patient education, including readability, cultural considerations, age-specific considerations, primary language, and literacy.[6]

Readability is an important factor in the consideration of printed educational materials. *Readability* refers to how easy or hard the literature is to read. Nearly 20% of the U.S. adult population have low literacy skills and read at or below the fifth-grade reading level.[40] Typical patient educational materials are written at or above the eighth- or ninth-grade reading level and may be out of reach for many readers.[5,41] If the patient or family is unable to read the material or understand its meaning, he or she cannot perform self-management tasks to maintain health. This sets the patient and the family up for failure and being labeled noncompliant.

Readability tools are designed to provide quick and easy assessment of the readability level of patient educational materials. However, these formulas do not assess the understandability of the material. Many formulas, such as the Simplified Measure of Gobbledygook (SMOG) and the Suitability Assessment of Materials (SAM) assessment tools, are available to assist practitioners in determining the readability of health educational materials. Selection of the appropriate readability formula depends on the type of information being presented. Additional tools may be found at www.readabilityformulas.com.

Providing written educational materials at the appropriate reading level is important so that the information can be easily read and understood by most patients and families.[42] To assist the nurse in overcoming literacy-related barriers to health education, it is recommended that patient educational materials be printed at or below the fifth-grade reading level.[40,43] Samples of health-related instructions at different reading levels are provided in Box 5.4.

Several situations present special challenges with regard to the use of printed patient education materials. The inability of a patient or family to read or understand the English language does not mean they cannot understand directions and treatment regimens. Multilingual, written educational materials are a necessity in any health care institution. Hodgdon states that "communication is 55% visual, 37% vocal, and 7% verbal or the actual message."[44] Including pictures, drawings, diagrams, charts, or tables in educational materials has been shown to enhance understanding and increase retention in patients with

---

BOX 5.4   Samples of Reading Levels

College Reading Level
Consult your physician immediately at the onset of chest discomfort, shortness of breath, or increased perspiration.

Twelfth-Grade Reading Level
Call your physician immediately if you experience chest discomfort, shortness of breath, or increased sweatiness.

Eighth-Grade Reading Level
Call your doctor immediately if you start having chest pain or shortness of breath or you feel sweaty.

Fourth-Grade Reading Level
Call your doctor right away if you start having chest pain, cannot breathe, or feel sweaty.

---

low literacy skills.[45] Materials translated into Braille or provided in audio format may be used for blind patients.

Many vendors supply printed materials for patient education, often translated into multiple languages. Common vendors include HERC Publishing, Pritchett and Hull, and Krames. National associations such as the American Cancer Society, the American Lung Association, and the American Heart Association also publish educational materials for patients. Each of the vendors has a website for easy viewing of sample patient education materials and pricing information. Prices for these materials vary from pennies per pamphlet to several dollars; some pamphlets by national organizations are available free of charge to the consumer. There are several items to consider when choosing standardized, printed educational materials. Read the entire pamphlet or booklet to determine appropriateness of the material for the desired patient population. Ask the vendor to supply the reading level of the material and the method used to determine it. Inquire about the frequency with which the printed material is updated to ensure that the patient or family members have the most recent edition.

Thoroughly read the document for inconsistent information or information that is incongruent with the treatment plan of a specific unit. For example, if the nurse educates the patient on a low-fat diet, but the pamphlet teaches only a low-salt diet, the patient may become confused and frustrated and not know which diet to follow at home. Another point to consider is whether the material contains information required by the institution and regulatory agencies such as The Joint Commission. Core measures outlined by The Joint Commission include certain items that must be included in discharge education and tracked by the institution. Some materials may not properly fit with a unit's plan for education and therefore are not appropriate for that particular institution. Printed material should be an adjunct to patient and family education and match what is taught and practiced in a specific facility.

When predeveloped educational materials do not meet the needs of the institution's patient population, an institution may decide to develop internal patient educational materials. Producing educational materials internally can be time-consuming and difficult.[12] Time must be spent determining content, readability, and design. Some simple rules when designing written patient education materials include (1) use a white background; (2) use pictures and graphics to illustrate major concepts; (3) use bullet points instead of paragraphs to reduce reading time and "word clutter"[43]; and (4) emphasize only key facts and desired behaviors, avoiding the addition of "nice to know" information that may distract the reader from the true message.

The practitioner must keep in mind that patients and families may receive a variety of educational materials during their hospital stay. Streamlining educational materials within an organization decreases inconsistency of information, increases the clarity of prescribed treatment, and helps to avoid duplication of efforts between disciplines and shifts. Although providing written materials may seem like a quick and easy educational method, the practitioner must still review the content with the patient or family to determine whether learning has occurred and whether there are any questions about the material.

Computers and Patient Education

Computer-assisted instruction. Computers offer self-directed learning, allowing the learner to go through the program at his or her own pace, spending as much or as little time as desired in one area of content. Computers stimulate all aspects of the adult learner—visual, auditory, and tactile. Although personal computers have become common, they may not be suitable for all patients because comfort levels with computer functions vary from person to person. The learner should be able to pay attention to the material being presented and not be preoccupied with learning how to manipulate the computer mouse. Touch screen technology, familiar to most individuals from grocery store checkout to the use of bank ATMs, can simplify the use and effectiveness of this mode of learning. Placing computer screens at the bedside provides the patient and family with on-demand learning materials whenever they are ready, willing, and able. However, the costs of computers and software may be prohibitive for hospitals as well as individuals.

Internet. Today's health care environment encourages participation in care decisions, and patients are turning to the Internet for information about symptoms, disease processes, and treatment alternatives.[46] New Internet tools, including wikis, blogs, and podcasts, are gaining increasing popularity. Wikis and blogs allow for questions and an exchange of information, and podcasts can provide convenient, current, just-in-time education.[47] However, the sheer volume of information available on the Internet hinders the patient's ability to select and obtain information that is accurate, reliable, and personally relevant. Because information on the Internet is not regulated or controlled for reliability or validity,[48,49] the nurse must be prepared to respond to the patient's need for information, to help him or her find, evaluate, and use the information available on the Internet.[42,46]

Communication

Communicating effectively is essential to obtaining positive outcomes for patient education. Speaking slowly and clearly and avoiding the use of slang or medical jargon is essential. Even when the patient and family speaks English, the stress of hospitalization, fear of health outcomes, and difficulty speaking of personal issues with a stranger can present a challenge to providing patient education. When the patient or family has limited English proficiency, the challenge becomes even greater. In many instances, a family member is called on to serve as interpreter. Although this may seem like an ideal solution, the family member may not have any better comprehension of the material being taught and thus is unable to adequately relay

---

BOX 5.5   Tips for Using an Interpreter

- Speak directly to the patient, not the interpreter.
- Position yourself so that you can maintain eye contact with the patient.
- Introduce the interpreter and clarify roles of others in the room.
- Nothing should be said that the patient should not hear.
- Pause after each complete thought to give interpreter time to translate.
- Plan ahead; let the interpreter know exactly the content and purpose of the session.
- Use the teach-back method to evaluate learning.
- Listen to the interpreter, who may identify cultural practice or norms that impede understanding.

From Techniques for educating with the aid of an interpreter. *Patient Education Management.* 2007;7:77.

---

the information. The use of professional interpreter services is preferable when the message is vital to a patient's health and well-being. Interpreter services are available through a variety of modes.[50] Some hospitals employ professional interpreters or provide special training for multilingual staff in effective interpretation. Telephonic interpretive services are offered by many vendors, and special phones with dual handsets are available for use. Emerging technology has given rise to video-on-demand interpretive services, such as those offered through the Language Access Network. Whichever method is used, interpretation can be a frustrating process. Box 5.5 describes helpful techniques to enhance the experience.[50,51]

All patients and families desire to be understood and have their concerns validated. This can be difficult for patients who are critically ill and whose ability to communicate to family and health care providers is impaired. Communication aids such as picture cards, picture boards, or word boards enhance the ability of the nurse to understand educational needs and communicate information. Augmentative and alternative communication systems may be considered for temporarily nonspeaking patients in the critical care unit. Technology known as an electronic voice output communication aid that has been available in the outpatient setting to help persons who cannot speak is becoming available in the critical care environment. A voice output communication aid is a prerecorded, human or digitized computer-generated voice message.[52] It can be beneficial for patients who are awake and alert but are unable to talk for reasons such as mechanical ventilation through an endotracheal tube or tracheostomy tube. Whole phrases, as opposed to pictures or single words, are communicated to the health care team; for example, "I am having pain."[52] This technology can assist the patient to communicate comfort needs, anxiety, and fears and to ask questions concerning care or progress. Intubated patients describe the inability of family members and caregivers to effectively understand their needs as an extremely stressful part of being in the critical care unit.[30] Augmentative and alternative communication systems can also assist the nurse to evaluate more effectively the outcome of education. Use of verbal, whole-sentence communication rather than traditional, nonverbal picture board communication has been found to decrease the guesswork in interpreting patient needs.[52]

Special Considerations
Older Adults

As individuals age, cognitive, physiologic, and psychological changes occur that must be considered when planning and implementing a teaching plan. It is the nurse's responsibility to understand the effects of aging and adjust teaching strategies to accommodate them.[53]

Cognitive effects of aging. Cognitive effects include processing information more slowly, a decrease in the ability to take in multiple messages, and difficulty understanding the abstract. When teaching an older adult, nurses should provide information slowly and deliberately to allow the patient time to process each concept. Information should be presented in two or three essential points and reviewed frequently. Nurses should avoid using vague terms, such as "several times a day" or "until better." Instead, the nurse must be very specific with amounts, times, and frequencies.

Physical effects of aging. Presbyopia, cataracts, glaucoma, and macular degeneration affect the vision of many older adults. Although additional lighting is necessary, it is also necessary to avoid direct sunlight, harsh lights, and using glossy paper. Colors in the blue end of the spectrum are difficult for an older adult to distinguish because of yellowing of the lens of the eye. When using written instructions or color-coded dosing, blues, greens, and purples should not be used.

High-pitched tones become more difficult to hear as an individual ages. Female nurses will need to make an effort to modulate their voices into the lower register so an older adult can hear better. In addition, careful enunciation of words containing higher pitched sounds such as "f", "s", "k", and "sh" may be necessary. Providing audio and video recordings will help reinforce learning.

Aging and associated comorbidities may result in fatigue, joint pain, or decreased dexterity. Learning can be facilitated by scheduling teaching sessions early in the day, keeping sessions short, and managing pain before learning.

Psychological effects of aging. Older adults often experience depression. Learning can be enhanced by selecting content that holds value and relevance to the individual. Nurses should choose content that is perceived by the learner as important in maintaining quality of life and should try to relate what they are teaching to the individual's previous life experiences.

Sedated and Unconscious Patients

Patient education should not be reserved for conscious and coherent patients only; it should be provided to the unconscious or sedated patients as well. Addressing the learning needs of this critically ill population of patients is challenging. These patients cannot communicate their educational needs, and they cannot interact and participate in the learning process. Although it is unknown what an unconscious or sedated patient hears or remembers, it is known that some sedated patients undergoing surgery remember discussions that took place among physicians and staff during the procedure. Therefore, one should not ignore unconscious or sedated patients during the education process. These patients may be unable to respond or participate, and the effectiveness of the teaching process cannot be evaluated, but providing information regarding environment, procedures, sensations, and time of day is benevolent and may help to decrease immediate physiologic stress.

Noncompliant Patients

Noncompliance, or an unwillingness to learn, does not necessarily mean that the patient is consciously choosing not to participate in his or her care or follow medical

instructions[54,55]. There are many other issues that can lead to noncompliance. The nurse must be alert for barriers that may prevent a willing patient from being compliant. Box 5.6 lists factors that may contribute to noncompliance or unwillingness to learn.[48]

STEP 4: EVALUATION

Evaluation is the final component in the patient and family education process. The intent of evaluation is to determine the effectiveness of the educational interventions. The nurse must use his or her clinical judgment and knowledge of adult learning principles to determine how well the learner has met the expected outcomes and objectives. The evaluation process is continual and assesses the entire teaching-learning interaction, including the level of learner interest in the session, willingness to learn the content, and level of participation during the encounter. Evaluation should be completed at the end of each teaching-learning encounter. This allows the nurse to immediately present positive and constructive feedback to the patient and family as well as revise the education plan to accommodate ongoing learning needs. It is also important to assess the response to teaching and determine whether follow-up education is required.

How to Evaluate

How does the nurse know if learning has occurred? Techniques such as verbalization of information, return demonstration, and physiologic measurement are common evaluation methods to determine the effectiveness of a teaching-learning encounter. Evaluation of knowledge retention can be completed by verbally questioning the learner. This method is known as teach-back. Teach-back is an interactive process that assists the nurse in determining whether the learner has retained the information taught. The nurse may ask the patient if he or she is able to list signs and symptoms of heart failure. Verbal questioning should occur immediately after the teaching event and throughout the hospitalization to assess knowledge retention. For example, the physician orders a new medication for the patient today, and the nurse educates that patient on the effects and side effects; the next day, the nurse may assess retention by asking the patient if he or she remembers the reason for taking the new medication. Common items that patients and families are asked to verbalize are reportable signs and symptoms, how to manage symptoms at home, when to take medication, how often medication should be taken, and who to call for questions or concerns.

Changes in attitude, beliefs, or lifestyle are often difficult to evaluate because learners can say they have changed their attitude when actually they have not. In this learning domain, the nurse must use his or her detective skills to assess whether the individual has accepted the prescribed treatment plan and modified behavior accordingly. Sometimes, the best way to evaluate a change in attitude is by observation and verbal questioning. An example is a patient who has been asked to comply with a low-cholesterol diet; a food diary the patient has kept as requested provides some evidence about what the patient has eaten. A wealth of information can also be obtained from the family concerning the patient's exhibited changes.

Physiologic evidence of the effectiveness of education can also be measured. Indicators such as blood cholesterol levels, blood pressure, heart rate, blood sugar levels, and weight can lead the practitioner to the conclusion that the patient and family may be having difficulties understanding or following through with the identified plan of care.[36] Adults generally want to comply with new expectations but often cannot for various reasons, such as a lack of money for medications or an inability to understand what is expected of them. These barriers must be explored and included in the education plan.

Observation and return demonstration is the evaluation of choice for the skills learning domain. For the patient and family members to be "checked off" on a particular skill, they should be able to perform it independently, using the nurse only as a resource for questions. Endotracheal suctioning, placing condom catheters, and performing dressing changes are examples of common tasks that patients and families may be asked to learn. Because of the increasingly complex care that patients require at home after discharge, these skills may be the entire focus of teaching before discharge. Not every teaching moment is a success, and the nurse need not feel guilty or like a failure when the learner has not achieved the desired objective. Revisiting and revising the goals and objectives during the teaching-learning session may be necessary to meet the ever-changing needs of the patient or family.

STEP 5: DOCUMENTATION

Documentation of education is necessary to communicate educational efforts to members of the health care team, patients and families, and regulatory agencies. The nurse should recognize that informal teaching at the bedside is education. It is important to record any information given to the patient on formal documents approved for use by each health care institution. In most institutions, formal education records are used to document education rendered by practitioners of any discipline involved in the care of a particular patient and family. These forms are communication tools used to indicate progress in the teaching-learning process from shift to shift, day to day, and discipline to discipline.[57] Documentation should include education from admission to discharge on topics ranging from orientation to the environment to acquisition of self-management skills for home care.

What Should Be Documented?

The complexity of information, demand by governing agencies, lawsuits, and the sheer volume of patients in and out of a unit are driving nurses to provide quality documentation of the education encounter.[55] Documentation of the teaching-learning process is multifaceted. The documentation form should "tell the story" of the education encounter from assessment to evaluation. Documentation of the education assessment should

include learning preferences; factors that impair ability, readiness, and willingness to learn; and actual or perceived learning needs. Information should be recorded on the interaction, material taught, supplemental materials distributed, response to the education, achievement of outcome, and any follow-up education or resources needed.

FACTORS THAT AFFECT THE TEACHING-LEARNING PROCESS

Many factors can produce barriers to a successful teaching-learning process. The physiologic, psychological, sociocultural, financial, and environmental factors previously discussed are known to affect the patient's and family's ability, willingness, and readiness to learn. Physical disabilities, impaired vision, and hearing loss affect the learner's ability to read materials, listen to instructions, or perform a technical task.[56] If a technical task is required, ensure that the patient or family member has the physical ability or manual dexterity to perform the required skill. Provision of eyeglasses and hearing aids is essential to improving participation in learning. Several other factors that have an impact on the teaching-learning process are as follows[5,12]:

- Lack of an accurate assessment
- Setting unrealistic goals
- Not involving the patient or the family in the process
- Overloading the learner with information
- Relying too heavily on resources
- Haphazard and nondirected teaching; lack of an education plan of care
- Teaching at the wrong time, hurried teaching, not paying attention to the learner
- Lack of trust and rapport between the teacher and learner
- Lack of communication among health care providers
- Language-related communication barriers

Although this list may seem overwhelming, it is important to be proactive and to remove as many of these barriers as possible. It takes less time and fewer resources to start with a structured education plan than it does to start over after the teaching-learning process has begun.

Barriers to the teaching-learning process exist for the patient or family and for the bedside nurse. Time constraints, decreased length of stay, and daily routines interrupt or impair the nurse's ability to communicate information to the patient and the family. Table 5.3 includes common barriers to the education process experienced by nurses. The patient's positive interactions and relationships with health care providers as well as a clear understanding of his or her illness, symptoms, and medications will promote adherence to the patient education plan.[51]

INFORMATIONAL NEEDS OF FAMILIES IN CRITICAL CARE

Family members and significant others of critically ill patients are integral to the recovery of their loved ones. When planning for the overall care of patients, nurses and other caregivers need to consider the informational and emotional support needs of this group.[58,59] Families of critically ill patients report their greatest need is for information.[58] Flexible visiting hours and informational booklets regarding the critical care experience are recommended to meet this need.[60,61]

TABLE 5.3   Barriers to Providing Education

Barrier	Example	Solution
Interruptions	Daily routines	Use all available teachable moments.
Distractions	Tasks; medication administration	Turn TV off; minimize noise.
	Phone calls	
	TV or other noise in patient's room	
Night shift	Sleeping patients	Plan education before bedtime.
Sedation or pain medications	Narcotic analgesic	Teach before administering medication.
Nurse unaware of what to teach	Diabetic education	Educate self.

Data from London F. *No Time to Teach.* Philadelphia: JB Lippincott; 1999; Rankin S, Stallings K. *Patient Education: Principles and Practice.* 4th ed. Philadelphia: JB Lippincott; 2001.

PREPARATION OF THE PATIENT AND FAMILY FOR TRANSFER FROM CRITICAL CARE

When patients are more stable, requiring less hemodynamic monitoring and close observation, they are frequently transferred to another level of care in a different geographic hospital setting. They may be transferred to an intermediate care unit (ie, step-down unit, intermediate care area, or telemetry). While on these units, patients receive optimal care to their level of requirement, a lower nurse-to-patient ratio, and less expensive technologic monitoring in a quieter environment.[55,56]

Transferring a patient from the critical care unit to a step-down unit may result in anxiety and stress.[62] Patients and families have become dependent on the monitors, equipment, constant nursing attention, and abundant information received while in the critical care unit. The patient has become secure knowing that immediate physiologic and emotional needs are being met. A strong bond has often developed between the staff and the family. Many patients and families are reluctant to give up that bond and believe that their needs will not be met as well on a step-down unit. To avoid anxiety and provide the patient and family with some control over the event, nurses need to prepare them for the transfer process. See nursing diagnosis "Relocation Stress Syndrome" in Appendix A.

Preparation for transfer should start after the patient has been stabilized and the life-threatening event that resulted in hospitalization has subsided. The stressor at this point is no longer the critical care environment but has become the unfamiliar step-down environment. Explanations about where the patient will be transferred, the reason for transfer, and the name of the nurse who will be providing care should be offered as soon as known. Before transfer, information about changes in care, expectations for self-care, and visiting hours should be provided to the patient and family. Family members should be contacted concerning exactly when the patient will be transferred so they can be present during the transfer or made aware of the patient's new location (see Table 5.2).

The education plan of care and tips learned by the critical care staff about the patient and family should be communicated to the step-down unit staff. Most patient transfers made from the critical care unit to a step-down unit are planned events. However, unplanned or unexpected transfers sometimes occur, usually when the critical care unit requires bed space for a more seriously ill patient. In this situation, the transfer occurs quickly during the day or often at night. Families may be present in the hospital or may have gone home for the evening. This sudden need to transfer the patient can produce as much anxiety as the initial event, primarily because the patient and family may not feel ready for the transfer or may think they have lost control of the situation. Providing the patient and family with concrete evidence of improvement, such as more favorable vital signs or the need for fewer medications or tubes, can assure them about improvement in the patient's condition before unplanned transfers occur. Increasing communication and providing consistent information to patients and families also increases satisfaction with care and services.[63]

CASE STUDY 5.1   Patient and Family Education

Brief Patient History

Mr. S is a 30-year-old Vietnamese-American man who is employed as a fisherman. Mr. S is married and has three children younger than 5 years. A few months earlier, he was diagnosed with type 1 diabetes mellitus after a 30-lb weight loss and a change in visual acuity. He has had two admissions for diabetic ketoacidosis in the past month.

Clinical Assessment

Mr. S was admitted to the critical care unit with diabetic ketoacidosis 2 days ago. His condition has been stabilized, and he is ready to be transferred to a nursing unit today. Mr. S states that he does not understand why "this keeps happening" because he takes his insulin if he plans on eating, although he does not always eat. His wife states that his blood sugar seems to be okay when he is at home, but that he gets into trouble when offshore.

Diagnostic Procedures

The following laboratory results were obtained on admission: blood glucose level of 620 mg/dL, carbon dioxide concentration of 11 mEq/L, and pH of 7.25. Ketones were identified in the urine and blood.

Assessment of learning needs identified a deficit in understanding regarding glucose monitoring and insulin requirements while away from home.

Medical Diagnosis

Mr. S is diagnosed with diabetic ketoacidosis resulting from noncompliance.

Questions

1. What major outcomes do you expect to achieve for this patient?
2. What problems or risks must be managed to achieve these outcomes?
3. What interventions must be initiated to monitor, prevent, manage, or eliminate the problems and risks identified?
4. What interventions should be initiated to promote optimal functioning, safety, and well-being of the patient?
5. What possible learning needs do you anticipate for this patient?
6. What cultural and age-related factors may have a bearing on the patient's plan of care?

SUMMARY

- A collaborative, well-organized, need-targeted education plan of care is essential to improving health outcomes and decreasing lengths of stay.
- The teaching-learning process is a dynamic, continuous activity that occurs throughout the entire hospitalization and may continue after the patient has been discharged.
- Information must be gathered on many factors that may affect the education process, including cultural or religious views of illness or death, emotional barriers, desire and motivation, physical or cognitive limitations, and barriers to effective communication.
- The learner's needs can be defined as gaps between what the learner knows and what the learner needs to know (eg, survival skills, coping skills, ability to make a care decision).
- Standardized education plans provide consistent interventions and outcomes; however, they must be individualized to meet the unique needs of the patient and family.
- The optimal environment for learning is one that is nonthreatening, comfortable, open, and honest.
- Determination of an appropriate teaching strategy is essential to meet the needs of the patient.
- Providing information regarding the environment, procedures, sensations, and time of day is important for patients who are unconscious and may help to decrease immediate physiologic stress.
- When planning for the overall care of patients, nurses must consider the informational needs and emotional support of family members.
- It is important to prepare patients and families for transfers to other units to decrease stress and anxiety related to going to a less intensively monitored environment.

ⓔ Visit the Evolve Site for additional study materials.

REFERENCES

1. The Joint Commission 2012 Comprehensive Accreditation Manual for Hospitals. Oakbrook Terrace, IL: The Joint Commission; 2004.
2. Fried T, et al. Primary care clinicians' experiences with treatment decision making for older persons with multiple conditions. JAMA Int Med. 2010;171(1):75-80.
3. Abubatig A, et al. Literature review: patients' and health care providers' perceptions of stressors in critical care units. Dimens Crit Care Nurs. 2013;32(1):22-27.
4. Bastable S. Nurse as Educator: Principles of Teaching and Learning for Nursing Practice. 4th ed. Boston, MA: Jones & Bartlett Publishers; 2013.
5. Rankin S, Stallings K, London F. Patient Education in Health and Illness: Issues, Principles and Practice. 5th ed. Philadelphia, PA: JB Lippincott; 2005.
6. Wei H, Camargo C. Patient education in the emergency department. Acad Emerg Med. 2000;7(6):710.
7. Briggs L, et al. Patient-centered advance care planning in special patient populations a pilot study. J Prof Nurs. 2004;20(1):47.
8. Moorhead S, et al, editors. Nursing Outcomes Classification (NOC). 5th ed. St Louis, MO: Mosby; 2012.
9. Hibbard J, et al. What the evidence shows about patient activation: better healthcare outcomes and care experiences: fewer data on costs. Health Affairs. 2013;32(2):207-214.
10. London F. No Time to Teach. 2nd ed. Philadelphia, PA: JB Lippincott; 2009.
11. Tallman K, et al. Living with advanced illness: longitudinal study of patient, family, and caregiver needs. Perm J. 2012;16(3):28-35.
12. Fidyk L, et al. Teaching nurses how to teach: strategies to enhance the quality of patient education. J Nurs Staff Dev. 2014;30(5):258–253.
13. Glittenburg J. A transdisciplinary, transcultural model for health care. J Trans Nurs. 2004;15(1):6.
14. Walsh S. Formulation of a plan of care for culturally diverse patients. Int J Nurs Terminol Classif. 1999;15(1):17.
15. Giger JM. Transcultural Nursing: Assessment and Interventions. 6th ed. St. Louis, MO: Mosby; 2012.
16. Suh EE. The model of cultural competence through an evolutional concept analysis. J Trans Nurs. 2004;15(2):93.
17. Blount KA, Moore LA. Medications and the elderly. Crit Care Nurs Clin North Am. 2002;14(1):111.
18. Knowles MS. The Modern Practice of Adult Education: From Pedagogy to Andragogy. New York, NY: Cambridge Books; 1988.
19. Price B. Six steps to teaching cancer patients. Cancer Nursing Practice. 2013;12(6):25-33.
20. Institute of Medicine. Health Literacy: A Prescription to End Confusion. Washington, DC: National Academies Press; 2004.
21. Egbert M, Nanna KM. Health literacy: challenges and strategies. http://nursingworld.org/MainMenuCategories/ANAMarketplace/ANAPeriodicals/OJIN/TableofContents/Vol142009/No3Sept09/Health-Literacy-Challenges.html Accessed April 28, 2012.
22. Glassman P. Health literacy. http://nnlm.gov/outreach/consumer/hlthlit.html Accessed April 28, 2012.
23. Berkman N, et al. Low health literacy and health outcomes: an updated systematic review. Ann Intern Med. 2011;155(2):97-107.
24. Moore V. Assessing health literacy. J Nurse Practitioners. 2012;8(3):243.
25. Leske JS. Protocols for practice: applying research at the bedside. Crit Care Nurs. 1998;18(4):92.
26. VanHorn E, et al. Family interventions during the trajectory of recovery from cardiac event: an integrative literature review. Heart Lung. 2002;31(3):186.
27. An K, et al. A cross-sectional examination of changes in anxiety early after acute myocardial infarction. Heart Lung. 2004;33(2):75.
28. Leske JS. Family stresses, strengths, and outcomes after critical injury. Crit Care Nurs Clin North Am. 2000;12(2):237.
29. Lazarus RS, Folkman S. Stress, Appraisal, and Coping. New York, NY: Springer; 1984.
30. Thomas L. Clinical management of stressors perceived by patients on mechanical ventilation. AACN Clin Issues Crit Care. 2003;14(1):73.
31. Laubach E. How to communicate with seriously ill patients. Nurs Manage. 2000;31(4):24H.
32. Nolen K, et al. Meeting the needs of family members of ICU patients. Crit Care Nurs Q. 2014;37(4):393-406.
33. Saunders R. Constructing a lesson plan. J Nurses Staff Dev. 2003;19(2):70.
34. Bulechek GM, et al, editors. Nursing Interventions Classification (NIC). 6th ed. St. Louis, MO: Mosby; 2013.
35. Benner C, et al. From Beginner to Expert: Excellence and Power in Clinical Nurse Practice. Menlo Park, CA: Addison-Wesley; 1984.
36. Clark P, Dunbar S. Family partnership intervention: a guide for family approach to care of patients with heart failure. AACN Clin Issues. 2003;14(4):467.
37. Garcia F, et al. "Ask tell ask" strategies to improve communication between nurses and patients and families in the intensive care unit (ICU). Presented at STTI 43rd Biennial Convention. Las Vegas: Nevada; November 7-11, 2015.
38. Abed M, et al. Video-assisted patient education to modify behavior: a systematic review. Patient Educ Couns. 2014;97:16-20.
39. Tuong W, et al. Videos to influence: a systematic review of effectiveness of video-based education in modifying health behaviors. J Behav Med. 2012;37(2):218-233.
40. Sheridan SL, et al. Interventions for individuals with low health literacy: a systematic review. J Health Commun. 2011;16(3):30-54.
41. Falvo D. Effective Patient Education: A Guide to Increased Adherence. Boston, MA: Jones & Bartlett Publishing; 2011.
42. Fegghi D, et al. Quality of online pediatric orthopaedic education materials. J Bone Joint Surg Am. 2014;96(23).
43. Hodgdon L. Visual Strategies for Improving Communication: Supports for School and Home. Troy, MI: QuirkRoberts Publishing; 2001.

44. Houts P, et al. The role of pictures in improving health communication: a review of research on attention. Patient Educ Couns. 2006;61:173.

45. Peregrin T. Picture this: visual cues enhance health education messages for people with low literacy skills. J Am Diet Assoc. 2010;110(5):S28.

46. Anderson A, et al. The Internet: friend or foe when providing patient education. Clin J Oncol Nurs. 2008;12(1):55-63.

47. Boulos M, et al. Wikis, blogs and podcasts: a new generation of Web-based tools for virtual collaborative clinical practice and education. BMC Med Educ. 2006;6:41.

48. Jones J. Patient education and the use of the Internet. Clin Nurs Spec. 2003;17(6):281.

49. Fahy E, et al. Quality of patient health information on the Internet: reviewing a complex and evolving landscape. Australas Med J. 2014;7(1):24-28.

50. Mikkelson H. The art of working with interpreters: a manual for health care professionals. http://www.acebo.com/pages/the-art-of-working-with-interpreters-a-manual-for-health-care-professionals Accessed April 28, 2012.

51. Techniques for educating with the aid of an interpreter. Patient Education Management. 2007:77.

52. Happ MB, et al. Electronic voice-output communication aids for temporarily non-speaking patients in a medical intensive care unit: a feasibility study. Heart Lung. 2004;33(2):92.

53. Speros C. More than words: promoting health literacy in older adults. Online J Issues Nurs. 2009;14(3).

54. Thomas M, editor. Lack of compliance may mean patients don't understand. Case Management Advisor. 2009;20(8):85.

55. Wu JR, et al. Factors influencing medication adherence in patients with heart failure. Heart Lung. 2008;37(1):8.

56. Bruccoliere T. How to make patient teaching stick. RN. 2000;63(2):34.

57. Russell C, Freiburghaus M. Heart transplant patient teaching documentation. Clin Nurs Spec. 2004;17(5):249.

58. Doering LV, et al. Recovering from cardiac surgery: what patients want to know. Am J Crit Care. 2002;11(4):333.

59. Henneman EA, et al. An evaluation of interventions for meeting the information needs of families of critically ill patients. Am J Crit Care. 1993;1(3):85.

60. Miracle VA, Hovenkamp G. Needs of families of patients undergoing invasive cardiac procedures. Am J Crit Care. 1994;3(3):155.

61. White SK, Edwards RJ. Visitation guidelines promote safe satisfying environments. Nurs Manage. 2006;37(8):21.

62. Radtke A. Telemetry monitoring: a preferred solution for intermediate care. Nurs Manage. 2006;37(12):52.

63. Mages ME. Helping patients, helping families. Healthc Exec. 2006;11(4):40.

6

Psychosocial Alterations and Management

Margaret Jordan Halter and Carrie Scotto

Patients are admitted to critical care units because they require urgent physiologic support. Living or dying is dependent on the use of technical interventions carried out by a skilled critical care team. However, when a person is seriously ill or injured, it is not only the body that suffers. Critical illness impacts the whole person—body, mind, and spirit. Psychological and spiritual variables have a significant impact on outcomes in physically compromised and vulnerable patients. Psychosocial interventions have the potential to support a patient's hope, energy, will to survive, and ability to meet life's challenges.

Critical care nurses provide care by communicating with compassion and understanding, practicing dignity-enhancing care, supporting patient coping, using a family-centered focus, and engaging spiritual resources. In a problem-oriented environment such as a critical care unit, nurses should remember that acute events also have the potential to reveal patient strengths and trigger a readiness for spiritual well-being and enhanced hope.

This chapter discusses the psychosocial challenges encountered by critically ill patients. We explore nursing diagnoses related to psychological, social, and spiritual health. Holistic nursing interventions help patients and family members cope effectively and thrive during a stressful experience. Providing meaningful person-to-person care also depends in part on the nurse's own emotional health. Therefore, a discussion of self-care is also included in this chapter.

STRESS

The term *stress* is often used to indicate a negative experience or internal tension. Yet an acute stress response is an essential and protective reaction to a stressor, designed to mobilize the body's response to threats for the purpose of survival. Stress is a nonspecific response to any demand placed on a person to adapt or change and can come from physical, emotional, social, spiritual, cultural, chemical, or environmental sources.[1]

The nursing diagnosis "stress overload" refers to excessive amounts and types of demands that require action. The stressors are experienced as a problem and contribute to the development of other problems.[2] Stress overload should be differentiated from other stress-related nursing diagnoses discussed in this chapter, including anxiety, fear, low self-esteem, hopelessness, powerlessness, spiritual distress, and ineffective coping. Stress overload does not occur because the patient or family members have coping deficits or psychological disorders. Rather, the stressors of critical illness are so numerous and severe that people become overwhelmed. The appropriate nursing response to patients at risk for stress overload is to reduce the number or types of stressors that patients experience.

To respond appropriately to patients at risk for stress overload, we should first be aware of the many stressors faced by critical care patients (Box 6.1). Normal life patterns are disrupted, and patients experience alterations in their bodily functions, social roles, job status, and finances. They are in strange, frightening, and restrictive environments. Critically ill patients experience distressing bodily reactions, lack of control, fear of medical equipment, loss of meaning, and relationship disturbances during and after treatment in a critical care unit.

Stress Response

Stress of any type—whether positive or negative, biologic, psychological, spiritual, or social—elicits the same physical responses. Classic stress theorists describe stress as a stimulus, a response, and a transaction. In his pioneering work, Selye[3] described the body's responses to a stressor. The general adaptation syndrome as described by Selye[3] is characterized by three stages: alarm reaction, resistance, and exhaustion.

An alarm reaction is initiated by the hypothalamus. When sensory and chemical information alerts the hypothalamus of danger, it responds by releasing corticotropin-releasing factor (CRF). Signaled by CRF, the pituitary gland releases the stress hormones cortisol and aldosterone. The sympathetic nervous division of the autonomic nervous system releases neurotransmitters and endocrine hormones associated with stress. Known as the "fight or flight" response, an alarm reaction triggers highly integrated cardiovascular and endocrine changes. These changes include elevations in blood pressure, respiratory rate, heart rate, systemic vascular resistance, and glucose production. Individuals also experience sweating, tremors, and nausea.

During the resistance stage, the person's systems fight back, which may lead to adaptation and a return of normal functioning. If adaptation fails and the stressors continue, exhaustion occurs. This stage is characterized by depleted reserves. Reversal of stress exhaustion can be accomplished by restoration of one's reserves through the use of medications, nutrition, and other stress reduction measures.

Nuernberger[4] described a process of shutting down in response to overstimulation of the parasympathetic nervous system. He labeled this survival tactic the general inhibition syndrome, or the "possum response." Defense mechanisms such as withdrawal, avoidance, and detachment are typical behaviors associated with this type of response.[5,6]

BOX 6.1   Common Stressors for Patients in Critical Care Units

- Threat of death
- Uncertainty about future and fear of permanent residual health deficits
- Pain, discomfort, and physical restrictions
- Lack of sleep
- Loss of autonomy and control over one's body, environment, privacy, and daily activities
- Unfamiliar environments with excessive light, noises, alarms, and distressing events
- Worry about finances, potential job loss, and stress on loved ones
- Separation from family, friends, and meaningful social roles and work
- Loss of dignity, embarrassing exposures, and a sense of vulnerability
- Boredom broken only by brief visits, threatening stimuli, and procedural touch
- Loss of ability to express oneself verbally when intubated
- Unfamiliar bodily sensations resulting from bed rest, medications, surgery, or symptoms
- Unanswered spiritual questions and concerns about meaning of the events and life

Individual Response to Stressors Depends on

- Individual's perception of stressor
- Acute or chronic nature of stressors
- Cumulative effect of multiple stressors
- Effectiveness of the individual's usual coping strategies and style
- Degree of social support

Both sympathetic and parasympathetic nervous system responses are innate and protective, but prolonged stimulation or imbalances in either response can be detrimental. Sustained or frequent sympathetic nervous system arousal places added physiologic burdens on a compromised critical care patient. In addition, an exhausted patient lacks the reserves necessary to recover from the demands of illness or injury. Prolonged parasympathetic imbalances are associated with diseases such as depression.

POSTTRAUMATIC STRESS DISORDER

Experiencing one or more traumatic events may trigger symptoms of posttraumatic stress disorder (PTSD). Nearly 25% of people surviving a critical illness and an intensive care unit stay subsequently exhibit symptoms of PTSD.[7] Although posttraumatic reactions may not be evident for weeks to months after an event, critical care nurses should be aware of the potential for complications of critical care unit stays. Nurses may recognize and reduce unnecessary stressors during a patient's stay, monitor for PTSD risk factors, and use interventions to reduce the occurrence of PTSD in critical care patients.

Classified as a trauma and stressor-related disorder, posttraumatic stress reactions involve a wide range of cardiovascular, neuromuscular, gastrointestinal, cognitive, emotional, mood, and memory responses. After an exposure to a traumatic event, people may experience intrusive recall of the distressing event. This recall is often triggered by a noise, sound, sight, smell, event, or memory. Nightmares and distressing memories during which a trauma is reexperienced provoke intense psychological and physiologic distress. People with PTSD can also exhibit numbing responses, including detachment, isolation,

restricted affect, and depression. In addition, PTSD may bring on periods of hyperactivity that can lead to sleep disturbances, hypervigilance, and nervous and repetitive behaviors. Cognitively, stress reactions lead to difficulty concentrating, poor executive function, and impaired decision making.

Griffiths and Jones[8] summarized 20 years of follow-up with critical care unit survivors. They discuss the importance of the quality and types of patients' memories of their critical care experience. Although most critical care patients have poor factual recall or amnesia related to their stay, they often live with delusional, paranoid, or nonfactual memories or create false substitute interpretations and experiences. These memories can cause problems as individuals attempt to construct a realistic understanding of their recovery.[9]

Family members are also at risk for developing posttraumatic stress reactions[10.] Prolonged periods of uncertainty, anxious waiting, disrupted sleep patterns, financial concerns, witnessing emergency interventions, and confronting fears of loss and death are profoundly unsettling. Kross et al[11] report both depression and higher rates of PTSD in family members of patients who die during a critical care unit stay.

Intensive care unit induced PTSD is largely unidentified and untreated. Critical care nurses can promote activities related to preventing posttraumatic stress reactions in patients and family members. Being aware of the possibility for stress overload in critical care settings is the first step. Care providers should then take steps to manage or eliminate as many of those stressors as possible. Often patients are unaware or uncertain of what has happened to them and their bodily function. Nurses should engage in encouraging and realistic discussions of the patient's experiences, explain events carefully, and talk openly about recovery timelines and the gradual process of regaining strength.

Certain populations are at greater risk for developing PTSD[8,12]. These populations include patients who are young, people who have delusional memories, and those individuals with preexisting psychiatric conditions. There is evidence that using lighter doses of sedation — keeping patients calm, but awake — may reduce the incidence of PTSD[13,14]

The process of identifying PTSD risk and symptoms is complex and multidimensional. Screening questionnaires have been developed and tested for initially evaluating risk for PTSD soon after discharge.[15]

Patient and family members usually recall and interpret the events, decisions, and time sequences involved in a critical care stay differently. Keeping a diary with photographs taken during a patient's stay in the critical care unit can help patients and family members reach a degree of shared common ownership of the experience[16]. Journal review helps patients understand what happened so that they can better come to terms with their illness and their recovery process.[17] In learning to live with the memories of critical care, patients benefit when they can construct a meaningful story.[18,19] The interventions described in this chapter are designed not only to support patients while they are in the unit but also to support patients' well-being over time, preparing them for the challenges of rehabilitation and recovery.

ANXIETY

Anxiety is a normal common subjective human response to a perceived or actual threat, which can range from a vague, generalized feeling of discomfort to a state of panic and loss of control. Feelings of anxiety are common in critically ill patients but are often undetected by care providers.[20] Anxiety and agitation in critical care patients can complicate patient recovery secondary to unplanned extubations,[21] episodes of shortness of breath, and behavioral changes.

The physiologic effects of anxiety can produce negative effects in critically ill patients by activating the sympathetic nervous system and hypothalamic-pituitary-adrenal axis. Anxiety elicits changes in the neurotransmitters in the brain that regulate mood—including acetylcholine, norepinephrine, dopamine, serotonin, and γ-aminobutyric acid—along with their corresponding receptors. The neurotransmitters' integration of these responses within the central nervous system relies on communication among the cerebral cortex, limbic system, thalamus, hypothalamus, pituitary gland, and reticular activating system. The cortex is involved with cognition, attention, and alertness, whereas emotional responses to stress are located in the limbic system. Corticotropin releasing factor (CRF) controls the endocrine response and the norepinephrine pathway that is active in regulating the sympathetic branch of the autonomic nervous system. A positive feedback loop between the CRF and the autonomic nervous system occurs when increased activation in one system influences the other system. It is also proposed that large amounts of circulating CRF can accelerate behavioral responses (ie, anxiety and hypersensitivity) to stressful stimuli.[6]

As anxiety levels increase, a patient experiences the physiologic effects of sympathetic nervous system stimulation with feelings of excitement and heightened awareness, followed by a diminishment of the perceptual field, problem-solving abilities, and coping skills. Panic attacks, a manifestation of severe anxiety common in critical care patients, can produce an acute stress response with tachycardia, hyperventilation, and dyspnea. Pharmacologic interventions for acute anxiety include the use of benzodiazepines, antihistamines, noradrenergic agents, antidepressants, and anxiolytics.[6]

The stressful experiences of having an acute or chronic illness, facing a real or anticipated loss, being admitted or discharged from a critical care unit, or requiring mechanical ventilation can trigger high degrees of patient anxiety.[22-24] Research also suggests that women, patients with less social support, and patients with longer critical care length of stay are at higher risk for developing anxiety on transfer out of the unit to a less intense level of care.[24] Whether the causes of anxiety are biochemical, genetic, emotional, or driven by the threats inherent in the situation, the critical care nurse should consider all contributing factors if interventions are to be effective.

Although rates of moderate to high anxiety exist in critical care patients, leading to higher complication rates,[25] valid and reliable methods to assess anxiety have not been put into practice. Critical care nurses most often rely on behavioral indicators, such as agitation and restlessness, and physiologic parameters, such as increased heart rate and blood pressure. Behavioral or vital sign changes do not provide consistently reliable indicators of anxiety and may lead to underestimation of the extent of anxiety in critical care patients.[23] The literature on anxiety in critical care patients cites more than 50 clinical indicators, many of which are nonspecific or can be associated with multiple causes.[26] Using valid scales for evaluating patients' self-perceived anxiety levels can be helpful in determining the level and extent of anxiety.[20] See also Appendix A, Nursing Management Plan: Anxiety.

Anxiety and Pain

Of particular importance in the critical care setting is the cyclic relationship between levels of anxiety and perceptions and tolerance of pain. Pain triggers anxiety, and increased anxiety intensifies pain experiences. This reciprocal relationship varies, depending on whether pain is produced by disease processes or invasive procedures, is acute or chronic in nature, or is anticipated. In critical care patients, pain experiences arise from many sources, including injured tissues, immobility, preexisting and chronic pain conditions, intubation, diagnostic or treatment procedures, bright lights, excessive noise, and interrupted sleep.

When pain or a discomfort such as nausea is severe enough, patients try to conserve energy and focus inwardly to gain control of their pain and anxiety. They may startle easily, become irritable, display anger, be vigilant and wary of caregivers, or be perceived as demanding. An overwhelmed patient often withdraws from interpersonal contact.[6,27] In situations of pain-induced anxiety, the nurse must identify the source of the pain, validate observations with the patient, and initiate pain management strategies. Medications such as theophylline, anticholinergics, dopamine, levodopa, salicylates, and steroids can also contribute to feelings of anxiety[27,28] (see Chapter 8).

ALTERATIONS IN SELF-CONCEPT

The stressors imposed by serious illness, trauma, and surgical procedures can cause disturbances in the patient's self-concept. Self-concept can be defined as the values, beliefs, and ideas that form a person's self-knowledge and influence relationships with others. One's self-concept is unique to the individual and is developed through perceptions of his or her own characteristics and abilities, goals, and ideals; interactions with others and the environment; and how those interactions are valued. One's self-concept also includes body image, self-esteem, and self-identity.[6,26]

People must make adjustments to their self-concept or role limitations when life circumstances necessitate change. Patients admitted to critical care settings may experience self-concept challenges, perceiving themselves to be viewed by others as a problem, as only their disease, or as a patient instead of as a person.[26] Patients in critical care units usually do not have time to adjust to their altered health status. They may exhibit early signs of a response to loss or disability, including shock, numbness, and avoidance of reality, and they may be unable to clearly understand the implications of the situation.[6,27] Self-concept constructs of particular relevance for critical care patients include body image, self-esteem, and identity disturbance.

Body Image

One's body is central to one's self-concept. Body image is the mental picture an individual has of his or her body and its physical functioning at a given time. Body image includes attitudes and feelings about one's appearance, body build, health, performance, ability, and gender. A person's body image develops over time, influenced by contact with people and the environment, emotional experiences, and fantasies. Body image is dynamic and changes based on present and past perceptions and experiences.[6,29]

When ill, inevitably a person comprehends that experience as being integral with his body. In their classic description of the impact of stress and coping on health and illness, Benner and Wrubel noted that a person does not just *have* a body; rather he or she *is* a body.[29] The experiences of being ill are "embodied" and are stored in bodily memory. Often bodily sensations in a state of illness do not make sense to the patient, which creates a cascade of stress responses.[30] Patients in critical care units are subjected to prolonged periods of lying in bed, position disorientation, sensory deprivation, muscle atrophy, changed metabolic patterns, mechanical ventilation, pain, profound weakness,[8] nutritional alterations, and medication-induced physical symptoms.

Disturbances in body image in critical care arise when the person fails to perceive or adapt to the changes that are imposed by the situation. In some instances, the person may feel betrayed by his or her body, which no longer seems normal. Body image issues often emerge and resolve over time, but critical care nurses begin the process of helping the patient live with a change in bodily appearance or function. A more keen awareness of the embodied nature of a patient's experiences helps nurses attune to the patient's bodily perceptions of all nursing activities. See Appendix A, Nursing Management Plan: Disturbed Body Image.

Self-Esteem

Self-esteem refers to how well one's behavior correlates with a sense of the ideal self and is most closely linked to one's sense of self-worth.[6] Maslow,[31] an early theorist of human flourishing, identified self-esteem as an important component in his hierarchy of human needs. Having high self-esteem helps a person deal with maturational and situational life crises more easily.

Self-esteem has been studied in a variety of contexts. Because nurses interact with patients so intimately and frequently, it is important that nurses develop a deeper appreciation of the impact of self-esteem on a patient's energy, recovery, and sense of self-efficacy. Illness robs a person of perspective, often leading to low self-esteem and feelings of powerlessness, helplessness, and depression.[32] Low self-esteem impairs one's ability to adapt. A patient may refuse to participate in self-care, exhibit self-destructive behavior, or become too compliant—asking no questions and permitting others to make all decisions.[32] A comprehensive approach to recovery includes the provision of ongoing supportive measures designed to help patients maintain self-esteem and a healthy body image. See Appendix A, Nursing Management Plan: Situational Low Self-Esteem.

Identity Disturbance

A personal identity disturbance, as a type of altered self-concept, is defined as an inability of a person to differentiate the self as a unique and separate human being from others within a social environment. The sense of depersonalization that accompanies identity disturbance engenders a high level of anxiety. Personal identity disturbance can result from the effects of psychoactive medications; biochemical imbalances in the brain; and organic brain disorders, dementia, traumatic brain injury, amnesia, or delirium (see Chapter 9). A careful nursing assessment, including the use of psychiatric or neurologic consultation, is essential in cases of identity disturbance. Disorientation and confusion, common in patients in critical care settings, are influenced by several factors, including the severity of the physical problem, chemical imbalances, sensory overload or deprivation, and previous illness or health care experiences.

RISK FOR COMPROMISED HUMAN DIGNITY

A sense of the dignity of the person underlies considerations of self-concept, body image, and self-esteem. The underlying purpose of all interactions with patients and family members is to bring them to restored health. When people are treated with dignity and respect, they are put in the best position to recover their health and well-being.[32]

When patients enter the health care system, including critical care units, they bring with them their diseases, defects, inadequacies, and shortcomings. Their bodily or psychological "failures" have brought them into relationship with health care providers. During a health care encounter, patients are subjected to intense physical, psychological, and lifestyle scrutiny. They feel literally and figuratively exposed. Patients' own disappointment and regrets are magnified when they experience the concern, effort, and emphasis placed on their failing health, leading to self-critical feelings.

Lazare's[33] insightful description of the shame and humiliation patients experience in medical encounters provoked an analysis of health care culture. Moral philosophers point to the "rules of cultural systems" as a source for the unintended but distressing experiences of shame, embarrassment, and humiliation experienced by patients and providers when giving and receiving medical care. The rules of cultural systems are notably present in critical care environments: objectification of the person (for more precise physiologic management), disempowerment, distancing the self from the experience of others, indifference, and dissociation. The authority of the medical model supersedes patient experiences, interpretations, and meanings.[34] The rules of cultural systems determine, in part, the behaviors of the people within a culture. Although health care providers do not intend to humiliate patients, they become accustomed to the cultural attitudes and circumstances that diminish patients' dignity on a daily basis.

A sense of dignity includes a person's positive self-regard, an ability to invest in and gain strength from one's own meaning in life, feeling valued by others, and how one is treated by caregivers. The model by Chochinov et al[35] for dignity-conserving care identifies sources of threats to dignity inherent in health care contexts, including the level of a person's independence and his or her symptom distress. Patients in most acute care settings, especially critical care, must by necessity give up the things that give them a sense of self: clothing, daily habits, and privacy. Their bodies are frequently exposed to people who inspect them for their pathology and irregularities. Often patients cannot communicate their preferences or give permission for assessments, tests, or interventions. Family members and friends have restricted access to patients because of environmental constraints. Stripped of everything that communicates personal identity, patients are known as their pathologies instead of as a person with a history and hopes for a future. When caregivers become more aware of their own feelings and humanity in an exchange, they are less often to unintentionally minimize patients' emotions and experiences.[33]

SPIRITUAL CHALLENGES IN CRITICAL CARE

Many of the psychosocial issues already discussed—stress, anxiety, self-concept, body image, self-esteem, coping, dignity, and relationships with others—are rooted in the spiritual dimension of life, the seat of a person's deepest meanings and ground of being. One's spiritual dimension encompasses the elements of life that provide meaning, purpose, hope, and connectedness to others and a higher power.[32,36,37] Providing spiritual care is essential for patient recovery in critical care units.

Spiritual Distress

Spiritual distress has been defined as a disruption in the life principle that pervades a person's entire being and that integrates and transcends one's biologic and psychosocial nature.[32] Threats of physiologic or psychological illness, prolonged pain, and suffering can challenge a person's spirituality. Separation from one's meaningful religious or spiritual practices and rituals, coupled with intense suffering, can induce spiritual distress for patients and their families.

Patients experiencing spiritual distress may question the meaning of suffering and death in relation to their personal belief system. They may wonder why the illness or injury has happened to them or may fear that what they have believed in has failed them in the time of greatest need. Some individuals in spiritual despair may question their existence, verbalize their wish to die, or display anger toward religious traditions. Unresolved spiritual distress is interpreted in the body as a stressor. Prolonged spiritual distress may lead to a sense of hopelessness, unwillingness to seek further treatment, or consent to therapeutic interventions or regimens.[32]

Hope and Hopelessness

Hope is a subjective, dynamic internal process essential to life. Considered to be a spiritual process, hope is an energy that arises out of a sense of being meaningfully connected to one's self, others, and powers greater than the self. With hope, a person is able to transition from a state of vulnerability to a point of being able to live as fully as possible.[38] The need for hope is stimulated by a demand to adapt or change in unexpected situations, as is the case for people who are critically ill.

The desire to maintain hope underlies many coping mechanisms. When people have hope and belief in their goals, they are empowered to engage in their own recovery with a sense of internal peace and freedom. Although hope has a future orientation, it also has a present orientation that impacts people in the here and now. We have come to understand, through observations of people in extreme circumstances, that an element of hope must be maintained for survival[39,40] and is an essential component in the successful treatment of illness.[41]

By contrast, hopelessness is a subjective state in which an individual sees extremely limited or no alternatives and is unable to mobilize energy on his or her own behalf.[26,31] Feelings of hopelessness can greatly hinder recovery. Conditions that increase a person's risk for feeling hopeless include a loss of dignity, long-term stress, loss of self-esteem, spiritual distress, and isolation, all of which can be present in a critical care experience. Patients who feel hopeless may be less involved in their recovery, withdraw from the support of others, and lack the energy and initiative to engage in increasing degrees of self-care.[31]

Loss of Control and Powerlessness

Many patients admitted to a critical care unit have experienced a rapid onset of illness or an injury and have not had time to adjust to the limits of their changed circumstances. They have to adapt quickly to a loss of control. The loss of control in critical care hospitalization can be as minor as not getting a preferred food or as serious as experiencing a radical loss of a sense of self.

Control, a person's ability to determine the use of time, space, and resources, becomes compromised in the critical care unit.

On admission to a hospital, people forfeit much of their independence as they become patients. Choice of clothing and use of other personal belongings are usually restricted in a critical care unit. Patients cannot decide who enters the room, who provides personal care, or who intrudes with painful treatments. Hospital rules are usually not open to modification.

Early research by Rotter[42] on human behavior and perception of control has been helpful in explaining the wide range of responses people have in situations in which they must give up control. Rotter suggested that a person's locus of control is internally or externally focused. Individuals who have an internal locus of control perceive themselves to be responsible for the outcome of events. Individuals with an external locus of control believe that their actions will have no effect on the outcome of a situation. Furthermore, as with any highly individualized concept, people vary in the amount of control they prefer.

Patients who have a pervasive sense that they can do nothing to change or control their circumstances are at risk for feeling powerless.[33] People who are critically ill can experience powerlessness because of the constraints of their health and the care environment, a loss of meaningful interpersonal interactions with their usual support system, inability to maintain cultural or religious beliefs and practices, or a helpless coping style. The degree of powerlessness a person experiences depends on his or her perceived sense of control, the type of loss that was experienced, and the availability of social support.

Powerlessness can be manifested by a refusal to participate in decision making, disengagement from plan of care, expressions of self-doubt, or a seeming lack of interest in recovery. Frustration, anger, and resentment over being dependent on others often occur and are exhibited in verbal expressions regarding dissatisfaction with care.[32] Poor interactions with health care providers who are perceived as imposing restrictions can make the situation worse. Patients may react aggressively, may try bargaining, or may refuse to comply with diagnostic and treatment regimens. Patients may lose sight of the areas of life over which they still maintain some influence because so much control has been taken from them.

Loss of control and powerlessness are also problematic as patients regain their health and are readied for transfer from the intensive care unit. Navigating the transition from dependence to independence has been identified as a source of distress for critically ill patients.[43] Many report a feeling of disconnection from caregivers and perceive this as a lack of sensitivity and caring. They feel abandoned by caregivers on whom they were recently dependent, and they worry they will not receive the care they need. See Appendix A, Nursing Management Plan: Powerlessness.

COPING WITH STRESS AND ILLNESS

Coping mechanisms are intentional processes used to adjust, adapt, and successfully meet life stressors. Each patient's response to stress is unique and depends on a variety of environmental factors and individual differences, including cognitive variables, the person's place in the life cycle, the degree of social support, and the person's perception of the nature of the stressor or loss.[6]

If a patient is coping effectively, he or she appears relatively comfortable with self and others, is able to form a valid appraisal of stressors, makes decisions consistent with his or her own preferences and values, and has access to needed resources. Effective coping mechanisms help a person maintain a perception of an acceptable degree of control and empower him or her to take necessary actions, share concerns, use healthy denial, and manage troublesome life challenges and uncertainties (see Chapter 10). Most people have a repertoire of coping mechanisms to manage stressful situations and life challenges. Coping mechanisms are learned and practiced over a lifetime and are based on the person's sense of the effectiveness of any given strategy for adapting to the stressor.[29]

Ineffective coping is defined as the impairment of a person's adaptive behaviors and problem-solving abilities when meeting life's demands and necessary roles. Manifestations of ineffective coping in critical illness include verbalization of an inability to cope, anxiety, and being unable to meet basic needs. The patient exhibits inappropriate use of defense mechanisms and has diminished problem-solving abilities. The patient may display apathy or destructive behavior toward self and others.

A person's coping mechanisms may or may not be effective, depending on the nature and seriousness of the challenge being faced, the person's prior experience with a similar situation, or the extent to which the coping mechanism can be used in a given situation. For example, a person may ordinarily cope with a distressing situation by careful problem analysis, information gathering, talking things over, and getting some refreshing sleep. That person may have a sense of ineffective coping when facing the lack of control characteristic of acute illness and critical care environments. This lack of control includes the inability to speak or process information, sleep interruptions, diminished access to resources, or limited time to make careful deliberations. Common effective coping responses can be problem focused, cognitively focused, or emotionally focused. Coping methods include physical exercise, meditation, prayer, healthful foods, social support, positive self-talk, reframing, time management, counseling, new skill building, and the use of spiritual and religious rituals.[6,28]

Use of Psychological Defense Mechanisms

The overuse of psychological defense mechanisms may give evidence of ineffective patient or family coping. Defense mechanisms are automatic self-protective measures developed in response to an internal or external stressor and may be evident when patients or family members feel out of control and unable to cope. Unrelenting anger, excessive protectiveness, distrust of others, extreme dependence or regression, psychological withdrawal, denial, or apathy concerning treatment goals may suggest that the stressors of the critical care experience have outstripped a person's coping abilities. Use of maladaptive measures may temporarily minimize anxiety but does not effectively or permanently resolve the conflict. Two common defense mechanisms especially evident in critical care settings are regression and denial.

Regression

Regression is an unconscious defense mechanism characterized by a retreat, in the face of stress, to behaviors characteristic of an earlier developmental level.[6] Regression allows a patient to give up former roles, autonomy, and privacy to become the passive recipient of medical and nursing care. On one hand, patients in critical care settings are expected to relinquish control and rely on others for even the most basic needs. To resist the care that others provide can jeopardize a patient's outcome. On the

other hand, favorable patient outcomes and a speedy recovery can be threatened when patients regress to the point of relinquishing all control and responsibility for themselves to others and become excessively dependent on others. Behaviors such as whining, clinging to staff, needing the nurse constantly at the bedside, and giving evidence of an inability to self-modulate feelings of anxiety or fear can interfere with patient recovery and negatively affect nurse-patient relationships.

When expectations related to patient or family participation in self-care must be challenged or changed, patients are best served when limits and responsibilities are mutually determined and set in a supportive manner. Responses to patients will be more understanding when nurses recall that regression has been encouraged and expected at certain phases of a critical care stay, fear and anxiety have been reinforced in critical care experiences, and usual coping mechanisms have been abandoned. Although regressive behaviors can be frustrating to caregivers, confrontations or reprimands should be avoided. Threatening responses from staff may worsen a situation in which the patient is already struggling with issues of dependence, autonomy, and self-worth.

Denial

Denial is defined as "conscious and unconscious attempts to disavow knowledge or the meaning of an event to reduce anxiety and fear."[2] Critically ill patients or their family members may use denial as a defense mechanism to protect against and manage an overwhelming sense of threat brought on by illness, injury, or impending death. As Weisman[38] noted in his classic work, denial has both protective and potentially detrimental functions.

The degree to which denial is used varies from person to person or may vary in the same person at different times. An inability to face the realities of a potential health problem leads some people to deny various aspects of their illness or the significance of potentially serious symptoms. Denial can lead to delayed treatment or lack of awareness of the danger of a symptom. Family members, unable to cope with a loved one's serious, irreversible illness, may focus only on the possibility of a full recovery. They resist having realistic discussions concerning goals of care, insist on repeated resuscitation attempts, or invest in home remodeling in anticipation of a homecoming. They may regard caregivers who try to discuss anything other than a full recovery as being negative or untrustworthy people.

Although it is common to be alert to the potentially negative aspects of ineffective denial, denial can serve as a valuable defense mechanism for people unable to absorb the full force of a loss or significant life change at a given time. Denial is protective in that sense and gives a person the psychological space and time needed to process and accept the realities of a highly distressing loss.

Nurses may find it particularly difficult to communicate with people who seem to be using denial to their own detriment. It may seem to the caregiver that the person would cope better by facing the realities of a situation and by taking the steps needed to go on with life. Depending on the need people have to protect against their changing realities, they may or may not be readily influenced by information that contradicts their beliefs. Patients or family members who give evidence of firm or fixed denial are best supported by caregivers who understand that their denial is protective at this time and who watch for cues that indicate a readiness to accept the reality of their situation.

Witnessing or responding therapeutically to problematic behavior can be challenging and uncomfortable, especially when the behavior seems to be directed at the caregiver. Critical care nurses should carefully evaluate their own response to what seems to be maladaptive behavior. Patients and family members are usually doing the best they can under very stressful circumstances and rely on the insight and understanding of caregivers who appreciate the complexities of stress, coping styles, and use of defensive mechanisms. A patient's stay in the critical care unit is only one phase in an often long journey to recovery from a serious health threat. Patients and family members need time to work through their experiences and often do so more effectively when they are given the support and encouragement they need during the acutely stressful events of being in a critical care unit. See Appendix A, Nursing Management Plan: Compromised Family Coping.

USEFUL PSYCHOSOCIAL SKILLS

Holistic Psychosocial-Spiritual Care

Critical care nurses possess sophisticated knowledge of anatomy and physiology, the pathophysiology of disease processes, and appropriate nursing interventions. In addition, a nurse who practices holistic critical care also needs the knowledge, wisdom, and skills to interpret the internal human responses to experiences of serious illness or injury. Attention to the whole patient is the ultimate goal of nursing care, and is vitally important for critical care patients, families, and nurses. Nightingale[44] believed that it was "unthinkable to consider sick humans as mere bodies who could be treated in isolation from their minds and spirits." Essential skills that underlie nursing interventions for psychosocial-spiritual care include using communication patterns based on compassion and care, practicing dignity-enhancing care, supporting patient coping, using a family-centered focus, and engaging spiritual resources.

Communicate With Compassion and Care

Caring, compassionate verbal and nonverbal communication patterns give substance to nursing activities that promote expert psychosocial-spiritual care interventions. Nelson et al[45] described the top challenges to providing care in the critical areas, especially for very seriously ill patients. None of the top challenges had to do with technical issues of medical management. Instead, the top challenges include

- Inadequate patterns of communication between the critical care team and family members
- Insufficient staff knowledge of effective communication
- Unrealistic family and provider expectations
- Family disagreements
- Lack of advance directives
- Voiceless patients
- Suboptimal space for having meaningful conversations.

Patients and family members rank their needs for communication with health care providers as one of the most important aspects of feeling cared for in the critical care setting,[46] especially in patients unable to speak.[47,48] Interviews with patients after critical care revealed that they believed that a nurse's caring attitude led to more positive memories of their experience. Patients also reported less stress when they perceived nurses to be caring, warm, and competent and when nurses communicated respect.[49] Many patients interpret a nurse's expressions of empathy and physical contact as evidence of caring and support.[47]

Sharing concerns with a caring and understanding listener often can relieve emotional or spiritual distress. Patients are consoled knowing that they are not alone when they sense that someone knows and cares about their feelings and experiences. Although the patient may share concerns with family members, he or she may be reluctant to upset loved ones and may find that talking to a nurse seems more appropriate and emotionally safer. A patient who copes by talking to others will benefit from a nurse who recognizes when the patient needs to talk and who knows how to listen.[48]

Nurses should not avoid difficult conversations. Patients need to talk about their fears and prefer conversations that balance their needs for honesty with their need to maintain hope.[48] It is also important to remember cultural differences in communicating with patients and family members. People in Western and American cultures expect and value honesty and truth telling in difficult situations. Patients and family members from other cultures may have taboos surrounding what should be discussed regarding the diagnosis and prognosis in serious illness.[50] Careful medical and nursing assessments, use of family and team conferences to foster communication, and enlisting the assistance of a spiritual counselor lead to more fruitful, understanding conversations in crisis and decision-making situations. Patients and family members in critical care areas need careful nurse-patient communication strategies (Box 6.2).

Trust

Effective verbal and nonverbal communication is essential for the development of trust in a nurse-patient relationship. Trust manifests itself in the belief of critical care patients that the people they depend on will get them through the illness and will be able to manage any untoward event that might occur. A patient needs to trust the nurse's competence in the physical

---

QSEN BOX 6.2   QSEN: Patient-Centered Care

Strategies for Communicating With Patients and Family Members

- Be patient. What is routine for caregivers can be stressful and new to patients and family members.
- Repeat information as many times as necessary. Stress reduces concentration, memory, and comprehension, especially in unfamiliar situations.
- Assess patient and family knowledge level and prior experience with critical care.
- Use understandable language and define medical terms, without talking down.
- Ask clarifying questions to help validate understanding.
- Use a welcoming, open communication style. Critical care units can feel intimidating to people unfamiliar with the environment.
- Offer frequent updates regarding the patient's condition, even if not asked.
- Engage in conversations of meaning with patients and family members, even if brief. Often critical care conversations are reduced to conveying only technical aspects of care.
- Honor privacy and provide space for family conferences.
- Speak to patients, even if they are unconscious. This conveys caring to family, and words may comfort the patient, even if there is no response.
- Use communication boards or other devices with patients unable to speak.
- Give patients time to respond and ask questions patients can likely answer easily.
- Speak slowly and look at patients when communicating. Gestures, lip movements, and facial expressions convey important messages.

and technical aspects of care and rely on what the nurse says. Patients are keen observers of their caregivers and read them well. Trust and hope are lessened when inappropriate information is given or nurses do not follow through on what they say. See also Appendix A, Nursing Management Plan: Impaired Verbal Communication.

Practice Dignity-Enhancing Care

"The capacity to give one's attention to a sufferer is a very rare and difficult thing; it is almost a miracle; it is a miracle."[51] The practice of care that enhances a patient's dignity is anchored in authentic human presence, the giving of one's whole attention and being to another person in a given moment. When authentically present, the nurse is able to go beyond relying only on scientific information and attunes himself or herself to a patient's needs, experiences, and emotions in a way that facilitates the patient's healing.[52]

Dignity-enhancing perspectives include the need a person has to maintain a continuity of the self; one's roles and legacy; and a sense of pride, hopefulness, control, acceptance, and resiliency. Dignity-enhancing care has four components: attitude, behaviors, compassion, and dialogue. Caregivers' first step in providing dignity-conserving care involves reflecting on the attitudes and assumptions they hold about other people and their situations. Attitudes, worldviews, and beliefs about a patient or family member influence your openness and ability to develop a trusting relationship.

Dignity-enhancing care is manifest in behaviors. Attending to the patient's physical appearance affirms the person's self-esteem and a healthy body image. Cleanliness and absence of body odors give patients a sense of worth. When providing physical care, provide privacy, respect social boundaries, and ask permission before touching when possible. Validate the patient by giving importance to the things that he or she cares about. Spending time with patients as they share their life stories helps the nurse know the patient better and facilitates the development of individualized interventions. Show respect for patients by calling them by their preferred names or titles to help reinforce the patient's self-concept and identity. Obtain the patient's permission to include others in private conversations.[53]

Compassion refers to the awareness of another person's suffering, coupled with a sincere intention to alleviate the suffering. In compassion, caregivers are able to identify with another person and recognize a shared humanity. Showing compassion can be simple, in acts of consideration, kindness, or a simple touch. Critical care nurses frequently touch people in the completion of procedures and caregiving activities. Keeping in mind individual and cultural differences, nurses should include nonprocedural touch in their care. The use of touch intended to communicate care and comfort can be an important part of patient healing and interpersonal connection.

Compassion is also evidenced in dialogue, the fourth element of dignity-conserving care. At the most basic level, patients and family members need timely updates, explanations, repetition of unfamiliar information, and thorough information sharing. At a deeper level, patients need to feel that they are heard by their caregivers and know that their personhood is valued and respected.

Support Patient Coping

A goal of expert psychosocial-spiritual care is to promote patient and family flourishing, empowering them to experience as much control and predictability as possible. As noted earlier, coping is a dynamic process involving cognitive and behavioral efforts to manage specific internal or external demands that are perceived to exceed the person's resources. The key to effective coping is to encourage the use of the best mix of strategies appropriate for a given situation.

Most adults cope by relying on their previously developed conscious and unconscious coping strategies and defense mechanisms, which are automatically triggered in a stressful situation. Teaching new coping skills to people who are experiencing acute psychological stress may be unrealistic. However, by using active listening skills and initiating conversations with patients and family members, the nurse can identify the coping resources, skills, and preferences that may be most helpful.

Helping Patients Maintain Control

One of the most effective ways to decrease the stress of being in a critical care environment is give patients as much control over their care and the environment as possible.[54] Allow patients to make decisions as they are able, such as how and when to administer personal hygiene, diet preferences, and the timing of nursing interventions. Inform patients and family members about daily activities, tests, or therapies; their purpose; and anticipated effects.

Critical care patients are often unable to see or turn around to witness what is going on in their environments. During treatments and procedures, provide the patient with explanations, brief discussions on what to expect, the anticipated time of a procedure, and descriptions of what is happening during an intervention. On one hand, the patient for whom control is important should be helped to maintain control in as many areas in life as possible. On the other hand, a patient must be given the opportunity to not exercise control if having too many choices provokes even greater stress.

Preparing the patient and family for transfer out of the critical care unit will help them to maintain a sense of control as they transition to a more independent environment. This requires the nurse to assess the knowledge and expectations of the patient and family about the change and provide realistic information about the new care setting.[42,55] The transfer should be framed as a positive first step toward going home, and the nurse should emphasize the progress and abilities of the patient.[54,56] A gradual reduction in the use of monitors and other technology a few days before discharge helps decrease the stress of the transition.[57,58] See Table 5.2.

Support Patient-Preferred Complementary Therapies

Patients and families enter health care settings with well-established practices and beliefs about managing stress; maintaining wellness, balance, and harmony in their lives; and knowing what methods best facilitate their bodies' own healing responses. Integrative health care practices involve a blending of allopathic medical health care methods with patient-identified complementary therapies.[59]

The type of complementary or integrative therapies used depends on a patient's preferences, coping style, physical capabilities, and personality type. Music therapy, relaxation, guided imagery, therapeutic massage, visualization, prayer, biofeedback, and mindfulness meditation are potentially useful for critically ill patients.[60] Significant decreases in anxiety and symptom distress have been attributed to tactile touch. Although more research is needed to support the value of complementary therapies on selected outcomes in critically ill hospitalized patients, early studies support their potential as therapeutic nursing interventions (see Chapter 1).

Creating Healing Environments

People are continuous with their environments. Alterations in the physical environment of critical care units can provide a sense of calm, enhance patient coping, and facilitate healing.[61] Nurses can make changes in care environments to give patients a greater sense of comfort and familiarity while they are in the unit.

Visiting policies. Although practices vary among critical care units, a more relaxed visitation policy humanizes the environment and facilitates healing. The American Association of Critical-Care Nurses (AACN) AACN Practice Alert[58] recommends giving unrestricted access of hospitalized patients to a chosen support person. Giving family members access to their loved ones enhances patient and family satisfaction and improves safety of care. Family members have insight into the patient's behaviors and preferences, especially with patients who are unable to communicate. Interacting with family members reduces patient anxiety and enhances a sense of control.[62] Including patients and family members in critical care interdisciplinary rounds has been shown to improve perceptions of accessibility and communication.[63]

Physical environment. Critical care areas are bright, loud, and busy. Close patient doors, turn off unnecessary equipment, and limit conversation at workstations. Music can promote relaxation in critical care areas when used during waking hours and with patient consent. Allow for natural sunlight if possible, and positioning patients so that they can see out of windows helps to maintain orientation to time.[61] Familiarize patient rooms by displaying photographs, cards, drawings, and favored items. Sleep deprivation is a serious concern in critical care environments. Group care activities to limit nighttime interruptions, and collaborate with laboratory and other staff to decrease sleep interruptions.[61] The use of earplugs during sleeping hours has been shown to improve patients' subjective experience of sleep.[64]

Provide Family-Centered Care

Family-centered care, an AACN practice standard for critical care, formalizes the patient and family as the unit of care. Family-centered care is based on the belief that patients and families should participate in decisions together and that patients need their families for love, understanding, and support while coping with critical illness.[54] The nurse's observable support of family members at the bedside gives the patient comfort. The patient determines who counts as family. Biologic or legal issues notwithstanding, it is the nature of the patient's relationships that determines the extent of interaction with others.

The elements essential to family-centered care include respect, collaboration, and support. Research demonstrates that family members of critical care patients want understandable information that is given in a timely manner. They want reassurance that their loved one is being monitored and is receiving the best care possible. Family members also need to be allowed access to their loved ones.[17,54] Some family members are reassured by helping with caregiving if this is acceptable to the patient.

Family members are particularly sensitive to a nurse's words and actions, making it essential that the nurse convey understanding and acceptance. The critical care nurse can observe the quality of the patient-family interaction and formulate interventions that will aid the family in supporting the patient.[54] The critical care nurse provides interventions aimed at supporting family members throughout the patient's stay in the unit.

Engage Spiritual Resources

A time of crisis can also lead to a time of positive spiritual renewal and readiness for an enhanced spiritual life. Spiritual and religious beliefs and practices often give patients and family members some measure of acceptance of an illness, a sense of mastery and control, strength to endure the stressors of illness, and a source of hope and trust beyond what medical interventions can provide. Transformative spiritual care strategies are particularly helpful in times of crisis and uncertainty. When faced with significant life challenges, people need resources to transcend their circumstances and know that no matter what happens, they will endure. Spiritual resources include faith in a higher power, support communities, a sense of hope and meaning in life, and religious practices. Patient and family spirituality affects their ability to cope with loss.[65]

Qualitative research by Cutcliffe[66] on critically ill patients' perspectives on hope revealed that hope is perceived as being directly related to help. That is, when patients know there is help, they feel more hopeful. They also described hope as closely interwoven with care. To feel cared for and cared about brings hope to critically ill patients. Hope was related to patients' sense of their personal future and was used as a coping resource. In each patient description of hope in Cutcliffe's study, the nurse plays a pivotal, potentially inspirational role. Nursing interventions that engender hope can be quite simple, quiet, and informal. Listening to patients' concerns, offering support, being present, enhancing dignity, and developing caring and trusting relationships with patients gives hope.[67] People hope for different things over the course of an illness. Listen for shifts in what patients hope for and find ways to help them meet their desired goals.

Although distinctions between spiritual and religious concerns are important to highlight,[68] many people find spiritual strength in their adherence to a particular religious tradition. They get inspiration to endure, hope, comfort, assurance, and confidence from the texts, rituals, and beliefs of their faith communities. Facilitate patient access to religious rituals, prayer, and scripture reading as hope-sustaining activities, and help patients make connections to their spiritual or cultural communities. Collaborate with the hospital's spiritual care department when you sense that a person has unmet or unaddressed spiritual questions or needs. Often a professional spiritual care provider is the best person to assess spiritual needs and plan helpful interventions. Spiritual and religious leaders can also provide valuable insights when discussing ethical decisions that may have implications for the person's values and beliefs.[68] Religious, spiritual, or philosophical practices can also directly inform diet, hygiene practices, and rituals surrounding birth, death, and medical interventions.

PATIENTS WITH PSYCHIATRIC DISORDERS

Patients admitted to critical care settings can have a preexisting mental health condition. Chronic depression, bipolar disorder, substance addiction, and self-destructive behaviors, including suicide attempts, can be the primary causes of a critical care hospitalization.[69] The critical care team should make every effort to continue medications for patients with mental health conditions during the critical care stay unless medically contraindicated. If the patient is unable to take oral medications, an alternative route should be found if possible. If psychotropic medications have been discontinued for medical reasons, discuss the need to resume those medications with the health care providers receiving the patient after discharge from the critical care unit.

Alcohol Withdrawal in Critical Care Settings

Nurses in any acute care setting must be alert to the symptoms of withdrawal from chemical substances, including alcohol, which can complicate recovery from the admitting diagnosis. In emergency admissions to a critical care unit, a full patient history of substance use frequently has not been uncovered. Investigators estimate that one in four patients admitted to general hospitals meet criteria for alcohol use disorder.[70] Without treatment, withdrawal from alcohol typically begins 3 hours to a few days after the last alcohol consumption.

The signs and symptoms of alcohol withdrawal are easily confused with other conditions. Patients may exhibit autonomic hyperactivity (eg, pulse of ≥100 beats/min, sweating), tremulousness, sleep disturbance, nausea and vomiting, agitation, and anxiety. Limited visual, tactile, and auditory hallucinations or illusions may also occur. Generalized tonic-clonic seizures are a serious symptom of alcohol withdrawal in some patients.

Alcohol withdrawal delirium is the most serious consequence of abstaining from alcohol. It is also known as delirium tremens. This delirium typically begins in 3 days but may take a week or more to manifest. Individuals who progress to this level are typically older and have other physical problems, particularly brain injury and liver disease. Symptoms include those previously identified in general withdrawal as well as other dramatic characteristics, including the following:

- Disorientation, confusion, and severe anxiety
- Longer lasting hallucinations (primarily visual)
- Profuse sweating
- Seizures
- High blood pressure
- Racing and irregular heartbeat
- Severe tremors
- Low-grade fever

Critical care nurses can quickly and accurately assess a patient's risk for alcohol withdrawal by using the Clinical Institute Withdrawal Assessment for Alcohol, revised.[71] This 10-item scale assesses for nausea and vomiting; tremors; paroxysmal (episodic) sweats; anxiety; agitation; tactile, auditory, and visual disturbances; headache; and orientation. Treatment protocols for alcohol withdrawal syndrome depend on the severity of the patient's symptoms.

Commonly used medications for withdrawal symptoms include the benzodiazepines, such as chlordiazepoxide and lorazepam. An anticonvulsant, carbamazepine, is also used for treating withdrawal symptoms and carries minimal risk of abuse. In the event of delirium occurring, benzodiazepines may be given intravenously. The β-adrenergic receptor antagonists and clonidine reduce sympathetic hyperactivity. Ondansetron and promethazine may be used for nausea. Thiamine, folic acid, and multivitamins should be added to intravenous fluids. (See also Chapter 33, Alcohol Screening Questionnaire, Box 33.1.)

Caring for Patients After Attempted Suicide

Nurses in critical care settings care for patients who have attempted suicide. It is especially important to practice dignity-enhancing care in these situations. Nurses should carefully consider their own attitudes concerning self-destructive behaviors. Caregivers can resent caring for a person whose critical condition is self-inflicted, while other patients want to live and are fighting for their lives. It helps to consider the degree of personal and spiritual distress the person must have experienced to bring him or her to the point of wanting life to end.

Suicidal behavior represents the extreme, maladaptive end of a continuum of self-protective responses to life's challenges.[6] While the patient is in the unit, primary nursing interventions include validating the patient's worth and self-esteem, helping him or her regulate emotional states and behaviors, and mobilizing the patient's social support, necessary for long-term recovery.[6]

Nurses also care for family members of persons who have attempted suicide. These individuals are often experiencing a significant family crisis and can have feelings of shame, guilt, or anger concerning the suicide attempt. Nurses should talk to family members in a private setting and establish an atmosphere of interested concern for their loved one.

Before the patient is discharged from the unit or hospital, nurses gather assessment data from family members, including information about the patient's medical and psychiatric history, history of previous suicide attempts, presence of a trigger for self-destructive behavior (eg, recent disagreement with someone or anniversary of a loss), presence of acute stressors, and availability of support systems. Family members should be encouraged to inform health care providers if the patient has stopped taking prescribed psychotropic medications or quit seeing a mental health provider and begin to make a plan for immediate follow-up care after discharge from the unit.[72]

NURSE SELF-CARE

Critical care nurses do amazing, life-giving work. The poet John O'Donohue[73] stated that nurses "stand like a secret angel between the bleak despair of illness and the unquenchable light of spirit that can turn the darkest destiny towards dawn." Critical care nurses possess the knowledge, skills, and professional attitude to help others in situations of uncertainty and suffering.

Considering the importance of the lifesaving work of critical care nurses, it is also important to recognize the need for consistent, intentional self-care. A nurse cannot give fully engaged, compassionate care to others when he or she is depleted. In critical care settings, nurses often witness prolonged, concentrated suffering. This can lead to feelings of frustration, anger, guilt, sadness, or anxiety. Frequent, intense, or prolonged exposure to grief and loss places nurses at risk for developing compassion fatigue, a physical, emotional, and spiritual exhaustion accompanied by emotional pain. The stressors of caregiving can lead to a decreased capacity to show compassion or empathize with people who are suffering.[74] Nurses also are at risk for developing PTSD reactions to the relentless stress and psychologically difficult work of caring for others in extreme situations.[74]

To avoid the extremes of either becoming overly involved in patients' suffering or detaching from them, nurses can use self-care activities to maintain balance. Nurses should first use self-reflection when they feel overwhelmed, considering the possible reasons for their feelings. There are often multiple causes for feeling overwhelmed, such as sadness about a particular patient, overwork, lateral hostility at work,[75,76] and disruptions in one's personal life. Reflection is an important first step because without awareness, it is difficult to identify possible solutions. Talking with friends, a spiritual care provider, or a close colleague can help the nurse recognize his or her own grief and reflect on the meaning of work.

Stress management techniques help to restore energy and enjoyment in caring for patients. Nurses who practice self-care are more likely to experience professional and personal growth and find more meaning in their work. Maintain physical health by eating well, exercising, engaging in relaxing activities, laughing, and getting enough sleep. Promote emotional health by participating in calming activities, such as meditation, daily gratitude reflections, deep breathing, walking, or listening to music.[77] Use self-transcendence (spiritual awareness) activities, such as journal writing, sharing stories, recognizing one's own positive contributions and unique gifts, and connecting with one's self.[77] Given the ongoing demands of critical care nursing, balance time at work with time for recreation and relaxation. Invest time in the people and activities that nurture the spirit. Learn from the courage exhibited by patients and family members, and, with good self-care, find joy and fulfillment in being a critical care nurse.

CASE STUDY 6.1 Patient With Psychosocial Needs

Brief Patient History
Ms. T is a 17-year-old woman who took an acetaminophen overdose after her boyfriend broke up with her. She states that she did not want to kill herself but just wanted to scare her boyfriend. Ms. T is having difficulty facing the need for a psychiatric evaluation and the potential for severe liver damage.

Clinical Assessment
Ms. T was admitted to the critical care unit from the emergency department in stable condition. She is awake; alert; and oriented to person, time, place, and situation. She is irritable, withdrawn, and wants to be left alone. Her parents stay at her bedside and share with the nurse their intense feelings of fear, confusion, and uncertainty concerning their daughter's serious psychological and physical condition.

Diagnostic Procedures
A psychiatric evaluation was completed, with the recommendation that Ms. T receive inpatient psychiatric care when medically stable.

Medical Diagnosis
Ms. T is diagnosed with acetaminophen toxicity and risk for hepatic failure.

Questions
1. What major outcomes do you expect to achieve for this patient?
2. What problems or risks must be managed to achieve these outcomes?
3. What interventions must be initiated to monitor, prevent, manage, or eliminate the problems and risks identified?
4. What interventions should be initiated to promote optimal functioning, safety, and well-being of the patient?
5. What possible learning needs do you anticipate for this patient?
6. What cultural and age-related factors may have a bearing on the patient's plan of care?

SUMMARY

- Critical care nurses consider connections between the body, mind, and spirit in providing holistic nursing care to critically ill patients.
- Patients in critical care settings must cope with many stressors. Each patient's response is unique and depends on various environmental factors and individual differences.
- A person's perceptions of self and relationships with others, of spiritual values, and of self-competency in social roles play a role in how he or she responds to stress or illness.
- Anxiety is a normal subjective response to a perceived or actual threat to self-integrity, which can range from a vague, generalized feeling of discomfort to a state of panic and loss of control.
- Disturbances in self-concept, body image, and self-esteem often accompany experiences of critical illness or injury.
- Spiritual distress, hopelessness, and powerlessness in critically ill patients can complicate recovery and should be addressed by critical care nurses.
- Each person has a preferred set of coping strategies for meeting life stressors.
- Dignity-enhancing care includes elements of attitude, behaviors, compassion, and dialogue.
- Supportive family members and friends provide a source of strength and hope for patients facing the stressors of a critical illness or injury.
- Spirituality provides patients with transcending practices for accepting what cannot be changed and for fostering hope and trust in self, others, and the transcendent.
- Critical care nurses should engage in self-care practices for their own wellness and to sustain meaning in their work with critically ill patients and their families.

ⓔ Visit the Evolve Site for additional study materials.

REFERENCES

1. Halter M, ed. Varcarolis' Foundations of Psychiatric Mental Health Nursing: A Clinical Approach. 7th ed. St. Louis, MO: Elsevier; 2013.
2. Herdman TH, Kamitsuru S, editors. NANDA International Nursing Diagnoses: Definitions and Classification, 2015-2017. Oxford, UK: Wiley Blackwell; 2014.
3. Selye H. Stress in Health and Disease. Boston, MA: Butterworth; 1976.
4. Nuernberger P. Freedom From Stress: A Holistic Approach. Honesdale, PA: The Himalayan International Institute of Yoga Science and Philosophy; 1981.
5. Lazarus R, Lazarus B. Passion and Reason: Making Sense of Emotions. New York, NY: Oxford University; 1994.
6. Stuart G. Principles and Practices of Psychiatric Nursing. 10th ed. St. Louis, MO: Mosby; 2012.
7. Johns Hopkins Medicine. PTSD common in ICU survivors. ScienceDaily, 20 April 2015. Retrieved on April 12, 2016 from www.sciencedaily.com/releases/2015/04/150420144753.htm.
8. Griffiths R, Jones C. Seven lessons from 20 years' of follow-up intensive care unit survivors. Curr Opin Crit Care. 2007;13:508.
9. Kiekkas P, et al. Psychological distress and delusional memories after critical care: a literature review. Int Nurs Rev. 2010;57:288.
10. Pillai L, et al. Can we predict intensive care relatives at risk for posttraumatic stress disorder? Indian J Crit Care Med. 2010;14(2):83.
11. Kross E, et al. ICU care associated with symptoms of depression and posttraumatic stress disorder among family members of patients who died in the ICU. Chest. 2011;139(4):795.
12. Wallen K, et al. Symptoms of acute post-traumatic stress disorder after intensive are. Am J Crit Care. 2008;17(6):534.

13. Rock L. Posttraumatic stress disorder after intensive care. CriticalCare Nurse. 2014;34(1):30.

14. Hoffman J. Nightmares after the ICU. New York Times. 2013. Retrieved from http://well.blogs.nytimes.com/2013/07/22/nightmares-after-the-i-c-u/?emc=eta1

15. Twigg E, et al. Use of a screening questionnaire for post-traumatic stress disorder (PTSD) on a sample of UK ICU patients. Acta Anaesthesiol Scand. 2007;52:202.

16. Garrouste-Orgeas M, et al. Impact of intensive care unit diary on psychological distress in patients and relatives. Critical Care Medicine. 2012;40(7):2033.

17. Haraldsson L, Lennart C, Conlon L, Henricson M. The experiences of ICU patients during follow-up sessions: a qualitative study. Intensive Crit Care Nurs. 2015;31(4):223-231.

18. Phillips C. Use of patient diaries in critical care. Nurs Stand. 2011;26(11):35.

19. Williams S. Recovering from the psychological impact of intensive care: how constructing a story helps. Nurs Crit Care. 2009;14(6):281.

20. Perpina-Galvan J, Richart-Martinez M. Scales for evaluating self perceived anxiety levels in patients admitted to intensive care units: a review. Am J Crit Care. 2009;18(6):571.

21. Jaber S, et al. A prospective study of agitation in a medical-surgical ICU: incidence, risk factors, and outcomes. Chest. 2005;128(4):2749.

22. Khalaila R, et al. Communication difficulties and psychoemotional distress in patients receiving mechanical ventilation. Am J Crit Care. 2011;20(6):470.

23. Chlan L, Savik K. Patterns of anxiety in critically ill patients receiving mechanical ventilator support. Nurs Res. 2011;60(3 Suppl):S50.

24. Brodsky-Israeli M, Ganz F. Risk factors associated with transfer anxiety among patients transferring from the intensive care unit to the ward. J Adv Nurs. 2011;67(3):510.

25. Ruz M, et al. Evidence that the brief symptom inventory can be used to measure anxiety quickly and reliably in patients hospitalized for acute myocardial infarction. J Cardiovasc Nurs. 2010;25(2):117.

26. Fortinash KM. The nursing process. In: Fortinash KM, Holoday-Worret PA, editors. Psychiatric Mental Health Nursing. 5th ed. St. Louis, MO: Mosby; 2012.

27. Doenges ME, Murr A, Moorhouse MF. Nurse's Pocket Guide: Diagnoses, Interventions, and Rationales. 12th ed. Philadelphia, PA: FA Davis; 2010.

28. Pasacreta JV, Minarik P, Nield-Anderson L. Anxiety and depression. In: Ferrell B, Coyle N, editors. Textbook of Palliative Nursing. 3rd ed. New York, NY: Oxford University Press; 2010.

29. Halter M, editor. Varcarolis' Foundations of Psychiatric Mental Health Nursing: A Clinical Approach. 7th ed. St. Louis, MO: Elsevier; 2013.

30. Fredriksen ST, Ringsberg K. Living the situation stress-experiences among intensive care patients. Intensive Crit Care Nurs. 2007;23:124.

31. Maslow H. Motivation and Personality. New York, NY: Harper & Row; 1954.

32. Ackley B, Ladwig G, editors. Nursing Diagnosis Handbook: An Evidence Based Guide to Planning Care. St. Louis, MO: Mosby; 2011.

33. Lazare A. Shame and humiliation in the medical encounter. Arch Intern Med. 1987;147:1653.

34. Malterud K, Hollnagel H. Avoiding humiliations in the clinical encounter. Scand J Prim Health Care. 2007;25:69.

35. Chochinov H, et al. Dignity in the terminally ill: a developing empirical model. Soc Sci Med. 2006;54(3):3433.

36. Tilsley A, et al. Identifying intensive care staff cultural, spiritual, and ethical beliefs to successfully implement a dying pathway: a two stage mixed methods sequential design. Aust Crit Care. 2015;28(1):38.

37. Timmins F, Kelly J. Spiritual assessment in intensive and cardiac care nursing. Nurs Crit Care. 2008;13(3):124-131.

38. Weisman A. On Death and Denying: A Psychological Study of Terminality. New York, NY: Behavioral Publications; 1972.

39. Amaert A, et al. Stroke patients in the acute care phase: role of hope in self-healing. Holist Nurs Pract. 2006;23(3):137.

40. Frankl V. Man's Search for Meaning. New York, NY: Washington Square Press; 1959.

41. Miller JF. Hope: a construct central to nursing. Nurs Forum. 2007;42(1):12-19.

42. Rotter JB. Generalized expectancies for internal versus external control of reinforcement. Psychol Monogr. 1966;80(1):1.

43. Ramsay P, et al. Intensive care survivors' experiences of ward-based care: Meleis' theory of nursing transitions and role development among critical care outreach services. J Clin Nurs. 2014;23(5-6):605-615.

44. Nightingale F. Notes on Nursing: What It Is and What It Is Not. New York, NY: D. Appleton and Company; 1860.

45. Nelson JE, et al. End of life care for the critically ill: a national intensive care unit survey. Crit Care Med. 2006;34:2547.

46. Happ M, et al. Nurse-patient communication interactions in the intensive care unit. Am J Crit Care Nurs. 2011;20(2):e28.

47. Stajduha K, et al. Patient perceptions of helpful communication in the context of advanced cancer. J Clin Nurs. 2010;19:2039.

48. Lowey S. Communication between the nurse and family caregiver in end of life care: a review of the literature. J Hosp Pall Nursing. 2008;10(1):35.

49. Grossbach I. Promoting effective communication for patients receiving mechanical ventilation. Crit Care Nurs. 2011;31(3):46.

50. Scheunermann L, et al. How clinicians discuss critically ill patients' preferences and values with surrogates: an empirical analysis. Crit Care Med. 2015;43(4):757-764.

51. Lipson M, Lipson A. Psychotherapy and the ethics of attention. Hast Cent Rep. 1996;26(1):17.

52. Newman M. Transforming Presence: The Difference That Nursing Makes. Philadelphia, PA: FA Davis; 2008.

53. Tulsky J. Interventions to enhance communication among patients, providers, and families. J Palliat Med. 2005;8(Suppl 1):S95.

54. Nolan K, Waren N. Meeting the needs of family members of ICU patients. Crit Care Nurs Q. 2014;37(4):393-406.

55. Garlow L, Day A, Payne C. Transitioning the complex trauma patient from the ICU: acute care nurses' perception of readiness. J Trauma Nurs. 2015;22(2):56-62.

56. Helder O, Verwiej J, van Staa A. Transition from neonatal intensive care unit to special care nurseries: experiences of parents and nurses. Pediatr Crit Care Med. 2012;13(3):305-311.

57. Haggstrom M, Asplund K, Kristiansen L. To reduce technology prior to discharge from intensive care—important but difficult. Scand J Caring Sci. 2012;27:506-515.

58. AACN Practice alert. Family visitation in the adult intensive care unit. Crit Care Nurse. 2016;36(1):e15-18. Retrieved on April 12, 2016 from http://www.aacn.org/wd/practice/docs/practicealerts/fam-visit-pa-feb2016ccn-pages.pdf?

59. Henricson M, et al. The outcome of tactile touch on stress parameters in intensive care: a randomized controlled trial. Complement Ther Clin Pract. 2008;14:244.

60. Austin D. The psychophysiological effects of music therapy in intensive care units. Paediatr Nurs. 2010;22(3):14.

61. Bazuin D, Cardon K. Creating healing intensive care unit environments: physical and psychological considerations in designing critical care areas. Crit Care Nurs. 2011;24(4):259.

62. Black P, et al. The effect of nurse-facilitated family participation in the psychological care of the critically ill patient. J Adv Nurs. 2011;67(5):1091.

63. Jacobowski N, et al. Communication in critical care: family rounds in the intensive care unit. Am J Crit Care. 2010;19(5):421.

64. Scotto C, et al. Earplugs improve patients' subjective experience of sleep in critical care. Nurs Crit Care. 2009;14(4):180-184.

65. Hodge D. Spiritual Assessment in Social Work and Mental Health Practice. New York, NY: Columbia University Press; 2015.

66. Cutcliffe J. Critically ill patients' perspectives of hope. Br J Nurs. 1996;26(5):687.

67. Tanis S, DiNapoli P. Paradox of hope in patients receiving palliative care: a concept analysis. Int J Human Caring. 2008;12(1):53.

68. Timmins F, et al. Supporting patients' and families' religious and spiritual needs in ICU: can we do more? Br Assoc Crit Care Nurs. 2015;20(3):115.

69. York L, Rayback S. Behavioral and psychological factors in critical care. In: Ahrens T, Prentice D, Kleinpell R, editors. Critical Care Nursing Certification. New York, NY: McGraw-Hill; 2010.

70. Repper-Delisi J. Successful implementation of alcohol withdrawal pathway in a general hospital. Psychomatics. 2008;39(4):292.

71. Nuss MA, et al. Utilizing CIWA-Ar to assess use of benzodiazepines in patients vulnerable to alcohol withdrawal syndrome. W V Med J. 2004;99:21.

72. National Suicide Prevention Lifeline. After attempt: a guide for talking care of your family member after treatment in the emergency department. http://www.suicidepreventionlifeline.org Accessed September 20, 2012.

73. O'Donohue J. To Bless the Space Between Us: A Book of Blessings. New York, NY: Doubleday; 2008.

74. Bush N. Compassion fatigue: are you at risk? Oncol Nurs Forum. 2009;26(1):24.

75. Mealer M, et al. The prevalence and impact of post-traumatic stress disorder and burnout syndrome in nurses. Depress Anxiety. 2009;26:1118.

76. Alspach G. Lateral hostility between critical care nurses: a survey report. Crit Care Nurs. 2008;28(2):13.

77. Showalter S. Compassion fatigue: what is it? Why does it matter? Recognizing the symptoms, acknowledging the impact, developing the tools to prevent compassion fatigue, and strengthen the professional already suffering from the effects. Am J Hosp Palliat Med. 2010;27(4):239.

7

Nutrition Alterations and Management

Kasuen Mauldin

Nutrition support is an essential component of providing comprehensive care to critically ill patients. Nutrition screening must be conducted on every patient, and a more thorough nutrition assessment is completed on any patient screened to be nutritionally at risk. Malnutrition can be related to any essential nutrient or nutrients. A serious type of malnutrition found frequently among hospitalized patients is protein-calorie malnutrition (PCM). Malnutrition is associated with a variety of adverse outcomes, including wound dehiscence, infections, pressure ulcers, respiratory failure requiring ventilation, longer hospital stays, and death. This chapter provides an overview of nutrient metabolism, nutrition status assessment, and implications of undernutrition for sick or stressed patients. Specifically, nutrition for each of the system alterations is discussed along with nursing management.

NUTRIENT METABOLISM

Nutrients are chemical substances found in foods that are needed for human life, growth, maintenance, and repair of body tissues. The main nutrients in foods are carbohydrates, proteins, fats, vitamins, minerals, and water. The process by which nutrients are used at the cellular level is known as *metabolism*. The energy-yielding nutrients or macronutrients are carbohydrates, proteins, and fats. For proper metabolic functioning, adequate amounts of micronutrients, such as vitamins, minerals (including electrolytes), and trace elements also must be supplied to the human body.

Energy-Yielding Nutrients
Carbohydrates
Through the process of digestion, carbohydrates are broken down into glucose, fructose, and galactose. After absorption from the intestinal tract, fructose and galactose are converted to glucose, the primary form of carbohydrate used by the cells. Glucose provides the energy needed to maintain cellular functions, including transport across cell membranes, secretion of specific hormones, muscle contraction, and synthesis of new substances. Most of the energy produced from carbohydrate metabolism is used to form adenosine triphosphate, the principal form of immediately available energy within all body cells. One gram of carbohydrate provides approximately 4 kcal of energy. For example, if a food contains 10 g of carbohydrates, 40 kcal (10 g × 4 kcal/g) of the total calories for that food comes from carbohydrates.

Inside the cell, glucose can be stored as glycogen or metabolized in a process called *glycolysis* for the subsequent release of energy. Liver and muscle cells have the largest glycogen reserves. In addition to glucose obtained from glycogen, glucose can be formed from lactate, amino acids, and glycerol. This process of manufacturing glucose from nonglucose precursors is called *gluconeogenesis*. Gluconeogenesis is carried out at all times, but it becomes especially important in maintaining a source of glucose in times of increased physiologic need and limited supply. Only the liver and, to a lesser extent, the kidney are capable of producing significant amounts of glucose for release into the blood for use by other tissues.

Proteins
Proteins are made up of chains of amino acids. Each amino acid consists of carbon, hydrogen, oxygen, and nitrogen in the form of one or more amine groups ($-NH_2$). Amino acids are the protein components that can be used by cells.

Proteins have important structural and functional duties within the body. Proteins provide the structural basis of all lean body mass, such as the vital organs and skeletal muscle. Proteins are important for visceral (cellular) functions, such as initiation of chemical reactions (eg, hormones, enzymes), transportation of other substances (eg, apoproteins, albumin), preservation of immune function (eg, antibodies), and maintenance of osmotic pressure (eg, albumin) and blood neutrality (eg, buffers). Some amino acids are used for energy, providing approximately 4 kcal per 1 gram.

Proteins are synthesized continuously, broken down into amino acids, and then resynthesized into new protein. This three-step process is called *protein turnover*. The rate of turnover is fastest (often only a few hours) in enzymes and hormones involved in metabolic activities. In very active tissues, such as those of the liver, kidney, and gastrointestinal (GI) mucosa, protein turnover occurs every few days. If necessary, 90% of the amino acids released by tissue breakdown can be reused, with the diet providing the remaining 10% of the amino acids needed for protein synthesis. In an injured or undernourished individual, many of the amino acids released by tissue breakdown may be used for gluconeogenesis. To preserve lean body mass, adequate energy must be supplied by the diet so that most of the amino acids from the diet and from tissue breakdown can be used for tissue synthesis, rather than gluconeogenesis.

Proteins, which often consist of hundreds or thousands of amino acids, are too large to be absorbed intact under normal circumstances. Through digestion, the proteins are broken down into amino acids and *dipeptides* or *tripeptides* (composed of two or three amino acids, respectively) that can be absorbed across the intestinal wall. Certain amino acids are *essential*; they cannot be produced by the body and must be supplied through the diet. Essential amino acids include valine, leucine, isoleucine, lysine, phenylalanine, tryptophan, threonine, and methionine, as well as histidine and arginine in infants. Other amino acids are nonessential and can be manufactured by the body under normal circumstances if the essential amino acids are in adequate supply. Some amino acids that may be nonessential in healthy adults become essential during illness. For example, histidine is an essential amino acid for adults with renal failure, and glutamine may be essential for individuals with trauma, sepsis, or other physiologic types of stress.

The amine group is essential for protein synthesis, but the nonamine portion of the molecule (ketoacid) is used in gluconeogenesis. If a ketoacid is used for gluconeogenesis, the amine group can be excreted in the urine as ammonia or urea. If the rate of gluconeogenesis rises, urinary nitrogen excretion also increases. In assessing protein nutrition, it is common to measure nitrogen balance, or the amount of nitrogen excreted compared with the amount consumed. Normally, most of the body's nitrogen losses are in the urine, and in determining nitrogen balance, urinary nitrogen excretion is measured (preferably over a 24-hour period). Nitrogen (protein) intake is recorded over the same period, and losses of nitrogen from feces and other routes (eg, sloughing of skin cells) are usually estimated.

Most healthy adults are in *nitrogen equilibrium*, meaning that they excrete the same amount of nitrogen that they consume. Individuals who excrete less nitrogen than they consume are said to be in *positive nitrogen balance*; this occurs during growth, pregnancy, and healing. Individuals who excrete more nitrogen than they consume are in *negative nitrogen balance*. Negative nitrogen balance is common in the early period after trauma or surgery. When the rate of gluconeogenesis is high, as may occur in a trauma patient who is initially too unstable to be fed, extensive loss of body proteins can occur. Losses include structural (eg, muscle) and visceral proteins. Visceral proteins, including immunoglobulins, albumin, and complement, are critical for survival. Therefore preservation of body protein is a key goal of nutrition support of critically ill patients.

Lipids (Fats)

Lipids include fatty acids, triglycerides (three fatty acids bound to a glycerol backbone), phospholipids (lipids containing phosphate groups), cholesterol, and cholesterol esters. Aside from their involvement in functions such as the maintenance of cell membranes and the manufacture of prostaglandins, lipids—primarily in the form of triglycerides—provide a stored source of energy. They are calorically dense molecules, providing more than twice the amount of energy (9 kcal) per gram as protein and carbohydrates. Most dietary lipids—consisting primarily of triglycerides—are too large to be absorbed intact and are partially broken down (hydrolyzed) in the intestine to form monoglycerides and diglycerides, which contain one or two fatty acids, respectively, bound to glycerol.

Bile salts produced in the liver are detergents, and they promote the formation of micelles, which are emulsions of fatty acids, monoglycerides, and bile salts. Long-chain fatty acids, which contain more than 12 carbon atoms, are very insoluble in water; they are found mainly in the interior of the micelle. The external portion of the micelle, which includes the glycerol part of the triglycerides, is more water soluble than the interior portion. This allows the micelle to cross the unstirred water layer that coats the intestinal absorptive surface.

Inside the intestinal cells, monoglycerides and long-chain fatty acids rejoin to form triglycerides, and they are surrounded by phospholipids and specific proteins to form chylomicrons.

These chylomicrons are transported out of the intestine through the lymphatic system, finally entering the blood circulation through the thoracic duct. Some of the chylomicrons are taken up by the liver, but most are directly transported to other tissues. Short-chain fatty acids (less than 8 carbon atoms long) and medium-chain fatty acids (8 to 12 carbon atoms long) are more water soluble than longer fatty acids; triglycerides containing these fatty acids can be absorbed without hydrolysis and are soluble enough to be transported to the liver through the portal vein, without chylomicron formation. Short-chain and medium-chain fatty acids have advantages in nutrition care of patients who have insufficient bile salt formation or inadequate intestinal surface area for absorption of long-chain fatty acids.

With the aid of the enzyme lipoprotein lipase, triglyceride-containing chylomicrons are broken down outside the cell and enter the cell as fatty acids and glycerol. Heparin stimulates lipoprotein lipase, and low doses of heparin are sometimes given to patients receiving intravenous lipid emulsions to improve lipid use. Insulin also stimulates the cellular uptake of triglycerides. Inside the cell, the fatty acids are oxidized (metabolized for energy) or reformed into triglycerides for storage. During an overnight fast, prolonged starvation, or metabolic stress when the carbohydrate supply is limited, the blood glucose level declines, and, consequently, insulin levels decrease. In response, a process called *lipolysis* causes the breakdown of intracellular triglycerides, which provides fatty acids for energy production and glycerol for gluconeogenesis.

The fatty acids released from adipose tissue can be used by the liver, heart, or other tissues. In the liver, fatty acids are broken down to ketones (β-hydroxybutyrate, acetoacetate, and acetone). In the absence of glucose, fatty acid breakdown and ketone production are increased. Ketones can be directly oxidized by skeletal muscle and used for energy. During prolonged starvation, the brain—which normally uses glucose—converts to using ketones as its primary energy source. This is a body defense mechanism to ensure a supply of energy when carbohydrate intake is low.

ASSESSING NUTRITION STATUS

The Joint Commission mandates nutrition screening be conducted on every patient within 24 hours of admission to an acute care center in the United States.[1] A brief questionnaire to be completed by the patient or significant other, the nursing admission form, or the physician's admission note usually provides enough information to determine whether the patient is at nutrition risk (Box 7.1). Any patient judged to be nutritionally at risk needs a more thorough nutrition assessment. The nutrition assessment process is continuous, with reassessments as a part of the overall nutrition care plan, as shown in Fig. 7.1.[2]

Nutrition assessment involves collection of four types of information: (1) anthropometric measurements; (2) biochemical (laboratory) data; (3) clinical signs (physical examination); and (4) diet and pertinent health history. This information provides a basis for (1) identifying patients who are malnourished or at risk of malnutrition; (2) determining the nutrition needs of individual patients; and (3) selecting the most appropriate methods of nutrition support for patients with or at risk of developing nutrition deficits. Nutrition support is the provision of specially formulated or delivered oral, enteral, or parenteral nutrients to maintain or restore optimal nutrition status.[3] The nutrition assessment can be performed by or under the supervision of a registered dietitian or by a nutrition care specialist (eg, nurse with specialized expertise in nutrition). Fig. 7.2 shows the route of administration of specialized nutrition support.

Assessment information must be evaluated in the context of the patient's overall clinical situation. Tracking multiple time points and trends in assessment data is more useful in determining nutrition status and intervention efficacy than looking at data from just one time point. Whenever possible, data should be measured rather than obtained from patient self-report or collected from family members. In addition, a team approach to nutrition assessment is key to ensuring the best quality of care. Members of the multidisciplinary team should work together in the nutrition care process from screening

for nutrition risk to providing and evaluating nutrition interventions. Effective team communication ensures that at-risk patients receive timely nutrition support and interventions that will improve clinical outcomes.

Anthropometric Measurements

Height and current weight are essential anthropometric measurements, and they should be measured rather than obtained through a patient or family report. The most important reason for obtaining anthropometric measurements is to be able to detect changes in the measurements over time (eg, track response to nutrition therapy). The patient's measurements may be compared with standard tables of weight-for-height or standard growth charts for infants and children. Another simple and reliable tool for interpreting appropriateness of weight for height for adults and older adolescents is the body mass index (BMI):

$$BMI = Weight \div height^2$$

Weight is measured in kilograms, and height is measured in meters. BMI values are independent of age and sex and are used for assessing health risk. The BMI can be classified as shown in Table 7.1.[4,5] Evidence that the associations between BMI, percent of body fat, and body fat distribution differ across populations suggests the possible need for developing different BMI cut-off values for different ethnic groups.[6] For example, alternative BMI classification cut-off values exist for Asians, who are at risk for obesity-related comorbidities at a lower BMI.[6]

It may be impossible to measure the height of some patients accurately. Total height can be estimated from arm span length or knee height.[7,8] To measure knee height, bend the knee 90 degrees, and measure from the base of the heel to the anterior surface of the thigh.

For men:

$$height (cm) = 64.19 - (0.04 \times age \ in \ years) + (2.02 \times knee \ height \ [cm])$$

For women:

$$height (cm) = 84.8 - (0.24 \times age \ in \ years) + (1.83 \times knee \ height \ [cm])$$

BOX 7.1 Patients Who Are at Risk for Malnutrition

Adults Who Exhibit Any of the Following
- Involuntary loss or gain of a significant amount of weight (>10% of usual body weight in 6 months, >5% in 1 month), even if the weight achieved by loss or gain is appropriate for height
- Chronic disease
- Chronic use of a modified diet
- Increased metabolic requirements
- Illness or surgery that may interfere with nutrition intake
- Inadequate nutrient intake for >7 days
- Regular use of three or more medications
- Poverty

Infants and Children Who Exhibit Any of the Following
- Low birth weight
- Small for gestational age
- Weight loss of 10% or more
- Weight-for-length or weight-for-height <5th percentile or >95th percentile
- Increased metabolic requirements
- Impaired ability to ingest or tolerate oral feedings
- Inadequate weight gain or significant decrease in an individual's usual growth percentile
- Poverty

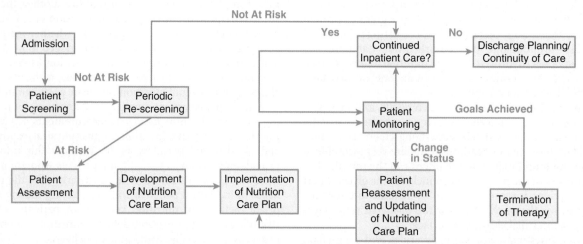

FIG. 7.1 Nutrition Care Process. (Redrawn from Mueller C, et al. A.S.P.E.N. Clinical guidelines, nutrition screening, assessment, and intervention in adults. *JPEN J Parenter Enteral Nutr.* 2011;35[1]:16-24.)

FIG. 7.2 Route of Administration of Specialized Nutrition Support. (Redrawn from Ukleja A, et al. Standards for nutrition support. *Nutr Clin Pract.* 2010;25[4]:403.)

TABLE 7.1 **Adult Body Mass Index Classifications**	
Classification	**BMI (kg/m²)**
Underweight	<18.5
Normal	18.5–24.99
Overweight	≥25
Pre-obese	25–29.99
Obese class I	30–34.99
Obese class II	35–39.99
Obese class III	≥40

BMI, body mass index.
From World Health Organization. Obesity: preventing and managing the global epidemic. Report of a WHO Consultation. *WHO Technical Report Series 894*. Geneva: World Health Organization; 2000.

During critical illness, changes in anthropometric measures such as weight are more likely to reflect changes in body water and its distribution. Good judgment must be used in interpreting anthropometric data. For example, edema may mask significant weight loss or underweight. Despite these limitations, weight remains an important measure of nutrition status, and any recent weight change must be evaluated. A woman who was obese 4 months earlier and has lost 15 kg (33 lb) since then may be at nutrition risk even if her current weight is appropriate for her height.

In addition to height and weight data, other measurements, such as arm muscle circumference, skin fold thickness, and body composition (proportion of fat and lean tissue, determined by bioelectric impedance or other methods), are sometimes performed, but these measurements are of limited use in assessing critically ill patients.[9]

Biochemical Data

A wide range of laboratory tests can provide information about nutrition status. The tests most often used in the clinical setting are summarized in Table 7.2. No diagnostic tests for evaluation of nutrition are perfect, and care must be taken in interpreting the results of the tests.[10] For example, many serum proteins sometimes used in nutrition assessment are now recognized to be more strongly affected by disease state rather than nutrient intake.

Clinical or Physical Manifestations

A thorough physical examination is an essential part of nutrition assessment. Box 7.2 lists some of the more common findings that may indicate an altered nutrition state. It is especially important for the nurse to check for signs of muscle wasting,

TABLE 7.2 Common Blood and Urine Tests Used in Nutrition Assessment

Test	Comments and Limitations
Serum Proteins	
Albumin or prealbumin	Levels decrease with protein deficiency and in liver failure. Albumin levels are slow to change in response to malnutrition and repletion. Prealbumin levels fall in response to trauma and infection.
Hematologic Values	
Anemia	
Normocytic (normal MCV, MCHC)	Common with protein deficiency
Microcytic (decreased MCV, MCH, MCHC)	Indicative of iron deficiency (can be due to blood loss)
Macrocytic (increased MCV)	Common in folate and vitamin B_{12} deficiency
Lymphocytopenia	Common in protein deficiency

MCH, mean corpuscular hemoglobin; *MCHC,* mean corpuscular hemoglobin concentration; *MCV,* mean corpuscular volume.

BOX 7.2 Clinical Manifestations of Nutrition Alterations

Manifestations That May Indicate Protein-Calorie Malnutrition
- Hair loss; dull, dry, brittle hair; loss of hair pigment
- Loss of subcutaneous tissue; muscle wasting
- Poor wound healing; decubitus ulcer
- Hepatomegaly
- Edema

Manifestations Often Present in Vitamin Deficiencies
- Conjunctival and corneal dryness (vitamin A)
- Dry, scaly skin; follicular hyperkeratosis, in which the skin appears to have gooseflesh continually (vitamin A)
- Gingivitis; poor wound healing (vitamin C)
- Petechiae; ecchymoses (vitamin C or K)
- Inflamed tongue, cracking at the corners of the mouth (riboflavin [vitamin B_2], niacin, folic acid, vitamin B_{12}, or other B vitamins)
- Edema; heart failure (thiamine [vitamin B_1])
- Confusion; confabulation (thiamine [vitamin B_1])

Manifestations Often Present in Mineral Deficiencies
- Blue sclerae; pale mucous membranes; spoon-shaped nails (iron)
- Hypogeusia, or poor sense of taste; dysgeusia, or bad taste; eczema; poor wound healing (zinc)

Manifestations Often Observed With Excessive Vitamin Intake
- Hair loss; dry skin; hepatomegaly (vitamin A)

BOX 7.3 Data Collection: Nutritional History

Inadequate Intake of Nutrients
- Alcohol abuse
- Anorexia, severe or prolonged nausea or vomiting
- Confusion, coma
- Poor dentition
- Poverty

Inadequate Digestion or Absorption of Nutrients
- Previous gastrointestinal operations, especially gastrectomy, jejunoileal bypass, and ileal resection
- Certain medications, especially antacids and histamine H_2-receptor antagonists (reduce upper small bowel acidity), cholestyramine (binds fat-soluble nutrients), and anticonvulsants

Increased Nutrient Losses
- Blood loss
- Severe diarrhea
- Fistulas, draining abscesses, wounds, decubitus ulcers
- Peritoneal dialysis or hemodialysis
- Corticosteroid therapy (increased tissue catabolism)

Increased Nutrient Requirements
- Fever
- Surgery, trauma, burns, infection
- Cancer (some types)
- Physiologic demands (pregnancy, lactation, growth)

loss of subcutaneous fat, skin or hair changes, and impairment of wound healing.

Diet and Health History

Information about dietary intake and significant variations in weight is a vital part of the history. Dietary intake can be evaluated in several ways, including a diet record, a 24-hour recall, and a diet history. The diet record, a listing of the type and amount of all foods and beverages consumed for some period (usually 3 days), is useful for evaluating the patient's intake in the critical care setting if the adequacy of intake is questionable. However, such a record reveals little about the patient's habitual intake before the illness or injury. The 24-hour recall of all food and beverage intake is easily and quickly performed, but it also may not reflect the patient's usual intake and has limited usefulness. The diet history consists of a detailed interview about the patient's usual intake, along with social, familial, cultural, economic, educational, and health-related factors that may affect intake. Although the diet history is time-consuming to perform and may be too stressful for acutely ill patients, it provides a wealth of information about food habits over a prolonged period and a basis for planning individualized nutrition education if changes in eating habits are desirable. Other information to include in a nutrition history is listed in Box 7.3.

Evaluating Nutrition Assessment Findings

A key part of the nutrition assessment process is using gathered patient information to estimate nutrient—specifically calorie or energy—needs. In the inpatient setting, working with the dietitian, estimated energy needs can be measured or calculated as described subsequently.

Determining Nutrition Needs

Various methods can be used in clinical practice to estimate caloric requirements. Indirect calorimetry, a method by which energy expenditure is calculated from oxygen consumption (Vo_2) and carbon dioxide production (Vco_2), is the most accurate method for determining caloric needs.[11,12] Indirect calorimetry is useful in patients suspected to have a high metabolic

TABLE 7.3 Estimating Energy Needs

Category	Description	Calories/kg	Calories/lb
Obese	More than 40% over ideal body weight or BMI >30	21	9.5
Sedentary	Relatively inactive individual without regular aerobic exercise; hospitalized patient without severe injury or sepsis	25–30	11–13.5
Moderate activity or injury	Individual obtaining regular aerobic exercise plus routine activities; patient with trauma or sepsis	30–35	13.5–16
Very active or severe injury	Manual laborer or athlete in very active training; patient with major burns or trauma	40	18

BMI, body mass index.

rate. This test can also analyze substrate use, which can be extrapolated from Vo_2 and Vco_2 during a steady state of respiration. The respiratory quotient (RQ) is equal to the Vco_2 divided by the Vo_2. Fat, protein, and carbohydrates each have a unique RQ, and RQ identifies which substrate is being preferentially metabolized and may provide target goals for calorie replacement.[12] For example, the RQ for the metabolism of fats is approximately 0.7, whereas the RQ for the metabolism of carbohydrates is 1.0. A mixed fuel diet results in an RQ of approximately 0.8.[12] The test can be performed on spontaneously breathing patients and on patients who require mechanical ventilation. Some ventilators are constructed so that they can perform indirect calorimetry. However, for most patients, indirect calorimetry requires the use of a metabolic cart, which is not available in all institutions. To maintain accuracy and reliability of measurement, several testing criteria must be met.[12] Information received from the metabolic cart is limited; measurements are conducted over a relatively brief period (often 20 to 30 minutes) and may not be representative of energy expenditure over the whole day.

Calorie and protein needs of patients are often estimated using formulas that provide allowances for increased nutrient use associated with injury and healing. Although indirect calorimetry is considered the most accurate method to determine energy expenditure, estimates using formulas have demonstrated reasonable accuracy.[13-15] Commonly used formulas for critically ill patients can be found in Appendix B. Some rules of thumb are available to provide a rough estimate of caloric needs so that nurses and other caregivers can quickly determine if patients are being seriously overfed or underfed (Table 7.3).

The goal of nutrition assessment is to obtain the most accurate estimate of nutrition requirements. Underfeeding and overfeeding must be avoided during critical illness. Overfeeding results in excessive production of carbon dioxide, which can be a burden in a patient with pulmonary compromise. Overfeeding increases fat stores, which can contribute to insulin resistance and hyperglycemia. Hyperglycemia increases the risk of postoperative infections in diabetic and nondiabetic patients.[16]

IMPLICATIONS OF UNDERNUTRITION FOR SICK OR STRESSED PATIENTS

Of hospitalized patients, 40% are at risk for malnutrition.[17-20] Although illness or injury is the major factor contributing to development of malnutrition, other possible contributing factors are lack of communication among the nurses, physicians, and dietitians responsible for the care of these patients; frequent diagnostic testing and procedures, which lead to interruption in feeding; medications and other therapies that cause anorexia, nausea, or vomiting and thus interfere with food intake; insufficient monitoring of nutrient intake; and inadequate use of supplements, tube feedings, or parenteral nutrition to maintain nutrition status.

Nutrition status tends to deteriorate during hospitalization unless appropriate nutrition support is started early and continually reassessed. Malnutrition in hospitalized patients is associated with a wide variety of adverse outcomes. Wound dehiscence, pressure ulcers, sepsis, infections, respiratory failure requiring ventilation, longer hospital stays, and death are more common among malnourished patients.[21-23] Decline in nutrition status during hospitalization is associated with higher incidences of complications, increased mortality rates, increased length of stay, and higher hospital costs.

It is rare for a patient to exhibit a lack of only one nutrient. Nutrition deficiencies usually are combined, with the patient lacking adequate amounts of protein, calories, and possibly vitamins and minerals.

Energy Deficiency
Protein-Calorie Malnutrition

Malnutrition results from the lack of intake of necessary nutrients or improper absorption and distribution of them as well as from excessive intake of some nutrients. Malnutrition can be related to any essential nutrient or nutrients, but a serious type of malnutrition found frequently among hospitalized patients is PCM. Poor intake or impaired absorption of protein and energy from carbohydrate and fat worsens the debilitation that may occur in response to critical illness. In PCM, the body proteins are broken down for gluconeogenesis, reducing the supply of amino acids needed for maintenance of body proteins and healing. Malnutrition can be caused by simple starvation—the inadequate intake of nutrients (eg, in a patient with anorexia related to cancer). It also can result from an injury that increases the metabolic rate beyond the supply of nutrients (hypermetabolism). In a seriously ill patient, if malnutrition occurs, usually it is the result of the combined effects of starvation and hypermetabolism. Two types of PCM are kwashiorkor and marasmus.

Kwashiorkor results in low levels of the serum proteins *albumin, transferrin,* and *prealbumin*; low total lymphocyte count; impaired immunity; loss of hair or hair pigment; edema resulting from low plasma oncotic pressure caused by a loss of plasma proteins; and an enlarged, fatty liver. Marasmus is recognizable by weight loss, loss of subcutaneous fat, and muscle wasting. In a person with marasmus, creatinine excretion in the urine is low, an indication of reduced muscle mass. Because PCM weakens muscles, increases vulnerability to infection, and can prolong hospital stays, the health care team should diagnose this serious disorder as quickly as possible so that an appropriate nutrition intervention can be implemented.

Metabolic Response to Starvation and Stress

To understand the development of malnutrition in the hospitalized patient, the nurse must understand the metabolic response to starvation and physiologic stress. Changes in endocrine status and metabolism together determine the onset and extent of malnutrition. Nutrition imbalance occurs when the demand for nutrients is greater than the exogenous nutrient supply. The major difference between a person who is starved and one who is starved and injured is that the latter has an increased reliance on tissue protein breakdown to provide precursors for glucose production to meet increased energy demands. Although carbohydrate and fat metabolism are also affected, the main concern is about protein metabolism and homeostasis.

During an acute, nonstressed fast, blood levels of glucose and insulin fall, and glucagon levels rise. Glucagon stimulates the liver to release glucose from its glycogen reserves, which become exhausted within a few hours. Glucagon also stimulates gluconeogenesis, and skeletal muscle provides a large amount of the substrates required for gluconeogenesis. As fasting progresses, fat becomes the primary source of fuel, and the blood ketone levels begin to increase. After the circulating ketone level rises, the brain is able to use ketones for 70% of its energy, decreasing the total body's reliance on glucose as an energy source. As gluconeogenesis from protein precursors decreases, protein breakdown and nitrogen excretion also slow. Some tissues, such as red blood cells, the renal medulla, and 30% of brain cells, are obligatory glucose users, and they continue to require a small amount of amino acids for gluconeogenesis. However, endogenous protein stores are spared from use for gluconeogenesis to a major extent, and protein homeostasis is partially restored.

Critically ill patients are at risk for a combination of starvation and the physiologic stress resulting from injury, trauma, major surgery, or sepsis. Starvation occurs because the person must have nothing by mouth (NPO) for surgical procedures, is unable to eat because of disease-related factors, or is hemodynamically too unstable to be fed. The physiologic stress causes an increased metabolic rate (hypermetabolism) that results in increased oxygen consumption and energy expenditure.

The hypermetabolic process results from increased catabolic hormone changes caused by the stressful event. The sympathetic nervous system is stimulated, causing the adrenal medulla to release catecholamines (epinephrine and norepinephrine). Other hormones released in response to stress include glucagon, adrenocorticotropic hormone, antidiuretic hormone, and glucocorticoids and mineralocorticoids (eg, cortisol, aldosterone). Cytokines are peptide messengers secreted by macrophages as part of the inflammatory response, and they serve as hormonal regulators of the immune system. Cytokine levels increase in response to sepsis and trauma. Important cytokines include tumor necrosis factor, cachectin, interleukin-1, and interleukin-6. All these hormonal changes cause nutrient substrates, primarily amino acids, to move from peripheral tissues (eg, skeletal muscle) to the liver for gluconeogenesis.

This mobilization of substrates occurs at the expense of body tissue and function at a time when the needs for protein synthesis (eg, wound healing, acute-phase proteins) also are high. Hyperglycemia results from the effects of increased catecholamines, glucocorticoids, and glucagon. The body relies on its protein stores to provide substrates for gluconeogenesis because glucose becomes the major fuel source. Loss of protein results in a negative nitrogen balance and weight loss. Catabolism may be unresponsive to nutrient intake.

Etiology-Based Approach in Defining Malnutrition

In 2012, the Academy of Nutrition and Dietetics and the American Society for Parenteral and Enteral Nutrition jointly released a consensus statement outlining recommendations for the identification and documentation of adult malnutrition in clinical practice.[24] The statement proposes an etiology-based approach in defining malnutrition that takes into account the role of inflammation. The three etiology-based malnutrition definitions for patients who have been identified as having compromised intake or loss of body mass are (1) starvation-related malnutrition without inflammation (eg, pure chronic starvation, anorexia nervosa); (2) chronic disease–related malnutrition with mild to moderate degree of inflammation (eg, organ failure, pancreatic cancer, sarcopenic obesity); and (3) acute disease–related or injury-related malnutrition with marked inflammatory response (eg, major infection, burns) (Fig. 7.3).[24] Two or more of the following six characteristics are currently recommended for the diagnosis of adult malnutrition: insufficient energy intake, weight loss, loss of muscle mass, loss of subcutaneous fat, localized or generalized fluid accumulation that may sometimes mask weight loss, and diminished functional status.[24] It is recommended that the above-listed characteristics be examined as a part of nutrition assessment and if identified should be documented at baseline and at frequent intervals during reassessments throughout the patient's hospital stay.

NUTRITION SUPPORT

Nursing Management of Nutrition Support

Nutrition support is an important aspect of care of critically ill patients. Maintenance of optimal nutrition status may prevent or reduce the complications associated with critical illness and promote positive clinical outcomes.[3] Critical care nurses play a key role in the delivery of nutrition support and must work closely with dietitians and physicians in promoting the best possible outcomes for their patients.

Nutrition support is the provision of oral, enteral, or parenteral nutrients. It is an essential adjunct in the prevention and management of malnutrition in critically ill patients.[3] The goal of nutrition support therapy is to provide enough support for body requirements, to minimize complications, and to promote rapid recovery. Critical care nurses must have a broad understanding of nutrition support, including the indications, prevention, and management of associated complications.

Oral Supplementation

Oral supplementation may be necessary for patients who can eat and have normal digestion and absorption but cannot consume enough regular foods to meet caloric and protein needs. Patients with mild to moderate anorexia, burns, or trauma sometimes fall into this category. To improve intake and tolerance of supplements, the critical care nurse can take several steps, as follows:
1. Collaborate with the dietitian to choose appropriate products, and allow the patient to participate in the selection process, if possible. Milkshakes and instant breakfast preparations are often more palatable and economical than commercial supplements. However, lactose intolerance is common among adults. Many disease processes (eg, Crohn disease, radiation enteritis, human immunodeficiency virus infection, severe gastroenteritis) can cause lactose intolerance. Individuals with this problem require commercial lactose-free supplements or milk treated with lactase enzyme.

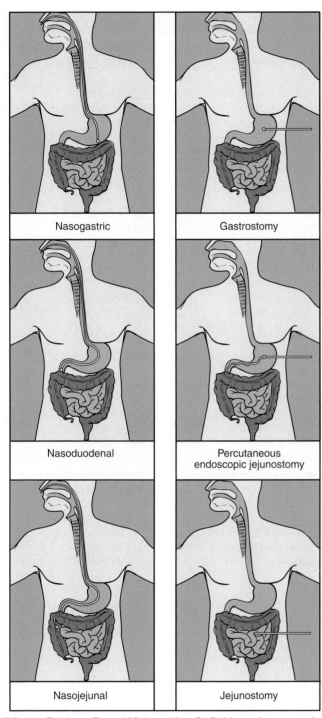

Nasogastric

Gastrostomy

Nasoduodenal

Percutaneous
endoscopic jejunostomy

Nasojejunal

Jejunostomy

FIG. 7.3 Etiology-Based Malnutrition Definitions, Incorporating the Role of Inflammation in Disease-Related Malnutrition. (From White JV, et al. Consensus statement of the Academy of Nutrition and Dietetics/American Society for Parenteral and Enteral Nutrition: characteristics recommended for the identification and documentation of adult malnutrition (undernutrition). *J Acad Nutr Diet.* 2012;112[5]:730-738.)

2. Offer to serve commercial supplements well chilled or on ice because this improves flavor.
3. Advise patients to sip formulas slowly, consuming no more than 240 mL over 30 to 45 minutes. These products contain easily digestible carbohydrates. If formulas are consumed too quickly, rapid hydrolysis of the carbohydrate in the duodenum can contribute to dumping syndrome, characterized by abdominal cramping, weakness, tachycardia, and diarrhea.

4. Record all supplement intake separately on the intake-and-output sheet so that it can be differentiated from intake of water and other liquids.

Enteral Nutrition

Enteral nutrition or tube feedings are used for patients who have at least some digestive and absorptive capability but are unable or unwilling to consume enough by mouth. When possible, the enteral route is the preferred method of feeding over total parenteral nutrition (TPN). The proposed advantages of enteral nutrition over TPN include lower cost, better maintenance of gut integrity, and decreased infection and hospital length of stay.[3] A review of the literature comparing enteral nutrition and TPN indicates that enteral nutrition is less expensive than TPN and is associated with a lower risk of infection.[3,25]

The GI tract plays an important role in maintaining immunologic defenses, which is why nutrition by the enteral route is thought to be more physiologically beneficial than TPN. Some of the barriers to infection in the GI tract include neutrophils; the normal acidic gastric pH; motility, which limits GI tract colonization by pathogenic bacteria; the normal gut microflora, which inhibit growth of or destroy some pathogenic organisms; rapid desquamation and regeneration of intestinal epithelial cells; the layer of mucus secreted by GI tract cells; and bile, which detoxifies endotoxin in the intestine and delivers immunoglobulin A to the intestine. A second line of defense against invasion of intestinal bacteria is the gut-associated lymphoid tissue.[26] The systemic immune defenses in the GI tract are stimulated by the presence of food within it. In animal models, resting the GI tract by providing TPN contributes to *bacterial translocation*, whereby bacteria normally found in the GI tract cross the intestinal barrier, are found in the regional mesenteric lymph nodes, and give rise to generalized sepsis. However, there is insufficient evidence in humans that TPN causes atrophy of the intestinal mucosa or that enteral nutrition prevents bacterial translocation.[27,28]

Patients who are experiencing severe stress that greatly increases their nutrition needs (caused by major surgery, burns, or trauma) often benefit from tube feedings. Table 7.4 lists different enteral formula types and the nutrition indications for using each one. Individuals who require elemental formulas because of impaired digestion or absorption or specialized formulas for altered metabolic conditions usually require tube feeding because the unpleasant flavors of the free amino acids, peptides, or protein hydrolysates used in these formulas are very difficult to mask if taken in orally.

Immune-enhancing formulas have emerged as a means to protect and stimulate the immune system. Some enterally delivered nutrients that may benefit critically ill patients include fiber, the amino acids glutamine and arginine, the omega-3 (n-3) fatty acids, and RNA.[29] Fiber is not digested by humans but can be metabolized by gut bacteria to yield short-chain fatty acids, the primary fuel of the colon cells. Glutamine is the major fuel of the small intestinal cells. It is considered a nonessential amino acid, but it becomes conditionally essential in illness. It has been shown to improve mortality and infectious morbidity in critically ill patients.[30-32] Arginine is involved in protein synthesis and is a precursor of nitric oxide, a molecule that stimulates vasodilation in the GI tract and heart and mediates hepatic protein synthesis during sepsis.[29] The omega-3 fatty acids, derived primarily from fish oils, are involved in synthesis of eicosanoids (molecules with hormone-like activity)—prostaglandins, prostacyclin, and leukotrienes—and may modulate the inflammatory response.

TABLE 7.4 Enteral Formulas

Formula Type	Nutrition Uses	Clinical Examples	Examples of Commercial Products (Manufacturer)
Formulas Used When GI Tract Is Fully Functional			
Polymeric (standard): Contains whole proteins (10%–15% of calories), long-chain triglycerides (25%–40% of calories), and glucose polymers or oligosaccharides (50%–60% of calories); most provide 1 calorie/mL	Inability to ingest food Inability to consume enough to meet needs	Oral or esophageal cancer Coma, stroke Anorexia resulting from chronic illness Burns or trauma	Ensure (Abbott) Osmolite 1 Cal (Abbott) Boost (Nestlé) Nutren 1.0 (Nestlé)
High-protein: Same as polymeric except protein provides about 25% of calories	Same as polymeric plus mild catabolism and protein deficits	Trauma or burns Sepsis	Promote (Abbott) Replete (Nestlé)
Concentrated: Same as polymeric except concentrated to 2 calories/mL	Same as polymeric but fluid restriction needed	Heart failure Neurosurgery COPD Liver disease	TwoCal HN (Abbott) Nutren 2.0 (Nestlé)
Formulas Used When GI Function Is Impaired			
Elemental or predigested: Contains hydrolyzed (partially digested) protein, peptides (short chains of amino acids) and/or amino acids, little fat (<10% of calories) or high MCT, and glucose polymers or oligosaccharides; most provide 1 calorie/mL	Impaired digestion and/or absorption	Short bowel syndrome Radiation enteritis Inflammatory bowel disease	Vital (Abbott) Peptamen (Nestlé)
Diets for Specific Disease States[a]			
Renal failure: Concentrated in calories; low sodium, potassium, magnesium, phosphorus, and vitamins A and D; low protein for renal insufficiency; higher protein formulas for dialyzed patients	Renal insufficiency Dialysis	Predialysis Hemodialysis or peritoneal dialysis	Nepro (Abbott) Suplena (Abbott) Renalcal (Nestlé) Novasource Renal (Nestlé)
Hepatic failure: Enriched in BCAA; low sodium	Protein intolerance	Hepatic encephalopathy	NutriHep (Nestlé)
Pulmonary dysfunction: Low carbohydrate, high fat, concentrated in calories	Respiratory insufficiency	Ventilator dependence	Pulmocare (Abbott) Nutren Pulmonary (Nestlé)
Glucose intolerance: High fat, low carbohydrate (most contain fiber and fructose)	Glucose intolerance	Individuals with diabetes mellitus whose blood sugar is poorly controlled with standard formulas	Glucerna (Abbott) Diabetisource (Nestlé) Glytrol (Nestlé)
Critical care, wound healing: High protein; most contain MCT to improve fat absorption; some have increased zinc and vitamin C for wound healing; some are high in antioxidants (vitamin E, beta-carotene); some are enriched with arginine, glutamine, or omega-3 fatty acids	Critical illness	Severe trauma or burns Sepsis	Oxepa (Abbott) Impact (Nestlé)

[a]These diets may be beneficial for selected patients; costs and benefits must be considered.
BCAA, branched chain–enriched amino acid; *COPD,* chronic obstructive pulmonary disease; *GI,* gastrointestinal; *MCT,* medium-chain triglyceride.

A variety of commercial enteral feeding products are available, some of which are designed to meet the specialized needs of critically ill patients. Products designed for stressed patients with trauma or sepsis are usually rich in glutamine, arginine, branched amino acids (a major fuel source, especially for muscle), and antioxidant nutrients, such as selenium and vitamins C, E, and A.[33] The antioxidants help to reduce oxidative injury to the tissues (eg, from reperfusion injury). Despite the fact that immune-enhancing formulas may reduce the incidence of infectious complications, the efficacy and safety of these formulas in critically ill patients have not been clearly demonstrated.[34-37]

Early enteral nutrition, administered with the first 24 to 48 hours of critical illness, has been advocated as a way to reduce septic complications and improve feeding tolerance in critically ill patients. Although studies[38] have shown a lower risk of infection and decreased length of stay with early enteral nutrition, the benefit of early enteral nutrition compared with enteral nutrition delayed a few days remains controversial.[3,39] Current guidelines support the initiation of nutrition support in critically ill patients who will be unable to meet their nutrient needs orally for a period of 5 to 10 days.[3] To avoid complications associated with intestinal ischemia and infarction, enteral nutrition must be initiated only after fluid resuscitation and adequate perfusion have been achieved.[40,41]

Critically ill patients may not tolerate early enteral feeding because of impaired gastric motility, ileus, or medications administered in the early phase of illness. This is particularly true for patients receiving gastric enteral feeding.[42] The assessment of enteral feeding tolerance is an important aspect of nursing care. Monitoring of gastric residual volume is a method used to assess enteral feeding tolerance. However, evidence suggests that gastric residuals are insensitive and unreliable markers of tolerance to tube feeding.[43] There is little evidence to support a correlation between gastric residual volumes and tolerance to feedings, gastric emptying, and potential aspiration. Except in selected high-risk patients, there is little evidence to support holding tube feedings in patients with gastric residual volumes less than 400 mL.[43] The gastric residual volume should be evaluated within the context of other GI symptoms. Prokinetic agents, including metoclopramide and erythromycin, have been used to improve gastric motility and promote early enteral nutrition in critically ill patients.[44-46]

Enteral feeding access. Achievement of enteral access is the cornerstone of enteral nutrition therapy. Several techniques can be used to facilitate enteral access. These include surgical methods, bedside methods, fluoroscopy, endoscopy, air insufflation, and prokinetic agents.[9] Placement of feeding tubes beyond the stomach (postpyloric) eliminates some of the problems associated with gastric feeding intolerance. However, placement of postpyloric feeding tubes is time-consuming and may be costly. Tubes with weights on the proximal end are available; they were originally designed for postpyloric feeding in the belief that that they would be more likely than unweighted tubes to pass spontaneously through the pyloric sphincter. However, randomized trials with the two types of tubes have shown that unweighted tubes are more likely to migrate through the pylorus than weighted tubes.[47] The weights sometimes cause discomfort while being inserted through the nares. Therefore unweighted tubes may be preferable.

After the tube is placed, the correct location must be confirmed before feedings are started and regularly throughout the course of enteral feedings. Radiographs are the most accurate way of assessing tube placement, but repeated radiographs are costly and can expose the patient to excessive radiation. After correct placement has been confirmed, marking the exit site of the tube to check for movement is helpful. Alternative methods for confirming tube placement have been researched that attempt to verify placement in the stomach or small intestine. An inexpensive and relatively accurate alternative method involves assessing the pH of fluid removed from the feeding tube; some tubes are equipped with pH monitoring systems. Assessing the pH in fluid aspirated from the feeding tube is an alternative method for confirming tube placement.[48]

Location and type of feeding tube. Decisions regarding enteral access should be determined based on GI anatomy, gastric emptying, and aspiration risk.[3] Nasal intubation is the simplest and most commonly used route for enteral access. This method allows access to the stomach, duodenum, or jejunum. Tube enterostomy—a gastrostomy or jejunostomy—is used primarily for long-term feedings (6 to 12 weeks or more) and when obstruction makes the nasoenteral route inaccessible. Tube enterostomies may also be used for patients who are at risk for tube dislodgment because of severe agitation or confusion. A conventional gastrostomy or jejunostomy is often performed at the time of other abdominal surgery. The percutaneous endoscopic gastrostomy tube has become extremely popular because it can be inserted at the bedside without the use of general anesthetics. Percutaneous endoscopic jejunostomy tubes are also used.

Postpyloric feedings through nasoduodenal, nasojejunal, or jejunostomy tubes are commonly used when there is a high risk of pulmonary aspiration because the pyloric sphincter theoretically provides a barrier that reduces the risk of regurgitation and

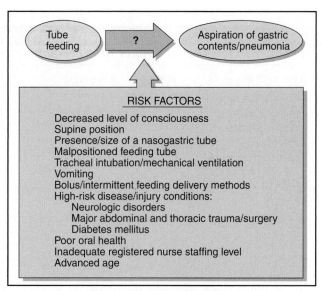

FIG. 7.4 Tube Feeding Sites.

aspiration.[49] However, some studies have demonstrated that gastric feeding is safe and not associated with an increased risk of aspiration.[50-52] Postpyloric feedings have an advantage over intragastric feedings for patients with delayed gastric emptying, such as patients with head injury, gastroparesis associated with uremia or diabetes, or postoperative ileus. Delivery of enteral nutrition into the small bowel is associated with improved tolerance,[53] higher calorie and protein intake,[54] and fewer GI complications.[41] Small bowel motility returns more quickly than gastric motility after surgery, and it is often possible to deliver transpyloric feedings within a few hours of injury or surgery.[49] Fig. 7.4 shows the locations of tube feeding sites.

Assessment and prevention of feeding tube complications. Nursing care of patients receiving enteral nutrition involves prevention and management of complications associated with the use of feeding tubes. Nursing management of these problems is summarized in Table 7.5. The skin around the feeding tube should be cleaned at least daily, and the tape around the tube should be replaced whenever loosened or soiled. Secure taping helps to prevent movement of the tube, which may irritate the nares or oral mucosa or result in accidental dislodgment. The tube must be taped in the dependent position to prevent unnecessary pressure and prevent necrosis. Commercially available attachment devices may be used to avoid inadvertent dislodgment.

To prevent mouth dryness, the patient is encouraged to breathe through the nose as much as possible. Frequent mouth care can clear the palate of unpleasant flavors from the formula and clean the teeth, tongue, and oral mucous membranes.

Dressings are used initially around gastrostomy insertion sites. The dressing is changed daily, and the skin is cleansed with soap and water. If leakage of gastric fluid occurs around a gastrostomy tube, the integrity of the gastrostomy balloon should be evaluated.[55] Karaya powder can be used to protect the peristomal skin from leakage. Fever, redness, purulent drainage, foul odor, or pain at the insertion site may indicate infection. Treatment may include application of a topical antibiotic ointment and daily cleansing with soap and water. Buried bumper syndrome may occur when the gastrostomy device disk, or bumper, is pulled tight against the abdominal wall. To prevent

QSEN   TABLE 7.5   QSEN: Patient Safety

Nursing Management of Enteral Tube Feeding Complications

Complication	Contributing Factors	Prevention or Correction
Pulmonary aspiration (signs and symptoms include tachypnea, shortness of breath, hypoxia, and infiltrate on chest radiographs)	Feeding tube positioned in esophagus or respiratory tract	Confirm proper tube placement before administering any feeding; check tube placement at least every 4–8 h during continuous feedings; consider intermittent feedings.
	Regurgitation of formula	Elevate the head to 30–45 degrees during feedings unless contraindicated; if the head cannot be raised, position the patient in lateral (especially right lateral, which facilitates gastric emptying) or prone position to improve drainage of vomitus from the mouth. Consider giving feeding into small bowel rather than stomach in high-risk patients. Metoclopramide may improve gastric emptying and decrease risk of regurgitation. Evaluate feeding tolerance every 2 h initially, then less frequently as condition becomes stable. Intolerance may be manifested by bloating, abdominal distention and pain, lack of stool and flatus, diminished or absent bowel sounds, tense abdomen, increased tympany, nausea and vomiting, residual volume >200 mL aspirated from NG tube or >100 mL aspirated from gastrostomy tube, although a high residual volume in the absence of other abnormal findings may not be grounds for stopping feedings (measuring residual volumes is a controversial practice; see tube occlusion below). If intolerance is suspected, abdominal radiographs may be obtained to check for distended gastric bubble, distended loops of bowel, or air-fluid levels.
Diarrhea	Medications with GI side effects (eg, antibiotics, digitalis, laxatives, magnesium-containing antacids, quinidine, caffeine)	Evaluate the patient's medications to determine their potential for causing diarrhea, and consult the pharmacist if necessary.
	Predisposing illness (eg, short bowel syndrome, inflammatory bowel disease)	Use continuous feedings; consider a formula with MCT and/or soluble fiber.
	Hypertonic formula or medications (eg, oral suspensions of antibiotics, potassium, other electrolytes), which can cause dumping syndrome	Evaluate formula administration procedures to ensure that feedings are not being given by bolus infusion; administer formula continuously or by slow intermittent infusion. Dilute enteral medications well.
	Bacterial contamination of formula	Use scrupulously clean technique in administering tube feedings; prepare formula with sterile water if there are any concerns about the safety of the water supply or if the patient is seriously immunocompromised; keep opened containers of formula refrigerated, and discard them within 24 h; discard enteral feeding containers and administration sets every 24 h; hang formula no more than 4–8 h unless it comes prepackaged in sterile administration sets.
	Fecal impaction with seepage of liquid stool around impaction	Perform a digital rectal examination to rule out impaction; see guidelines for prevention of constipation below.
	Lactose intolerance	Use lactose-free formula.
Constipation	Low-residue formula, creating little fecal bulk, lack of fiber	Consider using a fiber-containing formula; ensure fluid intake is adequate; stool softeners may be beneficial.
Tube occlusion	Medications administered by tube that physically plug the tube or coagulate the formula, causing it to clog the tube	If medications must be given by tube, avoid use of crushed tablets; consult with the pharmacist to determine whether medications can be dispensed as elixirs or suspensions. Irrigate tube with water before and after administering any medication; never add any medication to formula unless the two are known to be compatible.
	Sedimentation of formula	Irrigate tube every 4–8 h during continuous feedings and after every intermittent feeding. If residuals are measured, flush tube thoroughly after returning formula to the stomach because gastric juices left in tube may cause precipitation of formula. Instilling pancreatic enzymes into tube can remove or prevent some occlusions.
Gastric retention	Delayed gastric emptying related to head trauma, sepsis, diabetic or uremic gastroparesis, electrolyte balance, or other illness	The cause must be corrected if possible. Consult with the physician about use of postpyloric feedings or prokinetic agents to stimulate gastric emptying. Encourage the patient to lie in the right lateral position frequently, unless contraindicated.

GI, gastrointestinal; *MCT*, medium-chain triglyceride; *NG*, nasogastric.
Modified from Moore MC. *Pocket Guide to Nutritional Assessment and Care*. 6th ed. St. Louis: Mosby; 2009.

this, it is necessary to minimize tension on the disk. The tube may also become dislodged. A new gastrostomy tube needs to be reinserted within hours to prevent closure of the stoma.

Feeding tube occlusion. Regular irrigation helps to prevent feeding tube occlusion. Usually, irrigation with 20 to 30 mL of warm water every 3 to 4 hours during continuous feedings and before and after intermittent feedings and medication administration can maintain patency.[3] The volume of irrigant may have to be reduced for fluid restriction. Automatic enteral flush pumps are also available. Although cranberry juice or cola beverages are sometimes used in an effort to reduce the incidence of tube occlusion, water is the preferred irrigant because it has been shown to be superior in maintaining tube patency.[56] Tube occlusion may occur as a result of stagnant formula, inadequately crushed pills, or medication interactions with formula. Enteral infusion pumps should be used, and tubes should be flushed before feeding infusions are paused. Liquid medications or elixirs should be used when possible to avoid tube occlusion with pill fragments. The use of pancreatic enzymes in the feeding tube appears to reduce the risk of tube clogging and may be successful in removing a clog after it has formed.[56,57]

Aspiration. Pulmonary aspiration of enteral formulas and subsequent pneumonia is a serious complication of enteral feeding in critically ill patients. Risk factors for aspiration of enteral feeding include decreased level of consciousness, supine position, and swallowing disorders.[58] Fig. 7.5 shows the risk factors for aspiration in patients on tube feeds. To reduce the risk of pulmonary aspiration of formula during enteral feeding, the nurse must keep the head of the bed elevated unless contraindicated; temporarily stop feedings when the patient must be supine for prolonged periods; position the patient in the right lateral decubitus position when possible to encourage gastric emptying; use postpyloric feeding methods; keep the cuff of the endotracheal tube inflated as much as possible during enteral feeding, if applicable; and be alert to any increase in abdominal distention.

Two bedside methods have been used in the past to detect pulmonary aspiration of enteral feeding. One is the addition of blue dye to the enteral formula and observation of the patient for any dye-tinged tracheal secretions, and the other is glucose testing of tracheal secretions to detect the presence of the glucose-containing enteral formula. The glucose oxidase method may cause false-positive reactions if blood is present. It has a low sensitivity when low-glucose formulas are used, and it has questionable specificity.[59] There is no established protocol for blue dye testing. Although it has been used routinely in clinical practice for several years, there is no evidence to support its efficacy or safety. It lacks sensitivity and specificity in ruling out aspiration. Numerous clinical reports of systemic absorption of blue dye and adverse outcomes have been described.[60,61] Glucose oxidase testing and blue food coloring are not recommended as appropriate methods for detecting aspiration of enteral feedings.[60,62]

Gastrointestinal complications. Diarrhea is common in patients receiving enteral nutrition, with an incidence of 2% to 70%.[63] No single definition has been established for diarrhea. Current definitions include various stool frequencies, volumes, and weights.[64] Diarrhea in enterally fed critically ill patients has many factors. Common causes include medications, malabsorption, formula contamination, and low-fiber formulas. While the cause of diarrhea is being determined, nurses must provide adequate fluid and electrolyte replacement, maintain skin integrity, and administer antidiarrheal agents. To prevent complications, stool must be checked for infection, especially *Clostridium difficile*, before antidiarrheal medications can be administered.[65] Constipation is a complication of enteral feeding that may result from dehydration, bed rest, opioid administration, or lack of adequate fiber in enteral formulas. Pasty stools are normal in enterally fed patients. Bowel movements should be assessed daily. The nurse must ensure adequate fluid and fiber intake, promote optimal mobility, and administer laxatives and stool softeners as necessary.[66]

Formula delivery. Careful attention to administration of tube feedings can prevent many complications. Very clean or aseptic technique in the handling and administration of the formula can help prevent bacterial contamination and a resultant infection. When using cans of formula transferred to a feeding container, wash hands and tops of cans before opening, hang enough formula for just 8 hours of infusion, and do not add new formula to formula already hanging. Closed systems that use a prefilled sterile container that can be spiked with the enteral tube are also available.

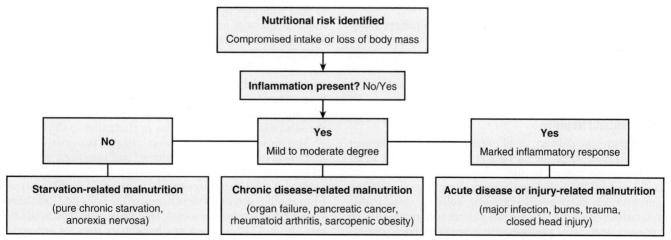

FIG. 7.5 Factors That Influence Aspiration in Tube-Fed Patients. (From Metheny NA. Risk factors for aspiration. *JPEN J Parenter Enteral Nutr.* 2002;26[6 suppl]:S26.)

Tube feedings may be administered intermittently or continuously. Bolus feedings, which are intermittent feedings delivered rapidly into the stomach or small bowel, are likely to cause distention, vomiting, and dumping syndrome with diarrhea. Instead of using bolus feedings, nurses can gradually drip intermittent feedings, with each feeding lasting 20 to 30 minutes or longer, to promote optimal assimilation. The question of which feeding schedule—continuous or intermittent—is superior for critically ill patients remains unanswered.

Adequacy of enteral nutrition. Critically ill patients have so many needs for care that it is easy to overlook the importance of nutrition. Many studies have shown that critically ill patients receive considerably less enteral nutrition than required.[67-70] This is a complication unique to enteral nutrition and is not observed with TPN. The discrepancy in nutrition intake has a variety of causes, including patient factors (eg, high residual volumes, emesis, abdominal distention), tube-related factors (eg, occlusion, malposition), and treatment-related factors (eg, interruptions caused by procedures, airway management, and medications).[68] Inadequate enteral nutrition delivery is also related to physicians' prescribing practices in the critical care unit.[70] The enteral delivery practices in the critical care unit and clinicians' concerns about aspiration may lead to inappropriate and prolonged interruptions in enteral feeding. Chest physiotherapy, suspicion of formula in the tracheobronchial secretions, and excessive gastric retention of formula are examples of appropriate reasons for stopping feedings. Evidence-based enteral nutrition delivery practices are needed for optimal nutrition outcomes in critically ill patients.

Tubing and catheter misconnections. Tubing and catheter or Luer connector (small device used in the connection of many medical components and accessories) misconnection errors have gained attention, with The Joint Commission issuing a *Sentinel Event Alert* in April 2006.[71] Examples of misconnection errors include misconnecting an enteric feeding tube into an intravenous catheter or injection of an intravenous fluid into a tracheostomy cuff inflation tube. These misconnection errors are potentially life-threatening, and increased awareness and precautions can improve patient safety. The following strategies should be followed to minimize risk for tubing and catheter misconnections[72]:

- Label all tubes and catheters, especially arterial, epidural, and intrathecal catheters.
- Trace lines back to their origins when initiating any new device or infusion.
- Standardize a line reconciliation process with patient hand-offs.
- Consider routing tubes and catheters with different purposes in different, standardized directions.
- Never use a standard Luer syringe for oral medications or enteric feedings.

Total Parenteral Nutrition

TPN refers to the delivery of all nutrients by the intravenous route. It is used when the GI tract is not functional or when nutrition needs cannot be met solely through the GI tract. Candidates for TPN include patients who have severely impaired absorption (eg, short bowel syndrome, collagen vascular diseases, radiation enteritis), intestinal obstruction, peritonitis, or prolonged ileus. Some postoperative, trauma, or burn patients may need TPN to supplement the nutrient intake that they are able to tolerate by the enteral route.

Types of parenteral nutrition. TPN involves administration of highly concentrated dextrose (25% to 70%), providing a rich source of calories. These highly concentrated dextrose solutions are hyperosmolar, up to 1800 mOsm/L, and must be delivered through a central vein.[73] Peripheral parenteral nutrition (PPN) has a glucose concentration of 5% to 10% and may be delivered safely through a peripheral vein. PPN solution delivers nutrition support in a large volume that cannot be tolerated by patients who require fluid restriction. It provides short-term nutrition support for a few days to less than 2 weeks.

Regardless of the route of administration, PPN and TPN provide glucose, fat, protein, electrolytes, vitamins, and trace elements. Although dextrose–amino acid solutions are commonly thought of as good growth media for microorganisms, they actually suppress the growth of most organisms usually associated with catheter-related sepsis except yeasts. However, because the many manipulations required to prepare solutions increase the possibility of contamination, TPN solutions are best used with caution. They should be prepared under laminar flow conditions in the pharmacy, with avoidance of additions on the nursing unit. Solution containers need to be inspected for cracks or leaks before hanging, and solutions must be discarded within 24 hours of hanging. An in-line 0.22-micron filter, which eliminates all microorganisms but not endotoxins, may be used in the administration of solutions. However, use of the filter cannot be substituted for good aseptic technique.

Nursing management of potential complications. Nursing management of patients receiving TPN includes catheter care, administration of solutions, prevention or correction of complications, and evaluation of patient responses to intravenous feedings. Table 7.6 describes nursing management of TPN complications. Evaluation of the patient's response is discussed later in this chapter.

Because TPN requires an indwelling catheter in a central vein, it carries an increased risk for sepsis and potential insertion-related complications, such as pneumothorax and hemothorax. Air embolism is also more likely with central vein TPN. Patients requiring multiple intravenous therapies and frequent blood sampling usually have multilumen central venous catheters, and TPN is often infused through these catheters.

Some clinical studies have reported that rates of catheter-related sepsis are higher with multilumen catheters; others have found no difference compared with single-lumen catheters.[74] Patients requiring multilumen catheters are likely to be very ill and immunocompromised, and scrupulous aseptic technique is essential in maintaining their multilumen catheters. The manipulation involved in frequent changes of intravenous fluid and obtaining blood specimens through these catheters increases the risk of catheter contamination. Peripherally inserted central catheters allow central venous access through long catheters inserted in peripheral sites. This reduces the risk of complications associated with percutaneous cannulation of the subclavian vein and provides an alternative to PPN.[75]

The indwelling central venous catheter provides an excellent nidus for infection. Catheter-related infections arise from endogenous skin flora, contamination of the catheter hub, seeding of the catheter by organisms carried in the bloodstream from another site, or contamination of the infusate. Good handwashing and scrupulous aseptic technique in all aspects of catheter care and TPN delivery are the primary steps for prevention of catheter-related infections. Other measures to reduce the incidence of catheter-related infections include using maximal barrier precautions (eg, cap, mask, sterile gloves, sterile drape) at the time of insertion, tunneling the catheter underneath the skin, use of a 2% chlorhexidine preparation for skin cleansing, no routine replacement of the central venous catheter for prevention of infection, and use of antiseptic-impregnated or antibiotic-impregnated central venous catheters.[76]

Metabolic complications associated with parenteral nutrition include glucose intolerance and electrolyte imbalance. Slow advancement of the rate of TPN (25 mL/h) to goal rate allows pancreatic adjustment to the dextrose load. Capillary blood glucose should be monitored every 4 to 6 hours. Insulin can be added to the TPN solution or can be infused as a separate drip to control glucose levels. Rapid cessation of TPN may not lead to hypoglycemia; however, tapering the infusion over 2 to 4 hours is recommended.[77]

Serum electrolytes are obtained on starting TPN. During critical illness, levels should be monitored and corrected daily and then weekly or twice weekly after the patient is more stable. The refeeding syndrome is a potentially lethal condition characterized by generalized fluid and electrolyte imbalance. It occurs as a potential complication after initiation of oral, enteral, or parenteral nutrition in malnourished patients. During chronic

QSEN   TABLE 7.6   QSEN: Patient Safety
Nursing Management of Total Parenteral Nutrition Complications

Complication	Clinical Manifestations	Prevention or Correction
Catheter-related sepsis	Fever, chills, glucose intolerance, positive blood culture	Use aseptic technique when handling catheter, IV tubing, and TPN solutions. Hang a bottle of TPN no longer than 24 h and lipid emulsion no longer than 12–24 h. Use an in-line 0.22-micron filter with TPN to remove microorganisms. Avoid drawing blood, infusing blood or blood products, piggybacking other IV solutions into TPN IV tubing, or attaching manometers or transducers through the TPN infusion line, if possible. If catheter-related sepsis is suspected, remove the catheter or assist in changing the catheter over a guidewire, and administer antibiotics as ordered.
Air embolism	Dyspnea, cyanosis, apnea, tachycardia, hypotension, "millwheel" heart murmur; mortality estimated at 50% (depends on quantity of air entering)	Use Luer-Lok connections; use an in-line air-eliminating filter. Have the patient perform a Valsalva maneuver during tubing changes; if the patient is on a ventilator, change tubing quickly at end expiration. Maintain occlusive dressing over catheter site for at least 24 h after removing catheter to prevent air entry through catheter tract. If air embolism is suspected, place the patient in left lateral decubitus and Trendelenburg positions (to trap air in the apex of the right ventricle, away from the outflow tract), and administer oxygen and CPR as needed; immediately notify physician, who may attempt to aspirate air from the heart.
Pneumothorax	Chest pain, dyspnea, hypoxemia, hypotension, radiographic evidence, needle aspiration of air from pleural space	Thoroughly explain the catheter insertion procedure to the patient because when a patient moves or breathes erratically, he or she is more likely to sustain pleural damage. Obtain a radiograph after insertion or insertion attempt. If pneumothorax is suspected, assist with needle aspiration or chest tube insertion, if necessary.
Central venous thrombosis	Edema of neck, shoulder, and arm on same side as catheter; development of collateral circulation on chest; pain in insertion site; drainage of TPN from the insertion site; positive findings on venography	Follow measures to prevent sepsis; repeated or traumatic catheterizations are most likely to result in thrombosis. If thrombosis is confirmed, remove the catheter, and administer anticoagulants and antibiotics, as ordered.
Catheter occlusion or semiocclusion	No flow or sluggish flow through the catheter	If the infusion is stopped temporarily, flush catheter with saline or heparinized saline. If the catheter appears to be occluded, attempt to aspirate the clot; if this is ineffective, the physician may order a thrombolytic agent such as streptokinase or alteplase (tPA) instilled in the catheter.
Hypoglycemia	Diaphoresis, shakiness, confusion, loss of consciousness	Infuse TPN within 10% of ordered rate; monitor blood glucose until stable. If hypoglycemia is present, administer oral carbohydrate; if the patient is unconscious or oral intake is contraindicated, the physician may order an IV bolus of dextrose.
Hyperglycemia	Thirst, headache, lethargy, increased urinary output	Administer TPN within 10% of ordered rate; monitor blood glucose level at least daily until stable. The patient may require insulin added to TPN if hyperglycemia is persistent; sudden appearance of hyperglycemia in a patient who was previously tolerating the same glucose load may indicate the onset of sepsis.
Hypertriglyceridemia	Serum triglyceride concentrations elevated (especially serious if >400 mg/dL); serum may appear turbid	Monitor serum triglycerides at baseline, 6 h after lipid infusion, and at least 3 times weekly until stable in patients receiving lipid emulsions; reduce lipid infusion rate or administer low-dose heparin with lipid emulsions as ordered if elevated levels are observed.

CPR, cardiopulmonary resuscitation; *IV*, intravenous; *tPA*, tissue plasminogen activator; *TPN*, total parenteral nutrition.
Modified from Moore MC. *Pocket Guide to Nutritional Assessment and Care.* 6th ed. St. Louis: Mosby; 2009.

starvation, several compensatory metabolic changes occur. The reintroduction of carbohydrates and amino acids leads to increased insulin production. This creates an anabolic environment that increases intracellular demand for phosphorus, potassium, magnesium, vitamins, and minerals.[78] These metabolic demands result in severe shifts from the extracellular compartment. Increased insulin levels also result in fluid retention. Severe hypophosphatemia, hypokalemia, and hypomagnesemia result in altered cardiac, GI, and neurologic function. In particular, hypophosphatemia causes a decrease in 2,3-diphosphoglycerate and limits the many reactions that require adenosine triphosphate. Hypophosphatemia and other electrolyte deficiencies may lead to respiratory failure, congestive heart failure, and dysrhythmias.

It is important to anticipate refeeding syndrome in patients who may be at risk. Patients with chronic malnutrition or underfeeding, chronic alcoholism, or anorexia nervosa, as well as patients maintained NPO for several days with evidence of stress, are at risk for refeeding syndrome.[79] In high-risk patients, nutrition support should be started cautiously at 25% to 50% of required calories and slowly advanced over 3 to 4 days as tolerated. Close monitoring of serum electrolytes before and during feeding is essential. Normal values do not always reflect total body stores. Correction of preexisting electrolyte imbalances are necessary before initiation of feeding. Continued monitoring and supplementation with electrolytes and vitamins are necessary throughout the first week of nutrition support.[79]

Lipid emulsion. Lipids or fat emulsions provide calories for energy and prevent essential fatty acid depletion. In contrast to dextrose–amino acid solutions, intravenous lipid emulsions provide a rich environment for the growth of bacteria and fungi, including *Candida albicans.* Lipid emulsions cannot be filtered through an in-line 0.22-micron filter because some particles in the emulsions have larger diameters than this. Lipids may be infused into the TPN line downstream from the filter. No other medications should be infused into a line containing lipids or TPN. Lipid emulsions are handled with strict asepsis, and they must be discarded within 12 to 24 hours of hanging. There is a trend toward mixing lipid emulsions with dextrose–amino acid TPN solutions; these are called three-in-one solutions or total nutrient admixtures. Consolidating the nutrients in one container is more economical and saves nursing time, although total nutrient admixture solutions may be less stable.[73]

Monitoring and Evaluation of Nutrition Support

A multidisciplinary approach is required in evaluating the effects of nutrition support on clinical outcomes. Assessment of response to nutrition support is an ongoing process that involves anthropometric measurements, physical examination, and biochemical evaluation. Daily monitoring of nutrition intake is an important aspect of critical care and is a key element in preventing problems associated with underfeeding and overfeeding. Daily weights and the maintenance of accurate intake-and-output records are crucial for evaluating nutrition progress and the state of hydration in the patient receiving nutrition support. Serum levels of electrolytes, calcium, phosphorus, and magnesium serve as a guide to the amount of these nutrients that must be supplied. Blood urea nitrogen and creatinine levels reflect the adequacy of renal function to handle nutrition support. Blood glucose is an indicator of the patient's tolerance of the carbohydrate, and prealbumin is an indicator of the adequacy of nutrition support. Serum triglyceride concentrations

(in patients receiving intravenous lipid emulsions) reflect the ability of the tissues to metabolize the lipids.

The Society of Critical Care Medicine and the American Society for Parenteral and Enteral Nutrition published "Guidelines for the Provision and Assessment of Nutrition Support Therapy in the Adult Critically Ill Patient." The publication is based on an extensive review of 307 articles and is intended for the care of critically ill adults who require a stay of more than 3 days in the critical care area. All practitioners who care for this target population are encouraged to become familiar with these evidence-based guidelines.[3]

It is within the scope of practice for critical care nurses to calculate caloric requirements and analyze daily caloric delivery, advocate for early nutrition support, and minimize feeding interruptions through careful patient assessment and interruption analysis. In addition to monitoring changes in weight and laboratory values, the nurse is the health care team member who has the most constant contact with the patient and who is highly qualified to evaluate feeding tolerance and adequacy of delivery.

NUTRITION AND CARDIOVASCULAR ALTERATIONS

Diet and cardiovascular disease may interact in various ways. Excessive nutrient intake—manifested by overweight or obesity and a diet rich in cholesterol and saturated fat—is a risk factor for development of arteriosclerotic heart disease. However, the consequences of chronic myocardial insufficiency can include malnutrition.

Nutrition Assessment in Cardiovascular Alterations

A nutrition assessment provides the nurse and other members of the health care team the information necessary to plan the patient's nutrition care and education. Common findings in the nutrition assessment of patients with cardiovascular disease are summarized in Box 7.4. The major nutrition concerns relate to appropriateness of body weight and the levels of serum lipids and blood pressure.

BOX 7.4 Common Findings in the Nutrition Assessment of Patients With Cardiovascular Disease

Anthropometric Measurements
- Overweight or obesity; underweight (cardiac cachexia)
- Abdominal fat: increased risk of cardiovascular disease with waist measurement >102 cm (>40 inches) for men and >88 cm (>35 inches) for women

Biochemical (Laboratory) Data
- Elevated total serum cholesterol, low-density lipoprotein cholesterol, and triglycerides

Clinical Findings
- Wasting of muscle and subcutaneous fat (cardiac cachexia)

Diet or Health History
- Sedentary lifestyle
- Excessive intake of saturated fat, cholesterol, salt, or alcohol
- Angina, respiratory difficulty, or fatigue during eating
- Medications that impair appetite (eg, digitalis preparations, quinidine)

Nutrition Intervention and Education in Cardiovascular Alterations

Myocardial Infarction

Short-term interventions. In the early period after a myocardial infarction, nutrition interventions and education are designed to reduce angina, cardiac workload, and risk of dysrhythmia. Meal size, caffeine intake, and food temperatures are some dietary factors that are of concern. Small, frequent snacks are preferable to larger meals for patients with severe myocardial compromise or postprandial angina.

If caffeine is included in the diet, its effects should be monitored. Because caffeine is a stimulant, it may increase heart rate and myocardial oxygen demand. In the United States and in most industrial nations, coffee is the richest source of caffeine in the diet, with approximately 150 mg of caffeine per 180 mL (6 fluid oz) of coffee. In comparison, the caffeine content of the same volume of tea or cola is approximately 50 mg or 20 mg, respectively. Very hot or very cold foods should be avoided because they can potentially trigger vagal or other neural input and cause cardiac dysrhythmias.

Long-Term Changes

The focus of nutrition and lifestyle interventions for a person who has had one myocardial infarction or is at increased risk for heart disease are directed at primary and secondary prevention strategies. These strategies include lifestyle interventions, such as decreased dietary intake of saturated fats, *trans* fats, and refined carbohydrates. Most of the education regarding these changes takes place in the rehabilitation period. However, during the acute phase of recovery, the patient and family may have an interest in learning more about risk reduction.

For an individual who is overweight or obese, gradual weight loss (0.45 to 0.9 kg [1 to 2 lb] per week) is the goal.[80] Weight loss can be achieved through moderate exercise (with the physician's approval) and reduction of dietary intake by 500 to 1000 kcal/day. Dietary guidelines from the American Heart Association support lipid-lowering therapy through adoption of a low-saturated-fat, low-refined-carbohydrate, and fiber-rich diet; maintenance of a healthy weight; and regular physical activity.[81] Recommendations include low-density lipoprotein cholesterol levels of 100 mg/dL or less as optimal and increased focus on the metabolic syndrome.[82,83] Metabolic syndrome is a group of risk factors (Table 7.7) associated with increased risk for cardiovascular disease and diabetes. The primary target for patients with metabolic syndrome is weight reduction reinforced with increased physical activity, as it is expected that lipid parameters and insulin resistance will be improved with changes in lifestyle habits.[84,85]

Elevated plasma levels of homocysteine, derived from the essential amino acid *methionine*, are a risk factor for heart disease. Homocysteine can damage the endothelium of the blood vessels, cause proliferation of smooth muscle in the vessel walls, and activate platelets and the coagulation cascade, contributing to thrombus formation. Adequate amounts of folic acid and vitamins B_6 and B_{12} are known to reduce homocysteine levels. Although elevated homocysteine levels remain a risk marker for heart disease, current research does not support treatment with folic acid and vitamins B_6 and B_{12} in lowering homocysteine levels to prevent risk of death from cardiovascular disease.[86]

For hypertensive cardiac disease, sodium chloride restriction is recommended. Some individuals have been shown to be more salt sensitive than others, and this salt sensitivity contributes to hypertension. Adoption of a healthy lifestyle is critical for the prevention of high blood pressure and is an indispensable part of the management of patients with hypertension.[87] A 10-lb weight loss reduces blood pressure. Adoption of the Dietary Approaches to Stop Hypertension (DASH)[88] eating plan also benefits blood pressure. The DASH diet is rich in fruits, vegetables, and low-fat dairy products with a reduced content of dietary cholesterol and reduced levels of saturated and total fat. It is rich in potassium and calcium content. Dietary sodium should be reduced to no more than 100 mmol/day (2.4 g of sodium). Alcohol intake should be limited to no more than 1 ounce (30 mL) of ethanol per day in men and no more than 0.5 ounce of ethanol in women.

Heart Failure

Nutrition intervention in heart failure is designed to reduce fluid retained within the body, reducing the preload. Because fluid accompanies sodium, limitation of sodium is necessary to reduce fluid retention. Specific interventions include limiting salt intake, usually to 2 g/day or less, and limiting fluid intake as appropriate.[89] If fluid is restricted, the daily fluid allowance is usually 1.5 to 2 L/day, which includes fluids in the diet and fluids given with medications and for other purposes (see "Heart Failure" in Chapter 14).

Cardiac Cachexia

Malnutrition is common in patients with heart failure. The term *cachexia* is derived from the Greek words *kakos*, meaning "bad," and *hexis*, meaning "condition." Cachexia is characterized by weight loss, anorexia, weakness, early satiety, and edema[90] and is seen in a variety of disorders, including cancer and heart failure. It is well recognized as an independent predictor of higher mortality in patients with heart failure.[91] Sodium and

TABLE 7.7	Metabolic Syndrome Definition[a]
Risk Factor	**Defining Level**
Elevated waist circumference	
Men	≥40 inches (≥102 cm)
Women	≥35 inches (≥88 cm)
Elevated triglycerides	≥150 mg/dL (≥1.7 mmol/L)
	or on medication treatment for elevated triglycerides
Reduced HDL cholesterol	
Men	<40 mg/dL (<1.03 mmol/L)
Women	<50 mg/dL (<1.3 mmol/L)
	or on medication treatment for reduced HDL cholesterol
Elevated blood pressure	≥130 mm Hg systolic or ≥85 mm Hg diastolic
	or on antihypertensive medication treatment in a patient with a history of hypertension
Elevated fasting glucose	≥100 mg/dL (≥5.6 mmol/L)
	or on medication treatment for elevated glucose

[a]Metabolic syndrome is diagnosed when 3 of 5 of the listed risk factors are present.
HDL, high-density lipoprotein.
Adapted from Grundy SM, et al. Diagnosis and management of the metabolic syndrome: an American Heart Association/National Heart, Lung, and Blood Institute scientific statement. *Circulation.* 2005;112:2735.

fluid restriction are appropriate interventions. It is important to concentrate nutrients into as small a volume as possible and to serve small amounts frequently, rather than three large meals daily, which may overwhelm the patient. The patient should be encouraged to consume calorie-dense foods and supplements.

Because the patient is likely to tire quickly and to experience anorexia (lack or loss of appetite), enteral tube feeding may be necessary. Most commonly used tube feeding formulas provide 1 calorie/mL, but more concentrated products are available to provide adequate nutrients in a smaller volume. The nurse must monitor the fluid status of these patients carefully when they are receiving nutrition support. Assessing breath sounds and observing for the presence and severity of peripheral edema and changes in body weight are performed daily or more frequently. A consistent weight gain of more than 0.11 to 0.22 kg (0.25 to 0.5 lb) per day usually indicates fluid retention rather than gain of fat and muscle mass.

NUTRITION AND PULMONARY ALTERATIONS

Malnutrition has extremely adverse effects on respiratory function, decreasing surfactant production, diaphragmatic mass, vital capacity, and immunocompetence. Patients with acute respiratory disorders find it difficult to consume adequate oral nutrients and can rapidly become malnourished. Individuals who have an acute illness superimposed on chronic respiratory problems are also at high risk. Nearly three-fourths of patients with chronic obstructive pulmonary disease have weight loss.[92] However, patients with undernutrition and end-stage chronic obstructive pulmonary disease often cannot tolerate the increase in metabolic demand that occurs during refeeding. They also are at significant risk for development of cor pulmonale and may fail to tolerate the fluid required for delivery of enteral or parenteral nutrition support. Prevention of severe nutrition deficits, rather than correction of deficits after they have occurred, is important in nutrition management of these patients (see "Acute Respiratory Failure" and "Long-Term Mechanical Ventilator Dependence" in Chapter 19).

Nutrition Assessment in Pulmonary Alterations

Common findings in nutrition assessment related to pulmonary alterations are summarized in Box 7.5. Patients with respiratory compromise are especially vulnerable to the effects of fluid volume excess and must be assessed continually for this complication, particularly during enteral and parenteral feeding.

Nutrition Intervention and Education in Pulmonary Alterations
Prevent or Correct Undernutrition and Underweight

The nurse and dietitian work together to encourage oral intake in undernourished or potentially undernourished patients who are capable of eating. Small, frequent feedings are especially important because a very full stomach can interfere with diaphragmatic movement. Mouth care should be provided before meals and snacks to clear the palate of the taste of sputum and medications. Administering bronchodilators with food can help to reduce the gastric irritation caused by these medications.

Many patients require enteral tube feeding or TPN because of anorexia, dyspnea, debilitation, or need for ventilatory

> **BOX 7.5 Common Findings in the Nutrition Assessment of Patients With Pulmonary Disease**
>
> **Anthropometric Measurements**
> - Underweight
>
> **Biochemical (Laboratory) Data**
> - Elevated Pco_2 related to overfeeding
>
> **Clinical Findings**
> - Edema, dyspnea, signs of pulmonary edema related to fluid volume excess
>
> **Diet or Health History**
> - Poor food intake related to dyspnea, unpleasant taste in the mouth from sputum production or bronchodilator therapy; endotracheal intubation preventing oral intake

support. It is especially important for the nurse to be alert to the risk of pulmonary aspiration in a patient with an artificial airway. To reduce the risk of pulmonary aspiration during enteral tube feeding, keep the patient's head elevated at least 45 degrees during feedings, unless contraindicated; keep the cuff of the artificial airway inflated during feeding, if possible; monitor the patient for increasing abdominal distention; and check tube placement before each feeding (if intermittent) or at least every 4 to 8 hours if feedings are continuous.

Avoid Overfeeding

Overfeeding of total calories or of carbohydrate or lipid alone can impair pulmonary function. Vco_2 increases when carbohydrate is relied on as the primary energy source. This is unlikely to be significant in a patient who is eating foods. Instead, it is an iatrogenic complication of TPN, in which glucose is often the predominant calorie source, or occasionally of tube feeding in a patient with a formula with very high carbohydrates. Excessive calorie intake can increase $Paco_2$ sufficiently to make it difficult to wean a patient from the ventilator. A balanced regimen with lipids and carbohydrates providing the nonprotein calories is optimal for a patient with respiratory compromise, and the patient needs to be reassessed continually to ensure that caloric intake is not excessive.[3]

Excessive lipid intake can impair capillary gas exchange in the lungs, although this is not usually sufficient to produce an increase in $Paco_2$ or decrease in Pao_2.[93] However, a patient with severe respiratory alteration may be further compromised by lipid overdose. If lipid intake is maintained at no more than 2 g/kg per day, lipid excess is rarely a problem. Serum triglyceride levels greater than 400 mg/dL may indicate inadequate lipid clearance and a need to decrease the lipid dosage.

Prevent Fluid Volume Excess

Pulmonary edema and failure of the right side of the heart, which may be precipitated by fluid volume excess, further worsen the status of a patient with respiratory compromise. Maintaining careful intake and output records allows for accurate assessment of fluid balance. Usually the patient requires no more than 35 to 40 mL/kg per day of fluid. For a patient receiving nutrition support, fluid intake can be reduced by using 20% lipid emulsions as a source of calories, by using tube feeding formulas that provide at least 2 calories/mL (the dietitian can recommend appropriate formulas), and by choosing oral supplements that are low in fluid. Additionally, powdered glucose polymers or powdered protein products can be used to increase caloric intake without increasing volume. The nurse plays a valuable role in continually reassessing the patient's state of hydration and alerting other team members to changes that may indicate the need for an increase or decrease in fluid intake.

NUTRITION AND NEUROLOGIC ALTERATIONS

Because neurologic disorders such as stroke and closed head injury tend to be long-term problems, good nutrition care is necessary to prevent nutrition deficits and promote well-being.

Nutrition Assessment in Neurologic Alterations

Nutrition-related assessment findings vary widely in patients with neurologic alterations, depending on the type of disorder present. Some common assessment findings are listed in Box 7.6.

Nutrition Intervention and Education in Neurologic Alterations

Prevention or Correction of Nutrition Deficits

Oral feedings. Patients with dysphagia or weakness of the swallowing musculature often experience the greatest difficulty in swallowing foods that are dry or thin liquids, such as water, that are difficult to control. For these patients, the nurse, the dietitian, and the speech therapist can work together to plan suitable meals and evaluate patient acceptance and tolerance (see "Stroke" in Chapter 23).

Soft, moist foods are usually easier to swallow than dry foods. An upright sitting position is preferable during meals, if possible, to allow gravity to facilitate effective swallowing. Water and other thin liquids may be especially difficult for a person with swallowing dysfunction to manage. Beverages may be thickened with commercial thickening products, with infant cereal, or with yogurt if the patient has difficulty swallowing thin fluids. Fruit nectars may be better tolerated than thinner juices.

The patient should not be rushed while eating because this may increase the risk of pulmonary aspiration. Providing small amounts of food at frequent intervals rather than larger amounts only at mealtimes may help the patient feel less need to hurry. Suction equipment should be kept available in case aspiration occurs. Dysphagia is frustrating and frightening for the patient and requires much understanding and patience by the family and caregivers.

Tube feedings or total parenteral nutrition. Patients who are unconscious or unable to eat because of severe dysphagia, weakness, ileus, or other reasons require tube feedings or TPN. Prompt initiation of nutrition support must be a priority in patients with neurologic impairments. Needs for protein and calories are increased by infection and fever, as may occur in a patient with encephalitis or meningitis. Needs for protein, calories, zinc, and vitamin C are increased during wound healing, as occurs in trauma patients and patients with pressure ulcers.

Patients with neurologic deficits are at increased risk for certain complications (particularly pulmonary aspiration) during tube feeding and require especially careful nursing management. Patients of most concern are (1) patients with an impaired gag reflex, such as some patients with cerebrovascular accident; (2) patients with delayed gastric emptying, such as patients in the early period after spinal cord injury and patients with head injury treated with barbiturate coma; and (3) patients likely to

---

BOX 7.6 Common Findings in the Nutrition Assessment of Patients With Neurologic Alterations

Biochemical (Laboratory) Data
- Hyperglycemia (with corticosteroid use)

Clinical Findings
- Wasting of muscle and subcutaneous fat related to disuse or to poor food intake

Diet or Health History
- Poor food intake related to altered state of consciousness, dysphagia or other chewing or swallowing difficulties, or ileus resulting from spinal cord injury or use of pentobarbital
- Hypermetabolism resulting from head injury
- Pressure ulcers

---

experience seizures. To help prevent pulmonary aspiration, the patient's head is kept elevated at an angle of 30 to 45 degrees, if not contraindicated; when elevation of the head is impossible, administering feedings with the patient in the prone or lateral position allows free drainage of emesis from the mouth and decreases the risk of aspiration (see "Aspiration Pneumonitis" in Chapter 19).

Administering phenytoin with enteral formulas decreases the absorption of the medication and the peak serum level achieved. A problem arises when a patient is receiving continuous enteral feedings and requires anticonvulsant therapy. One way to deal with the problem is stop the feeding for 1 to 2 hours before and after phenytoin administration.[94] Even when this practice is followed, the patient may require a higher phenytoin dosage than normal to maintain therapeutic serum concentrations. When continuous feedings are discontinued and the patient resumes eating meals or receives intermittent enteral feedings, the phenytoin dosage must be adjusted appropriately. Phenytoin levels should be monitored carefully in patients receiving enteral feedings. The infusion rate may need to be increased to account for the time that the enteral feeding is held for phenytoin administration.

Hyperglycemia is a common complication in patients receiving corticosteroids. Regular monitoring of blood glucose levels is an important part of care of such patients. They may require insulin to control hyperglycemia.

Prompt use of nutrition support is especially important for patients with head injuries because head injury causes marked catabolism, even in patients who receive barbiturates, which should decrease metabolic demands. Patients with head injury rapidly exhaust glycogen stores and begin to use body proteins to meet energy needs, a process that can quickly lead to PCM. The catabolic response is partly a result of corticosteroid therapy in patients with head injury. However, the hypermetabolism and hypercatabolism are also caused by dramatic hormonal responses to this type of injury.[95] Cortisol, epinephrine, and norepinephrine levels increase as much as seven times normal. These hormones increase the metabolic rate and caloric demands, causing mobilization of body fat and proteins to meet the increased energy needs. Patients with head injury undergo an inflammatory response and may be febrile, creating increased needs for protein and calories. Improvement in outcome and reduction in complications have been observed in patients with head injury who receive adequate nutrition support early in the hospital course[95,96] (see "Traumatic Brain Injuries" in Chapter 33).

Prevention of overweight and obesity. Many stable patients with neurologic disorders are less active than their healthy counterparts and require fewer calories. They may become overweight or obese if given normal amounts of calories for their age and gender. Within 1 or 2 months after spinal cord injury, substantial amounts of muscle atrophy and loss of body mass begin to occur as a result of denervation and disuse. Consequently, body weight and caloric needs decline. Ideal body weights for paraplegics and quadriplegics are less than ideal body weights for healthy adults of the same height.[97] Stable, rehabilitating paraplegics need approximately 27.9 calories/kg per day, and quadriplegics need approximately 22.7 calories/kg per day.[97,98] Patients with dysphagia or extreme swallowing musculature weakness may rely on very soft, easy-to-chew foods that are usually more dense in calories than bulky, high-fiber foods. They also may gain unneeded weight that will hamper their care and impede mobility. For these reasons, nutrition education of the patient with a spinal cord injury and family should include instruction about prevention of undesirable weight gain. Decreased use of high-fat foods (eg, dairy products—milkshakes, ice cream, butter, margarine, pastries) can help to reduce calorie intake. Fruits and vegetables without added fat or sauces are good choices because they are generally low in fat and supply fiber needed to help maintain regular bowel habits.

NUTRITION AND RENAL ALTERATIONS

Providing adequate nutrition care for patients with renal disease can be extremely challenging. Although renal disturbances and their treatments can markedly increase needs for nutrients, necessary restrictions in intake of fluid, protein, phosphorus, and potassium make delivery of adequate calories, vitamins, and minerals difficult. Thorough nutrition assessment provides the basis for successful nutrition management in patients with renal disease.

Nutrition Assessment in Renal Alterations

Some common assessment findings in individuals with renal disease are listed in Box 7.7.

Nutrition Intervention and Education in Renal Alterations

Nutrition needs of patients with renal disease are complex. The goal of nutrition intervention is to balance adequate calories, protein, vitamins, and minerals, while avoiding excesses of protein, fluid, electrolytes, and other nutrients with potential toxicity.

Protein

The kidney is responsible for excreting nitrogen from amino acids or proteins in the form of urea. When urinary excretion of urea is impaired in renal failure, blood urea nitrogen increases. Excessive protein intake may worsen uremia. However, patients with renal failure often have other physiologic stresses that increase protein or amino acid needs, such as losses because of dialysis, wounds, and fistulas; use of corticosteroid medications that exert a catabolic effect; increased endogenous secretion of catecholamines, corticosteroids, and glucagon, all of which can cause or aggravate catabolism; metabolic acidosis, which stimulates protein

---

BOX 7.7 Common Findings in the Nutrition Assessment of Patients With Renal Failure

Anthropometric Measurements
- Underweight (may be masked by edema)

Biochemical (Laboratory) Data
- Electrolyte imbalances
- Hypoalbuminemia related to protein restriction and amino acid losses in dialysis
- Anemia related to inadequate erythropoietin production and blood loss with hemodialysis
- Hypertriglyceridemia related to use of glucose as osmotic agent in dialysis and use of carbohydrates to supply needed calories

Clinical Findings
- Wasting of muscle and subcutaneous tissue (may be masked by edema)

Diet or Health History
- Poor dietary intake related to protein and electrolyte restrictions and alterations in taste

---

breakdown; and catabolic conditions, such as trauma, surgery, and sepsis.[99] Patients with acute kidney injury need adequate amounts of protein to avoid catabolism of body tissues.

Patients with stable acute kidney injury without evidence of fluid overload or electrolyte or acid-base disturbances can often be managed conservatively without dialysis. However, when renal function worsens, some form of renal replacement therapy is required to maintain homeostasis and prevent metabolic complications. Types of renal replacement therapy include peritoneal dialysis, intermittent hemodialysis, and continuous arteriovenous hemofiltration.[99] During hemodialysis, amino acids are freely filtered and lost, but proteins such as albumin and immunoglobulin are not. Proteins and amino acids are removed during peritoneal dialysis, creating a greater nutrition requirement for protein.[100,101] Protein needs may be higher, depending on the level of stress.[102] To limit catabolism, patients with acute kidney injury on dialysis therapy should receive approximately 1.5 to 2.0 g of protein/kg per day (with a maximum of 2.5 g of protein/kg per day), depending on catabolic rate, renal function, and dialysis losses.[3,103]

Fluid

A patient with renal insufficiency usually does not require a fluid restriction until urine output begins to diminish. Patients receiving hemodialysis are limited to a fluid intake resulting in a gain of no more than 0.45 kg (1 lb) per day on the days between dialysis. This generally means a daily intake of 500 to 750 mL plus the volume lost in urine. With the use of continuous peritoneal dialysis, hemofiltration, or hemodialysis, the fluid intake can be liberalized.[104] This more liberal fluid allowance permits more adequate nutrient delivery by oral, tube, or parenteral feedings. Enteral formulas containing 1.5 to 2 calories/mL or more provide a concentrated source of calories for tube-fed patients who require fluid restriction. Intravenous lipids, particularly 20% emulsions, can be used to supply concentrated calories for the patient receiving TPN. Intradialytic TPN can be given during hemodialysis sessions to some malnourished patients; it supplies an additional source of nutrients at a time when the fluid can be rapidly removed in dialysis.[100]

Energy (Calories)

Energy needs are not increased by renal failure, but adequate calories must be provided to avoid catabolism.[99,104] It is essential that the renal patient receive an adequate number of calories to prevent catabolism of body tissues to meet energy needs. Catabolism reduces muscle mass and other functional body tissues, and it releases nitrogen that must be excreted by the kidney. Adults with renal insufficiency need approximately 30 to 35 calories/kg per day to prevent catabolism and ensure that all protein consumed is used for anabolism rather than to meet energy needs.[104] After renal transplantation, when the patient usually receives large doses of corticosteroids, it is especially important to ensure that caloric intake is adequate (usually 25 to 35 calories/kg per day) to prevent undue catabolism.

Glucose in the peritoneal dialysate may be a significant source of calories and a contributing factor in hypertriglyceridemia. Approximately 70% of the glucose instilled during peritoneal dialysis to serve as an osmotic agent may be absorbed, and this must be considered part of the patient's carbohydrate intake. The glucose monohydrate dextrose, used in intravenous and dialysate solutions, supplies 3.4 calories/g. If the patient receives 4.25% glucose (4.25 g glucose/100 mL solution) in the dialysate, he or she receives the following:

$$42.5 \text{ g/L} \times 70\% \times 3.4 \text{ calories/g} = 101 \text{ calories/L of dialysate}$$

To help control hypertriglyceridemia, only approximately 30% to 35% of the patient's calories should come from carbohydrates, including glucose from the dialysate. The major portion of dietary carbohydrate should come from complex carbohydrates.

Consuming at least 20 to 25 g of fiber daily can help to control triglyceride levels. Sources of dietary fiber include cooked dried beans and peas (5 to 7 g fiber/0.5 cup); cereals containing whole grains (not 100% bran); berries, apples, oranges, pears, corn, and peas (3 to 5 g/serving); whole-grain breads; and most fruits and vegetables other than those listed previously (1 to 2 g/serving). Wheat bran is a good source of fiber (5 to 10 g/oz), but it is also a good source of phosphorus and may cause renal failure to progress more rapidly. For tube-fed patients, a formula containing dietary fiber can be chosen. To help control hypertriglyceridemia and to provide concentrated calories in minimal fluid, fat may need to supply 40% of the patient's calories.

Hypercholesterolemia is commonly found in patients with renal failure, and unsaturated fats and oils (corn, soybean, sunflower, safflower, cottonseed, canola, and olive) are preferred over saturated fats (primarily from meats and dairy products), which tend to raise cholesterol levels. The necessary restriction of meat, milk, and other protein foods in the diet helps lower intake of cholesterol and saturated fat. Intravenous lipids and the long-chain fats found in most commercial enteral formulas are primarily polyunsaturated.

Other Nutrients

Certain nutrients such as potassium and phosphorus are restricted because they are excreted by the kidney. The patient has no specific requirement for the fat-soluble vitamins A, E, and K because they are not removed in appreciable amounts by dialysis, and restriction generally prevents development of toxicity. Patients with end-stage renal disease may have decreased

---

> ### BOX 7.8 Common Findings in the Nutrition Assessment of Patients With Gastrointestinal Disease
>
> **Anthropometric Measurements**
> - Underweight related to malabsorption (from inadequate production of bile salts or pancreatic enzymes), anorexia, or poor intake (because of pain caused by eating)
>
> **Biochemical (Laboratory) Data**
> - Hypoalbuminemia (may result primarily from liver damage and not malnutrition)
> - Hypocalcemia related to steatorrhea
> - Hypomagnesemia related to alcohol abuse
> - Anemia related to blood loss from bleeding varices
>
> **Clinical Findings**
> - Wasting of muscle and subcutaneous fat
> - Confusion, confabulation, nystagmus, or peripheral neuropathy related to thiamine deficiency caused by alcohol abuse (Wernicke-Korsakoff syndrome)
>
> **Diet or Health History**
> - Steatorrhea

clearance of vitamin A, and levels should be monitored.[103] The needs for several water-soluble vitamins and trace minerals are increased in dialysis patients because they are small enough to pass freely through the dialysis filter. Vitamins and minerals should be supplemented as necessary.[104]

NUTRITION AND GASTROINTESTINAL ALTERATIONS

Because the GI tract is inherently related to nutrition, impairment of the GI tract and its accessory organs has a major impact on nutrition. Two of the most serious GI-related illnesses seen among critical care patients are hepatic failure and pancreatitis, and the following discussion focuses on these disorders.

Nutrition Assessment in Gastrointestinal Alterations

Some common assessment findings in individuals with GI disease are listed in Box 7.8.

Nutrition Intervention and Education in Gastrointestinal Alterations

Hepatic Failure

The liver is the most important metabolic organ, and it is responsible for carbohydrate, fat, and protein metabolism; vitamin storage and activation; and detoxification of waste products. Liver failure is associated with a wide spectrum of metabolic alterations. Because the diseased liver has impaired ability to deactivate hormones, levels of circulating glucagon, epinephrine, and cortisol are elevated. These hormones promote catabolism of body tissues and cause glycogen stores to be exhausted. Release of lipids from their storage depots is accelerated, but the liver has decreased ability to metabolize them for energy. Moreover, inadequate production of bile salts by the liver results in malabsorption of fat from the diet. Body proteins are used for energy sources, producing tissue wasting. Branched-chain amino acids (BCAAs)—leucine, isoleucine, and valine—are especially well used for energy, and their levels in the blood decline. Conversely, levels of aromatic amino acids (AAAs)—phenylalanine, tyrosine, and tryptophan—increase as a result of tissue catabolism and impaired ability of the liver to clear them from the blood. BCAAs are not as dependent on liver metabolism as the AAAs.[105] The AAAs are precursors for neurotransmitters (serotonin and dopamine) within the central nervous system. Rising levels of AAAs cause encephalopathy by promoting synthesis of false neurotransmitters that compete with endogenous neurotransmitters. The damaged liver cannot clear ammonia from the circulation adequately, and ammonia accumulates in the brain. The ammonia may contribute to the encephalopathic symptoms and to brain edema.[3,105]

Monitoring fluid and electrolyte status. Ascites and edema are caused by a combination of factors. Colloid osmotic pressure in the plasma decreases because of the reduction of production of albumin and other plasma proteins by the diseased liver, increased portal pressure caused by obstruction, and renal sodium retention from secondary hyperaldosteronism. To control the fluid retention, restriction of sodium (usually 2000 mg) and fluid (≤1500 mL daily) usually is necessary in conjunction with the administration of diuretics. Patients are weighed daily to evaluate the success of treatment. Physical status and laboratory data must be closely monitored for deficiencies of potassium; phosphorus; zinc; and vitamins A, D, E, and K.[3]

Provision of a nutritious diet and evaluation of response to dietary protein. PCM and nutrition deficiencies are common in patients with liver failure. The causes of malnutrition are complex and usually are related to decreased intake, malabsorption, maldigestion, and abnormal nutrient metabolism. Nutrition intervention is individualized and based on these metabolic changes. A diet with adequate protein helps to suppress catabolism and promote liver regeneration. Stable patients with cirrhosis usually tolerate 0.8 to 1 g of protein/kg per day. Patients with severe stress or nutrition deficits have increased needs—1.2 to 2 g of protein/kg per day.[105] Aggressive treatment with medications, including lactulose, neomycin, or metronidazole, is considered first-line therapy in the management of acute hepatic encephalopathy. Chronic protein restriction, which could lead to PCM, is not recommended as a long-term management strategy for patients with liver disease.[3,105]

Anorexia may interfere with oral intake, and the nurse may need to provide much encouragement to the patient to ensure intake of an adequate diet. Prospective calorie counts may need to be instituted to provide objective evidence of oral intake. Small, frequent feedings are usually better tolerated by an anorexic patient than three large meals daily. Soft foods are preferred because the patient may have esophageal varices that may be irritated by high-fiber foods. If patients are unable to meet their caloric needs, they may require oral supplements or enteral feeding. Small-bore nasoenteric feeding tubes can be used safely without increasing risk of variceal bleeding.[105] TPN should be reserved for patients who are absolutely unable to tolerate enteral feeding.[3] Diarrhea from concurrent administration of lactulose should not be confused with feeding intolerance.

A diet adequate in calories (at least 30 calories/kg daily) is provided to help prevent catabolism and to prevent the use of dietary protein for energy needs.[106] In cases of malabsorption, medium-chain triglycerides may be used to meet caloric needs.

Pancreatic enzymes may also be considered for malabsorption problems.

BCAA-enriched products have been developed for enteral and parenteral nutrition of patients with hepatic disease. These products may be used in patients with acute hepatic encephalopathy who do not tolerate standard diets or enteral formulas or who are unresponsive to lactulose. However, no substantial evidence exists showing that BCAAs are superior to standard formulas in regard to nitrogen balance or as treatment for encephalopathy.[3,105] A patient who undergoes successful liver transplantation is usually able to tolerate a regular diet with few restrictions. Intake during the postoperative period must be adequate to support nutrition repletion and healing; 1 to 1.2 g of protein/kg per day and approximately 30 calories/kg per day are usually sufficient. Immunosuppressant therapy (corticosteroids and cyclosporine or tacrolimus) contributes to glucose intolerance. Dietary measures to control glucose intolerance include (1) obtaining approximately 30% of dietary calories from fat, (2) emphasizing complex sources of carbohydrates, and (3) eating several small meals daily. Moderate exercise often helps to improve glucose tolerance.

Pancreatitis

The pancreas is an exocrine and endocrine gland required for normal digestion and metabolism of proteins, carbohydrates, and fats. Acute pancreatitis is an inflammatory process that occurs as a result of autodigestion of the pancreas by enzymes normally secreted by that organ. Food intake stimulates pancreatic secretion, increasing the damage to the pancreas and the pain associated with the disorder. Patients usually present with abdominal pain and tenderness and with elevations of pancreatic enzymes. A mild form of acute pancreatitis occurs in 80% of patients requiring hospitalization, and a severe form of acute pancreatitis occurs in the other 20%.[107] Patients with the mild form of acute pancreatitis do not require nutrition support and generally resume oral feeding within 7 days. Chronic pancreatitis may develop, and it is characterized by fibrosis of pancreatic cells. This results in loss of exocrine and endocrine function because of the destruction of acinar and islet cells. The loss of exocrine function leads to malabsorption and steatorrhea. In chronic pancreatitis, the loss of endocrine function results in impaired glucose intolerance.[107]

Prevention of further damage to the pancreas and preventing nutrition deficits. Effective nutrition management is a key treatment for patients with acute pancreatitis or exacerbations of chronic pancreatitis. The concern that feeding may stimulate the production of digestive enzymes and perpetuate tissue damage has led to the widespread use of TPN and bowel rest. Data suggest that for patients with severe pancreatitis, providing enteral nutrition support is more beneficial than prolonged bowel rest and provision of TPN.[3,108] Enteral nutrition infused into the distal jejunum bypasses the stimulatory effect of feeding on pancreatic secretion and is associated with fewer infectious and metabolic complications compared with TPN.[109,110]

The results of randomized studies comparing TPN with total enteral nutrition (or enteral tube feeding) indicate that total enteral nutrition is preferable to TPN in patients with severe acute pancreatitis, reducing costs and the risk of sepsis and improving clinical outcome.[109-111] Patients unable to tolerate total enteral nutrition should receive TPN, and some patients may require a combination of total enteral nutrition and TPN to meet nutrition requirements.[112,113] Low-fat enteral formulas and formulas with fat provided by medium-chain triglycerides are more readily absorbed than formulas that are high in long-chain triglycerides (eg, corn oil, sunflower oil).

When oral intake is possible, small, frequent feedings of low-fat foods are least likely to cause discomfort,[110] although the level of fat restriction should depend on the level of steatorrhea and abdominal pain the patient experiences.[108] For patients with chronic pancreatitis, pancreatic enzyme replacement therapy may be indicated.[108] Guidelines for the treatment of diabetes (discussed later) are appropriate for the care of patients with glucose intolerance or diabetes related to pancreatitis.

NUTRITION AND ENDOCRINE ALTERATIONS

Endocrine alterations have far-reaching effects on all body systems and affect nutrition status in a variety of ways. One of the most common endocrine problems in the general population and among critically ill patients is diabetes mellitus.

Nutrition Assessment in Endocrine Alterations

Because of the prevalence of patients with non–insulin-dependent diabetes mellitus (type 2 diabetes) among the hospitalized population and the association of type 2 diabetes with overweight, the nutrition problems most commonly identified in patients with endocrine alterations are overweight and obesity. Hyperglycemia and hyperlipidemia are other common findings in patients with diabetes.

Nutrition Intervention in Endocrine Alterations
Nutrition Support and Blood Glucose Control

Patients with insulin-dependent diabetes mellitus (type 1 diabetes) or endocrine dysfunction caused by pancreatitis often have weight loss and malnutrition as a result of tissue catabolism because they cannot use dietary carbohydrates to meet energy needs. Although patients with type 2 diabetes are more likely to be overweight than underweight, they also may become malnourished as a result of chronic or acute infections, trauma, major surgery, or other illnesses.[114] Nutrition support should not be neglected because a patient is obese, as PCM can develop in these patients. When a patient is not expected to be able to eat for at least 5 to 7 days or inadequate intake persists for that period, initiation of tube feedings or TPN is indicated. No disease process benefits from starvation, and development or progression of nutrition deficits may contribute to complications, such as pressure ulcers, pulmonary or urinary tract infections, and sepsis, which prolong hospitalization, increase the costs of care, and may result in death.

Blood glucose control is especially important in the care of surgical patients. Poorly controlled diabetes reduces immune function by impairing granulocyte adherence, chemotaxis, and phagocytosis.[115,116] In surveys of critically ill patients undergoing a variety of elective operations and coronary artery surgery,[115] glucose levels of 206 to 220 mg/dL or higher during the first 24 to 36 postoperative hours were associated with higher rates of nosocomial infection than lower glucose levels.[115,117] To maintain tight control of blood glucose, glucose levels are monitored regularly, usually several times a day, until the patient is stable. Patients unable to tolerate oral diets or enteral feeding may require TPN to meet nutrition requirements during acute

illness.[118] Regular insulin added to the solution is a common method of managing hyperglycemia in the patient receiving TPN. The dosage required may be larger than the patient's usual dose because some of the insulin adheres to glass bottles and plastic bags or administration sets. Multiple injections or, preferably, a continuous infusion of regular insulin may be used to maintain tight control of blood glucose in the enterally fed patient.[119] Although further study is needed, the following glucose goals are recommended: 80 to 120 mg/dL in critically ill patients in the critical care unit and 100 to 150 mg/dL for stable patients on the wards.[118]

In patients receiving enteral tube feedings, the postpyloric route (through a nasoduodenal, nasojejunal, or jejunostomy tube) may be the most effective because gastroparesis may limit tolerance of intragastric tube feedings.[120] Postpyloric feedings are given continuously because dumping syndrome and poor absorption may occur if feedings are given rapidly into the small bowel. Continuous enteral infusions are associated with improved control of blood glucose. Fiber-enriched formulas may slow the absorption of the carbohydrate, producing a more delayed and sustained glycemic response. Most standard formulas contain balanced proportions of carbohydrate, protein, and fats appropriate for diabetic patients. Specialized diabetic formulas have not shown improved outcomes compared with standard formulas.[119]

Severe Vomiting or Diarrhea in Patients With Type 1 Diabetes Mellitus

When insulin-dependent patients experience vomiting and diarrhea severe enough to interfere significantly with oral intake or result in excessive fluid and electrolyte losses, adequate carbohydrates and fluids must be supplied. Nausea and vomiting should be treated with antiemetic medication.[120] Delayed gastric emptying is common in diabetes and may improve with administration of prokinetic agents.[120] Small amounts of food or liquids taken every 15 to 20 minutes usually are the best tolerated by a patient with nausea and vomiting. Foods and beverages containing approximately 15 g of carbohydrate include ½ cup of regular gelatin, ½ cup of custard, ¾ cup of regular ginger ale, ½ cup of a regular soft drink, and ½ cup of orange or apple juice. Blood glucose levels should be monitored at least every 2 to 4 hours.

Nutrition Education in Diabetes

Optimal control of blood glucose in type 1 and type 2 diabetes is associated with a decreased risk of development of retinopathy, neuropathy, and other long-term complications.[114] Self-monitoring of blood glucose is essential in maintaining diabetic control, and nutrition is considered the most critical component of diabetes care in achieving blood glucose goals.[120] Meals are based on heart-healthy diet principles, according to which saturated fat and cholesterol are limited and protein accounts for 15% to 20% of total calories.[121] Most carbohydrate foods should be whole grains, fruits, vegetables, and low-fat milk.[122] Evidence-based medical nutrition therapy supports hospitals implementing a consistent carbohydrate meal plan for diabetic patients.[123] The meal plan is based on the amount of carbohydrate that is consistent from meal to meal each day. Although exact calorie levels are not specified, a typical daily menu provides approximately 1500 to 2000 calories with a range of three to five carbohydrate foods at each meal, each containing 15 g of carbohydrate.[122]

Careful monitoring of dietary intake and blood glucose levels is essential during critical illness to meet nutrition needs and maintain glucose control. Avoidance of overfeeding limits hyperglycemia and associated complications. Insulin can be adjusted to maintain blood glucose control based on frequent monitoring. Intensive insulin therapy has been shown to reduce mortality rates for critically ill surgical patients.[115] It is vital for the dietitian to work closely with the interdisciplinary team to determine feeding methods; appropriate enteral formulas; and the amounts of protein, lipid, and carbohydrate supplied in parenteral nutrition.[123]

CASE STUDY 7.1   Patient With Nutrition Issues

Brief Patient History

Mrs. S is a 49-year-old woman with end-stage cardiomyopathy. She and her husband have been restaurant owners for many years. She is anorexic and finds it difficult to eat solid foods, which is emotionally distressing for her and her family. She has lost 10 lb in the past month. Mrs. S was placed on the heart transplant list 6 months ago. She has agreed to hospitalization to optimize her medical management and nutrition status.

Clinical Assessment

Mrs. S is admitted to the critical care unit. A central line has been inserted for dobutamine therapy. A nutrition assessment has been completed by the dietitian that includes recommendations for frequent, small, calorie-dense, low-sodium feedings.

Diagnostic Procedures

Mrs. S is 5 feet 2 inches tall and weighs 90 lb. Her vital signs are as follows: blood pressure of 100/60 mm Hg, heart rate of 80 beats/min (sinus rhythm), respiratory rate of 20 breaths/min, and temperature of 98.2°F. Serum laboratory findings are as follows: hemoglobin level of 8.3 g/dL, prealbumin level of 14 mg/dL, sodium level of 125 mmol/L, potassium level of 3.3 mmol/L, chloride level of 94 mmol/L, carbon dioxide concentration of 26 mEq/L, calcium level of 8 mg/dL, magnesium level of 1.5 mg/dL, and B-type natriuretic peptide concentration of 500 pg/mL.

Medical Diagnosis

Mrs. S is diagnosed with cachexia resulting from end-stage cardiomyopathy.

Questions

1. What major outcomes do you expect to achieve for this patient?
2. What problems or risks must be managed to achieve these outcomes?
3. What interventions must be initiated to monitor, prevent, manage, or eliminate the problems and risks identified?
4. What interventions should be initiated to promote optimal functioning, safety, and well-being of the patient?
5. What possible learning needs do you anticipate for this patient?
6. What cultural and age-related factors may have a bearing on the patient's plan of care?

▌ S U M M A R Y

Nutrient Metabolism

- The major purposes of metabolism of the energy-yielding nutrients are the production of energy and the formation and preservation of lean body mass.

Assessing Nutrition Status

- Nutrition screening should be conducted on every patient, and a more thorough nutrition assessment should be completed on any patient screened to be nutritionally at risk.

Implications of Undernutrition for Sick or Stressed Patients

- Malnutrition can be related to any essential nutrient or nutrients, but a serious type of malnutrition found frequently among hospitalized patients is protein-calorie malnutrition. It is usually the result of the combined effects of starvation and hypermetabolism.
- The hypermetabolic process results from increased catabolic changes caused by a stressful event.
- Malnutrition is associated with various adverse outcomes, including wound dehiscence, pressure ulcers, infections, respiratory failure requiring ventilation, longer hospital stays, and death.

Nursing Management of Nutrition Support

- Whenever possible, the enteral route is the preferred method of feeding because of lower cost, better maintenance of gut integrity, and decreased infection and hospital stay.
- Oral supplementation may be necessary for patients who can eat and have normal digestion and absorption.
- Early enteral nutrition (within the first 24 to 48 hours of critical illness) reduces septic complications and improves feeding tolerance in critically ill patients.
- It is essential to check tube placement before feedings and regularly throughout the course of enteral feedings.
- Continued oral care is provided during the course of the enteral feedings.

Nutrition and Cardiovascular Alterations

- In the early period after a myocardial infarction, interventions are aimed at reducing angina, cardiac workload, and the risk of dysrhythmia; meal size, caffeine intake, and food temperatures are monitored closely.
- Interventions in heart failure are designed to reduce fluid retention, reducing the preload.
- Calorie-dense foods and supplements are provided to patients with cardiac cachexia.

Nutrition and Pulmonary Alterations

- Malnutrition has adverse effects on respiratory function, decreasing surfactant production, diaphragmatic mass, vital capacity, and immunocompetence.
- Because of anorexia, dyspnea, debilitation, or the need for ventilatory support, many patients require tube feeding or total parenteral nutrition.
- It is especially important to be alert to the risks of pulmonary aspiration in a patient with an artificial airway, keeping the head elevated 45 degrees during feedings, unless contraindicated, and keeping the cuff of the artificial airway inflated during feedings.

Nutrition and Neurologic Alterations

- Patients with dysphagia or weakness of the swallowing musculature often experience the greatest difficulty in swallowing foods that are dry or thin liquids, such as water, which are difficult to control.
- Beverages may be thickened with commercial thickening products, infant cereal, or yogurt; fruit nectars may be better tolerated than fruit juices.

- Prompt use of nutrition support is important for patients with head injuries because head injuries cause marked catabolism, and patients undergo an inflammatory response and may be febrile, increasing the need for proteins and calories.

Nutrition and Renal Alterations

- The goal of intervention is to balance adequate calories, protein, vitamins, and minerals, while avoiding excesses of proteins, fluid, electrolytes, and other nutrients with potential toxicities.
- Patients with acute kidney injury need adequate amounts of protein to avoid catabolism of body tissues.
- With the use of continuous peritoneal dialysis, hemofiltration, or hemodialysis, the fluid intake can be liberalized. This allows for more adequate nutrient delivery through oral, tube, or parenteral feedings.
- The need for several water-soluble vitamins and trace minerals is increased in dialysis patients because these nutrients are small enough to pass through the dialysis filter.

Nutrition and Gastrointestinal Alterations

- Ascites and edema in a patient with liver failure have many causes. There is decreased colloid osmotic pressure in the plasma because of reduced production of albumin and other plasma proteins, increased portal pressure caused by obstruction, and renal sodium retention from secondary hyperaldosteronism.
- Causes of malnutrition in liver failure are complex and related to decreased intake, malabsorption, maldigestion, and abnormal nutrient metabolism.
- In a patient with pancreatitis, concern that feeding may stimulate the production of digestive enzymes and perpetuate liver damage has led to the use of TPN and bowel rest.

Nutrition and Endocrine Alterations

- Blood glucose control is especially important in the care of surgical patients.
- Poorly controlled diabetes reduces immune function by impairing granulocyte adherence, chemotaxis, and phagocytosis.

Ⓔ Visit the Evolve site for additional study materials.

REFERENCES

1. Joint Commission on Accreditation of Healthcare Organizations. Comprehensive Accreditation Manual: CAMH for Hospitals: The Official Handbook. Chicago, IL: Joint Commission on Accreditation of Healthcare Organizations; 2011.
2. Mueller C, et al. A.S.P.E.N. Clinical guidelines nutrition screening, assessment, and intervention in adults. JPEN J Parenter Enteral Nutr. 2011;35(1):16-24.
3. McClave SA, et al. Society of Critical Care Medicine (SCCM) and American Society for Parenteral and Enteral Nutrition (ASPEN): Guidelines for the provision and assessment of nutrition support therapy in the adult critically ill patient. JPEN J Parenter Enteral Nutr. 2009;33(3):277.
4. World Health Organization. BMI classification. http://apps.who.int/bmi/index.jsp?introPage=intro_3.html Accessed October 23, 2015.
5. U.S. Department of Health and Human Services. Classification of overweight and obesity by BMI, waist circumference, and associated disease risks. https://www.nhlbi.nih.gov/health/educational/lose_wt/BMI/bmi_dis.htm Accessed October 23, 2015.
6. WHO expert consultation. Appropriate body-mass index for Asian populations and its implications for policy and intervention strategies. Lancet. 2004;363:157.
7. Prins A. Nutritional assessment of the critically ill patient. S Afr Clin Nutr. 2010;23(1).
8. Berger MM, et al. Stature estimation using the knee height determination in critically ill patients. e-SPEN, the European e-Journal of Clinical Nutrition and Metabolism. 2008;3(2):e84.
9. Simpson F, et al. Physical assessment and anthropometric measures for use in critical research conducted in critically ill patient populations: an analytic observational study. JPEN J Parenter Enteral Nutr. 2015;39(3):313-321.
10. Mahanna E, et al. Nutrition and metabolic support for critically ill patients. Curr Opin Anesth. 2015;28(2):131-138.
11. Academy of Nutrition and Dietetics. Evidence Analysis Library. What is the most accurate method for determination of resting metabolic rate (RMR) in critically ill patients? http://www.adaevidencelibrary.com. Accessed October 23, 2015.
12. Satchell MA. Nutrition in critical illness: calorimetry. Pediatric Critical Care Study Guide. 2012:452.
13. Academy of Nutrition and Dietetics. Evidence Analysis Library. Estimating RMR with predictive equations: what does the evidence tell us? http://www.adaevidencelibrary.com. Accessed October 23, 2015.
14. Academy of Nutrition and Dietetics. Evidence Analysis Library. If indirect calorimetry is unavailable or impractical, what is the best way to estimate resting metabolic rate (RMR) in obese adult critically ill patients? http://www.adaevidencelibrary.com. Accessed October 23, 2015.
15. Academy of Nutrition and Dietetics. Evidence Analysis Library. If indirect calorimetry is unavailable or impractical, what is the best way to estimate resting metabolic rate (RMR) in non-obese adult critically ill patients? http://www.adaevidencelibrary.com Accessed October 23, 2015.
16. Kwon S, et al. Importance of perioperative glycemic control in general surgery: a report from the Surgical Care and Outcomes Assessment Program. Ann Surg. 2013;257(1):8.
17. Kirkland LL, et al. Nutrition in the hospitalized patient. J Hosp Med. 2013;8(1):52-58.
18. Corkins MR, et al. Malnutrition diagnosis in hospitalized patients United States, 2010. JPEN J Parenter Enteral Nutr. 2014;38(2):186-195.
19. Barker LA, Gout BS, Crowe TC. Hospital malnutrition: prevalence, identification and impact on patients and the healthcare system. Int J Environ Res Public Health. 2011;8(2):514.
20. Joosten KFM, Hulst JM. Malnutrition in pediatric hospital patients: current issues. Nutrition. 2011;27(2):133.
21. Philipson TJ, et al. Impact of oral nutritional supplementation on hospital outcomes. Am J Manag Care. 2013;19(2):121-128.
22. Singer P, et al. The tight calorie control study (TICA-COS): a prospective, randomized, controlled pilot study of nutritional support in critically ill patients. Intensive Care Med. 2011;37(4):601-609.
23. Rubinson L, et al. Low caloric intake is associated with nosocomial bloodstream infections in patients in the medical intensive care unit. Crit Care Med. 2004;32:350.
24. White JV, et al. Consensus statement of the Academy of Nutrition and Dietetics/American Society for Parenteral and Enteral Nutrition: characteristics recommended for the identification and documentation of adult malnutrition (undernutrition). J Acad Nutr Diet. 2012;112(5):730-738.
25. Seres DS, et al. Advantages of enteral nutrition over parenteral nutrition. Therap Adv Gastroenterol. 2013;6(2):157-167.
26. Langkamp-Henken B. If the gut works, use it: but what if you can't? Nutr Clin Pract. 2003;18:449.
27. Barrett M, et al. Intestine, immunity, and parenteral nutrition in an era of preferred enteral feeding. Curr Opin Clin Nutr Metab Care. 2015;18(5):496-500.
28. Alpers DH. Enteral feeding and gut atrophy. Curr Opin Clin Nutr Metab Care. 2002;5(6):679.
29. Hayes GL, et al. Nutritional supplements in critical illness. AACN Adv Crit Care. 2011;22(4):301-316.
30. Casaer MP, Van den Berghe G. Nutrition in the acute phase of critical illness. N Engl J Med. 2014;370(13):1227-1236.

31. Bollhalder L, et al. A systematic literature review and meta-analysis of randomized clinical trials of parenteral glutamine supplementation. Clin Nutr. 2013;32(2):213-223.

32. Wischmeyer PE, et al. Parenteral glutamine supplementation in critical illness: a systematic review. Crit Care. 2014;18(2):R76.

33. Manzanares W, et al. Antioxidant micronutrients in the critically ill: a systematic review and meta-analysis. Crit Care. 2012;16(2):R66.

34. Evans DC, Hegazi RA. Immunonutrition in critically ill patients: does one size fit all? JPEN J Parenter Enteral Nutr. 2015;39(5):500-501.

35. Rice TW. Immunonutrition in critical illness: limited benefit, potential harm. JAMA. 2014;312(5):490-491.

36. Annetta MG, et al. Immunonutrients in critically ill patients: an analysis of the most recent literature. Minerva Anestesiol. 2016;82(3):320-331.

37. Hegazi RA, Wischmeyer PE. Clinical review: optimizing enteral nutrition for critically ill patients—a simple data-driven formula. Crit Care. 2011;15(6):234.

38. Rubinsky MD, Clark AP. Early enteral nutrition in critically ill patients. Dimens Crit Care Nurs. 2012;31(5):267-274.

39. Cahill NE, et al. When early enteral feeding is not possible in critically ill patients: results of a multicenter observational study. JPEN J Parenter Enteral Nutr. 2011;35(2):160-168.

40. Yang S, et al. Early enteral nutrition in critically ill patients with hemodynamic instability: an evidenced-based review and practical advice. Nutr Clin Pract. 2014;29(1):90-96.

41. Moore FA, Weisbrodt NW. Gut dysfunction and intolerance to enteral nutrition in critically ill patients. Nestle Nutr Workshop Ser Clin Perform Programme. 2003;8:149.

42. Davies AR, et al. A multicenter, randomized controlled trial comparing early nasojejunal with nasogastric nutrition in critical illness. Crit Care Med. 2012;40(8):2342-2348.

43. Kuppinger DD, et al. Use of gastric residual volume to guide enteral nutrition in critically ill patients: a brief systematic review of clinical studies. Nutrition. 2013;29(9):1075-1079.

44. Deane AM, et al. Randomized double-blind crossover study to determine the effects of erythromycin on small intestinal nutrient absorption and transit in the critically ill. Am J Clin Nutr. 2012;95(6):1396-1402.

45. Aderinto-Adike AO, Quigley EMM. Gastrointestinal promotility problems in critical care: a clinical perspective. J Dig Dis. 2014;15(7):335-344.

46. Neyens RR, et al. Prokinetic agents with enteral nutrition. Diet and Nutrition in Critical Care. 2015:1323-1332.

47. Lord LM, et al. Comparison of weighted vs. unweighted enteral feeding tubes for efficacy of transpyloric intubation. JPEN J Parenter Enteral Nutr. 1993;17(3):271.

48. Boeykens K, Steeman E, Duysburgh I. Reliability of pH measurement and the auscultatory method to confirm the position of a nasogastric tube. Int J Nurs Stud. 2014;51(11):1427-1433.

49. Davies AR, et al. A multicenter, randomized controlled trial comparing early nasojejunal with nasogastric nutrition in critical illness. Crit Care Med. 2012;40(8):2342-2348.

50. Esparza J, et al. Equal aspiration rates in gastrically and transpylorically fed critically ill patients. Intensive Care Med. 2001;27:660.

51. Neumann DA, DeLegge MH. Gastric versus small-bowel tube feeding in the intensive care unit: a prospective comparison of efficacy. Crit Care Med. 2002;30(7):1436.

52. Marik PE, Zaloga GR. Gastric versus postpyloric feeding: a systematic review. Crit Care. 2003;7(3):R46.

53. Davies AR, et al. Randomized comparison of nasojejunal and nasogastric feeding in critically ill patients. Crit Care Med. 2002;30(3):586.

54. Zhang Z, et al. Comparison of postpyloric tube feeding and gastric tube feeding in intensive care unit patients: a meta-analysis. Nutr Clin Pract. 2013;28(3):371-380.

55. Grant MJC, Martin S. Delivery of enteral nutrition. AACN Clin Issues. 2000;11(4):507.

56. Lord LM. Restoring and maintaining patency of enteral feeding tubes. Nutr Clin Pract. 2003;18:422.

57. Stumpf JL, et al. Efficacy of a Creon delayed-release pancreatic enzyme protocol for clearing occluded enteral feeding tubes. Ann Pharmacother. 2014;48(4):482-487.

58. Prabhakaran S, et al. Nasoenteric tube complications. Scand J Surg. 2012;101(3):147-155.

59. Metheny NA, Mills AC, Stewart BJ. Monitoring for intolerance to gastric tube feedings: a national survey. Am J Crit Care. 2012;21(2):e33-e40.

60. Maloney JP, Ryan TA. Detection of aspiration in enterally fed patients: a requiem for bedside monitors of aspiration. JPEN J Parenter Enteral Nutr. 2002;26(6):S34.

61. Lucarelli MR, et al. Toxicity of food drug and cosmetic blue no. 1 dye in critically ill patients. Chest. 2004;125(2):793.

62. McClave SA, et al. North American summit on aspiration in the critically ill patient: consensus statement. JPEN J Parenter Enteral Nutr. 2002;26(6):S80.

63. Whelan K, Schneider SM. Mechanisms, prevention, and management of diarrhea in enteral nutrition. Curr Opin Gastroenterol. 2011;27(2):152-159.

64. Majid HA, Emery PW, Whelen K. Definitions, attitudes, and management practices in relation to diarrhea during enteral nutrition: a survey of patients, nurses, and dietitians. Nutr Clin Pract. 2012;27(2):252-260.

65. Bernard AC, et al. Defining and assessing tolerance in enteral nutrition. Nutr Clin Pract. 2004;19(5):481.

66. Mostafa SM, et al. Constipation and its implications in the critically ill patient. Br J Anaesth. 2003;91(6):815.

67. Seron-Arbeloa C, et al. Enteral nutrition in critical care. J Clin Med Res. 2013;5(1):1.

68. Engel JM, et al. Enteral nutrition practice in a surgical intensive care unit: what proportion of energy expenditure is delivered enterally? Clin Nutr. 2003;22(2):187.

69. Krishnan JA, et al. Caloric intake in medical ICU patients: consistency of care with guidelines and relationship to clinical outcomes. Chest. 2003;124:297.

70. Kim H, et al. Why patients in critical care do not receive adequate enteral nutrition? A review of the literature. J Crit Care. 2012;27(6):702-713.

71. The Joint Commission. Sentinel Event Alert: Tubing misconnections—a persistent and potentially deadly occurrence. April 2006. http://www.joint commission.org/assets/1/18/SEA_36.PDF. Accessed November 21, 2015.

72. Aust MP. Tubing misconnections. Am J Crit Care. 2011;20(4):346.

73. Worthington P, et al. Parenteral nutrition for the acutely ill. AACN Clin Issues. 2000;11(4):559.

74. Krause R, et al. Which lumen is the source of catheter-related bloodstream infection in patients with multi-lumen central venous catheters? Infection. 2013;41(1):49-52.

75. Bourgeois FC, Lamagna P, Chiang VW. Peripherally inserted central catheters. Pediatr Emerg Care. 2011;27(6):556-561.

76. O'Grady NP, et al. Guidelines for the prevention of intravascular catheter-related infections. Am J Infect Control. 2011;39(4):S1-S34.

77. Speerhas R, et al. Maintaining normal blood glucose concentrations with total parenteral nutrition: is it necessary to taper total parenteral nutrition? Nutr Clin Pract. 2003;18:414.

78. Crook MA, et al. The importance of the refeeding syndrome. Nutrition. 2001;17:632.

79. Hearing SD. Refeeding syndrome. BMJ. 2004;328(7445):908.

80. Academy of Nutrition and Dietetics. Nutrition Care Manual website. Nutrition care > weight management > overweight and obesity > nutrition intervention. http://nutritioncaremanual.org Accessed November 21, 2015.

81. American Heart Association. The American Heart Association's Diet and Lifestyle Recommendations (08/2015). http://www.heart.org/HEART-ORG/GettingHealthy/NutritionCenter/HealthyEating/The-American-Heart-Associations-Diet-and-Lifestyle-Recommendations_UCM_305855_Article.jsp. Accessed November 21, 2015.

82. Lipsy RJ. The National Cholesterol Education Program Adult Treatment Panel III guidelines. J Managed Care Pharm. 2003;9(1 suppl):2.

83. Brewer HB. New features of the National Cholesterol Education Program Adult Treatment Panel III lipid-lowering guidelines. Clin Cardiol. 2003;26:19.

84. Grundy SM, et al. Diagnosis and management of the metabolic syndrome: an American Heart Association/National Heart, Lung, and Blood Institute scientific statement. Circulation. 2005;112:2735.

85. Ginsberg HN. Treatment for patients with the metabolic syndrome. Am J Cardiol. 2003;91(7):29.

86. Ebbing M, et al. Mortality and cardiovascular events in patients treated with homocysteine-lowering B vitamins after coronary angiography. JAMA. 2008;300:795.

87. Go AS, et al. An effective approach to high blood pressure control: a science advisory from the American Heart Association, the American College of Cardiology, and the Centers for Disease Control and Prevention. J Am Coll Cardiol. 2014;63(12):1230-1238.

88. Sacks FM, et al. Effects of blood pressure of reduced dietary sodium and the dietary approaches to stop hypertension (DASH) diet. N Engl J Med. 2001;344(1):3.

89. Academy of Nutrition and Dietetics. Nutrition Care Manual website. Nutrition care > cardiovascular disease > heart failure > nutrition prescription. http://nutritioncaremanual.org Accessed November 21, 2015.

90. Suzuki H, et al. Cancer cachexia—pathophysiology and management. J Gastroenterol. 2013;48(5):574-594.

91. Christensen HM, et al. Prevalence of cachexia in chronic heart failure and characteristics of body composition and metabolic status. Endocrine. 2013;43(3):626-634.

92. Cochrane WU, Afolabi OA. Investigation into the nutritional status, dietary intake and smoking habits of patients with chronic obstructive pulmonary disease. J Hum Nutr Diet. 2004;17(1):3.

93. Boisrame-Helms J, et al. Lipid emulsions for parenteral nutrition in critical illness. Prog Lipid Res. 2015;60:1-16.

94. Dickerson RN, et al. Adverse effects from inappropriate medication administration via a jejunostomy feeding tube. Nutr Clin Pract. 2003;18:402.

95. Ayodele-Adesanya TM, et al. Nutrition in traumatic brain injury: focus on the immune modulating supplements. In Sadaka F, editor. Traumatic Brain Injury [e-book]. InTech; 2014.

96. Wang X, et al. Nutritional support for patients sustaining traumatic brain injury: a systematic review and meta-analysis of prospective studies. PloS One. 2013;8(3):e58838.

97. Pellicane AJ, et al. Calorie and protein intake in acute rehabilitation in patients with traumatic spinal cord injury versus other diagnoses. Top Spinal Cord Inj Rehabil. 2013;19(3):229.

98. Aquilani R, et al. Energy expenditure and nutritional adequacy of rehabilitation paraplegics with asymptomatic bacteriuria and pressure sores. Spinal Cord. 2001;39:437.

99. Ikizler TA, et al. Prevention and treatment of protein energy wasting in chronic kidney disease patients: a consensus statement by the International Society of Renal Nutrition and Metabolism. Kidney Int. 2013;84(6):1096-1107.

100. Kellum JA, Lameire N. Diagnosis, evaluation, and management of acute kidney injury: a KDIGO summary (Part 1). Crit Care. 2012;17(1):204.

101. Case KO, et al. Nutrition support in the critically ill patient. Crit Care Nurs Q. 2000;22(4):75-89.

102. Scheinkestel CD, et al. Prospective randomized trial to assess caloric and protein needs of critically ill, anuric, ventilated patients requiring continuous renal replacement therapy. Nutrition. 2003;19:909.

103. Brown RO, Compher C. the American Society for Parenteral and Enteral Nutrition (ASPEN) Board of Directors. A.S.P.E.N. Clinical guideline: nutrition support in adult acute and chronic renal failure. J Parenter Enteral Nutr. 2010;34(4):366.

104. Cano NJM, et al. ESPEN guidelines on parenteral nutrition: adult renal failure. Clin Nutr. 2009;28(4):401-414.

105. Patton KM, Aranda-Michel J. Nutritional aspects in liver disease and liver transplantation. Nutr Clin Pract. 2002;17:332.

106. Saraf N. Nutritional management of acute and chronic liver disease. Hepatitis B Annual. 2008;5(1):117-133.

107. Khokhar AS, Seidner DL. The pathophysiology of pancreatitis. Nutr Clin Pract. 2004;19:5.

108. Academy of Nutrition and Dietetics. Nutrition Care Manual website. Nutrition Care > Gastrointestinal Disease > Liver, Gallbladder, and Pancreas Disease > Pancreatitis > Nutrition Intervention. http://nutrition caremanual.org. Accessed November 21, 2015.

109. Ong JPL, Fock KM. Nutritional support in acute pancreatitis. J Dig Dis. 2012;13(9):445-452.

110. Russell MK. Acute pancreatitis: a review of pathophysiology and nutrition management. Nutr Clin Pract. 2004;19:16.

111. Al-Omran M, et al. Enteral versus parenteral nutrition for acute pancreatitis. Cochrane Database Syst Rev. 2010:1.

112. Petrov MS, Pylypchuk RD, Uchugina AF. A systematic review on the timing of artificial nutrition in acute pancreatitis. Br J Nutr. 2009;101(6):787-793.

113. Talukdar R, Vege SS. Recent developments in acute pancreatitis. Clin Gastroenterol Hepatol. 2009;7(11):S3-S9.

114. Rodbard H, et al. Statement by an American Association of Clinical Endocrinologists/American College of Endocrinology consensus panel on type 2 diabetes mellitus: an algorithm for glycemic control. Endocr Pract. 2009;15(6):540-559.

115. Van den Berghe G, et al. Intensive insulin therapy in critically ill patients. N Engl J Med. 2001;345:1359.

116. Rassias AJ, et al. Insulin increases neutrophil count and phagocytic capacity after cardiac surgery. Anesth Analg. 2002;94:1113.

117. Umpierrez GE, et al. Hyperglycemia: an independent marker of in-hospital mortality in patients with undiagnosed diabetes. J Clin Endocrinol Metab. 2002;87:978.

118. McMahon MM. Management of parenteral nutrition in acutely ill patients with hyperglycemia. Nutr Clin Pract. 2004;19:120.

119. Charney P, Hertzler SR. Management of blood glucose and diabetes in the critically ill patient receiving enteral feeding. Nutr Clin Pract. 2004;19:129.

120. Jones MP. Management of diabetic gastroparesis. Nutr Clin Pract. 2004;19:145.

121. Evert AB, et al. Nutrition therapy recommendations for the management of adults with diabetes. Diabetes Care. 2014;37:S120-143.

122. American Diabetes Association. Nutrition recommendations and interventions for diabetes [position statement]. Diabetes Care. 2008;31(suppl 1):S61.

123. Clement S, et al. Management of diabetes and hyperglycemia in hospitals. Diabetes Care. 2004;27:553.

8

Pain and Pain Management

Céline Gélinas

Despite national and international efforts, guidelines, standards of practice, position statements, and many important discoveries in the field of pain management in the past 3 decades, critically ill patients experience moderate to severe pain at rest or during routine care.[1-3] For example, turning, endotracheal suctioning, tube or drain removal, wound care, and arterial line placement were identified as the most painful procedures by critically ill adults in previous studies.[2-4] Despite this situation, pain is undertreated in most critically ill patients.[5] Poor treatment of acute pain may lead to the development of serious complications[6,7] and chronic pain syndromes,[8-10] which may seriously impact the patient's functioning, quality of life, and well-being. Such evidence reinforces the importance of providing attention to pain in this specific context of care.

IMPORTANCE OF PAIN ASSESSMENT

Appropriate pain assessment is the foundation of effective pain treatment. Because pain is recognized as a subjective experience, the patient's self-report is considered the most valid measure for pain and should be obtained as often as possible.[11] In critical care, many factors, such as the administration of sedative agents, the use of mechanical ventilation, and altered levels of consciousness, may affect communication with patients.[12] These obstacles make pain assessment more complex. Nevertheless, except for being unable to speak, many mechanically ventilated patients can communicate that they are in pain by using head nodding, using hand motions, or seeking attention with other movements.[4,13] In such a situation, use of appropriate communication methods may reduce patients' distress associated with the presence of the endotracheal tube by enabling them to report the presence of pain or discomfort in a comprehensive way.[14]

Self-report pain intensity scales have been used with postoperative mechanically ventilated patients who were asked to point on the scale.[2,15] However, in a study of mechanically ventilated adults with various diagnoses (trauma, surgical, or medical), only one-third of mechanically ventilated patients were able to use a pain intensity scale.[15] With a greater degree of critical illness, providing a pain intensity self-report becomes more difficult because it requires concentration and energy. When the patient is unable to communicate in any way, observable behavioral indicators become unique indices for pain assessment and are part of clinical guidelines and recommendations developed in North America.[16,17] Pain is frequently encountered in critical care, and there is increased emphasis on the professional responsibility to manage the patient's pain effectively. The critical care nurse must understand the mechanisms, assessment process, and appropriate therapeutic measures for managing pain.

This chapter provides nurses with a better understanding of the physiology of pain. It also demonstrates strategies and tools that can be used for pain assessment and several methods for pain management in critically ill patients.

DEFINITION AND DESCRIPTION OF PAIN

Pain is described as an unpleasant sensory and emotional experience associated with actual or potential tissue damage or described in terms of such damage.[11,18] This definition emphasizes the subjective and multidimensional nature of pain. More specifically, the subjective characteristic implies that pain is whatever the person experiencing it says it is and that it exists whenever he or she says it does.[19] This definition also suggests that the patient is able to self-report. However, in the critical care context, many patients are unable to self-report their pain. Some authors[20] have proposed an alternative definition for nonverbal patients, in this case infants, but the same principle applies to any nonverbal population, stating that changes in behaviors caused by pain are valuable forms of self-report and should be considered as alternative measures of pain. Pain assessment must be designed to conform to the communication capabilities of the patient.

Components of Pain

The experience of pain includes sensory, affective, cognitive, behavioral, and physiologic components[21]:

The sensory component is the perception of many characteristics of pain such as intensity, location, and quality.

The affective component includes negative emotions such as unpleasantness, distress, and anticipation that may be associated with the experience of pain. Anxiety and fear can also be related to the experience of pain.

The cognitive component refers to the interpretation or the meaning of pain by the person who is experiencing it.

The behavioral component includes the strategies used by the person to express, avoid, or control pain.

The physiologic component refers to nociception and the stress response.

Types of Pain

Pain can be acute or chronic, with different sensations related to the origin of the pain ie, nociceptive or neuropathic.

Acute Pain

Acute pain has a short duration, it usually corresponds to the healing process (30 days), and it should not exceed 6 months. It implies tissue damage that is usually from an identifiable cause. If undertreated, acute pain may bring a prolonged stress response and lead to permanent damage to the patient's nervous system. In such a situation, acute pain can become chronic.[8,9]

Chronic Pain

Chronic pain persists for more than 6 months after the healing process from the original injury, and it may or may not be associated with an illness.[22] It develops when the healing process is incomplete or, as described earlier, when acute pain is poorly managed.[23] Both acute and chronic pain can have a nociceptive or neuropathic origin.[11]

Nociceptive Pain

Nociceptive pain arises from activation of nociceptors,[11] and it can be somatic or visceral. Somatic pain involves superficial tissues such as the skin, muscles, joints, and bones. Its location is well defined. Visceral pain involves organs such as the heart, stomach, and liver. Its location is diffuse, and it can be referred to a different location in the body.[24] Not all organs are sensitive to pain, and some can be damaged extensively without the patient feeling anything. For example, many diseases of the liver, lungs, or kidneys are completely painless, and the only symptoms felt are symptoms derived from the abnormal functioning of these organs. Relatively minor lesions in viscera such as the stomach, the bladder, or the ureters can produce excruciating pain, as these organs are abundantly innervated by sensory neurons that signal harmful events.[25]

Neuropathic Pain

Neuropathic pain arises from a lesion or disease affecting the somatosensory system.[11] The origin of neuropathic pain may be peripheral or central. Neuralgia and neuropathy are examples related to peripheral neuropathic pain, which implies damage of the peripheral somatosensory system. Central neuropathic pain involves the central somatosensory cortex and can be experienced by patients after a cerebral stroke. Neuropathic pain can be difficult to manage and frequently requires a multimodal approach (ie, combinations of several pharmacologic or nonpharmacologic treatments).[24]

Physiology of Pain
Nociception

Nociception represents the neural processes of encoding and processing noxious stimuli necessary, but not sufficient, for pain.[11] Pain results from the integration of the pain-related signal into specific cortical areas of the brain associated with higher mental processes and consciousness. In other words, pain is the conscious experience that emerges from nociception.[26] Four processes are involved in nociception[24]:

1. Transduction
2. Transmission
3. Perception
4. Modulation

The four processes are shown in Fig. 8.1, which integrates pain assessment with nociception, and in Fig. 8.2.

Transduction

Transduction refers to mechanical (eg, surgical incision), thermal (eg, burn), or chemical (eg, toxic substance) stimuli that damage tissues. In critical care, many nociceptive stimuli exist, including the patient's acute illness or condition, invasive technology used for the patient, and multiple interventions that have to be done. These stimuli, also called stressors, stimulate the liberation of many chemical substances, such as prostaglandins, bradykinin, serotonin, histamine, glutamate, and substance P. These neurotransmitters stimulate peripheral nociceptive receptors and initiate nociceptive transmission.

Transmission

As a result of transduction, an action potential is produced and is transmitted by nociceptive nerve fibers in the spinal cord that reach higher centers of the brain. This is called transmission, and it represents the second process of nociception. The principal nociceptive fibers are the A-delta (Aδ) and C fibers. Large-diameter, myelinated Aδ fibers that transmit well-localized, sharp pain are involved in "first pain" sensation, which leads to reflex withdrawal. Small-diameter, unmyelinated C fibers transmit diffuse, dull, aching pain, which is referred to as "second pain."[26] These fibers transmit the noxious sensation from the periphery through the dorsal root of the spinal cord. With the liberation of substance P, these fibers then synapse with ascending spinothalamic fibers to the central nervous system (CNS). These spinothalamic fibers are clustered into two specific pathways: neospinothalamic and paleospinothalamic pathways. Generally, the Aδ fibers transmit the pain sensation to the brain within the NS pathway, and the C fibers use the PS pathway.[27]

Through synapsing of nociceptive fibers with motor fibers in the spinal cord, muscle rigidity can appear because of a reflex activity.[28] Muscle rigidity can be a behavioral indicator associated with pain. It can contribute to immobility and decrease diaphragmatic excursion. This can lead to hypoventilation and hypoxemia. Hypoxemia can be detected by a pulse oximeter (Spo_2) and by monitoring of arterial partial pressure of oxygen (Pao_2). The interaction of a ventilated patient with the machine (eg, activation of alarms, fighting the ventilator) also may indicate the presence of pain.[29]

Perception

The pain message is transmitted by the spinothalamic pathways to centers in the brain, where it is perceived. Pain sensation transmitted by the neospinothalamic pathway reaches the thalamus, and the pain sensation transmitted by the paleospinothalamic pathway reaches the brainstem, hypothalamus, and thalamus.[27] These parts of the CNS contribute to the initial perception of pain. Projections to the limbic system and the frontal cortex allow expression of the affective component of pain.[30] Projections to the sensory cortex located in the parietal lobe allow the patient to describe the sensory characteristics of his or her pain, such as location, intensity, and quality.[30,31] The cognitive component of pain involves many parts of the cerebral cortex and is complex. These three components (affective, sensory, and cognitive) represent the subjective interpretation of pain. Parallel to this subjective process, certain facial expressions and body movements are behavioral indicators of pain occurring as a result of pain fiber projections to the motor cortex in the frontal lobe.

Modulation

Modulation is a process by which noxious stimuli that travel from the nociceptive receptors to the CNS may be enhanced or inhibited. Pain can be modulated by ascending and descending mechanisms. A typical example of ascending pain modulation is rubbing an injury site, which activates large A-beta (Aβ) fibers

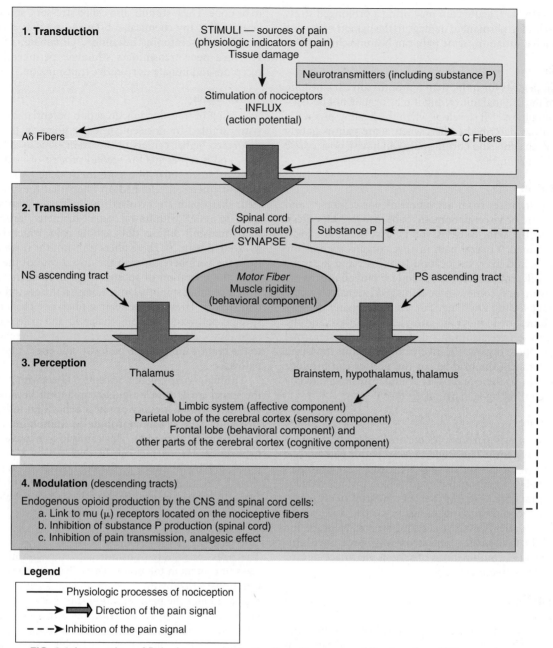

FIG. 8.1 Integration of Pain Assessment in the Four Processes of Nociception. CNS, central nervous system; NS, neospinothalamic pathway; PS, paleospinothalamic pathway. (Courtesy Céline Gélinas, Ingram School of Nursing, McGill University, Canada.)

in the periphery. Stimulation of these fibers activates inhibitory interneurons in the dorsal horn of the spinal cord, preventing nociceptive signal transmission from the periphery to the higher brain regions. The physiologic basis of this mechanism of pain modulation was elucidated by Melzack and Wall in 1965[32] and refers to the gate control theory. Analgesia may also be produced at the level of the spinal cord and brainstem (spinothalamic pathway) via the release of endogenous opioids and neurotransmitters. Endogenous opioids are naturally occurring morphine-like pentapeptides found throughout the nervous system and exist in three general classes: beta-endorphins, enkephalins, and dynorphins. These substances block neuronal activity related to nociceptive impulses by binding to opioid mu (μ) receptor sites in the central and peripheral nervous systems.[27]

In the ascending pain modulation mechanism, endogenous opioids may be produced in the brainstem, and the dorsal horn or exogenous opioids may be introduced by administration of an opioid analgesic. The released or introduced opioids bind to the mu-opioid receptors on nociceptive nerve fibers, blocking the release of substance P. In the descending pain modulation mechanism, the efferent spinothalamic nerve fibers that descend from the brain can inhibit the propagation of the pain signal by triggering the release of endogenous opioids in the brainstem and in the spinal cord. Serotonin and norepinephrine are important inhibitory neurotransmitters that act in the CNS. These substances are also released by the descending fibers of the descending spinothalamic pathway.[33] The use of distraction, relaxation, and imagery techniques can facilitate the release of

FIG. 8.2 **Four Processes of Nociception.** (From Jarvis C. *Physical examination & health assessment.* 6th ed. Philadelphia, Saunders; 2011.)

endogenous opioids and has been shown to reduce the overall pain experience.[34]

Summary

Nociception is an important physiologic mechanism of pain that can integrate many components of pain for its assessment. In transduction, stimuli are sources of pain that trigger the liberation of neurotransmitters. In transmission, diffusion of the action potential along the neospinothalamic pathway may lead to muscle rigidity—a reflex activity that can be observed as a behavioral indicator associated with pain. Muscle rigidity may also influence respiratory rate and amplitude and cause decrease in Spo₂. In perception, the patient's self-report of affective, sensory, and cognitive information can be obtained, and behavioral responses to pain may also be observed. Finally, in modulation, pain sensation may be attenuated by ascending and descending mechanisms.

Biologic Stress Response

A biologic stress response may be activated by pain, an obvious stressor. This stress response involves the nervous, endocrine, and immune systems in the hypothalamic-pituitary-adrenal axis.[35] The biologic stress response includes a short-term direct response, a midterm response, and a long-term indirect response. Stress mechanisms are depicted in Fig. 8.3.

Short-Term Direct Response

In the presence of a stressor such as pain, the hypothalamus releases corticotropin-releasing factor, which activates the sympathetic nervous system (SNS). Norepinephrine is then released from the terminals of sympathetic nerves, and epinephrine is released from the adrenal cortex. This mechanism constitutes the short-term direct stress response. The effects of these stress hormones allow observation of physiologic responses associated with activation of SNS. For example, increased blood pressure, increased heart rate, and increased respiratory rate are common signs of acute stress and may be associated with pain.[15,29,36] Pupil dilation also can be observed.[37]

If pain persists over time or injuries are located in the bladder or the intestines, the parasympathetic nervous system may be dominant. The blood pressure and heart rate may decrease rather than increase. The absence of pain-related indicators related to the activation of the SNS does not imply an absence of pain sensation.[38]

FIG. 8.3 Integration of Potential Physiologic Pain Indicators in the Biologic Stress Response.
ACTH, adrenocorticotropic hormone; CRF, corticotropin-releasing factor; IL, interleukin; TNF, tumor necrosis factor. (Courtesy Céline Gélinas, Ingram School of Nursing, McGill University, Canada.)

Midterm Indirect Response

At midterm, the corticotropin-releasing factor released from the hypothalamus stimulates the anterior pituitary to release adrenocorticotropic hormone and the posterior pituitary to release vasopressin, the antidiuretic hormone. Adrenocorticotropic hormone activates the adrenal cortex to release aldosterone and cortisol. Vasopressin and aldosterone increase sodium and water retention. This increases intravascular volume and decreases diuresis and increases blood pressure and cardiac preload. Cortisol also may contribute to systemic responses such as infection and hyperglycemia.

At midterm, pain may be associated with decreased diuresis, increased blood pressure, increased central venous pressure, and increased pulmonary artery occlusion pressure. However, changes in these parameters are not specific to pain, and their associations with pain are not supported by empiric data.

Long-Term Indirect Response

The stress hormones, specifically cortisol, have a long-term influence on the immune system in two ways: immunosuppression

and release of cytokines.[39] Cytokines may prolong by retroactivation the release of cortisol, which may exacerbate tissue damage, contributing to the chronic pain process.[23]

Summary

The biologic stress response allows observation of fluctuations in physiologic signs that represent a source of stress and may be associated with acute pain. The short-term signs are mainly related to SNS activation. Other signs, such as decreased diuresis and increased central venous pressure and pulmonary artery occlusion pressure, relate to the midterm indirect stress response. The immune system is involved in the long-term indirect response of stress. No acute pain indicators have been associated with this process. All the indicators identified within the biologic stress response are not specific to pain because they can be attributed to other distress conditions, homeostatic changes, and medications.[16]

Framework for Pain Assessment and Definition

As previously stated, self-report of pain is not always possible to obtain in critically ill patients, as many of them may be unable

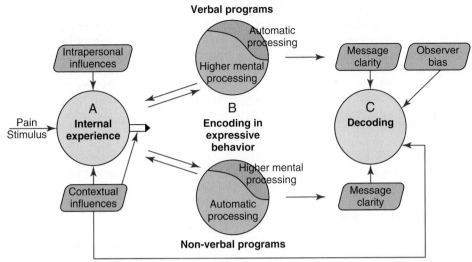

Verbal programs

FIG. 8.4 Communications Model of Pain. (Redrawn from Hadjistavropoulos T, Craig KD. A theoretical framework for understanding self-report and observational measures of pain: a communications model. *Behav Res Ther.* 2002;40:551.)

to communicate during their stay in the critical care unit. When the patient is unable to self-report, the expression of pain can be examined from the perspective of a communications model of pain.[40] The foundation of this model is that observational measures capture behaviors that are less subject to voluntary control and more automatic compared with self-report measures that depend on higher mental processes. Consequently, observational measures should be used to assess pain when the individual's self-report is unavailable, as is often the case in critically ill patients. This A → B → C model conceptualizes pain as an internal state (A) that may be encoded in particular features of expressive behaviors (B), allowing observers (in this case nurses) to draw inferences (C) about the nature of the sender's (ie, the patient) experience (Fig. 8.4).

More specifically, when an individual is exposed to a nociceptive stimulus known to be painful, information about real or potential tissue damage is transmitted and processed centrally into the brain. The processing of a nociceptive stimulus can be modulated by intrapersonal or contextual factors influencing the way information is integrated and consequently how pain is experienced in each individual. In critical care, intrapersonal factors that could potentially influence the processing of a nociceptive stimulus include the patient's sociodemographic characteristics, severity of critical illness or injury, level of sedation, and level of consciousness. Similarly, examples of contextual factors specific to the critical care unit environment that could influence the patient's pain experience include mechanical ventilation and administration of sedative and opioid agents. Taking into account the various intrapersonal and contextual factors, critically ill patients may express their pain through different patterns of verbal and nonverbal expressive modalities. The depicted pattern depends largely on the degree of impairment in the cortical areas of the brain associated with consciousness. Although some patients with a mild alteration of the level of consciousness may still have the capacity to self-report or express their pain with voluntary behaviors (eg, localization of the pain site), others with a severe alteration of the level of consciousness might respond to pain only through autonomic reactions such as reflex or fluctuations in physiologic signs. Whether patients are able to express their pain through self-report, voluntary behaviors, or autonomic reactions undoubtedly affects the clarity of the message and the capacity of nurses to identify the specific nature of patients' pain. Because behaviors are difficult to decode, educational training of nurses is necessary to support them in developing the competence of adequately assessing pain behaviors using observational measures.

PAIN ASSESSMENT

Pain assessment is an integral part of nursing care. Assessment is a prerequisite for adequate pain control and relief. As stated earlier, pain is a subjective, multidimensional concept that requires complex assessment. Many factors may alter verbal communication in critically ill patients, making pain assessment more challenging. This situation should not discourage nurses from assessing pain in these vulnerable patients because acute pain is a stressor that can exacerbate their condition.

Pain assessment has two major components: (1) nonobservable, or subjective, and (2) observable, or objective. The complexity of pain assessment requires the use of multiple strategies by critical care nurses. In the following sections, patient, health professional, and organizational barriers to pain assessment and management are addressed, and recommendations are proposed.

Subjective Component of Pain Assessment

Pain is known as a subjective experience. The subjective component of pain assessment refers to the patient's self-report about his or her sensorial, affective, and cognitive experience of pain. Because it is considered the most valid measure of pain, the patient's self-report must be obtained whenever possible.[16] A simple yes or no (presence versus absence of pain) is a valid self-report. Mechanical ventilation should not be a barrier for nurses to document patients' self-reports of pain. Many mechanically ventilated patients can communicate that they have pain or can use pain scales by pointing to numbers or symbols on the scale.[2,4,15] Attempts should be made to obtain a self-report before concluding that a patient is unable to self-report. More importantly, sufficient time should be allowed for the patient to respond with each attempt.[16]

If sedation and cognition levels allow the patient to give more information about pain, a multidimensional assessment can be documented. Multidimensional pain assessment tools including the sensorial, emotional, and cognitive components are available, such as the Brief Pain Inventory,[41] the Initial Pain Assessment Tool,[24] and the short-form McGill Pain Questionnaire.[42] However, because of the administration of sedative and analgesic agents in mechanically ventilated patients, the tool must be short enough to be completed. The short-form McGill Pain Questionnaire takes a few minutes to complete and has been used to assess mechanically ventilated patients who were in a stable condition.[2]

The patient's self-report of pain can also be obtained by questioning the patient using the mnemonic PQRSTU[43]:

P: Provocative and palliative or aggravating factors
Q: Quality
R: Region or location, radiation
S: Severity and other symptoms
T: Timing
U: Understanding

P: Provocative and Palliative or Aggravating Factors

The **P** in the mnemonic indicates what provokes or causes the patient's pain, what he or she was doing when the pain occurred, and what makes the pain worse or better. For example, deep breathing intensifying chest pain in the case of pericarditis is an illustration of an aggravating factor. Moderating factors that reduce or alleviate pain or discomfort are also important findings and may include resting to diminish burning chest pain that causes angina. Knowledge of any intensifying or alleviating conditions can contribute to the patient's plan of care throughout the continuum of care.

Q: Quality

The **Q** in the mnemonic refers to the quality of the pain or the pain sensation that the patient is experiencing. The patient may describe the pain as dull, aching, sharp, burning, or stabbing. This information provides the nurse with data regarding the type of pain the patient is experiencing (eg, somatic or visceral). The differentiation between types of pain may contribute to the determination of cause and management. A patient who has had open-heart surgery may complain of chest pain that is shooting or burning.[4] This information can lead the nurse to investigate for cutaneous or bone injuries as a result of a sternotomy. Another patient may describe a sharp thoracic pain that may lead the nurse to consider visceral pain as a result of pulmonary embolism. A verbal description of pain is important because it provides a baseline account, allowing the critical care nurse to monitor changes in the type of pain, which may indicate a change in the underlying pathology.

R: Region or Location, Radiation

R usually is easy for the patient to identify, although visceral pain is more difficult for the patient to localize.[24] If the patient has difficulty naming the location or is mechanically ventilated, ask the patient to point to the location on himself or herself or on a simple anatomic drawing.[44]

S: Severity and Other Symptoms

S, the severity or intensity of pain, is a measurement that has undergone much investigation. Many pain intensity scales are available, including the descriptive and numeric pain rating scales that are often used in the critical care environment (Fig. 8.5). Many critical care units use a specific pain intensity scale. The use of a single tool provides consistency of assessment and documentation. A visual format of a 0-to-10 self-report scale (ie, Numeric Rating Scale, Thermometer) has been found to be the most feasible in critically ill adults.[45,46] Asking the patient to grade his or her pain on a scale of 0 to 10 using a visual format is a consistent method and aids the nurse in objectifying the subjective nature of the patient's pain. However, the patient's tool preference should be considered.

The **S** in the mnemonic also refers to other symptoms accompanying the patient's pain experience, such as shortness of breath, nausea, and fatigue. Anxiety and fear are common emotions associated with pain.

T: Timing

The **T** in the mnemonic refers to documenting the onset, duration, and frequency of pain. This information can help to determine whether the origin of the pain is acute or chronic. The duration of pain can indicate the severity of the problem. For example, chest pain of less than 15 minutes' duration may be angina, and chest pain lasting more than 15 minutes may indicate a myocardial infarction.

U: Understanding

The **U** in the mnemonic is the patient's perception of the problem or cognitive experience of pain. Patients with known cardiac problems can tell the nurse whether their pain is the same as they had during myocardial infarction. Patients with a cerebral hemorrhage often describe experiencing the worst headache they have ever had.

Because of the patient's change in communication, lack of concentration , and the life-or-death immediacy of most actions in the critical care environment, pain assessment is often reduced to minimal information. Begin by asking, "Do

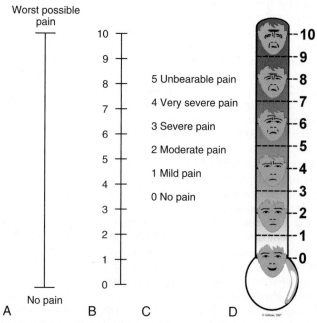

FIG. 8.5 Pain Intensity Scales (Vertical Format). (A) Visual analog scale (VAS). (B) Numeric Rating Scale (NRS). (C) Descriptive rating scale (DRS). (D) Faces Pain Thermometer. (Courtesy Céline Gélinas, Ingram School of Nursing, McGill University, Canada.)

you have pain?" The use of a simple yes or no question allows the patient to answer verbally or to indicate his or her response by nodding the head or by other signs. It is easier for mechanically ventilated patients to communicate with nurses in this way because they cannot express themselves verbally. Pain intensity and location also are necessary for the initial assessment of pain.

Observable or Objective Component of Pain Assessment

When the patient's self-report is impossible to obtain, nurses can rely on the observation of behavioral indicators, which are strongly emphasized in clinical recommendations and guidelines for pain management in nonverbal patients.[16,17] Fluctuations in vital signs should never be used alone but rather considered as a cue to begin further assessment for pain.[16,17]

Pain-related behaviors have been described in critically ill patients and were studied in the AACN Thunder Project II.[47] Patients who experienced pain during nociceptive procedures were three times more likely to have increased behavioral responses such as facial expressions, muscle rigidity, and vocalization than patients without pain. Similar observations were found in a study of 257 mechanically ventilated critically ill adult patients.[29] Patients who experienced pain during turning showed significantly more intense facial expressions (eg, grimacing), muscle rigidity, and less compliance with the ventilator (eg, fighting the ventilator) compared with patients without pain. Several behavioral scales have been developed for assessing pain in critically ill nonverbal adult patients.[48] The clinical guidelines of the Society of Critical Care Medicine (SCCM) recommend both the Behavioral Pain Scale (BPS)[49] and the Critical-Care Pain Observation Tool (CPOT)[50] for clinical use in medical, postoperative, and non–brain trauma critically ill adult patients unable to self-report.[17] The implementation of these scales in critical care units has led to enhanced nursing practices of pain assessment and management[51,52] and improved patient outcomes, including decreases in mechanical ventilation duration, infection rates, and adverse events.[53,54]

Behavioral Pain Scale

The BPS[49] shown in Table 8.1 was tested mostly in nonverbal mechanically ventilated patients with altered levels of consciousness.[48] CPOT validity is supported by the association of

significantly higher BPS scores during nociceptive procedures (eg, turning, endotracheal suctioning, peripheral venous cannulation) compared with rest or nonnociceptive procedures (eg, arterial catheter dressing change, compression stocking applications, eye care). The authors of the BPS determined a cut-off score greater than 5 for the presence of pain.[55] A positive association was also found between nurses' BPS ratings and conscious sedated patients' self-report of pain intensity during turning.[56] Good interrater reliability of BPS scores between several raters including nurses was reached. The BPS can be used quickly (2 to 5 minutes), and most clinicians were satisfied with its ease of use.[49,53]

Critical-Care Pain Observation Tool

The CPOT[50] shown in Table 8.2 was tested in verbal and nonverbal, critically ill adults.[48] Content validation was supported by critical care unit expert clinicians including nurses and physicians.[57] Validity of the CPOT use was supported with significantly higher CPOT scores during a nociceptive procedure (eg, turning with or without other care, endotracheal suctioning) compared with rest or a nonnociceptive procedure (eg, taking blood pressure, central catheter dressing change). Positive associations were found between the CPOT scores and the patient's self-report of pain. A cut-off score greater than 2 was established with the CPOT in postoperative adult patients in the critical care unit.[58] Similarly to the BPS, good interrater reliability of CPOT scores was achieved with nurses. Feasibility and clinical utility of the CPOT were positively evaluated by critical care nurses,[59] which was sustained at 12 months after implementation of the tool.[60] Nurses agreed that the CPOT was quick enough to be used in the critical care unit, simple to understand, easy to complete, and helpful for nursing practice. An online teaching video to learn how to use the CPOT at the bedside is available (see Table 8.2).

Use of Cut-Off Scores

A cut-off score refers to the score on a specific scale associated with the best probability of correctly ruling in or ruling out a patient with a specific condition—in this case pain. The use of a cut-off score with behavioral pain scales can help to identify when pain is highly likely to be present and guide nurses in determining whether or not an intervention to alleviate pain is required. Also, a cut-off score can help to evaluate the effectiveness of pain management interventions. Cut-off scores are established using a criterion (ie, a gold standard in the field). As mentioned previously, in the case of pain, the patient's self-report is known as the gold standard criterion.[11] Behavioral pain scores should be interpreted differently from the patient's self-report pain intensity scores. Although they both represent pain scores, they are measuring different dimensions of pain which are interrelated. More specifically, behavioral scores based on the nurse's observations are associated with the behavioral dimension of pain, and the patient's self-report of pain intensity relates to the sensory dimension of pain.[21] Although self-reported pain intensity scores and behavioral pain scores move in the same direction (ie, when one score increases, the other score increases as well), they are not equal scores.[16,48] Therefore it is important to know that behavioral pain scales only allow the detection of the presence versus absence of pain. Box 8.1 provides a case example showing how a cut-off score can be used in practice.

TABLE 8.1	Behavioral Pain Scale	
Item	**Description**	**Score**
Facial expression	Relaxed	1
	Partially tightened (eg, brow lowering)	2
	Fully tightened (eg, eyelid closing)	3
	Grimacing	4
Upper limbs	No movement	1
	Partially bent	2
	Fully bent with finger flexion	3
	Permanently retracted	4
Compliance with ventilation	Tolerating movement	1
	Coughing but tolerating ventilation for most of the time	2
	Fighting ventilator	3
	Unable to control ventilation	4
Total		3–12

From Payen JF, et al. Assessing pain in critically ill sedated patients by using a behavioral pain scale. *Crit Care Med.* 2001;29(12):2258.

TABLE 8.2   Critical Care Pain Observation Tool

Indicator	Score		Description
Facial expression	Relaxed, neutral	0	No muscle tension observed
	Tense	1	Presence of brow lowering, orbit tightening and levator contraction or any other change (eg, opening eyes or tearing during nociceptive procedures)
	Grimacing	2	All previous facial movements plus eyelid tightly closed (the patient may present with mouth open or biting the endotracheal tube)
Body movements	Absence of movements or normal position	0	Does not move at all (does not necessarily mean absence of pain) or normal position (movements not aimed toward the pain site or not made for the purpose of protection)
	Protection	1	Slow, cautious movements, touching or rubbing the pain site, seeking attention through movements
	Restlessness/ agitation	2	Pulling tube, attempting to sit up, moving limbs/ thrashing, not following commands, striking at staff, trying to climb out of bed
Compliance with the ventilator (intubated patients)	Tolerating ventilator or movement	0	Alarms not activated, easy ventilation
or	Coughing but tolerating	1	Coughing, alarms may be activated but stop spontaneously
	Fighting ventilator	2	Asynchrony: blocking ventilation, alarms frequently activated
Vocalization (nonintubated patients)	Talking in normal tone or no sound	0	Talking in normal tone or no sound
	Sighing, moaning	1	Sighing, moaning
	Crying out, sobbing	2	Crying out, sobbing
Muscle tension	Relaxed	0	No resistance to passive movements
	Tense, rigid	1	Resistance to passive movements
	Very tense or rigid	2	Strong resistance to passive movements, incapacity to complete them
Total	___ / 8		

1. The patient must be observed at rest for 1 minute to obtain a baseline value of the CPOT.
   1.1 Observation of patient at rest (baseline).
   The nurse looks at the patient's face and body to note any visible reactions for an observation period of 1 minute. The nurse gives a score for all items except for muscle tension. At the end of the 1-minute period, the nurse holds the patient's arm in both hands—she places one hand at the elbow and uses the other one to hold the patient's hand. Then she performs a passive flexion and extension of the upper limb and feels any resistance the patient may exhibit. If the movements are performed easily, the patient is found to be relaxed with no resistance (score 0). If the movements can still be performed but with more strength, then it is concluded that the patient is showing resistance to movements (score 1). If the nurse cannot complete the movements, strong resistance is felt (score 2). This can be observed in patients who are spastic.
2. Then the patient should be observed during painful procedures (eg, turning, wound care) to detect any changes in the patient's behaviors.
   2.2 Observation of patient during a painful procedure.
   While performing a procedure known to be painful, the nurse looks at the patient's face to note any reactions such as brow lowering or grimacing. These reactions may be brief or can last longer. The nurse also looks out for body movements. For instance, she looks for protective movements such as the patient trying to reach or touching the pain site (eg, surgical incision, injury site). In the mechanically ventilated patient, she pays attention to alarms and if they stop spontaneously or require that she intervenes (eg, reassurance, administering medication). It is important that the nurse auscultates the patient to check for the position of the endotracheal tube and the presence of secretions as these factors may influence this item without being indicative of pain. According to muscle tension, the nurse can feel if the patient is resisting against the movement or not. A score 2 is given when the patient is resisting against the movement and attempts to get on his/her back.
3. The patient should be evaluated before and at the peak effect of an analgesic agent to assess whether the treatment was effective or not in relieving pain.
4. The patient should be attributed the highest score observed during the observation period.
5. The patient should be attributed a score for each behavior included in the CPOT, and muscle tension should be evaluated last as it may lead to behavioral reactions not necessarily related to pain, but more to the actual stimulation. According to compliance with the ventilator, the nurse must check that the endotracheal tube is well positioned, and for the presence of secretions, which could lead to higher scores for this item.

An online teaching video funded and created by Kaiser Permanente Northern California Nursing Research (KPNCNR) to learn how to use the CPOT at the bedside is available at http://kpnursing.org/professionaldevelopment/index.html

Modified from Gélinas C, et al. Validation of the Critical-Care Pain Observation Tool (CPOT) in adult patients. *Am J Crit Care.* 2006;15:420. Figure of facial expressions courtesy of Céline GélinasIngram School of Nursing, McGill University, Canada.

Limitations Related to Use of Behavioral Pain Scales

Behavioral pain scales have been validated for pain assessment in critically ill patients, but they have some limitations. They are impossible to monitor in patients unable to respond behaviorally to pain, such as patients with paralysis or under the effects of neuromuscular blocking agents. Also, behavioral responses may be blurred with the administration of high doses of sedative agents.[15] Minimal behavioral responses to painful procedures were found in unconscious, mechanically ventilated critically ill adults who were more heavily sedated compared with conscious patients.[29]

In addition, behavioral pain scales developed for nonverbal critically ill patients may have to be adapted for patients with a brain injury and an altered level of consciousness, as they were found to exhibit different behavioral responses to pain.[29,61,62] Instead of grimacing, brain-injured patients with altered levels of consciousness seemed to react mostly by opening their eyes, showing face flushing, tearing, and exhibiting limb flexion when exposed to pain. Conscious brain-injured patients were more likely to exhibit brow lowering and touching the pain site in response to pain.[61,62] Further studies are needed to better understand how brain-injured patients react to painful procedures. The content of existing behavioral pain scales may need to be adjusted for use in this specific vulnerable group. When selecting a scale, nurses should make sure that is has been tested in a patient population and context in which they plan to use it. A scale can be shown to be valid only with a specific group of people and in a given context.[63] Until a validated behavioral pain scale is available for use in brain-injured critically ill patients, nurses should consult family members to better understand the patient's pain behaviors and their specific reactions at rest and during activity, or procedures should be documented in the chart.[16]

Physiologic Indicators

When patients cannot react behaviorally to pain, the only possible clues left for the detection of pain are physiologic indicators. Vital signs (ie, blood pressure, heart rate, respiratory rate) have received some attention; however, their validity in the pain assessment process is not supported. Although vital sign values generally increase during painful procedures,[15,29,36,37,49,64-67] they have also been found to decrease[68,69] or to remain stable.[70]

Moreover, vital signs are not consistently related to the patient's self-report of pain, and they are not predictive of pain.[15,29,65,67] In the American Society for Pain Management Nursing (ASPMN) recommendations[16] and the SCCM guidelines,[17] it is stated that vital signs should not be considered as primary indicators of pain because they can be attributed to other distress conditions, homeostatic changes, and medications. Instead, changes in vital signs should be considered a cue to begin further assessment of pain with appropriate tools.[16,17]

Besides vital signs, the pupil dilation reflex (PDR) has been studied in relation to the assessment of pain in the intensive care unit (ICU). It was first explored by Li et al[37] with 48 sedated and mechanically ventilated cardiac surgery patients in the ICU. Pupil size was found to increase significantly by 16% during a nociceptive procedure (ie, endotracheal suctioning or repositioning) and then returned to baseline 5 minutes after the procedure. PDR was also found to predict the presence of pain before surgical dressing changes in 37 ICU patients[71] as well as the need for analgesia before endotracheal suctioning in 34 sedated ICU patients.[72] Overall, such results suggest that PDR may be considered as a valid physiologic indicator in the pain assessment process. Further research is necessary.

Pain as a Vital Sign

Because pain is considered as another vital sign, including pain assessment with other routinely documented vital signs may help ensure that pain is assessed and controlled for in all patients on a regular basis. This approach can ensure that pain is detected and treatment implemented before the patient develops complications associated with unrelieved pain. The use of a pain flow sheet in critical care settings allows for a visible and ongoing pain assessment before and after an intervention for pain that is accessible to all clinicians involved in the assessment and management of pain.[73]

Patient Barriers to Pain Assessment and Management
Communication

The most obvious patient barrier to the assessment of pain in critical care patients is an alteration in the ability to communicate. A patient who is mechanically ventilated cannot verbalize a description of the pain. If the patient can communicate in any way, such as by head nodding or pointing, he or she may report the pain in that manner. If writing is possible, the patient may be able to describe the pain in detail. With patients unable to self-report, the nurse relies on validated behavioral pain scales such as the BPS[49] and the CPOT[50] to assess the presence of pain.[17]

The patient's family can contribute significantly in the assessment of pain. The family is intimately familiar with the patient's normal responses to pain and can assist the nurse in identifying clues. A family member's impression of a patient's pain should be considered in the pain assessment process of a critically ill patient.[16]

Altered Level of Consciousness and Unconsciousness

A patient who either is unconscious or has an altered level of consciousness presents a dilemma for all clinicians. Because pain relies on cortical response to provide recognition, the belief that the patient with a brain injury altering higher cortical function has no perception of pain may persist. Conversely, the inability to interpret the nociceptive transmission does not negate the transmission. Interviews by Lawrence[74] with 100 patients who recalled their experiences from a time when they were unconscious in critical care revealed that 25% of them could hear, understand, and respond emotionally to what was being said. Experts recommend assuming that patients who are unconscious or with an altered level of consciousness have pain and that they be treated the same way as conscious patients are treated when they are exposed to sources of pain.[16] It has been demonstrated that behavioral indicators of pain can be observed in reaction to a painful procedure in critically ill patients, no matter what their level of consciousness.[29] Moreover, it has been shown that some cortical activation related to pain perception is still present in unconscious patients in a neurovegetative state.[75] Knowing this, the critical care nurse can initiate a discussion with the other members of the health care team to formulate a plan of care for the patient's comfort.

Older Adult Patients

Many older adult patients do not complain much about pain. Misconceptions such as believing that pain is a normal consequence of aging or being afraid to disturb the health care team are barriers to pain expression for older adults.[24] Cognitive deficits and delirium present additional pain assessment barriers. Many older adult patients with mild to moderate cognitive impairments and even some with severe impairment are able to use pain intensity scales.[76-78] Vertical pain intensity scales are more easily understood by this group of patients and are recommended (see Fig. 8.5).[77] Older patients with cognitive deficits should receive repeated instructions and be given sufficient time to respond. When the self-report of pain is impossible to obtain, direct observation of pain-related behaviors is highly recommended in this population.[16,78] More than 24 behavioral tools have been developed for older patients with cognitive deficits.[79] The Pain Assessment Checklist for Seniors with Limited Ability to Communicate (PACSLAC),[80] Doloplus-2,[81] and the Pain Assessment in Advanced Dementia (PAINAD)[82] are recommended by experts.[78,83] However, these scales have not been validated in a critical care context.

Delirious Patients

Delirium is a form of transient cognitive impairment that is highly prevalent in critically ill patients.[17] Not much evidence is available on pain assessment tools that are valid for use in this specific clientele. An adapted version of the BPS (BPS-NI for Non-Intubated) was tested in 30 medical or surgical ICU patients with 84% being positive for delirium.[66] Higher BPS-NI scores were found during turning compared with rest and catheter dressing change, a nonnociceptive procedure, supporting its validity to discriminate between painful and nonpainful conditions. Findings with the CPOT in 40 delirious ICU patients were similar. Higher CPOT scores were found during painful procedures (ie, repositioning, endotracheal suctioning and dressing change of a wound) compared with a nonpainful procedure (ie, taking blood pressure).[84] Further testing of behavioral pain scales is encouraged to provide clinicians with valid tools for use in this challenging clientele. Adequate pain management is also important because pain is a modifiable factor of delirium.[85]

Neonates and Infants

Two-way verbal communication is impossible with critically ill infants, and this remains an important barrier to pain

assessment. The misconception that preterm neonates were incapable of pain sensation has persisted for a long time. Evidence supports that term and preterm neonates have the anatomic and functional capacity for pain sensation at birth.[86] One critical review examined more than 35 instruments used to assess pain in neonates and infants.[87] The Premature Infant Pain Profile (PIPP)[88] is the most recommended valid tool for pain assessment of infants, and it has been implemented in many clinical settings. The PIPP includes behavioral and physiologic indicators. The emphasis in pain assessment should be on behavioral indicators. Physiologic indicators should be interpreted with caution because they are also affected by disease, medications, and physiologic status.[16]

Cultural influences. Another barrier to accurate pain assessment is cultural influences on pain and pain reporting.[89] Cultural influences are compounded when the patient speaks a language other than that of the health team members. To facilitate communication, the use of a pain intensity scale in the patient's language is vital. The 0-to-10 numeric pain scales have been translated into many different languages.[24]

Although this chapter does not address specific cultural groups and their typical responses to pain, a few generalizations can be made. First, when assessing a patient from a cultural group different from your own, it should not be assumed the patient will have a specific response to pain or exhibit a particular behavior because of his or her culture. Patients have individual responses to pain. The health care practitioner may wrongfully assign or expect behaviors that a patient will not exhibit. A second consideration that is commonly overlooked is the role of pain in the life of the patient. The nurse must communicate with the patient or the family to ascertain what that role is.

Some cultures believe that God's test or punishment takes the form of pain. Persons with these cultural backgrounds do not necessarily believe that the pain should be relieved. Other cultures perceive pain as being associated with an imbalance in life. Persons from these cultures believe they need to manipulate the environment to restore balance to control pain.[89]

The complexities and intricacies of cultural beliefs require more extensive discussion than is possible here. It is important for the nurse to support, whenever possible, the special beliefs and needs of the patient and his or her family to provide the most therapeutic environment for healing to occur.

Lack of Knowledge

A relatively overlooked patient barrier to accurate pain assessment is the public knowledge deficit regarding pain and pain management. Many patients and their families are frightened by the risk of addiction to pain medication. They fear that addiction will occur if the patient is medicated frequently or with sufficient amounts of opioids necessary to relieve the pain. This concern is so powerful for some that they will deny or deliberately underreport the frequency or intensity of pain. Another misconception held by some patients is the expectation that unrelieved pain is simply part of a critical illness or procedure.[24] Many patients have no memory of receiving an explanation of their pain management plan.[90] With that in mind, it is important that the critical care nurse teach the family and the patient about the importance of pain control and the use of opioids in treating pain in critically ill patients.

Health Professional Barriers to Pain Assessment and Management

The health professional's beliefs and attitudes about pain and pain management are frequently a barrier to accurate and adequate pain assessment, and this can lead to poor management practices. Misconceptions and lack of knowledge exist regarding addiction, physiologic dependence, drug tolerance, and respiratory depression. Addiction rates for patients in acute pain who receive opioid analgesics are less than 1%. Some of the false beliefs that surround addiction result from a lack of knowledge about addiction and tolerance, and other concerns are related to the possible side effects of opioids.

Addiction and Tolerance

Addiction is defined by a pattern of compulsive drug use that is characterized by an incessant longing for an opioid and the need to use it for effects other than pain relief. Tolerance is defined as a diminution of opioid effects over time. Physical dependence and tolerance to opioids may develop if the medication is given over a long period. Physical dependence is manifested by withdrawal symptoms when the opioid is abruptly stopped. If this is an anticipated problem, withdrawal may be avoided by weaning the patient from the opioid slowly to allow the brain to reestablish neurochemical balance in the absence of the opioid.[24]

Respiratory Depression

Another concern of the health care professional is the fear that aggressive management of pain with opioids will cause critical respiratory depression. Opioids can cause respiratory depression, but this is rare. The incidence of respiratory depression is less than 2%.[91,92] Respiratory depression from the administration of opioids can be managed with diligent assessment practices, which are discussed later.

Organizational Barriers to Pain Assessment and Management

The organizational system influences pain and pain management practices as well as associated outcomes. Failure to make pain management a priority is the initial barrier. Failure to adopt standard pain assessment tools or to provide staff with sufficient time to assess and document pain and a lack of accountability for pain management practices are observed in some organizations. Evidence has demonstrated the lack of documentation of pain assessment and the undertreatment of pain in critical care settings.[5,93] The lack of collaboration between physicians and nurses is identified as a barrier to effective pain management.[94]

Because unrelieved pain is harmful to patients and increases the cost of care, it must be a priority for the health care organization. Every organization must analyze its pain management issues and practices and provide education about pain and pain management to staff. Now that pain is considered as the fifth vital sign, pain assessment must be included in documentation systems as a standard. Pain has to be assessed in all critically ill patients, regardless of their clinical condition or their level of consciousness. The implementation of pain assessment tools is essential so that the health care team can establish a common language of communication, which can facilitate interprofessional collaboration. There is an increased commitment to clinical practice guidelines and standards for pain assessment and management by organizations such as The Joint Commission (http://www.joint-commission.org), which have considerable influence in health care institutions. In addition, strategies to enhance collaboration

among health care professionals may include interdisciplinary care rounds or case reviews.[94,95] Patients have the right to be consulted about their pain care plan and should be involved in making decisions. The organization must continually evaluate outcomes and work to improve the quality of pain management.

PAIN MANAGEMENT

The management of pain in a critically ill patient is as multidimensional as the assessment. It is a multidisciplinary task. The control of pain can be pharmacologic, nonpharmacologic, or a combination of the two types of therapies. Pharmacologic pain management is predominantly used in critical care.

Pharmacologic Control of Pain

Pharmacologic management of pain has infinite variety in the critical care unit. Although this chapter is not an in-depth discussion of pharmacology, some commonly administered agents are discussed. Pain pharmacology is divided into three categories of action: opioid agonists, nonopioids, and adjuvants. Elements of the pain and analgesia practice guidelines[17] of the SCCM for the treatment of pain in critically ill adult patients are presented in Box 8.2. A care bundle for pain assessment and management in the critical care unit was created to facilitate the translation of the SCCM practice guidelines to the bedside. How pain is approached and managed is a progression or combination of the available agents, the type of pain, and the patient response to the therapy. Fig. 8.6 illustrates the analgesic action sites in relation to nociception.

BOX 8.2 Summary of Pain and Analgesia Guidelines

- Patients in critical care routinely experience pain at rest and with routine nursing care such as endotracheal suctioning or turning. Procedural pain is common in patients in critical care units.
  - Perform routine pain assessment in all patients.
  - In patients who are able to self-report their level of pain, use a numerical rating scale, usually 0-10.
  - In patients with intact motor skills who are unable to self-report their level of pain, behavioral pain scales should be used rather than vital signs to assess pain.
  - The BPS (scale 3-12) and CPOT (scale 0-8) are the most valid and reliable behavioral pain scales. A BPS >5 or a CPOT >2 indicates that the patient has significant pain.
  - Vital signs should be used only as a cue for further pain assessment.
- Treat pain within 30 minutes then reassess. Use intravenous opioids as first-line analgesic therapy for nonneuropathic pain, use nonopioid analgesics to reduce opioid side effects, and use either gabapentin or carbamazepine in conjunction with intravenous opioids for neuropathic pain.
- Preemptively treat procedural pain, especially before chest tube removal and similar procedures.
- Use thoracic epidural analgesia for abdominal aortic surgery. Suggest also using thoracic epidural analgesia for traumatic rib fractures. No evidence guides the use of lumbar epidural analgesia for abdominal aneurysm surgery or thoracic epidural analgesia for either intrathoracic or nonvascular abdominal surgical procedures. No evidence guides the use of regional versus systemic analgesia in medical ICU patients.
- Always treat pain before using sedation.
- Consider non-pharmacological adjunctive methods such as music of the patient's choice and relaxation techniques.

FIG. 8.6 Nociception and Analgesic Action Sites. BK, bradykinin; H, histamine; PG, prostaglandins; SP, substance P; 5HT, serotonin. (From McCaffery M, Pasero C. *Pain: Clinical Manual for Nursing Practice.* 2nd ed. St. Louis: Mosby; 1999.)

TABLE 8.3 Pharmacologic ManagementPain

Medication	Dosage	Onset (min)	Duration (h)	Available Routes	Properties	Side Effects and Comments
Morphine	1–4 mg IV bolus	5–10	3–4	PO, SL, R, IV, IM, SC, EA, IA	Analgesia, anti-anxiety	Standard for comparison
	1–10 mg IV infusion					Side effects: sedation, respiratory depression, euphoria or dysphoria, hypotension, nausea, vomiting, pruritus, constipation, urinary retention. M6G can accumulate in patients with renal failure or hepatic dysfunction
Fentanyl	25–100 mcg IV bolus	1–5	0.5–4	OTFC, IV, IM, TD, EA, IA	Analgesia, anti-anxiety	Same side effects as morphine
	25–200 mcg IV infusion					Rigidity with high doses
Hydromorphone (Dilaudid)	0.2–1 mg IV bolus	5	3–4	PO, R, IV, IM, SC, EA, IA	Analgesia, anti-anxiety	Same side effects as morphine
	0.2–2 mg IV infusion					
Codeine	15–30 mg IM, SC	10–20	3–4	PO, IM, SC	Analgesia (mild to moderate pain)	Lacks potency (unpredictable absorption; not all patients convert it to active form to achieve analgesia). Most common side effects: light-headedness, dizziness, shortness of breath, sedation, nausea, vomiting
Methadone (Dolophine)	5–10 mg IV	10	4–8	PO, SL, R, IV, SC, IM, EA, IA	Analgesia	Usually less sedating than morphine, but repeated doses can result in accumulation and can cause serious sedation (2–5 days)
Acetaminophen	650 mg maximum of 4 g/day	20–30	4–6	PO, R	Analgesia, antipyretic	Rare side effects. Hepatotoxicity
Ketorolac (Toradol)	15–30 mg IV	<10	6–8	PO, IM, IV	Analgesia, minimum antiinflammatory effect	Short-term use (<5 days). Side effects: gastric ulceration, bleeding, exacerbation of renal insufficiency. Use with care in older adult and renal failure patients

EA, epidural analgesia; *IA*, intrathecal analgesia; *IM*, intramuscular; *IV*, intravenous; *M6G*, morphine-6-glucuronide; *OTFC*, oral transmucosal fentanyl citrate; *PO*, oral; *R*, rectal; *SC*, subcutaneous; *SL*, sublingual; *TD*, transdermal.

Opioid Analgesics

The opioids most commonly used and recommended as first-line analgesics are the agonists. These opioids bind to mu receptors (transmission process) (see Fig. 8.6), which appear to be responsible for pain relief. Additional pharmacologic information is presented in Table 8.3. In the SCCM guidelines, opioids should be used as first-line therapy for treatment of nonneuropathic pain.[17]

Morphine. Morphine is the most commonly prescribed opioid in the critical care unit. Because of its water solubility, morphine has a slower onset of action and a longer duration compared with the lipid-soluble opioids (eg, fentanyl). Morphine has two main metabolites: morphine-3-glucuronide (M3G, inactive) and morphine-6-glucuronide (M6G, active). M6G is responsible for the analgesic effect but may accumulate and cause excessive sedation in patients with renal failure or hepatic dysfunction.[96] Morphine is available in a variety of delivery methods. It is the standard by which all other opioids are measured. It is also the agent that most closely mimics the endogenous opioids in the human pain modulation system.

Morphine is indicated for severe pain. It has additional actions that are helpful for managing other symptoms. Morphine dilates peripheral veins and arteries, making it useful in reducing myocardial workload. Morphine is also viewed as an antianxiety agent because of the calming effect it produces.

Many side effects have been reported with the use of morphine (see Table 8.3). The hypotensive effect can be particularly problematic in a patient who is hypovolemic. The vasodilation effect is potentiated in volume-depleted patients, and the hemodynamic status must be carefully monitored. Volume resuscitation restores blood pressure in the event of a prolonged hypotensive response.

A more serious side effect requiring diligent monitoring is the respiratory depressant effect. Opioids may cause this complication because they reduce the responsiveness of carbon dioxide chemoreceptors in the respiratory center located in the medulla.[97] Although infrequent, this effect can have significant sequelae for a critically ill patient. Many risk factors for opioid-induced respiratory depression have been identified.[92] Patients at risk include those with advanced age; obesity; sleep apnea; impaired renal, pulmonary, hepatic, or cardiac functioning; patients in whom pain is controlled after a period of poor control; opioid-naïve patients (ie, receiving opioids for less than a week); patients with concurrent use of CNS depressants; and those at postoperative day 1.[92] The critical care nurse must monitor the patient intensively to prevent this complication. Monitoring of patients receiving opioid analgesics is discussed in more detail later in this chapter. In addition to side effects common to all opioids, morphine may stimulate histamine release from mast cells, resulting in cardiac instability and allergic reactions.

Fentanyl. Fentanyl is a synthetic opioid preferred for critically ill patients with hemodynamic instability or morphine allergy. It is a lipid-soluble agent that has a more rapid onset than morphine and a shorter duration.[98] The metabolites of fentanyl are largely inactive and nontoxic, which makes it an effective and safe opioid. Fentanyl and hydromorphone are preferred in hemodynamically unstable patients and in patients with renal impairment.[98] It is available in intravenous, intraspinal, and transdermal forms. The transdermal form is commonly referred to as the "Duragesic patch" or the "72-hour patch."

Because the side effects of fentanyl are similar to the side effects of morphine, the nurse must monitor the hemodynamic and respiratory response carefully. When fentanyl is given by rapid administration and at higher doses, it has been associated with the additional hazard of bradycardia and rigidity in the chest wall muscles.[96,99] The use of transdermal fentanyl is rarely indicated in critically ill patients. The customary use of the "fentanyl patch" is for patients experiencing chronic pain or cancer pain; in critical care, it is used for patients who require extended pain control. Transdermal delivery requires 12 to 16 hours for onset of action, and the patch has a duration of action of 72 hours.[24] If this delivery method is used, the patient will require other opioid management until the transdermal fentanyl takes effect.

Hydromorphone. Hydromorphone is a semisynthetic opioid; the onset of action and duration are similar to morphine.[24] It is an effective opioid with multiple routes of delivery. It is more potent than morphine. Hydromorphone produces an inactive metabolite (ie, hydromorphone-3-glucuronide), making it the opioid of choice for use in patients with end-stage renal disease.[99]

Meperidine. Meperidine (Demerol) is a less potent opioid with agonist effects similar to those of morphine. It is considered the weakest of the opioids, and it must be administered in large doses to be equivalent in action to morphine. Because the duration of action is short, dosing is frequent. A major concern with this medication is the metabolite *normeperidine*, which is a CNS neurotoxic agent. At high doses in patients with kidney failure or liver dysfunction or in older adult patients, it may induce CNS toxicity including irritability, muscle spasticity, tremors, agitation, and seizures.[24] Although meperidine is useful in short-term specific conditions (eg, treating postoperative shivering[100]), it should not be used routinely for analgesia in the critical care unit.[98,99,101]

Codeine. Codeine has limited use in the management of severe pain. It is rarely used in the critical care unit. It provides analgesia for mild to moderate pain, and it is usually compounded with a nonopioid (eg, acetaminophen). To be active, codeine must be metabolized in the liver to morphine.[24] Codeine is available only through oral, intramuscular, and subcutaneous routes, and its absorption can be reduced in a critical care patient by altered gastrointestinal motility and decreased tissue perfusion.

Methadone. Methadone is a synthetic opioid with morphine-like properties but less sedation. It is longer acting than morphine and has a long half-life; this makes it difficult to titrate in critical care patients. Methadone lacks active metabolites, and routes other than the kidney eliminate 60% of the medication. This means that methadone does not accumulate in patients with kidney failure. Methadone can be used to treat chronic pain syndromes when patients experience tolerance with other opioids and may help facilitate the down-titration of opioid infusions in the critical care unit.[99] However, prolongation of the Q–T interval, which can lead to torsade de pointes, has been reported with its use.[96]

More potent opioids: remifentanil and sufentanil. Remifentanil and sufentanil are agonist opioids. The use of these potent medications has been studied in critically ill patients.

Remifentanil is 250 times more potent than morphine, and it has a rapid onset and predictable offset of action. For this reason, it allows a rapid emergence from sedation, facilitating the evaluation of the neurologic state of the patient after stopping the infusion.[102,103] As opposed to fentanyl, the use of remifentanil was associated with a lower incidence of postoperative delirium.[104]

Sufentanil is 7 to 13 times more potent than fentanyl and 500 to 1000 times more potent than morphine. It has more pronounced sedation properties than fentanyl and other opioids. Patients given sufentanil require minimal sedative agent doses to achieve an adequate sedation level. It has a rapid distribution and a high clearance rate, preventing accumulation when given for a long period.[105] Sufentanil has a longer emergence from sedation compared with remifentanil, but it has a longer analgesic effect after stopping its administration.[103]

Preventing and Treating Respiratory Depression

Respiratory depression is the most life-threatening opioid side effect. The risk of respiratory depression increases when other medications with CNS depressant effects (eg, benzodiazepines, antiemetics, neuroleptics, antihistamines) are concomitantly administered to the patient. Although no universal definition of respiratory depression exists, it is usually described in terms of decreased respiratory rate (fewer than 8 or 10 breaths/min), decreased SpO_2 levels, or elevated end-tidal carbon dioxide ($ETCO_2$) levels.[97] A change in the patient's level of consciousness or an increase in sedation normally precedes respiratory depression.

Monitoring. Guidelines on monitoring for patients receiving opioid analgesia were established by ASPMN.[97] In addition to assessing pain intensity as a targeted outcome of analgesia, regular sedation and respiratory assessments should be done. Valid and reliable sedation scales developed for use in critically ill patients should be employed. Respirations should be evaluated over 1 minute and qualified according to rate, rhythm, and depth of chest excursion. Technology-supported monitoring (eg, continuous pulse oximetry and capnography) can be useful in high-risk patients. More vigilant monitoring should be performed when patients may be at greater risk such as during the first 24 hours after surgery, after an increase in the dose of an opioid, or a change in opioid agent or route of administration. Pasero et al[106] suggested monitoring these parameters at least every 2 hours for the first 24 hours and every 4 hours thereafter in stable patients.

Snoring is a warning sign. It can be a sign of respiratory depression associated with airway obstruction by the tongue, leading to hypoxemia and possibly to cardiorespiratory arrest.[24] A patient snoring after administration of an opioid requires close observation by the critical care nurse.

Opioid reversal. Critical respiratory depression can be readily reversed with administration of the opioid antagonist *naloxone*.[24] The usual dose is 0.4 mg, which is mixed with 10 mL of normal saline (for a concentration of 0.04 mg/mL). Naloxone is normally given intravenously very slowly (0.5 mL over 2 minutes) while the patient is carefully monitored for reversal of the respiratory signs. Naloxone administration can be discontinued as soon as the patient is responsive to physical stimulation and able to take deep breaths. However, the medication should be kept nearby. Because the duration of naloxone is shorter than most opioids, another dose may be needed 30 minutes after the first dose. The nurse must monitor sedation and respiratory status and remind the patient to breathe deeply every 1 to 2 minutes until he or she becomes more alert. The benefits of reversing respiratory depression with naloxone must be carefully weighed against the risk of a sudden onset of pain and the difficulty achieving pain relief. To prevent this from occurring, it is important to provide a nonopioid medication for pain relief. Moreover, the use of naloxone is not recommended after prolonged analgesia because it can induce withdrawal and may cause nausea and cardiovascular complications (eg, dysrhythmias).

New Sedative With Analgesic Properties: Dexmedetomidine

Dexmedetomidine (Precedex) is a short-acting alpha-2 agonist that is indicated for short-term sedation of mechanically ventilated patients in the critical care unit.[107] Its mechanism of action is unique and differs from the mechanism of action of other commonly used sedatives in critical care. Compared with midazolam (Versed) or lorazepam (Ativan)—whose hypnotic effects act mainly on the limbic system, the cortex or both—the effect of dexmedetomidine is located in the locus caeruleus section of the brainstem. As a result, patients receiving dexmedetomidine intravenous infusions are calm and sleepy, yet they remain easily arousable.[108] For this reason, dexmedetomidine is ideal for mild to moderate sedation, often referred to as conscious sedation. Refer to Chapter 9 for details on dosage and administration.

Dexmedetomidine also possesses an analgesic property. The analgesic effects of dexmedetomidine are principally due to spinal antinociception via binding to nonnoradrenergic receptors (heteroreceptors) located on the dorsal horn neurons of the spinal cord.[107] Dexmedetomidine has been found to decrease postoperative opioid requirements in both adults and children.[109,110] These results suggest that dexmedetomidine could be of interest with respect to improving postoperative pain in critical care. Although dexmedetomidine is increasing in popularity for short-term sedation in the critical care unit, it is not without adverse effect. Inhibition of noradrenergic receptors in the brainstem and the spinal cord often causes hypotension and bradycardia.[108]

Nonopioid Analgesics

In the SCCM guidelines, the use of nonopioids in combination with an opioid is recommended to reduce opioid requirements and opioid-related side effects.[17] This strategy provides greater analgesic effect through action at the peripheral and central levels. Pharmacologic information is presented in Table 8.3.

Acetaminophen. Acetaminophen is an analgesic used to treat mild to moderate pain. It inhibits the synthesis of neurotransmitter prostaglandins in the CNS, and this is why it has no antiinflammatory properties.[111] Acetaminophen is metabolized by two pathways: major (nontoxic metabolite) and minor (toxic metabolite that is rapidly converted into a nontoxic form by glutathione). In an acetaminophen overdose, a larger amount is processed by the minor pathway which results in a larger quantity of toxic metabolites and may cause damage to the liver. Side effects are rare at therapeutic doses (total daily dose should not exceed 4 g in 24 hours). Nonopioids are rarely used alone in critically ill patients. The nurse must consider other products containing acetaminophen that the patient may receive when calculating the total daily dose of acetaminophen. Special care must be taken for patients with liver dysfunction, malnutrition, or a history of excess alcohol consumption; total dose of acetaminophen in these patients should not exceed 2 g/day.[17]

Nonsteroidal antiinflammatory drugs. The use of nonsteroidal antiinflammatory drugs (NSAIDs) in combination with opioids is indicated in patients with acute musculoskeletal and soft tissue inflammation.[24] The mechanism of action of NSAIDs is to block the action of cyclooxygenase (COX), the enzyme that converts arachidonic acid to prostaglandins. COX has two forms: COX-1 and COX-2. The production of prostaglandins (transduction process) is inhibited by blocking the action of COX (see Fig. 8.6). NSAIDs can be grouped as first-generation (COX-1 and COX-2 inhibitors such as aspirin, ibuprofen, naproxen, and ketorolac) or second-generation (COX-2 inhibitors such as celecoxib) agents. The inhibition of COX-1 is thought to be responsible for many of the side effects of NSAIDs, such as gastric ulceration, bleeding as a result of platelet inhibition, and acute renal failure. In contrast, the inhibition of COX-2 is responsible for the suppression of pain and inflammation.[111] Second-generation NSAIDs are associated with minimal risks of serious adverse effects, but their role in critically ill patients is unknown.[17]

Ketorolac is the most appropriate NSAID for use in the critical care setting. Not all critically ill patients are candidates for ketorolac therapy because of its side effects. Caution is advised for using ketorolac in older adults or in patients with kidney dysfunction because of their slower clearance rates. Because ketorolac is an NSAID, monitoring for clumping of platelets is of primary importance. Laboratory data should be evaluated for an increase in bleeding time, and the patient should be assessed for any signs of abnormal bleeding. Moreover, prolonged use of ketorolac for more than 5 days was associated with an increase in kidney failure and bleeding.[111] It is important to consider the concurrent use of opioids and NSAIDs to effect pain modification at both areas of transmission. This combination of agents often significantly reduces the amount of opioids required for effective pain management.

Other pharmacologic agents are used in the critical care unit. The most important factor to be considered in the management of pain with any pharmacologic agent is the careful assessment and reassessment of the patient's pain status during administration of the medication. The need to adjust the dosage, increase the frequency, or change the agent is based on assessment findings. The use of a pain flow sheet allows ongoing pain assessment and complete documentation of pain management in the critical care setting.

Adjuvants. Although not widely mentioned in the critical care literature, adjuvants can be helpful for pain relief in patients with complex pain syndromes such as neuropathic pain or for other specific purposes (eg, procedural pain). Anticonvulsants (eg, carbamazepine, phenytoin, gabapentin, pregabalin) are first-line analgesics for lancing neuropathic pain. The SCCM guidelines recommend the use of gabapentin or carbamazepine, in addition to intravenous opioids, for treatment of neuropathic pain.[17] Even if the specific mechanism for pain relief is unknown, analgesia probably results from the suppression of sodium ion (Na^+) discharges, reducing the neuronal hyperexcitability (action potential) in the transduction process (see Fig. 8.6).[24] Antidepressants are also considered as analgesics in various chronic pain syndromes such as headache, fibromyalgia, low back pain, neuropathy, central pain, and cancer pain. The analgesic dose is often lower than the dose required to treat depression. Antidepressant adjuvant analgesics are usually divided into two main groups: tricyclic antidepressants (eg, amitriptyline, imipramine, desipramine) and biogenic amine reuptake inhibitors (eg, venlafaxine, paroxetine, sertraline). The mechanism of analgesia most widely accepted is the ability of antidepressants to block the reuptake of neurotransmitters serotonin and norepinephrine in the CNS.[24] This increases the activity of the modulation process (see Fig. 8.6).

Ketamine. Anesthetics may be used to treat pain in the critical care setting. Ketamine is a dissociative anesthetic agent that has analgesic properties. It was traditionally used intravenously for procedural pain in burn patients. It is also available in enteral routes. Compared with opioids, ketamine has the benefit of sparing the respiratory drive, but it has many side effects related to the release of catecholamines and the emergence of delirium. For this reason, ketamine is not recommended for routine therapy in critically ill patients. Before administering ketamine, the dissociative state should be explained to the patient. *Dissociative state* refers to the feelings of separateness from the environment, loss of control, hallucinations, and vivid dreams. The use of benzodiazepines (eg, midazolam) can reduce the incidence of this unpleasant effect.[24]

Lidocaine. Lidocaine is another anesthetic that can be used for procedural and acute pain or for some patients with chronic neuropathic pain.[24] When used locally, anesthetics act through the transduction process (see Fig. 8.6).

Delivery Methods

The most common route for medication administration is the intravenous route by means of continuous infusion, bolus administration, or patient-controlled analgesia (PCA). Traditionally, the choice has been intravenous bolus administration. The benefits of this method are the rapid onset of action and the ease of titration. The major disadvantage is the increase and decrease of the serum level of the opioid, leading to periods of pain control with periods of breakthrough pain.[111]

Continuous infusion of opioids with an infusion pump provides constant blood levels of the ordered opioid; this promotes a consistent level of comfort. It is a particularly helpful method of administration during sleep because the patient awakens with an adequate level of pain relief. It is important that the patient be given the loading dose that relieves the pain and raises the circulating dose of the medication. After the basal rate is established, the patient maintains a steady state of pain control unless there is additional pain from a procedure, an activity, or a change in the patient's condition. In this situation, physician orders to administer additional boluses of opioid need to be available.

Patient-Controlled Analgesia

PCA is a method of medication delivery that uses the intravenous route and an infusion pump. It allows the patient to self-administer small doses of analgesics. Different opioids can be used, but the most extensively used is morphine. This method of medication delivery allows the patient to control the level of pain and sedation and to avoid the peaks and valleys of intermittent dosing by the health care professional. The patient can self-administer a bolus of medication the moment the pain begins, acting preemptively

Certain patients are not candidates for PCA. Patients with alterations in the level of consciousness or mentation are unable to understand the use of the equipment. Very elderly patients or patients with kidney failure or liver dysfunction may require careful screening for PCA.

Allowing the patient to self-administer opioid doses does not diminish the role of the critical care nurse in pain management. The nurse advises about necessary changes to the prescription and continues to monitor the effects of the medication and doses. The patient is closely monitored during the first 2 hours of therapy and after every change in the prescription. If the patient's pain does not respond within the first 2 hours of therapy, a total reassessment of the pain state is essential. The nurse monitors the number of boluses the patient delivers. If the patient is pressing the button to bolus medication more often than the prescription, the dose may be insufficient to maintain pain control. Naloxone must be readily available to reverse adverse opioid respiratory effects. Ideally, a patient undergoing an elective procedure requiring opioid analgesia postoperatively is instructed in the use of PCA during preoperative teaching. This allows the patient to become comfortable with the concept of self-medication before use.

Intraspinal Pain Control

Intraspinal anesthesia uses the concept that the spinal cord is the primary link in nociceptive transmission. The goal is to mimic the body's endogenous opioid pain modification system by interfering with the transmission of pain and providing an opioid receptor binding agent directly into the spinal cord. The hemodynamic status of the patient changes very little.

Intraspinal anesthesia is particularly appropriate for pain in the thorax, upper abdomen, and lower extremities. The two intraspinal routes are intrathecal and epidural (Fig. 8.7). Regardless of the route, the effects of the opioid agonist used are similar, and assessment parameters are the same as the assessment parameters used for other routes.

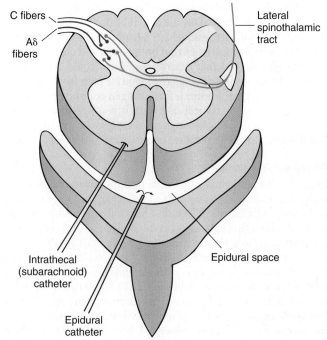

FIG. 8.7 Intraspinal Catheter Placement in a Spinal Cord Cross Section.

Intrathecal Analgesia

Intrathecal (subarachnoid) opioids are placed directly into the cerebrospinal fluid and attach to spinal cord receptor sites. Opioids introduced at this site act quickly at the dorsal horn. The dural sheath is punctured, eliminating the barrier for pathogens between the environment and the cerebrospinal fluid. This creates the risk of serious infections. The intrathecal route is usually reserved for intraoperative use. Single-bolus dosing provides short-term relief for short-lived pain (the pain of labor and delivery is well managed using this regimen). Side effects of intrathecal pain control include postdural puncture headache and infection.

Epidural Analgesia

Epidural analgesia is commonly used in the critical care unit after major abdominal surgery, nephrectomy, thoracotomy, and major orthopedic procedures. Per the SCCM guidelines, use of epidural analgesia should be considered for patients after surgery for abdominal aortic aneurysm and for patients with traumatic rib fractures.[17] Certain conditions preclude the use of this pain control method including systemic infection, anticoagulation, and increased intracranial pressure. Epidural delivery of opioids provides longer lasting pain relief with less dosing of opioids. When delivered into the epidural space, 5 mg of morphine may be effective for 6 to 24 hours compared with 3 to 4 hours when delivered intravenously. Opioids infused in the epidural space are more unpredictable than opioids administered intrathecally. The epidural space is filled with fatty tissue and is external to the dura mater. The fatty tissue interferes with uptake, and the dura mater acts as a barrier to diffusion, making diffusion rate difficult to predict.

The type of medication used determines the rapidity of medication diffusion. Hydrophilic medications (eg, morphine) are water soluble and penetrate the dura mater slowly, giving them a longer onset and duration of action. Lipophilic medications (eg, fentanyl) are lipid soluble; they penetrate the dura rapidly and have a rapid onset of action and a shorter duration of action.

The dura mater acts as a physical barrier and causes delay in diffusion of the medication. Compared with the intrathecal route, it allows more medication to be absorbed in the systemic circulation, requiring greater doses for pain relief. Medications delivered epidurally may be administered by bolus or by continuous infusion. Epidural analgesia is being used more often in the critical care environment, and it requires careful monitoring.

The nurse must assess the patient for respiratory depression. This phenomenon may occur early in the therapy or within 24 hours after initiation. The epidural catheter also puts the patient at risk for infection. The efficiency of this pain control method and the increased mobility of the patient do not diminish the nurse's responsibility to monitor and evaluate the outcomes of the pain management protocol in use.

Equianalgesia

When a modification of opioid is considered, the nurse must be aware of equianalgesic dosages. In doing any conversion, the goal is to provide equal analgesic effects with the new agents. This concept is referred to as *equianalgesia*. Morphine is the standard for the conversion of opioids. Prescribed dosages must take into account the patient's age and health status.[24] The critical care nurse must have access to a chart on the unit for easy referral to administer the correct dosages of opioids to critically ill patients. Because of the variety of agents and routes, the professional pain organizations have developed equianalgesia charts for use by health care professionals. All critical care units need to have an equianalgesic chart posted for easy reference. Box 8.3 presents a guide to using these charts. Table 8.4 provides the equianalgesic dose for different medications used in clinical practice. Table 8.5 presents an equianalgesic chart with oral nonopioid and opioid doses for mild to moderate pain.

BOX 8.3	Guide to Using Equianalgesic Charts

- Equianalgesic means approximately the same pain relief.
- The equianalgesic chart is a guideline. Doses and intervals between doses are titrated according to the individual's response.
- The equianalgesic chart is helpful when switching from one medication to another or when switching from one route of administration to another.
- Dosages in the equianalgesic chart for moderate to severe pain are not necessarily starting doses. The doses suggest a ratio for comparing the analgesia of one medication with another.
- For older patients, initially reduce the recommended adult opioid dose for moderate to severe pain by 25% to 50%.
- The longer the patient has been receiving opioids, the more conservative the starting dose of a *new* opioid should be.

TABLE 8.4 Equianalgesic Chart Approximate Equivalent Doses of Opioids for Moderate to Severe Pain			
Analgesic	Parenteral (IM, SC, IV) Route (mg)[a,b]	PO Route (mg)[a]	Comments
Mu Opioid Agonists			
Morphine	10	30	Standard for comparison; multiple routes of administration; available in immediate-release and controlled-release formulations; active metabolite M6G can accumulate with repeated dosing in renal failure
Codeine	130	200 NR	IM has unpredictable absorption and high side-effect profile; use PO for mild to moderate pain; usually compounded with nonopioid (eg, Tylenol No. 3)
Fentanyl	100 mcg/h parenterally and transdermally ≅ 4 mg/h morphine parenterally; 1 mcg/h transdermally ≅ 2 mg/24 h morphine PO	—	Short half-life, but at steady state, slow elimination from tissues can lead to prolonged half-life (up to 12 h); start opioid-naïve patients on no more than 25 mcg/h transdermally; transdermal fentanyl NR for acute pain management; available by oral transmucosal route

TABLE 8.4   Equianalgesic Chart Approximate Equivalent Doses of Opioids for Moderate to Severe Pain—cont'd

Analgesic	Parenteral (IM, SC, IV) Route (mg)[a,b]	PO Route (mg)[a]	Comments
Hydromorphone (Dilaudid)	1.5	7.5	Useful alternative to morphine; no evidence that metabolites are clinically relevant; shorter duration than morphine; available in high-potency parenteral formulation (10 mg/mL) useful for SC infusion; 3 mg rectal ≅ 650 mg aspirin PO; with repeated dosing (eg, PCA), it is more likely than 2–3 mg parenteral hydromorphone = 10 mg parenteral morphine
Levorphanol (Levo-Dromoran)	2	4	Longer acting than morphine when given repeatedly; long half-life can lead to accumulation within 2–3 days of repeated dosing
Meperidine	75	300 NR	No longer preferred as first-line opioid for management of acute or chronic pain because of potential toxicity from accumulation of metabolite, normeperidine; normeperidine has 15–20 h half-life and is not reversed by naloxone; NR in elderly patients or patients with impaired renal function; NR by continuous IV infusion
Methadone (Dolophine)	10	20	Longer acting than morphine when given repeatedly; long half-life can lead to delayed toxicity from accumulation within 3–5 days; start PO dosing on PRN schedule; in opioid-tolerant patients converted to methadone, start with 10%–25% of equianalgesic dose
Oxycodone	—	20	Used for moderate pain when combined with nonopioid (eg, Percocet, Tylox); available as single entity in immediate-release and controlled-release formulations (eg, OxyContin); can be used similar to PO morphine for severe pain
Oxymorphone (Numorphan)	1	10 rectal	Used for moderate to severe pain; no PO formulation
Agonist-Antagonist Opioids[c]			
Buprenorphine (Buprenex)	0.4	—	Not readily reversed by naloxone; NR for laboring patients
Butorphanol (Stadol)	2	—	Available in nasal spray
Dezocine (Dalgan)	10	—	
Nalbuphine (Nubain)	10	—	
Pentazocine (Talwin)	60	180	

[a]Duration of analgesia is dose dependent; the higher the dose, usually the longer the duration.

[b]IV boluses may be used to produce analgesia that lasts approximately as long as IM or SC doses. However, of all routes of administration, IV produces the highest peak concentration of the medication, and the peak concentration is associated with the highest level of toxicity (eg, sedation). To decrease the peak effect and reduce the level of toxicity, IV boluses may be administered more slowly (eg, 10 mg of morphine over a 15-min period), or smaller doses may be administered more often (eg, 5 mg of morphine every 1–1.5 h).

[c]Not recommended for severe, escalating pain. If used in combination with mu agonists, may reverse analgesia and precipitate withdrawal in opioid-dependent patients.

FDA, U.S. Food and Drug Administration; *IM*, intramuscular; *IV*, intravenous; *M6G*, morphine-6-glucuronide; *NR*, not recommended; *PCA*, patient-controlled analgesia; *PO*, per os (by mouth); *PRN*, pro re nata (as needed); *SC*, subcutaneous.

From Pasero C, McCaffrey M. *Pain Assessment and Pharmacologic Management*, St. Louis: Elsevier; 2011.

Nonpharmacologic Methods of Pain Management

Although numerous methods of pain management other than medications are mentioned in the critical care literature,[112] very few studies have been done to provide evidence of their effectiveness in the critical care setting. Nonpharmacologic methods can be used to supplement analgesic treatment, but they are not intended to replace analgesics. In most instances, these therapies may enhance the pharmacologic management of the patient's pain. Per the SCCM guidelines, administration of preemptive analgesic therapy or nonpharmacologic interventions, or both, is suggested to alleviate pain during invasive or potentially painful procedures in critically ill adult patients.[17]

Critical care nurses identify many barriers to the use of nonpharmacologic methods for pain management, including a lack of knowledge, training, and time.[113] Despite these barriers, more than 60% of critical care nurses are willing to use the methods to relieve their patients' pain. It is crucial that nurses be provided with the appropriate training and equipment required to apply nonpharmacologic methods for pain management in critically ill patients.

The key to success with any of these therapies is a comprehensive understanding of their mechanism of action so that the therapy matches the needs of the patient. Most of the following interventions require the patient's cooperation. There must be some commitment to the treatment on the part of the patient. When handled effectively, nonpharmacologic methods can assist in pain management.

Physical Techniques

Stimulating other non–pain sensory fibers (Aβ) in the periphery modifies pain transmission. These fibers are stimulated by thermal changes as in ice therapy and simple massage.

TABLE 8.5 Equianalgesic Chart Approximate Equivalent Doses of PO Nonopioids and Opioids for Mild to Moderate Pain

Analgesic	PO Dosage (mg)
Nonopioids	
Acetaminophen	650
Aspirin (ASA)	650
Opioids[a]	
Codeine	32–60
Hydrocodone[b]	5
Meperidine (Demerol)	50
Oxycodone[c]	3–5
Propoxyphene (Darvon)	65–100

[a]Often combined with acetaminophen; avoid exceeding maximum total daily dose of acetaminophen (4000 mg/day).
[b]Combined with acetaminophen (eg, Vicodin, Lortab).
[c]Combined with acetaminophen (eg, Percocet, Tylox); also available alone as controlled-release OxyContin and immediate-release formulations.
ASA, acetylsalicylic acid; *PO*, per os (oral).

Selected references for more information: McCaffery M, Pasero C. Acetaminophen and NSAIDS: adult dosing information. In Pasero C, McCaffery M. *Pain Assessment and Pharmacologic Management*. St. Louis: Mosby; 2011: 211; American Pain Society (APS). *Principles of Analgesic Use in the Treatment of Acute Pain and Cancer Pain*. 3rd ed. Glenview, IL: APS; 1992; and Kaiko R, et al. Analgesic efficacy of controlled-release (CR) oxycodone and CR morphine. *Clin Pharmacol Ther.* 1996;59:130.

Modified from Pasero C, McCaffery M. *Pain Assessment and Pharmacologic Management*. St. Louis: Elsevier; 2011.

Ice Therapy

Ice therapy was found to be helpful to reduce procedural pain in critically ill patients. In a study with 50 cardiac surgery patients in a critical care unit, a significant decrease in pain intensity was obtained after chest tube removal when ice packets were placed around the site for 10 minutes before removal of the chest tube.[114] The analgesic property of ice therapy was also studied by Demir and Khorshid[115] using a 20-minute application of cold packs before chest tube removal in the critical care unit. Pain intensity was significantly lower after chest tube removal in patients who received the cold packs and a dose of analgesic compared with a placebo and a control group.

Massage

The effect of massage on pain relief was explored in two randomized controlled trials of postoperative cardiac surgery patients after they were transferred from the critical care unit.[116,117] In these two studies, a significant decrease in pain intensity scores was obtained in patients who received a 20-minute massage intervention between postoperative day 2 and day 5 compared with a control group of patients who received standard care and a 20-minute quiet time during the same period. Similar findings were found in the critical care unit. In a more recent pilot randomized controlled trial[118] with 40 postoperative cardiac surgery patients, a decrease in pain intensity scores was observed in patients who were administered two to three 15-minute hand massage sessions during the first 24 hours after surgery compared with a control group of patients who did not receive hand massage but had the nurse holding their hands and reported no change in pain intensity.

Cognitive-Behavioral Techniques

Using the cortical interpretation of pain as the foundation, several interventions can reduce the patient's pain report including cognitive techniques such as relaxation, guided imagery, and music therapy.

Relaxation

Relaxation is a well-documented method for reducing the distress associated with pain. Although not a substitute for pharmacology, relaxation is an excellent adjunct for controlling pain. Relaxation decreases oxygen consumption and muscle tone, and it can decrease heart rate and blood pressure. Relaxation gives the patient a sense of control over the pain and reduces muscle tension and anxiety. Deep-breathing exercises may be helpful in patients who are not interested in relaxation therapy. In one study,[119] lower pain scores were found after chest tube removal in 40 critically ill patients executing deep breathing and receiving an analgesic compared with patients who received an analgesic only.

Guided Imagery

Guided imagery is a technique that uses the imagination to provide control over pain. It can be used to distract or relax. Guiding a patient to a place that is pain-free and relaxing takes a considerable time commitment on the part of the nurse. Although this may be difficult in the critical care environment, guiding a patient to a place in his or her imagination that is free from pain may be beneficial.[120]

Music Therapy

Music therapy is a commonly used intervention for relaxation. Music that is pleasing to the patient may have soothing effects, but its effects on reducing pain are controversial.[121] Ideally, the music should be supplied by a small set of headphones. It is important to educate the patient and family regarding the role of music in relaxation and pain control and to provide music of the patient's choice.

CASE STUDY 8.1 Patient With Pain

Brief Patient History

Ms. X has type 2 diabetes mellitus and peripheral arterial occlusive disease with neuropathy. Ms. X is disabled because of limited mobility and chronic pain associated with lower extremity claudication and neuropathic pain. She has been admitted for an elective right femoral to distal tibial bypass. Ms. X's chronic pain has been effectively managed with gabapentin (600 mg three times daily) and a 75-mcg fentanyl patch every third day. Ms. X reports that her pain patch is due to be changed the next day. Her diabetes mellitus has been effectively managed with diet and a combination of oral agents. Postoperatively, orders for pain management include her home regimen of gabapentin and fentanyl patch and an order for morphine for breakthrough pain.

Clinical Assessment

Ms. X is admitted to the critical care unit from the perianesthesia recovery room after an 8-hour surgical revascularization of the right lower extremity. She is awake; alert; and oriented to person, time, place, and situation. Ms. X is breathing through her mouth and taking shallow breaths. She complains of right lower extremity and bilateral foot pain. Her skin is warm and dry. Ms. X is able to move her toes on command, and lower extremity sensation to touch is intact; however, she is complaining of severe burning in both feet.

Diagnostic Procedures
Ms. X reports that her pain is a 10 on the Numeric Rating Scale. The Riker Agitation Sedation Scale score is 5.

Medical Diagnosis
The diagnosis is acute postoperative incisional pain superimposed on chronic neuropathic pain involving both lower extremities. Neuropathic pain is likely worsened because of missed doses of gabapentin.

Questions
1. What major outcomes do you expect to achieve for this patient?
2. What problems or risks must be managed to achieve these outcomes?
3. What interventions must be initiated to monitor, prevent, manage, or eliminate the problems and risks identified?
4. What interventions should be initiated to promote optimal functioning, safety, and well-being of the patient?
5. What possible learning needs do you anticipate for this patient?
6. What cultural and age-related factors may have a bearing on the patient's plan of care?

QSEN   QSEN: Informatics

Internet Resources
American Society for Pain Management Nursing (ASPMN): http://www.aspmn.org/
American Pain Society (APS): http://www.americanpainsociety.org
Canadian Pain Society (CPS): http://www.canadianpainsociety.ca
Canadian Pain Coalition (CPC): http://www.canadianpaincoalition.ca
Society of Critical Care Medicine (SCCM): http://www.sccm.org/

SUMMARY

- Pain in a critically ill patient is difficult to assess and manage. There are many sources of pain in the critical care setting, and the effects of unrelieved acute pain can have a significant impact on the patient's recovery.
- When possible, the patient's self-report of pain must be obtained. A simple yes or no communicated by head nodding from a mechanically ventilated patient is considered a valid self-report of pain.
- When the patient's self-report is unavailable, behavioral indicators are alternative measures of pain assessment; standardized tools (eg, BPS, CPOT) have been developed for assessment of pain in nonverbal critically ill patients.
- In some situations, behavioral indicators may be impossible to assess accurately, and the use of physiologic indicators is crucial. However, vital signs do not represent valid information for pain assessment. The pupil dilation reflex is being explored and may support nurses in the pain assessment process.
- The critical care nurse must collaborate with the multidisciplinary team to ensure that a plan of care for management of the patient's pain is developed. To fully participate, the nurse must have extensive knowledge of nonpharmacologic and pharmacologic therapies designed to achieve effective pain relief.

ⓔ Visit the Evolve site for additional study materials.

REFERENCES

1. Chanques G, et al. A prospective study of pain at rest: incidence and characteristics of an unrecognized symptom in surgical and trauma versus medical intensive care unit patients. *Anesthesiology*. 2007;107:858.
2. Puntillo KA, et al. Patients' perceptions and responses to procedural pain: results from Thunder Project II. *Am J Crit Care*. 2001;10:238.
3. Puntillo KA, et al. Determinants of procedural pain intensity in the intensive care unit. The Europain study. *Am J Respir Crit Care Med*. 2014;189:39-47.
4. Gélinas C. Management of pain in cardiac surgery ICU patients: have we improved over time? *Intensive Crit Care Nurs*. 2007;23:298.
5. Puntillo KA, et al. Practices and predictors of analgesic interventions for adults undergoing painful procedures. *Am J Crit Care*. 2002;11:415.
6. Dunwoody CJ, et al. Assessment, physiological monitoring, and consequences of inadequately treated acute pain. *Pain Manag Nurs*. 2008;9:S11.
7. Kehlet H. Surgical stress and postoperative outcome—from here to where? *Reg Anesth Pain Med*. 2006;31:47.
8. Joshi GP, Ogunnaike BO. Consequences of inadequate postoperative pain relief and chronic persistent postoperative pain. *Anesth Clin North Am*. 2005;23:21.
9. Kehlet H, et al. Persistent postsurgical pain: risk factors and prevention. *Lancet*. 2006;367:1618.
10. Nampiaparampil DE. Prevalence of chronic pain after traumatic brain injury: a systematic review. *JAMA*. 2008;300:711.
11. Loeser JD, Treede RD. The Kyoto protocol of IASP basic pain terminology. *Pain*. 2008;137:473.
12. Shannon K, Bucknall T. Pain assessment in critical care: what have we learnt from research. *Intensive Crit Care Nurs*. 2003;19:154.
13. Puntillo K, et al. Evaluation of pain in ICU patients. *Chest*. 2009;135:1069-1074.
14. Khalaila R, et al. Communication difficulties and psychoemotional distress in patients receiving mechanical ventilation. *Am J Crit Care*. 2011;20:470.
15. Gélinas C, Johnston C. Pain assessment in the critically ill ventilated adult: validation of the Critical-Care Pain Observation Tool and physiological indicators. *Clin J Pain*. 2007;23:497.
16. Herr K, et al. Pain assessment in the patient unable to self-report: position statement with clinical practice recommendations. *Pain Manag Nurs*. 2011;12:230-250.
17. Barr J, et al. Clinical practice guidelines for the management of pain, agitation, and delirium in adult ICU patients. *Crit Care Med*. 2013;41:263-306.
18. International Association for the Study of Pain (IASP) Subcommittee on Taxonomy. Pain terms: a list with definitions and notes on usage. *Pain*. 1979;6:249.
19. McCaffery M. *Nursing Management of the Patient With Pain*. 2nd ed. Philadelphia: JB Lippincott; 1979.
20. Anand KJS, Craig KD. New perspectives on the definition of pain. *Pain*. 1996;67:3.
21. McGuire D. Comprehensive and multidimensional assessment and measurement of pain. *J Pain Symptom Manage*. 1992;7:312.
22. International Association for the Study of Pain (IASP) Task Force on Taxonomy. *Classification of Chronic Pain*. Seattle: IASP Press; 1994.
23. Melzack R. Pain and stress: a new perspective. In: Gatchel RJ, Turk DC, eds. *Psychological Factors in Pain*. New York: Guilford Press; 1999.
24. Pasero C, McCaffery M. *Pain Assessment and Pharmacologic Management*. St Louis: Mosby; 2011.
25. Cervero F, Laird JMA. Visceral pain. *Lancet*. 1999;353:2145.
26. Marchand S. The physiology of pain mechanisms: from the periphery to the brain. *Rheum Dis North Am*. 2008;34:285.
27. Melzack R, Wall PD. *The Challenge of Pain*. 2nd ed. London: Penguin Books; 1996.
28. Carr DB, Goudas LC. Acute pain. *Lancet*. 1999;353:2051.
29. Gélinas C, Arbour C. Behavioral and physiological indicators during a nociceptive procedure in conscious and unconscious mechanically ventilated adults: similar or different? *J Crit Care*. 2009;24:628.e7.

30. Rainville P. Brain mechanisms of pain affect and pain modulation. *Curr Opin Neurobiol.* 2002;12:195.

31. Derbyshire SW, Osborn J. Modeling pain circuits: how imaging may modify perception. *Neuroimaging Clin N Am.* 2007;17:485.

32. Melzack R, Wall PD. Pain mechanisms: a new theory. *Science.* 1965;150:171.

33. Marks DM, et al. Serotonin-norepinephrine reuptake inhibitors for pain control: premise and promise. *Curr Neuropharmacol.* 2009;7:331.

34. Lorenz J, Minoshima S, Casey KL. Keeping pain out of mind: the role of the dorsolateral prefrontal cortex in pain modulation. *Brain.* 2003;126:5.

35. McCance KL, Huether SE. *Pathophysiology: the Biologic Basis for Disease in Adults and Children.* 6th ed. St. Louis: Mosby; 2010.

36. Arbour C, Gélinas C. Are vital signs valid indicators for the assessment of pain in cardiac surgery ICU adults? *Intensive Crit Care Nurs.* 2010;26:83.

37. Li DT, et al. Evaluations of physiologic reactivity and reflexive behaviors during noxious procedures in sedated critically ill patients. *J Crit Care.* 2009;24:472.e9.

38. Puntillo KA, et al. Relationship between behavioral and physiological indicators of pain, critical care self-reports of pain, and opioid administration. *Crit Care Med.* 1997;25:1159.

39. Rabin BS, et al. Bidirectional interaction between the central nervous system and the immune system. *Crit Rev Immunol.* 1989;9:279.

40. Hadjistavropoulos T, Craig KD. A theoretical framework for understanding self-report and observational measures of pain: a communication model. *Behav Res Ther.* 2002;40:551.

41. Daut RL, Cleeland CS. The prevalence and severity of pain in cancer. *Cancer.* 1982;50:1913.

42. Melzack R. The short form McGill Pain Questionnaire. *Pain.* 1987;30:191.

43. Jarvis C. *Physical Examination and Health Assessment.* 7th ed. Philadelphia: Saunders; 2016.

44. Puntillo KA. Pain management. In: Schell HM, Puntillo KA, eds. *Critical Care Nursing Secrets.* 2nd ed. Philadelphia: Hanley & Belfus; 2006.

45. Chanques G, et al. The measurement of pain in intensive care unit: comparison of 5 self-report intensity scales. *Pain.* 2010;151:711-721.

46. Gélinas C. The Faces Pain Thermometer: a new tool for critically ill adults [article in French]. *Perspect Infirm.* 2007;4:12-20.

47. Puntillo KA, et al. Pain behaviors observed during six common procedures: results from Thunder Project II. *Crit Care Med.* 2004;32:421.

48. Gélinas C, et al. A validated approach to evaluating psychometric properties of pain assessment tools for use in non-verbal critically ill adults. *Semin Respir Crit Care Med.* 2013;34:153-168.

49. Payen JF, et al. Assessing pain in critically ill sedated patients by using a behavioral pain scale. *Crit Care Med.* 2001;29:2258.

50. Gélinas C, et al. Validation of the Critical-Care Pain Observation Tool (CPOT) in adult patients. *Am J Crit Care.* 2006;15:420.

51. Gélinas C, et al. The impact of the implementation of the Critical-Care Pain Observation Tool on pain assessment/management nursing practices in the intensive care unit with nonverbal critically ill adults: a before and after study. *Int J Nurs Stud.* 2011;48:1495.

52. Rose L, et al. Behavioral pain assessment tool for critically ill adults unable to self-report pain. *Am J Crit Care.* 2013;22:246-254.

53. Chanques G, et al. Impact of systematic evaluation of pain and agitation in an intensive care unit. *Crit Care Med.* 2006;34:1691.

54. De Jong A, et al. Decreasing severe pain and serious adverse events while moving intensive care unit patients: a prospective interventional study (the NURSE-DO project). *Crit Care.* 2013;17(2):R74.

55. Payen JF, et al. Current practices in sedation and analgesia for mechanically ventilated critically ill patients: a prospective multicenter patient-based study. *Anesthesiology.* 2007;106(4):687-695.

56. Ahlers S, et al. The use of the behavioral pain scale to assess pain in conscious sedated patients. *Anesth Analg.* 2010;110:127.

57. Gélinas C, et al. Item selection and content validity of the Critical-Care Pain Observation Tool: an instrument to assess pain in critically ill nonverbal adults. *J Adv Nurs.* 2009;65:203.

58. Gélinas C, et al. Sensitivity and specificity of the Critical-Care Pain Observation Tool for the detection of pain in intubated adults following cardiac surgery. *J Pain Symptom Manage.* 2009;37:58.

59. Gelinas C. Nurses' evaluations of the feasibility and the clinical utility of the Critical Care Pain Observation Tool. *Pain Manag Nurs.* 2010;11:115.

60. Gélinas C, et al. Nurses' evaluations of the CPOT use at 12-month post-implementation in the intensive care unit. *Nurs Crit Care.* 2014;19:272-280.

61. Arbour C, et al. Detecting pain in traumatic brain injured patients exposed to common procedures in the ICU: typical or atypical behaviors? *Clin J Pain.* 2014;30(11):960-969.

62. Roulin MJ, Ramelet AS. Behavioral changes in brain-injured critical care adults with different levels of consciousness during nociceptive stimulation: an observational study. *Intensive Care Med.* 2014;40:1115-1123.

63. Streiner DL, Norman GR, Cairney J. *Health Measurement Scales: a Practical Guide to Their Development and Use.* 5th ed. Oxford: Oxford University Press; 2014.

64. Arroyo-Novoa CM, et al. Pain related to tracheal suctioning in awake acutely and critically ill adults: a descriptive study. *Intensive Crit Care Nurs.* 2008;24(1):20.

65. Boitor M, Lachance JF, Gélinas C. Validation of the Critical-Care Pain Observation Tool and vital signs in relation to the sensory and affective components of pain during mediastinal tube removal in postoperative cardiac surgery intensive care unit adults. *J Cardiovasc Nurs.* 2016;31(5):425.

66. Chanques G, et al. Assessing pain in non-intubated critically ill patients unable to self-report: an adaptation of the Behavioral Pain Scale. *Intensive Care Med.* 2009;35:2060-2067.

67. Kapoustina O, Echegaray-Benites C, Gélinas C. Fluctuations in vital signs and behavioral responses of brain surgery patients in the intensive care unit: are they valid indicators of pain? *J Adv Nurs.* 2014;70(11):2562-2576.

68. Arbour C, et al. Can vital signs fluctuations be used for pain assessment in nonverbal ICU patients with a traumatic brain injury? *Pain Res Treat.* 2014;2014:175794.

69. Young J, et al. Use of a behavioral pain scale to assess pain in ventilated, unconscious and/or sedated patients. *Intensive Crit Care Nurs.* 2006;22(1):32-39.

70. Siffleet J, et al. Patients' self-report of procedural pain in the intensive care unit. *J Clin Nurs.* 2007;16(11):2142-2148.

71. Lukaszewicz AC, et al. The relevance of pupillometry for evaluation of analgesia before noxious procedures in the intensive care unit. *Anesth Analg.* 2015;120(6):1297-1300.

72. Paulus J, et al. Pupillary reflex measurement predicts insufficient analgesia before endotracheal suctioning in critically ill patients. *Crit Care.* 2014;17(4):R161.

73. Gordon DB, et al. American Pain Society recommendations for improving the quality of acute and cancer pain management: american Pain Society Quality of Care Task Force. *Arch Intern Med.* 2005;165:1574.

74. Lawrence M. The unconscious experience. *Am J Crit Care.* 1995;4:227.

75. Laureys S, et al. Cortical processing of noxious somatosensory stimuli in the persistent vegetative state. *Neuroimage.* 2002;17:732.

76. Bjoro K, Herr K. Assessment of pain in the nonverbal or cognitively impaired older adult. *Clin Geriatr Med.* 2008;24:237.

77. Herr K. Pain assessment strategies in older adults. *J Pain.* 2011;3(Suppl 1): S3-S13.

78. Hadjistavropoulos T, et al. An interdisciplinary expert consensus statement on assessment of pain in older persons. *Clin J Pain.* 2007;23:S1.

79. Zwakhalen SM, et al. Pain in elderly people with severe dementia: a systematic review of behavioral pain assessment tools. *BMC Geriatr.* 2006;6:1.

80. Fuchs-Labelle S, Hadjistavropoulos T. Development and preliminary validation of the Pain Assessment Checklist for Seniors with Limited Ability to Communicate (PACSLAC). *Pain Manag Nurs.* 2004;5:37.

81. Wary B, Doloplus C. Doloplus-2, a scale for pain measurement [article in French]. *Soins Gerontol.* 1999;19:25.

82. Warden V, Hurley AC, Volicer L. Development and psychometric evaluation of the Pain Assessment in Advanced Dementia (PAINAD) scale. *J Am Med Dir Assoc.* 2003;4:9.

83. Herr K, Bursch H, Ersek M, et al. Use of pain-behavioral assessment tools in the nursing home: expert consensus recommendations for practice. *J Gerontol Nurs.* 2010;36:18.

84. Kanji S, et al. Validation of the critical care pain observation tool in critically ill patients with delirium: a prospective cohort study. *Crit Care Med.* 2016;44(5):943-947.

85. Graf C, Puntillo KA. Pain in the older adult in the intensive care unit. *Crit Care Clin.* 2003;19:749.

86. Anand KJS. The applied physiology of pain. In: Anand KJS, McGrath PJ, eds. *Pain in Neonates and Infants.* 3rd ed. Amsterdam: Elsevier; 2007.

87. Duhn LJ, Medves JM. A systematic integrative review of infant pain assessment tools. *Adv Neonatal Care.* 2004;4:126.

88. Stevens B, et al. Premature Infant Pain Profile: development and initial validation. *Clin J Pain.* 1996;12:13.

89. Davidhizar R, Giger JN. A review of the literature on care of clients in pain who are culturally diverse. *Int Nurs Rev.* 2004;51:47.

90. Carroll KC, et al. Pain assessment and management in critically ill postoperative and trauma patients: a multisite study. *Am J Crit Care.* 1999;8:105.

91. Cashman JN, Dolin SJ. Respiratory and haemodynamic effects of acute postoperative pain management: evidence from published data. *Br J Anaesth.* 2004;93:212.

92. Smith LH. Opioid safety: is your patient at risk for respiratory depression? *Clin J Oncol Nurs.* 2007;11:293.

93. Gélinas C, et al. Pain assessment and management in critically ill intubated patients: a retrospective study. *Am J Crit Care.* 2004;13:126.

94. Pasero C, et al. Structured approaches to pain management in the ICU. *Chest.* 2009;135:1665.

95. Rose L. Interprofessional collaboration in the ICU: how to define? *Nurs Crit Care.* 2011;16:5-10.

96. Devlin JW, Mallow-Corbett S, Riker RR. Adverse drug events associated with the use of analgesics, sedatives, and antipsychotics in the intensive care unit. *Crit Care Med.* 2010;38:S231.

97. Jarzyna D, et al. American Society for Pain Management Nursing guidelines on monitoring for opioid-induced sedation and respiratory depression. *Pain Manag Nurs.* 2011;12:118.

98. Brush DR, Kress JP. Sedation and analgesia for the mechanically ventilated patient. *Clin Chest Med.* 2009;30:131.

99. Devlin JW, Roberts RJ. Pharmacology of commonly used analgesics and sedatives in the ICU: benzodiazepines, propofol, and opioids. *Crit Care Clin.* 2009;25:431.

100. Ashley E, Given J. Pain management in the critically ill. *Br J Perioper Nurs.* 2008;18:504.

101. Erstad BL, et al. Pain management principles in the critically ill. *Chest.* 2009;135:1075.

102. Cavalière F, et al. A low-dose remifentanyl infusion is well tolerated for sedation in mechanically ventilated, critically ill patients. *Can J Anaesth.* 2002;49:1088.

103. Soltész S, et al. Recovery after remifentanyl and sufentanyl for analgesia and sedation of mechanically ventilated patients after trauma or major surgery. *Br J Anaesth.* 2001;86:763.

104. Radtke FM, et al. Remifentanyl reduces the incidence of post-operative delirium. *J Int Med Res.* 2010;38:1225.

105. Ethuin F, et al. Pharmacokinetics of long-term sufentanyl infusion for sedation in ICU patients. *Intensive Care Med.* 2003;29:1916.

106. Pasero C, et al. IV opioids range orders for acute pain management. *Am J Nurs.* 2007;107:62.

107. Gertler R, et al. Dexmedetomidine: a novel sedative-analgesic agent. *Proc (Bayl Univ Med Cent).* 2001;14:13.

108. Abramov D, Nogid B, Nogid A. The role of dexmedetomidine (Precedex) in the sedation of critically ill patients. *P and T.* 2005;30:158.

109. Pestieau SR, et al. High-dose dexmedetomidine increases the opioid-free interval and decreases opioid requirement after tonsillectomy in children. *Can J Anaesth.* 2011;58:540.

110. Ohtani N, et al. Perioperative infusion of dexmedetomidine at a high dose reduces postoperative analgesic requirements: a randomized control trial. *J Anesth.* 2011;25:872.

111. Lehne RA. *Pharmacology for Nursing Care.* 8th ed. Philadelphia: Elsevier; 2012.

112. Faigeles B, et al. Predictors and use of nonpharmacologic interventions for procedural pain associated with turning among hospitalized adults. *Pain Manag Nurs.* 2013;14(2):85.

113. Tracy MF, et al. Nurse attitudes towards the use of complementary and alternative therapies in critical care. *Heart Lung.* 2003;32:197.

114. Sauls J. The use of ice for pain associated with chest tube removal. *Pain Manag Nurs.* 2002;3:44.

115. Demir Y, Khorshid L. The effect of cold application in combination with standard analgesic administration on pain and anxiety during chest tube removal: a single-blinded, randomized, double-controlled study. *Pain Manag Nurs.* 2010;11:186.

116. Bauer BA, et al. Effect of massage therapy on pain, anxiety, and tension in cardiac surgical patients: a randomized study. *Complement Ther Clin Pract.* 2010;16:70.

117. Cutshall SM, et al. Effect of massage therapy on pain, anxiety, and tension in cardiac surgical patients: a pilot study. *Complement Ther Clin Pract.* 2010;16:92.

118. Boitor M, et al. Evaluation of preliminary effectiveness of hand massage therapy on postoperative pain of adults in the intensive care unit after cardiac surgery: a pilot randomized controlled trial. *Pain Management Nursing.* 2015;16(3):354-366.

119. Friesner SA, Curry DM, Moddeman GR. Comparison of two pain management strategies during chest tube removal: relaxation exercise with opioids and opioids alone. *Heart Lung.* 2006;35(4):269-276.

120. Good M, et al. Relief of postoperative pain with jaw relaxation, music and their combination. *Pain.* 1999;81:163.

121. Henry LL. Music therapy: a nursing intervention for the control of pain and anxiety in the ICU: a review of the research literature. *Dimens Crit Care Nurs.* 1995;14(6):295-304.

9

Sedation, Agitation, Delirium Management

Mary E. Lough

One of the challenges facing clinicians is how to provide a therapeutic healing environment for patients in the alarm-filled, emergency-focused critical care unit. Many critical care patients demonstrate agitation and discomfort caused by painful procedures, invasive tubes, sleep deprivation, fear, anxiety, and physiologic stress. Clinical practice guidelines have been developed by the Society of Critical Care Medicine (SCCM) to improve management of sedation, agitation, and delirium in critically ill patients.[1,2]

SEDATION

Sedation and Agitation Assessment Scales

The use of a validated scale is recommended to standardize assessments of agitation and sedation in a critically ill adult.[1] The Richmond Agitation-Sedation Scale (RASS)[3,4] and the Sedation-Agitation Scale (SAS) are two such scales (Table 9.1).[5] Because all individuals do not metabolize sedative medications at the same rate, the use of a standardized scale ensures that continuous infusions of sedatives such as propofol or dexmedetomidine are titrated to a specific goal. Collaboratively, the critical care team must determine which level of sedation is most appropriate for each individual patient.

Pain Assessment Scales

The first step in assessing an agitated patient is to rule out any sensations of pain.[1] Clinical assessment is more challenging when the patient is obtunded or has an artificial airway in place. If the patient can communicate, the verbal pain scale of 0 to 10 is very useful. If the patient is intubated and cannot vocalize, pain assessment becomes considerably more complex. The Behavioral Pain Scale (BPS) and the Critical-Care Pain Observation Scale (CPOT) are validated behavioral pain scales recommended for pain assessment in critically ill adults.[1] These pain scales are shown in Table 8.1 (BPS) and Table 8.2 (CPOT) in Chapter 8. Preemptive analgesia should be provided before painful procedures.[1] The SCCM guidelines recommend that all critically ill, intubated, mechanically ventilated patients have stated goals for analgesia and sedation.[1] The next step is to determine the minimum level of sedation required for an individual patient.[1]

Levels of Sedation

In the clinical setting, depth of sedation may also be referred to using general descriptive terms defined by the American Association of Anesthesiologists (Box 9.1).[6]

- *Light sedation* (minimal sedation) refers to pharmacologic relief of anxiety (anxiolysis) so that the patient is alert and can respond to verbal commands. (Approximates RASS −1 and SAS 3)
- *Moderate sedation* describes pharmacologic depression of patient consciousness. This is also known as procedural sedation, as this is often the target level when tubes or lines are to be inserted. (Approximates RASS −3 and SAS 3)
- *Deep sedation* describes pharmacologic depression of patient consciousness to where the patient cannot maintain an open airway. (Approximates RASS −4 and SAS 2)
- *General anesthesia* describes pharmacologic depression of patient consciousness using multiple medications, administered by a physician anesthesiologist or a nurse anesthetist. (Approximates RASS −5 and SAS 1)

When the patient has a depressed level of consciousness as a result of sedation (moderate, deep, or general anesthesia), vigilant monitoring of cardiac and respiratory function and vital signs is required. To ensure patient safety, in addition to the clinician performing the procedure, qualified clinicians who are able to monitor and recover the patient must be present. Additionally, the clinician administering the sedative medication must be qualified to manage the patient at whatever level of sedation or anesthesia is achieved.

Opioids and some antihistamine and antiemetic medications may produce a sedative effect. The nurse's responsibility to monitor the patient refers to the level of sedation regardless of the medications that are used.

Pharmacologic Management of Sedation

Achievement of the lightest possible sedation to provide comfort for an alert patient is now considered the standard in critical care.[7] To achieve this goal, it is necessary for all members of the clinical team to be familiar with the pharmacokinetics of frequently used categories of sedatives. Additionally, if the patient is experiencing pain, analgesia must be administered in addition to any sedative agents (see Chapter 8).[1] Sedative medications include benzodiazepines, sedative-hypnotic agents such as propofol, and the central alpha agonist dexmedetomidine (Table 9.2). At the present time, dexmedetomidine-based and propofol-based sedative regimens are recommended for routine sedation of mechanically ventilated adult patients.[1]

All sedatives are to be administered to a specific target level identified by a RASS or SAS level appropriate to the patient's clinical condition. A target level is specified every day and reevaluated whenever there is a change in sedation dosage or patient condition. One likely sedation goal is that the patient is awake and calm, specified as a target sedation level of RASS = 0 or SAS = 4. This describes a patient who follows simple

TABLE 9.1 Sedation Scales

Score	Description	Definition
Richmond Agitation-Sedation Scale (RASS)[a,b]		
+4	Combative	Overtly combative, violent, immediate danger to staff
+3	Very agitated	Pulls or removes tube(s) or catheter(s); aggressive
+2	Agitated	Frequent nonpurposeful movement; fights ventilator
+1	Restless	Anxious but movements not aggressive or vigorous
0	Alert and calm	
−1	Drowsy	Not fully alert, but has sustained awakening (eye opening/eye contact) to voice (>10 s)
−2	Light sedation	Briefly awakens with eye contact to voice (<10 s)
−3	Moderate sedation	Movement or eye opening to voice (but no eye contact)
−4	Deep sedation	No response to voice, but movement or eye opening to physical stimulation
−5	Unresponsive	No response to voice or physical stimulation
Sedation-Agitation Scale (SAS)[c]		
7	Dangerously agitated	Pulls at ETT, tries to remove catheters, climbs over bed rail, strikes at staff, thrashes side to side
6	Very agitated	Does not calm despite frequent verbal reminding of limits, requires physical restraints, bites ETT
5	Agitated	Anxious or mildly agitated, attempts to sit up, calms down to verbal instructions
4	Calm and cooperative	Calm, awakens easily, follows commands
3	Sedated	Difficult to arouse, awakens to verbal stimuli or gentle shaking but drifts off again; follows simple commands
2	Very sedated	Arouses to physical stimuli but does not communicate or follow commands; may move spontaneously
1	Unarousable	Minimal or no response to noxious stimuli; does not communicate or follow commands

[a]Sessler CN, et al. The Richmond Agitation-Sedation Scale: validity and reliability in adult intensive care unit patients. *Am J Respir Crit Care Med.* 2002;166:1338–1344.
[b]Ely EW, et al. Monitoring sedation status over time in ICU patients: reliability and validity of the Richmond Agitation-Sedation Scale (RASS). *JAMA.* 2003;289:2983–2991.
[c]Riker RR, et al. Prospective evaluation of the Sedation-Agitation Scale for adult critically ill patients. *Crit Care Med.* 1999;27:1325–1329.
ETT, endotracheal tube.

BOX 9.1 Levels of Sedation

Light Sedation (Minimal Sedation, Anxiolysis)
Medication-induced state during which patients respond normally to verbal commands. Although cognitive function and coordination may be impaired, ventilatory and cardiovascular functions are unaffected.

Moderate Sedation With Analgesia (Conscious Sedation, Procedural Sedation)
Medication-induced depression of consciousness during which patients respond purposefully to verbal commands, alone or accompanied by light tactile stimulation. No interventions are required to maintain a patent airway, and spontaneous ventilation is adequate. Cardiovascular function is usually maintained.

Deep Sedation and Analgesia
Medication-induced depression of consciousness during which patients cannot be easily aroused but respond purposefully after repeated or painful stimulation. The ability to maintain ventilatory function independently is impaired. Patients require assistance in maintaining a patent airway, and spontaneous ventilation may be inadequate. Cardiovascular function is usually maintained.

General Anesthesia
Medication-induced loss of consciousness during which patients are not arousable, even by painful stimulation. The ability to maintain ventilatory function independently is impaired, and assistance to maintain a patent airway is required. Positive pressure ventilation may be required because of depressed spontaneous ventilation or medication-induced depression of neuromuscular function. Cardiovascular function may be impaired.

Data from Joint Commission on Accreditation of Healthcare Organizations. *Comprehensive Accreditation Manual for Hospitals.* Oakbrook Terrace, IL: The Joint Commission; 2000; American Association of Anesthesiologists. Continuum of Depth of Sedation: Definition of General Anesthesia and Levels of Sedation/Analgesia. 1999; revised 2014. Available as: continuum-of-depth-of-sedation-definition-of-general-anesthesia-and-levels-of-sedation-analgesia.pdf at http://www.asahq.org September 21, 2016

verbal commands without agitation and who can sustain eye contact for at least 10 seconds, as described in Table 9.1. When the intent is to provide deep sedation, the target sedation level is specified as RASS = −4 to −5 or SAS = 1 to 2.[1] These target values describe a mechanically ventilated patient who is not responsive to a spoken voice and who does not respond purposefully to physical stimulation. If this is not the clinically intended level of consciousness, sedative infusions should be turned down or turned off.

Use of a target sedation number lowers the risk of unintentional oversedation (RASS −4 or −5; SAS 1 or 2). Prolonged oversedation is associated with negative sequelae, including pressure ulcers, thromboemboli, gastric ileus, nosocomial pneumonia, and delayed weaning from mechanical ventilation. Oversedation has also been linked to an increase in delirium and worse long-term cognitive outcomes.[8]

Benzodiazepines

Benzodiazepines have powerful amnesic properties that inhibit reception of new sensory information. Benzodiazepines do not confer analgesia. The most frequently used benzodiazepines are diazepam (Valium), midazolam (Versed), and lorazepam (Ativan). Previously a mainstay of sedation, benzodiazepines are no longer recommended for sedation of mechanically ventilated critically ill adults. Benzodiazepine-based sedative regimens are associated with worse patient outcomes, including longer duration of mechanical ventilation and delirium.[8]

Short-acting benzodiazepines (midazolam) are still helpful for the treatment of acute short-term agitation[1] because the intravenous onset of action is less than 3 minutes. However, when midazolam is administered for longer than 24 hours as a continuous infusion, the sedative effect is prolonged by its active metabolites. Longer acting benzodiazepines (lorazepam and diazepam) also have a role in the management of delirium tremens (described later) and seizures,[1] but these are different indications from routine sedation in critical illness.

The major unwanted side effects associated with benzodiazepines are dose-related respiratory depression and hypotension. If needed, flumazenil (Romazicon) is the antidote used to reverse benzodiazepine overdose in symptomatic patients.

TABLE 9.2   Pharmacologic Management
Sedation

Medication	Dosage	Action	Special Considerations
Benzodiazepines			
Diazepam	Loading dose IV: 5–10 mg/kg slowly Intermittent maintenance dose IV: 0.03–0.1 mg/kg every 30 min–6 h as needed	Anxiolysis Amnesia	Onset: 2–5 min after IV administration Side effects: hypotension, respiratory depression
		Sedation	Half-life: long (20–120 h); active metabolites also contribute to prolonged sedative effect Tolerance: physical tolerance develops with prolonged use, and higher doses of medication are required to achieve same effect over time; slow wean required from diazepam after continuous prolonged use; no active metabolites Phlebitis occurs with peripheral IV administration
Lorazepam	Loading dose IV: 0.02–0.04 mg/kg (≤2 mg) slowly	Anxiolysis	Onset: 15–20 min after IV administration
	Intermittent maintenance IV every 2–6 h: 0.02–0.6 mg/kg slowly	Amnesia	Side effects: hypotension, respiratory depression, propylene glycol–related acidosis, nephrotoxicity
	Continuous IV maintenance infusion: 0.01–0.1 mg/kg/h (≤10 mg/h)	Sedation	Half-life: relatively long (8–15 h) Tolerance: physical tolerance develops with use, and higher medication dosage is required to achieve same effect over time; slow wean required from lorazepam after continuous prolonged use Solvent-related acidosis and kidney failure occur at high doses
Midazolam	Loading dose IV: 0.01–0.05 mg/kg slowly over several minutes	Anxiolysis	Onset: 2–5 min after IV administration
	Continuous IV maintenance infusion: 0.02–0.1 mg/kg/h	Amnesia	Side effects: hypotension, respiratory depression
		Sedation	Half-life: 3–11 h; sedative effect is prolonged when midazolam infusion has continued for many days, owing to presence of active sedative metabolites; sedative effect is also prolonged in kidney failure Tolerance: physical tolerance develops with prolonged use, and higher medication dosages are required to achieve same effect over time; slow wean required from midazolam after prolonged use
Sedative-Hypnotics			
Propofol	Loading dose IV: 5 mcg/kg/min over 5 min Continuous IV maintenance infusion: 5–50 mcg/kg/min	Anxiolysis Amnesia	Onset: very rapid onset (1–2 min) after IV administration Side effects: hypotension, respiratory depression (patient must be intubated and mechanically ventilated to eliminate this complication), pain at injection site if administered via peripheral IV line; pancreatitis; hypertriglyceridemia, propofol-related infusion syndrome, allergic reactions
		Sedation	Half-life: 1–2 min when used as short-term agent; with prolonged continuous IV infusion, half-life extends to 50 ± 18.6 h Effective short-term anesthetic agent, useful for rapid "wake-up" of patients for assessment; if continuous infusion is used for many days, emergence from sedation can take hours or days; sedative effect depends on dose administered, depth of sedation, and length of time sedated Change IV infusion tubing every 6–12 h Requires dedicated IV catheter and tubing (do not mix with other medications) Monitor serum triglyceride levels
Central Alpha-Adrenergic Receptor Agonists			
Dexmedetomidine	Loading dose IV: 1 mcg/kg over 10 min Continuous IV maintenance infusion: 0.2–0.7 mcg/kg/h	Anxiolysis Analgesia	Onset: 5–10 min Side effects: Bradycardia, hypotension, loss of airway reflexes
		Sedation	Half life: 1.8–3.1 h No active metabolites Intermittent bolus dosing is not recommended Maintenance infusion is adjusted to achieve desired level of sedation

IV, intravenous.
From Barr J, et al. Clinical practice guidelines for the management of pain, agitation, and delirium in adult patients in the intensive care unit. *Crit Care Med*. 2013; 41:263–306.

Flumazenil should be used with caution in patients with benzodiazepine dependence because rapid withdrawal can induce seizures and other adverse side effects.[9]

Sedative-Hypnotic Agents

Propofol is a powerful sedative and respiratory depressant used for sedation in mechanically ventilated patients in critical care. It is immediately identifiable by its white milky appearance, always in a glass container. At high doses (greater than 100 to 200 mcg/kg per minute), propofol is intended to produce a state of general anesthesia in the operating room.[10] In the critical care unit, propofol is prescribed as a continuous infusion at lower doses (5 to 50 mcg/kg per minute) to induce sedation in critically ill patients.[10] Because propofol is lipid soluble, it quickly crosses cell membranes, including cells that comprise the blood–brain barrier. This allows rapid onset of sedation (approximately 30 seconds) with immediate loss of consciousness. In addition to a rapid onset of action, propofol has a very short half-life with initial use (2 to 4 minutes), is rapidly eliminated from the body (30 to 60 minutes), and does not have metabolites.[10] The short half-life makes propofol an ideal sedative for situations when a patient needs to be quickly awakened for a spontaneous awakening trial and spontaneous breathing trial or to assess neurologic status. Propofol is clinically effective and cost-effective because it can be titrated, or turned off, when a patient is mechanically ventilated and may decrease time to extubation. It is important to add an opiate to ensure adequate pain control and amnesia. Propofol is not a reliable amnesic, and patients sedated with only propofol can have vivid recollections of their experiences.

Risk of complications increases with long-term administration of propofol at high doses (greater than 4.00 mg/kg per hour for longer than 48 hours).[11] However, cases have been reported at lower dosages.[11] Propofol is delivered in a lipid-based emulsion, and side effects may be related to disruption of fatty acid metabolism, muscle injury, and release of toxic intracellular contents. The term *propofol-related infusion syndrome* describes metabolic acidosis, muscular weakness, rhabdomyolysis, myoglobinuria, acute kidney injury, and cardiovascular dysrhythmias. Metabolic acidosis is the most common sign with an estimated mortality of 50% based on published case reports.[11]

A rare benign effect of propofol infusion is green urine, seen in less than 1% of cases.[12] Urine discoloration occurs when the patient's liver cannot metabolize all of the propofol, and the remainder is excreted via the kidney. Propofol is not nephrotoxic, and the urine returns to a normal color when the medication is stopped. Other secondary side effects related to the fat-emulsion carrier include hyperlipidemia, hypertriglyceridemia, and acute pancreatitis. Serum triglycerides should be measured on all patients who receive propofol for longer than 48 hours.

Propofol is a lipid-based emulsion, a medium highly conducive to bacterial growth. For this reason, the manufacturer and the Centers for Disease Control and Prevention (CDC) recommend that the tubing be changed every 6 to 12 hours to prevent catheter-related infections.[13] Use of aseptic technique is mandatory.[14] Nursing vigilance is required to monitor sedation levels and to be alert for the rare but significant risk of propofol-related complications. Table 9.2 provides additional information.

Central Alpha Agonists

Two central alpha-adrenergic agonists with sedative properties are available. Clonidine is often prescribed as a Catapres patch, and dexmedetomidine (Precedex) is prescribed as a continuous infusion. Clonidine may be prescribed for patients experiencing alcohol withdrawal syndrome (see later).

Dexmedetomidine is an alpha-2 agonist that is approved by the US Food and Drug Administration for use as a short-term sedative (less than 24 hours) in mechanically ventilated patients. Sedation occurs when the medication activates postsynaptic alpha-2 receptors in the central nervous system in the brain. This activation inhibits norepinephrine release and blocks sympathetic nervous system fight-or-flight functions, leading to sedation. Sympathetic nervous system inhibition may cause hypotension and bradycardia. Analgesic effects occur because dexmedetomidine binds to alpha-2 receptors in the spinal cord. These unique mechanisms of action allow patients to be lightly sedated and also interactive, factors that are associated with a shorter time to extubation compared with traditional sedative regimens.[15] Dexmedetomidine may shorten the duration of delirium compared with other sedative agents.[16]

Dexmedetomidine is administered with a loading dose of 1.0 mcg/kg over 10 minutes, followed by a continuous infusion of 0.4 mcg/kg (range 0.2 to 0.7 mcg/kg per hour). Dexmedetomidine has a short half-life (6 minutes) and is eliminated from the body in approximately 2 hours. Elimination from the body is dramatically slowed if the patient has liver failure (see Table 9.2).

Many patients have other sedatives or opiates infusing in addition to dexmedetomidine, and the combination may potentiate the overall sedative effect. Monitoring of sedation level, blood pressure, heart rate, respiratory rate, and pulse oximetry is required. Dexmedetomidine confers sedation and analgesic effects without respiratory depression. Consequently patients can be extubated while still on a dexmedetomidine infusion. This can be helpful for patients who are anxious during ventilator weaning. Dexmedetomidine has also been used for patients on noninvasive mask ventilation.[17] Because of this favorable profile, dexmedetomidine use as a sedative agent has increased in critical care units.[18]

Daily Sedation Interruption

One strategy to avoid the pitfalls of sedative dependence and withdrawal is to turn off the sedative infusions once each day. This intervention has been given several names, including *sedation vacation* and *spontaneous awakening trial*. At a scheduled time, all continuously infusing sedatives are stopped. Sometimes analgesics are also stopped, depending on the hospital's protocol. The patient is allowed to regain consciousness for clinical assessment using a standardized instrument such as RASS or SAS (see Table 9.1).[19,20] The patient is carefully monitored, and when awareness is attained, an assessment of level of consciousness and neurologic function is performed. If the patient becomes agitated, it is essential that a protocol be in place for the nurse to restart the sedatives. One protocol scheduled the daily interruption of sedatives in the morning and recommended, after a full assessment, restarting the sedative and opiate infusions at 50% of the previous morning dose and adjusting upward until the patient is comfortable.[20]

Other protocols forgo infusions and use intermittent intravenous push "as-needed" sedatives and analgesics to manage pain and sedation. Another approach is to maintain the patient at a lighter level of sedation all the time rather than specifying specific times to stop the sedatives.[21]

TABLE 9.3	**Signs and Symptoms of Sedative or Analgesic Medication Withdrawal**[a]	
System	**Opiate Withdrawal**	**Benzodiazepine Withdrawal**[b]
Neurologic	Delirium, tremors, seizures	Agitation, anxiety, delirium, tremors, myoclonus, headache, seizures, fatigue, paresthesias, sleep disturbances
Sensory	Dilation of pupils, teary eyes, irritability, increased sensitivity to pain, sweating, yawning	Increased sensitivity to light/sound, sweating
Musculoskeletal	Cramps, muscle aches	Muscle cramps
Gastrointestinal	Vomiting, diarrhea	Nausea, diarrhea
Respiratory	Tachypnea	Tachypnea

[a]Data on propofol are limited, but withdrawal symptoms after prolonged use are similar to withdrawal symptoms of benzodiazepines.
[b]Not all symptoms are seen in all patients.

An important nursing responsibility is to prevent the patient from coming to harm during sedative or analgesic medication withdrawal (Table 9.3). If the patient is seriously agitated, it is vital to consult with the physician and pharmacist to establish an effective treatment plan that allows safe weaning from sedative medications (see Table 9.1).

AGITATION

Agitation describes hyperactive patient movements that range in intensity from slight restless hand and body movements to pulling out lines and tubes or physical aggression and self-harm. Some frequently encountered causes of agitation include pain, anxiety, delirium, hypoxia, ventilator dyssynchrony, neurologic injury, uncomfortable position, full bladder, sleep deprivation, alcohol withdrawal, sepsis, medication reaction, and organ failure. In the past, when a patient showed physical signs of agitation, a benzodiazepine sedative (lorazepam or midazolam) was quickly administered to reduce the patient's mental awareness and hyperactivity (see Table 9.2). However, because benzodiazepines have been shown to induce delirium, these medications are no longer recommended.[1] Haloperidol, an antipsychotic medication, can be administered for management of acute agitation.[22]

Agitation is assessed using a validated scale such as SAS or RASS (see Table 9.1). Standardized assessment scales allow clinicians to identify agitation in its milder forms and to potentially ameliorate the patient's symptoms. The goal is to treat the cause of the agitation rather than to overmedicate. When patients are dangerously agitated (SAS +7), are combative (RASS +4), or could endanger themselves or others, immediate sedation is warranted. In these extreme situations, a benzodiazepine is administered.[1]

DELIRIUM

Delirium is a global impairment of cognitive processes, usually of sudden onset, coupled with disorientation, impaired short-term memory, altered sensory perceptions (i.e., hallucinations), abnormal thought processes, and inappropriate behavior. Routine monitoring for delirium is recommended.[1] Delirium is more prevalent than generally recognized; it is difficult to diagnose in a critically ill patient and represents acute brain dysfunction caused by sepsis, critical illness, or dysfunction of other vital organs.[23] Greater than 50% of mechanically ventilated patients experience delirium.[23] Delirium increases hospital stay and mortality rates for patients who are mechanically ventilated.[1]

When patients are agitated, restless, and pulling at tubes and lines, they are often identified as being delirious. In this scenario,

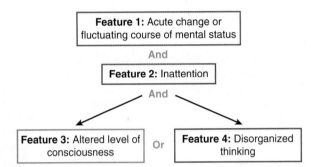

FIG. 9.1 Confusion Assessment Method for the ICU. Delirium is defined as positive in Feature 1 and Feature 2 and either Feature 3 or Feature 4. (Copyright 2002, E. Wesley Ely, MD, MPH, and Vanderbilt University. All rights reserved.)

delirium may be described as "ICU psychosis" or "sundowner syndrome." However, a delirious patient is not always agitated, and it is much more difficult to detect delirium when a patient is physically calm.

Specific scoring instruments are available to assess delirium, and two have been validated for use with mechanically ventilated critical care patients[1]: the Confusion Assessment Method for the Intensive Care Unit (CAM-ICU) (Figs. 9.1 and 9.2)[24,25] and the Intensive Care Delirium Screening Checklist (ICDSC) (Fig. 9.3).[26,27] Both instruments are used in tandem with RASS to exclude patients in coma and identify delirium. Coma is a known risk factor for development of delirium. Both CAM-ICU and ICDSC provide a structured format to evaluate delirium for verbal patients and for nonverbal and mechanically ventilated patients.

Pharmacologic Management of Delirium

Pharmacologic treatment of delirium is challenging.[1] The neuroleptic medication haloperidol (Haldol) has traditionally been administered to treat hyperactive delirium.[23] This antipsychotic agent stabilizes cerebral function by blocking dopamine-mediated neurotransmission at the cerebral synapses and in the basal ganglia. Electrocardiographic monitoring is recommended because haloperidol prolongs the Q–Tc interval, increasing the risk of ventricular dysrhythmias. Haloperidol and other antipsychotics should be avoided in patients who have a prolonged Q–Tc interval or a history of torsades de pointes.[1]

Atypical antipsychotics are sometimes administered to treat delirium associated with critical illness, although this class of medications has not yet been shown to prevent delirium.[28] These are medications that were developed to treat another condition such as schizophrenia or bipolar disorder. Haloperidol or other atypical antipsychotics are not administered prophylactically as

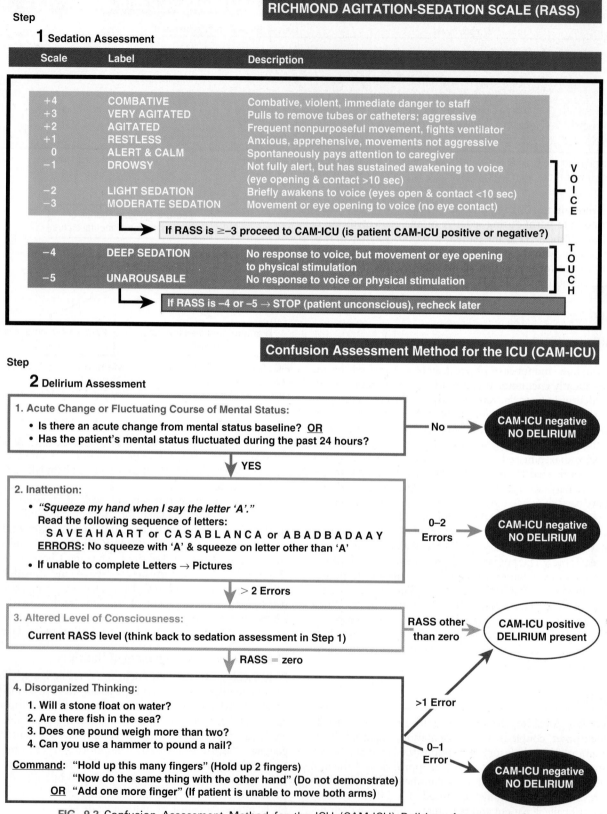

RICHMOND AGITATION-SEDATION SCALE (RASS)

Step
1 Sedation Assessment

Scale	Label	Description
+4	COMBATIVE	Combative, violent, immediate danger to staff
+3	VERY AGITATED	Pulls to remove tubes or catheters; aggressive
+2	AGITATED	Frequent nonpurposeful movement, fights ventilator
+1	RESTLESS	Anxious, apprehensive, movements not aggressive
0	ALERT & CALM	Spontaneously pays attention to caregiver
−1	DROWSY	Not fully alert, but has sustained awakening to voice (eye opening & contact >10 sec)
−2	LIGHT SEDATION	Briefly awakens to voice (eyes open & contact <10 sec)
−3	MODERATE SEDATION	Movement or eye opening to voice (no eye contact)

VOICE

If RASS is ≥−3 proceed to CAM-ICU (is patient CAM-ICU positive or negative?)

Scale	Label	Description
−4	DEEP SEDATION	No response to voice, but movement or eye opening to physical stimulation
−5	UNAROUSABLE	No response to voice or physical stimulation

TOUCH

If RASS is −4 or −5 → STOP (patient unconscious), recheck later

Confusion Assessment Method for the ICU (CAM-ICU)

Step
2 Delirium Assessment

1. Acute Change or Fluctuating Course of Mental Status:
- Is there an acute change from mental status baseline? <u>OR</u>
- Has the patient's mental status fluctuated during the past 24 hours?

→ No → **CAM-ICU negative NO DELIRIUM**

↓ **YES**

2. Inattention:
- *"Squeeze my hand when I say the letter 'A'."*
  Read the following sequence of letters:
  S A V E A H A A R T or C A S A B L A N C A or A B A D B A D A A Y
  <u>ERRORS:</u> No squeeze with 'A' & squeeze on letter other than 'A'
- If unable to complete Letters → Pictures

→ 0–2 Errors → **CAM-ICU negative NO DELIRIUM**

↓ **> 2 Errors**

3. Altered Level of Consciousness:
Current RASS level (think back to sedation assessment in Step 1)

→ RASS other than zero → **CAM-ICU positive DELIRIUM present**

↓ **RASS = zero**

4. Disorganized Thinking:
1. Will a stone float on water?
2. Are there fish in the sea?
3. Does one pound weigh more than two?
4. Can you use a hammer to pound a nail?

<u>Command:</u> "Hold up this many fingers" (Hold up 2 fingers)
     "Now do the same thing with the other hand" (Do not demonstrate)
<u>OR</u> "Add one more finger" (If patient is unable to move both arms)

→ >1 Error → **CAM-ICU positive DELIRIUM present**

→ 0–1 Error → **CAM-ICU negative NO DELIRIUM**

FIG. 9.2 Confusion Assessment Method for the ICU (CAM-ICU) Delirium Assessment. Step 1—Sedation Assessment; Step 2—Delirium Assessment. (Copyright 2002, E. Wesley Ely, MD, MPH, and Vanderbilt University. All rights reserved.)

The Intensive Care Delirium Screening Checklist (ICDSC)

1. Altered level of consciousness

(A) No response or (B) the need for vigorous stimulation in order to obtain any response signified a severe alteration in the level of consciousness precluding evaluation. If there is coma (A) or stupor (B) most of the time period, then a dash (—) is entered and there is no further evaluation for that period.

(C) Drowsiness or response to a mild to moderate stimulation implies an altered level of consciousness and scores 1 point.

(D) Wakefulness or sleeping state that could easily be aroused is considered normal and scores zero points.

(E) Hypervigilance is rated as an abnormal level of consciousness and scores 1 point.

2. Inattention

Difficulty in following a conversation or instruction, easily distracted by external stimuli, or difficulty in shifting focus scores 1 point.

3. Disorientation

Any obvious mistake in time, place, or person scores 1 point.

4. Hallucination, delusion, or psychosis

The unequivocal clinical manifestation of hallucination or of behaviour probably due to hallucination (eg, trying to catch a nonexistent object) or delusion or gross impairment in reality testing scores 1 point.

5. Psychomotor agitation or retardation

Hyperactivity requiring the use of additional sedative drugs or restraints in order to control potential danger (eg, pulling out IV lines, hitting staff), hypoactivity, or clinically noticeable psychomotor slowing scores 1 point.

6. Inappropriate speech or mood

Inappropriate, disorganized, or incoherent speech or inappropriate mood related to events or situation scores 1 point.

7. Sleep/wake cycle disturbance

Sleeping less than four hours, waking frequently at night (do not consider wakefulness initiated by medical staff or loud environment), or sleeping during most of the day scores 1 point.

8. Symptom fluctuation

Fluctuation of the manifestation of any item or symptom over 24 hours (eg, from one shift to another) scores 1 point.

How to Calculate a Score for the ICDSC*

Patient Evaluation	Day 1	Day 2	Day 3	Day 4	Day 5
Altered level of consciousness (A-E)*					
Inattention					
Disorientation					
Hallucination, delusion, psychosis					
Psychomotor agitation or retardation					
Inappropriate speech or mood					
Sleep-wake cycle disturbance					
Symptom fluctuation					
Total Score (0-8)					

*Level of Consciousness	Score
A: no response	–
B: response to intense and repeated stimulation (loud voice and pain)	–
C: response to mild or moderate stimulation	1
D: normal wakefulness	0
E: exaggerated response to normal stimulation	1
If **A** or **B**, do not complete patient evaluation for the period.	

Scoring System

The scale is completed based on information collected from each 8-hour shift or from the previous 24 hours. Obvious manifestation of an item = 1 point. No manifestation of an item or no assessment possible = 0 points. The score of each item is entered in the corresponding space and is 0 or 1. A total score of ≥4 on any given day has a 99% sensitivity for correlation with a psychiatric diagnosis of delirium.

*The ICDSC is also used in tandem with the RASS (see Table 9.1) to assess sedation-agitation in addition to delirium.

FIG. 9.3 Intensive Care Delirium Screening Checklist (ICDSC). The ICDSC is also used in tandem with the RASS scale (see Table 9.1) to assess sedation-agitation in addition to delirium. (From Bergeron N, et al. Intensive Care Delirium Screening Checklist: evaluation of a new screening tool. *Intensive Care Med.* 2001;27:859.)

prevention against delirium because there is no evidence that this reduces the incidence of delirium.[23]

Interventions to Prevent Delirium

Several research studies have shown that a "bundle" of interventions may prevent or reduce the duration of delirium in critical illness.[1] In mechanically ventilated patients, the interventions include spontaneous awakening trials, daily delirium monitoring, and early mobility.[29,30] Early mobility may also prevent the muscle weakness that accompanies long periods of bed rest during critical illness and may reduce the cognitive complications associated with prolonged illness that many patients experience.[30] Some critical care units have initiated sleep protocols to increase the opportunity for patients to sleep at night, dimming lights at night, ensuring there are periods of time when tubes are not manipulated, and clustering nursing care interventions to provide some uninterrupted rest periods.

ALCOHOL WITHDRAWAL SYNDROME AND DELIRIUM TREMENS

Critically ill patients who are alcohol dependent and were drinking before hospital admission are at risk of alcohol withdrawal syndrome (AWS).[31,32] AWS is associated with an increased risk of delirium, hallucinations, seizures, increased need for mechanical ventilation, and death. When hyperactive agitated delirium is caused by alcohol withdrawal, it is termed *delirium tremens* (DTs).[32] After hospital admission, approximately 50% of alcohol-dependent patients experience AWS-related symptoms with decreasing blood alcohol concentration.[32] Less than 5% experience severe complications such as DTs or a seizure.[31,32] Screening tools to identify alcohol dependence, such as the Alcohol Use Disorders Identification Test (AUDIT) shown in Table 33.1 in Chapter 33, are very helpful.[32] Management of alcohol withdrawal involves close monitoring of AWS-related agitation and administration of intravenous benzodiazepines, generally diazepam or lorazepam. Diazepam has the advantage of a longer half-life and high lipid solubility.[31] Lipid-soluble medications quickly cross the blood–brain barrier and enter the central nervous system to produce a sedative effect.[31,33] Benzodiazepines should be administered in response to increased signs of agitation associated with DTs, with dosage guided by a clinical protocol. This is described as an AWS symptom-triggered approach.[31,32] Adjunctive dexmedetomidine has been added to some protocols.[34] The severity of alcohol withdrawal can be assessed with a scale such as the Clinical Institute Withdrawal Assessment of Alcohol Scale (revised).[31] Multivitamins, including thiamine (vitamin B_1), are administered prophylactically to prevent additional neurologic sequelae.[31] Delirium related to alcohol withdrawal is pharmacologically managed very differently than delirium that is due to other causes. Long-acting benzodiazepines are the medications of choice in AWS.[31,33] In contrast, benzodiazepines are contraindicated for treatment of delirium from non–alcohol-related causes.

COLLABORATIVE MANAGEMENT

Collaborative management of anxiety, agitation, sedation, and delirium is a responsibility shared by all members of the health care team, as indicated by the clinical practice guidelines summarized in Box 9.2. Recognition of the problem is the first

step toward a solution to establish a more effective standard of patient care in management of sedation, analgesia, and delirium.

SUMMARY

- Use a validated sedation instrument (RASS or SAS) and titrate sedation medications to achieve the lightest possible level of sedation to prevent immobility-associated problems and delirium.
- Benzodiazepines are not recommended for routine sedation of mechanically ventilated adult patients.
- Dexmedetomidine and propofol are recommended for sedation of mechanically ventilated adult patients.
- Daily interruption of sedation and a spontaneous breathing trial are recommended for patients who are mechanically ventilated.

BOX 9.2   Evidence-Based Practice Summary of Guidelines for Assessment and Treatment of Agitation and Delirium

QSEN
- Agitation in critically ill patients may result from inadequately treated pain, anxiety, delirium, or ventilator dyssynchrony.
- Detection and treatment of pain, agitation, and delirium should be reassessed often in these patients.
- Patients should be awake and able to purposely follow commands to participate in their care unless a clinical indication for deeper sedation exists.

Agitation
- Depth and quality of sedation should be routinely assessed in all critical care patients.
- RASS and SAS are the most valid and reliable scales for assessing quality and depth of sedation in critically ill patients.
- Target lightest possible level of sedation and/or use daily sedative interruption.
- Use sedation protocols and checklists to facilitate sedation management.
- Suggest using analgesia-first sedation for intubated and mechanically ventilated critically ill patients.
- Suggest using nonbenzodiazepines for sedation (either propofol or dexmedetomidine) rather than benzodiazepines (either midazolam or lorazepam) in mechanically ventilated adult patients.

Delirium
- Delirium assessment should be routinely performed in all critically ill patients.
- CAM-ICU and ICDSC delirium monitoring tools are the most valid and reliable scales to assess delirium in mechanically ventilated patients.
- Mobilize critical care patients as early as possible to reduce incidence and duration of delirium and to improve functional outcomes.
- Promote sleep in critically ill patients by controlling light and noise, clustering patient care activities, and decreasing stimuli at night.
- Avoid use of antipsychotics in patients who are at risk for torsades de pointes.
- Suggest not using benzodiazepines in critically ill patients with delirium unrelated to alcohol/benzodiazepine withdrawal.

CSM-ICU, Confusion Assessment Method for the Intensive Care Unit; *ICDSC*, Intensive Care Delirium Screening Checklist; *RASS*, Richmond Agitation-Sedation Scale; *SAS*, Sedation-Agitation Scale.
From Barr J, et al. Clinical practice guidelines for the management of pain, agitation, and delirium in adult patients in the intensive care unit. *Crit Care Med.* 2013;41:263.

- Delirium can be hypoactive (withdrawn) or hyperactive (with agitation) and is a frequent complication of critical illness.
- Use a validated delirium assessment instrument (CAM-ICU or ICDSC) to identify delirium.
- Pharmacologic management of delirium most commonly includes treatment with haloperidol.
- Nonpharmacologic interventions to prevent delirium include provision of adequate sleep and early mobility.
- Delirium tremens is a complication of alcohol withdrawal syndrome.
- The benzodiazepines diazepam (Valium) and lorazepam (Ativan) are used in the treatment of delirium tremens.
- Ⓔ Visit the Evolve site for additional study materials.

CASE STUDY 9.1 Patient With Delirium

Brief Patient History

Mr. K is a 42-year-old Asian man who is in your city on a business trip. He is transported to your facility from his hotel because of a witnessed grand mal seizure. Paramedics administered lorazepam in the field. Mr. K's wife reports by phone that he is in good health and that she is not aware that he takes any medications regularly. She states that he recently quit drinking alcohol because of pressure from the family. She also comments that she thinks he takes alprazolam to calm his nerves once in a while.

Clinical Assessment

Mr. K is admitted to the critical care unit from the emergency department with hypertension, restlessness, mental confusion, paranoid ideations with rambling speech, and visual and auditory hallucinations. Mr. K's skin is warm and moist. Intravenous administration of thiamine, folic acid, multivitamins, and magnesium was begun in the emergency department. Physician orders were written for lorazepam every 6 hours and clonidine every 4 hours as needed for delirium-related symptoms.

Diagnostic Procedures

Mr. K's baseline vital signs are as follows: blood pressure of 190/92 mm Hg, heart rate of 130 beats/min (sinus tachycardia), respiratory rate of 26 breaths/min, and temperature of 98.8°F. Pulse oximetry oxygen saturation is 90% on 4 L/min oxygen using a nasal cannula. Assessment of delirium with the Confusion Assessment Method indicates the presence of acute and fluctuating change in mental status, inattention, and disorganized thinking. The Sedation-Agitation Scale score is 5. Serum and urine toxicology studies are negative for ethyl alcohol, cannabis, and opioids; urine is strongly positive for benzodiazepines. Sodium level is 135 mmol/L, potassium level is 4.3 mmol/L, chloride level is 84 mmol/L, carbon dioxide level is 26 mEq/L, calcium level is 8 mg/dL, magnesium level is 2.0 mg/dL, and gamma-glutamyltransferase level is 80 IU/L.

Medical Diagnosis

Mr. K is diagnosed with delirium tremens caused by alcohol and benzodiazepine withdrawal.

Questions

1. What major outcomes do you expect to achieve for this patient?
2. What problems or risks must be managed to achieve these outcomes?
3. What interventions must be initiated to monitor, prevent, manage, or eliminate the problems and risks identified?
4. What interventions should be initiated to promote optimal functioning, safety, and well-being of the patient?
5. What possible learning needs do you anticipate for this patient?
6. What cultural and age-related factors may have a bearing on the patient's plan of care?

REFERENCES

1. Barr J, et al. Clinical practice guidelines for the management of pain, agitation, and delirium in adult patients in the intensive care unit. *Crit Care Med.* 2013;41:263–306.
2. Barr J, Kishman Jr CP, Jaeschke R. The methodological approach used to develop the 2013 Pain, Agitation, and Delirium Clinical Practice Guidelines for adult ICU patients. *Crit Care Med.* 2013;41(9 suppl 1):S1–S15.
3. Sessler CN, et al. The Richmond Agitation-Sedation Scale: validity and reliability in adult intensive care unit patients. *Am J Respir Crit Care Med.* 2002;166:1338–1344.
4. Ely EW, et al. Monitoring sedation status over time in ICU patients: reliability and validity of the Richmond Agitation-Sedation Scale (RASS). *JAMA.* 2003;289:2983–2991.
5. Riker RR, Picard JT, Fraser GL. Prospective evaluation of the Sedation-Agitation Scale for adult critically ill patients. *Crit Care Med.* 1999;27:1325–1329.
6. American Association of Anesthesiologists (ASA). Continuum of Depth of Sedation: Definition of General Anesthesia and Levels of Sedation/Analgesia. 2014. Available at: https://www.asahq.org/quality-and-practice-management/standards-and-guidelines/search?q=moderate sedation. Accessed January 10, 2016.
7. Reade MC, Finfer S. Sedation and delirium in the intensive care unit. *N Engl J Med.* 2014;370:444–454.
8. Pandharipande PP, et al. Long-term cognitive impairment after critical illness. *N Engl J Med.* 2013;369:1306–1316.
9. Penninga EI, et al. Adverse events associated with flumazenil treatment for the management of suspected benzodiazepine intoxication—a systematic review with meta-analyses of randomised trials. *Basic Clin Pharmacol Toxicol.* 2016;118(1):37–44.
10. Whitcomb JJ, Huddleston MC, McAndrews KL. The use of propofol in the mechanically ventilated medical/surgical intensive care patient: is it the right choice? *Dimens Crit Care Nurs.* 2003;22:60–63.
11. Krajčov A, et al. Propofol infusion syndrome: a structured review of experimental studies and 153 published case reports. *Crit Care.* 2015;19:398.
12. Pedersen AB, Kobborg TK, Larsen JR. Grass-green urine from propofol infusion. *Acta Anaesthesiol Scand.* 2015;59:265–267.
13. O'Grady NP, et al. Guidelines for the prevention of intravascular catheter-related infections. *Am J Infect Control.* 2011;39(4 suppl 1):S1–S34.
14. King CA, Ogg M. Safe injection practices for administration of propofol. *AORN J.* 2012;95:365–372.
15. Keating GM. Dexmedetomidine: a review of its use for sedation in the intensive care setting. *Drugs.* 2015;75:1119–1130.
16. Djaiani G, et al. Dexmedetomidine versus propofol sedation reduces delirium after cardiac surgery: a randomized controlled trial. *Anesthesiology.* 2016;124(2):362–368.
17. Longrois D, et al. Sedation in non-invasive ventilation: do we know what to do (and why)? *Multidiscip Respir Med.* 2014;9:56.
18. Smithburger PL, et al. Patient predictors of dexmedetomidine effectiveness for sedation in intensive care units. *Am J Crit Care.* 2014;23:160–165.
19. Kress JP, et al. Daily interruption of sedative infusions in critically ill patients undergoing mechanical ventilation. *N Engl J Med.* 2000;342:1471–1477.
20. Girard TD, et al. Efficacy and safety of a paired sedation and ventilator weaning protocol for mechanically ventilated patients in intensive care (Awakening and Breathing Controlled trial): a randomised controlled trial. *Lancet.* 2008;371:126–134.
21. Mehta S, et al. Daily sedation interruption in mechanically ventilated critically ill patients cared for with a sedation protocol: a randomized controlled trial. *JAMA.* 2012;308:1985–1992.
22. Page VJ, et al. Effect of intravenous haloperidol on the duration of delirium and coma in critically ill patients (Hope-ICU): a randomised, double-blind, placebo-controlled trial. *Lancet Respir Med.* 2013;1:515–523.
23. Mehta S, et al. Prevalence, risk factors, and outcomes of delirium in mechanically ventilated adults. *Crit Care Med.* 2015;43:557–566.
24. Ely EW, et al. Evaluation of delirium in critically ill patients: validation of the Confusion Assessment Method for the Intensive Care Unit (CAM-ICU). *Crit Care Med.* 2001;29:1370–1379.

25. Ely EW, et al. Delirium in mechanically ventilated patients: validity and reliability of the confusion assessment method for the intensive care unit (CAM-ICU). *JAMA*. 2001;286:2703–2710.

26. Bergeron N, et al. Intensive care delirium screening checklist: evaluation of a new screening tool. *Intensive Care Med*. 2001;27:859–864.

27. Ouimet S, et al. Subsyndromal delirium in the ICU: evidence for a disease spectrum. *Intensive Care Med*. 2007;33:1007–1013.

28. Serafim RB, et al. Pharmacologic prevention and treatment of delirium in intensive care patients: a systematic review. *J Crit Care*. 2015;30:799–807.

29. Balas MC, et al. Critical care nurses' role in implementing the "ABCDE bundle" into practice. *Crit Care Nurse*. 2012;32:35–38. 40-37.

30. Balas MC, et al. Effectiveness and safety of the awakening and breathing coordination, delirium monitoring/management, and early exercise/mobility bundle. *Crit Care Med*. 2014;42:1024–1036.

31. Sarff M, Gold JA. Alcohol withdrawal syndromes in the intensive care unit. *Crit Care Med*. 2010;38(9 suppl):S494–S501.

32. Schuckit MA. Recognition and management of withdrawal delirium (delirium tremens). *N Engl J Med*. 2014;371:2109–2113.

33. Amato L, et al. Benzodiazepines for alcohol withdrawal. *Cochrane Database Syst Rev*. 2010;3:CD005063.

34. Bielka K, Kuchyn I, Glumcher F. Addition of dexmedetomidine to benzodiazepines for patients with alcohol withdrawal syndrome in the intensive care unit: a randomized controlled study. *Ann Intensive Care*. 2015;5:33.

End-of-Life Care

Caroline Etland

The end of life has become an important clinical topic in critical care, although requisite improvements in end-of-life care have been slow to follow. Because the primary purpose of admission of patients to a critical care unit is to provide aggressive, life-saving treatment, the death of a patient is generally regarded as a failure. Because our clinical culture emphasizes saving lives, the language that describes the end of life employs negative terminology, such as "forgoing life-sustaining treatments," "do not resuscitate (DNR)," and "withdrawal of life support." The phrase *withdrawal of care* should never be used, as it can cause families to think there will be no comfort measures or assistance provided after a decision is made to discontinue mechanical ventilation and other life-sustaining treatments.[1-3]

More accurate language has been used more recently in health care and popular literature to describe end-of-life decision making and medical interventions, such as *allow natural death* instead of "do not resuscitate" and *withholding of nonbeneficial treatment* in place of "futile care."[4] This shift toward more realistic descriptors reflects extensive recent research in health care, especially palliative care, and the effectiveness of goals-of-care discussions with patients with serious illnesses before crisis events. As trends in health care change, more evidence regarding timing and effectiveness of supportive care will be incorporated into treatment protocols and plans of care.

More attention is being given to the quality of the end-of-life experience of patients with serious illnesses, particularly patients who become critically ill. Research studies suggest that medical care for patients with advanced illness is characterized by inadequately treated physical distress; fragmented care systems; poor communication between physicians, patients, and families; and enormous strains on family caregiver and support systems.[5-7] In addition to health care system barriers to good end-of-life care, mainstream media has significantly influenced misconceptions about the success rate of medical interventions in seriously ill patients. A familiar media presentation of life and death in the hospital is a critical event in a patient who is resuscitated and immediately awakens with full capacity. In reality, treatment options are usually explained in rapid technical language, followed by a frightening question, "Do you want us to keep going?" or "Tell us what you want us to do." This heavy burden placed on family members means they must choose between treatment options, one of which may result in loss of their loved one.

The emphasis on patient autonomy as a valued ethical principle is deeply embedded in the health care system of the United States. Expert medical recommendations are offered to patients and families, and they often must determine in a brief space of time whether those recommendations are aligned with their personal values. Most nurses are familiar with the scenario of families of patients in the critical care unit being told how well one body organ is functioning and trying to reconcile this "good news" with another physician communicating a poor overall prognosis. Less often, families are provided with a longer term perspective that addresses the loss of functional status, decreased quality of life, and potential need for long-term care.

Adequate, realistic information about the limits of medicine and frailties of the body allow patients and families to make decisions that preserve a patient's dignity and respect individual autonomy. Hope is a powerful influence on decision making, and a shift from hope for recovery to hope for a peaceful death should be guided by clinicians with exemplary communication skills. Critical care nurses are often the interpreters of medical information and how it applies to personal preferences and values. The ability to respond realistically in accordance with the listener's values and culture is a learned skill. Many resources are available to further develop the necessary skills to better support patients and families through a critical care unit admission to discharge. The American Association of Critical-Care Nurses (AACN) has recognized the importance of this aspect of care in the critical care unit by developing protocols for palliative and end-of-life issues in the critical care unit and by identifying palliative and end-of-life care as a major advocacy initiative.[8,9] Several other key resources to enhance communication and elicit goals of care are discussed throughout this chapter.

This chapter focuses on the evidence available for the care rendered to the dying critical care patient and family through research reports and guidelines. One such report is from the National Consensus Project and the National Quality Forum,[10] in which the preferred practices of care for the imminently dying patient are discussed. Other reports that are specific to the critical care unit have been written by groups headed by Teno,[11] Nelson,[12] Glavan,[13] Beckstrand,[14] and Mularski.[15] In 2001, Curtis and Rubenfeld[16] provided a "how to" guide for critical care quality improvement to outline the process that can be used to improve end-of-life care in the intensive care unit (ICU) with these indicators. Death in the ICU has historically been a quality indicator of palliative care programs, However, White et al[17] suggested that death in the ICU as an end-of-life quality measure bears further examination to prevent "a bias against admitting patients with acute, potentially reversible illnesses for whom there is a relatively high risk of death." Health care organizations are encouraged to identify quality indicators specific to their patient population, services, resources, and culture to improve end-of-life care.

END-OF-LIFE EXPERIENCE IN CRITICAL CARE

Attention to the end of life of hospitalized patients has increased since the publication of the Study to Understand Prognoses and Preferences for Outcomes and Risks of Treatment (SUPPORT).[18] In this major report, more than 9000 seriously ill patients in five medical centers were studied. Despite an intervention to improve communication, shortcomings were found; aggressive treatment was common, only one-half of physicians knew their patients' preferences to avoid cardiopulmonary resuscitation (CPR), more than one-third of patients who died spent at least 10 days in a critical care unit, and family members of 50% of conscious patients reported moderate to severe pain at least one-half of the time.

Following closely after the publication of the SUPPORT study, the Institute of Medicine (IOM) released a report, *Approaching Death: Improving Care at the End of Life*,[19] followed by an updated report in 2014.[20] Based on the growth of palliative care programs as well as recent research on end-of-life care, the recommendations changed to highlight new priorities. Recommendations from the IOM reports are summarized in Table 10.1.

To describe the number of deaths in critical care units, Angus et al[21] reviewed hospital discharge data from six states and the National Death Index. Of the more than 500,000 deaths studied, 38.3% were in hospitals, and 22% occurred after admission to the critical care unit. Terminal admissions associated with critical care accounted for 80% of all terminal hospitalization costs. An analysis in 2014 revealed that although 90% of people would prefer to die in their own homes,[20] more than 20% received high-tech, aggressive care before they died.

TABLE 10.1 Comparison of Death in America Reports

Approaching Death Report (1997)	Dying in America Report (2014)
Patients with fatal illnesses and their family should receive reliable, skillful, and supportive care	Coordination of person-centered, family-oriented end-of-life care
Health professionals should improve care for dying patients	Improve clinician-patient communication, including robust advance care planning processes
Policymakers and consumers should work with health professionals to improve quality and financing of care	Improve access to palliative care training for physicians and nurses
Health profession education should include end-of-life content	Implement models of care to provide services that patients and families need that are not covered by existing insurance plans
Palliative care should be developed, possibly as a medical specialty	Implement culturally appropriate public education and public engagement strategies
Research on end of life should be funded	
The public should communicate more about the experience of dying and options available	

Adapted from Field and Cassel (1997)[19] and Dying in America (2014)[20]

Advance Directives

Although advance directives, also known as a *living will* or a *health care power of attorney*, were intended to ensure that patients received the care they desired at the end of life, the enactment of structures and processes to support completion of advance directives has been suboptimal. Completion rates in adults range from 16% to 36% overall with less than one-half of seriously or terminally ill patients having documented their wishes.[22] Most patients have expressed a desire to avoid "general life support" if dying or permanently unconscious, but few have expressed preferences regarding specific life-sustaining treatments; however, only about one-third of physicians are aware of the existence of advance directives in their patients.[23] In a large study of veterans, Silveria et al[24] found that veterans who had living wills or who had appointed a surrogate decision maker were much less likely to experience aggressive care at the end of life. Even when advance directives are present, the question arises about whether they are applicable for current care decisions; in other words, is this a terminal illness? The state of California has enacted legislation that requires physicians, nurse practitioners, and physician assistants to inform patients when a terminal illness is diagnosed and that they have a right to comprehensive information and counseling regarding end-of-life care.[25] This type of regulation supports discussion of wanted versus unwanted care at the time of diagnosis. However, many providers remain reluctant to document this information in the medical record.

Physician Orders for Life-Sustaining Treatment

The Physician Orders for Life-Sustaining Treatment (POLST)[26] is different from an advance directive. POLST forms are medical orders that are honored across all treatment settings and are especially important to emergency responders in the community. Also, they are completed by the patient and physician in the presence of a serious chronic illness and should be incorporated into medical orders on admission to the hospital or skilled nursing facility. POLST forms are more easily read than an advance directive in that the format is one of check boxes with specific directions. States that have approved use of POLST forms through legislation or specific regulations have witnessed a shift in proactive discussions of patients' wishes for life-sustaining treatment.[27,28]

Preventing unwanted life-sustaining treatment through ongoing communication between patient and provider impacts the critical care setting in several ways. Treatment decision making is supported when prior discussions have occurred between physicians, patients, and their loved ones regarding declining health and limits on intervention. Efficient resource utilization is maximized when inappropriate critical care unit admissions are prevented. Finally, moral distress of care providers is decreased when care is congruent with patient autonomy. Critical care nurses in states that recognize POLST forms need to be aware whether a regulatory mandate requires health care providers to honor the patient's wishes documented on the form or if the documentation is merely a guideline. Equally important is the need to identify the POLST form when it is presented and to communicate with medical staff to ensure that stated treatment wishes are incorporated into the plan of care and physician orders.

Advance Care Planning

Cultural influences in the United States discourage discussion of death. Planning for decisions to be made at a later date if one is unable to speak for one's self is a difficult process, but this knowledge helps family members to make the treatment decisions if a patient cannot communicate. Advance care planning for patients with chronic illness is advantageous for all involved.[29] A systematic review[30] of the effects of advance care planning on end-of-life care revealed that advance care planning decreases life-sustaining treatment, increases use of hospice and palliative care, and prevents hospitalization. When surrogates hear the patient's wishes for end-of-life care, they can be more knowledgeable and less conflicted when asked to make decisions that may result in a loved one's death during a serious illness (Box 10.1).

Communication of the patient's wishes between family members, primary care providers, and intensivists is critical. If patients have stated desires, they should be communicated when patients are entering or are transferred out of the critical care unit. If the patient has not specified his or her preferences, that information also is important and should be communicated to new health care providers; the level of care patients desire should be offered as appropriate. Families and care providers should be informed if patients decline aggressive care so that families will not be left with difficult decisions in emergency situations. Emotional support for the patient and the family is important as they discuss advance care planning in the critical care setting.

ETHICAL AND LEGAL ISSUES

Ethical and legal principles guide many of our decisions in caring for dying patients and their families. The patient is respected as autonomous and able to make his or her own decisions. The Patient Self-Determination Act supports the patient's right to control future treatment in the event the individual cannot speak for himself or herself. When the patient is unable to make decisions, the same respect is usually accorded to surrogates. In many cultures, however, "… individual identity is secondary to family identity, requiring individuals to prioritize family needs over individual needs."[31] Health care providers often struggle with this altered priority, and conflict can occur as a result. When clinicians are knowledgeable and respectful about a given culture and the process of decision making, greater trust is established, and decisions may be rendered more easily.

It can be helpful to analyze conflicted situations from a basis of ethical principles. Two of the basic principles underlying the provision of health care are beneficence and nonmaleficence.

BOX 10.1 Principles of a Good Death

- Anticipate and be able to prepare for a good death
- Retain some control
- Be afforded dignity and privacy
- Have symptom control including pain relief
- Choose place of death when possible
- Have access to information and expertise when necessary
- Have emotional and spiritual support
- Have access to hospice care
- Have control over who is present at death
- Respect the wishes of the dying patient through advance directives
- Have time to say good-bye
- Be able to die rather than pointlessly prolonging life

Adapted from Smith R. A good death. *BMJ*. 2000;320:129.

Beneficence is the principle of intending to benefit the other through one's actions. *Nonmaleficence* means to do no harm. Sometimes in end-of-life care, these two principles are in conflict, such as when resuscitation is attempted under beneficence but causes harm to the patient, especially if resuscitation was not desired by the patient. An equally troubling situation exists when the fear of liability drives decision making from the clinician's perspective. Medical recommendations for limitation of life-sustaining treatment or comfort care often result in conflict with surrogate decision makers. Developing more effective communication with patients and families is discussed later in this chapter.

COMFORT CARE

The decision to withdraw life-sustaining treatments and transition to comfort care at the end of life should be made with as much involvement of the patient as possible, including physical presence of the patient in decision making or procuring paper documents if the patient is unable to participate; the patient's wishes as understood from prior discussions with the patient should guide the decision about whether to withdraw treatment. Withholding and withdrawing treatment are considered to be morally and legally equivalent.[32] However, because families experience more stress in withdrawing treatments than in withholding them,[33] treatments should not be started that the patient would not want or that would not be of benefit.

The goal of withdrawal of life-sustaining treatments is to remove treatments that are not beneficial and may be uncomfortable. Any treatment in this circumstance may be withheld or withdrawn. After the goal of comfort has been chosen, each procedure and medication should be evaluated to see if it is necessary or causes discomfort. Treatments that cause discomfort do not need to be continued. Another defining question is whether treatments are prolonging the dying process. When disagreements arise, ethics consultations have been found to resolve conflicts regarding inappropriately prolonged, nonbeneficial, or unwanted treatments in the critical care unit, shifting the focus to more appropriate comfort care.[34]

Forgoing life-sustaining treatments is not the same as active euthanasia or assisted suicide. Killing is an action causing another's death, whereas allowing a person to die by withholding or withdrawing life-sustaining treatment is avoiding any intervention that interferes with a natural death after illness or trauma.[35]

Cardiopulmonary Resuscitation

CPR was originally developed for patients with coronary artery disease, and those patients are the most likely to survive resuscitation to discharge, as well as patients who experience cardiac arrest in the critical care unit.[36] The benefits of resuscitation may be overestimated for survival to discharge and for the more relevant outcome of resumption of baseline functional status. Researchers have found that the rate of overall survival to discharge after in-hospital CPR ranges from approximately 15% to 20%.[36] The survival rate for patients with cancer has increased because better treatment and support have transformed many cancers into chronic diseases.[37] It has also become evident that patients in the critical care unit have poor survival.[37] FitzGerald et al[38] found that functional status among almost half of the survivors of in-hospital CPR had deteriorated compared with their condition 2 months before the event. After 6 months, 30% of those patients had died, and two-thirds continued to lose function. Despite these dismal statistics, CPR is offered as an option without fully informing patients or families of the low possibility of survival, the pain and suffering involved during and after the procedure, and the potential for decline in functional status.

AACN[39] and the Emergency Nurses Association[40] have issued position statements recommending that families be allowed to be present during CPR and invasive procedures. Family presence is a significant source of support for the patient, and there may be a benefit to the family in observing the resuscitation that can aid in the grieving process when resuscitation is unsuccessful, by knowing that all was done that could be done (Box 10.2).

Impact of Do Not Resuscitate Orders

As a patient clinically declines and death approaches, the decision to initiate a DNR order is influenced by many factors including goals of care, comorbidities, pace of clinical decline, availability of surrogate decision makers, and provider practice patterns. Critical care nurses often initiate discussion of DNR status and play a key role in collaborating with physicians to identify which therapies remain useful to the patient.

Chang et al[41] studied the effect of DNR orders in two critical care units in Taiwan and found that even though a DNR order was issued late in the clinical course, life-sustaining interventions were reduced through discussions and consent by surrogate decision makers. Nurses in Korea did not change their nursing activities substantially after receiving a DNR order, continuing to focus on maintenance, preventive, and hygiene tasks.[42] They reported becoming more passive with

interventions such as central venous pressure monitoring, fluid and electrolyte balance, and reporting the patient's condition. However, the nurses were more active in communicating with the family. Results of these two studies from outside the United States highlight the challenges across the world with end-of-life care.

"DNR" and "withdrawal of life-sustaining treatment" are not synonymous. Nurses should demonstrate to families that loved ones are receiving aggressive comfort interventions as well as any treatments that remain part of the plan of care. Once a decision is made to withdraw life-sustaining treatment, comfort orders should be implemented before withdrawal of treatment. A best practice for minimizing pain and suffering of both patient and family is to use standardized order sets for consistency in practice.

Prognostication and Prognostic Tools

Most patients in the critical care unit have one or more chronic illnesses that greatly impact long-term recovery from major health events such as respiratory failure, myocardial infarction, or sepsis. Because humans and their course of illness can be unpredictable, physicians' ability to prognosticate the length of time before death is limited,[43] and the time to death usually is overestimated to patients and families as well as in the medical record.

Severity scoring systems belong to one of five classes: prognostic, disease-specific, single-organ failure, trauma scores, and organ dysfunction.[44] Two common tools for estimating critical care unit mortality are the Acute Physiology and Chronic Health Evaluation (APACHE) and multiple organ dysfunction score.[45,46] In addition to use of prognostic tools specific to the critical care unit, it makes sense to incorporate prognostic tools for chronic illnesses into overall decision making and the communication process with patients and families. Scoring diagnoses with a traditionally poor prognosis or a consistent trajectory of functional decline can be helpful in comparing current health status with the health status at the time of diagnosis. Loved ones of critically ill patients have witnessed the functional decline and may have hoped for improvement despite advancement of disease. Use of prognostic scales can add meaningful information to help patients and families make informed decisions. Some more commonly used prognostic scales are listed in Table 10.2.

Despite this information and these tools, uncertainty remains a major issue in decision making for physicians, patients, and families. Because of uncertainty and because a few patients who were never thought likely to survive actually return to a critical care unit, professionals are not always confident about issues of

BOX 10.2	End of Life Care: Fast Facts
Cardiopulmonary resuscitation and family presence at end of life	Fast Facts 23, 24, 179, 232, 233
Recommended prognosis for specific conditions	Fast Facts 13, 141, 143, 150, 183, 184, 234
Communication	Fast Facts 6, 11, 22, 64, 76, 77, 123
Decision making	Fast Facts 55, 193, 226, 229
Family meetings	Fast Facts 16, 222, 223, 225, 227
Effective use of hospice	Fast Facts 38, 139, 140
Pain management at end of life	Fast Facts 58, 106, 107, 126, 129, 142, 161, 260
Delirium at end of life	Fast Facts 1, 60, 160

For more information on recommended best practices, visit the Palliative Care Network of Wisconsin at http://www.mypcnow.org/fast-facts

TABLE 10.2   Selected Prognostic Scales

Prognostic Scale	Disease/Clinical Condition	Prognostic Scale	Disease/Clinical Condition
Palliative Prognostic Scale (PPS)	Any hospice population; palliative care patients	Lung Cancer Prognostic Model (LCPM)	Terminal lung cancer patients
Palliative Prognostic Index (PPI)	Terminal cancer patients	Dementia Prognostic Model (DPM)	Demographic, diagnosis, laboratory, and functional data on dementia residents
Palliative Prognostic Score (PaP)	Terminal cancer patients	Prognostic Index for One-Year Mortality in Older Adults (PIMOA)	Adults older than 70 years with previous stay in hospital
Seattle Heart Failure Model; Heart Failure Risk Scoring System (HFRSS)	Acute heart failure	Cancer Prognostic Scale (CPS)	Terminal cancer patients in progressive care unit
BODE Scale	Chronic obstructive pulmonary disease	Mortality Risk Index Score (MRIS)	New admission to nursing home

Adapted from Lau F, et al. A systematic review of prognostic tools for estimating survival time in palliative care. *J Palliat Care.* 2007;23(2):93.

survivability. Moreover, many families cling to small hopes of survival and recovery (see Box 10.2).

DECISION MAKING

Communication and Decision Making

Communication with the patient and family is critical. White et al[47] found that shared decision making about end-of-life treatment choices in physician-family conferences was often incomplete, especially among less educated families. Families were found to go through a process in their decision making in which they considered the personal domain (rallying support and evaluating quality of life), the critical care unit environment domain (awaiting the physicians and relating to the health care team), and the decision domain (arriving at a new belief and making and communicating the decision). Higher levels of shared decision making were associated with greater family satisfaction. Regardless of the health literacy of the patient or family, explanations of life-sustaining treatments such as CPR, ventilation, and tube feedings in simple language are necessary for effective communication. Many patients and families experience a "data dump" during communication with health care providers who focus on reporting vital statistics and odds of success. Several organizations have made available education handouts that explain life-sustaining treatments in realistic terms. These materials are in addition to discussions with a health care provider. Handouts are written at a low reading grade level and are available in several languages.[48,49] Focusing on improving critical care unit communication when patients are dying increases family satisfaction, decreases family stress, and decreases days of nonbeneficial treatment.[50]

Most physicians and nurses have not been taught how to conduct this type of dialogue in their training. There are many options to gain the training and experience necessary to shift the decision making from a purely clinical perspective to a more humanistic view. Programs such as Education in Palliative and End-of-life Care,[51] End-of-Life Nursing Education Consortium (ELNEC),[52] and Center to Advance Palliative Care Palliative Care Leadership Center[53] training are cost-effective methods to educate and support clinicians to communicate more effectively with patients and families at the end of life (see Box 10.2). Additional information on ethical and legal issues is provided in Chapters 2 and 3.

Patients

Patients' capacity for decision making is limited by illness severity and cognitive deficits accentuated by medications and the environment. When decision making is required, the patient is the first person to be approached if able to speak for himself or herself. When the patient is unable to safely make health care decisions because of disease progression or the therapy used for treatment, written documents such as a living will or a health care power of attorney should be obtained when possible. Additional information on power of attorney for health care can be found in the previous section on "Advance Care Planning." Without those documents, wishes of the patient should be ascertained from individuals closest to the patient. Some patients have neither capacity nor surrogates to assist in decision making; this was the case in 27% of deaths in one study.[54] In the absence of a surrogate decision maker, care decisions for unrepresented patients may be delayed, and discharge to another care setting can prove difficult. Only five states have

empowered existing institutional committees to make decisions for unrepresented patients, illustrating the need for transparent and fair processes to be developed.[55]

Families

Family members have reported dissatisfaction with communication and decision making, which has not improved dramatically in the last decade.[56] Increasing the frequency of communication and sharing concerns early in the hospitalization make subsequent discussions easier for the patient, family, and health professional. Families have commonly complained about infrequent physician communication,[57] unmet communication needs in the shift from aggressive to end-of-life care, and lacking or inadequate communication.[58] Sometimes families are not ready to receive the prognosis and engage in decision making. Communication seems to be the most common source of complaints in families across studies and should be at the center of efforts to improve end-of-life care.

Strategies to Support Decision Making
Daily Rounds

Having the entire critical care unit team present for morning rounds is one method of improving communication. However, a more recent study identified that there was low agreement among the health care team regarding patient care after daily rounds.[59] This finding points out the need for clear goals and collaboration among care providers to lessen the chance of miscommunication to families.

Family Meetings

Family meetings in the presence of the critical care team is another method used to arrive at a common understanding of the patient's prognosis and goals for future care. A research analysis of the amount of time families were able to speak in these meetings revealed that when families had greater opportunity to talk, their satisfaction with physician communication increased, and their ratings of conflict with the physician decreased.[60] Abbott et al[61] discussed families' descriptions 1 year after decisions about withdrawal of life support of conflict centering on communication and the behavior of the staff. After the patient's death, greater family satisfaction with withdrawal of life support was associated with the following measures[61,62]:

- Process of withdrawal of life support being well explained
- Withdrawal of life support proceeding as expected
- Patient appearing comfortable
- Family and friends being prepared
- Appropriate person initiating discussion
- Adequate privacy during withdrawal of life support
- Opportunity to voice concerns

Curtis et al[63] studied the process of family meetings and how to improve them to promote better end-of-life care for patients in the critical care unit and their families. They found that the missed opportunities that occur during these meetings were occasions to listen to family; to acknowledge and address emotions; and to pursue key tenets of palliative care such as patient preferences, surrogate decision making, and nonabandonment. How questions are asked of surrogates is extremely important. The question is not, "What do you want to do about (patient's name)?" but rather, "What would (patient's name) want if he knew he or she were in this situation?" These two questions have vastly different meanings and consequences for the patient and the family. The former question has a greater likelihood of engendering guilt. The latter question provides a sense of fulfilling the patient's wishes and respecting choices. This discussion is sometimes held during the family meeting, in which goals can be discussed. As families make decisions, they appreciate support for those decisions because the support can reduce the burden they experience. Sharma and Dy[56] reviewed valuable strategies for guiding clinical discussions and conducting family meetings that critical care nurses can use to focus discussions.

The health care team can reinforce the legitimacy of the family expressing feelings of disappointment, sadness, and loss. It is important that the family is made aware that the patient was more than a clinical disease and that he or she was recognized as an individual while in the critical care unit. In a German study, when relatives of critical care unit patients were provided with a brochure on bereavement and received proactive communication, they had lower negative scores on the Impact of Event Scale and on the Hospital Anxiety and Depression Scale.[64]

The Society of Critical Care Medicine (SCCM) recommends supporting the families of critical care unit patients.[65] SCCM presents 43 recommendations, including an endorsement of a shared decision-making model; family care conferencing; culturally appropriate requests for truth telling and informed refusal; spiritual support; staff education and debriefing; family presence at rounds and resuscitation; open and flexible visitation; family-friendly signs; and family support before, during, and after a death. One use of this guideline is to assess the level of family support for each critical care unit so that the most deficient recommendations could be addressed with quality-improvement actions. The categories used in this guideline are for general support of families of patients in the critical care unit. When cross-indexed with seven end-of-life domains,[66] the needs of a family with a dying patient are decision making, spiritual and cultural support, emotional and practical support of families including visitation and family preparation for death, and continuity of care (see Box 10.2).[67]

Cultural and Spiritual Influences on Communication

Cultural and spiritual influences on attitudes and beliefs about death and dying differ dramatically. The cultures of the predominant religions commonly seen in the surrounding community should be familiar to the local health care team. Globalization patterns in the last decade have altered the cultural and religious diversity of communities in the United States, necessitating that nurses partner more closely with spiritual care resources as well as community liaisons to better understand family structures and decision making. These differences may affect how the health care team is viewed, how decisions are made, whether aggressive treatment is preferred, how death is met, and how grieving will occur.[68,69] Patients who do not follow a particular religion should be assessed for their individual spiritual beliefs or lack thereof. Identifying sources of spiritual comfort strengthen the bond between caregivers, patients, or family. Satisfaction with critical care unit care has been associated with the extent to which the family is satisfied with their spiritual care, especially when the patient is near death.[70] Staff members' own attitudes about the specific practices of a culture should be carefully monitored[71] and tempered with respect and humility. Interpreters are necessary when the patient or the family members do not speak English. A cultural and religious assessment is warranted in all situations because cultural or religious affiliation does not imply that patients or families follow all of the tenets of that group.

Hospice Information

Although hospice care has been available for many years, patients and families often consider this method of care only in the last weeks or months of an end-stage illness, and they frequently view hospice care as "giving up," or outright abandonment. Health professionals can assist patients and families by providing information about the benefits of hospice, particularly regarding aggressive symptom management and family support. Some hospices are offering to partner with critical care units in the provision of end-of-life care and in the process of withdrawal of ventilatory support. Hospice care is an option that should be considered, especially in end-stage illness, and the benefit to surviving family members should be emphasized. In some circumstances, alert patients may express a wish to die at home. Hospice-to-home programs have demonstrated that granting this wish may be feasible with coordinated effort (see Box 10.2).

WITHDRAWAL OR WITHHOLDING OF TREATMENT

Discussions about the potential for impending death are never held early enough. The first discussion about prognosis often occurs in conjunction with the topic of the discontinuation of life support. Some family members dread such conversations but are grateful to discuss the uncertainty of their loved one's future. Physicians should give families time to adjust to this information and make preparations by providing early discussions about prognosis, goals of therapy, and the patient's wishes.[35]

Proactive Approach

When patients are admitted to the critical care unit with serious illnesses and are likely to die, a proactive approach to palliative care has been found to shorten critical care unit stays without a significant difference in mortality rates or discharge disposition.[72,73] The use of nonbeneficial resources decreases, and prolonged dying is avoided. Rapid response team daily rounds on non–critical care units have proven to be anecdotally effective in early identification of patients showing early signs of clinical deterioration. Communication with the provider at this time can avert an admission to a critical care unit, possible even averting a Code Blue event.

Patients with assistive cardiac devices present a different challenge in discussion of withdrawal of life support. These patients often are cognitively intact and consent to removal of technology that is keeping them alive. Wiegand and Kalowes[74] outlined issues surrounding discontinuation of cardiac devices as a preventive ethics approach with health care providers anticipating the need to shift goals of care and support patients and families through the process. To reduce confusion and distress among clinicians, protocols for discontinuation of organ-assistance devices are recommended as a standard of care.

Futility/Nonbeneficial Care Discussions

Nurses and physicians frequently disagree about the futility of interventions. Sometimes nurses consider withdrawal before physicians and patients do, and they then feel the care they are giving is unnecessary and possibly harmful. Nurses in one study were found to be more pessimistic but more often correct than physicians about the prognoses of dying patients, but the nurses also proposed treatment withdrawal for some very sick patients who survived.[75] Nurses described acknowledging futility and acting on the patient's distress, being ideally placed to advocate with specialists. At the same time, nurses describe the tension that can result in recommending palliative care or hospice to the medical staff.[76]

Steps Toward Comfort Care

Once a decision has been made to withdraw life-sustaining therapies, each intervention should be evaluated to determine if it still provides any benefit.[77] In a patient who has received life support for a prolonged time, a staged withdrawal of interventions such as removal of ventilator support via terminal weaning allows for better symptom control. For families, seeing a loved one look peaceful as life support is withdrawn ultimately helps with grief resolution in the future. Usually, routine interventions (eg, laboratory tests, imaging, cardiac monitoring) are removed first, followed by respiratory support devices. Withdrawal of specific treatments may have effects necessitating symptom management. Withdrawal of dialysis may cause dyspnea from volume overload, which may necessitate the use of opioids or benzodiazepines. Efforts to discontinue artificial feeding may be met with concern from the family because offering food has great social significance. It is essential to share information with family and providers regarding the potential benefits of withholding nutrition and fluids in the days immediately before death to prevent unnecessary suffering.[78] Critical care patients who survive withdrawal of life support measures may continue to remain in critical care for a period of time before dying or being transferred to a less acute setting. During this time, various symptoms may occur that can be distressing for patients, families, and nursing staff.

PALLIATIVE CARE

An important shift in care of terminally ill patients in the critical care unit has occurred with the growth of palliative care programs in the United States in the last decade.[79] The rapid expansion of this new specialty has decreased the mortality rate in critical care units for patients followed by palliative care services through transfer to lower acuity units as well as decreased the costs associated with higher acuity critical care beds, pharmacy, laboratory, and diagnostic costs. Studies by Morrison and colleagues[7] reviewed hospital and Medicare data to demonstrate that hospitals with palliative care services had significant cost savings compared with hospitals providing usual care. More recent initiatives such as the IPAL-ICU have demonstrated that a focus on lifesaving interventions can be integrated with palliative care concurrently, rather than one following the failure of another.[80]

Patients who are identified as being near the end of life require aggressive care for symptom management provided by a team of health professionals. Palliative care guidelines have been released by a consortium of organizations concerned with palliative care and end-of-life care, and they may provide guidance when the usual first-line treatments do not promote comfort for critically ill patients who are near death.[81] Strategies that are based on research evidence and expert opinion for specific conditions such as delirium, opioid dose escalation, and dyspnea at the end of life are outlined on the Palliative Care network of Wisconsin website, which provides access to evidence-based and expert-based Fast Facts that address a wide variety of clinical, ethical, and psychosocial problems that arise with the care of seriously ill and dying patients.[82] Publications such as the Quality Palliative Care guidelines and the IOM report *Improving Palliative Care for Cancer*[83] have stated that palliative care ideally begins at the time of diagnosis of a life-threatening illness and continues through cure or until death and into the family's bereavement period.

Symptom Management

It has long been in question whether critical care patients can accurately report their symptoms because of the effects of sedating medications, severe illness, and organ dysfunction. Kalowes[84] studied critical care unit patients with a diagnosis other than cancer during a daily wake-up and compared their report of symptoms with reports of their family members. Almost all patients had more than 10 symptoms, and there was 85.5% congruence between patient and family report of physiologic and psychological symptoms. Overall, patients experienced significant symptom burden near the end of life but received limited treatment to alleviate suffering.

Pain Management

Because many critical care patients are unconscious, assessment of pain and other symptoms becomes more difficult.[85] In sedated ventilated patients, especially patients receiving neuromuscular blocking medications, there is no systematic, reliable method to determine the presence or degree of pain.[86] Gélinas et al[87] recommends using signs of body movements, neuromuscular signs, facial expressions, or responses to physical examination for pain assessment in patients with altered consciousness (see Chapter 8).

Because opioids provide sedation, anxiolysis, and analgesia, they are particularly beneficial in ventilated patients. Morphine is the medication of choice, and there is no upper limit in dosing. However, in higher doses, morphine metabolites can cause myoclonus, hyperalgesia, and allodynia. In a paralyzed patient, this may not be detectable, but it can be uncomfortable on some level for the patient, perhaps evident in vital signs or response to ventilator settings. Careful assessment of patients' vital signs may reveal suspected discomfort that necessitates an opioid switch to hydromorphone (Dilaudid) or fentanyl. In nonventilated patients, sedation may cause respiratory depression, and nonopioids or specific anesthetic agents may be more appropriate. Antiinflammatory medications or neuroleptic agents often provide significant comfort for inflammatory conditions or neurologic pain.

Titration of intravenous infusions to achieve maximum effect with minimum sedation is an inexact science. Critical care nurses should assume that pain is present in an immobile patient and administer routine analgesics to prevent suffering. Jacobi et al[88] published a guideline for the sustained use of sedatives and analgesia (see Chapter 9).

Dyspnea

A systematic review and meta-analysis of cancer-related dyspnea interventions critically examined the common interventions used by many practitioners.[89] Dyspnea is best managed with close evaluation of the patient and the use of opioids, sedatives, and nonpharmacologic interventions (oxygen, positioning, and increased ambient air flow). Morphine reduces anxiety and muscle tension and increases pulmonary vasodilation but is ineffective when inhaled. Benzodiazepines, particularly midazolam, may be used in patients who are unable to take opioids or for whom the respiratory effects are minimal. Midazolam has been shown to be at least equally effective as morphine and, in some studies, superior to morphine.[90] Benzodiazepines and opioids should be titrated to effect. Oxygen did not prove to be superior in the studies reviewed, but ambient air movement of some sort often provides relief. Treatment efforts should be aimed at the patient's expression of dyspnea rather than at respiratory rates or oxygen levels.

Nausea and Vomiting

Nausea and vomiting are common and should be treated with antiemetics. The cause of nausea and vomiting may be intestinal obstruction or increased intracranial pressure. Treatment for decompression may be uncomfortable in dying patients, and its use should be weighed using a benefit-to-burden ratio. In certain circumstances, an intervention to provide percutaneous drainage for decompression may be used in a patient who is not imminently dying.

Fever and Infection

Fever and infection necessitate evaluation of the benefits of continuing antibiotics so as not to prolong the dying process. Management of fever with antipyretics may be appropriate for the patient's comfort, but other methods such as ice or hypothermia blankets should be balanced against the amount of distress the patient may experience.

Edema

Edema may cause discomfort, and diuretics may be effective if kidney function is intact. Dialysis is not warranted at the end of life. The use of fluids may contribute to the edema when kidney function is impaired and the body is slowing its functions.

Anxiety

Anxiety should be assessed verbally, if possible, or by changes in vital signs or restlessness. Benzodiazepines, especially midazolam with its rapid onset and short half-life, are frequently used. Minimizing noxious sounds and playing a patient's favorite music may help to soothe anxiety.

Delirium

Delirium is commonly observed in critically ill and dying patients. Haloperidol and benzodiazepines (eg, midazolam, lorazepam) have traditionally been used to manage delirium but have side effects that can be problematic. To ensure accurate trending of delirium, a standardized assessment tool such as the Confusion Assessment Method for the ICU is recommended to adequately assess delirium.[91] Evidence-based strategies to minimize and shorten the duration of delirium should be used.

Metabolic Derangement

Treatments for metabolic derangements, skin problems, anemia, and hemorrhage should be tempered with concerns for the patient's comfort. Only interventions promoting comfort should be performed. Patients do not necessarily feel better "when the laboratory values are right."

Near-Death Awareness

Two hospice nurses originally described the phenomenon of near-death awareness.[92] The same behaviors may be seen in conscious patients near death in the critical care unit. Having an awareness of the phenomenon enables more careful assessment of behaviors that may be interpreted as delirium, acid-base imbalance, or other metabolic derangements. These behaviors include communicating with someone who is not alive, preparing for travel, describing a place they can see, or even knowing when death will occur. Family members may find these behaviors disturbing but find comfort in understanding the phenomenon and in sharing these experiences with their loved one.

WITHDRAWAL OF MECHANICAL VENTILATION

A dramatic geographic variation exists in practices surrounding withdrawal of life-sustaining therapies. Some evidence suggests that this variation may be driven more by physicians' attitudes and biases than by factors such as patients' preferences or cultural differences. This inconsistency in care further complicates a difficult process. From clinical, ethical, and legal perspectives, standardized withdrawal from life-support order sets are recommended to direct and support nursing judgment in this complex and emotional clinical situation.

At the heart of the difficulty of conversations about withdrawal of life support is the pattern and selection of language to address the decision. Selph et al[93] taped end-of-life conversations between families and physicians and found that at least one supportive statement was provided 66% of the time during the discussion. In another study, 86% of nurses reported that they were involved in discussions of withdrawal of life-sustaining treatments and influenced the types of withdrawal interventions.[94] Recommendations for creating a supportive atmosphere during withdrawal discussions included the following:

- Taking a moment at the beginning of the conversation to inquire about the family's emotional state
- Acknowledging verbal and nonverbal expressions of emotion and using that to support families
- Acknowledging that most family members face a significant emotional burden when a loved one is critically ill or dying

During the family meeting in which a decision to withdraw life support is made, a time to initiate withdrawal is usually established. For example, a distant family member may need to arrive, and then the procedure will occur. When appropriate, the patient should be moved to a separate or special room. It is helpful if other staff members are alerted to the fact that a withdrawal is occurring. A neutral sign hung on the door or use of a special room may caution staff to avoid loud conversations and laughter, which is quite upsetting to grieving families. Nurses can support the family by suggesting specific measures to modify the environment and minimize symptoms that the family might perceive as suffering of their loved one.[95]

After the decision to remove ventilatory support is made and the family is gathered, the family should be told what the impending death will be like. When the patient is dependent on ventilatory support or vasopressors and that support is removed, death typically follows in minutes. The patient appears as if sleeping, and the usual signs of color and skin temperature changes will not be seen before death. The opposite is true if the patient is not ventilator dependent. When the patient is to be extubated at the beginning of the withdrawal process, the family should be prepared for respiratory noises and gasping respirations. These signs are less likely when the endotracheal tube is removed near the end of the withdrawal process, as is more commonly done. When assessing how prepared family members felt for what would happen during withdrawal of life support, Kirchhoff et al[95] found that families who did not receive preparatory information before the withdrawal of life support requested this information during interviews 2 to 4 weeks after the patient's death. Family members who received this recommended information reported they felt significantly more prepared. Providing information to families for the experience of withdrawal alerts them to what the patient may exhibit as death approaches, reducing the distress families may feel during the withdrawal process.

Pacemakers or implantable cardioverter-defibrillators should be turned off to prevent patient distress from their firing[96] and to avoid interfering with the pronouncement of death. Wiegand and Kalowes[74] provide detailed information about the conversations that should be held with the patient and how each of the specific devices are deactivated. Neuromuscular blocking agents should be discontinued before removal of ventilator support because paralysis precludes the assessment of the patient's discomfort and the means of the patient to communicate with loved ones.[86]

The removal of monitors is usually recommended. However, physicians and nurses may use the monitor to assess the distress of the patient during the withdrawal process and to adjust the amount of medication needed for symptom management. Families may glance at the monitor to verify that electrical activity has ceased because the appearance of death may be too subtle to detect. If not needed, monitors should be removed to make the room appear as normal as possible.

Sedation During Withdrawal of Life Support

Opioids and benzodiazepines are the most commonly administered medications because dyspnea and anxiety are the usual symptoms related to ventilator withdrawal. Campbell[97] stated that brain-dead patients do not require sedation and that patients with brainstem activity only may not show signs of distress or need sedation. von Gunten and Weissman[98] recommend sedating all patients, even patients who are comatose. Recommended dosing is a bolus intravenous dose of morphine (2 to 10 mg) and a continuous morphine infusion at 50% of the bolus dose per hour. An intravenous dose of midazolam (1 to 2 mg) is administered followed by an infusion at 1 mg/h.[98] The intent is to provide good symptom control, so doses accelerate until the patient's comfort is achieved. Additional medication should be available at the bedside for immediate administration if discomfort is observed in the patient. In one study, the use of opioids or benzodiazepines to treat discomfort after the withdrawal of life support did not hasten death in critically ill patients.[99] A standardized withdrawal order set with titration parameters minimizes variation and subjectivity among the physician's orders and the nurse's implementation of the orders.

Ventilator Settings

After the patient's comfort is achieved, ventilator settings are reduced. An experienced physician, a respiratory therapist, and a nurse should be present during this time. Ventilator alarms should be turned off. The method of withdrawal adopted is usually determined by the clinician's preference. The choice of terminal wean as opposed to extubation is based on considerations of access for suctioning, appearance of the patient for the family, how long the patient will survive off the ventilator, and whether the patient has the ability to communicate with loved ones at the bedside.

If terminal wean is used, positive end-expiratory pressure is reduced to normal, and then the mode is set to patient control. Next, the fraction of inspired oxygen is reduced to 0.21 (21%).

All these steps are taken slowly while observing the patient for distress or anxiety. If extubation is performed immediately rather than at the end of the terminal wean, the family should be prepared for airway compromise and the appearance of the patient.

All patients do not require the same ventilator weaning or extubation protocols. For example, Campbell[97] recommended turning off the ventilator and extubating patients who are brain dead, placing patients who have brainstem-only injuries on a T-piece, and using terminal weaning for patients with altered consciousness or who are conscious. The terminal wean offers the most control over secretions, respiratory noises, and gasping.

Terminal extubation of alert patients can be difficult, as there is uncertainty about the amount and type of medications to provide. Billings[100] outlined the issues surrounding the terminal extubation procedure. Patients indicating the desire to remove life support retain the need for comfort medications to control dyspnea and secretions until death. Some health care providers may believe this is a moral "gray area" and relate the process to assisted suicide. However, patients with decisional capacity may elect to discontinue life support, which has been supported by court decisions and bioethical opinion.

PROFESSIONAL ISSUES

Health Care Settings

Professional issues surround the provision of end-of-life and palliative care within traditional acute and clinical settings. In critical care units, care may be managed by an intensivist or by a committee of specialists, but seldom by the family physician who knows the patient. The use of consultants may be limited. Palliative care specialists may be available at certain times, but they are often considered "outsiders," although the trend to use this specialty service is increasing with the availability of programs in US hospitals. How the consultation is arranged may vary by institution. Turf issues should not compromise patient care. Having a clear plan for withdrawal and better preparation of the family may assist the professionals involved in feeling more comfortable with the care provided.[101] Expert nurses should advocate for vulnerable patients by communicating the patient's wishes and presenting a realistic picture to family members.[102]

Some interventions have been found to be helpful for health professionals in improving patient care. Although it did not improve nurses' assessment of patients' dying experience, a standardized order form for withdrawal was found to increase the amount of medications nurses administered for sedation.[103]

Emotional Support for the Nurse

Nurses who care for dying patients need to have their work valued as highly as other high-tech functions in the critical care unit. Critical care units usually have several nurses who are looked to by other staff to provide end-of-life care or to assist with withdrawal of life support. When several deaths occur close together, those nurses may be called on frequently. Some consideration in assignment should be given when a nurse has more than one death in a shift or a week. Taking a new admission is also difficult immediately after a death, and it can occur before the family has left the unit. Nurse administrators can provide some additional resources, debriefing, or time off when the burden has been high. Hearing supportive words from colleagues has been reported by critical care nurses as helpful in coping with the death of a patient.[104]

This issue is a serious one for critical care nurses because emotional and ethical distress can lead to burnout. Meltzer and Huckabay[105] found that the score on the emotional exhaustion subscale of the Maslach Burnout Inventory and the score on the frequency subscale on the Moral Distress Scale correlated for a group of 60 critical care nurses. Often, critical care nurses experience moral distress because of the severity of patients' illnesses as well as the requirement of technology to maintain vital organ function. Collaborative strategies for minimizing moral distress rely on the bedside nurse and critical care leadership to implement individual and organizational changes.[106]

Nurses experience moral distress when aggressive care is offered to patients who are not expected to benefit from it. These levels of distress are high and have implications for retention of highly skilled nurses.[107] One study showed that nurses' experience of moral distress and a negative ethical environment is more severe than that of their physician colleagues.[108] Developing a consensus about care was found to be the most helpful approach.[109] Nurses in this study had many suggestions when questioned about what could be done to improve end-of-life care, such as facilitating dying with dignity, having someone with patients who are dying, managing patients' symptoms, knowing and then following patients' wishes for end-of-life care, and promoting earlier cessation of treatment or not initiating aggressive treatment at all.

Until more recently, end-of-life content in nursing school curricula and textbooks was sparse, and continuing education was limited on this topic. ELNEC was created in 2000 to address gaps in education for nurses caring for dying patients.[52] Based on national reports, guidelines, recommendations, and research studies, ELNEC has grown into the premier source of end-of-life training for nurses all over the world. The Critical Care ELNEC course became available in 2006 and addressed topics focused on the critical care unit setting.

ORGAN DONATION

Legal Issues

The Social Security Act Section 1138 requires that hospitals have written protocols for the identification of potential organ donors.[110] The Joint Commission has a standard on organ donation, and legislation at state levels directs health care providers and organ recovery agencies.[111] Although an impending death marks a difficult time for family members, the nurse must notify the organ procurement official to approach the family with a donation request. These individuals have training to make a supportive request and are the ones to decide whether a family should not be approached based on the patient's disease. Organ donation may be appropriate in some cases, tissue donation remains a consideration. More information is available in Chapter 36.

Brain Death

Death may be pronounced when the patient meets a list of neurologic criteria. However, there are differences among hospital policies for certification of brain death, which may permit differences in the circumstances under which patients are pronounced dead in different US hospitals.[112] Families do not always understand the meaning of brain death, and they are less likely to donate organs when they believe the patient

will not be dead until the ventilator is turned off and the heart stops.[113] How these conversations are held will determine families' understanding and positively affect donation. Campbell[35] recommended not suggesting that the organs are alive while the brain is dead, but rather that the organs are functioning as a result of the machines used. Chapter 36 provides more information on the specifics of brain death.

FAMILY CARE

In this chapter, the term *family* means whatever the patient states is the family. An integral part of the patient-family dyad, families expect a cure for any condition the patient may have; they do not expect to receive bad news. They look for the good news in any message received from caregivers and are surprised when told that death is the only outcome possible.[95] Families need assistance in forming their expectations about outcomes. Ongoing communication about the patient's progress is preferable to waiting until the patient is near death and then communicating with the family. Most studies of families at this time are descriptive, and interventions need to be developed to help them.[114]

One intervention used with families at the end of life is a grieving or comfort cart. In one critical care unit,[115] the cart has a top drawer with English and Spanish versions of the Bible, Koran, and Book of Mormon and pamphlets about grief and bereavement. The lower portion of the cart holds paper cups, napkins, and condiments. Fresh coffee and tea are brewed on the unit and served with muffins and cookies from the cafeteria. Family responses have been positive because they do not want to leave the bedside despite their hunger. Another strategy is to provide nursing units with supplies including religious items and music to support the emotional and spiritual needs of families at the end of life.[116,117]

Waiting for Good News

Patients and families do not come to the critical care unit with the expectation of death. Even patients who have had previous admissions expect to be "saved." Having this in mind while talking to families may assist professionals in interpreting families' responses. Preparing families for changes in the patient as the health condition deteriorates helps them make plans. They need to know if other family members should be called, if someone should spend the night, or if financial arrangements should be changed before an impending death (eg, to enable the widow to have access to funds). Anticipated changes can be described to prepare families. Emotional support and grieving can be facilitated through discussion of the dying patient and their unique qualities and families' memories. Interactive patient education television services provide healing music and videos that help to create a more comfortable environment for families as they wait for the next step in the dying process. Families often play the patient's favorite music or movies. Many services also provide access to the Internet through which family pictures or videos can be accessed. Provision of these services can be beneficial before the patient dies through visiting a shared past, making the most of the present, and hoping for an end to the patient's suffering and healing for loved ones.

Families may refuse to forgo life-supporting treatments and want "everything done" for a variety of reasons. Effective communication throughout the hospitalization and information provided throughout the stay predispose the family to better acceptance of news as the patient deteriorates. Family satisfaction is increased when they feel supported during their decision making[118,119] or hear more empathic statements from physicians.

Families in Crisis

Families may experience a sense of crisis as emergencies occur or as the patient deteriorates and dies. Responses to the news of the death vary. Family members may show anger or be quiet, exhibit emotions or stoicism. Culture or religious beliefs may affect their response to news. It is helpful to ask if family members would like to see a chaplain or a social worker. Quiet and calm, some privacy, and support are always appreciated.

Family Presence During Cardiopulmonary Resuscitation

To be helpful, the family's presence during procedures or resuscitative attempts[39,40] should be coupled with staff support. Critical care nurses and emergency nurses have taken family members to the bedside for resuscitation or invasive procedures, but most did not have written policies for the family's presence.[120] Sometimes these experiences provide opportunities for the family to be supportive of the patient. At other times, the family may become more aware of what is involved in decisions they have made on behalf of the patient. Seeing the steps of resuscitation may make clearer the impact of decisions made or delayed.

Visiting Hours

Visiting in critical care units continues to be restricted[121] despite national calls for increases in patient or family control over the care.[122] Restricting visiting for dying patients in the critical care unit seems to be unconscionable. Providing visiting time to help family members say good-bye is important. Family members may have difficulty in seeing the person they knew among all the tubes. Coaching can be provided about how to approach the patient and about how the patient may still be able to hear despite appearing to be nonresponsive. Visitors should be permitted to the extent possible, while not interfering with other patients' privacy or rest. Children, unless they represent a significant source of infection, should be allowed to say good-bye, but they may need adult assistance in understanding the situation. Families may have religious or cultural ceremonies that are important for them to perform before the patient dies or experiences withdrawal of life support. These practices should be encouraged and facilitated as much as possible. Continuity of care by the same nurse is important, helping with families' closure and healing.

After Death

After the death, the family may wish to spend time at the bedside. Family members' time with the body should be unhurried and private. They need adequate room to sit and spend time. They can be asked if they need assistance or resources and whether they wish to be alone or have someone nearby. Frequently, the bed is needed for another patient, and juggling is required to ensure that the family has sufficient time even as another patient needs to be admitted. Supporting families after a death involves immediate bereavement support, information on what to do about the death, bereavement support for the future, contact with the family after death, and assessment of the quality of care the patient experienced.[123] Having material already prepared with the necessary after-death

information is quite helpful at this time. Most hospices offer bereavement support groups that are available to any member of the community free of charge, regardless of whether a loved one was enrolled in hospice. Nurses need to be aware of their own judgment on what is an appropriate response because individuals respond differently to the same news, even within the same family.

COLLABORATIVE CARE

The ability to provide collaborative, compassionate end-of-life care is the responsibility of all clinicians who work with critically ill patients. Interdisciplinary collaborative efforts are associated with improvement in care.[124] In 2008, the SCCM published a revised guideline, "Recommendations for End-of-Life Care in the Intensive Care Unit," to provide guidance for end-of-life care for the team.[125] The Evidence-Based Practice feature on end-of-life care provides a summary of the topics included (Box 10.3). The Robert Wood Johnson Foundation

---

QSEN BOX 10.3 QSEN: Guideline for End-of-Life Care in the Critical Care Unit

Key topics of the guidelines for end-of-life care in the critical care unit, based on research and expert panel review, are categorized.

Patient-Centered and Family-Centered Care and Decision Making: Comprehensive Ideal for End-of-Life Care
- Use legal standards for decision making
- Resolve conflict
- Communicate with families

Ethical Principles Related to Withdrawal of Life-Sustaining Treatment
- Withholding versus withdrawing
- Killing versus allowing to die
- Intended versus merely foreseen consequences

Practical Aspects of Withdrawing Life-Sustaining Treatments in Critical Care Unit
- Procedure
- Specific issues
- Use of paralytics

Symptom Management in End-of-Life Care
- Pain and dyspnea
- Delirium
- Medications used

Considerations at Time of Death
- Notification of death
- Brain death
- Organ donation
- Bereavement and support
- Needs of interdisciplinary team

Research, Quality Improvement, and Education
- Develop interventions likely to improve quality of care
- Develop education programs

Data from Truog RD, et al. Recommendations for end-of-life care in the intensive care unit: a consensus statement by the American Academy of Critical Care Medicine. *Crit Care Med*. 2008;36(3):953.

Critical Care End-of-Life Peer Workgroup[126] identified seven end-of-life care domains for use in the critical care unit:

1. Patient-centered and family-centered decision making
2. Communication
3. Continuity of care
4. Emotional and practical support
5. Symptom management and comfort care
6. Spiritual support
7. Emotional and organizational support for ICU clinicians

Individuals and groups[127,128] have developed websites for online tools to improve end-of-life care. Critical care unit staff can assess the quality of their care by assessing perceptions of families and staff, auditing documentation,[129] or making observations of care. The same attention should be directed toward improving end-of-life care that is directed toward skills of electrocardiogram interpretation or hemodynamic monitoring.

CASE STUDY 10.1   Patient at the End of Life

Brief Patient History

Mr. C is a 17-year-old, African American boy who was involved in a motor vehicle accident. He sustained a cervical fracture at the level of C2 that transected his spinal column and both vertebral arteries. Rescue breathing was begun in the field by bystanders, and he was intubated by paramedics en route to the hospital. Mr. C's parents state that they want everything possible done and that they have faith that God will heal their son.

Clinical Assessment

Mr. C is admitted to the critical care unit from the emergency department. He is ventilator dependent. His skin is warm and dry. He is unresponsive to verbal or painful stimuli, and there is no physical movement. Mr. C's family remains at the bedside 24 hours each day throughout the week. They converse with Mr. C, speaking about all the things they are going to do when he gets home.

Diagnostic Procedures

Mr. C's vital signs are as follows: blood pressure of 120/72 mm Hg, heart rate of 120 beats/min (sinus tachycardia), no spontaneous respiration, temperature of 97.8°F, and Glasgow Coma Scale score of 3. Computed tomography scan of the head showed a global ischemic infarct involving both ventricles, and electroencephalography revealed no detectable cortical activity.

Medical Diagnosis

Mr. C is diagnosed with brain death.

Questions

1. What major outcomes do you expect to achieve for this patient?
2. What problems or risks must be managed to achieve these outcomes?
3. What interventions must be initiated to monitor, prevent, manage, or eliminate the problems and risks identified?
4. What interventions should be initiated to promote optimal functioning, safety, and well-being of the patient?
5. What possible learning needs do you anticipate for this patient?
6. What cultural and age-related factors may have a bearing on the patient's plan of care?

SUMMARY

- End-of-life care requires knowledge and skill, similar to any other aspect of critical care unit care.
- Patient-centered and family-centered decision making is key.

- Communication skills are enhanced with additional training in end-of-life conversations.
- Family presence during procedures or resuscitative attempts should be coupled with staff support.
- Extended visiting times are needed to help family members say good-bye.
- Proactive control of symptoms is vital for the patient's comfort.

ⓔ Visit the Evolve site for additional study materials.

REFERENCES

1. Peden-McAlpine C, et al. Constructing the story: how nurses work with families regarding withdrawal of aggressive treatment in ICU – A narrative study. *Int J Nurs Stud.* 2015;52(7):1146.
2. Rabow MW, et al. End-of-life care content in 50 textbooks from multiple specialties. *JAMA.* 2000;283(6):771.
3. Kirchhoff KT, et al. Analysis of end-of-life content in critical care nursing textbook. *J Prof Nurs.* 2003;19(6):372.
4. Siegel MD. End of life decision making in the ICU. *Clin Chest Med.* 2009;30:181.
5. Prina LL. Funders' support for palliative and end of life care. *Health Affairs.* 2015;34(2):354.
6. Morrison RS, et al. The growth of palliative care programs in United States hospitals. *J Palliat Med.* 2005;8(6):1127.
7. Morrison RS, et al. Cost savings associated with U.S. hospital palliative care consultation programs. *Arch Intern Med.* 2008;168(16):1783.
8. Medina J, Puntillo K, eds. *AACN Protocols for Practice: palliative Care and End of Life Issues in Critical Care.* Boston: Jones & Bartlett; 2006.
9. AACN. Palliative and End of Life Advocacy Initiative. http://www.aacn.org/wd/practice/content/palliative-and-end-of-life-care.content?menu=practice. Accessed September 27, 2015.
10. National Consensus Project for Quality Palliative Care. Clinical Practice Guidelines for Quality Palliative Care, 2013. http://www.nationalconsensus project.org/. Accessed September 27, 2015.
11. Teno JM, et al. Bereaved family member perceptions of quality of end-of-life care in U.S. regions with high and low usage of intensive care unit care. *J Am Geriatr Soc.* 2005;53(11):1905.
12. Nelson JE, et al. End-of-life care for the critically ill: a national intensive care unit survey. *Crit Care Med.* 2006;34(10):2547.
13. Glavan BJ, et al. Using the medical record to evaluate the quality of end-of-life care in the intensive care unit. *Crit Care Med.* 2008;36(4):1138.
14. Beckstrand RL, et al. Providing a "good death": critical care nurses' suggestions for improving end-of-life care. *Am J Crit Care.* 2006;15(1):38.
15. Mularski RA, et al. Quality of dying in the ICU: ratings by family members. *Chest.* 2005;128(1):280.
16. Curtis JR, Rubenfeld GD, eds. *Managing Death in the Intensive Care Unit: the Transition From Cure to Comfort.* Oxford: Oxford University Press; 2001.
17. White DB, et al. Is dying in an ICU a sign of poor quality end of life care? *Am J Crit Care.* 2013;22(3):263.
18. SUPPORT Investigators. A controlled trial to improve care for seriously ill hospitalized patients. The Study to Understand Prognoses and Preferences for Outcomes and Risks of Treatments (SUPPORT). *JAMA.* 1995;274(20):1591.
19. Field MJ, Cassell CK, eds. *Approaching Death: improving Care at the End of Life.* Washington, DC: National Academy Press; 1997.
20. *Dying in America: Improving Quality and Honoring Individual Preferences Near the End of Life.* ; 2014. http://iom.nationalacademies.org/Activities/Aging/TransformingEndOfLife.aspx. Accessed September 27, 2015.
21. Angus DC, et al. Use of intensive care at the end of life in the United States: an epidemiologic study. *Crit Care Med.* 2004;32(3):638.
22. Department of Health and Human Services. Advance directives and advance care planning: report to Congress, August 2008. http://aspe.hhs.gov/basic-report/advance-directives-and-advance-care-planning-report-congress. Accessed October 4, 2015.

23. Nishimura A, et al. Patients who complete advance directives and what they prefer. *Mayo Clin Proc.* 2007;82(12):1480.

24. Silveria M, Kim S, Langa K. Advance directives and outcomes of surrogate decision making before death. *N Engl J Med.* 2015;362(13):1211.

25. California Legislative Information. AB-2139, Eggman. End of life care: patient notification. California. http://leginfo.legislature.ca.gov/faces/billNavClient.xhtml?bill_id=201320140AB2139. Accessed August 1, 2016.

26. *Center for Ethics in Health Care, Oregon Health Sciences University. History of the POLST paradigm initiative.* ; 2008. http://www.ohsu.edu/xd/education/continuing-education/center-for-ethics/ethics-programs/polst.cfm. Accessed August 1, 2016.

27. Hickman SE, et al. The consistency between treatments provided to nursing facility residents and orders on the Physician Orders for Life Sustaining Treatment form. *J Am Geriatr Soc.* 2011;59(11):2091.

28. Hickman SE, et al. A comparison of methods to communicate treatment preferences in nursing facilities: traditional practices versus the physician orders for life-sustaining treatment program. *J Am Geriatr Soc.* 2010;58(7):1241.

29. Briggs LA, et al. Patient-centered advance care planning in special patient populations: a pilot study. *J Prof Nurs.* 2004;20(1):47.

30. Brinkman-Stoppelenburg A, Rietjens J, van der Heide A. Effects of advance care planning on end of life care: a systematic review. *Palliat Med.* 2014;28(8):1000.

31. Adams H, et al. Integration of Latino/a values into palliative health care: a culture-centered model. *Palliat Support Care.* 2014;12:149.

32. Rubenfeld GD. Principles and practice of withdrawing life-sustaining treatments. *Crit Care Clin.* 2004;20(3):435.

33. Tilden V, et al. Family decision-making to withdraw life-sustaining treatments from hospitalized patients. *Nurs Res.* 2001;50(2):105.

34. Voigt LP, et al. Characteristics and outcomes of ethics consultations in an oncologic intensive care unit. *J Intensive Care Med.* 2014;(1):436.

35. Campbell ML. Forgoing Life-Sustaining Therapy: how to Care for the Patient Who Is Near Death. *Aliso Viejo, CA: AACN.* 1998.

36. Sandroni C, et al. Hospital cardiac arrest: incidence, prognosis, and possible measures to improve survival. *Intensive Care Med.* 2007;33:237.

37. Center to Advance Palliative Care. Fast Fact #179: CPR survival in the hospital setting. https://www.capc.org/fast-facts/179-cpr-survival-hospital-setting/. Accessed October 1, 2015.

38. FitzGerald JD, et al. Functional status among survivors of in-hospital cardiopulmonary resuscitation. SUPPORT investigators study to understand progress and preferences for outcomes and risks of treatment. *Arch Intern Med.* 1997;157(1):72.

39. American Association of Critical-Care Nurses. Family presence during CPR and invasive procedures. http://www.aacn.org/wd/practice/docs/practicealerts/fam-pres-resusc-pa-feb2016ccn-pages.pdf. Accessed August 1, 2016.

40. Emergency Nurses Association. Clinical Practice Guideline: family presence during invasive procedures and resuscitation. https://www.ena.org/practice-research/research/CPG/Documents/FamilyPresence-CPG.pdf. Accessed August 1, 2016.

41. Chang Y, Huang CF, Lin CC. Do-not-resuscitate orders for critically ill patients in intensive care. *Nurs Ethics.* 2010;17(4):445.

42. Park YR, Kim JA, Kim K. Changes in how ICU nurses perceive the DNR decision and their nursing activity after implementing it. *Nurs Ethics.* 2011;18(6):802.

43. Christakis NA, Lamont EB. Extent and determinants of error in doctors' prognoses in terminally ill patients: prospective cohort study. *BMJ.* 2004;320(7233):469.

44. Lau F, et al. A systematic review of prognostic tools for estimating survival time in palliative care. *J Palliat Care.* 2007;23(2):93.

45. Strand K, Flaatten H. Severity scoring in the ICU: a review. *Acta Anaesthesiol Scand.* 2008;52(4):467.

46. Marshall JC, et al. Multiple organ dysfunction score: a reliable descriptor of a complex clinical outcome. *Crit Care Med.* 1995;23(10):1638.

47. White DB, et al. Toward shared decision making at the end of life in intensive care units: opportunities for improvement. *Arch Intern Med.* 2007;167(5):461.

48. Coalition for Compassionate Care of California. Decision guides. http://capolst.org/polst-for-healthcare-providers/. Accessed October 4, 2015.

49. Family Caregiver Alliance. Fact and Tip Sheets. https://www.caregiver.org/fact-sheets. Accessed October 4, 2015.

50. Treece P. Communication in the intensive care unit about the end of life. *Adv Crit Care.* 2007;18(4):406.

51. EPEC. Education in palliative and end of life care. http://www.epec.net/. Accessed October 1, 2015.

52. American Association of Colleges of Nursing. End of Life Nursing Education Consortium (ELNEC). http://www.aacn.nche.edu/elnec. Accessed October 4, 2015.

53. Center to Advance Palliative Care. Palliative Care Leadership Centers. https://www.capc.org/palliative-care-leadership-centers/. Accessed October 4, 2015.

54. White DB, et al. Decisions to limit life-sustaining treatment for critically ill patients who lack both decision-making capacity and surrogate decision-makers. *Crit Care Med.* 2006;4(8):2053.

55. Pope TM. Making medical decisions for patients without surrogates. *N Engl J Med.* 2013;269(21):1976.

56. Sharma RK, Dy SM. Cross-cultural communication and use of the family meeting in palliative care. *Am J Hosp Palliat Med.* 2011;28(6):437.

57. Baker R, et al. Family satisfaction with end-of-life care in seriously ill hospitalized adults. *J Am Geriatr Soc.* 2000;48(Suppl 5):S61.

58. Curtis JR. Communicating about end-of-life care with patients and families in the intensive care unit. *Crit Care Clin.* 2004;20(3):363.

59. Have EC, Nap RE. Mutual agreement between providers in intensive care medicine on patient care after interdisciplinary care rounds. *J Intensive Care Med.* 2013;29(5):292.

60. Curtis JR, et al. The family conference as a focus to improve communication about end-of-life care in the intensive care unit: opportunities for improvement. *Crit Care Med.* 2001;29(Suppl 2):N26.

61. Abbott KH, et al. Families looking back: one year after discussion of withdrawal or withholding of life-sustaining support. *Crit Care Med.* 2001;29(1):197.

62. Keenan SP, et al. Withdrawal of life support: how the family feels, and why. *J Palliat Care.* 2000;16(Suppl):S40.

63. Curtis JR, et al. Missed opportunities during family conferences about end-of-life care in the intensive care unit. *Am J Respir Crit Care Med.* 2005;171(8):844.

64. Hartog CS, et al. End of life care in the intensive care unit: a patient-based questionnaire of intensive care unit staff perception and relatives psychological responses. *Palliat Med.* 2015;29(4):336.

65. Davidson JE, et al. Clinical practice guidelines for support of the family in the patient-centered intensive care unit: American College of Critical Care Task Force 2004-2005. *Crit Care Med.* 2007;35(2):605.

66. Clarke EB, et al. Quality indicators for end-of-life care in the intensive care unit. *Crit Care Med.* 2003;31(9):2255.

67. Kirchhoff KT, Faas AI. Family support at end of life. *AACN Adv Crit Care.* 2007;18(4):426.

68. Degenholtz HB, et al. Race and the intensive care unit: disparities and preferences for end-of-life care. *Crit Care Med.* 2003;31(Suppl 5):S373.

69. Lipson JG, et al. *Culture and Nursing Care: A Pocket Guide.* San Francisco: UCSF Nursing Press; 1996.

70. Wall RJ, et al. Spiritual care of families in the intensive care unit. *Crit Care Med.* 2007;35(4):1084.

71. Crawley LM. Racial, cultural, and ethnic factors influencing end-of-life care. *J Palliat Med.* 2005;8(Suppl 1):S58.

72. Campbell ML, Guzman JA. Impact of a proactive approach to improve end-of-life care in a medical ICU. *Chest.* 2003;123(1):266.

73. Norton SA, et al. Proactive palliative care in the medical intensive care unit: effects on length of stay for selected high-risk patients. *Crit Care Med.* 2007;35(6):1530.

74. Wiegand DL, Kalowes PG. Withdrawal of cardiac medications and devices. *AACN Adv Crit Care.* 2007;18(4):415.

75. Frick S, et al. Medical futility: predicting outcome of intensive care unit patients by nurses and doctors-a prospective comparative study. *Crit Care Med.* 2003;31(2):456.

76. Broom A, et al. Negotiating futility, managing emotions: nursing the transition to palliative care. *Qual Health Res*. 2015;25(3):299.
77. Truog RD, et al. Recommendations for end of life care in the intensive care unit: a consensus statement by the American College of Critical Care Medicine. *Crit Care Med*. 2008;36(30):953.
78. National Hospice and Palliative Care Organization. HPNA Position Statement: artificial nutrition and hydration in advanced illness. http://hpna.advancingexpertcare.org/wp-content/uploads/2015/08/Artificial-Nutrition-and-Hydration-in-Advanced-Illness.pdf. Accessed October 4, 2015.
79. Center to Advance Palliative Care. Palliative care programs continue rapid growth in U.S. hospitals becoming standard practice throughout the country. http://www.capc.org/news-and-events/releases/analysis-of-us-hospital-palliative-care-programs-2010-snapshot.pdf/file_view. Accessed March 4, 2012.
80. Center to Advance Palliative Care. The IPAL Project. https://www.capc.org/ipal/. Accessed October 1, 2015.
81. National Consensus Project for Quality Palliative Care. Clinical Practice Guidelines for Quality Palliative Care. http://www.nationalconsensusproject.org/Guidelines_Download2.aspx; 2013 Accessed October 4, 2015.
82. Center to Advance Palliative Care. Fast Facts and Concepts. https://www.capc.org/fast-facts/. Accessed October 4, 2015.
83. *Institute of Medicine. Improving Palliative Care for Cancer: summary and Recommendations*. Washington, DC: National Academy Press; 2001.
84. Kalowes P. *Symptom Burden at the End of Life in Patients With Terminal and Life Threatening Illness in Intensive Care Units. Doctoral dissertation*. San Diego: University of San Diego; 2007.
85. Mularski RA. Pain management in the intensive care unit. *Crit Care Clin*. 2004;20(3):381.
86. Weissman C. Sedation and neuromuscular blockade in the ICU. *Chest*. 2005;128(2):477.
87. Gélinas C, et al. Pain assessment and management in critically ill intubated patients: a retrospective study. *Am J Crit Care*. 2004;13(2):126.
88. Jacobi J, et al. Clinical practice guidelines for the sustained use of sedatives and analgesics in the critically ill adult. *Crit Care Med*. 2002;30(1):119.
89. Ben-Aharon I, et al. Interventions for alleviating cancer-related dyspnea: a systematic review and meta-analysis. *Acta Oncol*. 2012;51(8):996.
90. Fabbro ED, et al. Symptom control in palliative care, part III: dyspnea and delirium. *J Palliat Med*. 2006;9(2):422.
91. Vanderbilt University Medical Center. Confusion Assessment Method for the ICU (CAM-ICU): the Complete Training Manual. http://www.icudelirium.org/docs/CAM_ICU_training.pdf. Accessed October 1, 2015.
92. Callanan M, Kelley P. *Final Gifts: Understanding the Special Awareness, Needs, and Communications of the Dying*. New York: Bantam Books; 1997.
93. Selph RB, et al. Empathy and life support decisions. *J Gen Intern Med*. 2008;23(9):1311.
94. Kirchoff K, Kowalkowski J. Current practices for withdrawal of life support in intensive care units. *Am J Crit Care*. 2010;19(6):532.
95. Kirchhoff KT, et al. Preparing ICU families for withdrawal of life support: a pilot study. *Am J Crit Care*. 2008;17(2):113.
96. Goldstein NE, et al. Management of implantable cardioverter defibrillators in end-of-life care. *Ann Intern Med*. 2004;141(11):835.
97. Campbell ML. How to withdraw mechanical ventilation: a systematic review of the literature. *AACN Adv Crit Care*. 2007;18(4):397.
98. von Gunten C, Weissman DE. Symptom Control For Ventilator Withdrawal In The Dying Patient. Fast Facts And Concepts #34. http://www.mypcnow.org/fast-fact-index. Accessed August 1, 2016.
99. Chan JD, et al. Narcotic and benzodiazepine use after withdrawal of life support: association with time to death? *Chest*. 2004;126(1):286.
100. Billings A. Terminal extubation of the alert patient. *J Palliat Care*. 2011;14(7):800.
101. Rocker GM, et al. Canadian nurses' and respiratory therapists' perspectives on withdrawal of life support in the intensive care unit. *J Crit Care*. 2005;20(1):59.
102. Robichaux CM, Clark AP. Practice of expert critical care nurses in situations of prognostic conflict at the end of life. *Am J Crit Care*. 2006;15(5):480.
103. Treece PD, et al. Evaluation of a standardized order form for the withdrawal of life support in the intensive care unit. *Crit Care Med*. 2004;32(5):1141.
104. Kirchhoff KT, et al. Intensive care nurses' experiences with end-of-life care. *Am J Crit Care*. 2000;9(1):36.
105. Meltzer LS, Huckabay LM. Critical care nurses' perceptions of futile care and its effect on burnout. *Am J Crit Care*. 2004;13(3):202.
106. AACN. Position Statement on Moral Distress. http://www.aacn.org/WD/Practice/Docs/Moral_Distress.pdf. Accessed March 26, 2012.
107. Elpern EH, et al. Moral distress of staff nurses in a medical intensive care unit. *Am J Crit Care*. 2005;14(6):523.
108. Hamric AB, Blackhall LJ. Nurse-physician perspectives on the care of dying patients in intensive care units: collaboration, moral distress, and ethical climate. *Crit Care Med*. 2007;35(2):422.
109. Badger JM. Factors that enable or complicate end-of-life transitions in critical care. *Am J Crit Care*. 2005;14(6):513.
110. Social Security Administration. Hospital protocols for organ procurement and standards for organ procurement agencies, 2004: compilation of the Social Security laws. http://www.ssa.gov/OP_Home/ssact/title11/1138.htm; Accessed January 1, 2009.
111. The Joint Commission. Approved: revisions to Standard LD.3.1.10, Element of Performance 12, for critical access hospitals and hospitals. *Jt Comm Perspect*. 2007;27(6):14.
112. Powner DJ, et al. Variability among hospital policies for determining brain death in adults. *Crit Care Med*. 2004;32(6):1284.
113. Siminoff LA, et al. Families' understanding of brain death. *Prog Transplant*. 2003;13(3):218.
114. Wiegand DL. Families and withdrawal of life-sustaining therapy: state of the science. *J Fam Nurs*. 2006;12(2):165.
115. Whitmer M, et al. Caring in the curing environment. *J Hosp Palliat Nurs*. 2007;9(6):329.
116. Davidson J. Family-centered care: meeting the needs of patients' families and helping families adapt to critical illness. *Crit Care Nurse*. 2009;29(3):28.
117. Davidson J. Gap analysis of cultural and religious needs of hospitalized patients. *Crit Care Nurs Q*. 2008;31(2):119.
118. Gries CJ, et al. Family member satisfaction with end-of-life decision making in the ICU. *Chest*. 2008;133(3):704.
119. Stapleton RD, et al. Clinician statements and family satisfaction with family conferences in the intensive care unit. *Crit Care Med*. 2006;34(6):1679.
120. MacLean SL, et al. Family presence during cardiopulmonary resuscitation and invasive procedures: practices of critical care and emergency nurses. *Am J Crit Care*. 2003;12(3):246.
121. Kirchhoff KT, Dahl N. American Association of Critical-Care Nurses' national survey of facilities and units providing critical care. *Am J Crit Care*. 2006;15(1):13.
122. Berwick DM, Kotagal M. Restricted visiting hours in ICUs: time to change. *JAMA*. 2004;292(6):736.
123. Shannon S. Helping families cope with death in the ICU. In: Curtis JR, Rubenfeld GD, eds. *Managing Death in the Intensive Care Unit: the Transition from Cure to Comfort*. Oxford: Oxford University Press; 2001.
124. Baggs JG, et al. The dying patient in the ICU: role of the interdisciplinary team. *Crit Care Clin*. 2004;20(3):525.
125. Truog RD, et al. Recommendations for end-of-life care in the intensive care unit: a consensus statement by the American Academy of Critical Care Medicine. *Crit Care Med*. 2008;36(3):953.
126. Mularski RA. Proposed quality measures for palliative care in the critically ill: a consensus from the Robert Wood Johnson Foundation Critical Care Workgroup. *Crit Care Med*. 2006;34(11):S404.
127. Curtis JR. End of life care research program. http://depts.washington.edu/eolcare/currentprojects. Accessed April 14, 2012.
128. Promoting Excellence in End-of-Life Care. Innovative models and approaches for palliative care. http://www.promotingexcellence.org. Accessed March 15, 2012.
129. Kirchhoff KT, et al. Documentation on withdrawal of life support in adult patients in the intensive care unit. *Am J Crit Care*. 2004;13(4):328.

Cardiovascular Anatomy and Physiology

Mary E. Lough

ANATOMY

Discussion of the anatomy of the heart and blood vessels in this text begins on a macroscopic level with a description of the major structures and then progresses to the cellular and molecular levels for each structure.

Macroscopic Structure
Structures of the Heart

The thoracic case protects the heart, lungs, and great vessels. The heart is situated in the anterior thoracic cavity, just behind the sternum and above the diaphragm (Fig. 11.1A). Several important structures, including the esophagus, aorta, vena cava, and vertebral column, are located behind the heart. The position of the heart within the chest cavity is such that the chambers normally described as "right" and "left" are anterior and posterior. The right ventricle constitutes most of the anterior surface (closest to the chest wall) and the inferior surface (directly above the diaphragm). The left ventricle makes up the anterolateral (front and side) and posterior surfaces. The base of the heart is superior and includes the superior portion of the heart and the origin of the aorta, the vena cava, and the pulmonary arteries. The apex of the heart is inferior situated just above the diaphragm. A lateral view of the heart is shown in Fig. 11.1B. The increasing use of thoracic computed tomography in critical care has highlighted the anatomic inaccuracy of the terms *right ventricle* and *left ventricle* because these terms do not relate to the position of the heart in the chest when described in the standard anatomic position (ie, upright and facing the observer).[1]

Size and Weight of the Heart

Generally, the size of an individual's heart is about the size of that person's clenched fist. In an adult, this averages 12 cm in length and 8 to 9 cm in breadth at the broadest part. The weight of the normal heart averages 310 g in men and 255 g in women. No significant differences exist in ventricular wall thickness between men and women. Body weight is a better predictor of healthy heart weight than body surface area or height. Pathologic conditions such as hypertension increase the weight of the heart muscle because of ventricular hypertrophy.

Layers of the Heart

The four distinct layers of the heart are (1) the pericardium, (2) the epicardium, (3) the myocardium, and (4) the endocardium.

Pericardium. The heart and the origins of the great vessels are surrounded and enclosed by an outer covering known as the *pericardium.* The outermost *fibrous pericardium* is a thick envelope that is tough and inelastic. Ligaments anchor the outer pericardium to the diaphragm and the great vessels such that the heart is maintained in a fixed position within the thoracic cavity. The pericardium also provides a physical barrier to infection. Inside the fibrous layer is an inner, double-walled membrane described as the *serous pericardium.* The two layers are labeled "parietal" and "visceral." The *parietal pericardium* adheres to the tough, outer pericardium. The *visceral pericardium* is flexible, adheres directly to the heart, and folds with the surface contours of the heart. The *pericardial cavity* is the potential space between the visceral and parietal layers. The space between these two layers normally contains a small amount of pericardial fluid, which is secreted, resorbed, and serves as a lubricant between the layers so that the heart can beat and move without friction.[2] Pericardial fluid is produced as a plasma ultrafiltrate and is drained by the lymphatic system.[2] The fibrous, outer pericardial sac is noncompliant and unable to adapt to rapid increases in pericardial fluid volume and pressure. Inflammation of the sac is described as *pericarditis.*[3] The accumulation of excess fluid is described as a *pericardial effusion.* If the fluid collection in the sac impinges on ventricular filling, ventricular ejection, or coronary artery perfusion, removal of fluid may be necessary by *pericardiocentesis.*[3] The phrenic nerve provides sensory fibers to the pericardium. The pain that accompanies pericardial effusion and cardiac tamponade is sensed via phrenic nerve innervation.

Epicardial fat. In adults, a layer of adipose tissue is typically present beneath the myocardium and the visceral pericardium. This epicardial fat accumulates along the routes of the major coronary arteries and veins and increases the risk of coronary artery disease.[4] Autopsy data indicate that epicardial fat increases until age 20 to 40 years, but thereafter, the quantity does not depend on age. If a person is overweight or obese, usually more epicardial fat is present. Because obesity is endemic in modern society, epicardial fat is receiving more

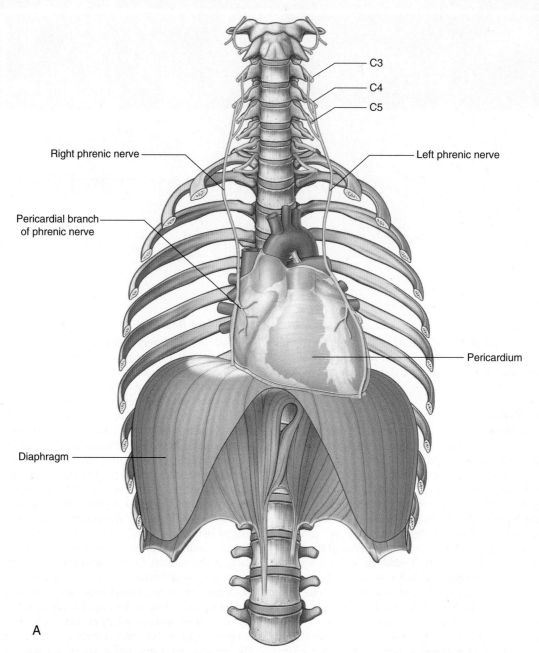

FIG. 11.1 (A) Heart situated on the diaphragm in the thoracic cavity, anterior view. (B) Lateral view of the heart in the thoracic cavity. (From Drake R, Vogl AW, Mitchell AWM. *Gray's Anatomy for Students*. 3rd ed. New York: Churchill Livingstone; 2015.)

attention. Epicardial fat is hypothesized to increase the risk of coronary artery disease because it contains smaller adipocytes compared with other fat deposits, has a different fatty acid composition, and has a higher protein content.[4] This composition facilitates the infiltration of free fatty acids and adipokines into coronary arteries. The fibrous, outer pericardium does not contain any fat deposits.

Epicardium. The epicardium is tightly adhered to the heart and the base of the great vessels as described earlier. The coronary arteries lie on the top of the visceral epicardium.

Myocardium. The next layer of the heart is the myocardium, a thick, muscular layer. This layer includes all of the atrial and ventricular muscle fibers necessary for contraction. The fibers are organized in a spiral formation that directs the force of

contraction toward the outflow tracts in a wringing motion from the apex toward the base. The arrangements of the myocardial fibers are shown in an anterior view of the heart (Fig. 11.2A), a posterior view of the heart (Fig. 11.2B), and a view from the apex of the heart (Fig. 11.2C).

Endocardium. The innermost layer of the heart is the endocardium, which is a thin layer of endothelium and connective tissue lining the inside of the heart. This layer is continuous with the endothelium of the great vessels to provide a continuous closed system. Disruption in the endothelium as a result of surgery, trauma, or congenital abnormality can predispose the endocardium to infection. Infective endocarditis is a devastating disease, which, if left untreated, can lead to massive valve damage or sepsis and death.[5]

FIG. 11.1, cont'd

FIG. 11.2 Layers of the Heart: Pericardium, Endocardium, Myocardium, Pericardium.

Cardiac Chambers

The human heart has four chambers: the right atrium, the right ventricle, the left atrium, and left ventricle. The circulating blood moves through the right side of the heart (right atrium, right ventricle) and through the pulmonary circulation and returns to the left side of the heart (left atrium and left ventricle) (Fig. 11.3).

The atria are thin-walled and normally low-pressure chambers. They function to receive blood from the vena cava and pulmonary arteries and to pump blood into their respective ventricles. Most atrial filling occurs passively from the vena cava and pulmonary veins (80%). Atrial contraction, also known as *atrial kick*, contributes approximately 20% of blood flow to ventricular filling at the end of diastole.

The ventricles are the primary pumping chambers of the heart. The healthy left ventricle is approximately 10 to 13 mm thick, and the interior chamber appears round in cross section. The left ventricular walls are much thicker than the right ventricle or the atria (Fig. 11.4). The right ventricle is approximately 3 mm thick, appears to have a triangular shape when viewed from the side, and has a crescent shape when viewed in cross

section (see Fig. 11.4). The right ventricle pumps blood into the low-pressure pulmonary circulation, which has a normal mean pressure of approximately 15 mm Hg. The left ventricle must generate tremendous force to eject blood into the aorta (normal mean pressure of approximately 100 mm Hg). Because of left ventricular wall thickness and the large force it must generate, the left ventricle is considered the major pump of the heart.

Cardiac Valves

Cardiac valves are composed of flexible, fibrous tissue. A normal valve has the translucent appearance of a rose petal. The valve structure allows blood to flow in only one direction. The opening and closing of the valves depend on the relative pressure gradients on either side of the valve. The four cardiac valves lie in an oblique plane of collagen described as the *fibrous skeleton*. Four adjacent rings of connective tissue contain and support the four cardiac valves (Fig. 11.5).

Mitral and tricuspid valves. The *atrioventricular* (AV) valves are named for their location between the atria and the ventricles. These are the tricuspid valve on the right and the mitral valve on the left. The mitral valve is described as having two leaflets, although the "leaflets" are a continuous tissue structure. The AV valves (mitral and tricuspid) are open during ventricular diastole (filling) (Fig. 11.5A). The *chordae tendineae* and *papillary muscles*, which attach to the tricuspid and mitral valves, provide stability and prevent backflow of blood into the atria during ventricular systole (contraction) (Fig. 11.5B). Papillary muscles arise from the ventricular myocardium and derive their blood supply from the coronary arteries. Each papillary muscle gives rise to approximately 4 to 10 main chordae tendineae, which divide into increasingly finer cords as they approach and attach to the valve leaflets in a variety of patterns.[6] The chordae tendineae are fibrous, avascular structures covered by a thin layer of endocardium (Fig. 11.6).

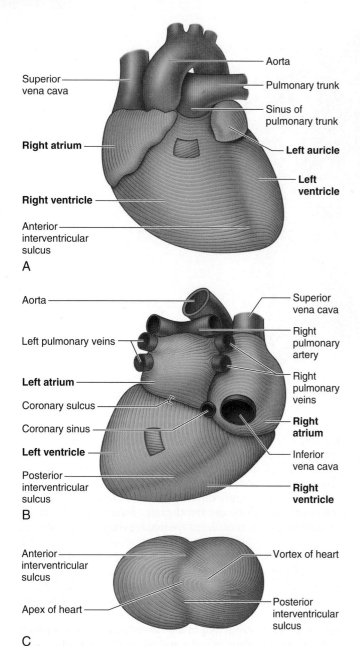

A

B

C

FIG. 11.3 Spiral Arrangement of Cardiac Muscles. (From Paulson F, Waschke J. *Sobotta Atlas of Human Anatomy*. Vol 2. 15th ed. Urban & Fischer; 2013.) (A) Anterior view of the heart showing spiral organization of myocardium. (B) Posterior view of the heart showing spiral organization of myocardium. (C) Spiral arrangement of the heart muscle from the apex.

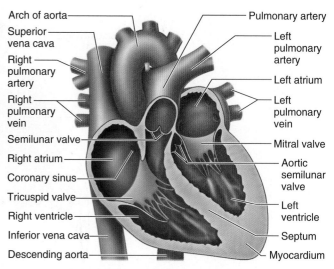

FIG. 11.4 Four chambers of the heart in cross section: Right atrium, right ventricle, left atrium, and left ventricle.

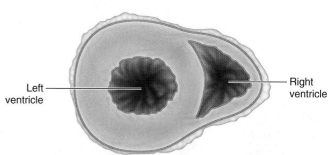

FIG. 11.5 Right and left ventricles in cross section.

Dysfunction of the chordae tendineae or of a papillary muscle may cause incomplete closure of an AV valve, which results in backflow of blood into the atrium. Degenerative disease of the valve leaflets is another cause of regurgitation of blood into the atrium. Valvular stenosis or regurgitation produces a murmur that can be auscultated with a stethoscope (see Chapter 12).

Aortic and pulmonary valves. The *semilunar valves* are names for three cup-like leaflets. The aortic valve (Fig. 11.7), is on the left side of the heart, and the pulmonic valve is on the right. These valves separate the ventricles from their respective outflow arteries (Table 11.1). During ventricular systole (contraction), the semilunar valves open, allowing blood to flow out of the ventricles. As systole ends and the pressure in the outflow arteries exceeds that of the ventricles, the semilunar valves close, preventing blood regurgitation back into the ventricles. In most individuals, the aortic valve has three leaflets. In less than 1% of the population, the aortic valve is bicuspid (two-leaflet valve), which increases susceptibility to aortic valve failure over time. Aortic valve dysfunction, from any cause, not only disrupts the valve leaflets but also pathologically alters the shape of the left ventricle.

Conduction System

To analyze electrical activity within the heart, it is helpful to understand the three main areas of impulse propagation and conduction: (1) the sinoatrial (SA) node; (2) the AV node; and (3) the conduction fibers within the ventricle, specifically the bundle of His, the bundle branches, and the Purkinje fibers (Fig. 11.8).

Sinoatrial node. The SA node is considered the natural pacemaker of the heart because it has the highest degree of automaticity, producing the fastest intrinsic heart rate (HR) (Table 11.2). The node is a spindle-shaped structure located near the entrance of the superior vena cava, on the posterior aspect of the right atrium. Normal variability in the position and shape of the node exists. The SA node is supplied from the right coronary system in approximately 60% of hearts and from the circumflex artery in approximately 40%.[7] The SA node contains two types of cells, the specialized *pacemaker cells*

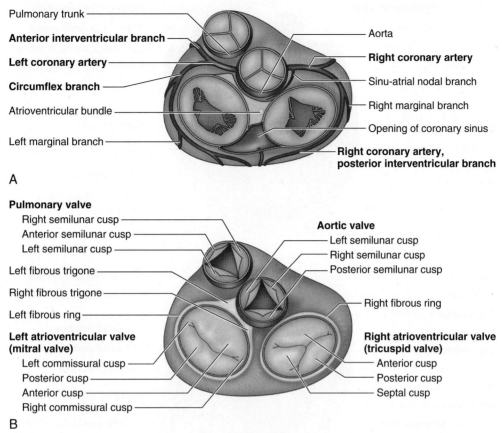

Pulmonary trunk

Anterior interventricular branch

Left coronary artery

Circumflex branch

Atrioventricular bundle

Left marginal branch

Aorta

Right coronary artery

Sinu-atrial nodal branch

Right marginal branch

Opening of coronary sinus

Right coronary artery, posterior interventricular branch

A

Pulmonary valve

Right semilunar cusp

Anterior semilunar cusp

Left semilunar cusp

Left fibrous trigone

Right fibrous trigone

Left fibrous ring

Left atrioventricular valve (mitral valve)

Left commissural cusp

Posterior cusp

Anterior cusp

Right commissural cusp

Aortic valve

Left semilunar cusp

Right semilunar cusp

Posterior semilunar cusp

Right fibrous ring

Right atrioventricular valve (tricuspid valve)

Anterior cusp

Posterior cusp

Septal cusp

B

FIG. 11.6 Heart Valve Movement During Diastole and Systole. (A) Mitral and tricuspid valves are open during diastole. (B) Aortic and pulmonic valves are open during systole.

found in the node center and the border zone cells. Both cell types have inherent pacemaker properties that allow automatic depolarization 60 to 100 times per minute to produce an electrical action potential. The cells in the nodal center are responsible for the pacemaking of the heart, whereas the intrinsic depolarization capability of the fibers in the border zone is depressed by surrounding atrial tissue. Once the center nodal cells depolarize, the impulse is conducted through the border zone via transmural activation toward the AV node.[8] An intraatrial conduction pathway known as *Bachmann's bundle* connects the superior right atrium to the superior left atrium.[9]

Atrioventricular node. The AV node is located posteriorly on the right side of the interatrial septum on the floor of the right atrium in an area known as *Koch's triangle*.[10] The AV node receives its blood supply from the first posterior septal branch of the right coronary artery in most hearts. The circumflex artery supplies the AV node in less than 10% of the population. Because the atria and ventricles are separated by nonconductive tissue, electrical impulses initiated in the atria are conducted to the ventricles only via the AV node. The AV node performs the following four essential functions to support cardiac conduction:

1. The AV node delays the conduction impulse from the atria (0.8 to 1.2 seconds) to provide time for the ventricles to fill during diastole.
2. The AV node controls the number of impulses that are transmitted from the atria to the ventricles. This prevents rapid irregular atrial heart rhythms from destabilizing the ventricular rhythm.

3. The AV node acts as a backup pacemaker if the faster SA node fails. Normally, the intrinsic AV nodal rate is slower than the SA nodal rate (see Table 11.2). When an impulse from the SA node arrives at the AV node, AV nodal tissue becomes depolarized, and the AV nodal pacemaker timing is reset. This prevents the AV node from initiating its own pacemaker impulse that would compete with the SA node.
4. The AV node can conduct retrograde (backward) impulses through the node. If the SA and AV pacemaker cells fail to fire, an electrical impulse may be initiated in the ventricles and conducted backward via the AV node. Retrograde conduction time is usually longer than antegrade (forward) conduction.

Bundle of his, bundle branches, and purkinje fibers. Electrical impulses are conducted in the ventricles through the bundle of His, the bundle branches, and the Purkinje fibers (see Fig. 11.8). These structures run through the subendocardium, down the right side of the interventricular septum. Approximately 12 mm from the AV node, the bundle of His divides into the right and left bundle branches. The right bundle branch continues down the right side of the interventricular septum toward the right apex. The left bundle branch is thicker than the right and takes off from the bundle of His at an almost right angle. It traverses the septum to the subendocardial surface of the left interventricular wall, where it divides into a thin anterior branch and a thick posterior branch. Functionally, when one of the left branches is blocked, it is referred to as a *hemiblock*. All the bundle branches are subject to conduction defects (bundle

Left superior pulmonary vein
Myocardium
Left auricle
Left fibrous ring
Great cardiac vein
Left atrioventricular orifice
Anterior papillary muscle
Chordae tendineae
Serous pericardium, visceral layer (epicardium)
Left ventricle
Apex of heart
A

Right pulmonary veins
Valve of foramen ovale
Left atrium, interatrial septum
Left inferior pulmonary vein
Left fibrous ring
Left atrioventricular valve, posterior cusp
Posterior papillary muscle
Myocardium
Interventricular septum, muscular part
Trabeculae carneae

Aortic bulb
Aortic sinus
Right coronary artery
Pulmonary trunk
Left semilunar cusp
Right auricle
Nodules of semilunar cusps
Right semilunar cusp
Posterior semilunar cusp
Interventricular septum, membranous part
Myocardium
Left ventricle
B

Lunula of semilunar valve
Left coronary artery
Left coronary artery, anterior interventricular branch
Left semilunar cusp
Chordae tendineae
Posterior papillary muscle
Left atrioventricular orifice
Left atrioventricular valve, anterior cusp
Anterior papillary muscle

FIG. 11.7 Mitral and Aortic Valves. (A) Mitral valve separates left atrium and left ventricle. (B) Aortic valve separates left ventricle and aorta

TABLE 11.1 Cardiac Valve Locations

Valve	Type	Situated Between
Tricuspid	Atrioventricular	Right atrium and right ventricle
Pulmonic	Semilunar	Right ventricle and pulmonary artery
Mitral	Atrioventricular	Left atrium and left ventricle
Aortic	Semilunar	Left ventricle and aorta

branch blocks) that give rise to characteristic changes in the 12-lead electrocardiogram.

The right bundle branch and the two divisions of the left bundle branch eventually divide into the Purkinje fibers, which have the fastest conduction velocity of all heart tissue. Purkinje fibers divide many times, terminating in the subendocardial surface of both ventricles. Conduction down the bundles and Purkinje fibers is followed by ventricular muscle depolarization (see Fig. 11.8).

Coronary Blood Supply

The coronary circulation consists of vessels that supply the heart structures with oxygenated blood (coronary arteries) and then return the blood to the general circulation (coronary veins). The right and left coronary arteries arise at the base of

the aorta, immediately above the aortic valve (Fig. 11.9). The coronary arterial openings are called the *coronary ostia* (plural). They traverse outside of the heart, above the epicardium, and in the natural grooves (sulci) between the chambers. To perfuse the thick heart muscle, branches from these main epicardial arteries penetrate deeply into the myocardial wall.

The *right coronary artery* (RCA) serves the right atrium and the right ventricle in most people. The sinus node artery, which supplies the SA node in approximately two-thirds of the population, arises from the RCA. The AV node is supplied via the RCA in 90% of the population. The term *dominant coronary artery* is used to describe the artery that supplies the posterior wall of the left ventricle. In most people, the RCA is dominant, supplying the posterior heart wall.

The *left coronary artery* system has several important branches. The *left main coronary artery* arises from the aortic root. It is a short but important artery that divides into two large arteries, the *left anterior descending* and the *circumflex* arteries, which serve the left atrium and most of the left ventricle (see Fig. 11.9). The left anterior descending artery travels in the sulcus over the anterior intraventricular septum. Septal perforator branches branch off at right angles to provide blood supply to the intraventricular septal muscle.

The coronary arteries are end-arteries; that is, they supply a discrete area of the myocardium. End-arteries are susceptible

1   Sinus node depolarization
    (no ECG signal)

2   Depolarization delay
    in AV node (PQ interval)

P   Atrial depolarization

Q   Depolarization of the
    ventricular septum

R   Depolarization of the distal
    third of the ventricular septum
    (vector in longitudinal cardiac axis)

S   Depolarization of remaining parts
    of the ventricles

ST Complete depolarization of
    ventricles (no potential difference
    = isoelectric)

T   Repolarization of ventricles

FIG. 11.8 Electrical Conduction System of the Heart Related to the Electrocardiogram *(ECG)* Waveform (PQRST). (From Paulson F, Waschke J. *Sobotta Atlas of Human Anatomy.* Vol 2. 15th ed. Urban & Fischer; 2013.)

TABLE 11.2	**Intrinsic Heart Pacemaker Rates**
Location	**Rate (beats/min)**
Sinoatrial node	60–100
Atrioventricular node	40–60
Purkinje fibers	15–40

to obstruction by atherosclerotic plaque or thrombus, which can result in loss of blood flow to the myocardial muscle normally supplied by that artery. Depending on the location of the obstruction, this can be fatal. Blockage of coronary arterial blood flow, especially in the left main coronary artery, usually results in death from massive infarction of the left ventricle. If the blocked artery supplies a smaller section of myocardium, the result may be infarction of a small area of myocardium, but not death. One of the mitigating factors when a coronary artery is partially obstructed or blocked is the extent of the coronary collateral circulation. The collateral circulation represents a rich branching vascular network and is variable among individual hearts. Collaterals are present at birth and become more prominent when a major coronary artery is blocked.[7]

Coronary veins. The coronary veins, which carry deoxygenated blood from the myocardium, are adjacent to the paths of the coronary arteries (Fig. 11.10). A significant difference is that the epicardial coronary veins ultimately join to form a large vein named the *coronary sinus* that travels along the posterior heart

between the sulcus of the left atrium and the left ventricle.[11] The deoxygenated blood flows into the back wall of the right atrium. Coronary venous blood then mixes with the systemic venous blood in the right atrium.

Physiologic cardiac shunts. A physiologic shunt occurs when deoxygenated blood (usually venous blood with reduced oxygen content) mixes with arterial oxygenated blood. In the heart, this is a normal physiologic process. The *thebesian veins* are small vessels that connect the capillary beds directly with the cardiac chambers via irregular endothelium-lined sinuses within the myocardium.[11] The thebesian veins add a small quantity of deoxygenated blood to the oxygenated blood in the left ventricle.

Major Cardiac Vessels
Aorta
The aorta is the largest artery in the body. It carries oxygenated blood from the left ventricle to the rest of the body. The aorta is separated from the left ventricle by the aortic valve. Just above the aortic valve are two small openings that represent the origins of the right and left coronary arterial systems known as the *coronary ostia.*[12]

Pulmonary Artery
The pulmonary artery carries deoxygenated blood from the right ventricle to the pulmonary arterioles. The pulmonary artery is separated from the right ventricle by the pulmonic valve. The main pulmonary artery divides into a right branch

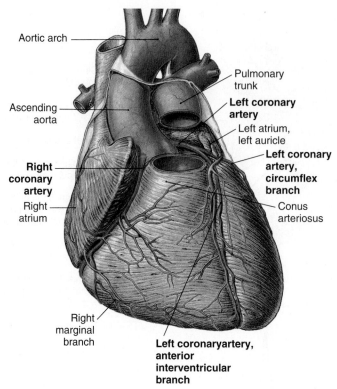

FIG. 11.9 Coronary Arteries; Anterior View of the Heart. (From Paulson F, Waschke J. *Sobotta Atlas of Human Anatomy*. Vol 2. 15th ed. Urban & Fischer; 2013.)

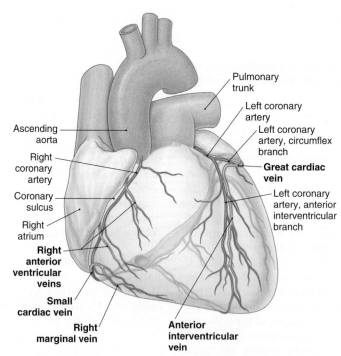

FIG. 11.10 Coronary Veins. Anterior view with posterior veins visible through the heart. (From Paulson F, Waschke J. *Sobotta Atlas of Human Anatomy*. Vol 2. 15th ed. Urban & Fischer; 2013.)

and a left branch, directing blood to the right and the left lung vasculature. The pulmonary artery is the only artery in the body that carries deoxygenated blood.

Pulmonary Veins

The four pulmonary veins return oxygenated blood from the lungs to the left atrium. These are the only veins in the body that carry oxygenated blood. The veins drain from the pulmonary vascular tree into the posterior wall of the left atrium. No valves inhibit the flow of blood into the left atrium. Blood flow is accomplished by simple hydrostatic pressure gradients. The pressure must be lower in the left atrium than in the pulmonary circulation for flow to occur in a forward direction.

Systemic Circulation

If the task of the heart is to generate enough pressure to pump the blood, it is the function of the vascular structures to act as conduits to carry vital oxygen and nutrients to each cell and to carry away waste products. The ability to exchange those nutrients and waste products at the cellular level is of primary importance. The vascular system acts not only as a conducting system for blood but also as a control mechanism for the pressure in the heart and vessels. The complex interplay between the heart and blood vessels maintains adequate pressure and velocity within this system for optimal functioning.

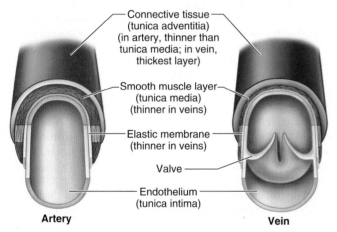

FIG. 11.11 Structure of blood vessels: arteries and veins.

Arterial system. Arteries are constructed of three layers (Fig. 11.11). (1) The *tunica externa*, also known as the *tunica adventitia*, comprises the outermost layer. It is composed largely of a connective tissue coat to provide strength and shape to the vessel. (2) The *tunica media*, or muscular middle layer, is made up of smooth muscle and elastic tissue. The muscular layer changes the lumen diameter as needed. (3) The innermost layer, or *tunica intima*, consists of a thin lining of endothelium and a small amount of elastic tissue. The smooth endothelial lining lowers resistance to the flowing bloodstream, minimizing the opportunity for platelet aggregation.

The intimal and the externa layers remain relatively constant in the vascular system, whereas the elastin and smooth muscle in the media vary in proportion, depending on the size and type of vessel (Fig. 11.12). The aorta contains the greatest amount of elastic tissue. This is necessary because of the sudden shifts in pressure created by the left ventricle. The arterioles, or smaller arteries, and precapillary sphincters have more smooth muscle than the larger arteries and aorta because they function to change the luminal diameter when regulating blood pressure and blood flow to tissues.

Blood flow and blood pressure. The pulsatile nature of arterial flow is caused by intermittent cardiac ejection and the stretch of the ascending aorta. The pressure wave initiated by left ventricular ejection (Fig. 11.13) travels considerably faster than blood itself. When an examiner palpates a pulse, it is the propagation of the pressure wave that is perceived.

In the normal arterial system, blood flow is described as laminar, or streamlined, because the fluid moves in one direction. However, differences exist in the linear velocities within a blood vessel. The layer of blood immediately adjacent to the vessel wall moves relatively slowly because of the friction created as it comes in contact with the motionless vessel wall. In contrast, the more central blood in the lumen travels more rapidly (Fig. 11.14). Clinical implications include conditions in which the vessel wall has an abnormality such as a small clot or plaque deposit. This disruption in the streamlined flow can set up eddy currents that may predispose the area to platelet aggregation and atherosclerosis.

Blood pressure measurement has several components. The *systolic blood pressure* (SBP) represents the ventricular volume ejection and the response of the arterial system to that ejection. The *diastolic blood pressure* (DBP) value indicates the ventricular resting state of the arterial system. The *pulse pressure* is the difference between the SBP and the DBP. The *mean arterial pressure* (MAP) is the mean value of the area under the blood pressure curve (Fig. 11.15).

FIG. 11.12 Blood Vessel Internal Diameter and Wall Thickness: Arteries, Veins, and Capillaries. (From Koeppen BM, Stanton BA. *Berne & Levy Physiology, Updated Edition.* 6th ed. St. Louis: Mosby; 2010.)

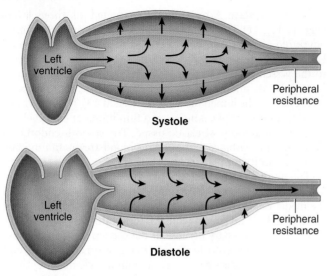

FIG. 11.13 Elastic and Recoil Properties of the Aorta.

FIG. 11.14 Laminar Blood Flow in an Artery.

FIG. 11.15 Arterial, Systolic, Diastolic, Pulse, and Mean Arterial Pressure. (From Berne RM, Levy MN. *Cardiovascular Physiology*. 8th ed. St. Louis: Mosby; 2001.)

Blood pressure may be measured in several ways. Direct measurement is accomplished by means of a catheter inserted into an artery. Blood pressure is measured in millimeters of mercury (mm Hg). The most common indirect method is by means of a stethoscope and sphygmomanometer (Fig. 11.16). Direct measurement is via direct cannulation of an artery as described in Chapter 13.

Vascular resistance is a reflection of arteriolar tone. The large amount of smooth muscle in the arterioles allows for relaxation or contraction of these vessels, which causes changes in the resistance and redistribution of blood flow

(Fig. 11.17). Resistance represents the opposition to flow caused by the blood vessels.

Most changes in resistance are caused by alterations in the tone of the arterial vessel walls, especially in the arterioles. The purpose of this mechanism is to maintain a constant blood pressure in the arterial system. The clinician can never assume that blood flow and blood pressure are identical. For example, poor blood flow to the tissues because of vasoconstricted peripheral arterioles causes the blood to back up and increases the blood pressure. A higher blood pressure is a compensatory mechanism but does not necessarily mean that tissue perfusion is adequate.

It is also possible to calculate the resistance within the systemic vascular system, described by the phrase *systemic vascular resistance*. When it occurs in the pulmonary circulation, it is termed *pulmonary vascular resistance*. These derived values are based on calculations from other hemodynamic parameters, as described in Chapter 13 and Appendix B.

Microcirculation. The *microcirculation* consists of arterioles, arterial capillaries, venous capillaries, and venules (Fig. 11.18). Oxygen, nutrients, hormones, and waste products are exchanged between the bloodstream and adjacent cells. Lymphatic capillaries remove fluid from tissues. The microcirculation has a vital role in the regulation of oxygen supply and demand at the tissue level. The density and anatomy of the microcirculation varies depending on the metabolic needs of each tissue or organ.

Precapillary sphincters are small cuffs of smooth muscle that control blood flow at the junction of the arterioles and the capillaries. The precapillary sphincters are innervated by norepinephrine released from the sympathetic nervous system (SNS) and epinephrine released by the adrenal medulla. They selectively control blood flow into capillary beds.

As blood reaches the capillary level, the pulsatile nature of arterial flow is dampened. Although the diameter of a capillary is less than that of an arteriole, the pressure and flow velocity in the capillary bed is low as a result of the large cross-sectional area of the branching capillary bed. The capillary consists of a single cell layer of endothelium and is devoid of muscle or elastin. This arrangement allows solutes to diffuse in and out of the capillaries unimpeded by mechanical barriers. The capillaries normally retain large structures such as red blood cells but are highly permeable to smaller solutes such as electrolytes.

Venous System

As blood leaves the capillary system, it passes through the venules and into the veins. Venules and veins contain elastic tissue, smooth muscle, and fibrous tissue (see Fig. 11.17). However, the veins contain a greater percentage of smooth muscle and fibrous tissue to accommodate the large venous volume and demand for reserve capacity. Veins are referred to as *capacitance vessels*, and most circulating blood is contained in the venous system (see Fig. 11.17). Approximately 75% of the total blood volume is found in the veins. This enables the body to tap into a large reserve during times of need. For example, when a person changes from a supine position to a sitting position, approximately 7 to 10 mL blood per kilogram of body weight pools in the legs. Potentially, cardiac output could decrease by 20%. However, normal arterial pressure and blood flow are maintained by a combination of reflex vasoconstriction and redistribution of blood from the venous capacitance vessels. In humans, these capacitance reservoirs are greatest in the spleen, liver, and intestines. Patients with decreased blood reserves, who are dehydrated or hypovolemic, require special

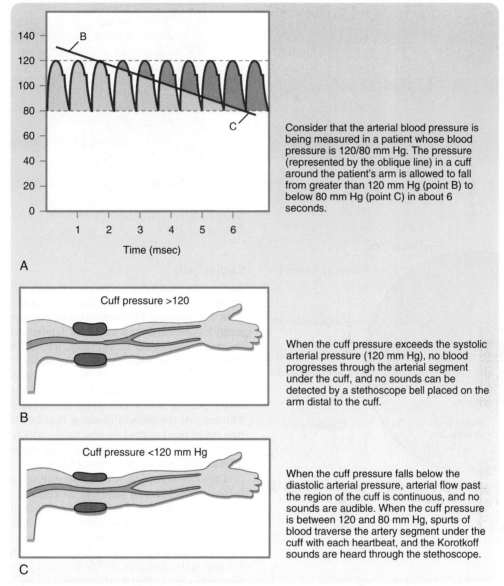

Consider that the arterial blood pressure is being measured in a patient whose blood pressure is 120/80 mm Hg. The pressure (represented by the oblique line) in a cuff around the patient's arm is allowed to fall from greater than 120 mm Hg (point B) to below 80 mm Hg (point C) in about 6 seconds.

Cuff pressure >120

When the cuff pressure exceeds the systolic arterial pressure (120 mm Hg), no blood progresses through the arterial segment under the cuff, and no sounds can be detected by a stethoscope bell placed on the arm distal to the cuff.

Cuff pressure <120 mm Hg

When the cuff pressure falls below the diastolic arterial pressure, arterial flow past the region of the cuff is continuous, and no sounds are audible. When the cuff pressure is between 120 and 80 mm Hg, spurts of blood traverse the artery segment under the cuff with each heartbeat, and the Korotkoff sounds are heard through the stethoscope.

FIG. 11.16 Blood Pressure Measurement With an Arm Cuff and Sphygmomanometer. (A) An example of a blood pressure waveform with a cuff pressure of 120/80 mm Hg. (B) When the arm cuff is inflated to a pressure above the systolic value (120 mm Hg), the artery is occluded and no sounds are audible. (C) When the pressure in the arm cuff is less than the systolic arterial pressure (120 mm Hg in this example) and above the diastolic pressure (80 mm Hg) Korotkoff sounds are audible using a stethoscope or Doppler. (From Koeppen BM, Stanton BA. *Berne & Levy Physiology, Updated Edition.* 6th ed. St. Louis: Mosby; 2010.)

caution during position changes, especially from the supine position to the standing position.

Microscopic Structure

To appreciate the unique pumping ability of the heart, the nurse must understand cardiac cell structure and function. This section reviews the anatomic mechanisms responsible for the contractile process in cardiac muscle cells.

Cardiac Fibers

Cardiac muscle fibers are typically found in a latticework arrangement. The fiber cells (myofibrils) divide, rejoin, and then separate again, but they retain distinct cellular walls and possess a single nucleus (Fig. 11.19).

Individual cardiac muscle cells, known as *myocytes*, are interlaced into a network of cardiac muscle fibers (Fig. 11.20A). Specialized junctional connector complexes called *intercalated disks* assist in propagation of depolarization. The *intercalated disks* are continuous with the *sarcolemma*, or cell membrane, and separate each myocardial cell from its neighbor (Fig. 11.20B). The point at which a longitudinal branch of one cell meets the branch of another is called a *tight junction* (or *gap junction*), which is contained within the intercalated disk. The gap junctions offer much less impedance to electrical flow than the sarcolemma does, so depolarization flows easily from one cell to another. The cardiac muscle is a functional syncytium: Depolarization initiated in any cardiac cell quickly spreads to all of the heart.

FIG. 11.19 Interconnecting Heart Muscle Fibers. (From Hall JE. *Guyton and Hall Textbook of Medical Physiology*. 13th ed. St Louis: Saunders; 2016.)

FIG. 11.17 Blood Pressure (A) and Blood Volume Percentage (B) Across the Cardiovascular System.

Cardiac Cells

Each cardiac cell contains many intracellular proteins that contribute to contraction. Two important contractile proteins are *actin* and *myosin*. These proteins abound in the cell in organized longitudinal arrangements. Under electron microscopy, the myosin filaments appear thick, whereas the actin filaments, which are almost twice as prevalent, appear thin. The actin filaments are connected to a *Z-line* on one end, leaving the other end free to interact with the myosin cross-bridges (Fig. 11.20). In the resting muscle cell, actin and myosin partially overlap. The ends of the myosin filament that overlap with actin have tiny projections named *myosin heads*, which contain a binding site for actin. For contraction to occur, the myosin heads must interact with actin to form cross-bridges.

The *sarcomere* is the functional unit of cardiac contraction. In the normal resting state, the sarcomere is approximately 2 to 2.2 mm long. Each sarcomere consists of a central *A-band* (thick filaments) and two halves of the *I-band* (thin filaments). The I-bands from two adjacent sarcomeres meet at the Z-line (also called a Z-band or Z-disk). The central portion of the A-band is the *M-band*, which does not contain actin. Myosin filaments are situated in the middle of the sarcomere and are attached to the Z-line of the sarcomere by the protein *titan* (Fig. 11.21). The thin filament is composed of the helical chains of the actin globular proteins that coil around a long filament of tropomyosin and three *troponin* proteins: (1) TnT, (2) TnC, and (3) TnI. The troponin complex is attached to actin at regularly spaced intervals.

Another extremely important intracellular structure necessary for successful contraction is the *sarcoplasmic reticulum*. Calcium ions are stored in the sarcoplasmic reticulum and released for use after depolarization (see Fig. 11.21).

Deep invaginations into the sarcomere are called *transverse tubules*, or *T-tubules*. T-tubules are essentially an extension of the cell membrane (sarcolemma); they conduct depolarization to structures deep within the cytoplasm such as the sarcoplasmic reticulum (see Fig. 11.21). Cardiac cells abound with mitochondria, which contain respiratory enzymes necessary for oxidative phosphorylation. This enables these cells to keep up with the tremendous energy requirements of repetitive contraction. When cardiac cells are damaged by trauma, ischemia, or infarction, myocardial cells release protein biomarkers such as troponin, which, when measured by laboratory analysis, can help determine the extent of injury (see Fig. 14.13 in Chapter 14).

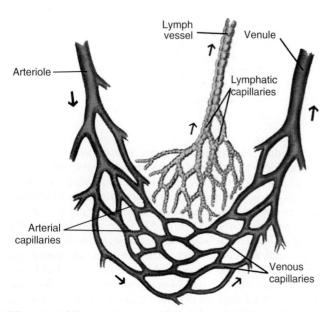

FIG. 11.18 Microcirculation With Branching Cross-Sectional Capillary Bed. (From Thompson JM, et al. *Mosby's Clinical Nursing*. 5th ed. St. Louis: Mosby; 2002.)

A

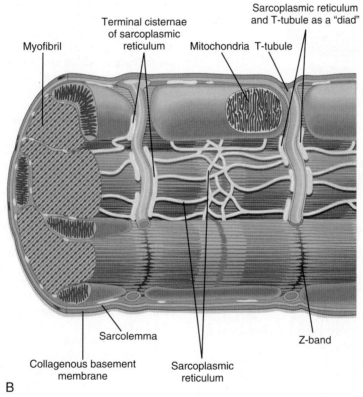

B

FIG. 11.20 (A) Photomicrograph of cardiac muscle cells (B) Sarcomere Within a Heart Muscle Cell Showing Intercalated Disks, Sarcoplasmic Reticulum and T-tubules. (From Koeppen BM, Stanton BA. *Berne & Levy Physiology, Updated Edition.* 6th ed. St. Louis: Mosby; 2010.)

PHYSIOLOGY

The electrical and mechanical properties of cardiac tissue have fascinated scientists for more than 100 years. These properties include excitability, conductivity, automaticity, rhythmicity, contractility, and refractoriness. This section relates these concepts specifically to cardiac cells (Table 11.3).

Electrical Activity

Transmembrane Potentials

Electrical potentials across cell membranes are present in essentially all the cells of the body. Cardiac cells are specialized for conduction of electrical impulses. This *electrical potential*, or *transmembrane potential*, refers to the relative electrical difference between the interior of a cell and the fluid surrounding the cell. *Ionic channels* are pores in cell membranes that allow for passage of specific ions at specific times or in response to specific signals.

Transmembrane potentials and ionic channels are extremely important in myocardial cells because they form the basis for electrical impulse conduction and muscular contraction. Knowledge of the normal structure and function of cardiac ion channels is increasingly important as a basis for understanding the genesis of lethal cardiac dysrhythmias and for the development of cardiac medications designed to treat these channelopathies.

Resting Membrane Potential

In a myocardial cell at rest, the normal resting membrane potential (RMP) is approximately −80 to −90 mV. This means that the interior of the cell is relatively negative compared with the exterior medium. The relative negativity of the cell interior is created by an uneven distribution of positively and negatively charged ions. When the cell is at rest, more positively charged ions are outside the cell than are inside the cell.

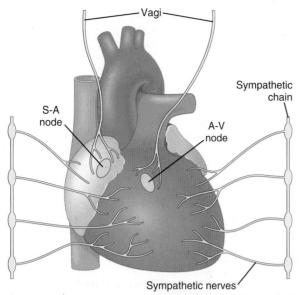

FIG. 11.21 Cardiac Muscle Depolarization and Repolarization. Role of calcium and adenosine triphosphate *(ATP)* in the sarcoplasmic reticulum. (From Hall JE. *Guyton and Hall Textbook of Medical Physiology.* 13th ed. St Louis: Saunders; 2016.)

TABLE 11.3 Heart Tissue Function Definitions

Term	Definition
Excitability	Ability of cell or tissue to depolarize in response to given stimulus
Conductivity	Ability of cardiac cells to transmit a stimulus from cell to cell
Automaticity	Ability of certain cells to spontaneously depolarize ("pacemaker potential")
Rhythmicity	Automaticity generated at regular rate
Contractility	Ability of cardiac myofibrils to shorten in length in response to electrical stimulus (depolarization)
Refractoriness	State of cell or tissue during repolarization, when cell or tissue cannot depolarize regardless of intensity of the stimulus or requires a much greater stimulus than is normally required

When the cell is at rest, the intracellular potassium ion (K^+) concentration is high, and the intracellular sodium ion (Na^+) level is low (Table 11.4). Calcium (Ca^{2+}) has a much higher concentration outside than inside the cell when the cell is at rest. These large differences in individual ion concentrations create chemical gradients. A *chemical gradient* describes the tendency of an ion to move from an area of higher solute concentration to an area of lower concentration. However, an *electrical gradient* is also present, which causes the positively charged ions to move to an area of relative negativity. An important factor influencing both gradients is *membrane permeability*, or the selectivity of the membrane to ionic movements. The cell membrane is approximately 50 times more permeable to K^+ than it is to Na^+. Because K^+ movement out of the cell results in greater negativity inside the cell, K^+ is the principal ion responsible for maintaining the negative RMP.

TABLE 11.4 Electrolyte Values in a Resting Myocardial Cell

	Extracellular Electrolyte Concentration (mEq/L)	Intracellular Electrolyte Concentration (mEq/L)
Potassium (K^+)	4	135
Sodium (Na^+)	145	10
Calcium (Ca^{2+})	2	0.1

Phases of the Action Potential

In a myocardial cell, when a sudden increase in permeability of the membrane to Na^+ occurs, it is followed by a rapid sequence of events that lasts a fraction of a second. This sequence of events is termed *depolarization*. The graphic representation of depolarization and repolarization is termed the *action potential (AP)* (Fig. 11.22). Ionic currents cause changes in electrical potentials, which are known as *AP phases 0, 1, 2, 3, and 4.* These phases give the AP a characteristic shape (Table 11.5; see Fig. 11.22).

Phase 0. The sodium crossing the cell membrane causes the cell to become depolarized and the interior of the cell to become more positive. At approximately −65 mV, the membrane reaches the threshold, the point at which the inward Na^+ current overcomes the efflux of K^+. This is accomplished by means of the fast Na^+ channels. With the fast Na^+ channels open, the inward rush of Na^+ is extremely rapid and briefly causes the inside of the cell to become slightly more positive than the outside of the cell. This series of events is graphically described as *phase 0* of the AP and is reflected in the overshoot of the AP, during which the charge is 20 to 30 mV (Fig. 11.23; see Fig. 11.22).

Phase 1. When the rapid influx of Na^+ is terminated, a brief period of partial repolarization occurs in *phase 1* as the AP slope returns toward zero as potassium leaves the cell (see Figs. 11.22 and 11.23).

Phase 2. The plateau that follows is described as *phase 2.* During this phase, the slow K^+ and Ca^{2+} channels open to allow the influx of Ca^{2+} and efflux of K^+. The Ca^{2+} entering the cell during *phase 2* causes cardiac contraction (see Figs. 11.22 and 11.23).

Phase 3. The repolarization phase is described as *phase 3,* and it depends on two processes. The first is the inactivation of the slow channels, which prevents further influx of Ca^{2+}. The other is the continued efflux of K^+ out of the cell. Both processes cause the intracellular environment to become more negative, reestablishing the RMP. Phase 3 is a gradual descent during which the interior of the cell becomes more negative relative to the outside (see Figs. 11.22 and 11.23).

Phase 4. In *phase 4,* the AP returns to an RMP of −80 to −90 mV. The excess Na^+ that entered the cell during depolarization is removed from the cell in exchange for K^+ by means of the Na^+-K^+ pump. This mechanism returns the intracellular concentrations of Na^+ and K^+ to the levels present before depolarization in preparation for the next depolarization (see Table 11.5, Fig. 11.22, and Fig. 11.23).

Fiber conduction and excitability. Different parts of the conduction system require different electrical currents and create individual transmembrane action potentials. As a local section of the cell becomes depolarized, reaches threshold, and completely depolarizes, it affects the adjacent area of the cell

FIG. 11.22 Cardiac Action Potentials. (A) Action potential phases 0 to 4 of a cardiac nonpacemaker cell. (B) Action potential of a cardiac pacemaker cell. (From Thompson JM, et al. *Mosby's Clinical Nursing.* 5th ed. St. Louis: Mosby; 2002.)

TABLE 11.5	Phases 0 Through 4 of a Cardiac Cell Action Potential		
Phase	**Description**	**Ionic Movement**	**Mechanisms**
0	Upstroke	Na^+ into cell	Fast Na^+ channels open
1	Overshoot	K^+ out of cell	Fast Na^+ channels close
2	Plateau	Ca^{2+} into cell, K^+ out of cell	Multiple channels (Ca^{2+}, Na^+, K^+) open to maintain membrane voltage
3	Repolarization	K^+ out of cell	Ca^{2+} and Na^+ channels close; K^+ channel remains open
4	Resting membrane potential	Na^+ out of cell, K^+ into cell	Na^+-K^+ pump

Ca^{2+}, calcium; K^+, potassium; Na^+, sodium.

and initiates depolarization in that area. The AP propagates down the cardiac fiber in a wave-like fashion (Fig. 11.24). This is analogous to a trail of gunpowder. When the gunpowder is lit at one end, a small area ignites, burns, and then ignites the area of gunpowder immediately adjacent to it and on down the line.

The time from the beginning of the AP until the fiber can accept another AP is called the *effective* or *absolute refractory period*. During this period, the cell cannot be depolarized regardless of the amount or intensity of the stimulus. This period lasts from the beginning of depolarization until the interior of the cell has repolarized to approximately −50 mV during phase 3. The absolute refractory period is immediately followed by the *relative refractory period*. At this time, the cell is not fully repolarized but could depolarize with a strong enough stimulus (Fig. 11.25). This period lasts from approximately −50 mV during phase 3 until the cell returns to RMP (phase 4); at that point, the cell is fully repolarized and is again ready to respond to the next stimulus. The concept of relative versus absolute refractory periods is useful for understanding the genesis of ventricular dysrhythmias (see Chapter 13). In brief, a cell cannot be stimulated to depolarize until it has at least partially recovered from the previous impulse. This is cardioprotective, as it means that an ectopic impulse cannot be propagated during the absolute refractory period.

Mechanical Activity
Excitation-Contraction Coupling
Electrical activity is the stimulus for mechanical contraction. As the myocardial cell is depolarized during phase 2 of the AP, extracellular Ca^{2+} ions enter the cytoplasm through the cell membrane via special Ca^{2+} channels. The entry of Ca^{2+} ions is the trigger for the release of Ca^{2+} stores from the sarcoplasmic reticulum (see Fig. 11.23). The cytoplasmic Ca^{2+} then binds with the regulatory TnC protein to induce a conformational change in TnI; this action induces a conformational change in TnT that moves the tropomyosin away from the myosin-binding site on actin. This permits actin to interact with myosin, releasing *adenosine diphosphate* (ADP) and an inorganic phosphate to provide the energy needed for myosin to slide along the actin molecule and initiate contraction. This mechanism is known as *cross-bridge cycling*. The result is myocardial contraction that spreads throughout the myocardium.

FIG. 11.23 Action Potential With Electrolyte Movement Across the Walls of the Myocardial Pacemaker Cells. (From Koeppen BM, Stanton BA. *Berne & Levy Physiology, Updated Edition.* 6th ed. St. Louis: Mosby; 2010.)

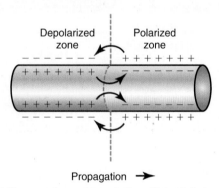

FIG. 11.24 Propagation of an Action Potential Across a Cell Wall.

FIG. 11.25 Refractory Periods. The effective (absolute) refractory period *(ERP)* extends from phase 0 from approximately −50 mV in phase 3. The remainder of the action potential is the relative refractory period *(RRP)*. (From Conover MB. *Understanding Electrocardiography.* 8th ed. St. Louis: Mosby; 2002.)

Once contraction has occurred, intracellular Ca^{2+} levels are lowered by two processes. Most Ca^{2+} is taken back up into the sarcoplasmic reticulum via a Ca^{2+} and magnesium (Mg^{2+})–dependent, adenosine triphosphate (ATP)–based process. In addition, the Na^+-Ca^{2+} exchange system located in the sarcolemma moves Ca^{2+} outside the cell. This decreases the concentration of Ca^{2+} in the cytoplasm, leading to muscular relaxation.

Cardiac Cycle

The term *cardiac cycle* refers to one complete mechanical cycle of the heartbeat, beginning with ventricular contraction and ending with ventricular relaxation (Fig. 11.26).

Atrial Systole

The atria fill by passive filling from the vena cavae (right atrium) and the pulmonary veins (left atrium). During diastole, the mitral and tricuspid valves are open, allowing for passive filling into the ventricles (see Fig. 11.5A). After electrical depolarization of the atria (p-wave), atrial contraction (atrial systole) is initiated, causing additional blood to enter the ventricular chamber. This is also referred to as *atrial kick*. The next action is the closure of the mitral and tricuspid valves.

Isovolumic Contraction

Ventricular depolarization from the QRS electrical stimulus depolarizes the septum and papillary muscles first. The ventricles then begin to tense, starting with the inner endocardium and traversing the myocardium toward the outer epicardium. This increases the pressure within the ventricular chambers. This is known as *isovolumic contraction* because even though the ventricular muscle is contracting, the volume of blood within the ventricles does not change. In Fig. 11.26, this is seen as a rapid increase in left ventricular pressure.

FIG. 11.26 Cardiac Cycle.

Ventricular Systole

Ventricular systole represents the ventricular ejection portion of the cardiac cycle. As ventricular tension increases, intraventricular pressures exceed the pressure in the aorta and pulmonary arteries, causing the aortic and pulmonic valves to open during systole (see Fig. 11.5B). The amount of blood ejected from the ventricles with each beat is called the *stroke volume* (SV). In a healthy heart, more than half of the total ventricular blood volume is ejected; the blood that remains in the ventricles is the *residual* or *end-systolic* volume.

The *ejection fraction* (EF) is the ratio of the SV ejected from the left ventricle per beat to the volume of blood remaining in the left ventricle at the end of diastole (left ventricular end-diastolic volume). EF is expressed as a percentage, and a normal value is 50% or greater. An EF of less than 35% indicates poor ventricular function (as in cardiomyopathy), poor ventricular filling, obstruction to outflow (as in some valve stenosis conditions), or a combination of these conditions.

Isovolumic Relaxation

The next phase is *isovolumic relaxation*, which occurs between the closure of the semilunar (aortic and pulmonic) valves and the opening of the AV (mitral and tricuspid) valves. All four valves are closed, and the pressure within the ventricular chamber falls to below atrial pressure without any change in intraventricular volume. At this point, the mitral and tricuspid valves open.

Ventricular Diastole

After the mitral and tricuspid valves open, most ventricular filling occurs. The next phase is a reduced ventricular filling period, during which blood flows passively from the periphery and the pulmonary vasculature into the ventricles. The last part of ventricular diastolic filling occurs during atrial contraction, also described as *atrial kick*. This provides approximately 20% of total ventricular filling in normal sinus rhythm. With this, the cycle is complete and ready to begin again with atrial systole (see Fig. 11.26).

Interplay of Heart and Vessels: Cardiac Output

Cardiac output (CO) is defined as the volume of blood ejected from the heart in 1 minute. The determinants of CO are HR in beats per minute (beats/min) and stroke volume (SV) in milliliters per beat (mL/beat). The equation is:

$$SV \times HR = CO$$

CO is usually expressed in liters per minute (L/min). Normal CO in adults is approximately 4 to 6 L/min at rest and increases with exercise. CO can be made specific to body size by using the person's height and weight to determine the cardiac index (CI). The CI is equal to CO divided by the individual's body surface area calculated from the height and weight. Body surface area is expressed in square meters (m^2); the normal range is 2.5 to 4.5 L/min per m^2. Changes in SV or HR can change CO. However, all three parameters must be individually assessed as described in the section on hemodynamics in Chapter 13.

For example, for a person with HR of 72 beats/min and SV of 70 mL/beat, the CI would be:

$$72 \text{ beats/min} \times 70 \text{ mL/beat} = 5.04 \text{ L/min}$$

If the HR were to change to 140 beats/min and the SV to 40 mL/beat in this person, the calculation would be:

$$140 \text{ beats/min} \times 40 \text{ mL/beat} = 5.6 \text{ L/min}$$

Although CO is higher, the faster HR would not be an improvement in this situation. The decreased SV in the second instance indicates that cardiac decompensation is imminent. SV as a value is influenced by three primary factors: (1) preload, (2) afterload, and (3) contractility (Fig. 11.27).

Preload

The concept of preload was introduced in the early 1900s when Starling described his findings in an isolated canine heart preparation. Starling found that as he increased the volume infused into a denervated heart, CO increased until it reached a point at which further infusion caused CO to decrease. This has become known as *Starling's law of the heart*, and it is graphically described as the *Starling curve* (Fig. 11.28). It can be described using as a foundation the discussion of the actin and myosin cross-bridges in the myofibril.[13] As the diastolic volume increases, it stretches the actin and myosin in their resting state. As contraction occurs, contractility increases as a result of the increased stretch. However, if the stretch is excessive and causes actin and myosin to be stretched beyond their cross-bridging limits (>2.2 mm), contractility decreases. This is the basis for Starling's curve. With the advent of intensive care units and sophisticated monitoring, this principle has acquired great significance in clinical practice. For example, after MI, the ability of the left ventricle to pump may be impaired. It is desirable to optimize the contractility of the remaining viable heart muscle by "stretching" it with added volume. However, if the intravascular volume exceeds the stretch limit, CO diminishes.

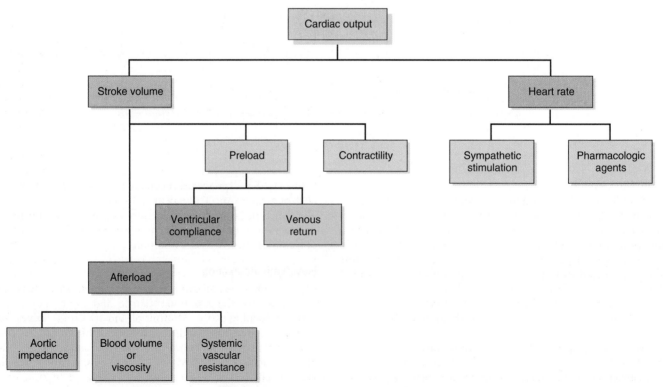

FIG. 11.27 Determinants of Cardiac Output.

Preload is the volume of blood in the left ventricle at the end of diastole. The pressure created by this volume is described as the *left ventricular end-diastolic pressure*. Factors affecting left ventricular preload include venous return to the heart, total blood volume, and atrial kick. Factors affecting the compliance (ability to stretch) of the ventricles are the stiffness and thickness of the muscular wall. One way to measure preload is through *pulmonary artery occlusion pressure*. Clinical application of pulmonary artery occlusion pressure is discussed in Chapter 13.

Afterload

Afterload can be defined as the ventricular wall tension or stress during systolic ejection. It is also described as a component of *systemic vascular resistance*. An increase in afterload usually means an increase in the work of the heart. Afterload is increased by factors that oppose ejection. Examples of increased afterload include aortic impedance (aortic stenosis), septal hypertrophy (obstruction in the outflow tract), vasoconstriction (increased systemic vascular resistance), and hypertension. Therapeutic management to decrease afterload is aimed at decreasing the work of the heart through the use of vasodilators to decrease the myocardial oxygen demand.

Contractility

Contractility refers to the heart's contractile force. It is also known as *inotropy*; this term breaks down to "ino" for strength and "tropy" for enhancing. Contractility can be increased by Starling's mechanism to increase stretch. It also is enhanced by the SNS that innervates the heart (Fig. 11.29) and by pharmacologic agents that mimic the SNS, known as *sympathomimetics* and described in Chapter 15.

Regulation of Heartbeat
Autonomic Nervous System Control

The *autonomic nervous system* (ANS) is composed of two competing neurologic systems of control, the parasympathetic nervous system (PNS) and the SNS.[14] The SNS and PNS operate

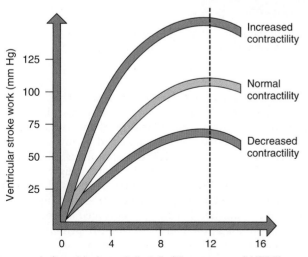

FIG. 11.28 Starling Curve. As the left ventricular end-diastolic pressure *(LVEDP)* increases, so does ventricular stroke work or contractility. When left ventricular filling pressure exceeds a maximal point, contractility and cardiac output diminish.

to create a balance and homeostasis between relaxation and "fight-or-flight" readiness (see Fig. 11.29). The parasympathetic system slows HR during periods of rest, and the sympathetic system increases HR in response to physiologic stress.[15] The effects of the divisions of the ANS on the heart are summarized in Table 11.6.

Parasympathetic fibers are concentrated near the SA and AV conduction tissue and in the atria. Specifically, this involves the right and left vagus nerves. Stimulation of the vagus nerve (parasympathetic nervous system) produces bradycardia as a result of hyperpolarization of phase 4 of the AP, which causes the slope to take longer to reach the threshold. As a consequence, sympathetic tone decreases.[14]

Sympathetic nerve fibers are subepicardial and follow the path of the major coronary arteries (shown in green in Fig. 11.29). Stimulation of sympathetic fibers directly alters ventricular function and increases HR and contractility. HR variability is a normal finding in a healthy heart.[16]

Intrinsic Regulation

Supplementing the ANS control of the heart are several reflexes that serve as feedback mechanisms to the brain. These reflexes maintain even blood flow, oxygenation, and perfusion in response to physiologic needs.

Baroreceptors. *Baroreceptors*, or pressure sensors, are located in the aortic arch and the carotid sinuses (Fig. 11.30). They are more sensitive to wall stretch than to the absolute blood pressure. As the receptors sense a change of shape in the arterial wall, usually from a change in pressure, the ANS is activated to raise HR (in the case of decreased pressure) or lower HR (in response to increased pressure). For example, a decrease in blood pressure alters the baroreceptor input to the vasomotor center in the medulla oblongata (brainstem), causing a reflex tachycardia. The baroreflex also initiates changes in venous tone to alter CO according to the need to increase or reduce blood return to the heart.

Chemoreceptors. Arterial *chemoreceptors*, known as *carotid* and *aortic bodies*, are located in the carotid arteries and at the bifurcation of the aortic arch and enjoy a rich capillary blood supply (see Fig 11.30). Their primary function is to maintain homeostasis during hypoxemia. Chemoreceptors signal changes in oxygen tension (Pao_2 <80 mm Hg) or a carbon dioxide tension ($Paco_2$) of greater than 40 mm Hg. They do not respond to changes in acid–base balance (pH), as changes in the pH level are detected by the central chemoreceptors in the brainstem (medulla oblongata). Information about changes in these parameters is communicated to the SNS via the brainstem. Stimulation of the carotid or aortic chemoreceptors normally causes an increase in respiratory rate and depth.

Right atrial receptors. The *Bainbridge reflex* is attributed to receptors in the right and left atria. When the pressure in the right atrium increases sufficiently to stimulate the stretch receptors, it causes a reflex tachycardia. The purpose of this reflex is possibly to protect the right side of the heart from an overload state and to quickly equalize filling pressures of the right and left sides of the heart.[17]

Natriuretic peptides. Another cardiac control mechanism involves the natriuretic peptide system (Fig. 11.31). The heart secretes two hormonal natriuretic peptides. The atrial myocardium secretes *atrial natriuretic peptide* in response to atrial stretch, and the ventricular myocardium secretes *brain natriuretic peptide* if stretch of the ventricular

FIG. 11.29 Autonomic Nervous System: Sympathetic and Parasympathetic Innervation of the Heart. (From Paulson F, Waschke J. *Sobotta Atlas of Human Anatomy.* Vol 2. 15th ed. Urban & Fischer; 2013.)

TABLE 11.6 Autonomic Nervous System Function in Heart Tissue

Function	Parasympathetic	Sympathetic
Automaticity	Decrease	Increase
Contractility	Decrease	Increase
Conduction velocity	Decrease	Increase
Chronotropy (rate)	Decrease	Increase

chamber occurs. Both peptides cause vasodilation, increase natriuresis (Na+ and water loss via the kidneys), and inhibit the SNS and the renin-angiotensin-aldosterone system (RAAS). Clinically, natriuretic peptide levels are measured to confirm a diagnosis of acute heart failure (see Fig. 13.86 in Chapter 13).

Renin-angiotensin-aldosterone system. The RAAS is activated by low blood pressure or intravascular volume depletion. The juxtaglomerular cells of the kidney, located near the afferent arteriole, are activated by low renal blood flow. As shown in Table 11.7, this stimulates release of the hormone renin. Renin converts the protein angiotensinogen to angiotensin I. When angiotensin I passes through the pulmonary vascular bed, it is activated by angiotensin-converting enzyme (ACE) to become angiotensin II. Angiotensin II is a powerful agent with two principal actions: (1) It activates peripheral vascular receptors to vasoconstrict the systemic arterial system and increase blood pressure, and (2) it activates the release of aldosterone from the adrenal glands (see Fig. 14.18 in chapter 14). Aldosterone works at the distal convoluted tubule in the kidney to retain sodium and, consequently, water. Many medications are used to

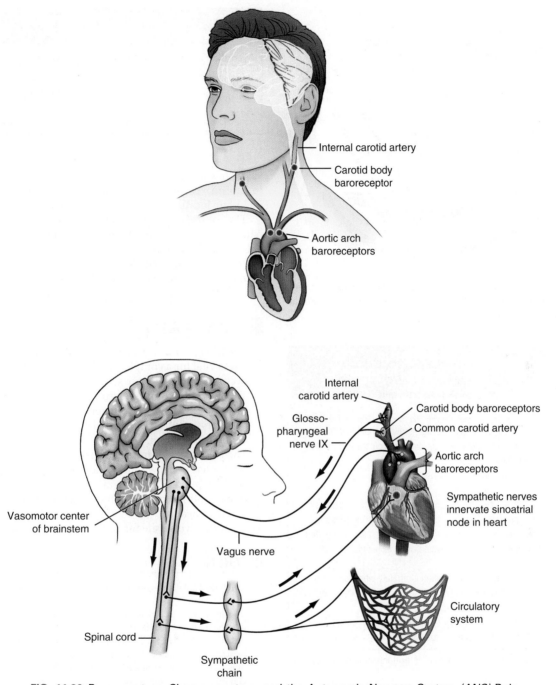

FIG. 11.30 Baroreceptors, Chemoreceptors, and the Autonomic Nervous System *(ANS)* **Role in Regulation of Heart Rate and Contractility.** (From Lough ME. Hemodynamic Monitoring: Evolving Technologies and Clinical Practice. St. Louis: Elsevier; 2015.)

manipulate the RAAS to manage symptoms of heart failure (see Table 14.8 in Chapter 14 and Table 15.21 in Chapter 15).

Respiratory influences. Normally, HR varies slightly with the respiratory cycle. The heart usually accelerates on inspiration and decelerates with exhalation (see "Sinus Dysrhythmia" in Chapter 14). Left ventricular SV decreases during normal inspiration.

Control of Peripheral Circulation
Intrinsic Control
Intrinsic, or local, control of the arterial peripheral circulation is most influential at the arteriolar level. Arterioles are the major

resistance vessels because of the amount of smooth muscle in the vessel walls. The arteriole has the potential for increasing or decreasing its lumen substantially. Several local factors influence this balance, including pharmacologic stimuli from locally released catecholamines, histamine, acetylcholine, serotonin, angiotensin, adenosine, and prostaglandins. These agents can be induced by various mechanisms such as tissue injury, hypoxemia, or hormones. For example, when red blood cells are exposed to hypoxia at the tissue level, they release the vasodilators nitric oxide and ATP to increase oxygen delivery. Other factors that influence circulation locally are temperature and carbon dioxide.

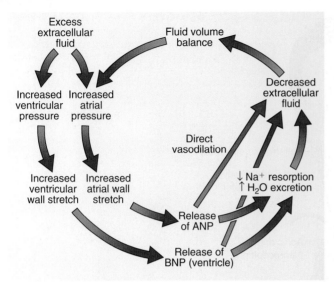

FIG. 11.31 Natriuretic Peptides. The release of atrial natriuretic peptide *(ANP)* from the atrium and brain natriuretic peptide *(BNP)* from the ventricle in response to volume overload.

TABLE 11.7 Renin-Angiotensin-Aldosterone and Antidiuretic Hormone Systems Maintain Fluid Balance

Hormone	Effect[a]
Renin ↓	Reduction in vascular volume or low arterial blood pressure stimulates renin release from juxtaglomerular cells near the kidney
Angiotensinogen ↓	Angiotensinogen is produced in the liver
Angiotensin I ↓	Lungs release ACE to convert angiotensin I to angiotensin II
Angiotensin II ↓	Angiotensin II activates peripheral vascular receptors to increase SVR and raise arterial blood pressure; angiotensin II release also stimulates adrenal glands to release aldosterone
	ADH is released from posterior pituitary when angiotensin II causes constriction of renal arterioles and when hypothalamus detects intracellular dehydration
Aldosterone	Aldosterone acts on kidney distal tubules to retain sodium; when salt is retained, so is water

ACE, angiotensin-converting enzyme; *ADH,* antidiuretic hormone; *SVR,* systemic vascular resistance.
[a]Overall effect is to increase intravascular volume and raise blood pressure.

Extrinsic Control

Extrinsic control is mediated by two major mechanisms: (1) the ANS and (2) peripheral vascular reflexes. The ANS exerts dual control over most organ systems via sympathetic (constriction) and parasympathetic (dilation) nerve fibers. Stimulation of the vasomotor center in the medulla causes increases in mean arterial pressure and HR by enhancing sympathetic outflow and possibly inhibiting parasympathetic outflow. Capacitance vessels (veins) contain up to 75% of the blood volume. Increases in venous tone (venoconstriction) increase the volume of blood returning to the right side of the heart to augment SV. The most richly innervated venous beds are those in splanchnic (spleen) and cutaneous (skin) circulations. The venous and arterial

TABLE 11.8 Medulla Oblongata Cardiovascular Actions

Medulla Oblongata Region	Effects
Dorsal lateral medulla (pressor region)	Vasoconstriction Cardiac acceleration Enhanced contractility
Ventromedial medulla (depressor region)	Direct spinal inhibition

vascular systems are interdependent; they dilate and constrict in unison. Table 11.8 summarizes the sympathetic receptors including location and effects of stimulation.

The control of peripheral circulation is achieved by a combination of intrinsic and extrinsic mechanisms. Additional influences include emotions, temperature, and humoral substances. For example, when red blood cells are exposed to hypoxia at the tissue level, they release the vasodilators nitric oxide and ATP to increase oxygen delivery.

SUMMARY

- Knowledge of normal cardiovascular anatomy and physiology is vital for a complete understanding of the changes that occur in cardiac disease states.
- The major anatomic structures of the heart include the pericardium, myocardium, endocardium, coronary arteries, coronary veins, atria, ventricles, heart valves, and electrical conduction system.
- The electrical conduction system, the mechanical events of the cardiac cycle, with the autonomic nervous system (ANS) and the preload volume in the veins act synergistically to ensure optimal cardiac output and hemodynamic stability in a state of health.
- ⓔ Visit the Evolve site for additional study materials.

REFERENCES

1. Dell'Italia LJ. Anatomy and physiology of the right ventricle. *Cardiol Clin.* 2012;30(2):167.
2. Vogiatzidis K, et al. Physiology of pericardial fluid production and drainage. *Front Physiol.* 2015;6:62.
3. Adler Y, et al. 2015 ESC Guidelines for the diagnosis and management of pericardial diseases: the Task Force for the Diagnosis and Management of Pericardial Diseases of the European Society of Cardiology (ESC) endorsed by: the European Association for Cardio-Thoracic Surgery (EACTS). *Eur Heart J.* 2015;36:2921.
4. Okura K, et al. Pericardial fat volume is an independent risk factor for the severity of coronary artery disease in patients with preserved ejection fraction. *J Cardiol.* 2015;65(1):37.
5. Baddour LM, et al. Infective endocarditis in adults: diagnosis, antimicrobial therapy, and management of complications: a scientific statement for healthcare professionals from the American Heart Association. *Circulation.* 2015;132(15):1435.
6. Gunnal SA, Wabale RN, Farooqui MS. Morphological study of chordae tendinae in human cadaveric hearts. *Heart Views.* 2015;16(1):1.
7. Zimarino M, et al. The dynamics of the coronary collateral circulation. *Nat Rev Cardiol.* 2014;11(4):191.
8. Guiraudon GM, Jones DL. Revisiting heart activation-conduction physiology, part I: atria. *J Interv Card Electrophysiol.* 2014;40(1):9.
9. Guiraudon GM, et al. Revisiting right atrial isolation rationale for atrial fibrillation: functional anatomy of interatrial connections. *J Interv Card Electrophysiol.* 2013;37(3):267.

10. Bartos DC, Grandi E, Ripplinger CM. Ion channels in the heart. *Compr Physiol*. 2015;5(3):1423.

11. Echeverri D, Cabrales J, Jimenez A. Myocardial venous drainage: from anatomy to clinical use. *J Invasive Cardiol*. 2013;25(2):98.

12. Loukas M, et al. The anatomy of the aortic root. *Clin Anat*. 2014;27(5):748.

13. Kobirumaki-Shimozawa F, et al. Cardiac thin filament regulation and the Frank-Starling mechanism. *J Physiol Sci*. 2014;64(4):221.

14. Shen MJ, Zipes DP. Role of the autonomic nervous system in modulating cardiac arrhythmias. *Circ Res*. 2014;114(6):1004.

15. Kapa S, DeSimone CV, Asirvatham SJ. Innervation of the heart: an invisible grid within a black box. *Trends Cardiovasc Med*. 2016;26(3):245.

16. Shaffer F, McCraty R, Zerr CL. A healthy heart is not a metronome: an integrative review of the heart's anatomy and heart rate variability. *Front Psychol*. 2014;5:1040.

17. Crystal GJ, Salem RM. The Bainbridge and the "reverse" Bainbridge reflexes: history, physiology, and clinical relevance. *Anesth Analg*. 2012;114(3):520.

12

Cardiovascular Clinical Assessment

Mary E. Lough

Physical assessment of a patient with cardiovascular disease is an important clinical skill to master. The process is systematic and detailed as described in this chapter. Bedside assessment allows the examiner to correlate all the other diagnostic studies to form a complete picture of the patient's cardiovascular status.[1]

HISTORY

Data collected from a thorough, thoughtful history taking contributes to both nursing and medical decisions about therapeutic interventions.[2] For a patient in acute distress, the history taking is shortened to just a few questions about the patient's chief complaint, precipitating events, and current medications (Box 12.1). For a patient who is not in obvious distress, the history focuses on the following four areas:

1. Review of the patient's present illness
2. Overview of the patient's general cardiovascular status, including previous cardiac diagnostic studies, interventional procedures, cardiac surgeries, and current medications (ie, cardiac, noncardiac, and over-the-counter medications)
3. Review of the patient's general health status, including family history of coronary artery disease (CAD), hypertension, diabetes, peripheral arterial disease, or stroke
4. Survey of the patient's lifestyle, including risk factors for CAD

One unique challenge in cardiovascular assessment is identifying when "chest pain" is of cardiac origin and when it is not. Almost 8 million patients come to hospital emergency departments with a chief complaint of chest pain.[3] Only approximately 10% of these patients are experiencing an acute cardiac event. In most cases, the chest pain is from another cause such as gastroesophageal reflux disease. For this reason, identifying the patients who are experiencing an acute coronary syndrome is crucial.[3]

The following safety information should always be considered:

- If any evidence of CAD or risk of heart disease exists, assume that the chest pain is caused by myocardial ischemia until proven otherwise.
- Questions to elicit the nature of the chest pain cover five basic areas: (1) quality of the pain, (2) location of the pain, (3) duration of the pain, (4) factors that provoke the pain, and (5) factors that relieve the pain. Questions that may help elicit this information are listed in Table 12.1.
- Little correlation may exist between the severity of chest discomfort and the gravity of its cause. This is a result of the subjective nature of pain and the unique presentation of ischemic disease in women, older patients, and patients with diabetes.

- Subjective descriptors vary greatly among individuals. Not all patients use the word "pain"; some may describe their problem as "pressure," "heaviness," "discomfort," or "indigestion."
- Other nonpainful symptoms that may signal cardiac dysfunction are dyspnea, palpitations, cough, fatigue, edema, ischemic leg pain, nocturia, cyanosis, and a history of syncope.

In the evaluation of acute chest pain, a 12-lead electrocardiogram to diagnose ST segment changes must be obtained within 10 minutes of arrival at an emergency department.[4]

PHYSICAL EXAMINATION

A comprehensive physical assessment is fundamental to arriving at an accurate diagnosis. A nurse who has developed the skills of *inspection*, *palpation*, and *auscultation* can be confident when assessing patients with cardiovascular disease.[1] *Percussion*, another physical assessment skill, is not employed when assessing the cardiovascular system.

Inspection

Face

The face is observed for skin color (ie, cyanotic, pale, or jaundiced) and for an apprehensive or painful expression. The patient's skin, lips, tongue, and mucous membranes are inspected for pallor or cyanosis. *Central cyanosis* is a bluish discoloration of the tongue and sublingual area. Central cyanosis is a medical emergency indicating hypoxemia. Pulse oximetry, arterial blood gas analysis, and treatment with 100% oxygen must be instituted immediately.

Thorax

The anterior thorax and posterior thorax are inspected for skeletal deformities that may displace the heart and cause cardiac compromise. The skin on the chest wall and abdomen is inspected for scars, bruises, wounds, and bulges associated with pacemaker or defibrillator implants. Respiratory rate, pattern, and effort are also observed and recorded.

Abdomen

The abdomen is assessed for signs of distention or ascites, which may be associated with right-sided heart failure. Abdominal adiposity is a known risk factor for CAD.

Nail Beds and Cyanosis

The nail beds are inspected for signs of discoloration or cyanosis. *Clubbing* in the nail bed is a sign associated with long-standing central cyanotic heart disease or pulmonary disease with

BOX 12.1   DATA COLLECTION

Cardiovascular History

Common Cardiovascular Symptoms
- Chest pains
- Palpitations
- Dyspnea
- Cough, hemoptysis
- Nausea
- Nocturia
- Edema
- Dizziness, syncope, visual changes
- Leg claudication (pain) or paresthesias
- Fatigue

Patient Lifestyle
- Baseline cognitive functioning
- Health habits
  - Use of tea and coffee, over-the-counter medication use, smoking, exercise, sleep, dietary habits
  - Use of illegal recreational drugs (eg, cocaine)
  - Use of alcohol (occasional, daily)
- Lifestyle pattern and responsibilities
- Working, relaxing, coping, cultural habits
- Social support systems
- Recent life changes within past 12 months
- Emotional state
- Evidence of psychological stress, anger, anxiety, depression
- Perception of illness and its meaning for the future

Cardiovascular Risk Factors
- Sex
- Age
- Cultural identity
- Family history of premature CAD (age 65 years or younger)
- Smoking history
- Hypertension
- Hyperlipidemia
- Sedentary lifestyle
- Diabetes mellitus
- Obesity
- Kidney failure

Medical History
Child
- Murmurs, cyanosis, streptococcal infections, rheumatic fever

Adult
- Diseases and abnormalities
  - Heart failure (right- or left-sided), CAD, heart valve disease, mitral valve prolapse, myocardial infarction, peripheral vascular disease (arterial or venous), diabetes mellitus, hypertension, hyperlipidemia, dysrhythmias, murmurs, endocarditis, visual defects, recent weight changes, psychiatric illnesses, thrombophlebitis, deep vein thrombosis, systemic or pulmonary emboli

- Surgical history
  - *Cardiovascular:* Coronary artery bypass grafting, valvular placement, peripheral vascular bypasses or repairs, pacemaker, defibrillator implant (ICD)
  - *Other body systems:* Neurologic, gastrointestinal, musculoskeletal, pulmonary, renal, immunologic, hematologic
- Allergies, especially to emergency medications (lidocaine, morphine), radiographic contrast agents, or iodine (shellfish)
- Recent dental work or infection

Family History
- CAD at age 65 years or younger
- Myocardial infarction
- Early death of unknown origin
- Hypertension
- Stroke
- Diabetes mellitus
- Lipid disorders
- Collagen vascular disease

Current Medication Use
- ACE inhibitors
- Anticoagulants
- Antidysrhythmics
- Antihypertensives
- Antiplatelet agents
- Angiotensin-receptor blockers
- Beta-blockers
- Calcium channel blockers
- Cholesterol-lowering agents
- Digitalis
- Diuretics
- Nitrates
- Hormone replacement therapy
- Oral contraceptives
- Potassium, calcium
- Nonprescription medications or herbal remedies

Cardiac Studies or Interventions Done in the Past
- Cardiac catheterization
- Electrophysiology study
- Cardiac ultrasound (echocardiogram)
- 12-lead electroencephalogram
- Exercise ECG (stress test)
- Myocardial imaging with radiographic isotopes (eg, thallium, dipyridamole, dobutamine)
- Thrombolytic therapy
- Percutaneous transluminal coronary angioplasty
- Atherectomy
- Stent placement
- Valvuloplasty

ACE, angiotensin-converting enzyme; *CAD,* coronary artery disease; *ECG,* electrocardiogram; *ICD,* implantable cardioverter defibrillator.

hypoxemia.[5] "Clubbing" of the nail refers to a nail that has lost the normal angle between the finger and the nail root; the nail becomes wide and convex. The terminal phalanx of the finger also becomes bulbous and swollen. Clubbing is rare and is a sign of severe central cyanosis (Fig. 12.1). *Peripheral cyanosis,* a bluish discoloration of the nail bed, is seen more commonly. Peripheral cyanosis results from a reduction in the quantity of oxygen in the peripheral extremities from arterial disease or decreased cardiac output. Clubbing never occurs as a result of peripheral cyanosis.

TABLE 12.1 Clarifying Chest Pain Symptoms by Asking Specific Questions

Determine	Typical Question
Location, radiation	Where is it?
	Does it move or stay in one place?
Quality	What is it like?
Quantity	How severe is it?
	How frequent is it?
	How long does it last?
Chronology	When did it begin?
	How has it progressed?
	What are you doing when it occurs?
	What do you do to get rid of it?
Associated findings	Do you feel any other symptoms at the same time?
Treatment sought and effect	Have you seen a physician in the past for this same problem?
	What was the treatment?
Personal	What do you think this is from?
Perception	Why do you think it happened now?

Clubbing of Nail Beds

Normal nail shows a slight angle between root of nail bed and finger.

Normal Finger and Nail Bed

Early clubbing shows loss of angle at root of nail bed. Fingertip is of normal size.

Early Clubbing

Moderate clubbing shows bulging of angle at root of nail bed. Distal finger/toe is enlarged.

Moderate Clubbing

Advanced clubbing shows bulging and widening of nail bed. Distal finger/toe is bulbous.

Advanced Clubbing

FIG. 12.1 Clubbing of Nail Beds.

Lower Extremities

Legs are inspected for signs of peripheral arterial disease or venous insufficiency. The visible signs of peripheral arterial vascular disease include pale, shiny legs with sparse hair growth. More recent guidelines indicate that many individuals, especially women, can have peripheral atherosclerosis without obvious signs or symptoms of arterial disease.[6] Venous disease is caused by failure of the valves in the veins causing bleeding into the surrounding tissues. Increasing pressure in the tissues causes edema, brown skin discoloration from red blood cell destruction, dependent rubor, and frequently nonhealing leg ulcers. A comparison of typical assessment findings in arterial and venous diseases is presented in Table 12.2.

Posture

Body posture can indicate the amount of effort it takes to breathe. For example, sitting upright to breathe may be necessary for a patient with acute heart failure. Leaning forward may be the least painful position for a patient with pericarditis.

Weight

Body weight in proportion to height is assessed to determine whether the patient is obese or cachectic.[7-9]

Mentation

The patient is observed for signs of confusion or lethargy that may indicate hypotension, low cardiac output, or hypoxemia.

Jugular Veins

The jugular veins of the neck are inspected for a noninvasive estimate of intravascular volume and pressure.[1] The internal jugular veins are observed for *jugular vein distention* (Fig. 12.2 and Box 12.2) caused by an elevation in *jugular venous pressure* (JVP). Elevated JVP can be observed as a sign without measurement. JVP is best observed in the right jugular vein.[1] The most common causes of JVP elevation are fluid volume overload and right ventricular failure. The right internal jugular vein can be palpated to permit noninvasive measurement of elevated central venous pressure (CVP) in centimeters (Fig. 12.3 and Box 12.3). Any elevation greater than 8 cm is considered high.[1] Bedside ultrasound can also be used to evaluate jugular vein distention and to estimate CVP.[10]

TABLE 12.2 Comparison of Arterial and Venous Disease in Legs

Signs and Symptoms	Peripheral Arterial Disease	Venous Insufficiency
Skin	Shiny dry appearance	Brown patches on skin at ankles and lower leg
	Pallor with elevation	Mottled rubor (brown/red) appearance especially when dependent
		Skin texture may be hard and fibrotic
		Flaking skin, dermatitis
Hair on leg	Decreased hair growth	Decreased hair growth
Ulcers on leg or foot	Foot or toe wounds (ulcers) that do not heal	Venous ulcers at ankle or lower leg
	Gangrene on toes	Moist with copious drainage
Nails	Slow nail growth	Normal
	Thick, opaque nails	
Varicose veins	No	Present
Temperature	Cold compared with rest of the body	Warm
Capillary refill	Slow (≥3 s)	Normal (<3 s)
Edema	None	Legs and feet are swollen and edematous
Pulses	Weak or absent	Normal
Pain	Burning sensation in feet	
	Leg cramps when walking: *intermittent claudication*	
	Leg cramps at rest: *ischemic claudication*	
	Numbness	
Associated conditions	Diabetes	
	Atherosclerotic disease	

FIG. 12.2 Assessment of Jugular Vein Distention. Applying light finger pressure over the sternocleidomastoid muscle, parallel to the clavicle, helps identify the external jugular vein by occluding flow and distending it. The finger pressure is released, and the patient is observed for true distention. If the patient's trunk is elevated to 30 degrees or more, jugular vein distention should not be present.

BOX 12.2 Procedure for Assessing Jugular Vein Distention

1. The patient reclines at 30- to 45-degree angle.
2. The examiner stands on the patient's right side and turns the patient's head slightly toward the left.
3. If the jugular vein is not visible, light finger pressure is applied across the sternocleidomastoid muscle just above and parallel to the clavicle. This pressure fills the external jugular vein by obstructing flow (see Fig. 12.2).
4. After the location of the vein has been identified, the pressure is released, and the presence of JVD is assessed.
5. Because inhalation decreases venous pressure, JVD should be assessed at end-exhalation.
6. Any fullness in the vein extending more than 3 cm above the sternal angle is evidence of increased venous pressure. Generally, the higher the sitting angle of the patient when JVD is visualized, the higher is the central venous pressure.
7. *Documentation:* JVD is reported by including the angle of the head of the bed at the time JVD was evaluated (eg, "Presence of JVD with head of bed elevated to 45 degrees").

JVD, jugular vein distention.

Abdominojugular Reflux

The *abdominojugular reflux sign* can assist with the diagnosis of right ventricular failure. This noninvasive test is used in conjunction with measurement of JVP. The procedure for assessing abdominojugular reflux is described in Box 12.4. A positive abdominojugular reflux sign is an increase in the JVP (CVP equivalent) of 4 cm or more sustained for at least 10 seconds.[1]

Thoracic Reference Points

The thoracic cage is divided with imaginary vertical lines (sternal, midclavicular, axillary, vertebral, and scapular), and the intercostal spaces are divided by imaginary horizontal lines to

FIG. 12.3 Position of Internal and External Jugular Veins. Pulsation in the internal jugular vein can be used to estimate central venous pressure. (Modified from Thompson JM, et al. *Mosby's Clinical Nursing.* 5th ed. St. Louis: Mosby; 2002.)

BOX 12.3　**Procedure for Assessing Central Venous Pressure**
1. The patient reclines in the bed. The highest point of pulsation in the internal jugular vein is observed during exhalation.
2. The vertical distance between this pulsation (top of the fluid level) and the sternal angle is estimated or measured in centimeters.
3. This number is added to 5 cm for an estimation of CVP; 5 cm is the approximate distance of the sternal angle above the level of the right atrium (see Fig. 12.3).
4. *Documentation:* The degree of elevation of the patient is included in the report (eg, "CVP estimated at 13 cm, using internal jugular vein pulsation, with head of bed elevated 45 degrees").

CVP, central venous pressure.

BOX 12.4　**Procedure for Assessing Abdominojugular Reflux**
1. Ask the patient to relax and breathe normally through an open mouth.
2. Measure JVD in the patient's right internal jugular vein, following the procedure described in Box 12.2.
3. Apply firm pressure of approximately 20–35 mm Hg to the patient's midabdomen for 15–30 s, and remeasure JVD during the compression.
4. Measure the right JVD a third time after compression is released.
5. Ask the patient not to tense or hold the breath during the test. (Doing so increases venous return to the heart and may produce a falsely positive result.)
6. A positive abdominojugular reflux is identified when abdominal compression causes a sustained JVD increase of 4 cm or more. This sign is indicative of right-sided heart failure.
7. A normal abdominojugular reflux is reported if there is no increase in JVD, a transient (<10 s) increase in JVD, or an increase in JVD less than or equal to 3 cm sustained throughout compression.

JVD, jugular vein distention.

serve as reference points in locating or describing cardiac findings (Fig. 12.4). The ribs are numbered from 1 (the first rib below the clavicle) to 12. The intercostal space below each rib is given the same number as the rib that lies above it. The second rib is the easiest to locate because it is attached to the sternum at the angle of Louis. This angle (also called the *sternal angle*) is the bony ridge on the sternum that lies approximately 2 inches below the sternal notch (see Fig. 12.4A). After the second rib has been located, it can be used as a reference point to count off the other ribs and intercostal spaces.

Apical Impulse

The anterior thorax is inspected for the *apical impulse*, sometimes referred to as the *point of maximal impulse*. The apical impulse occurs as the left ventricle contracts during systole and rotates forward, causing the left ventricular apex of the heart to hit the chest wall. The apical impulse is a quick, localized, outward movement normally located just lateral to the left midclavicular line at the fifth intercostal space in an adult patient (Fig. 12.5).[1] The apical impulse is the only normal pulsation visualized on the chest wall. In a patient without cardiac disease, point of maximal impulse may not be noticeable (see Fig. 12.5).

Palpation

Palpation is a technique that uses the sense of touch in the tips of the fingers and the palm of the hand.

Arterial Pulses

Seven pairs of bilateral arterial pulses are normally palpated. The examination incorporates bilateral assessment of the

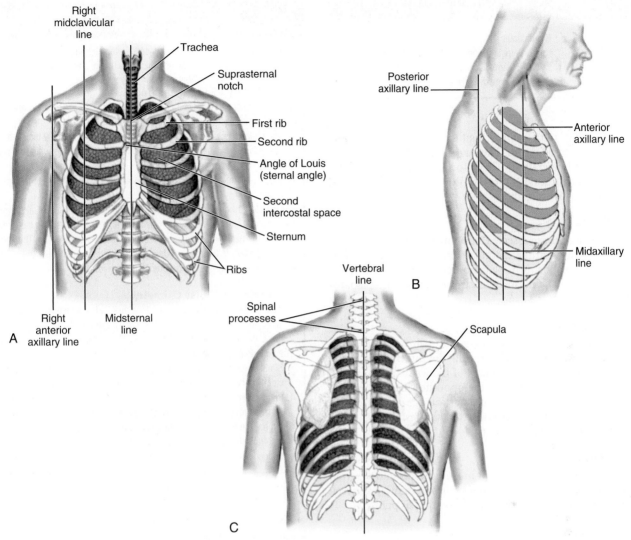

FIG. 12.4 Thoracic Landmarks. (A) Anterior thorax. (B) Right lateral thorax. (C) Posterior thorax.

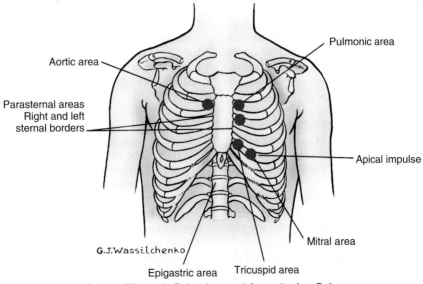

FIG. 12.5 Thoracic Palpation and Auscultation Points.

BOX 12.5 **Pulse Palpation Scale**

0	Not palpable
1+	Faintly palpable (weak and thready)
2+	Palpable (normal pulse)
3+	Bounding (hyperdynamic pulse)

---

carotid, brachial, radial, ulnar, popliteal, posterior tibial, and dorsalis pedis arterial pulses. The pulses are palpated separately and compared bilaterally to check for consistency. Pulse volume is graded on a scale of 0 to 3+ (Box 12.5). The abdominal aortic pulse can also be palpated.

Carotid Pulses

The carotid arteries are assessed at the medial midneck region. If blood flow through the carotid arteries is compromised by atherosclerotic plaque, firm palpation could cause total occlusion. The touch is light, and the carotid arteries are palpated gently and only one at a time.

Brachial, Ulnar, and Radial Pulses

The brachial pulse is assessed by gently palpating the inner aspect of the slightly bent elbow with the fingers. The radial pulse is palpated in the medial area of the wrist (thumb side). The ulnar artery is palpated at the opposite side of the wrist (little finger side). The radial and ulnar arterial pulses must be assessed before an arterial line is inserted; this test, known as the *Allen test*, is described in Box 12.6.

Femoral Pulses

The femoral arteries are palpated by pressing deeply into the groin beneath the inguinal ligament, approximately midway between the anterior superior iliac spine and the symphysis pubis.

Popliteal Pulses

The popliteal pulse is lightly palpated using the fingertips. The patient's leg is very slightly bent, and the clinician's two hands gently cup the patient's knee with the thumbs on top of the kneecap and the fingertips behind the knee.

Dorsalis Pedis and Posterior Tibial Pulses

The pulses of the lower leg and foot are assessed to determine blood flow to the limb and to assess adequacy of cardiac output to the extremities. The dorsalis pedis pulse is located on the upper aspect of the foot. The posterior tibial pulse is located behind the medial malleolus (inner ankle bone) of the lower leg.

Descending Aorta Pulse

When the patient is in the supine position, the abdominal aortic pulsation is located in the epigastric area and can be felt as a forward movement when firm fingertip pressure is applied above the umbilicus. If prominent or diffuse, the pulsation may indicate an abdominal aneurysm.

A diminished or absent pulse may indicate low cardiac output, arterial stenosis, or occlusion proximal to the site of the examination. An abnormally strong or bounding pulse suggests the presence of an aneurysm or an occlusion distal to the examination site. If a distal pulse cannot be palpated by using light finger pressure, a Doppler ultrasound stethoscope may enhance diagnostic accuracy. It is important to mark the location of the

---

BOX 12.6 **Procedure for Assessment of Arterial Blood Supply to the Hand: Allen Test**

Before a radial artery is punctured or cannulated, the Allen test is performed to assess blood flow to the hand and to ensure that it is adequate.

Allen Test by Visual Inspection
1. If the patient is alert and cooperative, he or she is asked to repeatedly make a tight fist to squeeze the blood out of the hand.
2. The radial artery is compressed with firm thumb pressure by the examiner.
3. The patient is requested to open the hand palm side up while the radial artery is still occluded.
4. Pressure is released, and the time it takes for color to return to the hand is noted.

If the ulnar artery is patent, color will return within 3 seconds. The patient may describe a tingling in the palm as blood flow returns. Delayed color return (a "failed" Allen test) implies that the ulnar artery is inadequate. This means the radial artery is the only reliable source of arterial blood flow to the hand, and therefore it must not be punctured or cannulated.

Allen Test With Pulse Oximetry
1. If the patient is unable to cooperate to make a fist, an alternative approach is to use a pulse oximeter that displays a pulse waveform.
2. Place the pulse oximeter on the patient's middle finger, and establish an adequate pulse amplitude display on the monitor.
3. Simultaneously compress the radial and ulnar arteries until the waveform clearly decreases or vanishes.
4. Release pressure off the ulnar artery only. If the ulnar artery is patent, the pulse amplitude recovers its normal appearance.
5. Repeat the procedure with the radial artery.
6. Arterial catheterization of the radial artery can be accomplished safely only if blood supply to the hand is adequate.

---

audible signal with an indelible ink marker pen for future evaluation of pulse quality.

Capillary Refill

Capillary refill assessment is an assessment technique that uses the patient's nail beds to evaluate arterial circulation to the extremity and determine overall perfusion. The nail bed is compressed to produce blanching, after which release of the pressure should result in the return of blood flow and baseline nail color in less than 2 seconds. Capillary refill time of greater than 5 seconds has been associated with more severe organ failure[11] and increased mortality.[12] Capillary refill is a standard component of the cardiovascular physical examination.

Edema

Edema is fluid accumulation in the extravascular spaces of the body. The dependent tissues within the legs and sacrum are particularly susceptible. Edema may be dependent, unilateral or bilateral, and pitting or nonpitting. The amount of edema is quantified by measuring the circumference of the limb or by pressing the skin of the feet, ankles, and shins against underlying bone. Edema is a symptom associated with several diseases, and further diagnostic evaluation is required to determine the cause. Although no universal scale for pitting edema exists, typical scales use a system ranging from 0 to 4+ (Table 12.3).

TABLE 12.3 Pitting Edema Scale

Scale	Edema	INDENTATION DEPTH English Units	Metric Units	Time to Baseline
0	None	0	0	
1+	Trace	0–0.25 inch	<6.5 mm	Rapid
2+	Mild	0.25–0.5 inch	6.5–12.5 mm	10–15 s
3+	Moderate	0.5–1 inch	12.5 mm–2.5 cm	1–2 min
4+	Severe	>1 inch	>2.5 cm	2–5 min

Auscultation
Blood Pressure Measurement

Blood pressure (BP) measurement is an essential component of every complete physical examination. More recent BP management guidelines specify antihypertensive medication treatment goals by age range.[13] For individuals who are age 60 years and older, a BP less than 150/90 mm Hg is the target. For individuals between age 30 and 59 years, a BP less than 140/90 mm Hg is the target.[13] In patients with chronic kidney disease or diabetes, the goal is a BP less than 140/90 mm Hg.[13]

These guideline BP targets have been challenged following the results of a breakthrough clinical trial that compared cardiovascular disease outcomes for 9300 patients whose systolic BP target was either 140 mm Hg or 120 mm Hg.[14,15] Patients were older than 50 years, did not have type 2 diabetes, and were representative of the general population of the United States.[16] On average, patients required two oral antihypertensive medications to reduce systolic BP to 140 mm Hg and required three oral antihypertensive medications to reduce systolic BP to 120 mm Hg.[15]

In the critical care setting, systemic BP can be measured directly or indirectly. Direct BP measurement is via an invasive arterial catheter. Indirect BP measurement is with a stethoscope and sphygmomanometer or electronic measuring devices. Ideally, indirect BP values closely reflect direct measurements (within 1 to 3 mm Hg). The following discussion reviews the essential elements of noninvasive BP monitoring.

Noninvasive blood pressure monitoring. The most common peripheral locations for BP monitoring are the bilateral brachial arteries. The pressure is measured in both arms to rule out subclavian arterial stenosis. Normally, the difference in pressure between the arms is less than 10 mm Hg. A difference of more than 15 mm Hg between the bilateral arm pressures suggests arterial obstruction on the side with the lower pressure and is found in approximately 5% of the population.[17] Asymmetry is documented so that all subsequent measurements can be made on the arm with the higher pressure.

Correct positioning of the extremity being measured is essential. BP can be measured in any position as long as the arm or the leg is at the level of the heart. Falsely elevated readings are obtained if the arm is at a level lower than the heart, and falsely low pressures are obtained when the arm is at a level higher than the heart.

Orthostatic hypotension. When a healthy person stands, 10% to 15% of the blood volume is pooled in the legs; this reduces venous return to the right side of the heart, which decreases cardiac output and lowers arterial BP. The fall in BP activates baroreceptors; the subsequent reflex increases in sympathetic outflow and parasympathetic inhibition lead to peripheral vasoconstriction, with increased heart rate and contractility.[18] Postural (orthostatic) hypotension occurs when the systolic BP falls 20 mm Hg or the diastolic BP falls 10 mm Hg with a change in position from sitting/supine to standing.[19] Orthostatic hypotension is usually accompanied by cerebral hypoperfusion identified by dizziness, lightheadedness, or syncope. If a patient experiences these symptoms, it is important to complete a full set of postural vital signs before increasing the patient's activity level (Box 12.7). The three most common causes of orthostatic vital sign changes (ie, decrease in BP and increase in heart rate) observed in critical care are as follows:

1. Intravascular volume depletion or fluid loss caused by bleeding, excessive diuresis, or fever
2. Inadequate vascular vasoconstrictor mechanisms to constrict the arterial bed, which can occur in older patients after prolonged immobility or as a result of spinal cord injury
3. Autonomic insufficiency caused by administration of pharmacologic agents such as beta-blockers, angiotensin-converting enzyme inhibitors, and calcium channel blockers

Blood pressure cuff size. Correct size and placement of the BP inflatable bladder (inside the nondistensible cuff) are crucial to obtaining an accurate BP measurement. The bladder-cuff should be long enough to encircle at least 80% of the width of the upper arm (or leg) in adults.[20] Cuffs that are too small can give falsely high readings, and cuffs that are too large can give falsely low readings. Box 12.8 lists the key points to observe when obtaining BP readings.

Korotkoff sounds. Obtaining systemic BP readings involves auscultation of *Korotkoff sounds,* the sounds created by turbulence of blood flow within a vessel caused by constriction of the BP cuff. The pressure in the cuff is inflated above the normal systolic pressure. As the pressure in the cuff is reduced, Korotkoff sounds change in quality and intensity. These sounds are divided into five stages. The systolic BP is the highest point at which initial tapping occurs. Diastolic BP is equated with the complete disappearance of Korotkoff sounds. Often, a muffling of diastolic sounds occurs before these sounds completely disappear. This has caused debate about which diastolic value to record. Because complete disappearance of Korotkoff sounds corresponds more closely to intraarterial catheter measurement, it is the value that should be recorded.

Auscultatory gap. In older patients with systolic hypertension, the presence of an *auscultatory gap* is common.[20] It is important to inflate the cuff to greater than the patient's normal systolic pressure to avoid this gap and underestimation of systolic BP. Use of an initial palpation estimate of the systolic BP taken before auscultation with a stethoscope is one recommended method to accurately determine the upper systolic BP.

BOX 12.7 Measurement of Postural (Orthostatic) Vital Signs

Guidelines
1. Record BP and HR in each position.
2. Do not remove cuff between measurements.
3. Record all associated signs and symptoms.
4. Clearly document patient position.

Lying   Sitting   Standing

Technique
1. Keep the patient as flat as possible for 10 min before the initial assessment.
2. *Patient supine:* Obtain initial BP and HR measurements.
3. *Patient sitting with legs hanging:* Measure immediately and after 2 min.

4. *Patient standing:* Measure immediately and after 2 min. If BP and HR are stable but orthostasis is suspected, BP and HR can be repeated every 2 min. This is rarely practical for a critically ill patient.

Results
Normal Changes
HR increases by 5–20 beats/min (transiently).
Systolic BP decreases by 10 mm Hg.
Diastolic BP decreases by 5 mm Hg.

Positive Orthostasis
Decrease in systolic BP by more than 20 mm Hg.
Decrease in diastolic BP by more than 10 mm Hg within 3 min.
BP, blood pressure; *HR*, heart rate.

BOX 12.8 Obtaining Accurate Blood Pressure Readings

- Compare right and left measurements.
- Position the extremity at the level of the heart.
- Document the position of the patient.
- Ensure proper cuff size.
- Measure readings at eye level at the top of the meniscus.

BOX 12.9 Procedure for Measuring Pulsus Paradoxus

Measurement With Sphygmomanometer
1. The patient should be lying supine in a comfortable position.
2. The breathing pattern should be of normal depth and rate to avoid excessive respiratory interference.
3. BP is measured following standard procedures (see Boxes 12.7 and 12.8). The sphygmomanometer cuff is inflated to a pressure greater than systolic BP, and Korotkoff sounds are auscultated over the brachial artery while the cuff is deflated at a rate of approximately 2–3 mm Hg per heartbeat.
4. The peak systolic BP during expiration (ie, pressure at which Korotkoff sounds are heard only during expiration) should be identified and then reconfirmed.
5. The cuff is deflated slowly to establish systolic BP at which Korotkoff sounds become audible during both inspiration and expiration.
6. If the auscultated difference between these two systolic BP values exceeds 10 mm Hg during quiet respiration, a paradoxical pulse is present.

Measurement by Waveform Analysis
1. A pulse oximetry sensor with a visible pulse waveform can be used as an additional measurement device.
2. In the critical care unit, an arterial waveform from an indwelling arterial catheter (if present) can be used to measure the difference in systolic BP between expiration and inspiration.

BP, blood pressure.

Automated blood pressure devices. Electronic automated devices are frequently used for measuring BP and have replaced the mercury sphygmomanometer in most environments. Mercury is a nondegradable environmental pollutant that is difficult to dispose of safely. For this reason, mercury sphygmomanometers have been phased out of use in most hospitals.

In general, auscultated readings (with a stethoscope) are considered to be more accurate than electronic oscillatory readings.[21] Devices placed on the arms or legs are considered accurate (as long as the cuff size is correct) for systolic measurement and trending of BP. Automatic BP cuff placement should be rotated frequently to avoid local skin irritation, especially when the automatic cuff is set to cycle frequently, such as every 15 minutes.

Pulse pressure. Pulse pressure describes the difference between systolic and diastolic values. The normal pulse pressure is 40 mm Hg (ie, the difference between a systolic BP of 120 mm Hg and a diastolic BP of 80 mm Hg). In a critically ill patient, a low BP is frequently associated with a narrow pulse pressure. For example, a patient with a BP of 90/72 mm Hg has a pulse pressure of 18 mm Hg. The narrowed pulse pressure is a temporary compensatory mechanism caused by arterial vasoconstriction resulting from volume depletion or heart failure. The narrow pulse pressure ensures that the mean arterial pressure (78 mm Hg in this example) remains in a therapeutic range to provide adequate organ perfusion.

In contrast, a hypotensive patient with sepsis who exhibits vasodilation has a wide pulse pressure and inadequate organ perfusion. If the BP is 90/36 mm Hg, the pulse pressure is 54 mm Hg, and the mean arterial pressure is an inadequate 54 mm Hg. In both of these examples, the systolic BP is the same (90 mm Hg); the difference in pulse pressure is a function of intravascular volume and vascular tone.

Pulsus paradoxus. In normal physiology, the strength of the pulse fluctuates throughout the respiratory cycle. When the "pulse" is measured using the SBP, the pressure is observed to decrease slightly during inspiration and to increase slightly during respiratory exhalation. The normal difference is 2 to 4 mm Hg. In some clinical conditions such as cardiac tamponade, the BP decline is abnormally large during inspiration. In general, an inspiratory decline of systolic BP greater than 10 mm Hg is considered diagnostic of *pulsus paradoxus*.[22] The techniques for measuring pulsus paradoxus using a sphygmomanometer, BP cuff, and pulse oximetry waveform are described in Box 12.9. If the patient is hypotensive, pulsus paradoxus is more accurately assessed in the critical care unit by monitoring a pulse oximetry waveform or an indwelling arterial catheter waveform.

Pulsus alternans. Pulsus alternans describes a regular pattern of pulse amplitude changes that alternate between stronger

BOX 12.10 Characteristics of First and Second Heart Sounds

First Heart Sound (S$_1$)	Second Heart Sound (S$_2$)	First Heart Sound (S$_1$)	Second Heart Sound (S$_2$)
High pitched	High pitched	Important to differentiate between split S$_1$ and S$_4$	↑ Split with inhalation
Loudest in mitral area (apex)	Loudest in aortic area (base)		
Split S$_1$	Split S$_2$	Occurs immediately before carotid upstroke	↓ Split with exhalation
Normal split less than 20 ms	Normal split less than 30 ms		
Split heard best in tricuspid area	Split heard best in pulmonic area		

↑, increased; ↓, decreased. *ms,* milliseconds.

G.J.Wassilchenko

FIG. 12.6 Transmission of Heart Sounds to Thorax and Their Relationship to Anatomic Position of Heart Valves.

and weaker beats. This finding is suggestive of end-stage left ventricular heart failure.

Vascular bruits. The carotid and femoral arteries are auscultated for bruits. A bruit, a high-pitched "sh-sh" sound, is an extracardiac vascular sound that vacillates in volume with systole and diastole. An abnormal bruit is produced as blood flows through a partially occluded vessel. Auscultation of a bruit can expedite the diagnosis of suspected arterial obstruction.

Normal Heart Sounds

Auscultation of the heart with a stethoscope is considered the most challenging part of the cardiac physical examination. Hand-held ultrasound devices increasingly are used at the bedside to augment cardiac auscultation findings.[23,24] A summary of the advice given by most experts to effectively acquire the skills of cardiac auscultation follows:

1. Auscultate systematically across the precordium.
2. Visualize the cardiac anatomy under each point of auscultation, expecting to hear the physiologically associated sounds.
3. Memorize the cardiac cycle to enhance the ability to hear abnormal sounds.
4. Practice, practice, practice.

First and second heart sounds. Normal heart sounds are referred to as the *first heart sound* (S$_1$) and the *second heart sound* (S$_2$). S$_1$ is the sound associated with mitral and tricuspid valve closure and is heard most clearly in the mitral and tricuspid areas. S$_2$ (aortic and pulmonic closure) can be heard best at the second intercostal space to the right and left of the sternum (see Fig. 12.5). Both sounds are high pitched and heard best with the diaphragm of the stethoscope (Box 12.10). Each sound is loudest in an auscultation area located downstream from the actual valvular component of the sound, as shown in Fig. 12.6.

Physiologic splitting of S$_1$ and S$_2$. Each normal heart sound has two components: right and left. Mitral valve closure and tricuspid valve closure are responsible for S$_1$, and aortic valve closure and pulmonic valve closure are responsible for S$_2$. All the components of the split sounds are high pitched and best heard with the diaphragm of the stethoscope (Fig. 12.7). Normally, sounds emitted from the left side are louder than sounds from the right because left ventricular contraction occurs milliseconds before right ventricular contraction. Physiologic splitting is accentuated by inspiration and usually disappears on expiration. This splitting is most easily detected on inspiration because there is an increased amount of blood return to the right side of the heart and a decreased amount of blood return to the left side of the heart. As a result, pulmonic valve closure is delayed because of the extra time needed for the increased blood volume to pass through the pulmonic valve, and aortic valve closure is early because of the relatively smaller amount of blood ejected from the left ventricle. The resulting heart sound is a split S$_2$ (the closure of each valve is audible because there is more time between left and right contractions) (see Fig. 12.7).

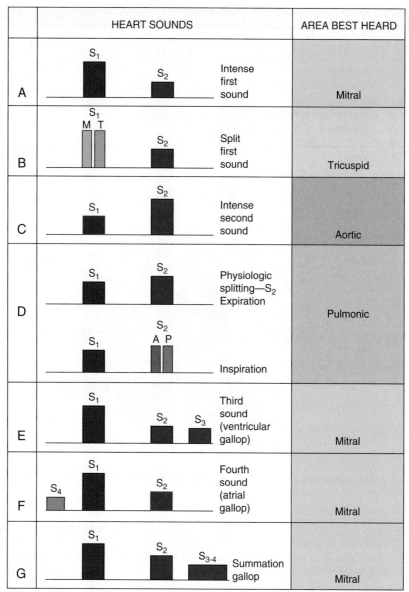

	HEART SOUNDS	AREA BEST HEARD
A	S_1 S_2 Intense first sound	Mitral
B	S_1 M T S_2 Split first sound	Tricuspid
C	S_1 S_2 Intense second sound	Aortic
D	S_1 S_2 Physiologic splitting—S_2 Expiration / S_1 S_2 A P Inspiration	Pulmonic
E	S_1 S_2 S_3 Third sound (ventricular gallop)	Mitral
F	S_4 S_1 S_2 Fourth sound (atrial gallop)	Mitral
G	S_1 S_2 S_{3-4} Summation gallop	Mitral

FIG. 12.7 Characteristics of Normal and Abnormal Heart Sounds and Auscultatory Area Where Each Is Best Heard.

Pathologic splitting of S_1 and S_2. A variety of abnormalities can alter the intensity and timing of split heart sounds. For example, during auscultation in the pulmonic area, a pathologic split is audible with a stethoscope if the pulmonic valve closure occurs after the aortic valve closure. Pathologic splitting of S_1 and S_2 is associated with specific cardiovascular conditions such as pulmonary hypertension, pulmonic stenosis, and right ventricular failure and with electrical conduction disturbances such as right bundle branch block and premature ventricular contractions.

Abnormal Heart Sounds

Third and fourth heart sounds. Abnormal heart sounds are known as the *third heart sound* (S_3) and the *fourth heart sound* (S_4); they are referred to as *gallops* when auscultated during an episode of tachycardia. These low-pitched sounds occur during diastole and are best heard with the bell of the stethoscope positioned lightly over the apical impulse. The characteristics

of S_3 and S_4 are described in detail in Box 12.11. The presence of S_3 may be normal in children, young adults, and pregnant women because of rapid filling of the ventricle in a young, healthy heart. However, S_3 in the presence of cardiac symptoms is an indicator of heart failure in a noncompliant ventricle with fluid overload.[25]

Auscultation of S_4 also leads the examiner to suspect heart failure and decreased ventricular compliance. Also referred to as an *atrial gallop*, S_4 occurs at the end of diastole (just before S_1), when the ventricle is full. It is associated with atrial contraction, also called *atrial kick*.

Heart Murmurs

Heart valve murmurs are prolonged extra sounds that occur during systole or diastole and are typically a sign of either ventricular dysfunction or *valvular heart disease*.[26] Murmurs are produced by turbulent blood flow through the chambers of the heart, from forward flow through narrowed or irregular valve

BOX 12.11   Characteristics of Third and Fourth Heart Sounds

Third Heart Sound (S₃)	Fourth Heart Sound (S₄)	Third Heart Sound (S₃)	Fourth Heart Sound (S₄)
Physiologic Causes	Related to diastolic motion and ventricular dilation with atrial contraction in late diastole	Ventricular dysfunction with increase in end-systolic volume (MI, heart failure, valvular disease, systemic or pulmonary hypertension)	Acute valvular regurgitation
Related to diastolic motion and rapid filling of ventricles in early diastole	May occur with or without cardiac decompensation	Hyperdynamic states (anemia, thyrotoxicosis, mitral or tricuspid regurgitation)	
Can be normal in children and young adults (<40 years old)	Ventricular hypertrophy with decrease in ventricular compliance (CAD, systemic hypertension, cardiomyopathy, aortic or pulmonary stenosis, increase in intensity with acute MI or angina)	Rhythmic Word Association "Kentucky": S₁, S₂, S₃	Rhythmic Word Association "Tennessee": S₄, S₁, S₂
		Synonyms	Synonyms
		Ventricular gallop	Atrial gallop
Pathologic Causes	Hyperkinetic states (anemia, thyrotoxicosis, arteriovenous fistula)	Protodiastolic gallop	Presystolic gallop

CAD, coronary artery disease; *MI*, myocardial infarction.

openings, or backward regurgitant flow through an incompetent valve. Murmurs occur in both systole and diastole. Most murmurs are caused by structural cardiac changes. The steps to auscultate effectively and accurately for cardiac murmurs are listed in Box 12.12. Murmurs are characterized by specific criteria as follows:

Timing: Place in the cardiac cycle (systole/diastole)

Location: Where the sound is auscultated on the chest wall (mitral or aortic area)

Radiation: How far the sound spreads across the chest wall

Quality: Whether the murmur is blowing, grating, or harsh

Pitch: Whether the tone is high or low

Intensity: Loudness is graded on a scale of 1 through 6; the higher the number, the louder the murmur (Box 12.13)

The four most common valvular murmurs auscultated in adults are briefly discussed in the following paragraphs. For more information on valvular anatomy, refer to Chapter 11; for information on valvular heart disease diagnostic procedures, see Chapter 13; and for valve-related therapeutic interventions, see Chapter 14.

Mitral stenosis. The term *mitral stenosis* refers to narrowing of the mitral valve orifice. This narrowing produces a low-pitched murmur, which varies in intensity and harshness depending on the degree of valvular stenosis. It occurs during diastole, is auscultated at the mitral area (fifth intercostal space, midclavicular line), and does not radiate. A prolonged duration of the murmur during diastole suggests that the mitral stenosis is severe.[1] As mitral stenosis progresses, left atrial enlargement occurs, often leading to atrial fibrillation and development of left atrial thrombi. The increased left atrial pressure increases pressure in the pulmonary vasculature. This causes a moist cough, decreased exercise tolerance, and breathlessness (dyspnea), especially with exercise.[26]

Mitral regurgitation. Mitral regurgitation is described as acute or chronic. Causes of acute mitral regurgitation include rupture of a papillary muscle after an acute myocardial infarction (MI) and rupture of one or more chordae tendineae. As a result, when the ventricle contracts during systole, a jet of blood is sent in a retrograde manner to the left atrium, causing a sudden increase in left atrial pressure, acute pulmonary edema, and low cardiac output and leading to cardiogenic shock.

BOX 12.12   Technique of Auscultation of Heart Sounds and Murmurs

1. Stethoscope
- Diaphragm
  - Larger surface area
  - Brings out higher frequency and filters out lower frequency
  - Use for listening to S₁/S₂ (split S₁/S₂), loud murmurs, pericardial friction rubs
- Bell
  - Smaller surface area
  - Filters out high-frequency sounds and accentuates low-frequency sounds
  - Rest lightly on area (or else it becomes a diaphragm)
2. Location: Heart sounds auscultated at *APTM*
   - *A:* Aortic area (second right ICS along sternal border)
   - *P:* Pulmonic area (second left ICS along sternal border)
   - *T:* Tricuspid area (fourth left ICS along sternal border)
   - *M:* Mitral area (fifth ICS at MCL)
3. "Know your bases"
- Base of the heart refers to the right and left second ICS beside the sternum S₂ where the aortic or pulmonic sounds are auscultated
- Apex or left ventricular area refers to the fifth ICS along the MCL
  - Most commonly referred to as PMI
  - Also referred to as mitral area
  - S₁ and mitral sounds are loudest here
- Erb's point: Second aortic area (third left ICS along sternal border); pericardial friction rubs are heard best here
4. Palpation
- Location
- Palpate carotid pulse (or watch ECG to identify S₁ and S₂)
5. Be quiet and patient
- Listen for S₁ and S₂ first, ignoring all other sounds
- Inching technique
- After you are sure which is S₁ or S₂, try to determine when the other sound comes in
- Is it systolic or diastolic?
- S₃ and S₄ are best heard with patient in left lateral decubitus position; note the location (suggests origin of sound)
- Note the timing (S₄ comes just before S₁, and S₃ comes just after S₂)
6. Interpret the sounds based on the clinical condition

ECG, electrocardiogram; *ICS*, intercostal space; *MCL*, midclavicular line; *PMI*, point of maximal impulse.

BOX 12.13 Grading of Cardiac Murmurs

Grade	Description
1	Very faint; may be heard only in quiet environment
2	Quiet but clearly audible
3	Moderately loud
4	Loud; may be associated with palpable thrill
5	Very loud; thrill easily palpable
6	Very loud; may be heard with stethoscope off the chest Thrill palpable and visible

Chronic primary mitral regurgitation is caused by deterioration of the valve structures (leaflets, chordae tendineae). It occurs in older adults from loss of valvular connective tissue and in younger adults from myxomatous degenerative valve changes associated with mitral prolapse.[26] The murmur of mitral regurgitation is auscultated in the mitral area and occurs during systole. It is high pitched and blowing, although the pitch and intensity vary depending on the degree of regurgitation. As mitral regurgitation progresses, the murmur radiates more widely. The murmur of mitral regurgitation can also occur when a dilated ventricle impedes the mitral valve from closing completely during systole.[26] One can detect the murmur with auscultation but not the cause of mitral regurgitation.

Aortic stenosis. The term *aortic stenosis* describes narrowing of the aortic valve orifice. As a result, the left ventricle faces increasing difficulty in ejecting blood to the aorta. The ventricle responds by increasing intraventricular pressure and adding muscle mass (left ventricular hypertrophy).[27] Over time, because of the pressure load and the increasingly restricted aortic valve outflow, the left ventricle fails and loses contractile force. The decreased blood volume entering the aorta during systole means that the coronary arteries do not fill efficiently, and chest pain is a common symptom of aortic stenosis. This chest pain can be difficult to differentiate from angina caused by CAD. Other symptoms include dizziness, syncope, and breathlessness secondary to left ventricular heart failure. After symptoms occur, the clinical course is poor unless the aortic valve is replaced. The murmur of aortic stenosis occurs during systole. It is auscultated at the aortic area (second intercostal space, right sternal border). Aortic stenosis produces a low-pitched murmur that does not radiate, although the tone of the murmur varies, depending on the degree of valvular obstruction. Because a strong correlation does not exist between the loudness of the murmur, clinical symptoms, and the severity of the stenosis, it is important to use transthoracic echocardiography to visualize the valve after an aortic stenosis murmur is detected.[26,28]

Aortic insufficiency. The term *aortic regurgitation* describes an incompetent aortic valve. Also commonly known as *aortic insufficiency*, it is often described in layperson's terms as a "leaking valve." After the left ventricle has ejected blood into the aorta, the valve normally closes, maintains a tight seal, and prevents blood from moving back into the left ventricle. If the valve cusps do not maintain this seal, the sound of blood flowing back into the left ventricle during diastole is heard as a decrescendo, high-pitched, blowing murmur. This early diastolic murmur is initially audible at the aortic area (second intercostal space, right sternal border), but as the aortic regurgitation progresses, it can be auscultated along the length of the left sternal border. As with all valvular murmurs, the pitch and intensity vary with the degree of regurgitation. Physical assessment findings are initially investigated noninvasively by echocardiography.[26] Invasive diagnostic testing subsequently may be required as described in Chapter 13. Box 12.14 lists expected abnormal findings at each of the key auscultation areas; Table 12.4 compares the features of the most common valvular murmurs.

Innocent Murmurs

In children, adolescents, and healthy young adults, systolic "high-flow" murmurs are common and are a result of vigorous ventricular contraction. These nonpathologic murmurs are termed *innocent murmurs*. They are always systolic, have a low to medium pitch (heard best with the bell of the stethoscope), and are of grade 1 to 2 intensity with a blowing quality. They are often heard best in the tricuspid area and do not radiate (Box 12.15).

Murmurs Associated With Myocardial Infarction

At the bedside, the nurse may be the first person to auscultate a new murmur. Holosystolic or pansystolic murmurs that can occur acutely as a complication of MI are good examples.

Papillary muscle rupture. The auscultation of a new, high-pitched, holosystolic, blowing murmur at the cardiac apex heralds mitral valve regurgitation resulting from papillary muscle dysfunction. This murmur may be soft (grade 1 or 2) and may occur only during ischemic episodes when papillary muscle contractility is impaired, but its presence is associated with persistent pain, ventricular failure, and higher mortality. If the murmur is loud (grade 5 or 6), harsh, and radiating in all directions from the apex, the papillary muscle or the chordae tendineae may have ruptured. The clinical auscultation of a new murmur is always confirmed by transthoracic or transesophageal echocardiography.[26] Papillary muscle rupture is an emergency situation requiring immediate medical and surgical intervention.

Ventricular septal rupture. Ventricular septal rupture is a rare emergency situation that can occur after an acute MI. Ventricular septal rupture describes a new opening in the septum between the two ventricles. It creates a harsh, holosystolic murmur that is loudest (by auscultation) along the left sternal border.[29] The murmur does not vary with respiration.[1] The clinical picture associated with acute ventricular septal rupture is that of acute ventricular failure and cardiogenic shock. Immediate diagnosis and treatment are necessary to prevent death.[29]

Cardiac Rubs

Pericardial friction rub. A *pericardial friction rub* is a sound that can occur 2 to 7 days after an MI. The friction rub results from pericardial inflammation (*pericarditis*). A pericardial friction rub can be auscultated in one-third of cases.[30] Classically, a pericardial friction rub is a grating or scratching sound that is both systolic and diastolic, corresponding with cardiac motion within the pericardial sac. It is often associated with chest pain, which can be aggravated by deep inspiration, coughing, swallowing, and changing position. It is important to differentiate pericarditis from acute myocardial ischemia, and the detection of a pericardial friction rub through auscultation can assist in this differentiation, leading to effective diagnosis and treatment.[30]

BOX 12.14 Auscultation of the Cardiac Valves

Aortic Area
- S_2 loud
- Aortic systolic murmur

Tricuspid Area
- S_1 split
- Right ventricular S_3 and S_4
- Tricuspid valve murmurs
- Murmur of ventricular septal defect

Pulmonic Area
- S_2 loud and split with inhalation

- Pulmonic valve murmurs

Mitral Area
- S_1 loud
- Left ventricular S_3 and S_4
- Mitral valve murmurs

Erb's Point
- S_2 split with inhalation
- Aortic diastolic murmur
- Pericardial friction rub

TABLE 12.4 Characteristics of Some Murmurs

Defects	Timing in Cardiac Cycle	Pitch; Intensity; Quality	Location; Radiation
Systolic Murmurs			
Mitral regurgitation	S_1 — S_2	High; harsh; blowing	Mitral area; may radiate to axilla
Tricuspid regurgitation	S_1 — S_2	High; often faint, but varies; blowing	Tricuspid RLSB, apex, LLSB, epigastric areas; little radiation
Ventricular septal defect	S_1 — S_2	High; loud; blowing	Left sternal border
Aortic stenosis	S_1 ◇ S_2	Chhhh hh; medium; rough, harsh	Aortic area to suprasternal notch, right side of neck, apex
Pulmonary stenosis	S_1 ◇ S_2	Low to medium; loud; harsh, grinding	Pulmonic area; no radiation
Diastolic Murmurs			
Mitral stenosis	Atrial kick S_2 — S_1	Low; quiet to loud with thrill; rough rumble	Mitral area; usually no radiation
Tricuspid stenosis	Atrial kick S_2 — S_1	Medium; quiet; louder with inspiration; rumble	Tricuspid area or epigastrium; little radiation
Aortic regurgitation	S_2 — S_1	High; faint to medium; blowing	Aortic area to LLSB and aorta; Erb's point
Pulmonic regurgitation	S_2 — S_1	Medium; faint; blowing	Pulmonic area; no radiation

LLSB, left lower sternal border; *RLSB*, right lower sternal border.

BOX 12.15 Description of Innocent Murmurs

- Always systolic
- Soft, short (grade 1 or 2, low pitched)
- Modified by change in position

- Normal S_2
- Most common at left sternal border

SUMMARY

- An accurate history from the patient or from a family member or significant other who knows the individual's current state of health is essential. Signs and symptoms experienced by the patient offer clues as to the underlying causes of the cardiac condition. If the patient exhibits obvious signs of acute distress (shortness of breath, pink-frothy sputum, hypotension, tachycardia, pallor, sweating) or complains of chest pain or pressure, the questions are brief and focused to quickly identify the immediate problem.
- Inspection is used to determine whether the patient is anxious or relaxed. Inspection is also employed to identify serious conditions such as cyanosis, clubbing of fingernails, or significant peripheral edema.
- Palpation of the major pulses is a routine part of the cardiovascular physical examination. Normally, pulses are equal bilaterally. The loss of a pulse on one side may indicate the presence of atherosclerotic arterial vascular disease.
- Auscultation of heart sounds and murmurs is a skill that takes time and practice to master. When performed skillfully, auscultation can reveal much about cardiac function and blood flow.

ⓔ Visit the Evolve site for additional study materials.

REFERENCES

1. Higgins JP. Physical examination of the cardiovascular system. *Int J Clin Cardiol.* 2015;2(1):1-7.
2. Foy AJ, Filippone L. Chest pain evaluation in the emergency department. *Med Clin North Am.* 2015;99(4):835-847.
3. Fanaroff AC, et al. Does this patient with chest pain have acute coronary syndrome? The rational clinical examination systematic review. *JAMA.* 2015;314(18):1955-1965.
4. Amsterdam EA, et al. 2014 AHA/ACC guideline for the management of patients with non-ST-elevation acute coronary syndromes: executive summary: a report of the American College of Cardiology/American Heart Association Task Force on Practice Guidelines. *Circulation.* 2014;130(25):2354-2394.
5. Tully AS, Trayes KP, Suddiford JS. Evaluation of nail abnormalities. *Am Fam Physician.* 2012;85(8):779-787.
6. Hirsch AT, et al. A call to action: women and peripheral artery disease: a scientific statement from the American Heart Association. *Circulation.* 2012;125:1449-1472.
7. Cornier MA, et al. Assessing adiposity: a scientific statement from the American Heart Association. *Circulation.* 2011;124:1996-2019.
8. Kushner RF, Ryan DH. Assessment and lifestyle management of patients with obesity: clinical recommendations from systematic reviews. *JAMA.* 2014;312(9):943-952.
9. Rao G, et al. Identification of obesity and cardiovascular risk in ethnically and racially diverse populations: a scientific statement from the American Heart Association. *Circulation.* 2015;132(5):457-472.
10. Pellicori P, et al. Revisiting a classical clinical sign: jugular venous ultrasound. *Int J Cardiol.* 2014;170(3):364-370.
11. Lima A, Bakker J. Clinical assessment of peripheral circulation. *Curr Opin Crit Care.* 2015;21(3):226-231.
12. Mrgan M, Rytter D, Brabrand M. Capillary refill time is a predictor of short-term mortality for adult patients admitted to a medical department: an observational cohort study. *Emerg Med J.* 2014;31(12):954-958.
13. James PA, et al. 2014 evidence-based guideline for the management of high blood pressure in adults: report from the panel members appointed to the Eighth Joint National Committee (JNC 8). *JAMA.* 2014;311(5):507-520.
14. Ambrosius WT, et al. The design and rationale of a multicenter clinical trial comparing two strategies for control of systolic blood pressure: the Systolic Blood Pressure Intervention Trial (SPRINT). *Clin Trials.* 2014;11(5):532-546.
15. SPRINT Research Group, et al. A randomized trial of intensive versus standard blood-pressure control. *N Engl J Med.* 2015;373(22):2103-2116.
16. Bress AP, et al. Generalizability of results from the Systolic Blood Pressure Intervention Trial (SPRINT) to the US adult population. *J Am Coll Cardiol.* 2016;67(5):463-472.
17. Singh S, et al. Prevalence of simultaneously measured interarm systolic blood pressure difference and its clinical and demographic predictors: a systemic review and meta-analysis. *Blood Press Monit.* 2015;20(4):178-185.
18. Stewart JM. Mechanisms of sympathetic regulation in orthostatic intolerance. *J Appl Physiol.* 2012;113(10):1659-1668.
19. Ricci F, De Caterina R, Fedorowski A. Orthostatic hypotension: epidemiology, prognosis, and treatment. *J Am Coll Cardiol.* 2015;66(7):848-860.
20. Aronow WS, et al. ACCF/AHA 2011 Expert Consensus Document on Hypertension in the Elderly: a report of the American College of Cardiology Foundation Task Force on Clinical Expert Consensus Documents. *Circulation.* 2011;123:2434-2506.
21. E.N.A. Emergency Nursing Resources Development Committee: emergency Nursing Resource: orthostatic vital signs. *J Emerg Nurs.* 2012;38(5):447-453.
22. Hamzaoui O, Monnet X, Teboul JL. Pulsus paradoxus. *Eur Respir J.* 2013;42(6):1696-1705.
23. Solomon SD, Sadana F. Point-of-care ultrasound in medical education—stop listening and look. *N Engl J Med.* 2014;370(12):1083-1085.
24. Frishman WH. Is the stethoscope becoming an outdated diagnostic tool? *Am J Med.* 2015;128(7):668-669.
25. Minami Y, et al. Third heart sound in hospitalised patients with acute heart failure: insights from the ATTEND study. *Int J Clin Pract.* 2015;69(8):820-828.
26. Nishimura RA, et al. 2014 AHA/ACC Guideline for the Management of Patients With Valvular Heart Disease: a report of the American College of Cardiology/American Heart Association Task Force on Practice Guidelines. *Circulation.* 2014;129(23):e521-e643.
27. Otto CM, Prendergast B. Aortic-valve stenosis—from patients at risk to severe valve obstruction. *N Engl J Med.* 2014;371(8):744-756.
28. Foppa M, Rao SN, Manning WJ. Doppler echocardiography in the evaluation of a heart murmur. *JAMA.* 2015;313(10):1050-1051.
29. Jones BM, et al. Ventricular septal rupture complicating acute myocardial infarction: a contemporary review. *Eur Heart J.* 2014;35(31):2060-2068.
30. Imazio M, Gaita F, LeWinter M. Evaluation and treatment of pericarditis: a systematic review. *JAMA.* 2015;314(14):1498-1506.

13

Cardiovascular Diagnostic Procedures

Mary E. Lough

Numerous cardiovascular diagnostic procedures are used in the diagnosis and management of critically ill patients. These are discussed under the major headings of "Hemodynamic Monitoring "Electrocardiography," "Laboratory Tests," and "Diagnostic Procedures."

HEMODYNAMIC MONITORING

Hemodynamic monitoring follows a spectrum of very invasive, moderately invasive, minimally invasive, and noninvasive methods (Fig. 13.1). Every method has advantages and disadvantages, and all require an understanding of the physiologic principles that guide diagnostic assessment and management. In clinical practice, there is tremendous variation in the technologies used depending on the setting and patient acuity. Some methods are based on pressure monitoring and others rely on visual displays. Hemodynamic technologies are discussed in this chapter following a more-invasive to less-invasive trajectory.[1-3]

Hemodynamic Monitoring Equipment

A traditional hemodynamic monitoring system has four component parts (Fig. 13.2):
1. An invasive catheter and high-pressure tubing connect the patient to the transducer.
2. The transducer receives the physiologic signal from the catheter and tubing and converts it into electrical energy.
3. The flush system maintains patency of the fluid-filled system and catheter.
4. The bedside monitor contains the amplifier with recorder, which increases the volume of the electrical signal and displays it on an oscilloscope and on a digital scale in millimeters of mercury (mm Hg).

Although many different types of invasive catheters can be inserted to monitor hemodynamic pressures, all such catheters are connected to similar equipment (see Fig. 13.2). However, there is variation in the way different hospitals configure their hemodynamic systems. The basic setup consists of the following:
- A bag of 0.9% sodium chloride (also known as normal saline) is used as a flush solution. In some hospitals, heparin is added as an anticoagulant. A pressure infusion cuff covers the bag of flush solution and is inflated to 300 mm Hg.
- The system contains intravenous (IV) tubing, three-way stopcocks, and an in-line flow device attached for continuous fluid infusion and manual flush. High-pressure tubing must be used to connect the invasive catheter to the transducer to prevent damping (flattening) of the waveform.
- A pressure transducer is used. Transducers are disposable and use a silicon chip.

Heparin

The use of the anticoagulant heparin added to the normal saline flush setup to maintain catheter patency is controversial.[4,5] Although many units do add heparin to flush solutions, other critical care units avoid heparin because of concern about development of heparin-induced antibodies that can trigger an autoimmune condition known as heparin-induced thrombocytopenia (HIT). This condition is sometimes described as a "heparin allergy" and, when present, is associated with a dramatic decrease in platelet count and thrombus formation. If heparin is used in the flush infusion, ongoing monitoring of the platelet count is recommended.[6]

Flush solutions, lines, stopcocks, and disposable transducers are changed every 96 hours per current US Centers for Disease Control and Prevention guidelines.[7] However, there is variation in practice among hospitals; some change the flush solutions every 24 hours. For this reason, it is essential to be familiar with the specific written procedures that concern hemodynamic monitoring equipment in each critical care unit. Dextrose solutions are not recommended as flush solutions in monitoring catheters.[7]

Calibration of Hemodynamic Monitoring Equipment

To ensure accuracy of hemodynamic pressure readings, two baseline measurements are necessary:
1. Calibration of the system to atmospheric pressure, also known as *zeroing the transducer*
2. Determination of the phlebostatic axis for transducer height placement, also called *leveling the transducer*[8]

Zeroing the Transducer

To calibrate the equipment to atmospheric pressure, referred to as zeroing the transducer, the three-way stopcock nearest to the transducer is turned simultaneously to open the transducer to air (atmospheric pressure) and to close it to the patient and the flush system. The monitor is adjusted so that "0" is displayed, which equals atmospheric pressure. Atmospheric pressure is not zero; it is 760 mm Hg at sea level. Using zero to represent current atmospheric pressure provides a convenient baseline for hemodynamic measurement purposes.

Some monitors also require calibration of the upper scale limit while the system remains open to air. At the end of the calibration procedure, the stopcock is returned to the closed position, and a closed cap is placed over the open port. At this point, the patient's waveform and hemodynamic pressures are displayed.

Disposable transducers are very accurate, and after they are calibrated to atmospheric pressure, drift from the zero baseline

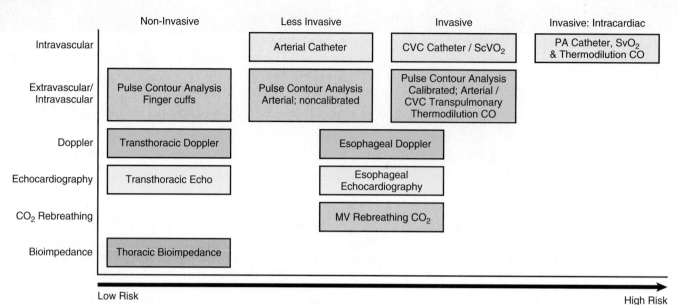

FIG. 13.1 Overview of options for hemodynamic monitoring in critical care from noninvasive to highly invasive, from low risk to high risk, and listing the different monitoring options that are available. Each of these monitoring options is discussed in the chapter. *CO,* Cardiac Output; *CO₂,* carbon dioxide; *CVC,* central venous catheter; *MV,* Mechanical Ventilation; *ScvO₂, SvO₂*

is minimal. Although in theory this means that repeated calibration is unnecessary, clinical protocols in most units require the nurse to calibrate the transducer at the beginning of each shift for quality assurance.

Phlebostatic Axis

The phlebostatic axis is a physical reference point on the chest that is used as a baseline for consistent transducer height placement. To obtain the axis, a theoretical line is drawn from the fourth sternal intercostal space, where it joins the sternum, to a theoretical line on the side of the chest that is one-half of the depth of the lateral chest wall.[8] This theoretical line approximates the level of the atria, as shown in Fig. 13.2. It is used as the reference mark for central venous pressure (CVP) and pulmonary artery (PA) catheter transducers. The level of the transducer "air reference stopcock" approximates the position of the tip of an invasive hemodynamic monitoring catheter within the chest.

Leveling the Transducer

Leveling the transducer is different from zeroing. This process aligns the transducer with the level of the left atrium. The purpose is to line up the *air–fluid interface* with the left atrium to correct for changes in *hydrostatic pressure* in blood vessels above and below the level of the heart.[8]

A carpenter's level or laser-light level can be used to ensure that the transducer is parallel with the phlebostatic axis reference point. When there is a change in the patient's position, the transducer must be leveled again to ensure that accurate hemodynamic pressure measurements are obtained.[8] Errors in measurement can occur if the transducer is placed below the phlebostatic axis because the fluid in the system weighs on the transducer, creating additional hydrostatic pressure, and produces a falsely high reading. For every inch the transducer is below the tip of the catheter, the fluid pressure in the system increases the measurement by 1.87 mm Hg. For example, if the transducer is positioned 6 inches below the tip of the catheter, this falsely elevates the displayed pressure by 11 mm Hg.

If the transducer is placed above this atrial level, gravity and lack of fluid pressure give an erroneously low reading. For every inch the transducer is positioned above the catheter tip, the measurement is 1.87 mm Hg less than the true value. If several clinicians are taking measurements, the reference point can be marked on the side of the patient's chest to ensure accurate measurements.

Patient Position During Hemodynamic Monitoring

The position of the patient during hemodynamic monitoring would not be an issue if critical care patients remained supine. However, the emphasis on raising the head of the bed above 30 degrees and frequent position changes to avoid pressure ulcers and bedside procedures mandate a reevaluation of transducer level with each position change.

Head of Bed Backrest Position

Nurse researchers have determined that the CVP, pulmonary artery pressure (PAP), and pulmonary artery occlusion pressure (PAOP)—also known as *pulmonary artery wedge pressure*—can be reliably measured at head of bed backrest positions from 0 (flat) to 60 degrees if the patient is lying on his or her back (supine).[8] If the patient is normovolemic and hemodynamically stable, raising the head of the bed usually does not affect hemodynamic pressure measurements. If the patient is so hemodynamically unstable or hypovolemic that raising the head of the bed negatively affects intravascular volume distribution, the first priority is to correct the hemodynamic instability and leave the patient in a lower backrest position. Most patients do not need the head of the bed to be lowered to 0 degrees to obtain accurate CVP, PAP, or PAOP readings.

Lateral Position

The landmarks for leveling the transducer are different if the patient is turned to the side. Researchers have evaluated hemodynamic pressure measurement readings with patients in the 30-degree and 90-degree lateral positions with the head

Normal saline and pressure bag

Bedside monitor

Macrodrip chamber

Electrical cable

High-pressure tubing

Fluid-filled tubing for flush

Invasive catheter

45

Roller clamp

30

Electrical connection

Disposable transducer

3-way stopcock (air reference)

Phlebostatic axis

Manual flush

0

Patient with invasive catheter

FIG. 13.2 The four parts of a hemodynamic monitoring system include an invasive catheter attached to high-pressure tubing to connect to the transducer; a transducer; a flush system, including a manual flush; and a bedside monitor.

of the bed flat, and they found the measurements to be reliable.[8] In the 30-degree angle position, the landmark to use for leveling the transducer is one-half of the distance from the surface of the bed to the left sternal border.[8] In the 90-degree right-lateral position, the transducer fluid–air interface was positioned at the fourth intercostal space at the midsternum. In the 90-degree left-lateral position, the transducer was positioned at the left parasternal border (beside the sternum).[8] It is important to know that measurements can be recorded in nonsupine positions, because critically ill patients must be turned to prevent development of pressure ulcers and other complications of immobility.

Intraarterial Blood Pressure Monitoring
Indications
Intraarterial blood pressure monitoring is considered lessinvasive than catheters placed into a central vein or through the cardiac chambers. Arterial blood pressure monitoring is indicated for any major medical or surgical condition that has the potential to alter blood pressure or cardiac output (CO), tissue perfusion, or fluid volume status. The system is designed for continuous measurement of three blood pressure parameters: systole, diastole, and mean arterial blood pressure (MAP). The direct arterial access is helpful in the management of patients with acute respiratory failure who require frequent arterial blood gas measurements.[4,9]

Catheters

The size of the catheter used is proportionate to the diameter of the cannulated artery. Catheters are most often inserted in the smaller arteries, using a "catheter-over-needle" unit in which the needle is used as a temporary guide for catheter placement. With this method, after the unit has been inserted into the artery, the needle is withdrawn, leaving the supple plastic catheter in place. To insert a catheter into a larger artery, the *Seldinger technique* is typically used, which involves the following steps:

1. Entry into the artery using a needle
2. Passage of a supple guidewire through the needle into the artery
3. Removal of the needle
4. Passage of the catheter over the guidewire
5. Removal of the guidewire, leaving the catheter in the artery

Insertion and Allen test. Several major peripheral arteries are suitable for receiving a catheter and for long-term hemodynamic monitoring. The most frequently used site is the radial artery. The femoral artery is a larger vessel that is also frequently cannulated. Other smaller arteries such as the dorsalis pedis, axillary, or brachial arteries are used only when other arterial access is unavailable.[4]

The major advantage of the radial artery is the supply of collateral circulation to the hand provided by the ulnar artery through the palmar arch in most people. Before radial artery cannulation, collateral circulation must be assessed by using Doppler flow or by the modified Allen test according to institutional protocol. In the Allen test, the radial and ulnar arteries are compressed simultaneously. The patient is asked to clench and unclench the hand until it blanches. One of the arteries is then released, and the hand should immediately flush from that side. The same procedure is repeated for the remaining artery.[4]

Nursing Management

Intraarterial blood pressure monitoring is designed for continuous assessment of arterial perfusion to the major organ systems of the body. MAP is the clinical parameter most often used to assess perfusion, as MAP represents perfusion pressure throughout the cardiac cycle. Because one-third of the cardiac cycle is spent in systole and two-thirds is spent in diastole, the MAP calculation must reflect the greater amount of time spent in diastole. This MAP formula can be calculated by hand or with a calculator, where diastole times 2 plus systole is divided by 3 as shown in the following formula:

$$\frac{(\text{Diastole} \times 2) + (\text{Systole} \times 1)}{3} = \text{MAP}$$

A blood pressure of 120/60 mm Hg produces a MAP of 80 mm Hg. However, the bedside hemodynamic monitor may show a slightly different digital number because bedside monitoring computers calculate the area under the curve of the arterial line tracing (Table 13.1).

Infection. Infection was once believed to be rare in arterial catheters because of the rapid arterial blood flow. New evidence suggests that arterial catheters are associated with the same risk of bloodstream infections as central venous catheters.[10] Therefore infection prevention measures must be just as meticulous for arterial catheters as for central catheters.[10]

Perfusion pressure. A MAP greater than 60 mm Hg is necessary to perfuse the coronary arteries. A higher MAP may be required to perfuse the brain and the kidneys. A MAP between 70 and 90 mm Hg is ideal for the cardiac patient to decrease left ventricular (LV) workload. After carotid endarterectomy or neurosurgery, a MAP of 90 to 110 mm Hg may be more appropriate to increase cerebral perfusion pressure. Systolic and diastolic pressures are monitored in conjunction with the MAP as a further guide to the accuracy of perfusion. If CO decreases, the body compensates by constricting peripheral vessels to maintain the blood pressure. In this situation, the MAP may remain constant, but the pulse pressure (difference between systolic and diastolic pressures) narrows. The following examples explain this point:

Mr. A: BP, 90/70 mm Hg; MAP, 76 mm Hg

Mr. B: BP, 150/40 mm Hg; MAP, 76 mm Hg

Both patients have a perfusion pressure of 76 mm Hg, but they are clinically very different. Mr. A is peripherally vasoconstricted, as is demonstrated by the narrow pulse pressure (90/70 mm Hg). His skin is cool to touch, and he has weak peripheral pulses. Mr. B has a wide pulse pressure (150/40 mm Hg), warm skin, and normally palpable peripheral pulses. Nursing assessment of a patient with an arterial line includes comparison of clinical findings with arterial line readings including perfusion pressure and MAP.

Pulse pressure. A clinical example of hemodynamic nursing assessment is presented. The patient is JW, 1 day after coronary artery bypass graft (CABG) surgery. JW recently has been weaned from dopamine and sodium nitroprusside and received an IV diuretic, 20 mg of furosemide (Lasix). He has voided 800 mL of urine via the urinary catheter during the past 2 hours. JW's MAP remains at 80 mm Hg, but his pulse pressure has narrowed by 30 mm Hg from 120/60 to 100/70 mm Hg. His heart rate (HR) has increased from 90 to 110 beats/min. This clinical situation is expected after furosemide administration, but the narrowed pulse pressure and increased HR may indicate hypovolemia. The nurse caring for JW will monitor the trend of the MAP. If the MAP begins to decrease and JW shows signs of a low CO, his physician will be notified. In most nonemergency situations, following the trend of the arterial pressure is more valuable than an isolated measurement.

Cuff blood pressure. If the arterial line becomes unreliable or dislodged, a cuff pressure can be used as a reserve system. In a normotensive, normovolemic patient, little difference exists between the arm cuff blood pressure and the intravascular catheter pressure, and differences of 5 to 10 mm Hg do not generally alter clinical management. The situation is different if the patient has a low CO or is in shock. The concern is that the cuff pressure may be unreliable because of peripheral vasoconstriction, and an arterial line is generally required. It is usual practice to compare a cuff pressure after the arterial line is inserted.[11]

Arterial Pressure Waveform Interpretation

As the aortic valve opens, blood is ejected from the left ventricle and is recorded as an increase of pressure in the arterial system. The highest point recorded is called *systole*. After peak ejection (systole), the force decreases, and the pressure falls. A notch (dicrotic notch) may be visible on the downstroke of this arterial waveform, representing closure of the aortic valve. The *dicrotic notch* signifies the start of blood flow into the arterial vasculature. The lowest point recorded is called *diastole*. A normal arterial pressure tracing is shown in Fig. 13.3. Electrical stimulation (QRS) is always first, and the arterial pressure tracing follows the initiating QRS complex.[12]

TABLE 13.1 Hemodynamic Pressures and Calculated Hemodynamic Values

Hemodynamic Pressure	Definition and Explanation	Normal Range
MAP	Average perfusion pressure created by arterial blood pressure during the cardiac cycle. The normal cardiac cycle is one-third systole and two-thirds diastole. These three components are divided by 3 to obtain the average perfusion pressure for the whole cardiac cycle.	70–100 mm Hg
CVP	Pressure created by volume in the right side of the heart. When the tricuspid valve is open, the CVP reflects filling pressures in the right ventricle. Clinically, the CVP is often used as a guide to overall fluid balance.	2–5 mm Hg 3–8 cm H_2O
LAP	Pressure created by the volume in the left side of the heart. When the mitral valve is open, the LAP reflects filling pressures in the left ventricle. Clinically, the LAP is used after cardiac surgery to determine how well the left ventricle is ejecting its volume. In general, the higher the LAP, the lower the ejection fraction from the left ventricle.	5–12 mm Hg
PAP	Pulsatile pressure in the pulmonary artery measured by an indwelling catheter.	
PAS		20–30 mm Hg
PAD		5–10 mm Hg
PAP_M		10–15 mm Hg
PAOP[a]	Pressure created by the volume in the left side of the heart. When the mitral valve is open, the PAOP reflects filling pressures in the pulmonary vasculature, and pressures in the left side of the heart are transmitted back to the catheter "wedged" into a small pulmonary arteriole.	5–12 mm Hg
CO	Amount of blood pumped out by a ventricle over 1 min. Clinically, it can be measured using the thermodilution CO method, which calculates CO in L/min.	4–6 L/min (at rest)
CI	CO divided by BSA, with tailoring of CO to individual body size. A BSA conversion chart is necessary to calculate CI, which is considered more accurate than CO because it is individualized to height and weight. CI is measured in L/min/m² of BSA.	2.2–4.0 L/min/m²
SV	Amount of blood ejected by the ventricle with each heartbeat, expressed in mL. Hemodynamic monitoring systems calculate SV by dividing CO (in L/min) by HR and then multiplying the answer by 1000 to change L to mL.	60–70 mL
SI	SV indexed to the BSA.	40–50 mL/m²
SVR	Mean pressure difference across the systemic vascular bed divided by blood flow. Clinically, SVR represents the resistance against which the left ventricle must pump to eject its volume. This resistance is created by the systemic arteries and arterioles. As SVR increases, CO falls. SVR is measured in Wood units or dyn • s • cm⁻⁵. If the number of Wood units is multiplied by 80, the value is converted to dyn • s • cm⁻⁵.	10–18 Wood units or 800–1400 dyn • s • cm⁻⁵
SVRI	SVR indexed to BSA.	2000–2400 dyn • s • cm⁻⁵
PVR	Mean pressure difference across pulmonary vascular bed divided by blood flow. Clinically, PVR represents the resistance against which the right ventricle must pump to eject its volume. This resistance is created by the pulmonary arteries and arterioles. As PVR increases, the output from the right ventricle decreases. PVR is measured in Wood units or dyn • s • cm⁻⁵. PVR is normally one-sixth of SVR.	1.2–3.0 Wood units or 100–250 dyn • s • cm⁻⁵
PVRI	PVR indexed to BSA.	225–315 dyn • s • cm⁻⁵
LCWI	Amount of work the left ventricle does *each minute* when ejecting blood. The hemodynamic formula represents pressure generated (MAP) multiplied by volume pumped (CO). A conversion factor is used to change mm Hg to kg-m. LCWI is always represented as an indexed volume (BSA chart). LCWI increases or decreases because of changes in pressure (MAP) or volume pumped (CO).	3.4–4.2 kg-m/m²
LVSWI	Amount of work the left ventricle performs with *each heartbeat*. The hemodynamic formula represents pressure generated (MAP) multiplied by volume pumped (SV). A conversion factor is used to change mL/mm Hg to g-m. LVSWI is always represented as an indexed volume. LVSWI increases or decreases because of changes in the pressure (MAP) or volume pumped (SV).	50–62 g-m/m²
RCWI	Amount of work the right ventricle performs *each minute* when ejecting blood. The hemodynamic formula represents pressure generated (PAP_M) multiplied by volume pumped (CO). A conversion factor is used to change mm Hg to kg-m. RCWI is always represented as an indexed value (BSA chart). Similar to LCWI, RCWI increases or decreases because of changes in the pressure (PAP_M) or volume pumped (CO).	0.54–0.66 kg-m/m²
RVSWI	Amount of work the right ventricle does *each heartbeat*. The hemodynamic formula represents pressure generated (PAP_M) multiplied by volume pumped (SV). A conversion factor is used to change mm Hg to g-m. RVSWI is always represented as an indexed value (BSA chart). Similar to LVSWI, RVSWI increases or decreases because of changes in the pressure (PAP_M) or volume pumped (SV).	7.9–9.7 g-m/m²

[a]Pulmonary artery occlusion pressure (PAOP) was formerly called *pulmonary capillary wedge pressure* (PCW or PCWP) or *pulmonary arterial wedge pressure* (PAWP).

BSA, body surface area; *CI*, cardiac index; *CO*, cardiac output; *CVP*, central venous pressure; *HR*, heart rate; *LAP*, left atrial pressure; *LCWI*, left cardiac work index; *LVSWI*, left ventricular stroke work index; *MAP*, mean arterial pressure; *PAD*, pulmonary artery diastolic; *PAOP*, pulmonary artery occlusion pressure; *PAP*, pulmonary artery pressure; *PAP_M*, mean pulmonary artery pressure; *PAS*, pulmonary artery systolic; *PVR*, pulmonary vascular resistance; *PVRI*, pulmonary vascular resistance index; *RCWI*, right cardiac work index; *RVSWI*, right ventricular stroke work index; *SI*, stroke volume index; *SV*, stroke volume; *SVR*, systemic vascular resistance; *SVRI*, systemic vascular resistance index.

Decreased arterial perfusion. Specific problems with heart rhythm can translate into poor arterial perfusion if CO decreases. Poor perfusion may be seen as a single, nonperfused beat after a premature ventricular contraction (PVC) (Fig. 13.4) or as multiple, nonperfused beats (Fig. 13.5). In ventricular bigeminy, every second beat is poorly perfused (Fig. 13.6). A disorganized atrial baseline resulting from atrial fibrillation creates a variable arterial pulse because of the differences in stroke volume (SV) between each beat

(Fig. 13.7). All these examples illustrate that when two beats are close together, the left ventricle does not have time to fill adequately, and the second beat is inadequately perfused or is not perfused at all.

Pulse deficit. A pulse deficit occurs when the apical HR and the peripheral pulse are not equal. In the critical care unit, this can be seen on the bedside monitor. Normally, there is one arterial upstroke for each QRS complex, and if there are more QRS complexes than arterial upstrokes, a pulse deficit

FIG. 13.3 Simultaneous ECG (A) and normal arterial pressure (B) tracings.

FIG. 13.4 Simultaneous ECG (A) and arterial pressure (B) tracings show normal arterial waveform with nonperfused premature ventricular contraction (PVC). The arterial waveform also shows evidence of pulsus paradoxus in a patient who is mechanically ventilated.

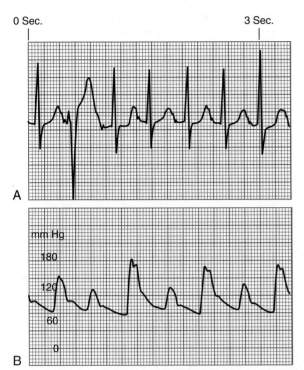

FIG. 13.5 Simultaneous ECG (A) and arterial pressure (B) tracings show pulsus alternans. A nonperfused premature ventricular contraction (PVC) is also present.

is present, as shown in Figs. 13.4 and 13.7. To identify a pulse deficit in an unmonitored patient, a stethoscope is placed over the apex of the heart. The heartbeat can be heard, but it cannot be felt as a radial pulse. To determine whether a pulse deficit is significant, it is necessary to evaluate the clinical impact on the patient and whether any change in MAP or pulse pressure has occurred. Generally, the more nonperfused beats, the more serious the problem.

Pulsus paradoxus. Pulsus paradoxus is a decrease of more than 10 mm Hg in the arterial waveform that occurs during inhalation (inspiration). It is caused by a fall in CO as a result of increased negative intrathoracic pressure during inhalation. As pressure within the thorax falls, blood pools in the large veins of the lungs and thorax, and SV is decreased. The procedure for identification of pulsus paradoxus is discussed in Chapter 12 (see Box 12.9).

In certain clinical conditions, the pulsus paradoxus is obvious and can be clearly seen on an arterial waveform. It can be used as a clinical diagnostic test in a patient with cardiac tamponade, pericardial effusion, or constrictive pericarditis.[13] Pulsus paradoxus commonly occurs in hypovolemic surgical patients who are mechanically ventilated with large tidal volumes (see Fig. 13.4).

Pulsus alternans. In pulsus alternans, every other arterial pulsation is weak. This sometimes occurs in individuals with advanced LV heart failure.

Damped waveform. If the arterial monitor shows a low blood pressure, it is important to determine whether it is a patient problem or a problem with the equipment, as described in Table 13.2. A low arterial blood pressure waveform is shown in Fig. 13.8. In this case, the digital readout correlated well with

FIG. 13.6 Simultaneous ECG (A) and arterial pressure (B) tracings show ventricular bigeminy. Every other ventricular beat is poorly perfused on the arterial pressure waveform. A well-perfused arterial pressure tracing is depicted (B) as the patient converts to normal sinus rhythm.

the patient's cuff pressure, confirming that the patient was hypotensive. This arterial waveform is more rounded, without a dicrotic notch, compared with the normal waveform in Fig. 13.3. A damped (flattened) arterial waveform is shown in Fig. 13.9. In this case, the patient's cuff pressure was significantly higher than the digital readout, representing a problem with equipment. A damped waveform occurs when communication from the artery to the transducer is interrupted and produces falsely lower values on the monitor and oscilloscope. Damping is often caused by a biofilm-fibrin "tail" that partially occludes the tip of the catheter, by kinks in the catheter or tubing, or by air bubbles in the system. Troubleshooting techniques (see Table 13.2) are used to find the origin of the problem and to remove the cause of damping.

Underdamped waveform. Another cause of arterial waveform distortion is *underdamping*, also called *overshoot* or *fling*. Underdamping is recognized by a narrow upward systolic peak that produces a falsely high systolic reading compared with the patient's cuff blood pressure, as shown in Fig. 13.10.

The overshoot is caused by an increase in dynamic response or increased oscillations within the system.

Fast-flush square waveform test. The dynamic response of the monitoring system can be verified for accuracy at the bedside by the *fast-flush square waveform test*, also called the *dynamic frequency response test*.[8] The nurse performs this test to ensure that the patient pressures and waveform shown on the bedside monitor are accurate.[8] The test makes use of the manual flush system on the transducer. Normally, the flush device allows only 3 mL of fluid per hour. With the normal waveform displayed, the manual fast-flush procedure is used to generate a rapid increase in pressure, which is displayed on the monitor oscilloscope. As shown in Fig. 13.11, the normal dynamic response waveform shows a square pattern with one or two oscillations before the return of the arterial waveform. If the system is overdamped, a sloped (rather than square) pattern is seen. If the system is underdamped, additional oscillations—or vibrations—are seen on the fast-flush square wave test. This test can be performed with any hemodynamic monitoring system. If air bubbles, clots,

FIG. 13.7 Simultaneous ECG (A) and arterial pressure (B) tracings show atrial fibrillation, which results in irregular atrial pulsations. The irregular pulsations create differences in beat-to-beat ventricular upstroke volume, resulting in diminished or absent ventricular output, as seen on the arterial waveform.

TABLE 13.2	Nursing Measures to Ensure Patient Safety and to Troubleshoot Problems With Hemodynamic Monitoring Equipment		
Problem	**Prevention**	**Rationale**	**Troubleshooting**
Overdamping of waveform	Provide continuous infusion of solution containing heparin through an in-line flush device (1 unit of heparin for each 1 mL of flush solution).	Ensure that recorded pressures and waveform are accurate because a damped waveform gives inaccurate readings.	Before insertion, completely flush the line and/or catheter. In a line attached to a patient, back flush through the system to clear bubbles from tubing or transducer.
Underdamping ("overshoot" or "fling")	Use short lengths of noncompliant tubing. Use fast-flush square wave test to demonstrate optimal system damping. Verify arterial waveform accuracy with the cuff blood pressure.	If the monitoring system is underdamped, the systolic and diastolic values will be overestimated by the waveform and the digital values. False high systolic values may lead to clinical decisions based on erroneous data.	Perform the fast-flush square wave test to verify optimal damping of the monitoring system.

TABLE 13.2   Nursing Measures to Ensure Patient Safety and to Troubleshoot Problems With Hemodynamic Monitoring Equipment—cont'd

Problem	Prevention	Rationale	Troubleshooting
Clot formation at end of the catheter	Provide continuous infusion of solution containing heparin through an in-line flush device (1 unit of heparin for each 1 mL of flush solution).	Any foreign object placed in the body can cause local activation of the patient's coagulation system as a normal defense mechanism. The clots that are formed may be dangerous if they break off and travel to other parts of the body.	If a clot in the catheter is suspected because of a damped waveform or resistance to forward flush of the system, gently aspirate the line using a small syringe inserted into the proximal stopcock. Flush the line again after the clot is removed, and inspect the waveform. It should return to a normal pattern.
Hemorrhage	Use Luer-Lock (screw) connections in line setup. Close and cap stopcocks when not in use.	A loose connection or open stopcock creates a low-pressure sump effect, causing blood to back into the line and into the open air. If a catheter is accidentally removed, the vessel can bleed profusely, especially with an arterial line or if the patient has abnormal coagulation factors (resulting from heparin in the line) or has hypertension.	After a blood leak is recognized, tighten all connections, flush the line, and estimate blood loss.
	Ensure that the catheter is sutured or securely taped in position.		If the catheter has been inadvertently removed, put pressure on the cannulation site. When bleeding has stopped, apply a sterile dressing, estimate blood loss, and inform the physician. If the patient is restless, an armboard may protect lines inserted in the arm.
Air emboli	Ensure that all air bubbles are purged from a new line setup before attachment to an indwelling catheter.	Air can be introduced at several times, including when CVP tubing comes apart, when a new line setup is attached, or when a new CVP or PA line is inserted. During insertion of a CVP or PA line, the patient may be asked to hold his or her breath at specific times to prevent drawing air into the chest during inhalation.	Because it is impossible to get the air back after it has been introduced into the bloodstream, prevention is the best cure.
	Ensure that the drip chamber from the bag of flush solution is more than one-half full before using the in-line, fast-flush system.	In-line, fast-flush devices are designed to permit clearing of blood from the line after withdrawal of blood samples.	If air bubbles occur, they must be vented through the in-line stopcocks, and the drip chamber must be filled.
	Some sources recommend removing all air from the bag of flush solution before assembling the system.	If the chamber of the intravenous tubing is too low or empty, the rapid flow of fluid will create turbulence and cause flushing of air bubbles into the system and into the bloodstream.	The LAP line setup is the only system that includes an air filter specifically to prevent air emboli.
Normal waveform with *low* digital pressure	Ensure that the system is calibrated to atmospheric pressure.	To provide a 0 baseline relative to atmospheric pressure.	Recalibrate the equipment if transducer drift has occurred.
	Ensure that the transducer is placed at the level of the phlebostatic axis.	If the transducer has been placed *higher* than the phlebostatic level, gravity and the lack of hydrostatic pressure will produce a false *low* reading.	Reposition the transducer at the level of the phlebostatic axis. Misplacement can occur if the patient moves from the bed to the chair or if the bed is placed in a Trendelenburg position.
Normal waveform with *high* digital pressure	Ensure that the system is calibrated to atmospheric pressure.	To provide a 0 baseline relative to atmospheric pressure.	Recalibrate the equipment if transducer drift has occurred.
	Ensure that the transducer is placed at the level of the phlebostatic axis.	If the transducer has been placed *lower* than the phlebostatic level, the weight of hydrostatic pressure on the transducer will produce a false *high* reading.	Reposition the transducer at the level of the phlebostatic axis.
			This situation can occur if the head of the bed was raised and the transducer was not repositioned. Some centers require attachment of the transducer to the patient's chest to avoid this problem.
Loss of waveform	Always have the hemodynamic waveform monitored so that changes or loss can be quickly noted.	The catheter may be kinked, or a stopcock may be turned off.	Check the line setup to ensure that all stopcocks are turned in the correct position and that the tubing is not kinked. Sometimes the catheter migrates against a vessel wall, and having the patient change position restores the waveform.

CVP, central venous pressure; *LAP,* left atrial pressure; *PA,* pulmonary artery.

FIG. 13.8 Simultaneous ECG (A) and arterial pressure (B) tracings show low arterial pressure waveform.

FIG. 13.9 Simultaneous ECG (A) and arterial pressure (B) tracings show damped arterial pressure waveform.

FIG. 13.10 Simultaneous ECG (A) and arterial pressure (B) tracings show the overshoot, or fling, caused by a heightened dynamic response in the monitoring system. The monitor recorded an arterial line blood pressure of 141/51 mm Hg. The patient's true blood pressure with a cuff was 110/54 mm Hg. The 110 mm Hg cuff systolic pressure is consistent with the arterial line tracing without "overshoot."

or kinks are in the system, the waveform becomes damped, or flattened, and this is reflected in the square waveform result.

This is an easy test to perform, and it should be incorporated into nursing care procedures at the bedside when the hemodynamic system is first set up, at least once per shift, after opening the system for any reason, and when there is concern about the accuracy of the waveform.[8] If the pressure waveform is distorted or the digital display is inaccurate, the troubleshooting methods described in Table 13.2 can be implemented. The nurse caring for a patient with an arterial line must be able to assess whether a low MAP or narrowed perfusion pressure represents decreased arterial perfusion or equipment malfunction.

Assessment of the arterial waveform on the oscilloscope, in combination with clinical assessment, and use of the square waveform test will yield the answer.

Hemodynamic monitoring alarms. All critically ill patients must have the hemodynamic monitoring alarms on and adjusted to sound an audible alarm if the patient should experience a change in blood pressure, HR, respiratory rate, or other significant monitored variable. A National Patient Safety Goal mandates reducing harm associated with clinical alarms. Alarm limits must be customized to the patient's physiologic baseline to reduce false-positive alarms.[14] The key issues concerning clinical monitor alarms are presented in Box 13.1.

Invasive Hemodynamic Monitoring

Invasive hemodynamic monitoring refers to monitoring situations where catheters are placed into central veins or pass through the right heart chambers (Fig. 13.1). This predominantly describes central venous catheters, pulmonary artery catheters, thermodilution cardiac output and continuous mixed-venous oxygen saturation monitoring. Some of the newer monitoring methods that combine arterial and central venous monitoring systems also are considered invasive (Fig. 13.1).

Central Venous Pressure Monitoring
Indications

CVP monitoring is indicated whenever a patient has a significant alteration in fluid volume (see Table 13.1). The CVP can be used as a guide in fluid volume replacement in hypovolemia and to assess the impact of diuresis after diuretic administration in the case of fluid overload. When a major IV line is required for volume replacement, a Central Venous Catheter (CVC) is used because large volumes of fluid can be delivered

Expected square wave test

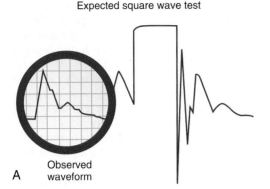

A Observed waveform

Overdamped

B Observed waveform

Underdamped

C Observed waveform

FIG. 13.11 Square Wave Test. (A) Expected square wave test result. (B) Overdamped. (C) Underdamped. (From Darovic GO. *Hemodynamic Monitoring: Invasive and Noninvasive Clinical Application.* 3rd ed. Philadelphia: Saunders; 2002.)

easily. Because of the risks associated with central lines during insertion and maintenance, this is considered an invasive form of hemodynamic monitoring.

Central Venous Catheters

The range of available CVC options includes single-lumen, double-lumen, triple-lumen, and quad-lumen infusion catheters, depending on the specific needs of the patient. CVCs are made from a variety of materials ranging from polyurethane to silicone; most are soft and flexible. Antimicrobial-impregnated or heparin-coated catheters have a lower rate of bloodstream infections.[7]

Insertion. The large veins of the upper thorax—subclavian (SC) and internal jugular (IJ)—are most commonly used for percutaneous CVC line insertion.[7] The femoral vein in the groin is used when the thoracic veins are not accessible. All three major sites have advantages and disadvantages.

Internal jugular vein. The IJ vein is the most frequently used access site for CVC insertion. Compared with the other thoracic veins, it is the easiest to canalize. If the IJ vein is unavailable, the external jugular vein may be accessed, although blood flow is significantly higher in the IJ vein, making it the preferred site. Another advantage of the IJ vein is that the risk of creating an iatrogenic pneumothorax is small. Disadvantages to the IJ vein are patient discomfort from the indwelling catheter when moving the head or neck and contamination of the IJ vein site from oral or tracheal secretions, especially if the patient is intubated or has a tracheostomy. This may be the reason why catheter-related infections are higher in the IJ than the SC position for indwelling catheters left in place for more than 4 days.

Subclavian vein. If the anticipated CVC dwelling time is prolonged (more than 5 days), the SC site is preferred. The SC position has the lowest infection rate and produces the least patient discomfort from the catheter. The disadvantages are that the SC vein is more difficult to access and carries a higher risk of iatrogenic pneumothorax or hemothorax, although the risk varies greatly depending on the experience and skill of the physician inserting the catheter.

Femoral vein. The femoral vein is considered the easiest cannulation site because there are no curves in the insertion route. The large diameter of the femoral vein carries a high blood flow that is advantageous for specialized procedures such as continuous renal replacement therapy or plasmapheresis. Because there is a higher rate of nosocomial infection with femoral catheters, this site is not recommended.[7] If a femoral venous access has been used, the CVC should be changed to either the SC or IJ location as soon as the patient is hemodynamically stable.[7]

During insertion of a catheter in the SC or IJ vein, the patient may be placed in a Trendelenburg position. Placing the head in a dependent position causes the IJ veins in the neck to become more prominent, facilitating line placement. To minimize the risk of air embolus during the procedure, the patient may be asked to "take a deep breath and hold it" any time the needle or catheter is open to air. The tip of the catheter is designed to remain in the vena cava and should not migrate into the right atrium. Because many patients are awake and alert when a CVC is inserted, a brief explanation about the procedure can minimize patient anxiety and result in cooperation during the insertion. This cooperation is important because CVC insertion is a sterile procedure and because the supine or Trendelenburg position may be uncomfortable for many patients. The electrocardiogram (ECG) should be monitored during CVC insertion because of the associated risk of dysrhythmias.

All CVCs are designed for placement by percutaneous injection after skin preparation and administration of a local anesthetic. Visualization of the vessel using bedside ultrasound before insertion is recommended to reduce CVC placement attempts.[7] A prepackaged CVC kit typically is used for the procedure. The standard CVC kit contains sterile towels, chlorhexidine and alcohol for skin preparation, a needle introducer, a syringe, guidewire, and a catheter. The Seldinger technique, in which the vein is located by using a "seeking" needle and syringe, is the preferred method of placement. A guidewire is passed through the needle, the needle is removed, and the catheter is passed over the guidewire. After the tip of the catheter is correctly placed in the vena cava, the guidewire is removed. Sterile IV tubing with solution is attached, and the catheter is sutured in place. A chest radiograph is obtained after upper thoracic CVC placement to verify placement and the absence of an iatrogenic hemothorax or pneumothorax, especially if the SC vein was accessed.

Central Venous Catheter Complications

The CVC is an essential tool in care of a critically ill patient, but it is associated with some risks, and it is the responsibility of all clinicians to be informed about these hazards and to follow hospital procedures to avoid iatrogenic complications. CVC complications include air embolus, catheter-associated thrombus formation, and infection.

Air embolus. The risk of air embolus, although uncommon, is always present for a patient with a central venous line in place. Air can enter during insertion through a disconnected or broken catheter by means of an open stopcock, or air can enter along the path of a removed CVC. This is more likely if the patient is in an upright position because air can be pulled into the venous system with the increase in negative intrathoracic pressure during inhalation. If a large volume of air is infused rapidly, it may become trapped in the right ventricular outflow tract, stopping blood flow from the right side of the heart to the lungs. Based on animal studies, this volume is approximately 4 mL/kg.[15] If the air embolus is large,

the patient experiences respiratory distress and cardiovascular collapse. An auscultatory clinical sign specifically associated with a large venous air embolism is the *mill wheel murmur*. A mill wheel murmur is a loud, churning sound heard over the middle chest, caused by the obstruction to right ventricular outflow. Treatment involves immediately occluding the external site where air is entering, administering 100% oxygen, and placing the patient on the left side with the head downward (left lateral Trendelenburg position). This position displaces the air from the right ventricular outflow tract to the apex of the heart, where the air may be aspirated by catheter intervention or gradually absorbed by the bloodstream as the patient remains in the left lateral Trendelenburg position. Precautions to prevent an air embolism in a CVP line include using only screw (Luer-Lock) connections, avoiding long loops of IV tubing, and using closed-top screw caps on the three-way stopcock.

Thrombus formation. Clot formation (thrombus) at the CVC site is common. Thrombus formation is not uniform; it may involve development of a *fibrin sleeve* around the catheter,[16] or the thrombus may be attached directly to the vessel wall. Other factors that promote clot formation include rupture of vascular endothelium, interruption of laminar blood flow, and physical presence of the catheter, all of which activate the coagulation cascade. The risk of thrombus formation is higher if insertion was difficult or there were multiple needlesticks. Gradual thrombus formation may lead to "sudden" CVC occlusion. Usually, it becomes more difficult to withdraw blood from the CVC, or the CVP waveform becomes intermittently damped over a period of hours or even 1 to 2 days and is reported as "needing frequent flushes" to remain patent. This situation is caused by the continued lengthening of a fibrin sleeve that extends along the catheter length from the insertion site past the catheter tip. Some catheters are heparin coated to reduce the risk of thrombus formation, although the risk of HIT does not make this a benign option. CVC complications can be additive; for example, the risk of catheter-related infection is increased in the presence of thrombi, where the thrombus likely serves as a culture medium for bacterial growth. Because of concerns over the development of HIT, many hospitals use a saline-only flush to maintain CVC patency.

Infection. Infection related to the use of CVCs is a major problem. The incidence of infection strongly correlates with the length of time the CVC has been inserted, with longer insertion times leading to higher infection rates.[7] CVC-related infection is identified at the catheter insertion site or as a bloodstream infection (septicemia). Systemic manifestations of infection can be present without inflammation at the catheter site. No decrease in bloodstream infections was found when catheters were routinely changed, and this practice is no longer recommended.[7] When a CVC is infected, it must be removed, and a new catheter must be inserted in a different site. If a catheter infection is suspected, the CVC should not be changed over a guidewire because of the risk of transferring the infection.[7]

Most infections are transmitted from the skin, and infection prevention begins before insertion of the CVC. Insertion guidelines state that the physician must use effective handwashing procedures, clean the insertion site with 2% chlorhexidine gluconate in 70% isopropyl, use sterile technique during catheter insertion, and maintain maximal sterile barrier precautions.[7] In most hospitals, the nurse is authorized to stop the procedure if these insertion infection control guidelines are not followed. A daily review to determine whether the central line is still required is recommended to ensure that CVCs are removed promptly when no longer needed (Box 13.2).[7] All clinicians must use good handwashing technique and follow aseptic procedures during site care and any time the CVC system is entered to withdraw blood, give medications, or change tubing.[7] Site dressings impregnated with chlorhexidine are recommended to reduce CVC infection rates.[7]

Nursing Management

In a critically ill patient, the CVC is used to monitor the CVP and waveform. The CVP catheter is used to measure the filling pressures of the right side of the heart. During diastole, when the tricuspid valve is open and blood is flowing from the right atrium to the right ventricle, the CVP accurately reflects right ventricular end-diastolic pressure. Normal CVP is 2 to 5 mm Hg (3 to 8 cm H_2O).

Central venous pressure—volume assessment. The time-honored practice of using the CVP value to assess central volume status has been challenged more recently.[17] A landmark systematic review of the literature revealed a weak relationship between the CVP measurement and blood volume.[17] Furthermore, a low CVP value was not always reliable in predicting who would respond to a fluid challenge.[17] Among patients with a CVP between 0 and 5 mm Hg, up to 25% do not respond to a fluid challenge as expected.[18] Overall, only approximately half of critically ill patients respond as expected to a fluid challenge.[17] In this situation, the clinician must look at other indices of poor tissue perfusion such as an elevated lactate level, low base deficit, or decreased urine output.[18]

Passive leg raise. Another method to assess fluid responsiveness is to passively raise and support the patient's legs to allow the venous blood from the lower extremities to flow rapidly into the vena cava and return to the right heart. This method has the advantage of not infusing any IV fluid.[19] If this maneuver significantly increases the CVP, this may suggest that the patient would have a positive response to an IV fluid bolus.[20] However, a change in the CVP value is not considered as reliable as using real-time monitoring of CO using a pulse wave analysis method as described later.[19]

Removal. Removal of the CVC usually is a nursing responsibility. Complications are infrequent, and the ones to anticipate are bleeding and air embolus. Recommended techniques to avoid air embolus during CVC removal include removing the catheter when the patient is supine in bed (not in a chair) and placing the patient flat or in reverse Trendelenburg position if the patient's clinical condition permits this maneuver. Patients with heart failure, pulmonary disease, and neurologic conditions with raised intracranial pressure should not be placed flat. If the patient is alert and able to cooperate, he or she is asked to take a deep breath to raise intrathoracic pressure during

---

QSEN BOX 13.2   QSEN: Patient Safety Alert

Prevention of Central Venous Catheter–Related Bloodstream Infections

1. Education, Training, and Staffing
   a. Nurses and other health care providers should receive education about indications for central venous catheter (CVC) use, maintenance, and infection prevention.
   b. Only trained personnel should insert and maintain CVCs.
   c. Adequate staffing levels in critical care units are associated with fewer catheter-related bloodstream infections (CRBSIs).
2. Selection of Catheters and Sites
   a. Use subclavian site rather than jugular or femoral insertion sites to minimize infection risk.
   b. Use ultrasound guidance to place CVCs.
   c. Remove any catheter that is no longer essential.
   d. If a CVC was placed in a medical emergency when aseptic technique was not assured, replace CVC within 48 h.
3. Hand Hygiene and Aseptic Technique
   a. Perform hand hygiene procedures by washing hands with soap and water or alcohol-based hand rub (ABHR) before and after palpating the CVC site, dressing the site, or any other intervention.
   b. New sterile gloves must be worn by the professional inserting the CVC.
   c. New sterile gloves must be donned before touching a new catheter for CVC exchange over a guidewire.
   d. Wear clean or sterile gloves when changing the catheter dressing.
4. Maximal Sterile Barrier Precautions
   a. For insertion, use maximal sterile barrier precautions including cap, mask, sterile gown, sterile gloves, and full-body drape.
5. Skin Preparation
   a. Prepare clean skin with greater than 0.5% chlorhexidine preparation with alcohol before CVC insertion.

b. Antiseptics should be allowed to dry according to the manufacturer's recommendation before CVC insertion.
6. Catheter Site Dressing Regimens
   a. Transparent, semipermeable polyurethane dressings permit continuous visualization of the CVC insertion site.
   b. Replace transparent dressings on CVC sites at least every 7 days.
   c. Monitor the site when changing the dressing or by palpation through an intact dressing.
   d. Replace catheter site dressing whenever the dressing becomes damp, loose, or soiled.
   e. Do not use topical antibiotic ointment or creams on insertion sites (except for dialysis catheters) because of increased fungal infection risk.
   f. Use a chlorhexidine-impregnated sponge dressing at CVC site if CRBSI rate is not decreasing by other means (no recommendation for other types of chlorhexidine dressings).
7. Patient Cleansing
   a. Use 2% chlorhexidine wash for daily skin cleaning to reduce CRBSIs.
8. Catheter Securement Device
   a. Use a sutureless catheter securement device to reduce catheter movement, which may reduce infection risk.
9. Antimicrobial Strategies
   a. Use an antimicrobial-impregnated CVC when catheters are expected to remain in place for longer than 5 days.
   b. Do not administer systemic antimicrobial prophylaxis to prevent CRBSIs.
   c. Do not routinely use anticoagulant therapy to prevent CRBSIs.
10. No Routine CVC Replacement
    a. Do not routinely replace CVCs.
    b. Do not replace CVCs on the basis of fever alone.

From O'Grady P, et al. Guidelines for the prevention of intravascular catheter-related infections. *Am J Infect Control.* 2011;39(4):S1-S34.

FIG. 13.12 Cardiac Events That Produce Central Venous Pressure Waveform With a, c, and v Waves. The a wave represents atrial contraction. The x descent represents atrial relaxation. The c wave represents the bulging of the closed tricuspid valve into the right atrium during ventricular systole. The v wave represents atrial filling. The y descent represents opening of the tricuspid valve and filling of the ventricle.

removal. After removal, to decrease the risk of air entering by a "track," an occlusive dressing is applied to the site. If bleeding at the site occurs after removal, firm pressure is applied. If a patient has prolonged coagulation times, fresh frozen plasma or platelets may be prescribed before CVC removal.

Patient position. To achieve accurate CVP measurements, the phlebostatic axis is used as a reference point on the body, and the transducer or water manometer zero must be level with this point. If the phlebostatic axis is used and the transducer or water manometer is correctly aligned, any head of bed position of up to 60 degrees may be used for accurate CVP readings for most patients.[8] Elevating the head of the bed is especially helpful for a patient with cardiopulmonary problems who cannot tolerate a flat position.

Central venous pressure waveform interpretation. The normal right atrial (CVP) waveform has three positive deflections—a, c, and v waves—that correspond to specific atrial events in the cardiac cycle (Fig. 13.12). The *a* wave reflects atrial contraction and follows the P wave seen on the ECG. The downslope of this wave is called the *x* descent and represents atrial relaxation. The *c* wave reflects the bulging of the closed tricuspid valve into the right atrium during ventricular contraction; this wave is small and not always visible but corresponds to the QRS–T interval on the ECG. The *v* wave represents atrial filling and increased pressure against the closed tricuspid valve in early diastole. The downslope of the v wave is named the *y* descent and represents the fall in pressure as the tricuspid valve opens and blood flows from the right atrium to the right ventricle.

Cannon waves. Dysrhythmias can change the pattern of the CVP waveform. In a junctional rhythm or following a PVC, the atria are depolarized after the ventricles when retrograde conduction to the atria occurs. This may be seen as a retrograde P wave on the ECG and as a large combined *ac* or *cannon wave* on the CVP waveform (Fig. 13.13). These cannon waves can

be easily detected as large pulses in the jugular veins. Other pathologic conditions, such as advanced right ventricular failure or tricuspid valve insufficiency, allow regurgitant backflow of blood from the right ventricle to the right atrium during ventricular contraction, producing large v waves on the right atrial waveform. In atrial fibrillation, the CVP waveform has no recognizable pattern because of the disorganization of the atria.

Specialized Central Venous Catheters

A CVC that incorporates a fiberoptic sensor to continuously measure central venous oxygen saturation ($Scvo_2$) can be used as a traditional CVC and additionally used to follow the trend of venous oxygen saturation.[21] The physiology underlying use of this fiberoptic technology is discussed later in sections on monitoring mixed venous oxygen saturation (Svo_2) and $Scvo_2$.

Pulmonary Artery Pressure Monitoring

The PA catheter is the most invasive of the critical care monitoring catheters (see Fig. 13.1). It is also known as a *right heart catheter* or *Swan-Ganz catheter* (named after the catheter's inventors). PA catheters are rarely used today except during and after open-heart surgery.[22] Concerns have also been raised about routine use of PA catheters for critically ill patients. The PA catheter is invasive. It previously seemed intuitive that the diagnostic information provided would confer a survival advantage over less invasive methods, but research has shown this is not the case. Consequently PA catheter use has decreased dramatically except in some cardiac surgery units.[1,2]

In noncardiac critical care units, the PA catheter has been replaced by less invasive technologies discussed later in this chapter.[19] One of the criticisms of the PA catheter is that the data it provides may result in overtreatment.[19]

FIG. 13.13 Simultaneous electrocardiogram (A) and central venous pressure (CVP) (B) tracings. The CVP waveform shows large cannon waves corresponding to the junctional beats or premature ventricular contractions *(bottom strip)*. As the patient converts to sinus rhythm, the CVP waveform has a normal configuration. ac, normal right atrial pressure tracing; c, cannon waves on CVP tracing; J, junctional rhythm followed by cannon waves on CVP waveform; PVC, premature ventricular contraction followed by cannon wave on CVP; S, sinus rhythm followed by normal CVP tracing with a, c, and v waves.

Indications

The thermodilution PA catheter is reserved for the most hemo-dynamically unstable patients for the diagnosis and evaluation of cardiogenic shock and management during and after heart surgery. The PA catheter can provide information about PA pressures (systolic, diastolic, mean), PAOP (wedge pressure), and CO. The location of the PA catheter provides access for measurement of mixed venous oxygen saturation.

Cardiac Output Determinants

CO is the product of HR multiplied by SV. SV is the volume of blood ejected by the heart during each beat (reported in milliliters).

$$HR \times SV = CO$$

The normal adult SV is 60 to 70 mL. The clinical factors that contribute to the heart's SV are preload, afterload, and contractility and may be monitored using the PA catheter (Fig. 13.14). Another contributor to CO is HR, which is usually recorded from the ECG leads.

Oxygen Supply and Demand

When the peripheral tissues need more oxygen (eg, during exercise or sepsis), the normal, healthy heart can augment HR and SV and greatly increase CO. In a critically ill patient, when the tissues require more oxygen, these normal mechanisms are often nonfunctional, and the critical care nurse assesses the need for and then optimizes hemodynamic function. The following discussion is intended to provide a basic understanding of the clinical factors that determine CO and the role of the critical care nurse in caring for the patient with an alteration in any of these factors.

Preload. Clinicians commonly describe the hemodynamic numbers related to preload as *filling pressures*. These values refer to the pressures resulting from the volumes in the atria and ventricles. These pressure numbers include pulmonary artery diastolic pressure (PADP) and PAOP (or wedge pressure),

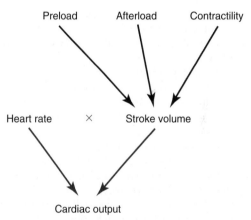

FIG. 13.14 Preload, afterload, and contractility contribute to stroke volume. Stroke volume × Heart rate = Cardiac output.

which measure preload in the left side of the heart, and CVP, which measures preload in the right side of the heart.

Preload is the *volume* in the ventricle at end-diastole. Because diastole is the filling stage of the cardiac cycle, the volume in the ventricle at end-diastole represents the presystolic volume available for ejection for that cardiac cycle. LV volume can be measured directly during cardiac catheterization, but it is not generally measured in the critical care unit. The principle is that the presence of blood within the ventricle creates pressures that can be measured by the PA catheter and transducer and can be displayed on the bedside monitor.

Estimation of preload. When the PA catheter is correctly positioned with the tip in one of the large branches of the PA, the only valve between the PA catheter tip and the left ventricle is the mitral valve. During diastole, when the mitral valve is open, no vascular obstruction exists between the tip of the PA catheter and the left ventricle (Fig. 13.15). The LV preload

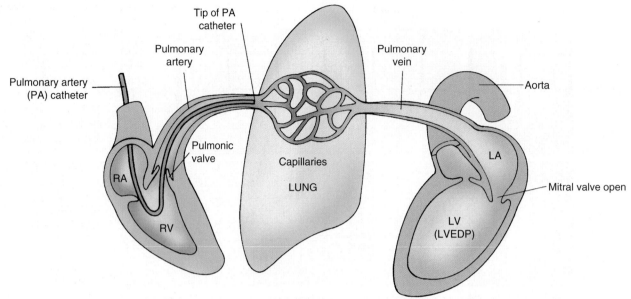

FIG. 13.15 Relationship of Pulmonary Artery Occlusion Pressure (PAOP) to Left Ventricular End-Diastolic Pressure (LVEDP). In most clinical situations, PAOP (ie, wedge pressure) accurately reflects LVEDP (ie, preload). During diastole, when the mitral valve is open, there are no other valves or other obstructions between the tip of the catheter and the left ventricle (LV). The pressure exerted by the volume in the LV is reflected through the left atrium (LA), through the pulmonary veins, and to the pulmonary capillaries. PA, pulmonary artery; RA, right atrium; RV, right ventricle.

volume creates left ventricular end-diastolic pressure (LVEDP). Using a PA catheter, preload is estimated by measuring the PAOP or "wedge" pressure. Normal left atrial pressure or PAOP is 5 to 12 mm Hg.

Frank-Starling law of the heart. The PAOP has clinical significance because a change in LV volume (preload) is reflected by a change in the measured PAOP (wedge pressure). Change in preload relies on the *Frank-Starling law of the heart.* This law states that the force of ventricular ejection is directly related to the following two elements:
1. Volume in the ventricle at end-diastole (preload)
2. Amount of myocardial stretch placed on the ventricle as a result

If the volume in the left ventricle is low, CO is also suboptimal. If IV fluids (volume) are infused, CO increases as LV volume and myocardial fiber stretch increase. This is true up to a point. Past this point, more fluid volume overdistends the ventricle and stretches the myocardial fibers so much that CO decreases. This scenario is seen clinically in the setting of acute heart failure with pulmonary edema. The increased volume in the overdistended left ventricle raises pressure in the left ventricle, left atrium, and pulmonary veins (that drain into the left atrium), and it ultimately raises pulmonary capillary pressures, measured as increased wedge pressure (PAOP). The impact of preload on CO is represented in Figs. 13.16 and 13.17 using the Frank-Starling curve as a model.

Ejection fraction. The relationship of preload to the CO is complex because not all of the preload volume is ejected with every heartbeat. The percentage of preload volume ejected from the left ventricle per beat is measured during cardiac catheterization and is described as the ejection fraction (EF). A normal EF in a healthy heart is 70%. In clinical practice, most cardiologists accept an EF value of greater than 50% as normal. The volume ejected from the left ventricle with each beat is known as the SV, which can be calculated at the bedside by dividing the CO by the HR per minute (SV = CO ÷ HR).

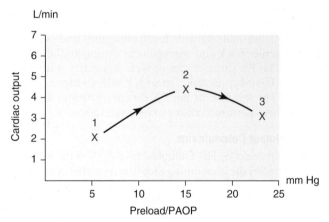

FIG. 13.16 Impact of Preload on Cardiac Output (CO). *1,* Poor cardiac output with low preload as a result of hypovolemia. *2,* Hypovolemia is corrected after administration of 2 L of intravenous fluid. The preload volume in the ventricle is increased, and pulmonary artery occlusion pressure (PAOP) has risen. Because of the increased fiber stretch from the increase in preload, CO also has risen. *3,* After infusion of an additional 2 L of intravenous solution, the myocardial fibers are overdistended, preload (PAOP) has increased, and CO has fallen as the volume in the left ventricle rises.

Cardiac dysfunction. A significant relationship exists between LVEDP and cardiac muscle dysfunction. As a general rule, the higher the pressure inside the left ventricle, the greater the degree of cardiac dysfunction. The pressure rises at end-diastole (end of filling) because the compromised ventricle cannot eject all of the preload blood volume. For example, in a patient with heart failure, the preload volume may be 100 mL. However, the SV ejected may be only 30 mL. The EF in this patient is 30% (normal EF is greater than 50%). The remaining preload volume (70 mL in this example) significantly elevates LV pressures. When the mitral valve opens at the beginning of

FIG. 13.17 Impact of Preload and Venodilation on Cardiac Output (CO). *1,* After an acute anterior wall myocardial infarction that has created significant left ventricular dysfunction, this patient has left ventricle (LV) pump failure with low CO and elevated filling pressures identified by an elevated pulmonary artery occlusion pressure (PAOP). One of the clinical problems faced by this patient is too much preload. *2,* After administration of diuretics to reduce volume and nitroglycerin to dilate the venous system, preload is reduced, and CO rises.

diastole, the pressure in the left atrium needs to be slightly higher than pressures in the left ventricle to allow filling. The 70 mL remaining in the ventricle produces high LV diastolic pressures. This elevates the left atrial filling pressure and consequently elevates the PAOP (wedge pressure). In this example, the left ventricle is overstretched by excessive preload, and CO is below normal. A plan of care for this patient includes decreasing LV preload through (1) restriction of IV and oral fluids, (2) venodilation, and (3) diuresis. The myocardial dysfunction leads to heart failure symptoms, which are discussed further in Chapter 14.

Pulmonary artery diastolic pressure and pulmonary artery occlusion pressure relationship. LVEDP can be estimated by indirect measures using the PA catheter. The most accurate is the PAOP method. The second method involves measuring PADP during diastole when the normal PADP is equal to or 1 to 3 mm Hg higher than the mean PAOP and LVEDP. It is physiologically impossible for the PAOP to be higher than the PADP. The clinician must recalibrate and troubleshoot the monitoring system if this appears to occur (see Table 13.2).

Pulmonary hypertension. Specific clinical conditions can alter the normal PADP/PAOP relationship (see Box 14.10 in Chapter 14).[23] In pulmonary hypertension, the pulmonary arterial systolic and diastolic pressures are independently raised above the LV pressures. In this clinical situation, the PADP does not accurately reflect function of the left side of the heart. The numeric difference between the PADP and the PAOP value is called a *gradient.* If a large gradient exists between the PAOP and PADP when the PA catheter is inserted, the patient has pulmonary hypertension (Table 13.3, illustration C). In addition to the echocardiogram and clinical assessment, the PA catheter is used in the diagnosis of pulmonary hypertension.[24,25]

Heart failure. In failure of the left side of the heart, the PAOP and PADP are elevated and approximately equal (see Table 13.3, illustration B). Left sided heart failure may also cause pulmonary hypertension. Over time, the damage to the lung vasculature occurs because of exposure to high LV pressure.

Mitral stenosis. Pathology of the mitral valve—stenosis or regurgitation—alters the accuracy of PAOP and PADP as parameters of LV function. In mitral valve stenosis, left atrial pressure and PAOP are increased and cause pulmonary congestion; however, these elevated values do not reflect the LVEDP because a stenotic mitral valve obstructs the normal path of blood flow from the left atrium to the left ventricle; this decreases LV preload and consequently lowers LVEDP. A nonstenotic mitral valve is essential for accurate readings because a narrowed mitral valve increases left atrial filling pressures in the presence of a normal LVEDP.

Mitral regurgitation. In patients with mitral regurgitation (MR), the mean PAOP (wedge pressure) reading is artificially elevated because of abnormal backflow of blood from the left ventricle to the left atrium during systole. The causes of MR are diverse because of the complex architecture of the mitral valve. In advanced heart failure, a dilated ventricle overstretches the valve anulus,[26] degenerative valve disease damages the valve leaflets,[27] and myocardial infarction (MI) can cause rupture of the papillary muscles or chordae tendineae.[28]

Acute MR is notable for very large v waves on the PAOP (wedge) tracing (see Table 13.3, illustration F). The size of the v wave is related to the amount of regurgitation during systole and the compliance of the left atrium. If MR is chronic and the left atrium is compliant and can stretch, the v waves may be small. In the setting of acute MR after infarction of a papillary muscle, the noncompliant or stiff atrium contributes to the development of large v waves on the wedge tracing if a PA catheter is used to monitor wedge pressure. Reading the PAOP tracing in the presence of MR is difficult. If the v waves are large (acute MR), they cannot be used to estimate LV preload. If the v wave is small (chronic MR), the mean PAOP may be used to estimate LV preload (LVEDP), which would be elevated. Echocardiography is increasingly used to confirm the presence of MR.

Afterload. Afterload is defined as the pressure the ventricle generates to overcome the resistance to ejection created by the arteries and arterioles. It is a calculated measurement derived from information obtained from the PA catheter. As a response to increased afterload, ventricular wall tension rises. After a decrease in afterload, wall tension is lowered. The technical name for afterload is *systemic vascular resistance* (SVR).

Systemic vascular resistance. Resistance to ejection from the left side of the heart is estimated by calculating the SVR. The formula, normally calculated by the bedside computer, is as follows:

$$SVR = \frac{MAP - CVP}{CO} \times 80$$

The normal value is 800 to 1200 dyn · sec · cm^{-5}. To index this value to the patient's body surface area, the cardiac index (CI) is placed in the formula in the same position as the CO. The critical care nurse frequently manipulates prescribed vasoactive medications to therapeutically alter SVR. In general, the lower the SVR value (arteries more dilated), the higher the CO.

Systemic vascular resistance and afterload reduction. Pharmacologic manipulation of SVR to improve cardiac performance is commonly used in critically ill patients. When the SVR is elevated, continuous infusions of vasodilators such as sodium nitroprusside or high-dose nitroglycerin may be used to reduce SVR.

TABLE 13.3 Clinical Interpretation of Pulmonary Artery Waveforms

PAP	Clinical Interpretation		WAVEFORM INTERPRETATION*
PAS	PAS pressure reflects the systolic pressure in the pulmonary vasculature. Waveform A is a normal waveform. The elevated values in pulmonary hypertension may be caused by idiopathic sources, some congenital heart defects, or lung disease.	A	
PAD	In a patient with healthy lung vasculature, PAD pressure reflects LVEDP, as shown in waveform B. Even if the patient experiences heart failure, PAOP and PAD increase together.	B	
	In the presence of acute respiratory distress syndrome or pulmonary hypertension, PAD pressure is not an accurate reflection of PAOP, as shown in waveform C.	C	
PAP$_M$	PAP$_M$ is used in the calculation of PVR and PVRI, as described in Table 13.1. High mean pressures can reflect cardiac or pulmonary disease. Low mean pressures reflect hypovolemia. Waveform D shows PAP$_M$ placement.	D	
PAOP[b]	In a healthy patient, PAOP reflects blood in the left ventricle at end diastole (LVEDP). The normal PAOP waveform is a left atrial waveform, as shown in waveform E.	E	
	If a patient has mitral valve regurgitation, v waves are larger than normal, increasing PAOP and possibly not reflecting true LVEDP, as shown in waveform F. PAOP is elevated in many cardiac disease states in which left ventricular function is compromised. PAOP is low in hypovolemic states.	F	

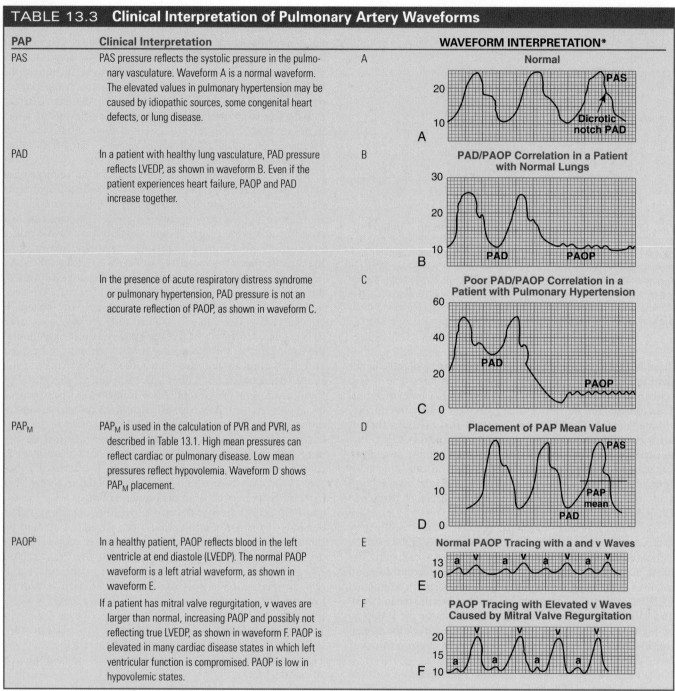

[a]Pressures on the y axis are given in mm Hg.
[b]Or pulmonary artery wedge pressure (PAWP).
LVEDP, left ventricular end-diastolic pressure; *PAD*, pulmonary artery diastolic; *PAOP*, pulmonary artery occlusion pressure; *PAP*, pulmonary artery pressure; *PAP$_M$*, mean pulmonary artery pressure; *PAS*, pulmonary artery systolic; *PVR*, pulmonary vascular resistance; *PVRI*, pulmonary vascular resistance index

If the SVR is extremely low (eg, less than 500 dyn • sec • cm^{-5}), as may occur in sepsis, the CO will be elevated, and MAP will be low. In this situation, volume and vasopressors are infused to increase MAP and SVR. After adequate volume resuscitation, the Surviving Sepsis Campaign guidelines recommend centrally administered dopamine, which increases MAP by affecting CO, or norepinephrine (Levophed), which increases MAP by vasoconstriction of the peripheral vasculature to increase SVR.[29]

Frequent assessment of the peripheral circulation is required when medications that increase SVR are used because excessive vasoconstriction can negatively affect tissue perfusion.

The following case can serve as an example. Mr. T had a large anterior wall MI 2 days ago. As a result, he has symptoms of acute heart failure, an elevated SVR of 1840 dyn • sec • cm^{-5}, and a low CO of 2.8 L/min. In a heart with decreased contractility after an acute MI, an SVR measurement above the normal range lowers CO. To optimize Mr. T's cardiac function, systemic vasodilators (afterload-reducing medications) are infused to lower the SVR into the normal range. After the administration of sodium nitroprusside (1 to 4 mcg/kg per minute), Mr. T's SVR decreased to 970 dyn • sec • cm^{-5}, and his CO increased to 4.1 L/min. In this situation, decreasing the SVR greatly increased the amount of blood ejected from the left ventricle.

For a person with a normal heart without cardiac dysfunction, an elevated SVR may have minimal impact on CO. The importance of SVR on CO is related to the functional quality of the myocardium. Whether the heart muscle is globally damaged (cardiomyopathy) or regionally damaged (MI), small changes in SVR can produce significant changes in CO.

Pulmonary vascular resistance. Resistance to ejection from the right side of the heart is estimated by calculating the pulmonary vascular resistance (PVR). The PVR value is normally one-sixth of the SVR. Normal PVR is 100 to 250 dyn • sec • cm^{-5}. The formula to calculate PVR is listed in Appendix B. Acute pulmonary hypertension, identified as a mean PA pressure greater than 25 mm Hg, can occur as a sequela of severe acute respiratory distress syndrome (ARDS).[30] The acute rise in PVR may cause the right ventricle to fail, although LV pressures generally remain within the normal range. Traditionally, a PA catheter was used to monitor vasodilator therapy and fluid management. However, because research trials have not shown a survival benefit for patients with ARDS who received this monitoring, a PA catheter is rarely used today.[19] In the latest ARDS guidelines, use of a PA catheter is not recommended.

Contractility. Many factors have an impact on contractility, including preload volume as measured by PAOP, SVR, myocardial oxygenation, electrolyte balance, positive and negative inotropic medications, and amount of functional myocardium available to contribute to contraction. These factors can have a positive inotropic effect, enhancing contractility, or a negative inotropic effect, decreasing contractility. Significant factors related to contractility that can be measured by the PA catheter include preload filling pressures, SVR, and CO. Additional contractility numbers can be calculated and are displayed in the hemodynamic profile on the bedside monitor. These include left and right ventricular stroke work index values. These values estimate the force of cardiac contraction (see Table 13.1).

Preload has an impact on contractility by means of Starling's mechanism. As volume in the ventricle rises, contractility increases. If the ventricle is overdistended with volume, contractility falls (see Figs. 13.16 and 13.17). SVR alters contractility by changes in resistance to ventricular ejection. If SVR is high, contractility is decreased. If SVR is low, contractility is augmented. Hypoxemia acts as a negative inotrope because the myocardium must have oxygen available to the cells to contract efficiently.

Optimizing contractility. IV medications such as dopamine, dobutamine, and milrinone are prescribed for their positive inotropic effect. The nurse considers the impact of these pharmacologic agents on contractility when following the trend of the patient's hemodynamic profile. No single hemodynamic number reflects contractility. However, if LV contractility is increased in response to treatment, this effect is frequently reflected by changes in PAOP (wedge pressure) and by an increase in CO.

Pulmonary Artery Catheters

The traditional PA catheter, invented by Swan and Ganz, has four lumens for measurement of right atrial pressure (similar to CVP), PA pressures, PAOP, and CO (Fig. 13.18A). Multifunction catheters may have additional lumens, which can be used for IV infusion (Fig. 13.18B) and to measure continuous Svo2, right ventricular volume, and continuous CO (Fig. 13.18C). Other PA catheters include transvenous pacing electrodes to pace the heart if needed.

The PA flow-directed catheter is 110 cm long. The most commonly used size is 7.5 or 8.0 Fr, although 5.0 and 7.0 Fr sizes are available. Each of the four lumens exits into the heart or pulmonary artery at a different point, graduated along the catheter length (see Fig. 13.18A).

Right atrial lumen. The proximal lumen is situated in the right atrium and is used for IV infusion, CVP measurement, withdrawal of venous blood samples, and injection of fluid for CO determinations. This port is often described as the *right atrial port.*

Pulmonary artery lumen. The distal PA lumen is located at the tip of the PA catheter and is situated in the pulmonary artery. It is used to record pressures within the artery and can be used for withdrawal of blood samples to measure mixed venous blood gases (eg, Svo2).

Balloon lumen. The third lumen opens into a balloon at the end of the catheter that can be inflated with 0.8 mL (7 Fr) to 1.5 mL (7.5 Fr) of air. The balloon is inflated during catheter insertion after the catheter reaches the right atrium to assist in forward flow of the catheter and to minimize right ventricular ectopy from the catheter tip. The balloon is also inflated to obtain the PAOP measurements when the PA catheter is correctly positioned in the pulmonary artery.

Thermistor lumen. The fourth lumen is a thermistor (temperature sensor) used to measure changes in blood temperature. It is located 4 cm from the catheter tip and is used to measure thermodilution CO.

Additional features. If continuous Svo2 is measured, the catheter has an additional fiberoptic lumen that exits at the tip of the catheter (see Fig. 13.18C). If cardiac pacing is used, two PA catheter methods are available. One type of catheter has three atrial (A) and two ventricular (V) pacing electrodes attached to the catheter so that when it is properly positioned, the patient can be connected to a pacemaker for atrioventricular (AV) pacing. The other catheter method uses a specific transvenous pacing wire that is passed through an additional catheter lumen and exits into the right ventricle if ventricular pacing is required. A right ventricular volumetric PA catheter is available that measures SV in the right ventricle.

Insertion

If a PA catheter is to be inserted into a patient who is awake, some brief explanations about the procedure are helpful to ensure that the patient understands what is going to happen. The initial insertion techniques used for placement of a PA catheter are similar to those described for CVC insertion. Because the PA catheter passes within the right heart chambers and pulmonary artery, the catheter insertion is monitored using fluoroscopy or waveform analysis on the bedside monitor (Fig. 13.19). In most insertions, the PA catheter floats into the right pulmonary artery.[31]

FIG. 13.18 Types of Pulmonary Artery Catheters. (A) Four-lumen catheter. (B) Five-lumen catheter that includes additional venous infusion port (VIP) into the right atrium. (C) Seven-lumen catheter that includes a VIP port and two additional lumens as well as a thermal filament for continuous cardiac output (CCO) and internal fiberoptic strands for continuous mixed venous oxygen saturation (Svo_2) monitoring (ie, optical module connector). An additional option is to combine the use of the CCO filament and the thermistor response time to calculate continuous right ventricular end-diastolic volume and right ventricular ejection fraction. (Copyright 2001 Edwards Lifesciences LLC. All rights reserved. Reprinted with permission of Edwards Lifesciences, Swan-Ganz is a trademark of Edwards Lifesciences Corporation, registered in the US Patent and Trademark Office.)

Before inserting the catheter into the vein, the physician—using sterile technique—tests the balloon for inflation and flushes the catheter with physiologic saline to remove any air. The PA catheter is then attached to the bedside hemodynamic line setup and monitor so that the waveforms can be visualized while the catheter is advanced through the right side of the heart (see Fig. 13.19). A larger introducer sheath (8.5 Fr)—which has

the tip positioned in the vena cava and has an additional IV side-port lumen—is often used to cannulate the vein first. This introducer sheath is known by several different names in clinical practice, including *sheath*, *cordis*, *introducer*, or *side port*. This introducer sheath remains in place, and the supple PA catheter is threaded through it into the vena cava and into the right side of the heart.

FIG. 13.19 Pulmonary Artery Catheter Insertion With Corresponding Waveforms.

Pulmonary Artery Waveform Interpretation

Each chamber of the heart has a distinctive waveform with recognizable characteristics. It is the responsibility of the critical care nurse to recognize each waveform displayed on the bedside monitor when the catheter enters the corresponding chamber during insertion and during routine monitoring.

Right atrial waveform. As the PA catheter is advanced into the right atrium during insertion, a right atrial waveform must be visible on the monitor, with recognizable a, c, and v waves (see Fig. 13.19). Normal mean pressure in the right atrium is 2 to 5 mm Hg. Before passage through the tricuspid valve, the balloon at the tip of the catheter is inflated for two reasons. First, it cushions the pointed tip of the PA catheter so that if the tip comes into contact with the right ventricular wall, it will cause less myocardial irritability and consequently fewer ventricular dysrhythmias. Second, inflation of the balloon assists the catheter to float with the flow of blood from the right ventricle into the pulmonary artery. Because of these features and the balloon, PA catheters are described as *flow-directional catheters.*

Right ventricular waveform. The right ventricular waveform is distinctly pulsatile, with distinct systolic and diastolic pressures. Normal right ventricular pressures are 20 to 30 mm Hg systolic and 0 to 5 mm Hg diastolic. Even with the balloon inflated, it is common for ventricular ectopy to occur during passage through the right ventricle. All patients who have a PA catheter inserted must have simultaneous ECG monitoring, with defibrillator and emergency resuscitation equipment nearby.

Pulmonary artery waveform. As the catheter enters the pulmonary artery, the waveform again changes. The diastolic pressure rises. Normal pressures in the pulmonary artery range from 20 to 30 mm Hg systolic over 10 mm Hg diastolic. A dicrotic notch, visible on the downslope of the waveform, represents closure of the pulmonic valve.

Pulmonary artery occlusion waveform (wedge). While the balloon remains inflated, the catheter is advanced into the wedge position. This maneuver produces the PAOP. The waveform decreases in size and is nonpulsatile, reflecting a normal left atrial tracing with a and v wave deflections. This is known as a *wedge tracing* because the balloon is "wedged" into a small pulmonary vessel, but it is technically described as the PAOP (see Fig. 13.19). The balloon occludes the pulmonary vessel so that the PA catheter tip and lumen are exposed only to left atrial pressure and are protected from the pulsatile influence of the right ventricle and PA. When the balloon is deflated, the catheter should spontaneously float back into the PA. When the balloon is reinflated, the wedge tracing should be visible. Normal PAOP ranges from 5 to 12 mm Hg.

After insertion, the introducer is sutured to the skin, and the catheter, which lies within the introducer, is secured with tape or with a specialized catheter securement device. A chest radiograph is taken to verify placement. If the catheter is advanced too far into the pulmonary bed, the patient is at risk for pulmonary infarction. If the PA catheter is not advanced sufficiently into the pulmonary artery, it will not be useful for PAOP readings. However, in many critical care units, if the patient's PADP and PAOP values are approximate (within 0 to 3 mm Hg), the PADP is reliably used to follow the trend of LV filling pressure (preload). This practice prevents possible trauma from frequent balloon inflation; in such a situation, the PA catheter is consciously pulled back into a safe position within the pulmonary artery so that wedging cannot occur.

After insertion of the catheter, the chest radiograph or fluoroscopy is used to verify the PA catheter position to ensure that it is not looped or knotted in the right ventricle and to rule out pneumothorax or hemorrhagic complications. A thin plastic sleeve is placed on the outside of the catheter when it is inserted to maintain sterility of the part of the PA catheter that exits from the patient. If the PA catheter is not in the desired position or if it migrates out of position, it can be repositioned. Use of this external sleeve on PA catheters has been associated with lower rates of bloodstream infection.[7]

Medical Management

Controversy exists in the medical community over the use of PA catheters, and rates of use have declined in response to lack of benefit demonstrated in clinical trials. Medical goals of hemodynamic monitoring include assessment of adequacy of perfusion in stable patients, early detection of decreased perfusion, titration of therapy to meet specific therapeutic outcomes, and differentiation of different organ system dysfunctions.

Nursing Management

The more knowledgeable the critical care nurse can become about use of the PA catheter, the more accurate and effective the nursing management interventions will be.[8] Factors that affect PA measurement are the head-of-bed backrest position and lateral body position relative to transducer height placement, respiratory variation, and use of positive end-expiratory pressure (PEEP).

Patient position. The patient does not need to be flat for accurate pressure readings to be obtained. In the supine position, when the transducer is placed at the level of the phlebostatic axis, a head-of-bed position from flat up to 60 degrees is appropriate for most patients.[8] PADP and PAOP measurements in the lateral position may be significantly different from measurements taken when the patient is lying supine. If there is concern about the validity of pressure readings in a particular patient, it is more reliable to take measurements with the patient on his or her back, with the head of bed elevated from flat to 60 degrees as tolerated. After a patient changes position, a stabilization period of 5 to 15 minutes is recommended before taking pressure readings.[8]

Respiratory variation. All PADP and PAOP (wedge) tracings are subject to respiratory interference, especially when the patient is on a positive-pressure, volume-cycled ventilator.[8] During the positive-pressure inhalation phase, the increase in intrathoracic pressure may "push up" the PA tracing, producing an artificially high reading (Fig. 13.20A). During inhalation with spontaneous breaths, negative intrathoracic pressure "pulls down" the waveform, producing an erroneously low measurement (Fig. 13.20B). To minimize the impact of respiratory variation, the PADP is read at end-expiration, which is the most stable point in the respiratory cycle when intrapleural pressures are close to zero. If the digital number fluctuates with respiration, a printed readout on paper can be obtained to verify true PADP. In some clinical settings, ECG signals or airway pressure and flow are recorded simultaneously with the PADP/PAOP tracing to identify end-expiration.[8]

Positive end-expiratory pressure. Some clinical diagnoses, such as ARDS, require the use of high levels of PEEP set with the ventilator to treat refractory hypoxemia. If a PEEP of greater than 10 cm H_2O is used, PAOP (wedge) and PAPs will be artificially elevated, and CO may be negatively affected. However, it is important NOT to disconnect a patient from the ventilator just to record PAP measurements because this will close alveoli, decrease the patient's oxygenation level, and may result in persistent hypoxemia.

Because patients remain on PEEP for treatment, they remain on it during measurement of PA pressures. In this situation, the trend of PA readings is more important than one individual measurement. The most important factor is not one individual measurement or the absolute number obtained; it is instead the trend of the measurements being used as a basis for clinical interventions to support and improve cardiopulmonary function in the critically ill.

Avoiding complications. Potential cardiac complications include ventricular dysrhythmias, endocarditis, valvular damage, cardiac rupture, and cardiac tamponade. Potential pulmonary complications include rupture of a PA, PA thrombosis, embolism or hemorrhage, and infarction of a segment of lung. The PA catheter tracing is continuously monitored to ensure that the catheter does not migrate forward into a spontaneous wedge or PAOP position. A segment of lung can infarct if the wedged catheter occludes a segment of the lung vasculature for a prolonged period. If the catheter is spontaneously wedged, the catheter must be gently pulled back out of the wedge position to prevent pulmonary infarction.

Infection is always a risk with a PA catheter. The risks are similar to those discussed in the section on CVCs (see Box 13.2).

Pulmonary artery catheter removal. PA catheters can be safely removed from the patient by critical care nurses competent in this procedure.[8] Removal is not usually associated with major complications. Rarely PVCs occur as the catheter is pulled through the right ventricle.[8]

Cardiac Output Measurement with a Pulmonary Artery Catheter

The PA catheter measures CO using an intermittent (bolus) or a continuous CO method.

Thermodilution cardiac output bolus method. The bolus thermodilution method is performed at the bedside and results in CO calculated in liters per minute. Three CO values that are within a 10% mean range are obtained at one time and are averaged to calculate CO. The thermodilution CO is very accurate when several injectate values are averaged.[32] A known amount, usually 10 mL, of room temperature physiologic saline solution is injected into the proximal lumen of the PA catheter. The injectate exits into the right atrium and travels with the flow of blood past the thermistor (temperature sensor) located at the distal end of the catheter in the PA. The injectate can be delivered by hand injection using individual syringes of saline. Frequently, a closed in-line system attached to a 500-mL bag of 0.9% saline is used as a reservoir to deliver the individual injections.

Cardiac output curve. The thermodilution CO method uses the indicator-dilution method, in which a known temperature is the indicator. It is based on the principle that the change in temperature over time is inversely proportional to blood flow. Blood flow can be diagrammatically represented as a CO curve on which temperature is plotted against time (Fig. 13.21A). Most hemodynamic monitors display this CO curve, which must then be interpreted to determine whether the CO injection is valid. The normal curve has a smooth upstroke, with a rounded peak and a gradually tapering downslope. If the curve has an uneven pattern, it may indicate faulty injection technique, and the CO measurement must be repeated. Patient movement or coughing also alters the CO measurement (Fig. 13.21B).

Injectate temperature. If the CO is within the normal range, it is equally accurate whether iced or room temperature injectate is used. However, if the CO values are extremely high or very low, iced injectate may be more accurate. To ensure accurate readings, the difference between injectate temperature and body temperature must be at least 10°C, and the injectate must be delivered within 4

FIG. 13.20 Pulmonary Artery (PA) Waveforms That Demonstrate the Impact of Mechanical Ventilation on PA Pressures. For accuracy, PA pressures are read at the end of exhalation. (A) In positive-pressure ventilation, the increase in intrathoracic pressure during inhalation "pushes up" the PA waveform, creating a falsely high reading. (B) In spontaneous breathing, the decrease in intrathoracic pressure during normal inhalation "pulls down" the PA waveform, creating a falsely low reading.

seconds, with minimal handling of the syringe to prevent warming of the solution. This is particularly important if iced injectate is used. With all delivery systems, the injectate is delivered at the same point in the respiratory cycle, usually end-exhalation.

Patient position and cardiac output. In a normovolemic, stable patient, reliable CO measurements can be obtained in a supine position (patient lying on his or her back) with the head of the bed elevated up to 60 degrees.[8] If the patient is hypovolemic or unstable, leaving the head of the bed in a flat position or only slightly elevated is the most clinically appropriate choice. CO measurements performed when the patient is turned to the side are not considered as accurate as measurements performed with the patient in the supine position.

Clinical conditions that alter cardiac output. Two clinical conditions produce errors in the thermodilution CO measurement: tricuspid valve regurgitation and ventricular septal rupture. If the patient has tricuspid valve regurgitation, the expected flow of blood from the right atrium to the pulmonary artery is disrupted by backflow from the right ventricle to the right atrium. This creates a lower CO measurement than the patient's actual output. If the person has an intracardiac left-to-right shunt, as occurs after ventricular septal rupture, the

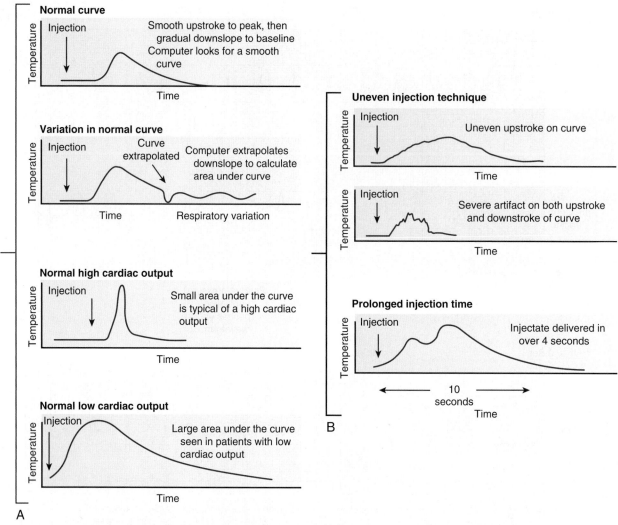

FIG. 13.21 (A) Variations in normal cardiac thermodilution bolus output curve. (B) Abnormal cardiac output (CO) curves produce erroneous CO values.

thermodilution CO measures the large right-to-left shunt volume and records a higher CO than the patient's true systemic output.

Continuous invasive cardiac output measurement. The bolus thermodilution method is reliable but performed intermittently. Continuous CO monitoring using a PA catheter is also frequently used in clinical practice. One method employs a thermal filament on the PA catheter to emit small energy signals (the indicator) into the bloodstream. These signals are then detected by the thermistor near the tip of the PA catheter. An indicator curve is created, and a CO value is calculated from these data.

Calculated hemodynamic profiles using a pulmonary artery catheter. For a patient with a thermodilution PA catheter in place, additional hemodynamic information can be calculated using routine vital signs, CO, and body surface area. These measurements are calculated using specific formulas that are indexed to a patient's body size.

The calculated values used in the hemodynamic profiles are described in Table 13.1. Clinical use of these profiles is described in two case studies. In Hemodynamic Profile 1 (Box 13.3), the example is a step-by-step interpretation of the hemodynamic profile to familiarize the reader with use of calculated values. In Hemodynamic Profile 2 (Box 13.4), the example uses only values indexed to body weight and illustrates the impact of treatment on these values over time.

Continuous Monitoring of Mixed Venous and Central Venous Oxygen Saturation

Indications

Continuous monitoring of venous oxygen saturation is indicated for a critically ill patient who has the potential to develop an imbalance between oxygen supply and metabolic tissue demand.[21,33-35] Continuous venous oxygen monitoring permits a calculation of the balance achieved between arterial oxygen supply (Sao_2) and oxygen demand at the tissue level by sampling desaturated venous blood from the PA catheter distal tip. This sample is called *mixed venous oxygen saturation* (Svo_2) because it is a mixture of all of the venous blood drained from many body tissues. The same fiberoptic technology has been used in combination with a fiberoptic triple-lumen CVC. In this situation, the venous blood is sampled from the superior vena cava, just above the right atrium, and the $Scvo_2$ is measured.

Under normal conditions, the cardiopulmonary system achieves a balance between oxygen supply and demand. The following four factors contribute to this balance[35]:

1. CO
2. Hemoglobin
3. Arterial oxygen saturation (Sao_2)
4. Tissue oxygen metabolism (Vo_2)

BOX 13.3   Hemodynamic Profile 1

Admission

Mr. SR has a medical history of cardiomyopathy and chronic obstructive pulmonary disease (COPD). He is admitted to a coronary care unit because of an exacerbation of biventricular heart failure. He has been complaining about anginal pain and shortness of breath. His nursing diagnoses are Decreased Cardiac Output and Impaired Gas Exchange.

Height	163 cm	PAD	27 mm Hg	PVR	322 dyn • s • cm^{-5}
Weight	79 kg	PAP$_M$	36 mm Hg	PVRI	612 dyn • s • cm^{-5}/m^2
BSA	1.9 m^2	PAOP	26 mm Hg	LCW	2.1 kg-m
		CVP	24 mm Hg	LCWI	1.1 kg-m/m^2
HR	104 beats/min	CO	2.48 L/min	LVSW	2.4 g-m
ABP		CI	1.31 L/min/m^2	LVSWI	10.7 g-m/m^2
Systolic	88 mm Hg	SV	23.8 mL	RCW	1.21 kg-m
Diastolic	51 mm Hg	SI	12.5 mL/m^2	RCWI	0.64 kg-m/m^2
MAP	63 mm Hg	SVR	1257 dyn • s • cm^{-5}	RVSW	11.7 g-m
PAS	55 mm Hg	SVRI	2388 dyn • s • cm^{-5}/m^2	RVSWI	6.2 g-m/m^2

Analysis of Hemodynamic Profile[a]

Profile	Analysis
HR (heart rate)	HR of 104 beats/min is above normal limits (normal, 60–100 beats/min).
ABP (arterial blood pressure)	Narrow pulse pressure of 88/51 mm Hg with low mean arterial pressure (MAP) of 63 mm Hg (normal MAP, 65–90 mm Hg).
PAP (pulmonary artery pressure)	Pulmonary artery pressures are elevated (55/27 mm Hg), consistent with diagnosis of cardiomyopathy, failure of left side of heart, and COPD (normal PAP, 25/10 mm Hg).
PAOP (pulmonary artery occlusion pressure)	Elevated PAOP (26 mm Hg), consistent with diagnosis of cardiomyopathy and failure of left side of heart (normal PAOP, 5–12 mm Hg).
CVP (central venous pressure)	Elevated CVP (24 mm Hg), consistent with diagnosis of cardiomyopathy, failure of right side of heart, and COPD (normal CVP, 4–6 mm Hg).
CO (cardiac output) and CI (cardiac index)	Poor CO and CI (CO, 2.48 L/min; CI, 1.31 L/min/m^2). Both values are below normal (normal CO, 4–6 L/min; normal CI, 2.2–4 L/min/m^2).
SV (stroke volume) and SI (stroke volume index)	SV and SI are low (SV, 23.8 mL; SI, 12.5 mL/m^2). These results would be anticipated from the low CO (normal SV, 60–70 mL; normal SI, 40–50 mL/min/m^2).
SVR (systemic vascular resistance) and SVRI (systemic vascular resistance index)	SVR and SVRI are at the upper normal range (SVR, 1257 dyn • s • cm^{-5}; SVRI, 2388 dyn • s • cm^{-5}/m^2). These values are not contributing to the low CO at this time (normal SVR, 800–1400 dyn • s • cm^{-5}; normal SVRI, 2000–2400 dyn • s • cm^{-5}/m^2).
PVR (pulmonary vascular resistance) and PVRI (pulmonary vascular resistance index)	PVR and PVRI are elevated (PVR, 322 dyn • s • cm^{-5}; PVRI 612 dyn • s • cm^{-5}/m^2). High PVR may be contributing to the low CO (normal PVR, 100–250 dyn • s • cm^{-5}; normal PVRI, 225–315 dyn • s • cm^{-5}/m^2).
LCWI (left cardiac work index) and LVSWI (left ventricular stroke work index)	Both LCWI and LVSWI are below normal (LCWI, 1.1 kg-m/m^2; LVSWI, 10.7 g-m/m^2), indicating that left ventricular myocardial damage may be present. This is consistent with Mr. SR's diagnosis of cardiomyopathy (normal LCWI, 3.4–4.2 kg-m/m^2; normal LVSWI, 50–62 g-m/m^2).
RCWI (right cardiac work index) and RVSWI (right ventricular stroke work index)	RCWI is normal, but RVSWI is below normal (RCWI, 0.64 kg-m/m^2; RVSWI, 6.2 g-m/m^2), indicating that right ventricular myocardial damage may be present. This is consistent with Mr. SR's diagnosis of cardiomyopathy and history of COPD (normal RCWI, 0.54–0.66 kg-m/m^2; normal RVSWI, 7.9–9.7 g-m/m^2).
Nursing impression	The hemodynamic data confirm the nursing clinical diagnosis of poor CO. The goal is to improve CO within the limits of Mr. SR's myocardial dysfunction and COPD. As CO improves and PA pressures decrease, the patient will have less pulmonary congestion, which will improve alveolar gas exchange.

[a]Formulas and normal values for the hemodynamic values are given in Table 13.1 and in Appendix B.
BSA, body surface area.

Three of these factors (CO, hemoglobin, and Sao$_2$) contribute to the supply of oxygen to the tissues. Tissue metabolism (Vo$_2$) determines oxygen consumption or the quantity of oxygen extracted at tissue level that creates the demand for oxygen (Fig. 13.22). The relationships of these factors to tissue oxygen utilization are illustrated in Fig. 13.23.

In addition to measurement of venous oxygen saturation, it is possible to calculate the quantity of oxygen (in mL/min) that is provided to the tissues by the cardiopulmonary system and to assess the amount of oxygen consumed by the body tissues. These calculations rely on principles of oxygen transport physiology and are the basis for calculation of Svo$_2$. These formulas are explained in greater detail in Table 13.4 and are listed in Appendix B.

Catheters

The type of catheter used to measure venous oxygen saturation is defined by where the fiberoptic tip is located—either at the tip of a CVC or on the distal tip of a PA catheter.

Svo$_2$ catheter. The pulmonary arterial Svo$_2$ catheter has the traditional four lumens plus a lumen containing two or three optical fibers. The fiberoptics are attached to an optical module that is connected to a small bedside computer. The optical module transmits a narrow band of light down one optical

BOX 13.4 Hemodynamic Profile 2

1. Admission

Mrs. JL has been admitted to the critical care unit with pulmonary edema. She has a history of anterior wall myocardial infarction and severe chronic obstructive pulmonary disease (COPD).

Height	159 cm	MAP	106 mm Hg	SI	9.9 mL/m^2
Weight	45.8 kg	PAS	53 mm Hg	SVRI	5351 dyn • s • cm^{-5}/m^2
BSA	1.40 m^2	PAD	27 mm Hg	PVRI	1046 dyn • s • cm^{-5}/m^2
		PAP$_M$	44 mm Hg	LCWI	1.9 kg-m/m^2
HR	131 beats/min	PAOP	27 mm Hg	LVSWI	14.3 g-m/m^2
ABP		CVP	19 mm Hg	RCW	0.78 kg-m/m^2
Systolic	160 mm Hg	CO	1.82 L/min	RCWI	5.9 g-m/m^2
Diastolic	80 mm Hg	CI	1.3 L/min/m^2		

Analysis of the Hemodynamic Profile[a]

In the above hemodynamic profile, notice the fast HR; high MAP; high PA and CVP filling pressures; low CI, SI, LVSWI, and RVSWI; and high SVRI and PVRI. These values are consistent with a diagnosis of failure of the left side of the heart causing pulmonary edema, which may lead to cardiogenic shock. Treatment is focused on increasing the CI by lowering SVRI and PVRI and using intravenous (IV) sodium nitroprusside and IV nitroglycerin in continuous infusion.

2. Three Hours Later

Height	159 cm	MAP	83 mm Hg	SI	16.5 mL/m^2
Weight	45.8 kg	PAS	41 mm Hg	SVRI	3088 dyn • s • cm^{-5}/m^2
BSA	1.40 m^2	PAD	26 mm Hg	PVRI	300 dyn • s • cm^{-5}/m^2
		PAP$_M$	33 mm Hg	LCWI	2.1 kg-m/m^2
HR	113 beats/min	PAOP	26 mm Hg	LVSWI	18.6 g-m/m^2
ABP		CVP	11 mm Hg	RCWI	0.84 kg-m/m^2
Systolic	104 mm Hg	CO	2.61 L/min	RVSWI	7.4 g-m/m^2
Diastolic	69 mm Hg	CI	1.86 L/min/m^2		

Analysis of Hemodynamic Profile 2

Results 3 hours after sodium nitroprusside administration showed improving hemodynamic values demonstrated as normal MAP and lower intracardiac filling pressures (PA and CVP). However, CI and SI remain low, and SVRI is above normal. Mrs. JL remains in severe left ventricular failure because of her low CI.

3. The Next Day

Height	159 cm	MAP	77 mm Hg	SI	22.5 mL/m^2
Weight	45.8 kg	PAS	31 mm Hg	SVRI	2423 dyn • s • cm^{-5}/m^2
BSA	1.40 m^2	PAD	15 mm Hg	PVRI	273 dyn • s • cm^{-5}/m^2
		PAP$_M$	23 mm Hg	LCWI	2.4 kg-m/m^2
HR	104 beats/min	PAOP	15 mm Hg	LVSWI	22.9 g-m/m^2
ABP		CVP	4 mm Hg	RCWI	0.74 kg-m/m^2
Systolic	111 mm Hg	CO	3.28 L/min	RVSWI	7.1 g-m/m^2
Diastolic	60 mm Hg	CI	2.34 L/min/m^2		

Analysis of Hemodynamic Profile 3

The next day, Mrs. JL's hemodynamic values have improved with continued use of sodium nitroprusside and nitroglycerin. The CI value is in the low-normal range, and SVRI and PVRI values are in the high-normal range. LVSWI remains low, reflecting the patient's compromised left ventricle from a prior anterior wall myocardial infarction.

[a]Formulas and normal values for the hemodynamic values are given in Table 13.1 and in Appendix B.
BSA, body surface area.

fiber. This light is reflected off the hemoglobin in the blood and returns to the optical module through the receiving fiberoptic. The Svo$_2$ signal is recorded on a continuous display.

Scvo$_2$ catheter. The central venous Scvo$_2$ technology is incorporated into a multilumen CVC. The fiberoptic catheter tip is positioned in a central vein, such as the superior vena cava. The technology used to measure the venous saturation is identical in both types of catheters, and the same continuous display module is used for both catheters.

The values obtained from the traditional PA (Svo$_2$) catheter and the central venous (Scvo$_2$) catheter are very similar, although the Scvo$_2$ values are slightly higher. The trend of parallel measurements (up or down as patient condition changes) is in the same direction in most cases. However, in severe sepsis, the Svo$_2$ reading may be significantly lower than the Scvo$_2$ value.[33]

Svo$_2$ or Scvo$_2$ calibration. The catheter is calibrated before insertion into the patient through a standardized color reference system, which is part of the catheter package. Insertion technique and sites are identical to those used for placement of conventional PA or CVC catheters. Waveform analysis or venous saturation measurement, or both, can be used for accurate placement. After the catheter is inserted, recalibration

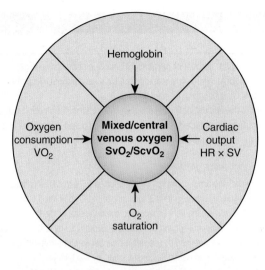

FIG. 13.22 Determinants of Venous Oxygen Saturation: Cardiac Output (CO), Hemoglobin (Hgb), Arterial Oxygen Saturation (SaO_2), and Tissue Oxygen Metabolism (VO_2). (From Lough, M.E. Hemodynamic Monitoring: *Evolving Technologies and Clinical Practice*, Philadelphia: Elsevier; 2016.)

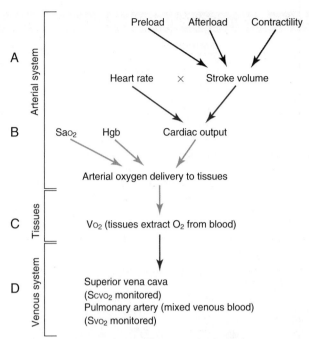

FIG. 13.23 Factors That Contribute to Mixed Venous Oxygen Saturation (SvO_2) Value. (A) Cardiac output (CO) is determined by heart rate (HR) × stroke volume (SV). (B) Oxygen saturation (SaO_2), hemoglobin (Hgb) level, and CO contribute to arterial oxygen delivery at the tissue level. (C) Tissues extract and use the oxygen carried in the blood. This process of cellular oxygen consumption is VO_2. (D) Blood returns to the superior vena cava (recorded as $ScvO_2$) and then to the pulmonary artery, where the mixed venous blood is recorded as SvO_2.

is unnecessary unless the catheter becomes disconnected from the optical module.

To recalibrate the fiberoptic module to verify accuracy when the catheter is already inserted in a patient, a mixed venous blood sample (SvO_2) or central venous sample ($ScvO_2$) must be withdrawn from the appropriate catheter tip and sent to the laboratory for oxygen saturation analysis.[33] In many critical care units, this is a standard daily procedure to ensure that readings used to guide patient care remain accurate.

Nursing Management

SvO_2 monitoring provides a continuous assessment of the balance of oxygen supply and demand for an individual patient. Nursing assessment includes evaluation of the SvO_2 or $ScvO_2$ value and evaluation of the four factors (SaO_2, CO, hemoglobin, and VO_2) that maintain the oxygen supply–demand balance.

Normal SvO_2 values. Normal SvO_2 is approximately 75% in a healthy individual (range, 60% to 80%). In critically ill patients, an SvO_2 value between 60% and 80% is evidence of adequate balance between oxygen supply and demand.

Normal $ScvO_2$ values. Normal values for the $ScvO_2$ catheter are slightly higher because the reading is taken before the blood enters the right heart chambers, where the *cardiac sinus* (vein) delivers venous blood drained from the myocardium into the right atrium. The heavily desaturated myocardial blood decreases the oxygen saturation slightly. For this reason, SvO_2 values are always slightly lower than $ScvO_2$ readings in the same patient.[33]

One clinical tip is to subtract 30 from the SaO_2, and the resulting value should represent an acceptable SvO_2. For example,

$$SaO_2 \text{ is } 100\% - 30\% = 70\% \text{ } SvO_2$$

$$SaO_2 \text{ is } 95\% - 30\% = 65\% \text{ } SvO_2$$

If the SvO_2 or $ScvO_2$ value changes by more than 10% and this change is maintained for more than 10 minutes, the clinician must determine which of the four factors is affecting SvO_2.

SvO_2 or $ScvO_2$ and arterial oxygen saturation. A change in SvO_2 or $ScvO_2$ may be caused by a change in SaO_2. If the SaO_2 is increased because supplemental oxygen is being administered, the SvO_2 also will increase. If the oxygen supply is disrupted and SaO_2 is decreased, SvO_2 will decrease. The SvO_2 can be decreased by any action or disease that reduces oxygen supply, including ARDS, endotracheal suctioning, removing a patient from the ventilator, or removing supplementary oxygen. Fig. 13.24 demonstrates a decrease in SvO_2 during suctioning in a patient with ARDS. Transient decreases in SvO_2 or $ScvO_2$ related to a nursing action such as endotracheal suctioning are not usually a cause for concern. Some patients may be slow to resaturate up to the presuction level of SvO_2 or $ScvO_2$. In this case, an appropriate nursing intervention is to wait until the venous oxygen saturation has again returned to baseline before initiating other nursing activities.

SvO_2 or $ScvO_2$ and cardiac output. A change in SvO_2 or $ScvO_2$ may be caused by an alteration in CO. Changes in one or more of the following four individual hemodynamic factors affect CO: preload, SVR, contractility, and HR (see Fig. 13.22). Fig. 13.25 shows an improvement in a patient's SvO_2 concentration from 70% to 80% after volume administration that increased preload (point A). This patient's CO later fell abruptly during a short run of ventricular tachycardia (VT) (point B). Any major loss of HR causes a decrease in CO. Alterations in contractility, preload, and afterload (SVR) also have the potential to alter CO.

Because CO is an important component of the continuous SvO_2 value, researchers investigated whether SvO_2 could be substituted for thermodilution CO as a monitoring tool. Studies of

TABLE 13.4 Calculations of Oxygen Transport Physiology

Name	Formula	Normal Value	Explanation
Arterial oxygen saturation (Sao$_2$)	$\dfrac{HgbO_2}{Hgb + HgbO_2} \times 100$	>96%	Sao$_2$ is determined by the amount of oxygen (O$_2$) bound to hemoglobin (Hgb), termed oxyhemoglobin (HgbO$_2$). HgbO$_2$ is divided by the total hemoglobin (Hgb + HgbO$_2$). Normally, 96% of O$_2$ is bound to hemoglobin.
Blood oxygen content	(O$_2$ dissolved) + (O$_2$ saturation)	19–20 mL/dL	Blood O$_2$ content is the amount of O$_2$ dissolved in 100 mL (1 dL) of blood. It can be calculated for arterial blood (Cao$_2$) and for venous blood (Cvo$_2$). Measured in units of mL/dL, it is the combination of dissolved O$_2$ (Pao$_2$) and O$_2$ saturation (Sao$_2$).
Cao$_2$ (arterial) Cvo$_2$ (venous)	(Po$_2$ × 0.003) + (1.34 × Hgb × Sao$_2$)	12–15 mL/dL	
Blood oxygen transport (ie, oxygen delivery)	CO × Cao$_2$ × 10 (arterial)	1000 mL/min	O$_2$ transport represents the amount (mL) of O$_2$ transported to or from the tissues each minute (mL/min). Arterial O$_2$ transport is a measure of the O$_2$ delivered to the tissues. Venous O$_2$ transport reflects the venous return to the right side of the heart.
	CO × Cvc$_2$ × 10 (venous)	750 mL/min	O$_2$ transport is calculated by multiplying the cardiac output (CO) by the O$_2$ content (Cao$_2$ or Cvo$_2$) and by the number 10. The difference between normal arterial and normal venous O$_2$ return represents O$_2$ consumption by the tissues.
Tissue oxygen consumption (Vo$_2$)	Arterial O$_2$ transport minus venous O$_2$ transport	250 mL/min	O$_2$ consumption is the amount of O$_2$ consumed by the tissues in 1 minute.
	(CO × Cao$_2$ × 10) – (CO × Cvo$_2$ × 10)		To calculate Vo$_2$, the arterial O$_2$ transport and venous O$_2$ transport values (calculated in mL/min) must be known. The difference is Vo$_2$.
Arterial-venous oxygen difference (a-v O$_2$ difference)	Arterial O$_2$ content minus venous O$_2$ content	3.0-5.5 mL/dL	The a-v O$_2$ difference is the difference between the arterial O$_2$ content (Cao$_2$) and the venous O$_2$ content (Cvo$_2$). Because Cao$_2$ and Cvo$_2$ are measured in mL/dL, the a-v O$_2$ difference is also measured in mL/dL.
	Cao$_2$ – Cvo$_2$		
Mixed venous oxygen saturation (Svo$_2$)	Arterial O$_2$ transport minus tissue O$_2$ consumption equals venous O$_2$ return	60%–80%	Svo$_2$ is the venous O$_2$ return that is bound (saturated) to hemoglobin. Saturation is measured as a percentage (%). The Svo$_2$ value is a function of the amount of O$_2$ delivered to the tissues minus the amount of O$_2$ consumed by the tissues (Vo$_2$) and is measured in mL/min. The higher the amount (mL) of O$_2$ in the venous return, the greater the hemoglobin saturation.
	(CO × Cao$_2$ × 10) – Vo$_2$		

FIG. 13.24 The Svo$_2$ value decreases during endotracheal (ET) suctioning. The ET suction decreases the oxygen saturation (Sao$_2$) level. The baseline Svo$_2$ value is low (60%) because the patient has acute respiratory distress syndrome and is hypoxemic.

adult patients after cardiac surgery and acute MI indicate that a sustained change in the Svo$_2$ value does not automatically mean there has been a change in CO. No consistent or reliable correlation was found between Svo$_2$ and CO. Instead, a change in Svo$_2$ indicates a need to check CO at the bedside to determine the cause of the change in venous oxygen saturation. The Svo$_2$ measurement is very sensitive and serves as an early warning for

changes in patient condition, whether or not the change is the result of an alteration in CO. Monitoring Svo$_2$ is an additional level of hemodynamic monitoring but does not replace thermodilution CO.

This principle is clearly illustrated in the Svo$_2$ Hemodynamic Profile 3 (Box 13.5), in which an increase in Svo$_2$ is not associated with a significant rise in CO. The rationale and explanation

10 AM   2 PM

FIG. 13.25 Impact of Changes in Cardiac Output (CO) on S_{VO_2} Values. *Point A:* Just before point A, S_{VO_2} readings are low because CO and pulmonary artery pressures were low as a result of excessive diuresis. Infusion of 500 mL of colloid solution and 1000 mL of lactated Ringer solution crystalloid increased S_{VO_2} level and improved CO, which rose to 3.7 L/min. *Point B:* A short run of ventricular tachycardia caused CO to fall abruptly to 2.5 L/min and decreased S_{VO_2} value. *Point C:* The beginning of an upward trend in S_{VO_2} is related to administration of fluids and to improvement in CO and in filling pressures. CO is now 3.4 L/min. The graph represents a 4-h printout; the space between each dotted line represents 20 min.

for this finding is also discussed in the section on assessment of oxygen consumption.

S_{VO_2} or S_{CVO_2} and hemoglobin. Hemoglobin is the transport mechanism for oxygen in the blood. If the hemoglobin level falls as a result of bleeding or red blood cell (RBC) destruction, the body maintains oxygen transport by increasing CO and using oxygen reserves in the venous blood return. The body can compensate efficiently for anemia. In a healthy person, the hemoglobin concentration must be extremely low before S_{VO_2} decreases. However, in an anemic patient with a compromised cardiovascular system who cannot adequately increase CO, S_{VO_2} or S_{CVO_2} declines as venous oxygen reserves are depleted.

S_{VO_2} or S_{CVO_2} and oxygen consumption. V_{O_2} describes the amount of oxygen the body tissues consume for normal function in 1 minute. If the body's metabolic demands increase because of exercise or increased metabolic rate, the body increases CO to augment oxygen supply and uses reserve oxygen in the venous system. Normal oxygen delivery to the tissues is 1000 mL (1 L) of oxygen per minute. At rest, a person may consume one-fourth of the available oxygen, or 250 mL of oxygen per minute. This leaves a venous oxygen reserve of 750 mL of oxygen per minute (see Table 13.4). For a normal individual, the combination of increased CO and use of considerable venous oxygen reserve provides adequate compensation for increased metabolic needs. However, for a critically ill patient with cardiac or respiratory dysfunction, an increase in activity leading to increased oxygen consumption may overwhelm the cardiopulmonary system and oxygen reserves.

In a critically ill patient, nursing procedures can increase V_{O_2} by 10% to 36% (Table 13.5). The critical care nurse can observe the effect of increased V_{O_2} during routine nursing care and under conditions that increase metabolic rate. Activities

such as turning, giving a backrub, or getting a patient out of bed are often accompanied by a sudden, temporary decrease in the patient's continuous S_{VO_2} or S_{CVO_2} reading. After the physical activity is finished, most patients resaturate up to their prior venous oxygen saturation level within a few minutes. In critically ill patients, it may take 5 minutes for resaturation (increase in S_{VO_2} or S_{CVO_2}) to occur. In this situation, the appropriate nursing action is to observe the patient clinically in conjunction with monitoring S_{VO_2} or S_{CVO_2} and to postpone additional maneuvers until the venous saturation has returned to baseline.

Many clinical conditions that dramatically increase V_{O_2} consumption are often seen in critical care units. Conditions such as sepsis, multiple-organ dysfunction syndrome, burns, head injury, and shivering can more than double the normal oxygen tissue requirements (see Table 13.5). Such dramatic increases in V_{O_2} translate into a low S_{VO_2} or S_{CVO_2} value, even if the CO is normal. This situation is demonstrated in Hemodynamic Profile 3, in which intense shivering resulted in increased tissue oxygen consumption and a low initial S_{VO_2} value (point A); after sedation, the S_{VO_2} value increased secondary to the normalization of tissue oxygen requirements (point B).

Normal S_{VO_2} or S_{CVO_2}. If S_{VO_2} or S_{CVO_2} is within the normal range of 60% to 80% and the patient is not clinically compromised, the nurse can assume that oxygen supply and demand are balanced for the patient. The situation becomes out of balance when a decrease in oxygen delivery (S_{AO_2}) occurs because of changes in CO or hemoglobin concentration, or an increase in oxygen demand (increased V_{O_2}) occurs.

Low S_{VO_2} or S_{CVO_2}. If S_{VO_2} or S_{CVO_2} falls below 60% and is sustained, the clinician must assume that oxygen supply is not equal to demand (Table 13.6). It is helpful to assess the cause of decreased S_{VO_2} or S_{CVO_2} in a logical sequence that reflects knowledge of the meaning of the venous saturation value. The following is one such assessment sequence:

1. Clinically assess the patient.
2. Assess whether the decreased S_{VO_2} or S_{CVO_2} is caused by low oxygen supply. Verify the effectiveness of the ventilator or oxygen mask, or check S_{AO_2} from arterial blood gas values.
3. Assess cardiac function by performing a CO measurement.
4. Assess hemoglobin value by checking recent laboratory results or by withdrawing a blood sample for laboratory analysis.
5. Assess whether the decreased S_{VO_2} or S_{CVO_2} is the result of a recent patient movement or nursing action that may have temporarily increased V_{O_2}.

The concept of target values has been helpful when designing protocols for hemodynamic monitoring. Target values for venous oximetry are S_{VO_2} of 70% or greater and S_{CVO_2} of 65% or greater. Patients with values below these targets are at greater risk for organ hypoperfusion and increased mortality. This was seen in a study of intraoperative and postoperative surgical patients, in whom S_{CVO_2} below 65% was associated with increased mortality.[33]

If S_{VO_2} or S_{CVO_2} falls below 40% and is maintained at this low value, the imbalance of oxygen supply and demand will be inadequate to meet tissue needs at the cellular level. At some point, the cells change from an aerobic to anaerobic mode of metabolism, which results in the production of lactic acid and is representative of a shock state in which cellular injury or cell death may result. At this point, every attempt must be made to determine the cause of the low S_{VO_2} or S_{CVO_2} and to correct the oxygen supply–demand imbalance.

BOX 13.5 Hemodynamic Profile 3

Mr. EH has just been admitted to the cardiovascular critical care unit after open heart surgery. At point A in the figure, he has an extremely low Svo_2 value of 40%. An Svo_2 value below 40% indicates that the oxygen supply is inadequate to meet the demands of the body tissues, resulting in metabolic acidosis. To determine the reason for the low Svo_2 level, values must be known for the hemoglobin (Hgb) level, arterial oxygen saturation (Sao_2), cardiac output (CO), and tissue oxygen consumption (Vo_2). Mr. EH's Hgb value is 11.6 g/dL (normal male Hgb, 13.5–18.0 g/dL), which is acceptable after major surgery; Sao_2 is 99.6% (normal, 97%), which is high because Mr. EH started receiving mechanical ventilation with 70% oxygen immediately after surgery; and CO is low at 3.15 L/min (normal, 4–6 L/min). Mr. EH is receiving dopamine (5 mcg/kg/min) for his low CO. He is cold and shivering because his body temperature is only 35.2°C after the surgery. Using the values of Hgb of 11.6 g/dL, Sao_2 of 99.6%, and CO of 3.15 L/min, it is possible to calculate the tissue oxygen consumption (Vo_2) for EH.

Arterial Supply   **Venous Return**

$$CO (Pao_2 \times 0.003) + (1.34 \times Hgb \times Sao_2) 10 - CO (Pvo_2 \times 0.0031) + (1.34 \times Hgb \times S\overline{v}o_2) 10 = \dot{V}o_2$$

To calculate arterial oxygen supply, the oxygen in the venous return, Vo_2, and the difference between the arterial (a) and venous (v) oxygen content (a-v O_2 difference), insert Mr. EH's values (in **boldface**) into the previous formula.

Arterial Supply	Venous Return	$\dot{V}o_2$	a-v O_2 Difference
3.15 (**354** × 0.003) + (1.34 × **11.6** × **0.99**) 10 −	**3.15** (**20** × 0.003) + (1.34 × **11.6** × **0.38**) 10		
3.15 (1.0 + 15.3) 10	**3.15** (0.06 + 5.90) 10		
3.15 (16.3) 10	**3.15** (5.90) 10		
505 mL/min (see illustration at top)	183 mL/min		= 322 mL/min 10.4 mL/dL

At point A in the figure, the arterial oxygen supply to the tissues is 505 mL/min (normal, 1000 mL/min), whereas the oxygen returned in the venous blood is only 183 mL/min (normal, 750 mL/min). Mr. EH's Vo_2 is elevated at 322 mL/min (normal, 250 mL/min). The clinical goals for this patient would be to (1) increase the CO and (2) use sedation or muscle relaxants to decrease oxygen consumption by controlling the patient's shivering. The difference between the oxygen content in the arterial (a) and the venous (v) blood (a-v O_2 difference) is very large at 10.4 mL/dL (normal, 3.5–5.0 mL/dL). These calculated values confirm the nursing diagnosis of Ineffective Tissue Perfusion with a decreased CO.

Two hours later, at point B in the figure, Mr. EH's Svo_2 has improved to a low-normal value of 60%. Additional inotropic medications have been administered. At this time, Hgb is 10.8 g/dL, Sao_2 is 99.6%, and CO remains low at 3.3 L/min. The improvement in Svo_2 has not been caused by a dramatic increase in CO. When Mr. EH's oxygen consumption is calculated at point B, it becomes evident that the decrease in physical activity after sedation with morphine to reduce shivering has improved the Svo_2. Mr. EH's values are in bold.

Arterial Supply   **Venous Return**

$$CO (Pao_2 \times 0.003) + (1.34 \times Hgb \times Sao_2) 10 - CO (Pvo_2 \times 0.003) + (1.34 \times Hgb \times S\overline{v}o_2) 10 = \dot{V}o_2$$

Arterial Supply	Venous Return	$\dot{V}o_2$	a-v O_2 Difference
3.3 (**266** × 0.003) + (1.34 × **10.8** × **0.99**) 10 −	**3.3** (**28** × 0.003) + (1.34 × **10.8** × **0.60**) 10		
3.3 (0.82 + 14.32) 10	**3.3** (0.86 + 8.6) 10		
3.3 (15.1) 1	**3.3** (9.4) 10		
498 mL/min	300 mL/min		= 198 mL/min 5.7 mL/dL

At point B in the figure, EH's arterial oxygen supply is still low at 498 mL/min, and the oxygen in his mixed venous blood return remains low at 300 mL/min. Vo_2 is now lower than normal (typical after sedation) at 198 mL/min. At this time, the a-v O_2 difference is almost within normal limits at 5.7 mL/dL. These findings are confirmed by the low-normal Svo_2 value of 60% at point B. This patient profile illustrates the point that tissue oxygen consumption (oxygen demand) can be as important as CO and oxygenation (oxygen supply) in determining Svo_2 in a patient with a compromised cardiovascular system.

See Table 13.1, Box 13.3, and Appendix B for explanations of abbreviations and of hemodynamic values.

TABLE 13.5 Alterations in Oxygen Consumption

Condition or Activity	% Increase Over Resting V_{O_2}	% Decrease Under Resting V_{O_2}
Clinical Conditions That Increase V_{O_2}		
Fever	10% (for each 1°C above normal)	
Skeletal injuries	10%–30%	
Work of breathing	40%	
Severe infection	60%	
Shivering	50%–100%	
Burns	100%	
Routine postoperative procedures	7%	
Nasal intubation	25%–40%	
Endotracheal tube suctioning	27%	
Chest trauma	60%	
Multiple-organ dysfunction syndrome	20%–80%	
Sepsis	50%–100%	
Head injury, with patient sedated	89%	
Head injury, with patient not sedated	138%	
Critical illness in emergency department	60%	
Nursing Activities That Increase V_{O_2}		
Dressing change	10%	
Electrocardiogram	16%	
Agitation	18%	
Physical examination	20%	
Visitor	22%	
Bath	23%	
Chest radiograph examination	25%	
Position change	31%	
Chest physiotherapy	35%	
Weighing on sling scale	36%	
Conditions That Decrease V_{O_2}		
Anesthesia		25%
Anesthesia in burn patients		50%

V_{O_2}, Oxygen consumption.
Modified from White KM, et al. The physiologic basis for continuous mixed venous oxygen saturation monitoring. *Heart Lung.* 1990;19(5 Pt 2):548.

In step with trends to limit the use of invasive monitoring catheters, the 2016 Surviving Sepsis guidelines for patients with severe sepsis or septic shock no longer recommend specific S_{cvO_2} targets.[36]

High S_{vO_2}. In certain clinical conditions, S_{vO_2} or S_{cvO_2} may increase to an above-normal level (greater than 80%). This occurs during times of low oxygen demand (decreased V_{O_2}), such as during anesthesia or hypothermia. In some cases of septic shock, the tissue cells cannot use the oxygen supplied to them, and the oxygen is not extracted from the blood at the tissue level. In this situation, the venous oxygen reserve remains elevated, and the S_{vO_2} or S_{cvO_2} value is higher than normal (see Table 13.6). If the S_{vO_2} PA catheter drifts into a wedged position, the S_{vO_2} increases because the fiberoptic tip of the catheter comes into contact with newly oxygenated blood.[33]

Less Invasive Hemodynamic Monitoring

Tremendous progress has been made in the development of less invasive methods of hemodynamic monitoring. The newer monitoring methods range from completely noninvasive to methods that, although less invasive than a PA catheter, involve insertion of intravascular catheters or esophageal probes to gather monitoring information (Table 13.7). All newer monitoring methods that estimate CO have been compared with the PA catheter thermodilution CO method.

The latest innovation is to provide a suite of hemodynamic monitoring options using similar technologies with different ranges of invasiveness as diagramed in Fig. 13.1. This range of hemodynamic options allows the critical care team to tailor the invasiveness and diagnostic capabilities of the monitoring system to the clinical needs of the patient.

Arterial Waveform–Based Hemodynamic Monitoring and Cardiac Output Methods

Arterial pressure–based systems are revolutionizing hemodynamic monitoring as proprietary technologies from different companies showcase new technologies with options ranging from noninvasive to invasive (see Fig. 13.1 and Table 13.7).

Finger cuff hemodynamic monitoring systems. Finger cuff systems are noninvasive and trend continuous blood pressure SV, stroke volume variation (SVV), and CO. These systems are designed for short-term use to monitor hemodynamic variables without inserting any lines. They are the first step in a suite of devices that use arterial waveform analysis (Fig. 13.26).[37] Finger-cuff devices may be particularly helpful during initial hemodynamic assessment or when invasive monitoring is not readily available.[3]

Arterial pulse analysis hemodynamic monitoring systems. Arterial waveform–based systems require insertion of an arterial catheter fitted with specialized sensors that use the arterial pressure and pulse waveform to provide real-time data. The systems use proprietary thermistors, software, and bedside computer systems (Fig. 13.27). The different technologies and the systems may be described as *pulse contour analysis*, *pulse wave analysis*, or *pulse power analysis*.[3] Arterial pressure–based systems trend continuous blood pressure, SV, SVV, pulse pressure variation, and CO. A significant advantage is that the patient does not have to be intubated or sedated to tolerate the monitoring system. Another advantage is that the CO values are recorded in real time and change with breathing pattern and fluid volume interventions. The SVV and CO values are sometimes referred to as *functional hemodynamics*.[38] This is because these values can be used in the assessment of *fluid volume responsiveness* using the *passive leg raise* maneuver (Fig. 13.28).[38] Real-time hemodynamic monitoring systems are especially well suited to this bedside examination. The increase in central blood volume as the legs are raised should increase SV and decrease SVV if a patient is fluid responsive (Fig. 13.29).

These systems are generally noncalibrated and considered minimally invasive.[39,40] In general, noncalibrated systems are reported to have lower levels of CO accuracy compared with bolus thermodilution methods.[39,40] However, the tradeoff is that noncalibrated systems offer a less invasive method of trending CO. Pulse waveform–based methods are less accurate with dysrhythmias because of the irregularity in the shape of the arterial waveform.[37,38]

TABLE 13.6 Measurements of Mixed Venous Oxygen Saturation

Svo$_2$ Measurement	Physiologic Basis for Changes in Svo$_2$/Scvo$_2$	Clinical Diagnosis and Rationale
High Svo$_2$ (80%–95%)	Increased oxygen supply	Patient receiving more oxygen than required by clinical condition
		Anesthesia, which causes sedation and decreased muscle movement
	Decreased oxygen demand	Hypothermia, which lowers metabolic demand (eg, during cardiopulmonary bypass)
		Sepsis caused by decreased ability of tissues to use oxygen at a cellular level
		False high-positive result because pulmonary artery catheter is wedged in a pulmonary arteriole (Svo$_2$ only)
Normal Svo$_2$/Scvo$_2$ (60%–80%)	Normal oxygen supply and metabolic demand	Balanced oxygen supply and demand
Low Svo$_2$/Scvo$_2$ (<60%)	Decreased oxygen supply caused by	Anemia or bleeding with compromised cardiopulmonary system
	Low Hgb	Hypoxemia resulting from decreased oxygen supply or lung disease
	Low Sao$_2$	Cardiogenic shock caused by LV pump failure
	Low CO	Metabolic demand exceeds oxygen supply in conditions that increase muscle movement and increase metabolic rate, including physiologic states such as shivering, seizures, and hyperthermia and nursing interventions such as being weighed on a bed scale and turning
	Increased Vo$_2$	

CO, cardiac output; *Hgb,* hemoglobin; *LV,* left ventricular; *Sao$_2$,* arterial saturation; *Scvo$_2$,* Central venous oxygen saturation; *Svo$_2$,* mixed venous oxygen saturation; *Vo$_2$,* oxygen consumption.

TABLE 13.7 Cardiac Output Measurement

Device Name	Probe Placement	Method	Cardiac Output Calculation	Clinical Issues
Noninvasive Methods				
Bioimpedance	External electrodes placed on the neck and chest	Thoracic electrical bioimpedance	1. A small alternating current is applied across the chest by skin electrodes.	Noninvasive
Pressure and Pulse Contour (ClearSight, Edwards Lifesciences, CA)	Fingers	External Finger Cuffs	2. Pulsatile changes in thoracic blood volume result in changes in electrical impedance. The rate of change of impedance during systole is measured and used to calculate CO. Pulsatile changes on finger arteries used to calculate BP, CO, SVV	Less accurate with low body temperature. One cuff used up to 8 hours on a finger. With 2 cuffs, change fingers each hour
Minimally Invasive Methods				
Pulse Contour Waveform Methods				
LiDCO (LiDCO Ltd., Cambridge, United Kingdom)	Requires a venous access catheter (central or peripheral) and an arterial catheter with a lithium-monitoring sensor attached (calibrated)	Pulse contour waveform analysis method (calibrated)	Independent calibration with a lithium dilution technique is initially required.	Easy to set up; uses conventional venous and arterial catheters
			1. A small, subtherapeutic dose of isotonic lithium chloride is injected through the venous catheter.	Can measure extravascular lung water for patients with pulmonary edema
			2. The lithium is detected at the arterial sensor (femoral artery), where a fixed flow pump ensures constant flow.	CO measurement is affected by artifact on arterial waveform and by irregular and damped arterial waveforms
			3. A concentration-time curve is produced for lithium before recirculation.	Can be used in conscious and in unresponsive patients
			4. CO is calculated based on lithium dose given and the measurement of area under the curve. A noncalibrated system is also available.	Requires calibration at least every 8 h to maintain accuracy; cannot be used in patients on lithium therapy because this interferes with calibration

TABLE 13.7 Cardiac Output Measurement—cont'd

Device Name	Probe Placement	Method	Cardiac Output Calculation	Clinical Issues
PiCCO (Pulsion Medical Systems, Munich, Germany)	Requires a central venous access catheter and uses a specialized arterial thermistor-tipped catheter in the femoral artery	Pulse contour waveform analysis method that uses transpulmonary thermodilution	1. A set volume of cold saline is injected through the central venous catheter. The arterial thermistor-tipped catheter detects the blood temperature change. 2. Continuous CO measurements are achieved by analyzing the systolic component of the arterial waveform. A noncalibrated system is also available.	CO measurement is affected by artifact on arterial waveform and irregular arterial waveforms Three calibrations are required initially, and frequent recalibration is required to maintain accuracy
FloTrac, Vigileo (Edward Lifesciences, Irvine, CA)	Requires a functional arterial catheter	Pulse contour waveform analysis method (does not require calibration)	1. Calculates CO by use of arterial pressure waveform analysis in conjunction with patient data (age, sex, height, weight). 2. Uses an internal proprietary algorithm based on the principle that pulse pressure (difference between systolic and diastolic pressure) is proportional to SV and inversely proportional to aortic compliance. 3. Aortic pressure is sampled at 100 Hz and is updated every 20 s.	Does not require external calibration, but requires zeroing of the transducer Lack of calibration procedures is controversial
Esophageal Probe Methods				
Esophageal Doppler	Ultrasound probe placed in the lower esophagus	SV is calculated by measurement of the aortic blood velocity in the descending thoracic aorta (by continuous wave Doppler) plus calculation of the cross-sectional area of the aorta; these values are used to calculate the CO.	1. Measurement of the aorta cross-sectional area, measured using M-mode ultrasound, and multiplying this value by blood velocity to calculate flow or CO. 2. The value of total CO is derived from a nomogram using aortic blood velocity, height, weight, and age.	Useful in the operating room or with deeply sedated patients Probe is stiff, and placement is not well tolerated by conscious patients
TEE	Ultrasound probe placed in esophagus	Probe placement allows imaging of LV outflow tract. SV is measured by Doppler.	1. LV outflow tract area is measured; this value is squared and multiplied by the velocity time interval of blood flow and HR. 2. LV SV can be measured, as can HR to use the SV × HR = CO formula.	Useful in the operating room or with deeply sedated patients Probe is stiff, and placement is not well tolerated by conscious patients Requires skill to accurately position probe to visualize LV outflow tract
Partial CO_2 Rebreathing Method				
NICO$_2$ (Philips, Respironics) Amsterdam, Netherlands	Addition of partial CO_2 rebreathing circuit to ventilator	Partial CO_2 rebreathing method	CO measurement is based on changes in respiratory CO_2 concentration obtained from a short period of rebreathing. CO_2 elimination is calculated by sensors that measure flow, airway pressure, and CO_2 concentration. These variables are used in the Fick partial rebreathing formula to calculate CO.	Can be used only in intubated and ventilated patients Specialized additional tubing setup on ventilator Cannot be used in patients who cannot tolerate hypercapnia (elevated CO_2) CO measurement altered by intrapulmonary shunt

CO, cardiac output; *CO$_2$*, carbon dioxide; *HR*, heart rate; *LV*, left ventricular; *SV*, stroke volume; *TEE*, transesophageal echocardiography.

Finger-cuff technologies

FIG. 13.26 Finger Cuff Arterial Pressure-Based Monitoring. Noninvasive systems that can measure blood pressure, heart rate and calculate stroke volume variation (SVV) and cardiac output (CO). From Lough, M.E. *Hemodynamic Monitoring: Evolving Technologies and Clinical Practice*, Philadelphia: Elsevier; 2016.

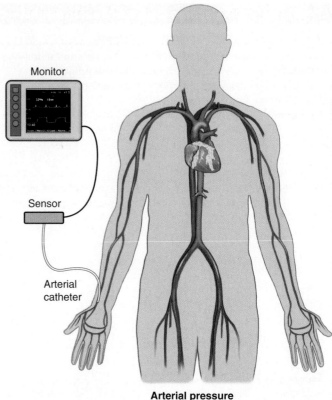

Arterial pressure

FIG. 13.27 Arterial Waveform and Pressure-Based Monitoring: Less invasive systems that use a specialized transducer and arterial catheter sensor to calculate Stroke Volume (SV), Stroke Volume Variation (SVV), Cardiac Output (CO) and Cardiac Index (CI). Both calibrated and noncalibrated hemodynamic systems are available. From Lough, M.E. Hemodynamic Monitoring: Evolving Technologies and Clinical Practice, Philadelphia: Elsevier; 2016.

FIG. 13.28 Passive Leg Raise in Intubated Patient. From Lough, M.E. *Hemodynamic Monitoring: Evolving Technologies and Clinical Practice*, Philadelphia: Elsevier; 2016.

The nursing management of an arterial catheter described in the earlier section on arterial pressure monitoring also applies here. If the arterial waveform is not pristine, the hemodynamic data will be compromised. The position of the transducer is also important. If the transducer level is misaligned by more than 4 inches (10 cm), inaccurate measurements can result.[41]

Transpulmonary thermodilution monitoring systems. Transpulmonary thermodilution monitoring systems are calibrated and more invasive, as they require both arterial and central venous access (Fig. 13.1). As explained earlier, the system may be described by specific *pulse analysis* terms depending on the manufacturer. Transpulmonary thermodilution systems are used when more exact (calibrated) information is required. The calibration methods vary from cold saline to lithium depending on the system used. Systems should be calibrated at least every 8 hours.[3]

To obtain a CO, using the transpulmonary thermodilution technique, a bolus of cold saline is injected into the CVC and measured at a femoral arterial thermistor-tipped catheter. Injectate temperature and transit time are used to generate a thermodilution temperature curve to calculate CO (Fig. 13.30).

The use of a CVC and an arterial catheter is invasive but avoids placing a catheter into the right heart chambers as with a PA catheter. Transpulmonary thermodilution systems also provide different data from the traditional PA catheter. The *extravascular lung water index* measures the volume and percentage of water in lung tissue; a higher value is a marker of pulmonary edema. Lung water content increases in conditions such as heart failure and ARDS. Higher lung water content is associated with higher

mortality. Knowledge of extravascular lung water may influence whether to administer diuretics or administer volume.

Pulse contour analysis enables the use of SVV to assess volume status. SVV measures the difference between the highest and lowest SV over the previous 30 seconds. The caveat is that for this to be considered truly accurate, the patient must be mechanically ventilated and not overbreathing the ventilator. This requirement restricts accurate SVV monitoring to patients during anesthesia, deep sedation, or pharmacologic paralysis.

Visual Hemodynamic Monitoring Methods

Transesophageal echocardiography. Traditionally, echocardiography would not have been described as a primary hemodynamic monitoring modality, although that view has changed in many settings. This is because transesophageal echocardiography (TEE) monitoring during cardiac surgery has increased, with more patients returning to the cardiac critical care unit with an esophageal probe in place.[42,43] Generally, surgical patients monitored with TEE are mechanically ventilated and anesthetized after surgery. Because of the close anatomic relationship between the heart and the esophagus, TEE produces images of very high quality of the heart chambers, heart valves, and thoracic aorta without the interference of the chest wall, bone, or air-filled lung (see Fig. 13.31). TEE has the advantage of displaying a real-time image of the heart in motion. This allows real-time assessment of LV cardiac contractility. Additional information specific to

FIG. 13.29 Stroke Volume Variation (SVV) in Response to a Volume Challenge. From Lough, M.E. *Hemodynamic Monitoring: Evolving Technologies and Clinical Practice,* Philadelphia: Elsevier; 2016.

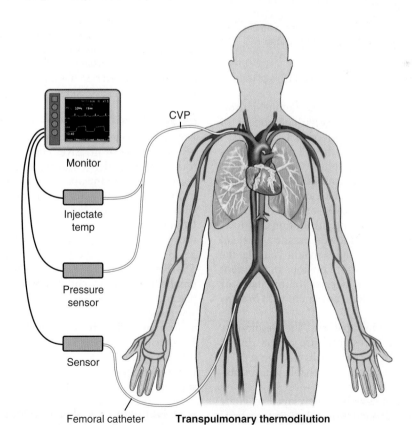

FIG. 13.30 Transpulmonary Thermodilution Arterial Waveform Pressure-Based Monitoring. More invasive calibrated systems that use an arterial catheter and central venous catheter (CVC) to obtain a transpulmonary thermodilution (TPTD) cardiac output (CVC through pulmonary vascular system to arterial catheter with sensor). From Lough, M.E. *Hemodynamic Monitoring: Evolving Technologies and Clinical Practice,* Philadelphia: Elsevier; 2016.

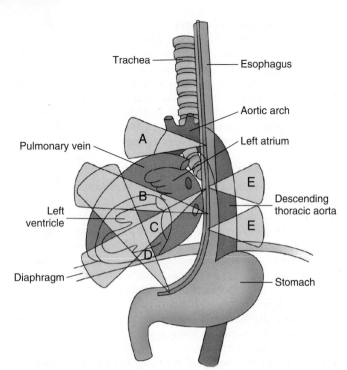

FIG. 13.31 Diagram of Common Scan Planes During a Transesophageal Echocardiogram (TEE) With a Two-Dimensional View. (A) Horizontal scan plane of the aortic arch and distal portion of aorta. (B) Basal short-axis (transverse), long-axis (sagittal), and short-axis views of both atria. (C) Four-chamber and left atrioventricular long-axis views. A sagittal scan plane can image a cross section of the left ventricle. (D) Transgastric, short-axis view of the left and right ventricles. (E) Transverse and sagittal scan sections of the descending aorta.

FIG. 13.32 Respiratory Changes in Intrathoracic Pressure on Inferior Vena Cava Diameter Viewed by Ultrasound. Respiratory intrathoracic pressure changes impact inferior vena cava (IVC) diameter. When a spontaneously breathing patient takes a deep breath (inhalation) or sniffs, the blood in the IVC rapidly enters the right atrium and the IVC decreases in diameter – a collapsed IVC is a sign of hypovolemia. In contrast, when a patient performs a Valsalva maneuverer, the IVC visibly fills up, with less blood going into the right atrium. **A1**. Exhalation (expiration), the IVC is at maximum diameter in a spontaneously breathing patient **A2**. Inhalation (inspiration) the IVC has collapsed indicating hypovolemia in a spontaneously breathing patient. **B1**. 2-D ultrasound of IVC from the subxiphoid view in a spontaneously breathing patient. **B2**. M-Mode ultrasound showing changes in the IVC diameter with breathing: Position **A** indicates exhalation (expiration); Position **B** indicates inhalation (inspiration). From Lough, M.E. Hemodynamic Monitoring: Evolving Technologies and Clinical Practice, Philadelphia: Elsevier; 2016.

noninvasive transthoracic echocardiography (TTE) is provided later on in this chapter.

Ultrasound-based hemodynamic monitoring. Handheld ultrasound has become an essential noninvasive component of beside hemodynamic assessment in many critical care units.[44] Critical care societies now recommend that all medical trainees learn the basic skills of ultrasonography.[44] One of the most useful ultrasound skills is the assessment of fluid volume status by examination of the inferior vena cava (IVC) during the respiratory cycle. In a mechanically ventilated patient, intrathoracic pressure is highest during inspiration and lowest at end-expiration. At the point of lowest pressure, preload volume is rapidly drawn into the right atrium causing the IVC to "collapse." This collapse is more obvious in a patient with hypovolemia. In a patient with normal volume status or hypervolemia, the IVC walls have less movement with breathing (Fig. 13.32).[44]

In a spontaneously breathing patient, the respiratory mechanics are different. The lowest pressure occurs during inspiration; with hypovolemia, the IVC walls may be seen to collapse.[44] This measure is considered less reliable in a spontaneously breathing patient.[45]

Many ultrasound protocols have been developed to guide clinical management. These validated protocols are often a first-line level of hemodynamic assessment in an unstable patient.

Ultrasound is a frequency greater than 20,000 Hz, which is above the range of human hearing. Ultrasound is reflected visibly at interfaces between tissues that have different densities. Protocols are used to ensure that all practitioners use ultrasound-guided diagnosis in a consistent manner. One of the earliest uses was in trauma where *focused assessment by sonography for trauma* (FAST) is used to evaluate intraabdominal blood. Chapter 33 has additional information about use of FAST for trauma assessment (See Fig. 33.16).

Doppler-Based Hemodynamic Monitoring Methods

Doppler offers another method to trend CO. This modality can be noninvasive or invasive. The esophagus is used as the monitoring site for patients who are deeply sedated or are under general anesthesia in the operating room. The esophageal Doppler probe is generally described as minimally invasive compared with a PA catheter (Fig. 13.33).[46] Insertion of the esophageal Doppler probe is similar to insertion of a gastric tube, although the probe is relatively inflexible and stiff.[46] The probe is inserted 35 to 40 cm from the teeth. The tip of the probe rests near T5-T6 on the vertebral column, where the esophagus typically is parallel with the descending aorta. When the probe is correctly placed, this method has a high degree of accuracy for CO measurement. Accurate CO values depend on correct placement and on the skill of the operator.[46]

Intermittent SV and CO information can also be obtained using a noninvasive transthoracic Doppler. This technique is more frequently used in pediatric and non–critical care settings.

Less Frequent Hemodynamic Monitoring Methods
Partial Carbon Dioxide Rebreathing Cardiac Output

A technique that is rarely used involves partial carbon dioxide (CO_2) rebreathing to estimate CO in mechanically ventilated patients. This technique involves the addition of an extra circuit (tubing loop) to the ventilator tubing where a sensor that uses

FIG. 13.33 Esophageal Doppler Probe with tip positioned in the esophagus, parallel to the descending aorta.

infrared light absorption measures CO_2, and a second sensor measures airflow in the circuit tubing to collect data during a breathing cycle. CO_2 production is calculated as the product of minute ventilation and CO_2 concentration. Arterial CO_2 content is derived from end-tidal CO_2 and the CO_2 dissociation curve. The differences in these values are then used to calculate the CO.[47] This system is rarely used in critical care and requires frequent calibration to maintain accuracy.

Thoracic Electrical Bioimpedance

Thoracic electrical bioimpedance is a noninvasive method of continuous CO measurement. Impedance cardiography works by emitting a low-voltage, high-frequency, alternating electrical current through the thorax by means of four skin electrodes. Two are placed at the base of the neck under the ear, and two are placed at the side of the chest in the midaxillary line at the midxyphoid level.[48] The sensing electrodes detect changes in electrical impedance within the thorax. Because blood flow through the thoracic aorta causes shifts in impedance, this information can be used to calculate SV and continuous CO. Use of thoracic electrical bioimpedance in the critical care setting is uncommon.

ELECTROCARDIOGRAPHY

Electrocardiography is a complex and vitally useful skill to master. Detailed evaluation of an ECG can provide a wealth of cardiac diagnostic information and often provides the basis on which other, definitive diagnostic tests are selected. The following sections discuss the many clinical factors that the critical care nurse considers when using ECG monitoring, specific dysrhythmias commonly encountered in clinical practice, and the skills needed for 12-lead ECG analysis. The intent is to provide a sound basis for understanding the value of the many clinical applications of electrocardiography.

Basic Principles of Electrocardiography

The ECG records electrical changes in heart muscle caused by an action potential. It does not record the mechanical contraction, which usually follows electrical depolarization immediately. A brief discussion of the cardiac action potential is provided to explain the concept that electrical changes occurring during electrical stimulation of the myocardial cell produce the deflections seen on the ECG tracing (Fig. 13.34).

Phase 0

During phase 0 (depolarization), the electrical potential changes rapidly from a baseline of −90 mV to +20 mV and stabilizes at approximately 0 mV. Because this is a significant electrical change, it appears as a wave on the ECG as the QRS complex.

Phases 1 and 2

During phases 1 and 2, an electrical plateau is created, and mechanical contraction occurs during this plateau. Because there is no significant electrical change, no waveform appears on the ECG (the recorded tracing is isoelectric with baseline).

Phase 3

During phase 3 (repolarization), the electrical potential again changes, this time a little more slowly, from 0 mV back to −90 mV. This is another major electrical event and is reflected on the ECG as a T wave.

Phase 4

During phase 4 (resting period), the chemical balance is restored by the sodium pump, but because positively charged ions are exchanged on a one-for-one basis, no electrical activity is generated, and no visible change occurs on the ECG tracing. For more information on the cardiac action potential, see "Phases of the Action Potential" in Chapter 12.

Electrocardiogram Leads

All electrocardiographs use a system of one or more leads. The basic three-lead system consists of three bipolar electrodes that are applied to the chest wall and labeled right arm (RA), left arm (LA), and left leg (LL). The term *bipolar* means that each created ECG lead has a positive and a negative pole. A third electrode acts as a ground. The function of the ground electrode is to prevent the display of background electrical interference on the ECG tracing. Electrodes do not transmit any electricity to the patient; rather, they sense and record intrinsic cardiac electrical activity from the body's surface. Lead wires can be disposable or reusable.[49] There is no difference in infection rates as long as the nondisposable ECG wires and connectors are thoroughly cleaned between each patient use.[50] The ECG electrode patch that touches the patient's skin is always disposable.

The positive electrode on the skin acts as a camera. If the wave of depolarization travels toward the positive electrode, an upward stroke, or *positive deflection*, is written on the ECG paper

FIG. 13.34 Correlation of Action Potential of a Ventricular Myocardial Cell With Electrical Events Recorded on Surface ECG. The ECG pattern is "silent" during phase 2 of the action potential. Mechanical contraction is occurring, but no significant electrical activity is present.

(Fig. 13.35A). If the wave of depolarization travels away from the positive electrode, a downward line, or *negative deflection*, is recorded on the ECG (Fig. 13.35B). When depolarization moves perpendicularly to the positive electrode, a biphasic complex occurs. Sometimes the complex may even appear almost flat, or isoelectric, if the electrical forces traveling in opposite directions are equal and have the effect of canceling each other (Fig. 13.35C). The size of the muscle mass being depolarized also has an effect, with the larger muscle mass (usually the left ventricle) having a greater influence on the tracing.

The wave of ventricular depolarization in the healthy heart travels from right to left and from head to toe. The appearance of the waveforms in different ECG leads depends on the location of the positive electrode.

12-Lead electrocardiogram. The standard 12-lead ECG provides a picture of electrical activity in the heart using 10 different electrode positions to create 12 unique views of electrical activity occurring within the heart.[51,52] A standard 12-lead ECG contains six limb lead images and six chest (precordial) lead images, and the correct placement of these leads is vitally important to avoid misdiagnosis. If a 12-lead ECG is being obtained, the limb electrodes are typically placed on the muscle of the limb avoiding bone, and the patient is asked to remain still. In the critical care unit, the electrodes are typically placed on the torso, near the origin of the limb, avoiding the clavicular bone (LA and RA) and the pelvic bone (LL and RL), as shown in Fig. 13.36A. This arrangement is used because patients wear the electrodes for hours or days, and limb movement would distort the electrical baseline. Practically, this means that ECG waveforms on the bedside monitor will not be identical to the waveforms obtained by a standard 12-lead ECG, for which the limb electrodes are placed directly on corresponding extremities.[51]

Standard limb leads. The limb lead tracings are obtained by placing electrodes on all four extremities: LA, RA, LL, and RL. Leads I, II, and III are *bipolar* limb leads that use limb lead electrodes paired as the positive and negative poles (see Fig. 13.36A). The electrodes are placed in a static position on the

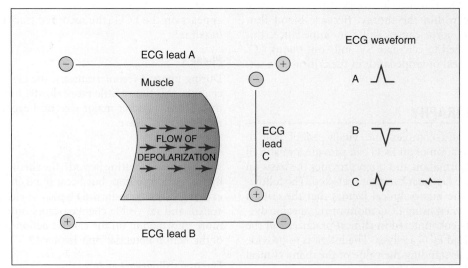

FIG. 13.35 Effect of Lead Position on ECG Tracing. (A) Flow of depolarization toward the positive electrode results in a positive deflection on the ECG. (B) Flow of depolarization away from the positive electrode results in a negative deflection on the ECG. (C) Flow of depolarization perpendicular to the positive electrode results in a biphasic or nearly isoelectric deflection on the ECG. This basic principle applies to the P wave and the QRS complex.

body, and the polarity is switched to achieve the desired view. This is done manually on the critical care bedside monitor or automatically by the electrocardiography machine when a 12-lead ECG is obtained:

Lead I—positive electrode at LA and negative electrode at RA
Lead II—positive electrode at LL and negative electrode at RA
Lead III—positive electrode at LL and negative electrode at LA

This configuration means that the three limb leads are linked in a circuit. The information obtained from the three limb leads is used to create a *central reference potential* that reflects the average potential of the RA, LA, and LL electrodes.[51] The central reference potential shown at the center of the electrode triangle in Fig. 13.36A is used to calculate the augmented vector leads.

Augmented vector leads. The *augmented vector leads*, labeled aVR, aVL, and aVF, are created from the derived electrode pairs previously described. These augmented leads have only one positive electrode (see Fig. 13.36A), with the calculated central

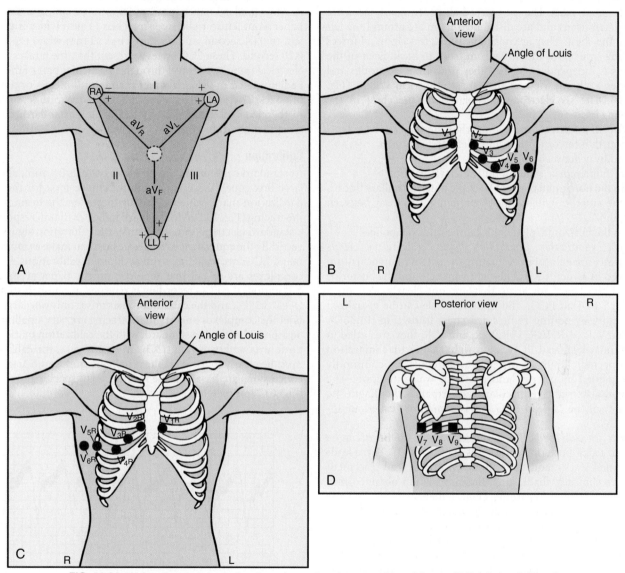

FIG. 13.36 (A) Standard limb leads. Leads are located on the extremities: right arm (RA), left arm (LA), and left leg (LL). The right leg electrode serves as a ground. Leads I, II, and III are bipolar, with each using a positive electrode and a negative electrode. Leads aVR, aVL, and aVF are augmented unipolar leads that use the calculated center of the heart as their negative electrode. (B) Precordial leads. V_1 to V_6 are the six standard precordial leads and are placed as follows: V_1, fourth intercostal space, right sternal border; V_2, fourth intercostal space, left sternal border; V_3, equidistant between V_2 and V_4; V_4, fifth intercostal space, left midclavicular line; V_5, anterior axillary line, same horizontal level as V_4; V_6, midaxillary line, same horizontal level as V_4. (C) The right precordial leads V_1R to V_6R are shown. They are not part of a standard 12-lead ECG but are used when a right ventricular infarction is suspected. Their placement is identical to V_3 to V_6 except that they are placed on the right side of the chest rather than on the left. (D) Posterior precordial leads V_7, V_8, and V_9 are placed on the patient's left posterior chest at the same horizontal level as V_4 (fifth intercostal space). V_7 is on the posterior axillary line, V_8 is on the scapular line, and V_9 is on the spinal border. These leads may be added to the standard 12-lead ECG when a posterior wall infarction is suspected.

reference potential (center of triangle) acting as a negative electrode. Under these circumstances, the ECG tracing obtained is ordinarily very small, so the machine enhances, or *augments*, it by adding enough voltage to render the waveform amplitudes roughly equivalent to the other lead views. The term *vector* refers to directional force. The augmented vector leads are used in the interpretation of myocardial injury and infarction. The limb leads and the augmented vector leads are derived from the four limb electrodes. They constitute the *frontal plane axis* of the 12-lead ECG.[53]

Precordial leads. The six precordial, or left chest, leads are labeled as V leads and are distributed in an arc around the left side of the chest. They are positioned to detect electrical forces traveling from right to left or from front to back. Each of the V leads is independent of the other precordial electrodes and provides a unique view of the cardiac electrical system (Fig. 13.36B). The six electrodes are placed on the chest in the following locations[51]:

V_1—fourth intercostal space at the right sternal border
V_2—fourth intercostal space at the left sternal border
V_3—midway between V_2 and V_4
V_4—fifth intercostal space in the midclavicular line
V_5—in the horizontal plane of V_4 at the anterior axillary line or, if the anterior axillary line is ambiguous, midway between V_4 and V_6
V_6—in the horizontal plane of V_4 at the midaxillary line

Right ventricular precordial leads. Additional leads sometimes are helpful in evaluating the extent of myocardium involved in an acute MI. The right ventricle and the posterior wall of the heart are areas that are not clearly seen on a standard 12-lead ECG. The right ventricle can be visualized more fully by adding right-sided chest leads (Fig. 13.36C). Labeled V_1R, V_2R, V_3R, V_4R, V_5R, and V_6R, they are added to the standard 12-lead ECG when right ventricular infarction is suspected. Right ventricular infarction is commonly accompanied by inferior and posterior wall infarction. The use of the six right ventricular leads expands the diagnostic accuracy of the 12-lead ECG and is sometimes called an *18-lead ECG*.

Posterior wall leads. The posterior wall of the heart can be assessed using posterior chest leads (Fig. 13.36D). These leads are labeled V_7, V_8, and V_9. Although posterior lead placement can be technically challenging, the information obtained may influence decisions regarding clinical management. The use of the posterior leads expands the diagnostic accuracy of the 12-lead ECG and can be described as a *15-lead ECG*.

Baseline distortion. The tracing must have a flat baseline, which is the portion of the tracing between the various waveforms. Two forms of artifact can distort the baseline: 60-cycle interference and muscular movement. The 60 cycle/s (Hertz) interference artifact (Fig. 13.37A) results from leakage of ambient electrical current in the immediate environment and appears as a generalized thickening of the baseline. It can usually be resolved by ensuring that all electrical equipment at the bedside is electrically grounded. Moving the offending device away from the patient may help, or occasionally it may be necessary to unplug one piece of equipment at a time until the offending device is found. Muscular movement (Fig. 13.37B) is displayed as a coarse, erratic disturbance of the baseline. In most cases, asking the patient to lie quietly while the ECG is being run is sufficient. If movement is caused by shivering or seizure activity, it is best to wait until the activity subsides before

obtaining the 12-lead ECG. When baseline tremor is caused by seizures or the tremor of Parkinson disease, resolution may be impossible. Electrical artifact disrupts accurate interpretation of the tracing and may mimic lethal ventricular dysrhythmias.

Electrocardiogram Analysis
Specialized Electrocardiogram Paper
ECG paper records the speed and magnitude of electrical impulses on a grid composed of small and large boxes (Fig. 13.38). Every large box contains 25 small (1 mm^2) boxes within it. At a standard paper speed of 25 mm/s, looking at the ECG paper from left to right, one small box (1 mm wide) is equivalent to 0.04 second, and one large box (5 mm wide) represents 0.20 second. These ECG boxes represent the time it takes for the electrical impulse to travel through a particular part of the heart and are stated in seconds rather than in millimeters or number of boxes. The vertical scale represents the magnitude, or force, of the electrical signal. The vertical scale is standardized to a specific calibration.

Calibration
At standard calibration, one small box equals 0.1 mm, and one large box equals 0.5 mm. It is important to look for the standardization mark, which is usually located at the beginning of the tracing (Fig. 13.39A). The mark indicates that in response to a standard electrical signal of 1 mV, the calibration signal rises vertically the equivalent of two large boxes to make a calibration mark. ECGs are sometimes run at different calibrations. If some complexes are so tall that they run off the paper at standard calibration, the ECG recording is repeated at one-half standard (Fig. 13.39B), and the calibration mark rises only one large box. If all the complexes on a standard tracing are very small, it may be repeated at double standard, with the calibration mark going up four large boxes (Fig. 13.39C). In any case, the calibration must be clearly marked on the tracing because some diagnostic conclusions are based on the magnitude of specific portions of the ECG complex.

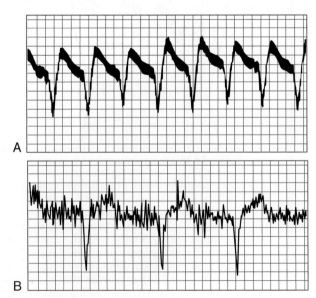

FIG. 13.37 (A) Artifact from 60-cycle interference. (B) Artifact caused by muscular movement.

Waveforms

The analysis of waveforms and intervals provides the basis for ECG interpretation (Fig. 13.40).

P wave. The P wave represents atrial depolarization.

QRS complex. The QRS complex represents ventricular depolarization, corresponding to phase 0 of the ventricular action potential. It is referred to as a *complex* because it consists of several different waves. The letter Q is used to describe an initial negative deflection; the first deflection from the baseline is labeled a Q wave only if it is negative. The letter R applies to any positive deflection from baseline. If there are two positive deflections in one QRS complex, the second is labeled R′ ("R prime") and is commonly seen in lead V₁ in patients with right bundle branch block (RBBB). The letter S refers to any subsequent negative deflections. Any combination of these deflections can occur and is collectively called the *QRS complex* (Fig. 13.41). The QRS complex duration is normally less than 0.10 second (2.5 small boxes).

T wave. The T wave represents ventricular repolarization, corresponding to phase 3 of the ventricular action potential. The onset of the QRS complex to approximately the midpoint or peak of the T wave represents an absolute refractory period, during which the heart muscle cannot respond to another stimulus no matter how strong that stimulus may be (Fig. 13.42). From the midpoint to the end of the T wave, the heart muscle is in the relative refractory period. The heart muscle has not yet fully recovered, but it can be depolarized again if a strong enough stimulus is received. This can be a particularly dangerous time for ventricular ectopy to occur, especially if any portion of the myocardium is ischemic because the ischemic muscle takes even longer to fully repolarize. This sets the stage for the disorganized, self-perpetuating depolarizations of various sections of the myocardium known as *ventricular fibrillation* (VF).

Intervals Between Waveforms

The intervals between waveforms are evaluated (see Fig. 13.40).

P–R interval. The P–R interval is measured from the beginning of the P wave to the beginning of the QRS complex. The P–R interval normally is 0.12 to 0.20 second long and represents the time between sinus node discharge and the beginning of ventricular depolarization. Because most of this period results from delay of the impulse in the AV node, the P–R interval is an indicator of AV nodal function.

In the electrophysiology laboratory and in some critical care units, these time values are described in milliseconds. There are 1000 ms in 1 second. Thus, the normal P–R interval value can also be written as 120 to 200 ms.

ST segment. The ST segment is the portion of the wave that extends from the end of the QRS complex to the beginning of the T wave. Its duration is not measured. Instead, its shape and location are evaluated. The ST segment is normally flat and at the same level as the isoelectric baseline. Any change from baseline is expressed in millimeters and may indicate myocardial ischemia (one small box equals 1 mm). ST segment

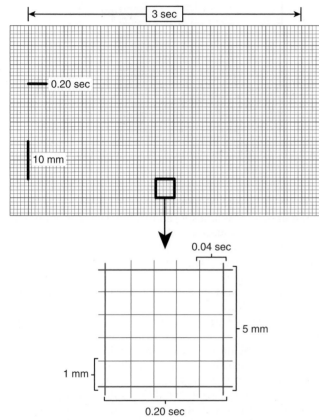

FIG. 13.38 ECG Graph Paper. The horizontal axis represents time, and the vertical axis represents the magnitude of voltage. Horizontally, each small box is 0.04 s, and each large box is 0.20 s. Vertically, each large box is 5 mm. Markings are present every 3 s at the top of the paper for ease in calculating heart rate.

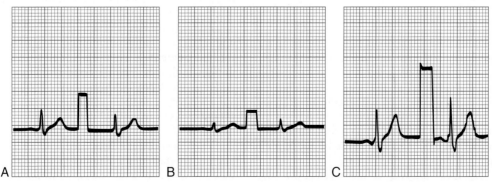

FIG. 13.39 (A) The machine is calibrated so that the normal standardization mark is 10 mm tall. (B) Half standardization is used when QRS complexes are too tall to fit on the paper. (C) Twice normal standardization is used when QRS complexes are too small to be adequately analyzed.

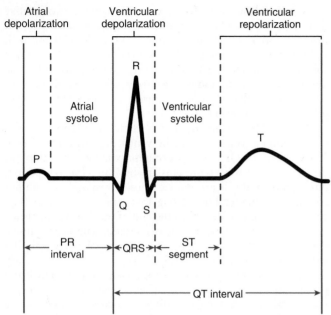

FIG. 13.40 Normal ECG Waveforms, Intervals, and Correlation With Events of Cardiac Cycle. The *P wave* represents atrial depolarization, followed immediately by atrial systole. The *QRS complex* represents ventricular depolarization, followed immediately by ventricular systole. The *ST segment* corresponds to phase 2 of the action potential, during which time the heart muscle is completely depolarized and contraction normally occurs. The *T wave* represents ventricular repolarization. The *P–R interval*, measured from the beginning of the P wave to the beginning of the QRS complex, corresponds to atrial depolarization and impulse delay in the atrioventricular (AV) node. The *Q–T interval*, measured from the beginning of the QRS complex to the end of the T wave, represents the time from initial depolarization of the ventricles to the end of ventricular repolarization.

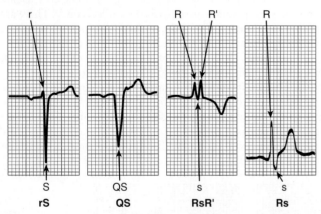

FIG. 13.41 Examples of QRS Complexes. Small deflections are labeled with lowercase letters, and uppercase letters are used for larger deflections. A second upward deflection is labeled R'.

elevation of 1 to 2 mm is associated with acute myocardial injury, preinfarction, and pericarditis. ST segment depression (decrease from baseline more of 1 to 2 mm) is associated with myocardial ischemia.[54] The ST segment must be monitored carefully in high-risk patients (described later).

Q–T interval. The Q–T interval is measured from the beginning of the QRS complex to the end of the T wave and indicates the total time interval from the onset of depolarization to the completion of repolarization. There is no established bedside monitoring lead recommended for measuring the Q–T

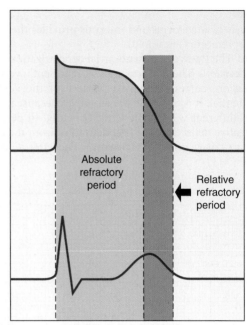

FIG. 13.42 Absolute and relative refractory periods are correlated with the cardiac muscle action potential and with an ECG tracing.

interval.[52] On the 12-lead ECG, the Q–T interval is usually the longest in precordial leads V_3 and V_4.[52] The important point is that each clinician measures the Q–T interval using the same ECG lead.[52] At a normal HR, the Q–T interval is less than one-half of the R–R interval when measured from one QRS complex to the next. However, the length of a Q–T interval depends on the HR and must be adjusted according to the HR to be evaluated in a clinically meaningful way.

Because the Q–T interval shortens at faster HRs and lengthens with slower HRs, it is often written as a "corrected" value (Q–Tc), meaning the Q–T value was mathematically corrected as if the HR were 60 beats/min. This allows comparison of the Q–Tc interval across a range of HRs. The Q–Tc interval is calculated by dividing the measured Q–T interval (in seconds) by the square root of the R–R cycle length (see Fig. 13.40).[52] The upper limit of normal for the Q–Tc interval is 0.48 second (480 ms) in women and less than 0.47 second (470 ms) in men.[52] A prolonged Q–T interval is significant because it can predispose the patient to the development of polymorphic VT, known also as *torsades de pointes*. A long Q–T interval can be congenital, as a result of genetic inheritance, or it can be acquired from an electrolyte imbalance or medications.[55,56] Many antidysrhythmic medications can prolong the Q–T interval, notably class Ia antidysrhythmics (quinidine, procainamide, disopyramide) and class III antidysrhythmics (amiodarone, dronedarone, ibutilide, dofetilide, sotalol). Not all high-risk medications are antidysrhythmics. The US Food and Drug Administration has added a "black box" warning and a requirement for Q–T interval monitoring for the antipsychotic medication haloperidol (Haldol), used in critical care for treatment of agitation and delirium.[57]

When medications associated with a high risk of torsades de pointes are started, it is important to record the premedication baseline Q–Tc interval and to continue to monitor the Q–Tc interval during treatment. The risk of torsades de pointes is increased with prolongation of the Q–Tc interval beyond 0.5 second (500 ms) or an increase of 60 ms compared with the baseline Q–Tc interval.[58]

Q–Tc interval monitoring is now an established practice in critical care. In a study of 900 cardiac patients, 18% were admitted with a Q–Tc interval longer than 500 ms, and more than one-third of this group were subsequently administered medications that prolong the Q–T interval.[59] Many patients with Q–Tc interval longer than 500 ms acquire multiple risk factors for torsades de pointes during their hospital stay.[56,59]

The risk of torsades de pointes is intensified with electrolyte abnormalities, including hypokalemia, hypomagnesemia, and hypocalcemia.[55] Risk increases in the presence of bradycardia, heart block with pauses, and premature beats with short-long-short cycles (Box 13.6).[55] Another risk factor may be genetics; 10% to 15% of patients with acquired long QT syndrome (medication induced) carry a genetic predisposition for the syndrome.[55]

Acute therapy is directed at increasing the HR, which shortens the Q–T interval, stopping culprit medications, and correcting electrolyte abnormalities. It may also include placement of a temporary pacemaker and administering IV magnesium, especially if serum levels of magnesium are low.

Ventricular Axis

Electrical impulses spread through cardiac muscle tissue in many directions at once when the ventricular muscle is depolarized. Using the 12-lead ECG, all these individual forces can be averaged to describe the overall direction that current is traveling, which is called the *mean vector*. This mean vector represents the general direction of the wavefront of depolarization within the heart. The mean vector can be plotted on a circular graph known as the *hexaxial reference system* (Fig. 13.43), and a degree value can be assigned to it. This degree represents the overall ventricular axis.[53]

Parameters for ventricular axis in degrees are −30 to +90 degrees.[53] Right-axis deviation is present if the heart's electrical axis falls between +90 and +180 degrees. Right-axis deviation can be further delineated as moderate right-axis deviation when it is between +90 and +120 degrees and marked right-axis deviation when it is between +120 and +180 degrees.[53]

Left-axis deviation is present if the axis falls between −30 and −90 degrees. Moderate left-axis deviation describes an axis between −30 and −45 degrees. Marked left-axis deviation describes an axis between −45 and −90 degrees.[53]

Fig. 13.43 shows how these points are located on the hexaxial reference system. If the axis plots in the upper left portion of the circle, also known as the *extreme quadrant* or *northwest quadrant*, it is called an *indeterminate axis*. This axis occurs rarely but can be seen when the wave of depolarization starts at the bottom of the ventricle—near the point of maximal impulse or apex of the ventricle—and spreads upward toward the atria. Clinically, this can be seen in beats of ventricular origin, such as PVCs and some pacemaker-initiated beats.

Calculating the ventricular axis. The ventricular axis is calculated using the six limb leads (leads I, II, III, aVR, aVL, aVF) in the following three steps (see ECG example in Fig. 13.44):

Step 1. Find the limb lead with the smallest QRS complex or the one that is the most *equiphasic* (equal portions above and below the baseline). In Fig. 13.45, lead aVF is the smallest.

Step 2. Using the hexaxial reference system (see Fig. 13.43), locate the lead that is perpendicular to the one that had the smallest complex. For example, perpendicular to lead aVF is lead I, so the mean vector lies parallel with lead I.

BOX 13.6   Risk Factors for Torsades De Pointes

Prolonged Q–Tc Interval
Q–Tc interval ≥500 ms

Medications
Use of Q–T interval–prolonging medications
Rapid intravenous infusion of Q–T interval–prolonging medications
Diuretics

Structural Heart Conditions
Heart failure
Myocardial infarction

Metabolic Conditions
Hypokalemia
Hypomagnesemia
Hypocalcemia
Liver failure with decreased medication metabolism

Bradycardia
Sinus bradycardia
Complete heart block
Incomplete heart block with pauses
Premature complexes leading to short-long-short cycles

Genetic Predisposition
Occult (latent) congenital Long QT Syndrome
Genetic polymorphisms (reduced repolarization reserve)

Age and Sex
Advanced age
Female sex
    Torsades de pointes risk increases with a higher number of risk factors, some of which may be clinically silent and difficult to detect.

From Drew BJ, et al. Prevention of torsade de pointes in hospital settings: a scientific statement from the American Heart Association and the American College of Cardiology Foundation. *Circulation.* 2010;121(8):1047.

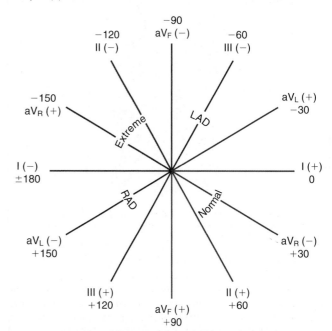

FIG. 13.43 Hexaxial Reference System. *LAD,* left-axis deviation; *RAD,* right-axis deviation.

Step 3. The third step is to determine whether the QRS complex is positive or negative in the lead parallel to the mean vector (in this case, lead I). If the QRS complex is positive, the mean vector is directed *toward* the positive electrode. If the QRS complex is negative, the mean vector is directed *away* from the positive electrode. In Fig. 13.45, the QRS complex deflection in lead I is upright or positive. The positive pole of lead I is at the right midpoint of the hexaxial reference system and corresponds to a numeric degree of zero, which is within the normal range (Box 13.7; see Fig. 13.45).

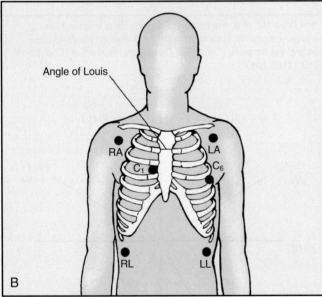

FIG. 13.44 (A) Three electrodes and lead-wire cables allow monitoring of three of the limb leads (I, II, and III). (B) In the multilead monitoring system, five electrodes and lead-wire cables allow monitoring of any of the six standard limb leads (I, II, III, aVR, aVL, or aVF) and any one precordial lead (V₁ or V₆). C₁ indicates the proper position of the chest electrode for monitoring lead V₁, and C₆ indicates the proper position of the chest electrode for monitoring V₆. Color-coded cable attachments allow quick identification and accurate electrode placement.

Cardiac Monitor Lead Analysis

During continuous cardiac monitoring, adhesive, pregelled electrodes are used to obtain an ECG tracing that is similar to one or more leads of a 12-lead ECG. At minimum, this requires three electrodes. One of the electrodes acts as a positive pole, one acts as a negative pole, and one acts as a ground. In most critical care units, five electrodes are used. Five electrode systems allow the clinician to monitor two leads simultaneously and permit selection of several different leads at any time through a lead selector switch on the monitor. Typical placement of the five electrodes in a multilead system is RA, LA, LL, and RL, with one chest lead that usually is placed in the V₁ position, as illustrated in Fig. 13.35.

The selection of an ECG monitoring lead is not a decision to be made casually or according to habit. The monitoring lead should be chosen taking into consideration the patient's clinical condition and recent clinical history.[52] If the patient has experienced ST segment elevation associated with acute coronary syndrome (ACS), percutaneous coronary intervention (PCI), or recent cardiac surgery, the leads that exhibited ST segment elevation should be used to guide selection of the optimal ECG monitoring leads.[52] The nurse verifies correct electrode placement and appropriate lead selection at the beginning of each shift.

Lead II

On a standard 12-lead ECG, lead II is formed by a positive electrode attached to the left leg, a negative electrode attached to the right arm, and a ground electrode attached to the right leg. It is

FIG. 13.45 Limb Leads of Normal ECG Illustrate Normal Axis of 0 Degrees.

BOX 13.7	**Steps in Determining the Axis**

1. Find the most isoelectric limb lead.
2. Using the hexaxial reference system, find the lead that is perpendicular to the lead identified in step 1.
3. Determine whether the QRS complex is positive or negative in the perpendicular lead.
4. Look at the corresponding positive or negative pole of the perpendicular lead on the hexaxial reference system.
5. The degree listed on the hexaxial reference system is the axis.

not practical to connect electrodes to the arms and legs during continuous monitoring, so the electrodes are placed on the torso near the origin of the limbs (see Fig. 13.44). In the critical care unit, most patients have at least five electrodes placed, and the lead is selected by choosing a lead selector button on the monitor. If the monitored heart has a normal electrical axis, lead II displays a waveform that is predominantly upright, with a positive P wave and positive QRS complex waveform (Fig. 13.46). P waves are usually easy to identify in lead II, and this lead is recommended for monitoring of atrial dysrhythmias. However, it is difficult to identify RBBB and left bundle branch block (LBBB) in lead II because this is a vertical lead that does not clearly display horizontal interventricular conduction changes. Lead II is also nondiagnostic in differentiating VT from supraventricular tachycardia (SVT) with aberrant conduction. More information on differentiating VT from wide complex SVT is provided later on in this chapter.

Lead V_1

The V_1 electrode is placed at the fourth intercostal space to the right of the sternal border. Most of the electrical activity of the heart is directed toward the left ventricle and away from the V_1 electrode. For this reason, the normal QRS complex in lead V_1 is mostly negative. Any abnormal electrical activity directed toward the right ventricle, such as in RBBB, results in an upright QRS complex, often in an RSR′ pattern.

A

0 Sec.   3 Sec.

B

FIG. 13.46 Monitoring Lead II. (A) Electrode placement. The negative electrode is placed below the right shoulder; the positive electrode is placed on the lower left torso, preferably below the rib cage; and the ground electrode is placed on the left shoulder. (B) Typical ECG tracing in lead II.

V_1 is the optimal lead to select if the critical care nurse needs to analyze ventricular ectopy. V_1 provides information to facilitate differentiation between RBBB versus LBBB pattern or to distinguish between VT and SVT with aberrant conduction, to determine whether PVCs originate in the right or left ventricle, and to clarify when ST segment changes are caused by the RBBB and when they are the result of ischemia. Lead V_1 is excellent for this purpose. More information on the criteria used to identify these rhythms using the V_1 lead is provided later on.

Electrocardiogram Lead Selection for Optimal Bedside Monitoring

In the early years of critical care nursing, the primary goals of cardiac monitoring were HR surveillance, detection of "warning" ventricular dysrhythmias (mostly PVCs), and early detection of lethal dysrhythmias (VF or asystole). Although these are still goals of ECG monitoring in the critical care unit, several more complex issues are now concerns. Not all wide QRS complex tachycardias are ventricular in origin; sometimes they are supraventricular with aberrant ventricular conduction. Many patients are undergoing reperfusion therapy involving PCI, stent, or fibrinolysis, and these patients require continuous monitoring for ST segment changes that may represent ischemia even in the absence of clinical symptoms. The nurse admitting a patient to the critical care unit or telemetry unit must make a well-planned choice of monitoring leads tailored to the patient's clinical needs. Accuracy of electrode placement is extremely important if these leads are to be used for specialized diagnostic purposes.[54] Upper limb electrodes are placed on the upper chest close to where the limb joins the torso. The lower limb electrodes are placed below the rib cage between the umbilicus and the midaxillary line.[54] Diagnostic accuracy is diminished if limb electrodes are moved too close to the heart.

Continuous Dysrhythmia Monitoring

Patients with serious cardiac diseases such as acute MI, heart failure, and cardiomyopathy are at risk for the development of bundle branch blocks (BBBs), complex ectopy, and wide complex tachycardias. These patients need to be monitored with a precordial lead that documents interventricular conduction changes. This is lead V_1. Some five-lead systems offer the clinician the choice of MCL_1 or V_1. The tracings in these two leads are not identical, and V_1 must always be chosen over MCL_1 because it has a higher diagnostic accuracy. The six frontal plane (limb and augmented lead) tracings also offer several monitoring choices that can be individualized to the clinical needs of the patient. Leads I and aVF are selected to detect a sudden change in ventricular axis. If ST segment monitoring is required, the lead is selected according to the area of ischemia. If the ischemic area is not unknown, leads V_3 and III are recommended to detect ST segment ischemia.[54] In inferior wall injury, leads II, III, and aVF are chosen; if lateral ischemia is present, lead I or aVL may be selected.

Continuous ST Segment Monitoring

A key responsibility of the critical care nurse is monitoring for ECG changes that signify myocardial ischemia.[54] At the bedside, this takes the form of continuous ST segment monitoring using the traditional bedside monitor and ECG electrodes. Increasingly, bedside monitoring systems incorporate ST segment analysis software to detect myocardial ischemia or injury. ST segment changes may be accompanied by classic symptoms such as chest pain, or they may be "silent," without any clinical symptoms except ST segment depression or elevation seen on the ECG monitor.[60] Risk of progression from silent ischemia to overt cardiac events has been documented in patients with diabetes mellitus.[61]

The best way to choose a lead for monitoring the ST segment to detect ischemia is to look at the patient's 12-lead ECG during an episode of ischemia, if available. The standard 12-lead ECG obtained in with an episode of chest pain or during a PCI will reveal the leads that best demonstrate ischemia in that patient.[52] Under normal (nonischemic) conditions, the ST segment is at the same level as the TP segment (segment of the isoelectric line that begins at the end of the T wave to the start of the next P wave),[62] also known as the *isoelectric line* (Fig. 13.47).

Patients at risk for *silent ischemia* include patients experiencing an acute coronary syndrome even if treated with fibrinolytics, nitrates, or anticoagulation therapy.[60] Patients undergoing a PCI are at risk for coronary artery repeat occlusion or spasm, reflected by ST segment changes similar to those seen during PCI balloon inflation. Any patient admitted to the critical care unit with a history of prior MI, angina, diabetes, or kidney failure is a candidate for ST segment monitoring.[52]

ST segment deviation can have nonischemic causes and can create a false-positive alarm. Common culprits include hyperkalemia, pericarditis, hypokalemia, hypomagnesemia, hypothermia, ventricular aneurysm, hypothyroidism, pulmonary infarction, and medications such as quinidine and digitalis. Patients with subarachnoid hemorrhage often demonstrate ST segment changes believed to be caused by excess release of norepinephrine from the myocardial sympathetic nerves. The degree of myocardial necrosis and ST segment elevation depends on the severity of neurologic injury.[63]

ST segment deviation is measured as the number of millimeters of ST segment vertical displacement from the isoelectric line or from the patient's baseline. Because ST segments may slope or arc, the best measurement position is 60 ms to the right of the J point (Fig. 13.48).[54] The J point is chosen to avoid monitoring the upstroke of the T wave. On the bedside monitor, ST segment elevation is displayed as a positive number, whereas ST segment depression is indicated as a

negative number (see Fig. 13.48). To be clinically significant, the J point of the ST segment must be displaced up or down from the isoelectric baseline by at least 1 or 2 mm (one or two small boxes on ECG paper), depending on the specific ECG lead being monitored.[64] Specific values for recognition of abnormal J point thresholds in different ECG leads are listed in Box 13.8.

When setting ST segment alarm parameters, the patient's condition is always considered. The alarm may be set at 1 mm above and below the baseline ST segment level in patients at high risk for ischemia. In stable, low-risk patients, the suggested setting is 2 mm above or below the isoelectric line.[52] The rationale for selection of wider ST segment alarm parameters in more stable patients is that this may reduce the number of false ST segment alarms.[52] Stable patients tend to be more active, and when patients change position, it can alter the isoelectric baseline; if there are too many false ST segment alarms, clinicians may be tempted to turn off or not pay attention to the alarm system. Poor electrode contact with the skin also is responsible for false ST segment change alarms, emphasizing the need for correct skin preparation before electrode placement.[52]

Some specific ECG patterns do not lend themselves to ST segment monitoring, particularly rhythms that are associated with a wide QRS complex and distortion of the ST

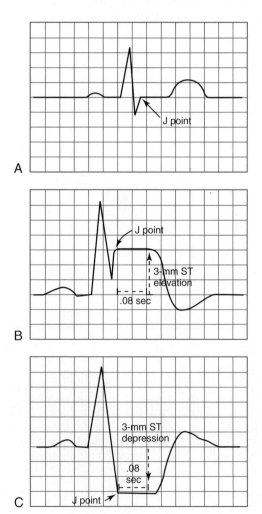

FIG. 13.48 (A) Normal position of J point. (B) A 3-mm ST segment elevation. (C) A 3-mm ST segment depression. ST segment changes are measured 60 to 80 ms (0.06 to 0.08 s) after the J point.

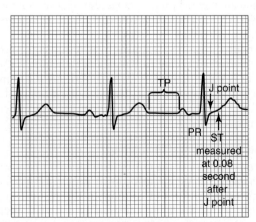

FIG. 13.47 The TP segment is used as the reference point for the isoelectric line if the heart rate is slow enough for the TP segment to be clearly seen. If not, the P–R interval can be used.

segment. This includes LBBB and RBBB, paced rhythms, and idioventricular rhythms. Other rhythms that make ST segment monitoring problematic include erratic atrial fibrillation or atrial flutter that obscures the isoelectric baseline.[52] When patients are moving in bed or walking, this distorts the ECG baseline, and continuous ST segment monitoring will be inaccurate.

Atrial Hypertrophy

Atrial chamber enlargement can be suspected from the 12-lead ECG because muscle size influences the ECG tracing. Atrial abnormalities may be identified by the size and shape of the P waves and are usually most obvious in lead II. Traditionally, wide, m-shaped P waves, classically seen in *left atrial hypertrophy*, were called *P mitrale* because left atrial hypertrophy is often caused by mitral stenosis (Fig. 13.49A). Tall, peaked P waves seen with *right atrial hypertrophy* were referred to as *P pulmonale* because this condition is often the result of chronic pulmonary disease (Fig. 13.48B). Current ECG guidelines emphasize that P wave abnormalities can be caused by many conditions and can occur without atrial enlargement. For this reason, the ECG is not considered definitive in the identification of atrial hypertrophy.[65] The less specific term *atrial abnormality* is suggested for P wave abnormalities when the underlying pathology is unknown.[65]

BOX 13.8 Abnormal J Point Thresholds Vary With Age, Sex, and Electrocardiogram Lead

Anterior, Lateral, and Inferior Wall Myocardial Infarction—J Point Threshold

For men older than 40 years, the threshold for abnormal J point elevation is 0.2 mV (2 mm) in leads V_2 and V_3 and 0.1 mV (1 mm) in all other leads.

For men younger than 40 years, the threshold for abnormal J point elevation in leads V_2 and V_3 is 0.25 mV (2.5 mm).

For women, the threshold for abnormal J point elevation is 0.15 mV (1.5 mm) in leads V_2 and V_3 and greater than 0.1 mV (1 mm) in all other leads.

Right Ventricular Wall Myocardial Infarction—J Point Threshold

For men and women, the threshold for abnormal J point elevation in V_3R and V_4R is 0.05 mV (0.5 mm) except for men younger than 30 years who have a lower threshold of 0.1 mV (1 mm).

Posterior Wall Myocardial Infarction—J Point Threshold

For men and women, the threshold for abnormal J point elevation in V_7 through V_9 should be 0.05 mV (0.5 mm).

J Point Depression

For men and women of all ages, the threshold for abnormal J point depression should be 0.05 mV (−0.5 mm) in leads V_2 and V_3 and −0.1 mV (−1 mm) in all other leads.

From Wagner GS, et al. AHA/ACCF/HRS recommendations for the standardization and interpretation of the electrocardiogram: Part VI: Acute ischemia/infarction: A scientific statement from the American Heart Association Electrocardiography and Arrhythmias Committee, Council on Clinical Cardiology; the American College of Cardiology Foundation; and the Heart Rhythm Society: Endorsed by the International Society for Computerized Electrocardiology. *Circulation.* 2009;119(10):e262.

Ventricular Hypertrophy

Ventricular hypertrophy describes an increase in the size and muscle mass of one or both ventricles. Because a larger muscle is being depolarized, a greater amount of electrical activity is recorded on the ECG during depolarization. In ventricular hypertrophy, the increased muscle mass results in increased QRS complex voltages, particularly in the precordial leads. Upright QRS complexes become taller, and negative QRS complexes become even more negative. The QRS complex often becomes slightly wider because it takes longer to depolarize a larger muscle. The QRS complex axis often shifts toward the enlarged ventricle because a greater portion of the total electrical activity of the heart occurs there. Although the 12-lead ECG can suggest hypertrophy, the echocardiogram is the most reliable diagnostic device because it can visualize ventricular wall thickness and motion.

Ischemia and Infarction

Ischemia occurs when the delivery of oxygen to the tissues is insufficient to meet metabolic demand. Cardiac ischemia in an unstable form occurs because of a sudden decrease in supply such as when the artery is blocked by a thrombus or when coronary artery spasm occurs.[66,67] Stable angina can occur when a stenotic coronary artery is unable to adapt to a sudden increase in demand created by exercise. Ischemia is by nature a transient process. The balance of supply versus demand is restored, and the cardiac muscle tissue recovers. Conversely, when the imbalance in myocardial oxygen demand/delivery becomes so great that the tissues can no longer survive, myocardial cells infarct and become necrotic. Many nursing and medical interventions are directed toward saving as much ischemic tissue as possible.

Infarction refers to the death and disintegration of muscle cells and their eventual replacement by fibrotic scar tissue. After infarction has occurred, the process cannot be reversed. Thus, careful ECG monitoring and swift intervention to restore myocardial perfusion before infarction can take place is critically important.

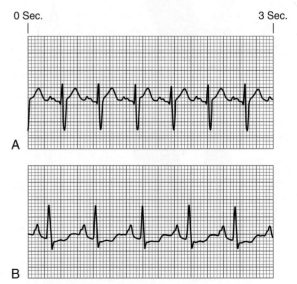

FIG. 13.49 Atrial Hypertrophy. (A) In left atrial hypertrophy, the P wave is broad and notched and is sometimes called *P mitrale* because it is often associated with mitral valve disease. (B) In right atrial hypertrophy, the P wave is tall and peaked and is sometimes called *P pulmonale* because it is often associated with pulmonary disease.

Electrocardiogram Changes Indicating Ischemia and Infarction

Ischemia and infarction cause changes in the way cardiac muscle cells respond to electrical stimuli. These changes can usually be seen in a 12-lead ECG tracing.

ST segment elevation is seen when the positive electrode lies directly over an area of transmural (full-wall thickness) injury (Fig. 13.50A). The ST segment changes on the surface ECG are caused by differences in voltage gradients between ischemic and healthy myocardium, referred to as *injury currents*.[64] This represents a preinfarction state, and interventions to unblock the occluded coronary artery must be initiated to prevent death of myocardium. ST segment elevation is a precursor to an ST elevation myocardial infarction (STEMI).[67]

Not every myocardial infarction is heralded by ST segment elevation. When the patient has an MI without ST segment elevation, it is described as a non–ST elevation (NSTEMI). The diagnosis can be considerably more challenging without the signature ST segment changes seen on the ECG.[66]

ST segment depression occurs when the reduction of blood flow is limited to the endocardium and some normal muscle tissue remains between the ischemic area and the positive electrode (Fig. 13.50B). ST segment depression is seen because the positive electrode is separated from the ischemic area by normal tissue. T waves most commonly flatten or become inverted.

Infarction involves necrosis (death) of muscle cells with eventual formation of scar tissue. These cells can no longer be depolarized when an impulse reaches them. If the infarction involves the epicardial (outer) layer of the heart muscle or the entire thickness of the heart wall (transmural lesion), the QRS complex changes. Abnormal Q waves typically develop in the leads overlying the affected area. Occasionally, the entire QRS complex becomes smaller without development of Q waves.

Non–Q Wave Infarction

Not every acute MI results in a pathologic Q wave on the 12-lead ECG. When the typical ECG changes are not present, the diagnosis depends on symptomatic clinical presentation, specific cardiac biomarkers (eg, cardiac troponin I, cardiac troponin T, creatine kinase-MB), and non-ECG diagnostic tests such as cardiac catheterization. STEMI is typically associated with a Q wave infarction. Conversely, NSTEMI is more likely to result in a non–Q wave infarction (See Fig. 14.12 in Chapter 14).

Infarct Location by 12-Lead Electrocardiogram

The location of the infarction can be roughly determined by noting the specific leads in which the ST segment and T wave changes are seen on the 12-lead ECG. Table 13.8 summarizes the anticipated 12-lead ECG changes.

Right ventricular infarction and posterior wall infarction are particularly difficult to identify on a standard 12-lead ECG because none of the standard leads directly view these areas. A right ventricular infarction may be suspected and investigated in the setting of an acute inferior wall myocardial infarction (MI).[68] To avoid missing this diagnosis, right-sided precordial leads (see Fig. 13.36B) can be placed, and a 12-lead ECG can be obtained for any patient with a suspected inferior right ventricular wall MI. Early identification of right ventricular infarct is important because it requires special management and carries a greater in-hospital mortality risk.[68] Nitrates and other vasodilatory agents, commonly administered in acute infarction of the left ventricle, can cause profound hypotension with negative effect on preload and CO when the infarcted area is in the right ventricle.[69]

A posterior wall infarction may be suspected in a patient with an acute inferior wall MI when there is ST segment depression in leads V_1, V_2, and V_3 on the standard 12-lead ECG. Tall, upright R waves may also be present. Posterior wall involvement can be verified by adding posterior precordial leads V_7, V_8, and V_9 (see Fig. 13.36D), although this is uncommon, mainly because the posterior leads have low voltage making changes difficult to see.

FIG. 13.50 (A) Acute transmural ischemia. The electrical forces *(arrows)* responsible for the ST segment are directed outward through the entire thickness of the heart muscle wall, causing ST segment elevation in leads directly over the ischemic area. (B) Acute subendocardial ischemia. The electrical forces responsible for the ST segment are deviated toward the inner layer of the heart, resulting in ST segment depression in leads directly over that area of the heart muscle wall.

TABLE 13.8 Electrocardiogram Changes During Myocardial Infarction

Location of Infarction	Artery Involved	Leads Involved	ECG Changes[a]
Anterior wall	LAD	V_{3-4}	Q waves, ST ↑,T ↓
Inferior wall	RCA or LCx	II, III, aVF	Q waves, ST ↑,T ↓
Ventricular septum	LAD	V_{1-2}	Q waves, ST ↑,T ↓
Lateral wall	LCx	V_{5-6}, I, aVL	Q waves, ST ↑,T ↓
Posterior wall	RCA or LCx	V_{1-3} (ant[a]); V_{7-9} (post[b])	Tall, upright R; ST ↓; upright T with ST ↑ V_{7-9}
Right ventricle	Proximal RCA	V_4R (right[c])	ST ↑

[a]See Fig. 13.36B for ECG lead placement.
[b]See Fig. 13.36D for ECG lead placement.
[c]See Fig. 13.36C for ECG lead placement.

Infarct Progression on Electrocardiogram

When blood flow in a coronary artery is suddenly occluded, the entire area of heart muscle normally perfused by that artery becomes ischemic. Collateral arterioles usually exist, which overlap and supply the perimeter of this area and may prevent necrosis of some of the affected tissue. At the center of the ischemic area, collateral blood flow is minimal or does not exist at all. Within a few hours, this tissue begins to die. On the ECG tracing, this process is illustrated as follows: Within minutes of the onset of infarction, ST segment elevation occurs in the leads directly overlying the affected heart wall. This ST segment elevation persists for a period of hours to 1 day, gradually becoming less severe. Within the first few hours, T waves may become tall and symmetric. They are known as hyperacute T waves, and they indicate acute ischemia. Meanwhile, usually within 4 to 24 hours from the onset of the infarction, abnormal Q waves begin to develop in the affected leads, and T waves begin to invert. Sometimes, instead of Q waves developing, the R waves become smaller. This still indicates necrosis of muscle tissue. The ST segments become isoelectric again in a few days, and the T wave becomes symmetric and deeply inverted in the affected leads. The T waves usually return to normal within several days. The Q waves may persist for the remainder of the patient's life, or they may get smaller over time and disappear altogether in some individuals. Table 13.9 summarizes the timing of these changes.

Intraventricular Conduction Defects

Intraventricular conduction defects are the result of an abnormal pathway of conduction through the ventricles. Normally, conduction spreads rapidly from the AV node to the bundle of His and down the right and left bundle branches. The right bundle branch is long and thin and terminates in a mass of Purkinje fibers, which spread the wave of depolarization into surrounding right ventricular muscle. After only a short distance, the left bundle branch divides into the left anterior fascicle, the left posterior fascicle, and many people have an additional left septal fascicle near the septum (Fig. 13.51). The terms *fascicle* and bundle are often used interchangeably when describing anatomy of the conduction system. Each of these fascicles causes depolarization of separate areas of the left ventricle. If any part of the conduction system fails, the muscle cells in that area still depolarize but not as quickly. Depolarization must then spread from cell to cell, a slower process than activation through specialized conduction pathways.

On the ECG, intraventricular conduction defects cause a widening of the QRS complex because of the slower spread of depolarization. The affected muscle tissue begins the slower cell-to-cell depolarization just as the other areas in the ventricle are almost finished. This later depolarization is then tacked onto the end of the normal QRS complex, making it prolonged and altering its shape.

Any part of the conduction system can be affected. The term *bundle branch block* refers to complete interruption of conduction through the right bundle or the entire left bundle branch.

Right and Left Bundle Branch Blocks

The chest leads are the most useful in identifying complete RBBB and LBBB. V_1 and V_6 are the best leads from which to identify forces traveling in a horizontal direction because they are located on the right and left sides of the heart, respectively. Fig. 13.52A shows the normal sequence of ventricular activation and the usual shape of the QRS complex in V_1 and V_6.

Right bundle branch block. In complete RBBB, the QRS complex is wider than 0.12 second (120 ms) (Fig. 13.52B). This is because the right ventricle is not activated through the normal rapid conduction system. Instead, it must be activated slowly, from one cell to the next. Electrical forces that are not counterbalanced by opposing forces from the left side of the heart travel toward the right at the end of the ventricular activation. The septum is depolarized first in a normal manner from left to right. Next, the wave of depolarization spreads through the left ventricle and is recorded in lead V_1 as a tiny negative deflection. The final portion of the QRS complex is wide and upright, indicating final electrical forces traveling toward the right. This represents right ventricular depolarization that occurs after LV depolarization is almost complete. In V_1, this QRS complex represents a classic pattern that is labeled rsR' in V_1.[53] The ST segment, representing repolarization, is also abnormal and makes recognition of ST segment changes related to ischemia difficult to detect by ECG monitoring. The presence of a RBBB is associated with a higher risk of cardiac events.[70]

In lead V_6, the positive electrode is on the left side of the chest, and the waveforms are reversed. The final forces of the QRS complex are negative because they are traveling toward the right and away from the positive electrode of V_6. The final negative deflection in V_6 is smaller than the final upright deflection in lead V_1 because the positive electrode in V_6 is at a greater distance from the right ventricle.

TABLE 13.9	Timing of Electrocardiogram Changes	
Time Frame	**ECG Change**
Immediate	ST segment elevation in leads over area of infarction
Within a few hours	Giant, upright T waves
Several hours	ST segment normalizes; T waves invert symmetrically
Several hours to days	Q waves or reduced R waves; voltage may remain low permanently

ECG, electrocardiogram.

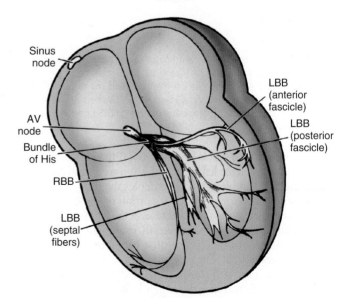

FIG. 13.51 Cardiac Conduction System. AV, atrioventricular; LBB, left bundle branch; RBB, right bundle branch. (Modified from Conover MB. *Understanding Electrocardiography.* 8th ed. St. Louis: Mosby; 2002.)

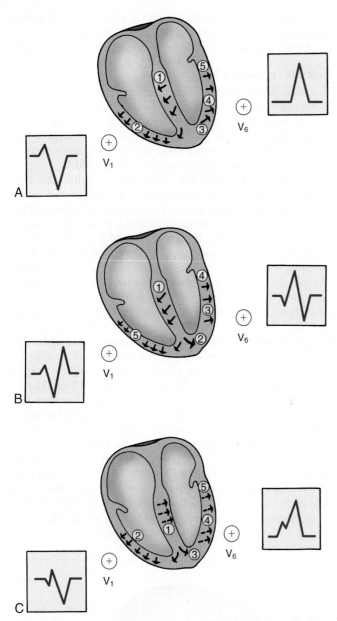

FIG. 13.52 (A) Sequence of ventricular depolarization and resulting QRS complex, as seen in leads V_1 and V_6. (B) Sequence of ventricular depolarization for a right bundle branch block and resulting QRS complex, as seen in leads V_1 and V_6. (C) Sequence of ventricular depolarization for a left bundle branch block and resulting QRS complex, as seen in leads V_1 and V_6.

Left bundle branch block. In complete LBBB (Fig. 13.52C), the conduction through the left ventricle must spread from cell to cell, which results in a prolonged QRS complex duration, longer than 0.12 second (120 ms).[53] Because a portion of the common left bundle normally initiates depolarization of the septum, the septum is depolarized in an abnormal direction, from right to left. In lead V_1, this is recorded as an initial negative deflection. Next, the right ventricle is depolarized, which is identified as a small upright notch in the QRS complex as the forces travel briefly toward the positive electrode of V_1. Sometimes this notch is absent. The final forces travel toward the left as the left ventricle is being depolarized. The left ventricle is a very large muscle mass, and these final electrical forces are large and wide. In lead V_1, the final deflection is a deep, negative deflection (S wave), whereas in lead V_6, these final forces inscribe a tall, upright deflection (R wave).

The presence of an LBBB makes diagnosis of an acute anterior wall MI extremely difficult because the change in repolarization masks ST segment elevation. Perhaps related to this difficulty in interpreting injury, patients with ACS in the presence of LBBB have double the in-hospital mortality risk compared with patients with ACS but without LBBB.[71]

BBBs may be recognized at the bedside if the patient is being monitored with leads V_1 and V_6. However, definitive diagnosis of BBB should be made via a 12-lead ECG. A BBB exists when the P wave is followed by a QRS complex that is wider than 0.12 second (120 ms) with other features of the block.[53] The presence of the P wave indicates that the QRS complex did not originate from the ventricles. One quick method to determine which bundle branch is blocked is to look at the last part of the QRS complex just before it returns to the baseline in leads V_1 and V_6. If upright in V_1 and negative in V_6, an RBBB exists. If negative in V_1 and upright in V_6, an LBBB is present.

Hemiblocks

Hemiblocks involve conduction failure of only part of the left bundle branch. In left anterior fascicular block, also called *left anterior hemiblock*, LV depolarization begins in the left posterior fascicle and spreads anteriorly through Purkinje fibers distal to the block. The QRS complex is of normal duration, meaning it is less than 0.12 second. However, the frontal plane axis changes dramatically and becomes more negative than −30 degrees, indicating left-axis deviation (axis between −45 degrees and −90 degrees) (Boxes 13.9 and 13.10).[53,72] Anterior hemiblock is a relatively frequent finding in patients with arterial hypertension or cardiomyopathy (see Box 13.10).

Left posterior fascicular block is also a hemiblock and is also known by the term *left posterior hemiblock.* The QRS complex duration is within normal limits (less than 0.12 second).[53] The block in the posterior fascicle changes the normal conduction pathway so that the anterior portion of the left ventricle is depolarized first. Conduction spreads slowly to the right, inferiorly and posteriorly. The axis then swings entirely in the other direction and becomes greater than +90 degrees, indicating right-axis deviation (axis between 90 degrees and 180 degrees).[53] Isolated posterior hemiblock is rare, and it is almost always associated with concomitant RBBB.[72]

Bifascicular Block

Blockage of either of the two branches of the LV conduction system plus RBBB constitutes a *bifascicular block.* Any combination of these conduction disturbances can occur and can evolve into complete heart block. Normally, bifascicular block (hemiblock plus RBBB) is well tolerated, and no intervention is necessary. The exception is bifascicular block that develops during an acute MI, in which the evolving infarct may warrant placement of a temporary pacemaker prophylactically in case conduction tissue ischemia progresses to complete heart block.

Dysrhythmia Interpretation

In clinical practice, the terms *dysrhythmia* and *arrhythmia* often are used interchangeably. The question of which word is the more accurate one is often discussed. Both terms are correct, and either may be used in practice. In this textbook, dysrhythmia is the more commonly used term. A dysrhythmia is any disturbance in the normal cardiac conduction pathway. Dysrhythmias can be detected on a 12-lead ECG, but they often occur only sporadically. For this reason, patients in a critical care unit are monitored continuously using a single-lead or

BOX 13.9 Causes of Left-Axis Deviation

- Normal variation
- Mechanical shifts: exhalation; high diaphragm caused by pregnancy, ascites, or abdominal tumor
- Left anterior hemiblock
- Left ventricular hypertrophy
- Wolff-Parkinson-White syndrome
- Hyperkalemia
- Cardiomyopathy

BOX 13.10 Causes of Right-Axis Deviation

- Normal variation
- Mechanical shifts: inhalation, emphysema
- Left posterior hemiblock
- Right ventricular hypertrophy
- Lateral wall myocardial infarction
- Right bundle branch block
- Dextrocardia

dual-lead system, and rhythm strips are recorded each shift and any time the patient's heart rhythm changes. Dysrhythmias occur frequently in cardiac and noncardiac critically ill patients. A systematic approach to assess a rhythm disturbance is an indispensable skill. Steps to accurately interpret a rhythm strip are introduced first, followed by specific criteria to evaluate common dysrhythmias encountered in clinical practice.

Heart Rate Determination

The first thing to assess when evaluating a rhythm strip is the ventricular rate. Regardless of the dysrhythmia involved, the ventricular rate holds the key to whether the patient can tolerate the dysrhythmia (ie, maintain adequate blood pressure, CO, and mentation). If the ventricular rate is consistently greater than 200 or less than 30, emergency measures must be started to correct the rate. A detailed analysis of the underlying rhythm disturbance can proceed later, when the immediate crisis is over. The three methods for calculating rate (Fig. 13.53A) are as follows:

1. Number of R–R intervals in 6 seconds times 10 (ECG paper is usually marked at the top in 3-second increments, making a 6-second interval easy to identify)
2. Number of large boxes between QRS complexes divided into 300
3. Number of small boxes between QRS complexes divided into 1500

In a healthy heart, the atrial rate and the ventricular rate are the same. However, in many dysrhythmias, the atrial and ventricular rates are different, and both must be calculated. To find the atrial rate, the P–P interval, instead of the R–R interval, is used in one of the three methods listed for determining rate.

The choice of method for calculating the HR depends on the regularity of the rhythm. If the rhythm is irregular, the first method (R–R intervals in 6 seconds × 10) is the only method that can be used (Fig. 13.53B). If the rhythm is regular, it is more accurate to use the second or third method. The second method can be easier to use when two consecutive R waves fall exactly on dark lines, and it provides a rapid estimate of rate. The third method is recommended when both R waves do not fall exactly on dark lines.

Rhythm Determination

The term *rhythm* refers to the regularity with which the P waves or R waves occur. Calipers assist in determining rhythm. One point of the calipers is placed on the beginning of one R wave, and the other point is placed on the next R wave. Leaving the calipers "set" at this interval, each succeeding R–R interval is checked to be sure it is the same width as the first one measured.

In describing the rhythm, three terms are used. If the rhythm is *regular*, the R–R intervals are the same ±10%. For example, if there are 20 small boxes in an R–R interval, an R wave could be off by two small boxes, but the rhythm would still be considered regular. If the rhythm is *regularly irregular*, the R–R intervals are not the same, but some sort of pattern is involved, which could be grouping, rhythmic speeding up and slowing down, or any other consistent pattern (Fig. 13.54). If the rhythm is *irregularly irregular*, the R–R intervals are not the same, and no pattern can be found.

P Wave Evaluation

The P wave is analyzed by answering the following questions: First, is the P wave present or absent? Second, is it related to the QRS complex? It is expected that one P wave will be in front of every QRS. Sometimes, two, three, or four P waves may be in front of every QRS complex. If this pattern is consistent, the P wave and QRS are still related, although not on a 1:1 basis.

P–R Interval Evaluation

The duration of the P–R interval, which normally is 0.12 to 0.20 second (120 to 200 ms), is measured first. This is measured from the start of a visible P wave to the beginning of the next QRS complex (see Fig. 13.47). All P–R intervals on the strip are verified to be sure they have the same duration as the original interval.

QRS Complex Evaluation

The entire ECG strip must be evaluated to ascertain that the QRS complexes are consistently the same shape and width. The normal QRS complex duration is 0.06 to 0.10 second (60 to 110 ms). Any QRS longer than 0.10 second is considered abnormal. If more than one QRS shape is visible on the strip, each QRS complex must be measured. The QRS is measured from where it leaves the baseline to where it returns to the baseline (see Fig. 13.55).

Q–T Interval Evaluation

The length of the Q–T interval varies with the HR. The Q–T interval is shorter when the HR is faster. A Q–T interval corrected for HR (Q–Tc interval) that is longer than 0.50 second (500 ms) is of concern, as discussed earlier in the section on Q–T interval.

Sinus Rhythms

The cardiac cycle begins when an impulse originates in the sinus node. As the wave of depolarization spreads through the atria, a P wave is inscribed on the ECG. The impulse is delayed briefly in the AV node, which corresponds to the P–R interval on the ECG. After leaving the AV node, the wave of depolarization spreads rapidly through the bundle of His and the bundle branches and causes ventricular depolarization, which is recorded as a QRS complex by the ECG. Contraction immediately follows depolarization. Contraction is terminated by repolarization, which is demonstrated as a T wave on the ECG.

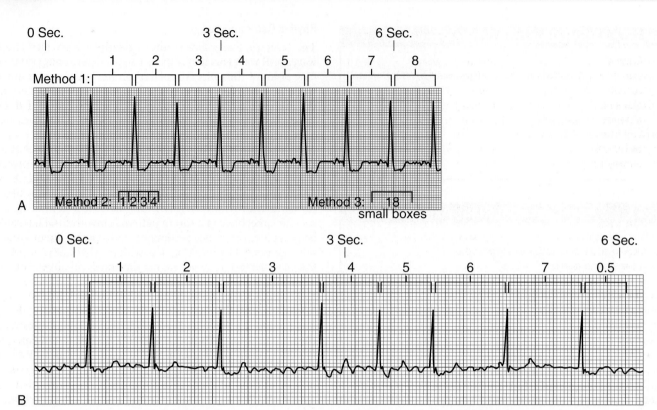

FIG. 13.53 (A) Calculation of heart rate if the rhythm is regular. Method 1: Number of R–R intervals in 6 s multiplied by 10 (eg, 8 × 10 = 80/min). Method 2: Number of large boxes between QRS complexes divided into 300 (eg, 300 ÷ 4 = 75/min). Method 3: Number of small boxes between QRS complexes divided into 1500 (eg, 1500 ÷ 18 = 84/min). (B) Rate calculation if the rhythm is irregular. Only method 1 can be used (eg, 7.5 intervals × 10 = 75/min).

FIG. 13.54 (A) Regularly irregular rhythm is irregular but has a consistent pattern in that every other beat is premature. (B) Irregularly irregular rhythm is irregular with no consistent pattern.

FIG. 13.55 P–R Interval Measurement, From the Beginning of the P wave to the Beginning of the QRS Complex. The P–R interval on this tracing is 0.20 s; the QRS complex duration illustrates normal and abnormal intervals. The narrow QRS complexes measure 0.08 s, which is normal. The wide QRS complexes measure 0.20 s and are caused by ventricular ectopy.

Normal Sinus Rhythm

If all the events described for sinus rhythms occur in their normal sequence with normal rates and intervals, the patient is in normal sinus rhythm. The criteria for normal sinus rhythm are as follows:

Rate. The intrinsic rate of the sinus node is 60 to 100 beats/ min. *Intrinsic rate* is the normal rate at which a pacemaker site in the heart depolarizes automatically with no outside influences, such as medications, fever, or exercise. In normal sinus rhythm, the rate must be whatever is normal for the sinus node (60 to 100 beats/min).

Rhythm. The rhythm must be regular ±10%.

P wave. P waves must be present, and only one must precede every QRS complex.

P–R interval. The P–R interval represents delay in the AV node. In normal sinus rhythm, the P–R interval is 0.12 to 0.20 second.

QRS complex. Size and shape do not matter in this complex because it depends on lead placement and gain adjustments on the monitor. However, all QRS patterns must look alike. If conduction through the ventricles is normal, the QRS complex duration is 0.06 to 0.10 second. Fig. 13.56 is an example of normal sinus rhythm in V_1.

Sinus Bradycardia

Sinus bradycardia meets all the criteria for normal sinus rhythm except that the rate is less than 60 beats/min (Table 13.10). It is normally seen in well-trained athletes at rest or in other individuals during sleep. Other conditions in which sinus bradycardia occurs include vagal stimulation, increased intracranial pressure, medication therapy with digoxin or beta-blockers, and ischemia of the sinus node caused by an acute MI. Sinus bradycardia usually is not treated unless the patient displays symptoms of hypoperfusion, such as hypotension, dizziness, chest pain, or changes in level of consciousness.

Sinus Tachycardia

Sinus tachycardia meets all the criteria for normal sinus rhythm except that the rate is greater than 100 beats/min (see Table 13.10). Rates may be 180 to 200 beats/min in healthy young adults during strenuous exercise. However, in the critical care setting, bed rest is prescribed for most patients. It is wise to be skeptical of any "sinus tachycardia" with a rate greater than 150 beats/min and to search for a triggering focus other than the sinus node. For example, atrial flutter waves may be difficult to see at first glance because of baseline distortion caused by the high ventricular rate (Fig. 13.57).

FIG. 13.56 Normal Sinus Rhythm. The rate is 70, and the rhythm is regular. One P wave is present before each QRS complex. The P–R interval is 0.18 s and does not vary throughout the strip. The QRS complex duration is 0.08 s. All evaluation criteria are within normal limits.

Sinus tachycardia can be caused by a wide variety of factors, such as exercise, emotion, pain, fever, hemorrhage, shock, heart failure, and thyrotoxicosis.[73] Illegal stimulant drugs such as cocaine, Ecstasy, and amphetamines can raise the resting HR significantly. Many medications used in critical care can also cause sinus tachycardia; common culprits are aminophylline, dopamine, hydralazine, atropine, and catecholamines such as epinephrine. Tachycardia is detrimental to anyone with ischemic heart disease because it decreases the time for ventricular filling, decreases SV, and compromises CO. Tachycardia increases heart work and myocardial oxygen demand, while decreasing oxygen supply by decreasing coronary artery filling time.

If the cause of the tachycardia can be determined, such as fever or pain, the cause is treated rather than trying to lower the HR directly. Several medications are available to decrease the HR if needed. Calcium channel blockers and beta-blockers are widely used for this purpose. However, a word of caution is warranted. CO is determined by both HR and SV. If an injured heart can no longer maintain an adequate SV, HR can be increased to maintain CO and supply an adequate blood flow to vital body tissues. If a medication is administered to force the sinus node to slow, severe and relatively immediate heart failure can result. The sinus node is controlled by many neural and humoral influences in the body, and the rate is set to try to meet the perceived demands; a close examination of the reason for the tachycardia is mandatory before treatment decisions are made.

Sinus Dysrhythmia

Sinus dysrhythmia, commonly called *sinus arrhythmia* in clinical practice, meets all the criteria for normal sinus rhythm except that the rhythm is irregular (see Table 13.10). This irregularity coincides with the respiratory pattern; HR increases with inhalation and decreases with exhalation (Fig. 13.58). Sinus dysrhythmia often occurs in children and young adults, and the incidence decreases with age. No treatment is required. To avoid being misled by other rhythm disturbances, the examiner must look at all P waves closely to verify that they are the same shape and that the P–R intervals are constant.

Atrial Dysrhythmias

Atrial dysrhythmias originate from an ectopic focus in the atria somewhere other than the sinus node. The ectopic impulse occurs prematurely, before the normal sinus impulse occurs. The premature atrial depolarization may initiate a normal QRS complex, an abnormal or aberrant pattern, or an SVT. Huge advances have been made in the understanding of the pathogenesis and management of atrial dysrhythmias.

TABLE 13.10	Sinus Rhythms			
Parameter	**Normal Sinus Rhythm**	**Sinus Bradycardia**	**Sinus Tachycardia**	**Sinus Dysrhythmia**
Rate	60–100 beats/min	<60 beats/min	>100 beats/min	Variable
Rhythm	Regular	Regular	Regular	Irregular; respiratory variation
P wave	Present, with 1 per QRS complex	Present, with 1 per QRS complex	Present, with 1 per QRS complex	Present, with 1 per QRS complex
P–R interval	0.12–0.20 s and constant	0.12–0.20 s and constant	0.12–0.20 s and constant	0.12–0.20 s and constant
QRS complex	0.06–0.10 s	0.06–0.10 s	0.06–0.10 s	0.06–0.10 s

Premature Atrial Contractions

Premature atrial contractions (PACs) are isolated early beats from an ectopic focus in the atria. The underlying rhythm is usually sinus. The regular sinus rhythm is interrupted by an early, abnormally shaped atrial P wave. The early atrial wave usually looks different from the sinus P wave and may be inverted. The P–R interval may be longer, shorter, or the same as the P–R interval of a sinus impulse. The QRS complex that follows the ectopic atrial P wave can vary in shape depending on the degree of refractoriness of the AV node.

Normal, narrow QRS complex. If the atrial impulse arrives in the AV node after the AV node is fully repolarized, the impulse is conducted to the ventricles as a normal QRS complex. If the ventricles are also fully repolarized, conduction through the bundle branches is expected, and a normal QRS complex is recorded on the ECG (Fig. 13.59A).

Wide QRS complex. Occasionally, the early ectopic P wave can be conducted through the AV node, but part of the conduction pathway through the ventricular bundle branches is blocked. Because the right bundle branch normally has the longest refractory period, it is usually the right bundle branch that is still blocked when the early impulse arrives. This produces a QRS that is wider than 0.12 second (120 ms) or wider than three small boxes on the ECG paper, with a shape consistent with RBBB (Fig. 13.59B). Conduction through the ventricles that is different from normal is referred to as *aberrant.* Consequently, these early, abnormally conducted PACs are described as *aberrantly conducted PACs.*

Pause with no QRS complex. The ectopic P wave sometimes arrives so early that the AV node is still in its absolute refractory period. In this case, the wave of depolarization does not move past the AV node, and no QRS complex follows. All that is seen on the ECG is an early, abnormal P wave fol-lowed by a pause until the next sinus P wave occurs (Fig. 13.59C). This is called a *nonconducted PAC.* Usually, these P waves are so early that they are superimposed on the T wave of the previous beat, making them difficult to find. The pause that follows is still clearly seen. Whenever an unexpected pause occurs in a rhythm, the T wave preceding the pause must be examined very carefully and compared with other T waves on the same strip to locate distortions that may reveal a hidden early P wave.

PACs can occur in individuals with normal hearts. PACs are accentuated by emotional upheaval, nicotine, caffeine, and digitalis. Mitral valve prolapse is associated with an increased frequency of atrial dysrhythmias. Heart failure can cause PACs because of increased pressure within the atria. As atrial pressure begins to rise, the atrial walls are stretched, causing irritability of atrial cells and the occurrence of PACs.

Supraventricular Tachycardia

SVT describes a varied group of dysrhythmias that originate above the AV node. SVT is not a specific term; it includes sinus tachycardia, atrial tachycardia, multifocal atrial tachycardia, atrial flutter, atrial fibrillation, and junctional tachycardia. Each of these entities has a distinct pathophysiology, specific therapy, and expected outcome. SVT may also be described as a *narrow complex tachycardia,* defined as a QRS complex that is less than 0.12 second (120 ms).[73] After the specific dysrhythmia is identified, it usually is referred to by a specific name, such as atrial fibrillation with a rapid ventricular response. SVT describes a rapid, sustained atrial or junctional tachycardia when the exact mechanism is unknown. Women are affected by episodic SVT at approximately twice the rate of men.

In an acute situation, a rapid dysrhythmia may be difficult to identify precisely. SVT can cause hemodynamic instability. It is important to differentiate VT from SVT; the focus then can be directed toward rate control until the acute situation is resolved and hemodynamic stability is restored. At that point, a more careful analysis is needed to determine the specific dysrhythmia responsible for the SVT. The differentiation of wide complex SVT from VT requires specific knowledge of the relevant ECG criteria (discussed later).

SVT is not always benign. Approximately 14% of people with SVT report that they have experienced syncope (lost consciousness) while driving, and 50% have experienced symptoms of near-syncope.[73] Medications are used to limit the SVT rate and prevent "blackouts" or syncope. SVT that is persistent for weeks or months may lead to a tachycardia-mediated cardiomyopathy. A baseline 12-lead ECG is helpful, and a 12-lead ECG should be obtained during the palpitations when possible.[73]

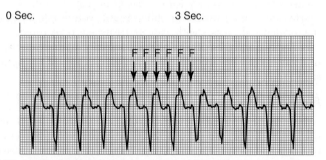

FIG. 13.57 Although the tracing may be confused with sinus tachycardia, it is atrial flutter with 2:1 conduction. It is difficult to see the extra flutter waves (F) that are hidden in the QRS complexes.

FIG. 13.58 Sinus Dysrhythmia. The heart rate is increased during inspiration and decreased during expiration.

Supraventricular Tachycardia With Aberrant Conduction

If the QRS complex in SVT is wider than 0.12 second, it is important to differentiate between SVT with aberrant conduction and VT (discussed later). SVT with aberrant conduction includes SVT with a BBB and SVT that uses an anomalous congenital additional fiber (accessory pathway), such as Wolff-Parkinson-White syndrome. Patients with SVT with aberrant conduction are frequently misdiagnosed, and evaluation by a specialist is highly recommended.[73]

Paroxysmal Supraventricular Tachycardia

Paroxysmal means starting and stopping abruptly. *Paroxysmal supraventricular tachycardia* (PSVT) refers to the sudden interruption of sinus rhythm by an atrial ectopic focus that fires repetitively at a rate of 150 to 250 beats/min and eventually stops as suddenly as it began (Fig. 13.60).

The rhythm of PSVT is perfectly regular because the reentry loop has a specific length; each circuit through the loop requires exactly the same amount of time to complete. Reentry within the atria itself or involving the AV node is the mechanism responsible for most SVTs, including PSVT. Other common

FIG. 13.59 Premature Atrial Contractions (PACs). (A) Normally conducted PAC. The early P wave is indicated by the *arrow*, and the QRS complex that follows has a normal shape and duration. (B) Nonconducted (blocked) PACs. The early P waves are indicated by *arrows*. They distort the T waves, making them appear peaked compared with the normal T waves seen after the third and fourth QRS complexes. (C) Right bundle branch block aberration after a PAC.

underlying mechanisms include abnormal automaticity and triggered activity. P waves are present and abnormally shaped, although they may be difficult to identify, as they often blend in with the previous T wave because of the rapid rate. It is most helpful if the beginning of the PSVT run is captured and recorded on ECG paper because the early, abnormal P wave is often easiest to identify in front of the first beat of the run. The P–R interval should be the same for each cycle in the run, but it will probably be different from the P–R interval of the patient's own normal sinus rhythm. As with PACs, the QRS complex is usually normal because after the impulse passes through the AV node, conduction through the ventricles follows the usual pathway (Table 13.11). However, in PSVT (as discussed for SVT), aberrant conduction, often in the form of LBBB or RBBB, can occur with a wide QRS complex (greater than 0.12 second); this creates difficulty in differentiating relatively benign PSVT from its more serious counterpart, VT.

Because of refractoriness in the AV node, sometimes not all of the ectopic P waves are conducted to the ventricles. Usually, at least every other P wave conducts a QRS complex, described as a 2:1 ratio, but occasionally the conduction may drop to three P waves for every QRS complex (3:1 ratio).

PSVT has essentially the same causal factors as PACs. PSVT has greater clinical significance because it may be sustained for long periods and because it occurs at such a rapid rate. As stressed in the discussion of sinus tachycardia, rapid rates decrease ventricular filling time, increase myocardial oxygen consumption, and decrease oxygen supply. Heart failure, angina, or MI can result. PSVT usually responds rapidly to medical management, which initially includes the use of vagal maneuvers.[73] Vagal maneuvers used in critical care include the following:

Valsalva maneuver. The patient is asked to "bear down," as if going to the bathroom.

Carotid sinus massage. It is performed on only one side of the neck over the carotid artery by a physician on a patient with a monitored ECG and avoided on older patients who may have atherosclerotic disease of the carotid arteries.

If vagal maneuvers are unsuccessful at terminating the PSVT, the next step usually is the use of IV medications if the patient is hemodynamically stable. The IV medication of choice to briefly block conduction through the AV node is adenosine (Adenocard).[73] In PSVT, adenosine alone is often sufficient to restore normal sinus rhythm, but if not, it will unmask the ectopic P waves and confirm or provide strong clues to diagnose the SVT. The usual dose is 6 mg given intravenously by rapid push, followed by a normal saline-flush. If the 6 mg adenosine does not create a temporary AV block or restore sinus rhythm, a 12-mg IV dose is administered. Potential dysrhythmic side effects of adenosine include a 1% to 15% chance of initiating atrial fibrillation. Adenosine should be used with caution in patients with severe asthma or chronic obstructive pulmonary disease (COPD).

Other IV medications that may be used to slow the rate in PSVT are amiodarone (Cordarone), a class III antidysrhythmic with a rapid onset and a short half-life.[73] Alternatively, diltiazem, a class IV calcium channel blocker in the nondihydropyridine group, can be administered. The action of these medications is to slow conduction through the AV node.[73] Other medications for short and ongoing management are also available.[73] If IV medications do not convert the PSVT or sustained SVT or if the patient becomes hemodynamically unstable, the next step is electrical cardioversion.[73]

FIG. 13.60 Paroxysmal Supraventricular Tachycardia. The atrial rate during tachycardia is 158 beats/min. The run starts and stops abruptly.

TABLE 13.11   Atrial Dysrhythmias

Parameter	Paroxysmal Supraventricular Tachycardia	Multifocal Atrial Tachycardia	Atrial Flutter	Atrial Fibrillation
Rate				
Atrial	150–250 beats/min	100–160 beats/min	250–350 beats/min	>350 beats/min (unable to count it)
Ventricular	Same or less	Same	250–350 beats/min, one-half or less	100–180 beats/min (uncontrolled); <100 beats/min (controlled)
Rhythm	Regular	Irregular	Atrial, regular; ventricular, may or may not be regular	Irregularly irregular
P wave	Present; abnormally shaped	Present; 3 or more different shapes	F waves	Fibrillatory baseline
P–R interval	May be normal or prolonged	Variable	Conduction ratio: flutter waves per QRS complex	Absent
QRS complex	0.06–0.10 s	0.06–0.10 s	0.06–0.10 s	0.06–0.10 s

Focal Atrial Tachycardia

Focal atrial tachycardia occurs when there is a nonsinus focus that is firing rapidly.[73] This dysrhythmia can be managed with the same medications used for other atrial dysrhythmias (amiodarone, diltiazem, verapamil, beta-blockers), with flecainide or propafenone used in patients without structural heart disease.[73] Focal atrial tachycardia can be permanently eliminated using catheter ablation.[73]

Multifocal Atrial Tachycardia

Multifocal atrial tachycardia (MAT) refers to numerous irritable atrial foci that intermittently fire and generate an impulse (Fig. 13.61). The atrial rate is greater than 100 beats/min but usually does not exceed 160 beats/min. The atrial feature that distinguishes MAT on the ECG is that there are at least three different P wave shapes, indicating at least three different irritable foci within the atria. MAT is always irregular and is frequently misdiagnosed and confused with atrial fibrillation. MAT is most commonly seen in older patients with COPD.[74] COPD causes chronic pulmonary hypertension, which in turn causes chronically elevated right ventricular and right atrial pressures. The abnormally high right atrial pressure causes stretching of the right atrial muscle cells and chronic irritability. Pharmacologic management of recurrent symptomatic MAT includes beta-blockers or verapamil.[73] Additionally, treatment is focused on management of the underlying disorder, generally COPD or heart valve disease. When the underlying cause cannot be resolved, MAT is described as refractory to treatment. There is no role for electrical cardioversion or catheter ablation.[73]

Atrial Flutter

Atrial flutter is recognized on the ECG by the *sawtooth* atrial pattern. These sawtooth-shaped atrial wavelets are not P waves; they are more appropriately called F waves (atrial flutter waves), as shown in Fig. 13.62. The AV node does not allow conduction of all these impulses to the ventricles.

Pathogenesis of atrial flutter. Atrial flutter can be started by any isolated atrial impulse, but to be maintained, the atrial flutter requires a *reentry circular pathway* around macroscopic structures in the atria. Typically, these structures are in the right atrium and in 75% of cases involve the vena cava and the tricuspid valve in an area known as the *cavotricuspid isthmus.*[73] The *reentry loop* can circle counterclockwise around the tricuspid valve or circle the inferior vena caval opening or encircle the IVC and the tricuspid valve. To maintain a viable, self-perpetuating reentry pathway, the loop must avoid the sinoatrial node and be large enough to always meet tissue that is ready to be depolarized (accept a new electrical stimulus). The atrial reentry rate in atrial flutter is typically between 250 beats/min and 330 beats/min, producing the classic sawtooth or flutter wave pattern.[73] The atrial flutter wavelet always appears regular because the circuit is always the same length and requires exactly the same amount of time to complete the reentry loop.

Atrial and ventricular rates in atrial flutter. When evaluating the rate of atrial flutter, it is important to calculate both atrial and ventricular rates. The ventricular rhythm is regular if the same number of flutter waves occurs between each QRS complex—in other words, if the degree of block at the AV node remains constant. Sometimes, the refractoriness in the AV node changes from beat to beat, resulting in an irregular

FIG. 13.61 Multifocal Atrial Tachycardia (MAT). There are several differently shaped P waves, and the P–R intervals vary.

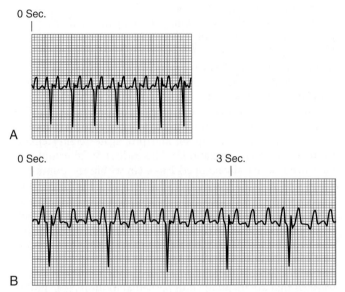

FIG. 13.62 (A) Initial strip shows atrial flutter with 2:1 conduction through the atrioventricular (AV) node. (B) During carotid sinus massage, the AV conduction rate is decreased, revealing the flutter waves more clearly.

ventricular response. When describing atrial flutter, the term *P–R interval* no longer applies; instead, a conduction ratio, such as 3:1 or 4:1 (ratio of atrial waves to QRS complexes) is used. In normal sinus rhythm, measuring the P–R interval allows evaluation of the speed of conduction through the AV node; in atrial flutter, the number of flutter waves that bombard the AV node before one is allowed to pass through to the ventricles is a measure of AV nodal conduction. After the impulse has passed the AV node, conduction through the ventricles is unaltered. The QRS complex duration remains normal or at least the same as it was in normal sinus rhythm (see Table 13.11). Atrial flutter and atrial fibrillation often coexist in the same patient.[73]

The major factor underlying atrial flutter symptoms is the ventricular response rate. If the atrial rate is 300 beats/min and the AV conduction ratio is 4:1, the ventricular response rate is 75 beats/min and should be well tolerated. However, if the atrial rate is 300 beats/min but the AV conduction ratio is 2:1, the corresponding ventricular rate of 150 beats/min may cause angina, acute heart failure, or other signs of cardiac decompensation. An atrial rate of 250 beats/min with a 1:1 AV conduction ratio yields a ventricular response rate of 250 beats/min; the patient is extremely symptomatic, and emergency measures are needed to decrease the ventricular rate.

Sometimes it is difficult to identify the flutter waves, especially if the conduction ratio is 2:1. Vagal maneuvers or adenosine can be useful diagnostic tools to allow better visualization of the flutter waves (see Fig. 13.62A). Vagal maneuvers or IV adenosine cannot terminate atrial flutter but do create a temporary AV block to permit visualization of the atrial waveform and thereby facilitate accurate diagnosis, as seen in Fig. 13.62B.

Atrial flutter management. Antidysrhythmic medications are prescribed in two ways to treat atrial flutter: to convert the rhythm to sinus rhythm (rhythm control) and to slow conduction through the AV node (rate control). The most effective medications for rhythm control are amiodarone, dofetilide and sotalol; flecainide or propafenone can be used in the absence of structural heart disease. Medications that slow conduction through the AV node are used to control the ventricular rate, including calcium channel blockers (diltiazem, verapamil) and beta-blockers.[73] Amiodarone shares both properties. It can slow conduction through the AV node and convert the atrial dysrhythmia. Amiodarone is preferred when the atrial flutter creates hemodynamic instability.[73] If at any time a patient with atrial flutter becomes hemodynamically unstable, electrical cardioversion is the recommended emergency intervention.[73]

Nonpharmacologic interventions to convert atrial flutter to sinus rhythm are the most effective; they include catheter ablation and electrical synchronized cardioversion. If atrial flutter has been present for more than 48 hours, one-third of patients will have thrombi in the atria, and anticoagulation is mandated before pharmacologic or electrical cardioversion.[73]

For patients with atrial flutter unrelated to an acute disease process, permanent termination of the atrial flutter circuit can be achieved by *radiofrequency catheter ablation.*[75] Catheter ablation is used to create a line of conduction block across one or more sections of the reentry pathway. The most frequent location in atrial flutter is a narrow band of tissue between the IVC and the tricuspid anulus known as the *cavotricuspid isthmus.*[73] Table 15-16 in Chapter 15 contains additional information on antidysrhythmic medications for the treatment of atrial dysrhythmias.

Atrial Fibrillation

Atrial fibrillation is the most frequently encountered dysrhythmia in the developed world (Fig. 13.63). This dysrhythmia affects 2.7 million to 6.1 million adults in the United States; this number is expected to double in the next 25 years.[76] Treatment of atrial fibrillation adds approximately $8700 per patient per year in health care costs.[76] When first detected, atrial fibrillation may be described as *paroxysmal* (duration less than 7 days from onset), *persistent* (duration more than 7 days), or *long-standing persistent* (duration more than 12 months). When all attempts at conversion to sinus rhythm have failed and there is an acceptance by the patient that atrial fibrillation is not reversible, it is described as *permanent* atrial fibrillation (Fig. 13.64).[75,76] The etiology of atrial fibrillation is either associated with structural heart disease such as a mitral valve stenosis or described as *non-valvular atrial fibrillation.*[76]

Atrial fibrillation may be classified under the broad category of SVT because the HR is rapid and many patients have symptoms of hypotension and breathlessness during paroxysmal atrial fibrillation when uncontrolled by medication. Uncoordinated atrial electrical activity leads to a rapid deterioration in atrial mechanical function. The ECG tracing in atrial fibrillation is notable for an uneven atrial baseline that lacks clearly defined P waves and instead shows rapid oscillations or fibrillation wavelets that vary in size, shape, and frequency. The atrial fibrillation waves are particularly visible in the inferior ECG leads II, III, and AVF.

The ventricular response to atrial fibrillation is influenced by several factors, including the efficiency of the AV node, autonomic nervous system activity (ie, the level of sympathetic and parasympathetic [vagus nerve] tone), presence of medications that increase or slow conduction through the AV node–bundle branch conduction system, and various structural heart conditions such as cardiomyopathy and heart failure.[76] Atrial fibrillation displays irregular R–R intervals (different timing

FIG. 13.63 Atrial Fibrillation. The ventricular rhythm is irregularly irregular.

intervals between the QRS complexes) that do not show any logical pattern. The ability of the AV node and bundle branches to conduct or block the fibrillating atrial impulses is key to the appearance of the QRS complex on the surface ECG. In atrial fibrillation, the QRS complex shape is usually narrow and normal in appearance as long as the pathway through the ventricles is intact after the impulse leaves the AV node. The AV node acts as a filter to protect the ventricles from the hundreds of atrial impulses that occur each minute, although the AV node does not receive all these atrial impulses. When the atrial muscle tissue immediately surrounding the AV node is in a refractory state, impulses generated in other areas of the atria cannot reach the AV node, which helps to explain the wide variation in R–R intervals during atrial fibrillation (see Table 13.11).

Pathogenesis of atrial fibrillation. The pathogenesis of atrial fibrillation has traditionally been ascribed to random electrical foci firing in the atria. Research using high-density atrial mapping, high-speed video recordings, and ECG analysis has uncovered distinct spatial organization within the atria.[76] Atrial fibrillation involves several reentry circuits within the atria, and in some cases, they originate at specific anatomic sites. The four pulmonary veins that drain into the left atrium are a trigger site for early atrial foci to initiate and propagate reentry circuits to maintain atrial fibrillation.[76] The earliest atrial ectopic foci have been electrically mapped 2 to 4 cm within the pulmonary veins. The affected pulmonary veins contain thin myocardial sleeves that project into the pulmonary veins from the left atrium. This ectopic tissue resembles discontinuous finger-like projections approximately 5 mm thick that extend 4.5 cm into one or more pulmonary veins. The tissue ultimately becomes part of the venous wall. The spread of atrial fibrillation to the rest of the atria is thought to occur through multiple reentry *wavelets* that are maintained in perpetual motion by a "mother rotor," or dominant reentry circuit, which functions at a higher frequency, drives the atrial fibrillation, and originates from the ectopic pulmonary vein tissue.

When a single focus can be identified, it is possible to encircle that area and isolate that site using radiofrequency catheter ablation. Several different catheter ablation designs are used to

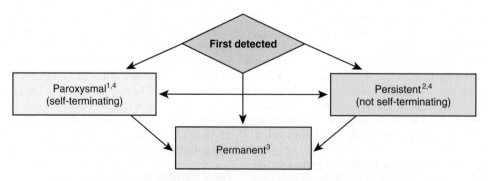

[1]Episodes that generally last less than or equal to 7 days (most less than 24 h).
[2]Usually more than 6 days.
[3]Cardioversion failed or not attempted.
[4]Both paroxysmal and persistent AF may be recurrent.

FIG. 13.64 Patterns of New-Onset Atrial Fibrillation. (From Fuster V, et al. ACC/AHA/ESC 2006 guidelines for the management of patients with atrial fibrillation: A report of the American College of Cardiology/American Heart Association Task Force on Practice Guidelines and the European Society of Cardiology Committee for Practice Guidelines [Writing Committee to revise the 2001 guidelines for the management of patients with atrial fibrillation]: Developed in collaboration with the European Heart Rhythm Association and the Heart Rhythm Society. *Circulation.* 2006;114[7]:e257.)

isolate foci that originate in the four pulmonary veins—encircling all four veins together or isolating individual pulmonary veins or in pairs.[76,77]

The atria demonstrate other pathologic changes in atrial fibrillation, typically atrial fibrosis and loss of atrial muscle mass.[76] Any change in atrial architecture increases the risk of atrial fibrillation.[76] An enlarged atrium is an independent risk factor for atrial fibrillation. Additionally, ongoing atrial fibrillation can contribute to pathologic atrial enlargement.

It is probable that there are several different types of atrial fibrillation involving different mechanisms. As electrophysiologic mapping techniques become more advanced, the mystery surrounding the origins of atrial fibrillation will become clearer. Although atrial fibrillation may look disorganized on the ECG baseline tracing, an electrical pattern exists within the atria. Knowledge of this pattern will ultimately lead to treatments that can help cure or control atrial fibrillation.

Atrial fibrillation risk factors. Atrial fibrillation is encountered most frequently in older adults. Less than 1% of adults younger than 60 years have atrial fibrillation.[76] In contrast, almost one-third of adults older than 80 years have atrial fibrillation.[76] Atrial fibrillation is the most common cardiac dysrhythmia in the United States and is responsible for most dysrhythmia-related hospital admissions. There are known risk factors that increase the risk of developing atrial fibrillation, notably structural heart disease, including hypertension, ischemic heart disease, hyperlipidemia, and heart failure. Other disease states associated with higher risk include diabetes mellitus, chronic kidney disease, anemia, arthritis, and COPD.[76]

Atrial fibrillation management. Debate continues about the most effective treatment approach for atrial fibrillation, as shown in the algorithm to treat new-onset atrial fibrillation (Fig. 13.65). In the past, the gold standard goal has been to convert the patient out of atrial fibrillation back to sinus rhythm. However, for many older adults, remaining out of atrial fibrillation is an unattainable goal. The major therapeutic decision is whether it is possible to achieve *rhythm* control or ventricular *rate* control.[78] The risk of stroke increases fivefold with atrial fibrillation.[76] Therefore, all patients with atrial fibrillation require anticoagulation to prevent development of atrial thrombi, thrombotic embolism, and stroke.[76]

Rhythm control. For a hospitalized patient with new-onset atrial fibrillation with unstable hemodynamic values, the primary focus is generally on rhythm control (conversion to sinus rhythm) using antidysrhythmic medications or electrical cardioversion. Emergency medications used to convert atrial fibrillation to sinus rhythm, also known as a *chemical cardioversion*, include amiodarone and ibutilide. Antidysrhythmic medications used long-term to maintain sinus rhythm include amiodarone, dronedarone, disopyramide, flecainide, propafenone, quinidine, sotalol, and dofetilide. Selection of the optimal medication depends on whether or not the patient has underlying structural heart disease.[76,78,79] Even with medication therapy, recurrence of atrial fibrillation is likely. Electrical cardioversion may be successful in converting the atria to sinus rhythm if attempted within a few days or weeks of the onset of atrial fibrillation. Success is less likely if atrial fibrillation has existed for a long time.[76]

Rate control. The most frequently prescribed medications used to control the ventricular rate in atrial fibrillation include calcium channel blockers, beta-blockers, and digoxin. These medications work to slow conduction through the AV node. They have no impact on the fibrillating atria. In the past, it was assumed that rate control was an inferior strategy because the patient stayed in atrial fibrillation, lost "atrial kick," and was presumed to have an increased risk of embolic stroke. Two multicenter trials have altered that perception: the *Atrial Fibrillation Follow-up: Investigation of Rhythm Management* (AFFIRM) and the *RAte Control vs. Electrical Cardioversion for Persistent Atrial Fibrillation* (RACE). These two trials found similar morbidity, mortality, and quality of life in patients treated with rhythm conversion or rate control. For long-term management of permanent atrial fibrillation, rate control is the recommended approach, and therapeutic anticoagulation to prevent embolic stroke is mandatory.[80] Antidysrhythmic medications used to manage atrial fibrillation are listed in Table 15.17 in Chapter 15.

Stroke Risk Assessment and Antithrombotic Therapy in Atrial Fibrillation

Atrial fibrillation, because of the development of thrombi in the atria, greatly increases the risk of embolic stroke. Several scoring mechanisms have been developed to help predict which patients with atrial fibrillation require prophylactic anticoagulation.

CHADS2

The acronym *CHADS2* is an easy-to-remember risk assessment tool used to predict stroke risk in atrial fibrillation and to guide antithrombotic therapy (Box 13.11). The letters stand for *c*ardiac failure, *h*ypertension, *a*ge, *d*iabetes, *s*troke (double points).[80] The score ranges from 0 to 6. For a score of 0, no treatment or aspirin is recommended; for a score of 1, aspirin or warfarin is recommended; for a score between 2 and 6, anticoagulation with warfarin is recommended.[80] Newer oral anticoagulants in clinical use including dabigatran (Pradaxa), a thrombin inhibitor, and rivaroxaban, a factor Xa inhibitor, are prescribed for atrial fibrillation in patients with higher CHAD2 scores.[81] In cases of serious bleeding, idarucizumab (Praxbind) is a specific antidote for dabigatran.[82,83] It is either administered as a bolus or infused over 5 minutes to quickly normalize coagulation times.[82,83]

CHA2DS2-VASc

Other scoring systems such as the CHA2DS2-VASc have expanded the risk factor profile to include acute heart failure, hypertension, age 75 years or older (double points), diabetes, stroke (double points), vascular disease, age 65 to 74 years, and sex (female).[81,84]

Electrical and chemical (medication-induced) forms of cardioversion entail the threat of precipitating emboli into the systemic circulation. During atrial fibrillation, the atria do not contract effectively, and blood may pool and promote clots that attach to the atrial walls (mural thrombi). If cardioversion is successful and normal sinus rhythm is restored, the atria again contract forcibly and, if thrombus formation has occurred, may send clots traveling through the pulmonary or systemic circulation. The atrial fibrillation antithrombotic recommendations described earlier, apply equally to patients with atrial flutter.[80,84]

To prevent embolic stroke, it is important to pay attention to the *48-hour rule*. Patients who have been in atrial fibrillation for 48 hours or longer (how long may be unknown) must be

FIG. 13.65 Management of New-Onset Atrial Fibrillation. (From Fuster V, et al. ACC/AHA/ESC 2006 guidelines for the management of patients with atrial fibrillation: A report of the American College of Cardiology/American Heart Association Task Force on Practice Guidelines and the European Society of Cardiology Committee for Practice Guidelines [Writing Committee to revise the 2001 guidelines for the management of patients with atrial fibrillation]: Developed in collaboration with the European Heart Rhythm Association and the Heart Rhythm Society. *Circulation.* 2006;114[7]:e257.)

BOX 13.11   CHADS2 Score

Letter	Risk Factor	Score
C	Chronic heart failure	1
H	Hypertension	1
A	Age >75 years	1
D	Diabetes mellitus	1
S	Stroke or TIA	2

The CHADS2 score is used to predict the risk of having a stroke in atrial fibrillation. A higher score is associated with a higher risk of embolic stroke. CHADS2 minimum score is 0; CHADS2 maximum score is 6.

Score of 0: no treatment or aspirin

Score of 1: aspirin or warfarin

Score of 2–6: warfarin

---

adequately anticoagulated with an oral vitamin K antagonist (warfarin) to achieve a target international normalized ratio (INR) of 2.0 to 3.0 for at least 3 weeks before elective cardioversion.[80] After successful cardioversion, patients should be anticoagulated for an additional 4 weeks.[80] Advancements in antithrombotic therapies have resulted in several newer oral agents in addition to warfarin. The medications dabigatran, rivaroxaban, and apixaban are available specifically for prevention of stroke in patients with nonvalvular atrial fibrillation.[80]

These three antithrombotic agents do not require routine anticoagulation monitoring.

TEE is helpful in identifying the presence or absence of thrombi in fibrillating atria and is recommended as a screening tool before elective cardioversion.[80] It is especially helpful for patients in atrial fibrillation for less than 48 hours who, in the absence of atrial thrombi, may undergo cardioversion without anticoagulation.[80] TEE is described in more detail in the section on transesophageal echocardiography later in this chapter. Patients who experience episodes of rapid atrial fibrillation for only a few hours or days at a time and then convert back to sinus rhythm spontaneously (paroxysmal atrial fibrillation) are also at risk for embolic stroke.

Surgical Procedures to Manage Atrial Fibrillation

The Cox-Maze III procedure (typically called the maze procedure) is an open-heart surgical operation. The surgery is suitable for only a tiny fraction of the patients who have atrial fibrillation, usually those who have *lone atrial fibrillation,* meaning without other structural heart disease. This surgery is designed to permanently cure atrial fibrillation by "cut and sew" insertion of strategic scar lines into the atria. The success rate, measured as freedom from atrial fibrillation, is 75% to 95% up to 15 years after surgery.[81,84] The surgical maze procedure is now rarely performed. It has been replaced by catheter-based techniques that create lines of conduction block (scar) around the pulmonary veins.[86]

TABLE 13.12   Junctional Rhythms

Parameter	Junctional Escape Rhythm	Accelerated Junctional Rhythm	Junctional Tachycardia
Rate	40–60 beats/min	60–100 beats/min	>100 beats/min
Rhythm	Regular	Regular	Regular
P waves	May be present or absent; inverted in lead II	May be present or absent; inverted in lead II	May be present or absent; inverted in lead II
P–R interval	<0.12 s	<0.12 s	<0.12 s
QRS complex	0.06–0.10 s	0.06–0.10 s	0.06–0.10 s

Catheter Procedures to Manage Atrial Fibrillation

The goal of radiofrequency catheter ablation is to reduce clinical symptoms associated with atrial fibrillation. Based on the results of published studies, 57% of patients have reduced symptoms after ablation even without antidysrhythmic medications.[86] When multiple ablation procedures are performed, the success rate increases to 71% without antidysrhythmic medications and to 77% with antidysrhythmics.[86]

Junctional Dysrhythmias

Only certain areas of the AV node have the property of automaticity. The entire area around the AV node is collectively called the *junction*; impulses generated there are called *junctional* impulses. After an ectopic impulse arises in the junction, it spreads in two directions at once. One wave of depolarization spreads upward into the atria and depolarizes them, causing the recording of a P wave on the ECG. This is called *retrograde (backward) conduction*, and the P wave is inverted when viewed in lead II. At the same time, another wave of depolarization spreads downward into the ventricles through the normal conduction pathway, producing a normal QRS complex. This is called *antegrade (forward) conduction*. Depending on timing, the P wave (1) may be seen in front of the QRS complex, with a short P–R interval of less than 0.12 second; (2) may be obscured entirely by the QRS complex; or (3) may immediately follow the QRS complex.

Premature Junctional Contraction

If only a single ectopic impulse originates in the junction, it is simply called a *premature junctional contraction.* On the ECG, the rhythm is regular from the sinus node except for one early QRS complex of normal shape and duration. The P wave can be entirely absent. If a P wave can be found, it very closely precedes or follows the QRS complex. In lead II, the P wave appears inverted (having a negative deflection) because the atria are being depolarized from the AV node upward, which is the opposite direction from the wave of depolarization that occurs when triggered by the sinus node. If the P wave appears before the QRS complex, the P–R interval is less than 0.12 second. Premature junctional contractions have virtually the same clinical significance as PACs. However, if the patient is receiving digoxin, digitalis toxicity may be suspected. Although digoxin slows conduction through the AV node, it also increases automaticity in the junctional area.

Junctional Escape Rhythm

Sometimes the junction becomes the dominant pacemaker of the heart (Table 13.12). The intrinsic rate of the junction normally is 40 to 60 beats/min. The intrinsic rate of the sinus node is 60 to 100 beats/min. Under normal conditions, the junction never has a chance to escape and depolarize the heart because

it is overridden by the sinus node. However, if the sinus node fails, the junctional impulses can depolarize completely and pace the heart. This is called a *junctional escape rhythm*, and it is a protective mechanism to prevent asystole in the event of sinus node failure. Generally, a junctional escape rhythm (Fig. 13.66) is well tolerated hemodynamically, although efforts must be directed toward restoring sinus rhythm. A pacemaker sometimes is inserted as a protective measure because of concern that the AV junction may also fail.

Junctional Tachycardia and Accelerated Junctional Rhythm

A junctional rhythm can also occur at a faster rate (see Table 13.12). As with sinus rhythm, the term *tachycardia* is reserved for rates greater than 100 beats/min. *Junctional tachycardia* is a narrow complex rhythm that arises from the AV junction nearer to the His bundle area. The rate is rapid (120 to 220 beats/min).[73] This is an uncommon rhythm in adults with the exception of digoxin toxicity in a patient taking digoxin (see later).[73] Junctional tachycardia may cause hemodynamic compromise, depending on the rate and the patient's underlying cardiac reserve.

When the junctional rate is greater than 60 beats/min and less than 100 beats/min, it is described as an *accelerated junctional rhythm*. Blood pressure is usually maintained in an accelerated junctional rhythm because the HR is within the normal range to provide adequate diastolic filling time.

Digitalis toxicity is always a concern in patients taking this medication because digoxin enhances automaticity of the AV node. With digitalis toxicity, the optimal strategy is to measure the digoxin serum level and withhold digoxin until the dysrhythmia resolves. When digitalis toxicity is life-threatening, the fastest acting antidote is *digoxin immune Fab*.[87]

Ventricular Dysrhythmias

Ventricular dysrhythmias result from an ectopic focus in any portion of the ventricular myocardium. The usual conduction pathway through the ventricles is not used, and the wave of depolarization must spread from cell to cell. As a result, the QRS complex is prolonged and is always greater than 0.12 second. The width of the QRS complex, not the height, is important in the diagnosis of ventricular ectopy.

Premature Ventricular Contractions

A PVC is a single ectopic impulse originating in the ventricles. Some PVCs are very small in height but remain wider than 0.12 second. If there is doubt, a different lead is evaluated. The shape of the QRS complex depends on the location of the ectopic focus. If the ectopic focus is in the right ventricle, the impulse spreads from right to left, and the QRS complex resembles an LBBB pattern because the left ventricle is the last to be depolarized. In V_1, this is a wide negative QRS complex (Fig. 13.67A).

FIG. 13.66 Junctional Escape Rhythm. The ventricular rate is 38 beats/min. P waves are absent, and the QRS complex has a normal width.

If the ectopic focus is in the LV free wall, the wave of depolarization spreads from left to right (Fig. 13.67B).

Because the ectopic focus may be any cell in the ventricle, the QRS complex can manifest in an unlimited number of shapes or patterns. If all the ventricular ectopic beats look the same in a particular lead, they are called *unifocal*, which means that they probably all result from the same irritable focus (Fig. 13.68A). Conversely, if the ventricular ectopic beats are of various shapes in the same lead, they are called *multifocal* (Fig. 13.68B). Multifocal ventricular ectopic beats are more serious than unifocal ventricular ectopic beats because they indicate a greater area of irritable myocardial tissue and are more likely to deteriorate into VT or ventricular fibrillation. In general, ventricular dysrhythmias have more serious implications than atrial or junctional dysrhythmias and occur only rarely in healthy individuals.

A PVC originates in a ventricular cell that has become abnormally permeable to sodium, usually as a result of damage of one kind or another. Because of this new permeability to sodium, the cell reaches depolarization threshold before an impulse is received from the sinus node. After the depolarization threshold is reached, the cell automatically depolarizes, initiating total ventricular depolarization. Ordinarily, the ventricular impulse does not conduct back through the AV node; the sinus node is not disturbed and continues to depolarize the atria, resulting in a normal P wave. Conduction from the sinus node does not proceed into the ventricles if they are in a refractory state. Assuming there is no further ventricular ectopy, the next sinus beat conducts normally through the AV node and into the ventricles.

Compensatory pause. If the interval from the last normal QRS complex preceding the PVC to the next one is exactly equal to two complete cardiac cycles (Fig. 13.69A), a compensatory pause is present. Because this does not usually occur in PACs or premature junctional contractions, when present, it is diagnostic of ventricular ectopy. If the normal sinus P wave that occurs immediately after the PVC finds the ventricles sufficiently recovered to accept another impulse, a normal QRS complex results, and the PVC is sandwiched between two normal beats (Fig. 13.69B). This PVC is referred to as *interpolated* (meaning "between"). Interpolated PVCs usually occur when the PVC is very early or the normal sinus rate is relatively slow.

The ventricular impulse occasionally spreads backward across the AV node to depolarize the atria. When this occurs, the sinus node is reset, and no full compensatory pause occurs.

Describing ventricular ectopy. PVCs can develop concurrently with any supraventricular dysrhythmia. It is not sufficient to describe a patient's rhythm as "frequent PVCs" or even "frequent unifocal PVCs." The underlying rhythm must always

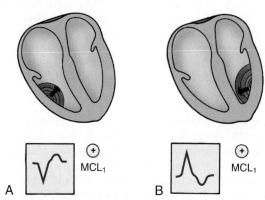

FIG. 13.67 (A) Right ventricular premature ventricular contraction (PVC). The spread of depolarization is from right to left, away from the positive electrode in lead V$_1$, resulting in a wide, negative QRS complex. (B) Left ventricular PVC. The spread of depolarization is from left to right, toward the positive electrode in lead V$_1$ (MCL$_1$). The QRS complex is wide and upright.

FIG. 13.68 (A) Unifocal premature ventricular contractions (PVCs). (B) Multifocal PVCs.

FIG. 13.70 Ventricular Bigeminy.

FIG. 13.71 R-on-T Phenomenon.

FIG. 13.69 (A) Premature ventricular contraction (PVC) with fully compensatory pause. The interval between the two sinus beats that surround the PVC (R_1 and R_2) is exactly two times the normal interval between sinus beats (R_3 and R_4). The fully compensatory pause occurs because the sinus node continues to pace despite the PVC. The sinus P wave *(arrow)* is hidden in the ST segment of the PVC. This P wave did not conduct through to the ventricles because they had just been depolarized and were still in the absolute refractory period. (B) Interpolated PVC. The PVC falls between two normal QRS complexes without disturbing the rhythm. The R–R interval between sinus beats remains the same.

be described first, such as "sinus bradycardia with frequent unifocal PVCs" or "atrial fibrillation with occasional multifocal PVCs." Timing of PVCs can also be described. When a PVC follows each normally conducted beat, *ventricular bigeminy* is present (Fig. 13.70). If a PVC follows every two normal beats, it is called *ventricular trigeminy.*

In individuals with underlying heart disease, PVCs or episodes of self-terminating VT are potentially malignant. Nonsustained VT is defined as three or more consecutive premature ventricular beats at a rate faster than 110 beats/min lasting less than 30 seconds.

Premature ventricular contraction timing. The timing of PVCs can be important, especially if myocardial ischemia is present. The relative refractory period, represented on the ECG by the last half of the T wave, is a particularly vulnerable time for ectopy to occur because repolarization is incomplete. Repolarization is even more delayed in ischemic tissue so that various portions of the ventricular muscle are not repolarized simultaneously. If a PVC occurs at this critical point when only a part of the muscle is repolarized, individual segments of muscle can depolarize separately from each other, resulting in VF. This is called the *R-on-T phenomenon* (Fig. 13.71).

Two consecutive PVCs are described as a *couplet,* and three consecutive PVCs are called a *triplet* or a *three-beat run of ventricular tachycardia.* More than three consecutive PVCs are considered VT, but it is still useful to state how many beats of VT occurred if the run was short (ie, lasting less than 20 beats).

Causes of premature ventricular contractions. PVCs can result from many causes. They have been known to occur, although rarely, in healthy individuals with no evidence of heart disease. The critical care nurse has an important role in identifying factors that may be causing or at least contributing to PVCs. Acute ischemia is the most dangerous cause of ventricular ectopy. Ischemia causes cell membrane permeability to change, giving rise to early depolarization and the initiation of ectopic impulses. Ventricular ectopy that occurs during an acute ischemic event may require treatment with IV amiodarone or other antidysrhythmic medications.

Metabolic abnormalities are common causes of PVCs. Hypokalemia, hypoxemia, and acidosis predispose the cell membrane to instability and may cause ventricular ectopy. Treatment is directed toward identifying the metabolic disturbance and correcting it. Arterial blood gas values and serum potassium and magnesium levels are obtained if no recent results are available. The ability of oxygen and potassium values to change very rapidly in a critically ill patient must not be underestimated. If PVCs develop during suctioning of an intubated patient, a few additional breaths of 100% oxygen usually are sufficient to restore adequate oxygenation and to eliminate the ventricular ectopy.

Any form of structural heart disease can lead to ventricular ectopy. Patients with cardiomyopathy or ventricular aneurysms can have chronic, severe ventricular ectopy, which may prove to be refractory to antidysrhythmic agents. Invasive procedures, such as insertion of a PA catheter or cardiac catheterization, can cause PVCs by mechanically irritating the ventricular muscle. In these situations, the ectopy usually resolves with removal or advancement of the catheter.

Certain medications can cause ventricular ectopy. Digitalis toxicity may precipitate PVCs, which are resistant to conventional antidysrhythmic therapy. Some class I antidysrhythmic medications can cause more serious dysrhythmias than the dysrhythmias they were intended to treat. This is called a *prodysrhythmic effect* (also described as a *proarrhythmic effect*), and it can sometimes be fatal. Class 1a medications prolong the Q–T interval by lengthening the ventricular refractory period. This is a therapeutic effect, but when the Q–T interval prolongation becomes excessive, a characteristic form of polymorphic VT called *torsades de pointes* develops (Fig. 13.72). In this dysrhythmia, VT is very rapid, and QRS complexes appear to twist in a spiral pattern around the baseline. Torsades de pointes results in hemodynamic instability because of the extremely rapid rate. If torsades de pointes is not terminated, death ensues. Sometimes torsades de pointes stops spontaneously, although the patient may experience a syncopal episode or seizure at the time of the dysrhythmia. Risk factors for development of torsades de pointes are listed in Box 13.6 earlier in the chapter.

Premature ventricular contraction management. Not all ventricular ectopy requires treatment. In individuals without significant underlying heart disease, PVCs do not represent an increased risk for sudden death and are considered benign. If the patient complains of palpitations, therapy includes reassurance and assessment of electrolyte levels and any medications that increase ventricular irritability. During an acute MI, antidysrhythmic medications such as amiodarone or beta-blockers may be used to decrease the risk of isolated PVCs progressing to VT. In contrast, if a patient with PVCs has a healthy heart, antidysrhythmic medications, specifically medications that increase the incidence of VT, are used as a last resort because of the risk of prodysrhythmia. Chapter 15 provides further information about antidysrhythmic medications (see Table 15.16).

Idioventricular rhythms. Sometimes an ectopic focus in the ventricle can become the dominant pacemaker of the heart (Table 13.13). If the sinus node and the AV junction fail, the ventricles depolarize at their own intrinsic rate of 20 to 40 times per minute. This is called an *idioventricular rhythm* and is a naturally protective mechanism. Rather than trying to abolish the ventricular beats, the aim of treatment is to increase the effective HR and reestablish dominance of a higher pacing site such as the sinus node or the AV junction. Usually a temporary pacemaker is used to increase the HR until the underlying problems that caused failure of the other pacing sites can be resolved.

An *accelerated idioventricular rhythm* (AIVR) occurs when a ventricular focus assumes control of the heart at a rate greater than its intrinsic rate of 40 beats/min but less than 100 beats/min (Fig. 13.73). Although relatively benign in and of itself, this rhythm must be closely observed for any increase in rate, and the patient must be observed for hemodynamic deterioration. Usually, AIVR is not treated pharmacologically if well tolerated with a stable blood pressure, although a transvenous temporary pacemaker should be inserted electively as a precaution against sudden hemodynamic deterioration. IV lidocaine must never be administered to a patient with an idioventricular rhythm because it suppresses the ventricular pacemaker and converts the rhythm to asystole.

Ventricular tachycardia. VT is caused by a ventricular pacing site firing at a rate of 100 times or more per minute, usually maintained by a reentry mechanism within the ventricular tissue (Fig. 13.74). The complexes are wide, and the rhythm may be slightly irregular, often accelerating as the tachycardia continues (see Table 13.13). In most cases, the sinus node is not affected and it continues to depolarize the atria on schedule. P waves can sometimes be seen on the ECG tracing. They are not related to the QRS complex and may even appear to conduct a normal impulse to the ventricles if their timing is just right. A brief episode is termed *nonsustained VT* for a duration less than 30 seconds.

If the sinus impulse and the ventricular ectopic impulse meet in the middle of the ventricles, a fusion beat results. Fusion beats are narrower than ventricular beats and look like a cross between the patient's sinus QRS complex and the ventricular ectopic QRS complex (Fig. 13.75). When present, P waves and fusion beats are helpful in verifying the diagnosis of VT as opposed to SVT. Differentiation between VT and SVT was discussed earlier.

Most VT occurs in the presence of structural cardiac disease, such as myocardial ischemia, congenital heart disease, valvular

0 Sec.   3 Sec.   6 Sec.

FIG. 13.72 Torsades de Pointes.

TABLE 13.13   Ventricular Rhythms

Parameter	Idioventricular Rhythm	Accelerated Idioventricular Rhythm	Ventricular Tachycardia	Ventricular Fibrillation
Rate	20–40 beats/min	40–100 beats/min	>100 beats/min	None
Rhythm	Usually regular	Usually regular	Usually regular	Irregular
P waves	Absent or retrograde	Absent or retrograde	Absent or retrograde	None
PR interval	None	None	None	None
QRS complex	>0.12 s	>0.12 s	>0.12 s	Fibrillatory waves

dysfunction, and cardiomyopathy. Other triggers include drug toxicities, electrolyte disturbances, and certain antidysrhythmic medications (prodysrhythmia). VT is a life-threatening dysrhythmia and must be treated quickly. The rapid ventricular rate decreases blood pressure, and the patient may lose consciousness. The loss of the synchronized timing of atrial contraction, which normally adds volume to the ventricles just before contraction and enhances the force of contraction, is lost, greatly reducing CO. If not terminated quickly, VT is likely to degenerate into VF and death.

How VT is clinically managed depends on whether the patient is stable or unstable as well as whether a pulse and adequate blood pressure are present. Pulseless VT is a life-threatening condition. The patient loses consciousness and needs immediate cardiopulmonary resuscitation and defibrillation as described in the American Heart Association protocols for advanced cardiac life support. Patients with stable or wide complex "slow VT" who have an HR below 150 beats/min, palpable pulse, and stable blood pressure may be treated pharmacologically with the IV antidysrhythmics amiodarone, procainamide, or sotalol (beta-blocker with class III antidysrhythmic properties) as described in the advanced cardiac life support protocols.

After the acute episode is over, patients who have already experienced sustained VT or cardiac arrest continue to be at risk for sudden cardiac death. An extensive clinical evaluation of these patients is warranted including cardiac catheterization and electrophysiologic testing with programmed ventricular stimulation. Therapy is aimed at preventing a recurrence of sustained VT or VF. It may include treating the underlying cause, administering antidysrhythmic medications, performing ablation of the reentrant pathway within the ventricle, or inserting an implantable cardioverter defibrillator (ICD).

ICDs can be programmed to deliver several bursts of overdrive pacing to terminate stable VT before cardioversion. This has the advantage of being more comfortable for the patient because it prevents the discomfort of an internal shock if overdrive pacing is successful. Most patients with an ICD are also managed with antidysrhythmic medications. Antitachycardia (overdrive) pacing is an effective treatment if combined with defibrillation backup. It is risky without defibrillator support, as one of the complications of antitachycardia pacing is acceleration of the VT toward a faster pulseless VT, polymorphic VT, or even VF. Chapter 15, provides more information on ICDs (see Fig. 15.10).

Ventricular Fibrillation

VF is the result of chaotic electrical activity in the ventricles from repetitive, small areas of reentry or a series of rapid discharges from various foci within the ventricular myocardium. This electrical activity causes the ventricles to be unable to contract completely and effectively. The ventricles merely quiver, and no forward flow of blood occurs. Without forward flow, no palpable pulse or audible apical heart tones are present. Clinically, VF is indistinguishable from asystole (absence of electrical activity). On the ECG, VF appears as a continuous, undulating pattern without clear P wave, QRS complex, or T wave (Fig. 13.76). When VF occurs in the setting of an acute ischemic event and is accompanied by a significant amount of myocardial damage, the survival rate is poor. Resuscitation is often unsuccessful; recurrence rates are high for patients who are resuscitated. VF is seen on the ECG as large, erratic undulations of the baseline (coarse VF) or as a mild tremor (fine VF). In VF, the patient does not have a pulse, no blood is being pumped forward, and defibrillation is the only definitive therapy. Defibrillation is more likely to be successful with coarse VF. Antidysrhythmic

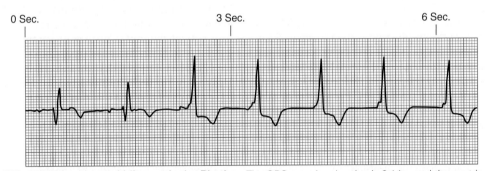

FIG. 13.73 Accelerated Idioventricular Rhythm. The QRS complex duration is 0.14 s, and the ventricular rate is 65 beats/min.

FIG. 13.74 Ventricular Tachycardia.

FIG. 13.75 Ventricular Fusion Beat (arrows). The QRS complex duration is only 0.08 s, and the shape represents the normal QRS complex and the previous PVC.

medications such as IV amiodarone are administered if initial attempts at defibrillation fail. As with any cardiac arrest situation, supportive measures such as cardiopulmonary resuscitation, intubation, and correction of metabolic abnormalities are performed concurrently with definitive therapy.

Differential Diagnosis of Wide QRS Complex Tachycardia

Wide complex tachycardias may be caused by different mechanisms, including the following:

1. VT
2. SVT with aberrancy secondary to conduction slowing in the bundle branch system
3. SVT with anterograde conduction over an accessory pathway
4. Ventricular paced rhythm

VT is the most common reason for a sudden-onset wide complex tachycardia. The challenge is to recognize the atypical *supraventricular* wide complex tachycardia when the trigger is an ectopic atrial or junctional focus arising from an irritable site above the ventricles.[88] Typical SVT has a narrow QRS complex (less than 0.12 second duration) because the electrical impulse enters the ventricle through the AV node and continues down the normal conduction pathway by means of the bundle branches through the ventricles. VT always has a wide QRS complex (longer than 0.12 second) because the impulse begins somewhere within the ventricles and must spread slowly, moving from cell to cell, without the benefit of the usual conduction pathways. It is easy to distinguish between typical SVT and VT by QRS complex width alone. However, not all SVTs result in a narrow QRS complex. An SVT manifests with a wide QRS complex in three situations:

1. The patient may already have an RBBB or LBBB, resulting in a wide QRS rhythm even during sinus rhythm. If the patient develops an atrial or junctional tachycardia, the shape of the bundle branch block is unchanged, and the QRS complex is still wide.
2. A supraventricular impulse may arrive in the ventricles so early that only part of the conduction system is repolarized. One of the bundle branches is still refractory, causing the wave of depolarization to spread abnormally (aberrantly) through the ventricles and resulting in a wide QRS complex.
3. Occasionally, an anatomic variant occurs in which the patient has a small strip of muscle tissue connecting the atria with the ventricles and bypassing the AV node. This is called an *accessory pathway* or *bypass tract*, the most common of which occurs in Wolff-Parkinson-White syndrome.[73] This does not pose a hemodynamic problem in normal sinus rhythm, although it sometimes causes subtle ECG changes that make it easier to be detected. However, when rapid atrial dysrhythmias occur, they can be conducted directly to a portion of the ventricular myocardium without the normal AV delay. Depolarization through the ventricles then proceeds from cell to cell rather than through the normal and efficient pathway of the conduction system, resulting in a wide QRS complex tachycardia that closely resembles VT.

Significance of ventricular tachycardia and supraventricular tachycardia. Standard treatment for VT includes administration of IV amiodarone. In contrast, SVT is treated with a variety of medications that work by blocking the AV node conduction pathway—diltiazem, verapamil, amiodarone, or digoxin.[73] A problem occurs if the SVT has occurred as a result of the presence of an accessory pathway and the narrow complex tachycardia is treated with verapamil or other medications that block the AV node but do not block the Wolff-Parkinson-White accessory pathway.[73] This can result in an extremely fast wide complex tachycardia through the accessory pathway with acute, severe hypotension or loss of consciousness requiring immediate cardioversion. For this reason, it is important to be sure of the cause of the tachycardia in individuals who are relatively hemodynamically stable before treatment is initiated.

Regardless of the site of origin, a rapid wide QRS complex tachycardia may not be well tolerated, largely because of the fast HR that prevents adequate ventricular filling during diastole as well as increasing myocardial oxygen demand while decreasing time available for coronary artery filling. Hemodynamic deterioration is evidenced by syncope, severe hypotension, or ischemic symptoms. In this case, emergency external cardioversion must be performed regardless of whether the tachycardia is of ventricular or supraventricular origin. Correct diagnosis of a wide QRS complex tachycardia may have an impact on the long-term management of a patient as well. If atrial flutter or fibrillation is determined to be the underlying mechanism, long-term treatment probably includes amiodarone or a betablocker to reduce the HR response when these dysrhythmias occur.[73] If VT is determined to be the underlying mechanism in a patient without a history of ventricular dysrhythmias, a careful search for the cause (eg, hypoxemia, electrolyte imbalance, excess sympathetic stimulation, ischemia) is warranted. Depending on the clinical situation, the patient may require long-term antidysrhythmic therapy. If there is a history of VT or sudden cardiac death and the patient is already on antidysrhythmic therapy, a recurrent episode of VT indicates that the current treatment regimen is ineffective and the therapy needs to be changed.

Clinical differentiation of ventricular tachycardia from supraventricular tachycardia. Contrary to popular belief, hemodynamic stability or instability does not help to differentiate between VT and SVT with a wide QRS complex. In theory, SVT is better tolerated, especially if atrial contraction is still occurring before each ventricular contraction (AV synchrony). However, clinically this is often variable. VT may be well tolerated, especially if the rate is less than 150 beats/min. Some patients can be in sustained VT for hours without significant hemodynamic compromise. Conversely, because AV synchrony is lost in atrial fibrillation or atrial flutter and the ventricular response rate may be very rapid, ventricular filling and CO can be severely compromised.[73]

Careful physical examination can be valuable in determining the source of the tachycardia. The jugular venous pulse can be assessed for the presence of cannon a waves. When the atria contract at the same time as ventricular systole, the AV valves

0 Sec.   3 Sec.

FIG. 13.76 Ventricular Fibrillation.

are closed, and the blood in the atria is forced to regurgitate into the venous system. This is seen as a very large pulsation in the jugular vein. If it occurs sporadically (not with every beat), it is a sign of AV dissociation, or independent beating of the atria and ventricles. Heart sounds provide another diagnostic clue. Variation of the intensity of the first heart sound (S_1) from beat to beat favors VT because this is also indicative of AV dissociation.

The most reliable bedside method of diagnosing a wide QRS complex tachycardia is through careful analysis of the ECG. HR and heart rhythm are evaluated first, although they are not the only diagnostic indicators. The QRS complex width is measured in more than one lead because the lead with the widest QRS complex is the most reliable indicator of true QRS complex duration. It is assumed that some portion of the QRS complex is isoelectric in leads where the QRS complex appears to be narrow. QRS complex widths of less than 0.14 second (140 ms) favor SVT with aberrant conduction, whereas a width greater than 0.14 second in an RBBB pattern or greater than 0.16 second (160 ms) in an LBBB pattern favors VT.[88]

The tracing is examined closely for the presence of P waves. If P waves can be identified and they do not correlate on a 1:1 basis with the QRS complexes, AV dissociation exists and strongly suggests VT. Although P waves may be found in any lead, they are generally most readily visible in leads V_1 or II. When the sinus node remains in control of the atria and a ventricular ectopic focus is in control of the ventricles, it is likely that at some point the timing will be coordinated, and, by chance, the sinus impulse will conduct through the AV node and begin to depolarize the ventricles just as the ventricular ectopic focus fires. The resulting QRS complex is a fusion beat (see Fig. 13.75), which resembles a blend of the patient's normal QRS complex and the wide QRS complex of the ventricular dysrhythmia. The presence of fusion beats also strongly suggests VT.

Another helpful diagnostic criterion for VT is a QRS complex axis in the northwest quadrant of −90 degrees to −180 degrees

(Fig. 13.77). An axis in this quadrant means that the wave of depolarization is directed upward and to the right, exactly the opposite of normal ventricular depolarization. Even when ventricular conduction is abnormal, as in BBBs, ventricular depolarization begins at the level of the AV junction and spreads downward toward the apex, although conduction disturbances direct the current flow more to the right or left than normal. Although not all VT rhythms have an axis in the extreme or northwest quadrant, when this axis is present, it confirms the diagnosis of VT. Fig. 13.78 shows how this abnormal axis can be identified from a five-lead ECG bedside monitor by observing the shape of the QRS complex in leads I and aVF.

The shape of the QRS complex in the right precordial lead V_1 and the left precordial lead V_6 can be diagnostic of VT or SVT with aberrant conduction. Fig. 13.78 summarizes these QRS complex patterns. If the QRS complex is entirely positive from V_1 through V_6 or entirely negative, the diagnosis is VT. This phenomenon is known as *precordial concordance*.

Nursing management. Proper electrode placement and appropriate lead selection have already been discussed but cannot be overemphasized. In addition to correct lead placement and selection, every effort must be made to record the wide QRS complex tachycardia on a standard 12-lead ECG. Emergency treatment must not be delayed if the patient is hemodynamically unstable, but documenting the dysrhythmia by recording a "stat" 12-lead ECG must be given a high priority if time permits. VT and SVT are often nonsustained, and waiting for a physician's order or the arrival of a technician to perform the test could result in failure to document the AV conduction disturbance.

The sinoatrial node normally triggers electrical depolarization in the heart. From there, the impulse travels through the right atrium to the AV node. The left atrium is depolarized by a conduction fiber known as *Bachmann bundle* that connects the right and left atria. The electrical impulse is briefly delayed in the AV node to allow the atria to contract and the mitral and tricuspid valves to close before the impulse is conducted to the bundle of His, the bundle branches, and the Purkinje fibers.

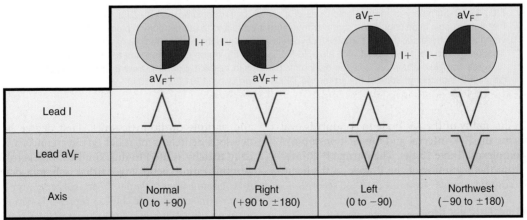

FIG. 13.77 Determination of QRS Complex Axis Quadrant by Noting Predominant QRS Complex Polarity in Leads I and aVF. Normal axis: If QRS complex during tachycardia is primarily positive in both leads I and aVF, the axis falls within the normal quadrant from 0 to 90 degrees. Right-axis deviation: If the QRS complex is primarily negative in lead I and positive in lead aVF, right-axis deviation is present. Left-axis deviation: If the QRS complex is predominantly positive in lead I and negative in lead aVF, left-axis deviation is present. *Indeterminate axis:* If the QRS complex is primarily negative in both leads I and aVF, a markedly abnormal "indeterminate," or "northwest," axis is present that is diagnostic of ventricular tachycardia. (From Drew B. Bedside electrocardiographic monitoring: State of the art for the 1990s. *Heart Lung.* 1991;20[6]:610.)

V₁ OR MCL₁	V₆ OR MCL₆
VENTRICULAR	
Monophasic R	Biphasic rS with R:S ratio <1
Taller left peak	Monophasic Q
Biphasic RS	Notched QS
Biphasic qR	Biphasic qR
Any one of the following in V₁ *or* V₂: (a) R >30 ms (b) Slurred or notched S descent (c) QRS onset to S nadir >60 ms	QRS onset to predominant peak (or nadir) ≥0.07 sec.
SUPRAVENTRICULAR WITH BUNDLE BRANCH BLOCK OR ABERRATION	
Bimodal rR' or Triphasic rsR'	Triphasic qRs with R:S ratio >1
All of the following in V₁ *and* V₂: (a) R ≤30 ms or no R (b) Straight S descent (c) QRS onset to S nadir ≤ 60 ms	QRS onset to predominant peak (or nadir) ≤0.05 sec.
UNHELPFUL QRS MORPHOLOGIES	
Slurred or notched taller right peak	Monophasic R
	Taller left or right peak
	Biphasic Rs with R:S ratio >1

*Tachycardias with a right bundle branch block pattern in V₁ only

FIG. 13.78 Summary of morphologic clues in V₁ or MCL₁ *(left column)* and in V₆ or MCL₆ *(right column)* that are valuable in distinguishing supraventricular tachycardia with bundle branch block or aberration from ventricular tachycardia. If wide-complex tachycardia with taller right peak pattern (ie, unhelpful morphology) develops in a patient monitored with a single MCL₁ lead, the nurse changes leads to determine whether the wide complex falls into one of the diagnostic patterns in V₆ (MCL₆). (From Drew B. Bedside electrocardiographic monitoring: State of the art for the 1990s. *Heart Lung.* 1991;20[6]:610.)

On the ECG, the ability of the AV node to conduct is evaluated by measuring the P–R interval and the relationship of P waves to QRS complexes (Table 13.14). The normal P–R interval, measured from the beginning of the P wave to the beginning of the QRS complex, ranges from 0.12 to 0.20 second.

First-Degree Atrioventricular Block

When all atrial impulses are conducted to the ventricles but the P–R interval is greater than 0.20 second, a condition known as *first-degree AV block* exists (Fig. 13.79). First-degree AV block can be chronic or acute, and it may be caused by a multitude of conditions. Long-standing first-degree block may occur related to fibrosis and sclerosis of the conduction system, lack of blood supply to the conduction system secondary to coronary artery disease (CAD), valvular heart disease, myocarditis,

and various cardiomyopathies. First-degree heart block that develops acutely is of much greater concern. Causes include drug toxicity related to digoxin, beta-blockers, or amiodarone administration; acute myocardial ischemia or MI; hyperkalemia; edema after valvular heart surgery; and increased vagal tone. First-degree AV block represents slowed conduction through the AV node. If the associated QRS complex is narrow, it is likely that the only conduction abnormality is in the AV node. However, if the associated QRS complex is widened, it is likely that there is also damage to the bundle branches as a result of sclerosis, ischemia, or infarction.

Second-Degree Atrioventricular Block

Second-degree AV block can be broadly defined as a condition in which some atrial impulses are conducted to the ventricles,

TABLE 13.14   Atrioventricular Block

Parameter	First-Degree	Second-Degree Mobitz I (Wenckebach)	Second-Degree Mobitz II	Third-Degree (Complete)
P–R interval	>0.20 s and constant	Increases with each consecutively conducted P wave	Constant	Varies randomly
P waves	1 P wave for each QRS complex	Intermittently not conducted, yielding more P waves than QRS complexes	Intermittently not conducted, yielding more P waves than QRS complexes	P waves independent and not related to QRS complexes
QRS complex	0.06–0.10 s	0.06–0.10 s	May be normal, but usually coexists with BBB (>0.12 s)	0.06–0.10 s if junctional escape pacemaker activates ventricles >0.12 s if ventricular escape pacemaker activates ventricles

BBB, bundle branch block.

FIG. 13.79 First-Degree Atrioventricular Block. The P–R interval is prolonged to 0.44 s.

but others are "blocked" at the AV node. This description of intermittent AV conduction covers two patterns with markedly different clinical significance: Second-degree AV block is divided into Mobitz type I (also known as *Wenckebach block*) and Mobitz type II.

Mobitz type I. In Mobitz type I block, the AV conduction times progressively lengthen until a P wave is not conducted. This typically occurs in a pattern of *grouped beats* and is observed on the ECG by a gradually lengthening P–R interval, until ultimately the final P wave in the group fails to conduct. In Mobitz type I, the QRS complex is generally of normal width and appearance. Several criteria must be present for Mobitz I (Wenckebach) to be diagnosed, as follows:

1. The sinus node is functional and generates impulses that conduct to the AV node at a constant rate. On the ECG, the measured P–P interval is regular.
2. As each successive atrial impulse arrives earlier into the *relative refractory period* of the impaired AV node, more time is needed to conduct the impulse. On the ECG, this is seen as an incremental increase in the length of each P–R interval. The R–R interval usually becomes shorter with each beat.
3. The P–R interval is shortest in the first beat.
   a. The initial P–R interval is often, but not always, of normal length. If first-degree block coexists, the initial P–R interval will be prolonged, but this initial P–R interval will still have the shortest measured interval of the group.
   b. The initial P–R interval is shorter because the AV node has experienced a "rest" or longer recovery time secondary to the final nonconducted P wave in the group, as subsequently described.
4. The final P wave of the group is not conducted. The atrial impulse arrives during the absolute refractory period of the AV node and is not conducted. This is seen on the ECG by a P wave that is *not* followed by a QRS complex (Fig. 13.80).

Mobitz I block has a specific, repeating pattern that catches the eye. The expected groups are 3:2, 4:3, or 5:4. For example, if four P waves are conducted to the ventricles and the fifth one is not, a 5:4 conduction ratio is present (five P waves to four QRS complexes). The nonconducted P wave ends a group. After the pause, the cycle repeats itself. The P–R interval typically lengthens the most with the second beat of the cycle.

Mobitz type I does not generally cause significant hemodynamic compromise as long as the ventricular HR is maintained. However, in the presence of ischemia and infarction, it may progress to a more severe level of block. If Mobitz type I occurs in the setting of an acute inferior wall infarction, close observation and occasionally placement of a temporary pacemaker as a precautionary measure are warranted.

Mobitz type II. Mobitz type II block is always anatomically located below the AV node in the bundle of His, in the bundle branches, or in the Purkinje fibers. This results in an all-or-nothing situation with respect to AV conduction. Sinus P waves are or are not conducted. When conduction does occur, all P–R intervals are the same. Because of the anatomic location of the block, the P–R interval is constant and the QRS complexes are wide on the surface ECG (Fig. 13.81).

Mobitz II block is more ominous clinically than Mobitz I and may progress to complete AV block. If the block involves the Purkinje fibers, an escape rhythm may not develop. For this reason, it is important to prepare for *transcutaneous cardiac pacing* (TCP) by bringing the TCP device (often combined with a defibrillator) to the bedside as a precaution. TCP refers to external pacing from outside the chest wall. When pacing is required, two large pacing electrodes are placed on the chest. There is always a diagram on the machine showing where to place the pads on the chest. Consider the possibility that the patient will need a temporary transvenous pacemaker inserted and possibly require a permanent pacemaker before hospital discharge.

2:1 Conduction. Occasionally, only every other P wave is conducted through the AV node (Fig. 13.82). This pattern may indicate Mobitz type I or Mobitz type II because consecutive conduction of P waves—which reveal a lengthening or constant P–R interval—does not occur. In Mobitz I, the conduction ratios may have decreased from 4:3 to 3:2 to 2:1, but the site and type of block have not changed. The change in conduction ratio may be caused by an increase in atrial rate, or it may change spontaneously.

In 2:1 conduction, it is impossible to be certain whether the block is Mobitz type I or type II from the surface ECG. If it occurs along with other Mobitz I ratios, it is probably still Mobitz I. If

FIG. 13.80 Mobitz type I (Wenckebach) Second-Degree Atrioventricular Block. The P–R intervals gradually increase from 0.36 to 0.46 s until a P wave is not conducted to the ventricles.

FIG. 13.81 Mobitz Type II Second-Degree Atrioventricular Block. The P–R intervals remain constant.

FIG. 13.82 A 2:1 Atrioventricular (AV) Block. Because no two consecutive P waves are conducted, it is impossible to determine with certainty whether this is a Mobitz I or Mobitz II second-degree AV block.

it is an isolated occurrence with no other strips for comparison, the QRS complex width and the P–R interval offer valuable clues to the site of the block. In Mobitz I, the QRS complex is usually normal, and the P–R interval is usually prolonged. In Mobitz II, the QRS complex is usually wide, and the P–R interval is usually normal. During an acute inferior MI, Mobitz type I AV block with 2:1 conduction is much more common than type II.

Third-Degree Atrioventricular Block

Third-degree, or complete, AV block is a condition in which no atrial impulses can conduct from the atria to the ventricles. This condition is also described by the terms *complete heart block* or *AV dissociation* to indicate that different cardiac pacemakers control the atrial rate and the ventricular rate. The block can be located at the level of the AV node or below the node within the bundle of His or the bundle branches. It can be caused by infarction, digitalis toxicity, or age-related degeneration of the conduction system in older patients. It is hoped that a junctional focus or ventricular focus depolarizes spontaneously at its intrinsic rate of 20 to 40 beats/min and that ventricular contraction continues. If not, asystole occurs; there is no pulse, and death results if pacemaker support is not immediate.

On the ECG, P waves are present and usually occur at regular intervals. If a junctional focus is pacing the heart, normal QRS complexes are present but occur at a rate and timing interval totally independent of the P waves. The P–R intervals vary widely because the P wave and QRS complex are not related to each other. If a ventricular focus is pacing the heart, the QRS complex is wide and unrelated to the P waves (Fig. 13.83).

Management of Atrioventricular Block

Clinically, the consequences of AV block range from benign to life-threatening. First-degree AV block is seldom of immediate concern but bears close observation for progression

of the conduction disturbance. Second-degree Mobitz I (Wenckebach) is usually benign as long as the patient is not bradycardic. If hemodynamic compromise is present or deemed likely, a temporary pacemaker can be inserted prophylactically. Second-degree Mobitz II is more serious and often precedes complete AV block. Use of a temporary pacemaker is recommended, but its insertion can be elective if the patient remains hemodynamically stable. Complete heart block causes AV dissociation and is associated with a low CO that requires use of a pacemaker. In complete heart block, the patient may exhibit cannon waves as the dissociated atria contact against closed AV valves and create a "wave" on the atrial pressure waveform. An example of this phenomenon is shown in Fig. 13.13. If the patient is hemodynamically unstable, external TCP can be used to maintain an adequate ventricular rate until a transvenous or permanent pacemaker can be inserted.

LABORATORY TESTS

Laboratory assessment of cardiovascular status is obtained through studies of blood serum. Accurate interpretation of these laboratory studies, along with the clinical picture, enables the critical care team to diagnose, treat, and assess the response to therapeutic interventions.

Laboratory studies of blood serum are performed to assess the following:
1. Electrolyte levels that can alter cardiac muscle contraction
2. Cardiac biomarkers that reflect myocardial cellular integrity or infarction
3. Hematologic status to evaluate risk of anemia and infection
4. Coagulation times
5. Serum lipid levels
6. Status of other organ systems that can secondarily affect cardiac function

0 Sec.   3 Sec.

FIG. 13.83 Third-Degree (Complete) Heart Block.

Electrolytes

Potassium

During depolarization and repolarization of nerve and muscle fiber, potassium and sodium exchange occurs intracellularly and extracellularly. The potassium gradient across the cell membrane determines conduction velocity and helps confine pacing activity to the sinus node. Excess or deficiency of potassium can alter myocardial muscle function. Normal serum potassium levels are 3.5 to 4.5 mEq/L.

Hyperkalemia. Elevated serum potassium, called *hyperkalemia*, can be caused by various conditions including excess potassium administration, extensive skeletal muscle destruction (rhabdomyolysis), tumor lysis syndrome, and kidney failure. Some medications may induce hyperkalemia including potassium-sparing diuretics, angiotensin-converting enzyme inhibitors, and angiotensin receptor blockers.[89] Hyperkalemia can elicit significant changes in the ECG because it decreases AV conduction velocity, slows ventricular depolarization, and accelerates repolarization. As the serum levels of potassium rise, tall, narrow peaked T waves are usually, although not uniquely, associated with early hyperkalemia and are followed by prolongation of the P–R interval, loss of the P wave, widening of the QRS complex, heart block, and asystole (Fig. 13.84A). Severely elevated serum potassium (greater than 8 mEq/L) causes a wide QRS complex tachycardia, as shown in the 12-lead ECG in Fig. 13.84B. If not corrected, severe hyperkalemia can lead to VF or cardiac standstill. Evidence of hyperkalemia is not always visible on the ECG. Furthermore, research has shown that ECG waveform changes are not a sensitive indicator of elevated potassium levels. When hyperkalemia is suspected, it is safer to draw serial serum potassium levels than to rely on the ECG waveform alone.

This life-threatening condition can be acutely managed with IV insulin to drive the potassium inside the cell and temporarily out of the plasma. Glucose is usually administered at the same time to avoid hypoglycemia as a secondary complication. Potassium is permanently removed from the bloodstream by cation-exchange resin products, such as Kayexalate, placed into the gastrointestinal tract or is removed directly from the blood by hemodialysis.[90] Coexisting low serum sodium, calcium, or pH levels potentiate the cardiac effects of hyperkalemia.

Hypokalemia. A low serum potassium (K+) level, called *hypokalemia* (less than 3.5 mEq/L), is commonly caused by diuretic therapy with insufficient replacement, gastrointestinal losses, and some medications.[90] Hypokalemia is also reflected by changes on the ECG (Fig. 13.85). The earliest ECG change is often PVCs, which can deteriorate into VT or VF without appropriate potassium replacement.

Hypokalemia impairs myocardial conduction and prolongs ventricular repolarization; this can be seen by a prominent U wave (a positive deflection after the T wave on the ECG). The U wave is not totally unique to hypokalemia, but its presence is a signal for the clinician to check the serum potassium level. In the critical care unit, where patients are receiving diuretics or have gastric tubes to suction, the serum potassium level is checked frequently by the critical care nurse and replaced intravenously to normal levels to prevent dysrhythmias. Great care must be taken with IV potassium replacement to ensure that it is diluted sufficiently and administered slowly to prevent accidental overdose. Potassium is a high-alert medication, and additional safety procedures are recommended for replacement of this electrolyte (Box 13.12). Table 13.15 lists electrolyte values that affect cardiac contractility.

Calcium

Calcium (Ca^{2+}) is an important cation in the body. Calcium metabolism is controlled by many factors, including normal parathyroid hormone function, calcitonin, and vitamin D acting on target organs such as the kidney, bone, and gastrointestinal tract. Calcium is an important mediator of many cardiovascular functions because of its effect on vascular tone, myocardial contractility, and cardiac excitability.

Serum calcium values can be recorded in three ways, depending on the hospital laboratory: milliequivalents per liter (mEq/L), milligrams per deciliter (mg/dL), or millimoles per liter (mmol/L). In the bloodstream, approximately 50% of calcium is biologically active and is known as *ionized calcium*.[91] The remaining calcium is bound to protein (primarily albumin) and inorganic ions such as sulfate and phosphate. Calcium is not biologically active in its bound state.[91] The normal values for total and ionized serum calcium levels are listed in Table 13.15. The normal serum concentration of ionized calcium is maintained within very narrow limits; changes in ionized calcium level are responsible for the clinical effects of hypercalcemia and hypocalcemia. The only accurate way to determine the level of ionized calcium—described as physiologically active, unbound, or free—is to measure the ionized serum value with a laboratory assay.[91] The mathematically calculated values that extrapolate from total calcium and serum albumin levels have been shown to be inaccurate and should not be used with critically ill patients.[92]

Hypercalcemia. Hypercalcemia is defined as increased amounts of ionized calcium (greater than 4.8 mg/dL or 1.30 mmol/L) or increased amounts of total serum calcium (greater than 10.5 mg/dL or 2.60 mmol/L). Serum calcium levels are increased by bone tumors; primary hyperparathyroidism caused by elevated parathyroid hormone levels; excessive intake of supplemental calcium and vitamin D, usually in oral antacids; hypomagnesemia; and as a complication of kidney failure from decreased excretion of calcium. Hypercalcemia affects many organs; causes smooth muscle relaxation; and can lead to neurologic changes such as lethargy, confusion, and even coma. Cardiovascular effects of elevated serum calcium include strengthening contractility and shortening ventricular repolarization, demonstrated on the ECG by a shortened Q–Tc interval. Rhythm disturbances may include bradycardia; first-degree, second-degree, and third-degree heart block; and BBB. Hypercalcemia can potentiate the effects of digitalis and cause hypertension.[93]

Management of symptomatic hypercalcemia involves promotion of calcium excretion by diuretics and infusion of high-volume physiologic saline at 200 to 300 mL/h if tolerated by the heart, lungs, and kidneys. Patients who cannot tolerate this clinical regimen may receive hemodialysis using a low-calcium dialysate.

Hypocalcemia. Hypocalcemia is defined as an ionized calcium level below normal (less than 1.05 mmol/L) or a low total serum calcium level. Hypocalcemia (measured by ionized calcium) is a common finding and was found in 55% of critically ill patients on admission to the critical care unit in one study.[92] The more severe the patient's illness, the greater the risk of developing hypocalcemia.[92] Transfusions of blood from the blood bank lower serum calcium levels because the citrate used as an anticoagulant in banked blood binds to the calcium.[93] This is called *citrate chelation.* If citrate is used during hemodialysis or plasmapheresis, it has the same calcium-binding (chelating) effect. Phosphate also binds to calcium and can lower the serum calcium level. Metabolic alkalosis often coexists with hypocalcemia. The cardiovascular effects of hypocalcemia include decreased myocardial contractility, decreased CO, and hypotension. Rhythm disturbances with severe hypocalcemia are variable, ranging from bradycardia to VT and asystole. When ionized calcium is low, the ECG may show a prolonged Q–Tc interval (Fig. 13.86). A prolonged Q–Tc predisposes a patient to torsades de pointes, a life-threatening ventricular dysrhythmia.

Management of hypocalcemia, especially when ionized calcium is low, involves infusion of IV calcium chloride or IV calcium gluconate.[93]

- Calcium chloride provides 27 mg of elemental calcium/mL (272 mg in 10 mL).

- Calcium gluconate provides 9 mg of elemental calcium/mL (90 mg in 10 mL).

Magnesium

Magnesium (Mg^{2+}) is essential for many enzyme, protein, lipid, and carbohydrate functions in the body and is critical for the production and use of energy.[94] The body stores most magnesium in bone (50% to 60%), muscle, and soft tissues, with less than 1% present in blood.[94] As with other electrolytes, the ionized portion of serum magnesium is the biologically active component that is available for biochemical processes. Only 2% of clinical laboratories in the United States measure ionized magnesium[94]; routine blood tests measure total serum magnesium.[94] Serum magnesium can be reported in units of mEq/L, mg/dL, or mmol/L, depending on the laboratory running the analysis. The normal serum range is 1.5 to 2 mEq/L, 1.8 to 2.4 mg/dL, or 0.7 to 1.1 mmol/L. Normal reference values vary between hospital laboratories.

Hypermagnesemia. Hypermagnesemia is rare in critical care patients. It results from kidney failure, tumor lysis syndrome, or iatrogenic overtreatment.

Hypomagnesemia. Hypomagnesemia is defined as a total serum magnesium concentration less than 1.5 mEq/L. It is commonly associated with other electrolyte imbalances, most notably alterations in potassium, calcium, and phosphorus. Low serum magnesium levels can result from many causes. In the critical care unit, aggressive diuresis with loop diuretics can lower serum levels.[94] Diarrhea can be a significant cause of magnesium loss because lower gastrointestinal fluids contain up to 15 mEq/L of magnesium; vomiting or gastric suction causes less depletion because upper gastrointestinal fluids contain

FIG. 13.84 Effects of Hyperkalemia on ECG. (A) Stages in hyperkalemia from normal potassium levels to plasma levels of 8 mEq/L. At approximately 6 mEq/L, the P wave flattens, the QRS complex broadens, and the ST segment disappears, with the S wave flowing into the tall, tented T wave. (B) A 12-lead ECG of a patient with a serum potassium level of 9.1 mEq/L.

Hypokalemia

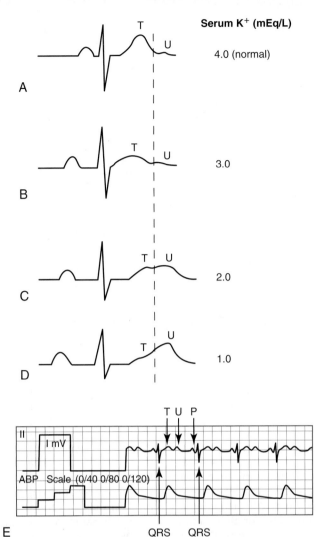

FIG. 13.85 Effects of Hypokalemia on the ECG. (A) At a normal serum concentration of 3.5 to 4.5 mEq/L, the amplitude of the T wave is appreciably greater than that of the U wave. (B) By the time the serum potassium level has decreased to 3 mEq/L, the amplitudes of the T and U waves are approaching each other. (C–D) With a further decrease in the level of potassium, the U wave begins to tower over and fuse with the T wave. (E) ECG tracing from a patient with a serum potassium of 2.6 mEq/L shows a prominent U wave.

approximately 1 mEq/L). Another cause of magnesium depletion is rapid administration of citrated blood products, which results in citrate chelation. The citrate is added to banked blood as an anticoagulant, and it binds to magnesium. Insufficient dietary magnesium intake and chronic alcohol abuse are also risk factors. Hypomagnesemia can also occur in patients who take proton-pump inhibitor medications to reduce production of gastric acid. This condition improves when the proton-pump inhibitors are stopped. In chronic hypomagnesemia, serum levels are replenished from the bone stores.[94]

In hypomagnesemia, the ECG changes are similar to changes seen with hypokalemia and hypocalcemia: prolonged P–R and Q–Tc intervals, presence of U waves, T wave flattening, and widened QRS complex. Cardiac dysrhythmias may be supraventricular or ventricular and include the polymorphic ventricular rhythm torsades de pointes. In cardiac arrest with pulseless VT with torsade de pointes, administer IV magnesium, 1 to 2 g diluted in 10 mL solution (5% dextrose or normal saline), over 15 minutes.[95] It is important to evaluate kidney function when administering magnesium to avoid precipitating hypermagnesium states.

Cardiac Biomarker Studies
Cardiac Biomarkers in Acute Coronary Syndrome
Cardiac biomarkers are proteins that are released from damaged myocardial cells.[96] When myocardial cells are damaged, they release detectable proteins into the bloodstream so that an increase in biomarkers can be correlated with heart muscle injury. The biomarkers that are routinely measured include cardiac troponin I and cardiac troponin T. Table 13.16 summarizes the cardiac biomarkers related to myocardial injury and MI. In many hospitals, the laboratory turnaround time for results of quantitative cardiac biomarkers is approximately 60 minutes. If point-of-care testing at the bedside is used, the results are rapidly available.[96]

Troponin T and troponin I. The troponins are biomarkers for myocardial damage. The elevation of troponin I and troponin T occurs 3 to 6 hours after acute myocardial damage.[96] Troponin levels are measured at symptom onset in the hospital or when the patient comes to the emergency department. Serial troponin values are measured 3 hours and 6 hours later.[96]

Because troponin I is found only in cardiac muscle, it is a highly specific biomarker for myocardial damage. A newer development is the advent of high-sensitivity troponin I monitoring. The advantage to using a more sensitive biomarker test is that more patients with ACS will be identified, although this will not eliminate the requirement for astute clinical assessment

---

QSEN BOX 13.12   **QSEN: Patient Safety Alert**

Medication Administration

1. Accurate Patient Identification
   - Use at least two patient identifiers (not the patient's room number) when taking blood samples or administering medications or blood products. Examples include the patient's name or date of birth.
2. Effective Communication Among Caregivers
   - An organizational method to decrease the number of medication errors is the use of *computerized physician order entry.*
   - Hospitals should have a process for taking verbal or telephone orders that requires a verification "read back" of the complete order by the person receiving the order.

- The Institute of Safe Medication Practices (ISMP) maintains a list of medications with similar-sounding names, as name confusion can lead to medication errors. The list is available on the ISMP website at https://www.ismp.org/tools/confuseddrugnames.pdf. Medication errors can be reported to the Medication Errors Reporting Program.
- Standardize the abbreviations, acronyms, and symbols used throughout the organization, including a list of abbreviations, acronyms, and symbols not to use.
- Examples of problematic abbreviations include "U" for units and "μg" for micrograms. When handwritten, a capital U can be mistaken for a zero (0);

Continued

QSEN BOX 13.12   QSEN: Patient Safety Alert—cont'd

Medication Administration

in numerous case reports, an insulin dosage written in U was interpreted as 0. Using the abbreviation "µg" instead of "mcg" for micrograms is also problematic; when handwritten, the Greek letter µ can look like an "m." The error-prone abbreviations list is available on the ISMP website at https://www.ismp.org/tools/errorproneabbreviations.pdf

- Use of trailing zeros (eg, 2.0 versus 2) and use of a leading decimal point without a leading zero (eg, .2 instead of 0.2) are dangerous prescription-writing practices. Misinterpretation has caused 10-fold dosing errors.

3. High-Alert Medication Safety
- Remove concentrated electrolytes (including, but not limited to, potassium chloride [KCl], potassium phosphate, and hypertonic sodium chloride) from patient care units.
- Standardize and limit the number of medication concentrations available in the organization.
- In the first 2 years after enacting a *sentinel event reporting mechanism*, the most common category was medication errors, and the most frequently implicated medication was KCl. The Joint Commission reviewed 10 incidents of patient death resulting from misadministration of KCl. Eight deaths were the result of direct infusion of concentrated KCl. In six of the eight cases, KCl was mistaken for another medication, primarily because of similarities in packaging and labeling. Most often, KCl was mistaken for sodium chloride, heparin, or furosemide (Lasix).
- The Joint Commission suggests that health care organizations *not* make concentrated KCl available outside the pharmacy unless appropriate, specific safeguards are in place.

- A list of high-alert medications is available on the ISMP website at http://www.ismp.org.

4. Infusion Pump Safety
- Ensure free-flow protection on all general-use and patient-controlled analgesia intravenous (IV) infusion pumps used in the organization.
- Infusion pumps that do not provide protection from the free flow of IV fluid or medication into the patient are hazardous.
- *Free flow* occurs when IV solution flows freely under the force of gravity without being controlled by the infusion pump. Free flow typically occurs after the administration set is temporarily removed from the pump to transfer a patient to another area, change a patient's gown, or place a patient on a radiography table. Clinicians can greatly reduce this risk by using administration sets with set-based anti–free-flow mechanisms that prevent gravity free flow by closing off the IV tubing to prohibit flow when the administration set is removed from the pump.

5. Hospital Safety
- The Joint Commission develops Hospital National Patient Safety Goals each year that incorporate medication safety requirements. This information is available on The Joint Commission website at http://www.joint-commission.org/standards_information/npsgs.aspx.

More information can be accessed on the following websites of safety organizations:

http://www.ismp.org
http://www.jointcommission.org
http://www.usp.org

TABLE 13.15   Chemistry Values That Affect Cardiac Contractility and Conduction

Electrolyte	NORMAL RANGES[a]		
	mEq/L	mg/dL	mmol/L
Potassium (K⁺)	3.5–4.5		3.50–4.50
Ionized calcium (Ca)		4.0–5.0	1.00–1.30
Total calcium (Ca²⁺)		8.5–10.5	2.00–2.60
Magnesium (Mg²⁺)	1.5–2.0	1.8–2.4	0.70–1.10

[a]Laboratory values may be reported as mEq/L, mg/dL, or mmol/L. Each measurement parameter used produces a different value. Some electrolytes are reported with more than one reference value. Different clinical laboratories use different reference values, and the cited reference values may vary slightly between hospital laboratories.

because of the many other conditions associated with elevated troponin levels.[66] A negative high-sensitivity troponin result eliminates acute MI as a diagnosis in 99% of cases.[66]

Natriuretic Peptide Biomarkers in Heart Failure

Natriuretic peptides are biomarkers that provide additional information for accurate evaluation of a patient with acute shortness of breath.[97] It can be difficult to identify whether a breathless patient has a primary pulmonary problem or has symptoms of acute heart failure with pulmonary edema. Cardiac natriuretic peptides are used to help make the correct diagnosis. In decompensated heart failure, ventricular distention from volume overload or pressure overload causes

myocytes in the ventricle to release B-type natriuretic peptide (BNP). Several laboratory assays are commercially available to measure BNP including a point-of-care test, a central laboratory test for BNP, and a different laboratory test to measure the N-terminal fragment of pro-BNP (NTpro-BNP).[97] BNP has a half-life of approximately 20 minutes, whereas NTpro-BNP has a longer half-life of 1 to 2 hours. Some clinical laboratories stratify NTpro-BNP by age. The choice of test generally depends on what is available in the hospital clinical laboratory.

With greater ventricular wall stress, more natriuretic peptide is released from the myocardium, reflected as an elevated BNP level. The BNP value is combined with the physical examination, 12-lead ECG, and chest radiograph to increase the accuracy of heart failure diagnosis (Fig. 13.87). A symptomatic patient with a BNP level less than 100 pg/mL or NTpro-BNP less than 300 pg/mL is unlikely to be in heart failure. Conversely, a patient with a BNP level greater than 400 pg/dL is almost definitely in heart failure. BNP is an excellent test to rule out acute heart failure. The challenge lies in interpreting the results of patients with a BNP level of 100 to 400 pg/mL, sometimes described as the *gray zone*. This gray zone highlights the importance of using a spectrum of clinical and diagnostic tests. As the symptoms of heart failure are successfully treated, the BNP level usually decreases toward the normal range.

There are some caveats to the use of natriuretic peptides as biomarkers principally because they are not unique to the heart. Natriuretic peptides are also released from the endothelium and from the kidney, and this can alter the measured BNP levels.

0 Sec. 3 Sec. 6 Sec.

FIG. 13.86 Abnormal Q–T Prolongation in a Hypocalcemic Patient. A 50-year-old woman was admitted to the critical care unit with a diagnosis of alcoholic liver disease and malnourishment. Total calcium concentration is 5.1 mg/dL, and the albumin level is 1.3 mg/dL. The Q–T interval (0.55 s) is markedly prolonged for the heart rate (HR) (100 beats/min). The Q–T interval varies with the HR and can be corrected (Q–T$_c$) as if the HR were 60 beats/min using the formula $\sqrt{QT/RR} = Q - T_c$. The Q–T$_c$ should be 0.44 s or less. The Q–T$_c$ in the ECG tracing shown is 0.55 s. Hypocalcemia lengthens ventricular repolarization. A quick method for assessing the Q–T interval is to remember that it is usually less than half of the R–R interval. If it is more than one half of the R–R interval, it is prolonged. (From Yucha CB, Toto KH. Calcium and phosphorus derangements. *Crit Care Nurs Clin North Am.* 1994;6[4]:747.)

TABLE 13.16 Serum Biomarkers After Acute Myocardial Infarction

Serum Biomarker	Time to Initial Elevation (h[a])	Peak Elevation[b] (h[a])	Return to Baseline (days[a])
Cardiac troponin I	3–12	24	5–10
Cardiac troponin T	3–12	12–48	5–14
CK-MB[c]	3–12	24	2–3

[a]Time periods represent average reported values.
[b]Does not include patients who have had reperfusion therapy.
[c]The creatine kinase (CK) enzyme consists of two subunits, the brain type (B) and the muscle type (M).

Filtration by the kidney is one of the mechanisms by which BNP is cleared from the bloodstream. BNP levels are higher in patients with kidney failure, especially if the glomerular filtration rate is less than 60 mL/min/1.7 m^2.

Hematologic Studies

Hematologic laboratory studies that are routinely ordered for the management of patients with altered cardiovascular status are RBC or erythrocyte level, hemoglobin level, hematocrit level, and white blood cell (WBC) or leukocyte level.

Red Blood Cells

The normal amount of RBCs in a person varies with age, sex, environmental temperature, altitude, and exercise. Men produce 4.5 to 6 million RBCs/mm^3, whereas the normal level for women is 4 to 5.5 million RBCs/mm^3. *Anemia* is the clinical condition that occurs when insufficient RBCs are available to carry oxygen to the tissues. *Polycythemia* is the condition that occurs when excess RBCs are produced.

Hemoglobin

Hemoglobin levels normally range from 14 to 18 g/dL in men and from 12 to 16 g/dL in women.

Hematocrit

The hematocrit is the volume percentage of RBCs in whole blood. The value is 40% to 54% for men and 38% to 48% for women.

FIG. 13.87 Brain Natriuretic Peptide (BNP) Algorithm in the Diagnosis of Heart Failure (HF).

White Blood Cells

Most inflammatory processes that produce necrotic tissue within the heart muscle, such as rheumatic fever, endocarditis, and MI, increase the WBC level. WBCs are also known as leukocytes, and a WBC test may be called a serum leukocyte count. The normal WBC level for men and women is 5000 to 10,000 cells/mm^3. The WBC level also increases in response to infection.

Platelets

The normal platelet count is 150,000 to 400,000 cells/mm^3. Less commonly, the normal platelet count range is written as 150 to 400 × 10^9/L. Normally, the platelet count is the only laboratory value that is reported. There is no routine test available for critical care patients that can evaluate platelet functionality. Platelets are important because they are the first cells to be activated when the coagulation system is stimulated. Many medications inhibit platelet function and make the platelets "slippery" so that they do not clump together to activate the clotting process. The antiplatelet action of a medication sometimes is its intended role, such as with aspirin used to prevent ACS, and it can be an unintended side effect. A low platelet count is called *thrombocytopenia*.

Blood Coagulation Studies

Coagulation studies are ordered to determine blood-clotting effectiveness. Anticoagulants—most notably heparin, direct thrombin inhibitors, warfarin, and platelet inhibitory agents—are administered daily in critical care units for many clinical reasons. It is essential to understand the laboratory tests that are used to monitor the effectiveness of therapeutic anticoagulation.

Prothrombin time. Most coagulation study results are reported as the length of time in seconds it takes for blood to form a clot in the laboratory test tube. The *prothrombin time* is not directly used to determine the therapeutic dosage of warfarin (Coumadin) necessary to achieve anticoagulation. Because the prothrombin time is not standardized between laboratories, the result of this test is reported as a standardized *international normalized ratio* (INR).[98]

International normalized ratio. The INR was developed by the World Health Organization (WHO) in 1982 to standardize PT results among clinical laboratories worldwide. Table 13.17 shows target INR ranges for different cardiovascular conditions that require anticoagulation. A target INR of 2.5 (range, 2.0 to 3.0) is desirable.[99,100]

When a patient is first started on warfarin, it can take 72 hours or more to achieve a therapeutic level of anticoagulation. This is because the half-life of prothrombin is 36 to 42 hours. This delay in anticoagulation effectiveness also occurs if a patient is being converted from heparin-based anticoagulation—monitored by activated partial thromboplastin time—to warfarin-based anticoagulation (monitored by INR). To ensure a safe transition, a period of 48 to 72 hours is required to obtain a therapeutic INR value before the heparin is discontinued.

Activated partial thromboplastin time. The activated partial thromboplastin time is used to measure the effectiveness of IV or subcutaneous ultrafractionated heparin therapy.[98] Coagulation monitoring is required with ultrafractionated heparin, although not with subcutaneous low-molecular-weight heparin because of lower levels of plasma protein binding. In cases of overanticoagulation with heparin, the antidote is protamine sulfate.

Activated clotting time. The *activated clotting time* (ACT) is a *point-of-care test* that is performed outside of the laboratory setting in areas such as the cardiac catheterization laboratory, operating room, or critical care unit. Normal and therapeutic values for ACT coagulation studies are shown in Table 13.17.

Serum Lipid Studies

Four primary blood lipid levels are important in evaluating an individual's risk of developing or having progression of CAD: total cholesterol, low-density lipoprotein cholesterol (LDL-C), triglycerides, and high-density lipoprotein cholesterol (HDL-C). When levels of cholesterol low-density lipoproteins (LDLs) and triglycerides are elevated or the level of high-density lipoproteins (HDLs) is low, the patient is considered at risk for developing or having progression of CAD and is offered intensive interventions involving diet therapy, exercise prescription, and medication therapy.[101-104] The following lipid biomarkers are frequently ordered together as a "lipid panel."

Total Cholesterol

Cholesterol is a fat-like substance (lipid) that is present in cell membranes, is produced by the liver, and is a precursor of bile

TABLE 13.17 Normal and Therapeutic Coagulation Values

Test	Clinical Condition	Normal Value	Therapeutic Anticoagulant Target Value
INR	Normal coagulation	<1.0	
INR	Atrial fibrillation		2.0–3.0
INR	Treatment of DVT/PE		2.0–3.0
INR	Mechanical heart valves		2.0–3.0
aPTT	Normal coagulation	28–38 s	1.5–2.5 × normal
PTT	Normal coagulation	60–90 s	1.5–2.0 × normal
ACT[a]	Normal coagulation	0–120 s	150–300 s

[a]ACT is normal, but therapeutic values may vary with type of activator used.

ACT, activated coagulation time; *aPPT,* activated partial thromboplastin time; *DVT,* deep vein thrombosis; *INR,* international normalized ratio; *PE,* pulmonary embolism; *PTT,* partial thromboplastin time.

acids and steroid hormones. The cholesterol level in the blood is determined partly by genetics and partly by acquired factors such as diet, calorie balance, and level of physical activity. Cholesterol in excess amounts (greater than 200 mg/dL) in the serum forces the progression of atherosclerosis (atherogenesis). Table 13.18 lists the desirable lipid levels to lower the risk of CAD and to reduce morbidity and mortality in patients with established CAD.

Low-Density Lipoproteins

Approximately 60% to 70% of the total serum cholesterol is carried in the bloodstream, complexed as LDL-C. The LDL-C and total serum cholesterol levels are directly correlated with risk for CAD, and high levels of each are significant predictors of future acute MI in individuals with established coronary artery atherosclerosis. LDL-C is the major atherogenic lipoprotein and is the primary target for cholesterol-lowering efforts.[103] Guidelines recommend maintaining an LDL-C level below 130 mg/dL for a patient with no history of atherosclerotic disease. A patient with known CAD but who is not high risk should aim for an LDL-C level below 100 mg/dL. The recommended target LDL-C level for high-risk patients with CAD or diabetes is 70 mg/dL.[102,104]

Very-Low-Density Lipoproteins and Triglycerides

Very-low-density lipoproteins contain 10% to 15% of the total serum cholesterol along with most of the triglycerides in fasting serum.

High-Density Lipoproteins

HDLs are particles that carry 20% to 30% of the total serum cholesterol. A low HDL-C level (less than 35 mg/dL) is another independent significant risk factor for CAD. Several studies also support the finding that HDL-C helps protect against atherogenesis, and a level greater than 50 mg/dL may act as a shield against the risk of CAD. Low HDL-C levels are often associated with elevated triglyceride levels.[102,104]

Triglycerides

Triglycerides are another form of lipid in the bloodstream that is normally included in the lipid assessment panel. The normal fasting level is less than 100 mg/dL.[102] Elevated triglyceride levels are associated with diabetes mellitus and an increased risk of atherosclerotic disease.

TABLE 13.18 Desirable Lipid Levels

Lipid	Desirable Level
Total cholesterol	<200 mg/dL
	<130 mg/dL without CAD
LDL-C	<100 mg/dL with CAD but not considered high risk
	<70 mg/dL with CAD and considered at high risk for future coronary events
Triglycerides	<100 mg/dL
HDL-C	>40 mg/dL (male)
	>50 mg/dL (female)

CAD, coronary artery disease; *HDL-C*, high-density lipoprotein cholesterol; *LDL-C*, low-density lipoprotein cholesterol.
Data from the Executive Summary of the Third Report of the National Cholesterol Education Program (NCEP) Expert Panel on Detection, Evaluation, and Treatment of High Blood Cholesterol in Adults (Adult Treatment Panel III). *JAMA*. 2001;285(19):2486; and Grundy SM, et al. Implications of recent clinical trials for the National Cholesterol Education Program (NCEP) Adult Treatment Panel III (ATP III) Guidelines. *Circulation*. 2004;110:227.

DIAGNOSTIC PROCEDURES

Cardiac Catheterization and Coronary Arteriography

Cardiac catheterization and coronary arteriography are routine diagnostic procedures for patients with known or suspected heart disease. Clinical indications for cardiac catheterization include ACS, heart failure with a history suggestive of coronary artery or valvular heart disease, and congenital heart disease. Cardiac catheterization is used to confirm physical findings and to provide a baseline for medical or surgical therapy.[105,106]

Left-Heart Cardiac Catheterization

During catheterization of the left side of the heart, hemodynamic pressure measurements are taken in the aortic root, the left ventricle, and the left atrium.[107] Radiopaque contrast dye is used to visualize the left ventricle (ventriculogram). This information is also used to calculate the LV EF. The coronary arteries are visualized, and contrast dye is injected directly into each arterial system. The general term for vessel imaging is *angiogram* (veins and arteries), but the more specific term used to describe visualization of the coronary arteries is *arteriogram*.

Right-Heart Cardiac Catheterization

Catheterization of the right side of the heart is performed using a thermodilution PA catheter. Information obtained includes hemodynamic pressure measurements in the right atrium, the right ventricle, the PA, and the PA occlusion wedge position as well as the measurement of CO, calculated hemodynamic values, and oxygen saturations and an angiogram of the right-heart chambers using radiopaque contrast dye.

Procedure

Before catheterization, the patient meets with the cardiologist to discuss the purpose, benefit, and risks of the study. For many patients, cardiac catheterization is the first major invasive procedure after a diagnosis of possible heart disease. The patient is often very anxious and has many questions. It is important that nursing and medical staff fully answer patients' questions about the catheterization experience.

The morning of the procedure the patient fasts except for ingesting prescribed cardiac medications. Light premedication is given before the patient goes to the catheterization laboratory. If there is a history of allergy, an antihistamine or corticosteroid may be administered to prevent an anaphylactic reaction to the radiopaque contrast dye. Throughout the cardiac catheterization, the patient remains awake and alert. He or she is positioned on a hard table with a C-shaped camera arm overhead or to the side. This arm can be positioned to view the heart from several different angles.

Prevention of contrast-induced nephropathy. In patients with an elevated serum creatinine, sodium bicarbonate or NS is administered to protect the kidneys from the damaging effects of the contrast medium.[108] *N*-acetylcysteine has not been shown to be effective. Up to 10% of acute kidney injuries in the hospital occur as a result of procedures that use IV contrast dye.

Cardiac catheterization catheters, which are available in a variety of designs and sizes, are placed in the femoral vein and artery after the patient receives a local anesthetic. The choice of catheters is based on the cardiologist's experience and the diagnostic study required. The femoral artery is used to catheterize the left side of the heart, including the coronary arteries. The femoral vein is frequently used as the access vessel to pass catheters to the right side of the heart. During the study, the patient receives heparin systemically to reduce the risk of emboli. Many patients also receive nitroglycerin to control chest pain, particularly when the coronary arteries are full of contrast material during the coronary arteriographic procedure. The patient may also experience bradycardia or hypotension at this time. To move the contrast dye more quickly and minimize the vagal effect on HR and blood pressure, the patient may be asked to cough. If bradycardia persists, atropine or occasionally a transvenous pacemaker may be used. If hypotension continues, IV fluids are administered as a bolus. At the end of the study, the femoral catheters are removed from the vessels. After catheterization, when the patient is stable, the cardiologist meets with the patient and family to discuss the findings and plan of care.

Nursing Management

Femoral artery site care. After the diagnostic catheters (and the sheaths through which they are inserted) are removed from the femoral artery and vein, pressure is applied to the femoral vessels until bleeding has stopped. After catheterization, the patient remains flat for up to 6 hours (varies by institutional protocol and catheter size) to allow the femoral arterial puncture site to form a stable clot. Most bleeding occurs within the first 2 to 3 hours after the procedure. During this time, the groin site is checked frequently for evidence of bleeding or hematoma. Three methods may be used to control bleeding at the femoral arterial puncture site after catheter or sheath removal. The most basic method is manual pressure, in which a clinician holds pressure directly on the vein or artery until bleeding stops. The second method uses external mechanical compression over the site (C-clamp or FemoStop [St. Jude Medical, Sweden]). The third method is for the cardiologist to use an *arteriotomy closure device* at the end of the catheterization procedure. One closure device is designed to suture the artery closed as the sheath is removed; another option is placement of a collagen plug into the track of the sheath insertion site. All these methods are effective. After routine diagnostic cardiac catheterization procedures, there is no difference in the rate of femoral arterial site complications for the different methods. The patient is asked to lie still and not to bend at the hip. It usually takes approximately 40 minutes for a stable clot to form, but it can take longer in some patients, including patients with a large body surface area.

Peripheral pulses. The peripheral pulses located distal to the arterial access site are monitored closely by the critical care nurse. If the femoral artery has been used, dorsal pedal and posterior tibial pulses are assessed. If an alternative access site such as the radial artery is used, the radial pulse is assessed. Pulses are assessed every 15 minutes for the first hour after the catheterization and every 30 minutes to 1 hour thereafter. The limb corresponding to the catheterization site is assessed for changes in color, temperature, pain, or paresthesia to detect early evidence of acute arterial occlusion.

Rehydration. The patient is encouraged to drink large amounts of clear liquids, and the IV fluid rate is increased to 100 mL/h. Fluid is given for rehydration because the radiopaque contrast material acts as an osmotic diuretic. Rehydration is also used to prevent *contrast-induced nephropathy* or damage to the kidney from the contrast dye used to visualize the heart structures. Patients who have elevated blood urea nitrogen or creatinine levels before catheterization are at risk for acute kidney failure from the dye. For these patients, the quantity of contrast material is consciously limited, and fluid boluses are given to preserve kidney function.

Angina. The patient is assessed for chest pain after the procedure. Sublingual nitroglycerin usually is sufficient to relieve the pain, discomfort, or pressure. Not all patients describe their angina as "pain," and many other descriptors such as "pressure" may be used. Patients are encouraged to use the 0-to-10 pain scale to quantify the angina. A 12-lead ECG must be obtained immediately to identify the coronary arteries involved, and the cardiologist is notified. If the chest pain persists, this may indicate that a clot has formed in a coronary artery, and the patient may need to return to the cardiac catheterization laboratory for an interventional cardiology procedure. Chapter 15 provides more information about PCI in the section on catheter interventions for coronary artery disease (see Fig. 15.11, Fig. 15.12, Fig. 15.13).

Dysrhythmias. Dysrhythmias are always a concern after an invasive cardiovascular diagnostic procedure. They result from the underlying cardiac disease and the low potassium levels that can occur after excessive diuresis.

Patient Education

Because of the invasive nature of cardiac catheterization, many patients express considerable anxiety. Relevant information concerns the sensory details of the procedure, such as lying flat and immobile on a hard table for many hours and sometimes experiencing a feeling of warmth when the dye is injected. Pain is uncommon because opiate analgesics and sedative medications are always provided. Information about possible outcomes—positive and negative—and possible complications must be provided to the patient. Postcatheterization requirements such as lying still and drinking large quantities of fluids are explained. The basic information can be provided using written and audiovisual material, but it is vital to individualize the content and answer any specific concerns or questions. Patients are also asked to report any other unusual symptoms, such as chest pain or nausea.

Electrophysiology Study
Indications

An electrophysiology study (EPS) is an invasive diagnostic tool used to record intracardiac electrical activity. A person may have an EPS performed because of a history of a syncopal episode (loss of consciousness); rapid wide complex tachycardia; or other cardiac electrical problems not diagnosed by noninvasive diagnostic studies such as the 12-lead ECG, treadmill stress test, signal-averaged ECG, or Holter monitoring. An EPS is performed in a specially equipped cardiac catheterization laboratory.

Before the EPS, written and verbal education is provided to the patient and family to increase their sense of security and to decrease stress and anxiety. All antidysrhythmic medications are discontinued several days before the study so that any ventricular dysrhythmias may be readily induced during the EPS. Anticoagulants, especially warfarin, are also stopped before EPS. Premedication is administered before the study to induce a relaxed state, and the patient is conscious during the procedure and receives sedative agents (eg, midazolam or propofol) at regular intervals. The patient fasts 6 hours before the EPS and during the procedure lies supine on a hard table with a C-shaped or U-shaped camera arm to the side or directly overhead to verify the position of the EPS catheters in the heart.

Electrophysiology equipment for stimulation of dysrhythmias and monitoring is usually positioned nearby. A peripheral IV access line and surface ECG leads are placed, and electrophysiology catheters are inserted into the femoral vein and advanced to the right side of the heart under fluoroscopy. These catheters, similar to pacing catheters, are placed at specific anatomic sites within the heart to record the earliest electrical activity. The catheter placements are demonstrated in Fig. 13.88, with catheter tip positions shown at the following locations:
1. High right atrium near the sinoatrial node
2. AV node
3. Coronary sinus behind the left atrial/ventricular border
4. Bundle of His near the tricuspid valve
5. Right ventricle near the apex

During EPS, *programmed electrical stimulation* is used to trigger the dysrhythmia. This technique delivers pulses of two to four early paced beats via a specific catheter to the selected area of myocardium. During the EPS, the electrophysiologist looks for a site of early electrical activation that stimulates the myocardium before the sinoatrial node. The goal of an EPS is to discover the origin of dysrhythmias that cannot be evaluated from the surface ECG alone.

Atrial measurements. Typical measurements during EPS include sinus node recovery time and sinoatrial conduction time plus atrial pacing to measure the atrial and AV node refractory periods. Coronary sinus pacing is used to induce left atrial tachydysrhythmias. Atrial pacing usually is performed after the ventricular study to reduce the risk of putting the patient into atrial fibrillation or flutter because of retrograde conduction up the bundle of His and AV node.

Ventricular measurements. Programmed electrical stimulation is used to induce the ventricular dysrhythmia, especially in patients who have experienced sustained or nonsustained VT or survived a sudden cardiac death episode. To measure the retrograde V-to-A interval and stimulate the myocardium, the right ventricular catheter is selected to rapidly pace the right ventricle; the catheter then is moved to the right ventricular outflow tract (near the pulmonary valve), and the pacing stimulation is repeated. This protocol produces VT in most patients with a known history of VT or VF.

After the dysrhythmia is induced and diagnosed, it can be converted to normal sinus rhythm by 10 to 15 paced beats delivered at a rate faster than the VT or by cardioversion and defibrillation plus IV antidysrhythmic medications. At the end of the study, all the electrophysiology catheters are removed before the patient returns to the nursing unit.

Implantable cardioverter defibrillators. When a follow-up EPS is required for a patient with an ICD, the device can substitute for the electrophysiology catheters. The ICD has sensing leads, pace termination, backup bradycardia pacing, and cardioversion and defibrillation capabilities. The EPS can be performed by the external ICD programmer in the EPS laboratory. The ICD generator and leads perform programmed electrical stimulation in a manner similar to a full EPS. Chapter 15 provides more information on the therapeutic uses of ICDs.

Chest Radiography
Basic Principles and Technique

Chest radiography is the oldest noninvasive method for visualizing images of the heart, and it remains a frequently used and valuable diagnostic tool. Information about cardiac anatomy and physiology can be obtained with ease and safety at a relatively low cost. In the critical care unit, the nurse may be the first person to view the chest radiograph of an acutely ill patient. Critical care nurses also have an important role in ensuring the quality of the film through proper positioning and instruction of the patient. For these reasons, it is crucial to understand the basics of chest radiography techniques and interpretation as they apply to the cardiovascular and pulmonary systems.

Tissue densities. As x-rays travel through the chest from the emitting tube to the film plate, they are absorbed to various degrees by the tissues through which they pass (Table 13.19).

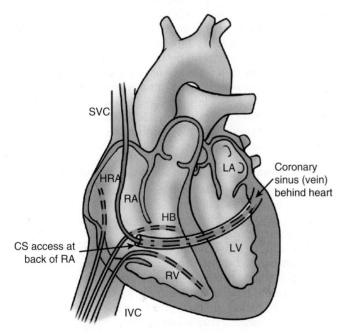

Placement of catheters in the heart in an electrophysiology study.

FIG. 13.88 Catheter Placement Within the Heart During an Electrophysiology Study. LA, left atrium; LV, left ventricle; RA, right atrium.

Very dense tissue, such as bone, absorbs almost all the x-rays, leaving the film unexposed, or white. The heart, aorta, and pulmonary vessels and the blood they contain are moderately dense structures, appearing as gray areas on the radiographic film. These vascular structures are surrounded by air-filled lung that allows the greatest penetration of x-rays, resulting in fully exposed (black) areas on the film. Thoracic structures can be studied best by examining their borders. Two structures with the same density, when located next to each other, have no visible border. If a structure is located next to a contrasting density (eg, vascular structures next to an air-filled lung), even subtle changes in size and shape can be seen.

Standard views. In most institutions, a standard radiographic examination of the heart and lungs consists of posteroanterior and left lateral films. The standard film is taken in the radiology department with the patient in an upright position; the film exposed during a deep, sustained inhalation; and the x-ray tube aimed horizontally 6 feet from the film. This is referred to as a *posteroanterior film* because the beam traverses the patient from posterior to anterior.

Portable chest radiography. Because most patients in critical care units are too ill to go to the radiology department, chest radiographs are routinely obtained by using portable radiographic machines with the patient sitting upright or lying supine, depending on the patient's clinical condition and the judgment of the nurse. The film plate is placed behind the patient's back, and an anteroposterior projection is used, in which the x-ray beam enters from the front of the chest. For the supine film, with the patient lying flat on the bed, the x-ray tube can be only approximately 36 inches from the patient's chest because of ceiling height and radiographic equipment construction. This results in a lower quality film from a diagnostic standpoint because the images of the heart and great vessels are magnified and not as sharply defined. Whenever possible, the upright (anteroposterior) film is preferred to the supine (flat) one, as it provides a more accurate image, it shows more of the lung because the diaphragm is lower, and the thoracic structures appear sharper and less magnified.

Nursing interventions to produce optimal chest radiograph. The critical care nurse can have a big impact on the quality of the radiographic film. Several key elements must be considered, as follows:

• The radiograph is taken when the patient has taken a deep breath (inspiration). During exhalation, the lungs are less full of air, which can make the lung tissue appear cloudy as if there is additional lung water. The heart also appears larger during exhalation. This could lead to an erroneous diagnosis of heart failure. Alert patients are encouraged to take in a deep breath and hold it while the exposure is obtained. For patients receiving mechanical ventilatory

TABLE 13.19	**Intrathoracic Structure Radiographic Densities**	
Metal or Bone (White)	**Fluid (Gray)**	**Air (Black)**
Ribs, clavicle, sternum, spine	Blood	Lung
Calcium deposits	Heart	
Surgical wires or clips	Veins	
Prosthetic valves	Arteries	
Pacemaker wires	Edema	

support, the exposure must be timed to coincide with maximal inhalation.

- It is important to remove extrinsic tubing and other movable objects from the patient's thorax to permit optimal visualization of the chest. Hands or arms should not be across the chest while the radiograph is obtained.
- The patient should sit upright in bed if the clinical condition permits this position. Upright radiograph views have a sharper focus because the distance from the patient to the x-ray tube is closer to the standard 72 inches (6 feet).
- The nurse should ensure that the patient is straight in the bed rather than turned or twisted; this permits clearer visualization of the major thoracic structures.

Indications

There is considerable debate over the optimal frequency of the routine chest radiograph in the critical care unit. The American College of Radiology expert panel made the following recommendations for portable radiographic machines used in the critical care unit:

1. Daily chest radiographs are recommended for patients with acute cardiopulmonary problems and patients receiving mechanical ventilation.
2. Patients who require cardiac monitoring but are otherwise stable need an admission radiograph only.
3. A chest radiograph is obtained when a new thoracic device is placed or there is a specific question about the patient's cardiopulmonary status that the radiograph could address.

Chest Radiograph Analysis: Lines and Tubes

Evaluation of a chest film is a systematic process. All thoracic invasive tubes and lines must be located and identified. Major thoracic structures including the lungs, pleural space, mediastinum, diaphragm, and vascular structures are assessed and compared with previous films, if available. Variations from previous films can alert the clinician to possible complications and provide information about the patient's hemodynamic status.

Central venous catheter. CVCs are seen on the chest film as moderately radiopaque tubes extending centrally from an SC, IJ, or femoral vein insertion site. The ideal location of the catheter tip is within the superior vena cava above the right atrium. CVC misplacement during insertion may result in inadvertent arterial cannulation and extravascular placement with pneumothorax or hemothroax.[109]

Pulmonary artery catheter. A chest radiograph is required after insertion of a PA catheter, also known as a Swan-Ganz catheter. The primary clinical reason for the chest radiograph is to determine the position of the tip of the PA catheter. To wedge correctly, the catheter tip (balloon deflated) must rest in the right or left pulmonary artery and not extend beyond the hilum of the lung.[109]

Endotracheal tube. A chest radiograph is always requested after endotracheal intubation because physical examination is not sufficiently sensitive to determine endotracheal tube position. The tip of the endotracheal tube should be 2 to 4 cm above the *carina*—the anatomic location where the trachea divides into the right main bronchus and left main bronchus. Inadvertent intubation of the right bronchus is the most common malposition.[109]

Enteric tube. Because the consequences of delivering enteral nutrition into a nongastric space are so severe, a chest radiograph is required after placement and before beginning tube feeds.

Chest tube. Chest tubes contain a radiopaque line that makes them clearly visible on the chest radiograph. Chest tubes are located within the pleural or mediastinal space. Pulmonary chest tubes are placed to treat pneumothorax or hemothorax. Most pneumothoraces in the critical care unit are iatrogenic (eg, ventilator barotrauma) or traumatic (eg, complication of CVC placement), or they occur after cardiothoracic surgery. Approximately 10% of chest tubes are malpositioned.[109]

Intraaortic balloon catheter. An intraaortic balloon pump (IABP) provides mechanical support for the failing heart. The catheter that is evaluated on the chest radiograph is a 26- to 28-mm inflatable balloon that surrounds a catheter inserted into the descending aorta, usually percutaneously through the femoral artery. A chest radiograph must be obtained immediately after insertion to evaluate the position of the IABP catheter. The distal tip of the IABP catheter contains a small radiopaque marker that is helpful in determining its position on the chest film. The tip of the IABP catheter must lie below the origin of the left subclavian artery in the descending thoracic aorta (just below the aortic arch). Even when inserted properly, there is a risk of aortic dissection. Aortic dissection is a life-threatening complication. It can be seen on the chest radiograph as a loss of sharpness of the borders of the descending thoracic aorta.

Pacemaker or implantable defibrillator. A *pacemaker* and ICD are cardiovascular devices that can be visualized on a chest film. There is considerable variety in the range of pacing electrodes that are encountered in critical care patients. If the pacemaker is permanently implanted, the entire system is seen on the chest film. If it is only a temporary pacemaker, the pulse generator is external to the body and is not seen on the chest radiograph. The pacing electrodes are radiopaque and look like white wires extending transvenously into the right side of the heart. Pacing wires sutured on the epicardium during cardiac surgery are visible on the right atrium or right ventricle, or both. Patients with a history of heart failure may have an additional pacing wire inserted into the coronary sinus (vein) to pace the left ventricle in addition to a right ventricular wire (biventricular pacing). Table 13.20 summarizes the most common cardiovascular devices and their correct position as seen on the chest radiograph.

Chest Radiograph Analysis: Cardiac and Pulmonary Factors

A wealth of physiologic data can be gleaned from a chest radiograph. To be valid, this information must be interpreted in the context of a thorough physical examination and clinical knowledge of the patient's condition.

Heart size. Comparison of the cardiothoracic ratio (Fig. 13.89) can be used to assess heart size. The normal heart size is less than one-half of the diameter of the chest viewed on the radiograph. Patients with chronic heart failure often have cardiomegaly (enlarged heart), which can dramatically occupy much of the thoracic diameter on the film.

Pulmonary edema. Pulmonary edema is a common finding in critically ill patients. "Wet lungs" appear on the chest radiograph as white, dense, cloudy areas and may accentuate pulmonary vascular markings. Pulmonary edema shows up

TABLE 13.20 Cardiovascular Devices

Device	Function	Position
Pulmonary artery catheter	Measures pulmonary artery occlusion pressure and right-heart pressures	Tip in right or left pulmonary artery
Central venous catheter	Central venous pressure measurement, venous access	Superior vena cava
Left atrium catheter	Left atrial pressure	Left atrium
Mediastinal chest tubes	Mediastinal fluid evacuation	Anterior mediastinum, posterior pericardium
Pacemaker leads	Cardiac pacing	Over right heart
Intraaortic balloon catheter	Assists left ventricular function	Tip just below top of aortic arch

FIG. 13.89 Determining the cardiothoracic ratio is a technique for estimating heart size on a posteroanterior chest radiograph. Normally, the cardiac diameter is 50% or less of the thoracic diameter when measured during full inhalation. The width of the vascular pedicle (arrows) is a more accurate indicator of systemic blood volume. C, maximal cardiac diameter; T, maximal thoracic diameter measured to the inside of the ribs.

very clearly on the chest radiograph, although in the absence of a clinical history the radiograph is insufficient to determine if the pulmonary edema is from a cardiac or a pulmonary cause. If the pulmonary edema is caused by heart failure, sometimes described as *hydrostatic pulmonary edema*, the fluid may be in a "bat-wing" distribution, with the white areas concentrated in the hilar region (origin of the major pulmonary vessels). However, as heart failure progresses, the quantity of fluid in the alveolar spaces increases, and the white, fluffy appearance is seen throughout the lung.

If the pulmonary edema is caused by ARDS, also known as *noncardiogenic pulmonary edema*, the fluid is randomly distributed. It may be described as diffuse bilateral infiltrates.[109]

Pneumonia. Hospital-acquired pneumonia is a serious iatrogenic complication that may be detected on a chest radiograph. For a mechanically ventilated patient, the risk is increased because the normal oropharyngeal defenses are bypassed by intubation. This leaves the patient vulnerable for development of *ventilator-associated pneumonia*. On the chest radiograph, any appearance of a new or progressive opacity (dense, white area) is a cause for concern and should be clinically investigated. More comprehensive information on pneumonia is provided in Chapter 19.

Pneumothorax. Pneumothorax, or air within the pleural cavity, is diagnosed by chest radiography. The pleura normally are not visible because they are adjacent to the chest wall. As the pneumothorax increases in size, the nurse can see the edge of the pleura as the trapped air separates it from the chest wall. The "pneumo" (air) appears black within the pleura. There are no lung markings in the pleural area, and the collapsed lung appears increasingly dense (gray or white). The biggest risk is development of a *tension pneumothorax* that will shift the mediastinal structures. This is also visible on a chest radiograph.

Digital Radiography

Digital radiography systems are the norm in hospitals. In a digital radiograph, the image is divided into discrete elements (pixels) that are assigned a specific value and are available for display on a computer screen. Digital systems have many advantages. No film development is necessary; the image can be expanded to show greater detail. Digital systems can be used for computer-assisted diagnosis, where computer analysis of the image is used to detect and quantify pathologic findings. If a baseline film has been digitally recorded, the baseline film can be "subtracted" from the current film, highlighting any areas of change, such as increased heart size or new pulmonary infiltrates.

Ambulatory Electrocardiography

Before coming to the critical care unit, a patient might have had other ECG tests to determine the degree of cardiovascular disease. *Ambulatory electrocardiography* is a technique that records the ECG of patients while they perform their usual activities. It is designed to document abnormal cardiac rhythms that occur randomly or that are induced by specific circumstances such as emotional stress or physical activity. Clinical indications include palpitations, dizziness, syncope, and pacemaker evaluation. Two types of recording systems are available: *continuous* and *intermittent*. Many intermittent systems have a short memory loop that permits capture of recent antecedent ECG rhythms that may have precipitated the symptoms of concern.

Continuous Electrocardiogram Recording Systems

Holter monitors are the most widely used continuous recording systems. The patient wears skin electrodes and carries a small box that contains a digital recorder. The monitor is carried by a shoulder strap or clipped to a belt or pocket for 24 hours or longer and then is returned to the hospital or clinic for reading. This is a totally noninvasive procedure with no adverse effects. All Holter monitors record at least two leads to minimize inaccurate interpretation caused by artifact.

Most systems have an event marker, which the patient can press to indicate the onset of symptoms. The patient is asked to keep a diary of activities, symptoms, and any medications that are taken.

Continuous recording systems are the most thorough form of ambulatory electrocardiography because they record every heartbeat for 24 hours. They do not require active participation of the patient (although a detailed patient log is helpful) and do not miss asymptomatic ECG changes or dysrhythmias that may be accompanied by a loss of consciousness. When dysrhythmias occur that correlate with symptoms or symptoms occur in the absence of dysrhythmias, one of the primary goals of Holter monitoring has been achieved. Most patients do not have typical symptoms daily. If no significant dysrhythmias or symptoms occur during the 24-hour monitoring period, the test is unhelpful. The only activities that are restricted while wearing a Holter monitor are activities that would get the chest electrodes or monitor wet, eliminating swimming and taking a shower or tub bath.

Intermittent Electrocardiogram Recording Systems

A portable monitor that does not record the ECG continuously can also be used to diagnose dysrhythmias. These may also be described as *event monitors*. The patient wears electrodes, but the device is not constantly recording. The patient is instructed to press a button when experiencing symptoms to initiate the recording manually in real time. The big advantages of the intermittent recording system are the ability to wear the recorder for weeks and the ability to trigger recording when symptoms such as heart palpitations occur.[110]

Implantable electrocardiogram recording systems. For patients whose symptoms are not diagnosed with the traditional methods or who require longer periods of follow-up to diagnose syncope or intermittent dysrhythmias, a small, continuous *implantable loop recorder* may be inserted under the skin of the upper chest. The recorder is approximately 2 inches by 1 inch by 1 inch. Insertion takes approximately 20 minutes under local anesthetic. It is especially useful if prior short-term ambulatory ECG recordings have failed to reveal an underlying problem. The inserted loop recorder continuously monitors the ECG rhythm for up to 14 months. After a syncopal episode (loss of consciousness), the patient or a family member places a small, handheld activator on the chest wall over the loop recorder to capture the most recent ECG data. The stored ECG is subsequently analyzed to determine whether the syncopal episode was caused by a dysrhythmia. At this point, after a diagnosis is made, the implantable loop recorder can be safely removed.

Internet remote electrocardiogram monitoring. Patients with ICDs or permanent pacemakers can have their device monitored by an Internet-based, remote monitoring system. The patient dials a prearranged phone number to send the information to a protected site. The information is downloaded by the dysrhythmia nurse or electrophysiologist to a secure Internet web page in the clinical setting. The clinician can view all the programmable details plus any dysrhythmic events or malfunction of the ICD or pacemaker.

Stress Tests: Exercise With Electrocardiogram Monitoring

Exercise stress testing is a noninvasive test. It consists of an ECG tracing during a period of *physiologic stress* on the heart muscle and its blood supply to uncover and diagnose ischemia that is not apparent at rest. Physiologic stress is created by asking the patient to walk on a treadmill or to ride a stationary bicycle.[111]

Physiology of exercise on the cardiovascular system. Exercise places unique demands on the cardiovascular system. Systemic oxygen consumption increases markedly, requiring the heart to increase CO to meet these demands. Myocardial contractility increases, resulting in greater SV and systolic blood pressure. HR is increased as a result of circulating catecholamines. Normally, as HR and SV rise, CO is increased dramatically, and the tissue needs for oxygen are met. This enhanced myocardial performance is not without a penalty. Even at rest, the heart muscle extracts 70% of the oxygen available in the circulating blood. When the myocardial demand for oxygen increases during exercise, coronary blood flow must increase to maintain an adequate oxygen supply. In patients with CAD, coronary blood flow cannot increase sufficiently to meet the high metabolic needs of the myocardium during exercise, and ischemia results.

Stress test protocols. Exercise is performed using a treadmill on which the speed and slope can be varied or using a stationary bicycle. Numerous protocols have been developed using a treadmill. Two popular ones are the *Bruce protocol*, in which the grade and speed are varied every 3 minutes, and the *Balke protocol*, in which speed remains constant and grade is gradually increased every minute. Regardless of the protocol used, the ECG is monitored continuously. Blood pressure is also measured and recorded every minute.[111]

Heart rate criteria in treadmill stress test. The treadmill test is stopped when a target level, based on the patient's maximal stress test HR, is reached. The maximal predicted HR is estimated using the following formula[111]:

$$220 - \text{Patient's age}$$

Increasing the HR to 85% to 90% of the predicted maximum is preferred, and this level of exercise is sufficient in most patients to unmask any significant CAD. The diagnostic value of the test is based on the maximal HR achieved, *not* on the length of time that the patient remains on the treadmill. A well-trained athlete may be able to stay on the treadmill for 15 minutes, whereas an older or sedentary person may tolerate it for only 3 to 5 minutes; however, if 85% of the predicted maximal HR is achieved, both tests are equally diagnostic. A person who is taking beta-blockers may be unable to reach his or her age-adjusted targeted HR because of the bradycardic effect of this class of medications.

The exercise test workload is described as a metabolic equivalent (MET) of oxygen consumption.[111] The definition of 1 MET is 3.5 mL of oxygen per kilogram per minute at rest for a 70-kg, 40-year-old man. The stress test result may be described as "poor exercise tolerance" (less than 5 MET) or "good exercise tolerance" (10 to 11 MET). To put these numbers into a clinical perspective, patients with heart disease who achieved less than 5 MET during an exercise test were four times more likely to die compared with patients who achieved 10 MET or more.[71]

Clinical reasons to stop treadmill test. The test may be aborted before maximal HR is reached if symptoms occur. Reasons to halt the test include the development of moderate to severe angina (chest pain), signs of pallor or poor perfusion, and the patient asking to stop the test. Other signs that can alert the nurse to stop the test include ST segment elevation equal to or greater than 1.0 mm (one small box), ST depression equal to or greater than 2.0 mm (2 small boxes), cardiac dysrhythmias or a marked shift in ventricular axis, and increased symptoms such as breathlessness or fatigue and a fall in blood pressure of 10 mm Hg or more from baseline. Blood pressure is expected to rise during exercise, but a systolic blood pressure greater than

250 mm Hg or a diastolic blood pressure greater than 115 mm Hg is an indication to stop the test.[111]

Signal-Averaged Electrocardiogram

The *signal-averaged electrocardiogram* (SAECG) is used to identify late potentials within the QRS complex. These low-amplitude waveforms cannot be detected on a standard surface ECG but can be recorded as an SAECG. Late potentials indicate slow conduction within the ventricular myocardium that can be a substrate for ventricular dysrhythmias and put the individual at risk for sudden cardiac death.

SAECG is a noninvasive test. The patient lies in a supine position and is asked to keep muscle movement to a minimum. Cardiac electrode leads are applied to the anterior and posterior chest walls, and the leads are connected to an SAECG computer. This computer produces a high-resolution, high-magnification ECG signal. This "noise-free" ECG is analyzed for QRS complex duration and for the presence, duration, and measurement of late myopotentials. After computer analysis, the SAECG is described as negative (normal) or positive (abnormal). A positive SAECG in combination with other specific indicators is a predictor of increased risk for sudden cardiac death.

Many patients with a positive SAECG (abnormal) produce a normal SAECG when placed on antidysrhythmic medications. The SAECG is not analyzed in isolation. It is used in conjunction with other cardiac diagnostic tests, including the electrophysiology study. It is a helpful adjunct to the EPS but does not replace it.

Echocardiography

Echocardiography uses *waves of ultrasound* to obtain and display images of cardiac structures. Normal human hearing occurs at a sound frequency of 20 to 20,000 cycles per second (Hz). Ultrasound uses sound frequencies above 20,000 Hz. Ultrasound is reflected best at interfaces between tissues that have different densities. In the heart, these are the blood, cardiac valves, myocardium, and pericardium. Because all these structures differ in density, their borders can be seen on the echocardiogram. Echocardiography is used to detect structural heart abnormalities such as mitral valve stenosis and regurgitation, prolapse of mitral valve leaflets, aortic stenosis and insufficiency, hypertrophic cardiomyopathy, atrial septal defect, thoracic aortic dissection, cardiac tamponade, and pericardial effusion.

Transthoracic Echocardiography

When transthoracic echocardiography (TTE) is performed, the patient is in a supine, left lateral, or semirecumbent position. The position used depends on the patient's clinical condition and on which structures are to be examined. A transducer is placed on the skin, with lubricant between the transducer and the skin to improve contact and reduce artifact. The active element in the transducer is a piezoelectric crystal. *Piezoelectric* refers to the ability to transform electrical energy into mechanical energy (in this case, sound energy). The transducer emits ultrasound waves and receives a signal from the reflected sound waves. Periods of sound transmission alternate with periods of sound reception.

Ultrasonic waves do not travel through air very well, and they cannot penetrate very dense structures such as bone. In adults, the transducer is usually placed in the third or fourth intercostal space to the left of the sternum because at that point the pericardium is in direct contact with the chest wall, and the ultrasonic waves are not obstructed by air or bone. Other positions are sometimes used if the standard location does not provide adequate visualization of the cardiac structures. In the critical care unit, the echocardiograph machine is usually brought to the bedside. The lighting in the room can be dimmed to improve the visual clarity of the images displayed on the screen.

Nursing care consists of monitoring the patient during the procedure, which is usually performed by an echocardiography technician. TTE is completely noninvasive; the nurse explains this and the purpose of the test to the patient and family. The procedure is not uncomfortable, but it may be tiring for certain patients because of the length of the procedure, which is usually 30 to 60 minutes.

Echocardiography
Motion-Mode Echocardiography

In motion-mode (M-mode) TTE, a thin beam of ultrasound is directed through the heart (Fig. 13.90A). Each interface is represented by a dot, and when recorded over time (similar to an ECG tracing), each dot becomes a line on an oscilloscope. A strip-chart recording can be made of this tracing as the heart beats. Heart motion is recorded over time, and a typical M-mode echo is shown in Fig. 13.90B. M-mode echocardiograms are particularly useful in detecting small pericardial effusions and cardiac tamponade.

Two-Dimensional and Three-Dimensional Echocardiograms

The two-dimensional echocardiogram uses crystals in the transducer to create a cross-sectional imaging plane. Sections of the heart are then viewed from numerous different angles (Fig. 13.91). The picture is displayed on an oscilloscope, and digital photographs are taken to serve as a permanent record. The two-dimensional echocardiogram images a whole "slice" of the heart at once and is used for direct measurement of LV volumes and wall mass. The two-dimensional slice also permits visualization of the cardiac structures in relation to each other and readily identifies valvular dysfunction and wall-motion abnormalities after MI. A more recent innovation is the three-dimensional echocardiogram. It produces a more realistic image of structures such as the mitral valve.

Phonocardiogram

Phonocardiography is combined with echocardiography to evaluate valvular dysfunction. A phonocardiogram (*phono* [sound], *cardio* [heart], and *gram* [recording]) provides a graphic display of the sounds that occur in the heart and great vessels. The transducer is placed on the chest wall to record heart sounds that correspond to auscultation with a traditional stethoscope. Chapter 12 provides more information on heart sounds (see Fig. 12.6) and heart murmurs (Table 12.4).

Color-Flow Doppler Echocardiography

Doppler echocardiography provides a special kind of echocardiogram that assesses blood flow. It uses a pulsed or continuous wave of ultrasound that records frequency shifts of reflected sound waves, showing velocity and direction of blood flow relative to the transducer. Doppler signals are usually displayed in color. Known as *color-flow mapping* or *imaging*, this technique analyzes Doppler signals from multiple intracardiac sites simultaneously. The Doppler tracing for each site is displayed in a

FIG. 13.90 (A) Schematic representation of cardiac structures traversed by two echo beams. (B) Normal, M-mode echocardiogram at the level of the aorta, aortic valve leaflets, and left atrium. *AMVL*, anterior mitral valve leaflet; *Ao*, aorta; *AV*, aortic valve; *IVS*, interventricular septum; *LA*, left atrium; *LV*, left ventricle; *PMVL*, posterior mitral valve leaflet; *PPM*, posterior papillary muscle; *T*, transducer. ([B] from Kinney M, et al. *Andreoli's Comprehensive Cardiac Care.* 8th ed. St. Louis: Mosby; 1995.)

color-coded format superimposed on a real-time two-dimensional echocardiographic image. Flow toward the transducer is displayed in one color, whereas flow away from the transducer is displayed in a contrasting color. The brightness of the color varies to signify different flow velocities.

Doppler echocardiography is especially useful in individuals with valvular heart disease. The blood flow associated with regurgitation and stenosis can be detected, and estimates can be made of the severity of the disease. Doppler can accurately estimate right ventricular systolic pressure. When several valves are involved, the Doppler technique can clarify the extent of damage to the individual valves. Other uses for Doppler echocardiography include evaluation of congenital shunts, measurement

of volume flow and CO, and assessment of new structural abnormalities after acute MI. By measuring flow velocity in the right ventricular outflow tract, mean PAP can be estimated.

Transesophageal Echocardiography

TEE is a technique in which the transducer (single-plane, biplane, or multiplane device) is mounted on a flexible shaft similar to an endoscope and advanced into the esophagus, from where cardiac structures can be clearly visualized. The multiplane transducer has a single array of crystals that can be rotated in a 180-degree arc, requiring less manipulation of the probe within the esophagus. Because of the close anatomic relationship between the heart and the esophagus, TEE produces

FIG. 13.91 Two-Dimensional Echocardiogram. *Several sections of the heart can be viewed at one time, and it is easier to see the relationships of the chambers. LA, left atrium; LV, left ventricle; MV, mitral valve; PV, pulmonary vein; RV, right ventricle; TV, tricuspid valve. (From Kinney M, et al.* Andreoli's Comprehensive Cardiac Care. *8th ed. St. Louis: Mosby; 1995.)*

high-quality images of intracardiac structures and the thoracic aorta without the interference of the chest wall, bone, or air-filled lung.

The insertion procedure is similar to upper gastrointestinal endoscopy. The patient is asked to fast for a minimum of 6 hours before TEE to prevent nausea and vomiting. For an elective TEE, medication is usually given to inhibit salivary secretions, reducing the risk of aspiration. Analgesic and sedative agents are administered to reduce fear and anxiety and to provide retrograde amnesia. Routine antibiotic prophylaxis against bacteremia and endocarditis is unnecessary, although it is considered for high-risk patients such as patients with prosthetic valves, previous endocarditis, or very poor dentition. The pharyngeal region is anesthetized with 2% viscous lidocaine and 10% lidocaine spray to lessen the gag reflex and prevent retching and laryngospasm. The patient is usually placed in the left lateral decubitus position, although the supine position can be used in the critical care setting if necessary. A soft bite block is inserted between the teeth to prevent damage to the echoscope. As the echoscope is inserted, the patient is asked to swallow. The echoscope is advanced to 25 cm from the mouth, and

imaging is begun (Fig. 13.31). TEE is also used intraoperatively during cardiac surgery for monitoring valve repair and replacement. The images obtained by TEE are superior to transthoracic views in a variety of ways. The entire thoracic aorta can be visualized clearly. Both atrial chambers are clearly seen with TEE, and the left atrial appendage is particularly well visualized, making TEE the procedure of choice for detection of left atrial thrombus. Diagnosis and quantification of atrial septal defects is possible with this method, and the addition of Doppler capabilities allows assessment of atrial shunting. TEE is useful in evaluating patients with valvular disorders, including infective endocarditis to visualize vegetations on the valve leaflets.

Manipulation of the TEE probe within the esophagus can cause a vasovagal response, producing bradycardia and hypotension. The most serious risk of the procedure is esophageal bleeding. Individuals with liver cirrhosis or esophageal varices and patients on a heparin drip are also at risk for esophageal bleeding. During TEE, the patient's vital signs are closely monitored with ECG, blood pressure, and clinical observation. If esophageal entry is difficult, it cannot be forced. Emergency resuscitation equipment must be present in case of a severe vasovagal episode (eg, bradycardia, hypotension). Suction equipment must be at the bedside in the event that the patient vomits or has difficulty handling oral secretions.

Stress Echocardiography

Stress echocardiography is often used in the outpatient setting to identify stable angina. It provides a very accurate picture of the ischemic impact of CAD on the myocardium.[112] Stress echocardiography can diagnose regional (ischemia) and global (cardiomyopathy) abnormalities.[112] It may also be used after MI to evaluate the impact of necrosis on viable wall tissue. Physiologic stress from increased exercise creates an imbalance between myocardial oxygen supply and demand. This causes ischemia and eventually results in wall-motion abnormalities, which are detectable with an echocardiogram. Stress can be applied to the heart by physical and pharmacologic means.[112] One of two methods of physical exertion usually is employed: The patient can exercise on a treadmill or a stationary bicycle. The protocols used for physical echocardiographic stress testing are very similar to the protocols used in the ECG stress test setting previously described (Table 13.21).

Dobutamine stress test. When patients are unable to exercise to raise the HR sufficiently to evaluate myocardial response, pharmacologic agents may be used. Dobutamine, a beta-1 agonist, is most frequently used and is discussed here. However, alternative agents may be selected to provoke accelerated HRs for the study, including the vasodilators adenosine and dipyridamole as well as regadenoson (an adenosine A2A receptor agonist). Choice of agent is based on the patient's concomitant disease states and clinical status.

Pharmacologic stress is most frequently incited with a dobutamine infusion beginning at 5 mcg/kg per minute and increasing as needed to 40 or 50 mcg/kg per minute to achieve 85% of maximal HR.[112] Dobutamine causes myocardial ischemia through a dramatic increase in myocardial oxygen demand by an increase in HR, contractility, and systemic blood pressure. Potential side effects include hypotension, hypertension, dysrhythmias, nausea, headache, anxiety, and tremor. Atropine is also administered if the dobutamine infusion alone does not cause an adequate increase in HR. Because of the potential risks of dobutamine stress echocardiography, it is recommended that

TABLE 13.21	Stress Testing Methods		
Test Parameters	**Stress Electrocardiography**	**Stress Echocardiography**	**Stress Radionuclide Imaging**
Exercise stress test	3-, 5-, or 12-lead ECG leads are attached to the chest and limbs to monitor the ECG *during* exercise protocol.	Patient exercises according to protocol.	Radiopharmaceutical (thallium-201 or technetium-99m) is injected before exercise.
		Echocardiogram is recorded immediately *after* exercise.	Patient exercises according to the protocol.
			Heart is scanned *after* exercise to view uptake of radiotracer.
Pharmacologic stress test	Patient is at rest. IV medications stimulate HR and contractility:	Patient is at rest. IV medications stimulate HR and contractility:	Patient is at rest. IV medications simulate exercise:
	Dosage starts with dobutamine at 5 mcg/kg/min and is increased as needed to increase HR. ECG pattern is monitored during the medication infusions. Other medications include adenosine, regadenoson, and dipyridamole.	Dosage starts with dobutamine at 5 mcg/kg/min and is increased as needed to increase HR. Echocardiogram is recorded during and after the medication infusions. Other medications include adenosine, regadenoson, and dipyridamole.	Dosage starts with dobutamine 5 mcg/kg/min and is increased as needed to increase HR. Radionuclide image is scanned during and after pharmacologic stress. Other medications include adenosine, regadenoson, and dipyridamole.
Clinical indications	Used to rule out CAD.	Useful for patients with LBBB, RBBB, and implanted pacemaker because the wall motion is visualized directly.	Helpful for patients with LBBB, RBBB, and implanted pacemaker
	Not as helpful if patient has a distorted ECG pattern at baseline owing to LBBB, RBBB, or internal ventricular pacemaker because ST segment changes are obscured.		It is useful before CABG to determine if bypass graft will supply blood to an ischemic area. There is no benefit in grafting an artery to an infarcted area.
Clinical outcome of a positive test result	Chest pain develops.	Chest pain develops.	Areas of the heart that do not take up radiotracer are called *cold spots*. A cold spot is ischemic or infarcted tissue.
	ST segment ECG pattern changes.	Wall-motion abnormalities are visualized.	A follow-up scan later the same day (or the next day with some radiotracers) shows whether the cold spot has filled in; if yes, the area is ischemic; if it remains cold, the area is infarcted.

CABG, coronary artery bypass graft; *CAD,* coronary artery disease; *ECG,* electrocardiogram; *HR,* heart rate; *IV,* intravenous; *LBBB,* left bundle branch block; *RBBB,* right bundle branch block.

qualified physicians be engaged in at least 100 studies a year to maintain competence.

Intravascular Ultrasound

Intravascular ultrasound is used as an adjunct diagnostic technique during coronary angiography or during a percutaneous coronary procedure. A miniature, flexible ultrasound catheter that incorporates a high-frequency transducer (20 to 40 MHz) provides high-resolution images of the coronary arterial wall. This technology is not an alternative to angiography but is used as a complementary diagnostic technique. Intravascular ultrasound permits an anatomic view of the interior of the coronary artery. The cardiologist can visualize the exact location of atherosclerotic plaque or see if a coronary stent has deployed (expanded) correctly against the vessel wall.

Intracardiac Ultrasound

The use of intracardiac ultrasound is increasing. Flexible ultrasound catheters can be directed into the atria and ventricles. Diagnostic uses include direct visualization of intracardiac structures, replacement for TEE during interventional or selected surgical procedures, and views of the atrial or ventricular septum during a repair procedure.

Magnetic Resonance Imaging

Magnetic resonance imaging (MRI) is a noninvasive imaging technique that can obtain specific biochemical information from body tissue without the use of ionizing radiation. The procedure does not present any known hazard to living cells. In many respects, the image created is superior to radiography and ultrasonography because bone does not interfere with MRI.

Indications

Cardiac MRI can provide information about tissue integrity, cardiac wall-motion abnormalities, aneurysms, EF, CO, patency of proximal coronary arteries, and flow rates through coronary artery bypass grafts. MRI is useful in diagnosing complications of MI such as pericarditis or pericardial effusion, valvular dysfunction, ventricular septal rupture, aneurysm, and intracardiac thrombus.

Blood that is actively flowing does not emit a magnetic resonance signal; it provides a natural dark contrast material in the lumen of proximal coronary arteries. As a result, abnormalities of lumen size such as narrowing—which may provide evidence of obstruction—can be visualized.

How Magnetic Resonance Imaging Works

The physics behind MRI scanning is complex, but the basic concept is simple. Certain atoms within molecules act as tiny bar magnets with north and south poles. The nuclei spin around this axis like a spinning top. Under normal conditions, these small atomic magnets are arranged at random. If a patient is placed within a strong magnetic field, many of the nuclei line up in the same direction as the magnetic force. When a radiofrequency wave is sent, some of the nuclei absorb this energy, causing them to fall out of alignment and wobble like a gyroscope that is winding down. This wobbling out of alignment is called *resonance.* The process of returning to alignment with the magnetic field after the radiofrequency signal is turned off is called *relaxation.* These energy changes can be detected and recorded by the scanner.

Each type of atom has its own unique resonance and relaxation pattern. The easiest one to record is the hydrogen ion, although other atoms such as phosphorus, sodium, and carbon are being studied. Because there are two hydrogen ions per molecule of water, MRI is especially sensitive to changes in tissue water content. Myocardial ischemic injury results in predictable increases in regional myocardial water content, allowing differentiation between normal and ischemic tissue. Infarction leading to myocardial scarring results in tissue with a decreased water content, which can be identified on an MRI scan as an area of decreased signal intensity.

MRI works well for structures that have little or no motion, such as the brain. Cardiac applications have been limited because of the constant motion of the heart. In an attempt to overcome this limitation, various gating or slicing techniques have been used to time the images at exact phases of the cardiac cycle. The gating can be timed from the R wave of the ECG or from the arterial pulse tracing. Either method is satisfactory as long as the patient is in normal sinus rhythm. With any irregularity of the rhythm, the gating technique becomes much less helpful.

Metal Objects

MRI is a safe procedure. The main hazard is related to the presence of metal substances in the environment. Because the magnetism used is approximately 40,000 times stronger than the magnetic field of the earth, metal objects such as IV line poles, infusion pumps, or oxygen tanks can become projectiles if they come close enough to the magnet's pull. No metal objects are permitted in the area of the MRI scanner. The patient must be asked about the presence of any metallic implants (pacemaker) or other metal (residual bullet or shrapnel) that may be moved by the magnetic force during the scan. Aneurysm clips are composed of ferromagnetic materials and can experience significant torque when exposed to the magnetic field. Another consideration is that exposure to the strong magnetic field may cause a cardiac pacemaker or ICD to turn off or switch modes.

Challenges With Magnetic Resonance Imaging

MRI has significant limitations that affect patients in the critical care setting. One of the challenges is that patients must leave the unit and be transported to the nuclear medicine laboratory for MRI. Standard ventilators, monitoring equipment, and infusion pumps cannot be used because these machines contain metal parts. Special ventilators with nonmagnetic accessories are available as well as nonmetal ECG, pulse oximetry sensors, and infusion pumps.

The narrow size of the magnet bore (tube or tunnel) requires the patient to lie flat and motionless for long periods. The close quarters inside the magnet bore tend to provoke claustrophobia in anyone already predisposed to it, and sedation may be required. A claustrophobic patient needs considerable reassurance and education before lying supine and motionless inside the MRI tube. A more recent innovation is the use of open MRI scanners. The MRI tube is open at both ends so that the patient's head is not enclosed while the body is scanned.

Cardiac Radionuclide Imaging Studies

Several types of radionuclide imaging tests are available. As with diagnostic ECG and echocardiography, many of the radionuclide tests can be performed both at rest and during exercise.

Purpose of Radionuclide Scans

The purpose of a radionuclide scan is to determine whether there is a perfusion defect in cardiac muscle. A scan is indicated for a patient with chest pain and known or suspected CAD. The radionuclide scan is especially helpful for a patient who has a coexisting LBBB or a permanent pacemaker where the QRS complex shape is distorted. Both situations make interpretation of acute angina challenging to interpret accurately on the 12-lead ECG. This has opened a window of opportunity for radionuclide imaging, in which the myocardial ability to receive blood flow is visualized directly.

A radionuclide scan adds to the information that has been gained from a cardiac catheterization study and a 12-lead ECG. Coronary artery anatomy and patency is important because regional myocardial blood supply is always from a specific coronary artery and any blockage of an artery can lead to a discrete myocardial perfusion defect, meaning that the blood supply to this area is decreased (ischemic) or absent (infarcted). Although coronary arteriography defines the anatomy of the coronary arteries, it does not show whether the arteries perfuse the cardiac muscle.

Radionuclide Isotopes

The radioisotopes used in cardiac diagnostic imaging are very different from the radioisotopes used in oncology for tumor ablation. Diagnostic isotopes have a short half-life (minutes to hours) and are used in very small amounts to minimize radioactivity risk. Patients do not need to be isolated, and no specific precautions are required for blood, urine, stool, or other body fluids.

Thallium-201. Thallium-201 (^{201}Tl) is a low-energy radioactive isotope. It is an analogue of potassium and acts like potassium when injected into the bloodstream. Because thallium is similar to potassium, it is absorbed from the bloodstream by cardiac muscle cells as part of the sodium-potassium adenosine triphosphatase (ATPase) pump. Thallium uptake depends on two factors: the patency of the coronary arteries and the amount of healthy myocardium with a functional sodium-potassium ATPase pump. Areas of infarcted myocardium (dead tissue) do not take up thallium. After thallium has been injected, a specialized scintillation camera and associated computer system are used to scan the myocardium.

Technetium-99m. Technetium-99m (^{99m}Tc) is also used frequently. It is often attached to other trace substances for diagnostic imaging (^{99m}Tc-sestamibi or ^{99m}Tc-tetrofosmin).[113] These substances may be described as *radiopharmaceuticals.*[113] ^{99m}Tc tracers are highly suited to imaging myocardium during

ACS because the tracers do not redistribute over time (they remain in myocardium), allowing a second scan to be performed many hours later if needed.[113] In clinical practice, this is seldom practical, and use of radiopharmaceuticals in emergency situations is rare outside of research studies.[113] These tests are used when the patient's hemodynamic and cardiac condition is stable.

Stress Test Radionuclide Scan

A stress test radionuclide scan is conducted in a specialized nuclear medicine department. The walls of the testing space are normally lined with lead to prevent any radioactivity dispersal to other areas. A patent IV line is required. A radioisotope flow agent (^{201}Tl or ^{99m}Tc) is injected into the bloodstream before exercise to permit identification of perfused versus nonperfused (cold) areas. After the physical activity, a specialized perfusion-scanning camera is used to scan the heart. As with the other cardiac stress tests, the options to increase the HR and myocardial blood flow are physical exercise by the patient or infusion of a medication to achieve the same effect (see Table 13.21).

Exercise radionuclide scan procedure. Before the *exercise radionuclide scan*, the procedure is fully explained to the patient, including a description of the equipment (ECG monitoring equipment, cardiovascular exercise treadmill or stationary bicycle, and an Anger gamma scintillation camera). The patient is usually fasting because the scan involves vigorous exercise. Vasodilating medications that may alter the uptake of the radioisotope (nitrates, theophylline, and related medications) are held (not taken by the patient) before any baseline study. Other medications that will not affect the outcome of the study can be taken as usual. A patent IV line is inserted before the test. In the laboratory, the patient is asked to exercise vigorously for 1 minute or more or until angina or fatigue develops. At this point, the isotope is injected into the bloodstream. After the injection, the patient is asked to exercise vigorously for another minute to stress the heart and circulate the radioisotope. As soon as possible after exercise (within 10 minutes), the patient is asked to lie on the examination table for the first perfusion scan by the scintillation camera. The camera examines the heart from three angles—anterior, left anterior oblique, and left lateral oblique—to increase accuracy. On the camera screen, the heart image looks like a circle with a hole (doughnut shape). The myocardium appears, but the fluid-filled center does not.

Pharmacologic radionuclide scan procedure. A patient who cannot tolerate a radionuclide exercise stress test can undergo a pharmacologic radionuclide test at rest. The test can be performed with ^{201}Tl or ^{99m}Tc. In the absence of physical exercise, a dobutamine infusion is used to increase coronary artery and myocardial blood flow.[113] Maximal contractility is achieved with dobutamine at approximately 10 mcg/kg per minute for normal hearts. The goal is to drive the HR to the 85% maximal HR predicted for that individual; if needed, atropine is added to achieve the desired HR. After the first scan, the patient is removed from the scanner, and the HR is allowed to return to baseline. After approximately 5 to 10 minutes, the patient is asked to return to the scanner to ensure the LV wall motion has also returned to baseline.

Radionuclide test results. If no perfusion defect is seen, the test is complete for that patient. If a perfusion defect (dark area) is observed in the myocardium, the patient is asked to

return for a repeat scan 2 to 4 hours later or the next day, depending on the radioisotope tracer that was used. If a perfusion defect is present 4 hours later, the area is infarcted. This is sometimes described as a *cold spot* or as a *fixed lesion*. If the perfusion defect has taken up the radioisotope since the first test (redistribution), the area is ischemic. An ischemic defect is amenable to reperfusion therapy such as coronary artery bypass graft or a catheter-based procedure to open a coronary artery.

Computed Tomography Angiography

Computed tomography is employed to calculate the Coronary Artery Calcium Score(CACS).[114] The quantity of calcium in atherosclerotic plaque is measured using electron-beam or multidetector computed tomography, then the CACS is calculated. A score less than 100 is considered low risk, whereas a score greater than 300 indicates high risk of a future coronary event. Clinically, the CACS is considered along with other risk factor information to evaluate individual risk from atherosclerotic coronary disease.

SUMMARY

Hemodynamic Monitoring

- Hemodynamic monitoring is one of the major reasons patients are admitted to the critical care unit.
- Hemodynamic monitoring of CO is in transition from invasive (PA catheter) to less invasive systems or noninvasive (ultrasound/Doppler) methods.
- Continuous monitoring of venous oxygen saturation (Svo_2 and $Scvo_2$) is indicated for a critically ill patient who has the potential to develop an imbalance between oxygen supply and metabolic tissue demand.

Electrocardiography

- Accurate ECG lead placement and interpretation of ECG rhythms in the context of a clinical diagnosis yields relevant information that contributes to optimal patient outcomes. This includes recognition of ischemia and infarction on a 12-lead ECG and knowledge of atrial dysrhythmias, ventricular dysrhythmias, and heart blocks.

Laboratory Tests

- Laboratory studies required in cardiac care include electrolyte levels (potassium, sodium, calcium), cardiac biomarkers (troponin and creatine kinase-MB), hematologic status (hemoglobin, hematocrit, WBC, platelets), coagulation times (INR, activated partial thromboplastin time), serum lipid levels (LDL-C, HDL-C, triglycerides), and laboratory values associated with the status of other organ systems that can secondarily affect cardiac function.

Diagnostic Procedures

- Specialized diagnostic studies include cardiac catheterization to assess the ventricular chambers and pressures, angiography to assess the coronary arteries, and EPS to assess the heart's electrical system.
- Interpretation of the chest radiograph is used to noninvasively locate catheters, tubes, and implantable devices and to detect complications such as pulmonary edema, pneumonia, and pneumothorax.

- Echocardiography is frequently used in the critical care unit for rapid assessment of change in cardiac function; use has increased as this technology has become smaller and more portable.
- Ambulatory ECG tests include Holter monitoring, treadmill stress tests, signal-averaged ECG, MRI, and computed tomography.

ⓔ Visit the Evolve site for additional study materials.

REFERENCES

1. Ahmad T, et al. Variation in haemodynamic monitoring for major surgery in European nations: secondary analysis of the EuSOS dataset. *Perioper Med (Lond)*. 2015;4:8.
2. Judge O, et al. Current use of the pulmonary artery catheter in cardiac surgery: a survey study. *J Cardiothorac Vasc Anesth*. 2015;29(1):69–75.
3. Vincent JL, et al. Perioperative cardiovascular monitoring of high-risk patients: a consensus of 12. *Crit Care*. 2015;19:224.
4. Lough ME. Arterial pressure monitoring. In: Lough ME, ed. *Hemodynamic Monitoring: evolving Technologies and Clinical Practice*. Philadelphia: Elsevier; 2016.
5. Robertson-Malt S, et al. Heparin versus normal saline for patency of arterial lines. *Cochrane Database Syst Rev*. 2014;(5):CD007364.
6. Linkins LA, et al. Treatment and prevention of heparin-induced thrombocytopenia. Antithrombotic Therapy and Prevention of Thrombosis, 9th ed: American College of Chest Physicians Evidence-Based Clinical Practice Guidelines. *Chest*. 2012;141(2 suppl):e495S–e530S.
7. O'Grady NP, et al. Guidelines for the prevention of intravascular catheter-related infections. *Am J Infect Control*. 2011;39(4 suppl 1):S1–S34.
8. AACN Practice Alert Pulmonary Artery/Central Venous Pressure. *Crit Care Nurse*. 2016;36(4):e12–e18.
9. Saugel B, Dueck R, Wagner JY. Measurement of blood pressure. *Best Pract Res Clin Anaesthesiol*. 2014;28(4):309–322.
10. O'Horo JC, et al. Arterial catheters as a source of bloodstream infection: a systematic review and meta-analysis. *Crit Care Med*. 2014;42(6):1334–1339.
11. Lakhal K, et al. Noninvasive monitoring of blood pressure in the critically ill: reliability according to the cuff site (arm, thigh, or ankle). *Crit Care Med*. 2012;40(4):1207–1213.
12. Esper SA, Pinsky MR. Arterial waveform analysis. *Best Pract Res Clin Anaesthesiol*. 2014;28(4):363–380.
13. Hamzaoui O, Monnet X, Teboul JL. Pulsus paradoxus. *Eur Respir J*. 2013;42(6):1696–1705.
14. The Joint Commission (TJC). National Patient Safety Goals; 2016. http://www.jointcommission.org/standards_information/npsgs.aspx Accessed March 16th 2016.
15. Wang AZ, et al. The differences between venous air embolism and fat embolism in routine intraoperative monitoring methods, transesophageal echocardiography, and fatal volume in pigs. *J Trauma*. 2008;65(2):416–423.
16. Sinno MC, Alam M. Echocardiographically detected fibrinous sheaths associated with central venous catheters. *Echocardiography*. 2012;29(3):E56–59.
17. Marik PE, Baram M, Vahid B. Does central venous pressure predict fluid responsiveness? A systematic review of the literature and the tale of seven mares. *Chest*. 2008;134(1):172–178.
18. Kupchik N, Bridges E. Critical analysis, critical care: central venous pressure monitoring: what's the evidence? *Am J Nurs*. 2012;112(1):58–61.
19. Monnet X, Teboul JL. Passive leg raising: five rules, not a drop of fluid! *Crit Care*. 2015;19:18.
20. Lakhal K, et al. Central venous pressure measurements improve the accuracy of leg raising-induced change in pulse pressure to predict fluid responsiveness. *Intensive Care Med*. 2010;36(6):940–948.
21. Christensen M. Mixed venous oxygen saturation monitoring revisited: thoughts for critical care nursing practice. *Aust Crit Care*. 2012;25(2):78–90.
22. Marik PE. Obituary: pulmonary artery catheter 1970 to 2013. *Ann Intensive Care*. 2013;3(1):38.
23. Opitz CF, et al. Pulmonary hypertension: hemodynamic evaluation. Updated recommendations of the Cologne Consensus Conference 2011. *Int J Cardiol*. 2011;154(suppl 1):S13–S19.
24. Rosenkranz S, Preston IR. Right heart catheterisation: best practice and pitfalls in pulmonary hypertension. *Eur Respir Rev*. 2015;24(138):642–652.
25. Haynes A. Hemodynamic management in right heart failure and pulmonary hypertension. In: Lough ME, ed. *Hemodynamic Monitoring: evolving Technologies and Clinical Practice*. Philadelphia: Elsevier; 2016.
26. Asgar AW, Mack MJ, Stone GW. Secondary mitral regurgitation in heart failure: pathophysiology, prognosis, and therapeutic considerations. *J Am Coll Cardiol*. 2015;65(12):1231–1248.
27. De Bonis M, et al. Treatment and management of mitral regurgitation. *Nat Rev Cardiol*. 2012;9(3):133–146.
28. Kutty RS, Jones N, Moorjani N. Mechanical complications of acute myocardial infarction. *Cardiol Clin*. 2013;31(4):519–531. vii-viii.
29. Timmerman R. Vasoactive hemodynamic medications. In: Lough ME, ed. *Hemodynamic Monitoring: evolving Technologies and Clinical Practice*. Philadelphia: Elsevier; 2016.
30. Price LC, et al. Pathophysiology of pulmonary hypertension in acute lung injury. *Am J Physiol Lung Cell Mol Physiol*. 2012;302(9):L803–L815.
31. Tempe DK, et al. Where does the pulmonary artery catheter float: transesophageal echocardiography evaluation. *Ann Card Anaesth*. 2015;18(4):491–494.
32. Giraud R, et al. Reproducibility of transpulmonary thermodilution cardiac output measurements in clinical practice: a systematic review. *J Clin Monit Comput*. 2016; http://dx.doi.org/10.1007/s10877-016-9823-y.
33. Leeper B. Venous oxygen monitoring. In: Lough ME, ed. *Hemodynamic Monitoring: evolving Technologies and Clinical Practice*. Philadelphia: Elsevier; 2016.
34. Walley KR. Use of central venous oxygen saturation to guide therapy. *Am J Respir Crit Care Med*. 2011;184(5):513–520.
35. Squara P. Central venous oxygenation: when physiology explains apparent discrepancies. *Crit Care*. 2014;18(6):579.
36. Singer M, et al. The Third International Consensus Definitions for Sepsis and Septic Shock (Sepsis-3). *JAMA*. 2016;315(8):801–810.
37. Headley J. Arterial waveform and pressure-based hemodynamic monitoring. In: Lough ME, ed. *Hemodynamic Monitoring: evolving Technologies and Clinical Practice*. Philadelphia: Elsevier; 2016.
38. Hofer CK, Rex S, Ganter MT. Update on minimally invasive hemodynamic monitoring in thoracic anesthesia. *Curr Opin Anaesthesiol*. 2014;27(1):28–35.
39. Peeters Y, et al. Hemodynamic monitoring: to calibrate or not to calibrate? Part 1. Calibrated techniques. *Anaesthesiol Intensive Ther*. 2015;47(5):487–500.
40. Bernards J, et al. Hemodynamic monitoring: to calibrate or not to calibrate? Part 2. Non-calibrated techniques. *Anaesthesiol Intensive Ther*. 2015;47(5):501–516.
41. He HW, et al. The effect of variable arterial transducer level on the accuracy of pulse contour waveform-derived measurements in critically ill patients. *J Clin Monit Comput*. 2016;30(5):569–575; http://dx.doi.org/10.1007/s10877-016-9823-y.
42. Sidebotham DA, et al. Intraoperative transesophageal echocardiography for surgical repair of mitral regurgitation. *J Am Soc Echocardiogr*. 2014;27(4):345–366.
43. Ender J, Sgouropoulou S. Value of transesophageal echocardiography (TEE) guidance in minimally invasive mitral valve surgery. *Ann Cardiothorac Surg*. 2013;2(6):796–802.
44. Turner EE, Tarabichi Y, Puri N. Ultrasonography-based hemodynamic monitoring. In: Lough ME, ed. *Hemodynamic Monitoring: evolving Technologies and Clinical Practice*. Philadelphia: Elsevier; 2016.
45. Airapetian N, et al. Does inferior vena cava respiratory variability predict fluid responsiveness in spontaneously breathing patients? *Crit Care*. 2015;19:400.
46. Philips R. Doppler based hemodynamic monitoring. In: Lough ME, ed. *Hemodynamic Monitoring: evolving Technologies and Clinical Practice*. Philadelphia: Elsevier; 2016.
47. Young BP, Low LL. Noninvasive monitoring cardiac output using partial CO_2 rebreathing. *Crit Care Clin*. 2010;26(2):383–392.

48. Malfatto G, et al. Transthoracic impedance accurately estimates pulmonary wedge pressure in patients with decompensated chronic heart failure. *Congest Heart Fail*. 2012;18(1):25–31.

49. Albert NM, et al. Differences in alarm events between disposable and reusable electrocardiography lead wires. *Am J Crit Care*. 2015;24(1):67–73.

50. Albert NM, et al. Infection rates in intensive care units by electrocardiographic lead wire type: disposable vs reusable. *Am J Crit Care*. 2014;23(6):460–467. quiz 468.

51. Kligfield P, et al. Recommendations for the standardization and interpretation of the electrocardiogram: part I: the electrocardiogram and its technology: a scientific statement from the American Heart Association Electrocardiography and Arrhythmias Committee, Council on Clinical Cardiology; the American College of Cardiology Foundation; and the Heart Rhythm Society: endorsed by the International Society for Computerized Electrocardiology. *Circulation*. 2007;115(10):1306–1324.

52. Drew BJ, et al. Practice standards for electrocardiographic monitoring in hospital settings: an American Heart Association scientific statement from the Councils on Cardiovascular Nursing, Clinical Cardiology, and Cardiovascular Disease in the Young: endorsed by the International Society of Computerized Electrocardiology and the American Association of Critical-Care Nurses. *Circulation*. 2004;110(17):2721–2746.

53. Surawicz B, et al. AHA/ACCF/HRS recommendations for the standardization and interpretation of the electrocardiogram: Part III: Intraventricular conduction disturbances: a scientific statement from the American Heart Association Electrocardiography and Arrhythmias Committee, Council on Clinical Cardiology; the American College of Cardiology Foundation; and the Heart Rhythm Society: endorsed by the International Society for Computerized Electrocardiology. *Circulation*. 2009;119(10):e235–e240.

54. American Association of Critical Care Nurses (AACN): ST segment monitoring: AACN Practice Alert. http://www.aacn.org/wd/practice/docs/practicealerts/st-segment-monitoring.pdf?menu=aboutus. Accessed March 16, 2016.

55. Drew BJ, et al. Prevention of torsade de pointes in hospital settings: a scientific statement from the American Heart Association and the American College of Cardiology Foundation. *Circulation*. 2010;121(8):1047–1060.

56. Pickham D, et al. High prevalence of corrected QT interval prolongation in acutely ill patients is associated with mortality: Results of the QT in Practice (QTIP) Study. *Crit Care Med*. 2012;40(2):394–399.

57. Muzyk AJ, et al. Examination of baseline risk factors for QTc interval prolongation in patients prescribed intravenous haloperidol. *Drug Saf*. 2012;35(7):547–553.

58. Sommargren CE, Drew BJ. Preventing torsades de pointes by careful cardiac monitoring in hospital settings. *AACN Adv Crit Care*. 2007;18(3):285–293.

59. Tisdale JE, et al. Prevalence of QT interval prolongation in patients admitted to cardiac care units and frequency of subsequent administration of QT interval-prolonging drugs: a prospective, observational study in a large urban academic medical center in the US. *Drug Saf*. 2012;35(6):459–470.

60. Conti CR, Bavry AA, Petersen JW. Silent ischemia: clinical relevance. *J Am Coll Cardiol*. 2012;59(5):435–441.

61. Zellweger MJ, et al. Progression to overt or silent CAD in asymptomatic patients with diabetes mellitus at high coronary risk: main findings of the prospective multicenter BARDOT trial with a pilot randomized treatment substudy. *JACC Cardiovasc Imaging*. 2014;7(10):1001–1010.

62. Rautaharju PM, et al. AHA/ACCF/HRS recommendations for the standardization and interpretation of the electrocardiogram: part IV: the ST segment, T and U waves, and the QT interval: a scientific statement from the American Heart Association Electrocardiography and Arrhythmias Committee, Council on Clinical Cardiology; the American College of Cardiology Foundation; and the Heart Rhythm Society: endorsed by the International Society for Computerized Electrocardiology. *Circulation*. 2009;119(10):e241–e250.

63. Behrouz R, Sullebarger JT, Malek AR. Cardiac manifestations of subarachnoid hemorrhage. *Exp Rev Cardiovasc Ther*. 2011;9(3):303–307.

64. Wagner GS, et al. AHA/ACCF/HRS recommendations for the standardization and interpretation of the electrocardiogram: part VI: acute ischemia/infarction: a scientific statement from the American Heart Association Electrocardiography and Arrhythmias Committee, Council on Clinical Cardiology; the American College of Cardiology Foundation; and the Heart Rhythm Society: endorsed by the International Society for Computerized Electrocardiology. *Circulation*. 2009;119(10):e262–e270.

65. Hancock EW, et al. AHA/ACCF/HRS recommendations for the standardization and interpretation of the electrocardiogram: part V: electrocardiogram changes associated with cardiac chamber hypertrophy: a scientific statement from the American Heart Association Electrocardiography and Arrhythmias Committee, Council on Clinical Cardiology; the American College of Cardiology Foundation; and the Heart Rhythm Society: Endorsed by the International Society for Computerized Electrocardiology. *Circulation*. 2009;119(10):e251–e261.

66. Amsterdam EA, et al. 2014 AHA/ACC guideline for the management of patients with non-ST-elevation acute coronary syndromes: executive summary: a report of the American College of Cardiology/American Heart Association Task Force on Practice Guidelines. *Circulation*. 2014;130(25):2354–2394.

67. O'Gara PT, et al. 2013 ACCF/AHA guideline for the management of ST-elevation myocardial infarction: executive summary: a report of the American College of Cardiology Foundation/American Heart Association Task Force on Practice Guidelines. *Circulation*. 2013;127(4):529–555.

68. Goldstein JA. Acute right ventricular infarction. *Cardiol Clin*. 2012;30(2):219–232.

69. Peters A, Lakhter V, Bashir R. Under-pressure: right ventricular infarction. *Am J Med*. 2015;128(9):966–969.

70. Bussink BE, et al. Right bundle branch block: prevalence, risk factors, and outcome in the general population: results from the Copenhagen City Heart Study. *Eur Heart J*. 2013;34(2):138–146.

71. Morrow DA. Cardiovascular risk prediction in patients with stable and unstable coronary heart disease. *Circulation*. 2010;121(24):2681–2691.

72. Elizari MV, Chiale PA. The electrocardiographic features of complete and partial left anterior and left posterior hemiblock. *J Electrocardiol*. 2012;45(5):528–535.

73. Page RL, et al. 2015 ACC/AHA/HRS Guideline for the Management of Adult Patients With Supraventricular Tachycardia: a Report of the American College of Cardiology/American Heart Association Task Force on Clinical Practice Guidelines and the Heart Rhythm Society. *Circulation*. 2016;133:e471–e505.

74. Goudis CA, et al. Electrocardiographic abnormalities and cardiac arrhythmias in chronic obstructive pulmonary disease. *Int J Cardiol*. 2015;199:264–273.

75. Prystowsky EN, Padanilam BJ, Fogel RI. Treatment of atrial fibrillation. *JAMA*. 2015;314(3):278–288.

76. January CT, et al. 2014 AHA/ACC/HRS guideline for the management of patients with atrial fibrillation: A report of the American College of Cardiology/American Heart Association Task Force on practice guidelines and the Heart Rhythm Society. *Circulation*. 2014;130(23):e199–e267.

77. Latchamsetty R, Morady F. Catheter ablation of atrial fibrillation. *Cardiol Clin*. 2014;32(4):551–561.

78. Sardar MR, Saeed W, Kowey PR. Antiarrhythmic drug therapy for atrial fibrillation. *Cardiol Clin*. 2014;32(4):533–549.

79. Zimetbaum P. Antiarrhythmic drug therapy for atrial fibrillation. *Circulation*. 2012;125(2):381–389.

80. You JJ, et al. Antithrombotic therapy for atrial fibrillation: antithrombotic Therapy and Prevention of Thrombosis, 9th ed: American College of Chest Physicians Evidence-Based Clinical Practice Guidelines. *Chest*. 2012;141(2 suppl):e531S–e575S.

81. Camm AJ, et al. Guidelines for the management of atrial fibrillation: the Task Force for the Management of Atrial Fibrillation of the European Society of Cardiology (ESC). *Eur Heart J*. 2010;31(19):2369–2429.

82. Pollack CV, et al. Idarucizumab for dabigatran reversal. *N Engl J Med*. 2015;373(6):511–520.

83. Eikelboom JW, et al. Idarucizumab: the antidote for reversal of dabigatran. *Circulation*. 2015;132(25):2412–2422.

84. Camm AJ, et al. 2012 focused update of the ESC Guidelines for the management of atrial fibrillation: an update of the 2010 ESC Guidelines for the management of atrial fibrillation. Developed with the special contribution of the European Heart Rhythm Association. *Eur Heart J*. 2012;33(21):2719–2747.

85. Vadmann H, et al. Atrial flutter and thromboembolic risk: a systematic review. *Heart.* 2015;101(18):1446–1455.

86. Calkins H. Catheter ablation to maintain sinus rhythm. *Circulation.* 2012;125(11):1439–1445.

87. Roberts DM, et al. Pharmacological treatment of cardiac glycoside poisoning. *Br J Clin Pharmacol.* 2016;81(3):488–495.

88. Alzand BS, Crijns HJ. Diagnostic criteria of broad QRS complex tachycardia: decades of evolution. *Europace.* 2011;13(4):465–472.

89. Raebel MA. Hyperkalemia associated with use of angiotensin-converting enzyme inhibitors and angiotensin receptor blockers. *Cardiovasc Ther.* 2012;30(3):e156–e166.

90. Kovesdy CP. Management of hyperkalemia: an update for the internist. *Am J Med.* 2015;128(12):1281–1287.

91. Baird GS. Ionized calcium. *Clin Chim Acta.* 2011;412(9-10):696–701.

92. Steele T, et al. Assessment and clinical course of hypocalcemia in critical illness. *Crit Care.* 2013;17(3):R106.

93. Kelly A, Levine MA. Hypocalcemia in the critically ill patient. *J Intensive Care Med.* 2013;28(3):166–177.

94. de Baaij JH, Hoenderop JG, Bindels RJ. magnesium in man: implications for health and disease. *Physiol Rev.* 2015;95(1):1–46.

95. Neumar RW, et al. part 8: adult advanced cardiovascular life support: 2010 American Heart Association Guidelines for Cardiopulmonary Resuscitation and Emergency Cardiovascular Care. *Circulation.* 2010;122(18 Suppl 3):S729–S767.

96. Amundson BE, Apple FS. Cardiac troponin assays: a review of quantitative point-of-care devices and their efficacy in the diagnosis of myocardial infarction. *Clin Chem Lab Med.* 2015;53(5):665–676.

97. Maisel A, et al. The potential role of natriuretic peptide-guided management for patients hospitalized for heart failure. *J Card Fail.* 2015;21(3):233–239.

98. Tripodi A, Lippi G, Plebani M. How to report results of prothrombin and activated partial thromboplastin times. *Clin Chem Lab Med.* 2016;54(2):215–222.

99. Holbrook A, et al. Evidence-based management of anticoagulant therapy: antithrombotic Therapy and Prevention of Thrombosis, 9th ed: american College of Chest Physicians Evidence-Based Clinical Practice Guidelines. *Chest.* 2012;141(2 suppl):e152S–e184S.

100. Whitlock RP, et al. Antithrombotic and thrombolytic therapy for valvular disease: antithrombotic Therapy and Prevention of Thrombosis, 9th ed: american College of Chest Physicians Evidence-Based Clinical Practice Guidelines. *Chest.* 2012;141(2 suppl):e576S–e600S.

101. Smith S, et al. AHA/ACCF Secondary Prevention and Risk Reduction Therapy for Patients With Coronary and Other Atherosclerotic Vascular Disease: 2011 update. A Guideline From the American Heart Association and American College of Cardiology Foundation. *Circulation.* 2011;124:2458–2473.

102. Miller M, et al. Triglycerides and cardiovascular disease: a scientific statement from the American Heart Association. *Circulation.* 2011;123:2292–2333.

103. Grundy SM, et al. Implications of recent clinical trials for the National Cholesterol Education Program Adult Treatment Panel III guidelines. *Circulation.* 2004;110(2):227–239.

104. Stone NJ, et al. 2013 ACC/AHA guideline on the treatment of blood cholesterol to reduce atherosclerotic cardiovascular risk in adults: a report of the American College of Cardiology/American Heart Association Task Force on Practice Guidelines. *J Am Coll Cardiol.* 2014;63(25 Pt B):2889–2934.

105. Patel MR, et al. ACCF/SCAI/AATS/AHA/ASE/ASNC/HFSA/HRS/SCCM/SCCT/SCMR/STS 2012 Appropriate Use Criteria for Diagnostic Catheterization: a Report of the American College of Cardiology Foundation Appropriate Use Criteria Task Force, Society for Cardiovascular Angiography and Interventions, American Association for Thoracic Surgery, American Heart Association, American Society of Echocardiography, American Society of Nuclear Cardiology, Heart Failure Society of America, Heart Rhythm Society, Society of Critical Care Medicine, Society of Cardiovascular Computed Tomography, Society for Cardiovascular Magnetic Resonance, and Society of Thoracic Surgeons. *J Am Coll Cardiol.* 2012;59(22):1995–2027.

106. Sanborn TA, et al. ACC/AHA/SCAI 2014 health policy statement on structured reporting for the cardiac catheterization laboratory: a report of the American College of Cardiology Clinical Quality Committee. *Circulation.* 2014;129(24):2578–2609.

107. Nishimura RA, Carabello BA. Hemodynamics in the cardiac catheterization laboratory of the 21st century. *Circulation.* 2012;125(17):2138–2150.

108. Stacul F, et al. Contrast induced nephropathy: updated ESUR Contrast Media Safety Committee guidelines. *Eur Radiol.* 2011;21(12):2527–2541.

109. Bentz MR, Primack SL. Intensive care unit imaging. *Clin Chest Med.* 2015;36(2):219–234. viii.

110. Hendrikx T, et al. Intermittent short ECG recording is more effective than 24-hour Holter ECG in detection of arrhythmias. *BMC Cardiovasc Disord.* 2014;14:41.

111. Fletcher GF, et al. Exercise standards for testing and training: a scientific statement from the American Heart Association. *Circulation.* 2013;128(8):873–934.

112. Douglas PS, et al. ACCF/ASE/AHA/ASNC/HFSA/HRS/SCAI/SCCM/SCCT/SCMR 2011 Appropriate Use Criteria for Echocardiography. A Report of the American College of Cardiology Foundation Appropriate Use Criteria Task Force, American Society of Echocardiography, American Heart Association, American Society of Nuclear Cardiology, Heart Failure Society of America, Heart Rhythm Society, Society for Cardiovascular Angiography and Interventions, Society of Critical Care Medicine, Society of Cardiovascular Computed Tomography, and Society for Cardiovascular Magnetic Resonance Endorsed by the American College of Chest Physicians. *J Am Coll Cardiol.* 2011;57(9):1126–1166.

113. Hendel RC, et al. ACCF/ASNC/ACR/AHA/ASE/SCCT/SCMR/SNM 2009 Appropriate Use Criteria for Cardiac Radionuclide Imaging: a Report of the American College of Cardiology Foundation Appropriate Use Criteria Task Force, the American Society of Nuclear Cardiology, the American College of Radiology, the American Heart Association, the American Society of Echocardiography, the Society of Cardiovascular Computed Tomography, the Society for Cardiovascular Magnetic Resonance, and the Society of Nuclear Medicine. *Circulation.* 2009;119(22):e561–e587.

114. Grayburn PA. Interpreting the Coronary-Artery Calcium Score. *N Engl J Med.* 2012;366(4):294–296.

14

Cardiovascular Disorders

Annette Haynes

Cardiovascular disease remains the leading cause of death in the United States. In 2012, the overall rate of mortality attributable to cardiovascular disease (CVD) was 229.6 per 100,000.[1,2] From 2001 to 2011, the mortality rate attributable to CVD declined by 30.8%.[1] In the United States, someone dies as a result of a cardiac event every 40 seconds.[1] CVD causes one in three deaths in the United States, and one in nine death certificates mentions heart failure. One in three people has some form of CVD.[1] The American Heart Association (AHA) has evolved from focusing only on prevention of disease to an emphasis on cardiovascular health with a healthy lifestyle, maintaining health factors, and population-level health promotion. A healthy lifestyle includes a healthy diet, appropriate energy intake, physical activity, and not smoking. Health factor goals throughout the life span include optimal blood lipid levels, blood pressure (BP), and glucose levels. Population-level health promotion aims to improve the cardiovascular health of the public. The seven metrics of a healthy lifestyle and health factors are the basis of the 2020 Impact goals to improve cardiovascular health for all Americans by 20% and decrease deaths from CVD and stroke by 20% by 2020.

Cardiovascular operations and procedures increased by 28% between 2000 and 2010. In 2011, the estimated annual medical costs of CVD and stroke including direct costs and lost future productivity were $320.1 million.[1] The critical care nurse is in a unique position to assist with educating the public on a daily basis about CVD and the risk factors that are modifiable with changes in habits or lifestyles. An understanding of the pathology of CVD processes and clinical management allows the critical care nurse to anticipate and plan interventions. This chapter focuses on cardiac disorders commonly seen in the critical care environment.

CORONARY ARTERY DISEASE

Description and Etiology

The biggest contributor to cardiovascular system–related morbidity and mortality is *coronary artery disease* (CAD). *Atherosclerosis* is a progressive disease that affects arteries throughout the body. In the heart, atherosclerotic changes are clinically known as CAD. This disease process is also known by the term *coronary heart disease* (CHD) because other heart structures ultimately become involved in the disease process. The atherosclerotic vascular changes that lead to CAD may begin in childhood. Research and epidemiologic data collected during the past 50 years have demonstrated a strong association between preventable risk factors and nonpreventable risk factors and the development of CAD,[1,2] also delineated as *nonmodifiable* and *modifiable coronary risk factors* (Box 14.1). The nonmodifiable risk factors include age, family history, race, and whether male or female. The salient modifiable risk factors for CAD include: diabetes (see Table 14.1), Hyperlipidemia (see Table 14.2), Hypertension (see Table 14.3), cigarette smoking, obesity, and physical inactivity (see Box 14.2).[1-16] Other risk factors include elevated C-Reactive protein (see Table 14.4) a marker of inflammation and two CAD disease-risk equivalents: chronic kidney disease and diabetes. See Box 14.3 for a summary of all of the currently recommended target levels to prevent and manage CAD risk.

Women and Heart Disease

Substantial progress has been made in the awareness, treatment, and prevention of CVD in women.[17] In 2011, CVD still caused approximately more than one-third of female deaths in the United States.[1] After age 65 years, a higher percentage of women than men have hypertension. Average body weight continues to increase, with nearly two out of every three women in the United States older than age 20 years being overweight or obese.[17] The average age for first acute myocardial infarction (MI) in men is 65 years; in women, it is 71.8 years.[1] The incidence of CVD is two to three times higher among postmenopausal women than among women who are premenopausal.[1] In the past, it seemed logical to prescribe *hormone replacement therapy* (HRT) to treat the symptoms of menopause.[18] Current 2011 guidelines do not recommend the use of HRT for primary or secondary prevention of CVD.[18] Data from the Framingham Heart Study indicate the lifetime risk for CVD is more than one in two for women.[19,20] Women lag 10 years behind men for total CHD risk and more than 20 years for MI and sudden death. In the 2011 update of *Effectiveness Based Guidelines for the Prevention of CVD in Women,*[17] a new algorithm for risk classification in women was adopted that stratified women's risk into the following three categories:

- *At high risk:* Documented CHD, CVD, peripheral artery disease (PAD), abdominal aortic aneurysm, diabetes mellitus, end-stage or chronic kidney disease, or 10-year predicted risk for CHD greater than 10%.
- *At risk:* Cigarette smoking; systolic BP 120 mm Hg or greater, diastolic BP 80 mm Hg or greater, or treated hypertension; total cholesterol 200 mg/dL or greater, high-density lipoprotein (HDL) C less than 50 mg/dL, or treated for dyslipidemia; obesity, particularly central adiposity; poor diet; physical inactivity; family history of premature CVD occurring in first-degree relatives in men younger than 55 years old or women younger than 65 years old; metabolic syndrome; evidence of advanced subclinical atherosclerosis (eg, coronary calcification, carotid plaque, or thickened intimal mean thickness); systemic autoimmune collagen vascular disease

BOX 14.1 Modifiable and Nonmodifiable Coronary Artery Disease Risk Factors

Nonmodifiable Risk Factors
- Age
- Sex
- Family history
- Race

Modifiable Risk Factors
- Elevated serum lipids
- Hypertension
- Cigarette smoking
- Prediabetes or diabetes mellitus
- Diet high in saturated fat, cholesterol, and calories
- Elevated homocysteine level
- Metabolic syndrome
- Obesity
- Physical inactivity
- Postmenopause (modification is controversial)

TABLE 14.1 Fasting Blood Glucose and Risk for Coronary Artery Disease

Blood Glucose Level	Fasting Plasma Glucose Level[a] (mg/dL)
Normal	70–100
Prediabetes	101–125
Diabetes	≥126

[a]Values greater than normal increase the risk for coronary artery disease and kidney failure.

TABLE 14.2 Treatment of Blood Cholesterol to Decrease Atherosclerotic Cardiovascular Risk Disease[4]

Patient Characteristics	Intensity of Statins Needed
Age ≤ 75 y and no safety concerns	High-intensity statin
Age > 75 y or safety concerns	Moderate-intensity statin
Primary Prevention for LDL-C >190 mg/dL	
Age >21 y	High-intensity statins to achieve 50% decrease in LDL-C; consider nonstatin therapy
Diabetes; age 40–75 y; LDL-C 70–189 mg/dL	Moderate-intensity statins; high-intensity statins when 10-y ASCVD risk is ≥7.5%
No diabetes; age 40–75 y; LDL-C 70–189 mg/dL	Moderate-intensity statins; if 10-y ASCVD risk is ≥7.5%, moderate- to high-intensity statins; if 10-y ASCVD risk is 0.5%–7.5%, moderate-intensity steroids
Other Factors to Consider	
LDL-C ≥160 mg/dL	Family history; premature ASCVD; Hs-CRP ≥2; CAC Agatston score >300; ABI <0.9; or lifetime ASCVD risk
LDL-C <190 mg/dL	Age <40 y or >75 y; or <5% 10-y ASCVD risk
Clinical ASCVD Risk Factors	
ACS	
History of MI	
Stable or unstable angina	
Coronary or other arterial revascularization	
Stroke	
TIA	
PAD	

ABI, ankle-brachial index; *ACS,* acute coronary syndrome; *ASCVD,* atherosclerotic cardiovascular disease; *CAC,* coronary artery calcium; *HDL-D,* high-density lipoprotein cholesterol; *hsCRP,* high-sensitivity C-reactive protein; *LDL-C,* low-density lipoprotein cholesterol; *MI,* myocardial infarction; *PAD,* peripheral artery disease; *TIA,* transient ischemic attack.

(eg, lupus or rheumatoid arthritis); history of preeclampsia, gestational diabetes, or pregnancy-induced hypertension; or poor exercise tolerance with treadmill testing.

- *Ideal cardiovascular health:* Framingham risk score less than 10%, absence of major CVD risk factors, and engagement in a healthy lifestyle.[1,17]

In 2011, these guidelines added an acknowledgment of several 10-year risk equations for the prediction of 10-year global CVD risk, such as the updated Framingham CVD risk profile and the Reynolds risk score for women.[17,19]

The AHA defined a new concept of ideal cardiovascular health in women as follows:
- Absence of clinical CVD and presence of all ideal levels of total cholesterol (less than 200 mg/dL)
- BP less than 120/80 mm Hg
- Fasting blood glucose less than 100 mg/dL
- Adherence to healthy behaviors
- Lean body mass index less than 25 kg/m²
- Participation in physical activity at recommended levels
- Cessation of smoking
- Pursuit of eating pattern as suggested by *Dietary Approaches to Stop Hypertension* (DASH diet)[20]

Almost 400,000 women die of CVD annually in the United States. Mortality rates for women after an acute MI are higher than for men: 26% compared with 19%. The risk factors hypertension, diabetes mellitus, alcohol intake, and physical inactivity are more strongly associated with acute MI in women than in

TABLE 14.3 Hypertension Management Guidelines[14]

General Population (No Diabetes or CKD)		Diabetes or CKD Present	
Age ≥60 y	Age <60 y	All ages; diabetes present; no CVD	All ages; CKD present with or without diabetes
BP goal: SBP <150; DBP <90	BP goal: SBP <140; DBP <90	BP goal: SBP <140; DBP <90	BP goal: SBP <140; DBP <90

[a]BP values greater than normal increase the risk for coronary artery disease and heart failure. All BP values are reported in mm Hg.
BP, blood pressure; *CKD,* chronic kidney disease; *CVD,* cardiovascular disease; *DBP,* diastolic blood pressure; *SBP,* systolic blood pressure.

BOX 14.2   Detailed Coronary Artery Disease Risk Factors

Age

- Coronary artery disease (CAD) disease generally first manifests after age 45 y.
- Men tend to develop CAD symptoms 5–10 y earlier than women.
- Rate of cardiovascular disease (CVD) in women increases after age 75 y.
- CAD rate is 2–3 times greater in postmenopausal women compared with premenopausal women.

Family History

- Positive family history is defined as a close blood relative who has a myocardial infarction (MI) or stroke before age 60 y.
- Family history suggests genetic or lifestyle predisposition for development of CAD.
- Patients with CAD family history have a 50% greater risk of having an MI.

Diabetes Mellitus

- Elevated blood glucose is a known risk factor for development of vascular inflammation associated with atherosclerosis.
- The American Diabetes Association recommends use of the hemoglobin A_{1c} test with a threshold of 6.5% or greater, fasting blood glucose 126 mg/dL or greater, or 2-h plasma glucose 200 mg/dL during an oral glucose tolerance test to diagnose diabetes.
- Diabetics have increased risk of developing CAD and worse clinical outcomes after acute coronary syndrome (ACS) events.
- See Table 14.1 for fasting blood glucose levels and risk for CAD.

Physical Activity

- A sedentary lifestyle has negative effects regardless of age, sex, body mass index (BMI), and smoking status.
- Regular vigorous physical activity using large muscle groups promotes adaptation to aerobic exercise, which can prevent development of CAD and reduce symptoms in patients with established CVD.
- Exercise, decreased low-density lipoprotein (LDL) and triglyceride levels, and increased high-density lipoprotein (HDL) cholesterol reduce insulin resistance at the cellular level, lowering the risk for developing type 2 diabetes.
- Lifelong physical activity is necessary to prevent atherosclerotic CAD and stroke.

Obesity

- BMI greater than 30 kg is considered obese.
- Two-thirds of US adults are overweight.
- Obesity is associated with a sedentary lifestyle, calories consumed, and portion size.
- Normal BMI is 18.5–25 kg/m (Weight$_{kg}$/Height$_m$) ÷ Height$_m$

Fat Pattern Distribution

- Higher weight carried in the abdominal area has greater risk of CAD.
- Large waist (apple body shape)—excess abdominal adiposity—indicates added fat around the abdominal organs.
- Smaller waist and larger hips (pear body shape) is associated with lower risk of CAD.
- Goal waist measurements are less than 40 inches for men and less than 35 inches for women.

High-Fat Diet

- A diet rich in saturated fats leads to elevated cholesterol levels.
- A low-fat, high-fiber diet and increased physical activity are the first line of treatment.
- If these are ineffective, lipid-lowering medications are indicated.

- Less than 50% of patients prescribed reduction therapy take their medications.
- Only one-third of treated patients reach their LDL target value.

Hyperlipidemia

- Hyperlipidemia causes severe atherosclerosis and development of CAD.
- Total cholesterol is the sum of HDL, LDL, and VLDL cholesterol (goal <200 mg/dL)

HDL (Goal >40 mg/dL for Men; >50 mg/dL for Women)

- HDL is known as "good cholesterol"; higher serum level protects against atherosclerotic events.
- HDL promotes efflux of cholesterol from cells.
- It has antiinflammatory and antioxidant effects on the arterial wall.[6]

LDL (Goal <100 mg/dL)

- LDL is known as "bad cholesterol" because high serum levels are associated with increased risk of ACS, stroke, and peripheral artery disease.
- LDL initiates atherosclerosis by infiltrating the vessel wall and inflammatory vessel effects.
- Initial efforts to decrease LDL are based on weight loss, smoking cessation, low-fat diet, physical exercise, and maintaining normal body size.
- If lifestyle changes are not effective in decreasing LDL, the medication category of choice is statins.
- See Table 14.2 for lipid guidelines and risk for CAD.

Triglycerides (Ideal Goal <100 mg/dL)

- Triglyceride level greater than 150 mg/dL increases risk for heart disease and stroke.
- Mean triglyceride level in men older than 20 y is 108.8 mg/dL.

Lipoprotein(a) (Goal <30 mg/dL)

- Lp(a) is one of the lipid particles that makes up total LDL value.
- Lp(a) is described verbally as "LP little a"
- It is manufactured in the liver and circulates bound to a large glycoprotein called apolipoprotein A.
- It is elevated in the presence of inflammation.
- Lp(a) stimulates atheroma and clot formation in inflamed arteries.
- Elevated Lp(a) is the most frequently encountered genetic lipid disorder in families with premature CAD.
- Medication treatment is high doses (1500–2000 mg/day) of extended-release nicotinic acid (niacin).

Metabolic Syndrome

- Metabolic syndrome refers to clustering of risk factors associated with CVD and type 2 diabetes.
- Approximately one-third of people in the United States have metabolic syndrome.
- Risk factors include:
  - Fasting plasma glucose greater than 100 mg/dL or taking medications to lower elevated blood glucose.
  - HDL cholesterol less than 40 mg/dL in men and less than 50 mg/dL in women.
  - Triglycerides greater than 150 mg/dL or taking medications to lower elevated triglycerides.
  - Waist circumference greater than 40 inches (102 cm) in men or greater than 35 inches (88 cm) in women.
  - Blood pressure (BP) greater than 130 mm Hg systolic or greater than 85 mm Hg diastolic or taking antihypertensive medications.

BOX 14.2   Detailed Coronary Artery Disease Risk Factors—cont'd

Cigarette Smoking

- Smoking unfavorably alters lipid profile by decreasing HDL and increasing LDL and triglyceride levels.
- The greater number of cigarettes smoked per day, the greater risk of developing CAD, acute MI, and stroke.
- Smoking less than 5 cigarettes per day increases risk.
- Smokers are 2–4 times more likely to develop CAD compared with nonsmokers.[1]
- Passive, secondhand smoke exposure also increases CVD risk for nonsmoking adults with up to 30% increased risk of coronary heart disease.
- Of US adults, 20% are current smokers.
- Within 1 y of giving up cigarettes, an ex-smoker's risk of developing CAD decreases significantly.
- Nicotine is addictive, and giving up smoking is difficult.
- People need tremendous support to be able to "kick the habit."

Hypertension

- Hypertension is defined as systolic BP greater than 120 mm Hg and/or diastolic BP greater than 90 mm Hg.
- Increased systolic pressure damages endothelium, leading to vascular inflammation and plaque development.
- Hypertension is known as the silent killer because 28% of patients without CAD and 51% of patients with CVD are unaware of having hypertension.
- Initial treatments aim at lifestyle changes including physical activity, low sodium diet, limiting alcohol intake, and achieving normal body weight.
- Most patients are started on a diuretic; if this is insufficient, an angiotensin-converting enzyme inhibitor, angiotensin receptor blocker, beta-blocker, or calcium channel blocker may be added.
- Most patients require at least two medications from different classifications to normalize their BP.
- See Table 14.3 for BP guidelines and CAD risk.

Risk Equivalents for CAD

- Medical conditions in which patients have as much risk of experiencing a coronary event as if they already had CAD include:
  - Chronic kidney disease—risk for death from acute MI rises as serum creatinine level increases
  - Diabetes mellitus
  - Peripheral artery disease
  - Cerebrovascular disease

TABLE 14.4   C-Reactive Protein and Risk for Coronary Artery Disease

Category	hs-CRP Level[a] (mg/L)
Low risk (normal)	<1
Moderate risk	1–3
High risk	>3

hs-CRP, high-sensitivity C-reactive protein.

*Values >1 mg/dL increase the risk for coronary artery disease, but test results are not valid in the presence of infection or other inflammatory condition. Normal values may vary slightly between clinical laboratories; however, values <1 mg/dL are usually considered normal. A test result >10 mg/L suggests a noncoronary source of inflammation or infection. Based on data from Ramasamy I. Biochemical markers in acute coronary syndrome. *Clin Chim Acta*. 2011;412:1279.

men.[17,21] Many reasons contribute to the higher mortality from acute MI in women, including waiting longer to seek medical care, having smaller coronary arteries, being older when symptoms occur, and experiencing very different symptoms from those of men of similar age.[19,20]

Vascular Inflammation

The link between vascular inflammation and atherosclerotic disease is well established[22] (see the section on "Pathophysiology of Coronary Artery Disease"). Research to identify prognostic and sensitive inflammatory markers is ongoing.

C-Reactive Protein

The inflammatory marker most frequently cited is *C-reactive protein* (CRP). It is measured as high-sensitivity CRP (hs-CRP).[22] CRP is associated with an increased risk for development of other cardiovascular risk factors including diabetes, hypertension, and weight gain. The higher the hs-CRP value, the greater the risk of a coronary event, especially if all

other potential causes of systemic inflammation such as infection can be ruled out. Value ranges for hs-CRP are shown in Table 14.4. If other systemic inflammatory conditions such as bronchitis or urinary tract infection are present, the hs-CRP test loses all predictive value. CRP and other inflammatory markers are used to estimate the probability of future acute coronary events.[22-25] During acute coronary syndrome (ACS) events, there is widespread activation of neutrophils in the cardiac circulation (measured from the coronary sinus), which suggests that inflammation is not limited to one unstable plaque.[22]

Coronary Artery Disease Risk Equivalents

Certain medical conditions are risk equivalents of CAD. A *risk equivalent* means the person has the same risk of having an acute MI as if he or she already had CHD. Two noncardiac medical conditions considered risk equivalents for CAD are diabetes mellitus and chronic kidney disease.[26] PAD and cerebrovascular disease are atherosclerotic conditions that are also considered CAD risk equivalents.[26]

Multifactorial Risk

CAD has multifactorial causation; the greater the number of risk factors, the greater the risk of developing CAD. The best time for an individual to make lifestyle changes is *before* the symptoms of CAD occur. Patients with two or more risk factors or with one or more CAD risk-equivalent diseases have the greatest potential to benefit from risk factor reduction and lifestyle change.[26] The major risk factors for developing CAD have been extensively documented in large epidemiologic studies and include smoking, family history, adverse lipid profile, and elevated BP.

Primary Versus Secondary Prevention of Coronary Artery Disease

If a person has symptoms of CAD or has previously had an ACS event, the goal of any lifestyle change or medication is called *secondary prevention,* or preventing another heart attack.[11] If an individual matches the risk profile described previously but does *not* have symptoms of CAD or has *not* had an acute MI, the treatment plan is described as *primary prevention.* The constellation of cardiac risk factors is well established and can predict development of CAD for most populations in the developed world.

Pathophysiology of Coronary Artery Disease

CAD is a progressive atherosclerotic disorder of the coronary arteries that results in narrowing or complete occlusion. *Atherosclerosis* affects the medium-sized arteries that perfuse the heart and other major organs. Normal arterial walls are composed of three layers: (1) the *intima* (inner lining), (2) the *media* (middle muscular layer), and (3) the *adventitia* (outer coat).

Development of Atherosclerosis

Atherosclerosis is a chronic inflammatory disorder that is characterized by an accumulation of macrophages and T lymphocytes in the arterial intimal wall. A high low-density lipoprotein (LDL) cholesterol concentration is one of the triggers of vascular inflammation. The inflammation injures the wall, allowing the LDL cholesterol to move into the vessel wall below the endothelial surface. Blood monocytes adhere to endothelial cells and migrate into the vessel wall. Within the artery wall, some monocytes differentiate into macrophages that unite with and then internalize LDL cholesterol. The *foam cells* that result are the marker cells of atherosclerosis.

Elevated LDL cholesterol levels promote low-level endothelial inflammation, which allows lipoproteins to infiltrate the intimal vessel wall. After it has infiltrated under the endothelium, LDL cholesterol tends to stay within the vessel wall rather than return to the circulation. This contrasts with the actions of HDL cholesterol, which enters the vessel wall, helps efflux cholesterol from cells, and then returns to the circulation.[6] The actions of HDL cholesterol may help minimize the number of foam cells in the artery wall.[6]

Atherosclerotic Plaque Rupture

When a mature atherosclerotic plaque develops, it is not uniform in composition. It has a lipid liquid center filled with procoagulant factors. A connective tissue *fibrous cap* covers the top of the fluid lipid center.[2] The abrupt rupture of this cap allows procoagulant lipids to flood into the vessel lumen and rapidly form a coronary thrombosis, as shown in Table 14.5. As the enlarging clot blocks blood flow through the coronary artery, an MI will occur unless adequate collateral circulation from other coronary vessels occurs. Symptoms and suggested cardiac interventions at appropriate stages in development of CAD are listed in Table 14.5.

Plaques that are likely to rupture are saturated with macrophages and other inflammatory cells. These *vulnerable plaques* are usually not obstructive and are situated at bends or branch points in the arterial tree.[3] It is unknown what factors cause the fibrous cap to rupture or erode. As deep fissures in the cap expose the procoagulant factors to the blood plasma, an unstoppable cycle is put into motion. When platelets in the bloodstream are exposed to collagen, necrotic debris, von Willebrand factor, and thromboxane, a clot is formed and can occlude the coronary artery. Highly fibrotic plaques do not rupture. The type of atherosclerotic plaque that is prone to rupture has a weak fibrous cap and a large amount of liquid cholesterol within the core (see Table 14.5).

Plaque Regression

A reduction in blood cholesterol decreases atherosclerotic plaque size by decreasing the amount of liquid cholesterol within the plaque core.[5] Lowering cholesterol levels does not change the dimensions of the fibrous or calcified portions of the plaque. However, lower cholesterol levels reduce vascular inflammation and make vulnerable plaque less likely to rupture.

Acute Coronary Syndrome

The term *acute coronary syndrome* is used to describe the array of clinical presentations of CAD that range from unstable angina to acute MI (Fig. 14.1).[1,3] An acute MI is generally described by patients as a "heart attack." This section discusses stable manifestations of CAD (stable angina) and acute manifestations described as an ACS (unstable angina and acute MI). Fig. 14.1 is a concept map of ACS.

Angina

Angina pectoris, or chest pain, caused by myocardial ischemia is not a separate disease but rather a symptom of CAD. It is caused by a blockage or spasm of a coronary artery, leading to diminished myocardial blood supply. The lack of oxygen causes myocardial ischemia, which is felt as chest discomfort, pressure, or pain. Angina may occur anywhere in the chest, neck, arms, or back, but the most commonly described location is pain or pressure behind the sternum. The pain often radiates to the left arm but can also radiate down both arms and to the back, shoulder, jaw, or neck (Fig. 14.2). Angina symptoms are not the same for all individuals. Many patients may describe pressure or discomfort rather than pain, and presenting symptoms can be highly individualized, as described in Box 14.3. Patients and families must be taught that angina does not always present in the dramatic heart attack scenario, as often portrayed on television and in movies, in which the person clutches the throat or chest and exhibits extreme distress.[2,3]

Angina symptom equivalents. Men and women should be informed of angina symptom equivalents such as unexpected shortness of breath; breaking out in a cold sweat; or sudden fatigue, nausea, or lightheadedness.[21]

Women and angina. Many women experience a variety of symptoms before an acute MI and during the acute event, as shown in Box 14.4.[19,20] The recognition and publicity about the fact that many women have atypical symptoms but do not experience "crushing chest pain" is important to understand to avoid a woman's symptoms being trivialized by clinicians.[19] It is vital that women are made aware of the *angina symptom equivalents* of unexplained shortness of breath; breaking out in a cold sweat; or sudden fatigue, nausea, or lightheadedness.[2,26] More women die every year in the United States of ACS compared with men, a fact that is largely unknown by health care providers.[19,20]

Stable angina. Stable angina is predictable and caused by similar precipitating factors each time; typically, it is exercise induced. Patients become used to the pattern of this type of angina and may describe it as "my usual chest pain." Pain control should be achieved within 5 minutes of rest and by taking sublingual nitroglycerin. Ischemia and chest pain occur

TABLE 14.5 **Coronary Artery Disease: Pathogenesis, Symptoms, Diagnosis and Management Timeline**

	Pathology of CAD	Symptoms of CAD	Diagnosis of CAD	Management of CAD
	Normal coronary artery seen in young healthy children	No symptoms	None	• Healthy lifestyle. • Obesity prevention.
	Fatty streaks on intima of aorta and coronary arteries in many young adults.	No symptoms	None	• Preventative measures with a focus on a healthy lifestyle.
	Atherosclerotic plaque increases in size but does not occlude blood flow.	• No symptoms • Most adults are unaware they have CAD	None	• Cardiac risk factor management.
	Atherosclerotic plaque occludes more than 70% of coronary artery lumen. Stable cap on lipid plaque interior.	STABLE ANGINA • Chest pain or pressure with exertion or exercise.	• ECG stress test. • Elective coronary arteriogram.	• Aggressive risk factor management. • Sub-lingual nitroglycerin for angina. • Elective PCI with stent.
	Atherosclerotic plaque becomes fibrous and calcified. Plaque has a large pro-coagulant lipid core. Cap has thinned with cracks allowing platelets and fibrin to aggregate.	UNSTABLE ANGINA / ACS • Change in chest pain/pressure symptoms. • Chest pain/pressure at rest. • Symptoms not relieved by NTG.	• 12 Lead ECG. • Coronary arteriogram. • Biomarkers.	• Emergency PCI with stent. • Aggressive risk factor management. • Aggressive risk factor management.
	Atherosclerotic cap ruptures and the procoagulant lipid core is released forming a thrombosis that blocks blood flow.	STEMI or NSTEMI • Abrupt onset of chest pain or pressure or symptoms at rest. • Angina not relieved by NTG • Sudden shortness of breath, cold sweat.	• Emergency 12 Lead ECG. • Emergency coronary arteriogram. • Biomarkers.	• Emergency PCI with stent. • Aggressive risk factor management.

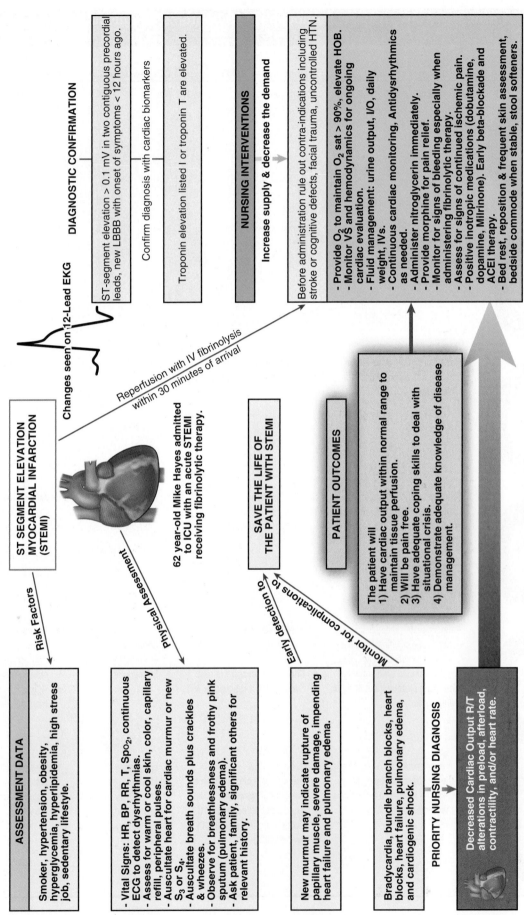

ASSESSMENT DATA

Smoker, hypertension, obesity, hyperglycemia, hyperlipidemia, high stress job, sedentary lifestyle.

- Vital Signs: HR, BP, RR, T, Spo₂, continuous ECG to detect dysrhythmias.
- Assess for warm or cool skin, color, capillary refill, peripheral pulses.
- Auscultate heart for cardiac murmur or new S₃ or S₄.
- Auscultate breath sounds plus crackles & wheezes.
- Observe for breathlessness and frothy pink sputum (pulmonary edema).
- Ask patient, family, significant others for relevant history.

New murmur may indicate rupture of papillary muscle, severe damage, impending heart failure and pulmonary edema.

Bradycardia, bundle branch blocks, heart blocks, heart failure, pulmonary edema, and cardiogenic shock.

PRIORITY NURSING DIAGNOSIS

Decreased Cardiac Output R/T alterations in preload, afterload, contractility, and/or heart rate.

ST SEGMENT ELEVATION MYOCARDIAL INFARCTION (STEMI)

62 year-old Mike Hayes admitted to ICU with an acute STEMI receiving fibrinolytic therapy.

SAVE THE LIFE OF THE PATIENT WITH STEMI

PATIENT OUTCOMES

The patient will
1) Have cardiac output within normal range to maintain tissue perfusion.
2) Will be pain free.
3) Have adequate coping skills to deal with situational crisis.
4) Demonstrate adequate knowledge of disease management.

DIAGNOSTIC CONFIRMATION

ST-segment elevation > 0.1 mV in two contiguous precordial leads, new LBBB with onset of symptoms < 12 hours ago.

Confirm diagnosis with cardiac biomarkers

Troponin elevation listed I or troponin T are elevated.

Changes seen on 12-Lead EKG

Reperfusion with IV fibrinolysis within 30 minutes of arrival

NURSING INTERVENTIONS

Increase supply & decrease the demand

Before administration rule out contra-indications including stroke or cognitive defects, facial trauma, uncontrolled HTN.

- **Provide O₂ to maintain O₂ sat > 90%, elevate HOB.**
- **Monitor VS and hemodynamics for ongoing cardiac evaluation.**
- **Fluid management: urine output, I/O, daily weight, IVs.**
- **Continuous cardiac monitoring, Antidysrhythmics as needed.**
- **Administer nitroglycerin immediately.**
- **Provide morphine for pain relief.**
- **Monitor for signs of bleeding especially when administering fibrinolytic therapy.**
- **Assess for signs of continued ischemic pain.**
- **Positive inotropic medications (dobutamine, dopamine, Milrinone). Early beta-blockade and ACEI therapy.**
- **Bed rest, reposition & frequent skin assessment, bedside commode when stable, stool softeners.**

Risk Factors

Physical Assessment

Early detection to

Monitor for complications to

FIG. 14.1 Concept Map for Acute Coronary Syndrome. Concept maps created by © DEANNE A. BLACH, MSN, RN. *ACEI*, Angiotensin receptor blockers I; *BP*, Blood Pressure; *CO*, Cardiac Output; *EkG*, Electrocardiogram; *HOB*, Head of Bed; *HR*, Heart Rate; *HTN*, Hypertension; *O₂ Sat*, Oxygen saturation; *RR*, Respiratory rate; *R/T*, Related To; *S/S*, Signs and Symptoms; *SPO₂*, Saturation of Hemoglobin with Oxygen Measured by Pulse Oximetry; *STEMI*, ST Segment Elevation Myocardial Infarction; *T*, Temperature; *U/O*, Urine Output.

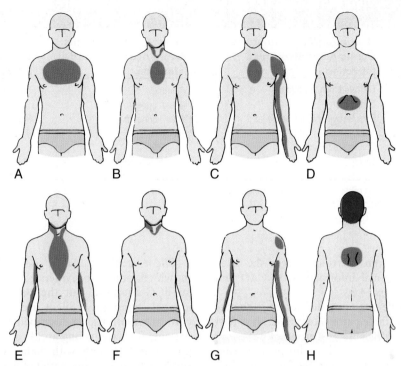

FIG. 14.2 Common Sites for Anginal Pain. (A) Upper part of chest. (B) Beneath sternum, radiating to neck and jaw. (C) Beneath sternum, radiating down left arm. (D) Epigastric. (E) Epigastric, radiating to neck, jaw, and arms. (F) Neck and jaw. (G) Left shoulder. (H) Intrascapular.

BOX 14.3   Characteristics of Angina Pectoris

Location
- Beneath sternum, radiating to neck and jaw
- Upper chest
- Beneath sternum, radiating down left arm
- Epigastric
- Epigastric, radiating to neck, jaw, and arms
- Neck and jaw
- Left shoulder, inner aspect of both arms
- Intrascapular

Duration
- Less than 5 min (stable)
- Longer than 5 min or worsening symptoms without relief from rest or sublingual nitroglycerin indicates preinfarction symptoms (unstable)

Quality
- Sensation of pressure or heavy weight on the chest
- Feeling of tightness like a vise
- Visceral quality (deep, heavy, squeezing, aching)
- Burning sensation

- Shortness of breath, with feeling of suffocation
- Most severe pain ever experienced

Radiation
- Medial aspect of left arm
- Jaw
- Left shoulder
- Right arm

Precipitating Factors
- Exertion or exercise
- Cold weather
- Exercising after large, heavy meal
- Walking against the wind
- Emotional upset
- Fright, anger
- Coitus

Medication Relief
- Usually within 45 s to 5 min after sublingual nitroglycerin administration

BOX 14.4   Cardiovascular Symptoms Experienced by Women Before Acute Myocardial Infarction

Generalized Symptoms Before Acute Myocardial Infarction	Discomfort/Pain Symptoms During Acute Myocardial Infarction	Generalized Symptoms Before Acute Myocardial Infarction	Discomfort/Pain Symptoms During Acute Myocardial Infarction
Unusual fatigue	Centered high in chest	Vomiting	Both arms
Dizzy or faint	Left breast	Loss of appetite	Top of shoulders
Hot, flushed	Back/between shoulder blades	New vision problems	Right arm or shoulder
Indigestion	Neck/throat	Headache	Jaw/teeth
Heart racing	Generalized chest	Coughing	
Numbness in hands/fingers	Leg(s)	Choking sensation	

From McSweeney JC. Preventing and experiencing ischemic heart disease as a woman: State of the science. A scientific statement from the American Heart Association. *Circulation.* 2016;133:1302.

when myocardial demand from exertion exceeds the fixed blood oxygen supply. Additional information on CAD and stable angina is provided in Box 14.5.

Unstable angina. Unstable angina is defined as a change in a previously established stable pattern of angina. It is part of the continuum of ACS. Unstable angina usually is more intense than stable angina, may awaken the person from sleep, or may necessitate more than nitrates for pain relief. A change in the level or frequency of symptoms requires immediate medical evaluation. Severe angina that persists for more than 5 minutes, worsens in intensity, and is not relieved by one nitroglycerin tablet is a medical emergency, and the patient or a family member must call 911 immediately.[27] The 911 (Emergency Medical Services [EMS]) system is available to 90% of the population of the United States.[28] Family and friends are discouraged from driving a person experiencing unstable angina to the hospital and instead are urged to call 911. Patients should be instructed never to drive themselves but to contact the EMS by calling 911.

Unstable angina is an indication of atherosclerotic plaque instability. It can signal atherosclerotic plaque rupture and thrombus formation that can lead to MI. A patient who comes to the emergency department with recent-onset unstable angina but who has nonspecific or nonelevated ST segment changes on a 12-lead electrocardiogram (ECG) may be admitted to the critical care unit to rule out MI. If the symptoms are typical of MI, it is important to treat the patient according to the latest published guidelines because not all patients who experience MI have ST segment elevation on the 12-lead ECG.[16,27]

Variant angina. Variant angina, or Prinzmetal angina, is caused by a dynamic obstruction from intense vasoconstriction of a coronary artery.[29] Spasm can occur with or without atherosclerotic lesions. Variant angina commonly occurs when the individual is at rest, and it is often cyclic, occurring at the same time every day. Smoking, alcohol use, and illegal stimulant drug (cocaine) use may precipitate spasm. A definitive diagnosis of variant angina is made during a cardiac catheterization study. Signs of spasm include ST segment elevation and chest pain. Coronary artery spasm can occur with or without CAD. The prognosis is excellent when no significant coronary artery stenosis exists. Coronary artery spasm is treated with nitroglycerin or calcium channel blockers to vasodilate the coronary arteries.

Silent ischemia. Silent ischemia describes a situation in which objective evidence of ischemia is observed on an ECG monitor, but the person does not complain of anginal symptoms. Silent ischemia can occur in many clinical situations, as described in Box 14.6. One-third of patients who are having an MI do not report chest pain as a symptom.[26] Patients with diabetes are at particular risk for silent ischemia. Many patients who had type 2 diabetes for more than 10 years have developed *autonomic neuropathy,* which decreases their ability to experience chest pain. Patients with diabetes may misinterpret angina symptom equivalents such as nausea, vomiting, and diaphoresis as signaling a disruption in glucose control rather than a sign of myocardial ischemia.

Medical Management

Accurate assessment of chest pain symptoms is essential if unstable angina is to be recognized and treated effectively. Factors to consider when assessing chest pain are listed in Box 14.7. An important reason to ask questions about the chest pain is to differentiate between stable and unstable angina. The change from stable to unstable angina is potentially life-threatening for the patient. If the ST segments are elevated or a newly documented left bundle branch block (LBBB) is seen on the 12-lead ECG, the patient should be treated for acute MI.[2] However, if these classic ECG signs are missing and the chest pain continues, the current pharmacologic treatment of choice is aspirin (if the patient cannot tolerate aspirin, a thienopyridine such as clopidogrel can be given). Patients with definite unstable angina or non–ST segment elevation myocardial infarction (NSTEMI) should receive dual antiplatelet therapy on admission if an invasive strategy is imminent. A glycoprotein (GP) IIb/IIIa inhibitor or direct thrombin inhibitor such as bivalirudin is administered; a loading dose of clopidogrel is given at least 6 hours before the procedure. Patients undergoing noninvasive treatment should receive aspirin and a thienopyridine (clopidogrel, prasugrel, or ticagrelor) for 1 month and ideally up to 1 year. If symptoms persist, diagnostic angiography is performed. A stress test should be performed on patients who are not undergoing invasive therapy for unstable angina or NSTEMI; if the stress test is negative, the GP IIb/IIIa inhibitor can be discontinued and unfractionated heparin (UFH) administered for 48 hours.

QSEN BOX 14.5 QSEN: Evidence-Based Practice

Coronary Artery Disease and Stable Angina

Strong evidence exists that the following lifestyle interventions help to prevent coronary artery disease (CAD).

- Diet:
  - Diet low in salt and high in fiber, fruit, vegetables, and grains.
  - All dietary fat less than 30% of total calories; saturated fat less than 7%.
  - Limit glucose in diet (simple sugars).
  - Limit calories if overweight.
  - Omega-3 fatty acids included in diet.
- Exercise:
  - Start by walking more often and increase physical exercise from there.
  - Refer to cardiac rehabilitation program.
- Obesity:
  - Achieve healthy body weight.
- Addiction:
  - Stop cigarette smoking.
  - Avoid exposure to environmental (secondhand) tobacco smoke at home and at work.
  - Limit alcohol intake.

Strong evidence exists that the following diagnostic procedures help the patient with angina.

- When a patient presents with chest pain, quickly obtaining a detailed history of symptoms, focused physical examination, and risk factor assessment can help determine whether the probability of CAD is low, intermediate, or high.
- Initial laboratory tests include hemoglobin, fasting blood glucose, lipid panel, and cardiac enzymes.
- Obtain a baseline 12-lead electrocardiogram (ECG) at rest, even if chest pain is not present.
- Obtain a 12-lead ECG during an episode of chest pain.
- Obtain a chest radiograph if symptoms of heart failure are present.
- Obtain an exercise 12-lead ECG if the patient's condition is stable and symptoms suggest CAD or if the patient's condition is stable with complete left bundle branch block or right bundle branch block that makes the ECG difficult to interpret for ischemia.
- Obtain cardiac echocardiography for a patient with a systolic murmur suggestive of aortic stenosis.
- Use cardiac echocardiography to determine the extent of left ventricular (LV) hypertrophy or dysfunction.
- Stress cardiac echocardiography is recommended for patients with greater than 1 mm of ST segment depression at rest (stress may be induced by physical exercise or by pharmacologic stimulation).
- Coronary angiography (typically as part of a cardiac catheterization procedure) is recommended for patients at high risk for adverse coronary events.

Initial Pharmacologic and Lifestyle Treatment Recommendations

- The goal of treatment is to eliminate chest pain.
- The 10 most important elements of CAD and stable angina management can be remembered using the following A-to-E mnemonic:
  - *A*—Aspirin and antianginal medications: Prescribe daily, low-dose (75–325 mg) aspirin, oral nitrates, and sublingual nitroglycerin for episodes of angina.
  - *B*—Beta-blockers and blood pressure: Use angiotensin-converting enzyme inhibitors and beta-blockers to decrease blood pressure to less than 140/90 mm Hg if no other CAD risk factors are present and to less than 130/80 mm Hg if diabetes or kidney disease is present.

  - *C*—Cholesterol and cigarettes: Obtain a fasting lipid profile. Recommend diet or lipid reduction medication therapy (statin) to lower low-density lipoprotein cholesterol (LDL-C) to less than 100 mg/dL (<70 mg/dL if achievable), increase high-density lipoprotein cholesterol to more than 40 mg/dL for men or more than 50 mg/dL for women, and reduce triglycerides to less than 150 mg/dL. Recommend adding plant stanols or sterols (2 g/day) or viscous fiber (>10 g/day), or both, to diet to further lower LDL-C; add dietary omega-3 fatty acids in the form of fish or capsule (1 g/day). Always ask about tobacco use, and strongly recommend smoking cessation; encourage nicotine replacement therapy (nicotine patches or gum) as needed.
  - *D*—Diet and diabetes: Prescribe a low-fat, calorie-appropriate diet and provide nutritional consultation as needed to achieve a fasting blood glucose level of 70–100 mg/dL and hemoglobin A_{1c} of less than 6.5%.
  - *E*—Education and exercise: Provide education about risk factor modification and the CAD disease process; recommend daily exercise for 30–60 min (ideal) or at least seven times each week (minimum of 5 days per week). A body mass index between 18.5 kg/m^2 and 24.9 kg/m^2 and waist circumference less than 40 inches for men or less than 35 inches for women should be recommended. Treat depression, if present. HRT is not recommended as a treatment for symptoms of coronary heart disease. Influenza vaccination is recommended.

Interventional and Surgical Recommendations for Stable High-Risk Patients

Patients are risk stratified according to their symptoms and the results of cardiac diagnostic tests.

- Percutaneous catheter intervention (PCI):
  - PCI is more frequently performed than open heart surgery for relief of anginal symptoms.
- Coronary artery bypass graft surgery:
  - For patients with left main occlusion or multivessel disease.
  - For patients with two-vessel disease who have significant proximal left anterior descending coronary artery stenosis and an LV ejection fraction less than 50%.

References

Anderson JL, et al. 2011 ACCF/AHA focused update incorporated into the ACC/AHA 2007 guidelines for the management of patients with unstable angina/non-ST-elevation myocardial infarction: a report of the American College of Cardiology Foundation/American Heart Association Task Force on Practice Guidelines. *Circulation.* 2011;123:e426.

Fihn SD, et al. 2012 ACCF/AHA/ACP/AATS/PCNA/SCAI/STS guideline for the diagnosis and management of patients with stable ischemic heart disease: a report of the American College of Cardiology Foundation/American Heart Association Task Force on Practice Guidelines, and the American College of Physicians, American Association for Thoracic Surgery, Preventive Cardiovascular Nurses Association, Society for Cardiovascular Angiography and Interventions, and Society of Thoracic Surgeons. *Circulation.* 2012;126(25):e354.

Mosca L, et al. Effectiveness-based guidelines for the prevention of cardiovascular disease prevention in women—2011 update: a guideline from the American Heart Association. *Circulation.* 2011;123:1243.

Wright SR, et al. 2011 ACC/AHA focused update of the guidelines for the management of patients with unstable angina/non-ST elevation myocardial infarction: a report from the American College of Cardiology/American Heart Association Task Force on Practice Guidelines developed in collaboration with the American College of Emergency Physicians, Society for Cardiovascular Angiography and Interventions, and Society for Thoracic Surgeons. *J Am Coll Cardiol.* 2011;57:1920.

Nursing Management

Nursing management of a patient with CAD and angina incorporates a variety of nursing diagnoses (Box 14.8). Nursing interventions focus on early identification of myocardial ischemia, control of chest pain, recognition of complications, maintenance of a calm environment, and patient and family education.

Recognizing Myocardial Ischemia

Complaints of chest discomfort (angina) must be evaluated quickly because angina is an indicator of myocardial ischemia (see Box 14.7). The patient is asked to rate the intensity of the chest discomfort on a scale of 0 to 10. Pain levels must be assessed with sensitivity to differences in cultural manifestations of pain. The term *chest pain* is not to be used exclusively because some patients describe their angina as "pressure" or "heaviness." It is important to document the characteristics of the pain and the patient's heart rate and rhythm, BP, respirations, temperature, skin color, peripheral pulses, urine output, mentation, and overall tissue perfusion. A 12-lead ECG is used to identify the area of ischemic myocardium. The major concern is that the chest pain may represent preinfarction angina, and early identification is essential so that the patient can be immediately treated. Treatment may include transfer to the cardiac catheterization laboratory for a coronary arteriogram and opening of a blocked artery. If the hospital does not have a cardiac catheterization laboratory, GP IIb/IIIa receptor blockers may be infused to prevent the evolution of the acute MI before transfer.[2,16]

Relieving Chest Pain

In the critical care unit, control of angina is achieved by a combination of supplemental oxygen, nitrates, analgesia, and surveillance of angina and of the effects of pharmacologic therapy.

- *Oxygen:* All patients with acute ischemic pain are administered supplemental oxygen to increase myocardial oxygenation. Pulse oximetry is used to guide therapy and maintain oxygen saturation above 90% unless the patient has a history of chronic obstructive pulmonary disease and is a carbon dioxide retainer.
- *Nitrates:* A combination of intravenous and sublingual nitroglycerin is used to vasodilate the coronary arteries and decrease pain. After nitrate administration, the critical care nurse closely observes the patient for relief of chest pain, for return of the ST segment to baseline, and for the potential development of unwanted side effects such as hypotension and headache. Administration of a nitrate is avoided if the systolic BP is less than 90 mm Hg. Medication interactions with nitrates are another potential cause for concern. The phosphodiesterase inhibitor medication *sildenafil* is prescribed for several conditions including pulmonary hypertension (PH) (Revatio) and erectile dysfunction (Viagra). Sildenafil and nitrates in combination may contribute to a precipitous fall in BP.[3]
- *Analgesia:* Morphine (2 to 4 mg given intravenously) is the analgesic opiate of choice for preinfarction angina. It relieves pain and decreases fear and anxiety. After administration, the critical care nurse assesses the patient for pain relief and the development of unwanted side effects such as hypotension and respiratory depression.[2,16]
- *Aspirin:* Chewing an oral non–enteric-coated aspirin (162 to 325 mg) at the beginning of chest pain has been shown to reduce mortality. The nonenteric formulation is preferred because it increases absorption in the mouth when chewed, not swallowed.[2,16]

Maintaining a Calm Environment

Patients admitted to a critical care unit with unstable angina experience extreme anxiety and fear of death. The critical care nurse is faced with the challenge of ensuring that the elements of a calm environment to alleviate the patient's fear and anxiety are maintained, while being ready at all times to respond to an acute emergency such as a cardiac arrest or to assist with emergency intubation or insertion of hemodynamic monitoring catheters. Additional aspects of acute cardiac care are listed in Box 14.9.

BOX 14.9 PATIENT EDUCATION PLAN

Coronary Artery Disease and Angina

The patient should be able to teach back the following topics:

- Angina: Describe signs and symptoms such as pain, pressure, and heaviness in chest, arms, or jaw.
- Preinfarction or unstable angina: Any chest pain that is not relieved by a sublingual nitroglycerin (NTG) tablet taken 5 min apart × 3 doses provides a reason to call 911 (emergency services).
- Use of the 0–10 pain scale: Notify critical care nurse or emergency personnel of any changes in pain intensity.
- Use of sublingual NTG for angina: Pain intensity should decrease on pain scale after NTG administration. At home, NTG must be kept in a dark, airtight container, or it loses its potency. To ensure potency, the NTG supply must be replaced approximately every 6 months. Active NTG has a slight burning sensation when placed under the tongue.
- Avoid Valsalva maneuver.
- Risk factor modification tailored to the patient's individual risk factor profile:
  - Decrease fat intake to 30% of total calories a day.
  - Stop smoking.
  - Reduce salt intake.
  - Control hypertension.
  - Treat diabetes and control blood glucose levels (if patient has diabetes).
  - Increase physical activity; achieve ideal body weight.
- Intention to attend a cardiac rehabilitation program.
- Medication teaching about indications and side effects.
- Follow-up care after discharge.
- Symptoms to report to a health care professional.
- Discussion of how to handle emotional stress and anger.

Patient Education

In the critical care unit, the patient's ability to retain educational information is severely affected by stress and pain. Patient education topics that should be discussed when the clinical condition has stabilized are listed in Box 14.9. It is essential to teach avoidance of the Valsalva maneuver, which is defined as forced expiration against a closed glottis. This can be explained to the patient as "bearing down" during defecation or breath holding when repositioning in bed. The Valsalva maneuver causes an increase in intrathoracic pressure, which decreases venous return to the right side of the heart and can be associated with low BP and symptomatic bradycardia.

After the anginal pain is controlled, longer term education of the patient and the family can begin. Points to cover include (1) risk factor modification, (2) signs and symptoms of angina, (3) when to call the physician, (4) medications, and (5) dealing with emotions and stress. However, because the acute hospital length of stay for uncomplicated angina is usually less than 3 days, referral to a cardiac rehabilitation program for a controlled exercise program and risk factor modification after discharge may be the most helpful teaching intervention a critical care nurse can provide. Clinical practice guidelines for the management of CAD and stable angina are listed in Box 14.6 earlier in the chapter.

MYOCARDIAL INFARCTION

Description and Etiology

Myocardial infarction is the term used to describe irreversible myocardial necrosis (cell death) that results from an abrupt decrease or total cessation of coronary blood flow to a specific area of the myocardium. In the hospital, this is often referred to as an *acute MI*, indicating the sudden onset and the life-threatening nature of the event. Increasingly, an acute MI is described in relation to whether ST segment elevation is seen on a diagnostic 12-lead ECG. It may be labeled an *acute NSTEMI*[16] or an *acute STEMI* (ST segment elevation MI).[2]

Three mechanisms can block the coronary artery and are responsible for the acute reduction in oxygen delivery to the myocardium: (1) plaque rupture, (2) new coronary artery thrombosis, and (3) coronary artery spasm close to the ruptured plaque.

Myocardial tissue can best be salvaged within the first 2 hours (120 minutes) after the onset of anginal symptoms, as illustrated in Fig. 14.3.[30] The earlier the myocardium is revascularized, the better the chances of survival. However, many people do not seek treatment until the acute phase has passed or delay seeking treatment because of denial of symptoms.

Pathophysiology

Ischemia

The outer region of the infarcted myocardial area is the *zone of ischemia*, or penumbra, as illustrated in Fig. 14.4. It is composed of viable cells. Priority interventions are targeted to save this viable muscle. Repolarization in this zone is temporarily impaired but eventually is restored to normal. Repolarization of the cells in this area manifests as T wave inversion on the ECG (Fig. 14.5B).

Injury

The infarcted zone is surrounded by injured but still potentially viable tissue in an area known as the *zone of injury* (see Fig. 14.4). Cells in this area do not fully repolarize because of the deficient blood supply. This is recorded on the ECG as elevation of the ST segment (Fig. 14.5C).

Infarction

The area of dead muscle (necrosis) in the myocardium is known as the *zone of infarction* (see Fig. 14.4). On the ECG, evidence of this zone is seen as new pathologic Q waves, which reflect a lack of depolarization from the cardiac surface involved in the MI (Fig. 14.5D). As healing takes place, the cells in this area are replaced by scar tissue.

Q Wave Myocardial Infarction

MIs are classified according to the location on the myocardial surface and the muscle layers affected. Not all infarctions cause necrosis in all layers, as shown in Fig. 14.6. A transmural MI involves all three cardiac layers—*endocardium, myocardium,* and *epicardium.* A transmural (full-thickness) MI usually provokes significant ECG changes (see Fig. 14.5). This is also described as a *Q wave MI.* Not every acute MI produces a recognizable series of Q waves on the 12-lead ECG. Some patients who had a demonstrated Q wave on a 12-lead ECG as a result of an acute MI lose the Q wave months or years later. The reasons for this are unknown, but it may represent the development of collateral circulation.

Twelve-Lead Electrocardiogram Changes

The ECG changes produced by an MI demonstrate alteration in myocardial depolarization (QRS complex) and repolarization (ST segment). The changes in repolarization are seen by the presence of new Q waves. These new, pathologic Q waves are deeper and wider than the tiny Q waves found on a normal 12-lead ECG.[3,16]

EMS on Scene

- EMS arrival on scene as FMC
- Prehospital 12-lead ECG by EMS to diagnose STEMI

- EMS transport directly to a PCI-Capable hospital with FMC-to-PCI device goal of ≤90 minutes
- Activate hospital PCI team when en route to hospital

- Onset of symptoms
- Call 911

Non-PCI Capable Hospital

- Immediate interhospital transport to a PCI-Capable hospital for patients with STEMI
- Goal is FMC-to-PCI device time of ≤120 minutes.
- When unavoidable time delays will make the FMC-to-PCI device time longer than 120 minutes, fibrinolysis should be selected as the method of reperfusion for patients without contraindications.
- IV fibrinolysis should start within 30 minutes of arrival.

PCI-Capable Hospital

- When a patient is initially seen at a PCI-Capable hospital, the goal is a door-to-PCI device time of under 90 minutes.

Goal is Total Ischemic Time ≤ 120 Minutes

FIG. 14.3 Evaluation of Prehospital Chest Pain and Acute Coronary Syndrome and Treatment Options. The first step is to call 911 (green arrow). Transport to a PCI-capable hospital is always the optimal first choice when available (red arrows). Transport to a non-PCI-capable hospital is considered when other options are unavailable (yellow arrow and yellow box). *ECG*, electrocardiogram; *EMS*, emergency medical services; *FMC*, first medical contact; *PCI*, percutaneous coronary intervention; *STEMI*, ST segment elevation myocardial infarction.

Zone of ischemia
Zone of injury
Zone of infarction

Reciprocal Changes Shown on Opposite Side

LEFT VENTRICLE

FIG. 14.4 Zone of ischemia, zone of injury, and zone of infarction are shown through electrocardiogram waveforms and reciprocal waveforms corresponding to each zone.

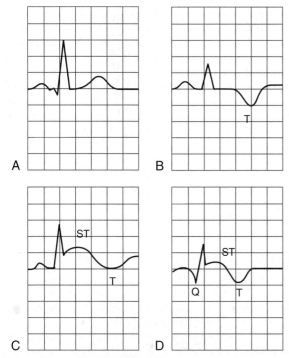

FIG. 14.5 Electrocardiogram (ECG) Changes Indicative of Ischemia, Injury, and Infarction (Necrosis) of the Myocardium.
(A) Normal ECG. (B) Ischemia indicated by inversion of the T wave. (C) Ischemia and current of injury indicated by T wave inversion and ST segment elevation. The ST segment may be elevated above or depressed below the baseline, depending on whether the tracing is from a lead facing toward or away from the infarcted area and depending on whether epicardial or endocardial injury occurs. Epicardial injury causes ST segment elevation in leads facing the epicardium. (D) Ischemia, injury, and myocardial necrosis. The Q wave indicates necrosis of the myocardium.

TABLE 14.6 New York Heart Association Functional Classification of Heart Failure

Class	Definition
I	Normal daily activity does not initiate symptoms
II	Normal daily activities initiate onset of symptoms, but symptoms subside with rest
III	Minimal activity initiates symptoms; patients are usually symptom-free at rest
IV	Any type of activity initiates symptoms, and symptoms are present at rest

TABLE 14.7 Correlations Among Ventricular Surfaces, Electrocardiogram Leads, and Coronary Arteries

Surface of Left Ventricle	ECG Leads	Usually Involved
Inferior	II, III, aVF	Right coronary artery
Lateral	V_5–V_6, I, aVL	Left circumflex artery
Anterior	V_2–V_4	Left anterior descending artery
Anterior lateral	V_1–V_6, I, aVL	Left main coronary artery
Septal	V_1–V_2	Left anterior descending artery
Posterior	V_1–V_2	Left circumflex or right coronary artery (reciprocal changes)
	V_7–V_9 (direct)	

I lateral	aVR	V_1 septal	V_4 anterior
II inferior	aVL lateral	V_2 septal	V_5 lateral
III inferior	aVF inferior	V_3 anterior	V_6 lateral

ECG, electrocardiogram.

Myocardial Infarction Location

The location of infarction is determined by correlating the ECG leads with Q waves and the ST segment and T wave abnormalities (Table 14.6). The ECG manifestations that are used to diagnose MI and pinpoint the area of damaged ventricle include inverted T waves, ST segment elevation, and pathologic Q waves in specific lead groupings, as described subsequently.

Anterior wall infarction. Anterior wall infarction results from occlusion of the proximal left anterior descending artery (Table 14.7). ST segment elevation is expected in leads V_1 through V_4 on the 12-lead ECG, as shown in Fig. 14.7. If the left main coronary artery is occluded, the ECG manifestations will involve almost all precordial leads V_1 through V_6 and leads I and aVL (see Table 14.7). These specific groups of ECG changes that help locate the part of the heart that is experiencing infarction are called *indicative changes.* A large anterior wall MI may be associated with left ventricular pump failure, cardiogenic shock, or death.

Left lateral wall infarction. Left lateral wall infarction occurs as a result of occlusion of the circumflex coronary artery. On a 12-lead ECG, new Q waves and ST segment T wave changes are seen in leads I, aVL, V_5, and V_6 (Fig. 14.8). In reality, few patients present with only lateral wall ECG changes, and some

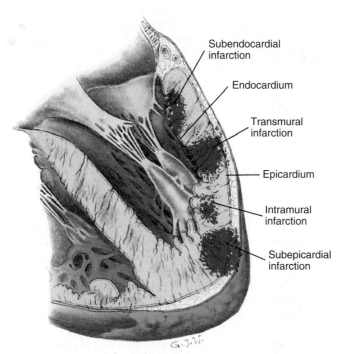

FIG. 14.6 Location of Infarctions in Myocardium.

Subendocardial infarction
Endocardium
Transmural infarction
Epicardium
Intramural infarction
Subepicardial infarction

anterior wall leads (V_3 and V_4) may show evidence of injury or infarction.

Inferior wall infarction. Inferior wall infarction occurs with occlusion of the right coronary artery. This infarction manifests by ECG changes in leads II, III, and aV_F (Fig. 14.9). Conduction disturbances are expected with an inferior wall MI and are related to the anatomy of the coronary arterial supply. Because the right coronary artery perfuses the sinoatrial node in slightly more than half of the population and supplies the proximal bundle of His and the atrioventricular (AV) node in more than 90% of individuals, heart block and other conduction disturbances should be anticipated.

Right ventricular infarction. Infarction of the right ventricle occurs when a blockage occurs in a proximal section of the right coronary artery. This places the entire right ventricle and inferior wall at risk. Right ventricular ischemia can be demonstrated in one-half of inferior wall STEMIs, although only 10% to 15% show the hemodynamic abnormalities associated with classic infarction of the right ventricle. If massive infarction occurs, the patient can experience cardiogenic shock, which carries a mortality rate of more than 50% in this population.[31]

The ECG leads on the 12-lead ECG also correlate with the coronary arteries. Leads can also be placed on the right side of the chest to assist in the diagnosis of right ventricular infarction and posteriorly to show a posterior infarction. To detect a right ventricular infarction, specific ECG lead placement is used. Electrodes are placed over the right precordium (chest) in a mirror image of the conventional left-sided leads. It is important to write R on the 12-lead ECG (eg, V_1R through V_6R) in front of the recorded right ventricular chest leads to ensure that the lead location is clear. The limb leads are not affected. Fig. 13.36C in Chapter 13 shows the correct position of the right-sided precordial leads used to diagnose an acute right ventricular MI. The ECG voltage is much lower in the V_1R through V_6R leads; when detected, ST segment elevation is usually seen in V_4R (Fig. 14.10).[2] The right ventricle has a very thin wall, which means that ST segment elevation is detected only in the right ventricular leads during the acute phase of the infarction.

Posterior wall infarction. Infarction in the posterior wall can occur because of a blockage in the right coronary artery or in the circumflex artery. This occurs because both arteries supply this section of the heart, although the right coronary artery is generally the dominant vessel. A posterior wall MI is difficult to detect but may be identified by specific leads placed in the left scapular area or by very tall R waves in leads V_1 and V_2 (Fig. 14.11). Fig. 13.36D in Chapter 13 shows the correct placement of the left posterior leads used to diagnose an acute posterior MI.

Non–ST Segment Elevation Myocardial Infarction

The 12-lead ECG is a highly useful diagnostic tool. For many years, it was considered the gold standard when diagnosing acute MI. However, the ST segment is not elevated in every acute MI. One reason for the lack of ST segment elevation may be that the infarction and subsequent necrosis are not full-thickness lesions. Because some of the muscle in the area can still be depolarized, ST segment elevation may not occur. This type of MI is also less likely to develop Q waves on a subsequent 12-lead ECG after the acute phase has passed. This situation is diagnostically known as an NSTEMI.[27] This condition has previously been described by several names

including nontransmural MI, non–Q wave MI, and subendocardial MI. Because patients who sustain an NSTEMI do have CAD, it is important that they be treated aggressively to minimize the size of the infarcted area. Without the visual clue of ST segment elevation on the 12-lead ECG, the patients cannot receive immediate intravenous fibrinolytic agents, but they can be appropriately managed in an interventional catheterization laboratory and receive GP IIb/IIIa inhibitor therapy, as illustrated in the timeline in Fig. 14.3. The 12-lead ECG plays a vital role in identifying the treatment plan for a patient with ACS. Visualizing ST segment elevation when present is helpful. Patients without ST segment elevation may still be at risk for becoming unstable and should be monitored (Fig. 14.12). In this case, the definitive diagnosis may be made in the cardiac catheterization laboratory or by elevation of specific cardiac biomarkers.

Cardiac Biomarkers During Myocardial Infarction

Cardiac biomarkers are released in the presence of damage and necrosis of the myocardium. These biomarkers are also called *cardiac enzymes.* To confirm the diagnosis of acute MI, the serum biomarkers troponin I or troponin T are measured by a blood test. Troponins begin to rise within 3-4 hours of STEMI and are detectable for 7-10 days. Creatine kinase–muscle/brain (CK-MB) is another cardiac biomarker that may be measured. If the coronary artery is opened by fibrinolytic therapy or a percutaneous catheter intervention (PCI), the biomarkers exhibit a more rapid increase and dramatic decrease (Fig. 14.13). Information on biomarkers is also presented in Table 13.16 in Chapter 13.

Complications of Acute Myocardial Infarction

Many patients experience complications occurring early or late in the post-MI course. These complications may result from electrical dysfunction or from a cardiac contractility problem. Electrical dysfunctions include bradycardia, bundle branch blocks, and various degrees of heart block. Pumping complications can cause heart failure, pulmonary edema, and cardiogenic shock. The presence of a new murmur in a patient with an acute MI warrants special attention, as it may indicate rupture of the papillary muscle. The murmur can be indicative of severe damage and impending complications such as heart failure and pulmonary edema.

Sinus bradycardia. Sinus bradycardia (heart rate less than 60 beats/min) occurs frequently in patients who sustain an acute MI. It is more prevalent with an inferior wall infarction in the first hour after STEMI. Symptomatic bradycardia with hypotension and low cardiac output is treated with atropine (0.5 to 1.0 mg by intravenous push), repeated every 3 to 5 minutes to a maximum dose of 0.03 mg/kg (eg, 2 mg for a person who weighs 70 kg) per Advanced Cardiac Life Support guidelines.

Sinus tachycardia. Sinus tachycardia (heart rate greater than 100 beats/min) most often occurs with an anterior wall MI. Anterior infarctions impair left ventricular pumping ability, reducing the ejection fraction and the stroke volume. In an attempt to maintain cardiac output, the heart rate increases. Sinus tachycardia is corrected by treating the underlying cause, as it greatly increases myocardial oxygen consumption, leading to further ischemia.

Atrial dysrhythmias. Premature atrial contractions occur frequently in patients who sustain an acute MI. Atrial fibrillation

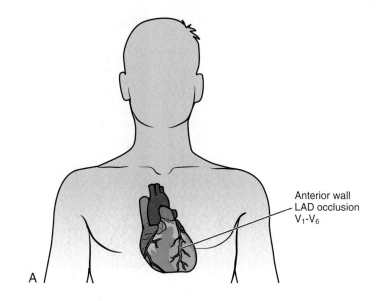

Anterior wall
LAD occlusion
V_1-V_6

A

LIMB LEADS		PRECORDIAL LEADS	
Lead I	AV_R	V_1	V_4
Lead II	AV_L	V_2	V_5
Lead III	AV_F	V_3	V_6

B

Example of an Acute Anterior Wall MI

C

FIG. 14.7 Changes Seen on 12-Lead Electrocardiogram (ECG) With Anterior Wall Myocardial Infarction (MI). (A) Infarction location on the cardiac wall. (B) ECG leads with expected ST segment elevation. (C) A 12-lead ECG from a patient experiencing left anterior wall MI. LAD, left anterior descending artery.

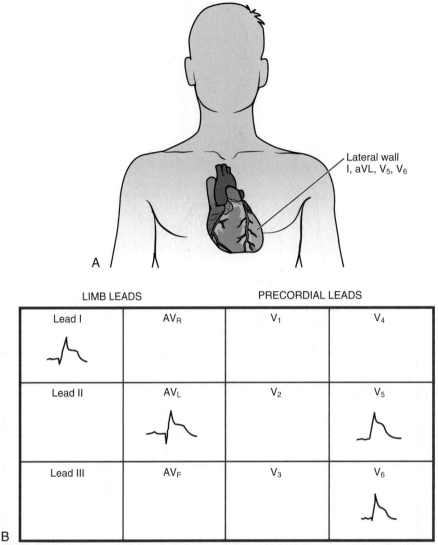

LIMB LEADS   PRECORDIAL LEADS

Lead I	AV$_R$	V$_1$	V$_4$
Lead II	AV$_L$	V$_2$	V$_5$
Lead III	AV$_F$	V$_3$	V$_6$

FIG. 14.8 Changes Seen on 12-Lead Electrocardiogram (ECG) With Lateral Wall ST Segment Elevation Myocardial Infarction. (A) Infarction location on the cardiac wall. (B) ECG leads with expected ST segment elevation.

(AF) is also common and may occur spontaneously or may be preceded by premature atrial contractions. With the onset of AF, the loss of organized atrial contraction decreases cardiac output by up to 20%. Patients with new-onset or preexisting AF have higher morbidity rates than patients without AF during an ACS event. Patients with ACS and new-onset AF experience a greater number of in-hospital adverse events such as reinfarction, shock, pulmonary edema, bleeding, and stroke. Management of AF includes rate control and rhythm control.[32]

Ventricular dysrhythmias. Premature ventricular contractions are seen in almost all patients within the first few hours after MI. They are initially controlled through administration of oxygen to reduce myocardial hypoxia and by correcting acid–base or electrolyte imbalances. In the setting of an acute MI, premature ventricular contractions are pharmacologically treated if they have the following characteristics: frequent (more than 6 per minute), closely coupled (R-on-T phenomenon), multiform shapes, and occurrence in bursts of three or more, increasing the risk of sustained ventricular tachycardia (VT). Ventricular fibrillation (VF) is a life-threatening dysrhythmia are associated with high mortality in acute MI. Beta-blockers are prescribed after acute MI to decrease mortality from ventricular dysrhythmias.

Atrioventricular heart block during myocardial infarction. Heart block can occur in 6% to 14% of patients with STEMI, and these patients have increased mortality rates. In STEMI, AV block most often occurs after an inferior wall MI. Because the right coronary artery supplies the AV node in 90% of the population, right coronary artery occlusion leads to ischemia and infarction of the AV node cells. The development of sudden heart block has become much less common because most patients receive fibrinolysis or undergo PCI to open the occluded vessel. In most cases, transcutaneous pacing is the primary intervention; transvenous pacemakers are used less frequently.

Ventricular aneurysm after myocardial infarction. A ventricular aneurysm (Fig. 14.14) is a noncontractile, thinned left ventricular wall that results from an acute transmural infarction. It most often occurs in the setting of an acute left anterior descending artery occlusion with a wide area

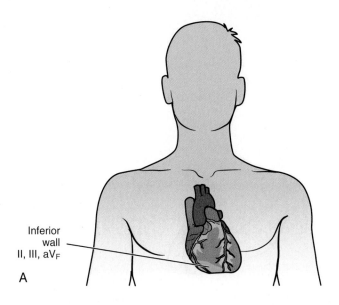

Inferior
wall
II, III, aV_F

A

LIMB LEADS   PRECORDIAL LEADS

Lead I	aV_R	V_1	V_4
Lead II	aV_L	V_2	V_5
Lead III	aV_F	V_3	V_6

B

Example of an Acute Inferior Wall MI

C

FIG. 14.9 Changes Seen on 12-Lead Electrocardiogram (ECG) With Inferior Wall Myocardial Infarction (MI). (A) Infarction location on the cardiac wall. (B) ECG leads with expected ST segment elevation. (C) A 12-lead ECG from a patient experiencing inferior wall MI.

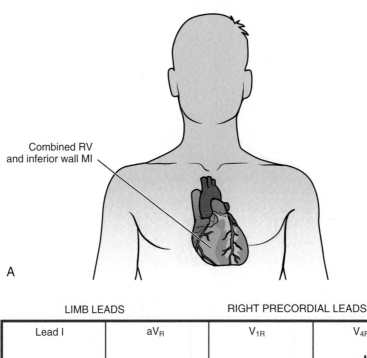

LIMB LEADS   RIGHT PRECORDIAL LEADS

Lead I	aV$_R$	V$_{1R}$	V$_{4R}$
Lead II	aV$_L$	V$_{2R}$	V$_{5R}$
Lead III	aV$_F$	V$_{3R}$	V$_{6R}$

FIG. 14.10 Changes Seen on 12-Lead Electrocardiogram (ECG) With Inferior Right Ventricular (RV) ST Segment Elevation Myocardial Infarction. (A) Picture of an RV wall MI. (B) Acute inferior wall MI, with the right coronary artery (RCA) occluded.

of infarcted myocardium. The most effective prevention is early reperfusion of the myocardium, accomplished by opening the thrombosed coronary artery. The most common complications of a ventricular aneurysm are acute heart failure, systemic emboli, angina, and VT. Treatment is directed toward management of these complications and surgical repair by left ventricular aneurysmectomy. The affected area may be described as *hypokinetic* (contracts poorly), *akinetic* (noncontractile scar tissue), or *dyskinetic* (scar tissue that moves in the opposite direction to the normal contractile myocardium). The prognosis depends on the size of the aneurysm, the level of overall left ventricular dysfunction, and the severity of coexisting CAD.

Ventricular septal rupture after myocardial infarction. Rupture of the ventricular septal wall after MI is a rare but potentially lethal complication of an acute anterior wall MI (Fig. 14.15). *Ventricular septal rupture,* also known as *acquired ventricular septal defect,* is an abnormal communication between the right and left ventricle. Studies report this complication occurs in less than 0.2% to 3.9% of all MIs, and the incidence has declined

because most patients with STEMI have the blocked coronary artery opened through PCI or fibrinolysis within a short time frame after diagnosis.[33] Nevertheless, rupture of the ventricular septum carries an extremely high mortality rate. Mortality rates between 35% and 73% are typical.[33] Most patients with septal rupture also have signs and symptoms of cardiogenic shock. Ventricular septal rupture manifests as severe chest pain, syncope, hypotension, and sudden hemodynamic deterioration caused by shunting of blood from the high-pressure left ventricle into the low-pressure right ventricle through the new septal opening. A holosystolic murmur (often accompanied by a thrill) can be auscultated and is best heard along the left sternal border. Rupture of the septum is a medical and surgical emergency. The patient's condition is stabilized with vasodilators and an intraaortic balloon pump (IABP) to decrease afterload. The goal of afterload reduction in this patient population is to decrease the amount of blood being shunted to the right side of the heart and consequently to increase the flow of blood to the systemic circulation. Survival improves if the septal rupture is very small and the patient's condition is sufficiently stable to wait for scar

Example of an Acute Inferior Wall and RV Wall MI. Shows ST elevation in leads II, III, AV$_F$, and reciprocal changes (ST depression) in anterior and lateral leads.

#1

Reciprocal changes seen in V$_1$, V$_2$, V$_3$, V$_4$, I, and aVL, which provides a clue as to the extent of the MI.
Angiographic changes associated with an occlusion of the RCA.
These findings can range from:
  - Proximal occlusion (near origin of RCA) that will produce inferior MI, posterior MI, and RV MI
  - Middle RCA occlusion that will produce posterior and inferior MI
C - Distal RCA occlusion that will produce inferior wall MI

Example of an Acute RV MI in right precordial leads.

#2

ECG shows ST elevation in right precordial leads (V$_3$R to V$_6$R), indicating RV wall injury/infarct.
  Note limb leads are identical in both ECGs.

D   **These two 12-lead ECGs are from the same patient with RV MI.**

FIG. 14.10, cont'd (C) Example of an acute inferior RV wall MI with conventional 12-lead ECG. (D) Example of an acute RV wall MI with a right-sided 12-lead ECG. Both 12-lead ECGs are taken from the same patient.

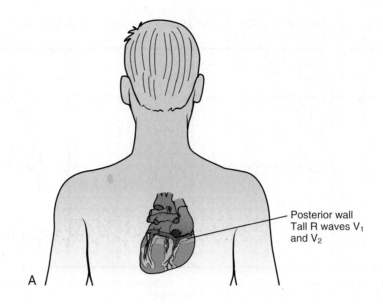

Posterior wall
Tall R waves V₁
and V₂

A

B

FIG. 14.11 Changes Seen on 12-Lead Electrocardiogram (ECG) With ST Segment Elevation Myocardial Infarction (STEMI). (A) Infarction location on the cardiac wall. (B) ECG leads with expected ST segment elevation in posterior wall STEMI.

FIG. 14.12 Acute Coronary Syndrome: STEMI, NSTEMI, Unstable Angina, Electrocardiography Changes Over Time.

tissue to form before surgical repair. When the septal opening is large, the massive left-to-right shunt across the septum makes the chances of survival dismal with or without surgery.[33]

Papillary muscle rupture after myocardial infarction. Papillary muscle rupture can occur when the infarct involves the area around one of the papillary muscles that support the mitral valve. Infarction of the papillary muscles results in ineffective mitral valve closure, and blood is forced back into the low-pressure left atrium during ventricular systole. The rupture may be partial or complete. Complete rupture is catastrophic and precipitates severe acute mitral regurgitation, cardiogenic shock, and high risk of death.

Partial rupture (Fig. 14.16) also results in mitral regurgitation, but the condition can be stabilized with aggressive medical management using an IABP and vasodilators. Urgent surgical intervention is required to replace the mitral valve.[34]

Cardiac wall rupture after myocardial infarction. The incidence of cardiac wall rupture has two peak times. The first occurs within the first 24 hours, and the second occurs between 3 and 5 days after infarction when leukocyte scavenger cells are removing necrotic debris, thinning the myocardial wall. The onset is sudden and usually catastrophic. Bleeding into the pericardial sac results in cardiac tamponade, cardiogenic shock, pulseless electrical activity, and death. Survival is rare. If rupture occurs in the hospital, emergency pericardiocentesis is required to relieve the tamponade until a surgical repair can

be attempted. The best prevention is early reperfusion of the myocardium.

Pericarditis after myocardial infarction. Pericarditis is inflammation of the pericardial sac. It can occur during or after acute MI. The damaged epicardium becomes rough and inflamed and irritates the pericardium lying adjacent to it, precipitating pericarditis. Pain is the most common symptom of pericarditis, and a pericardial friction rub is the most common initial sign. The friction rub is best auscultated with a stethoscope at the sternal border and is described as a grating, scraping, or leathery scratching. Pericarditis frequently produces a pericardial effusion.[35] After the effusion occurs, the friction rub may disappear. On a 12-lead ECG, pericarditis may manifest as elevation of the ST segment in all the typically upright leads.[36] Pericarditis is treated with nonsteroidal antiinflammatory drugs, aspirin, and rest. Pericarditis that occurs as a late complication of acute MI is known as *Dressler syndrome.*

Heart failure and acute myocardial infarction. Many patients with acute STEMI also have acute heart failure on admission to the hospital. These patients have often waited longer to come to the hospital and are older and more likely to be female. Compared with patients with acute MI but not heart failure, these patients have a higher risk of adverse in-hospital events and have longer lengths of stay and higher in-hospital mortality rates. More detailed information about heart failure is presented later in this chapter.

FIG. 14.13 Cardiac Biomarkers During ST Elevation Myocardial Infarction and the Impact of Early Reperfusion. ACS, Acute Coronary Syndrome, CK-MB, Creatinine-Kinase: Muscle/Brain; MI, Myocardial Infarction; PCI, Percutaneous Coronary Intervention; STEMI, ST segment elevation myocardial infarction; TnC, Troponin C; TnI, Troponin I; TnT, Troponin T;

Medical Management

Quality outcomes research shows that compliance with the guidelines developed by the American College of Cardiology (ACC) and the AHA decreases in-hospital mortality after acute MI.[37] When the AHA/ACC guidelines for treatment of STEMI or NSTEMI are followed, patients admitted to hospitals have an 8.3% in-hospital mortality rate compared with a 15.3% mortality rate in patients treated at hospitals where the most recent guidelines are not fully used.[37] The guidelines are research based and are designed to improve the outcome of patients admitted to the hospital with acute MI. Clinical guidelines address the issues of interventions to open the coronary artery, anticoagulation, prevention of dysrhythmias, intensive glucose control, and prevention of ventricular remodeling after STEMI. To facilitate

rapid coronary artery revascularization in STEMI, local hospitals are encouraged to develop a coordinated patient transfer strategy between PCI-capable and non–PCI-capable hospitals, as illustrated in Fig. 14.3.[2]

Recanalization of Coronary Artery

The essential immediate interventions for a patient with an acute STEMI are fibrinolytic therapy or PCI to open the occluded artery.[2] All clinical guidelines emphasize the need for patients with symptoms of ACS to be rapidly triaged and treated.[2]

Anticoagulation

In the acute phase after STEMI, heparin is administered in combination with fibrinolytic therapy to recanalize (open) the

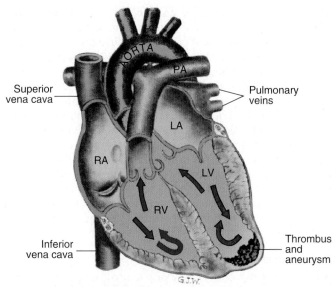

FIG. 14.14 Ventricular Aneurysm After Acute Myocardial Infarction. LA, left atrium; LV, left ventricle; PA, pulmonary artery; RA, right atrium; RV, right ventricle.

FIG. 14.16 Papillary Muscle Rupture After Acute Myocardial Infarction. LA, left atrium; LV, left ventricle; PA, pulmonary artery; RA, right atrium; RV, right ventricle.

FIG. 14.15 Ventricular Septal Rupture After Acute Myocardial Infarction. LA, left atrium; LV, left ventricle; PA, pulmonary artery; RA, right atrium; RV, right ventricle.

coronary artery.[2] For patients who will receive fibrinolytic therapy, an initial heparin bolus of 60 units/kg (maximum 5000 units) is given intravenously, followed by a continuous heparin drip at 12 units/kg per hour (maximum 1000 units/h) to maintain an activated partial thromboplastin time (aPTT) between 50 and 70 seconds (1.5 to 2.0 times control) for 48 hours or until revascularization.[2]

It is also prudent to administer intravenous UFH or subcutaneous low-molecular-weight heparin (LMWH) if the patient is at risk for thrombus development. For patients with known heparin-induced thrombocytopenia, as an alternative to

LMWH or UFH, a third class of antithrombotic medications is available—direct antithrombotic agents (eg, hirudin, bivalirudin, argatroban). Patients at risk for thrombotic emboli include patients with an anterior wall infarction, AF, previous embolus, cardiomyopathy, or cardiogenic shock.

Dysrhythmia Prevention

The antidysrhythmic with the best safety record after STEMI is amiodarone. Beta-blockers are another class of antidysrhythmics that are recommended for all patients after STEMI. Beta-blockers prevent ventricular dysrhythmias, lower BP, and prevent reinfarction especially in patients with left ventricular dysfunction.[2]

Prevention of Ventricular Remodeling

Many patients are at risk for development of heart failure after STEMI. Vasodilating medications (angiotensin-converting enzyme inhibitors [ACEIs] or angiotensin II receptor blockers [ARBs]) can stop or limit the ventricular remodeling that leads to heart failure. Ventricular remodeling refers to progressive changes in the size, architecture, and shape of the myocardium and occurs because of an injury such as MI. Ventricular remodeling is modulated by catecholamines and activation of neurohormonal compensatory mechanisms. The heart chamber walls ultimately become dilated, thinned, and poorly contractile. An ACEI or, if it is not tolerated, an ARB is indicated for all patients after STEMI.[2] Information about the clinical effects of heart failure is provided later in this chapter.

Nursing Management

Nursing management of a patient with an acute MI incorporates a variety of nursing diagnoses (Box 14.10). Nursing interventions focus on achieving a balance between myocardial oxygen supply and demand, preventing complications, and providing patient and family education.

Balance of Myocardial Oxygen Supply and Demand

In the acute period, if severe heart muscle damage has occurred, myocardial oxygen supply is increased by the administration of

BOX 14.10 NURSING DIAGNOSES

Myocardial Infarction

- Acute Pain related to transmission and perception of cutaneous, visceral, muscular, or ischemic impulses, p. 1010
- Decreased Cardiac Output related to alterations in preload, p. 1015
- Decreased Cardiac Output related to alterations in afterload, p. 1015
- Decreased Cardiac Output related to alterations in contractility, p. 1016
- Decreased Cardiac Output related to alterations in heart rate or rhythm, p. 1016
- Activity Intolerance related to cardiopulmonary dysfunction, p. 1006
- Risk for Decreased Cardiac Tissue Perfusion, p. 1041
- Disturbed Sleep Pattern related to fragmented sleep, p. 1023
- Anxiety related to threat to biologic, psychologic, or social integrity, p. 1012
- Ineffective Coping related to situational crisis and personal vulnerability, p. 1036
- Powerlessness related to lack of control over current situation or disease progression, p. 1038
- Deficient Knowledge related to lack of previous exposure to information, p. 1020 (see Box 14.12, Patient Education Plan for Myocardial Infarction)

BOX 14.11 Clinical Manifestations of Acute Myocardial Infarction

- Tachycardia with or without ectopy
- Bradycardia
- Normotension or hypotension
- Tachypnea
- Diminished heart sounds, especially S_1
- If left ventricular dysfunction present, may have S_3, S_4, or both
- Systolic murmur
- Pulmonary crackles
- Pulmonary edema
- Air hunger
- Orthopnea
- Frothy sputum
- Decreased cardiac output
- Decreased urine output
- Decreased peripheral pulses
- Slow capillary refill
- Restlessness
- Confusion
- Anxiety
- Agitation
- Denial
- Anger

supplemental oxygen to prevent tissue hypoxia. This imbalance manifests as many clinical signs (Box 14.11). Cardiac medications play an increasingly important role in balancing supply and demand, and the critical care nurse administers and monitors the effectiveness of these agents. For a patient with a low cardiac output, positive inotropic medications such as dobutamine, dopamine, or both may be administered. Milrinone, a phosphodiesterase inhibitor, which increases contractility by improving sarcolemma calcium uptake and causes positive inotropic effects in the myocardium, may be prescribed.

In contrast to dobutamine and dopamine, milrinone does not compete for receptor sites in patients taking beta-blockers. These inotropic agents are used to increase cardiac contractility in the healthy areas of the heart (increasing oxygen supply), while avoiding damage to the recently infarcted areas. Myocardial oxygen supply can be further enhanced by the use of coronary artery vasodilators. Nitroglycerin is often administered for the first 48 hours to increase vasodilation and prevent myocardial ischemia. Research evidence supports the administration of early beta-blockade therapy to decrease myocardial workload and to prevent dysrhythmias. However, if the patient is in cardiogenic shock, beta-blockers are withheld until the cardiac output has improved.[2] Other interventions to decrease cardiac work and myocardial oxygen consumption include bed rest with bedside commode privileges when the patient is clinically stable.

Prevention of Complications

A thorough grasp of the range of potential complications that can occur after STEMI is essential. Cardiac monitoring for early detection of ventricular dysrhythmias is ongoing. Assessment for signs of continued ischemic pain is important because angina is a warning sign of the myocardium being at risk. In response to angina, a 12-lead ECG is obtained to determine if an extension of the infarct exists, nitroglycerin is administered, and the physician is notified immediately so that interventions may be initiated to limit the size of the MI. Heart failure is a serious complication after STEMI. When the patient's BP is stable, treatment with ACEIs is initiated. These vasodilators are used to prevent left ventricular remodeling and dilation that occurs in many patients after acute MI. Hypotension is a potential complication of ACEIs, especially with the first dose. It is an important nursing responsibility to monitor BP and patient symptoms after taking an ACEI. Surveillance to detect obvious and subtle signs of bleeding is also a priority because so many patients with acute MI receive antiplatelet, anticoagulant, and fibrinolytic medications.[2,16,27]

In the first 24 hours after an MI, diet is progressed as tolerated. Preventing hospital-acquired pneumonia and deep vein thrombosis (DVT) is facilitated by early mobilization and raising the head of the bed 30 degrees or more. An upright position facilitates decrease in venous return, lowering of preload, and decrease in the workload of the myocardium. The patient is taught to avoid increasing intraabdominal pressure (Valsalva maneuver). Stool softeners may be given to the patient to lessen the risk of constipation from analgesics and bed rest and to decrease the risk of straining. Providing a calming and quiet environment that focuses on the well-being of the patient assists in the recovery phase.

Depression After Myocardial Infarction

Depression is a condition that occurs across a wide spectrum of human experience. Depression is a risk factor for development of CAD and impedes recovery after acute MI.[38] Key symptoms of depression mentioned frequently by cardiac patients are fatigue, change in appetite, and sleep disturbance.

Patient Education

After the acute phase of an MI, patient and family education becomes a priority. Education focuses on the following key elements: (1) risk factor reduction, (2) manifestations of angina, (3) when to call a physician or emergency services,

Myocardial Infarction

The patient should be able to teach back the following topics:

- Pathophysiology of coronary artery disease, angina, and acute myocardial infarction.
- Angina: Describe signs and symptoms such as pain, pressure, or heaviness in chest, arms, or jaw.
- Use of 0–10 pain scale: Notify critical care nurse or emergency personnel of any changes in chest pain intensity.
- Avoid Valsalva maneuver.
- Risk factor modification tailored to the patient's individual risk factor profile:
  - Decrease daily fat intake to less than 30% of total calories.
  - Reduce total serum cholesterol to less than 200 mg/dL.
  - Reduce low-density lipoprotein cholesterol to less than 70 mg/dL.
  - Stop smoking.
  - Reduce salt intake.
  - Control hypertension.
  - Control diabetes (if patient has diabetes).
  - Increase physical activity.
  - Achieve ideal body weight, if overweight.
- Referral to cardiac rehabilitation program.
- Medication teaching about indications and side effects.
- Follow-up care after discharge.
- Symptoms to report to a health care professional.
- Discussion of how to handle emotional stress and anger.

(4) medications, and (5) resumption of physical and sexual activities (Box 14.12). It is recommended that a referral be made to a cardiac rehabilitation program to reinforce education that was initiated during hospitalization.[2,39] Clinical practice guidelines for multidisciplinary care of a patient with an acute MI are listed in Box 14.13.

SUDDEN CARDIAC DEATH

Description

Of the patients who die suddenly each year of CHD, 50% of men and 64% of women have no previous symptoms of the disease. Of sudden cardiac deaths (SCDs), 70% to 89% occur in men, and the annual incidence is three to four times higher in men than in women; however, this disparity decreases with advancing age. People who have had an MI with symptoms that last less than 1 hour or occur in a hospital emergency department have an SCD rate four to six times higher than that of the general population. SCD represents approximately 5% of the total annual mortality rate for all causes.[40]

When the onset of symptoms is rapid, the most likely mechanism of SCD is VT, which degenerates into VF. Despite aggressive cardiopulmonary resuscitation (CPR) initiated outside the hospital, few individuals who sustain an out-of-hospital cardiac arrest survive to hospital discharge. Strategies that have been shown to improve resuscitation survival involve huge community-wide programs to teach laypersons CPR and how to use an automated external defibrillator. These programs assist with survival to hospital discharge.[1,41]

Etiology

Most SCD incidents occur in patients with preexisting ventricular dysfunction resulting from cardiac disease. Specific SCD risk factors include extensive coronary atherosclerosis with or without a history of acute MI; dilated or hypertrophic cardiomyopathy; valvular heart disease; autonomic nervous system abnormalities; electrical system abnormalities such as AV block, Wolff-Parkinson-White syndrome, long QT syndrome, or Brugada syndrome; and taking medications that prolong the Q–T interval.[41,42,43] An ejection fraction less than 30% and a history of ventricular dysrhythmias are powerful predictors of SCD. Other risk factors are listed in Box 14.14. Many individuals are unaware of their risk or have not considered other risk factors.

Medical Management

Depending on the length of time the patient was unconscious as a result of the cardiac arrest, cognitive defects may be present because of the lack of cerebral blood flow and resultant hypoxia. The cardiac arrest may also have damaged the myocardium and other tissues. Therapy is tailored to the needs of the patient.[44,45] For comatose patients at high risk for hypoxic brain injury after cardiac arrest, therapeutic hypothermia is initiated to preserve brain function. In the Framingham study, women experienced SCD at half the rate of men and were on average 6 to 10 years older than men when they experienced the event.[40] Prevention focuses on identification and treatment of high-risk cardiac patients (see sections on "Implantable Cardioverter Defibrillator" and "Antidysrhythmic Medications" in Chapter 15).

HEART FAILURE

Description and Etiology

The number of patients with heart failure is increasing in the United States. Almost 6 million adults (older than age 18 years) in the United States have heart failure. It is estimated that by 2030, an additional 3 million more people will be diagnosed with heart failure.[1] Fig. 14.17 is a concept map of heart failure.

Pathophysiology

Heart failure is a response to cardiac dysfunction, a condition in which the heart cannot pump blood at a volume required to meet the body's needs. Any condition that impairs the ability of the ventricles to fill or eject blood can cause heart failure. CAD with resultant necrotic damage to the left ventricle is the underlying cause of heart failure in most patients. Other major conditions that lead to heart failure include valvular dysfunction, infection (myocarditis or endocarditis), cardiomyopathy, and uncontrolled hypertension.[46] Hypertension is the precursor of heart failure in men and women.[1]

Assessment and Diagnosis

Heart failure is typically classified on the basis of New York Heart Association (NYHA) criteria. Patients are assigned into four groups, I through IV, according to the severity of symptoms and degree of patient activity eliciting symptoms (see Table 14.6). Research-based clinical guidelines suggest adding a second level of classification that emphasizes the progressive nature of heart failure through stages identified by increasing distress and intensified clinical interventions (Table 14.8).[47] Heart failure can manifest in many different ways, depending on how far ventricular remodeling and dysfunction have advanced. Heart failure may be discovered because of a known clinical syndrome such as acute MI or because of decreased exercise tolerance, fluid retention, or admission to the critical care unit for

QSEN BOX 14.13 **QSEN: Evidence-Based Practice**

Acute Coronary Syndrome and Acute Myocardial Infarction (Non-STEMI and STEMI)

Prevention of Acute Coronary Syndrome

The term *acute coronary syndrome* (ACS) is used to define the life-threatening consequences of coronary artery disease (CAD), notably unstable angina, non–ST segment elevation myocardial infarction (non-STEMI), and ST segment elevation myocardial infarction (STEMI):

- *Unstable angina* is a term that denotes chest pain that is not relieved by sublingual nitroglycerin or rest within 5 min.
- Non-STEMI is an acute myocardial infarction (MI) *without* ST segment elevation on the 12-lead electrocardiogram (ECG).
- STEMI is an acute MI *with* ST segment elevation on the 12-lead ECG.

All recommendations are class I, meaning that there is strong research evidence to support these recommendations.

Recommendations That Decrease Risk of Developing Non-STEMI and STEMI

- Primary care providers should evaluate CAD risk factors for all patients every 3–5 y using a validated risk assessment scoring tool.
- The 10-y risk of ACS and acute MI should be assessed for all patients who have more than two major risk factors through the use of evidence-based risk assessment tools.
- An intensive risk factor modification program is recommended for patients with established CAD or high-risk equivalents such as diabetes or chronic kidney disease.

Recommendations About Emergency ACS Symptoms

- A patient who has previously diagnosed CAD should take one sublingual nitroglycerin dose, and the patient (if alone) or a friend or relative should call 911 if chest pain or discomfort is unrelieved or worsening in 5 min.
- The same recommendation applies to a patient without known CAD. If pain is unrelieved with rest or worsening at 5 min, the patient (if alone) or a friend or relative should call 911.
- Patients with chest discomfort should be transported to the hospital by ambulance rather than be driven by a friend or relative.
- Family members should be advised to take a cardiopulmonary resuscitation (CPR) course before an ACS emergency occurs. This course teaches CPR skills, demonstrates use of an automated external defibrillator (AED), and educates participants about the "chain of survival" concept.

Recommendations for Prehospital EMS Paramedic First Responders

- First responders such as emergency medical services (EMS) paramedics can provide early defibrillation and advanced cardiac life support (ACLS) for patients in cardiac arrest.
- EMS personnel should administer 162–325 mg of nonenteric aspirin (chewed, not swallowed) to patients with chest pain and suspected STEMI.
- A prehospital fibrinolysis protocol is reasonable for patients with STEMI if there are physicians in the ambulance or if there is a well-organized EMS service with full-time paramedics plus 12-lead ECG transmission capability and online medical direction.
- Patients older than 75 y and patients with cardiogenic shock should be transported to a hospital with the capability to provide fibrinolytics, emergency percutaneous coronary intervention (PCI), or emergency coronary artery bypass graft (CABG) surgery.
- Patients with STEMI who have a contraindication to fibrinolytic therapy should be brought to a hospital with the capability to provide emergency PCI or CABG surgery. At the scene, the door-to-departure time should be *less than 30 min*. PCI should be initiated *within 90 min* after initial medical contact.

Recommendations for Initial Emergency Clinical Management

- Hospitals should establish multidisciplinary teams to facilitate rapid triage of patients who present to the emergency department (ED) with chest pain.

- Use of written protocols is recommended to standardize care. An immediate cardiology consultation is advised if the patient's symptoms fall outside the written protocol.

STEMI

- *Fibrinolytics for STEMI:* Time from coming into contact with the health care system (paramedics or ED) to receiving fibrinolytics should be *less than 30 min*. A brief, focused neurologic examination to determine prior stroke or presence of cognitive defects is necessary before administration of fibrinolytics.
- *PCI for STEMI:* Time from coming into contact with the health care system (paramedics or ED) to balloon inflation PCI should be *less than 90 min*.

Non-STEMI

- If the level of risk for a patient with non-STEMI is not immediately apparent, a "chest pain unit" within the ED permits close surveillance by competent clinicians without immediate hospital admission.
- Glycoprotein IIb/IIIa inhibitors for non-STEMI, in addition to aspirin and heparin, are indicated if cardiac catheterization or PCI is planned.
- PCI may be indicated for non-STEMI.

Recommendations for Initial Emergency Physical Assessment

Vital Signs

- Heart rate, blood pressure, respiratory rate, temperature, oxygen saturation with pulse oximetry (SpO_2), and ECG monitoring to detect presence of dysrhythmias are obtained.

Physical Assessment

- Assess for warm or cool skin, color, capillary refill, and peripheral pulses.
- Auscultate heart for cardiac murmur or new S_3 or S_4.
- Auscultate lungs for air entry plus crackles and wheezes.
- Observe for breathlessness and frothy pink sputum (pulmonary edema).
- Ask patient, family, or significant others for relevant history.

Recommendations for Emergency Diagnostics

12-Lead ECG

- For all patients with chest discomfort or angina-equivalent symptoms, a 12-lead ECG should be obtained and shown to the ED physician within 10 min after the patient's arrival in the ED.
- If the first ECG is normal, but the patient continues to have symptoms of chest pain or discomfort, the 12-lead ECG should be repeated at 5- to 10-min intervals, *or* continuous 12-lead ECG monitoring can be used.
- In patients with inferior wall infarction, right ventricular infarction must be suspected and right-sided ECG leads recorded. V_4R is the diagnostic lead of choice to diagnose ST segment elevation in the right ventricle.

Laboratory Studies

- Laboratory tests should be performed as part of the general management of STEMI but should not delay the administration of reperfusion therapy.

Cardiac Biomarkers

- Measurement of cardiac-specific troponins is recommended for patients with coexistent skeletal muscle injury. Clinicians are advised not to wait for results of the biomarker assay before initiating reperfusion therapy. Point-of-care (handheld) biomarker assay results can be used for rapid determination of treatment, but subsequent biomarker assays should be done by quantitative laboratory analysis.

Imaging Studies

- *Portable chest radiograph:* Obtaining a chest radiograph must not delay reperfusion therapy unless a major complication such as aortic dissection is suspected.

Acute Coronary Syndrome and Acute Myocardial Infarction (Non-STEMI and STEMI)

- *Portable echocardiography (transthoracic echocardiogram or transesophageal echocardiogram) or magnetic resonance imaging:* A scan should be obtained to distinguish aortic dissection from STEMI for patients in whom the symptoms are unclear.

Recommendations for Care
Prevent Hypoxia
- Supplemental oxygen is administered to maintain oxygen saturation greater than 90%.

Coronary Vasodilation
- Sublingual nitroglycerin (0.04 mg every 5 min × 3 doses) is administered. If chest pain or discomfort is ongoing, start a peripheral intravenous (IV) line. Administer IV nitroglycerin for relief of chest pain, control of hypertension, or relief of pulmonary congestion.

Pain Control
- Intravenous morphine sulfate (2–4 mg) is administered; dosage can be increased by 2- to 8-mg IV increments at 5- to 15-min intervals for STEMI pain control.

NSAIDs
- Discontinue nonsteroidal antiinflammatory drugs (NSAIDs; except for aspirin), both nonselective and cyclooxygenase 2 selective agents, at time of presentation with STEMI because of increased risk of mortality, reinfarction, hypertension, heart failure, and myocardial rupture associated with NSAID use.

Aspirin
- Aspirin 162 mg is chewed by patient for rapid buccal absorption.

Beta-Blockers
- Oral beta-blocker therapy is administered to patients with STEMI who do not have contraindications to beta blockade, regardless of fibrinolytic or primary PCI reperfusion.
- Contraindications for beta blockade with STEMI include signs of heart failure, low cardiac output, cardiogenic shock risk, heart block or prolonged P–R interval (>0.24 s), and active asthma or reactive airways disease.
- While considering the options for reperfusion, beta-blockers are given if the patient has tachycardia or hypertension; otherwise, they are started as soon as possible after STEMI.

Angiotensin-Converting Enzyme Inhibitors
- Oral angiotensin-converting enzyme inhibitors (ACEIs) are indicated within the first 24 h after STEMI unless contraindicated.

Recommendations for Emergency Interventions for STEMI
Fibrinolytic Medications
- Fibrinolytic medications are administered to patients with STEMI (if PCI is unavailable) with ST segment elevation greater than 0.1 mV (1 mm or one small box) in two contiguous precordial (chest) leads *or* two adjacent limb leads, new left bundle branch block (LBBB) or presumed new LBBB, and onset of symptoms less than 12 h earlier.
- Before administration of fibrinolytic therapy, rule out neurologic contraindications.
- Rule out facial trauma, uncontrolled hypertension, or ischemic stroke within the last 3 months.
- If contraindications to fibrinolysis are present, PCI is the preferred method of reperfusion.

PCI
- Emergency diagnostic coronary angiography should be performed to identify blocked coronary artery before PCI.

- Emergency PCI is recommended over fibrinolytic therapy if symptom onset was longer than 3 h ago.
- Emergency PCI can be performed within 12 h after symptom onset for patients with new LBBB or presumed new LBBB.
- Emergency PCI balloon inflation should be done within 90 min after arrival at the hospital.

Cardiac Surgery
Emergency CABG surgery is undertaken for specific indications in STEMI:
- Failed PCI with persistent pain or hemodynamic instability.
- Recurrent ischemia refractory to medical therapy in patients with suitable anatomy who are not candidates for PCI.
- Post-MI ventricular septal rupture or papillary muscle rupture, both of which frequently lead to cardiogenic shock.
- Cardiogenic shock less than 36 h after MI, in patients younger than 75 y with ST segment elevation, or in patients with new LBBB who have multivessel or left main disease.
- Recurrent ventricular dysrhythmias in patients with 50% or greater left main coronary artery lesion or triple-vessel disease or both.

Recommendations for Secondary Prevention of Complications
Medications
- ACEIs to prevent ventricular remodeling.
- Beta-blockers to prevent ventricular dysrhythmias.
- Diuretics if heart failure has developed.
- Antihyperlipidemics if total cholesterol, low-density lipoprotein cholesterol, or triglycerides are elevated.

Recommendations for Management of Complications After STEMI
Cardiogenic Shock
- Intraaortic balloon pump for patients with hypotension (blood pressure of 90 mm Hg or systolic blood pressure of 30 mm Hg below baseline).

Ventricular Arrhythmias
- Ventricular fibrillation (VF) or pulseless ventricular tachycardia (VT) is managed by standard ACLS criteria.
- Patients with hemodynamically significant VT more than 2 days after STEMI who have ongoing ventricular dysrhythmias are considered for implantation of an implantable cardioverter defibrillator (ICD).
- Patients with an ejection fraction (EF) between 30% and 40% at 1 month after STEMI should undergo an electrophysiology study; if they are inducible to VT/VF, an ICD is recommended to reduce risk of sudden cardiac death (SCD).
- Patients with an EF of less than 30% at 1 month after STEMI are at high risk for SCD.

AV Block
- Transvenous pacemaker (emergency) or permanent pacemaker (later elective) is inserted for symptomatic second-degree or third-degree atrioventricular block.
- All patients who require permanent pacing after STEMI should also be evaluated for ICD indications.

Provide Relevant Education
Medications
- Provide written and verbal instructions about medication dosages, administration, and side effects.

Emergency Information
- Give the patient and family information about calling 911 if pain/angina-equivalent symptoms persist or worsen after 5 min.

Continued

QSEN BOX 14.13   QSEN: Evidence-Based Practice—cont'd

Acute Coronary Syndrome and Acute Myocardial Infarction (Non-STEMI and STEMI)

- Family members of high-risk patients are advised to take a CPR class and learn about AEDs.

Risk Factors
- Provide education to reduce risk factors including education on smoking cessation, hypertension control, weight control, normal blood glucose, low-fat diet, and normal lipid panel.
- Patients are advised to increase physical activity.
- Women are advised to avoid new hormone replacement therapy.

Cardiac Rehabilitation
- Participation in a cardiac rehabilitation program will help the patient continue the process of risk factor and lifestyle modification.

References

Anderson JL, et al. 2011 ACCF/AHA focused update incorporated into the ACC/AHA 2007 guidelines for the management of patients with unstable angina/non-ST-elevation myocardial infarction: a report of the American College of Cardiology Foundation/American Heart Association Task Force on Practice Guidelines. *Circulation*. 2011;123:e426.

O'Gara PT, et al. 2013 ACCF/AHA guideline for the management of ST-elevation myocardial infarction: a report of the American College of Cardiology Foundation/American Heart Association Task Force on Practice Guidelines. *Circulation*. 2013;127(4):e362.

Wright SR, et al. 2011 ACC/AHA focused update of the guidelines for the management of patients with unstable angina/non ST elevation myocardial infarction: a report of the American College of Cardiology/American Heart Association Task Force on Practice Guidelines developed in collaboration with the American College of Emergency Physicians, Society for Cardiovascular Angiography and Interventions, and Society for Thoracic Surgeons. *J Am Coll Cardiol*. 2011;57:1920.

BOX 14.14   Causes of Sudden Cardiac Death

Acquired SCD Risk

Most patients with sudden cardiac death (SCD) are older adults and have a history of coronary artery disease (CAD), myocardial infarction (MI), and subsequent heart failure.
- Heart failure:
  - Ejection fraction less than 30%.
  - Heart structure is abnormal (systolic or diastolic ventricular dysfunction).
  - CAD and a history of MI that has produced scar tissue is the most common cause of ventricular tachycardia (VT)/ventricular fibrillation (VF) leading to SCD.
- Cardiomyopathy (dilated or ischemic):
  - Patients who are inducible for VT/VF in electrophysiology study (EPS) are at highest risk.
  - Risk is decreased by implantation of an implantable cardioverter defibrillator (ICD) and antidysrhythmic medication therapy.

Genetic SCD Risk

Genetic cardiovascular disease accounts for 40% of SCD in young adults.
- Brugada syndrome:
  - Electrocardiogram (ECG) signs: Coved-type ST segment elevation (>2 mm) in right precordial leads, although ECG variations also occur.
  - Heart structure appears normal.
  - High risk of VT or VF in otherwise young healthy adults.
  - VT/VF often occurs at night or at rest.
  - Represents 4% of all SCD; average age is 41 y.

- Represents up to 20% of genetic SCD patients.
- Hereditary: Autosomal-dominant genetic transmission.
- Five times more common in men.
- Patients who are inducible in EPS are at increased risk.
- Risk reduced by implantation of an ICD.
- Wolff-Parkinson-White (WPW) syndrome:
  - Congenital accessory conduction pathway connects atria and ventricles.
  - Accessory pathway is *in addition* to the normal conduction system.
  - Accessory pathway allows very rapid transmission of impulses leading to "preexcitation" of the ventricle that can degenerate into VT/VF, especially if atrial dysrhythmias are present.
  - WPW syndrome is usually identified when the patient is a teenager or young adult.
  - WPW syndrome is often recognized during exercise by palpitations or breathlessness.
  - Cure is possible in many cases by radiofrequency ablation of the accessory pathway.
- Hypertrophic cardiomyopathy (HCM):
  - Risk of VT/VF with exercise exists.
  - The obstructive form of HCM can be cured in many cases by alcohol ablation of the enlarged ventricular septum.
  - For other patients with HCM, the risk is reduced by implantation of an ICD.
- Long QT syndrome:
  - Risk of VT/VF with exercise exists.
  - Risk is reduced by implantation of an ICD.

an unrelated condition.[47] For patients with fluid retention, the most reliable clinical sign of fluid volume overload is jugular venous distention.[46,47] The procedure used to estimate jugular venous distention is described in Fig. 12.2 in Chapter 12.

The first step in the diagnosis is to determine the underlying structural abnormality creating the ventricular dysfunction and symptoms. Various imaging tests are available to visualize cardiac anatomy, and laboratory tests are used to evaluate the impact of hormonal or electrolyte imbalance. The results of these tests permit the cardiology team to design a treatment plan to control symptoms and possibly correct the underlying cause. All patients do not have the same type of heart failure.

Left Ventricular Failure

Failure of the left ventricle is defined as a disturbance of the contractile function of the left ventricle, resulting in a low cardiac output state. This leads to vasoconstriction of the arterial bed that increases systemic vascular resistance (SVR), a condition also described as "high afterload," and creates congestion and edema in the pulmonary circulation and alveoli. Patients presenting with left ventricular failure have one of the following: (1) decreased exercise tolerance, (2) fluid retention, or (3) discovery made during examination of noncardiac problems.[47] Clinical manifestations of left ventricular failure include decreased peripheral perfusion with weak or diminished pulses; cool, pale extremities; and, in later stages, peripheral cyanosis

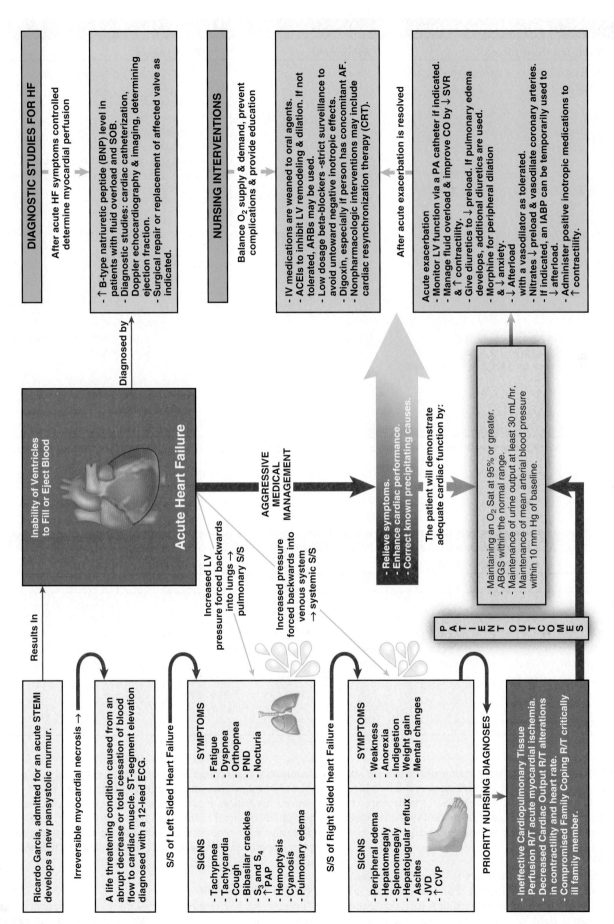

DIAGNOSTIC STUDIES FOR HF

After acute HF symptoms controlled determine myocardial perfusion

- ↑ B-type natriuretic peptide (BNP) level in patients with fluid overload and SOB.
- Diagnostic studies: cardiac catheterization, Doppler echocardiography & imaging, determining ejection fraction.
- Surgical repair or replacement of affected valve as indicated.

NURSING INTERVENTIONS

Balance O₂ supply & demand, prevent complications & provide education

- IV medications are weaned to oral agents.
- ACEIs to inhibit LV remodeling & dilation. If not tolerated, ARBs may be used.
- Low dosage beta-blockers -strict surveillance to avoid untoward negative inotropic effects.
- Digoxin, especially if person has concomitant AF.
- Nonpharmacologic interventions may include cardiac resynchronization therapy (CRT).

After acute exacerbation is resolved

Acute exacerbation
- Monitor LV function via a PA catheter if indicated.
- Manage fluid overload & improve CO by ↓ SVR & ↑ contractility.
- Give diuretics to ↓ preload. If pulmonary edema develops, additional diuretics are used.
- Morphine for peripheral dilation & ↓ anxiety.
- ↓ Afterload with a vasodilator as tolerated.
- Nitrates ↓ preload & vasodilate coronary arteries.
- If indicated, an IABP can be temporarily used to ↓ afterload.
- Administer positive inotropic medications to ↑ contractility.

Diagnosed by

Inability of Ventricles to Fill or Eject Blood

Acute Heart Failure

Results In

Ricardo Garcia, admitted for an acute STEMI develops a new pansystolic murmur.

Irreversible myocardial necrosis →

A life threatening condition caused from an abrupt decrease or total cessation of blood flow to cardiac muscle. ST-segment elevation diagnosed with a 12-lead ECG.

S/S of Left Sided Heart Failure

Increased LV pressure forced backwards into lungs → pulmonary S/S

Increased pressure forced backwards into venous system → systemic S/S

SYMPTOMS
- Fatigue
- Dyspnea
- Orthopnea
- PND
- Nocturia

SIGNS
- Tachypnea
- Tachycardia
- Cough
- Bibasilar crackles
- S₃ and S₄
- ↑ PAP
- Hemoptysis
- Cyanosis
- Pulmonary edema

S/S of Right Sided heart Failure

SYMPTOMS
- Weakness
- Anorexia
- Indigestion
- Weight gain
- Mental changes

SIGNS
- Peripheral edema
- Hepatomegaly
- Splenomegaly
- Hepatojugular reflux
- Ascites
- JVD
- ↑ CVP

AGGRESSIVE MEDICAL MANAGEMENT

- Relieve symptoms.
- Enhance cardiac performance.
- Correct known precipitating causes.

The patient will demonstrate adequate cardiac function by:

- Maintaining an O₂ Sat at 95% or greater.
- ABGS within the normal range.
- Maintenance of urine output at least 30 mL/hr.
- Maintenance of mean arterial blood pressure within 10 mm Hg of baseline.

PATIENT OUTCOMES

PRIORITY NURSING DIAGNOSES

- Ineffective Cardiopulmonary Tissue Perfusion R/T acute myocardial ischemia.
- Decreased Cardiac Output R/T alterations in contractility and heart rate.
- Compromised Family Coping R/T critically ill family member.

FIG. 14.17 Concept Map for Acute Heart Failure. *ABGs,* Arterial Blood Gases; *BNP,* B-type natriuretic peptide; *CO,* Cardiac Output; *CRT,* Cardiac resynchronization therapy; *CVP,* Central Venous Pressure; *HF,* Heart Failure; *IABP,* Intra-aortic Balloon Pump; *JVD,* Jugular Vein Distention; *LV,* Left Ventricular; *O₂ Sat,* Oxygen saturation; *PAP,* Pulmonary Artery Pressure; *R/T,* Related To; *SOB,* Shortness of Breath; *S/S,* Signs and Symptoms; *SVR,* Systemic Vascular Resistance. Concept maps created by © DEANNE A. BLACH, MSN, RN.

TABLE 14.8 Progression of Heart Failure

Stage	Structural Heart Disorder	Symptoms	Management
A	No, but at risk because of hypertension, CAD, diabetes mellitus	None	Preventive treatment of known risk factors: • Hypertension • Lipid disorders • Cigarette smoking • Diabetes mellitus • Discourage alcohol and illicit drug use
B	Yes, but without symptoms; previous MI, family history of CM; asymptomatic valvular disease or CM	None	Treat all risk factors; if indicated, use the following: • ACEIs • Beta-blockers
C	Yes, with prior or current symptoms	Shortness of breath; fatigue; reduced exercise tolerance	Treat all risk factors and HF symptoms: • Diuretics • ACEIs • Beta-blockers • Digitalis • Dietary salt restriction
D	Yes, with refractory HF symptoms despite maximal specialized interventions (pharmacologic, medical, nursing); recurrent hospitalization for HF symptoms	Marked symptoms at rest despite maximal medical therapy	Refractory HF requires interventions from previous stages (A–C), plus the following: • Continuous IV inotropic support • Mechanical assist devices • Heart transplantation • Hospice care

ACEI, angiotensin-converting enzyme inhibitor; *CAD,* coronary artery disease; *CM,* cardiomyopathy; *HF,* heart failure; *IV,* intravenous; *MI,* myocardial infarction.

Modified from Hunt SA, et al. ACC/AHA 2005 guideline update for the diagnosis and management of chronic heart failure in the adult: A report of the American College of Cardiology/American Heart Association Task Force on Practice Guidelines. *Circulation.* 2005;112(12):e154.

TABLE 14.9 Clinical Manifestations of Right-Sided and Left-Sided Heart Failure

LEFT VENTRICULAR FAILURE		RIGHT VENTRICULAR FAILURE	
Signs	Symptoms	Signs	Symptoms
Tachypnea	Fatigue	Peripheral edema	Weakness
Tachycardia	Dyspnea	Hepatomegaly	Anorexia
Cough	Orthopnea	Splenomegaly	Indigestion
Bibasilar crackles	Paroxysmal nocturnal dyspnea	Hepatojugular reflux	Weight gain
Gallop rhythms (S_3 and S_4)	Nocturia	Ascites	Mental changes
Increased pulmonary artery pressures		Jugular venous distention	
Hemoptysis		Increased central venous pressure	
Cyanosis		Pulmonary hypertension	
Pulmonary edema			

(Table 14.9). Over time, with progression of the disease state, the fluid accumulation behind the dysfunctional left ventricle elevates pulmonary pressures, contributes to pulmonary congestion and edema, and produces dysfunction of the right ventricle resulting in failure of the right side of the heart.

Right Ventricular Failure

Failure of the right side of the heart is defined as ineffective right ventricular contractile function. Pure failure of the right ventricle may result from an acute condition such as a pulmonary embolus or a right ventricular infarction, but it is most commonly caused by failure of the left side of the heart. The common manifestations of right ventricular failure are jugular venous distention, elevated central venous pressure, weakness, peripheral or sacral edema, hepatomegaly (enlarged liver), jaundice, and liver tenderness. Gastrointestinal symptoms include poor appetite, anorexia, nausea, and an uncomfortable feeling of fullness (see Table 14.9).[47]

Systolic Heart Failure

The term *systolic dysfunction* describes an abnormality of the heart muscle that markedly decreases contractility during systole (ejection) and lessens the quantity of blood that can be pumped out of the heart. Patients with a diagnosis of systolic heart failure (SHF) have signs and symptoms of heart failure combined with a below-normal ejection fraction. Left ventricular systolic dysfunction is the classic picture that most clinicians consider when thinking about heart failure. In addition to the signs and symptoms of left heart failure (described earlier), the patient has a low ejection fraction. It is still debated how low the ejection fraction has to be to qualify as SHF, but the value usually is less than 50%; some clinicians cite values less than 45% or 40%.[48] Symptoms of SHF include dyspnea, exercise intolerance, and fluid volume overload.

CAD and its sequelae represent the underlying cause in two-thirds of patients with systolic heart failure.[47] The remaining patients with systolic dysfunction have *nonischemic cardiomyopathy* (described as *dilated cardiomyopathy* [DCM]),[47] which results from an identifiable cause, such as hypertension, thyroid disease, cardiac valvular disease, alcohol use, or myocarditis.[47] If the cause is unknown, systolic dysfunction is described as *idiopathic dilated cardiomyopathy*. SHF increases with age. Clinical findings that are required to make a diagnosis of SHF include the following:

- Signs and symptoms of heart failure
- Left ventricular systolic dysfunction with an ejection fraction below normal

In systolic heart failure, the ventricular chambers change their shape, a detrimental development termed *ventricular remodeling*. The negative impact on the cardiac cells is different from the dysfunction and loss of myocytes from myocardial ischemia and infarction.

Significant hemodynamic changes occur as systolic dysfunction progresses. In systolic heart failure, the left ventricular end-diastolic volume is high, which increases the left ventricular end-diastolic pressure compared with a normal heart. The increase in intracardiac volume and pressure causes an increase in left atrial and pulmonary venous pressures. This means that all blood flowing into the heart through the pulmonary vascular bed is exposed to increased hydrostatic pressure, which is necessary to fill the congested heart. The increase in pulmonary vascular pressure causes transudation of fluid from the pulmonary capillaries into the alveolar interstitium, and this fluid is ultimately forced through the walls of the alveoli, causing pulmonary edema. The pulmonary complications of heart failure are described in greater detail later. The elevated left heart pressures eventually raise pressures in the right side of the heart and lead to secondary right heart failure.

Diastolic Heart Failure

The term *diastolic dysfunction* describes an abnormality of the heart muscle that makes it unable to relax, stretch, or fill during diastole. Diastolic heart failure (DHF), also known as heart failure with preserved ejection fraction, is caused by left ventricular dysfunction.[49] DHF is treated differently from SHF. Studies have shown that patients with DHF have a preserved ejection fraction defined as 40% to 50%.[49] Principal causes are similar to SHF (described earlier): CAD, myocardial ischemia, AF, advanced age (older than 75 years), obesity, hypertension, and diabetes mellitus.[49] Some conditions that are known to markedly alter diastolic function include hypertrophic cardiomyopathy (HCM), restrictive cardiomyopathy, and infiltrative diseases such as amyloidosis and neoplastic infiltrate. The incidence of DHF is highest among patients older than 75 years,

and the condition disproportionately affects older women. It is postulated that the process of aging impacts diastolic function negatively, imposing stiffness and fibrosis on the cardiac muscle and cardiovascular vessels.

Clinical findings that are required to make a diagnosis of DHF include the following:[49]

- Signs and symptoms of heart failure
- Normal or only mildly abnormal left ventricular systolic dysfunction
- Abnormal left ventricular relaxation, filling, diastolic distensibility, or diastolic stiffness

Normally, diastole is the filling stage of the cardiac cycle when the ventricle relaxes completely. The abnormal hemodynamics of DHF can be elicited by diagnostic tests such as cardiac catheterization and a stress echocardiogram (see "Stress Echocardiography" and Table 13.21 in Chapter 13). An ejection fraction above the range of 40% to 50% is considered normal for this population.

In DHF, the left ventricular end-diastolic pressure is high, whereas the left ventricular end-diastolic volume is paradoxically low compared with normal hearts.[49] Another diagnostic clue is that many patients with DHF have normal intracardiac pressures at rest, but during exercise, the left ventricular end-diastolic pressure and pulmonary vascular pressure rise rapidly. This occurs because the noncompliant, stiff ventricle cannot increase stroke volume during exercise; cardiac output remains low, even though physical demand is high. Patients with DHF often experience a sudden increase in BP and sinus tachycardia during exercise; they are exercise intolerant and experience fatigue, dyspnea, pulmonary venous congestion, and pulmonary edema.[49]

Systolic Diastolic Heart Failure Versus Diastolic Heart Failure

It is impossible to accurately determine whether a patient has SHF or DHF from clinical assessment alone.[47] Both types of heart failure produce similar signs and symptoms. The level of symptoms and quality of life vary among individuals and between men and women, even when the ejection fraction and presumed cardiac dysfunction are the same. This variation may occur because most symptoms come from the neurohormonal compensatory mechanisms (described later) rather than the cardiac output. An elevated B-type natriuretic peptide (BNP) level (greater than 100 pg/mL) is very useful to diagnose heart failure in patients with fluid overload and shortness of breath.[47,49,50] The BNP value tends to be higher in patients with a diagnosis of SHF compared with patients with DHF, although the difference is not reliable enough to be used to differentiate the two types of heart failure in clinical practice.[47] The more severe the heart failure, the higher the BNP level. The primary use of the BNP test is to determine whether the patient has heart failure.

The definitive diagnosis of the type of heart failure is often made using Doppler echocardiography. A two-dimensional echocardiogram coupled with Doppler flow studies to determine whether abnormalities of the myocardium, heart valves, or pericardium are present and which chambers are involved is the single most powerful diagnostic test in the evaluation of patients with heart failure. Calculation of the ejection fraction can be determined using Doppler echocardiography or during a cardiac catheterization. These diagnostic tests also show that some patients exhibit combined SHF and DHF.[47,49]

It is impossible to distinguish whether a patient has SHF or DHF simply by looking at the medications they are prescribed. The same medications are used to treat the two types of heart failure, although the underlying rationales may be different.[47-49] For example, beta-blockers are used in DHF to slow the heart rate, to prolong diastole to give more time for ventricular filling, and to modify the ventricular response to exercise, especially for patients who have a preserved ejection fraction.[49] When beta-blockers are prescribed for treatment of SHF, the intent is to preserve long-term inotropic (contractile) function and prevent ventricular remodeling.[47] Diuretics are used to treat both types of heart failure, although a smaller dosage is generally needed in DHF.[47,49] ACEIs and ARBs are also used to treat both types of heart failure. The medications used to treat heart failure are further discussed in Chapter 15 (see Table 15.21).

Acute Heart Failure Versus Chronic Heart Failure

Acute or chronic heart failure is determined by the rapid progression of the syndrome, the presence and activation of compensatory mechanisms, and the presence or absence of fluid accumulation in the interstitial space (see Table 14.8). In clinical practice guidelines, the terms *acute* and *chronic* have replaced the older term *congestive heart failure* because not all heart failure involves pulmonary congestion. However, congestive heart failure is still commonly used to describe patients in clinical practice.

Acute heart failure has a sudden onset, with no compensatory mechanisms. The patient may experience acute pulmonary edema, low cardiac output, or cardiogenic shock. Patients with chronic heart failure are hypervolemic, have sodium and water retention, and have structural heart chamber changes such as dilation or hypertrophy.[47]

Chronic heart failure is an ongoing process, with symptoms that may be made tolerable by medication, diet, and a reduced activity level. The deterioration into acute heart failure can be precipitated by the onset of dysrhythmias, acute ischemia, sudden illness, or cessation of medications. This may necessitate admission to a critical care unit. Hypertension is the primary precursor of heart failure in women, whereas CHD, specifically MI, is the primary cause of heart failure in men.[47]

Neurohormonal Compensatory Mechanisms in Heart Failure

When the heart begins to fail and the cardiac output is no longer sufficient to meet the metabolic needs of tissues, the body activates several major compensatory mechanisms: the sympathetic nervous system, the renin-angiotensin-aldosterone system (RAAS), and, if hypertension is present, the development of ventricular hypertrophy (see Table 14.8). This process ultimately reshapes the ventricle in a process described as *ventricular remodeling*. These pathophysiologic processes and the pharmacologic measures taken to limit ventricular remodeling are described in this section.

The sympathetic nervous system compensates for low cardiac output by increasing heart rate and BP. As a result, levels of circulating catecholamines are increased, leading to peripheral vasoconstriction. In addition to increasing BP and heart rate, catecholamines cause shunting of blood from nonvital organs such as the skin to vital organs such as the heart and brain. This mechanism, although initially helpful, may become a negative factor if elevation of heart rate increases myocardial oxygen demand, while shortening the amount of time for diastolic filling and coronary artery perfusion.

Activation of the RAAS in heart failure promotes fluid retention.[47] The RAAS is activated by low cardiac output that causes the hormone renin to be secreted by the kidneys. A physiologic chain of events is then set in motion that leads to volume overload. The renin acts on angiotensinogen in the bloodstream and converts it to angiotensin I; when angiotensin passes through the lung tissues, it is activated by angiotensin-converting enzyme, an enzyme that converts angiotensin I to angiotensin II, a powerful vasoconstrictor that increases SVR, BP, and the workload of the left ventricle; the increased SVR further decreases cardiac output. The mineralocorticoid hormone aldosterone is released from the adrenal glands and stimulates sodium retention via the distal tubules of the kidney. In response to the low cardiac output, the renal arterioles constrict, decrease glomerular filtration, and increase reabsorption of sodium from the proximal and distal tubules. To break the RAAS cycle of fluid retention in heart failure, two types of medications are prescribed to interrupt the steps. To inhibit the conversion of angiotensin I to angiotensin II, an ACEI is prescribed (see Table 15.21 in Chapter 15). These agents prevent arterial vasoconstriction, decrease BP and SVR, and decrease the amount of ventricular remodeling that often occurs with heart failure. A medication that inhibits angiotensin II directly may be prescribed instead. The medications in this category are ARBs.[47] Spironolactone (Aldactone) is a medication from a different category that is also prescribed to break the RAAS cycle. Spironolactone is a mineralocorticoid receptor antagonist that inhibits (blocks) the retention of sodium from the distal tubules of the kidney.[51] Fig. 14.18 depicts the mechanism of action by which these medications act on the RAAS.

Ventricular hypertrophy is the final compensatory mechanism. It is also strongly associated with preexisting hypertension. Because myocardial hypertrophy increases the force of contraction, hypertrophy helps the ventricle overcome an increase in afterload. When this mechanism is no longer efficient for the ventricle, it will remodel by dilation.

Ventricular remodeling occurs as a result of the previously described mechanisms. The shape of the ventricle is changed, or is remodeled, to resemble a round bowl. A dilated ventricle has poor contractility and is enlarged without hypertrophy. Research trial evidence indicates that synergistic use of medications from different categories—ACEI or ARB, spironolactone, and beta-blockade—can halt or reduce the progression of heart failure remodeling.[47-49,51]

Pulmonary Complications of Heart Failure

The clinical manifestations of acute heart failure result from tissue hypoperfusion and organ congestion and are progressive. The severity of clinical manifestations increases as heart failure worsens. Initially, manifestations appear only with exertion, but eventually, they also occur at rest.[47,49]

Shortness of Breath in Heart Failure

The patient experiences the feeling of shortness of breath first with exertion, but as heart failure worsens, symptoms are also present at rest. A diagnostic blood test is available to assist clinicians in differentiating whether a patient's shortness of breath is caused by cardiac failure or by pulmonary complications. BNP, a cardiac neurohormone released by the ventricles in response

Organs involved	Pathophysiology	Medication actions

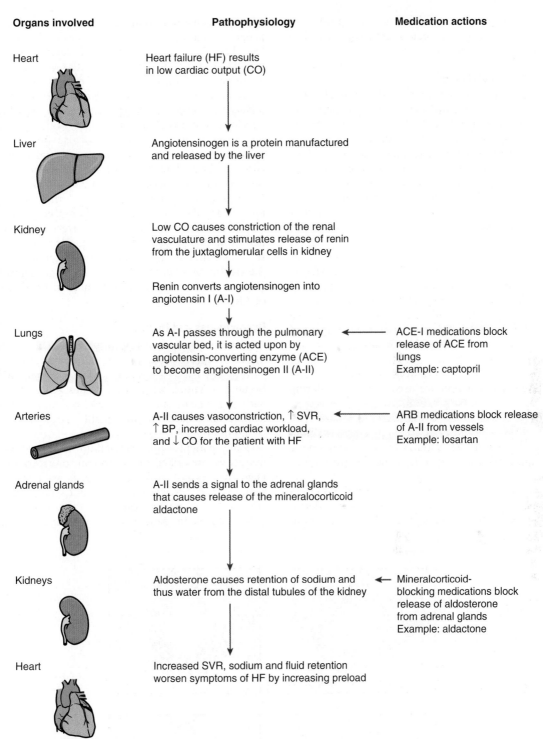

Heart — Heart failure (HF) results in low cardiac output (CO)

Liver — Angiotensinogen is a protein manufactured and released by the liver

Kidney — Low CO causes constriction of the renal vasculature and stimulates release of renin from the juxtaglomerular cells in kidney

Renin converts angiotensinogen into angiotensin I (A-I)

Lungs — As A-I passes through the pulmonary vascular bed, it is acted upon by angiotensin-converting enzyme (ACE) to become angiotensinogen II (A-II) ← ACE-I medications block release of ACE from lungs
Example: captopril

Arteries — A-II causes vasoconstriction, ↑ SVR, ↑ BP, increased cardiac workload, and ↓ CO for the patient with HF ← ARB medications block release of A-II from vessels
Example: losartan

Adrenal glands — A-II sends a signal to the adrenal glands that causes release of the mineralocorticoid aldactone

Kidneys — Aldosterone causes retention of sodium and thus water from the distal tubules of the kidney ← Mineralcorticoid-blocking medications block release of aldosterone from adrenal glands
Example: aldactone

Heart — Increased SVR, sodium and fluid retention worsen symptoms of HF by increasing preload

FIG. 14.18 Renin-Angiotensin-Aldosterone System, Its Role in Heart Failure, and Medication Actions.

to volume expansion and pressure overload, is elevated in DHF and SHF. Heart failure increases left ventricular wall tension because of the excess preload in the ventricles. When the BNP blood level is greater than 100 pg/mL, the dyspnea is most likely related to cardiac failure rather than pulmonary failure.[47,50] The more severe the heart failure, the higher the BNP value.[50] If the patient has concomitant kidney disease the BNP will be also elevated because of the kidney failure. BNP greater than 200 pg/mL

is required to diagnose heart failure.[47,50] Breathlessness in heart failure is described by the following terms:
- *Dyspnea:* Sensation of shortness of breath from pulmonary vascular congestion and decreased lung compliance.
- *Orthopnea:* Difficulty breathing when lying flat because of an increase in venous return that occurs in the supine position.
- *Paroxysmal nocturnal dyspnea:* Severe form of orthopnea in which the patient awakens from sleep gasping for air.

- *Cardiac asthma:* Dyspnea with wheezing, a nonproductive cough, and pulmonary crackles that progress to the gurgling sounds of pulmonary edema.

Pulmonary Edema in Heart Failure

Pulmonary edema, or protein-laden fluid in the alveoli, inhibits gas exchange by impairing the diffusion pathway between the alveolus and the capillary (Fig. 14.19A). It is caused by increased left atrial and ventricular pressures and results in an excessive accumulation of serous or serosanguineous fluid in the interstitial spaces and alveoli of the lungs. The formation of pulmonary edema has two stages. The first stage is not as severe and is characterized by interstitial edema, engorgement of the perivascular and peribronchial spaces, and increased lymphatic flow (Fig. 14.19B). The later stage is characterized by alveolar edema resulting from fluid moving into the alveoli from the interstitium (Fig. 14.19C). Eventually, blood plasma moves into the alveoli faster than the lymphatic system can clear it, interfering with diffusion of oxygen, depressing the arterial partial pressure of oxygen (Pao_2), and leading to tissue hypoxia (Fig. 14.19D).

Patients experiencing heart failure and pulmonary edema are extremely breathless and anxious and have a sensation of suffocation. They expectorate pink, frothy sputum and feel as if they are drowning. They may sit bolt upright, gasp for breath, or thrash about. The respiratory rate is elevated, and accessory muscles of ventilation are used, with nasal flaring and bulging neck muscles. Respirations are characterized by loud inspiratory and expiratory gurgling sounds. Diaphoresis is profuse, and the skin is cold, ashen, and sometimes cyanotic. This reflects low cardiac output, increased sympathetic stimulation, peripheral vasoconstriction, and desaturation of arterial blood.

Arterial blood gases in pulmonary edema. Arterial blood gas values are variable. In the early stage of pulmonary edema, respiratory alkalosis may be present because of hyperventilation, which eliminates carbon dioxide. As the pulmonary edema progresses and gas exchange becomes impaired, acidosis (pH less than 7.35) and hypoxemia ensue. A chest radiograph usually confirms an enlarged cardiac silhouette, pulmonary venous congestion, and interstitial edema.

Cardiogenic pulmonary edema versus noncardiogenic pulmonary edema. In the critical care unit, when a patient develops pulmonary edema, it is often a challenge to determine whether the cause is cardiac, known as *cardiogenic pulmonary edema*, or pulmonary or systemic in origin. The latter is referred to as *noncardiogenic pulmonary edema* or, more commonly, *acute respiratory distress syndrome* (ARDS). Options to determine the cause of the pulmonary edema include use of the serum BNP level or insertion of a pulmonary artery catheter. The pulmonary artery catheter is used to determine the patient's pulmonary artery occlusion pressure. It is essential to understand the different causes because the treatment of each form of pulmonary edema is specific. Chapter 20 provides more information on the management of ARDS.

Dysrhythmias and Heart Failure

A ventricular ejection fraction less than 30% and the presence of NYHA class III or IV heart failure are strongly associated with ventricular dysrhythmias and an increased risk for death.[52] Because sustained VT or VF initiates SCD, high-risk patients with severe heart failure are prescribed antidysrhythmic medications and have an implantable cardioverter defibrillator (ICD) inserted.[52]

Many patients with heart failure also have AF. Digoxin is frequently prescribed for AF to control ventricular heart rate. Digoxin does not prolong life, but it makes patients feel less symptomatic. Digoxin may also work synergistically with specific beta-blockers (eg, carvedilol) and make the symptoms more tolerable for patients with severe heart failure.[47]

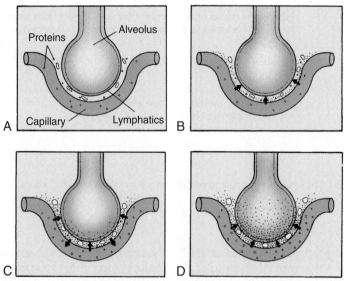

FIG. 14.19 As Pulmonary Edema Progresses, It Inhibits Oxygen and Carbon Dioxide Exchange at the Alveolar Capillary Interface. (A) Normal relationship. (B) Increased pulmonary capillary hydrostatic pressure causes fluid to move from the vascular space into the pulmonary interstitial space. (C) Lymphatic flow increases in an attempt to pull fluid back into the vascular or lymphatic space. (D) Failure of lymphatic flow and worsening of left-sided heart failure results in further movement of fluid into the interstitial space and the alveoli.

Medical Management

The goals of the medical management of heart failure are to relieve symptoms, enhance cardiac performance, and correct known precipitating causes.

Relief of Symptoms and Enhancement of Cardiac Performance

In the acute phase of advanced heart failure, the patient may have a pulmonary artery catheter in place so that left ventricular function can be monitored closely. Control of symptoms involves management of fluid overload and improvement of cardiac output by decreasing SVR and increasing contractility. Diuretics are administered to decrease preload and to eliminate excess fluid from the body.[47] If pulmonary edema develops, additional diuretics are used. Morphine is given to facilitate peripheral dilation and decrease anxiety. Afterload is decreased by vasodilators such as sodium nitroprusside (Nipride) and nitroglycerin. Sodium nitroprusside is a balanced vasodilator medication that relaxes arterial resistance and venous capacitance vessels. By reducing both preload and afterload, it can relieve congestion and improve cardiac output, particularly in patients with increased SVR. It is useful in favorably redistributing total left ventricular stroke volume in patients with either mitral or aortic insufficiency such that regurgitant flow is reduced while forward flow is increased.[46] Nitrates are used to decrease preload and vasodilate the coronary arteries if CAD is an underlying cause of the acute heart failure. For some patients, an IABP is temporarily required.[46] Contractility is initially increased by continuous infusion of positive inotropic medications (dopamine) or by combination inodilators such as dobutamine or milrinone.

After the acute exacerbation is resolved, the patient is transitioned to oral agents and weaned off the intravenous medications. Before transition out of the critical care unit, the patient with heart failure receives ACEIs to inhibit left ventricular chamber remodeling and slow left ventricular dilation. If the patient does not tolerate ACEIs, ARBs may be substituted.[46-49] Low-dose beta-blockers such as carvedilol may also be prescribed, although strict surveillance is required to anticipate and avoid untoward negative inotropic effects.[47] Digoxin may be added to the regimen, especially if the patient has concomitant AF.[47] Nonpharmacologic interventions that are increasingly used include *cardiac resynchronization therapy* (CRT).[53-55] CRT is biventricular pacing, where the right and left ventricles each have a pacing lead in contact with the myocardium. In patients with heart failure, CRT has a beneficial effect on clinical symptoms, exercise capacity, and systolic left ventricular performance.[53-55]

Correction of Precipitating Causes

After symptoms of heart failure are controlled, diagnostic studies such as cardiac catheterization, echocardiography, and diagnostic imaging tests to determine myocardial perfusion are undertaken to uncover the cause of the heart failure and tailor long-term management to treat the cause. Some structural problems such as valvular disease may be amenable to surgical correction.

Palliative Care for End-Stage Heart Failure

In 2004, a consensus statement on palliative and supportive care in advanced heart failure was published.[56] Heart failure is a progressive disease, and patients do not recover.[56,57] At a point in the trajectory of heart failure, many patients with NYHA class IV heart failure become candidates for palliative care.[56] The primary aim of palliative care is symptom management and relief of suffering. Fundamental to all symptom management strategies for heart failure is the optimization of medications according to current guidelines.[47,49] The most common symptoms of advanced heart failure are dyspnea, pain, and fatigue.[56,57]

Nursing Management

Nursing management of a patient with heart failure incorporates a variety of nursing diagnoses (Box 14.15). Nursing management interventions are designed to achieve optimal cardiopulmonary function, promote comfort and emotional support, monitor the effectiveness of pharmacologic therapy, ensure nutritional intake is sufficient, and provide patient and family education.

Optimizing Cardiopulmonary Function

The patient's ECG is evaluated for dysrhythmias that may be present as a result of medication toxicity or electrolyte imbalance. Patients with heart failure are prone to digoxin toxicity because of decreased renal perfusion and electrolyte imbalances. Breath sounds are auscultated frequently to determine the adequacy of respiratory effort and to assess for onset or worsening of pulmonary congestion. Oxygen is administered through a nasal cannula to relieve dyspnea. Diuretics or vasodilators are used to decrease excessive preload and afterload.[47,49] If the patient is not hypotensive, morphine may be administered to decrease hyperventilation and anxiety. If the patient's ventilatory status worsens, the nurse must be prepared for endotracheal intubation and mechanical ventilation. Obtaining daily weights is important until the weight stabilizes at a "dry" weight. Generally, the daily weight is used in fluid management, and a weekly weight is optimally used for tracking body weight (eg, muscle, fat).

Promoting Comfort and Emotional Support

During periods of breathlessness, activity must be restricted. Bed rest usually is prescribed for the patient, who is positioned with the head of the bed elevated to allow for maximal lung expansion. The arms can be supported on pillows so that no undue stress is placed on the shoulder muscles. The legs may be placed in a dependent position to encourage venous pooling, decreasing venous return. Rest periods must be carefully

---

◎ BOX 14.15 NURSING DIAGNOSES

Acute Heart Failure

- Impaired Gas Exchange related to ventilation/perfusion mismatching or intrapulmonary shunting, p. 1030
- Decreased Cardiac Output related to alterations in preload, p. 1015
- Decreased Cardiac Output related to alterations in contractility, p. 1016
- Decreased Cardiac Output related to alterations in heart rate or rhythm, p. 1016
- Activity Intolerance related to cardiopulmonary dysfunction, p. 1006
- Anxiety related to threat to biologic, psychologic, or social integrity, p. 1012
- Ineffective Coping related to situational crisis and personal vulnerability, p. 1036
- Deficient Knowledge related to lack of previous exposure to information, p. 1020 (see Box 14.16, Patient Education Plan for Acute Heart Failure)

planned and adhered to, and independence within the patient's activity prescription must be fostered. Vital signs are recorded before an activity is begun and after it is completed. Signs of activity intolerance such as dyspnea, fatigue, sustained increase in pulse, and onset of dysrhythmias are documented and reported to the physician. Activity is gradually increased according to the patient's tolerance. Skin breakdown is a risk because of the combination of bed rest, inadequate nutrition, peripheral edema, and decreased perfusion to the skin and subcutaneous tissue. Frequent position changes and mobilization can help to provide comfort and prevent this complication.

Monitoring Effects of Pharmacologic Therapy

Patients experiencing acute heart failure require aggressive pharmacologic therapy.[46-49] The critical care nurse must know the action, side effects, therapeutic levels, and toxic effects of diuretics and venodilators used to decrease preload, positive inotropic agents used to increase ventricular contractility, vasodilators used to decrease afterload, and any antidysrhythmics used to control heart rate and prevent dysrhythmias. The patient's hemodynamic response to these agents is closely monitored. Fluid intake and output balances are tabulated daily or hourly in the critical care unit.

Nutritional Intake

Patients experiencing heart failure often have decreased appetite and nausea, so small, frequent meals may be more appropriate than the standard three large meals. Food must be as tasty as possible; favorite foods and foods from home may be incorporated into the diet as long as the foods are compatible with nutritional restrictions such as low levels of sodium to decrease the risk of fluid retention. Each patient must be assessed for nutritional imbalance individually. Not all patients with heart failure have the same nutritional needs.

Patient Education

The nurse assesses the patient's and family's understanding of the pathophysiology and individual risk factor profile for heart failure. Primary topics of education include (1) the importance of a daily weight, (2) fluid restrictions, (3) written information about the multiple medications used to control the symptoms of heart failure, (4) physical activity, and (5) when to call a health care provider (Box 14.16).[47,58,59] Many patients with a diagnosis of heart failure also require education about lifestyle changes such as smoking cessation, weight loss, energy conservation, and how to incorporate exercise and sodium restriction into their daily lives.[47,58,59] Achieving the optimal outcomes for a patient with heart failure requires contributions from a team of educated health care clinicians (Box 14.17).[47,58,59]

CARDIOMYOPATHY

Description and Etiology

Cardiomyopathy is a disease of the heart muscle (*cardio-* [heart], *-myo-* [muscle], and *-pathy* [pathology]). Cardiomyopathies are classified on the basis of structural abnormalities and genotype if known. Cardiomyopathies are categorized as *extrinsic,* caused by external factors such as hypertension, ischemia, inflammation, or valvular dysfunction, or as *intrinsic,* corresponding to myocardial diseases without identifiable external causes.[60,61] The two main forms of primary cardiomyopathies are HCM and DCM. Most cases of HCM and 20% to 50% of cases of DCM are familial,

---

BOX 14.16   PATIENT EDUCATION PLAN

Acute Heart Failure

The patient should be able to teach back the following topics:

- Heart failure: Pathophysiology of heart failure.
- Fluid balance: Low-salt diet to reduce fluid retention; intake and output measurement; signs of fluid overload such as peripheral edema.
- Daily weight: Increase or loss of 1–2 lb in a few days is a sign of fluid gain or loss, not true weight gain or loss.
- Breathlessness: Increasing shortness of breath, wheezing, and sleeping upright on pillows or in a recliner are symptoms that must be monitored and reported to a health care professional.
- Activity: Activity conservation with rest periods as heart failure progresses.
- Medications: As medications are complex, information must be given in writing and orally:
  - Preload: Purpose of diuretics, increased urine output, and control of fluid volume.
  - Afterload: Purpose of vasodilators or angiotensin-converting enzyme inhibitors in decreasing workload of the heart.
  - Heart rate: Purpose of digoxin is to control atrial fibrillation, a frequent dysrhythmia in heart failure.
  - Contractility: With the exception of digoxin, no oral contractility medications are approved by the US Food and Drug Administration.
  - Anticoagulation: Patients with distended atria and enlarged ventricles or with atrial fibrillation may be prescribed an anticoagulant such as warfarin (Coumadin); risks of bleeding, importance of correct dosages, prothrombin times, international normalized ratio, and nutritional-pharmacologic interactions are emphasized.
- Follow-up care.
- Symptoms to report to a health care professional.

---

showing a genetic disposition.[61] Cardiomyopathy categories are hypertrophic, restrictive, and dilated, as illustrated in Fig. 14.20.

Hypertrophic Obstructive Cardiomyopathy

HCM is a genetically inherited disease that affects the myocardial sarcomere.[61] As HCM progresses, the left ventricle becomes stiff, noncompliant, and hypertrophied, sometimes in an asymmetric fashion.[60] HCM occurs in two forms. A well-known but less frequent manifestation is a stiff, noncompliant myocardial muscle with left ventricular hypertrophy and hypertrophy of the upper ventricular septum. This left ventricular septal hypertrophy obstructs outflow through the aortic valve, especially during exercise (see Fig. 14.20A). It also pulls the papillary muscle out of alignment, causing mitral regurgitation. Other patients with HCM have generalized left ventricular hypertrophy, but the septum is not more enlarged than the rest of the myocardium.[60] HCM causes significant diastolic dysfunction because the muscle-bound, stiff, noncompliant heart muscle does not allow adequate filling during diastole.

Two advances in diagnostic medicine have propelled understanding of the differences between these two forms of HCM. *Two-dimensional transthoracic echocardiography* (TTE) is often useful as the first diagnostic test to identify HCM.[60] TTE enables visualization of septal anatomy, septal movement, and ventricular wall thickness and motion. The second advance is *diagnostic genetics.* Genetic testing for HCM usually is performed at a center with expertise in this area.[60] HCM is inherited as an autosomal dominant trait, and the clinical expression is caused by mutations in any 1 of 10 genes. Each gene encodes different

QSEN BOX 14.17 **QSEN: Evidence-Based Practice**

Heart Failure

A collaborative heart failure management team provides an integrated approach to care to achieve clinical stability for the patient.

1. Ensure systematic assessment and management:
   - To achieve an absence of "congestion" and to stabilize patient's condition at the best "stage" possible when in the hospital (see Tables 14.6 and 14.8).
   - To maintain same stability once discharged home and to avoid hospital readmission.
2. Counsel and educate patient and family after discharge from hospital. Patients and families should understand the following:
   - Heart failure disease process.
   - Heart failure medications, dosages, medication schedule, medication side effects.
   - Fluid balance related to salt-restriction diet (2 g/day of sodium), daily weight, diuretic regimen.
   - When to call health care provider.
   - Risk of additional complications: sudden cardiac death; progressive heart failure; need for other cardiac procedures (pacemaker, implantable cardioverter-defibrillator, percutaneous coronary intervention) or cardiac surgery (coronary artery bypass graft, valve replacement); mechanical assist device or heart transplantation, as needed by some patients.
   - Purpose of advance directive for health care decisions.
3. Promote patient compliance with treatment regimen:
   - Patient needs support from concerned companions and health care professionals.
   - Patient should remain physically active and involved with life.
4. Facilitate hospital discharge; implement outpatient models of health care delivery:
   - Close communication between inpatient and outpatient health care providers is essential.

Reference

Yancy CW, et al. 2013 ACCF/AHA guideline for management of heart failure. *J Am Coll Cardiol.* 2013;62(16):e147.

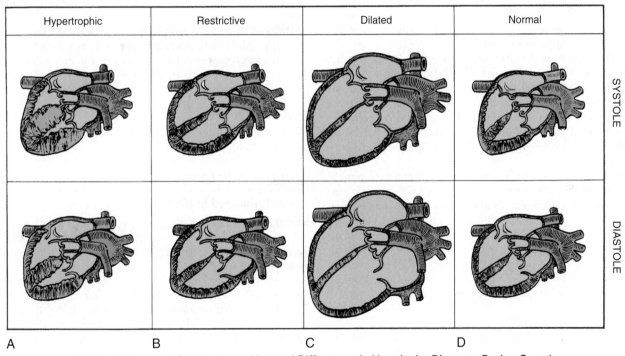

Hypertrophic	Restrictive	Dilated	Normal	
				SYSTOLE
				DIASTOLE
A	B	C	D	

FIG. 14.20 Types of Cardiomyopathies and Differences in Ventricular Diameter During Systole and Diastole Compared With a Normal Heart. (A) Hypertrophic. (B) Restrictive. (C) Dilated. (D) Normal.

protein components of the myocardial sarcomere.[60] Genetic analysis is an area of ongoing research that will undoubtedly help clarify other aspects of HCM within the next decade.

Symptoms are similar to symptoms seen with heart failure, with the addition of myocardial ischemia, supraventricular tachycardia, VT, syncope, and stroke.[60,61] Symptoms usually are more intense with physical exercise, especially in the obstructive form of HCM, in which the aortic outflow tract is obstructed by the enlarged left ventricular septum. Because a known association exists between HCM and SCD, limitation of physical activity may be recommended. Causes of SCD are thought to stem from ventricular dysrhythmias and AF.[60] The atrial dysrhythmias are related to increased age and atrial enlargement. Pharmacologic management includes beta-blockers to decrease left ventricular workload, medications to control and prevent atrial and ventricular dysrhythmias, anticoagulation if AF or left ventricular thrombi are present, and medications to manage heart failure. Interventional procedures include insertion of an ICD to decrease the risk of SCD and percutaneous alcohol ablation of the intraventricular septum to decrease the size of the septal wall.[60,61]

Dilated Cardiomyopathy

DCM is characterized by gross dilation of both ventricles without muscle hypertrophy (see Fig. 14.20C). Several distinct causes of DCM exist. DCM has both primary and secondary causes and is the most common cause of heart failure. DCM results from valvular, ischemic, toxic, metabolic, infectious, and systemic causes.[62]

Ischemic dilated cardiomyopathy. Ischemic DCM results from repeated myocardial injury or infarction resulting in reduction of ejection fraction. It is the most common cause of DCM in the United States. The patient has signs and symptoms of SHF and a low ejection fraction.[60,62] Treatment consists of the use of ACEIs in symptomatic and asymptomatic patients and beta-blockers and digoxin in symptomatic patients.

Idiopathic dilated cardiomyopathy. When the cause of DCM is unknown, it is called *idiopathic DCM.* In some cases, the occurrence is linked to genetic inheritance. Scientific advances in molecular genetics permit detailed studies of families with a high incidence of DCM. It is thought that 10% to 50% of *familial idiopathic DCM* cases reflect genetic transmission. In affected families, various genetic mutations occur in the gene that codes for the sarcomere contractile protein in the heart. The heritable trait can be expressed as an autosomal dominant or recessive inheritance pattern. Preliminary research indicates that the genetic picture is highly individual for different family groups, even if the clinical picture appears similar.

Other causes of dilated cardiomyopathy. Many other nonischemic, nongenetic causes of DCM exist. Injury can be caused by valvular heart dysfunction that has placed extreme pressure or volume on the chambers, and viral or bacterial infections such as myocarditis can lead to inflammatory changes that permanently remodel the heart.[62] Other noncardiac causes include infiltration by systemic collagens as in amyloidosis or sarcoidosis.[62]

In DCM, the myocardial muscle fibers contract poorly, resulting in global left ventricular dysfunction, low cardiac output, atrial and ventricular dysrhythmias, blood pooling that leads to ventricular thrombi and embolic episodes, refractory heart failure, and premature death. The goals of medical management of DCM are similar to the goals for systolic heart failure: improvement of pump function, removal of excess fluid, control of heart failure symptoms, anticipation and management of complications, and prevention of SCD.

Restrictive Cardiomyopathy

RCM is the least commonly encountered cardiomyopathy in developed countries (see Fig. 14.20B). As with the other cardiomyopathies, RCM can be idiopathic or can have a known cause. RCMs involve abnormalities of diastolic function with preserved systolic function. DHF, low cardiac output, dyspnea, orthopnea, and liver engorgement are the most common clinical manifestations of RCM. An elevated jugular venous pressure, S_4, and late S_3 may be present. Both ventricles are typically small with decreased volumes and large atria. The atrial septum and cardiac valves may be thickened, and pericardial effusion may be present. Medical management is aimed at improving symptoms and preventing tachycardia. Diuretics reduce pulmonary pressure and fluid volume relieving dyspnea. Nitrates can also provide relief. Patients are advised to reduce sodium intake, weigh daily, and restrict water intake. ACEIs and ARBs improve stroke volume and reduce myocardial oxygen demand.[47,48]

◎ BOX 14.18 NURSING DIAGNOSES

Cardiomyopathy

- Decreased Cardiac Output related to alterations in preload, p. 1015
- Decreased Cardiac Output related to alterations in afterload, p. 1015
- Decreased Cardiac Output related to alterations in contractility, p. 1016
- Decreased Cardiac Output related to alterations in heart rate or rhythm, p. 1016
- Impaired Gas Exchange related to ventilation/perfusion mismatching or intrapulmonary shunting, p. 1030
- Activity Intolerance related to cardiopulmonary dysfunction, p. 1006
- Anxiety related to threat to biologic, psychologic, or social integrity, p. 1012
- Powerlessness related to lack of control over current situation or disease progression, p. 1038
- Deficient Knowledge related to lack of previous exposure to information, p. 1020 (see Box 14.19, Patient Education Plan for Cardiomyopathy)

Nursing Management

Nursing management of a patient with cardiomyopathy incorporates a variety of nursing diagnoses related to the symptoms of heart failure. These nursing diagnoses are reviewed in Box 14.18. Nursing interventions are individualized according to the type of cardiomyopathy and are focused on achievement of a stable fluid balance, monitoring the effects of pharmacologic therapy, safely increasing mobility, and providing patient and family education. As with heart failure, a collaborative team of compassionate, knowledgeable professionals is required to provide effective care and education for these challenging patients.[63]

Patient Education

Education is tailored to the type of cardiomyopathy and to any associated conditions (Box 14.19).

PULMONARY HYPERTENSION

Description and Etiology

PH is a progressive, ultimately fatal disease of the pulmonary vasculature. PH results from progressive narrowing of the small pulmonary vessels resulting in an increase in pulmonary vascular resistance. Pulmonary artery hypertension (PAH) is the largest subdivision of this complex disease.[64,65] PAH is a disease of the small pulmonary arteries that is characterized by vascular proliferation, inflammation, and remodeling.[64,65] If untreated, PH progresses to right ventricular failure and death.[64] It is discussed with cardiovascular disease that target the arteries because it affects arterial vessels. PH may arise as an isolated condition or be associated with other diseases.

World Health Organization Classification of Pulmonary Hypertension

The World Health Organization (WHO) classification of PH was most recently updated in 2013 at the Fifth World Symposium of Pulmonary Hypertension. This updated model groups disorders according to similarities in pathophysiology and treatment (Table 14.10).[66] Some of the causes of PH likely to be seen in a critical care unit are discussed in this section. Whatever the cause, the presence of PH significantly increases morbidity and mortality of any underlying cardiac or pulmonary disease. PH is a serious and frequently life-threatening condition that requires aggressive treatment.[67]

BOX 14.19 PATIENT EDUCATION PLAN

Cardiomyopathy

The patient should be able to teach back the following topics:
Cardiomyopathy produces symptoms of heart failure; patient education covers many of the same issues discussed for heart failure.

- Cardiomyopathy: Explain pathophysiology of cardiomyopathy and heart failure.
- Fluid balance: Low-salt diet to reduce fluid retention; intake and output measurement; signs of fluid overload such as peripheral edema.
- Daily weight: Increase or loss of 1–2 lb in a few days is a sign of fluid gain or loss, not true weight gain or loss.
- Breathlessness: Increasing shortness of breath, wheezing, and sleeping upright on pillows are symptoms that must be monitored and reported to a health care professional.
- Activity: Activity conservation with rest periods as heart failure progresses.
- Medications: As medications are complex, information must be given in writing and orally:
  - Preload: Purpose of diuretics, increased urine output, and control of fluid volume.
  - Afterload: Purpose of vasodilators or angiotensin-converting enzyme inhibitors in decreasing the workload of the heart.
  - Heart rate: Purpose of digoxin is to control atrial fibrillation, a frequent dysrhythmia in heart failure; purpose of amiodarone is to control ventricular and atrial dysrhythmias, which are common in heart failure.
  - Contractility: With the exception of digoxin, no oral contractility medications are approved by US Food and Drug Administration
  - Decrease sympathetic response: Purpose of carvedilol (beta-blocker) is to lower cardiac response to adrenergic stimulation.
  - Anticoagulation: Patients with distended atria, enlarged ventricles, or atrial fibrillation may be prescribed anticoagulants such as warfarin (Coumadin) or aspirin or both; risk of bleeding, importance of correct dosages, prothrombin times, international normalized ratio, and nutritional-pharmacologic interactions are emphasized.
- Follow-up care.
- Symptoms to report to a health care professional.

TABLE 14.10 World Health Organization Classification of Pulmonary Hypertension

Group 1	PAH
	Idiopathic PAH
	Heritable *BMPR2, ALK1*, endoglin (with or without hereditary hemorrhagic telangiectasia)
	Associated PAH induced by medications, unknown drugs, and toxins
	Connective tissue diseases
	HIV infection
	Portal hypertension
	Congenital heart disease
	Schistosomiasis
	Chronic hemolytic anemia
	Persistent pulmonary hypertension of the newborn
Group 1′	Pulmonary venoocclusive disease, pulmonary capillary hemangiomatosis, or both
Group 2	PH from left heart disease
	Systolic dysfunction
	Diastolic dysfunction
	Valvular disease
Group 3	PH from lung diseases, hypoxia, or both
	Chronic obstructive pulmonary disease
	Interstitial lung disease
	Other pulmonary diseases with mixed restrictive and obstructive pattern
	Sleep-disordered breathing
	Alveolar hypoventilation disorders
	Chronic exposure to high altitude
	Developmental abnormalities
Group 4	Chronic thromboembolic PH
Group 5	PH with unclear mechanisms, multifactorial mechanisms, or both
	Hematologic disorders: Myeloproliferative disorders, splenectomy
	Systemic disorders: Sarcoidosis, pulmonary Langerhans cell histiocytosis, lymphangioleiomyomatosis, neurofibromatosis, vasculitis
	Metabolic disorders: Glycogen storage disease, Gaucher disease, thyroid disorders
	Other: Tumoral obstruction, fibrosing mediastinitis, chronic kidney failure on dialysis

HIV, human immunodeficiency virus; *PAH*, pulmonary artery hypertension; *PH*, pulmonary hypertension.
Simmoneau G, et al. Updated clinical classification of pulmonary hypertension. *J Am Coll Cardiol*. 62(25):D34, 2013.

Functional Classification of Pulmonary Hypertension

A functional classification describes a grouping of physical symptoms that limit a patient's activity as a result of his or her disease condition. The AHA has used a functional classification for heart failure symptoms for many years (see Table 14.6). The NYHA heart failure classification was used for PAH symptoms until 2003, when a disease-specific functional classification was developed (Table 14.11). The premise is the same as the NYHA classification, with the understanding that a higher number means that the patient is more symptomatic, has greater limitation of activity, and risks higher mortality. The functional classification level strongly predicts mortality and is used to guide PAH therapy.[68]

Idiopathic Pulmonary Artery Hypertension

If the cause of PH is unknown, it is called idiopathic PAH and is classified as WHO group I (see Table 14.10). Idiopathic PAH is characterized by the following features (Fig. 14.21):
- Intimal endothelial cell proliferation and medial thickening as a result of vascular smooth muscle cell proliferation
- Muscularization of precapillary arterioles
- Angioproliferative plexiform lesions of the endothelial cells develop from proliferation and fibrosis of the endothelium and increase obstruction

Idiopathic PAH is rare, with an incidence of approximately three to six cases per 1 million people per year. It has a female-to-male ratio of almost 3:1 with the previous mean age at diagnosis 37 years.[64] More recently, PAH is more frequently diagnosed in older patients (50 to 65 ± 15 years old).[69] PH has an insidious onset, and diagnosis is difficult because of the nonspecific nature of the symptoms (eg, dyspnea, fatigue). Frequently, by the time a firm diagnosis is made, the patient is highly symptomatic with anginal chest pain, near-syncope or syncope, and right ventricular heart failure.[70] Without treatment, patients with PAH had estimated median survival rates at 1, 3, and 5 years of 68%, 48%, and 34%. Treatment increases survival by 20% to 30%, with PAH 3-year survival increasing to 83%.[71]

Medications, illegal drugs, and toxin-induced PAH include agents with identified risk of inducing PAH. The first identified

TABLE 14.11 World Health Organization Functional Classification of Pulmonary Hypertension

Class	Symptoms
I	Patients with PH but without resulting limitation of physical activity; ordinary physical activity does not cause undue dyspnea of fatigue, chest pain, or near syncope
II	Patients with PH resulting in slight limitation of physical activity; they are comfortable at rest; ordinary physical activity causes undue dyspnea or fatigue, chest pain, or near syncope
III	Patients with PH resulting in marked limitation of physical activity; they are comfortable at rest; less than ordinary activity causes undue dyspnea or fatigue, chest pain, or near syncope
IV	Patients with PH with inability to carry out any physical activity without symptoms; these patients manifest signs of right heart failure; dyspnea and/or fatigue may be present at rest; discomfort is increased by any physical activity

PH, pulmonary hypertension.
From Zamanian RT, et al. Current clinical management of pulmonary arterial hypertension. *Circ Res*. 2014;115:131.

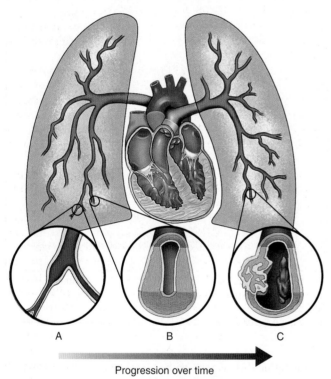

FIG. 14.21 Pulmonary Hypertension Progression Over Time. Pulmonary Hypertension is a progressive disease. (A) Vasoconstriction. (B) Hypertrophy and hyperplasia of all three layers of the small pulmonary arteries. (C) Development of plexiform vascular lesions and localized thrombosis contribute to progressive narrowing of the peripheral pulmonary vessels. From Lough, M.E. Hemodynamic Monitoring: Evolving Technologies and Clinical Practice, Philadelphia: Elsevier; 2016.

group included aminorex and fenfluramine derivatives used for weight loss. Since these agents were removed from the market, other agents, including toxic rapeseed oil, St. John's wort, and antiobesity agents containing phenylpropanolamine, have been identified as increasing the risk for developing IPAH.[66]

Amphetamine use is a likely risk for developing PAH, with methamphetamine demonstrating a strong relationship to IPAH.[66,67] The risk of developing PAH increases with exposure to toxic drug or environmental stimuli.

Heritable Pulmonary Artery Hypertension

Heritable PAH, previously known as *familial pulmonary artery hypertension*, is a condition with genetic mutations classified in WHO group I (see Table 14.10). Several genes associated with heritable PAH have been confirmed, including bone morphogenetic protein receptor type 2 (*BMPR2*), actin receptor-like kinase type 1 (*ALK1*), caveolin 1 (*CAV1*), Potassium Two Pore Domain Channel Subfamily K Member 3 (*KCNK3*), and endoglin (*ENG*).[67] *BMPR2* is the associated genetic abnormality in 70% of these cases.[67] Transmission of the *BMPR2* mutation leads to alteration of apoptosis (programmed cell death) that favors cellular proliferation.[67] In families with this gene, the children of patients have a 50% risk of inheriting the gene. However, not everyone who inherits the gene will exhibit the signs and symptoms of the disease, the reasons for which are not understood.[67] In heritable PAH, the pathogenesis of PAH is thought to be caused by multiple genetic and environmental stimuli. This has led to the development of a "multiple-hit hypothesis." This hypothesis predicts that modifier genes and environmental stimuli influence primary gene abnormalities such as the *BMPR2* mutation to develop into clinically evident PAH.[70]

Associated Pulmonary Artery Hypertension

Associated PAH may be related to other risk factors or conditions. This is classified as a WHO group I disease (see Table 14.10). Associated PAH includes many conditions associated with lesions in the small pulmonary muscular arterioles (eg, collagen vascular disease, human immunodeficiency virus infection, portal hypertension, congenital systemic-to-pulmonary shunts, schistosomiasis, chronic hemolytic anemia).

Pulmonary Venoocclusive Disease and Pulmonary Capillary Hemangiomatosis

Pulmonary venoocclusive disease and pulmonary capillary hemangiomatosis are included in IPAH because of pathologic similarities. These conditions are relocated from previous classification groups and renamed *Group 1′* because they have similar pathologic changes. Similar clinical presentation, risk factors, and familial association suggest that this subgrouping represents different components of a single disease spectrum.[66,67]

Pulmonary Hypertension Caused by Left Heart Disease

PH that results from left heart disease is classified as a WHO group II condition (see Table 14.10). This is the most common form of PH, with systolic dysfunction, diastolic dysfunction, and valvular disease composing distinct etiologies.[65,66] Pulmonary venous hypertension causes PH by a mechanism different from those of other forms of PH. It occurs as a result of elevated pressures in the left side of the heart that subsequently raise the pulmonary venous pressure. Patients with pulmonary venous hypertension have a history of CAD, acute MI, valvular disease, heart failure, or DCM. PH develops initially as a passive process of back-pressure that produces upstream elevation in the pulmonary venous and ultimately pulmonary artery pressure (PAP). Prolonged pressure elevation leads to an increase in pulmonary arteriolar resistance and persistent vascular changes.[65,67]

Pulmonary Hypertension Associated With Lung Disease or Hypoxemia

Chronic lung disease is often associated with hypoxemia and may entrain PH. In this group, which is classified as WHO group III (see Table 14.10), PH is caused by alveolar hypoxia secondary to lung disease, impaired control of breathing, or chronic exposure to high altitude.[66] All patients with PH feel short of breath with exercise, but patients with chronic obstructive pulmonary disease or interstitial lung disease (cystic fibrosis, pulmonary fibrosis, and emphysema) are breathless even at rest. All patients with obstructive pulmonary disease have worse survival rates when PH progresses.[66] Pulmonary function tests and sleep apnea studies are performed as part of the diagnostic work-up for patients with PAH and lung disease.[67]

Chronic Thromboembolic Pulmonary Hypertension

PAH that results from chronic thromboembolic conditions, such as chronic thromboembolic pulmonary hypertension, is classified as WHO group IV (see Table 14.10). PAH can occur acutely in response to a large pulmonary embolus that blocks flow to the pulmonary vascular bed. PAH can also occur after multiple microembolic thrombi that obstruct the smaller pulmonary arteries. Chronic thromboembolic pulmonary hypertension has an incidence of up to 4% after acute pulmonary emboli.[65,66] If the risk of pulmonary emboli is recognized in a patient with hypercoagulability, this condition is potentially preventable. When PH is diagnosed, guidelines recommend that a ventilation/perfusion scan be performed to determine the presence or absence of pulmonary emboli.[67] Treatment in a center of excellence with experience in pulmonary thromboendarterectomy is highly recommended for this condition, as skill in the procedure and required support systems are essential.[67,68]

Pulmonary Hypertension With Unclear and Multifactorial Mechanisms

Group V in the WHO classification (see Table 14.10) comprises miscellaneous conditions, including hematologic disorders (myeloproliferative disorders, splenectomy) systemic disorders (sarcoidosis, neurofibromatosis, vasculitis), metabolic disorders (glycogen storage disease, Gaucher disease, thyroid disorders), and other disorders (tumoral obstruction, fibrosing mediastinitis, chronic kidney failure).

Pathophysiology

The pulmonary vascular bed is normally a high-flow, low-pressure, low-resistance system that easily adjusts to changes in cardiac output, oxygen demand, and exercise.[64] In the presence of PH these characteristics are lost. Progressive and sustained elevation of pulmonary pressures with increased pulmonary vascular resistance leads to increased pressure on the right ventricle, increased right ventricular workload, right ventricular hypertrophy, heart failure, and death.

The three major components in the pathogenesis of chronic PH are (1) endothelial dysfunction and vasoconstriction, (2) vascular remodeling, and (3) thrombosis. A fourth component is the development of plexiform lesions that irreversibly obliterate the pulmonary arterioles (see Fig. 14.21).[64] Impaired endothelial cell function results in vasoconstriction caused by a decrease in endothelial cell–derived nitric oxide (NO), a decrease in prostacyclin, and an increase in the vasoconstrictor endothelin. This results in thrombi within the pulmonary arterioles from increased thrombosis and diminished thrombolysis.

Overproduction of substances that cause vasoconstriction such as thromboxane and endothelin or a decrease in endothelial factors that cause vasodilation, specifically endothelial prostacyclin and NO, or a combination of these factors, may be the catalyst.[67]

Assessment and Diagnosis

The diagnosis of PH is difficult. PH is often a diagnosis of exclusion when all other diagnostic theories are exhausted. The clinical symptoms of PH are nonspecific in the early stages of the disease and reflect the inability of the pulmonary vascular bed to accommodate increased cardiac output with exercise. These factors support findings that symptoms are often present more than 2 years before diagnosis.[70]

Physical Assessment

The severity of PH clinical symptoms is classified using WHO pulmonary hypertension functional classes I to IV (see Table 14.10). This classification is similar to the NYHA classification for heart failure.[67] Physical examination clues that reveal right ventricular failure include elevated jugular venous pressure, a palpable right ventricular heave, hepatomegaly, ascites, and peripheral edema. Auscultation of heart sounds reveals a prominent pulmonic component to S_2 and a holosystolic blowing murmur from tricuspid regurgitation. Pulmonary edema suggests left ventricular dysfunction or a noncardiac cause such as ARDS.[68]

Signs and symptoms early in PAH include fatigue and shortness of breath caused by impaired oxygen transport and reduced cardiac output. Later symptoms include syncope from systemic hypotension as a result of low cardiac output and angina from the underfilled right and left ventricles. Patients may have intestinal edema, which can cause constipation, abdominal pain, malabsorption, and anorexia.[68]

Diagnostic tests that can assist with PAH diagnosis include a 12-lead ECG, echocardiogram, and right-sided cardiac catheterization. The most helpful noninvasive test is the echocardiogram. Echocardiography can estimate right atrial pressure and PAP, and it can determine the degree of right ventricular dysfunction.[67,68] Signs of significant disease include right ventricular dilation and hypertrophy; septal bowing into the left ventricle, creating a D-shaped left ventricle; right ventricular hypokinesis; tricuspid regurgitation; right atrial enlargement; and a dilated inferior vena cava.

The 12-lead ECG is a noninvasive test that may show right-axis deviation and right ventricular hypertrophy resulting from PAH. The 12-lead ECG is an adjunct test that can indicate strain on the right ventricle, but it cannot diagnose PH when used alone.

The most helpful invasive diagnostic test is right-sided cardiac catheterization because it can provide verifiable numbers. To diagnose PAH, the mean PAP must be greater than 25 mm Hg at rest.[67] Precise analysis of mixed venous oxygen saturation (Svo_2) during insertion and passage of the pulmonary artery catheter through the cardiac chamber can allow diagnosis of intracardiac shunts. A pulmonary artery occlusion pressure less than 15 mm Hg rules out left ventricular heart disease.[67] Information on diagnostic use of the pulmonary artery catheter and Svo_2 is included in the section on "Hemodynamics" in Chapter 13.

The ability of the pulmonary vessels to vasodilate in response to administration of a pulmonary artery vasodilator, called a *positive vasoreactivity test,* is an important component of the cardiac catheterization study when used to diagnose PAH. Vasoactive medications used in the test include inhaled NO (iNO), intravenous adenosine, or intravenous epoprostenol (prostacyclin). The ability of the pulmonary vasculature to dilate determines how helpful pharmacologic pulmonary artery vasodilators are likely to be. A positive response includes a reduction in mean PAP of at least 10 mm Hg to achieve a mean PAP less than 40 mm Hg with an increased or unchanged cardiac output. Only approximately 10% to 20% of patients with PH have a positive response to vasodilators.[67]

If diagnostic tests are performed when PH is advanced, the PAP may almost equal the systemic aortic pressure, and the pulmonary arterioles may not vasodilate in response to vasodilator medications. In this scenario, the enlarged right ventricle puts pressure on the intraventricular septum and compresses the left ventricle. The smaller, compressed left ventricle results in greatly reduced left ventricular stroke volume and cardiac output.[67,68]

Formal assessment of exercise tolerance is important for evaluation and ongoing treatment of PAH. The *6-minute walk distance* (6MWD) and a variety of treadmill exercise tests are used for this evaluation. In the 6MWD, the patient walks as far as possible for 6 minutes. The distance walked in 6 minutes has a strong association with mortality among patients with IPAH.[67] Evaluation of serial 6MWD tests can monitor the severity, response to treatment, or progression of the disease.

Medical Management

Medical management focuses on early diagnosis, use of appropriate pharmacologic therapies, and prevention of complications. Goals of therapy include alleviation of symptoms, improvements in quality of life, and survival. Improvements are measured by changes in functional class and exercise tolerance.[68] Clinical practice guidelines for this complex and progressive disease recommend referral to a medical center specializing in the management of PH.[67]

Medications

Table 14.12 lists PH medications. Most patients are maintained on multiple medications that include oral endothelin receptor antagonists, phosphodiesterase-5 inhibitors, pulmonary vasodilators, prostacyclin derivatives, calcium channel blockers (early stage only), anticoagulants, diuretics, and oxygen. Fig. 14.22 provides an example of how these medications can be combined as part of the treatment regimen.[72,73]

Calcium channel blockers improve survival of patients with PH who demonstrate a significantly positive vasoreactivity test result during right-sided cardiac catheterization (responders).[72] Long-acting calcium channel blockers include nifedipine, diltiazem, and amlodipine.[73] Most patients with PH are nonresponders and are more effectively managed with one of the following newer medications developed specifically to treat PH.[74]

Endothelin receptor antagonists are used for treating PH. Endothelin 1 is a potent vasoconstrictor and smooth muscle mitogen capable of inducing smooth muscle cell hypertrophy. Two types of endothelin receptors are endothelin A, which causes vasoconstriction and smooth muscle proliferation, and endothelin B, which causes vasodilation and is involved in clearance of endothelin. Bosentan (Tracleer) is an oral endothelin receptor antagonist.[72] Bosentan is approved for WHO classes III and IV. In IPAH and scleroderma-related disorders, it improves symptoms, functional class, hemodynamics, and exercise capacity measured by 6MWD.[72] Ambrisentan (Letairis) is useful in treating IPAH and PH resulting from connective tissue disease and congenital heart disease. It improves symptoms, time to clinical worsening, exercise capacity, and functional class.[72] Macitentan and riociguat are two new oral agents added to the updated guidelines treatment algorithm. Macitentan is a new endothelin receptor antagonist that improved both morbidity and mortality in studies.[73] Riociguat works as a stimulator of soluble guanylate cyclase that induces cyclic guanosine monophosphate (cGMP) release. This affects the NO pathway, increasing vasodilation and resulting in improved exercise tolerance and pulmonary hemodynamics.[73]

Phosphodiesterase inhibitors are designed to inhibit the degradation of cGMP. These medications promote pulmonary vasodilation and decrease vascular smooth muscle cell proliferation. Sildenafil and tadalafil (Adcirca) are potent inhibitors of phosphodiesterase-5; both agents are used to treat erectile dysfunction and are an effective treatment option for PAH.[74] Started as monotherapy, sildenafil is also used as part of a multimedication treatment regimen.[72,74]

NO is a potent *vasodilator* that dilates the pulmonary vasculature in ventilated lung units. It improves oxygenation and reduces PAP.[74,75] In critically ill mechanically ventilated patients, iNO is useful especially in combination with dobutamine or milrinone. Abrupt withdrawal of iNO can lead to methemoglobinemia, nitrogen dioxide production, and rebound PH with hemodynamic collapse, which limits iNO use.

Prostacyclins are potent vasodilators that affect the pulmonary and systemic circulations, and they have antiproliferative and antiplatelet aggregatory effects.[72,74] Prostacyclin analogue medications are known as *prostanoids*. The four prostanoid medications approved by the US Food and Drug Administration are (1) epoprostenol (Flolan), (2) treprostinil (Remodulin), (3) iloprost (Ventavis), and (4) inhaled treprostinil (Tyvaso).[72-75]

- *Epoprostenol:* In patients with advanced PH and right ventricular failure, long-term therapy with intravenous epoprostenol can be lifesaving. Epoprostenol therapy is started in the hospital and continued long-term at home. Epoprostenol has a short elimination half-life of less than 5 minutes.[72] Patients who are critically ill and have functional class IV symptoms should be started on epoprostenol because it is the most rapidly effective therapy.[69,72] Epoprostenol provides a sustained survival benefit of 62.8% at 3 years compared with 35.4% with historical controls.[69]

- *Treprostinil:* A more recently approved prostanoid, treprostinil sodium is administered by a subcutaneous or intravenous infusion catheter and pump and has a half-life of 3 to 4 hours. Subcutaneous administration is safe and effective and avoids the risks associated with the indwelling catheter. However, it is associated with injection site pain, which may not be tolerated. These prostacyclin analogues do not cure PH, but all vasodilate the pulmonary vascular bed, control symptoms, and prolong life in responsive patients.

- *Iloprost:* Iloprost is an inhaled prostanoid administered with an ultrasonic nebulizer 6 to 12 times each day. Iloprost has a serum half-life of 20 to 25 minutes. Studies show that it provides improved functional class, exercise capacity, and pulmonary hemodynamics.[75] Studies on long-term use and use as combination therapy with oral agents have demonstrated safety and efficacy.

TABLE 14.12 Pharmacology

Pulmonary Hypertension Medications

Medication	Dosage	Action	Special Considerations
Endothelin Receptor Antagonist			
Bosentan (Tracleer)	62.5–125 mg PO bid	Blocks vasoconstriction and smooth muscle proliferation	Monitor LFTs
Ambrisentan (Letairis)	5–10 mg PO daily	NO pathway leads to vasodilation	Monitor LFTs
Macitentan (Opsumit)	10 mg PO daily		
Riociguat (Adempas)	0.5–2.5 mg PO tid		
Phosphodiesterase-5 Inhibitors			
Sildenafil (Revatio)	5–20 mg PO tid	Pulmonary vasodilation and decreases smooth muscle proliferation	Concomitant use with nitrates can result in irreversible hypotension
	IV bolus 2.5 mg or 10 mg tid		
Tadalafil (Adcirca)	40 mg PO daily		
Pulmonary Vasodilator			
Inhaled NO (iNO)		Dilates pulmonary vasculature	Abrupt withdrawal results in rebound pulmonary hypertension; NO production leads to methemoglobinemia
Prostacyclin Derivative			
Epoprostenol (Flolan)	Start at 2–4 ng/kg/min continuous IV infusion	Dilates pulmonary and peripheral vessels; antiproliferative, antiplatelet	Rebound pulmonary hypertension if abruptly discontinued or dose decreased
(Veletri)	20–40 ng/kg/day		Flolan needs to be refrigerated or covered with ice bags for short half-life; Veletri is stable at room temperature
Treprostinil (Remodulin)	20–80 ng/kg/mg continuous SC/IV infusion		Pain at injection site
(Tyvaso oral inhalation)	3 inhalations (18 mcg) 4–9 times/day		
Iloprost	2.5–5 mcg (6-9 inhalations) nebulized qid		Hemoptysis
Anticoagulant			Maintain INR with oral vitamin K antagonist therapy
Calcium Channel Blocker			
Nifedipine	120–240 mg/day	Vasodilator	Can cause hypotension; useful *only* in vasoreactor-positive patients
Diltiazem	240–720 mg/day		
Amlodipine	Up to 20 mg/day		
Diuretics		Decrease volume overload	Monitor electrolytes and kidney function closely

bid, two times a day; *INR*, international normalized ratio; *IV*, intravenous; *LFT*, liver function test; *NO*, nitric oxide; *PO*, by mouth; *qid*, four times a day; *SC*, subcutaneous; *tid*, three times a day.

- *Tyvaso (inhaled treprostinil):* Tyvaso is the most recent analogue studied with successful results in treatment of PH. Tyvaso improved 6MWD when used in combination therapy with bosentan or sildenafil therapy.[75,76] Tyvaso is an inhaled prostanoid administered with a handheld nebulizer four times daily.

Anticoagulation is an essential component of pharmacologic management. Risk factors for venous thromboembolism (VTE) such as heart failure, right ventricular dysfunction, low stroke volume and decreased arterial pulse pressure, a sedentary lifestyle, and a thrombophilic predisposition are found in PH. Warfarin (Coumadin) improves survival in patients with IPAH and associated PAH. The usual target international normalized ratio (INR) of 2 to 3 is reduced to 1.5 to 2.5 when warfarin is used with prostacyclin analogues.[72,74]

Diuretics are used to prevent right ventricular volume overload, edema, ascites, and malabsorption associated with bowel edema. Serum electrolytes and kidney function are closely monitored.[72]

Supplemental oxygen use is a key component of therapy for chronic PH.[67,68] Chronic hypoxemia from impaired cardiac output results in mixed venous desaturation. Hypoxemia can also be related to right-to-left shunting through patent foramen ovale or heart defects.[67] Oxygen inhalation decreases PAP and improves cardiac output. Hypoxia is a potent pulmonary vasoconstrictor. Oxygen saturation is preferably maintained above 90%.[68]

SYMPTOMATIC PULMONARY ARTERIAL HYPERTENSION

Oral anticoagulants
Diuretics
Oxygen
Digoxin
Supervised rehabilitation

← General treatment measures →

Avoid excess exercise
Birth control
Psychologic and
social support
Infection prevention

Acute vasoreactivity test

ACUTE RESPONDER
WHO FC I-IV

Oral CCB

Sustained response

Continued responder   Nonresponder

NONRESPONDER

FC II	FC III	FC IV
Ambrisentan	Ambrisentan	Ambrisentan
Bosentan	Bosentan	Bosentan
Sildenafil	Sildenafil	Sildenafil
Tadalafil	Tadalafil	Tadalafil
	Epoprostenol IV	Epoprostenol IV
	Iloprost inh	Iloprost inh
	Treprostinil SC	Treprostinil SC
	Treprostinil IV	Treprostinil IV
	Treprostinil inh	Treprostinil inh
		Initial combo treatment

Sequential combo therapy

Prostanoids

PDE-5 ⇌ ERA

Atrial septostomy and/or lung transplantation

FIG. 14.22 Combination Medication Therapy Used to Treat Pulmonary Artery Hypertension. CCB, calcium channel blocker; ERA, endothelin receptor antagonist; FC, functional class; inh, inhalation; IV, intravenous; PDE-5, phosphodiesterase-5; SC, subcutaneous; WHO, World Health Organization. (Based on Badesch DB, et al. Diagnosis and assessment of pulmonary arterial hypertension. *J Am Coll Cardiol.* 2009;54[1]:S55.)

For patients who are refractory to pharmacologic management, a heart-lung transplant may be an option.[67,73] Detailed information on heart-lung transplantation is provided in Chapter 36.

Nursing Management

Nursing management of a patient with PH incorporates a variety of nursing diagnoses related to the symptoms of breathlessness and right-sided heart failure. These nursing diagnoses are reviewed in Box 14.20. Nursing interventions are individualized according to how advanced the symptoms of PH are. Interventions focus on lowering PAP, administering pharmacologic therapy, monitoring the effects and safety of all medications, treating pain that can occur at the site of injection (with epoprostenol or treprostinil), and providing patient and family education.

Patient Education

If the cause for PH is known, the patient should receive education before discharge. All patients should be provided with a written medication list with the name and purpose of all their medications. Specific education topics include (1) the use and care of a handheld nebulizer, tunneled intravenous catheter, or subcutaneous pump for medication administration; (2) infection control; and (3) sterile preparation of the prostacyclin analogue medication. Providing the patient with the name of the health care professional to contact for questions related to PH is also important (Box 14.21). A collaborative team of empathetic, educated professionals is essential to provide effective care for these challenging patients (Box 14.22).

◎ BOX 14.20 NURSING DIAGNOSES
Pulmonary Artery Hypertension

- Impaired Gas Exchange related to ventilation/perfusion mismatching or intrapulmonary shunting, p. 1030
- Activity Intolerance related to cardiopulmonary dysfunction, p. 1006
- Decreased Cardiac Output related to alterations in afterload (pulmonary), p. 1015
- Decreased Cardiac Output related to alterations in preload, p. 1015
- Decreased Cardiac Output related to alterations in contractility, p. 1016
- Decreased Cardiac Output related to alterations in heart rate or rhythm, p. 1016
- Risk for Infection, p. 1046
- Anxiety related to threat to biologic, psychologic, or social integrity, p. 1012
- Ineffective Coping related to situational crisis and personal vulnerability, p. 1036
- Deficient Knowledge related to lack of previous exposure to information, p. 1020 (see Box 14.21, Patient Education Plan for Pulmonary Artery Hypertension)

✳ BOX 14.21 PATIENT EDUCATION PLAN
Pulmonary Artery Hypertension

The patient should be able to teach back the following topics:
- Pathophysiology of pulmonary artery hypertension and disease process.
- Symptoms: Dyspnea at rest or, more commonly, with exertion.
- Activity conservation with scheduled rest periods.
- Medications: Purpose, side effects, special considerations.
  - Epoprostenol (Flolan): Intravenous (IV) by pump, half-life of 2–3 min.
  - Treprostinil (Remodulin): IV or subcutaneous (SC) by pump, half-life of 3 h.
  - Iloprost (Ventavis) and epoprostenol (Veletri): Inhalation.
  - Bosentan (Tracleer): Oral.
  - Sildenafil (Viagra): Oral concomitant use with nitrates contraindicated, as may result in profound hypotension.
- Pain management at insertion site of IV or SC catheter.
- Use of handheld nebulizer for inhaled iloprost or treprostinil (Tyvaso).
- Anticoagulation: Purpose of international normalized ratio; monitoring of skin, gums, urine, and stool for signs of bleeding; precautions to prevent bleeding when on anticoagulation (eg, use soft toothbrush, use electric razor when shaving, avoid contact sports).
- Follow-up care after discharge.
- Symptoms to report to a health care professional.

QSEN BOX 14.22 QSEN: Evidence-Based Practice
Pulmonary Artery Hypertension

Recommendations for Early Detection and Screening for Pulmonary Artery Hypertension
- Relatives of patients with heritable pulmonary artery hypertension (PAH) are recommended to undergo prenatal genetic testing before any pregnancy.
- Pregnancy is not recommended for female patients with PAH.
- If PAH is suspected, a 12-lead electrocardiogram (ECG) is required as an early screening test to rule out other possible cardiac anomalies; the ECG is not diagnostic for PAH.
- If PAH is suspected, a chest radiograph can reveal features supportive of a PAH diagnosis.
- If PAH is suspected, Doppler echocardiography is recommended to noninvasively evaluate right ventricular systolic pressures and to assess for anatomic abnormalities such as right atrial or right ventricular enlargement, left ventricular involvement, and intracardiac shunting.

Recommendations for Diagnostic Tests to Further Evaluate Pulmonary Artery Hypertension
- In patients with unexplained PAH, testing for connective tissue disease and human immunodeficiency virus infection is recommended.
- In patients with probable connective tissue PAH, a ventilation-perfusion scan is recommended to identify perfusion blocks and severity of disease progression.
- Pulmonary function tests are recommended to rule out other causes of lung disease.
- Lung biopsy is not recommended; it carries a high risk and low diagnostic yield.
- Right-sided heart catheterization is recommended, as is acute vasoreactivity testing using a short-acting agent such as intravenous (IV) epoprostenol, IV adenosine, or inhaled nitrous oxide.
- Serial assessments of functional class and endurance on a 6-min walk are recommended.

Recommendations for General Management of Pulmonary Artery Hypertension
- Anticoagulation with warfarin (Coumadin) should be considered.
- Diuretics should be administered, as indicated.
- Supplemental oxygen should be used as necessary to maintain oxygen saturation values higher than 90% at all times.
- Referral to a center that specializes in treatment of PAH is strongly recommended.

Recommendations for Medications to Treat Pulmonary Artery Hypertension
- A calcium channel blocker is recommended for patients with positive vasoreactivity testing.
- All patients should be considered for long-term therapy with a combination of the following medications (see Fig. 14.22):
  - Endothelin receptor antagonists
    Bosentan (oral)
    Ambrisentan (oral)
    Macitentan (oral)
  - Soluble guanylate cyclase sensitizer
    Ricioguat
  - Phosphodiesterase inhibitors
    Sildenafil
    Tadalafil
  - Prostanoids
    Epoprostenol (IV)
    Treprostinil (subcutaneous, IV, inhaled)
    Iloprost (inhaled)
- Patients with PAH in functional class IV are candidates for long-term treatment with IV epoprostenol.

References
Galie N, et al. 2015 ESC/ERS guidelines for the diagnosis and treatment of pulmonary hypertension. *Eur Heart J.* 2016;37:67.
Zamanian RT, et al. Current clinical management of pulmonary arterial hypertension. *Circ Res.* 2014;115:131.

ENDOCARDITIS

Description and Etiology

Endocarditis is an inflammation on the endothelial surface of the heart, specifically thrombotic-fibrin vegetation on the cardiac valves. This irritation can be related to infectious or noninfectious sources.[77] Although most commonly associated with valve leaflets, chordae, chamber walls, paraprosthetic tissue, implanted shunts, conduits, and fistulas may also be affected.[77] The older term *bacterial endocarditis* has been replaced by the term *infectious endocarditis* (IE) because nonbacterial organisms can be the infective source of the endothelial inflammation. The incidence of IE has not declined over the past 30 years, with 10,000 to 20,000 cases reported each year.[77] IE is the fourth most common cause of life-threatening infectious syndromes (after urosepsis, pneumonia, and intraabdominal sepsis). The risk of acquiring IE is higher among patients with congenital heart disease, valvular heart disease, and prosthetic heart valves. Approximately 75% of patients have a preexisting structural abnormality of the involved cardiac valve. Increasing incidence of invasive health care interventions such as implantable pacemakers and ICDs, body piercings, intravenous drug abuse (IVDA), and an increase in the number of older patients with degenerative valve disease increase the numbers at risk for IE.[77] Involvement of right heart valves is highly suspicious for IVDA.[78] Among intravenous drug abusers, the incidence of IE is 60 times that of age-matched controls.[79]

Development of IE depends on the following events:[78]

- Presence of a nonbacterial thrombotic lesion on a cardiac valve or endothelium
- Bacteremia (bacteria in bloodstream)
- Bacteria attaching to the nonbacterial thrombotic lesion
- Proliferation of bacteria on and within the lesion that may develop into a vegetation

Research suggests the source of the organism is less likely to be related to a specific invasive procedure such as a urogenital procedure or dental work. Rather, IE results from the confluence of multiple daily bacteremic events in the presence of a susceptible cardiac lesion.[78]

Pathophysiology

IE results from a bacterial or fungal organism in the bloodstream that successfully colonizes the cardiac endothelium. IE is fatal if not treated. Bacterial organisms, typically streptococci, staphylococci, and enterococci, are the most common pathogens. An increase in multidrug-resistant organisms has led to increased numbers of patients, more serious complications, and higher mortality rates.[78] Sites where endocarditis vegetations occur often correlate with aberrant intracardiac flow caused by valvular damage or septal defects. After the vegetations have colonized, organisms multiply at a rapid rate inside a protective platelet-fibrin casing that sequesters the infection.[79]

Assessment and Diagnosis

Diagnosis must be made as soon as possible to initiate treatment and identify patients at high risk for complications. Diagnosis is guided by classic manifestations of bacteremia or fungemia, evidence of active valvulitis, peripheral emboli, and immunologic vascular phenomena.

Modified Duke Criteria

The 2015 AHA scientific statement on IE supports use of the modified Duke criteria for diagnosis, early identification, and treatment of IE. This system stratifies patients with suspected IE into three categories: (1) definite cases, (2) possible cases, and (3) rejected cases (Table 14.13). A definite diagnosis of IE requires two major criteria, one major and three minor criteria, or five minor criteria. A possible diagnosis of IE requires one major and one minor criteria, or three minor criteria.[77-79]

Blood Cultures

Initial symptoms include fever sometimes accompanied by rigor (shivering), fatigue, and malaise; up to 50% of patients report myalgias and joint pain.[77] Blood cultures are drawn during periods of elevated temperature to detect the infective organism. At least 10 mL of venous blood should be placed in each of the blood culture containers to ensure that the organism will be detected.[79] Culture-negative endocarditis occurs in up to one-third of cases and usually is related to prior antibiotic use or infection by a "fastidious" organism, which does not proliferate under conventional laboratory culture conditions.[78] White blood cell counts are typically elevated, and the symptoms are identified in the Duke criteria (see Table 14.13).

Chest Radiograph

Cough and pleuritic chest pain are present in 40% to 60% of cases. The first noninvasive test is often a chest radiograph to detect nodular infiltrates, cardiomegaly, and enlarged pulmonary vessels.

Echocardiogram

The other essential noninvasive test is an echocardiogram of the heart valves to visualize vegetations. TTE may be performed initially, but transesophageal echocardiography is more valuable because of the clarity of the heart valve images. Transesophageal echocardiography is more sensitive in detection of vegetations and abscesses.[77,78] Color-flow

TABLE 14.13 **Modified Duke Criteria**	
Major Criteria[a]	**Minor Criteria[a]**
Blood culture positive for IE	Predisposition: Patients with a heart condition or an injectable drug user
Evidence of endocardial involvement	Fever: Temperature >38°C
	Vascular phenomena: Major arterial emboli, septic pulmonary infarcts, mycotic aneurysm, intracranial hemorrhage, conjunctival hemorrhages, and Janeway lesions
	Immunologic phenomena: Glomerulonephritis, Osler nodes, Roth spots, and rheumatoid factor
	Microbial evidence: Positive blood culture that does not meet any major criterion or serologic evidence of active infection with organism consistent with IE

[a]A *definite* diagnosis of IE requires two major criteria, one major and three minor criteria, or five minor criteria. A *possible* diagnosis of IE requires one major and one minor criteria, or three minor criteria.
IE, infective endocarditis.
Data from Baddour LM, et al. Infective endocarditis in adults: Diagnosis, antimicrobial therapy, and management of complication. *Circulation.* 2015;132:1435; and Nishimura RA, et al. 2014 AHA/ACC guideline for the management of patients with valvular heart disease guidelines. *J Am Coll Cardiol.* 2014;63(22):e57.

mapping is especially useful to visualize the severity of valvular regurgitation.

Complications

Heart failure is the most frequent complication of IE and the most frequent cause of death. Embolic complications are the second most common complication, occurring in 22% to 50% of IE cases; 65% of the emboli occur in the central nervous system (CNS) and can cause a stroke. Pulmonary embolism (PE) occurs in 66% to 75% of IVDA cases that involve vegetations on the tricuspid valve. Other organs affected by emboli include liver, spleen, kidney, abdominal mesenteric artery, and peripheral vessels. Septic emboli may be visible on the fingers and toes. Rate of emboli formation rapidly declines with appropriate intravenous antimicrobial administration.[78] Risk of death increases with the development of emboli and decreased arterial perfusion to vital organs. Even with appropriate treatment, mortality risk is almost 40% at 1 year.[80] Clinical manifestations of IE that may be discovered on physical examination are listed in Box 14.23.

Medical Management

Treatment requires prolonged intravenous therapy with adequate doses of antimicrobial agents tailored to the specific IE microbe and patient circumstances. The antibiotic management of native valve endocarditis is frequently different from treatment of prosthetic valve endocarditis or IVDA endocarditis. Antibiotic treatment, administered in high doses intravenously, is prolonged and may involve combination therapy.[77-80] Best outcomes are achieved if therapy is initiated before hemodynamic compromise.

In many cases, antimicrobial medications are insufficient to cure the IE. Cardiac surgery to excise the damaged native or prosthetic valve is required for persistent vegetation, valve dysfunction, perivalvular extension, and aggressive fungal or antibiotic-resistant bacteria. Valve surgery usually is delayed until the patient is stable.[77] Early surgery is indicated for patients demonstrating signs of heart failure or for persistent symptomatic infection lasting longer than 5 to 7 days with appropriate antimicrobial treatment.[80] An increasing number of patients with uncomplicated IE are being discharged earlier than in the past and are continuing intravenous antimicrobial therapy at home with a surgically or peripherally implanted long-term central venous catheter.

Nursing Management

Nursing management of a patient with IE incorporates a variety of nursing diagnoses (Box 14.24). Nursing interventions focus on timely antimicrobial administration to resolve the infection, prevent complications, provide pain medication, and individualize patient education.

Resolving the Infection

IE requires a long course (usually 4 to 6 weeks) of intravenous antibiotics. Treatment is begun in the hospital and continued at home with an indwelling central catheter after the patient is in stable condition. Nursing assessment includes monitoring for signs of worsening infection such as persistent temperature elevation, malaise, weakness, easy fatigability, night sweats, or new emboli on hands or feet (see Box 14.24).

Preventing Complications

Complications occur in 20% to 50% of patients with IE.[80] The nursing assessment is attuned to the early detection of changes such as shortness of breath or chest pain with hemoptysis. As valvular dysfunction accelerates, acute heart failure develops. Cardiac assessment includes auscultation of heart sounds to detect the presence of or change in a cardiac murmur. Murmurs can be caused by worsening heart failure or by pulmonary emboli. Changes in level of consciousness, visual changes, or complaints of headache should always be reported immediately because of the risk of emboli. Evaluation of liver and kidney function is essential to monitor the health of those organs because of the risk of emboli. Because of the complex and prolonged antibiotic therapy required for treating IE, adverse medication reactions are another important consideration.

Patient Education

A patient with IE needs to know the manifestations of infection, how to take an oral temperature, and what medical procedures increase risk for recurrence of IE. A written list of all medications must be supplied (Box 14.25). It is essential to reinforce to patients the necessity to provide a comprehensive endocarditis history to their other health care providers such as the dentist or the podiatrist.[77] The known intravenous drug abuser has a unique set of challenges to overcome. Multidisciplinary support for the patient to meet the challenge of opiate withdrawal and psychologic dependence is essential to prevent a relapse. Many clinicians participate in the care of a patient with IE (Box 14.26).

BOX 14.23 Clinical Manifestations of Endocarditis

- Fever
- Splenomegaly
- Hematuria
- Petechiae
- Cardiac murmurs
- Easy fatigability
- Osler nodes[a]
- Splinter hemorrhages in nail beds
- Roth spots[b]

[a]Small, raised, tender areas most commonly found in pads of fingers and toes.

[b]Round or oval spots consisting of coagulated fibrin; seen in the retina and lead to hemorrhage.

BOX 14.24 NURSING DIAGNOSES

Endocarditis

- Decreased Cardiac Output related to alterations in preload, p. 1015
- Decreased Cardiac Output related to alterations in afterload, p. 1015
- Decreased Cardiac Output related to alterations in contractility, p. 1016
- Decreased Cardiac Output related to alterations in heart rate or rhythm, p. 1016
- Activity Intolerance related to cardiopulmonary dysfunction, p. 1006
- Acute Pain related to transmission and perception of cutaneous, visceral, muscular, or ischemic impulses, p. 1010
- Risk for Infection, p. 1046
- Anxiety related to threat to biologic, psychologic, or social integrity, p. 1012
- Deficient Knowledge related to lack of previous exposure to information, p. 1020 (see Box 14.25, Patient Education Plan for Endocarditis)

VALVULAR HEART DISEASE

Description and Etiology

The term *valvular heart disease* describes structural and functional abnormalities of single or multiple cardiac valves. The result is an alteration in blood flow across the valve. The two types of valvular lesions are *stenotic* and *regurgitant*. These are described in this section with reference to the specific cardiac valves involved.

Admission of patients with valvular disease to the critical care unit is generally related to surgical replacement or an exacerbation of heart failure. In the past, most valvular lesions in the United States were rheumatic in origin, and damage was a direct result of group A beta-hemolytic streptococcal pharyngitis. As a result of aggressive treatment of "strep throat," this has become a rare problem. Valve lesions now more commonly occur in patients with congenital disorders and older patients. These patients are more likely to present with symptoms of heart failure and degenerative valve changes.[80] These changes may be described as myxomatous leaflet, degeneration, or annular calcification.[80]

Pathophysiology

Mitral Valve Stenosis

The term *mitral valve stenosis* describes a progressive narrowing of the mitral valve orifice. The primary cause is rheumatic endocarditis with rare occurrences related to congenital malformations. Mitral stenosis occurs in twice as many women as men.[80] Symptoms occur when the normal valve size is reduced to 2 cm^2 or less. Symptoms occur at rest when the valve area is reduced to less than 1 cm^2.[80] Narrowing is caused by aging valve tissue or by acute rheumatic valvulitis (Table 14.14A). The diffuse valve leaflets fibrose and fuse, reducing mobility and thickening the chordae tendineae. As a result, the mitral valve can no longer open or close passively in response to left atrial and ventricular pressure changes. Blood flow across the valve is impeded. Mitral stenosis increases the risk of developing AF because of the high pressures in the left atrium that stimulate left atrial remodeling and enlargement. Development of AF significantly increases symptoms and may increase the need for surgical replacement of the valve.

✳ BOX 14.25   PATIENT EDUCATION PLAN

Endocarditis

The patient should be able to teach back the following topics:

- Pathophysiology of endocarditis
- Medications: Importance of long-term intravenous antibiotics for eradication
- Temperature: Daily temperature monitoring
- Infection control: Prophylactic antibiotics related to dental work or other invasive procedures after current medical crisis is controlled
- Activity tolerance: Increase activity as tolerated and rest periods as needed
- Heart failure: If symptoms of heart failure are present, education is provided on fluid and sodium restriction, fluid balance, diuretic management, daily weight, and controlling breathlessness
- Follow-up care after discharge
- Symptoms to report to a health care professional

QSEN BOX 14.26   QSEN: Evidence-Based Practice

Infective Endocarditis and Infective Endocarditis Prophylaxis

Diagnosis of IE

The Modified Duke Criteria are recommended to guide diagnosis of infective endocarditis (IE) (see Table 14.13). Endocarditis prophylaxis is recommended for patients with the following:

- Prosthetic heart valve with a history of IE.
- Valve repair.
- Complex cyanotic congenital heart disease.
- Congenital valve malformation such as bicuspid aortic valve.
- Hypertrophic cardiomyopathy with latent or resting obstruction.
- Mitral valve prolapse with valvular regurgitation and/or thickened valve leaflets.
  Special considerations apply for patients with prosthetic valve and IE.
- Patients with a risk for IE who have unexplained fever for more than 48 h should have at least two sets of blood cultures obtained from different sites.
- Surgical valve replacement is indicated for patients with IE of a prosthetic valve who present in heart failure.

Antimicrobial Therapy

Antimicrobial therapy administered for IE is characterized by four features:

1. It is prolonged.
2. It is bactericidal.
3. It is intravenous (IV).
4. It is high dosage.
   At least two sets of blood cultures are obtained every 24–48 h until the infection is cleared from the bloodstream. IV antimicrobial therapy is continued after hospital discharge in the home setting.

Complications From IE

- Emboli from infected heart valves occur in 22%–50% of IE cases, and 65% of embolic events involve the central nervous system. The rate of embolic events decreases significantly during and after 2–3 weeks of appropriate antimicrobial therapy.
- Acute heart failure has the greatest impact on overall prognosis.

Complications From Antibiotics

- Toxicity from the high doses of antibiotics may impair kidney function or vestibular function (balance).
- Diarrhea and colitis can be caused by a reaction to the antibiotic therapy or by overgrowth by *Clostridium difficile*.

Indications for Surgery

- Removal of infected device.
- Increase in size of valve vegetation despite appropriate antimicrobial therapy.
- Mitral or aortic regurgitation with acute heart failure unresponsive to medical therapy.
- One or more embolic events during the first 2 weeks of antimicrobial therapy.

References

Habib G, et al. 2015 ESC guidelines for the management of infective endocarditis. The Task Force for the Management of Infective Endocarditis of the European Society of Cardiology (ESC). *Eur Heart J.* 2015;36(42):2921.
Nishimura RA, et al. 2014 AHA/ACC guideline for the management of patients with valvular heart disease guidelines. *J Am Coll Cardiol.* 2014;63(22):e57.

TABLE 14.14 Valvular Dysfunction

	Pathophysiology	Clinical Manifestations	Physical Signs
Mitral Valve Stenosis A. RA LA RV LV Mitral valve stenosis ↓ indicates stenosis A	Left atrium must generate more pressure to propel blood beyond lesion; rise in left atrial pressure and volume reflected retrograde into pulmonary vessels; right ventricular hypertrophy; right ventricular failure	Dyspnea on exertion; fatigue and weakness; pronounced respiratory symptoms (eg, orthopnea, paroxysmal nocturnal dyspnea); mild hemoptysis with bronchial capillary rupture; susceptibility to pulmonary infections	• Chest radiograph: Pulmonary congestion, redistribution of blood flow to upper lobes • ECG: Atrial fibrillation and other atrial dysrhythmias • Auscultation: Diastolic murmur, accentuated S_1, opening snap • Catheterization: Elevated pressure gradient across valve; increased left atrial pressure, pulmonary artery occlusion pressure, and pulmonary artery pressure; low cardiac output
Mitral Valve Regurgitation B. RA LA RV LV Mitral valve regurgitation indicates backward flow from a valve that is leaking or regurgitant B	LV dilation and hypertrophy; left atrial dilation and hypertrophy	Weakness and fatigue; exertional dyspnea; palpitations; severe symptoms precipitated by LV failure, with consequent low output and pulmonary congestion	• Chest radiograph: Left atrial and LV enlargement, variable pulmonary congestion • ECG: P mitrale, LV hypertrophy, atrial fibrillation • Auscultation: Murmur throughout systole • Catheterization: Opacification of left atrium during LV injection, v waves, increased left atrial and LV pressures • Variable elevations of pulmonary pressures
Aortic Valve Stenosis C. RA LA RV LV Aortic valve stenosis ↑ indicates stenosis C	LV hypertrophy; progressive failure of ventricular emptying; pulmonary congestion; failure of right side of heart, with systemic venous congestion; sudden cardiac death	Exertional dyspnea; exercise intolerance; syncope; angina; heart failure (LV failure)	• Chest radiograph: Poststenotic aortic dilation, calcification • ECG: LV hypertrophy • Auscultation: Systolic ejection murmur • Catheterization: Significant pressure gradient, increased LV end-diastolic pressure

TABLE 14.14   Valvular Dysfunction—cont'd

	Pathophysiology	Clinical Manifestations	Physical Signs
Aortic Valve Regurgitation D. Aortic valve regurgitation **indicates backward flow from a valve that is leaking or regurgitant** D	Increased volume load imposed on LV; LV dilation and hypertrophy	Fatigue; dyspnea and exertion; palpitations	• Chest radiograph: Boot-shaped elongation of cardiac apex • ECG: LV hypertrophy • Auscultation: Diastolic murmur • Catheterization: Opacification of LV during aortic injection • Peripheral signs: Hyperdynamic myocardial action and low peripheral resistance
Tricuspid Valve Stenosis E. Tricuspid valve stenosis ↓ **indicates stenosis** E	Right atrium must generate higher pressure to eject blood beyond lesion; right atrial dilation; systemic venous engorgement; increased venous pressure	Venous distention; peripheral edema; ascites; hepatic engorgement; anorexia	• Chest radiograph: Right atrial enlargement • ECG: Right atrial enlargement (P pulmonale) • Auscultation: Diastolic murmur • Catheterization: Elevated right atrial pressure with large a waves; pressure gradient across tricuspid valve
Tricuspid Valve Regurgitation F. Tricuspid valve regurgitation **indicates backward flow from a valve that is leaking or regurgitant** F	Right ventricular hypertrophy and dilation	Decreased cardiac output; neck vein distention; hepatic engorgement; ascites; edema; pleural effusions	• Chest radiograph: Right atrial and ventricular enlargement • ECG: Right ventricular hypertrophy and right atrial enlargement, atrial fibrillation • Auscultation: Murmur throughout systole • Catheterization: Elevated right atrial pressure and v waves

ECG, electrocardiogram; *LV,* left ventricular; *P mitrale,* m-shaped P waves that occur in left atrial hypertrophy and are often caused by mitral stenosis; *P pulmonale,* tall, peaked P waves that occur in right atrial hypertrophy and are often caused by chronic pulmonary disease.

Mitral Valve Regurgitation

Mitral valve regurgitation may result from rheumatic disease, aging of the valve, endocarditis, collagen vascular disease, or papillary muscle dysfunction (see Table 14.14B). In mitral regurgitation, the valve anulus, leaflets, chordae tendineae, and papillary muscles all may be dysfunctional, or the dysfunction may be isolated to just one component of the valve. Mitral valve regurgitation results in a retrograde flow of blood into the left atrium with each ventricular contraction. It is always described as chronic or acute because of the very different impact on the left-sided chambers.

In chronic mitral valve regurgitation, the left atrium has dilated to accommodate the additional regurgitant volume, whereas the left ventricle has hypertrophied (increased muscle) to maintain an adequate stroke volume and cardiac output.[81] In contrast, acute mitral valve regurgitation is precipitated by chordae tendineae or papillary muscle rupture resulting from an acute MI or IE.[80] This is a medical emergency. The left atrium cannot accommodate the sudden increase in volume and pressure, and use of an IABP and inotropic and afterload-reducing pharmacologic support are often required to increase forward output and to reduce pulmonary congestion.[80,82] After the patient's condition has stabilized, surgical replacement or repair of the incompetent valve is performed.[80] A transcatheter mitral valve repair may be considered for a patient with chronic severe MR and NYHA class III or IV symptoms. Studies of percutaneous mitral valve repair using the MitraClip (Abbot Vascular) device reduced severity of MR, improved symptoms, and led to reverse left ventricular remodeling.[80,83]

Aortic Valve Stenosis

The term *aortic valve stenosis* describes a narrowing of the aortic valve area. It can result from aging, rheumatic valvulitis, or deterioration of a congenital bicuspid valve (see Table 14.14C).[80,84] The pathologic hallmarks are inflammation, fibrous valvular thickening, and tissue calcification resembling bone formation.[80] When the aortic valvular opening is reduced to less than 1.5 cm^2, the condition is classified as mild. Cardiac catheterization or Doppler echocardiography can identify a gradient of less than 25 mm Hg across the valve.[80] *Gradient* represents the difference in systolic pressure between the left ventricle and the aorta. A significant pressure difference is a diagnostic hallmark of valvular stenosis. If the valve orifice has narrowed to 1 cm^2 or less, the gradient will be greater than 40 mm Hg, and the diagnosis will be upgraded to severe aortic valve stenosis.[80] The impedance of left ventricular ejection into the aorta results in increased left ventricular systolic pressure, left ventricular hypertrophy, and eventually left ventricular dilation. When symptoms such as angina, dyspnea, syncope, and other indicators of heart failure develop, it is critical to intervene to prevent further damage to the left ventricle. Aortic valve replacement is usually indicated. Congenitally abnormal valves may require replacement by the fourth to sixth decades, and the degenerative changes are often tolerated until approximately 72 years of age.[80] For patients with severe aortic stenosis and too high a surgical risk, percutaneous transcatheter aortic valve replacement procedures have proven safe and effective.[85,86] Studies of these percutaneous procedures have demonstrated decreased mortality, improved quality of life, and cost-effectiveness.[80,85,86]

Aortic Valve Regurgitation

Aortic regurgitation, also known as *aortic insufficiency*, may occur as a result of rheumatic fever, systemic hypertension, Marfan syndrome, syphilis, rheumatoid arthritis, aging valve tissue, discrete subaortic stenosis, or percutaneous interventions such as balloon dilation or transcatheter aortic valve replacement (Table 14.14D).[80] Aortic valve incompetence results in a reflux of blood back into the left ventricle during ventricular diastole. To accommodate this extra volume, the left ventricle initially dilates and then enlarges in an attempt to empty more completely and to meet the needs of the peripheral circulation. Aortic valve replacement is recommended for symptomatic patients with well-preserved or moderate left ventricular dysfunction.[80]

Tricuspid Valve Stenosis

Tricuspid valve stenosis is rarely an isolated lesion (Table 14.14E). It often occurs in conjunction with mitral or aortic disease or congenital disease (Epstein anomaly). Its origin most often is rheumatic fever or a complication of IVDA and resultant IE.[80] Tricuspid valve stenosis increases the pressure and work of the usually low-pressure right atrium, resulting in right atrial hypertrophy. The right atrium dilates in an attempt to accommodate the residual right atrial volume and the incoming venous return. As a result, systemic venous congestion occurs—the consequences of which include jugular venous congestion, liver failure, hepatomegaly, ascites, and peripheral edema.

Tricuspid Valve Regurgitation

Tricuspid valve regurgitation usually results from advanced failure of the left side of the heart that eventually affects the right side of the heart, severe PH, or as a complication of IE. Other causes include carcinoid, rheumatoid arthritis, radiation therapy, trauma, and Marfan syndrome (see Table 14.14F).[80]

Pulmonary Valve Disease

Pulmonary valve disease is an uncommon disorder in adults. It is most often related to congenital anomalies and produces failure of the right side of the heart.[80,87] Acquired cases are most often related to carcinoid or rheumatic fever pathologies. Initial symptoms include dyspnea, and symptoms of severe heart failure occur with disease progression. Balloon valvuloplasty has proven successful for treatment of these patients.[80] more recent studies have proved percutaneous pulmonary valve and valve conduits as successful replacements for the pulmonary valve apparatus.[87-89]

Mixed Valvular Lesions

Many persons have *mixed valvular lesions* as an element of stenosis and regurgitation. Mixed lesions can accentuate the severity of a condition. For example, when combined, aortic stenosis and aortic regurgitation increase left ventricular volume and pressure and multiply the degree of left ventricular work.

Medical Management

Management of valvular disorders includes pharmacologic therapy to control symptoms of heart failure and cardiac surgical repair or replacement of the affected valve.[80] When surgery is not feasible, balloon dilation is a rare option selected for patients too ill to undergo a major cardiac surgical procedure.[80] Percutaneous valve devices including stent valves and mitral clips are being evaluated as a less invasive alternative.[80,85,86,88,89]

Nursing Management

Nursing management of a patient with valvular heart disease incorporates a variety of nursing diagnoses (Box 14.27). Nursing management interventions focus on achievement of

Valvular Heart Disease

- Decreased Cardiac Output related to alterations in preload, p. 1015
- Decreased Cardiac Output related to alterations in afterload, p. 1015
- Decreased Cardiac Output related to alterations in contractility, p. 1016
- Decreased Cardiac Output related to alterations in heart rate or rhythm, p. 1016
- Activity Intolerance related to cardiopulmonary dysfunction, p. 1006
- Deficient Knowledge related to lack of previous exposure to information, p. 1020 (see Box 14.28, Patient Education Plan for Valvular Heart Disease)

Valvular Heart Disease

The patient should be able to teach back the following topics:
- Pathophysiology of valvular disease.
- Infection control: Prophylactic antibiotics related to dental work or other invasive procedures.
- Heart failure: If symptoms of heart failure are present, education is provided on fluid and sodium restriction, fluid balance, diuretic management, daily weight, and controlling breathlessness.
- Surgery: If open-heart surgery was performed, information about postsurgical recovery is provided.
- Medications: Medications may be complex, and information must be given in writing and orally:
  - Preload: Purpose of diuretics, increased urine output, and control of fluid volume.
  - Afterload: Purpose of vasodilators or angiotensin-converting enzyme inhibitors in decreasing the workload of the heart.
  - Heart rate: Purpose of digoxin is to control the rate in atrial fibrillation, a frequent dysrhythmia in heart failure.
  - Contractility: With the exception of digoxin, no oral contractility medications are approved by US Food and Drug Administration.
  - Anticoagulation: Patients with distended atria, enlarged ventricles, atrial fibrillation, or mechanical valves may be prescribed anticoagulants such as warfarin (Coumadin); risks of bleeding, importance of correct dosages, prothrombin times, international normalized ratio, and nutritional-pharmacologic interactions are emphasized.
- Follow-up care after discharge.
- Symptoms to report to a health care professional.

adequate cardiac output, maintenance of fluid balance, and patient and family education.

Cardiac Output

Low cardiac output is a common finding in patients with valvular heart disease. It can occur because of decreased forward flow through a stenotic valve, bidirectional flow across an incompetent valve, or associated heart failure. Vital signs and the effect of positive inotropic and afterload-reducing agents are assessed and documented. If the patient has hemodynamic catheters inserted, cardiac output and hemodynamic parameters are measured and evaluated. Patient care activities are carefully planned to provide adequate rest periods to prevent fatigue.

Fluid Balance

Fluid status is evaluated by auscultation of breath sounds for crackles, heart sounds for presence of S_3, daily weights to trend a "sudden weight gain," and presence of peripheral edema. The appearance of pulmonary crackles or an S_3 heart sound confirms volume overload. The jugular vein is assessed for signs of increased distention. Diuretics and vasodilators are administered to counteract excess fluid retention. The patient is weighed daily, and fluid intake and output are monitored and recorded.

Patient Education

Education for a patient with acute or chronic heart failure caused by valvular dysfunction includes (1) information related to diet, (2) fluid restrictions, (3) the actions and side effects of heart failure medications, (4) the need for prophylactic antibiotics before undergoing any invasive procedures, and (5) when to call the health care provider to report a negative change in cardiac symptoms (Box 14.28).

Many patients also require information about valvular heart surgery or percutaneous replacement procedures. Achieving optimal outcomes for a patient with valve disease requires contributions from a team of educated health care clinicians. Collaborative multidisciplinary priorities are listed in Box 14.29. In Chapter 15 the section on Valvular Surgery provides more information on surgical management.

ATHEROSCLEROTIC DISEASES OF THE AORTA

Description

Two aortic conditions are described—aortic aneurysm and aortic dissection. Both disease states are the result of progressive atherosclerotic disease and systemic arterial hypertension.

Aortic Aneurysm

An *aortic aneurysm* is a localized dilation of the arterial wall that results in an alteration in vessel shape and blood flow. There are two types of vascular aneurysms (Fig. 14.23A and B). Aortic aneurysm is diagnosed most commonly in older adults. Abdominal aortic aneurysm is four times more common compared with thoracic aneurysm.

Aortic Dissection

An *aortic dissection* occurs when a column of blood separates the vascular layers. This creates a false lumen, which communicates with the true lumen through a tear in the intima (Fig. 14.23C).

Etiology

Of patients with an aortic aneurysm, 90% have a history of systemic hypertension. Other causes of aortic aneurysm include atherosclerotic changes in the thoracic and abdominal aorta, blunt trauma, Marfan syndrome, pregnancy, and injury or dissection.

Assessment and Diagnosis

An aortic aneurysm does not always produce symptoms. It may be detected during routine abdominal examination as a palpable, pulsatile mass located in the umbilical region of the abdomen to the left of the midline. A thoracic aneurysm may be identified on a routine chest radiograph. An aortic dissection is usually identified emergently by the onset of acute pain.

Aortic Aneurysm

An aneurysm less than 4 cm in diameter can be managed on an outpatient basis with frequent BP monitoring and ultrasound testing to document any changes in the size of the aneurysm. Management includes weight loss, smoking cessation, and

QSEN BOX 14.29   QSEN: Evidence-Based Practice

Valvular Heart Disease

Class I recommendations with strong evidence are provided.

Recommendations for Detection and Surveillance of Valvular Disease by Echocardiography

- Echocardiography is noninvasive and is used for all initial diagnostic and serial follow-up evaluations.

Recommendations for Aortic Stenosis

- Echocardiography is the primary diagnostic tool.
- Coronary arteriography is used before aortic valve replacement (AVR) if coronary artery disease (CAD) is suspected.
- AVR is recommended for symptomatic patients with severe aortic stenosis; AVR can be combined with coronary artery bypass graft (CABG) surgery when CAD is present.

Recommendations for Aortic Regurgitation

- Echocardiography is the primary diagnostic tool.
- Cardiac catheterization is used if noninvasive tests are inconclusive.
- AVR is indicated for symptomatic patients with severe AR regardless of left ventricular (LV) systolic function.
- AVR is indicated for nonsymptomatic patients with severe AR with LV systolic dysfunction (ejection fraction <0.5 [50%]); AVR can be combined with CABG surgery if CAD is present.

Recommendations for Mitral Stenosis

- Echocardiography is the primary diagnostic tool.
- Anticoagulation is indicated in patients with mitral stenosis (MS) and atrial fibrillation (paroxysmal, persistent, or permanent) and in patients with MS in sinus rhythm with a prior embolic event or left atrial thrombus.
- Cardiac catheterization if noninvasive tests are inconclusive.
- Mitral valve repair (preferable) or mitral valve replacement is indicated for symptomatic (New York Heart Association functional class III or IV) moderate or severe MS if percutaneous mitral balloon valvuloplasty is contraindicated.

Recommendations for Mitral Regurgitation

- Echocardiography is the primary diagnostic tool.
- Cardiac catheterization if noninvasive tests are inconclusive or if additional hemodynamic measurements are required.
- Mitral valve repair is the operation of choice over valve replacement in most patients with chronic mitral regurgitation.

See Box 14.26 for recommendations related to management of patients with valve disease and prosthetic valves.

References

Nishimura RA, et al. 2014 AHA/ACC guideline for the management of patients with valvular heart disease guidelines. *J Am Coll Cardiol.* 2014;63(22):e57.

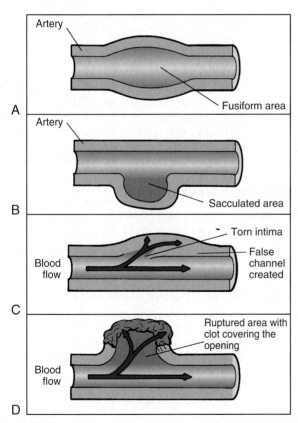

FIG. 14.23 Four Types of Vascular Injury. (A) In a fusiform aneurysm, an entire segment of an artery is dilated, taking on a spindle or bulbous shape. Fusiform aneurysms occur most often in the abdominal aorta and result from atherosclerosis. (B) A sacculated aneurysm involves only one side of an artery and usually is located in the ascending aorta. (C) Dissection occurs because of a tear in the intima, resulting in the shunting of blood between the intima and media of a vessel. (D) A pseudoaneurysm can result from arterial trauma from an arterial introducer sheath or intraaortic balloon catheter, when the arterial opening does not heal normally and is covered by a clot that may rupture at any time.

hypertension control. An aortic aneurysm larger than 5 cm in diameter requires evaluation for surgical repair or placement of an aortic stent to eliminate the risk of rupture (see Chapter 15).

Aortic Dissection

Aortic dissections are classified according to the site of the tear. Two classification systems are used in clinical practice. These use the letters A and B or the numerals I, II, or III, as shown in Fig. 14.24. The classic clinical presentation is the sudden onset of intense, severe, tearing pain, which may be localized initially in the chest, abdomen, or back. As the aortic tear (dissection) extends, pain radiates to the back or distally toward the lower extremities. Many patients have hypertension on initial presentation, and the focus is on control of BP and early operation. Higher surgical mortality is found among patients who present with shock, hypotension, and signs of poor organ perfusion.[90]

The International Registry of Aortic Dissection records indicate that acute aortic dissection is more common in men (72%) than in women (32%), but because women present at an older age and after greater delay, they have higher in-hospital mortality rates. The female mortality rate is twice that of an age-matched population of men.[91] Risk of aneurysm rupture and likelihood of poor outcome after rupture is greater with women.[91] Morbidity and mortality associated with aortic dissection increase with advancing age.[90]

Cardiovascular warning signs may include severe hypertension, fleeting peripheral pulses, limb ischemia, or a new murmur indicative of aortic regurgitation. The most frequent acute neurologic changes include altered mental status and coma.[90] An ascending aortic dissection produces pain in the central chest or midscapular region of the back. A descending aortic dissection usually manifests with pain that radiates down the back, abdomen, or legs. The location of the dissection may be estimated according to the site of pain, although this does not eliminate the need for diagnostic procedures.

The two most helpful initial diagnostic tests are TTE and computed tomography (CT) because both permit rapid visualization of the thoracic structures. A chest radiograph is helpful only if the mediastinum is already widened. Diagnostic findings that identify high-risk patients include a widened mediastinum or an excessively dilated aorta. The definitive invasive diagnostic procedure is an aortogram (aortic angiogram with radiopaque contrast agent).[92]

Medical Management

Medical management of an aortic aneurysm depends on what symptoms are seen and on hemodynamics. If the patient is stable, management is focused on controlling hypertension and educating the patient about the need for corrective surgery before the aneurysm is more than 5 cm wide. If the patient is seen with an acute aortic dissection, management involves immediate control of hypertension with intravenous medications and control of pain with opiates.[90] Progression of the dissection is evaluated by the patient's report of worsening or new pain. If the patient presents with hypotension or in cardiogenic shock, BP support measures to maintain tissue perfusion are initiated. In such cases, emergency surgery may be performed. Surgery is usually required for dissections that involve the ascending aorta to prevent death from cardiac tamponade. This includes type A or type I and type II dissections (see Fig. 14.24).[92,93] The surgical procedure includes resection of the affected area, followed by graft placement and restoration

FIG. 14.24 Aortic Dissection. (A) Separation of vascular layers. (B) Classification of aortic dissection. (Modified from Price SA, Wilson LM. *Pathophysiology: Clinical Concepts of Disease Processes*. 5th ed. St. Louis: Mosby; 1997.)

of blood flow to major branches of the aorta. The aortic valve is replaced if the dissection involves the valve. Dissections that involve the descending aorta (type B or type III) do not always require surgery.[92]

Nursing Management

Nursing management of a patient with an aortic aneurysm or aortic dissection incorporates a variety of nursing diagnoses (Box 14.30). Nursing interventions are directed toward control of hypertension, pain control, and education of the patient and family.

Hypertension Management

The cardiovascular status is assessed hourly, including monitoring BP in both arms, checking peripheral pulses bilaterally, auscultating for an aortic murmur, and monitoring the ECG for ischemic changes or dysrhythmias. Patients usually require an arterial line and receive potent antihypertensive medications such as labetalol, which combines beta-blocking activity to reduce cardiac output and lower BP and peripheral alpha-blocking activity to vasodilate the arteries and decrease BP.

Pain Control

Acute pain is a classic sign of aortic dissection. Opiates and sedatives are administered to control pain, decrease anxiety, and increase comfort. Because these medications can mask the pain of further dissection, they are administered judiciously. The patient's neurovascular status is assessed hourly. Documentation includes the presence and distribution of pain, pallor, paresthesia, paralysis, and movement of the limb.

Patient Education

In the acute period, education is limited to an explanation of the critical care environment and the importance of BP control. If additional procedures such as aortography, CT, or surgery are to be performed, the critical care nurse assists with these explanations (Box 14.31). Recommendations for prevention and treatment of atherosclerotic aortic aneurysm and dissection are listed in Box 14.32.

PERIPHERAL ARTERY DISEASE

Description

Peripheral vascular disease is divided into PAD and peripheral venous disease. Venous disease is a chronic condition

---

◎ BOX 14.30   NURSING DIAGNOSES

Aortic Aneurysm and Aortic Dissection

- Decreased Cardiac Output related to alterations in preload, p. 1015
- Acute Pain related to transmission and perception of cutaneous, visceral, muscular, or ischemic impulses, p. 1010
- Risk for Ineffective Peripheral Tissue Perfusion, p. 1044
- Risk for Decreased Cardiac Tissue Perfusion, p. 1041
- Risk for Infection, p. 1046
- Anxiety related to threat to biologic, psychologic, or social integrity, p. 1012
- Risk for Ineffective Renal Perfusion, p. 1045
- Activity Intolerance related to cardiopulmonary dysfunction, p. 1006
- Deficient Knowledge related to lack of previous exposure to information, p. 1020 (see Box 14.31, Patient Education Plan for Aortic Aneurysm and Aortic Dissection)

✳ BOX 14.31 PATIENT EDUCATION PLAN

Aortic Aneurysm and Aortic Dissection

The patient should be able to teach back the following topics:

- Pathophysiology of atherosclerotic aortic disease: Aortic aneurysm or aortic dissection.
- Hypertension control: Hypertension increases the risk of aneurysm rupture or aortic dissection.
- Pain control: Use of 0–10 pain scale; information about availability of pain medications for acute pain.
- Preprocedure teaching for aortic angiogram, computed tomography scan, or transesophageal echocardiogram.
- Preoperative teaching for aortic surgical repair.
- Risk factor modification: After the acute episode, if the cause of the aortic aneurysm or aortic dissection is atherosclerosis, an individual risk factor profile is developed for each patient; strategies to discuss include decrease daily fat intake to less than 30% of total calories, achieve total blood cholesterol level of less than 200 mg/dL, stop smoking, reduce salt intake, control hypertension, treat diabetes if patient has diabetes, increase physical activity, achieve and maintain ideal body weight.
- Symptoms to report to a health care professional: Pain, signs and symptoms of infection.
- Follow-up care after discharge.

---

that is managed on an outpatient basis and does not require admission to a critical care unit. In contrast, PAD may require critical care admission for an acute thrombotic occlusion or after a vascular surgical procedure. PAD can occur in any peripheral artery. It is especially painful in the arteries that supply the lower extremities. The following descriptions relate to PAD.

Etiology

Atherosclerosis is a common cause of chronic arterial occlusion in older adults. PAD affects less than 4% of people younger than 40 years but has an impact on almost 22% of adults older than 70 years.[94] Risk factors are the same for PAD and CAD. Most patients with PAD have at least one risk factor that predisposes them to development of CAD.[94,95] Diabetes, smoking, hypertension, hyperlipidemia, and male gender increase the risk of peripheral artery occlusion.[94,96] As with CAD, the presence of kidney disease increases the incidence of concomitant PAD.

Pathophysiology

The most commonly affected vessels in the lower extremities are the superficial femoral artery and the popliteal artery in the legs, followed by the distal aorta and iliac arteries.

QSEN BOX 14.32 QSEN: Evidence-Based Practice

Aortic Aneurysm and Aortic Dissection

Recommendations for Prevention of Atherosclerotic Aortic Aneurysm and Dissection

- Hypertension is a major risk factor. There are no specific recommendations related to blood pressure (BP) control and aortic disease. Reduction of BP to less than 130/80 mm Hg is consistent with recommendations for other atherosclerotic diseases (coronary and cerebrovascular).
- Cigarette smoking is a major risk factor for aortic disease; smoking cessation is essential.
- Routine use of statins has been found to decrease the aneurysm rupture rate and may be effective in decreasing abdominal aortic aneurysm (AAA) growth rate.
- Aortic dissection also occurs as a complication of blunt chest trauma from high-speed motor vehicular trauma.

Recommendations for Treatment of Aortic Dissection

- Admission to the critical care unit for monitoring of heart rate and BP.
- Reduction of systolic BP using intravenous (IV) beta-blockers (esmolol) or beta-blocker plus alpha-blocker combination (labetalol). Beta-blockers are recommended because they reduce the force of blood ejected from the ventricle against the weakened aortic wall.
- If further systolic BP reduction is necessary, IV vasodilators (sodium nitroprusside) are added in addition to beta-blockers.
- Intubation and mechanical ventilation are recommended if profound hemodynamic instability exists.
- Pain relief (morphine sulfate) and sedation are recommended.
- Diagnosis of aortic dissection is made by clinical signs and location of the site of the tear and false lumen. Computed tomography is the most common diagnostic test in an emergency. Magnetic resonance imaging is often used for chronic stable dissections. Transthoracic echocardiography followed by transesophageal echocardiography may also be used.
- Treatment recommendations depend on the classification of the dissection:

- Type A (type I, type II) dissections that involve the aortic arch are repaired surgically to prevent aortic rupture or cardiac tamponade.
- Type B (type III) dissections are recommended for medical treatment. Surgery or endovascular repair is recommended only in cases of persistent chest pain, aortic expansion, periaortic hematoma, or mediastinal hematoma.
- Type A aortic dissection is a high-risk diagnosis with an overall hospital mortality rate of 25%. Patients with type A dissections who are admitted to the hospital with hypotension have a higher risk of adverse events.

Recommendations for Treatment of Elective Abdominal Aortic Aneurysm

- Formation of AAA or dissection before the sixth decade of life is uncommon.
- Based on current evidence, a 5.5-cm aneurysm diameter is the best threshold for repair in the "average" male patient. Vascular surgery experts recommend that women have elective repair of an aneurysm 4.5–5 cm. Individual anatomy, patient age, and physical size must also be considered.
- Until the results of long-term randomized trials are available, the choice between endoluminal repair (stent) and open abdominal surgery depends on patient and physician preferences.

References

Feldman M, Shah M, Elefteriades A. Medical management of acute type A aortic dissection. *Ann Thorac Cardiovasc Surg*. 2010;15(5):286.

Grootenboer N, et al. Systematic review and meta-analysis of sex differences in outcome after intervention for abdominal aortic aneurysm. *Br J Surg*. 2010;97(8):1169.

Hiratzka L, et al. 2010 ACCF/AHA/AATS/ACR/SCA/SCAO/SIR/STS/SVM guidelines for the diagnosis and management of patients with thoracic aortic disease. *Circulation*. 2010;121(13):e266.

Moll FL, et al. Management of abdominal aortic aneurysms. Clinical practice guidelines for the European Society of Vascular Surgery. *Eur J Vasc Endovasc Surg*. 2011;41:S1.

Assessment and Diagnosis
Ankle-Brachial Index

The ankle-brachial index (ABI) is a noninvasive test used to estimate the severity of arterial disease in the leg by comparing it with the measured arterial pressure in the arm. The systolic BP is measured on the arm and on the leg (just above the ankle). A cuff is used to occlude the pressure, and the systolic BP is measured at the posterior tibial pulse and the dorsalis pedis pulse locations.[97] The systolic BP can be palpated with the fingers or auscultated using a handheld 5- to 7-MHz Doppler device. To calculate the ABI, the arm systolic BP is divided into the ankle systolic BP number.[97] A normal ABI value is between 0.9 and 1.0, signifying that the peripheral arteries are normal. Patients with an ABI value between 0.71 and 0.9 have mild PAD; patients with an ABI between 0.41 and 0.7 have moderate PAD; and patients with an ABI less than 0.4 have severe PAD.[95,97] Generally, as the ABI value decreases, symptoms of peripheral ischemia increase.

Intermittent Claudication

Arterial occlusion obstructs blood flow to the distal extremity. The lack of blood flow produces ischemic muscle pain known as *intermittent claudication.* This cramping, aching pain while walking is often the first symptom of PAD. The pain is relieved by rest and may remain stable in occurrence and intensity for many years. Symptoms do not occur until more than 75% of the vessel lumen is occluded.

As with other atherosclerotic conditions, PAD is typically asymptomatic until the disease process is well advanced. Clinicians who rely on history of leg pain alone severely underestimate PAD in the early stages. Only approximately 10% of the population with PAD has classic symptoms of intermittent claudication (leg pain associated with PAD). Up to 50% of patients with PAD are asymptomatic, and 40% have a variety of leg symptoms different from classic claudication.[98] The ABI can be used as a screening tool to detect the presence of PAD before symptoms occur.[97,98] Prevention measures can then be discussed with the patient.

Rest Pain

As PAD progresses, patients may develop pain at rest. Pain at rest threatens the viability of the limb and requires immediate catheter or surgical intervention to relieve the blockage and restore circulation to the extremity.

Acute Occlusion

The symptoms of acute occlusion from thrombosis are sudden onset of severe pain, loss of pulses, collapse of superficial veins, coldness, pallor, and impaired motor and sensory function. As with rest pain, acute occlusion requires immediate intervention to open the artery.

Atrophic Tissue Changes

Skin changes associated with PAD include thickening of the nails and drying of the skin. Hair loss is common on the lower leg, feet, and toes. Pallor and a temperature gradient may be present as a line of demarcation between areas that have adequate arterial perfusion and areas that have poor perfusion. Wasting of muscle or soft tissue may be seen. As atherosclerotic arterial disease progresses, skin ulcerations and gangrene can occur.

Medical Management

Medical therapy is geared toward controlling or eliminating risk factors, providing effective foot care, and suggesting alterations in lifestyle to promote rest and pain relief. Pharmacologic management may include the use of anticoagulants, vasodilators, or antiplatelet agents.[99] If these therapies do not produce positive results, the patient may be a candidate for percutaneous transluminal angioplasty, stent placement, or vascular bypass surgery. Percutaneous transluminal angioplasty or stent placement is effective if the lesion (blockage) is discrete and localized. However, if the arterial disease is diffuse, bypass surgery is usually performed. If gangrene (cell death) is present, limb or partial limb amputation is required.

Nursing Management

Nursing management of a patient with PAD incorporates a variety of nursing diagnoses (Box 14.33). Nurses assess the quality of the peripheral artery pulses, intervene to maintain skin integrity and control pain, and educate the patient and family about peripheral vascular disease.

Arterial Pulses

Assessments of peripheral pulses, limb color, and temperature are critical in the evaluation of an ischemic limb. Arterial pulses are typically diminished, transiently present (intermittent vessel spasm), or absent distal to the site of occlusion. Patients with diabetes have a much higher incidence of peripheral vascular disease (arterial and venous) compared with the general population. Most hospitals use a standard scale to improve documentation of pulses. If the pulse cannot be palpated, Doppler ultrasonography may be used to assess blood flow.

Skin Integrity

Care is taken to protect the limb from injury and development of pressure ulcers. Healing is often impaired because of poor arterial blood flow or diabetes. Feet may be protected from injury by cotton or lamb's wool placed between the toes or by a bed cradle. However, for an acute ischemic limb, removal of the thrombus is the only treatment that can salvage ischemic tissue.

Pain Control

The term *intermittent claudication* refers to pain during exercise in the presence of PAD. Leg pain that occurs after exercise, caused by increased muscle oxygen demand, can be effectively managed by stopping the exertion. However, pain at rest (without exercise) is a warning sign of an anoxic limb. The pain of an acute ischemic limb is extreme, and morphine is used for pain control. Ultimately, removal of the arterial obstruction is the only method to eliminate the pain.

ⓞ BOX 14.33 NURSING DIAGNOSES
Peripheral Artery Disease

- Acute Pain related to transmission and perception of cutaneous, visceral, muscular, or ischemic impulses, p. 1010
- Risk for Ineffective Peripheral Tissue Perfusion, p. 1044
- Activity Intolerance related to prolonged immobility or deconditioning, p. 1006
- Anxiety related to threat to biologic, psychologic, or social integrity, p. 1012
- Powerlessness related to lack of control over current situation or disease progression, p. 1038
- Deficient Knowledge related to lack of previous exposure to information, p. 1020 (see Box 14.34, Patient Education Plan for Peripheral Artery Disease)

✱ BOX 14.34 PATIENT EDUCATION PLAN

Peripheral Artery Disease

The patient should be able to teach back the following topics:

- Pathophysiology of peripheral artery disease.
- Daily inspection and care of feet and legs.
- Avoidance of trauma to feet or legs.
- Increase walking distance gradually.
- Risk factor modification: After the acute episode, if the cause of peripheral artery disease is atherosclerosis, an individual risk factor profile is developed for each patient; strategies to discuss include decrease daily fat intake to less than 30% of total calories, achieve total blood cholesterol level of less than 200 mg/dL, stop smoking, reduce salt intake, control hypertension, control diabetes if patient has diabetes, increase physical activity, achieve and maintain ideal body weight.
- Preprocedure teaching about angiogram, percutaneous angioplasty, or stent placement in the lower extremities.
- Risks and benefits of fibrinolytic therapy for acute peripheral artery occlusion.
- Preoperative teaching for revascularization surgery.
- Rehabilitation education, if amputation is indicated.
- Medications:
  - Antithrombotic therapy: Usually aspirin to decrease platelet adhesiveness.
  - Low-density lipoprotein cholesterol lipid-lowering agents: 3-hydroxy-3-methylglutaryl coenzyme A reductase inhibitors.
  - Antihypertensive agents: Antihypertensive medications and how to self-monitor blood pressure.
- Symptoms to report to a health care professional: Pain (chest or legs), leg or foot trauma.
- Follow-up care after discharge.

Patient Education

Education topics include risk factor modification that emphasizes similar lifestyle changes to those recommended for patients with CAD including smoking cessation, promoting exercise, maintenance of ideal body weight, inspection of the feet and legs, foot care, avoidance of foot trauma, and medications. Many patients with PAD underestimate their risk of stroke or acute MI and do not understand that the risk factors for PAD are the same risk factors for all cardiovascular atherosclerotic diseases.[95] Walking is good exercise for increasing blood flow to the lower extremities and is highly recommended for patients with PAD.[98]

If a surgically implanted prosthetic bypass graft is in place, teaching must include information about IE precautions. If the patient has diabetes, education about diabetes management is included in the teaching plan. Box 14.34 lists the salient points to include when teaching patients and families about PAD. Symptoms of PAD are listed in Box 14.35.

CAROTID ARTERY DISEASE

Description

The bifurcation of the carotid arteries is a common site of atherosclerotic plaque development (Fig. 14.25). Because these arterioles carry the blood supply to the brain, when they are obstructed, the presenting symptoms are neurologic. Treating carotid artery disease, a readily treatable obstruction, can prevent a stroke. Blood supply to the brain is provided by two separate arterial systems: (1) the vertebral arteries and (2) the internal carotid arteries, whose branches anastomose to form

QSEN BOX 14.35 QSEN: Evidence-Based Practice

Peripheral Artery Disease

Peripheral artery disease (PAD) affects 8 million men and women age 40 y and older in the United States. An international multidisciplinary group of clinicians summarized evidence from clinical trials to begin the process of developing clinical guidelines.

Recommendations to Increase Awareness of PAD and Its Consequences

- Patients who are at highest risk of developing PAD are patients who smoke cigarettes, have diabetes, and are older. In screening asymptomatic patients in high-risk groups, 30%–50% of patients have PAD and do not know it.
- Other PAD risk factors include hypertension, hyperlipidemia, male sex, elevated C-reactive protein levels, elevated plasma fibrinogen levels, elevated blood glucose, prior myocardial infarction (MI), heart failure, and history of transient ischemic attack or stroke.
- Patients with symptomatic PAD had a four to five times increased risk of stroke and a 20%–60% increased risk of MI with a twofold to sixfold increased risk of death from coronary heart disease compared with patients without PAD.
- Many patients are unaware of the link between PAD and cardiac and cerebrovascular atherosclerotic disease.

Recommendations to Improve Identification of Patients With Symptomatic PAD

- Because PAD is asymptomatic in the early stages of the disease, the ankle-brachial index (ABI) is recommended as a screening tool in high-risk patients. (See text for information on how to measure the ABI.)

- If the diagnosis is not made until the patient complains of intermittent claudication (pain with walking), the disease is already at an advanced stage.

Recommendations to Treat Risk Factors Associated With PAD

- Smokers should stop smoking. This is not easy to do. Physician advice with frequent follow-up and pharmacologic therapy (nicotine replacement and bupropion) demonstrate 1-y success rates of 5%, 16%, and 30%.
- If the patient is hyperlipidemic, a normal lipid panel needs to be achieved: Reduce total serum cholesterol to less than 200 mg/dL and low-density lipoprotein cholesterol to less than 70 mg/dL.
- Studies have not specifically examined the effect of controlling hypertension and diabetes on rates of PAD. However, extrapolating from the cardiac literature, researchers recommend reducing blood pressure to less than 130/80 mg Hg and maintaining blood glucose within the normal range (70–110 mg/dL; hemoglobin A_{1c} ≤7%).
- Low-dose aspirin or another platelet inhibitor medication is recommended.
- Exercise rehabilitation is recommended with promotion of daily walking. The goal is to increase the ability of the patient to walk longer distances without leg pain.

References

Alonso-Coello P, et al. Antithrombotic therapy in peripheral artery disease: antithrombotic therapy and prevention of thrombosis, 9th ed. American College of Chest Physicians evidence-based clinical guidelines. *Chest.* 2012;141:e669S.

Kearon C, et al. Antithrombotic therapy for VTE diseases, antithrombotic therapy and prevention of thrombosis, 9th ed. American College of Chest Physicians evidence-based clinical practice guidelines. *Chest.* 2012;141(suppl 2):e419S.

the circle of Willis. Any abrupt interruption in circulation for 4 to 6 minutes can produce permanent brain damage. When circulation to an area is impaired gradually, collateral circulation is often able to develop and maintain an adequate supply of blood to that area of the brain. Abrupt interruption in blood supply leads to an area of brain tissue becoming ischemic and often permanently damaged.

Etiology

The most common cause of carotid artery disease is atherosclerosis.[100] Uncommon causes include fibromuscular dysplasia, irradiation, and arteritis. The risk factors for development of atherosclerotic carotid artery disease and stroke are similar to those for CAD and PAD. Patients with any of these conditions must be educated about the other disease processes. Modifiable risk factors include uncontrolled hypertension (systolic BP greater than 160 mm Hg), AF, smoking, diabetes with uncontrolled blood glucose levels, and hyperlipidemia.[100] Women taking HRT after menopause also have an increased risk of stroke.[100] The incidence of carotid stenosis increases with age. Asymptomatic carotid artery stenosis with greater than 50% occlusion is present in 22% to 28% of men and women older than 50 years, and the risk of stroke doubles with each successive decade after age 55 years. The presence of coexisting CAD also increases the incidence of stroke, with a relative risk of 1.73 for men and 1.55 for women.[100]

The major mechanisms by which atherosclerosis in the carotid arteries creates ischemic symptoms are embolization and thrombosis. Ulcerated carotid lesions with accumulated platelet and fibrin produce thrombi that travel along with cholesterol deposits to become emboli to the brain. Stenotic areas in the carotid arteries are prone to thrombosis because of sluggish

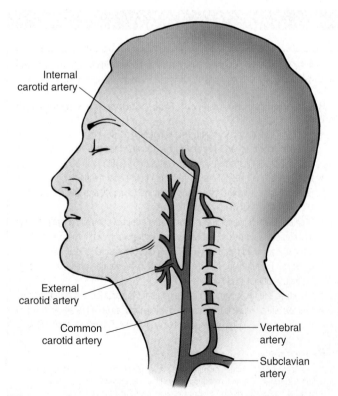

FIG. 14.25 Common, Internal, and External Carotid Arteries. Atherosclerotic plaque develops in the common carotid artery at the bifurcation into the internal and external carotid arteries. Plaque can develop in the common, internal, and external carotid arteries.

flow across the lesions. Doppler studies can examine the carotid arteries noninvasively. If a stroke is suspected, an emergency CT scan of the head is the appropriate diagnostic test.[100]

Carotid artery disease can remain asymptomatic for many years. After emboli are dislodged, the manifestations of carotid artery disease are neurologic and include hemiparesis, dysphasia, dysarthria, global aphasia, diplopia, vertigo, syncope, confusion, and monocular blindness. Neurologic symptoms that resolve completely within a short time are classified as *transient ischemic attacks* (TIAs). Symptoms that do not resolve are described as ischemic strokes.[100] If a patient has recently experienced a TIA, the risk of stroke is increased by more than 10% in the first 22 days, with the risk increasing 17% in the first 90 days.[1,100] Additional information on the neurologic management of the patient experiencing a stroke is provided in Chapter 23.

Medical Management

Medical management is focused on reducing the atherosclerotic risk factors that can be controlled by the patient. This includes regulation of hypertension, smoking cessation, seeking medical attention for treatable cardiac abnormalities such as AF, reducing weight, and reducing the cholesterol level to less than 200 mg/dL. Antithrombotic therapy (warfarin, aspirin, or other antiplatelet therapy) must be prescribed for patients with AF with a comprehensive individualized assessment of the relative risk of embolism versus the risk of bleeding complications.[100]

Asymptomatic patients who have carotid stenosis pose a quandary. In these patients, the risk of stroke needs to be weighed against the risks of surgery—specifically, the increased risk of stroke during surgery. Current clinical guidelines suggest that patients with carotid stenosis greater than 60% would benefit from carotid surgical endarterectomy when performed by a surgeon with a history of operative morbidity and mortality rates of less than 3%.[100] The role of stent placement in the carotid artery has also shown similar success with skilled interventionalists.[101,102] Patients with carotid artery stenosis need to be informed about the risks involved with any procedure and their risk for future cerebrovascular events, such as stroke.

Nursing Management

Several nursing diagnoses are associated with management of a patient with carotid artery disease (Box 14.36). Nursing management is focused on assessment of adequate cerebral perfusion, represented by vital signs, respiratory pattern, level of consciousness, pupil reaction, pupil size, and possible cranial nerve deficits manifested by difficulty in swallowing, loss of gag reflex, changes in speech, and loss of facial symmetry. The National Institutes of Health Stroke Scale is used to predict patient outcome on initial and ongoing assessment of TIA and stroke-related symptoms. The nurse educates the patient and family about the causes of the current event and provides information on preventing further cerebrovascular events.

Neurologic Assessment

Neurologic assessment of a patient with carotid artery disease is divided into two parts: (1) level of consciousness, mental alertness, and cerebral perfusion and (2) cranial nerve function. A neurologic assessment is performed to ensure that

BOX 14.36 NURSING DIAGNOSES

Carotid Artery Disease

- Acute Pain related to transmission and perception of cutaneous, muscular, or ischemic impulses, p. 1010
- Risk for Ineffective Cerebral Tissue Perfusion, p. 1042
- Anxiety related to threat to biologic, psychologic, or social integrity, p. 1012
- Deficient Knowledge related to lack of previous exposure to information, p. 1020 (see Box 14.37, Patient Education Plan for Carotid Artery Disease)

❋ BOX 14.37 PATIENT EDUCATION PLAN

Carotid Artery Disease

The patient should be able to teach back the following topics:
- Pathophysiology of atherosclerotic carotid artery disease.
- Pathophysiology of embolic stroke (emboli from carotid artery).
- Warning signs of impending stroke.
- Risk factor modification: After the acute episode, if the cause of carotid artery disease is atherosclerosis, an individual risk factor profile is developed for each patient; strategies to discuss include decrease daily fat intake to less than 30% of total calories, achieve total blood cholesterol level of less than 200 mg/dL, stop smoking, reduce salt intake, control hypertension, control diabetes if patient has diabetes, increase physical activity, achieve and maintain ideal body weight.
- Signs and symptoms to report to a health care professional.
- Follow-up care after discharge.

the patient has not experienced a TIA or stroke. Questions to ascertain level of consciousness relate to time and place and reason for hospital admission. Mental alertness is assessed by the patient's ability to respond to these and other questions. The person is asked to move all four limbs on command. To assess specific cranial nerves, the patient is asked to make a grimace, which should demonstrate bilateral facial symmetry; to stick out the tongue to ensure it is midline; and to swallow and speak, which should be done without difficulty (see "Cranial Nerves" in Chapter 21 and "Rapid Neurologic Examination" in Chapter 22).

Patient Education

If a patient who has known carotid artery disease and has not had a cerebrovascular event is admitted to a critical care unit, preventive education is essential. It is important to discuss the mechanism of stroke in carotid artery disease. A stroke is most often caused by an embolic thrombus that has traveled in the bloodstream to a specific area of the brain. The thrombus may have originated in the atria during an episode of AF or in the carotid arteries. In the carotid arteries, a thrombus can develop across the narrowed carotid artery lumen, reducing flow and causing widespread cerebral hypoperfusion. Many patients who have atherosclerotic carotid artery disease also have CAD or PAD and diabetes or hypertension.[100] The major areas of patient education are listed in Box 14.37. Recommendations for prevention of carotid artery disease are listed in Box 14.38.

QSEN BOX 14.38 QSEN: Evidence-Based Practice

Carotid Artery Disease

Recommendations for Prevention of Carotid Artery Disease
- Smokers should stop smoking and avoid exposure to environmental tobacco smoke (secondhand tobacco smoke); smoking doubles the risk of stroke.
- Achieve a normal blood pressure (BP), preferably less than 120/80 mm Hg, for individuals at high risk of stroke. Oral antihypertensive medications are prescribed if the target BP is not met with diet and exercise alone. Reduction of BP greatly reduces stroke incidence.
- Achieve and maintain normal weight. The target weight-to-height ratio is a body mass index (BMI) between 18.5 kg/m^2 and 24.9 kg/m^2. Obesity is defined as a BMI above 25 kg/m^2. Obese patients are also identified as having a large waist circumference—more than 40 inches for men or more than 35 inches for women.
- Have serum lipids checked, and attain a normal lipid profile. Many patients are prescribed lipid-lowering medications to achieve the following goals:
  - Total cholesterol below 200 mg/dL.
  - Low-density lipoprotein cholesterol below 70 mg/dL if patient has cardiovascular disease risk factors (all patients with carotid artery disease are likely to fall in this category), diabetes, or kidney disease.
  - Triglycerides below 150 mg/dL.
- Normal fasting blood glucose level should be between 70 mg/dL and 110 mg/dL. If the patient has diabetes, hemoglobin A$_{1c}$ should be near normal or less than 7%.
- A healthy diet should be instituted. Reduce saturated fat and add fruits and vegetables. Add omega-3 fatty acids as part of the treatment regimen to lower elevated triglycerides.
- Regular exercise is essential. The optimal goal is 30–60 min daily or at least three times weekly.

Recommended Medications for Carotid Artery Disease
- Aspirin (50–325 orally each day) or other platelet-inhibitor medications are recommended. The combination of aspirin plus extended-release dipyridamole and clopidogrel monotherapy are acceptable options for initial antiplatelet therapy.
- The statin class of medications is recommended to aggressively lower lipid levels.
- Antihypertensive medications are used to lower BP into normal range.

Recommended Interventions for Carotid Artery Disease
Asymptomatic Patients
- Medical therapy without revascularization is recommended for low-grade carotid stenosis, which is defined as a carotid artery narrowed to less than 60% in asymptomatic patients.
- Carotid endarterectomy and optimal medical therapy are recommended for carotid stenosis greater than 60% in asymptomatic patients with low operative risk.

Symptomatic Patients
- Medical therapy without revascularization is recommended for low-grade carotid stenosis, defined as a carotid artery narrowed to less than 50% in patients with symptoms.
- Carotid endarterectomy and optimal medical therapy are recommended for carotid stenosis greater than 50% in patients with symptoms.

References
Goldstein LB, et al. Guidelines for the primary prevention of stroke: a guideline for healthcare professionals from the American Heart Association/American Stroke Association. *Stroke.* 2011;42(2):517.

Gurm HS, et al. Long-term results of carotid stenting versus endarterectomy in high-risk patients. *N Engl J Med.* 2008;358(15):1572.

VENOUS THROMBOEMBOLISM

Description

VTE comprises two related conditions: (1) DVT and (2) PE. DVT is a clot (thrombus) that forms in a large vein in the leg, pelvis, and, less commonly, the arm. It is often accompanied by inflammation, pain, tenderness, and redness at the site of the thrombus. The concern is that the thrombus may migrate as a VTE through the venous circulation to the pulmonary vascular bed, causing a PE, development of PH, or death.[103,104]

Etiology

At least 900,000 episodes of VTE leading to hospitalization and 300,000 related deaths occur in the United States annually.[104] Patients in the critical care unit face additional risks from invasive procedures, immobility, and vascular inflammation. Other risk factors for VTE include advanced age, obesity, immobility, trauma, spinal cord injury, active cancer, major surgery, pregnancy, family history, heart failure, and sepsis.[104] VTE incidence is similar for men and women, unless a woman is taking HRT or a contraceptive pill, which increases her risk. Inherited coagulation disorders and hypercoagulability, also called *genetic thrombophilia,* confer a propensity for clotting and increase the DVT risk profile in patients with this genetic inheritance.[104] In the critical care population, the incidence of DVT is 28% to 32% with rates of 60% to 70% in the trauma and stroke populations.[103]

Three major predisposing factors are traditionally described as Virchow's triad: (1) stasis of blood, (2) endothelial injury, and (3) hypercoagulability. Theories on the role of inflammation are adding to the risk profile of thrombosis generation.[103] Two of these three conditions usually must be present for thrombosis to occur. Patients in critical care units generally have one or more risk factors that predispose them to the development of a venous thrombus. A hospitalized patient has more than a 100-fold increased incidence of acute VTE compared with the general public.[104] The incidence of DVT increases with age and markedly increases the patient's risk of fatal PE (see "Pulmonary Embolism" in Chapter 19).

Assessment and Diagnosis

Development of DVT may be insidious. Many patients with DVT are asymptomatic. Pain, if present, is described as an aching or throbbing sensation, which worsens with ambulation. A positive Homans sign, which is pain in the calf on dorsiflexion of the foot, heightens the suspicion of a DVT but is not considered a reliable marker. If DVT is present in the upper extremity, the entire arm swells. Other clinical manifestations include redness with swelling, increased skin temperature, dilation of superficial veins, and mottling and cyanosis caused by stagnant blood flow. In patients in the critical care unit, symptoms are often masked by intubation, sedation, and altered levels of consciousness.

Venous Ultrasound and D-Dimer

When DVT is suspected, noninvasive venous ultrasonography typically is performed to evaluate vein patency.[103] If the thrombus is large and the vein is easy to visualize, the presence of a DVT can be confirmed by this method alone. However, when the results of ultrasound are inconclusive, the addition of the D-dimer blood test increases diagnostic accuracy. The D-dimer test measures the presence of cross-linked fibrin derivatives in the serum. It is a sensitive marker of thrombosis but it lacks specificity. If the normal D-dimer serum value is elevated, it signifies the presence of clots, but the thrombi could be located anywhere in the body. Ultrasonography can help localize the DVT. Together, these two tests represent a useful and powerful diagnostic strategy.[103] When the D-dimer value is normal (not elevated), a DVT (or other thrombosis) can safely be ruled out.

Diagnosis of Pulmonary Embolism

If PE is suspected, a CT scan of the thorax may be obtained. Contrast-enhanced CT arteriography is faster and has greater sensitivity and specificity for detecting emboli in the pulmonary arteries.[105] A ventilation-perfusion scan is most likely to be diagnostic in the absence of disease, but it is less helpful in critically ill patients. A normal perfusion scan result effectively rules out acute PE.[105]

Current guidelines recommend evaluating the risk factors for each patient on an individual basis. Maintaining a high index of suspicion and using thromboprophylaxis for at-risk patients is essential. If VTE is suspected, clinical assessment, venous ultrasound, and D-dimer assay results confirm or negate the presence of VTE.[105]

Medical Management

Prevention of Venous Thromboembolism

Major therapeutic emphasis is placed on prophylaxis for critically ill patients at high risk for VTE.[104] Preventive measures include prophylactic anticoagulation with subcutaneous LMWH or UFH, increasing mobility, and use of sequential compression devices placed on the lower extremities. Normally, the simple action of walking helps return blood to the right side of the heart and prevents venous stasis that may lead to development of venous thrombi. For critically ill patients, immobility is often imposed because of severity of the illness. After they become stable, most patients are assisted out of bed and helped to walk to restore the circulatory pump.

Management of Diagnosed Venous Thromboembolism

Initially, the patient is confined to bed rest with elevation of the limb, and anticoagulation therapy is initiated. Analgesics are prescribed to reduce discomfort.

Anticoagulation

Anticoagulants are prescribed to reduce further clotting. The risks and benefits of therapeutic anticoagulation are discussed with the patient and family before therapy begins. In the acute phase, VTE can be treated with intravenous heparin or subcutaneous LMWH. Subsequently, oral warfarin may be used. Antiplatelet therapy with aspirin or other medications is added to prevent VTE recurrence. Antiplatelet therapy alone does not provide protection against development of VTE.[104] Anticoagulation with rivaroxaban (orally active direct factor Xa inhibitor) is also an option.[104] None of the aforementioned antithrombotics dissolves the existing clot, but these medications can prevent new thrombi from forming. Lytic therapy usually is reserved for massive PE. Patients receiving anticoagulation therapy require careful assessment for bleeding tendencies, including obtaining frequent bleeding studies—aPTT or INR. Stool and urine are tested for the presence of occult blood; gums are inspected for bleeding; and when endotracheal suctioning is required, it is important to be gentle and to assess for the presence of blood in the aspirate. After the patient begins to ambulate, custom-fitted, below-the-knee elastic stockings are ordered.[104] Complaints or observation of dyspnea or chest

Venous Thromboembolism

- Activity Intolerance related to prolonged immobility or deconditioning, p. 1006
- Acute Pain related to transmission and perception of cutaneous, visceral, muscular, or ischemic impulses, p. 1010
- Powerlessness related to lack of control over current situation or disease progression, p. 1038
- Anxiety related to threat to biologic, psychologic, or social integrity, p. 1012
- Deficient Knowledge related to lack of previous exposure to information, p. 1020 (see Box 14.40, Patient Education Plan for Venous Thromboembolism)

Venous Thromboembolism

The patient should be able to teach back the following topics:
- Pathophysiology of deep vein thrombosis.
- Discuss risk of pulmonary embolus and need for antiembolism stockings or pneumatic compression devices on legs; avoid trauma to legs; report any chest pain, breathlessness, or increased respiratory rate.
- Medications: Anticoagulants (heparin or warfarin [Coumadin]) to prevent formation of new thrombus at the site; aspirin to decrease platelet aggregation.

pain must be quickly evaluated to assess the risk of PE. Medical management with anticoagulants is adequate for most patients; however, patients at risk for PE (patients with cancer, bleeding disorders, or spinal cord injury) may require surgical intervention for protection. Possible procedures include venous embolectomy and insertion of an inferior vena cava filter.[103]

Nursing Management

Several nursing diagnoses are used in the management of a patient with VTE (Box 14.39). The focus of nursing management is to prevent the development of DVT. For patients with DVT, interventions include rest of the affected extremity, prevention of complications that may result from VTE, and monitoring anticoagulant therapy.

Activity With Deep Vein Thrombosis

Previously, it was thought that physical activity should be limited in a patient who has developed a DVT to prevent dislodgment of emboli. Findings from more recent studies with support from updated treatment guidelines indicate during the acute phase, self-care activities need not be limited once anticoagulation is initiated, and graduated ambulation is encouraged.[103] Range-of-motion exercises can be performed with any unaffected limb. The patient is instructed to avoid bending at the knees or hips because this impedes venous return. Antiembolism stockings that have been custom-fitted can be used. It is unclear when it is safe to resume normal activity such as walking after DVT. It is usually resumed after a Doppler study shows no evidence of DVT in the extremity and after symptoms have abated. Prevention strategies become important because the patient remains at risk for a recurrence. In general, early ambulation after surgery or other procedures and avoidance of bed rest are the most effective prevention strategies.

Risk of Pulmonary Embolism

The patient with a VTE is closely monitored for signs of PE and instructed to report immediately any chest pain, dyspnea, hemoptysis, or tachypnea. Risk factors for VTE are almost identical to risk factors for PE. For patients who must remain immobile because of their clinical condition, external pneumatic compression devices, antiembolism stockings, and low-dose heparin are commonly used.[103]

Anticoagulation

Anticoagulant therapy is monitored by obtaining daily coagulation values—aPTT if the patient is receiving intravenous heparin and daily INR if the patient is receiving warfarin.[104] Although the American College of Clinical Pharmacology clinical practice guidelines limit routine coagulation monitoring recommendations for LMWH to anti–factor Xa levels in pregnant women only, this approach may be expanded to all patients in the future.[104] Signs of bleeding are monitored, and symptoms are treated promptly. For a critically ill patient, hemoglobin levels and hematocrit are monitored daily, and stools are assessed for occult blood. Avoidable mechanical trauma is minimized. The alert patient should be instructed to use a soft toothbrush and, if needed, an electric razor.

Patient Education

Patient education emphasizes VTE prevention for all patients who are immobile in the critical care unit for any length of time. This includes explanations about activity prophylaxis such as early ambulation after major surgery, external pneumatic compression boots, and low-dose heparin.

For patients who have a diagnosed DVT, education is focused on identifying symptoms to report, avoidance of trauma to the limb, and elevation of the limb to decrease venous pooling and increase blood flow. If the patient is on anticoagulation medications, the risks and benefits of this therapy are discussed as well as the risk of VTE and pulmonary embolus. The patient is instructed to report any chest pain, shortness of breath, or respiratory distress (Box 14.40). A collaborative team of clinicians who are aware of current clinical recommendations is essential to provide effective care for all critical care patients at risk for VTE (Box 14.41).

HYPERTENSIVE EMERGENCY

Description

Hypertensive emergency is relatively uncommon. It is seen in less than 1% of patients who have hypertension, but when present, it is life-threatening and demands early recognition and management to minimize morbidity and mortality. It was formerly known as *hypertensive crisis* or *malignant hypertension*. With the advent of so many categories of antihypertensive medications, this condition can be effectively managed in the critical care setting. The following two forms of acute hypertension are recognized:
- *Hypertensive emergencies* pose a risk of end-organ damage and are life-threatening conditions. The target organ can be the heart (acute MI), the brain (stroke), or the kidney (kidney failure).
- *Hypertensive urgencies* are characterized by a serious elevation in BP but do not put the patient at risk for end-organ damage.[106]

Etiology

Hypertensive emergency may occur in patients with no history of hypertension or can be precipitated by noncompliance with

BOX 14.41 **QSEN: Evidence-Based Practice**

Venous Thromboembolism

Summary of Evidence-Based Recommendations for VTE Prevention

Strong evidence exists for the following:

- For highest risk patients, combine pharmacologic and mechanical prevention methods.
- All patients admitted to the critical care unit must be assessed for risk of venous thromboembolism (VTE).
- Most critically ill patients require thromboprophylaxis.
- Aspirin *alone* should not be used for VTE prophylaxis for any patient group.
- Pharmacologic thromboprophylaxis with low-dose unfractionated heparin *or* low-molecular-weight heparin (subcutaneous administration), fondaparinux *or* rivaroxaban.
- Oral vitamin K agonists (warfarin) used to achieve a target international normalized ratio (INR) of 2.5 (INR range, 2–3).
- Mechanical prophylaxis: Graduated compression stockings or intermittent pneumatic compression devices.
- Patients at highest risk for VTE include patients undergoing open urologic surgery, gynecologic surgery, or total hip or knee procedures; all trauma patients with at least one risk factor; and medical patients with acute heart failure or acute respiratory failure; others included in this group are immobile patients confined to bed who have at least one risk factor.

Reference

Kearon C, et al. antithrombotic therapy for VTE disease: antithrombotic therapy and prevention of thrombosis, 9th ed: American College of Chest Physicians Evidence-Based Clinical Practice Guidelines. *Chest.* 2012;141(suppl 2):e419s.

TABLE 14.15 **Hypertensive Emergencies**

Emergency	Possible Causes
Cardiovascular Compromise	
Chest pain	Unstable angina, myocardial infarction, aortic dissection
Acute heart failure	Myocardial infarction, severe hypertension
Hypertension after vascular surgery	Aortic aneurysmectomy, carotid endarterectomy, coronary artery bypass grafting
CNS Compromise	
Papilledema	Increased intracranial pressure—mass lesion Malignant hypertension—any cause
Headache, agitation, lethargy, confusion	Hypertensive encephalopathy—any cause, subarachnoid hemorrhage, stroke
Coma	Stroke, advanced hypertensive encephalopathy, trauma, tumor
Seizures	Advanced hypertensive encephalopathy, CNS tumor, eclampsia, stroke (less common)
Focal neurologic deficit	Stroke, CNS tumor, hypertensive encephalopathy
Acute kidney failure	Malignant hypertension, vasculitis, scleroderma, glomerulonephritis
Catecholamine excess	Pheochromocytomas, MAOI in combination with certain medications and foods; abrupt withdrawal of antihypertensive medications such as clonidine, guanabenz, or beta-blockers

CNS, central nervous system; *MAOI,* monoamine oxidase inhibitor.

or inadequate medication therapy. In patients with no known history of hypertension, causes of hypertensive emergency include the following:

1. Acute kidney failure.
2. Acute CNS events: Hypertension frequently accompanies subarachnoid hemorrhage, intracerebral hemorrhage, or a stroke.
3. Acute aortic dissection: Hypertension frequently precedes dissection.
4. Pregnancy-induced eclampsia: Intense arterial vascular constriction, which increases BP and decreases blood supply to the placenta.
5. Pheochromocytoma: An adrenal tumor that produces epinephrine and norepinephrine and increases BP as a result of the circulating catecholamines.
6. Drug-induced hypertension: Illegal drugs, particularly cocaine or amphetamines.
7. Medication-food interactions: Hypertensive response to tyramine-containing foods or beverages (beer or aged cheese) or during treatment with a monoamine oxidase inhibitor, which is now rare because most patients are prescribed other antidepressant medications.

Pathophysiology

The exact trigger of a hypertensive crisis is often unknown. However, most patients have diagnosed hypertension before the event, and the sudden rise in BP is often related to the underlying disease process. Clinical manifestations of hypertensive emergency are listed in Table 14.15.

Assessment and Diagnosis

Hypertensive emergency can manifest as any of the following symptoms, depending on the target organ involved:

1. CNS compromise, identified by headache, blurred vision, change in level of consciousness, or coma
2. Cardiovascular compromise, identified by the chest pain of ACS or aortic dissection
3. Acute kidney failure, identified by a sudden absence of urine output
4. Catecholamine excess

Worsening of symptoms may indicate hypertensive encephalopathy. Diagnostic studies include BP measurement in both arms and placement of an intraarterial line for close monitoring of BP. A 12-lead ECG reading is taken to evaluate for evidence of STEMI or left ventricular hypertrophy.

Medical Management

Hypertensive Emergencies

Hypertensive emergencies are defined as an acute BP elevation greater than 180/120 mm Hg complicated by impending or progressive target organ dysfunction.[106] Hypertensive emergencies with the risk of end-organ damage necessitate admission of the patient to the critical care unit, where intravenous antihypertensive therapy can be administered and BP can be monitored continuously with an arterial line. Several intravenous medications in different medication classes are available for acute reduction of BP. Ideally, the medication should be targeted to the specific condition.

Sodium nitroprusside is frequently the first medication used to lower BP in hypertensive emergency. Sodium nitroprusside is useful because of its half-life of seconds. It is unsuitable for long-term use because of development of a metabolite that causes cyanide-like toxicity.[106,107] Labetalol and esmolol are effective short-acting beta-blockers. Beta-blockers are especially effective if aortic dissection is present. For patients with heart failure, the intravenous ACEI enalaprilat lowers BP. The vasodilator nitroglycerin is used for patients with hypertension who have chest pain. For patients with kidney dysfunction, the dopamine D_1 receptor antagonist fenoldopam may be used to lower BP and increase blood flow to the kidneys.[106] Hydralazine is the intravenous agent of choice in eclampsia because it does not cross the placental barrier. The calcium channel blocker nicardipine and the combination alpha-beta blocker labetalol are less likely to decrease cerebral blood flow and have been used in patients with CNS compromise.[106] Sometimes combinations of the above-mentioned agents are more effective in hypertension control. The intravenous diuretic furosemide (Lasix) is useful in patients with fluid retention.[106, 107]

Initial goals of therapy in hypertensive emergencies limit reducing mean arterial BP by no more than 20% to 25% over a period of several minutes to several hours.[106] Variability depends on the target organ that is affected. When the brain is the target organ, cerebral hypoperfusion can occur if BP is lowered too rapidly. Guidelines for treating stroke do not recommend a rapid reduction of BP. If the BP is excessively high, the aim is to reduce by not more than 20% to 15% in the first 24 hours.[106] BP spontaneously decreases during the first 10 days after a stroke.[106] For a patient with CAD experiencing a hypertensive emergency, the need to maintain adequate diastolic BP to allow for coronary artery filling is paramount.[106, 107] If vasodilator therapy decreases the diastolic pressure too much—when coronary artery filling occurs—myocardial ischemia may result. The question of how much to decrease the BP in a hypertensive emergency is not simply a matter of reading the number on the monitor from the patient's arterial line; it involves an assessment of the underlying pathology and an appreciation of the physiologic requirements of the affected target organ. The section on "Vasodilator Medications" in Chapter 15 provides more information on specific agents.

Hypertensive Urgencies

Hypertensive urgencies may not necessitate admission to a critical care unit because organ damage is not evident and the patient may be treated with rapid-acting oral antihypertensive agents. Many medication categories are available, including ACEIs, ARBs, calcium channel blockers, and beta-blockers.[107] A loop diuretic (eg, furosemide) often is prescribed in addition to the antihypertensive agents when the patient has fluid retention.

Nursing Management

The focus of nursing management for a patient with hypertensive crisis is to return the BP to the desired range without introducing other complications as a result of therapy. After hypertension is controlled, the nurse identifies the factors that resulted in this life-threatening condition. Several nursing diagnoses are associated with hypertensive crisis (Box 14.42).

During the acute phase, the patient is observed closely for clinical manifestations in other organ systems including the neurologic, cardiac, and renal systems. Neurologic compromise may be manifested by mental confusion, stupor, seizures, coma, or stroke. Cardiac compromise may be exhibited by aortic

---

BOX 14.42 NURSING DIAGNOSES
Hypertensive Emergency

- Risk for Ineffective Cerebral Tissue Perfusion, p. 1042
- Risk for Ineffective Peripheral Tissue Perfusion, p. 1044
- Anxiety related to threat to biologic, psychologic, or social integrity, p. 1012
- Deficient Knowledge related to lack of previous exposure to information, p. 1020 (see Box 14.43, Patient Education Plan for Hypertensive Emergency)

BOX 14.43 PATIENT EDUCATION PLAN
Hypertensive Emergency

The patient should be able to teach back the following topics:
- Pathophysiology of hypertensive crisis.
- Normal and abnormal blood pressure values.
- Self-monitoring of blood pressure at home.
- Connection between hypertension and other atherosclerotic diseases such as coronary artery disease, peripheral artery disease (PAD), and cerebrovascular disease.
- Warning signs of a "heart attack" or myocardial infarction.
- Warning signs of a "brain attack" or stroke.
- Warning signs of intermittent claudication or PAD.
- Risk factors modification: After the acute episode, if the cause of carotid artery disease is atherosclerosis, an individual risk factor profile is developed for each patient; strategies to discuss include decrease daily fat intake to less than 30% of total calories, achieve total blood cholesterol level of less than 200 mg/dL, stop smoking, reduce salt intake, control hypertension, control diabetes if patient has diabetes, increase physical activity, achieve and maintain ideal body weight.
- Medications: Antihypertensive medications, rationale, and side effects.
- Signs and symptoms to report to a health care professional.
- Follow-up care after discharge.

---

dissection, myocardial ischemia, or dysrhythmias. Acute kidney failure may not be evident immediately, but urine output, blood urea nitrogen, and serum creatinine values are evaluated over several days to determine whether the kidneys were affected by the hypertensive episode. When short-acting intravenous antihypertensive agents are administered, BP is closely monitored. If potent antihypertensive medications such as sodium nitroprusside or labetalol are being used, an arterial line must be inserted, and the medications must be infused through an infusion pump.[106]

Patient Education

Patient education during the acute phase of a hypertensive emergency is limited to an explanation of the need to control BP and the purpose of the equipment used in the critical care unit. After the hypertensive crisis is resolved, the focus of education is on lifestyle changes to modify risk factors. Hypertension is emphasized as a risk factor for atherosclerotic disease of the heart, brain, and peripheral artery system. A more complete discussion of hypertension as a cardiovascular risk factor is provided at the beginning of this chapter. The major points to discuss with the patient are listed in Box 14.43. Management of hypertensive emergencies and urgencies is presented in Box 14.44.

QSEN BOX 14.44   QSEN: Evidence-Based Practice

Hypertensive Emergencies

Definition

Hypertensive emergency is defined as an acute blood pressure (BP) elevation greater than 180/120 mm Hg complicated by impending or progressive target organ dysfunction.

Recommendations

- Early identification of hypertensive emergency in the emergency department and admission to a critical care unit is recommended.
- Patients with hypertensive emergency should have continuous BP monitoring.
- Intravenous (IV) medications are used to reduce BP (not necessarily to normal) to prevent or limit target organ damage.
- Initial goal is to reduce BP by no more than 25%. For example, reduce systolic blood pressure (SBP) to 160 mm Hg and diastolic blood pressure (DBP) to 100–110 mm Hg in the 2–6 h after admission.
- Decreasing BP gradually is recommended to avoid cerebral, coronary, or kidney ischemia.
- Medications that cause rapid falls in BP are not recommended in the management of acute hypertensive emergency. For this reason, short-acting nifedipine is *not* endorsed (sublingual or IV).
- Further gradual reductions in BP can be achieved in the following 24–48 h.

Special Situations: Hypertension and Acute Ischemic Stroke

- For patients admitted with an ischemic stroke, no clinical evidence exists to support rapid reduction in BP.
- For patients with SBP greater than 220 mm Hg or DBP between 120 mm Hg and 140 mm Hg, BP should be lowered cautiously by 10%–15% only.

- If DBP is greater than 140 mm Hg, sodium nitroprusside is recommended to cautiously lower SBP by approximately 10%.
- If SBP is greater than 185 mm Hg or DBP is greater than 110 mm Hg, the use of thrombolytic therapy (tissue plasminogen activator [tPA]) is contraindicated within the first 3 h after an acute ischemic stroke. BP must be lowered before administration of tPA.
- Careful monitoring of the patient for signs of neurologic deterioration related to the lower BP is mandatory in all situations.

Special Situation: Hypertension and Aortic Dissection

- Patients with aortic dissection should have SBP lowered to <100 mm Hg if tolerated.

Ultimate Blood Pressure Target Goal

- The goal of therapy for all patients is a target BP of 140/90 mm Hg or lower before discharge from the hospital. Some patients require oral medications to achieve this target.
- Target BP is 130/80 mm Hg or lower for patients with known hypertension, kidney failure, diabetes, or cardiovascular disease. Almost all patients with these conditions require oral medications to achieve their target BP. Many patients require two or more oral medications.

References

James PA, et al. 2014 Evidence-based guideline for the management of high blood pressure in adults. Report from the panel members appointed to the Eighth Joint National Committee (JNC8). *JAMA*. 2014;311(5):507.
Papadopoulos D, et al. Hypertension crisis. *Blood Press*. 2010;19:328.

SUMMARY

- The number of patients with cardiovascular disease in the United States continues to grow.
- Considerable research and clinical progress have clarified the diagnosis and management of many cardiac conditions.
- Atherosclerosis provides a common link among CAD, atherosclerotic aortic disease, PAD, and carotid artery disease. The risk factors and general management strategies for all these diseases are the same.
- STEMI, NSTEMI, aortic aneurysm, aortic dissection, and embolic stroke are acute manifestations of chronic disease progression.
- Heart failure is a consequence of damaged heart muscle that results from MI, cardiomyopathy, valve disease, or hypertension.

Coronary Artery Disease

- Progressive atherosclerotic buildup in coronary arteries results in narrowing of lumens and decreasing flow.
- Medical management focuses on lifestyle changes and symptom management including anticoagulants and vasodilators to increase flow.
- Nursing management focuses on treating symptoms and providing patient education.

Acute Coronary Syndrome

- ACS is an umbrella term for the clinical presentation of ischemic coronary artery events.

- Medical management includes vasodilators and anticoagulation.
- Nursing management focuses on managing pain and symptoms, maintaining a calm environment, and providing patient and family education.

Myocardial Infarction

- MI is irreversible myocardial necrosis secondary to an abrupt decrease of total blood flow through coronary arteries.
- Medical management focuses on reestablishing flow through the arteries and preventing ventricular remodeling.
- Nursing management focuses on improving myocardial oxygen supply or decreasing demands, preventing complications, and providing patient and family education.

Cardiomyopathy

- Cardiomyopathy is a disease caused by structural abnormalities of the heart that affect cardiac function.
- Medical management focuses on relieving symptoms and preventing arrhythmias.
- Nursing management focuses on maintaining fluid balance, monitoring medication effects, improving mobility, and providing patient and family education.

Sudden Cardiac Death

- SCD refers to sudden death without previous symptoms of disease. The mechanism is most likely ventricular tachycardia that evolves to ventricular fibrillation.

- Medical management focuses on using hypothermia after a cardiac arrest procedure to protect the brain and rhythm management with probable insertion of an implantable cardioverter defibrillator device.
- Nursing management focuses on monitoring treatment effects, preventing complications, and providing patient and family education.

Heart Failure
- Heart failure is a response to cardiac dysfunction that results in impaired ability to eject blood from the ventricle.
- Medical management focuses on relieving symptoms, enhancing cardiac performance, and correcting the precipitating cause.
- Nursing management focuses on supporting optimal cardiopulmonary function, promoting comfort, providing emotional support, and providing patient and family education.

Pulmonary Hypertension
- PH is a progressive sustained increase in pulmonary pressures with resultant right heart failure and ultimately death.
- Medical management focuses on multidrug therapies and prevention of complications.
- Nursing management focuses on managing symptoms, providing education on multidrug treatments including intravenous site care, and developing extended support systems.

Endocarditis
- IE is an infection on the endocardial surface of the heart, heart valves, or both.
- Medical management requires prolonged treatment with intravenous antibiotics. Some patients require excision of the involved valve for eradication of infection.
- Nursing management includes monitoring for worsening symptoms and providing patient education on the need for prolonged medication for treatment including intravenous site care.

Valvular Heart Disease
- Valvular heart disease comprises structural and functional abnormalities of cardiac valves.
- Medical management includes medications to control symptoms and surgical interventions to repair or replace involved valves.
- Nursing management focuses on titrating medications to improve flow through involved valves, monitoring patient symptoms and responses to treatment, and organizing patient care activities to prevent fatigue.

Atherosclerosis of the Aorta
- Aortic disease results from progressive atherosclerosis and hypertension and includes aneurysmal and local dilation of the wall and aortic dissection where blood separates the vascular layers.
- Medical management depends on symptoms and hemodynamics. Corrective surgery is indicated for aneurysms more than 5 cm wide. Acute dissection requires immediate control of hypertension and pain, and surgical correction is required for dissection of the ascending aorta.
- Nursing management focuses on monitoring for changes in cardiovascular status and administering medications for significant BP reduction and pain control.

Peripheral Artery Disease
- PAD includes chronic venous disease and acute arterial changes.
- Medical management focuses on controlling or eliminating risk factors; pharmacologic management including anticoagulants, vasodilators, and antiplatelets; and surgical interventions including percutaneous transluminal coronary angioplasty, stent placement, or vascular bypass.
- Nursing care includes assessment of pulses, maintenance of skin integrity, and pain control.

Carotid Artery Disease
- Carotid artery disease results in obstruction of the major arterial supply to the brain.
- Medical management focuses on limiting risks and performing surgical endarterectomy when obstruction is greater than 60%.
- Nursing management focuses on monitoring neurologic assessment and educating patients and family about stroke symptoms.

Venous Thromboembolism
- VTE includes DVT and PE with clot formation and obstruction of large vessels.
- Medical management focuses on prevention and treatment with anticoagulation.
- Nursing management focuses on prevention with activity started as soon as possible for critically ill patients and monitoring the effects of anticoagulation.

Hypertensive Emergency
- Hypertensive emergency is defined as acute BP elevation greater than 180/120 mm Hg and may include symptoms of CNS or cardiovascular compromise, acute kidney failure, or catecholamine excess.
- Medical management is aimed at use of appropriate medications to initially decrease BP by no more than 20% to 25% over several hours.
- Nursing management is focused on close monitoring of symptoms with judicious use of BP-lowering medications.
- ⓔ Visit the Evolve site for additional study materials.

REFERENCES

1. Mozaffarian D, et al. american Heart Association. Heart disease and stroke statistics—2015 update: a report from the American Heart Association. *Circulation.* 2015;131:e290-e322.
2. O'Gara PT, et al. 2013 ACCF/AHA Guideline for the management of ST-elevation myocardial infarction: a report of the American College of Cardiology Foundation/American Heart Association Task Force on Practice Guidelines. *Circulation.* 2013;127(4):e362.
3. Fihn SD, et al. 2012 ACCF/AHA/ACP/AATS/PCNA/SCAI/STS guideline for the diagnosis and management of patients with stable ischemic heart disease: a report of the American College of Cardiology Foundation/American Heart Association Task Force on Practice Guidelines, and the American College of Physicians, American Association for Thoracic Surgery, Preventive Cardiovascular Nurses Association, Society for Cardiovascular Angiography and Interventions, and Society of Thoracic Surgeons. *Circulation.* 2012;126(25):e354-e471.
4. Yusef S, et al. INTERHEART Study Investigators. Effect of potentially modifiable risk factors associated with myocardial infarction in 52 countries (The INTERHEART Study): case-control study. *Lancet.* 2004;364(9438):937.

5. Stone NJ, et al. 2013 ACC/AHA guideline on treatment of blood choles-terol to reduce atherosclerotic cardiovascular risk in adults: a report of the American College of Cardiology/American Heart Association Task Force on Practice Guidelines. *J Am Coll Cardiol*. 2014;63(25):2889-2934.

6. Arora S, Patra SK, Saini R. HDL—a molecule with multifaceted role in coronary artery disease. *Clin Chim Acta*. 2016;452:66-81.

7. Miller M, et al. Triglycerides and cardiovascular disease: a scientific state-ment from the American Heart Association. *Circulation*. 2011;123:2292-2333.

8. Eckel RH, et al. 2013 Guidelines on lifestyle management to reduce cardiovascular risk. *J Am Coll Cardiol*. 2014;63(25):2960-2984.

9. Fox CS. Update on prevention of cardiovascular disease in adults with type 2 diabetes mellitus in light of recent evidence: a scientific statement from the American Heart Association and the American Diabetes Associ-ation. *Diabetes Care*. 2015;38:1777-1803.

10. Goff DC, et al. 2013 ACC/AHA guideline on assessment of cardiovas-cular risk. A report of the American College of Cardiology/American Heart Association Task Force on Practice Guidelines. *J Am Coll Cardiol*. 2013;63(25):2935-2959.

11. Smith SC, et al. AHA/ACC secondary prevention and risk reduction therapy for patients with coronary and other atherosclerotic vascular dis-ease. 2011 Update: a guideline from the American Heart Association and American College of Cardiology Foundation. *Circulation*. 2011;24:2458.

12. Rosendorff C, et al. Treatment of hypertension in patients with coronary artery disease. A scientific statement from the American Heart Associa-tion, American College of Cardiology, and American Society of Hyper-tension. *Hypertension*. 2015;65:1372-1407.

13. Grundy SM. Pre-diabetes, metabolic syndrome, and cardiovascular risk. *J Am Coll Cardiol*. 2012;59(7):635-643.

14. James PA. 2014 Evidence-based guideline for the management of high blood pressure in adults. Report from the panel members appointed to the Eighth Joint National Committee (JNC8). *JAMA*. 2014;311(5):507-520.

15. Sargent RP, et al. Reduced incidence of admissions for myocardial in-farction associated with public smoking ban: before and after study. *BMJ*. 2004;328(7446):977.

16. Wright SR, et al. 2011 ACC/AHA focused update of the guidelines for the management of patients with unstable angina/non-ST-elevation myocar-dial infarction: a report of the American College of Cardiology/American Heart Association Task Force on Practice Guidelines developed in collab-oration with the American College of Emergency Physicians, Society for Cardiovascular Angiography and Interventions, and Society for Thoracic Surgeons. *J Am Coll Cardiol*. 2011;57:1920.

17. Mosca L, et al. Effectiveness-based guidelines for the prevention of cardiovascular disease in women—2011 update: a guideline from the American Heart Association. *Circulation*. 2011;123:1243-1262.

18. Anderson GL, et al. Effects of conjugated equine estrogen in postmeno-pausal women with hysterectomy: The Women's Health Initiative randomized controlled trial. *JAMA*. 2004;291(14):1701.

19. Mehta LS, et al. Acute myocardial infarction in women. A scientific statement from the American Heart Association. *Circulation*. 2016;133:916-947.

20. McSweeney JC. Preventing and experiencing ischemic heart disease as a woman: State of the science. A scientific statement from the American Heart Association. *Circulation*. 2016;133:1302-1331.

21. Lloyd-Jones DM, et al. On behalf of the American Heart Association Strategic Planning Task Force and Statistics Committee. Defining and setting national goals for cardiovascular health promotion and disease reduction: The American Heart Association's Strategic Impact Goal through 2020 and beyond. *Circulation*. 2010;121:586.

22. Soeki T, Sata M. Inflammatory biomarkers and atherosclerosis. *Int Heart J*. 2016;57(2):134-139.

23. Kavousi M, et al. Evaluation of newer risk markers for coronary heart disease. A cohort study. *Ann Intern Med*. 2012;156:438.

24. Adamcova M, et al. Cardiac troponins—translational biomarkers in car-diology: Theory and practice of cardiac troponin high-sensitivity assays. *Biofactors*. 2016;42(2):133-148.

25. Lupton JR, et al. Serum homocysteine is not independently associated with an atherogenic lipid profile: The Very Large Database of Lipids (VLDL-21) study. *Atherosclerosis*. 2016;249:59-64.

26. Greeland P, et al. 2010 ACCF/AHA guideline for cardiovascular risk in asymptomatic adults. A report of the American College of Cardiology Foundation/American Heart Association Task Force on Practice Guide-lines. Writing Committee Members. *Circulation*. 2010;122:e584.

27. Anderson JL, et al. 2011 ACCF/AHA focused update incorporated into the ACC/AHA 2007 guidelines for the management of patients with unstable angina/non-st-elevation myocardial infarction: a report of the American College of Cardiology Foundation/American Heart Associa-tion Task Force on Practice Guidelines. *Circulation*. 2011;123:e426.

28. Goldberg RJ, et al. Community trends in the use and characteristics of persons with acute myocardial infarction who are transported by emer-gency medical services. *Heart Lung*. 2012;41(4):323.

29. Bayes de Luna A, et al. Prinzmetal angina: ECG changes and clinical considerations: a consensus paper. *Ann Noninvasive Electrocardiol*. 2014;19(5):442-453.

30. Levine GN, et al. 2011 ACC/AHA/SCAI guideline for percutaneous coro-nary intervention: executive summary: a report of the American College of Cardiology Foundation/American Heart Association Task Force on Practice Guidelines and the Society for Cardiovascular Angiography and Interventions. *Circulation*. 2011;124:2574.

31. Goldstein JA. Acute right ventricular infarction. *Cardiol Clin*. 2012;30(2):219.

32. Wann SL, et al. 2011 ACC/AHA/HRS focused update on the man-agement of patients with atrial fibrillation (update on dabigatran). A report of the American College of Cardiology Foundation/American Heart Association Task Force on Practice Guidelines. *Circulation*. 2011;123:1140.

33. Novak M, et al. Ventricular septal rupture—a critical condition as a complication of acute myocardial infarction. *JCCM*. 2015;1(4):162-166.

34. Meris A, et al. Mechanisms and predictors of mitral regurgitation after high-risk myocardial infarction. *J Am Soc Echocardiogr*. 2012;25(5):535.

35. Seferović PM, et al. Pericardial syndromes: an update after the ESC guidelines 2004. *Heart Fail Rev*. 2013;18(3):255-266.

36. Kloos JA. Characteristics, complications, and treatment of acute pericar-ditis. *Crit Care Nurs Clin North Am*. 2015;27(4):483.

37. Krumholz HM, et al. Patterns of hospital performance in acute myocar-dial infarction and heart failure 30-day mortality and readmission. *Circ Cardiovasc Quality Outcomes*. 2009;5(2):407.

38. O'Neil A, et al. Depression as a predictor of work resumption following myocardial infarction (MI): a review of recent research evidence. *Health Qual Life Outcomes*. 2010;8:95.

39. Thomas RJ, et al. AACVPR/ACCF/AHA 2010 update: performance measures on cardiac rehabilitation for referral to cardiac rehabilitation/secondary prevention services. A report of the American Association of Cardiovascular and Pulmonary Rehabilitation and the American College of Cardiology Foundation/American Heart Association Task Force on Performance Measures. *Circulation*. 2010;122:1342-1350.

40. Fox CS, et al. Temporal trends in coronary heart disease mortality and sudden cardiac death from 1950 to 1999: The Framingham Heart Study. *Circulation*. 2004;110(5):522.

41. Fishman GI, et al. Sudden cardiac death prediction and prevention: Report from a National Heart, Lung, and Blood Institute and Heart Rhythm Society workshop. *Circulation*. 2010;122:2335-2348.

42. Baye de Luna A, et al. Current electrocardiographic criteria for diagnosis of Brugada pattern: a consensus report. *J Electrocardiol*. 2012;45:433-442.

43. Probst V, et al. Long term prognosis of patients diagnosed with Brugada syndrome. Results from the FINGER Brugada syndrome registry. *Circulation*. 2010;121:635-643.

44. Priori SG, et al. 2015 ESC guidelines for the management of patients with ventricular arrhythmias and the prevention of sudden cardiac death. *Eur Heart J*. 2015;36:2793-2867.

45. Ghani A, et al. Sex based differences in cardiac arrhythmias, ICD utiliza-tion and cardiac resynchronization therapy. *Neth Heart*. 2011;19(1):35.

46. Greenberg B. Acute decompensated heart failure: treatment and chal-lenges. *Circulation*. 2012;76(3):532.

47. Yancy CW, et al. 2013 ACCF/AHA guideline for management of heart failure. *J Am Coll Cardiol*. 2013;62(16):e147.

48. Paul S, Page 2nd RL. Foundations of pharmacotherapy for heart failure with reduced ejection fraction. Evidence meets practice, Part 1. *J Cardiovasc Nurs.* 2016;31(2):101-113.

49. Kozik A, Wilczek K, Polonski L. Management of diastolic heart failure. *Cardiol J.* 2010;17(6):558-565.

50. Kociol RD, et al. Admission, discharge, or change in B-type natriuretic peptide and long-term outcomes: Data from Organized Program to Initiate Lifesaving Treatment in Hospitalized Patients with Heart Failure (OPTIMIZE-HF) linked to Medicare claims. *Circ Heart Fail.* 2011;4:628.

51. Butler J, et al. Update on aldosterone antagonists use in heart failure with reduced left ventricular ejection fraction. Heart Failure Society of America Guidelines Committee. *J Card Fail.* 2012;18:265.

52. Prasad R, Pugh PJ. Drug and device therapy for patients with chronic heart failure. *Expert Rev Cardiovascular Ther.* 2012;10(3):313.

53. Sing PJ, Gras D. Biventricular pacing: current trends and future strategies. *Eur Heart J.* 2012;33:305.

54. Arshad A, et al. Cardiac resynchronization therapy is more effective in women than in men: The MADIT-CRT (Multicenter Automatic Defibrillator Implantation Trial with Cardiac Resynchronization Therapy) trial. *J Am Coll Cardiol.* 2011;57:813.

55. Linde C, Ellenbogen K, McAllister FA. Cardiac resynchronization therapy (CRT): clinical trials, guidelines, and target populations. *Heart Rhythm.* 2012;8(suppl):S3.

56. Gadoud A, Jenkins SM, Hogg KJ. Palliative care for people with heart failure: Summary of current evidence and future direction. *Palliat Med.* 2013;27(9):822-828.

57. Shah AB, et al. Failing the failing heart: a review of palliative care in heart failure. *Rev Cardiovasc Med.* 2013;14(1):41-48.

58. Evangalista LS, et al. Health literacy and the patient with heart failure: implications for patient care and research. A consensus statement of the Heart Failure Society of America. *J Card Fail.* 2010;16:9.

59. White M, et al. Is "teach-back" associated with knowledge retention and hospital readmission in hospitalized heart failure patients? *J Cardiovasc Nurs.* 2013;28(2):137-146.

60. Gersh BJ, et al. 2011 AHA/ACC Guideline for the Diagnosis and Treatment of Hypertrophic Cardiomyopathy. A report of the American College of Cardiology Foundation/American Heart Association Task Force on Practice Guidelines. *Circulation.* 2011;124:e783.

61. Friedrich FW, Carrier L. Genetics of hypertrophic and dilated cardiomyopathy. *Curr Pharm Biotechnol.* 2012;13(13):2467.

62. Kelkar AA, et al. Mechanisms contributing to the progression of ischemic and nonischemic dilated cardiomyopathy. *J Am Coll Cardiol.* 2015;66(18):2038-2047.

63. Gary SF, et al. ACCF/AHA/ACP/HFSA/ISHLT 2010 clinical competence statement on management of patients with advanced heart failure and cardiac transplant. *Circulation.* 2010;122:644.

64. Shah SJ. Pulmonary hypertension. *JAMA.* 2012;308(13):1366.

65. Rosenkranz S. Pulmonary hypertension 2015: current definitions, terminology, and novel treatment options. *Clin Res Cardiol.* 2015;104:197-207.

66. Simmoneau G, et al. Updated clinical classification of pulmonary hypertension. *J Am Coll Cardiol.* 2013;62(25):D34-D41.

67. Galie N, et al. 2015 ESC/ERS guidelines for the diagnosis and treatment of pulmonary hypertension. *Eur Heart J.* 2016;37:67-119.

68. Zamanian RT, et al. Current clinical management of pulmonary arterial hypertension. *Circ Res.* 2014;115:131-147.

69. Waxman AB, Zamanian RT. Pulmonary arterial hypertension: new insights into the optimal role of current and emerging prostacyclin therapies. *Am J Cardiol.* 2013;111(suppl):1A-16A.

70. Brown LM, et al. Delay in recognition of pulmonary arterial hypertension: Factors identified from the REVEAL registry. *Chest.* 2011;140(1):19.

71. Keogh A, et al. Survival after the initiation of combination therapy in patients with pulmonary arterial hypertension: An Australian collaborative report. *Intern Med J.* 2011;41(3):235.

72. Iheagwara NL, Thomas TF. Pharmacologic treatment of pulmonary hypertension. *US Pharm.* 2010;35(8):HS11.

73. Hill NS, Cawley MJ, Heggen-Peay CL. New therapeutic paradigms and guidelines in the management of pulmonary arterial hypertension. *J Manag Care Spec Pharm.* 2016;22(3a):s3-S21.

74. Anderson JR, Nawarskas JJ. Pharmacotherapeutic management of pulmonary arterial hypertension. *Cardiol Rev.* 2010;18(3):148.

75. Gupta V, Ahsan F. Inhalation therapy for pulmonary hypertension: current status and future prospects. *Crit Rev Ther Drug Carrier Syst.* 2010;27(4):313-370. 27.

76. McLaughlin VV, et al. Addition of inhaled treprostinil to oral therapy for pulmonary arterial hypertension. *J Am Coll Cardiol.* 2010;55(18):1915.

77. Luttenberger K, DiNapoli M. Subacute bacterial endocarditis: making the diagnosis. *Nurs Pract.* 2011;36(3):31-38.

78. Baddour LM, et al. Infective endocarditis in adults: diagnosis, antimicrobial therapy, and management of complication. *Circulation.* 2015;132:1435-1485.

79. Habib G, et al. 2015 ESC guidelines for the management of infective endocarditis. The Task Force for the Management of Infective Endocarditis of the European Society of Cardiology (ESC). *Eur Heart J.* 2015;36(42):2921-2964.

80. Nishimura RA, et al. 2014 AHA/ACC guideline for the management of patients with valvular heart disease: a report of the American College of Cardiology/American Heart Association Task Force on Practice Guidelines. *J Am Coll Cardiol.* 2014;63(22):e57-185.

81. Foster E. Mitral regurgitation due to degenerative mitral-valve disease. *N Engl J Med.* 2010;363(2):156.

82. Romeo F, et al. The outcome of intra-aortic balloon pump support in acute myocardial infarction complicated by cardiogenic shock according to the type of revascularization: a comprehensive meta-analysis. *Am Heart J.* 2013;165:679-692.

83. Jilaihawi H, Hussaini A, Kar S. Mitraclip: a novel percutaneous approach to mitral valve repair. *Biomed Biotech.* 2011;12(8):633.

84. Siu SC, Silverside CK. Bicuspid aortic valve. *J Am Coll Cardiol.* 2010;55(2):2789.

85. Horne A. Transcatheter aortic valve replacement: historical perspective, current evidence, and future directions. *Am Heart J.* 2014;168:414-423.

86. Makkar RR, et al. Transcatheter aortic-valve replacement for inoperable severe aortic stenosis. *N Engl J Med.* 2012;336(18):1696.

87. Fitzgerald KP. The pulmonary valve. *Cardiol Clin.* 2011;29(2):223.

88. Ansari MM, et al. Percutaneous pulmonary valve implantation, present status and evolving future. *J Am Coll Cardiol.* 2015;66(20):2246-2255.

89. Asnes J, Hellenbrand WE. Evaluation of the Melody Transcatheter pulmonary valve and Ensemble delivery system for the treatment of dysfunctional right ventricle to pulmonary artery conduits. *Expert Rev Med Devices.* 2015;12(6):653-665.

90. Moll FL, et al. Management of abdominal aortic aneurysms. Clinical practice guidelines for the European Society of Vascular Surgery. *Eur J Vasc Endovasc Surg.* 2011;41:S1.

91. Grootenboer N, et al. Systematic review and meta-analysis of sex differences in outcome after intervention for abdominal aortic aneurysm. *Br J Surg.* 2010;97(8):1169.

92. Hiratzka L, et al. 2010 ACCF/AHA/AATS/ ACR/SCA/SCAO/SIR/STS/ SVM guidelines for the diagnosis and management of patients with thoracic aortic disease. *Circulation.* 2010;121(13):e266.

93. Feldman M, Shah M, Elefteriades A. Medical management of acute type A aortic dissection. *Ann Thorac Cardiovasc Surg.* 2010;15(5):286.

94. Tendara M, et al. ESC guidelines on the diagnosis and treatment of peripheral artery disease. *Eur Heart J.* 2011;32:2851.

95. Olin JW, et al. ACCF/AHA/ACR/ACAI/SIR/SVM/SVN/SVS 2010 performance measures for adults with peripheral artery disease. *Vasc Med.* 2010;15(6):481.

96. Argacha JF, et al. Acute effects of passive smoking on peripheral vascular function. *Hypertension.* 2008;51(6):1506.

97. McDermott MM, et al. The ankle-brachial index is associated with the magnitude of impaired walking endurance among men and women with peripheral arterial disease. *Vasc Med.* 2010;15(4):251.

98. Murphy TP, et al. Supervised exercise versus primary stenting for claudication resulting from aortoiliac peripheral artery disease: Six-month outcomes from the claudication: exercise versus endoluminal revascularization (CLEVER) study. *Circulation.* 2011;125(1):130.

99. Alonso-Coello P, et al. Antithrombotic therapy in peripheral artery disease: antithrombotic therapy and prevention of thrombosis, 9th ed: American College of Chest Physicians evidence-based clinical guidelines. *Chest.* 2012;141(suppl 2):e669S.

100. Goldstein LB, et al. Guidelines for the primary prevention of stroke: a guideline for healthcare professionals from the American Heart Association/American Stroke Association. *Stroke.* 2011;42(2):517.

101. Mantese VA, et al. The Carotid Revascularization Endarterectomy versus Stenting Trial (CREST): stenting versus carotid endarterectomy for carotid disease. *Stroke.* 2010;41:S31.

102. Gurm HS, et al. Long-term results of carotid stenting versus endarterectomy in high-risk patients. *N Engl J Med.* 2008;358(15):1572.

103. Chan CM, Shorr AF. Venous thromboembolic disease in the intensive care unit. *Semin Respir Crit Care Med.* 2010;30(1):39.

104. Kearon C, et al. Antithrombotic therapy for VTE diseases, antithrombotic therapy and prevention of thrombosis, 9th ed: American College of Chest Physicians evidence-based clinical practice guidelines. *Chest.* 2012;141(suppl 2):e419S.

105. Tapson VF. Acute pulmonary embolism. *N Engl J Med.* 2008;358(10):1037.

106. Papadopoulos D, et al. Hypertension crisis. *Blood Press.* 2010;19:328.

107. James PA, et al. 2014 Evidence-based guideline for the management of high blood pressure in adults. Report from the panel members appointed to the Eighth Joint National Committee (JNC8). *JAMA.* 2014;311(5):507-520.

15

Cardiovascular Therapeutic Management

Joni L. Dirks and Julie Waters

PACEMAKERS

Pacemakers are electronic devices that can be used to initiate the heartbeat when the intrinsic electrical system of the heart cannot effectively generate a rate adequate to support cardiac output. Pacemakers may be used temporarily, either supportively or prophylactically, until the condition responsible for the rate or conduction disturbance resolves. They also may be used on a permanent basis if the patient's condition persists despite adequate interventions. The use of permanent pacemakers as a form of device-based therapy has expanded significantly.[1]

This section emphasizes temporary pacemakers because the critical care nurse is responsible for preventing, assessing, and managing pacemaker malfunctions when these devices are used in the clinical setting. A brief discussion of permanent pacemakers is provided, and similarities between implanted and temporary pacemakers are presented where appropriate.

Indications for Temporary Pacing

The clinical indications for instituting temporary pacemaker therapy are similar regardless of the cause of the rhythm disturbance that necessitates the placement of a pacemaker (Box 15.1). The causes range from ischemia and electrolyte imbalances to sequelae related to acute myocardial infarction (MI) or cardiac surgery.

Therapeutic Indications

Dysrhythmias that are unresponsive to medications and result in compromised hemodynamic status are a definite indication for pacemaker therapy. The goal of therapy in the case of brady-dysrhythmia is to increase the ventricular rate and enhance cardiac output. Alternatively, overdrive pacing can be used to decrease the rate of a rapid supraventricular or ventricular rhythm. This rapid pacing of the heart (ie, overdrive pacing) functions to prevent the breakthrough ectopy that can result from a slow rate or to interrupt an ectopic focus and allow the natural pacemaker to regain control. Temporary pacing may be used in the treatment of symptomatic bradycardia or progressive heart block that occurs as a result of myocardial ischemia, medication overdose, or illegal drug toxicity. After cardiac surgery, temporary pacing may be used to improve a transiently depressed, rate-dependent cardiac output. Conduction disturbances that occur after valvular surgery can be managed effectively with temporary pacing.

Diagnostic Indications

Several diagnostic uses for temporary pacing have evolved. Electrophysiology studies (EPS) are performed in cardiac catheterization laboratories equipped with specialized pacing equipment. During EPS, catheters with pacing electrodes are used to diagnose a patient's potential for dysrhythmias.[2] The electrodes are used to induce dysrhythmias in patients with recurrent symptomatic tachydysrhythmias; this allows the physician to closely evaluate the particular dysrhythmia and determine appropriate therapy. For patients whose tachydysrhythmia is found to be refractory to conventional antidysrhythmic therapy, radiofrequency (RF) current catheter ablation of the responsible tissue can be done safely and effectively in the electrophysiology laboratory. After a mapping procedure has localized the site of dysrhythmia formation, short bursts of RF current are delivered through the catheter, destroying the offending tissue with heat. Ablation has been shown to be an effective treatment for patients with symptomatic supraventricular tachycardias (SVTs) that result from atrioventricular (AV) node reentry or accessory pathways, such as Wolff-Parkinson-White syndrome.[3,4] Catheter ablation may also be used as a therapeutic strategy for selected patients with atrial fibrillation (AF).[5]

Intracardiac electrograms—recordings of cardiac electrical activity obtained from pacing electrodes—may provide useful diagnostic information. The atrial electrogram is an amplified recording of atrial activity that can be obtained through the use of an atrial pacing electrode or an esophageal pill electrode and a standard electrocardiogram (ECG) machine. It may be used after cardiac surgery to facilitate the diagnosis of supraventricular dysrhythmias in patients with temporary atrial epicardial wires already in place.[6]

Pacemaker System

A pacemaker system is a simple electrical circuit consisting of a pulse generator and a pacing lead (an insulated electrical wire) with one, two, or three electrodes.

Pacing Pulse Generator

The pulse generator is designed to generate an electrical current that travels through the pacing lead and exits through an electrode (exposed portion of the wire) that is in direct contact with the heart. This electrical current initiates a myocardial depolarization. The current then seeks to return by one of several pathways to the pulse generator to complete the circuit.

The power source for a temporary external pulse generator is a standard alkaline battery inserted into the generator. Implanted permanent pacemaker batteries are usually long-lived lithium cells.

Pacing Lead Systems

The pacing lead used for temporary pacing may be bipolar or unipolar. In a bipolar system, two electrodes (positive and negative) are located within the heart, whereas in a unipolar system, only one electrode (negative) is in direct contact with the myocardium. In both systems, the current flows from the negative terminal of the pulse generator, down the pacing lead to the negative electrode, and into the heart. The current is then picked up by the positive electrode (ground) and flows back up the lead to the positive terminal of the pulse generator.

BOX 15.1 **Indications for Temporary Pacing**

- Bradydysrhythmias
  - Sinus bradycardia and arrest
  - Sick sinus syndrome
  - Heart blocks
- Tachydysrhythmias
  - Supraventricular
  - Ventricular
- Permanent pacemaker failure
- Support of cardiac output after cardiac surgery
- Diagnostic studies
  - Electrophysiology studies
  - Atrial electrograms

The bipolar lead used in transvenous pacing has two electrodes on one catheter (Fig. 15.1). The distal, or negative, electrode is at the tip of the pacing lead and is in direct contact with the heart, usually inside the right atrium or right ventricle. Approximately 1 cm from the negative electrode is a positive electrode. The negative electrode is attached to the negative terminal, and the positive electrode is attached to the positive terminal of the pulse generator, either directly or by means of a bridging cable (see Fig. 15.1B).

An epicardial lead system is often used for temporary pacing after cardiac surgery. The bipolar epicardial lead system has two separate insulated wires (one negative and one positive electrode) that are loosely secured with sutures to the cardiac chamber to be paced. Both leads are in contact with the myocardial tissue, so either wire may be used as the negative, or pacing, electrode. The remaining wire is then used as the positive, or ground, electrode.

A unipolar pacing system (epicardial or transvenous) has only one electrode (the negative electrode) making contact with the heart. For a permanent pacemaker, the positive electrode can be created by the metallic casing of the subcutaneously implanted pulse generator (Fig. 15.2), or, as is the case with a unipolar epicardial lead system, the positive electrode can be formed by a piece of surgical steel wire sewn into the

FIG. 15.1 Components of a Temporary Bipolar Transvenous Catheter. (A) Single-chamber temporary (external) pulse generator. (B) Bridging cable. (C) Pacing lead. (D) Enlarged view of pacing lead tip. (A reproduced with permission of Medtronic, Inc.)

subcutaneous tissue of the chest or the metal portion of a surface ECG electrode.

Because the unipolar pacing system has a wide sensing area as a result of the relatively long distance between the negative and positive electrodes, it has better sensing capabilities than a bipolar system. However, this feature makes the unipolar system more susceptible to sensing extraneous signals, such as the electrical artifacts created by normal muscle movements (ie, myopotentials) or by external electromagnetic interference (EMI), which may result in inappropriate inhibition of the pacing stimulus. This problem is of more concern in permanent pacing systems, in which the "can" of the pacemaker generator may be used as a part of the pacing circuit. Because the can is located near a large muscle mass, upper body movement can result in the inappropriate sensing of myopotentials.[7]

Pacing Routes

Several routes are available for temporary cardiac pacing (Box 15.2). Permanent pacing usually is accomplished transvenously, although when a thoracotomy is otherwise indicated, as in cardiac surgery, the physician may elect to insert permanent epicardial pacing wires.

Transcutaneous cardiac pacing involves the use of two large skin electrodes, one placed anteriorly and the other posteriorly on the chest, connected to an external pulse generator. It is a rapid, noninvasive procedure that nurses can perform in the emergency setting and is recommended in the advanced cardiac life support algorithm for the treatment of symptomatic bradycardia that does not respond to atropine.[8] Improved technology related to stimulus delivery and the development of large electrode pads that help disperse the energy have helped reduce the pain associated with cutaneous nerve and muscle stimulation. Discomfort may still be an issue for some patients, particularly when higher energy levels are required to achieve capture. This route is typically used as a short-term therapy until the situation resolves or another route of pacing can be established.

The insertion of temporary epicardial pacing wires has become a routine procedure during many cardiac surgical cases. Ventricular and, in many cases, atrial pacing wires are loosely sewn to the epicardium. The terminal pins of these wires are pulled through the skin before the chest is closed. If both chambers have pacing wires attached, the atrial wires exit subcostally to the right of the sternum, and the ventricular wires exit in the same region but to the left of the sternum. These wires can be removed several days after surgery by gentle traction at the skin surface with minimal risk of bleeding.[9]

Temporary transvenous endocardial pacing is accomplished by advancing a pacing electrode wire through a vein, often the subclavian or internal jugular vein, and into the right atrium or right ventricle. Insertion can be facilitated through direct visualization with fluoroscopy or by the use of a standard ECG. In some cases, the pacing wire is inserted through a special pulmonary artery catheter by means of a port that exits in the right atrium or right ventricle.

Five-Letter Pacemaker Codes

In the 1960s, pacemaker terminology was limited to *fixed-rate* and *demand* pacing; *AV sequential* pacing was introduced in the early 1970s. Although these terms are still useful for understanding pacemaker function (Box 15.3), the continued expansion of functional capabilities of pulse generators has made it necessary to develop a more precise classification system. In 1974, the Inter-Society Commission for Heart Disease adopted a three-letter code for describing the various pacing modalities available. The code has since undergone several revisions, including the addition of two more letters representing programming characteristics and multisite pacing functions, to accommodate the development of newer devices that are rate responsive or that pace from more than one site within the atria and the ventricles. The current five-letter code is described in Table 15.1.[10] The original three-letter code is adequate to describe temporary pacemaker function.

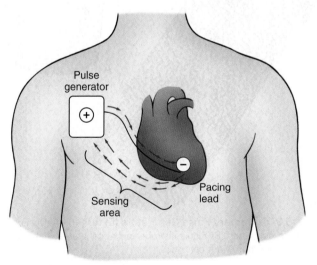

FIG. 15.2 Components of a Permanent Unipolar Transvenous Pacing System.

TABLE 15.1   NASPE/BPEG Generic Code

Position I: Chambers Paced	Position II: Chambers Sensed	Position III: Response to Sensing	Position IV: Rate Modulation	Position V: Multisite Pacing
0 = None	0 = None	0 = None	0 = None	0 = None
A = Atrium	A = Atrium	T = Triggered	R = Rate modulation	A = Atrium
V = Ventricle	V = Ventricle	I = Inhibited		V = Ventricle
D = Dual (A + V)	D = Dual (A + V)	D = Dual (T + I)		D = Dual (A + V)

BPEG, British Pacing and Electrophysiology Group; *NASPE,* North American Society of Pacing and Electrophysiology.
Modified from Bernstein AD, et al. The Revised NASPE/BPEG generic pacemaker code for antibradycardia, adaptive-rate and multisite pacing. *Pacing Clin Electrophysiol.* 2002;25:260.

TABLE 15.2   Examples of Temporary Pacing Modes

Pacing Mode	Description
Asynchronous	
A00	Atrial pacing, no sensing
V00	Ventricular pacing, no sensing
D00	Atrial and ventricular pacing, no sensing
Synchronous	
AAI	Atrial pacing, atrial sensing, inhibited response to sensed P waves
VVI	Ventricular pacing, ventricular sensing, inhibited response to sensed QRS complexes
DVI	Atrial and ventricular pacing, ventricular sensing; both atrial and ventricular pacing are inhibited if spontaneous ventricular depolarization is sensed
DDD	Both chambers are paced and sensed; inhibited response of pacing stimuli to sensed events in their respective chambers; triggered response to sensed atrial activity to allow for rate-responsive ventricular pacing

FIG. 15.3 Temporary Pulse Generators (External). (A) Dual-chamber pulse generator. (B) Single-chamber pulse generator. (Reproduced with permission of Medtronic, Inc.)

The original code is based on three categories, each represented by a letter. The first letter refers to the cardiac chamber that is paced. The second letter designates which chamber is sensed, and the third letter indicates the pacemaker's response to the sensed event. These three letters are used to describe the mode of pacing. For example, a VVI pacemaker paces the ventricle when the pacemaker fails to sense an intrinsic ventricular depolarization, but sensing of a spontaneous ventricular depolarization inhibits ventricular pacing. A VOO pacemaker paces the ventricle at a fixed rate and has no sensing capabilities. In DDD pacing, atrial and ventricular leads are used for pacing and sensing. In response to sensed activity, the pacemaker inhibits the pacing stimulus; a sensed P wave in the atrium inhibits the atrial spike, and a sensed R wave in the ventricle inhibits the ventricular pacing spike. A sensed P wave may also be used to trigger a ventricular pacing stimulus if normal conduction through the AV node is impaired. Table 15.2 lists temporary pacing modes.

Physiologic pacing has traditionally been used to describe modes in which the normal physiologic, or sequential, relationship between atrial and ventricular stimulation and contraction is maintained. AV synchrony increases the volume in the ventricle before contraction and helps to improve cardiac output. This may be achieved with atrial pacing in patients who have an intact conduction system or by dual-chamber pacing when atrial-to-ventricular conduction is impaired (ie, during heart block). More recently, physiologic pacing has evolved to include the maintenance of ventricular synchrony. Strategies to achieve this include minimizing the use of ventricular pacing and simultaneous pacing of both the right ventricle and the left ventricle.[11]

Pacemaker Settings

The controls on all external temporary pulse generators are similar. Their functions must be thoroughly understood so that pacing can be initiated quickly in an emergency situation and troubleshooting can be facilitated if problems with the pacemaker arise.

The *rate control* (Fig. 15.3) regulates the number of impulses that can be delivered to the heart per minute. The rate setting depends on the physiologic needs of the patient, but it usually is maintained between 60 and 80 beats/min. Pacing rates for overdrive suppression of tachydysrhythmias may greatly exceed

---

BOX 15.4 Determining Temporary Pacemaker Pacing Threshold

1. Adjust pacemaker rate setting so that patient is 100% paced. It may be necessary to increase the pacing rate to achieve this setting.
2. Gradually decrease the output (milliampere) setting until 1:1 capture is lost. The pacing threshold is the point at which capture is lost.
3. Slowly increase the output setting until 1:1 capture is reestablished. With a properly positioned pacing electrode, the pacing threshold should be less than 1 mA.
4. Set the output setting two to three times higher than measured threshold because thresholds tend to fluctuate over time.
5. If a dual-chamber pulse generator is being used, evaluate pacing thresholds for the atrial and ventricular leads separately.

BOX 15.5 Determining Temporary Pacemaker Sensitivity Threshold

1. Set sensitivity control to its most sensitive setting.
2. Adjust the pulse generator rate to 10 beats/min less than patient's intrinsic rate (flash indicator should flash regularly).
3. Reduce the generator output to the minimal value to eliminate the risk of competing with the intrinsic rhythm.
4. Gradually increase the sensitivity value until the sense indicator stops flashing and the pace indicator starts flashing.
5. Decrease sensitivity until the sense indicator begins to flash again; this is the sensitivity threshold.
6. Adjust the sensitivity setting on the generator to half of threshold value; restore the generator output and rate to their original values.

---

these values. Some generators have special controls for overdrive pacing that allow for rates of 800 stimuli per minute. If the pacemaker is operating in a dual-chamber mode, the ventricular rate control also regulates the atrial rate.

The *output dial* regulates the amount of electrical current, measured in milliamperes (mA), that is delivered to the heart to initiate depolarization. The point at which depolarization occurs, called *threshold*, is indicated by a myocardial response to the pacing stimulus (ie, capture). Threshold can be determined by gradually decreasing the output setting until 1:1 capture is lost. The output setting is then slowly increased until 1:1 capture is reestablished; this threshold to pace is less than 1 mA with a properly positioned pacing electrode. The output is set two to three times higher than threshold because thresholds tend to fluctuate over time. Box 15.4 details the procedure for measuring pacing thresholds. Separate output controls for atrium and ventricle are used with a dual-chamber pulse generator.

The *sensitivity control* regulates the ability of the pacemaker to detect the heart's intrinsic electrical activity. Sensitivity is measured in millivolts (mV) and determines the size of the intracardiac signal that the generator will recognize. If the sensitivity is adjusted to its most sensitive setting—a setting of 0.5 to 1 mV—the pacemaker can respond even to low-amplitude electrical signals coming from the heart. Turning the sensitivity to its least sensitive setting (ie, adjusting the dial to a setting of 20 mV or to the area labeled *async*) results in inability of the pacemaker to sense any intrinsic electrical activity and causes the pacemaker to function at a fixed rate. A sense indicator (often a light) on the pulse generator signals each time intrinsic cardiac electrical activity is sensed. A pulse generator may be designed to sense atrial activity or ventricular activity, or both. Box 15.5 describes the procedure for measuring sensitivity. The sensitivity is set at half of the value of the sensitivity threshold to ensure that all appropriate intrinsic cardiac signals are sensed. For example, if the measured sensitivity threshold is 3.0 mV, the generator is set at 1.5 mV. The sensing ability of the pacemaker can be quickly evaluated by observing for a change in pacing rhythm in response to spontaneous depolarizations.

The *AV interval control* (available only on dual-chamber generators) regulates the time interval between the atrial and ventricular pacing stimuli. This interval is analogous to the P–R interval that occurs in the intrinsic ECG. Proper adjustment of this interval to between 150 and 250 ms preserves AV synchrony and permits maximal ventricular stroke volume and enhanced cardiac output. Because the AV interval is limited by the length

of the cardiac cycle, new temporary generators automatically adjust the AV delay based on the programmed heart rate.[6]

Temporary dual-chamber pacemakers have other settings that are required in the DDD mode (see Fig. 15.3B). The *lower rate*, or *base rate*, determines the rate at which the generator will pace when intrinsic activity falls below the set rate of the pacemaker. The *upper rate* determines the fastest ventricular rate the pacemaker will deliver in response to sensed atrial activity. This setting is needed to protect the patient's heart from being paced in response to rapid atrial dysrhythmias. There also is an *atrial refractory period*, programmable from 150 to 500 ms, which regulates the length of time, after a sensed or paced ventricular event, during which the pacemaker cannot respond to another atrial stimulus. An emergency button is also available on most models to allow for rapid initiation of asynchronous (DOO) pacing during an emergency.

On all temporary pacemakers, an on/off switch is provided with a safety feature that prevents the accidental termination of pacing. On new generators, there is also a locking feature to prevent unintended changes to the prescribed settings.

Pacing Artifacts

All patients with temporary pacemakers require continuous ECG monitoring. The pacing artifact is the spike that is seen on the ECG tracing as the pacing stimulus is delivered to the heart. A *P wave* is visible after the pacing artifact if the atrium is being paced (Fig. 15.4A). Similarly, a *QRS complex* follows a ventricular pacing artifact (Fig. 15.4B). With dual-chamber pacing, a pacing artifact precedes both the P wave and the QRS complex (Fig. 15.4C).

Not all paced beats look alike. For example, the artifact (spike) produced by a unipolar pacing electrode is larger than the artifact produced by a bipolar lead (Fig. 15.5). The QRS complex of paced beats appears different, depending on the location of the pacing electrode. If the pacing electrode is positioned in the right ventricle, a left bundle branch block pattern is displayed on the ECG. A right bundle branch block pattern is visible if the pacing stimulus originates from the left ventricle.

Pacemaker Malfunctions

Most pacemaker malfunctions can be categorized as abnormalities of pacing or of sensing. Problems with pacing can involve failure of the pacemaker to deliver the pacing stimulus, a pacing stimulus that fails to depolarize the heart, or an incorrect number of pacing stimuli per minute.

FIG. 15.4 Pacing Examples. (A) Atrial pacing. (B) Ventricular pacing. (C) Dual-chamber pacing. Each *asterisk* represents a pacemaker impulse.

FIG. 15.5 Bipolar and Unipolar Pacing. (A) Bipolar pacing artifact. (B) Unipolar pacing artifact. (Modified from Conover MB. *Understanding Electrocardiography.* 8th ed. St. Louis: Mosby; 2003.)

Pacing Abnormalities

Failure of the pacemaker to deliver the pacing stimulus results in disappearance of the pacing artifact, even if the patient's intrinsic rate is less than the set rate on the pacer. This can occur intermittently or continuously and can be attributed to failure of the pulse generator or its battery, a loose connection between the various components of the pacemaker system, broken lead wires, or stimulus inhibition as a result of EMI. Tightening connections, replacing the batteries or the pulse generator itself, or removing the source of EMI may restore pacemaker function.

If the pacing stimulus fires but fails to initiate a myocardial depolarization, a pacing artifact will be present but will not be followed by the expected P wave or QRS complex, depending on the chamber being paced (Fig. 15.6). This *loss of capture* most often can be attributed to displacement of the pacing electrode or to an increase in threshold (electrical stimulus necessary to elicit a myocardial depolarization) as a result of medications, metabolic disorders, electrolyte imbalances, or fibrosis or myocardial ischemia at the site of electrode placement. In many cases, increasing the output (mA) elicits capture. For transvenous leads, repositioning the patient on his or her left side may improve lead contact and restore capture.

Pacing can occur at inappropriate rates. For example, impending battery failure in a permanent pacemaker can result in a gradual decrease in the paced rate, also referred to as *rate drift*. Inappropriate stimuli from a pacemaker may result in pacemaker-mediated tachycardia; this usually is caused by sensing of inappropriate signals in a dual-chamber pacemaker that is in a trigger mode, such as DDD. The tachycardia can be terminated by placing a magnet over the generator to transiently suspend sensing.[12]

Sensing Abnormalities

Sensing abnormalities include undersensing and oversensing.

Undersensing. Undersensing is the inability of the pacemaker to sense spontaneous myocardial depolarizations. Undersensing results in competition between paced complexes and the heart's intrinsic rhythm. This malfunction is manifested on the ECG by pacing artifacts that occur after or are unrelated to spontaneous complexes (Fig. 15.7). Undersensing can result in the delivery of pacing stimuli into a relative refractory period of the cardiac depolarization cycle (see Fig. 11.25 in Chapter 11). A ventricular pacing stimulus delivered into the downslope of the T wave (R-on-T phenomenon) is a real danger with this type of pacer aberration because it may precipitate a lethal dysrhythmia. The nurse must act quickly to determine the cause and initiate appropriate interventions. The cause often can be attributed to inadequate wave amplitude (height of the P or R wave). If this is the case, the situation can be promptly remedied by increasing the sensitivity by moving the sensitivity dial toward its lowest setting. Other possible causes include inappropriate (asynchronous) mode selection, lead displacement or fracture, loose cable connections, and pulse generator failure.

Oversensing. Oversensing occurs as a result of inappropriate sensing of extraneous electrical signals that leads to unnecessary

FIG. 15.6 Pacemaker Malfunction: Failure to Capture. Atrial pacing and capture occur after pacer spikes 1, 3, 5, and 7. The remaining pacer spikes fail to capture the tissue, resulting in loss of the P wave, no conduction to the ventricles, and no arterial waveform. Each *asterisk* represents a pacemaker impulse.

FIG. 15.7 Pacemaker Malfunction: Undersensing. After the first two paced beats, a series of intrinsic beats occurs; the pacemaker unit fails to sense these intrinsic QRS complexes. These spikes do not capture the ventricle because they occur during the refractory period of the cardiac cycle. Each *asterisk* represents a pacemaker impulse.

triggering or inhibition of stimulus output, depending on the pacer mode. The source of these electrical signals can range from tall peaked T waves to EMI in the critical care environment. Because most temporary pulse generators are programmed in demand modes, oversensing results in unexplained pauses in the ECG tracing as the extraneous signals are sensed and inhibit pacing. Moving the sensitivity dial toward 20 mV (less sensitive) often stops the pauses. With permanent pacemakers, a magnet may be placed over the generator to restore pacing in an asynchronous mode until appropriate changes in the generator settings can be programmed.

Medical Management

The physician determines the pacing route based on the patient's clinical situation. Transcutaneous pacing typically is used in emergent situations until a transvenous lead can be secured. If the patient is undergoing heart surgery, epicardial leads may be electively placed at the end of the operation. The physician places the transvenous or epicardial pacing lead or leads, repositioning them as needed to obtain adequate pacing and sensing thresholds. Decisions regarding lead placement may later limit the pacing modes available to the clinician. For example, to perform dual-chamber pacing, both atrial and ventricular leads must be placed. However, in an emergency, interventions are focused on establishing ventricular pacing, and atrial lead placement may not be feasible. After lead placement, the initial settings for output and sensitivity are determined, the pacing rate and mode are selected, and the patient's response to pacing is evaluated.

Nursing Management

Nursing responsibilities in the care of a patient with a temporary pacemaker are associated with several nursing diagnoses and can be combined into four primary areas: assessment and prevention of pacemaker malfunction, protection against microshock, surveillance for complications such as infection, and patient education.

Prevention of Pacemaker Malfunction

Continuous ECG monitoring is essential to facilitate prompt recognition of and appropriate intervention for pacemaker malfunction. Proper care of the pacing system can prevent pacing abnormalities.

The temporary pacing lead and bridging cable must be properly secured to the body with tape to prevent accidental displacement of the electrode, which can result in failure to pace or sense. The external pulse generator can be secured to the patient's waist with a strap or placed in a telemetry bag for a mobile patient. If the patient is on a regimen of bed rest, the pulse generator can be suspended with twill tape from an intravenous pole mounted overhead on the ceiling. This positioning prevents tension on the lead while the patient is moved (given adequate length of bridging cable) and alleviates the possibility of accidental dropping of the pulse generator.

The nurse inspects for loose connections between the leads and pulse generator on a regular basis. Replacement batteries and pulse generators must always be available on the unit. Although the battery has an anticipated life span of 1 month, it probably is sound practice to change the battery if the pacemaker has been operating continually for several days. Newer generators provide a low-battery signal 24 hours before complete loss of battery function occurs to prevent inadvertent interruptions in pacing. The pulse generator must always be labeled with the date on which the battery was replaced.

It is important to be aware of all sources of EMI within the critical care environment that may interfere with the pacemaker's function. Sources of EMI in the clinical area include electrocautery, defibrillation current, radiation therapy, magnetic resonance imaging (MRI) scanners, and transcutaneous electrical nerve stimulation units.[13] In most cases, if EMI is suspected of precipitating pacemaker malfunction, conversion to the asynchronous mode (fixed rate) can maintain pacing until the cause of the EMI is removed.

Microshock Protection

Because the pacing electrode provides a direct, low-resistance path to the heart, the nurse takes special care while handling the external components of the pacing system to avoid conducting stray electrical current from other equipment. Even a small amount of stray current transmitted through the pacing lead could precipitate a lethal dysrhythmia. The possibility of microshock can be minimized by wearing gloves when handling the pacing wires and by proper insulation of terminal pins of pacing wires when they are not in use (Box 15.6). The latter precaution can be accomplished by the use of caps provided by the manufacturer or by improvising with a plastic syringe or section of disposable rubber glove. The wires are taped securely to the patient's chest to prevent accidental electrode displacement.

Infection Risk

Infection at the lead insertion site is a rare but serious complication associated with temporary pacemakers. The site is carefully inspected for purulent drainage, erythema, and edema, and the patient is observed for signs of systemic infection. Site care is performed according to the institution's policies and procedures. Although most infections remain localized, endocarditis can occur in patients with endocardial pacing leads. A less common complication associated with transvenous pacing is myocardial perforation, which can result in rhythmic hiccoughs or cardiac tamponade.

Patient Education

Patient teaching for a patient with a temporary pacemaker emphasizes the prevention of complications (Box 15.7). The patient is instructed not to handle any exposed portion of the lead wire and to notify the nurse if the dressing over the insertion site becomes soiled, wet, or dislodged. The patient also is advised not to use any electrical devices brought in from home that could interfere with pacemaker functioning. Patients with temporary transvenous pacemakers need to be taught to restrict movement of the affected extremity to prevent lead displacement.

QSEN BOX 15.6   QSEN: Patient Safety Alert

Prevention of Microshock

- Wear gloves when handling pacing wires
- Secure all connections between pulse generator, pacing cable, and leads
- Insulate lead tips with nonconducting materials when not attached to generator (manufacturer's cap, finger cot, plastic syringe)
- Keep dressings and pacing equipment dry
- Ensure all electrical equipment is properly grounded
- Use battery-operated shavers

Permanent Pacemakers

Almost 400,000 permanent pacemakers are implanted annually in the United States, and critical care nurses are likely to encounter these devices in their clinical practice.[14] Implanted pacemakers were originally designed to provide an adequate ventricular rate in patients with symptomatic bradycardia. Today, the goal of pacemaker therapy is to simulate, as much as possible, normal physiologic cardiac depolarization and conduction. Sophisticated generators permit rate-responsive pacing, effecting responses to sensed atrial activity (DDD) or to various physiologic sensors (body motion or minute ventilation). For patients who do not have a functional sinus node that can increase their heart rate, rate-responsive pacemakers may improve exercise capacity and quality of life.[15] Table 15.3 describes the types of rate-responsive pacing generators in clinical use. The concept of physiologic pacing continues to evolve because studies have indicated that pacing initiated from the right ventricular (RV) apex—even in a dual-chamber mode—may promote heart failure in patients with permanent pacemakers.[16] Further research has been conducted to identify alternative sites for pacing and modes that can maximize intrinsic AV conduction and minimize ventricular pacing.[17]

A patient who undergoes implantation of a permanent pacemaker is usually in the hospital for less than 24 hours. Longer lengths of stay are expected for patients with serious comorbidities such as MI or cardiogenic shock. Technologic advances in the computer industry have had a major impact on permanent pacemakers. Microprocessors have allowed for the development of increasingly smaller generators despite the incorporation of more complex features. Today's generators are smaller, more energy efficient, and more reliable than previous models. A modern pacemaker is shown in Fig. 15.8. A more recent enhancement has been the release of a pacemaker that is compatible with MRI.[18] Studies are underway to evaluate a leadless pacing system that consists of a self-contained unit placed in the RV via the femoral vein.[19,20] A rapidly expanding role for permanent pacemakers has been the use of these devices as a type of nonpharmacologic therapy for treatment of conditions such as heart failure and AF.

Cardiac Resynchronization Therapy

Approximately one-third of patients with severe heart failure have ventricular conduction delays (prolonged QRS duration or bundle branch block). These conduction delays have been shown to create a lack of synchrony between the contractions of the left ventricle and right ventricle. The hemodynamic consequences of this dyssynchrony include impaired ventricular filling with decreased ejection fraction, cardiac output, and mean arterial pressure.[21] Cardiac resynchronization therapy (CRT) uses atrial pacing plus stimulation of both the left ventricle and the right ventricle (biventricular pacing) in an attempt to optimize atrial and ventricular mechanical activity. The CRT device uses three pacing leads, one each in the right atrium and the right ventricle and a specially designed transvenous lead that is inserted through the coronary sinus to pace the left ventricle. Because many patients with heart failure are also at risk for sudden cardiac death, biventricular pacing is available on many implantable cardioverter defibrillators (ICDs). Numerous clinical trials have shown that CRT improves symptoms, functional status, and mortality in patients with moderate to advanced heart failure and helps prevent progression of heart failure in patients with fewer symptoms.[22] The greatest benefit appears to be in patients with a confirmed left bundle branch block and a QRS duration greater than 150 ms.[23]

Atrial Fibrillation Suppression

The incidence of AF is increasing, and it is a common comorbidity in patients requiring a pacemaker. Atrial pacing has been proposed as a possible preventive therapy for this dysrhythmia

---

BOX 15.7 PATIENT EDUCATION PLAN

Temporary Pacemaker

The patient should be able to teach back the following topics:
- Description of pacemaker therapy
- Care of pacemaker system
  Minimize handling of leads or cables
  Notify nurse if dressing becomes wet or loose
- Activity restrictions (minimize upper extremity movement with transvenous leads)
- Electrical safety precautions (no electric razors)
- Symptoms to report (dizziness)

TABLE 15.3 Permanent Pacemaker Rate-Response Pacing Modes

Pulse Generator	Description
AAIR	AAI features plus rate-responsive pacing; used for patients with symptomatic bradycardia who have a paceable atrium and intact atrioventricular conduction
VVIR	VVI features plus rate-responsive pacing; used for patients with atrium that is unpaceable as a result of chronic atrial fibrillation or other atrial dysrhythmia
DDDR	DDD features plus rate-responsive pacing; used for patients with symptomatic bradycardia in which the atrium is paceable but atrioventricular conduction is, or may become, unreliable

FIG. 15.8 Permanent Pacemaker (Medtronic Revo MRI SureScan). (Reproduced with permission of Medtronic, Inc.)

in selected patients. Atrial pacing in patients with bradycardia has been shown to reduce the recurrence of AF, especially compared with ventricular pacing. Programming that promotes intrinsic conduction, such as a longer AV delay, and implanting pacemakers that have specific algorithms to minimize ventricular pacing have been most effective.[11] Another promising therapy is the use of pacemakers that can quickly deliver antitachycardia pacing to terminate AF in response to a sensed change in the rate or regularity of the atrial rhythm.[24]

Medical Management

Permanent pacemakers may be implanted with the patient under local anesthesia in the cardiac catheterization laboratory. Transvenous leads usually are inserted through the cephalic or subclavian vein and positioned in the right atrium or right ventricle, or both, with fluoroscopic guidance. Satisfactory lead placement is determined by testing the stimulation and sensitivity thresholds with a pacing system analyzer. The leads are then attached to the generator, which is inserted into a surgically created pocket in the subcutaneous tissue below the clavicle. Ongoing assessment of pacemaker function after discharge can now be performed remotely, using wireless technology via the Internet or a cellular network. Remote monitoring reduces the number of clinic visits and provides early detection of patient or device problems.[25]

Nursing Management

Nursing management for patients after permanent pacemaker implantation includes monitoring for complications related to insertion and for pacemaker malfunction. Postoperative complications are rare but include cardiac perforation and tamponade, pneumothorax, hematoma, lead displacement, and infection.[26]

The process for identification of permanent pacemaker malfunction is the same as the process described previously for temporary pacemakers. To evaluate pacemaker function, the nurse must know at least the pacemaker's programmed mode of pacing and the lower rate setting. With permanent pacemakers, settings are adjusted noninvasively through a specialized programmer that uses pulsed magnetic fields or an RF signal. If a pacemaker problem is suspected, ECG strips are obtained, and the physician is notified so that the pacemaker settings can be reprogrammed as needed. If the patient experiences symptoms of decreased cardiac output, he or she may require support with temporary transcutaneous pacing until the problem is corrected.

The foregoing discussion provides an introduction to the basic concepts of pacemaker therapy. However, nurses who care for patients with permanent or temporary pacemakers must be familiar with ever more sophisticated modes of pacemaker function. Only by keeping pace with current technology can the nurse accurately interpret pacer function and safely and effectively care for patients with pacemakers.

IMPLANTABLE CARDIOVERTER DEFIBRILLATORS

An ICD is an electronic device that is used in the treatment of tachydysrhythmias. ICDs are capable of identifying and terminating life-threatening ventricular dysrhythmias. Initially, an ICD was recommended only for patients who had survived an episode of cardiac arrest caused by ventricular fibrillation (VF) or ventricular tachycardia (VT) or in whom lethal arrhythmias could be induced during EPS. This secondary prevention was supported by randomized clinical trials that found improved survival with an ICD compared with treatment with antidysrhythmic medications.[1] The use of ICDs has since expanded to primary prevention of sudden cardiac death in high-risk patients, identified by heart failure classification (New York Heart Association class III or class IV) and a low left ventricular ejection fraction (less than 30% to 35%). At the present time, more than 80% of ICDs are implanted for primary prevention, resulting in almost 100,000 implants per year in the United States.[14,27]

Implantable Cardioverter Defibrillator System

The ICD system consists of leads and a generator and is similar to a pacemaker but with some key differences. The leads contain not only electrodes for sensing and pacing but also integrated defibrillator coils capable of delivering a shock. The generator is larger, to accommodate a more powerful battery and a high-voltage capacitor, along with the microprocessor. It is surgically placed in the subcutaneous tissue of the pectoral region in the upper chest (Fig. 15.9). The early model generators could defibrillate or cardiovert only lethal dysrhythmias. The current generation of devices delivers a tiered therapy, with options for programmable antitachycardia pacing, bradycardia backup pacing, low-energy cardioversion, and high-energy defibrillation. With tiered therapy, antitachycardia pacing is used as the first line of treatment in some cases of VT. If the VT can be pace-terminated successfully, the patient will not receive a shock from the generator and may not even realize that the ICD terminated the dysrhythmia. If programmed bursts of pacing do not terminate the VT, the ICD will cardiovert the rhythm. If the dysrhythmia deteriorates into VF, the ICD is programmed to defibrillate at a higher energy. If the dysrhythmia terminates spontaneously, the device will not discharge. Occasionally, the electrical rhythm may deteriorate to asystole or a slow idioventricular rhythm; in such cases, the bradycardia backup pacing function is activated.

Product development for ICDs has resulted in dual-chamber devices with leads in both atria and ventricles. The introduction of atrial leads allows for dual-chamber pacing to optimize hemodynamic performance and atrial sensing to discriminate more accurately between atrial tachycardia and VT to decrease the incidence of inappropriate shocks. ICDs may also incorporate triple-lead systems (leads in one atrium and both ventricles) to allow for CRT and defibrillation in one device. Other developments in ICD technology include improved diagnostic and telemetry functions, such as the ability to provide real-time electrograms obtained from the ICD electrodes or the ability to perform remote device interrogation using cellular or wireless technology.[28]

Insertion of Implantable Cardioverter Defibrillator

The ICD has progressed in both programmable functions and insertion technique. Initially, all ICDs were implanted surgically during open-heart surgery or via thoracotomy, with electrode patches attached directly to the heart. The current smaller generators, combined with the use of transvenous leads, obviate the need for major surgery. Transvenous electrode leads are inserted into the subclavian vein and advanced into the right side of the heart, where contact with the endocardium is achieved. To improve defibrillation efficacy, an additional subcutaneous patch may be placed with some models.

A

B

1 PACING

In most cases of ventricular tachycardia, the ICD can restore normal heart rhythm with painless pacing therapy.

2 CARDIOVERSION

If dysrhythmia continues, the ICD automatically delivers low-energy synchronized shocks. Mild discomfort.

3 HIGH-ENERGY DEFIBRILLATION

High-energy shock therapy for ventricular fibrillation, designed to stop the heart and instantly reset the rhythm. This feels like a sudden "kick in the chest."

C

FIG. 15.9 Placement of Implantable Cardioverter Defibrillator (ICD) With a Transvenous Lead System. (A) The generator is placed in a subcutaneous "pocket" in the pectoral region. The pacing, cardioversion, and defibrillation functions all are contained in a lead (or leads) inserted into the right atrium and ventricle. (B) Example of a dual-chamber ICD (Medtronic Gem II DR) with tiered therapy and pacing capabilities. (C) Tiered therapy is designed to use increasing levels of intensity to terminate ventricular dysrhythmias. (B reproduced with permission of Medtronic, Inc.)

The endocardial leads are connected to the generator by tunneling through the subcutaneous tissue, and thoracotomy is avoided. Procedural complications are infrequent but may include hematoma, pneumothorax, cardiac tamponade, or lead dislodgment.[29] A subcutaneous ICD has been introduced more recently that consists of a generator implanted in the left axillary area and a single subcutaneous lead for detection of ventricular dysrhythmias and delivery of therapy.[30] Although this device is unable to provide pacing therapies, it may provide an alternative for patients who lack vascular access and avoid complications related to transvenous lead placement.

Medical Management

Medical management in a patient with an ICD begins before implantation with a thorough evaluation of the patient's risk for dysrhythmia and underlying cardiac function. Numerous noninvasive studies are available to help identify patients at risk for sudden cardiac death, including ambulatory monitoring, autonomic reflex testing, and heart rate variability studies. Some patients may undergo EPS to determine the origin of the dysrhythmia and the effect of antidysrhythmic agents in suppressing or altering the rate of the dysrhythmia. Further assessment of cardiac status is made to determine whether additional interventions (eg, revascularization, CRT) are indicated to improve cardiac function. This part of the work-up may include cardiac catheterization, stress testing, and echocardiography. Based on the evaluation, decisions are made regarding the implantation approach (eg, thoracotomy at the time of surgery, nonthoracotomy) and the type of therapy required (eg, antitachycardia pacing, cardioversion, defibrillation).

An electrophysiologist performs the initial programming of the device at the time of implantation. Defibrillation efficacy of the ICD is generally assessed by inducing the dysrhythmia and then evaluating the ability of the device to terminate it. Modern ICDs are more reliable and offer higher energy levels than in the past, so some providers now omit testing and just program a high-output (30 J or more) setting for defibrillation. Bypassing defibrillation testing avoids the risks involved in inducing a lethal rhythm, especially in older patients with multiple comorbidities.[31] This practice is likely to increase, as a more recent clinical trial found no improvement in shock efficacy or clinical outcomes in patients who underwent defibrillation testing at the time of implant.[32] Other adjustments in programming may be performed to decrease unnecessary shocks including aggressive use of antitachycardia pacing and withholding shocks for SVT or nonsustained ventricular rhythms. These strategies are important because studies indicate that 17% of shocks may be inappropriate, resulting in unnecessary pain, reduced quality of life, and potential myocardial damage.[33] After it has been determined that the ICD functions appropriately, further follow-up can be conducted on an outpatient basis, with remote monitoring options to monitor the number of discharges and the battery life of the device.[28]

Nursing Management

If the ICD system was implanted during open-heart surgery, postoperative nursing management is similar to that for any patient undergoing cardiac surgery. If an endocardial lead system is implanted, nursing management is less intense, and the hospital stay is shorter. The nursing management of a patient with an ICD includes assessing for dysrhythmias and monitoring for complications related to insertion. In the case of a ventricular dysrhythmia, it is important to know the type of ICD implanted, how the device functions, and whether it is activated (ie, "on"). If the patient experiences a shockable rhythm, the nurse should be prepared to defibrillate in the event that the device fails. During external defibrillation, the paddles or patches should not be placed directly over the ICD generator, as long as this can be accomplished without delay of defibrillation.[34] For recurring shocks, patients should be assessed for underlying causes such as electrolyte imbalance, ischemia, or worsening heart failure.[12] Most patients continue to take some antidysrhythmic medications to decrease the number of shocks required and to slow the rate of the tachycardia. Complications associated with a permanent ICD include infection from the implanted system, broken leads, and sensing of supraventricular tachydysrhythmias resulting in unneeded discharges.

Patient Education

To facilitate a positive psychologic adjustment to the ICD, education of the patient and family about the device is vital (Box 15.8). Preoperative teaching for a patient with an ICD includes information about how the device works and what to expect during the implantation procedure. After implantation, education is focused on aspects of living with an ICD. Patients need information pertaining to device follow-up, technology used for remote monitoring, and instructions about what to do if they experience a shock. Many institutions have successfully used family support groups for this patient population. Finally, because the ICD is an adjunctive treatment rather than a cure for heart failure, patients need to understand the importance of continued risk factor modification and prescribed medications.

FIBRINOLYTIC THERAPY

Fibrinolytic therapy is an important clinical intervention for patients experiencing acute ST segment elevation MI. Before the introduction of fibrinolytic agents, medical management of acute MI was focused on decreasing myocardial oxygen

---

✴ BOX 15.8 PATIENT EDUCATION PLAN

Implantable Cardioverter Defibrillator

Before discharge, the patient should be able to teach back the following topics:

- Pathophysiology of the underlying disease process including sudden cardiac death, ventricular dysrhythmias, and heart disease
- Information regarding how the implantable cardioverter defibrillator is programmed to function
- Actions to take if a shock occurs
- Importance of continuing antidysrhythmic and heart failure medications
- Activity limitations related to driving and avoiding strong magnetic fields
- Signs and symptoms of device failure
- Follow-up schedule for remote monitoring and office visits
- Cardiopulmonary resuscitation training for family members

---

demands to minimize myocardial necrosis and preserve ventricular function. Today, efforts to limit the size of the infarction are directed toward timely reperfusion of the jeopardized myocardium through restoration of blood flow in the culprit vessel (the open artery theory). Two options are available for opening the artery—fibrinolytics and mechanical intervention. Although mechanical catheter-based intervention has been proven to yield better outcomes when performed in a timely fashion, only 40% of US hospitals are estimated to have this capability.[35] For this reason, fibrinolytic therapy continues to play a role in the treatment of acute MI.

The use of fibrinolytic therapy is predicated on the theory that the significant event in an acute coronary syndrome (eg, unstable angina, acute MI) is the rupture of an atherosclerotic plaque with thrombus formation (Fig. 15.10). The thrombus, which is composed of aggregated platelets bound together with fibrin strands, occludes the coronary artery, depriving the myocardium of oxygen previously supplied by that artery. The administration of a fibrinolytic agent results in lysis of the acute thrombus, resulting in recanalization, or opening, of the obstructed coronary artery and restoration of blood flow to the affected tissue. In addition to restoring perfusion, adjunctive measures (anticoagulants and antiplatelet therapy) are taken to prevent further clot formation and repeat occlusion.

ELIGIBILITY CRITERIA

Certain criteria have been developed, based on research findings, to determine the patient population that would most likely benefit from the administration of fibrinolytic therapy. Patients with recent onset of chest pain (less than 12 hours' duration) and persistent ST segment elevation (greater than 0.1 mV in two or more contiguous leads) are considered candidates for fibrinolytic therapy.[36] Patients who present with bundle branch blocks that may obscure ST segment analysis and a history suggesting acute MI are also considered candidates for therapy (see "Myocardial Infarction" in Chapter 14, specifically Figure 14.3). The goal of therapy is to administer fibrinolytic therapy within 30 minutes after presentation ("door to needle") because early reperfusion yields the greatest benefit.[37]

Exclusion criteria are usually based on the increased risk of bleeding incurred from the use of fibrinolytics. Patients who have stable clots that might be disrupted by fibrinolytic therapy (recent surgery, facial or head trauma,) usually are not considered

FIG. 15.10 Thrombus formation and site of action of medications used in the treatment of acute myocardial infarction. (A) Site of action of antiplatelet agents such as aspirin, thienopyridines, and glycoprotein IIb/IIIa inhibitors. (B) Heparin bonds with antithrombin III and thrombin to create an inactive complex. (C) Fibrinolytic agents convert plasminogen to plasmin, an enzyme responsible for degradation of fibrin clots.

BOX 15.9 **Fibrinolytic Therapy Selection Criteria**

- No more than 12 h from onset of chest pain and preferably within 30 min of diagnosis of ST segment elevation myocardial infarction
- ST segment elevation on electrocardiogram or new-onset left bundle branch block
- Ischemic chest pain unresponsive to sublingual nitroglycerin
- No conditions that might cause a predisposition to hemorrhage

---

candidates for fibrinolytic therapy. Other common criteria for the use of fibrinolytic therapy are presented in Box 15.9.

At the present time, fibrinolytic therapy is not indicated for patients with unstable angina or non–ST segment elevation acute coronary syndrome.[38] It is believed that these conditions result from plaque rupture with the formation of only a partially occlusive thrombus. Fibrinolysis breaks up the clot and releases thrombin, and this can paradoxically increase the material necessary for further thrombosis.[36] Instead, these patients are treated with antiplatelet agents (eg, aspirin, clopidogrel, glycoprotein [GP] IIb/IIIa inhibitors) and antithrombin medications (eg, heparin).

Fibrinolytic Agents

Four fibrinolytic agents are currently available for intravenous treatment of acute ST segment elevation MI. All these agents stimulate lysis of the clot by converting inactive plasminogen to plasmin, an enzyme responsible for degradation of fibrin (see Fig. 15.10). The first-generation fibrinolytic agents (eg, streptokinase, urokinase) had their primary effect on circulating plasminogen. Newer fibrinolytic agents (eg, alteplase, reteplase, tenecteplase) have a greater effect on clot plasminogen than on circulating plasminogen and are considered clot selective. Currently approved fibrinolytic agents are compared in Table 15.4. Because patients with an area of plaque disruption are still at risk for clot formation and reocclusion, fibrinolytic therapy is used in conjunction with anticoagulants and antiplatelet agents. Current guidelines recommend that anticoagulant therapy be administered for a minimum of 48 hours after reperfusion. Unfractionated heparin traditionally has been used, but low-molecular-weight heparin and fondaparinux are also acceptable options and are preferred when anticoagulation is planned for more than 48 hours after fibrinolytic therapy.[39] Antiplatelet therapy with clopidogrel is recommended for 14 days, and aspirin should be continued indefinitely.[37]

TABLE 15.4 Pharmacologic Management
Fibrinolytic Agents for Use in Acute Myocardial Infarction

Medication	Dosage	Actions	Special Considerations
Clot-Specific			
tPA (alteplase)	IV: 100 mg over 90 min with first 15 mg given as a bolus over 2 min (dose is adjusted based on weight for patients ≤67 kg)	Binds to fibrin at clot and promotes activation of plasminogen to plasmin	Anticoagulants are given concurrently. Aspirin and clopidogrel are begun with administration and continued daily.
rPA (reteplase)	IV: 10 units given as a bolus over 2 min, repeated in 30 min	Binds to fibrin at clot and promotes activation of plasminogen to plasmin	Anticoagulants are given concurrently. Aspirin and clopidogrel are begun with administration and continued daily.
Tenecteplase (TNKase)	IV: 30–50 mg based on body weight, given as a single bolus	Binds to fibrin at clot and promotes activation of plasminogen to plasmin	Anticoagulants are given concurrently. Aspirin and clopidogrel are begun with administration and continued daily.
Non–Clot-Specific			
Streptokinase (SK)	IV: 1.5 million units given over 60 min	Catalyzes conversion of plasminogen to plasmin, which causes lysis of fibrin; has systemic lytic effects	May cause allergic reactions and hypotension. Anticoagulants are given concurrently. Aspirin and clopidogrel are begun with administration and continued daily.

IV, intravenous; *rPA*, recombinant plasminogen activator; *tPA*, tissue plasminogen activator.

Streptokinase

Streptokinase is a fibrinolytic agent derived from beta-hemolytic streptococci, which, when combined with plasminogen, catalyzes the conversion of plasminogen to plasmin, the enzyme responsible for clot dissolution in the body. Because streptokinase is a bacterial protein, it can produce various allergic reactions, including anaphylaxis. In addition, the fibrinolytic action of streptokinase is systemic (non–clot specific) and prolonged (half-life of 20 to 25 minutes), increasing the risk for bleeding complications. Because of these issues, streptokinase is no longer widely used in the United States.

Tissue Plasminogen Activator

Tissue plasminogen activator (tPA), or alteplase (Activase), is a naturally occurring enzyme (ie, nonantigenic) that is clot specific and has a very short half-life (3 to 4 minutes). It converts plasminogen to plasmin after binding to the fibrin-containing clot. This clot-specific action results in an increased concentration and activity of plasmin at the site of the clot, where it is needed. Several different intravenous dosing regimens have been proposed and tested in the clinical setting, but accelerated-dose tPA is considered the most effective means of establishing early patency of the occluded vessel.[40]

Recombinant Plasminogen Activator

Recombinant plasminogen activator, or reteplase, is a variant of the natural human enzyme tPA. Reteplase is less fibrin selective and has a longer half-life than tPA, making it suitable for bolus administration rather than as a continuous infusion. This new-generation plasminogen activator is given as a double bolus and then followed with adjunctive therapies. In contrast to tPA, reteplase does not require weight-based dosing. Studies have shown that reteplase is as effective as tPA in the treatment of acute MI and is easier to administer.[41]

Tenecteplase

Tenecteplase (TNKase) is the newest of the fibrinolytic agents. It is a genetically engineered variant of alteplase with slower plasma clearance and better fibrin specificity. Studies have shown that tenecteplase is as effective as alteplase, and the two agents have similar rates of bleeding complications.[41] Tenecteplase requires only a single bolus injection, which may help facilitate more rapid treatment both inside and outside the hospital. Although the need for weight-based dosing is a potential disadvantage of this medication, tenecteplase is the most widely used fibrinolytic agent in the United States at the present time.[42]

Outcomes of Fibrinolytic Therapy

The benefit of fibrinolytic therapy correlates with the degree of restoration of normal blood flow in the infarct-related artery. Coronary artery patency is defined by angiographic perfusion grades developed by the Thrombolysis in Myocardial Infarction (TIMI) study group in 1985 (Box 15.10).[43] Achievement of TIMI grade 3 flow is associated with the best long-term survival. Studies also indicate that rapid restoration of normal blood flow, within 90 minutes after treatment, results in improved left ventricular (LV) function and reduced mortality. The three fibrin-specific fibrinolytics have been shown to achieve TIMI 3 flow in 50% to 60% of patients at 90 minutes.[41] Fibrinolytic therapy continues to evolve, and medication dose ranges and regimens are subject to change when research findings are updated.

Fibrinolytic agents target the fibrin portion of the clot; other treatment strategies focus on the platelet portion of the clot (see Fig. 15.10). Oral antiplatelet agents (aspirin and clopidogrel)

BOX 15.10 **Flow in Infarct-Related Artery as Described in Thrombolysis in Myocardial Infarction Trial**

Perfusion Grades	Flow in the Infarct-Related Artery
TIMI 3	Normal or brisk flow through coronary artery
TIMI 2	Partial flow, slower than in normal vessels
TIMI 1	Sluggish flow with incomplete distal filling
TIMI 0	No flow beyond point of occlusion

TIMI, Thrombolysis in Myocardial Infarction Trial.
Modified from The TIMI Study Group. The thrombolysis in myocardial infarction (TIMI) trial: phase I findings. *N Engl J Med.* 1985;312:932.

BOX 15.11 **Noninvasive Evidence of Reperfusion**

- Cessation of chest pain
- Reperfusion dysrhythmias, primarily ventricular
- Return of elevated ST segments to baseline
- Early and marked peaking of creatine kinase and troponins

---

are administered in conjunction with fibrinolytics. The effectiveness of combining intravenous antiplatelet agents (GPIIb/IIIa receptor antagonists) with a lower dose of a fibrinolytic has been evaluated in clinical trials. Combination therapy provided reperfusion rates equivalent to rates obtained with a fibrinolytic alone but was associated with an increased risk of bleeding.[44]

Evidence of Reperfusion

Several phenomena may be observed after reperfusion of an artery that has been completely occluded by a thrombus (Box 15.11). Although recognition of these noninvasive markers of recanalization is important for assessing the patient's response to fibrinolytic therapy, they are less reliable than angiography in determining whether reperfusion has been successful.

Pain and Reperfusion Dysrhythmias

One possible sign of reperfusion is the abrupt cessation of chest pain as blood flow is restored to the ischemic myocardium. Another potential indicator of reperfusion is the appearance of various "reperfusion dysrhythmias." A variety of dysrhythmias can occur—premature ventricular contractions, bradycardias, heart block, VT—but accelerated idioventricular rhythms have shown the best correlation with reperfusion.[45] Reperfusion dysrhythmias are usually self-limiting or nonsustained, and aggressive antidysrhythmic therapy is not required. However, vigilant monitoring of the patient's ECG is essential because dysrhythmias associated with ongoing ischemia could deteriorate rapidly and may necessitate emergency treatment.

ST Segment

Another noninvasive marker of recanalization is rapid return to baseline of the elevated ST segments, which indicates restoration of blood flow to previously ischemic myocardial tissue. A monitoring lead should be chosen that clearly demonstrates ST segment elevation before initiation of therapy (see "Continuous ST Segment Monitoring" in Chapter 13).[46] The inability to achieve 50% resolution of the ST segment elevation within 60 to 90 minutes of administering the medication is generally considered an indication of failure of fibrinolytic therapy.[37]

Cardiac Biomarkers

Serial measurement of serum biomarkers may serve as further evidence of successful reperfusion after fibrinolytic therapy. Cardiac-specific creatine kinase and troponin increase rapidly and then decrease markedly after reperfusion of the ischemic myocardium. This phenomenon is called *washout* because it is thought to result from the rapid readmission of substances released by damaged myocardial cells into the circulation after restoration of blood flow (see "Cardiac Biomarker Studies" in Chapter 13, and Fig. 14.13 in Chapter 14.).

Residual Coronary Artery Stenosis

Fibrinolytic therapy has been determined to be a successful strategy for reopening occluded coronary arteries in the setting of acute MI. It limits infarct size, salvaging myocardium and significantly reducing morbidity and mortality associated with cardiogenic shock and VF. However, residual coronary artery stenosis resulting from the atherosclerotic process remains, even after successful fibrinolysis. Subsequent prevention of reocclusion is critical to preserving myocardial function and preventing the risk of late complications. Therefore, fibrinolytic therapy is recognized as an emergency procedure to restore patency until more definitive therapy can be initiated to effectively reduce the degree of stenosis. Current guidelines recommend that patients who receive fibrinolytic therapy be transferred to a facility capable of performing interventional catheter-based procedures and undergo routine angiography within the first 3 to 6 hours to allow for additional intervention as warranted.[47]

Nursing Management

Nursing management of patients undergoing fibrinolytic therapy begins with identifying potential candidates. In many institutions, checklists are used to facilitate the rapid identification of patients who are candidates for fibrinolytics. The nurse prepares the patient for fibrinolytic therapy by starting intravenous lines and obtaining baseline laboratory values and vital signs. Throughout the administration of the fibrinolytic agent, assessment of the patient continues for clinical indicators of reperfusion and complications related to therapy.

The most common complication related to thrombolysis is bleeding, which is due to the fibrinolytic therapy itself and anticoagulation therapy that patients routinely receive to minimize the possibility of rethrombosis. The nurse must continually monitor for clinical manifestations of bleeding (Box 15.12). Mild gingival bleeding and oozing around venipuncture sites is common and not a cause of concern. Should serious bleeding occur, such as intracranial or internal bleeding, all fibrinolytic and antithrombotic therapies are discontinued, and volume expanders or coagulation factors, or both, are administered.

In addition to accurate assessment of the patient for evidence of bleeding, nursing management includes preventive measures to minimize the potential for bleeding. For example, handling of the patient is limited, injections are avoided if possible, and additional pressure is provided to ensure hemostasis at venipuncture and arterial puncture sites. Intravenous lines

BOX 15.12 Signs of Inadequate Hemostasis Related to Fibrinolytic Therapy

- Bleeding or hematoma at puncture sites
- Hematuria, hematemesis, hemoptysis, melena, epistaxis
- Bruising or petechiae (pinpoint hemorrhages)
- Flank ecchymoses with complaints of low back pain (suggestive of retroperitoneal bleeding)
- Gingival bleeding
- Change in neurologic status (intracranial bleeding)
- Deterioration in vital signs, decreased hematocrit values (internal bleeding)

✴ BOX 15.13 PATIENT EDUCATION PLAN

Fibrinolytic Therapy

Before discharge, the patient should be able to teach back the following topics:
- Pathophysiology of atherosclerosis
- Risk factor management
- Description of fibrinolytic agent and how it works
- Measures to minimize bleeding and bruising associated with fibrinolytic therapy
- Recognition and actions to take for recurrent ischemic symptoms
- Information regarding prescribed medications (antiplatelet agents, anticoagulants)

are placed before lytic therapy is administered, and a heparin lock may be used for obtaining laboratory specimens during treatment.

Patient Education

Education for the patient receiving fibrinolytic therapy includes information regarding the actions of fibrinolytic agents, with emphasis on precautions to minimize bleeding (Box 15.13). For example, the patient is cautioned against vigorous toothbrushing and told to refrain from using straight-edge razors. Information is provided regarding ongoing risk factor management in the prevention of atherosclerotic coronary artery disease (CAD).

CATHETER-BASED INTERVENTIONS FOR CORONARY ARTERY DISEASE

During the past 3 decades, the use of catheter-based procedures to open coronary arteries blocked or narrowed by CAD has expanded dramatically. These procedures are collectively referred to as *percutaneous coronary intervention* (PCI). Advances in device technology, along with more effective anticoagulant and antiplatelet regimens, have reduced complication rates and improved procedural outcomes. As a result, elective PCI is increasingly performed as a short-stay or outpatient procedure.[48] In the setting of emergency PCI associated with acute myocardial ischemia, patients are hospitalized for a period of time depending on the cardiovascular work-up that is required.

Percutaneous transluminal coronary angioplasty (PTCA), frequently abbreviated to *balloon angioplasty,* was introduced in 1977 as an alternative to coronary surgical revascularization. PTCA avoided many of the risks associated with cardiac

FIG. 15.11 Percutaneous Transluminal Coronary Angioplasty (PTCA). PTCA is used to open a stenotic vessel occluded by atherosclerosis.

surgery (general anesthesia, sternotomy, extracorporeal circulation, and mechanical ventilation), but its success was hampered by complications related to the procedure (acute closure, dissection) and restenosis or renarrowing of the vessel after the procedure. Continued research led to the development of new interventional devices to overcome the limitations of conventional angioplasty and further expanded the use of catheter-based interventions. Current PCI procedures include PTCA, atherectomy, and stent implantation as well as many adjunctive devices used to facilitate successful revascularization in coronary vessels.

Indications for Catheter-Based Interventions

Indications for catheter-based interventions have been considerably broadened since the initial application of PTCA. Previously, only patients with single-vessel CAD were considered for PTCA, whereas patients with multivessel disease, including patients who have previously undergone saphenous vein or internal mammary artery (IMA) grafting, may now be candidates for catheter-based intervention. PCI was previously considered a rescue procedure to reduce a severe stenosis that persisted after fibrinolytic therapy, but it is now preferred as the initial treatment method for acute MI (primary PCI).[37]

Earlier restrictions regarding the characteristics and location of the atherosclerotic lesion have also changed with operator experience and improved technology. Distal, moderately calcified, and bifurcation stenoses are considered suitable for PCI. Left main coronary artery lesions, although considered high risk, can be successfully treated under certain conditions. It is now possible to traverse and dilate a totally occluded vessel.[49] Lesion morphology related to shape, size, location, and amount of calcification has been more clearly defined through clinical experience and is used to guide the selection of specific catheter-based interventions.

Percutaneous Transluminal Coronary Angioplasty

PTCA involves the use of a balloon-tipped catheter that, when advanced through an atherosclerotic lesion (atheroma), can be inflated intermittently for the purpose of dilating the stenotic area and improving blood flow through it (Fig. 15.11). The high inflation pressure of the balloon stretches the vessel wall, fractures the plaque, and enlarges the vessel lumen. After balloon deflation, the vessel exhibits some degree of elastic recoil, resulting in a residual stenosis of approximately 30%. In a successful angioplasty procedure, the stenosis is reduced to less than 50% of the vessel lumen diameter.[49]

Although PTCA has relatively high success rates in initially opening occluded vessels, the technique by itself has major limitations, including the risk of acute vessel closure and a high frequency of restenosis. In the early application of angioplasty, acute closure occurred in 8% of patients as a result of dissection of the vessel wall and associated thrombus formation or vessel spasm. Restenosis occurred in more than one-third of patients who underwent PTCA within the first 6 months and was diagnosed when patients experienced a recurrence of anginal symptoms. Studies showed that restenosis was influenced by the final lumen diameter achieved by the procedure, the severity of elastic recoil of the vessel walls in response to the balloon inflation, and the amount of intimal hyperplasia that occurred as the vessel healed over the treated area. Patient characteristics such as a history of diabetes or unstable angina were also found to increase the risk of restenosis.

In the current era of PCI, design enhancements have led to low-profile angioplasty catheters that are able to traverse tortuous anatomy and noncompliant balloons that prevent overdistention of the vessel.[50] Another modification has been the cutting balloon—a device that produces incisions in the plaque before the balloon is dilated. Even with these improvements, PTCA is rarely used alone as an intervention except to treat lesions in very small coronary arteries.[50] Nevertheless, PTCA remains an essential adjunctive technique in PCI for predilating vessels and for deploying and expanding intracoronary stents.

Atherectomy

Atherectomy is the excision and removal of the atherosclerotic plaque by cutting, shaving, or grinding. Initially, it was thought that removing (rather than compressing) the atherosclerotic plaque would decrease the rate of restenosis. Despite significant improvements in initial procedural success, atherectomy failed to significantly reduce the rate of restenosis. Atherectomy is useful for removing plaque in heavily calcified lesions, to help increase wall compliance and facilitate angioplasty and stent placement. In the current era, atherectomy devices are used in less than 5% of PCI procedures.[51]

The most frequently used atherectomy device in coronary vessels is the Rotablator. This device has a high-speed, rotating, diamond-coated burr that drills through the plaque, creating tiny particles (Fig. 15.12). The particulate matter is carried through the bloodstream and disposed of by the reticuloendothelial system. Rotational atherectomy can increase procedural success for PCI performed on calcified bifurcation lesions and chronic total occlusions.[51] However, the use of this device is also associated with an increased risk of procedural complications, including vasospasm, perforation, and transient vessel occlusion.[52]

Adjunctive Devices

Initial devices for performing PCI were designed to optimize flow at the point of the lesion or blockage within the coronary artery. However, despite evidence of procedural success on angiography, some patients still exhibited signs of compromised distal perfusion. This "no reflow" phenomenon is believed to be caused by distal embolization of atherosclerotic plaque or thrombus at the time of the procedure.[40] Several adjunctive tools have been developed to help protect the microvasculature during PCI procedures. Embolic protection devices consist of balloons or filters that are positioned beyond the lesion to trap and remove debris that might be released during the intervention. One type of distal filter is shown in Fig. 15.13. Thrombectomy catheters are used to decrease the

FIG. 15.12 Rotational Atherectomy Catheter.

Distal embolic filter

FIG. 15.13 Embolic Protection Device.

risk of thrombotic emboli by removing large thrombi from the vessel before the intervention. These devices are recommended for use in PCI performed on saphenous vein grafts and may be helpful in native vessels when primary PCI is performed for ACS.[53]

Coronary Stents

A major development in the field of interventional cardiology has been the coronary stent prosthesis. A stent is a metal structure that is introduced into the coronary artery over a guidewire and expanded into the vessel wall at the site of the lesion. Bare metal stents were first used to treat acute or threatened vessel closure after failed PTCA. The stent acted as a scaffold to tack dissection flaps against the vessel wall and provided mechanical support to minimize elastic recoil. Subsequent studies confirmed the clinical benefits of stents, which led to elective coronary stent placement as a primary procedure. Stent implantation was initially limited to large vessels (greater than 3 mm) with proximal, discrete lesions. Improvements in stent design and operator technique allow for deployment in smaller vessels with diffuse disease, vessels with lesions at bifurcations, and vessels with thrombus. Multiple stents may be implanted sequentially within a vessel to fully cover the area of the lesion. Stents are the predominant form of PCI at the present time and are used in more than 90% of all interventional procedures.[14]

FIG. 15.14 The intracoronary stent is a balloon-expandable stent.

Numerous stents are available. They are composed of various types of metal (stainless steel, titanium, cobalt chromium) and come in a variety of configurations (eg, mesh, coil). Although initially composed of metal alone, contemporary stents incorporate various polymer coatings and medications in an effort to improve long-term patency of the vessel. Most stents are balloon expandable (Fig. 15.14).

Stent Thrombosis

Early use of stents was hampered by a high incidence of subacute stent thrombosis—abrupt occlusion of a previously patent vessel secondary to clot formation. This thrombosis tended to occur during the first 2 to 14 days after stent placement and resulted in MI in most cases.[50] Later it was found that stent thrombosis was due in part to inadequate stent expansion within the vessel—which could be remedied by applying high-pressure balloon inflations within the stent during deployment. In addition, antiplatelet therapy was found to be more important than anticoagulation in preventing stent thrombosis.[54] Because platelet activation is a complex process involving multiple pathways, combination therapy with two or more agents has proven most effective. The current standard of care for PCI typically includes dual antiplatelet therapy with aspirin and a thienopyridine. These oral agents are administered before the procedure and continued at discharge.[55] Clopidogrel, a second-generation thienopyridine, has been studied extensively but may be ineffective in 26% of patients.[56] Prasugrel and ticagrelor are newer agents that offer a faster onset of action, higher levels of platelet inhibition, and lower incidence of resistance.[57] Oral antiplatelet agents are described in Table 15.5.

GPIIb/IIIa inhibitors, which are more potent intravenous antiplatelet agents, may also be used during PCI procedures, primarily in high-risk patients.[36] These medications act on the GPIIb/IIIa receptors on the platelet membrane to inhibit the final phase of platelet aggregation and prevent platelets from binding with fibrinogen. Abciximab (ReoPro) was the first of the GPIIb/IIIa inhibitors to be approved by the US Food and Drug Administration (FDA) as an adjunct to PTCA for the prevention of abrupt closure of arteries in high-risk patients. Two additional agents, eptifibatide (Integrilin) and tirofiban (Aggrastat), were subsequently approved. Intravenous antiplatelet agents are described in Table 15.6.

In-Stent Restenosis

Stents have been shown to decrease the incidence of restenosis compared with balloon angioplasty, most likely as a result of achieving the largest possible lumen diameter at the time of the intervention. Successful stent implantation should result in less than 10% residual stenosis and optimally as close to zero as possible. However, stents have not proved to be a cure for restenosis as was once hoped. Restenosis within the stent is caused by intimal hyperplasia and can occur in a diffuse pattern throughout the stent, as discrete lesions within the body of the stent, or at the stent margins. In contrast to thrombosis, restenosis is a gradual process that generally occurs within the first 6 to 12 months and manifests clinically as recurrent angina. The incidence of in-stent restenosis requiring reintervention is approximately 20% within the first year after implantation of a bare metal stent.[58] Factors that increase the risk of in-stent restenosis are listed in Box 15.14.

Drug-Eluting Stents

In an effort to minimize restenosis, drug-eluting stents (DES) were developed. These stents have polymer coatings impregnated with medications that are released slowly into the endothelium at the site of stent placement to inhibit cellular proliferation. The first generation of DES to receive FDA approval were coated with sirolimus (an immunosuppressive medication used to prevent organ transplant rejection) and paclitaxel (an anticancer agent).[50] In initial trials, DES were found to decrease the 6-month restenosis rate to less than 10%, and they soon became the predominant stent. Later studies demonstrated similar efficacy between bare metal stents and DES in long-term outcomes (stent thrombosis, MI, or death) and raised concerns regarding the possibility of late stent thrombosis (greater than 1 year) with DES.[54] Because DES delay endothelialization, dual antiplatelet therapy must be continued for a longer period to prevent stent thrombosis. Second-generation stents, which incorporate thin struts, biocompatible polymers, and different medications, have improved safety and efficacy compared with early stents.[59] Studies have found that the incidence of stent thrombosis is much lower with second-generation everolimus-eluting stents compared with bare metal stents over a 2-year follow-up period.[60] Bare metal stents and DES are compared in Table 15.7.

TABLE 15.5 Pharmacologic Management

Oral Antiplatelet Agents

Medication	Dosage	Action	Special Considerations
Aspirin	81–325 mg	Inhibits synthesis of thromboxane A_2 resulting in irreversible inhibition of platelet activation	Lower doses are recommended when given with other antithrombotics.
Clopidogrel (Plavix)	300–600 mg loading dose	Irreversibly inhibits ADP $P2Y_{12}$ platelet receptor to block platelet activation	Onset of action 2–4 h.
	75–150 mg maintenance		Should be held 5–7 days before elective surgery to decrease risk of bleeding.
			Some patients may have a genetic resistance to clopidogrel, resulting in inadequate platelet inhibition.
Prasugrel (Effient)	60 mg loading dose	Irreversibly inhibits ADP $P2Y_{12}$ platelet receptor to block platelet activation	Onset of action 15–30 min.
	10 mg daily maintenance		Should be held 5–7 days before elective surgery to decrease risk of bleeding.
			Contraindicated in patients with prior TIA or stroke; not recommended in patients age >75 y.
Ticagrelor (Brilinta)	180 mg loading dose	Reversibly inhibits ADP $P2Y_{12}$ platelet receptor to block platelet activation	Onset of action 30 min.
	90 mg twice daily maintenance		Should be held 5 days before elective surgery to decrease risk of bleeding.
			Contraindicated in patients with history of ICH or severe hepatic impairment.
			Maintenance aspirin dose >100 mg reduces effectiveness.

ADP, adenosine diphosphate; *ICH*, intracranial hemorrhage; *TIA*, transient ischemic attack.

TABLE 15.6 Pharmacologic Management

Intravenous Antiplatelet Agents

Medication	Dosage	Action	Special Considerations
Abciximab (ReoPro)	ACS: 0.25 mg/kg IVP, then 10 mcg/min until PCI (continue infusion for minimum of 18 h to maximum of 26 h) PCI: 0.25 mg/kg IVP, then 0.125 mcg/kg/min × 12 h	Inhibits GPIIb/IIIa receptors responsible for platelet aggregation	Used concomitantly with aspirin and anticoagulants. May affect platelet function for 48 h after infusion.
Eptifibatide (Integrilin)	ACS: 180 mcg/kg IV bolus, followed by continuous infusion of 2 mcg/kg/min up to 72 h PCI: 180 mcg/kg IV bolus immediately before PCI (repeat after 10 min) followed by continuous infusion of 2 mcg/kg/min for 12–24 h	Reversibly binds to GPIIb/IIIa platelet receptor and inhibits platelet aggregation	Concomitant aspirin and anticoagulants may be administered. Platelet function returns to baseline within 6–8 h. Contraindicated in patients with significant kidney dysfunction.
Tirofiban (Aggrastat)	ACS: 25 mcg/kg within 5 min, then continued at 0.15 mcg/kg/min for up to 18 h	Reversibly binds to GPIIb/IIIa platelet receptor and inhibits platelet aggregation	Platelet function returns to baseline within 4–8 h. Dosage should be reduced in patients with kidney dysfunction.

ACS, acute coronary syndrome; *GP*, glycoprotein; *IV*, intravenous; *IVP*, intravenous push; *PCI*, percutaneous coronary intervention.

Procedure

PCI is performed in the cardiac catheterization laboratory under fluoroscopy. Patients typically receive antiplatelet therapy (a thienopyridine and aspirin) before beginning the procedure. An introducer catheter, or sheath, is inserted percutaneously into an artery to provide access to the coronary arteries. The femoral artery is used most commonly in the United States and has the advantage of being able to accommodate large catheters. However, access via the radial artery (transradial access) is increasing because studies show that it results in lower rates of bleeding and vascular complications and is associated with earlier ambulation and increased patient satisfaction.[61] In some cases, a venous sheath is inserted and used to perform a right heart catheterization or to insert a pacing catheter, or both. A catheter with pacing capabilities may be indicated if dilation of the right coronary artery or circumflex artery is anticipated because the blood supply to the conduction system of the heart may be interrupted, requiring emergency pacing.

The patient is systemically anticoagulated to prevent clots from forming on or in any of the catheters. Unfractionated heparin has been used traditionally, initiated with a weight-based

BOX 15.14 Risk Factors for In-Stent Restenosis

Patient Factors
- Age
- Diabetes mellitus
- Chronic kidney failure

Anatomic Factors
- Longer lesions (>20 mm)
- Small vessel diameter (<3 mm)
- Complex, branched lesions

Procedural Factors
- Inadequate stent expansion
- Stent design (bare metal stent vs drug-eluting stent)
- Gaps in sequential placement

TABLE 15.7 Comparison of Bare Metal and Drug-Eluting Stents

Characteristics	Bare Metal Stent	Drug-Eluting Stent
Restenosis rate (at 6 months)	15%–20%	5%–10%
Cost	$	$$$
Duration of dual antiplatelet therapy	Minimum of 1 month for non-ACS patients, at least 12 months for stents implanted for ACS	Minimum of 12 months for either non-ACS or ACS patients and longer if tolerated
Recommended lesion features	Short lesions <20 mm	Longer lesions >20 mm
	Large vessel diameter >3 mm	Small vessel diameter <3.5 mm

ACS, acute coronary syndrome.

bolus and then titrated to achieve a target activated clotting time. Other anticoagulants may be selected based on physician preference or if the patient cannot tolerate heparin. Some of these newer agents have been shown to decrease the risk of bleeding complications compared with unfractionated heparin.[62] Options for anticoagulant agents are described in Table 15.8.

A special guiding catheter, designed to engage the coronary ostia, is inserted through the arterial sheath and advanced in a retrograde manner through the aorta. Nitroglycerin, calcium channel blockers, or adenosine may be given at this time to prevent coronary artery spasm and to maximize coronary vasodilation during the procedure.[63] A guidewire is then advanced down the coronary artery and negotiated across the occluding atheroma. The balloon catheter is advanced over this guidewire and positioned across the lesion. The balloon is inflated and deflated repetitively until evidence of dilation is demonstrated on an angiogram (Fig. 15.15). For lesions that do not respond well to angioplasty, additional plaque or thrombus removal may be done with an adjunctive device.

In most procedures, vessel dilation is followed by deployment of an intracoronary stent. A stent is positioned at the target site, the stent is expanded, and the catheter is removed, leaving the stent in place. Intravascular ultrasound is used by many clinicians to evaluate the vessel lumen diameter after stent deployment to ensure optimal expansion.[64] Information obtained by ultrasound provides a better estimate of residual plaque than information provided by angiography because contrast material may surround the latticework of the stent, giving the appearance of a large lumen even when the stent is not fully open. To facilitate early sheath removal, heparin or other anticoagulants are usually discontinued immediately after the procedure. Sheaths are removed when the activated clotting time returns to normal in heparinized patients or sooner if other anticoagulants or a vascular closure device is used. If GPIIb/IIIa inhibitors were initiated during the procedure, they may be continued for 12 to 24 hours, depending on the agent used. Dual antiplatelet therapy with aspirin and a thienopyridine (clopidogrel, prasugrel, or ticagrelor) is routinely prescribed at discharge. Recommendations for thienopyridine

TABLE 15.8 Pharmacologic Management

Anticoagulants

Medication	Dosage	Action	Special Considerations
Unfractionated Heparin			
Heparin sodium	Initial bolus 60 units/kg (maximum dose 4000 units), followed by 12 units/kg/h infusion	Enhances activity of antithrombin III, a natural anticoagulant, to prevent clot formation	Effectiveness of treatment may be monitored by aPTT or ACT.
			Response is variable because of binding with plasma proteins. Effects may be reversed with protamine sulfate. Risk of developing HIT. Should not be given to patients already receiving therapeutic SC enoxaparin.
Low-Molecular-Weight Heparin			
Enoxaparin (Lovenox)	30 mg IV bolus, followed by 1 mg/kg SC every 12 h For patients already on SC dosing, an additional bolus of 0.3 mg/kg is given if last dose was >8 h before PCI	Enhances activity of antithrombin III	More predictable response than heparin because enoxaparin is not largely bound to protein. No need for aPTT or ACT monitoring.
			Lower risk of HIT than with UFH. Significant reduction in dosage needed when CrCl <30 mL/min. Administer within 30 min of initiation of fibrinolytic therapy.

TABLE 15.8 Pharmacologic Management—cont'd

Medication	Dosage	Action	Special Considerations
Direct Thrombin Inhibitors			
Bivalirudin (Angiomax)	0.75 mg/kg IV bolus, followed by infusion at 1.75 mg/kg/h during PCI. If infusion continued >4 h, rate is decreased to 0.2 mg/kg/h	Directly inhibits thrombin	May be administered alone or in combination with GPIIb/IIIa inhibitors. Produces dose-dependent increase in aPTT and ACT. Coagulation times return to baseline within 1 h after stopping infusion. Dose should be reduced for patients with kidney dysfunction. No reversal agent is available. May be used instead of UFH for patients with HIT.
Argatroban	Loading dose of 100 mcg/kg IV bolus over 1 min, followed by infusion of 1–3 mcg/kg/min	Directly inhibits thrombin	May be used instead of UFH for patients with HIT. ACT is monitored during PCI; aPTT is used during prolonged infusion. Abrupt discontinuation may lead to rebound hypercoagulable state.
Factor Xa Inhibitor			
Fondaparinux (Arixtra)	2.5 mg IV, followed by 2.5 mg SC once daily	Selective inhibitor of factor Xa	May be used in conjunction with fibrinolytics. For PCI, must be administered with another anticoagulant (ie, UFH) to prevent catheter thrombosis. Long half-life (>17 h). Contraindicated in patients with kidney failure.

ACT, activated clotting time; *aPTT,* activated partial thromboplastin time; *CrCl,* creatinine clearance; *GP,* glycoprotein; *HIT,* heparin-induced thrombocytopenia; *IV,* intravenous/intravenously; *MI,* myocardial infarction; *PCI,* percutaneous coronary intervention; *SC,* subcutaneous/subcutaneously; *UFH,* unfractionated heparin.

FIG. 15.15 (A) Coronary arteriogram of an acute proximal total occlusion of the right coronary artery. The patient had sudden onset of chest pain at home and was emergently admitted to the cardiac catheterization laboratory. (B) The same vessel as in (A) after successful coronary atherectomy and intracoronary fibrinolytic therapy to open the occluded artery. Symptoms of chest pain resolved after the procedure.

administration vary based on the type of stent used (see Table 15.7), whereas aspirin is continued indefinitely.

Acute Complications

The incidence of serious cardiac complications after PCI, including coronary spasm, coronary artery dissection, and acute coronary thrombosis, has decreased significantly with improvements in technology. Stents have proved efficacious in the repair of coronary dissections, decreasing the need for emergency bypass surgery. Acute thrombosis has decreased with the established use of dual antiplatelet agents. Bleeding and complications at the site of vascular cannulation (hematoma, compromised blood flow to the involved extremity, and retroperitoneal bleeding with femoral access) occur infrequently but are associated with increased morbidity and lengthened hospitalization.[65] Other complications that can occur in the period immediately after PCI include contrast-induced kidney failure, dysrhythmias, and vasovagal response (hypotension, bradycardia, and diaphoresis) during manipulation or removal of introducer sheaths.

Nursing Management

Nursing management after PCI focuses on accurate assessment of the patient's condition and prompt intervention. The nurse at the bedside is in a unique position to continuously monitor for clinical manifestations of potential problems and to take quick and appropriate action to minimize the deleterious effects of complications related to the interventional catheter procedure.

Angina

It is essential that the nurse observe the patient for recurrent angina or ST segment elevation, which are clinical indicators of myocardial ischemia. Monitoring leads should be selected that will reflect ischemia in the vessels that were treated during the intervention. Angina after a coronary interventional procedure may be caused by transient coronary vasospasm, or it may signal a more serious complication—acute thrombosis. In any case, the nurse must act quickly to assess for manifestations of myocardial ischemia and initiate clinical interventions as indicated. The physician usually orders intravenous nitroglycerin to be titrated to alleviate chest pain. Continued angina despite maximal vasodilator therapy usually rules out transient coronary vasospasm as the source of ischemic pain, and a return to the cardiac catheterization laboratory must be considered.

Prevention of Contrast-Induced Acute Kidney Injury

Patients undergoing PCI are exposed to significant amounts of contrast dye, with its associated nephrotoxicity. Protective strategies may be implemented before the procedure, especially for patients with evidence of baseline kidney impairment. This may include hydration and infusion of sodium bicarbonate before the procedure.[66] Although an early study indicated that administration of N-acetylcysteine (Mucomyst) might be beneficial, current guidelines do not recommend it for prevention of contrast-induced acute kidney injury.[64] After PCI, hydration is important to maintain adequate flow through the kidneys. Intravenous fluids are administered, and patients are encouraged to take oral fluids as tolerated. Whenever possible, nephrotoxic drugs, such as nonsteroidal antiinflammatory drugs and metformin, should be withheld for 48 to 72 hours after the procedure.[67]

Vascular Site Care

While the sheath is in place or after its removal, bleeding or hematoma at the insertion site may occur secondary to the effects of anticoagulation. The nurse observes the patient for bleeding or swelling at the puncture site and for changes in vital signs (hypotension, tachycardia) that could indicate hemorrhage. If a femoral approach was used, the nurse also assesses the patient for back pain, which can indicate retroperitoneal bleeding from the internal arterial puncture site.

Peripheral ischemia can also occur secondary to cannulation of the vessel, so nursing care includes frequent assessment of the adequacy of circulation to the involved extremity (Box 15.15). After obtaining radial access, peripheral circulation may be assessed by monitoring the plethysmography

---

QSEN BOX 15.15 QSEN: Patient Safety Alert

Peripheral Ischemia

- Maintain head of bed 30 degrees or lower for femoral access
- Keep cannulated extremity straight (use immobilizer or splint as needed)
- Monitor distal perfusion (pulse strength, capillary refill) frequently
- Assess color, sensation, and temperature in involved extremity

---

waveform from a pulse oximeter probe placed on the thumb of the affected extremity.[68] The patient is instructed to keep the limb straight and minimize movement. For femoral access, the head of the bed is not elevated more than 30 degrees while the sheath is in place (to prevent dislodgment) and for a period of time after its removal (to prevent bleeding). For brachial or radial access, a splint may be used to prevent flexion of the arm or wrist. Additional activity restrictions vary depending on the size and location of the sheath, type of anticoagulation prescribed, methods used to achieve hemostasis, and institutional protocols. After sheath removal, direct pressure is applied to the puncture site for 15 to 30 minutes until hemostasis is achieved. If direct pressure is inadequate or the patient is at higher risk for bleeding, a C-clamp or other compression device may be used to apply continuous pressure for 1 to 2 hours to ensure adequate hemostasis. Patients usually are allowed to resume ambulation 2 to 4 hours after the procedure or sooner if a vascular closure device is employed.[69,70]

Many products have been introduced to facilitate adequate hemostasis at the femoral access site after sheath removal. Active closure devices use mechanical sutures, collagen plugs, or metal clips to close the vessel when the sheath is removed. Advantages of these devices include a reduced time to hemostasis regardless of the patient's level of anticoagulation, earlier ambulation, and increased patient comfort.[71] The Perclose closure device contains needles and sutures that are used to suture the artery closed after the interventional procedure (Fig. 15.16). Angio-Seal is a vascular hemostatic device that uses a collagen plug to seal the arterial puncture site. Gentle pressure is maintained over the puncture site for approximately 5 minutes, until hemostasis is achieved. The StarClose vascular closure device consists of a tiny circumferential nitinol (nickel and titanium) clip that is applied to the surface of the vessel to close the femoral artery at the end of the procedure.

Reports of complications and increased cost have limited the use of active closure devices.[65] To avoid these complications, numerous products have been developed to enhance manual compression and shorten the time required to achieve hemostasis. Some of these devices rely on the delivery of prothrombotic materials by a patch, whereas others increase local pressure over the puncture site. These devices do not offer immediate closure but may decrease the time to ambulation.[71] Vascular closure systems are compared in Table 15.9.

Patient Education

In most cases, patients undergoing elective angioplasty, atherectomy, or stent procedures are hospitalized for less than 24 hours. All patients require education about their medication regimen and about risk factor modification (Box 15.16). Because of the short hospital stay, the nurse often has time to do little more than identify the offending risk factors and initiate basic

Percutaneous Vascular Surgical Device

Marker lumens

Back-bleeding indicates intraluminal needle position.

Sheath loaded with 4 needles carrying sutures

Subcutaneous layer

Artery

Marker port

A

Needle

Suture

Needles are deployed through artery wall as device handle is pulled upward.

B

Square knots are tied in each suture and delivered to the artery surface with a knot pusher. Complete hemostasis is achieved with percutaneous vascular surgery.

Knot pusher

Subcutaneous layer

C

FIG. 15.16 Example of Percutaneous Vascular Surgical Device Used to Close Femoral Artery After Catheter-Based Interventions for Coronary Artery Disease. (A) Insertion of the device into the femoral artery. (B) After the interventional procedure, the device is removed by pulling upward to allow the needles in the device to close the artery. (C) The sutured artery is secured with a knot pusher. (Courtesy Perclose, Inc., Redwood City, CA.)

instruction. Patients are referred to local cardiac rehabilitation centers for more extensive teaching and follow-up to facilitate understanding and compliance with risk factor modification.

Another point of instruction that must be addressed is the patient's knowledge deficit related to discharge medications. Patients are sent home on a regimen of antiplatelet medications and medications for secondary prevention, such as lipid-lowering agents and blood pressure medications. A nitrate such as isosorbide may be prescribed to promote vasodilation, or, if the patient has demonstrated evidence of a vasospastic component to the disease, calcium channel blockers may be used. It is essential that the patient clearly understands the rationale

for therapy and the potential side effects of each medication. Patients also need to understand the importance of compliance with antiplatelet therapy, as premature discontinuation of these agents is associated with increased risk of death as a result of stent thrombosis.[54]

Percutaneous Valve Repair
Balloon Valvuloplasty
Percutaneous catheter technology has also been adapted to allow for nonsurgical interventions for valvular heart disease. Balloon valvuloplasty, also known as balloon commissurotomy, is an accepted alternative to surgical repair for patients with

TABLE 15.9   Vascular Closure Devices

Technology and Examples	Description	Comments
Patch		
Chito-Seal	Patches that contain materials to promote clotting are applied directly to the puncture site, along with manual compression.	Less expensive than active closure devices.
Clo-Sur P.A.D.		No foreign material is left in the patient.
D-Stat Syvek Patch		
Suture		
Perclose A-T	Sutures deployed through the sheath are used to close arteriotomy site.	Allows for immediate reaccess through site if needed (see Fig. 15.16).
ProGlide		Device failure may require surgical repair
Prostar XL		
Plug or Sealant		
Angio-Seal	Placement of a procoagulant sealant such as collagen or thrombin is used to close the artery.	Reaccess must be done 1 cm above the previous arterial access site to avoid dislodging the sealant.
ExoSeal	Angio-Seal also includes an intravascular suture to anchor the collagen plug in place.	Extrusion of sealant into the vessel may compromise the arterial lumen.
Mynx	The Exoseal deploys an absorbable sealant made of polyglycolic acid.	Components are absorbed within 30–90 days, depending on the sealant used.
Vascade	The Mynx system uses a balloon catheter to inject a polyethylene glycol sealant into the puncture site tract.	
Clip or Staple		
StarClose	Circumferential staples or clips are deployed at the site of the arteriotomy to close the vessel.	Extravascular clip does not compromise artery lumen.

✱ BOX 15.16   PATIENT EDUCATION PLAN

Percutaneous Transluminal Coronary Angioplasty, Coronary Atherectomy, and Stent Placement

Before discharge, the patient should be able to teach back the following topics:

- Pathophysiology of atherosclerosis
- Risk factor modification (diet, exercise, smoking cessation, weight loss)
- Information about prescribed medications (eg, antiplatelet agents, antihypertensives, nitrates, calcium channel blockers, lipid-lowering medications)
- Symptoms to report to the health care professional (chest pain, shortness of breath, bleeding or drainage from the access site)
- Follow-up appointments

---

mitral valve stenosis. This procedure has a limited role in aortic stenosis because it provides only short-term improvement and is associated with high morbidity and mortality. Current guidelines recommend balloon valvuloplasty for aortic stenosis only as a bridge to surgery or transcatheter valve replacement (discussed later) in patients with severe symptoms.[72]

Balloon valvuloplasty is performed in the cardiac catheterization laboratory by placing a balloon across the stenotic valve and inflating it to reduce stenosis. Regurgitant flow can result, particularly after mitral valvuloplasty, and may lead to the need for emergent valve replacement if severe. The risks of balloon valvuloplasty are similar to the risks inherent in most catheterization procedures and include cardiac perforation, thromboembolic events, dysrhythmias, and vascular complications caused by the sheath. Nursing management after the procedure is similar to nursing management for other percutaneous cardiac catheter procedures.

Transcatheter Aortic Valve Replacement

Transcatheter aortic valve replacement (TAVR) is a transformational therapy for patients who have severe aortic stenosis but who are extremely high-risk surgical candidates or who are inoperable because of associated comorbidities.[72,73] TAVR can be done with spinal or general anesthesia in a hybrid equipped cardiac surgery operating room. The procedure consists of positioning a bioprosthetic valve that has been loaded on a stent within the native aortic valve and then expanding the stent to anchor the valve within the aortic annulus.[74] Different approaches are used to deploy the device, but once it is in place, contrast medium is used to ensure correct positioning of the catheter valve across the aortic annulus.

Although TAVR has been shown to have excellent clinical outcomes in high-risk patients, the multiple comorbid diseases often present in this group require nursing care to focus on preventing the complications associated with these conditions. Postoperative assessment includes monitoring hemodynamics and fluid balance, observing for signs of stroke and kidney injury, and identifying rhythm disturbances that may require backup pacing or medical interventions.[75] Vascular access complications can be significant after TAVR and require very tight control of blood pressure along with vigilance in monitoring for signs of bleeding, arterial rupture, cardiac tamponade, and limb ischemia.[74] Recommendations are for patients to be treated with dual antiplatelet therapy for a minimum of 6 months to prevent thromboembolism and ensure that the valve is endothelialized.[74]

CARDIAC SURGERY

Nursing management of a patient undergoing cardiac surgery is demanding but exciting work that requires the talents of an experienced team of critical care nurses. This section introduces basic cardiac surgical techniques along with principles of cardiopulmonary bypass (CPB) and highlights the key points about postoperative care of adult patients who require valve replacement or coronary artery revascularization.

Coronary Artery Bypass Graft Surgery

Since its introduction almost 50 years ago, coronary artery bypass graft (CABG) surgery has proved to be safe and effective in relieving angina symptoms and improving survival in most patients. Although there has been a great deal of evolution

FIG. 15.17 Saphenous Vein Graft. (Leg illustration from Moser D, Riegel B. *Cardiac Nursing: A Companion to Braunwald's Heart Disease.* Philadelphia: Saunders; 2007.)

involving less invasive techniques, improved pharmacologic therapy, and expanded education regarding lifestyle modifications, CABG surgery continues to have an important role in the treatment of CAD. Information on "Coronary Artery Disease" is presented in Chapter 14, and "Catheter-Based Interventions for Coronary Artery Disease" are discussed earlier in this chapter.

Surgical revascularization has been shown to be more efficacious than PCI in patients with multivessel or left main coronary disease.[76] Bypass surgery may allow for more complete revascularization because it can be used on vessels that are not amenable to treatment with a percutaneous approach, such as vessels with total occlusions or excessive tortuosity. However, as medical therapy and surgical procedures continue to evolve, updated studies and evaluations are required to guide optimal treatment.

Myocardial revascularization involves the use of a conduit, or channel, designed to bypass an occluded coronary artery. Surgeons must evaluate which conduits would provide the best graft patency and long-term outcomes for their patients. The long saphenous vein graft is the most frequently used conduit for CABG surgery. Saphenous vein grafting involves the anastomosis of an excised portion of the saphenous vein proximal to the aorta and distal to the coronary artery below the obstruction (Fig. 15.17). Endoscopic vein harvesting has been associated with decreased length of hospital stay and increased patient satisfaction but has also been linked to a possible risk of early graft failure and so requires further research.[77] Graft patency has increased with improved harvesting techniques, adjunctive medication strategies (statins and antiplatelet agents), and aggressive risk factor modification such as smoking cessation.[78,79]

Use of arterial conduits has dramatically improved long-term graft patency. The IMA, which usually remains attached to its origin at the subclavian artery, is swung down and anastomosed distal to the coronary artery (Fig. 15.18). Either the right IMA or the left IMA may be used as a conduit. The IMA is currently recommended as the conduit of choice for CABG

FIG. 15.18 Internal Mammary Artery Graft.

surgery, with a standard practice of attaching the left internal mammary artery to the artery that supplies the largest myocardial territory, most often the left anterior descending artery.[80,81] Emergency CABG surgery may preclude the use of the IMA because of the extra time required to mobilize the artery and the inability to effect cardioplegia (heart paralysis) through this conduit. Current recommendations also include the use of radial artery grafts in certain scenarios.[80] Conduits used for myocardial revascularization are compared in Table 15.10.

TABLE 15.10   Conduits Used for Coronary Artery Bypass Grafts

Type of Graft	Advantages	Disadvantages
Saphenous vein	Easily harvested	Long-term patency still to be determined
	Length allows for multiple grafts	Requires at least two anastomosis sites
	No anatomic limitations to graft sites	
Internal mammary artery	Proven patency rates	Requires extensive dissection
	Requires only one anastomosis	Not accessible for emergency bypass
		Associated with increased chest wall discomfort postoperatively
		Anatomic limitations to bypassing some areas of the heart
Radial artery	Improved patency rates	Requires adequate collateral flow to hand through the ulnar artery
	Easily harvested	May be associated with higher rates of vasospasm
		Requires two anastomosis sites

FIG. 15.19 (A) Mechanical bileaflet valve. (B) Prosthetic tissue valve. (C) Mechanical bileaflet valve (St. Jude). (D) Starr-Edwards ball-and-cage valve. A–C depict valves currently in use; the ball-and-cage valve (D) is no longer in clinical use. (A courtesy St. Jude Medical.)

Valvular Surgery

Valvular disease results in various hemodynamic dysfunctions that can usually be managed medically as long as the patient remains symptom-free. There is reluctance to intervene surgically early in the course of this disease because of the surgical risks and long-term complications associated with prosthetic valve replacement. However, these consequences must be weighed against the possibility of irreversible deterioration in LV function that may develop during the compensated asymptomatic phase (see "Valvular Heart Disease" and Table 14.14. in Chapter 14).

Surgical therapy for aortic valve disease consists primarily of aortic valve replacement, although repairs may be done for selected regurgitant valves.[72] Three surgical procedures are available to treat mitral valve disease: commissurotomy, valve repair, and valve replacement. Commissurotomy is performed for mitral stenosis; the fused leaflets are incised, and calcium deposits are débrided to increase valve mobility. Repair of damaged leaflets may be accomplished with pericardial patches. In the setting of mitral regurgitation, valve repair may include reshaping of the leaflets and the use of a ring to reduce the size of the dilated mitral annulus, enhancing leaflet coaptation (annuloplasty). Although it is technically more demanding, valve repair is preferred over valve replacement to avoid the complications inherent with a prosthetic valve—the risk of thromboembolic events and the need for long-term anticoagulation.[82] If reconstruction of the mitral valve is impossible, it is replaced.

The two categories of prosthetic valves are mechanical valves and biologic valves, or tissue valves. *Mechanical valves* are made from combinations of metal alloys, pyrolytic carbon, Dacron, and Teflon and have rigid occluding devices (Fig. 15.19). Their construction renders them highly durable, but all patients with mechanical valves require anticoagulation to reduce the incidence of thromboembolism. *Biologic valves* are constructed from animal or human cardiac tissue and have flexible occluding mechanisms. Because of their low thrombogenicity, tissue valves offer the patient freedom from therapeutic anticoagulation. However, their durability is limited by their tendency toward early calcification. Various valvular prostheses are described in Box 15.17.

The choice of a valvular prosthesis depends on many factors. Because mechanical valves are more durable, they may be preferred for a young person who is anticipated to have a relatively long life span ahead. Similarly, a bioprosthesis (tissue valve) may be chosen for an older adult patient; the valve has a reduced longevity, but this disadvantage is offset by the older patient's shorter life expectancy.[72] For patients with medical contraindications to anticoagulation and for patients whose past compliance with medications has been questionable, a tissue valve may be selected.[83] Technical considerations, such as the size of the annulus (or the anatomic ring in which the valve

BOX 15.17 Classification of Prosthetic Cardiac Valves

Mechanical Valves
Tilting-disk: A free-floating, lens-shaped disk mounted on a circular sewing ring
- Medtronic Hall
- Omniscience
- Bjork-Shiley Monostrut

Bi-leaflet: Two semicircular leaflets, mounted on a circular sewing ring that opens centrally
- St. Jude Medical
- CarboMedics
- On-X/ATS

Biologic or Tissue Valves (Bioprostheses)
Porcine heterograft: A porcine aortic valve mounted on a semiflexible stent and preserved in glutaraldehyde
- Hancock
- Carpentier-Edwards
- Toronto Stentless (St. Jude)
- Free Style Stentless (Medtronic)

Homograft: A human heart valve (aortic or pulmonic) harvested from a donated heart and cryopreserved; may or may not be mounted on a support ring

TABLE 15.11 Physiologic Effects of Cardiopulmonary Bypass

Effects	Causes
Intravascular fluid deficit (hypotension)	Third spacing
	Postoperative diuresis
	Sudden vasodilation (medications, rewarming)
Third spacing (weight gain, edema)	Decreased plasma protein concentration
	Increased capillary permeability
Myocardial depression (decreased cardiac output)	Hypothermia
	Increased SVR
	Prolonged CPB pump run
	Preexisting heart disease
	Inadequate myocardial protection
Coagulopathy (bleeding)	Systemic heparinization
	Mechanical trauma to platelets
	Decreased release of clotting factors from liver as a result of hypothermia
Pulmonary dysfunction (decreased lung mechanics and impaired gas exchange)	Decreased surfactant production
	Pulmonary microemboli
	Interstitial fluid accumulation in lungs
Hemolysis (hemoglobinuria)	Red blood cells damaged in pump circuit
Hyperglycemia (rise in serum glucose concentration)	Decreased insulin release
	Stimulation of glycogenolysis
Hypokalemia (low serum potassium concentration)	Intracellular shifts during bypass and postoperative diuresis
Hypomagnesemia (low serum magnesium concentration)	Postoperative diuresis resulting from hemodilution
Neurologic dysfunction (decreased level of consciousness, motor/sensory deficits)	Inadequate cerebral perfusion
	Microemboli to brain (air, plaque fragments, fat globules)
Hypertension (transient increase in blood pressure)	Catecholamine release and systemic hypothermia causing vasoconstriction

CPB, cardiopulmonary bypass; *SVR,* systemic vascular resistance.

sits), can also influence the choice of valve; for example, a bioprosthesis may be too big for a small aortic root. The trend has been toward bioprosthesis implantation, which may increase the opportunities for TAVR implantations in the future.[84]

Cardiopulmonary Bypass

CPB is a mechanical means of circulating and oxygenating a patient's blood, while diverting most of the circulation from the heart and lungs during cardiac surgical procedures. The extracorporeal circuit consists of cannulas that drain off venous blood; an oxygenator that oxygenates the blood; and a pump head that propels the arterialized blood back to the ascending aorta, which has been cross-clamped to prevent the back flow of blood into the heart.

Several adjunctive strategies are used to facilitate circulation and oxygenation while the patient is on bypass (on-pump). The patient is systemically heparinized before initiation of bypass to prevent clotting within the bypass circuit. After the patient is taken off the CPB machine, protamine sulfate is given to reverse the effects of the heparin.

Rapidly stopping the heart in diastole by perfusing the coronary arteries with a potassium cardioplegic (heart-paralyzing) agent assists with intraoperative myocardial protection. The cardioplegia solution must be reinfused at regular intervals during CPB to keep the heart in an arrested state so that the surgeon can operate while the heart is stopped as well as to minimize myocardial oxygen requirements.

Systemic hypothermia during bypass can reduce tissue oxygen requirements to 50% of normal, which affords the major organs additional protection from ischemic injury. Lowering the body temperature to approximately 28°C (82.4°F) is accomplished through a heat exchanger incorporated into the pump. The blood is warmed to normal body temperature before bypass is discontinued.

The technique of hemodilution is also used to enhance tissue oxygenation by improving blood flow through the systemic and pulmonary microcirculation during bypass. *Hemodilution* refers to the dilution of the patient's own (autologous) blood with the isotonic crystalloid solution used to prime the circuit. This hemodilution enhances capillary perfusion by reducing blood viscosity (stickiness) and decreasing the risk of microthrombi formation. At the completion of CPB, the large quantities of "pump blood" that remain in the bypass circuit can be collected and used for initial postoperative volume replacement.

Numerous clinical sequelae can result from CPB (Table 15.11). Knowledge of these physiologic effects allows the nurse to anticipate problems and intervene effectively in the postoperative period.

Off-Pump Coronary Artery Bypass Graft Surgery

Some surgeons may elect to perform off-pump CABG (OP-CABG) surgery with the goal of avoiding the potential complications associated with CPB and cross-clamping of the

◎ BOX 15.18 NURSING DIAGNOSES

Open Heart Surgery

- Decreased Cardiac Output related to alterations in preload, p. 1015
- Decreased Cardiac Output related to alterations in afterload, p. 1015
- Decreased Cardiac Output related to alterations in contractility, p. 1016
- Decreased Cardiac Output related to alterations in heart rate or rhythm, p. 1016
- Impaired Gas Exchange related to ventilation-perfusion mismatching or intrapulmonary shunting, p. 1030
- Ineffective Airway Clearance related to excessive secretions or abnormal viscosity of mucus, p. 1034
- Activity Intolerance related to cardiopulmonary dysfunction, p. 1006
- Deficient Fluid Volume related to absolute loss, p. 1019
- Risk for Infection, p. 1046
- Acute Pain related to transmission and perception of cutaneous, visceral, muscular, or ischemic impulses, p. 1010
- Anxiety related to threat to biologic, psychologic, or social integrity, p. 1012
- Disturbed Sleep Pattern related to fragmented sleep, p. 1023
- Deficient Knowledge related to lack of previous exposure to information, p. 1020 (see Box 15.20, Patient Education for Open Heart Surgery)

aorta. OP-CABG surgeries account for approximately 15% to 20% of all CABG procedures in the United States.[85] Several techniques are used to stabilize the operative area during an OP-CABG procedure. Immobilization devices that use compression or suction to create an immobile area have been developed to stabilize cardiac wall motion at the site of the anastomosis. Medications that temporarily decrease the heart rate (eg, esmolol, diltiazem) or cause transient cardiac asystole (eg, adenosine) may also be used to further limit cardiac motion.

Despite the fact that the OP-CABG procedure was developed to decrease complications associated with CPB, there are no convincing data that OP-CABG surgery is superior to on-pump CABG surgery. Long-term graft patency, complete revascularization, and overall survival may be better with conventional CABG surgery.[86] The use of OP-CABG surgery has been shown to reduce the rates of transfusions, reoperation for perioperative bleeding, respiratory complications, and acute kidney injury.[87] The OP-CABG procedure may be most beneficial in patients with significant comorbid conditions, in patients with contraindications to CPB, and in patients in whom aortic atherosclerosis precludes cross-clamping.

Postoperative Management

Medical and nursing management of the postoperative cardiac surgery patient often overlaps. The physician prescribes therapeutic interventions and identifies specific hemodynamic end points to maintain adequate organ perfusion and oxygen delivery. The nurse is responsible for applying these therapies to maintain the patient's hemodynamic parameters within the desired range. In most institutions, standard protocols are used to facilitate the postoperative nursing diagnoses and management of cardiac surgical patients (Box 15.18).

Cardiovascular Support

Postoperative cardiovascular support often is indicated because of a low-output state resulting from preexisting heart disease, a prolonged CPB pump run, inadequate myocardial protection, or some combination of these factors. Cardiac output can be

maximized by adjustments in heart rate, preload, afterload, and contractility.

Heart Rate. In the presence of low cardiac output, the heart rate can be appropriately regulated via temporary pacing or medication therapy. Temporary atrial or ventricular epicardial pacing is usually instituted when the heart rate decreases to less than 60 beats/min and the patient is hypotensive, requiring a supportive rate of 80 to 100 beats/min. In the case of tachycardia, intravenous beta-blockers (esmolol) or calcium channel blockers (diltiazem) may be used in the acute postoperative period to slow supraventricular rhythms. Electrolyte disturbances such as hypokalemia, hypomagnesemia, hypocalcemia, and hypercalcemia must be closely monitored and corrected to prevent postoperative dysrhythmias.

Atrial fibrillation occurs in approximately one-third of patients after cardiac surgery, with a peak occurrence in the first 2 to 3 days after surgery. This rhythm may induce hemodynamic compromise, prolong hospitalization, and increase the patient's risk of stroke. Prophylactic administration of beta-blockers is recommended to decrease the incidence of AF and its clinical sequelae; amiodarone is an alternative for patients who have contraindications to beta-blockers.[80] Ventricular arrhythmias are uncommon, so ongoing ischemia should be suspected and investigated.

Preload. In most patients, reduced preload is the cause of low postoperative cardiac output. The most common causes of decreased preload are hypovolemia from bleeding, fluid shifts caused by the systemic inflammatory response, increased vascular capacitance with rewarming, and elevated cardiac preload requirements.[88] Appropriate volume resuscitation immediately postoperatively is one of the most important interventions and should be a first-line therapy for hemodynamic instability. To enhance preload, volume may be administered in the form of crystalloid, colloid, or packed red cells. Crystalloids are preferred for fluid resuscitation; the type of crystalloid depends on institutional preference.[88] Traditionally, preload has been evaluated by intermittent pressure readings obtained from catheters placed in the right atrium or pulmonary artery. A growing body of research suggests that static indices such as central venous pressure and pulmonary artery occlusion pressure have a very weak relationship with the patient's intravascular volume and are not helpful in predicting if a patient will respond to fluid resuscitation.[89] Dynamic measures of preload responsiveness (ie, pulse pressure variation and systolic pressure variation) have been shown to more accurately predict an increase in cardiac output in response to a volume challenge in patients in the postoperative period after CABG surgery, although there are still many limitations to these measures.[90] Excessive fluid administration can also lead to adverse events. Approximately 2 to 3 L of crystalloid should suffice for most patients.

Afterload. Patients who have had cardiac surgery may demonstrate postoperative hypertension. Although it is transient, postoperative hypertension can precipitate or exacerbate bleeding from the mediastinal chest tubes. The high systemic vascular resistance (SVR) (afterload) resulting from the intense vasoconstriction can increase LV workload. Vasodilator therapy with intravenous sodium nitroprusside or nitroglycerin often is used to reduce afterload, control hypertension, and improve cardiac output. Increased afterload may be partially due to the peripheral vasoconstrictive effects of hypothermia, which can be managed with careful rewarming.

A significant percentage of patients experience hypotension after CPB secondary to peripheral vasodilation. This condition is believed to occur in part because of the systemic inflammatory response to CPB. Therapy for hypotension after cardiac surgery usually includes volume loading and vasopressors. Typical vasopressor agents include norepinephrine and vasopressin in patients with excessive vasodilation. Phenylephrine should be used cautiously because it increases afterload and decreases graft flow.[89]

Contractility. If the adjustments in heart rate, preload, and afterload fail to produce significant improvement in cardiac output, contractility can be enhanced with positive inotropic support or an intraaortic balloon pump (IABP) to augment circulation (discussed later). There is a great deal of variability in the choice of vasoactive agents used with few data guiding decision making. Epinephrine, norepinephrine, dopamine, and dobutamine are commonly used inotropic catecholamines.

Temperature Regulation

Hypothermia can contribute to depressed myocardial contractility, vasoconstriction, and ventricular dysrhythmias in a patient who has undergone cardiac surgery. Hypothermia may also contribute to postoperative bleeding because the functioning of clotting factors is depressed during hypothermia. After surgery, patients may be rewarmed with the use of warm blankets or forced-air warming devices. Excessive temperature elevations must be avoided with the goal of maintaining a target body temperature of 36°C to 37°C (96.8°F to 98.6°F).

Control of Bleeding

Postoperative bleeding from the mediastinal chest tubes can be caused by inadequate hemostasis, disruption of suture lines, or coagulopathy associated with CPB or hypothermia. Blood conservation strategies should be used to limit the number of transfusions, as the administration of packed red blood cells has been independently associated with increased complications and increased mortality.[80] At the present time, blood transfusions are not recommended for a hemoglobin greater than 10 g/dL, but transfusions are reasonable in most postoperative patients whose hemoglobin is less than 7 g/dL.[91]

Although no exact definition exists for excessive bleeding, amounts greater than 200 mL/h often require further interventions. Clotting factors (fresh frozen plasma, fibrinogen, and platelets), protamine, or desmopressin may be administered. Medications used in the treatment of postoperative bleeding are described in Table 15.12. To help guide the selection of appropriate factors or medications, thromboelastography may be used to determine which part of the clotting cycle is deficient. Because blood pressure drives bleeding, the systolic blood pressure should be targeted to no higher than 90 to 100 mm Hg.[86] Using therapeutic positive end-expiratory pressure to reduce excessive postoperative bleeding is not well established.[91] Rewarming the patient reverses the depressed manufacture and release of clotting factors that results from hypothermia. However, persistent mediastinal bleeding—usually greater than 500 mL in 1 hour or 300 mL/h for 2 consecutive hours despite normalization of clotting studies—is an indication for reexploration of the surgical site.

Chest Tube Patency

Chest tube stripping to maintain patency of the tubes is controversial because of the high negative pressure generated by

TABLE 15.12 Medications Used to Treat Postoperative Bleeding

Medication	Dose	Action and Side Effects
Aminocaproic acid (Amicar)	Loading dose: 4–5 g over 1 h, followed by continuous infusion of 1 g/h for 8 h or until bleeding is controlled	Inhibits conversion of plasminogen to plasmin to prevent fibrinolysis, helping to stabilize clots
Desmopressin acetate (DDAVP)	0.3 mcg/kg IV over 20–30 min	Improves platelet function by increasing levels of factor VIII Side effects include facial flushing, tachycardia, headache, and hypotension
Protamine sulfate	25–50 mg IV slowly over 10 min	Neutralizes anticoagulant effect of heparin Can cause hypotension, bradycardia, and allergic reactions

IV, intravenously.

routine methods of stripping. It is believed to result in tissue damage that can contribute to bleeding. This risk must be carefully weighed against the real danger of cardiac tamponade if blood is not effectively drained from around the heart. Chest tube stripping often is advocated in instances of excessive postoperative bleeding. However, the technique of "milking" the chest tubes is advisable for routine postoperative care because this technique generates less negative pressure and decreases the risk of bleeding.

Cardiac Tamponade

Cardiac tamponade is a potentially lethal complication that may occur after surgery if blood accumulates in the mediastinal space, impairing the heart's ability to pump. Signs of tamponade include elevated and equalized filling pressures (eg, central venous pressure, pulmonary artery diastolic pressure, pulmonary artery occlusion pressure), decreased cardiac output, decreased blood pressure, jugular venous distention, pulsus paradoxus, muffled heart sounds, sudden cessation of chest tube drainage, and a widened cardiac silhouette on radiographs. A bedside echocardiogram may be done to confirm tamponade. Interventions for tamponade may include emergency sternotomy in the critical care unit or a return to the operating room for surgical evacuation of the clot.

Pulmonary Care

Mechanical ventilation is used initially to provide adequate alveolar oxygenation and ventilation in the postoperative period. Protocols that facilitate early extubation (less than 6 hours after surgery) have been implemented in most institutions and have been shown to decrease pulmonary complications after cardiac surgery.[88] Early extubation requires a multidisciplinary approach that incorporates anesthesiologists, surgeons, nurses, and respiratory therapists. Potential candidates must be identified before surgery so that the anesthetic regimen supports early extubation.

After surgery, patients are evaluated for hemodynamic stability, adequate control of bleeding, normothermia, and the ability to follow commands. Once these criteria have been met, most institutions have a weaning protocol to follow that often involves a spontaneous breathing trial to evaluate the patient's readiness for extubation. Patients who exhibit hemodynamic instability or intraoperative complications or who have underlying pulmonary disease may require longer periods of mechanical ventilation. After extubation, supplemental oxygen is administered, and patients are medicated for incisional pain to facilitate aggressive pulmonary toilet and early mobility, which is essential to help prevent postoperative complications.[92]

Neurologic Complications

The neurologic dysfunction often seen in patients who have undergone cardiac surgery has been attributed to decreased cerebral perfusion, cerebral microemboli, hypoxia, and the systemic inflammatory response. The dysfunction can range from subtle cognitive changes to signs of acute stroke. The risk of delirium is increased in cardiac surgery patients, especially older adults, and is associated with increased mortality and reduced quality of life and cognitive function.[93,94] Nursing staff can play a critical role in the prevention and recognition of delirium. Nonpharmacologic interventions involve reorienting patients, providing visual and hearing aids, early mobilization, sleep promotion, and judicious use of medications known to potentiate delirium.[95] Pharmacologic treatment of delirium with antipsychotics has little evidence to support its use.[94,96] Liberalization of visitation policies to allow family members a prolonged presence at the bedside is also highly desirable.

Infection

Postoperative fever is common after CPB. However, persistent temperature elevation to greater than 101°F (38.3°C) must be investigated. Sternal wound infections and infective endocarditis are the most devastating infectious complications, but leg wound infections, pneumonia, and urinary tract infections also

can occur. Infection rates are greater in patients with diabetes, malnutrition, chronic diseases, and obesity as well as patients requiring emergent or prolonged surgery. Using a continuous insulin infusion to maintain blood glucose concentrations less than or equal to 180 mg/dL, while avoiding hypoglycemia, may reduce the incidence of adverse events, including deep sternal wound infections.[80]

Acute Kidney Injury

Acute kidney injury is recognized as a significant problem after cardiac surgery because of a very complex pathogenesis. Prevention of acute kidney injury by avoiding renal insults is still the mainstay of management.[97] Kidney dysfunction in the postoperative period requires frequent monitoring of urine output and serum creatinine levels. Because of fluid retention, diuresis is often required to help mobilize fluids from the interstitial to the intravascular space and may be done with the administration of medications or may be allowed to occur naturally. The patient's potassium levels may be depleted with the diuresis, requiring that levels be closely monitored and replaced.

Guidelines for Coronary Artery Bypass Graft Surgery

The American College of Cardiology and the American Heart Association have developed a set of clinical practice guidelines for care of patients undergoing CABG surgery.[80] These guidelines are designed to support clinical decision making with research evidence (Box 15.19).

Patient Education

Patient education includes information related to the surgical procedure, risk factor management, and prevention of atherosclerosis. Patients who have undergone valve surgery may also require information regarding the need for antibiotic prophylaxis before invasive procedures and specific instructions pertaining to their anticoagulation regimen (Box 15.20).

QSEN　BOX 15.19　QSEN: Evidence-Based Practice

Coronary Artery Bypass Graft Surgery

A summary is provided of evidence and evidence-based review recommendations for management of patients undergoing coronary artery bypass graft (CABG) surgery.

Strong Evidence to Support the Following
Coronary Artery Bypass Graft Surgery for Patients

- Emergency CABG surgery is indicated for patients with acute myocardial infarction (MI) when primary percutaneous coronary intervention (PCI) has failed or cannot be performed, coronary anatomy is suitable for CABG surgery, and persistent ischemia and/or hemodynamic instability refractory to nonsurgical therapy is present.
- Emergency CABG surgery is indicated for patients undergoing surgical repair of postinfarction mechanical complications of MI, patients with cardiogenic shock, or patients with life-threatening ventricular dysrhythmias in the presence of left main stenosis or three-vessel coronary artery disease (CAD).
- CABG surgery is indicated for patients undergoing noncoronary cardiac surgery if 50% or greater stenosis of left main or 70% or greater stenosis of other major coronary arteries.
- CABG surgery is indicated for patients with significant (50% or greater) stenosis of left main coronary artery.
- CABG surgery is indicated for patients with significant (70% or greater) stenosis in three major coronary arteries or in the proximal left anterior descending (LAD) artery plus one other major coronary artery.

- CABG surgery or PCI is indicated in patients with one or more significant (70% or greater) coronary artery stenoses with unacceptable angina despite guideline-directed medical therapy.
- Patients undergoing CABG surgery who have at least moderate aortic stenosis should undergo aortic valve replacement.
- Patients undergoing CABG surgery who have severe ischemic mitral valve regurgitation not likely to resolve with revascularization should undergo mitral valve repair or replacement.

Anesthetic Considerations

- Anesthetic management should be directed toward early postoperative extubation and accelerated recovery of low-risk to medium-risk patients.

Bypass Graft Conduits

- If possible, the left internal mammary artery (LIMA) should be used to bypass the LAD artery.

Antiplatelet Therapy

- Aspirin should be administered preoperatively, if not previously prescribed, initiated within 6 h postoperatively and continued indefinitely.
- In elective cases, clopidogrel and ticagrelor should be discontinued 5 days before surgery, and prasugrel should be discontinued for at least 7 days.

QSEN BOX 15.19 **QSEN: Evidence-Based Practice—cont'd**

Coronary Artery Bypass Graft Surgery

Management of Hyperlipidemia
- All patients should receive statin therapy unless contraindicated.

Blood Glucose Management
- Continuous intravenous insulin is administered to maintain early postoperative blood glucose concentration 180 mg/dL or less, while avoiding hypoglycemia to reduce adverse events.

Dysrhythmia Management
- Beta-blockers should be administered for at least 24 h before CABG surgery, reinstituted as soon as possible after surgery, and prescribed at discharge unless contraindicated to reduce the incidence and clinical sequelae of atrial fibrillation.

Angiotensin-Converting Enzyme Inhibitors and Angiotensin Receptor Blockers
- Angiotensin-converting enzyme inhibitors and angiotensin receptor blockers should be instituted or restarted postoperatively and continued indefinitely for patients with left ventricular ejection fraction (LVEF) 40% or less, hypertension, diabetes, or chronic kidney disease.

Smoking Cessation
- All patients who smoke should receive educational counseling and be offered smoking cessation therapy during hospitalization for CABG surgery.

Cardiac Rehabilitation
- Cardiac rehabilitation should be offered to all eligible patients after CABG surgery.

Reduction in Risk of Infection
- Antibiotics should be administered preoperatively in all patients to reduce the risk of postoperative infection.

Bleeding and Transfusions
- Aggressive attempts at blood conservation are indicated to reduce the need for red blood cell transfusions.

Moderate Evidence to Support the Following
Coronary Artery Bypass Graft Surgery for Patients
- CABG surgery is indicated in patients with multivessel CAD with recurrent angina or MI within the first 48 h of ST segment elevation MI presentation as an alternative to a more delayed strategy.
- CABG surgery or PCI is indicated for selected patients age 75 y or older with ST segment elevation or left bundle branch block who are suitable for revascularization regardless of the time interval from MI to the onset of shock.
- Emergency CABG surgery is indicated after failed PCI to retrieve a foreign body in a crucial anatomic location or for hemodynamic compromise in patients with impairment of the coagulation system and without previous sternotomy
- CABG surgery is indicated in patients with significant (70% or greater) stenosis in two major coronary arteries with extensive myocardial ischemia or target vessels supplying a large area of viable myocardium.
- CABG surgery is indicated in patients with mild to moderate left ventricular systolic dysfunction (LVEF 35% to 50%) and significant (70% or greater stenosis) multivessel CAD or proximal LAD stenosis with viable myocardium present.
- CABG surgery is indicated in patients with complex three-vessel CAD (SYNTAX score greater than 22) with or without involvement of the proximal LAD artery who are good candidates for CABG surgery.

- CABG surgery is preferred over PCI to improve survival in patients with multivessel CAD and diabetes mellitus, particularly if a LIMA graft can be anastomosed to the LAD artery.
- Patients undergoing CABG surgery who have moderate ischemic mitral valve regurgitation not likely to resolve with revascularization should undergo mitral valve repair or replacement.

Hybrid Coronary Revascularization
- The planned combination of LIMA-to-LAD artery grafting and PCI of one or more non-LAD coronary arteries is reasonable for (1) limitations to CABG surgery such as heavily calcified proximal aorta or poor target vessels for CABG surgery, (2) lack of suitable graft conduits, and (3) unfavorable LAD artery for PCI.

Antiplatelet Therapy
- Clopidogrel 75 mg daily is a reasonable alternative in patients who cannot take aspirin.

Beta-Blockers
- Preoperative beta-blockers, particularly in patients with an ejection fraction greater than 30%, can reduce the risk of in-hospital mortality.
- Preoperative beta-blockers can reduce the incidence of perioperative myocardial ischemia.

Emotional Dysfunction and Psychosocial Considerations
- Cognitive-behavioral therapy or collaborative care for patients with clinical depression after CABG surgery can be beneficial to reduce objective measures of depression.

Carotid Artery Disease
- For patients with a previous transient ischemic attack or stroke and significant (50% to 99%) carotid artery stenosis, carotid revascularization should be considered in conjunction with CABG surgery. Sequence and timing (staged or simultaneous) should be determined by the relative magnitude of cerebral and myocardial dysfunction.

Infection Prevention
- Leukocyte-filtered blood can be useful to reduce the rate of overall perioperative infection and in-hospital death.

Adjuncts to Myocardial Protection
- Insertion of an intraaortic balloon pump is reasonable to reduce the mortality rate in patients undergoing CABG surgery who are considered to be at high risk (eg, LVEF less than 30% or left main CAD).
- Assessment of cardiac biomarkers in the first 24 h after CABG surgery may be considered.

Dysrhythmia Management
- For patients who cannot take beta-blockers, amiodarone is an alternative to reduce the incidence of postoperative atrial fibrillation.
- Digoxin and nondihydropyridine calcium channel blockers can be useful to control the ventricular rate in the setting of atrial fibrillation but are not indicated for prophylaxis.

Reference
Hillis LD, et al. 2011 ACCF/AHA guideline for coronary artery bypass graft surgery: Executive summary: A report of the American College of Cardiology Foundation/American Heart Association Task Force on Practice Guidelines. *Circulation.* 2011;124(23):2610.

Technical Advances

Minimally Invasive Cardiac Surgery

Continuously evolving techniques have expanded the options for patients undergoing cardiac surgery, with a general transition from surgical to minimally invasive (minithoracotomy and small port) therapies along with percutaneous approaches. Replacement or repair of the mitral valve via a small right thoracotomy, a "mini-mitral," is one of the most common minimally invasive cardiac surgeries.[98] Minimally invasive direct coronary artery bypass graft surgery and endoscopic coronary artery bypass both use a small left anterior thoracotomy for off-pump bypass of the left anterior descending artery with left internal mammary artery. Development of robotic surgical technology now allows surgeons to view computer-enhanced images while manipulating instruments through a totally endoscopic port-only approach using robotic arms. This approach has been especially popular for mitral valve procedures but can also be used for CABG surgery.[99] Hybrid operating rooms allow for coronary revascularization by combining catheter-based procedures with surgical interventions to treat CAD, with the idea of capitalizing on the benefits of each. Minimally invasive procedures have many of the same patient complications as conventional methods do but with a few modifications. Rib retraction can cause significant pain issues, single lung ventilation can lead to increased atelectasis, and femoral access for perfusion can lead to an increase in the incidence of lower leg ischemia; because of the small incisions that complicate intraoperative hemostasis, concern for bleeding should have a lower threshold.[86]

Surgical Treatment of Cardiac Dysrhythmias

Several surgical techniques have been developed for the control of refractory AF with the goal of maintaining sinus rhythm. These techniques are usually performed on patients who need open heart surgery for another reason, such as a CABG or valve replacement procedure. The Cox-Maze procedure involves a series of scars that are made in the atrial tissue to create an electrical maze that disrupts the reentrant pathways and directs the sinus impulse through the AV node. The procedure also includes surgical isolation of the pulmonary veins, which are thought to be responsible for initiation of AF, and removal of the left and right atrial appendages. The goal of treatment is not only to prevent the recurrence of atrial tachydysrhythmias but also to restore sinus rhythm and AV synchrony, if possible. The Cox-Maze procedure is the gold standard for the surgical treatment of AF.[100] Catheter ablation during cardiac surgery may use RF energy or less often cryoablation and microwave energy, as it is faster and easier than the "cut-and-sew" surgical maze procedure. Modifications of the procedure have led to less invasive thoracoscopic versions performed off-pump. Patients require continued monitoring for arrhythmias, as AF is common for months afterward while the scar tissue fully matures. If the sinus node is no longer functioning, a pacemaker may be implanted to restore an AV sequential rhythm. Even after successful treatment of AF with the surgical approach, long-term anticoagulation is required in many patients.[100]

Although future trends in the surgical management of cardiac disease are difficult to predict, the critical care nurse must continue to be prepared to meet the challenge of providing a high level of nursing management at the bedside. A solid knowledge base and keen assessment skills are prerequisites for the accurate anticipation of problems and prompt intervention necessary to stabilize the patient and prevent the occurrence of life-threatening complications.

MECHANICAL CIRCULATORY SUPPORT

Mechanical circulatory support (MCS) is used in the treatment of heart failure when conventional pharmacologic therapy has proved ineffective. The primary goals of MCS are to decrease myocardial workload and maintain adequate perfusion to vital organs. If the acute heart failure is reversible, a short duration of ventricular assistance is used to allow the myocardium time to recover. If the condition is irreversible, MCS may be used as a bridge to heart transplantation for qualified candidates or as destination therapy for patients who have no other surgical options.

Intraaortic Balloon Pump

The IABP is the most commonly used temporary percutaneous left ventricular assist device (LVAD) for supporting failing circulation (Box 15.21). The evidence for many of the long

---

✳ BOX 15.20 PATIENT EDUCATION PLAN

Open Heart Surgery

Before discharge, the patient should be able to teach back the following topics:

- Pathophysiology of disease (coronary artery or valvular disease)
- Risk factor modification to prevent coronary artery disease (smoking cessation, regular exercise, weight loss)
- Postoperative incisional care
- Activity limitations (no lifting, pushing, or pulling anything heavier than 10 lb for 6 to 8 weeks; no driving for 6 to 8 weeks)
- Recommended exercise progression after surgery
- Recommended diet after surgery
- Information regarding prescribed medications (including prescribed pain medication)
- Anticipated mood changes after surgery
- Follow-up appointment for clinic or primary physician
- Additional information for patients with valve procedures
- Symptoms of endocarditis
- Antibiotic prophylaxis before invasive procedures
- Information regarding anticoagulant therapy and follow-up

BOX 15.21 Indications for Use of Intra-Aortic Balloon Pump

- Failure to wean from cardiopulmonary bypass
- Unstable angina refractory to medications
- Recurrent angina after acute myocardial infarction (MI)
- Hemodynamic support for high-risk percutaneous coronary intervention and coronary artery bypass graft surgery
- Complications of acute MI
  - Cardiogenic shock
  - Papillary muscle dysfunction or rupture with mitral regurgitation
  - Ventricular septal rupture
- Refractory ventricular dysrhythmias
- Septic shock
- Bridge to definitive therapy: Cardiac transplantation or ventricular assist device

accepted indications continues to be reevaluated to establish which clinical settings would be advantageous to use IABP.[101-105] The intraaortic balloon (IAB) catheter consists of a single, sausage-shaped polyurethane balloon that is wrapped around the distal end of a vascular catheter and positioned in the descending thoracic aorta just distal to the takeoff of the left subclavian artery. "Counterpulsation" is the key mechanism for the IABP. Its therapeutic effects are based on the hemodynamic principles of diastolic augmentation and afterload reduction (Box 15.22).

Initially, as the balloon is inflated in diastole concurrent with aortic valve closure, the blood in the aortic arch above the level of the balloon is displaced retrograde (backward) toward the aortic root, augmenting diastolic coronary arterial blood flow and increasing myocardial oxygen supply (Fig. 15.20A). The blood volume in the aorta below the level of the balloon is propelled forward toward the peripheral vascular system, which may enhance systemic perfusion. Subsequently, the deflation of the balloon just before the opening of the aortic valve creates a potential space or vacuum in the aorta, toward which blood flows unimpeded during ventricular ejection (Fig. 15.20B). This decreased resistance to LV ejection, or decreased afterload, facilitates ventricular emptying and reduces myocardial oxygen demands. The overall physiologic effect of IABP therapy is an improvement in the balance between myocardial oxygen supply and demand. Contraindications to IABP include aortic aneurysm, significant aortic valve insufficiency, and severe peripheral vascular disease.[106,107]

Medical Management

The IAB may be inserted in the operating room, the cardiac catheterization laboratory, or the critical care unit. The IAB catheter is usually inserted percutaneously through the femoral artery and advanced to the correct position in the descending thoracic aorta. The physician may insert the balloon through an introducer sheath or perform a sheathless insertion to minimize the degree of vessel occlusion created by the catheter. If percutaneous catheter placement is not feasible, the catheter may be placed through surgical cutdown or by a direct thoracic approach. After insertion, the balloon is attached to the console and filled with the prescribed volume of helium, and pumping is initiated.

Nursing Management

The management of the pumping console and its timing functions may be performed by the nurse caring for the patient or delegated to specially trained personnel. Multiple factors may affect the efficacy of the IABP including position of the balloon within the aorta; balloon displacement volume; inflation and deflation timing; signal quality; the patient's cardiac function; and hemodynamic variables, which include circulating blood volume, blood pressure, and vascular resistance.[108] Clinicians need to be aware of these factors to adequately assess for and ensure optimal IABP performance.

Balloon Catheter Position

The balloon catheter must be maintained in proper position to optimize its effectiveness and minimize complications. The balloon may migrate proximally and occlude the left subclavian artery or the carotids, or it may move distally, compromising renal and mesenteric circulation. Careful assessment of the left radial pulse, level of consciousness, urinary output, and gastrointestinal symptoms is essential. Measures to prevent accidental displacement of the balloon catheter include ensuring that the IAB is secured to the patient's skin, that the patient maintains complete bed rest with the head of the bed elevated no more than 30 degrees, and that any flexion of the involved hip is avoided.

BOX 15.22 Physiologic Effects of Intraaortic Balloon Pump

Increased
- Coronary blood flow
- Cardiac output
- Urine output
- Improved mentation

Decreased
- Signs of myocardial ischemia: Angina, ST segment changes, ventricular dysrhythmias
- Afterload
- Preload
- Myocardial oxygen demand
- Pulmonary congestion
- Heart rate

Balloon inflated

Balloon deflated

A

B

FIG. 15.20 Mechanisms of Action of Intraaortic Balloon Pump. (A) Diastolic balloon inflation augments coronary blood flow. (B) Systolic balloon deflation decreases afterload.

Timing

The IABP depends on proper timing to ensure optimal hemodynamic benefits.[109] Although systems now adjust the timing automatically, clinicians must still be aware of how to set the timing, understand the method used, and evaluate its effects. The ECG and arterial pressure tracings are constantly monitored to verify the timing and effect of balloon counterpulsation (Fig. 15.21). For counterpulsation to occur, the pump must receive a trigger signal to identify the beginning and end of the cardiac cycle. The trigger can be the R wave of the ECG, the upstroke of the arterial pressure waveform, or a pacemaker spike.[106]

Dysrhythmias

Dysrhythmias can adversely affect the timing of balloon inflation and deflation, so rhythm disturbances must be detected and treated promptly. Current IABPs have automatic timing features that use internal algorithms to adjust inflation and deflation in response to changes in the patient's heart rate or rhythm. Catheters are also available that incorporate a fiberoptic sensor to enhance the quality of the arterial waveform, which allows beat-to-beat adjustments to improve timing accuracy.

Vascular Complications

One complication of IABP support is lower extremity ischemia resulting from occlusion of the femoral artery by the catheter itself or by emboli caused by thrombus formation on the balloon (see Box 15.15). Although ischemic complications have decreased with sheathless insertion techniques and the introduction of smaller balloon catheters (7 Fr vs 9.5 Fr), evaluation of peripheral circulation remains an important nursing assessment. The presence and quality of peripheral pulses distal to the catheter insertion site are assessed frequently, along with color, temperature, and capillary refill of the involved extremity. Signs of diminished perfusion must be reported immediately. Anticoagulation (eg, heparin infusion) may be prescribed to decrease the incidence of thrombosis. Other vascular complications associated with IABP include acute aortic dissection and the development of pseudoaneurysms at the catheter insertion site.

Balloon Perforation

Another potential complication of IABP therapy is balloon perforation. Perforation occurs because of repeated contact of the balloon membrane with calcified plaque in the aorta as the balloon inflates and deflates. The patient is monitored for evidence of a balloon leak, such as a gas leak alarm from the pump console or the presence of blood in the IAB tubing. If a balloon leak is detected, pumping is stopped, and the physician is immediately notified so that the balloon can be removed. If the balloon is not promptly removed or pumping is attempted after the perforation, the IAB may become entrapped as the blood hardens within the catheter, creating a mass. If this occurs, the balloon must be surgically removed.

Preventing Further Complications

Log rolling, in which the patient is moved from side to side every 2 hours, is used to maintain skin integrity and to prevent pulmonary atelectasis. Because thrombocytopenia may occur as a result of mechanical destruction of the platelets by the pumping action of the balloon, platelet counts are closely monitored, and the patient is observed for evidence of bleeding. Because infection of the insertion site is a potential complication, the dressing is changed in accordance with the hospital policy for other invasive lines.

Psychologic Needs

The psychologic needs of the patient on IABP therapy must be considered. Sleep deprivation is common and is related in part to the continuous nursing management requirements for the patient and the noise level in the unit, including the sounds made by the balloon pumping device. Anxiety related to fear of nonrecovery and loss of control because of forced immobility is common.

Weaning

Weaning from the IABP is considered after hemodynamic stability has been achieved with no—or only minimal—pharmacologic support. Weaning is accomplished by reducing the ratio of augmented to nonaugmented beats from 1:1 to 1:2 or 1:3 as tolerated. Another, less common weaning method involves a gradual decrease in balloon volume. To prevent thrombus formation on the balloon surface, the IABP must remain at a minimal pumping ratio (or volume) until its removal.

Patient Education

Patient education for a patient with an IAB is presented in Box 15.23. Many IABP manufacturers provide helpful educational booklets designed for patients and families.

Temporary Mechanical Circulatory Support Devices

If unable to correct perfusion derangements with IABP insertion, if an IABP is contraindicated, or if the patient is too unstable to attempt an IABP placement, alternative MCS strategies should be employed. Several temporary ventricular assist device (VAD) systems are available including pneumatic pumps, axial flow pumps, and centrifugal pumps

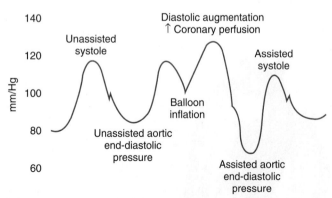

FIG. 15.21 Timing and Effect of Balloon Counterpulsations. Timing is adjusted by synchronizing balloon inflation with the dicrotic notch on the arterial waveform, resulting in an elevated diastolic pressure. Inflation is maintained throughout diastole to augment coronary perfusion. Deflation occurs just before the next systole, resulting in a reduced systolic pressure and decreased afterload.

BOX 15.23   PATIENT EDUCATION PLAN

Intraaortic Balloon Pump

The patient should be able to teach back the following topics:
- Description of an intraaortic balloon pump and how it works
- Activity restrictions (minimize leg movement)
- Symptoms to report to the health care professional (pain in the back, leg, or chest)

(Table 15.13). With no specific data to guide device selection, it is primarily a choice of the surgeon and institution. Many VADs cannot be placed in the intensive care unit, which limits how quickly therapy can be initiated. Another consideration is that many VADs provide only single ventricular support, which would necessitate a second device in the setting of biventricular failure.

Extracorporeal Membrane Oxygenation System

Mechanical cardiopulmonary support is termed *extracorporeal membrane oxygenation* (ECMO) and is being used with increasing frequency in critical care units to treat refractory cardiogenic shock and failure to wean from CPB. There are two types of ECMO—venoarterial and venovenous. Both types provide respiratory support, but only venoarterial ECMO provides hemodynamic support. Venoarterial ECMO can be initiated quickly at the bedside by either a direct right atrial cannulation (via a preexisting sternotomy) or peripherally using a percutaneous technique (Fig. 15.22). Once the patient is connected to the ECMO circuit and hemodynamic parameters are satisfactory, vasoactive drugs can be weaned to minimal levels to allow the myocardium to rest. Anticoagulation is required for most venoarterial ECMO support because of the risk of venous and arterial thromboembolization. However, consideration must also be given to the fact that bleeding is the most common complication, often requiring transfusions after placement.[110] Staff must be highly trained to maintain the ECMO circuit and monitor for other complications such as cardiac tamponade, multiorgan failure, sepsis, limb ischemia, and pulmonary complications. Major limitations of ECMO include its limited availability, short duration of usage, required support of highly trained personnel, and complications related to vascular access.[101] Once evidence of cardiac function has returned, weaning trials can be conducted to assess if the patient can be maintained with conventional support.

Long-Term Ventricular Assist Devices

The VAD is designed to support or replace a failing natural heart with flow assistance. Newer generation continuous-flow VADs have taken the place of first-generation pulsatile-flow VADs because of their small size and superior survival rates, which rival survival rates of cardiac transplant.[111,112]

VADs are currently indicated for three types of clinical applications. The first category of patients includes patients who continue to demonstrate persistent heart failure despite aggressive medical therapy but who have the potential for regaining normal heart function if the heart is given time to rest. This category, called *bridge to recovery*, consists of patients who have acute postsurgical myocardial dysfunction, are in refractory cardiogenic shock after acute MI, or have acute viral myocarditis. The second category, called *bridge to transplantation*, includes patients with decompensated chronic heart failure who need circulatory support until heart transplantation can be performed. The third category, called *destination therapy*, includes patients with severe heart failure who are not candidates for heart transplantation and for whom all other medical options have been exhausted. Several VADs have received FDA approval for destination therapy or bridge to transplant, and many other devices are in clinical trials.

TABLE 15.13 Ventricular Assist Devices		
Type	**Indications**	**Description**
Temporary		
CentriMag	Short-term univentricular or biventricular support	Continuous-flow pump that produces blood flow from 0–10 L/min.
		Blood flow is produced by rotation of a magnetically suspended impeller, eliminating contact between components.
		Placed either through an open chest or by percutaneous methods.
Impella LP 2.5 and Impella LP 5.0	Short-term left ventricular support	Continuous-flow pump that has a percutaneously inserted catheter, allowing flows of 2.5 L/min or 5 L/min for the version that requires a surgical cutdown for implantation.
		The catheter is placed retrograde across the aortic valve to pull blood from the left ventricle, which is returned to ascending aorta.
TandemHeart	Short-term left or right ventricular support	Percutaneously inserted device that provides continuous flow up to 5 L/min.
		LVAD: Inflow is obtained from a catheter positioned in the left atrium (by a transseptal approach), and outflow is through the femoral artery.
		RVAD: Inflow is obtained from a catheter positioned in the right atrium, and outflow is through the pulmonary artery.
		Device allows for transport to a center for long-term therapy.
Long-Term		
HeartWare	Long-term left ventricular support as bridge to transplantation or destination therapy	A continuous flow rotary pump with centrifugal design that produces nonpulsatile flow.
	FDA approved for bridge to transplant	Its small size allows for placement above the diaphragm in the pericardial space.
		The pump has no points of mechanical contact, which reduces damage to red blood cells.
HeartMate II	Long-term left ventricular support	An electrically driven rotary pump that produces nonpulsatile flow
	FDA approved for bridge to transplantation and destination therapy	Smaller size allows for implantation in patients with body surface area <1.5 m².
		Anticoagulation and antiplatelet therapy are required.

FDA, US Food and Drug Administration; *LVAD,* left ventricular assist device; *RVAD,* right ventricular assist device.

Central Venous to Arterial ECMO Circuit

Return cannula

Drainage cannula

Oxygenator

Pump

Ascending aorta

Right atrium

Inferior vena cava

Descending aorta

A

Peripheral Venous to Arterial ECMO Circuit

Oxygenator

Pump

Inferior vena cava

Femoral artery

Femoral vein

Drainage cannula

B

Return cannula

FIG. 15.22 Extracorporeal Membrane Oxygenation (ECMO): Central (A) and peripheral (B) placement of an extracorporeal membrane oxygenation (ECMO) circuit. (Modified from Hung M et al. Extracorporeal membrane oxygenation coming to an ICU near you. *Journal of the Intensive Care Society.* 13(1):2012;12(1):31-38.)

There is no single ideal system, so device selection is based on individual VAD capabilities and institutional preference (see Table 15.13). All devices consist of a blood pump, cannula, controller, and some type of power source. Percutaneous VADs allow for rapid, minimally invasive, short-term support for patients in cardiogenic shock until recovery occurs or a long-term device can be placed (Fig. 15.23). Implantable MCS is used for bridge to transplant or destination therapy.[101,105] An LVAD is used most commonly because LV failure occurs more often than RV failure (Fig. 15.24). Use of biventricular support may be needed in the acute phase because RV failure often follows LV failure.[111] Inlet cannulas that divert blood from the heart to the LVAD for LV support are placed in the left atrium or the LV apex, with the outlet cannula attached to the ascending aorta or femoral artery. For the right VAD, the inlet cannula would be placed on the right side with the outlet cannula in the pulmonary artery. An additional option for biventricular failure is the total artificial heart, which can be used for bridge to transplant.[101] Flow rates between 1 and 10 L/min are used by the different devices to maintain adequate cardiac output while decreasing ventricular workload.

FIG. 15.23 Impella Ventricular Assist Device. Blood is pulled into the catheter from the left ventricle and returned to the ascending aorta.

FIG. 15.24 Left Ventricular Assist Device (LVAD) System.

Nursing Management

Nursing diagnoses and management for a patient with a VAD include monitoring for hemodynamic changes and for complications related to the device. The same interventions that are used for cardiac surgery patients to optimize cardiac output by manipulation of heart rate, preload, afterload, and contractility apply to patients with a VAD. Adequate filling volumes are essential to maintain pump flow. Afterload reduction may be needed to improve output from the unassisted ventricle when univentricular support is used. Although complication rates vary among the different models, complications common to all types of VADs include bleeding, infection, thromboembolism, heart failure, arrhythmias,

---

and device failure.[104,111] On physical examination, patients with continuous-flow VADs may not have palpable pulses; this can make measurement of blood pressure difficult and will require an invasive arterial catheter for the initial postoperative period. An occlusive pressure obtained by Doppler at the brachial artery is the best reflection of mean arterial pressure.[111,113] Arterial blood gas analysis may be required because pulse oximetry may be unreliable with little or no pulse.[111] Nurses must often rely on basic assessments such as circulation, mentation, and urine output to determine if the patient is receiving adequate support.

Device Failure

Although the incidence of device failure continues to decrease, it is a life-threatening event because of the nature of this therapy. VAD designs vary considerably, and troubleshooting methods for device failure are unique to each device. The nurse must be aware of signs of device malfunction as well as patient factors (volume status, dysrhythmias, RV failure) that may affect VAD function.

Anticoagulation

Anticoagulation protocols vary with the device, individual patient, and institution. Both antiplatelet agents and warfarin are commonly used. Although bleeding is the most frequent complication, thrombotic events can also be a problem leading to stroke and device failure.[111] Coagulation studies must be frequently monitored during support.

Infection

Patients with a VAD are at considerable risk for localized and septicemic infections. Infectious risks are posed by the presence of invasive catheters and the surgically implanted VAD. Infection is prevented by the use of strict aseptic technique with all invasive tubing and dressing changes. Site care varies, depending on institutional protocols and the type of VAD that is used. Nurses monitor patients for infection by measuring temperatures, inspecting insertion sites and incisions, and obtaining daily leukocyte counts. If an infection is suspected, pan-cultures (blood, urine, and sputum) are taken to guide appropriate antibiotic therapy.

Patient Education

The rapid and acute nature of cardiogenic shock limits the nurse's ability to prepare patients and families for VAD insertion. Despite the critical nature of the illness, nurses explain the reason for the use of the VAD and provide information about the critical care environment and equipment (Box 15.24). The number of patients with VADs discharged to home continues to increase. These patients and their families require education related to care of the device and reinforcement on the components of heart failure management.

VASCULAR SURGERY

Vascular surgery may be used as a treatment for arterial occlusive disease or to correct structural abnormalities such as aneurysms. With the evolution in endovascular technology, many patients with vascular disease can now be effectively treated with percutaneous procedures. The choice between an open surgical procedure and an endovascular intervention depends on many factors, including the type and location of the vascular lesion, life expectancy, comorbid conditions, and patient preference. Because atherosclerosis is a diffuse disease that affects both the peripheral vessels and the coronary arteries, patients undergoing arterial vascular surgery are at high risk for perioperative cardiac events. The nursing care of patients after vascular surgery focuses not only on observations for surgical complications such as hematoma or reocclusion but also on prompt recognition and appropriate treatment of complications that may arise from the impact of the procedure on preexisting cardiac, pulmonary, or kidney disease.

Carotid Endarterectomy

Carotid endarterectomy may be beneficial in both symptomatic and asymptomatic patients with stenoses greater than 50% to 70% at low risk for surgical perioperative complications.[114,115] The procedure is performed through a neck incision that allows for visualization of the vessel. The plaque is removed, and the vessel is closed directly or with a patch composed of saphenous vein or a prosthetic material. A Jackson-Pratt drain may be placed at the end of the procedure to minimize hematoma formation. Complications after carotid endarterectomy include perioperative MI, cerebral ischemia or infarction, bleeding, and cranial nerve damage.

Postoperative Nursing Management

Patients require 12 to 24 hours of intensive nursing assessment in the period immediately after carotid endarterectomy. Complications are rare but may be life-threatening and require rapid intervention. Serial assessments are performed, and the surgeon is promptly notified of significant changes in the patient's status.

Neurologic Assessment

Frequent neurologic assessments are performed as the patient awakens from anesthesia and then hourly for the first 12 hours. These assessments should include level of consciousness, orientation, pupil response, motor function, and evaluation of cranial nerve function (eg, swallowing or gag reflexes, hoarseness, tongue movement, facial drooping). Compression, traction, or inadvertent severing can damage nerves that lie in or near the surgical field. The most common injuries are damage to the laryngeal and hypoglossal nerves. Most cranial nerve dysfunction resolves within a short time.[116]

Bleeding

Bleeding is assessed by observation of the dressing for drainage or swelling and measurement of output from the neck drain, if present. If hematoma formation occurs internally, it may impinge on the trachea, so the patient is also monitored for signs of a compromised airway. In addition to monitoring respiratory rate and oxygen saturation, the nurse assesses the patient for tracheal deviation and for symptoms of upper airway obstruction such as stridor or wheezing. A small venous hematoma may respond to manual pressure, but larger arterial hematomas that expand rapidly require emergent return to the operating room for reexploration and evacuation.

Cardiovascular Monitoring

Continuous ECG monitoring with ST segment monitoring is used to detect myocardial ischemia after carotid endarterectomy. Bradycardia is common as a result of baroreceptor stimulation during the operative procedure but is usually hemodynamically tolerated as long as the patient's blood pressure is adequate. Manipulation of the carotid bulb during surgery often results in hemodynamic instability in the immediate postoperative period. An arterial line is usually placed to allow for prompt detection and treatment of hypotension or hypertension. Adequate blood pressure control in the postoperative period is of paramount importance. Hypertension increases the risk of bleeding at the suture line and is typically treated with short-acting vasodilators such as sodium nitroprusside. Relative hypotension compared with the patient's baseline value results in inadequate cerebral perfusion and potential neurologic deficits, so vasopressors such as phenylephrine may be used to maintain an adequate blood pressure.

Carotid Stents

Although carotid endarterectomy has been the gold standard for treatment of patients with significant carotid artery stenosis, carotid stent placement is increasingly used as an alternative.[117] This procedure is performed with the use of local anesthesia and percutaneous cannulation similar to that used in coronary stent placement. The use of embolic protection devices to trap and remove embolic particles generated during the procedure improves neurologic outcomes.[117] Clinical trials have demonstrated equivalent outcomes between the two procedures in symptomatic patients and improved outcomes with the use of stents in asymptomatic patients.[118]

Nursing care of patients after carotid stent placement is similar to care provided after carotid endarterectomy. Patients require intensive nursing for a brief time to allow for frequent neurologic assessments and treatment of hemodynamic instability.[119] Patients are also monitored for potential complications related to vascular access sheaths.

Abdominal Aortic Aneurysm Repair

An abdominal aortic aneurysm is usually repaired when endovascular stent placement is not an option; the aneurysm is 5 cm or larger, causing symptoms, or rapidly expanding. Repair is done to prevent the high mortality associated with abdominal aneurysm rupture. Repair involves insertion of a prosthetic graft to support the portion of the vessel weakened by the aneurysm. Graft placement is done via either an open surgical procedure or a less invasive endovascular approach.

Surgical Repair

Surgery is performed with the patient under general anesthesia and involves access through a midline abdominal incision or a flank incision (retroperitoneal approach). Clamping of the aorta proximal and distal to the dilated area isolates the aneurysm. The aneurysmal portion of the aorta is replaced with a prosthetic graft, which is then enclosed within the aneurysmal sac.

Postoperative complications include myocardial ischemia or infarction, bleeding, acute kidney injury, and distal embolization.[120] Rarely, colon or spinal cord ischemia may occur because of interruption of blood flow during aortic cross-clamping or embolization. After the surgical procedure, patients are monitored in the critical care unit for 24 to 48 hours with a total hospital length of stay of approximately 5 days.

Postoperative Management

Nursing assessment of vital signs and assessment of peripheral perfusion are performed frequently in the early postoperative period. Continuous ECG monitoring with ST segment analysis is used to detect myocardial ischemia. An arterial line is placed to allow for prompt detection and treatment of hypotension or hypertension. Hypertension increases the risk of bleeding at the suture lines and is often treated with short-acting vasodilators such as sodium nitroprusside. Hypotension may result in compromised perfusion to organs or the extremities and is treated with volume replacement and vasopressors as needed. Hourly assessment of urine output is performed to evaluate kidney function. If urine output is less than 30 mL/h, diuretics may be used after correction of hypovolemia. The dressing is assessed for bleeding, and potential signs of internal hemorrhage from the graft site (hypotension, complaints of back pain) are further evaluated with serial hematocrit measurements. Patients without preoperative pulmonary conditions may be rapidly weaned from ventilatory support, with supplemental oxygen given as needed to maintain oxygen saturation in the normal range.

Endovascular Stent Grafts

Endoluminal placement of stent grafts provides a less invasive approach for repair of an abdominal aortic aneurysm. In this procedure, a sutureless vascular graft is implanted into the abdominal aorta through a femoral arteriotomy. The stent isolates the aneurysmal wall from intraluminal blood pressure to prevent further expansion or rupture of the aneurysm. This procedure can be performed with the patient under epidural anesthesia with minimal blood loss and a shorter length of stay. Initially introduced as an alternative for patients who would otherwise be deemed inoperable because of comorbid conditions, this procedure is now performed in most elective cases.[121] Although the operative mortality and morbidity may be less with endovascular stents, randomized studies have shown no significant difference in long-term survival between open surgical and endovascular interventions in patients with abdominal aortic aneurysm.[122] In addition, follow-up surveillance is essential after stent placement because late complications such as endoleak and device migration can occur, necessitating reintervention.[123]

Peripheral Vascular Procedures

Arteriosclerosis obliterans is a condition in which atherosclerosis produces progressive obstruction of medium to large arteries. These lesions commonly occur at bifurcations of the abdominal aorta and the iliac, femoral, popliteal or tibial, and peroneal arteries. Progression of peripheral artery disease can lead to critical limb ischemia. This condition may initially manifest as intermittent claudication, but if left untreated, it can progress to rest pain, ulceration, or even gangrene. Initial treatment focuses on lifestyle modification, such as smoking cessation, exercise therapy, adequate diabetic control, effective treatment of hypertension, and management of dyslipidemia. Pharmacologic interventions such as antiplatelet and antithrombotic agents may be used. If these strategies fail, patients may be considered for revascularization via surgical bypass or a percutaneous intervention (angioplasty, atherectomy, or stent placement). Regardless of the type of procedure selected, inflow is always established first—through repair of vascular defects that compromise flow into the femoral vessels. If symptoms persist, this is followed by repair of outflow lesions in vessels in the lower leg.[124]

Because there are many endovascular and surgical options available for the treatment of peripheral artery disease, treatment decisions can be complicated. The risks of the procedure need to be weighed against the anticipated benefits including long-term patency and options for further treatment if needed. Consensus guidelines have been issued that include treatment recommendations based on lesion morphology, but practice continues to evolve with improvements in technology and operator expertise.[125]

Surgical Revascularization

Surgical revascularization uses graft material to bypass the diseased portion of the vessel, improving distal blood flow. Procedures are usually performed under general anesthesia, although regional anesthesia may be used in some cases. Conduits available for peripheral vascular bypass include vein grafts (reversed saphenous vein, arm vein, or human umbilical vein) and synthetic grafts made of polytetrafluoroethylene. As in CABG surgery, the type of conduit used has an impact on the patency rate of the graft. Although synthetic grafts perform well in larger vessels (higher flow), veins are preferred in smaller vessels because of better patency rates.[126] Types of peripheral vascular procedures are shown in Fig. 15.25.

Percutaneous Interventions

Percutaneous interventions used in the coronary arteries—angioplasty, atherectomy, and stent placement—can be performed to treat occlusion or narrowing in the peripheral vasculature as well. Similar advances in catheter design and the development of intravascular stents have resulted in a dramatic increase in the number of endovascular procedures performed for peripheral artery disease. No longer limited to the treatment of short, focal stenoses or for poor surgical candidates, these devices are now routinely used as first-line therapy. Atherectomy is employed more often because the diameter of peripheral vessels can more easily accommodate the larger catheters required for these procedures. Intravascular stents may be used in combination with percutaneous transluminal angioplasty, depending on lesion morphology and location. Mechanical movement of the leg can increase the incidence of stent fracture and poor endothelialization, limiting use in some areas.[127] Complications of interventional vascular procedures include hematoma formation at the site of the arteriotomy, formation of a pseudoaneurysm, distal embolization, and thrombotic occlusion.

Acute occlusion of a peripheral artery may occur as a result of local thrombosis, emboli, trauma, or compression. Left untreated, the resultant ischemia may lead to amputation of the affected limb. Catheter-based interventions that may be used to recanalize acutely occluded arteries include intraarterial infusions of fibrinolytic medications and the use of thrombectomy devices to fragment and remove the clot. If these interventions are unsuccessful, revascularization may be performed. In the setting of limb-threatening ischemia, surgical intervention is associated with increased mortality as well as increased rates of amputation in the year after the procedure.[128]

FIG. 15.25 Peripheral Arterial Bypass Procedures. (A) aortoiliac bypass, (B) aortobifemoral bypass, (C) femoropopliteal bypass, (D) femorotibial bypass.

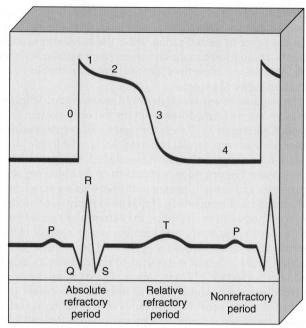

FIG. 15.26 Phases of the Cardiac Action Potential and Their Relationship to Refractory Periods of the Heart. *Phase 0,* depolarization with rapid influx of sodium. *Phase 1,* rapid repolarization with rapid efflux of potassium ions and decreased sodium conductance. *Phase 2,* plateau with slow influx of sodium and calcium ions. *Phase 3,* repolarization with continued efflux of potassium ions. *Phase 4,* resting phase with restoration of ionic balance by sodium and potassium pumps.

to detect episodes of myocardial ischemia throughout the perioperative period.

EFFECTS OF CARDIOVASCULAR MEDICATIONS

Multiple medications are used in the treatment of critically ill cardiovascular patients. The critical care nurse is responsible for preparation and administration of these pharmacologic therapies and often is required to titrate the dose on the basis of the patient's hemodynamic response. The medications used to treat cardiovascular disease are rapidly changing and expanding as more is learned about the pathophysiology of cardiac disease and as improved formulas are developed by pharmaceutical companies. The critical care nurse who has a general understanding of the mechanisms of action of the various pharmacologic classifications can readily apply this knowledge to new medications within the same classification. This section provides a concise review of medications commonly administered to support cardiovascular function in the critical care setting. The emphasis is on intravenously administered medications that are used for acute rather than long-term management of cardiovascular conditions.

Antidysrhythmic Medications

Antidysrhythmic medications comprise a diverse category of pharmacologic agents used to terminate or prevent an array of abnormal cardiac rhythms. These agents are commonly classified according to their primary effect on the action potential of cardiac cells (Fig. 15.26). The classification scheme shown in Table 15.14 is the most commonly used system. Classification of newer agents is more difficult because some of these agents have characteristics of more than one class, and others have no characteristics of the current system.

Nursing Management. The primary focus of nursing care in the immediate postprocedural period is assessment of the adequacy of perfusion to the affected limb and identification of complications. Pulse checks are performed frequently, and the physician is notified of any decrease in the strength of the Doppler signal. Adequate blood pressure is essential to maintain perfusion through the repaired vessel or graft. Because distal perfusion is compromised in these patients, nursing measures to prevent skin breakdown (eg, sheepskin, frequent repositioning, foot cradles) are implemented. If the repair was performed above the renal arteries, kidney function may be impaired as a result of interruption of renal blood flow during the procedure. Therefore, urine output is assessed hourly and supported with fluids and diuretics as needed. Because patients with peripheral vascular disease are at high risk for cardiac events, ST segment monitoring is performed

TABLE 15.14 Classification of Antidysrhythmic Agents

Class	Action	Medications
I	Blocks sodium channels (stabilizes cell membrane)	
IA	Blocks sodium channels and delays repolarization, lengthening duration of the action potential	Quinidine Procainamide Disopyramide
IB	Blocks sodium channels and accelerates repolarization, shortening duration of the action potential	Lidocaine Mexiletine
IC	Blocks sodium channels and slows conduction through His-Purkinje system, prolonging QRS duration	Flecainide Propafenone
II	Blocks beta-receptors	Esmolol Metoprolol Propranolol
III	Slows repolarization and prolongs duration of the action potential	Amiodarone Dronedarone Dofetilide Ibutilide Sotalol
IV	Blocks calcium channels	Diltiazem Verapamil

TABLE 15.15 Effects of Adrenergic Receptors

Receptor	Location	Response to Stimulation
Alpha	Vessels of skin, muscles, kidneys, and intestines	Vasoconstriction of peripheral arterioles
Beta-1	Cardiac tissue	Increased heart rate Increased conduction Increased contractility
Beta-2	Vascular and bronchial smooth muscle	Vasodilation of peripheral arterioles Bronchodilation

Class I

Class I agents are sodium channel blockers that decrease the influx of sodium ions through "fast" channels during phase 0 depolarization. This prolongs the absolute (effective) refractory period, decreasing the risk of premature impulses from ectopic foci. These medications also depress automaticity by slowing the rate of spontaneous depolarization of pacemaker cells during the resting phase (phase 4).

Class I antidysrhythmic medications can be subdivided further into three groups according to their potency as sodium channel inhibitors and their effect on phase 3 repolarization. Class IA agents—quinidine, procainamide, and disopyramide—block both the fast sodium channels and phase 3 repolarization, prolonging the action potential duration. Clinically, this may result in measurable increases in the QRS duration and lengthening of the Q–T interval. All class IA agents may depress myocardial contractility, with disopyramide having the most potent negative inotropic effect. Medications in class IB have only a moderate effect on sodium channels and accelerate phase 3 repolarization to shorten the action potential duration; lidocaine and mexiletine belong in this group. Class IC agents are the most potent sodium channel blockers and have little effect on repolarization. Class IC agents increase the P–R and QRS intervals. Flecainide and propafenone are included in this group. Both of these agents are proarrhythmic and have negative inotropic effects, which limits their use in patients with heart failure.[129]

Class II

Class II agents are beta-adrenergic blockers (beta-blockers). They inhibit dysrhythmias mediated by the sympathetic nervous system by competing with endogenous catecholamines for available receptor sites. As a result, spontaneous depolarization during the resting phase (phase 4) is depressed, and

AV conduction is slowed. Antidysrhythmic medications in this class can be further subdivided into cardioselective agents (agents that block only beta-1-receptors) and noncardioselective agents (agents that block both beta-1- and beta-2-receptors). Knowledge of the effects of adrenergic-receptor stimulation allows for anticipation of both the therapeutic responses brought about by beta-blockade and the potential adverse effects of these agents (Table 15.15). For example, bronchospasm can be precipitated by noncardioselective beta-blockers in a patient with chronic obstructive pulmonary disease caused by blockade of the effects of beta-2-receptors in the lungs. Beta-blockers also are negative inotropes and must be used cautiously in patients with LV dysfunction. Although numerous beta-blockers are marketed, only esmolol, metoprolol, and propranolol are available as intravenous agents for the treatment of acute dysrhythmias. Of these, esmolol (Brevibloc) offers significant advantages for critically ill patients because of its short half-life (approximately 9 minutes). It is used in the treatment of SVTs, such as AF and atrial flutter.

Class III

Class III agents include amiodarone, dronedarone, dofetilide, ibutilide, and sotalol. These agents block potassium channels to slow the rate of phase 3 repolarization, increasing the effective refractory period and the action potential duration. Although their effects on the action potential are similar, these medications differ greatly in their mechanism of action and their side effects. Intravenous amiodarone was originally approved for the treatment of serious ventricular dysrhythmias refractory to other medications. Because of its effectiveness, it is now used for both atrial and ventricular dysrhythmias.[130] Dronedarone is similar to amiodarone but has fewer extracardiac side effects. Dofetilide (Tikosyn) is a newer class III antidysrhythmic agent used for the conversion to and maintenance of normal sinus rhythm in patients with highly symptomatic AF or atrial flutter. Because dofetilide prolongs the refractoriness of both atrial and ventricular tissue, prolongation of the Q–T interval can occur and is associated with an increased risk of torsades de pointes. As a result, therapy with dofetilide is initiated in a hospital setting with mandatory ECG monitoring.[129] Ibutilide (Covert) is a short-term antidysrhythmic agent used for the rapid conversion of acute AF or atrial flutter to sinus rhythm. Ibutilide is administered as a 10-minute infusion in a carefully monitored clinical setting. The most serious side effect of ibutilide is its potential for inducing life-threatening dysrhythmias, especially torsades de pointes.[129] Sotalol not only blocks potassium channels but also has properties of a noncardioselective beta-blocker and should be used cautiously in patients with heart failure.

Class IV

Class IV agents are calcium channel blockers that inhibit the influx of calcium through slow calcium channels during the plateau phase (phase 2). This effect occurs primarily in tissue in which slow calcium channels predominate, primarily the sinus and AV nodes and the atrial tissue. Verapamil was the first medication in this category available as an intravenous antidysrhythmic. It depresses sinus and AV node conduction and is effective in terminating SVTs caused by AV nodal reentry. Diltiazem (Cardizem) has become available in intravenous form and is thought to be as effective as verapamil in treating supraventricular dysrhythmias, with fewer hypotensive side effects. Because accessory pathways are not affected by calcium channel blockade, both of these agents must be avoided when treating AF or flutter in patients with Wolff-Parkinson-White syndrome.[8]

Unclassified Antidysrhythmics

Adenosine (Adenocard) is an antidysrhythmic agent that remains unclassified under the current system. Adenosine occurs endogenously in the body as a building block of adenosine triphosphate. Given in intravenous boluses, adenosine slows conduction through the AV node, causing transient AV block. It is used clinically to convert SVTs and to facilitate differential diagnosis of rapid dysrhythmias. Because of its short half-life, adenosine is administered intravenously as a rapid bolus, followed by a saline flush. The bolus is delivered as centrally as possible so that the medication reaches the heart before it is metabolized. Side effects are transient because adenosine is rapidly taken up by the cells and is cleared from the body within 10 seconds.

Magnesium is also unclassified under the present system. Although its action as an antidysrhythmic agent is not entirely understood, clinical studies suggest that it may reduce the incidence of both ventricular and supraventricular dysrhythmias in selected patient populations.[131] It is considered the treatment of choice in patients with torsades de pointes. For acute treatment, 1 to 2 g of magnesium is administered over 1 to 2 minutes. In patients with confirmed hypomagnesemia, this bolus may be followed with repeated infusions.[132]

Side Effects

Antidysrhythmic medications carry the risk of serious side effects, some of which can be life-threatening. The major side effects of intravenous antidysrhythmic agents are listed in Table 15.16. The most severe complication is the potential for a prodysrhythmic effect. This may result in worsening of the underlying dysrhythmia, the occurrence of a new dysrhythmia, or the development of a bradydysrhythmia. For example, torsades de pointes is a prodysrhythmia caused by many medications that prolong the Q–T interval on the ECG. Because the

TABLE 15.16 Pharmacologic Management
Selected Antidysrhythmic Agents

Medication	Dosage	Actions	Special Considerations
Adenosine	6 mg IV rapid push; if unsuccessful, repeat with 12 mg over 1–2 s; follow with IV fluid 10 mL flush (NS or D_5W)	Blocks AV node to terminate SVT, PSVT	Transient; flushing, dyspnea, hypotension
Digoxin	0.5–1 mg loading dose in divided doses; maintenance dose of 0.125–0.375 mg daily	Conversion and/or rate control in SVT, AFib, AF	Bradycardia, heart block Toxicity: CNS and GI symptoms
Diltiazem	Bolus dose of 0.25 mg/kg IV over 2 min, followed by infusion of 5–15 mg/h	Conversion and/or rate control in SVT, AFib, AF	Bradycardia, hypotension, AV block
Esmolol	Loading dose of 500 mcg/kg over 1 min, followed by infusion of 50 mcg/kg/min for 4 min; repeat procedure every 5 min, increasing infusion by 25–50 mcg/kg/min to maximum of 200 mcg/kg/min	Conversion and/or rate control in SVT, AFib, AF Also used to decrease rate of sinus tachycardia	Hypotension, bradycardia, heart failure
Ibutilide	0.010–0.025 mg/kg infused over 10 min (may repeat once) or 1 mg diluted in 50 mL infused over 10 min (may repeat once)	Conversion of AFib, AF	Minimal side effects except for rare polymorphic VT (torsades de pointes)
Verapamil	5–10 mg IV, may repeat in 15–30 min	Conversion and/or rate control in SVT	Hypotension, bradycardia, heart failure
Lidocaine	1–1.5 mg/kg bolus, followed by continuous infusion of 1–4 mg/min	Treatment of ventricular dysrhythmias (PVCs, VT, VF)	CNS toxicity, nausea, vomiting with repeated doses
Amiodarone	*VT/VF arrest:* 300 mg IV push; may repeat with 150 mg in 3–5 min (maximum dose, 2.2 g/24 h) *Pulsatile VT, AFib, AF:* 150 mg IV over 10 min, followed by 360 mg over 6 h (1 mg/min); maintenance infusion of 0.5 mg/min	Treatment of atrial (AFib, AF, SVT) and ventricular (PVCs, VT, VF) dysrhythmias	Hypotension, abnormal liver function tests
Procainamide	Loading dose of 12–17 mg/kg at a rate of 20 mg/min, followed by infusion of 1–4 mg/min	Treatment of atrial (AF, SVT) and ventricular (PVCs, VT) dysrhythmias	Hypotension, GI effects Widening of QRS and Q–T lengthening

AF, atrial flutter; *AFib,* atrial fibrillation; *AV,* atrioventricular; *CNS,* central nervous system; D_5W, 5% dextrose in water; *GI,* gastrointestinal; *IV,* intravenous/intravenously; *NS,* normal saline; *PSVT,* paroxysmal supraventricular tachycardia; *PVCs,* premature ventricular contractions; *ST,* sinus tachycardia; *SVT,* supraventricular tachycardia; *VF,* ventricular fibrillation; *VT,* ventricular tachycardia.

development of a prodysrhythmia is unpredictable, the nurse plays an important role in evaluating ECG changes, monitoring serum medication levels, and assessing patient symptoms. Antidysrhythmic agents may also alter the amount of energy required for defibrillation and pacing. For example, increases in the dose of an antidysrhythmic medication may increase the amount of output (mA) required to depolarize the myocardium.

Treatment of Atrial Fibrillation

More than 5 million people in the United States have AF, and extensive research has been done on the treatment of this disorder.[14] The goals of pharmacologic therapy for AF include reestablishing and maintaining sinus rhythm, decreasing the rapid ventricular response during episodes of AF, and preventing the risk of thromboembolism. Table 15.17 reviews current medications used in the treatment of AF. Results of several large clinical trials suggest that rate control is equivalent to restoration of sinus rhythm in terms of mortality, with less incidence of adverse medication effects.[133] Although warfarin has been the traditional choice for antithrombotic therapy, the FDA has approved new anticoagulant agents for embolism prophylaxis in patients with nonvalvular AF. Dabigatran (Pradaxa) is a direct thrombin inhibitor, whereas rivaroxaban and apixaban effect anticoagulation through inhibit factor Xa. These agents have advantages over warfarin in that they have fewer medication interactions and do not require routine monitoring.[134] However, concerns have been raised over possible risks of life-threatening hemorrhage because none of these drugs has an antidote. In addition, dabigatran should not be used in patients with a mechanical heart valve.[135]

Inotropic Medications

Critically ill patients with compromised cardiac function often require medications to enhance myocardial contractility (positive inotropes). Clinically available inotropes include cardiac

---

TABLE 15.17	Medications Used for Atrial Fibrillation	
Treatment Goal	**Classification and Medications**	**Special Considerations**
Conversion or maintenance of sinus rhythm	Class IA	Class IA agents prolong Q–T intervals and may cause torsades de pointes.
	Quinidine	Rate control should be achieved before initiation of therapy.
	Procainamide (Pronestyl)	
	Disopyramide (Norpace)	
	Class IC	Class IC agents are prodysrhythmic in patients with CAD or previous MI and should be avoided in these patients.
	Flecainide (Tambocor)	
	Propafenone (Rythmol)	
	Class III	Amiodarone and sotalol also have beta-blocking properties and may help with rate control.
	Amiodarone (Cordarone)	Treatment with dofetilide requires careful monitoring for prodysrhythmic effects.
	Dofetilide (Tikosyn)	Ibutilide is an IV agent and is used for conversion only.
	Dronedarone (Multaq)	
	Ibutilide (Corvert)	
	Sotalol (Betapace)	
Control of ventricular rate	Beta-blockers	IV esmolol may be used in acute settings to control ventricular rate.
	Esmolol (Brevibloc)	Oral agents are used for maintenance therapy.
	Metoprolol (Lopressor)	Beta-blockers provide good rate control during exercise.
	Propranolol (Inderal)	
	Calcium channel blockers	Intravenous calcium channel blockers may be used in emergency situations, followed by oral agents for maintenance therapy.
	Diltiazem (Cardizem)	
	Verapamil (Isoptin)	
	Digitalis compounds	Digoxin does not effectively control rate with exercise, so it may be used in combination with other medications.
	Digoxin (Lanoxin)	
Prevention of thromboembolism	Anticoagulants	Heparin may be used in emergency situations, before cardioversion.
	Heparin	Warfarin is used long-term, with monitoring to achieve INR of 2–3.
	Warfarin (Coumadin)	Dabigatran is an oral direct thrombin inhibitor approved to reduce risk of thromboembolism in patients with nonvalvular AFib.
		Dabigatran does not require routine anticoagulant monitoring.
	Dabigatran (Pradaxa)	
	Rivaroxaban (Xarelto)	Rivaroxaban and apixaban are factor Xa inhibitors approved to reduce risk of thromboembolism in patients with nonvalvular AFib.
	Apixaban (Eliquis)	Rivaroxaban and apixaban do not require routine anticoagulant monitoring.
	Antiplatelet agents	Aspirin may be used in patients with contraindications to warfarin or in low-risk patients younger than 65 y.
	Aspirin	

AFib, atrial fibrillation; *CAD*, coronary artery disease; *INR*, international normalized ratio; *IV*, intravenous; *MI*, myocardial infarction.

glycosides, sympathomimetics, and phosphodiesterase inhibitors. These agents increase myocardial contractility, resulting in improved cardiac output, more complete emptying of the ventricles, and decreased filling pressures.

Cardiac Glycosides

Cardiac glycosides include digitalis and its derivatives. Although these medications have been used for centuries, their slow onset of action and risk of toxicity make them more appropriate for management of chronic heart failure. Because digoxin also causes slowing of the sinus rate and a decrease in AV conduction, it may be administered intravenously in the acute care setting to control supraventricular dysrhythmias.

Sympathomimetic Agents

Sympathomimetic agents stimulate adrenergic receptors, simulating the effects of sympathetic nerve stimulation. Included in this category are naturally occurring catecholamines (epinephrine, dopamine, and norepinephrine) and synthetic catecholamines (dobutamine and isoproterenol). The cardiovascular effects of these medications, which vary according to their selectivity for specific receptor sites, are often dose dependent as well. Table 15.18 describes the cardiovascular effects of sympathomimetic agents at various dosages.

Dopamine (Intropin) is one of the most widely used medications in the critical care setting. It is a chemical precursor of norepinephrine, which, in addition to both alpha-receptor and beta-receptor stimulation, can activate dopaminergic receptors in the renal and mesenteric blood vessels. The actions of dopamine are dose related, although there is some overlap in effect.[136] At low dosages of 1 to 2 mcg/kg per minute, dopamine stimulates dopaminergic receptors, causing renal and mesenteric vasodilation. The resultant increase in renal perfusion increases urinary output. However, this increase in urine output does not confer protection against the development of acute kidney injury. Moderate dosages result in stimulation of beta-1-receptors to increase myocardial contractility and improve cardiac output. At dosages greater than 10 mcg/kg per minute, dopamine predominantly stimulates alpha-receptors, resulting in

vasoconstriction that often negates both the beta-adrenergic and the dopaminergic effects.

Dobutamine (Dobutrex) is a synthetic catecholamine with predominantly beta-1-adrenergic effects. It also produces some beta-2 stimulation, resulting in mild vasodilation. Dobutamine is as effective as dopamine in increasing myocardial contractility and is useful in the treatment of heart failure, especially in hypotensive patients who cannot tolerate vasodilator therapy. The usual dosage range is 2 to 20 mcg/kg per minute, titrated on the basis of hemodynamic parameters.

Epinephrine (Adrenalin) is produced by the adrenal gland as part of the body's response to stress. This agent has the ability to stimulate both alpha-receptors and beta-receptors, depending on the dose administered (see Table 15.18). At doses of 1 to 2 mcg/min, epinephrine binds with beta-receptors to increase heart rate, cardiac conduction, contractility, and vasodilation, increasing cardiac output. As the dosage is increased, alpha-receptors are stimulated, resulting in increased vascular resistance and increased blood pressure. At these doses, the impact of epinephrine on cardiac output depends on the ability of the heart to pump against the increased afterload. Epinephrine accelerates the sinus rate and may precipitate ventricular dysrhythmias in the ischemic heart. Other side effects include restlessness, angina, and headache.

Norepinephrine (Levophed) is similar to epinephrine in its ability to stimulate beta-receptors and alpha-receptors, but it lacks the beta-2 effects of epinephrine. At low infusion rates, beta-1-receptors are activated to produce increased contractility, augmenting cardiac output. At higher doses, the inotropic effects are limited by marked vasoconstriction mediated by alpha-receptors. Clinically, norepinephrine is used most often as a vasopressor to elevate blood pressure in shock states.[137]

Isoproterenol (Isuprel) is a pure beta-receptor stimulant with no alpha-adrenergic effects. It produces dramatic increases in heart rate, conduction, and contractility through beta-1 stimulation and vasodilation through beta-2 stimulation. Isoproterenol also produces vasodilation of the pulmonary arteries and bronchodilation. It greatly increases the automaticity of cardiac cells and frequently precipitates dysrhythmias,

TABLE 15.18 Physiologic Effects of Sympathomimetic Agents

| Medications | Dosage | RECEPTOR ACTIVATED[a] | | | | CARDIOVASCULAR EFFECTS | | |
		Alpha	Beta-1	Beta-2	Dopa	CO	HR	SVR
Dobutamine	<5 mcg/kg/min	0	↑↑↑	↑	0	↑↑	↑	↓↓
	5–20 mcg/kg/min	0	↑↑↑	↑↑	0	↑↑↑	↑↑↑	↓↓
Dopamine	<3 mcg/kg/min	0	↑	↑	↑↑↑	0/↑	0/↑	0
	3–10 mcg/kg/min	↑↑	↑↑↑	↑	↑↑↑	↑↑↑	↑	↑
	11–20 mcg/kg/min	↑↑↑	↑↑↑	↑	↑↑	↑↑	↑↑	↑↑↑
Epinephrine	<2 mcg/min	0	↑	↑↑	0	0/↑	0/↑	↓
	2–8 mcg/min	↑↑	↑↑↑	↑↑	0	↑↑↑	↑↑	↑
	9–20 mcg/min	↑↑↑	↑↑↑	↑↑	0	↑↑	↑↑	↑↑↑
Isoproterenol	1–7 mcg/min	0	↑↑↑	↑↑↑	0	↑↑↑	↑↑↑	↓↓↓
Norepinephrine	<2 mcg/min	↑↑↑	↑↑	0	0	↑	0/↑	↑↑↑
	2–16 mcg/min	↑↑↑↑	↑↑	0	0	↓	↑	↑↑↑↑
Phenylephrine	10–100 mcg/min	↑↑↑↑	0	0	0	0	↓	↑↑↑

[a]See Table 15.14 for actions of receptors.

0, no effect; *↑*, increased (number of arrows indicates degree of effect); *↓*, decreased (number of arrows indicates degree of effect); *CO*, cardiac output; *HR*, heart rate; *SVR*, systemic vascular resistance.

such as premature ventricular contractions and VT. These effects limit its usefulness in most patients and it is rarely used.

Phosphodiesterase Inhibitors

Medications in this classification inhibit the enzyme phosphodiesterase, resulting in increased levels of cyclic adenosine monophosphate and intracellular calcium. Phosphodiesterase inhibitors are both inotropic agents and potent vasodilators (inodilators). Improvement in cardiac output occurs as a result of increased contractility and decreased afterload. Milrinone (Primacor), a second-generation drug in this category, is used in the treatment of patients with acute decompensated heart failure. Milrinone can cause hypotension and may induce atrial and ventricular dysrhythmias (premature ventricular contractions, VT) in some patients.[138]

Vasodilator Medications

Vasodilators are pharmacologic agents that improve cardiac performance by various degrees of arterial or venous dilation, or both. The goal of vasodilator therapy may be reduction of preload or afterload, or both. Afterload reduction is accomplished by vasodilation of arterial vessels. This results in decreased resistance to LV ejection and may improve cardiac output without increasing myocardial oxygen demands. Reduction of preload is accomplished by dilation of venous vessels to increase capacitance. This results in decreased filling pressures for a failing heart. These medications may be classified into four groups on the basis of mechanism of action (Table 15.19).

Direct Smooth Muscle Relaxants

Direct-acting vasodilators include sodium nitroprusside, nitroglycerin, and hydralazine. These medications produce relaxation of vascular smooth muscle through the activation of nitric oxide, which results in decreased peripheral vascular resistance. Hypotension may occur as a result of peripheral vasodilation, and headaches may be caused by cerebral vasodilation. Compensatory mechanisms can occur in response to the decrease in blood pressure. These mechanisms include baroreceptor activation that causes reflex tachycardia and activation of the renin-angiotensin-aldosterone system (see Fig. 14.18 in Chapter 14), with resultant sodium and water retention.

Sodium nitroprusside (Nipride) is a potent, rapidly acting venous and arterial vasodilator that is particularly suitable for rapid reduction of blood pressure in hypertensive emergencies and perioperatively. It also is effective for afterload reduction in the setting of severe heart failure. Sodium nitroprusside is administered by continuous intravenous infusion, with the dosage titrated to maintain the desired blood pressure and SVR. Prolonged administration can result in thiocyanate toxicity, manifested by nausea, confusion, and tinnitus.[139]

Intravenous nitroglycerin (Tridil) causes both arterial and venous vasodilation, but its venous effect is more pronounced. It is used in the critical care setting for the treatment of acute heart failure because it reduces cardiac filling pressures, relieves pulmonary congestion, and decreases cardiac workload and oxygen consumption. Nitroglycerin dilates the coronary arteries and is a useful adjunct in the treatment of unstable angina and acute MI. The initial dosage is 5 mcg/min, and the infusion is titrated upward to achieve the desired clinical effect: a reduction or elimination of chest pain, decreased pulmonary artery occlusion pressure (wedge pressure), or a decrease in blood pressure. The most common side effects of this medication are hypotension, reflex tachycardia, and headache. Nitroglycerin becomes less effective with prolonged infusions, as tolerance develops within 24 to 48 hours.[139]

Hydralazine (Apresoline) is a potent arterial vasodilator. It is not given as a continuous infusion; rather, it is administered in slow intravenous doses of 5 to 10 mg every 4 to 8 hours. Occasionally, hydralazine is given as an intermediate agent during the transition between weaning of a continuous infusion and initiation of oral antihypertensive medications. The major side effect is reflex tachycardia mediated by the sympathetic nervous system. Hydralazine has been used for treatment of preeclampsia because only minimal amounts cross the placenta,

TABLE 15.19 Pharmacologic Management
Selected Vasodilator Agents

Medication	Dosage	Action	Special Considerations
Sodium nitroprusside (Nipride)	0.25–6 mcg/kg/min IV infusion	Potent arterial and moderate venous dilation	May cause hypotension and reflex tachycardia, thiocyanate toxicity with prolonged infusions, or kidney dysfunction
Nitroglycerin (Tridil)	5–300 mcg/min IV infusion	Potent venodilator, with arterial effects at higher doses	May cause headache, reflex tachycardia, hypotension
Calcium Channel Blockers			
Clevidipine (Cleviprex)	1–2 mg/h IV infusion, titrated to 32 mg/h (500 mg/24 h)	Potent arterial dilator, with no effect on venous capacitance (preload)	Hypotension, reflex tachycardia, nausea, vomiting, rebound hypertension
Nicardipine (Cardene)	5 mg/h IV, titrated to 15 mg/h	Potent arterial dilator, no effect on preload	Hypotension, headache, reflex tachycardia
ACEIs			
Enalaprilat (Vasotec)	0.625 mg IV over 5 min, then every 6 h	Moderate dilation of arteries and veins	Hypotension, elevation of liver enzymes
Alpha-Adrenergic Blockers			
Labetalol (Normodyne)	20–80 mg IV bolus every 10 min, then 1–2 mg/min infusion	Moderate dilation of arteries and veins	Orthostatic hypotension, bronchospasm, AV block
Phentolamine (Regitine)	1–5 mg IV slowly every 6 h	Moderate dilation of arteries and veins	Hypotension, tachycardia

ACEIs, angiotensin-converting enzyme inhibitors; *AV,* atrioventricular; *IV,* intravenous/intravenously; *PO,* by mouth.

but newer agents such as nicardipine or labetalol are preferred because of a more predictable response.[139]

Calcium Channel Blockers

Calcium channel blockers are a chemically diverse group of medications with differing pharmacologic effects, based on their classification (Table 15.20). Nifedipine (Procardia), nicardipine (Cardene), and clevidipine (Cleviprex) are dihydropyridines. Medications in this group of calcium channel blockers (with the suffix "-pine") are used primarily as arterial vasodilators. These agents reduce the influx of calcium in the arterial resistance vessels. Coronary and peripheral arteries are affected. They are used in the critical care setting to treat hypertension. Nicardipine was the first available intravenous calcium channel blocker and as such could be more easily titrated to control blood pressure. Because this medication has vasodilatory effects on coronary and cerebral vessels, it has proven beneficial in treating hypertension in patients with CAD or ischemic stroke. Side effects of nicardipine are related to vasodilation and include hypotension, reflex tachycardia, flushing, and headache.

Clevidipine is a newer short-acting calcium channel blocker that allows for even more precise titration of blood pressure in the management of acute hypertension. Advantages of this agent include its short half-life (approximately 1 minute), rapid onset of action, predictable dose response, and minimal effect on heart rate.[139] Because clevidipine is mixed in a phospholipid emulsion, it can cause allergic reactions in patients with allergies to soybeans or eggs.

Diltiazem (Cardizem) is from the benzothiazine group of calcium channel blockers. Verapamil (Calan, Isoptin) is part of the phenylalkylamine group. The different classifications account for the differing actions of these calcium channel blockers. These medications dilate coronary arteries but have little effect on the peripheral vasculature. They are used in the treatment of angina, especially angina with a vasospastic component, and as antidysrhythmics in the treatment of SVTs.

Angiotensin-Converting Enzyme Inhibitors

Angiotensin-converting enzyme inhibitors (ACEIs) produce vasodilation by blocking the conversion of angiotensin I to angiotensin II. Because angiotensin is a potent vasoconstrictor, limiting its production decreases vascular resistance. In contrast to the direct vasodilators, ACEIs do not cause reflex tachycardia or induce sodium and water retention. However, these medications may cause a profound fall in blood pressure, especially in patients who are volume-depleted. Blood pressure must be monitored carefully, especially at the initiation of therapy.

ACEIs are used in patients with heart failure to decrease SVR (afterload) and pulmonary artery occlusion pressure (preload). Most of these agents are available only in an oral form. Enalaprilat is available in an intravenous form and may be used to decrease afterload in more emergent situations.

Angiotensin Receptor Blockers

Angiotensin receptor blockers prevent the vasoconstrictive effects of angiotensin II through direct blockade at the receptor site, producing hemodynamic effects similar to ACEIs. These agents may be used as an alternative in patients who cannot tolerate ACEIs because of side effects, such as cough.[140] At the present time, angiotensin receptor blockers are available only in oral form.

Alpha-Adrenergic Blockers

Peripheral adrenergic blockers block alpha-receptors in arteries and veins, resulting in vasodilation. Orthostatic hypotension is a common side effect and may result in syncope. Long-term therapy also may be complicated by fluid and water retention.

Labetalol (Normodyne), a combined peripheral alpha-blocker and cardioselective beta-blocker, is used in the treatment of acute stroke and hypertensive emergencies.[141] Because the blockade of beta-1-receptors permits the decrease of blood pressure without the risk of reflexive tachycardia and increased cardiac output, labetalol is also useful in the treatment of acute aortic dissection.[142]

Phentolamine (Regitine) is a nonselective peripheral alpha-blocker that deceases blood pressure through arterial vasodilation. It is administered by slow intravenous push 1 to 5 mg every 6 hours to reduce blood pressure. Phentolamine is used only in very specific circumstances for catecholamine-induced

TABLE 15.20 Pharmacologic Management

Classification of Calcium Channel Blockers

Medication	Dosage	Actions	Special Considerations
Dihydropyridines			
Nicardipine (Cardene)	5 mg/h IV, titrated to 15 mg/h	Short-term control of hypertension	Hypotension, reflex tachycardia, headache, flushing
Nifedipine (Procardia)	10–30 mg PO	Hypertension	Hypotension, reflex tachycardia, headache
Clevidipine (Cleviprex)	1–2 mg/h IV infusion, titrated to 32 mg/h	Short-term control of hypertension	Hypotension, reflex tachycardia, nausea, vomiting, rebound hypertension
Benzothiazepines			
Diltiazem (Cardizem)	Bolus dose of 0.25 mg/kg IV over 2 min, followed by infusion of 5–15 mg/h	Treatment of SVT, AFib, AF, angina	Bradycardia, hypotension, atrioventricular block
Phenylalkylamines			
Verapamil (Calan, Isoptin)	5–10 mg IV, may repeat in 15–30 min	Treatment of AF, PSVT	Hypotension, bradycardia, heart failure

AF, atrial flutter; *AFib,* atrial fibrillation; *IV,* intravenous/intravenously; *PO,* by mouth; *PSVT,* paroxysmal supraventricular tachycardia; *SVT,* supraventricular tachycardia.

hypertension or toxicities related to ingestion of illegal drugs (eg, cocaine). Phentolamine is the medication of choice to control blood pressure and sweating caused by *pheochromocytoma,* an epinephrine-secreting tumor that can arise from the adrenal medulla.[139]

Phentolamine also is used to treat the *extravasation of dopamine* or other vasopressors into peripheral tissues. If this occurs, 5 to 10 mg is diluted in 10 mL normal saline and administered intradermally into the infiltrated area as soon as possible following extravasation.

Dopamine Receptor Agonists

Fenoldopam (Corlopam) is a unique type of vasodilator, a selective, specific dopamine (D_1) receptor agonist. Fenoldopam is a potent vasodilator that affects peripheral, renal, and mesenteric arteries. It is administered by continuous intravenous infusion beginning at 0.01 mcg/kg per minute and titrated up to the desired blood pressure effect, with a maximum recommended dose of 1.6 mcg/kg per minute. It can be administered as an alternative to sodium nitroprusside or other antihypertensives in the treatment of hypertensive emergencies. Fenoldopam can be used safely in patients with kidney dysfunction.[139]

Vasopressors

Vasopressors are sympathomimetic agents that mediate peripheral vasoconstriction through stimulation of alpha-receptors (see Table 15.15). This results in increased SVR and elevates blood pressure. Some of these medications (epinephrine and norepinephrine) also have the ability to stimulate beta-receptors. Vasopressors are not widely used in the treatment of critically ill cardiac patients because the dramatic increase in afterload is taxing to a damaged heart. Occasionally, vasopressors may be used to maintain organ perfusion in shock states. For example, phenylephrine (Neo-Synephrine) or norepinephrine (Levophed) may be administered as a continuous intravenous infusion to maintain organ perfusion by increasing SVR in cases of severe sepsis or septic shock.

Vasopressin, also known as antidiuretic hormone, has become popular in the critical care setting for its vasoconstrictive effects. At higher doses, vasopressin directly stimulates V1 receptors in vascular smooth muscle, resulting in vasoconstriction of capillaries and small arterioles. A one-time dose of 40 units intravenously was previously administered for treatment of cardiac arrest, but new advanced cardiac life support guidelines suggest it offers no advantages over administration of epinephrine alone.[143] In septic shock, vasopressin levels have been reported to be lower than anticipated for a shock state. Vasopressin continuous infusion of 0.03 unit/min may be added to the norepinephrine infusion in refractory shock per sepsis guidelines.[144] Patients must be assessed for side effects such as heart failure caused by the antidiuretic effects and monitored for increased risk of ischemia in the myocardium, spleen, and periphery. Vasopressin should be infused through a central line to avoid the risk of peripheral extravasation and resultant tissue necrosis. Placement of an arterial line is recommended in shock states to monitor blood pressure and SVR.

Medication Treatment of Heart Failure

More than 6 million Americans have heart failure, making it a major chronic health issue.[14] The goals of treatment in heart failure include alleviating symptoms, slowing the progression of the disease, and improving survival. Findings from numerous randomly controlled clinical trials have resulted in guidelines for the pharmacologic treatment of heart failure.[140]

More information about heart failure is available in Chapter 14. Table 15.21 reviews medications currently recommended for treatment of heart failure. Types of medications that have been found to worsen heart failure should be avoided including most antidysrhythmics, calcium channel blockers, and nonsteroidal antiinflammatory drugs.[21]

TABLE 15.21 Medications Used for Heart Failure

Classification and Medications	Mechanism of Action	Effects	Special Considerations
ACEIs			
Captopril (Capoten)	Interfere with RAAS by preventing conversion of angiotensin I to angiotensin II	Decrease afterload	Agents appear equivalent in treatment of heart failure
Enalapril (Vasotec)		Decrease preload	Monitor closely for hypotension when initiating therapy
Fosinopril (Monopril)		Reverse ventricular remodeling	May be contraindicated in patients with elevated creatinine, indicating kidney failure
Lisinopril (Prinivil) Perindopril (Aceon) Quinapril (Accupril) Ramipril (Altace) Trandolapril (Mavik)			
Angiotensin Receptor Blockers			
Candesartan (Atacand)	Interfere with RAAS by blocking effect of angiotensin II at the angiotensin II receptor site	Decrease afterload	Used as primary therapy or as an alternative for patients who cannot tolerate ACEIs because of side effects such as severe cough
Losartan (Cozaar)		Decrease preload	Can also be used in combination with ACEI for systolic dysfunction; monitor renal function and serum potassium levels
Valsartan (Diovan)		Reverse ventricular remodeling	

Continued

TABLE 15.21 Medications Used for Heart Failure—cont'd

Classification and Medications	Mechanism of Action	Effects	Special Considerations
Beta-Blockers			
Metoprolol succinate (Toprol XL)	Counteract SNS response activated in heart failure by blocking receptor sites	Slow heart rate	Not initiated during decompensated stage of heart failure
Bisoprolol (Zebeta)	Metoprolol and bisoprolol are cardioselective beta-blockers, whereas carvedilol blocks alpha- and beta-receptor sites	Prevent dysrhythmias	Use cautiously in patients with reactive airway disease, poorly controlled diabetes, bradydysrhythmias, or heart block
Carvedilol (Coreg)		Decrease blood pressure	Carvedilol dose is increased slowly, while monitoring for symptoms caused by vasodilation such as dizziness or hypotension
		Reverse ventricular remodeling	
Aldosterone Antagonists			
Spironolactone (Aldactone)	Counteract effects of aldosterone, which include sodium and water retention	Decrease preload	May increase serum potassium
Eplerenone (Inspra)		Decrease myocardial hypertrophy	
Inotropes			
Digoxin (Lanoxin)	Affects Na⁺,K⁺-ATPase pump in myocardial cells to increase the strength of contraction	Increases contractility	Risk of toxicity is increased with hypokalemia
		Increases cardiac output	
		Prevents atrial dysrhythmias	

ACEIs, Angiotensin-converting enzyme inhibitors; *Na⁺,K⁺-ATPase,* sodium-potassium adenosine triphosphatase; *RAAS,* renin-angiotensin-aldosterone system; *SNS,* sympathetic nervous system.

SUMMARY

Pacemakers
- Pacemakers are electronic devices that can be used to initiate a heartbeat when the heart's intrinsic electrical system cannot generate a rate adequate to support cardiac output.
- The goal of therapy with either a temporary or a permanent pacemaker is to simulate normal physiologic cardiac depolarization and conduction.
- Nursing responsibilities for patients with pacemakers include assessment and prevention of pacemaker malfunction, protection against microshock, surveillance for complications, and patient education.

Implantable Cardioverter Defibrillators
- An ICD is an electronic device that is used to terminate life-threatening ventricular dysrhythmias, through pacing, cardioversion, or defibrillation.
- Nursing management of a patient with an ICD includes assessing for dysrhythmias, monitoring for complications, and patient education.

Fibrinolytic Therapy
- Fibrinolytic therapy is used to restore blood flow through an occluded coronary artery in patients with an acute ST segment elevation MI.
- Nursing care for patients receiving fibrinolytic agents includes identifying appropriate candidates for therapy, administering the fibrinolytic agent, assessing for evidence of reperfusion, and monitoring for bleeding complications.

Catheter-Based Interventions for Coronary Artery Disease
- PCI refers to procedures that use catheters to open blocked or narrowed coronary arteries; procedures include balloon angioplasty, atherectomy, and stent implantation.
- Antiplatelet therapy is considered an essential adjunct to PCIs to help maintain vessel patency during and after the procedure.
- Complications associated with PCIs include coronary artery spasm, dissection, and thrombosis; contrast-induced kidney injury; and bleeding at the vascular access site.
- Percutaneous valve repair offers an alternative to surgery for high-risk patients.

Cardiac Surgery
- CABG surgery provides myocardial revascularization by using a conduit to bypass an occluded coronary artery.
- Valvular surgery is used either to repair a cardiac valve or to replace it with a mechanical or biologic valve.
- CPB is an extracorporeal circuit used to circulate and oxygenate a patient's blood during some cardiac surgical procedures.
- Complications associated with CPB include intravascular fluid deficits, myocardial depression, coagulopathy, pulmonary dysfunction, hemolysis, hyperglycemia, electrolyte disturbances, neurologic dysfunction, and hypertension.
- Postoperative nursing management for cardiac surgery patients includes optimizing cardiac function (heart rate,

CASE STUDY 15.1   Patient With a Cardiac Problem

Brief Patient History

Mrs. G is a 54-year-old African American woman who has been having intermittent indigestion for the past month. She has a history of hypertension and hyperlipidemia. She was admitted as an inpatient on a medical floor for management of her blood pressure and is scheduled to undergo endoscopy tomorrow. Mrs. G suddenly becomes diaphoretic and complains of nausea and epigastric pain.

Clinical Assessment

The rapid response team is called to evaluate Mrs. G. When the team arrives at her bedside, she continues to complain of pain, which now radiates to her neck and back. She has some slight shortness of breath and is vomiting.

Diagnostic Procedures

The admission electrocardiogram shows ST segment elevation in leads II, III, and AVF. Baseline vital signs are as follows: blood pressure of 160/90 mm Hg, heart rate of 98 beats/min (sinus rhythm), respiratory rate of 18 breaths/min, temperature of 99°F, and oxygen saturation of 94%.

Medical Diagnosis

Mrs. G is diagnosed with an inferior myocardial infarction.

Questions

1. What major outcomes do you expect to achieve for this patient?
2. What problems or risks must be managed to achieve these outcomes?
3. What interventions must be initiated to monitor, prevent, manage, or eliminate the problems and risks identified?
4. What interventions should be initiated to promote optimal functioning, safety, and well-being of the patient?
5. What possible learning needs do you anticipate for this patient?
6. What cultural and age-related factors may have a bearing on the patient's plan of care?

QSEN   QSEN: Informatics

Internet Resources

Centers for Disease Control and Prevention Heart Disease Educational Material for Patients
http://www.cdc.gov/heartdisease/materials_for_patients.htm

National Heart, Lung, and Blood Institute Health Information for the Public: Heart and Vascular Diseases
http://www.nhlbi.nih.gov/health/resources/heart

American Heart Association Consumer and Patient Education Materials
Caregiver Resources Introduction: Caring for Someone After Heart Surgery
http://www.heart.org/HEARTORG/Caregiver/Resources/CaringforSomeoneAfterHeartSurgery/Caring-for-Someone-After-Heart-Surgery_UCM_301857_Article.jsp#.Vq7FE1KoPI4

About Arrhythmia
http://www.heart.org/HEARTORG/Conditions/Arrhythmia/AboutArrhythmia/About-Arrhythmia_UCM_002010_Article.jsp#.Vq7FaVKoPI4

Prevention and Treatment of Arrhythmia
http://www.heart.org/HEARTORG/Conditions/Arrhythmia/PreventionTreatmentofArrhythmia/Prevention-Treatment-of-Arrhythmia_UCM_002026_Article.jsp#.Vq7GM1KoPI4

Devices for Arrhythmia
http://www.heart.org/HEARTORG/Conditions/Arrhythmia/PreventionTreatmentofArrhythmia/Devices-for-Arrhythmia_UCM_301994_Article.jsp#.Vq7GmFKoPI4

preload, afterload, and contractility), temperature regulation, control of bleeding, and monitoring for complications.

Mechanical Circulatory Assist Devices

- Mechanical circulatory assist devices are used in the treatment of heart failure to decrease myocardial workload and maintain adequate perfusion to vital organs.
- Indications for an IABP include failure to wean from CPB, unstable or recurrent angina, complications of acute MI, hemodynamic support for high-risk interventions, septic shock, and as a bridge to definitive therapy.
- Nursing interventions for patients with an IABP include monitoring for and preventing complications, assessing for proper timing, evaluating hemodynamic changes, and providing patient education.
- VADs can be used on a temporary basis as a bridge to recovery or transplant or as permanent destination therapy.
- Nursing management for a patient with a VAD consists of monitoring for hemodynamic changes and complications related to device failure, bleeding, infection, and thromboembolism.

Vascular Surgery

- Vascular surgery may be performed to treat arterial occlusive disease or to correct structural abnormalities such as aneurysms.
- Many patients with vascular disease can be effectively treated with percutaneous procedures (ie, angioplasty, atherectomy, endovascular stents) rather than open surgical repair.
- Nursing care focuses on observing for vascular complications such as hematoma or reocclusion and the prompt recognition and treatment of complications arising from comorbidities such as cardiac, pulmonary, and kidney disease.

Effects of Cardiovascular Medications

- Multiple medications are used in the treatment of critically ill patients, and the nurse is responsible for administration, titration, and monitoring for side effects.
- Antidysrhythmic medications are used to terminate or prevent abnormal cardiac rhythms and are classified according to their primary effect on the action potential of cardiac cells.
- Inotropic agents increase myocardial contractility resulting in improved cardiac output, more complete emptying of the ventricles, and decreased filling pressures.
- Vasodilators have varying effects on arterial and venous dilation and can be used to reduce preload, afterload, or both.
- Vasopressors mediate peripheral vasoconstriction, which results in an increase in SVR and elevates blood pressure.
- Goals of pharmacologic treatment of heart failure include alleviating symptoms, slowing the progression of the disease, and improving survival.

ⓔ Visit the Evolve site for additional study materials.

REFERENCES

1. Samii SM. Indications for pacemakers, implantable cardioverter-defibrillators and cardiac resynchronization devices. *Med Clin N Am.* 2015;99:795.
2. Mahida S, et al. Role of electrophysiological studies in predicting risk of ventricular arrhythmia in early repolarization syndrome. *J Am Coll Cardiol.* 2015;65:151.
3. Mainigi SK, et al. Usefulness of radiofrequency ablation of supraventricular tachycardia to decrease inappropriate shocks from implantable cardioverter-defibrillators. *Am J Cardiol.* 2012;109:231.
4. Shenasa M, Shenasa H, Soleimanieh M. Paroxysmal supraventricular tachycardias: atrioventricular nodal reentrant tachycardia and atrioventricular reentrant tachycardias. *Card Electrophysiol Clin.* 2014;6:483.
5. Haegeli LM, Calkins H. Catheter ablation of atrial fibrillation: an update. *Eur Heart J.* 2014;35:2454.
6. Ley SJ, Koulakis D. Temporary pacing after cardiac surgery. *AACN Adv Crit Care.* 2015;26(3):275.
7. Stone ME, et al. Perioperative management of patients with cardiac implantable electronic devices. *Br J Anaesth.* 2011;107(Suppl 1):i16.
8. Neumar RW, et al. Part 1: Executive summary: 2015 American Heart Association guidelines update for cardiopulmonary resuscitation and emergency cardiovascular care. *Circulation.* 2015;132(Suppl 2):S315.
9. Mahon L, et al. Cardiac tamponade after removal of temporary epicardial pacer wires. *Am J Crit Care.* 2012;21(6):432.
10. Bernstein AD, et al. The revised NASPE/BPEG generic pacemaker code for antibradycardia, adaptive-rate and multi-site pacing. *Pacing Clin Electrophysiol.* 2002;25:260.
11. Gillis AM, et al. HRS/ACCF Expert consensus statement on pacemaker device and mode selection. *J Am Coll Cardiol.* 2012;60:682.
12. Allison MG, Mallemat HA. Emergency care of patients with pacemakers and defibrillators. *Emerg Med Clin N Am.* 2015;33:653.
13. Beinart R, Nazarian S. Effects of external electrical and magnetic fields on pacemakers and defibrillators: from engineering principles to clinical practice. *Circulation.* 2013;128:2799.
14. Mozzafarian D, et al. Heart disease and stroke statistics—2015 update: a report from the American Heart Association. *Circulation.* 2015;131:e29.
15. Xiong WW, Benditt DG. Physiologic sensors in pacemakers: how do they work and how many do we need? *Electrophysiol Clin.* 2013;5:303.
16. Tracy LF, et al. 2012 ACCF/AHA/HRS focused update of the 2008 guidelines for device-based therapy of cardiac rhythm abnormalities. *Circulation.* 2012;126:1784.
17. Vardas PE, et al. New developments in cardiac pacemakers. *Circulation.* 2012;127:2343.
18. Mitka M. First MRI-safe pacemaker receives conditional approval from FDA. *JAMA.* 2011;305(10):985.
19. Knops RE, et al. Chronic performance of a leadless cardiac pacemaker: 1-year follow-up of the LEADLESS trial. *J Am Coll Cardiol.* 2015;65:1497.
20. Miller MA, et al. Leadless cardiac pacemakers: back to the future. *J Am Coll Cardiol.* 2015;66(10):1179.
21. Yancy CW, et al. 2013 ACCF/AHA guideline for the management of heart failure: executive summary. *Circulation.* 2013;128:1810.
22. Chatergee NA, Singh JP. Cardiac resynchronization therapy: past, present and future. *Heart Fail Clin.* 2015;11:287.
23. Stavrakis S, Lazzara R, Thadani U. The benefit of cardiac resynchronization therapy and QRS duration: a meta-analysis. *J Cardiovasc Electrophysiol.* 2012;23:163.
24. Padeletti L, et al. New-generation atrial antitachycardia pacing (reactive ATP) is associated with reduced risk of persistent or permanent atrial fibrillation in patients with bradycardia: results from the MINERVA randomized multicenter trial. *Heart Rhythm.* 2015;12(8):1717.
25. Freeman V, Saxon L. Remote monitoring and outcomes in pacemaker and defibrillator patients: big data saving lives? *J Am Coll Cardiol.* 2015;65(24):2612.
26. Gold MR. Are leadless pacemakers a niche or the future of device therapy? *J Am Coll Cardiol.* 2015;65(15):1505.
27. Swerdlow CD, Wang PJ, Zipe DP. Pacemaker and implantable cardioverter-defibrillators. In: Mann DL, et al., eds. *Braunwald's Heart Disease.* 10th ed. Philadelphia: Saunders; 2015:721.
28. Wilson D, Herweg B. New technology for implantable cardioverter defibrillators. *Card Electrophysiol Clin.* 2014;6:261.
29. Persson R, et al. Adverse events following implantable cardioverter defibrillator implantation: a systematic review. *J Interv Card Electrophysiol.* 2014;40:191.
30. Lewis G, Gold MR. Clinical experience with subcutaneous implantable cardioverter-defibrillators. *Nat Rev Cardiol.* 2015;12(7):398.
31. Russo AM, et al. Patient, physician, and procedural factors influencing the use of defibrillation testing during initial implantable cardioverter defibrillator insertion: findings from the NCDR. *Pacing Clin Electrophysiol.* 2013;36:1152.
32. Healey JS, et al. Cardioverter defibrillator implantation without induction of ventricular fibrillation: a single-blind, non-inferiority, randomized controlled trial (SIMPLE). *Lancet.* 2015;385:785.
33. Tan VH, et al. Impact of programming strategies aimed at reducing nonessential implantable cardioverter defibrillator therapies on mortality a systematic review and meta-analysis. *Circ Arrhythm Electrophysiol.* 2014;7:164.
34. Link MS, et al. Part 6: Electrical therapies—automated external defibrillators, defibrillation, cardioversion, and pacing: 2010 American Heart Association Guidelines for Cardiopulmonary Resuscitation and Emergency Cardiovascular Care. *Circulation.* 2010;122(Suppl 3):S706.
35. Langabeer JR, et al. Growth in percutaneous coronary intervention capacity relative to population and disease prevalence. *J Am Heart Assoc.* 2013;2(6):e000370.
36. Lincoff AM. Managing acute coronary syndromes: decades of progress. *Cleve Clin J Med.* 2014;81(4):233.
37. O'Gara PT, et al. 2013 ACCF/AHA guideline for the management of ST-elevation myocardial infarction: a report of the American College of Cardiology Foundation/American Heart Association Task Force on Practice Guidelines. *Circulation.* 2013;127(4):e362.
38. Amsterdam EA, et al. 2014 ACC/AHA guideline for the management of patients with non-ST-elevation acute coronary syndromes: a report of the American College of Cardiology/American Heart Association Task Force on Practice Guidelines. *Circulation.* 2014;130:e344–e426.
39. Mega JL, Morrow DA. ST elevation myocardial infarction management. In: Mann DL, et al., ed. *Braunwald's Heart Disease: A Textbook of Cardiovascular Medicine.* 10th eds. Philadelphia: Saunders; 2015:1095.
40. Thomas JL, French WJ. Current state of ST-segment myocardial infarction: evidence-based therapies and optimal patient outcomes in advanced systems of care. *Cardiol Clin.* 2014;32:371.
41. Chakrabarti AK, et al. Newer pharmaceutical agents for STEMI interventions. *Intervent Cardiol Clin.* 2012;1(4):429.
42. Gibson CM, Levin T. Characteristics of fibrinolytic (thrombolytic) agents and clinical trials in acute ST elevation myocardial infarction. *UpToDate.* March 13, 2014. www.uptodate.com. Accessed October 19, 2015.
43. The TIMI Study Group. The Thrombolysis In Myocardial Infarction (TIMI) trial: phase I findings. *N Engl J Med.* 1985;312:932.
44. Dauerman HL, Sobel BE. Toward a comprehensive approach to pharmacoinvasive therapy for patients with ST segment elevation acute myocardial infarction. *J Thromb Thrombolysis.* 2012;34:180.
45. Levin T, Gibson CM. Fibrinolytic therapy in acute ST elevation myocardial infarction: initiation of therapy. *UpToDate.* August 14, 2014. www.uptodate.com. Accessed September 11, 2015.
46. American Association of Critical Care Nurses. *AACN practice alert: ST segment monitoring*; 2009. http://www.AACN.org Accessed September 20, 2015.
47. Welsford M, et al. Part 5: Acute coronary syndromes: 2015 International consensus on cardiopulmonary resuscitation and emergency cardiovascular care with treatment recommendations. *Circulation.* 2015;132(Suppl 2):S146.
48. Gilchrist IC. Same day discharge after elective percutaneous intervention. *Curr Cardiol Rep.* 2014;16:470.
49. Harold JG, et al. ACCF/AHA/SCAI 2013 update of the clinical competence statement of coronary artery interventional procedures. *J Am Coll Cardiol.* 2013;62:357.
50. Mauri L, Bhatt DL. Percutaneous coronary intervention. In: Mann DL, et al., eds. *Braunwald's Heart Disease.* 10th ed. Philadelphia: Saunders; 2015:1245.

51. Tomey MI, Kini AS, Sharma SK. Current status of rotational atherectomy. *JACC Cardiovasc Interv.* 2014;7:345.

52. Wasiak J, et al. Percutaneous transluminal rotational atherectomy for coronary artery disease. *Cochrane Database Syst Rev.* 2012;(12):CD003334.

53. Sturm E, Goldberg D, Goldberg S. Embolic protection devices in saphenous vein graft and native vessel percutaneous intervention: a review. *Current Cardiol Rev.* 2012;8:192.

54. Claessen BE, et al. Stent thrombosis: a clinical perspective. *JACC Cardiovasc Interv.* 2014;7:1082.

55. Kim SJ, Giugliano RP, Jang IK. Adjunctive pharmacologic therapy in percutaneous coronary intervention: Part I: Antiplatelet therapy. *Coron Artery Dis.* 2011;22:100.

56. St. Laurent PS. Acute coronary syndromes: new and evolving therapies. *Crit Care Nurs Clin N Am.* 2011;23:559.

57. Clark MG, et al. Managing the acute coronary syndrome patient: evidence based recommendations for anti-platelet therapy. *Heart Lung.* 2015;44:141.

58. McDonald RA, et al. Reducing in-stent restenosis: therapeutic manipulation of miRNA in vascular remodeling and inflammation. *J Am Coll Cardiol.* 2015;65:2314.

59. Siontis GC, et al. Percutaneous coronary interventional strategies for treatment of in-stent restenosis: a network analysis. *Lancet.* 2015;386:655.

60. Palmerini T, et al. Stent thrombosis with drug-eluting and bare-metal stents: evidence from a comprehensive network meta-analysis. *Lancet.* 2012;379:1393.

61. Mamas MA, et al. Baseline bleeding risk and arterial access site practice in relation to procedural outcomes after percutaneous coronary intervention. *J Am Coll Cardiol.* 2014;64:1554.

62. Kim SJ, Giugliano RP, Jang IK. Adjunctive pharmacologic therapy in percutaneous coronary intervention: Part II: anticoagulant therapy. *Coron Artery Dis.* 2011;22:113.

63. Claessen BE, et al. Vasoactive and antiarrhythmic drugs during percutaneous coronary intervention. *Intervent Cardiol Clin.* 2013;2:665.

64. Levine GN, et al. 2011 ACCF/AHA/SCAI guideline for percutaneous coronary intervention and executive summary. *Circulation.* 2011;124:2574.

65. Ndrepepa G, Kastrati A. Bleeding complications in patients undergoing percutaneous coronary interventions: current status and perspective. *Coron Artery Dis.* 2014;25:247.

66. Dirkes S. Acute kidney injury: not just acute renal failure anymore? *Crit Care Nurse.* 2011;31(1):37.

67. Bashore TM, et al. 2012 American College of Cardiology Foundation/Society for Cardiovascular Angiography and Interventions expert consensus document on cardiac catheterization laboratory standards update. *J Am Coll Cardiol.* 2012;59:2221.

68. Bonnett C, et al. Preventing radial artery occlusion by using reserve Barbeau assessment: bringing evidence-based practice to the bedside. *Crit Care Nurse.* 2015;35:77.

69. Merriweather N, Sulzbach-Hokes L. Managing risk of complications at femoral vascular access sites in percutaneous coronary intervention. *Crit Care Nurse.* 2012;32:316.

70. Mohammady M, et al. Bed rest duration after sheath removal following percutaneous coronary interventions: a systematic review and meta-analysis. *J Clin Nurs.* 2013;23:1476.

71. Krishnasamy VP, et al. Vascular closure devices: technical tips, complications, and management. *Tech Vasc Interv Radiol.* 2015;18:100.

72. Nishimura RA, et al. 2014 AHA/ACC guideline for the management of patients with valvular heart disease: executive summary. *Circulation.* 2014;129:2440.

73. Holmes DR, et al. 2012 ACCF/AATS/SCAI/STS expert consensus document on transcatheter aortic valve replacement. *Ann Thorac Surg.* 2012;93:1340.

74. McRae ME, Rodger M. Transcatheter aortic valve implantation outcomes. *J Cardiovasc Nurs.* 2014;27(3):270.

75. Panos AM, George EL. Transcatheter aortic valve implantation options for treating severe aortic stenosis in the elderly. *Dimens Crit Care Nurs.* 2014;33(2):49.

76. Weintraub WS, et al. Comparative effectiveness of revascularization strategies. *N Engl J Med.* 2012;366(16):1467.

77. Kempfert J, et al. Current perspectives in endoscopic vessel harvesting for coronary artery bypass grafting. *Expert Rev Cardiovasc Ther.* 2011;9(11):1481.

78. Hayward P, et al. Comparable patencies of the radial artery and right internal thoracic artery or saphenous vein beyond 5 years: results from the Radial Artery Patency and Clinical Outcomes trial. *J Thorac Cardiovasc Surg.* 2010;139:60.

79. Kim FY, et al. Saphenous vein graft disease: review of pathophysiology, prevention and treatment. *Cardiol Rev.* 2013;21:101.

80. Hillis LD, et al. 2011 ACCF/AHA guideline for coronary artery bypass surgery: A report of the American College of Cardiology Foundation/American Heart Association task force on practice guidelines. *Circulation.* 2011;124(23):e652.

81. Bello S, et al. Conduits for coronary artery bypass surgery: the quest for the second best. *J Cardiovasc Med.* 2011;12(6):411.

82. Piaschyk M, et al. A journey through heart valve surgery. *Crit Care Nurs.* 2011;23:587.

83. Huang G, Rahimtoola S. Prosthetic heart valve. *Circulation.* 2011;123:2602.

84. Dvir D, et al. Transcatheter aortic valve implantation in failed bioprosthetic surgical valves. *JAMA.* 2014;312(2):162.

85. Bakaeen FG, et al. Trends in use of off-pump coronary artery bypass grafting: results from the Society of Thoracic Surgeons Adult Cardiac Surgery Database. *J Thorac Cardiovasc Surg.* 2014;148:856.

86. Stephens RS, Whitman GJ. Postoperative critical care of the adult cardiac surgical patient: Part II: procedure-specific considerations, management of complications, and quality improvement. *Crit Care Med.* 2015;43:1995.

87. Lamy A, et al. Off-pump or on-pump coronary-artery bypass grafting at 30 days. *N Engl J Med.* 2012;366:1489.

88. Stephens RS, Whitman GJ. Postoperative critical care of the adult cardiac surgical patient: Part I: routine postoperative care. *Crit Care Med.* 2015;43:1477.

89. Kupchik N, Bridges E. Central venous pressure monitoring: What's the evidence? *Am J Nurs.* 2012;112(2):58.

90. Kramer A, et al. Pulse pressure variation predicts fluid responsiveness following coronary artery bypass surgery. *Chest.* 2004;126(5):1563.

91. Ferraris VA, et al. Update to the Society of Thoracic Surgeons and the Society of Cardiovascular Anesthesiologists blood conservation clinical practice guidelines. *Ann Thorac Surg.* 2011;91:944.

92. Bigeleisen PE, Goehner N. Novel approaches in pain management in cardiac surgery. *Curr Opin Anesthesiol.* 2015;28:89.

93. Koster S. Consequences of delirium after cardiac operations. *Ann Thorac Surg.* 2012;93:705.

94. Barr J, et al. American College of Critical Care Medicine: clinical practice guidelines for the management of pain, agitation, and delirium in adult patients in the intensive care unit. *Crit Care Med.* 2013;41:263.

95. Allen J, Alexander E. Prevention, recognition, and management of delirium in the intensive care unit. *AACN Adv Crit Care.* 2012;23(1):5.

96. Mu JL, Lee A, Joynt GM. Pharmacologic agents for the prevention and treatment of delirium in patients undergoing cardiac surgery: systematic review and meta-analysis. *Crit Care Med.* 2015;43:194.

97. Gaffney AM, Sladen RN. Acute kidney injury in cardiac surgery. *Curr Opin Anesthesiol.* 2015;28:50.

98. Grossi EA, et al. Evolution of operative techniques and perfusion strategies for minimally invasive mitral valve repair. *J Thorac Cardiovasc Surg.* 2012;143:S68.

99. Mandal K, et al. Robotically assisted minimally invasive mitral valve surgery. *J Thorac Dis.* 2013;5(Suppl 6):S694.

100. Calkins H, et al. 2012 HRS/EHRA/ECAS expert consensus statement on catheter and surgical ablation of atrial fibrillation: recommendations for patient selection, procedural techniques, patient management and follow-up, definitions, endpoints, and research trial design. *J Heart Rhythm.* 2012;9(4):632.

101. Peura JL, et al. Recommendations for the use of mechanical circulatory support: device strategies and patient selection. *Circulation.* 2012;126:2648.

102. Ihdayhid AR, et al. Intra-aortic balloon pump: indications, efficacy, guidelines and future directions. *Curr Opin Cardiol.* 2014;29:285.

103. Thiele H, et al. Intraaortic balloon support for myocardial infarction with cardiogenic shock. *N Engl J Med.* 2012;367(14):1287.

104. Toeg HD, et al. An update on mechanical circulatory support for heart failure therapy. *Curr Opin Cardiol.* 2014;29:167.

105. Feldman D, et al. The 2013 International Society for Heart and Lung Transplantation guidelines for mechanical circulatory support; executive summary. *J Heart Lung Transplant.* 2013;32(2):157.

106. Trost JC, Hillis D. Intra-aortic balloon counterpulsation. *Am J Cardiol.* 2006;97:1391.

107. Moon C. Peroperative intraaortic balloon pumping in high-risk cardiac surgery patients. *Dimens Crit Care Nurs.* 2012;31(4):223.

108. Hanlon-Pena PM, Quaal S. Intra-aortic balloon pump timing: review of the evidence supporting current practice. *Am J Crit Care.* 2011;20(4):323.

109. Hanlon-Pena PM, Quaal S. Resource document: evidence supporting current practice in timing assessment. *Am J Crit Care.* 2011;20(4):e99.

110. Loforte A, et al. Peripheral extracorporeal membrane oxygenation system as salvage treatment of patients with refractory cardiogenic shock: preliminary outcome evaluation. *Artif Organs.* 2012;36(3):E53.

111. Pratt AK, et al. Left ventricular assist device management in the ICU. *Crit Care Med.* 2014;41(1):158.

112. McIlvennan CK, et al. Clinical outcomes after continuous-flow left ventricular assist device. *Circ Heart Fail.* 2014;7:1003.

113. Bennett MK, et al. Ideal methodology to assess systemic blood pressure in patients with continuous-flow left ventricular assist devices. *J Heart Lung Transplant.* 2010;29:593.

114. Kernan WN, et al. Guidelines for the prevention of stroke in patients with stroke and transient ischemic attack: a guideline for healthcare professionals from the American Heart Association/American Stroke Association. *Stroke.* 2014;45:2160.

115. Meschia JF, et al. Guidelines for the primary prevention of stroke: a guideline for healthcare professionals from the American Heart Association/American Stroke Association. *Stroke.* 2014;45:3754.

116. Knutson JA, et al. Carotid artery endarterectomy: a multidisciplinary approach to improving resource utilization and quality assurance. *J Vasc Nurs.* 2013;31:84.

117. White CJ. Carotid artery stenting. *J Am Coll Cardiol.* 2014;64:722.

118. Chaturvedi S, Sacco RL. How recent data have impacted the treatment of internal carotid artery stenosis. *J Am Coll Cardiol.* 2015;65:1134.

119. Treat-Jacobson DJ, et al. Society for Vascular Nursing clinical practice guideline (CPG) for carotid artery stenting. *J Vasc Nurs.* 2013;31:32.

120. Chadi SA, et al. Trends in management of abdominal aortic aneurysms. *J Vasc Surg.* 2012;55(4):924.

121. Mohan PP, Hamblin MH. Comparison of endovascular and open repair of ruptured abdominal aortic aneurysm in the United States in the last decade. *Cardiovasc Intervent Radiol.* 2014;7:337.

122. Jackson RS, Chang DC, Freischlag JA. Comparison of long-term survival after open vs endovascular repair of intact abdominal aortic aneurysm among Medicare beneficiaries. *JAMA.* 2012;307(15):1621.

123. Buckley SD, Buckley CJ. Endovascular aortoiliac aneurysm repair: surgical progress through new treatment paradigms and innovative endograft design. *AORN J.* 2014;100(3):271.

124. Rooke TW, et al. 2011 ACCF/AHA Focused update of the guideline for the management of patients with peripheral artery disease (updating the 2005 guideline). *Circulation.* 2011;124:2020.

125. Norgren L, et al. Inter-society consensus for the management of peripheral arterial disease (TASC II). *J Vasc Surg.* 2007;45(Suppl S):S5.

126. Shamoun FE, Fankhauser GT, Mookadam M. Vascular medicine: aortic and peripheral arterial disease. *Prim Care Clin Office Pract.* 2013;40:169.

127. Bujak M, Gamberdella J, Mena C. Management of atherosclerotic aortoiliac occlusive disease. *Intervent Cardiol Clin.* 2014;3:531.

128. Kempe K, et al. Results of surgical management of acute thromboembolic lower extremity ischemia. *J Vasc Surg.* 2014;60:702.

129. Sardar MR. Antiarrhythmic drug therapy for atrial fibrillation. *Cardiol Clin.* 2014;32:533.

130. Samarin MJ, Mobrien KM, Oliphant CS. Continuous intravenous antiarrhythmic agents in the intensive care unit: strategies for safe and effective use of amiodarone, lidocaine, and procainamide. *Crit Care Nurs Q.* 2015;38:329.

131. Tracy C, Boushahri A. Managing arrhythmias in the intensive care unit. *Crit Care Clin.* 2014;30:365.

132. Drew BJ, et al. Prevention of torsade de pointes in hospital settings: a scientific statement from the American Heart Association and the American College of Cardiology Foundation. *Circulation.* 2010;121:1047.

133. Halsey C, Chugh A. Rate versus rhythm control for atrial fibrillation. *Cardiol Clin.* 2014;32:521.

134. Straznitskas A, Giarratano M. Emergent reversal of oral anticoagulation: review of current treatment strategies. *AACN Adv Crit Care.* 2014;25:5.

135. January CT, et al. 2014 AHA/ACC/HRS guideline for the management of patients with atrial fibrillation: a report of the American College of Cardiology/American Heart Association task force on practice guidelines and the Heart Rhythm Society. *Circulation.* 2014;130:e199.

136. Jentzer JC, et al. Pharmacotherapy update on the use of vasopressors and inotropes in the intensive care unit. *J Cardiovasc Pharmacol Ther.* 2015;20(3):249.

137. Kanter J, DeBlieux P. Pressors and inotropes. *Emerg Med Clin North Am.* 2014;32:823.

138. Francis GS, Bartos JA, Adatya S. Inotropes. *J Am Coll Cardiol.* 2014;63(20):2069.

139. Adabeyo O, Rogers RL. Hypertensive emergencies in the emergency department. *Emerg Med Clin North Am.* 2015;33:539.

140. Buonocore D, Wallace E. Comprehensive guideline for care of patients with heart failure. *AACN Adv Crit Care.* 2014;25:151.

141. Miller J, et al. Management of hypertension in stroke. *Ann Emerg Med.* 2014;64:248.

142. Suzuki T. Type-selective benefits of medications in treatment of acute aortic dissection (from the International Registry of Acute Aortic dissection [IRAD]). *Am J Cardiol.* 2012;109:122.

143. Callaway CW, et al. Part 4: advanced life support: 2015 International consensus on cardiopulmonary resuscitation and emergency cardiovascular care science with treatment recommendations. *Circulation.* 2015;132(Suppl 1):S84.

144. Dellinger RP, et al. Surviving sepsis campaign: international guidelines for management of severe sepsis and septic shock 2012. *Crit Care Med.* 2013(41):580.

16

Pulmonary Anatomy and Physiology

Kathleen M. Stacy

The pulmonary system consists of the thorax, conducting airways, respiratory airways, and pulmonary blood and lymph supply. The primary functions of the pulmonary system are ventilation and respiration. *Ventilation* is the movement of air in and out of the lungs. *Respiration* is the process of gas exchange by means of movement of oxygen from the atmosphere into the bloodstream and movement of carbon dioxide from the bloodstream into the atmosphere. The anatomic structures that constitute the pulmonary system are intimately related to function, and structural abnormalities can readily translate into pulmonary disorders. An applicable knowledge of anatomy and physiology is imperative in caring for a patient with pulmonary dysfunction.

THORAX

The thorax contains the major organs of respiration and consists of the thoracic cage, lungs, pleura, and muscles of ventilation. Together, these structures form the ventilatory pump, which performs the work of breathing.

Thoracic Cage

The thoracic cage is a cone-shaped structure that is rigid but flexible so as to protect the underlying structures and to accommodate inhalation and exhalation. The cage consists of 12 thoracic vertebrae, each with a pair of ribs. Posteriorly, each rib is attached to its own vertebra, but anteriorly, attachment varies (Fig. 16.1). The first seven pairs of ribs are attached directly to the sternum. The 8th, 9th, and 10th pairs are attached by cartilage to the ribs above. Because the 11th and 12th ribs have no anterior attachment, they sometimes are referred to as *floating ribs*. The second rib is attached to the sternum at the angle of Louis, which is the raised ridge that can be felt just below the suprasternal notch.[1]

Lungs

The lungs are cone-shaped organs that have a total volume of approximately 3.5 to 8.5 L. The superior portion is known as the *apex*, and the inferior portion is known as the *base*. The apical portion of each lung rises a few centimeters above the clavicle (see Fig. 16.1). Each lung is firmly attached to the thoracic cavity at the hilum and at the pulmonary ligament.[2]

Lobes and Segments

The lungs are divided into lobes and segments (Fig. 16.2), with the lobes being separated by pleural membrane–covered fissures. The right lung, which is larger and heavier than the left, is divided into upper, middle, and lower lobes. The left lung is divided into only an upper and a lower lobe.[2] A portion of the left lung, the lingula, corresponds anatomically with the right middle lobe. The horizontal fissure divides the right upper lobe from the right middle lobe. The oblique fissure divides the right upper and middle lobes from the lower lobe and the left upper lobe from the lower lobe. The lobes are divided into 18 segments, each of which has its own bronchus branching immediately off a lobar bronchus. There are 10 segments in the right lung and 8 in the left lung.[1]

Mediastinum

The area between the two lungs, the mediastinum, contains the heart, great vessels, lymphatics, and esophagus. A portion of the mediastinal area contains the root of the lungs, also known as the hilum, in which the visceral and parietal pleural membranes form a sheath around the main stem bronchi, the major blood vessels, and the nerves that enter and exit the lungs.[2]

Pleura

The pleura is a thin membrane that lines the outside of the lungs and the inside of the chest wall. The visceral pleura adheres to the lungs, extending onto the hilar bronchi and into the major fissures. The parietal pleura lines the inner surface of the chest wall and mediastinum.[2] The two pleural surfaces are separated by an airtight space, which contains a thin layer of lubricating fluid. Pleural fluid allows the visceral and parietal pleural membranes to glide against each other during inhalation and exhalation.[1,3] The pleural space has the capacity to hold much more fluid than its normal volume of a few milliliters.[1]

Intrapleural Pressure

The pleural space has a pressure within it called the *intrapleural pressure*, which differs from the intrapulmonary (pressure within the lungs) and atmospheric pressures.[4] Under normal conditions, intrapleural pressure is less than intrapulmonary pressure and less than atmospheric pressure, with a normal range of -4 to -10 cm H_2O during exhalation and inhalation, respectively.[3] A deep inhalation can generate intrapleural pressures of -12 to

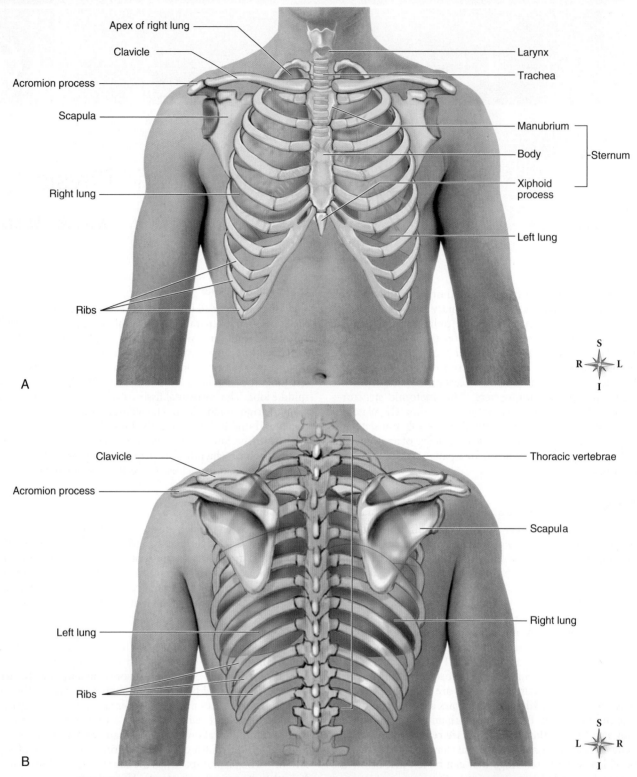

FIG. 16.1 Bony Structures of the Chest. These structures form a protective and expandable cage around the lungs and heart. (A) Anterior view. (B) Posterior view. (Adapted from Thompson JM, Wilson SF. *Health Assessment for Nursing Practice.* St. Louis: Mosby; 1996. In Patton KT, Thibodeau GA, eds. *Anatomy and Physiology.* 8th ed. St. Louis: Mosby; 2013.)

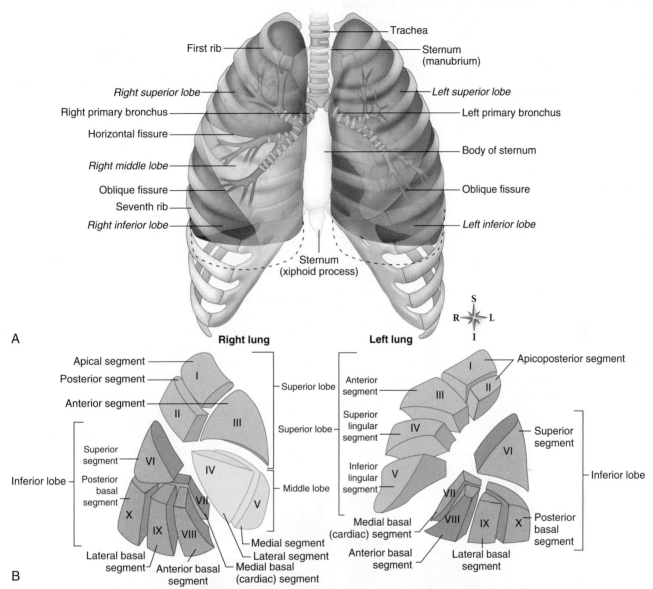

Trachea
Sternum (manubrium)
First rib
Right superior lobe
Left superior lobe
Right primary bronchus
Left primary bronchus
Horizontal fissure
Body of sternum
Right middle lobe
Oblique fissure
Oblique fissure
Seventh rib
Right inferior lobe
Left inferior lobe
Sternum (xiphoid process)

A   **Right lung**   **Left lung**

S
R ✴ L
I

Apical segment
Posterior segment
Anterior segment
Superior lobe
Anterior segment
Apicoposterior segment
Superior lobe
Superior lingular segment
Superior segment
Posterior basal segment
Inferior lobe
Middle lobe
Inferior lingular segment
Inferior lobe
Superior segment
Posterior basal segment
Lateral basal segment
Anterior basal segment
Medial basal (cardiac) segment
Medial segment
Lateral segment
Medial basal (cardiac) segment
Anterior basal segment
Lateral basal segment

B

FIG. 16.2 Lobes and Segments of the Lungs. (A) Anterior view of the lungs, bronchi, and trachea. (B) Expanded diagram showing the bronchopulmonary segments. (From Patton KT, Thibodeau GA, eds. *Anatomy and Physiology*. 8th ed. St. Louis: Mosby; 2013.)

−18 cm H_2O. This negative intrapleural pressure results from forces within the chest wall that exert pressure to pull the parietal pleura outward and away from the visceral pleura, whereas the elastic fibers within the lungs exert pressure to pull the visceral pleura inward away from the parietal pleura. The constant pull of the two pleural membranes in opposite directions causes the pressure within the space to be subatmospheric.[4] The negative pressure in the pleural space keeps the lungs inflated (Box 16.1). If atmospheric pressure enters the pleural space, all or part of a lung will collapse, producing a pneumothorax.[1]

Muscles of Ventilation

The muscles of ventilation (Fig. 16.3) are governed by the regulatory activity of the central nervous system, which sends messages to the muscles to stimulate contraction and relaxation. This muscular activity controls inhalation and exhalation. Muscles that increase the size of the chest are called *muscles of*

inhalation; muscles that decrease the size of the chest are called *muscles of exhalation*.[5]

Inhalation

The main muscle of inhalation is the diaphragm. The diaphragm is a dome-shaped, fibromuscular septum that separates the thoracic and abdominal cavities and is connected to the sternum, ribs, and vertebrae. During normal, quiet breathing, the diaphragm does approximately 80% of the work of breathing. On inhalation, the diaphragm contracts and flattens, pushes down on the viscera, and displaces the abdomen outward. Diaphragmatic contraction also lifts and expands the rib cage to some extent.[1,5,6]

The action of the diaphragm is governed by the medulla, which sends its impulses through the phrenic nerve. The phrenic nerve arises from the cervical plexus through the fourth cervical nerve, with secondary contributions by the third and

The lungs stay inflated because the pressure surrounding them (intrapleural) is always less than the pressure within them (intrapulmonary).

Why Is the Intrapleural Pressure Less Than the Intrapulmonary Pressure?

The intrapleural pressure is always (1) less than intrapulmonary pressure, (2) less than atmospheric pressure, and (3) considered negative because of the pull of the two pleural membranes in opposite directions. The parietal pleura is pulled outward by forces within the chest wall, whereas the visceral pleura is pulled inward by the force of the elastic fibers within the lungs.

Why Do the Two Pleural Membranes Pull in Opposite Directions?

The parietal pleura, attached to the chest, is pulled outward because the elastic fibers within the intercostal muscles exert outward pressure on the ribs. These fibers are in a relaxed state when the rib cage is fully expanded, such as during a deep inhalation. The visceral pleura is attached to the lungs and is pulled inward because the elastic fibers within the lungs that are responsible for elastic recoil exert pressure to make the lungs smaller. Elastic fibers in the lung are in a relaxed position only when the lung is at its smallest configuration, as occurs with a pneumothorax. Because of the opposite pull of the chest wall and the lung and because the pleural membranes are attached to these structures, there is a constant pull of the two membranes in opposite directions. The subatmospheric pressure that results within the pleural space and the greater-than-atmospheric intrapulmonary pressure within the lungs allows the lungs to remain inflated. Anything that causes the pressure within the pleural space to rise to atmospheric pressure or above will cause the lung to collapse—a pneumothorax.

fifth cervical nerves. For this reason and because the diaphragm does most of the work of inhalation, trauma involving levels C3 to C5 causes ventilatory dysfunction.[5]

Muscles that lift the rib cage are other muscles of inhalation. The most important of these are the external intercostal muscles, which elevate the ribs and expand the chest cage outward. The scalene, anterior serratus, and sternocleidomastoid muscles also participate to elevate the first two ribs and sternum.[1,5,6]

Exhalation

Exhalation in the healthy lung is a passive event requiring very little energy. Exhalation occurs when the diaphragm relaxes and moves back up toward the lungs. The intrinsic elastic recoil of the lungs assists with exhalation. Because exhalation is a passive act, there are no true muscles of exhalation other than the internal intercostal muscles, which assist the inward movement of the ribs. However, exhalation becomes a more active event during exercise, requiring some participation of the accessory muscles of ventilation. Several muscles of the abdomen are thought to contribute to active exhalation.[4,5]

Accessory Muscles

The accessory muscles of ventilation usually are considered to be muscles that enhance chest expansion during exercise but that are not active during normal, quiet breathing. These muscles include the scalene, sternocleidomastoid, and other chest and back muscles, such as the trapezius and the pectoralis major.[1,5,6]

CONDUCTING AIRWAYS

The conducting airways consist of the upper airways, the trachea, and the bronchial tree. The conducting airways warm and

FIG. 16.3 Muscles of Ventilation. (From Wilkin RL, et al, eds. *Egan's Fundamentals of Respiratory Care.* 8th ed. St. Louis: Mosby; 2003.)

humidify the inhaled air, act as a protective mechanism that prevents the entrance of foreign matter into the gas exchange areas, and serve as a passageway for air entering and leaving the gas exchange regions of the lungs.[1-3]

Upper Airways

The upper airways consist of the nasal and oral cavities, the pharynx, and the larynx (Fig. 16.4). Their main contribution to ventilation is the conditioning of inspired air. *Conditioned air* is air that has been warmed, humidified, and cleansed of some irritants. Warming and humidifying, which are essential to prevent irritation of the lower airways, occur mainly within the nose by means of a dense vascular network that lines the nasal passages. The air is cleansed by the coarse hairs that line the nasal passages and filter large inhaled particles.[1,3]

Epiglottis

The epiglottis is located in the upper airways. The epiglottis protects the lower airways by closing the opening to the trachea during swallowing so that food passes into the esophagus and not the trachea. The epiglottis is a thin, leaf-shaped, elastic cartilage that is located directly posterior to the root of the tongue and attached to the thyroid cartilage (see Fig. 16.4). The epiglottis opens widely during inhalation, permitting air to pass through the trachea into the lower airways.[1]

Trachea

The trachea is a hollow tube approximately 11 cm (4.5 inches) long and 2.5 cm (1 inch) in diameter (Fig. 16.5). The trachea begins at the cricoid cartilage and ends at the bifurcation (major carina) from which the two main stem bronchi arise. The carina is positioned approximately at the level of the aortic arch, the fifth thoracic vertebra,[7] or just below the level of the angle of Louis.[1] The trachea consists of smooth muscle supported anteriorly by 16 to 20 C-shaped, cartilaginous rings. They prevent tracheal collapse during bronchoconstriction and strong coughing. The posterior wall of the trachea lies contiguous with the anterior wall of the esophagus. Having no cartilaginous support, this wall is composed only of muscle tissue, which is separated from the anterior esophageal wall by loose connective tissue (see Fig. 16.5, inset).[1]

Bronchial Tree

The two main stem bronchi are structurally different (see Fig. 16.5). The left bronchus is slightly narrower than the right, and because of its position above the heart, the left bronchus angles

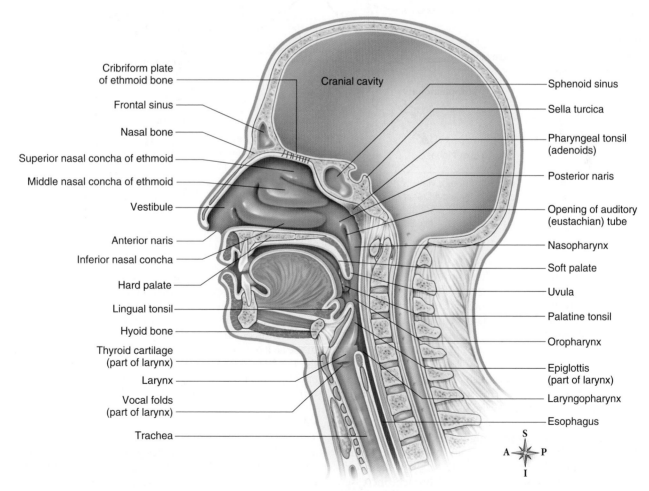

FIG. 16.4 Upper Respiratory Tract. In this midsagittal section through the upper respiratory tract, the nasal septum has been removed to reveal the turbinates (nasal conchae) of the lateral wall of the nasal cavity. The three divisions of the pharynx (nasopharynx, oropharynx, and laryngopharynx) are also visible. (From Patton KT, Thibodeau GA, eds. *Anatomy and Physiology.* 8th ed. St. Louis: Mosby; 2013.)

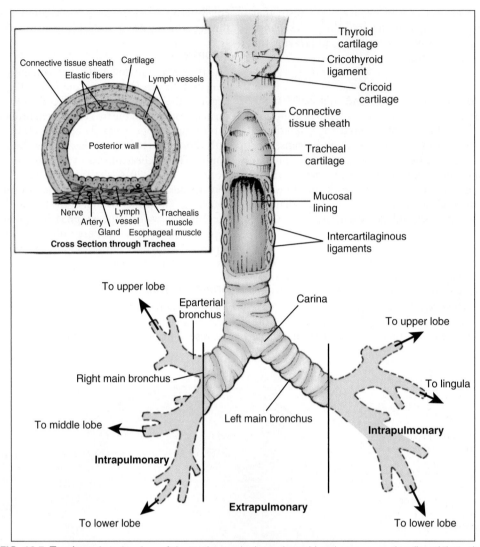

FIG. 16.5 Trachea. Anterior view of the trachea and primary bronchi and a cross section *(inset)* through a part of the trachea, including a C-shaped cartilaginous element. (From Martin DE. *Respiratory Anatomy and Physiology.* St. Louis: Mosby; 1988.)

directly toward the left lung at approximately 45 to 55 degrees from the midline. The right bronchus is wider and angles at 20 to 30 degrees from the midline. Because of this angulation and the forces of gravity, the most common site of aspiration of foreign objects is through the right main stem bronchus into the lower lobe of the right lung.[2,3]

Bronchi

Each branching of the tracheobronchial tree produces a new generation of tubes (Fig. 16.6). The main stem bronchi are the first generation; the next branch, the five lobar bronchi, is the second generation. The third generation includes the 18 segmental bronchi. The fourth through approximately the ninth generations are referred to as the small bronchi, beginning with the subsegmental bronchi. In these bronchi, diameters decrease; however, because the number of bronchi increases with each generation, the total cross-sectional area increases with each generation. This great increase in the cross-sectional area of the lung is significant because it allows easy ventilation despite decreasing airway lumens.[1]

Bronchioles

The final subdivision of the conducting airways is the bronchioles. These tubes have a diameter less than 1 mm and have no connective tissue and cartilage within their walls. However, their walls do contain smooth muscle.[2] When smooth muscle constriction occurs, these airways may close completely because of the lack of structural support. The terminal bronchioles form the last branch of the conducting airways, after which the gas exchange areas of the lungs begin. There are more than 32,000 terminal bronchioles.[1]

Defense System

The main defense system within the airways is the mucociliary escalator, or mucous blanket, a combination of mucus and cilia. The mucus, which floats atop the cilia (Fig. 16.7), traps foreign particles. Ciliary movement propels the entire mucous blanket and any trapped particles upward toward the pharynx at an average speed of 1 mm/min in the smaller bronchioles and 12 mm/min in the larger airways and trachea. After the pharynx is reached, the mucus is swallowed or cleared. The submucous

Conducting Airways				Respiratory Unit
Trachea	Segmental bronchi	Subsegmental bronchi (bronchioles)		Alveolar ducts
		Nonrespiratory	Respiratory	
Generations	8	16	24	26

FIG. 16.6 Conducting and Respiratory Airways. Note escalating branching with increasing generations. (From Thompson JM, et al, eds. *Mosby's Clinical Nursing.* 5th ed. St. Louis: Mosby; 2002.)

FIG. 16.7 Cilia. Scanning electron micrograph of the luminal surface and cilia of a bronchiole from a healthy man (×2000). (From Ebert RV, Terracio MJ. Observation of the secretion on the surface of the bronchioles with the scanning electron microscope. *Am Rev Respir Dis.* 1975;112:491.)

glands of the airways produce approximately 100 mL of mucus per day, with all but approximately 10 mL resorbed through the bronchial lining. The mucociliary escalator is so efficient that almost no particles larger than 3 μm reach the alveoli.[8]

The cough reflex is another protective mechanism in the lungs. Excessive amounts of foreign particles in the trachea and bronchi can initiate the cough reflex. Once initiated, the rapid expulsion of air carries away any foreign particles with it.[9]

RESPIRATORY AIRWAYS

The respiratory airways consist of the respiratory bronchioles and the alveoli. The respiratory airways also are known as the *terminal respiratory units*, or the *acini*. Gas exchange takes place in these areas of the lungs.

Respiratory Bronchioles

Each terminal bronchiole gives rise to two respiratory bronchioles, with each branching two to four more times.[2] The respiratory bronchioles form the transition zone of the lungs, acting as conducting airways and gas exchange units. While air is moving through them, alveolar outpouchings on their surfaces allow gas exchange to take place (see Fig. 16.6).[1]

Alveoli

Each respiratory bronchiole gives rise to several alveolar ducts, which terminate in clusters of 10 to 16 alveoli (see Fig. 16.6). Each terminal respiratory unit contains approximately 100 alveolar ducts and 2000 alveoli.[2] The alveolus is the primary site of gas exchange and the end point in the respiratory tract. The two lungs contain approximately 300 million alveoli. The alveoli comprise several types of cells, including type I and II alveolar epithelial cells and alveolar macrophages.[1,3]

Type I Alveolar Epithelial Cells

Type I alveolar epithelial cells constitute approximately 90% of the total alveolar surface within the lungs (Fig. 16.8). They are the chief structural cells of the alveolar wall and play a major role in the maintenance of the gas-blood barrier and gas exchange. Type I cells are extremely susceptible to injury and become inflamed when exposed to inhaled toxins.[1]

Collateral air passages. A variety of collateral air passages are located within the lower regions of the lungs. Within the walls of the type I cells are the pores of Kohn (Fig. 16.9), which allow collateral movement of air between alveoli. The canals of Lambert are collateral air pathways that exist between the alveoli and the respiratory and terminal bronchioles. They are of particular benefit when a respiratory bronchiole is blocked or collapsed because they allow gas to pass into alveoli distal to the blockage.

FIG. 16.8 Type 1 Alveolar Epithelial Cell. Detail of an alveolar surface composed chiefly of type I alveolar epithelial cells (scale: 1 cm of picture width = 3.46 μm). (From Martin DE. *Respiratory Anatomy and Physiology*. St. Louis: Mosby; 1988.)

FIG. 16.9 Pores of Kohn. Scanning electron micrograph of the surface of a human alveolus shows the pores of Kohn *(P)* and a macrophage *(arrow)* (×1500). (Courtesy M.S. Wang, MD.)

Collateral air passages are of significant benefit in any pathologic condition of the lung that results in obstruction of airflow into a portion of the lungs. However, these pores and canals also allow the movement of microorganisms through lung tissue.[1,2]

Type II Alveolar Epithelial Cells

Type II alveolar epithelial cells occur in much greater numbers than type I cells, but because of their minute size, they constitute a smaller portion of the total alveolar wall. After injury to the alveolar wall, type II cells rapidly divide to line the surface; later, they transform into type I cells. The most important function of the type II cells is their ability to produce, store, and secrete pulmonary surfactant (Fig. 16.10).[1,3]

Surfactant. Surfactant is a phospholipid composed of fatty acids bound to lecithin. Similar to other surfactants, such as detergents and soaps, pulmonary surfactant functions to lower surface tension of the alveoli. With detergents and

FIG. 16.10 Type II Alveolar Epithelial Cell. Note presence of brush microvilli on all except the bald top of the round luminal surface. Type II cells produce surfactant (scale: 1 cm of picture width = 0.85 μm). (From Martin DE. *Respiratory Anatomy and Physiology*. St. Louis: Mosby; 1988.)

soaps, this decrease in surface tension cleans clothes, whereas within the lungs, surfactant stabilizes the alveoli, increases lung compliance, and eases the work of breathing. When pulmonary disease disrupts the normal synthesis and storage of surfactant, the lungs become less compliant, and the work of breathing increases. Severe loss of surfactant results in alveolar instability and collapse and impairment of gas exchange.[10]

Defense System

Alveolar macrophages are monocytes that originate in the bone marrow and are released into the bloodstream (Fig. 16.11).[1-3] On entering the pulmonary capillary circulation, they move through the capillary membrane wall into the interstitial space and through to the alveoli. In the alveoli, the monocytes transform into macrophages and assume a phagocytic role. They move from alveolus to alveolus through the pores of Kohn, keeping the alveoli clean and sterile through phagocytosis and microbial killing activity, which includes the secretion of hydrogen peroxide, lysozyme, and other substances that kill microorganisms.[2,3]

PULMONARY BLOOD AND LYMPH SUPPLY

Two vascular systems and one lymphatic system make up the pulmonary blood and lymph supply. The pulmonary circulation is the vascular system that forms the gas exchange network surrounding the alveoli. The bronchial circulation is the vascular system that perfuses the tracheobronchial tree.[1]

Pulmonary Circulation

The pulmonary circulatory system begins at the pulmonary artery, which receives venous blood from the right side of the heart. The pulmonary artery then divides into left and right

FIG. 16.11 Alveolar Macrophage. Scanning electron micrograph of a healthy human lung shows an alveolar macrophage *(Ma)* attached to the epithelium partly by filopodia *(FP)* and forming an undulating membrane *(U)* in the direction of forward movement to the left. Several capillaries *(C)* are evident, and a type II alveolar epithelial cell *(EP2)* can be seen in the background (original magnification ×3700.) (From Gehr P, et al. The normal human lung: ultrastructure and morphometric estimation of diffusion capacity. *Respir Physiol.* 1978;32[2]:121.)

branches and continues to branch until it forms the capillaries that surround the alveoli (Fig. 16.12). After gas exchange takes place, the blood is returned to the left side of the heart through the pulmonary veins.[1,2]

Pulmonary Artery Pressures

The pulmonary circulation is by far the largest vascular bed within the body, and it is the only one that receives the entire cardiac output. Just as the systemic circulation has a systolic and a diastolic blood pressure, so does the pulmonary circulation. However, because of the relative lack of smooth muscle within the vessels of the pulmonary circulation, the pressures are vastly lower than within the systemic circulation.[1,3] Pulmonary artery systolic pressure ranges from 15 to 30 mm Hg, pulmonary artery diastolic pressure ranges from 4 to 12 mm Hg, and pulmonary artery mean pressure ranges from 9 to 18 mm Hg.[11] Because of the low pulmonary artery pressures, right ventricular wall thickness needs to be only approximately one-third of left ventricular wall thickness. However, just as hypertension can occur within the systemic circulation, hypertension also can occur within the pulmonary circulation.[12]

Alveolar-Capillary Membrane

The vessels of the alveolar-capillary membrane form a network around each alveolus that is so dense it forms an almost continuous sheet of blood covering the alveoli.[2] The interior diameter of each capillary segment is just large enough to allow red blood cells to squeeze by in single file so that their cell membranes touch the capillary walls (Fig. 16.13).[3] In this way, oxygen and carbon dioxide need not pass through significant amounts of plasma when diffusing into and out of the alveoli, making a highly efficient vehicle for gas exchange. Each red blood cell spends approximately three-fourths of a second in the alveolar-capillary network and is exposed to the alveolar gas of two or three alveoli.[1] In that short time, hemoglobin is brought from its normal venous blood saturation

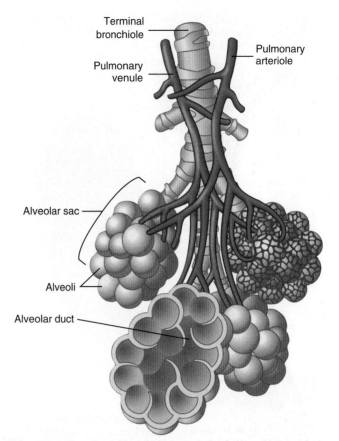

FIG. 16.12 Terminal Ventilation and Perfusion Units of the Lung. (Modified from Patton KT, Thibodeau GA, eds. *Anatomy and Physiology.* 8th ed. St. Louis: Mosby; 2013.)

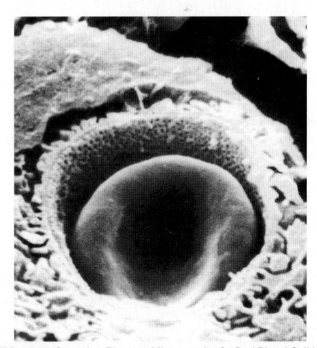

FIG. 16.13 Scanning Electron Micrograph of a Red Blood Cell in a Capillary. Note the diameters of both are similar. In many instances, the red blood cells course through even smaller capillaries, often through capillaries that are one-half of the diameter of the red blood cell. This is possible because the cells are pliable, mainly as a result of their biconcave disk shape. (From Martin DE. *Respiratory Anatomy and Physiology.* St. Louis: Mosby; 1988.)

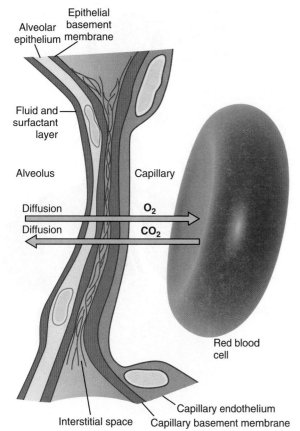

FIG. 16.14 Layers of the Alveolar-Capillary Membrane. (From Hall JE, ed. *Guyton and Hall Textbook of Medical Physiology.* 13th ed. Philadelphia: Saunders; 2016.)

level of 75% to its arterial saturation of more than 96%.[3] Hemoglobin levels have been shown to reach normal within only a 0.25-second exposure to alveolar gas; under conditions such as in tachycardia, in which the red blood cells spend less time within the pulmonary capillary network, normal oxygenation can still occur.[3]

Membrane Layers

The alveolar-capillary membrane is less than 0.5 μm thick[13] and is composed of several layers of cells: alveolar epithelium, alveolar basement membrane, interstitial space, capillary basement membrane, and capillary endothelium (Fig. 16.14). Oxygen and carbon dioxide traverse easily across these layers, which present no barrier to diffusion because the membrane is very thin.[3]

Bronchial Circulation

The bronchial circulation, also known as the *systemic blood supply to the lungs*, is the system that perfuses the tracheobronchial tree, the visceral pleura, interstitial and connective tissue, some arteries and veins, lymph nodes, and the nerves within the thoracic cavity. The bronchial arteries that perfuse structures in the left side of the thorax branch off the aorta, and the arteries that perfuse the right-sided structures branch from the intercostal, subclavian, or internal mammary artery. After perfusing the specific lung structures, most of the venous blood returns to the right side of the heart; however, some venous blood from the bronchial circulation returns directly into the pulmonary veins and the left atrium.[14]

Physiologic Shunting

The left atrium normally contains pure oxygenated blood, with a hemoglobin saturation level of 100%. The mixing of venous blood from the bronchial circulation with the oxygenated blood in the left atrium decreases the saturation of left atrial blood to 96% to 99%. For this reason, while a person is breathing room air, the oxygen saturation of arterial blood is less than 100%. The dumping of venous blood into the left atrium is known as an *anatomic shunt*. The thebesian veins, which drain the right coronary circulation, are also responsible for the addition of venous blood to the left atrium. These two systems constitute the normal anatomic shunt, which accounts for approximately 3% to 5% of the total cardiac output.[15]

Lymphatic Circulation

The lungs are more richly supplied with lymphatic tissue than any other organ, perhaps because of their constant exposure to the external environment. The lymphatic vessels parallel much of the pulmonary vasculature and the tracheobronchial tree to the level of the terminal and respiratory bronchioles. Lymphatic vessels also are located within the connective tissue of lung parenchyma and within the pleural membranes. These vessels eventually drain into the primary lymph nodes located at the hila of the lungs. The lymphatic system in the lungs serves two purposes. As part of the immune system, the lymphatic system is responsible for removing foreign particles and cell debris from the lungs and for producing antibody-mediated and cell-mediated immune responses. The lymphatic system also is responsible for removing fluid from the lungs and for keeping the alveoli clear.[1-3]

VENTILATION

Air moves into and out of the lungs because of the difference between intrapulmonary pressure (pressure inside the lungs) and atmospheric pressure (Fig. 16.15). The movement of air into the lungs is known as *inhalation* (see Fig. 16.15), and the movement of air out of the lungs is known as *exhalation* (Fig. 16.16). At the command of the central nervous system, the muscles of ventilation contract, the thorax and lungs expand, and intrapulmonary pressure decreases. When the pressure falls below atmospheric pressure, air enters the lungs, and inhalation occurs. At the end of inhalation, the muscles of ventilation relax, the thorax contracts and the lungs are compressed, and intrapulmonary pressure increases. When the pressure rises above atmospheric pressure, air exits the lungs, and exhalation occurs.[4,16]

Work of Breathing

The work of breathing is the amount of work that must be performed to overcome the elastic and resistive properties of the lungs. The elastic properties are determined by lung recoil, chest wall recoil, and the surface tension of the alveoli. The resistive properties are determined by airway resistance.[1,16,17] Normally, the work of breathing occurs during inhalation, but even exhalation can be a strain when lung recoil, chest wall recoil, or airway resistance is abnormal.[4,16]

During normal, quiet ventilation, only 1% to 2% of basal oxygen consumption is required by the pulmonary system.[17] During heavy exercise, the amount of energy required by the pulmonary system can become progressively greater. The work of breathing can be a factor that limits exercise in a patient with

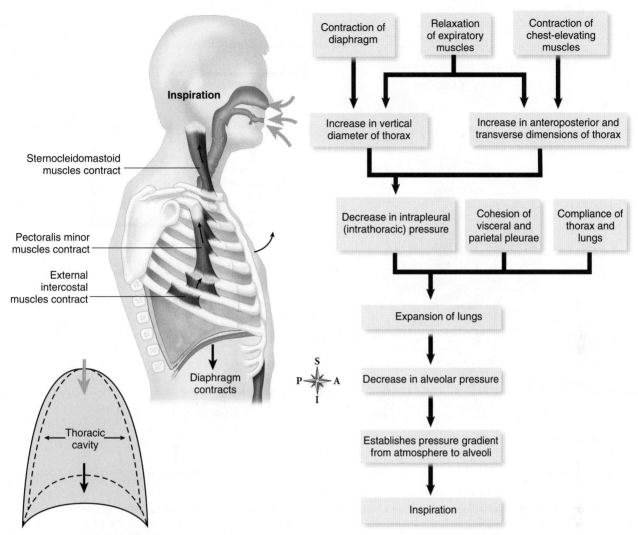

FIG. 16.15 Mechanism of Inspiration. Note the role of the diaphragm and the chest-elevating muscles (pectoralis minor and external intercostals) in increasing thoracic volume, which decreases pressure in the lungs and draws air inward. (From Patton KT, Thibodeau GA, eds. *Anatomy and Physiology.* 8th ed. St. Louis: Mosby; 2013.)

pulmonary disease. Pathologic conditions of the pulmonary system can drastically change the energy requirement for ventilation. Pulmonary diseases that decrease lung compliance (eg, atelectasis, pulmonary edema), decrease chest wall compliance (eg, kyphoscoliosis), increase airway resistance (eg, bronchitis, asthma), or decrease lung recoil (eg, emphysema) can increase the work of breathing so much that one-third or more of the total body energy is used for ventilation (Box 16.2).[4,16]

Pulmonary Volumes and Capacities

Pulmonary ventilation can be described in terms of volumes and capacities (Fig. 16.17). Tidal volume(V_T) is the amount of air inhaled and exhaled with each breath. Inspiratory reserve volume (IRV) is the maximum amount of air that can be inhaled over and above the normal tidal volume. Expiratory reserve volume(ERV) is the maximum amount of air that can be exhaled beyond the normal tidal volume. The residual volume (RV) is the amount of air left in the lungs after a complete exhalation. Inspiratory capacity(IC) is the sum of the tidal volume and the inspiratory reserve. Functional residual

capacity(FRC) is the sum of the expiratory reserve volume and the residual volume. Vital capacity(VC) is the sum of the inspiratory reserve volume, the tidal volume, and the expiratory reserve volume. Total lung capacity (TLC) is the sum of all four volumes and represents the maximal amount of air that can be inhaled.[3,16]

Physiologic Dead Space

The portion of total ventilation that participates in gas exchange is known as *alveolar ventilation*. The portion of ventilation that does not participate in gas exchange is known as *wasted ventilation*. The areas in the lungs that are ventilated but in which no gas exchange occurs are known as *dead space regions*. The conducting airways are referred to as *anatomic dead space* because they are ventilated but not perfused and therefore are unable to participate in gas exchange. Some ventilation goes to unperfused alveoli. Without perfusion, gas exchange cannot take place, and the ventilation is wasted. These unperfused alveoli are known as *alveolar dead space*. Anatomic dead space plus alveolar dead space is called *physiologic dead space*.[3,15,16]

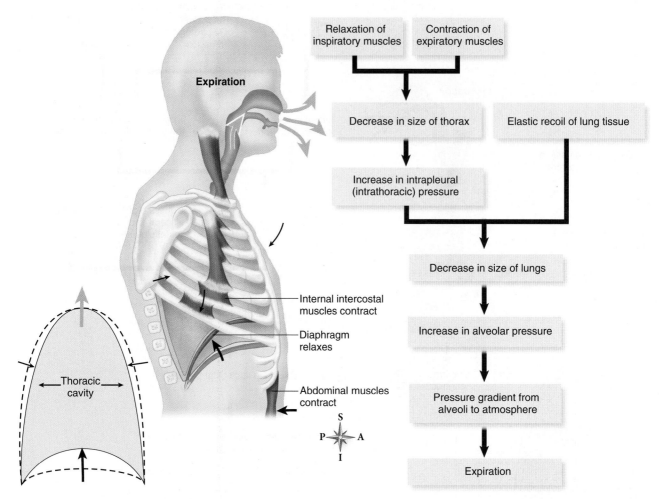

FIG. 16.16 Mechanism of Expiration. Note that relaxation of the diaphragm plus contraction of chest-depressing muscles (internal intercostals) reduces thoracic volume, which increases pressure in the lungs and pushes air outward. (From Patton KT, Thibodeau GA, eds. *Anatomy and Physiology.* 8th ed. St. Louis: Mosby; 2013.)

BOX 16.2 How Lung Disease Can Alter Ventilation

Normal muscular action of the diaphragm, flexibility of the rib cage, elasticity of the lungs, and airway diameter are instrumental in allowing easy inhalation and exhalation. Any interference with these actions impairs normal ventilation. Pulmonary diseases can be categorized as obstructive or restrictive, depending on how the underlying cause affects normal ventilation.

Restrictive diseases limit lung or chest wall movement and include diffuse interstitial lung fibrosis, atelectasis, kyphoscoliosis, and severe chest wall pain. These conditions can be acute or chronic, and because they restrict lung or chest wall expansion, or both, patients have smaller tidal volumes but an increased ventilatory rate to maintain minute ventilation.

Obstructive diseases impede normal airflow. Classic examples are emphysema, in which airflow is decreased because of a decrease in lung recoil, and asthma, in which airflow is decreased because of diffuse airway narrowing. Emphysema results in lungs that inflate easily but, lacking the normal elastic recoil, do not compress to assist with exhalation. Patients with emphysema may have little difficulty inhaling but struggle to exhale.

Regulation of Ventilation

Regulation of ventilation by the brain is complex and not completely understood. Ventilation is regulated by a triad comprising a controller (located within the central nervous system), a group of effectors (muscles of ventilation), and various sensors that include chemoreceptors (central and peripheral) and mechanoreceptors (located in chest wall and lungs). Efferent nerve fibers convey impulses from the controller to the effectors, whereas afferent nerve fibers carry impulses from some of the sensors to the controller (Fig. 16.18).[18]

Controller

The central nervous system houses what is known as the *controller of ventilation.* The controller is not located in one specific area; rather, it is in several areas that work together to provide coordinated ventilation. The brainstem regulates automatic ventilation, the cerebral cortex allows voluntary ventilation, and neurons housed in the spinal cord process information from the brain and from the peripheral receptors, allowing them to send final information to the muscles of ventilation.[18]

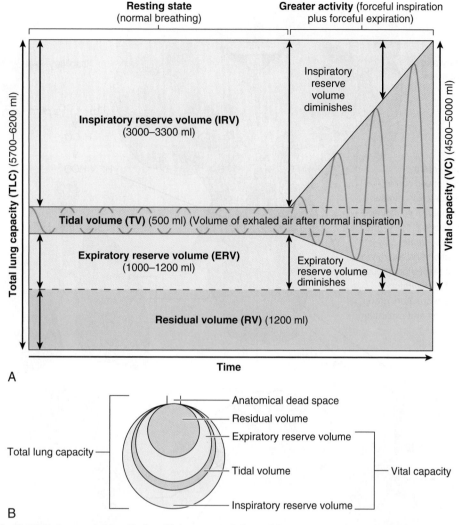

Resting state (normal breathing)

Greater activity (forceful inspiration plus forceful expiration)

Total lung capacity (TLC) (5700–6200 ml)

Inspiratory reserve volume (IRV) (3000–3300 ml)

Inspiratory reserve volume diminishes

Vital capacity (VC) (4500–5000 ml)

Tidal volume (TV) (500 ml) (Volume of exhaled air after normal inspiration)

Expiratory reserve volume (ERV) (1000–1200 ml)

Expiratory reserve volume diminishes

Residual volume (RV) (1200 ml)

Time

A

Total lung capacity

Anatomical dead space
Residual volume
Expiratory reserve volume
Tidal volume
Inspiratory reserve volume

Vital capacity

B

FIG. 16.17 Pulmonary Ventilation Volumes and Capacities. (A) Spirogram. (B) Pulmonary volumes (at rest) represented as relative proportions of an inflated balloon. During normal, quiet respirations, the atmosphere and lungs exchange approximately 500 mL of air *(TV)*. With forcible inspiration, approximately 3300 mL more air can be inhaled *(IRV)*. After a normal inspiration and normal expiration, approximately 1000 mL more air can be forcibly expired *(ERV)*. Vital capacity is the amount of air that can be forcibly expired after a maximal inspiration and indicates the largest amount of air that can enter and leave the lungs during respiration. Residual volume is the air that remains trapped in the alveoli.

Brainstem. In the brainstem, the medulla oblongata and the pons are involved in ventilation. Four different groups of neurons are thought to participate in the regulation of inhalation and exhalation. The dorsal respiratory group, located in the medulla, is responsible for the basic rhythm of ventilation. Cells in this area are thought to fire automatically and trigger inhalation. The pneumotaxic center in the pons is responsible for limiting inhalation and triggering exhalation. This response also facilitates control of the rate and pattern of respiration. The ventral respiratory group, located in the medulla, is responsible for inspiration and expiration during periods of increased ventilation. The apneustic center in the lower pons is thought to work with the pneumotaxic center to regulate the depth of inspiration.[18]

Cerebral cortex. The cerebral cortex functions by allowing voluntary ventilation to override the automatic controls of the medulla and pons. Voluntary ventilatory control is most important during behavioral states such as crying, laughing, singing, and talking. During these states, voluntary control may override the automatic control, which responds chiefly to chemical stimuli and to changes in lung inflation.[3,18]

Effectors

The effectors of ventilation are the muscles of ventilation (see Fig. 16.3). In considering their function in the control of ventilation, the most important issue is that they function in a coordinated fashion. The central nervous system regulates this function.[18]

Sensors

The main sensors for the regulation of ventilation are the central and peripheral chemoreceptors (see Fig. 16.18). These chemoreceptors respond to changes in the chemical composition of the blood or other fluid around them. Other sensors that are found in the lung include the irritant receptors, stretch receptors, and the juxtacapillary receptors (J-receptors).[3,18]

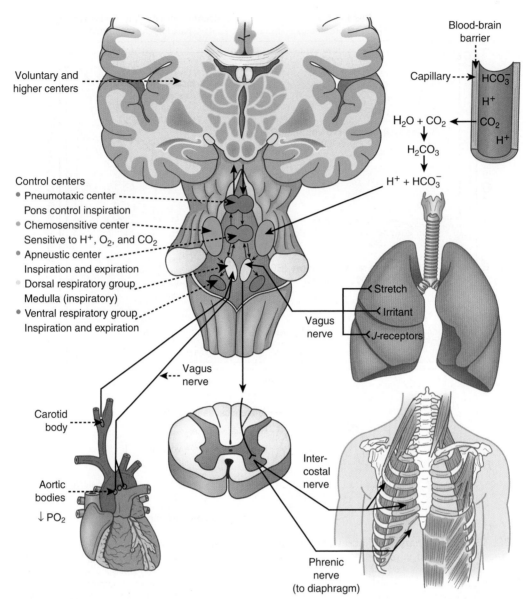

FIG. 16.18 Respiratory Control System. (From McCance KL, et al, eds. *Pathophysiology: The Biologic Basis for Disease in Adults and Children.* 7th ed. St. Louis: Mosby; 2014.)

Central chemoreceptors. The central chemoreceptors are located near the ventral surface of the medulla in the chemosensitive area (see Fig. 16.18). These chemoreceptors are surrounded by cerebral extracellular fluid and respond primarily to changes in the hydrogen ion concentration of that fluid. Ventilation increases when the hydrogen ion concentration rises and decreases when the hydrogen ion concentration falls. A rise in the partial pressure of carbon dioxide ($Paco_2$) causes the movement of carbon dioxide across the blood-brain barrier into the cerebrospinal fluid, stimulating the movement of hydrogen ions into the extracellular fluid of the brain. These hydrogen ions then stimulate the chemoreceptors, and ventilation is increased. The increase in ventilation causes exhalation of excess carbon dioxide, the $Paco_2$ decreases, and ventilation returns to normal. Central chemoreceptors are not affected by changes in the partial pressure of oxygen (Pao_2).[18]

Peripheral chemoreceptors. The peripheral chemoreceptors are located above and below the aortic arch and at the bifurcation of the common carotid arteries (see Fig. 16.18). The most important action of the peripheral chemoreceptors is their response to changes in the Pao_2 because they are the primary receptors that increase ventilation in response to arterial hypoxemia. Immediate hyperventilation, one of the principal compensatory mechanisms in response to hypoxemia, is governed by these chemoreceptors. The peripheral chemoreceptors also respond to changes in $Paco_2$ and hydrogen ion concentration. An increase in either $Paco_2$ or hydrogen ion concentration results in an increase in ventilation. Studies indicate that the peripheral chemoreceptors probably are more involved with short-term response to carbon dioxide, whereas the central chemoreceptors are responsible for the long-term response to carbon dioxide.[18]

Other receptors. Irritant receptors lie between airway epithelial cells, and they stimulate bronchoconstriction and hyperpnea in response to inhaled irritants. Stretch receptors, which are located in the airways, are stimulated by changes

Inspired air
$PO_2 = 159$ mm Hg
$PCO_2 = 0.3$ mm Hg
$PH_2O = 3.7$ mm Hg
$PN_2 = 597$ mm Hg

Expired air
$PO_2 = 127$ mm Hg
$PCO_2 = 28$ mm Hg
$PH_2O = 21$ mm Hg
$PN_2 = 584$ mm Hg

Pulmonary artery

Pulmonary vein

From heart and systemic circulation values

$PO_2 = 40$ mm Hg
$PCO_2 = 46$ mm Hg
$PH_2O = 47$ mm Hg
$PN_2 = 573$ mm Hg

$PO_2 = 104$ mm Hg
$PCO_2 = 40$ mm Hg
$PH_2O = 47$ mm Hg
$PN_2 = 569$ mm Hg

CO_2

O_2

To heart and systemic circulation values

$PO_2 = 100$ mm Hg
$PCO_2 = 40$ mm Hg
$PH_2O = 47$ mm Hg
$PN_2 = 573$ mm Hg

Tissues

$PO_2 = 40$ mm Hg
$PCO_2 = 46$ mm Hg
$PH_2O = 47$ mm Hg
$PN_2 = 573$ mm Hg

FIG. 16.19 **Process of Respiration.** (From McCance KL, et al, eds. *Pathophysiology: The Biologic Basis for Disease in Adults and Children.* 7th ed. St. Louis: Mosby; 2014.)

in lung volume. They inhibit inhalation and are thought to protect the lung from overinflation (Hering-Breuer reflex). J-receptors lie in the alveolar walls close to the capillaries. They are stimulated by engorgement of the pulmonary capillaries and an increase in the interstitial fluid volume. Stimulation of the J-receptors is thought to cause rapid, shallow breathing.[19]

RESPIRATION

Respiration refers to the movement of oxygen and carbon dioxide. Gas exchange that takes place at the lung level through the alveolar-capillary membrane is referred to as *external respiration.* The diffusion of gases in and out of the cells at the tissue level is referred to as *internal respiration.*[3]

Diffusion

Oxygen and carbon dioxide move throughout the body by diffusion. Diffusion moves molecules from an area of high concentration to an area of low concentration. The difference in the concentrations of the gases is referred to as the *driving pressure.* The greater the driving pressure of the gas through the membrane, the greater the rate of diffusion.[3] Within the lungs, diffusion occurs because of the difference in the driving pressure between the pulmonary capillaries and the alveoli. Oxygen is in high concentration within the alveoli and exerts a higher driving pressure compared with the pulmonary capillaries;

therefore oxygen moves by diffusion from the alveoli into the pulmonary capillaries. Carbon dioxide is in higher concentration and has a higher driving pressure within the pulmonary capillaries compared with the alveoli; therefore carbon dioxide diffuses out of the capillaries into the alveoli, where carbon dioxide is exhaled (Fig. 16.19). The driving pressure of oxygen is lower at higher altitudes because the effects of gravity on the gases are lessened,[20] and the driving pressure of oxygen is higher when supplemental oxygen is administered.[21]

In addition to the driving pressure of gases, several other factors affect the rate of diffusion, such as the thickness of the alveolar-capillary membrane,[3] the surface area of the membrane,[22] and the diffusion coefficient of the gas.[21] An increase in the thickness of the alveolar-capillary membrane (eg, pulmonary edema, fibrosis)[3] or a decrease in the surface area of the membrane (eg, pneumonectomy, lobectomy, pulmonary embolus, emphysema)[22] decreases the rate of diffusion. The diffusion coefficient of each gas is determined by its solubility. The higher the diffusion coefficient, the faster the gas diffuses. Carbon dioxide has a much higher diffusion coefficient than oxygen, and carbon dioxide diffuses 20 times more rapidly than oxygen.[21]

VENTILATION/PERFUSION RELATIONSHIPS

Ventilation ($\dot{V}$) and perfusion ($\dot{Q}$) should be equally matched at the alveolar-capillary membrane level for optimal gas exchange to take place, but because of normal regional variations in the distribution of ventilation and perfusion, this is not the case. Normally, alveolar ventilation is approximately 4 L/min, and pulmonary capillary perfusion is approximately 5 L/min. The normal ventilation/perfusion ratio (V̇/Q̇) is 4:5, or 0.8.[15,21]

Distribution of Ventilation

The distribution of ventilation throughout the lungs is uneven as result of a variety of factors, including the configuration of the thorax and the effects of gravity on intrapleural pressure. The thorax allows more lung expansion at the base than at the apex, which permits more ventilation to the base and limits ventilation to the apex. Gravity also produces regional variations in intrapleural pressure. At rest, the negative intrapleural pressure at the apex is greater than at the base, and alveoli in the apexes are larger and have more air left in them at the end of expiration. Because the alveoli are larger, they are less compliant and more difficult to inflate. On inhalation, the alveoli at the base expand more because they have less pressure to overcome.[3,15,16] In an upright person, the base of the lung receives approximately four times more ventilation than the apex.[16] In a supine person, gravity produces the same effects in the dependent zones of the lungs (posterior regions).[3,15,16]

Distribution of Perfusion

The distribution of perfusion through the lungs is related to gravity and intraalveolar pressures. Because of the effects of gravity, the pressure in the capillaries in the lungs is higher in the bases than in the apexes. This promotes preferential blood flow to the gravity-dependent areas of the lungs. Intraalveolar

pressures also vary throughout the different regions of the lungs, with the highest pressure in the apexes and the lowest pressure in the bases. In some areas of the lungs, the intraalveolar pressure has the potential of exceeding capillary hydrostatic pressure, resulting in an absence of blood flow to these areas. On the basis of this concept, the lung can be divided into three zones. Zone 1 is the nondependent portion of the lung, which has the potential of no perfusion. Zone 2 is the middle portion of the lung, which receives various degrees of blood flow. Zone 3 is the gravity-dependent area of the lung, which receives a constant blood flow (Fig. 16.20).[3,15]

Ventilation/Perfusion Mismatch

Various factors can affect the matching of ventilation to perfusion in the lungs, and their relationship can be considered as a continuum (Fig. 16.21). At one end of the continuum, the alveolus is receiving ventilation but is not receiving any perfusion and is unable to participate in gas exchange. This situation is referred to as *alveolar dead space*. On the other end of the continuum, the alveolus is receiving perfusion but is not receiving any ventilation and is unable to participate in gas exchange. This situation is referred to as *intrapulmonary shunting*. In this case, the blood is returned to the left side of the heart unoxygenated.[21] An infinite number of ventilation/perfusion mismatches exist between these two extremes. Situations in which ventilation exceeds perfusion (V̇/Q̇ >0.8) are considered to be *dead space producing*, whereas situations in which perfusion exceeds ventilation (V̇/Q̇ <0.8) are considered to be *shunt producing*. Although minor mismatching of ventilation may not

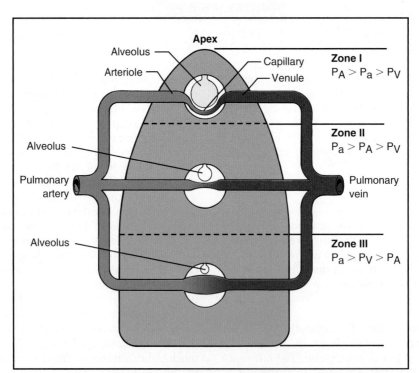

FIG. 16.20 Effects of Gravity and Alveolar Pressure on Pulmonary Blood Flow. Note three lung zones. In zone I, alveolar pressure *(PA)* is greater than arterial and venous pressure, and no blood flow occurs. In zone II, arterial pressure *(Pa)* exceeds alveolar pressure, but alveolar pressure exceeds venous pressure *(PV)*. Blood flow occurs in this zone, but alveolar pressure compresses the venules (venous ends of the capillaries). In zone III, both arterial and venous pressures are greater than alveolar pressure, and blood flow fluctuates, depending on the difference between arterial and venous pressures. (From McCance KL, et al, eds. *Pathophysiology: The Biologic Basis for Disease in Adults and Children.* 7th ed. St. Louis: Mosby; 2014.)

significantly affect gas exchange, significant alterations in the relationship result in hypoxemia.[15,21]

Hypoxic Vasoconstriction

The distribution of perfusion is affected by the amount of oxygen in the alveoli. Although most blood vessels in the body dilate in response to hypoxia, the pulmonary vessels constrict when the Pao_2 is less than 60 mm Hg. This event, known as *hypoxic vasoconstriction*, usually occurs when a portion of the

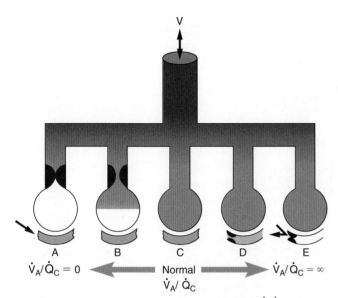

FIG. 16.21 Continuum of Ventilation/Perfusion ($\dot{V}/\dot{Q}$) Relationships. (A) Intrapulmonary shunting. (B) $\dot{V}/\dot{Q}$ mismatching is a shunt-producing situation. (C) Normal $\dot{V}/\dot{Q}$ ratio. (D) $\dot{V}/\dot{Q}$ mismatching is a dead space–producing situation. (E) Alveolar dead space. (From Misasi RS, Keyes JL. Matching and mismatching ventilation and perfusion in the lung. *Crit Care Nurse.* 1996;16[3]:23.)

pulmonary capillaries perfuses unventilated or underventilated alveoli. Hypoxic vasoconstriction is thought to be a compensatory response used to limit the return of unoxygenated blood to the left side of the heart. If the response is prolonged and generalized throughout the lungs, pulmonary hypertension results.[3]

GAS TRANSPORT

Gas transport refers to the movement of oxygen and carbon dioxide to and from the tissue cells. The transportation vehicle is the bloodstream, which is moved by the pumping action of the heart (cardiac output). At the tissue level, oxygen and carbon dioxide move into and out of the cell by diffusion. Oxygen diffuses into the cell because of the pressure gradient that exists between oxygen in the capillary and oxygen in the cell (Fig. 16.22A). Carbon dioxide diffuses into the capillary because of the pressure gradient that exists between carbon dioxide in the cell and carbon dioxide in the capillary (Fig. 16.22B).[3]

Oxygen Content

Oxygen is transported to the tissues by the blood in two ways: dissolved in plasma (Pao_2) or bound to hemoglobin molecules (oxygen saturation). Most of the oxygen is transported by hemoglobin, with the portion of oxygen dissolved in plasma equal to approximately 3% of the total oxygen within the blood.[23] The pressure exerted by the oxygen dissolved in plasma is important because this oxygen diffuses across the capillary membrane into the cells first and serves as the vehicle for the unloading of the oxygen from the hemoglobin molecule. As dissolved oxygen leaves the plasma and diffuses into the cells, the molecules of oxygen move off the hemoglobin molecule, dissolve into the plasma, and diffuse into the cells.[20] For this process to begin, a pressure gradient must exist between the oxygen level in the capillary and the oxygen level in the cell.

FIG. 16.22 Internal Respiration. (A) Diffusion of oxygen from a tissue capillary into a tissue cell. (B) Diffusion of carbon dioxide from a tissue cell into a tissue capillary.

Factors shifting curve to the left
1. ↑ pH
2. ↓ Pco$_2$
3. ↓ Temperature
4. ↓ 2, 3-DPG:
     a. Hexokinase deficiency
     b. Hypothyroidism
     c. Bank blood
5. Some congenital hemoglobinopathies:
     a. Hemoglobin Ranier
     b. Hemoglobin Hiroshima
     c. Hemoglobin San Francisco
6. Carboxyhemoglobin

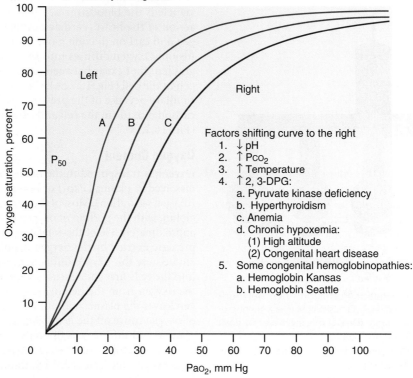

FIG. 16.23 Oxyhemoglobin Dissociation Curve. (A) Curve is shifted to the left because of hemoglobin's increased affinity for oxygen. (B) Standard oxyhemoglobin dissociation curve. (C) Curve is shifted to the right because of hemoglobin's decreased affinity for oxygen. (Modified from Kinney MR, et al, eds. *AACN's Clinical Reference for Critical Care Nursing.* 4th ed. St. Louis: Mosby; 1998.)

Oxygen Content Formula

The amount of oxygen in the arterial blood can be calculated using the arterial oxygen content (Cao$_2$) formula. The amount of oxygen in the venous blood can be calculated using the venous oxygen content (Cvo$_2$) formula (see Appendix B).[23]

Oxyhemoglobin Dissociation Curve

The relationship between dissolved oxygen and hemoglobin-bound oxygen is plotted as the oxyhemoglobin dissociation curve (Fig. 16.23). The sigmoid shape of the oxyhemoglobin dissociation curve illustrates several essential points about the relationship between the two ways oxygen is carried. The steep lower portion of the curve, at Pao$_2$ levels of 10 to 60 mm Hg, shows that the peripheral tissues can withdraw large amounts of oxygen from the hemoglobin molecule with only a small change in Pao$_2$, preserving the gradient for the continued unloading of hemoglobin.[20,23] The area at Pao$_2$ levels of 60 to 100 mm Hg is called the *flat upper portion* of the curve. This portion shows that the saturation of hemoglobin remains high even as the Pao$_2$

declines. For example, in a healthy person, a Pao$_2$ of 60 mm Hg yields an oxygen saturation level of 89%, whereas a Pao$_2$ of 100 mm Hg yields an oxygen saturation level of 98%. The large drop in Pao$_2$ (from 100 to 60 mm Hg) causes only a small drop in oxygen saturation (from 98% to 89%).[21,23]

Shifts in oxyhemoglobin dissociation curve. Under normal circumstances, hemoglobin has a steady and predictable affinity for oxygen. The combination of oxygen and hemoglobin based on this affinity is responsible for the position of the oxyhemoglobin dissociation curve in which a given Pao$_2$ yields a predictable oxygen saturation.[20,23] Occasionally, events occur that alter the affinity hemoglobin has for oxygen. These events include changes in pH, Paco$_2$, temperature, and 2,3-diphosphoglycerate (2,3-DPG) levels (Box 16.3). When this affinity is altered, the position of the oxyhemoglobin dissociation curve shifts (see Fig. 16.23). Shifts in the position of the curve mean there is a change in the way oxygen is taken up by the hemoglobin molecule at the alveolar level and a change in the way oxygen is delivered at the tissue level.[21,23]

BOX 16.3   What Is 2,3-DPG?

2,3-Diphosphoglycerate (2,3-DPG), an organic phosphate found primarily in red blood cells, has the ability to alter the affinity of hemoglobin for oxygen. When the level of 2,3-DPG increases within the red blood cells, hemoglobin's affinity for oxygen is decreased (a shift in the oxyhemoglobin curve to the right), making more oxygen available to the tissues. Increased synthesis of 2,3-DPG is an important component of the adaptive responses in healthy individuals to an acute need for more tissue oxygen. Tissue hypoxia stimulates production of 2,3-DPG, and increased amounts have been found in patients with anemia, right-to-left shunts, or acute heart failure and in individuals residing at high altitudes.

A decrease in the amount of 2,3-DPG is detrimental to tissue oxygenation because it causes hemoglobin's affinity for oxygen to increase (a shift in the oxyhemoglobin curve to the left). Decreased 2,3-DPG levels occur with hypophosphatemia, septic shock, and the use of banked blood. Blood preserved with acid citrate dextrose loses most of its red cell 2,3-DPG within several days. Blood preserved with citrate phosphate dextrose maintains its 2,3-DPG levels for several weeks. Transfusion of blood with a low level of 2,3-DPG cannot be beneficial for tissue oxygenation until the 2,3-DPG level is restored, which may take 18–24 hours.

Shift to the right. When the curve is shifted to the right (see Fig. 16.23, curve C), there is a lower oxygen saturation level for any given Pao_2; in other words, hemoglobin has less affinity for oxygen. Although the saturation level is lower than expected, a right shift enhances oxygen delivery at the tissue level because hemoglobin unloads more readily. Factors that cause this change in oxygen-hemoglobin affinity and shift the curve to the right include fever, increased $Paco_2$, acidosis, and increased 2,3-DPG levels.[21,23]

Shift to the left. When the curve is shifted to the left (see Fig. 16.23, curve A), the reverse occurs. There is a higher arterial saturation for any given Pao_2 because hemoglobin has an increased affinity for oxygen. Although the saturation level is higher, oxygen delivery to the tissues is impaired because hemoglobin does not unload as easily. Factors that contribute to this effect include hypothermia, alkalemia, decreased $Paco_2$, and decreased 2,3-DPG levels.[21,23]

Abnormalities of Hemoglobin

Hemoglobin carries approximately 97% of the total amount of oxygen held within the bloodstream. This great carrying capacity depends on hemoglobin that is normal in amount and molecular structure. Most hemoglobin abnormalities affect the oxygen-carrying capability of this molecule. The most common abnormality involving hemoglobin is a decrease in amount of hemoglobin. This can be an acute or a chronic (anemia) situation. Abnormal hemoglobin structure also can pose problems, such as hemoglobin S, which is responsible for sickle cell anemia. Hemoglobin S has less affinity for oxygen than normal hemoglobin. Normal hemoglobin can become abnormal hemoglobin under certain conditions. Methemoglobin and carboxyhemoglobin are two examples. Methemoglobin occurs when the iron atoms within the hemoglobin molecule are oxidized from the ferrous state to the ferric state. Methemoglobin does not carry oxygen. Carboxyhemoglobin occurs when carbon monoxide combines with hemoglobin. Carbon monoxide uses the same binding site as oxygen and has a much greater affinity for hemoglobin.[21]

Carbon Dioxide Content

Carbon dioxide, one of the end products of aerobic cellular metabolism, is produced continuously within the cells. On its way from the cells to the lungs, carbon dioxide is transported within the plasma and the erythrocytes. Carbon dioxide is transported, physically dissolved as the $Paco_2$ (5%), bound to blood proteins (including hemoglobin) in the form of carbaminohemoglobin compounds (5% to 1%), and combined with water to form carbonic acid (8% to 9%), some of which dissociates into hydrogen ions and bicarbonate. In the lungs, these methods of carbon dioxide carriage are reversed as the carbon dioxide leaves the plasma and erythrocytes for exhalation.[21]

SUMMARY

Anatomy

- The pulmonary system consists of the thorax, conducting airways, respiratory airways, and pulmonary blood and lymph supply.
- The thorax consists of the thoracic cage, lungs, pleura, and muscles of ventilation, and its major function is to form the ventilatory pump and perform the work of breathing.
- The conducting airways consist of the upper airways, the trachea, and the bronchial tree, and their major functions are to warm and humidify the inhaled air, to prevent the entrance of foreign matter into the gas exchange areas, and to serve as a passageway for air entering and leaving the gas exchange regions of the lungs.
- The respiratory airways consist of the respiratory bronchioles and the alveoli, and their major function is gas exchange.
- The pulmonary circulation is the vascular system that forms the gas exchange network surrounding the alveoli, and the bronchial circulation is the vascular system that perfuses the tracheobronchial tree.
- The lymphatic system is responsible for removing foreign particles and cell debris from the lungs, for producing antibody-mediated and cell-mediated immune responses, for removing fluid from the lungs, and for keeping the alveoli clear.

Physiology

- The primary functions of the pulmonary system are ventilation and respiration.
- Ventilation is the movement of air in (inhalation) and out (exhalation) of the lungs.
- The work of breathing is the amount of work that must be performed to overcome the elastic and resistive properties of the lungs.
- Respiration is the process of gas exchange.
- External respiration takes place at the lung level through the alveolar-capillary membrane.
- Internal respiration is the diffusion of gases in and out of the cells at the tissue level.
- Ⓔ Visit the Evolve site for additional study materials.

REFERENCES

1. Fischman CL, Rodriguez NE. The respiratory system. In: Kacmarek RM, Stoller JK, Heuer AJ, eds. *Egan's Fundamentals of Respiratory Care.* ed 11. St Louis: Elsevier; 2017.
2. Albertine KH. Anatomy of the lungs. In: Broaddus VC, et al., ed. *Murray and Nadel's Textbook of Respiratory Medicine.* ed 6. Philadelphia: Elsevier; 2016.
3. Brashers VL. Structure and function of the pulmonary system. In: McCance KL, et al., ed. *Pathophysiology: The Biologic Basis for Disease in Adults and Children.* ed 7. St. Louis: Mosby; 2014.

4. Charalampidis C, et al. Pleura space anatomy. *J Thorac Dis.* 2015;7(Suppl 1):S27–S32.

5. Nason LK, et al. Imaging of the diaphragm: anatomy and function. *Radiographics.* 2012;32(2):E51–E70.

6. Benditt JO, McCool FD. The respiratory system and neuromuscular diseases. In: Broaddus VC, et al., eds. *Murray and Nadel's Textbook of Respiratory Medicine.* ed 6. Philadelphia: Elsevier; 2016.

7. Minnich DJ, Mathisen DJ. Anatomy of the trachea, carina, and bronchi. *Thorac Surg Clin.* 2007;17(4):571–585.

8. Antunes MB, Cohen NA. Mucociliary clearance—a critical upper airway host defense mechanism and methods of assessment. *Curr Opin Allergy Clin Immunol.* 2007;7(1):5.

9. Pitts T. Airway protective mechanisms. *Lung.* 2014;192(1):27–31.

10. Enhorning G. Surfactant in airway disease. *Chest.* 2008;133(4):975–980.

11. Polanco PM, Pinsky MR. Practical issues of hemodynamic monitoring at the bedside. *Surg Clin N Am.* 2006;86(6):1431–1456.

12. Smith CS, et al. Care of the patient with pulmonary arterial hypertension. *Dimens Crit Care Nurs.* 2015;34(6):340–347.

13. Powell PL, Wagner PD, West JD. Ventilation, blood flow, and gas exchange. In: Broaddus VC, et al., eds. *Murray and Nadel's Textbook of Respiratory Medicine.* ed 6. Philadelphia: Elsevier; 2016.

14. Charana NB, Thompson WH, Carvalho P. Functional anatomy of bronchial veins. *Pulm Pharmacol Ther.* 2007;20(2):100–103.

15. Misasi RS, Keyes JL. Matching and mismatching ventilation and perfusion in the lung. *Crit Care Nurse.* 1996;16(3):23–27.

16. Mireles-Cabodevila E, Chatburn RL. Ventilation. In: Kacmarek RM, Stoller JK, Heuer AJ, eds. *Egan's Fundamentals of Respiratory Care.* ed 11. St. Louis: Elsevier; 2017.

17. Henderson W, Pare PA, Ayas NT. Respiratory system mechanics and energetics. In: Broaddus VC, et al., eds. *Murray and Nadel's Textbook of Respiratory Medicine.* ed 6. Philadelphia: Elsevier; 2016.

18. Dempsey JA, Smith CA. Pathophysiology of human ventilatory control. *Eur Respir J.* 2014;44(2):495–512.

19. Hainsworth R. Cardiovascular control from cardiac and pulmonary vascular receptors. *Exp Physiol.* 2014;99(2):312–319.

20. Moore LG, Charles SM, Julian CG. Humans at high altitude: hypoxia and fetal growth. *Respir Physiol Neurobiol.* 2011;178(1):181–190.

21. Cohen Z. Gas exchange and transport. In: Kacmarek RM, Stoller JK, Heuer AJ, eds. *Egan's Fundamentals of Respiratory Care.* ed 11. St. Louis: Elsevier; 2017.

22. Hébert PC, et al. Physiologic aspects of anemia. *Crit Care Clin.* 2004;20(2):187–212.

23. MacIntyre NR. Tissue hypoxia: implications for the respiratory clinician. *Respir Care.* 2014;59(10):1590–1596.

17

Pulmonary Clinical Assessment

Kathleen M. Stacy

Assessment of a patient with pulmonary dysfunction is a systematic process that incorporates an inquiry into the chronology of the present illness, better known as the *history*, and an investigation of the current physical manifestations, better known as the *focused clinical assessment*. The purpose of the assessment is twofold: first, to recognize changes in the patient's pulmonary status that necessitate nursing or medical intervention and, second, to determine the ways in which the patient's pulmonary dysfunction is interfering with his or her self-care activities. After completion, the assessment serves as the foundation for developing the management plan for the patient. The assessment process can be brief or can involve a detailed history and examination, depending on the nature and immediacy of the patient's situation. Whatever the setting, the nurse should develop and practice a sequential pattern of assessment to avoid omitting portions of the examination.

HISTORY

Taking a thorough and accurate history is an essential part of the assessment process. The patient's history provides the foundation and direction for the rest of the assessment. The overall goal of the patient interview is to expose key clinical manifestations that will facilitate the identification of the underlying cause of the illness. This information then assists in the development of an appropriate management plan.

The initial presentation of the patient determines the rapidity and direction of the interview. For a patient in acute distress, the history is curtailed to just a few questions about the patient's chief complaint and precipitating events. For a patient in no obvious distress, the history focuses on five areas: (1) review of the patient's present illness, (2) overview of the patient's general respiratory status, (3) examination of the patient's general health status, (4) survey of the patient's family and social background, and (5) description of the patient's current symptoms.[1] Specific items included in each of these areas are outlined in the Box 17.1.

Symptoms that are common in a patient with a pulmonary disorder include dyspnea, cough, wheezing, edema, palpitations, fatigue, chest pain, hemoptysis, and sputum abnormalities. Information is elicited regarding the location, onset and duration, characteristics, setting, aggravating and alleviating factors, associated symptoms, and efforts to treat the symptoms. If the cough is productive, the patient is asked questions about the color, amount, odor, and consistency of the sputum.[2-5]

FOCUSED CLINICAL ASSESSMENT

Four techniques are used in physical assessment: inspection, palpation, percussion, and auscultation. *Inspection* is the process of looking intently at the patient. *Palpation* is the process of touching the patient to judge the size, shape, texture, and temperature of the body surface or underlying structures. *Percussion* is the process of creating sound waves on the surface of the body to determine abnormal density of any underlying areas. *Auscultation* is the process of concentrated listening with a stethoscope to determine characteristics of body functions.

Inspection

Inspection of the patient focuses on three areas: (1) observation of the tongue and sublingual area, (2) assessment of chest wall configuration, and (3) evaluation of respiratory effort. If possible, patients are positioned upright, with their arms resting at their sides.[3] Inspection usually begins during the interview.[2]

Tongue and Sublingual Area

The patient's tongue and sublingual area is observed for a blue, gray, or dark purple tint or discoloration indicating the presence of central cyanosis. *Central cyanosis* is a sign of hypoxemia, or inadequate oxygenation of the blood, and is considered to be a life-threatening condition. Central cyanosis occurs when the amount of reduced hemoglobin (unsaturated hemoglobin) exceeds 5 g/dL. The fingers and toes may also appear discolored, an indication of the presence of peripheral cyanosis.[6]

Chest Wall Configuration

The size and shape of the patient's chest wall are assessed for an increase in the anteroposterior diameter and for structural deviations. Normally, the ratio of anteroposterior diameter to lateral diameter ranges from 1:2 to 5:7 (Fig. 17.1A).[2,4,5] An increase in the anteroposterior diameter is suggestive of chronic obstructive pulmonary disease.[2,4,5] The shape of the chest is inspected for any structural deviations. Some more frequently seen abnormalities are pectus excavatum, pectus carinatum, barrel chest, and spinal deformities. In *pectus excavatum* (funnel chest), the sternum and lower ribs are displaced posteriorly, creating a funnel or pit-shaped depression in the chest. This abnormality causes a decrease in the anteroposterior diameter of the chest and may interfere with respiratory function. In *pectus carinatum* (pigeon breast), the sternum projects forward, causing an increase in the anteroposterior diameter of the chest. The *barrel chest* also results in an increase in anteroposterior diameter of the chest and is characterized by displacement of the sternum forward and the ribs outward (Fig. 17.1B). Spinal

BOX 17.1   DATA COLLECTION

Pulmonary History

Common Pulmonary Symptoms

Cough
- Onset and duration
  - Sudden or gradual
  - Episodic or continuous
- Characteristics
  - Dry or wet
  - Hacking, hoarse, barking, or congested
  - Productive or nonproductive
- Sputum
  - Present or absent
  - Frequency of production
  - Appearance—color (eg, clear, mucoid, purulent, blood-tinged, mostly bloody), foul odor, frothy
  - Amount
- Pattern
  - Paroxysmal
  - Related to time of day, weather, activities, talking, or deep breathing
  - Change over time
- Severity
  - Causes fatigue
  - Disrupts sleep or conversation
  - Produces chest pain
- Associated symptoms
  - Shortness of breath
  - Chest pain or tightness with breathing
  - Fever
  - Upper respiratory tract signs (eg, sore throat, congestion, increased mucus production)
  - Noisy respirations or hoarseness
  - Gagging or choking
  - Anxiety, stress, or panic reactions
- Efforts made to treat
  - Prescription or nonprescription medications
  - Vaporizers
  - Effective or ineffective

Shortness of Breath or Dyspnea on Exertion
- Onset and duration
  - Sudden or gradual
  - Gagging or choking episode a few days before onset
- Pattern
  - Related to position—improves when sitting up or with head elevated; number of pillows used to alleviate problems
  - Related to activity—exercise or eating; extent of activity that produces dyspnea
  - Related to other factors—time of day, season, or exposure to something in the environment
  - Harder to inhale or harder to exhale
- Severity
  - Extent activity is limited
  - Breathing itself causes fatigue
  - Anxiety about getting enough air
- Associated symptoms
  - Pain or discomfort—exact location in respiratory tree
  - Cough, diaphoresis, swelling of ankles, or cyanosis
- Efforts made to treat
  - Prescription or nonprescription medications

- Oxygen
- Effective or ineffective

Chest Pain
- Onset and duration
  - Gradual or sudden
  - Associated with trauma, coughing, or lower respiratory tract infection
- Associated symptoms
  - Shallow breathing
  - Uneven chest expansion
  - Fever
  - Cough
  - Radiation of pain to neck or arms
  - Anxiety about getting enough air
- Efforts made to treat
  - Heat, splinting, or pain medication
  - Effective or ineffective

Pulmonary Risk Factors
- Tobacco use—current and past
  - Type of tobacco—cigarettes, cigars, pipes, or smokeless
  - Duration and amount—age started, inhale when smoking, amount used in the past and present
  - Pack years—number of packs per day multiplied by number of years patient has smoked
  - Efforts to quit—previous attempts and current interest
- Work environment
  - Nature of work
  - Environmental hazards—chemicals, vapors, dust, pulmonary irritants, or allergens
  - Use of protective devices
- Home environment
  - Location
  - Possible allergens—pets, house plants, plants and trees outside the home, or other environmental hazards
  - Type of heating
  - Use of air conditioning or humidifier
  - Ventilation
  - Stairs to climb

Medical History

Child
- Infectious respiratory diseases
  - Strep throat
  - Mumps
  - Tonsillitis
- Asthma
- Cystic fibrosis
- Immunizations

Adult
- Previous diagnosis of pulmonary disorders—dates of hospitalization
- Chronic pulmonary disease—date, treatment, and compliance with therapy
  - Tuberculosis
  - Bronchitis
  - Emphysema
  - Bronchiectasis
  - Asthma
  - Sinus infection

BOX 17.1   DATA COLLECTION—cont'd

Pulmonary History

- Other chronic disorders—cardiovascular, cancer, musculoskeletal, neurologic, immune
  - Obstruction of one or both nares
  - Mouth breathing often necessary (especially at night)
  - History of nasal discharge
  - Compromised immune system function
- Nosebleed
- Sleep apnea
  - Obstructive
  - Central
- Previous tests
  - Allergy testing
  - Pulmonary function tests
  - Tuberculin and fungal skin tests
  - Chest radiographs

Surgical
- Thoracic trauma
- Thoracic surgery
- Nasal surgery or injury

Family History
- Tuberculosis
- Cystic fibrosis
- Emphysema
- Allergies
- Asthma
- Atopic dermatitis
- Smoking by household members
- Malignancy

Current Medication Use
- Inhalators
- Steroids
- Antibiotics
- Immunizations
  - Pneumococcal (Pneumovax)
  - Influenza

FIG. 17.1 Chest Wall Configuration. (A) Normal configuration. (B) Increased anteroposterior diameter. Note the contrast in the angle of the slope of the ribs. (From Kacmarek RM, et al, eds. *Egan's Fundamentals of Respiratory Care.* 10th ed. St. Louis: Mosby; 2013.)

deformities, such as *kyphosis*, *lordosis*, and *scoliosis*, also may be present and can interfere with respiratory function.[7]

Respiratory Effort

The patient's respiratory effort is evaluated for rate, rhythm, symmetry, and quality of ventilatory movements.[2] Normal breathing at rest is effortless and regular and occurs at a rate of 12 to 20 breaths/min.[3] There are a number of abnormal respiratory patterns (Fig. 17.2). Some more commonly seen patterns in patients with pulmonary dysfunction are tachypnea, hyperventilation, and air trapping. *Tachypnea* is manifested by an increase in the rate and decrease in the depth of ventilation. *Hyperventilation* is manifested by an increase in the rate and depth of ventilation. Patients with chronic obstructive pulmonary disease often experience obstructive breathing, or *air trapping*. As the patient breathes, air becomes trapped in the lungs, and ventilations become progressively more shallow until the patient actively and forcefully exhales.[8]

Additional Assessment Areas

Other areas assessed are patient position, active effort to breathe, use of accessory muscles, presence of intercostal retractions, unequal movement of the chest wall, flaring of nares, and pausing midsentence to take a breath.[2,4,5] The presence of iatrogenic features, such as chest tubes, central venous lines, artificial airways, and nasogastric tubes, is identified as these features may affect assessment findings.

Palpation

Palpation of the patient focuses on three areas: (1) confirmation of the position of the trachea, (2) assessment of thoracic expansion, and (3) evaluation of fremitus. The thorax is assessed for any areas of tenderness, lumps, or bony deformities. The anterior, posterior, and lateral areas of the chest are evaluated in a systematic fashion.[2]

Position of the Trachea

The position of the patient's trachea is confirmed at midline and is assessed by placing the fingers in the suprasternal notch and moving upward (Fig. 17.3).[8] Deviation of the trachea to either side may indicate a pneumothorax, unilateral pneumonia, diffuse pulmonary fibrosis, a large pleural effusion, or severe atelectasis. With atelectasis, the trachea shifts to the same

FIG. 17.2 Patterns of Respiration. (From Ball JW, et al. *Seidel's Guide to Physical Examination.* 8th ed. St. Louis: Mosby; 2015.)

FIG. 17.3 Position of the Trachea. (From Ball JW, et al. *Seidel's Guide to Physical Examination.* 8th ed. St. Louis: Mosby; 2015.)

side as the problem; with pneumothorax, the trachea shifts to the opposite side of the problem.[7]

Thoracic Expansion

The patient's thoracic expansion is assessed for the degree and symmetry of movement and is assessed by placing the hands on the anterolateral chest with the thumbs extended along the costal margin, pointing to the xiphoid process, or on the posterolateral chest with the thumbs on either side of the spine at the level of the 10th rib (Fig. 17.4). The patient is instructed to take a few normal breaths and then a few deep breaths. Chest movement is assessed for equality, which signifies symmetry

of thoracic expansion.[3,7,8] Asymmetry is an abnormal finding that can occur with pneumothorax, pneumonia, or other disorders that interfere with lung inflation. The degree of chest movement is felt to ascertain the extent of lung expansion. The thumbs should separate 3 to 5 cm during deep inspiration.[5,8] Lung expansion of a hyperinflated chest is less than expansion of a normal chest.[5,8]

Tactile Fremitus

The patient is assessed for tactile fremitus to identify, describe, and localize any areas of increased or decreased fremitus. Tactile fremitus refers to the palpable vibrations felt through the chest wall when the patient speaks and is assessed by placing the palmar surface of the hands against opposite sides of the chest wall and having the patient repeat the word "ninety-nine" (Fig. 17.5). The hands are moved systematically around the thorax until the anterior, posterior, and both lateral areas have been assessed.[7,8] If only one hand is used, the hand is moved from one side of the chest to the corresponding area on the other side of the chest until all areas have been assessed.[8]

Tactile fremitus varies from patient to patient and depends on the pitch and intensity of the voice. Fremitus is described as normal, decreased, or increased. With normal fremitus, vibrations can be felt over the trachea but are barely palpable over the periphery.[2] With decreased fremitus, there is interference with the transmission of vibrations. Examples of disorders that decrease fremitus include pleural effusion, pneumothorax, bronchial obstruction, pleural thickening, and emphysema. With increased fremitus, there is an increase in the transmission of vibrations. Examples of disorders that increase fremitus include pneumonia, lung cancer, and pulmonary fibrosis.[5]

FIG. 17.4 Thoracic Expansion. (A) Position of the hands for palpation of posterior thorax excursion. (B) As the patient inhales, movement of chest excursion separates the nurse's thumbs. (From Perry AG, Potter PA, Ostendorf WR. *Clinical Nursing Skills and Techniques.* 7th ed. St. Louis: Mosby; 2014.)

FIG. 17.5 Tactile Fremitus. Simultaneous application of the fingertips of both hands to compare sides. (From Barkauskas V, Baumann L, Darling-Fisher CS. *Health and Physical Assessment.* 3rd ed. St. Louis: Mosby; 2002.)

Percussion

Percussion of the patient focuses on two areas: (1) evaluation of the underlying lung structure and (2) assessment of diaphragmatic excursion. Although the technique is not used

FIG. 17.6 Underlying Lung Structures. (From Barkauskas V, Baumann L, Darling-Fisher CS. *Health and Physical Assessment.* 3rd ed. St. Louis: Mosby; 2002.)

often, percussion is a useful method for confirming suspected abnormalities.

Underlying Lung Structure

The patient's underlying lung structure is evaluated to estimate the amounts of air, liquid, or solid material present. This assessment is performed by placing the middle finger of the nondominant hand on the chest wall. The distal portion, between the last joint and the nail bed, is then struck with the middle finger of the dominant hand. The hands are moved systematically and side to side around the thorax to compare similar areas until the anterior, posterior, and both lateral areas have been assessed (Fig. 17.6). Five tones can be elicited: resonance, hyperresonance, tympany, dullness, and flatness. These tones are distinguished by differences in intensity, pitch, duration, and quality. Table 17.1 describes the different percussion tones and their associated conditions.[3,7]

Diaphragmatic Excursion

The patient is assessed for diaphragmatic excursion to evaluate the movement of the diaphragm. This assessment is accomplished by measuring the difference in the level of the diaphragm on inspiration and expiration and is performed by instructing the patient to inhale and hold the breath. The posterior chest is percussed downward, over the intercostal spaces, until the dull sound produced by the diaphragm is heard. The spot is marked. The patient is then instructed to take a few breaths in and out, exhale completely, and then hold his or her breath. The posterior chest is percussed again, and the new area of dullness over the diaphragm is located and marked. The difference between the two spots is identified and measured (Fig. 17.7). Normal diaphragmatic excursion is 3 to 5 cm.[8] Diaphragmatic excursion is decreased in ascites, pregnancy, hepatomegaly, and emphysema and is increased in pleural effusion and disorders that elevate the diaphragm, such as atelectasis or paralysis.[7]

Auscultation

Auscultation of the patient focuses on three areas: (1) evaluation of normal breath sounds, (2) identification of abnormal

TABLE 17.1 Percussion Tones

Tone	Description	Condition
Resonance	Intensity: Loud Pitch: Low Duration: Long Quality: Hollow	Normal lung Bronchitis
Hyperresonance	Intensity: Very loud Pitch: Very low Duration: Long Quality: Booming	Asthma Emphysema Pneumothorax
Tympany	Intensity: Loud Pitch: Musical Duration: Medium Quality: Drumlike	Large pneumothorax Emphysematous blebs
Dullness	Intensity: Medium Pitch: Medium-high Duration: Medium Quality: Thudlike	Atelectasis Pleural effusion Pulmonary edema Pneumonia Lung mass
Flatness	Intensity: Soft Pitch: High Duration: Short Quality: Extremely dull	Massive atelectasis Pneumonectomy

FIG. 17.7 Diaphragmatic Excursion. Excursion distance is usually 3–5 cm. (From Ball JW, et al. *Seidel's Guide to Physical Examination.* 8th ed. St. Louis: Mosby; 2015.)

breath sounds, and (3) assessment of voice sounds. Auscultation requires a quiet environment, proper positioning of the patient, and a bare chest.[9] Breath sounds are best heard with the patient in the upright position.[5]

Normal Breath Sounds

The patient's breath sounds are auscultated to evaluate the quality of air movement through the lungs and to identify the presence of abnormal sounds. This assessment is performed by placing the diaphragm of the stethoscope against the chest wall and instructing the patient to breathe in and out slowly with his or her mouth open.[2] Breath sounds are assessed during both inspiration and expiration. Auscultation is done in a systematic sequence: side-to-side, top-to-bottom, posteriorly, laterally,

and anteriorly (Fig. 17.8).[5] Normal breath sounds are different, depending on their location. There are three categories: vesicular, bronchovesicular, and bronchial. Fig. 17.9 describes the characteristics of normal breath sounds and their associated conditions.[2,5,9]

Abnormal Breath Sounds

Abnormal breath sounds are identified after normal breath sounds have been clearly delineated. There are three categories of abnormal breath sounds: absent or diminished breath sounds, displaced bronchial breath sounds, and adventitious breath sounds. Table 17.2 describes the various abnormal breath sounds and their associated conditions.[2,5,9]

An *absent* or *diminished breath sound* indicates that there is little or no airflow to a particular portion of the lung (a small segment or an entire lung).[9] *Displaced bronchial breath sounds* are normal bronchial sounds heard in the peripheral lung fields instead of over the trachea. This condition is usually indicative of fluid or exudate in the alveoli.[9] *Adventitious breath sounds* are extra or added sounds heard in addition to the other sounds previously discussed. They are classified as crackles, rhonchi, wheezes, and friction rubs.

Crackles, also called *rales*, are short, discrete popping or crackling sounds produced by fluid in the small airways or alveoli or by the snapping open of collapsed airways during inspiration. They can be heard on inspiration and expiration and may clear with coughing.[2,5,9] Crackles can be further classified as fine, medium, or coarse, depending on pitch.[3,5]

Rhonchi are coarse, rumbling, low-pitched sounds produced by airflow over secretions in the larger airways or narrowing of the large airways. They are heard mainly on expiration and sometimes can be cleared with coughing. Rhonchi can be further classified as bubbling, gurgling, or sonorous, depending on the characteristics of the sound.[9]

Wheezes are high-pitched, squeaking, whistling sounds produced by airflow through narrowed small airways. They are heard mainly on expiration but may be heard throughout the ventilatory cycle. Depending on their severity, wheezes can be further classified as mild, moderate, or severe.[9]

A *pleural friction rub* is a creaking, leathery, loud, dry, coarse sound produced by irritated pleural surfaces rubbing together and is usually heard best in the lower anterolateral chest area during inspiration and expiration. Pleural friction rubs are caused by inflammation of the pleura.[2,5]

Voice Sounds

Assessment of voice sounds is particularly useful in detecting lung consolidation or lung compression. Three abnormal types of voice sounds are bronchophony, whispering pectoriloquy, and egophony.[9]

Bronchophony describes a condition in which the spoken voice is heard on auscultation with higher intensity and clarity than usual. Normally, the spoken word is muffled when heard through the stethoscope. Bronchophony is assessed by placing the diaphragm of the stethoscope against the posterior side of the patient's chest and instructing the patient to say "ninety-nine." When the sound heard is clear, distinct, and loud, bronchophony is present.[9]

Whispering pectoriloquy describes a condition of unusually clear transmission of the whispered voice on auscultation. Normally, the whispered word is unintelligible when heard through the stethoscope. Whispering pectoriloquy is assessed by placing the stethoscope against the posterior side of the

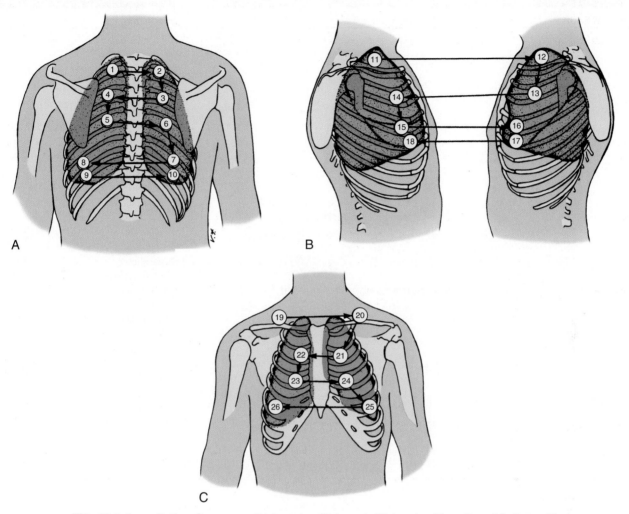

FIG. 17.8 Auscultation Sequence. (A) Posterior. (B) Lateral. (C) Anterior. (From Perry AG, Potter PA, Ostendorf WR. *Clinical Nursing Skills and Techniques.* 7th ed. St. Louis: Mosby; 2014.)

BREATH SOUND	PITCH	INTENSITY	LOCATION	DIAGRAM OF SOUND
Vesicular or normal breath sounds	Low	Soft	Peripheral lung areas	
Bronchovesicular	Moderate	Moderate	Around upper part of sternum, between scapulae	
Bronchial	High	Loud	Over trachea	

FIG. 17.9 Characteristics of Normal Breath Sounds. (From Kacmarek RM, et al, eds. *Egan's Fundamentals of Respiratory Care.* 10th ed. St. Louis: Mosby; 2013.)

TABLE 17.2 Abnormal Breath Sounds

Abnormal Sound	Description	Condition
Absent breath sounds	No airflow to particular portion of lung	Pneumothorax
		Pneumonectomy
		Emphysematous blebs
		Pleural effusion
		Lung mass
		Massive atelectasis
		Complete airway obstruction
Diminished breath sounds	Little airflow to particular portion of lung	Emphysema
		Pleural effusion
		Pleurisy
		Atelectasis
		Pulmonary fibrosis
Displaced bronchial sounds	Bronchial sounds heard in peripheral lung fields	Atelectasis with secretions
		Lung mass with exudates
		Pneumonia
		Pleural effusion
		Pulmonary edema
Crackles (rales)	Short, discrete popping or crackling sounds	Pulmonary edema
		Pneumonia
		Pulmonary fibrosis
		Atelectasis
		Bronchiectasis
Rhonchi	Coarse, rumbling, low-pitched sounds	Pneumonia
		Asthma
		Bronchitis
		Bronchospasm
Wheezes	High-pitched, squeaking, whistling sounds	Asthma
		Bronchospasm
Pleural friction rub	Creaking, leathery, loud, dry, coarse sounds	Pleural effusion
		Pleurisy

patient's chest and instructing the patient to whisper "one, two, three." When the sound heard is clear and distinct, whispering pectoriloquy is present.[9]

Egophony describes a condition in which the voice sounds increase in intensity and develop a nasal bleating quality on auscultation. Egophony is assessed by placing the stethoscope against the posterior side of the patient's chest and instructing the patient to say "e-e-e." When the "e" sound changes to an "a" sound, egophony is present.[2,4,9]

ASSESSMENT FINDINGS OF COMMON DISORDERS

Table 17.3 presents various common pulmonary disorders and their associated assessment findings.

TABLE 17.3 Assessment Findings With Associated Lung Conditions

Condition[a]	Breath Sounds	Description	Inspection	Palpation	Percussion	Auscultation
Normal Lung	Inspiration > Expiration Pitch: Low Intensity: Soft Adventitious sounds: None	Tracheobronchial tree and alveoli are clear; pleurae are thin and close together; chest wall is mobile	Good, symmetric rib and diaphragmatic movement Anteroposterior diameter < transverse diameter Respirations 12–20 breaths/min and regular	Trachea: Midline Expansion: Adequate, symmetric Tactile fremitus: Moderate and symmetric No lesions or tenderness	Resonant Diaphragmatic excursion: 3–5 cm	Breath sounds: Vesicular Vocal resonance: Muffled Adventitious sounds: None except for a few transient crackles at bases
Asthma Bronchospasm	Inspiration = Expiration Pitch: Moderate Intensity: Soft Adventitious sounds: Expiratory sibilant wheezes	Asthma is characterized by intermittent episodes of airway obstruction caused by bronchospasm, excessive bronchial secretion, or edema of bronchial mucosa; resultant airway resistance, especially during expiration, produces symptoms of wheezing, dyspnea, and chest tightness	Cyanosis Air trapping with audible wheezing Use of accessory muscles of respiration Increased respiratory rate	Tactile fremitus: Decreased	Hyperresonant	Breath sounds: Distant Vocal resonance: Decreased Adventitious sounds: Wheezes

Continued

TABLE 17.3 Assessment Findings With Associated Lung Conditions—cont'd

Condition[a]	Description	Inspection	Palpation	Percussion	Auscultation	Breath Sounds
Atelectasis Collapsed portion of lung	Atelectasis is collapse of alveolar lung tissue, and findings reflect presence of small, airless lung; this condition is caused by complete obstruction of draining bronchus by tumor, thick secretions, or aspirated foreign body or by compression of lung	Less chest motion on affected side; Affected side retracted, with ribs appearing close together; Cough; Rapid, shallow breathing	Trachea: Shifted to affected side; Expansion: Decreased on affected side; Tactile fremitus: Decreased or absent	Dull to flat over collapsed lung; Hyperresonant over remainder of affected hemithorax	Breath sounds: Decreased or absent; Vocal resonance: Varies in intensity, usually reduced or absent in affected area; Adventitious sounds: Fine, high-pitched crackles may be heard over terminal portion of inspiration	Inspiration > Expiration; Over empty area: Pitch: Low or absent; Intensity: Soft or absent; Adventitious sounds: Fine, high-pitched crackles over terminal portion of inspiration if bronchus patent; Over consolidated lung: Bronchial breath sounds, crackles, and wheezes
Bronchiectasis	Bronchiectasis is abnormal dilation of bronchi or bronchioles, or both (coughing)	If mild, respirations are normal; If severe, tachypnea; Less expansion of affected side; Cough with purulent sputum	Trachea: Midline or deviated toward affected side; Expansion: Decreased on affected side; Tactile fremitus: Increased	Resonant or dull	Breath sounds: Usually vesicular; Vocal resonance: Usually muffled; Adventitious sounds: Crackles	Inspiration > Expiration; Pitch: Low; Intensity: Soft; Adventitious sounds: Crackles (sometimes disappear after)

Condition	Description	Signs	Findings
Bronchitis, acute	Acute bronchitis is inflammation of bronchial tree characterized by partial bronchial obstruction and secretions or constrictions; it results in abnormally deflated portions of lung	If severe, tachypnea and cyanosis; Rasping cough with mucoid sputum	Tactile fremitus: Normal to increased; Resonant; Breath sounds: Vesicular; Inspiration ≥ Expiration; Pitch: Low; Intensity: Soft; Adventitious sounds: Localized crackles, expiratory sibilant wheezes; Vocal resonance: Moderate; Adventitious sounds: Localized crackles, sibilant wheezes
Emphysema	Emphysema is a permanent hyperinflation of lung beyond terminal bronchioles, with destruction of alveolar walls; airway resistance is increased, especially on expiration	Dyspnea with exertion; Barrel chest; Tachypnea; Use of accessory muscles of respiration	Expansion: Limited; Tactile fremitus: Decreased; Resonant to hyperresonant; Diaphragmatic excursion: Decreased; Breath sounds: Decreased intensity; often prolonged expiration; Inspiration = Expiration; Pitch: Low to very low; Intensity: Soft to very soft; Vocal resonance: Muffled or decreased; Adventitious sounds: Occasional wheezes; often fine crackles in late inspiration; Adventitious sounds: Occasional rhonchi and/or sibilant wheezes; fine inspiratory crackles

Continued

TABLE 17.3 Assessment Findings With Associated Lung Conditions—cont'd

Condition[a]	Breath Sounds	Description	Inspection	Palpation	Percussion	Auscultation
Pleural Effusion and Thickening	Inspiration > Expiration Pitch: Low to absent Intensity: Soft to absent Adventitious sounds: Occasional pleural friction rub	Pleural effusion is collection of fluid in pleural space; if pleural effusion is prolonged, fibrous tissue may also accumulate in pleural space; clinical picture depends on amount of fluid or fibrosis present and rapidity of development; fluid tends to gravitate to most dependent areas of thorax, and adjacent lung is compressed	Tachypnea Decrease in definition of intercostal spaces on affected side Dyspnea	Trachea: Deviation toward normal side Expansion: Decreased on affected side Tactile fremitus: Decreased or absent	Dull to flat No diaphragmatic excursion on affected side	Breath sounds: Decreased or absent Vocal resonance: Muffled or absent; if fluid compresses lung, sounds may be bronchial over compression, and bronchophony, egophony, and whisper pectoriloquy may be present Adventitious sounds: Pleural friction rub sometimes present
Pneumonia With Consolidation	Inspiration = Expiration Pitch: High	Pneumonia with consolidation occurs when alveolar air is replaced by fluid or tissue; physical findings depend on amount of parenchymal tissue involved	Tachypnea Guarding and less motion on affected side	Expansion: Limited on affected side Tactile fremitus: Usually increased, but may be weak if bronchus leading to affected area is plugged	Dull to flat	Breath sounds: Increased in intensity; broncho-vesicular or bronchial breath sounds over affected area Vocal resonance: Increased bronchophony, egophony, whisper pectoriloquy present

Pneumothorax

Pneumothorax implies air in pleural space

1. Closed type: Air in pleural space does not communicate with air in lung

2. Open type: Air in pleural space freely communicates with air in lung; air in pleural space is atmospheric

3. Tension type: Air in pleural space communicates with air in lungs only on inspiration; air pressure in pleural space is greater than atmospheric pressure

Physical signs depend on degree of lung collapse and presence or absence of pleural effusion

Restricted lung expansion on affected side

If large, tachypnea

Bulging in intercostal spaces on affected side

Cyanosis

Trachea: Deviated toward normal side

Expansion: Decreased on affected side

Tactile fremitus: Absent

Hyperresonant

Decreased diaphragmatic excursion

Breath sounds: Usually decreased or absent; if open pneumothorax, have amorphous quality

Vocal resonance: Decreased or absent

Adventitious sounds: None

Inspiration > Expiration

Pitch: Low to absent

Intensity: Soft to absent

Adventitious sounds: None

Intensity: Loud

Adventitious sounds: Inspiratory crackles in terminal third of inspiration

Adventitious sounds: Inspiratory crackles in terminal third of inspiration

Pulmonary Fibrosis, Diffuse

Pulmonary fibrosis is presence of excessive amount of connective tissue in lungs; consequently, lungs are smaller than normal and less compliant; lower lobes are usually affected most

Dyspnea on exertion

Tachypnea

Thoracic expansion diminished

Cyanosis

Trachea: Deviated to most affected side

Resonant to dull

Breath sounds: Reduced or absent, bronchovesicular or bronchial

Vocal resonance: Increased, whisper pectoriloquy may be present

Adventitious sounds: Crackles on inspiration

Inspiration = Expiration

Pitch: Low to absent

Intensity: Soft to absent

Adventitious sounds: Crackles

aAlthough some disease conditions are bilateral, one diseased lung and one normal lung are illustrated for each condition to provide contrast. When an abnormality is illustrated, the pathologic condition is illustrated on the left side, and the normal lung is illustrated on the right side.
From Barkauskas V, Baumann L, Darling-Fisher CS. *Health and Physical Assessment.* 3rd ed. St. Louis: Mosby; 2002.

SUMMARY

History

- A review of the patient's current illness and symptoms, including the presence or absence of shortness of breath, chest pain, and cough, is an essential part of the patient's medical history.
- As the patient's condition permits, additional information is obtained regarding his or her general respiratory status; general health status; and family and social background, including tobacco use, work environment, and home environment.

Focused Clinical Assessment

- Inspection focuses on the tongue and sublingual area, chest wall configuration, and respiratory effort.
- Palpation focuses on position of the trachea, thoracic expansion, and fremitus (normal, decreased, or increased).
- Percussion (when performed) focuses on underlying lung structure and diaphragmatic excursion.
- Auscultation focuses on the presence or absence of normal breath sounds (vesicular, bronchovesicular, and bronchial), abnormal breath sounds (diminished or absent breath sounds, displaced bronchial breath sounds, and adventitious breath sounds), and voice sounds (bronchophony, whispering pectoriloquy, and egophony).

- Adventitious breath sounds are classified as crackles, rhonchi, wheezes, and friction rubs.
- Auscultation is done in a systematic fashion—side-to-side, top-to-bottom, posteriorly, laterally, and anteriorly.
- Ⓔ Visit the Evolve site for additional study materials.

REFERENCES

1. Baid H. The process of conducting a physical assessment: a nursing perspective. *Br J Nurs.* 2006;15(13):710–714.
2. Simpson H. Respiratory assessment. *Br J Nurs.* 2006;15(9):484–488.
3. Reinke LF. Respiratory assessment. In: Geiger-Bronksy M, Wilson DJ, eds. *Respiratory Nursing: A Core Curriculum.* New York: Springer; 2008.
4. Finesilver C. Pulmonary assessment: what you need to know. *Prog Cardiovasc Nurs.* 2003;18(2):83–92.
5. Kallet RH. Bedside assessment of the patient. In: Kacmarek RM, Stoller JK, Heuer AJ, eds. *Egan's Fundamentals of Respiratory Care.* 11th ed. St. Louis: Elsevier; 2017.
6. Higginson R, Jones B. Respiratory assessment in critically ill patients: airway and breathing. *Br J Nurs.* 2009;18(8):456. 458–461.
7. Davis JL, Murray JF. History and physical examination. In: Broaddus VC, et al., ed. *Murray and Nadel's Textbook of Respiratory Medicine.* 6th ed. Philadelphia: Saunders; 2016.
8. Ball JW, et al. *Seidel's Guide to Physical Examination.* 8th ed. St. Louis: Mosby; 2015.
9. Wilkins RL, Hodgkin J, Lopez B. *Fundamentals of Lung and Heart Sounds.* 3rd ed. St. Louis: Mosby; 2004.

18

Pulmonary Diagnostic Procedures

Jeanne M. Maiden

To complete the assessment of a critically ill pulmonary patient, the patient's laboratory studies and diagnostic tests are reviewed. Although many procedures exist for diagnosing pulmonary disease, their application in a critically ill patient is limited. Only studies and tests that are used in the critical care setting are presented here. Bedside monitoring devices are also discussed.

LABORATORY STUDIES

Arterial Blood Gases

Interpretation of arterial blood gas (ABG) levels can be difficult, especially if the nurse is under pressure to do it quickly and accurately. One method that can help ensure accuracy when analyzing ABG levels is to follow the same steps of interpretation each time. A specific method to be used each time that blood gas values must be interpreted is presented here (Box 18.1).

Steps for Interpretation of Blood Gas Levels

Step 1. Look at the Pao_2 level, and answer this question: Does the Pao_2 show hypoxemia? The Pao_2 is a measure of the partial pressure (P) of oxygen dissolved in arterial (a) blood plasma. Sometimes, Pao_2 is shortened to Po_2. It is reported in millimeters of mercury (mm Hg). The Pao_2 reflects 3% of total oxygen in the blood.[1,2]

The normal range of Pao_2 values for individuals breathing room air at sea level is 80 to 100 mm Hg. However, the normal range is age dependent for infants and for adults 60 years old or older. The normal level for infants breathing room air is 50 to 70 mm Hg.[1] The normal level for adults 60 years old or older decreases with age as changes occur in the ventilation/perfusion ($\dot{V}/\dot{Q}$) matching in the aging lung.[1,3] The correct Pao_2 for older adults can be ascertained as follows: 80 mm Hg (the lowest normal value) minus 1 mm Hg for every year of age more than 60 years. Using this formula, a 65-year-old individual can have a Pao_2 of 75 mm Hg (80 mm Hg − 5 mm Hg = 75 mm Hg) and still be within the normal range. An acceptable range for an 80-year-old person (20 years older than 60 years) is 60 mm Hg (80 mm Hg − 20 mm Hg = 60 mm Hg).

At any age, a Pao_2 lower than 40 mm Hg represents a life-threatening situation that necessitates immediate action.[1,2] A Pao_2 value less than the predicted lowest value indicates hypoxemia, which means that a lower-than-normal amount of oxygen is dissolved in plasma.[1,2]

The Pao_2 level is analyzed before the levels of other blood gas components. A Pao_2 of less than 40 mm Hg severely compromises tissue oxygenation and requires immediate administration of supplemental oxygen or mechanical ventilation, or both. The test results for the Pao_2 level can be analyzed quickly. If the Pao_2 level is more than the lowest value for the patient's age, the Pao_2 is considered normal.

Step 2. Look at the pH level, and answer this question: Is the pH on the acid or alkaline side of 7.40? The pH is the hydrogen ion (H^+) concentration of plasma. Calculation of pH is accomplished by using the arterial partial pressure of carbon dioxide ($Paco_2$) and the plasma bicarbonate level (HCO_3^-). The formula used is the Henderson-Hasselbalch equation (see Appendix B).[1,2]

The normal pH of arterial blood is 7.35 to 7.45, and the mean is 7.40. If the pH level is less than 7.40, it is on the acid side of the mean. A pH level less than 7.35 is known as *acidemia*, and the overall condition is called *acidosis*. If the pH level is greater than 7.40, it is on the alkaline side of the mean. A pH level greater than 7.45 is known as *alkalemia*, and the overall condition is called *alkalosis*.[1,2]

Step 3. Look at the $Paco_2$ level, and answer this question: Does the $Paco_2$ show respiratory acidosis, alkalosis, or normalcy? The $Paco_2$ is a measure of the partial pressure of carbon dioxide dissolved in arterial blood plasma, and it is reported in millimeters of mercury (mm Hg). The $Paco_2$ is the acid–base component that reflects the effectiveness of ventilation in relation to the metabolic rate.[1,2] In other words, the $Paco_2$ value indicates whether the patient can ventilate well enough to rid the body of the carbon dioxide produced as a consequence of metabolism.

The normal range for $Paco_2$ is 35 to 45 mm Hg. This range does not change as a person ages. A $Paco_2$ value greater than 45 mm Hg defines *respiratory acidosis*, which is caused by alveolar hypoventilation. Hypoventilation can result from chronic obstructive pulmonary disease (COPD), oversedation, head trauma, anesthesia, drug overdose, neuromuscular disease, or hypoventilation with mechanical ventilation.[2]

Ventilatory failure results when the $Paco_2$ level exceeds 50 mm Hg. Acute ventilatory failure occurs when the $Paco_2$ level is greater than 50 mm Hg and the pH level is less than 7.30. Ventilatory failure is referred to as *acute* because the pH is abnormal, not allowing enough time for the body to compensate by returning the pH to the normal range. Chronic ventilatory failure is defined as a $Paco_2$ value greater than 50 mm Hg and a pH level greater than 7.30.[1]

A $Paco_2$ value that is less than 35 mm Hg defines *respiratory alkalosis*, which is caused by alveolar hyperventilation. Hyperventilation can result from hypoxia, anxiety, pulmonary embolism, pregnancy, and hyperventilation with mechanical ventilation or as a compensatory mechanism for metabolic acidosis.[4]

Step 4. Look at the HCO_3^- level, and answer this question: Does the HCO_3^- show metabolic acidosis, alkalosis, or normalcy? Bicarbonate (HCO_3^-) is the acid–base component that reflects

BOX 18.1 Interpretation of Arterial Blood Gases

Step 1
Look at the arterial partial pressure of oxygen (Pao$_2$) level, and answer this question: Does the Pao$_2$ level show hypoxemia?

Step 2
Look at the pH level, and answer this question: Is the pH level on the acid or alkaline side of 7.40?

Step 3
Look at the arterial partial pressure of carbon dioxide (Paco$_2$) level, and answer this question: Does the Paco$_2$ level show respiratory acidosis, alkalosis, or normalcy?

Step 4
Look at the bicarbonate (HCO$_3^-$) level, and answer this question: Does the HCO$_3^-$ level show metabolic acidosis, alkalosis, or normalcy?

Step 5
Look again at the pH level, and answer this question: Does the pH show a compensated or an uncompensated condition?

BOX 18.2 Uncompensated Arterial Blood Gas Values

	Example 1		Example 2
Pao$_2$:	90 mm Hg	Pao$_2$:	90 mm Hg
pH:	7.25	pH:	7.25
Paco$_2$:	50 mm Hg	Paco$_2$:	40 mm Hg
HCO$_3^-$:	22 mEq/L	HCO$_3^-$:	17 mEq/L
Interpretation: Uncompensated respiratory acidosis		*Interpretation:* Uncompensated metabolic acidosis	

BOX 18.3 Compensated Arterial Blood Gas Values

	Example 1		Example 2
Pao$_2$:	90 mm Hg	Pao$_2$:	90 mm Hg
pH:	7.37	pH:	7.42
Paco$_2$:	60 mm Hg	Paco$_2$:	48 mm Hg
HCO$_3^-$:	38 mEq/L	HCO$_3^-$:	35 mEq/L
Interpretation: Compensated respiratory acidosis with metabolic alkalosis. (Acidosis is considered the main disorder, and alkalosis is the compensatory response because the pH is on the acid side of 7.40.)		*Interpretation:* Compensated metabolic alkalosis with respiratory acidosis. (Alkalosis is considered the main disorder, and acidosis is the compensatory response because the pH is on the alkaline side of 7.40.)	

kidney function. The HCO$_3^-$ level is reduced or increased in the plasma by renal mechanisms. The normal range is 22 to 26 mEq/L.[2,4]

An HCO$_3^-$ level of less than 22 mEq/L defines *metabolic acidosis*, which can result from ketoacidosis, lactic acidosis, renal failure, or diarrhea. The cumulative effect is a gain of acids or a loss of base. An HCO$_3^-$ level that is greater than 26 mEq/L defines *metabolic alkalosis*, which can result from fluid loss from the upper gastrointestinal tract (vomiting or nasogastric suction), diuretic therapy, severe hypokalemia, alkali administration, or steroid therapy.[2,4]

Step 5. Look again at the pH level, and answer this question: Does the pH show a compensated or an uncompensated condition? If the pH level is abnormal (less than 7.35 or greater than 7.45), the Paco$_2$ value or the HCO$_3^-$ level, or both, will also be abnormal. This is an *uncompensated* condition because the body has not had enough time to return the pH to its normal range.[2,5] Box 18.2 provides two examples of uncompensated ABG values. If the pH level is within normal limits and the Paco$_2$ value and the HCO$_3^-$ level are abnormal, the condition is *compensated* because the body has had enough time to restore the pH to within its normal range.[2,5]

Differentiating the primary disorder from the compensatory response can be difficult. The primary disorder is the abnormality that caused the pH level to shift initially and is determined according to the pH level; the primary disorder is considered to be the one on whichever side of 7.40 the pH level occurs.[4] Box 18.3 provides two examples of compensated ABG values. Partial compensation may be present and is evidenced by abnormal pH, Paco$_2$, and HCO$_3^-$ levels, indications that the body is attempting to return the pH to its normal range.[4]

Table 18.1 summarizes the changes in the acid–base components that accompany various acid–base disorders.[4,5] In addition to the parameters previously discussed, other factors must be considered when reviewing a patient's ABG levels, including oxygen saturation, oxygen content, base excess and deficit, and anion gap analysis. Table 18.2 summarizes conditions that may potentiate acid–base abnormalities.[2,5]

Oxygen Saturation

Oxygen saturation is a measure of the amount of oxygen bound to hemoglobin compared with the maximal capability of hemoglobin for binding oxygen. It can be assessed as a component of the ABGs (Sao$_2$) or can be measured noninvasively using a pulse oximeter (Spo$_2$).[1] Oxygen saturation is reported as a percentage or as a decimal; normal values are greater than 95% when the patient is on room air. Normally, the saturation level cannot reach 100% (on room air) because of physiologic shunting.[1] However, when supplemental oxygen is administered, oxygen saturation may approach 100% so closely that it is reported as 100%.

Proper evaluation of the oxygen saturation level is vital. For example, an Sao$_2$ of 97% means that 97% of the available hemoglobin is bound with oxygen. The word *available* is essential to evaluating the Sao$_2$ level because the hemoglobin level is not always within normal limits, and oxygen can bind only with what is available. A 97% saturation level associated with 10 g/dL of hemoglobin does not deliver as much oxygen to the tissues as does a 97% saturation level associated with 15 g/dL of hemoglobin. Assessing only the Sao$_2$ level and finding it within normal limits does not ensure that the patient's oxygenation status is normal. The hemoglobin level must also be evaluated before a decision on oxygenation status can be made.[1,5]

Oxygen Content

Oxygen content (Cao$_2$) is a measure of the total amount of oxygen carried in the blood, including the amount dissolved in plasma (measured by the Pao$_2$) and the amount bound to the hemoglobin molecule (measured by the Sao$_2$). Cao$_2$ is reported

TABLE 18.1 Arterial Blood Gas Assessment

Disorder	pH	$Paco_2$ (mm Hg)	HCO_3^- (mEq/L)
Respiratory Acidosis			
Uncompensated	<7.35	>45	22–26
Partially compensated	<7.35	>45	>26
Compensated	7.35–7.39	>45	>26
Respiratory Alkalosis			
Uncompensated	>7.45	<35	22–26
Partially compensated	>7.45	<35	<22
Compensated	7.41–7.45	<35	<22
Metabolic Acidosis			
Uncompensated	<7.35	35–45	<22
Partially compensated	<7.35	<35	<22
Compensated	7.35–7.39	<35	<22
Metabolic Alkalosis			
Uncompensated	>7.45	35–45	>26
Partially compensated	>7.45	>45	>26
Compensated	7.41–7.45	>45	>26
Combined (or mixed) respiratory and metabolic acidosis	<7.35	>45	<22
Combined (or mixed) respiratory and metabolic alkalosis	>7.45	<35	>26

HCO_3^-, bicarbonate; $Paco_2$, arterial partial pressure of carbon dioxide.

TABLE 18.2 Acid-Base Disorders

Disorders	Potential Cause
Respiratory acidosis	Chronic obstructive pulmonary disease
	Acute airway obstruction
	Central nervous system depression
	Sedatives
	Anesthetics
	Opioids
	Trauma
	Spinal cord
	Brain
	Chest wall
	Neuromuscular disease
	Poliomyelitis
	Myasthenia gravis
	Guillain-Barré syndrome
	Hypoventilation with mechanical ventilation
Respiratory alkalosis	Hypoxia
	Anxiety
	Fear
	Pain
	Stimulants
	Pulmonary embolism
	Hyperventilation with mechanical ventilation
Metabolic acidosis	Lactic acidosis
	Ketoacidosis
	Renal failure (uremia)
	Rhabdomyolysis
	Ingestion of acids (methanol, salicylates, ethylene glycol)
	Diarrhea
	Renal tubular acidosis
	Ileostomy
	Pancreatic fistula
Metabolic alkalosis	Steroid therapy
	Vomiting
	Gastrointestinal suction
	Diuretic therapy
	Hypokalemia
	Hypovolemia
	Hypochloremia
	Sodium bicarbonate intake

in milliliters of oxygen carried per 100 mL of blood. The normal value is 20 mL of oxygen per 100 mL of blood. To calculate the oxygen content, the Pao_2, the Sao_2, and the hemoglobin level are used (see Appendix B). A change in any one of these parameters affects the Cao_2.[1,5]

The value of assessing the Cao_2 is best illustrated by the examples in Table 18.3. The ABG parameters that are used most commonly to evaluate oxygenation status (Pao_2 and Sao_2) are both normal. Assessing only the Pao_2 and the Sao_2 would lead to the invalid conclusion that Patient B's oxygenation status is normal. However, consideration of the hemoglobin level and the Cao_2 reveals that the oxygenation of Patient B's blood is significantly abnormal.

Base Excess and Base Deficit

Base excess and base deficit reflect the nonrespiratory contribution to acid–base balance and are reported in milliequivalents per liter (mEq/L) above or below the normal range of −2 mEq/L to +2 mEq/L. A negative base level is reported as a *base deficit*, which correlates with *metabolic acidosis*, whereas a positive base level is reported as a *base excess*, which correlates with *metabolic alkalosis*.[1,4,5]

Classic Shunt Equation and Oxygen Tension Indices

The efficiency of oxygenation can be assessed by measuring the degree of intrapulmonary shunting that occurs in a patient at

any one time, using the classic shunt equation and oxygen tension indices. *Intrapulmonary shunting* (QS/QT [the portion of cardiac output not exchanging with alveolar blood divided by the total cardiac output]) refers to venous blood that flows to the lungs without being oxygenated because of nonfunctioning alveoli.[1] Other names for this condition include shunt effect, low $\dot{V}/\dot{Q}$, wasted blood flow, and venous admixture.[1,5]

Direct determination of intrapulmonary shunting requires the use of the classic shunt equation (see Appendix B), which is invasive and cumbersome. A shunt greater than 10% is considered abnormal and indicative of a shunt-producing disorder. A shunt greater than 30% is a serious and potentially life-threatening condition, which requires pulmonary intervention.[1]

Often, intrapulmonary shunting is estimated by using the oxygen tension indices. One advantage to these methods is the ease of performance, although they have been found to be unreliable in critically ill patients.[1] An estimate

TABLE 18.3 Oxygenation Status

Patient	Pao$_2$ Level (mm Hg)	Sao$_2$ Level (%)	Hgb (g/dL)	Cao$_2$ (mL/dL)
A	100	97	15	19.8
B	100	97	10	13.3

Cao$_2$, arterial oxygen content; *Hgb*, hemoglobin; *Pao$_2$*, arterial partial pressure of oxygen; *Sao$_2$*, arterial oxygen saturation.

TABLE 18.4 Calculation of Intrapulmonary Shunting

Fio$_2$	Pao$_2$ Level (mm Hg)	Pao$_2$ Level (mm Hg)	Pao$_2$/Fio$_2$	a/A RATIO (%)	A-a Gradient (mm Hg)
0.21	40	97	190	41	57
0.50	80	300	160	27	220
1.0	150	610	150	25	460

A, alveolar; *a*, arterial; *Fio$_2$*, fraction of inspired oxygen; *Pao$_2$*, arterial partial pressure of oxygen.
Modified from Murray JF, Nadel JA, eds. *Textbook of Respiratory Medicine.* Philadelphia: Saunders; 1988.

of intrapulmonary shunting can be determined by computing the difference between the alveolar and arterial oxygen concentrations. Normally, alveolar (A) and arterial (a) Po$_2$ values are approximately equal. When they are not, it indicates that venous blood is passing malfunctioning alveoli and returning unoxygenated to the left side of the heart.[1] The most common oxygen tension indices used to estimate intrapulmonary shunting are the Pao$_2$/Fio$_2$ ratio, the Pao$_2$/Pao$_2$ ratio, and the A-a gradient (P[A – a]o$_2$).

Pao$_2$/Fio$_2$ Ratio

The Pao$_2$/Fio$_2$ ratio is clinically the easiest formula to calculate because this formula does not call for the computation of the alveolar Po$_2$. Normally, the Pao$_2$/Fio$_2$ ratio is greater than 286; the lower the value, the worse the lung function.[1,5]

Pao$_2$/Pao$_2$ Ratio

The Pao$_2$/Pao$_2$ ratio (arterial/alveolar oxygen ratio) is normally greater than 60%. The disadvantage to using this formula is that this formula calls for the computation of the alveolar Po$_2$ (see Appendix B), but the advantage is that this formula is unaffected by changes in the Fio$_2$, as long as the underlying lung condition is stable.[1,5]

Alveolar-Arterial Gradient

The A-a gradient (P[A – a]o$_2$) is normally less than 20 mm Hg on room air for patients younger than 61 years. This estimate of intrapulmonary shunting is the least reliable clinically, but it is used often in clinical decision making. A major disadvantage to using this formula is that it is greatly influenced by the amount of oxygen the patient is receiving.[1,5]

Serial determinations of the estimates of intrapulmonary shunting provide the practitioner with objective data on which to base clinical decisions.[1] Table 18.4 shows the change in intrapulmonary shunting in hypoxemic patients using the previously described oxygen tension indices to estimate severity of shunting.

Dead Space Equation

The efficiency of ventilation can be measured using the clinical dead space (Vd/Vt) equation (see Appendix B). The formula measures the fraction of tidal volume not participating in gas exchange. A dead space value greater than 0.6 indicates a dead space–producing disorder and is considered abnormal. The major limitations to using this formula are that it requires the measurement of exhaled carbon dioxide to complete and that the work of breathing by patients must remain stable during the collection.[1,6]

Sputum Studies

Careful analysis of sputum specimens is crucial for rapid identification and treatment of pulmonary infections. The most difficult aspect of sputum examination is proper collection of the specimen. Collection of a good sputum sample requires a conscious, cooperative, and sufficiently hydrated patient.[7] When the patient has difficulty producing sputum, heated, nebulized saline may help to loosen secretions for expectoration.[7] Chest physiotherapy combined with nebulization improves the success rate. Collection of a sputum specimen is best done in the morning because a greater volume of secretions is present as a result of nighttime pooling. Brushing the teeth and rinsing the oropharyngeal airway is recommended to reduce contamination before collecting a sample.[2,7,8]

Many critically ill patients cannot cough effectively, and sputum collection by other means is required. These methods include tracheobronchial aspiration, transtracheal aspiration, and fiberoptic bronchoscopy with a protected brush catheter. Because each method has its own benefits and risks, the patient's clinical condition determines the appropriate technique.

Many critically ill patients have endotracheal or tracheostomy tubes already in place. Collecting sputum specimens from these patients requires special attention to technique (Box 18.4). Deep specimens are obtained to avoid collecting specimens that contain resident upper airway flora that may have migrated down the tube. Colonization of the lower airways with upper airway flora can occur within 48 hours of intubation.[7-9]

After a sputum specimen is obtained, the sputum is examined for volume, physical properties, mucopurulence, and color. Next, a microscopic examination is done to identify the source of the specimen. If a bacterial infection is suspected, a Gram stain is performed, followed by culture and sensitivity assessments.[7-9]

DIAGNOSTIC PROCEDURES

Bronchoscopy

Fiberoptic bronchoscopy is a relatively safe procedure done at the bedside, and it is most often used as a diagnostic and therapeutic tool (Fig. 18.2). Diagnostic indications include hemoptysis, infectious pneumonia, difficult intubation, pulmonary injury after chest trauma, acute burn inhalation injury, aspiration lung injuries, and acute upper airway obstruction. Therapeutic indications include aspiration of foreign bodies; removal of obstructing secretions; atelectasis; difficult intubation; and resection of small, benign growths from the airway.[2,10]

Before bronchoscopy, a complete medical history is obtained, and a thorough examination, including a chest x-ray examination, is performed.[2] Preprocedural evaluation of the patient includes clotting studies (prothrombin time, partial thromboplastin time, and platelet count) and evaluation of the ABG levels.[2] Hypoxemic patients need supplemental oxygen during

BOX 18.4 Procedure Sputum Specimen Collection

1. Clear the endotracheal or tracheostomy tube of all local secretions, avoiding deep airway penetration.
2. Attach a sputum trap to a sterile suction catheter, and advance the catheter into the trachea while trying to avoid contact with the endotracheal tube or tracheostomy tube (Fig. 18.1).
3. After the catheter is fully advanced, apply suction until secretions return to the sputum trap. When enough secretions are collected, discontinue suctioning, and remove the catheter.
4. Do not apply suction while the catheter is being withdrawn because this can contaminate the sample with sputum from the upper airway. Do not flush the catheter with sterile water because this dilutes the sample.
5. If the catheter becomes plugged with secretions, place it in a sterile container, and send it to the laboratory. The specimen must be transported immediately or refrigerated if a delay is necessary.

FIG. 18.2 Flexible Fiberoptic Bronchoscopy. The catheter is introduced into a small airway. Bronchial alveolar lavage is performed by injecting and withdrawing small amounts of sterile normal saline solution, gently aspirating after each instillation. Specimens are sent to the laboratory for analysis. (From Malarkey LM, McMorrow ME. *Saunders Nursing Guide to Laboratory and Diagnostic Tests.* St. Louis: Saunders; 2005.)

FIG. 18.1 Specimen Container. (From Kacmarek RM, et al, eds. *Egan's Fundamentals of Respiratory Care.* 10th ed. St. Louis: Mosby; 2013.)

the procedure. The patient must have no oral intake for 6 to 8 hours before bronchoscopy to reduce the risk of aspiration.[2,11]

Although a topical anesthetic can be used alone, the anesthetic is usually supplemented by an intravenous sedative or analgesic, or both. A benzodiazepine for sedative effects and an opioid analgesic are administered intravenously during the procedure.[2,10] Preprocedural medications for a diagnostic bronchoscopy may include atropine and intramuscular codeine. Atropine lessens the vasovagal response and reduces the secretions, whereas codeine decreases the cough reflex. When bronchoscopy is performed therapeutically to remove secretions, the patient has decreased cough and gag reflexes, which may impair secretion clearance.[2,10] Maintenance of the airway is essential to prevent complications.

Complications of the procedure may be related to the procedure itself, the anesthetic, or an ancillary procedure. Minor complications include laryngospasm, bronchospasm, epistaxis, fever, vomiting, altered pulmonary mechanics, and hemodynamic instability. Major complications include anaphylaxis, infection, hypotension, cardiac dysrhythmias, pneumothorax, hemorrhage, respiratory failure, hypoxemia, and cardiopulmonary arrest.[2,10]

Thoracentesis

Thoracentesis is a simple, usually uncomplicated procedure done at the bedside for the removal of fluid or air from the pleural space (Fig. 18.3). A thoracentesis is used most often as a diagnostic measure; it may also be performed therapeutically for the drainage of a pleural effusion or empyema.[2,12] No absolute contraindications to thoracentesis exist, although there are some risks that may contraindicate the procedure in all but emergency situations. These risk factors include unstable hemodynamics, coagulation defects, mechanical ventilation, the presence of an intraaortic balloon pump, and patients who are uncooperative. In most clinical situations, diagnostic thoracentesis can be delayed until these risk factors are eliminated.[12]

The patient is placed in a sitting position with legs over the side of the bed and with hands and arms supported on a padded overbed table. If the patient's condition precludes sitting, the side-lying position with the back flush with the edge of the bed and the affected side down can be used.[12] The patient is cautioned not to move or cough during the procedure.[12] During

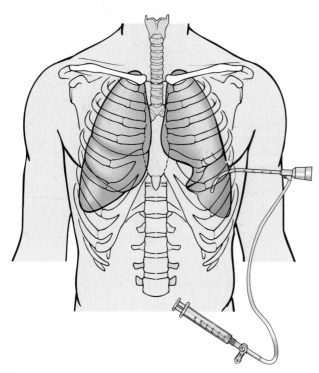

FIG. 18.3 Thoracentesis. The needle has penetrated the fluid-filled pleural space to remove fluid. (From Lewis S, et al. *Medical-Surgical Nursing: Assessment and Management of Clinical Problems.* 9th ed. St. Louis: Mosby; 2014.)

the thoracentesis, the site of the needle insertion is usually determined by previous chest x-ray examination, ultrasonography, computed tomography scan, or chest percussion. A local anesthetic is used to minimize the patient's discomfort during insertion of the thoracentesis needle.[12]

Complications associated with thoracentesis include pain, pneumothorax, and reexpansion pulmonary edema. Pneumothorax can occur as a result of introduction of air into the pleural space, puncture of the lung, or rupture of the visceral pleura.[2,12] Reexpansion pulmonary edema can occur when a large amount of effusion fluid (approximately 1000 to 1500 mL) is removed from the pleural space. Removal of the fluid increases the negative intrapleural pressure, which can lead to edema when the lung does not reexpand to fill the space. The patient experiences severe coughing and shortness of breath. The onset of these symptoms is an indication to discontinue the thoracentesis.[13]

Bedside Pulmonary Function Tests

Pulmonary function tests (PFTs) are designed to quantify respiratory function and are an essential component of a thorough pulmonary evaluation. PFTs are used for a variety of purposes, including preoperative assessment, evaluating lung mechanics, diagnosing and tracking pulmonary diseases, and monitoring therapy. Results are individualized according to age, sex, and body size.[2,6,14]

A complete PFT consists of four components: lung volumes, mechanics of breathing, diffusion, and ABGs. PFTs may take 2 hours to complete. Because of the severity of illness encountered in the critical care area, all four components are rarely completed. Most often, measurements of pulmonary function in a critically ill patient are limited to areas that give the

practitioner information about the patient's need for or ability to wean from mechanical ventilation. This section covers the areas tested most often at the bedside of critically ill patients.

Measurement of lung volumes and capacities (Box 18.5) provides valuable information about the origin of a disease process. Four lung volumes and four lung capacities can be measured. Measurement of volumes at the bedside is limited to tidal volume and vital capacity. A vital capacity of 10 to 15 mL/kg usually is a minimally accepted value for weaning, with a respiratory rate of less than 24 breaths/min.[2,6]

Assessment of the mechanics of breathing includes measurement of the flow of gas, lung and chest compliance, respiratory muscle strength, and tissue resistance. In the critical care area, dynamic and static compliance are measured at the bedside. *Compliance* is a measure of the distensibility of the lungs (how easily they are inflated). Dynamic compliance is measured during the breathing cycle. A value of 46 to 66 mL/cm H_2O is normal (see Appendix B). Measurement of dynamic compliance does not differentiate among resistance forces. Conditions that increase resistance alter the dynamic compliance value. Dynamic compliance decreases with any decrease in lung compliance or increase in airway resistance, as occurs with bronchospasm and retained secretions. Static compliance is measured under no-flow conditions so that resistance forces are removed. Static compliance decreases with any decrease in lung compliance, as occurs with pneumothorax, atelectasis, pneumonia, pulmonary edema, and chest wall restrictions. A normal range is 57 to 85 mL/cm H_2O (see Appendix B).[14]

Assessment of inspiratory muscle strength can be evaluated through the measurement of maximal inspiratory pressure (MIP) and negative inspiratory pressure. Both should be more negative than −20 to −25 cm H_2O. Other names for these tests are negative inspiratory effort, peak inspiratory pressure (PIP), and peak inspiratory force. Assessing the maximal inspiratory pressure and negative inspiratory pressure requires a cooperative patient, and the values can provide useful information about spontaneous breathing ability. Maximal expiratory presssure (MEP) can be measured to test the ability to cough in patients with neuromuscular dysfunction. Other common methods used to assess respiratory muscle strength are

TABLE 18.5 Bedside Pulmonary Function Tests

Test	Description
Respiratory rate (f)	Number of breaths per minute
Tidal volume (VT)	Volume of air exhaled after a normal resting inhalation
Minute ventilation (VE)	Volume of air expired per minute (tidal volume respiratory rate = minute ventilation)
Maximal voluntary ventilation (MVV)	Maximal amount of air that can be moved into and out of the lungs in 1 minute
Forced vital capacity (FVC)	Maximal amount of air that can be forcefully exhaled from the lungs after maximal inhalation
Maximal inspiratory pressure (MIP)	Maximal negative pressure generated on inhalation
Maximal expiratory pressure (MEP)	Maximal positive pressure generated on exhalation
Peak expiratory flow rate (PEFR)	Maximal flow rate achieved during forced exhalation
Forced expiratory flow at midpoint of vital capacity (FEF$_{25\%-75\%}$)	Measure of average flow rate during the middle 50% of exhalation
Forced expiratory flow at 1 second (FEV$_1$)	Volume of air exhaled during the first second of forced exhalation

maximum voluntary ventilation (MVV), minute ventilation VE, and breathing pattern.[14]

Dynamic PFTs are designed to evaluate the function of the respiratory muscles, thorax, and lungs. These tests are timed breathing studies that evaluate the degree of respiratory impairment and include forced vital capacity (FVC), peak expiratory flow rate (PEFR), forced expiratory volume in 1 second (FEV$_1$), and forced expiratory volume divided by forced vital capacity (FEV$_1$/FVC). Forced expiratory flow (FEF$_{25\%-75\%}$) is the mean rate of airflow over the middle half of the FVC and is a good index of airway resistance. When these studies are performed at the bedside, they require the use of spirometry for volume measurement. The tests can be performed with intubated or nonintubated patients. In an intubated patient, the spirometer is attached to the end of the endotracheal tube. In a nonintubated patient, a nose clip is placed on the patient, and the patient is instructed to breathe through a spirometer tube. The patient is seated on the side of the bed if possible.[2,6,14] Each of these parameters is described in Table 18.5.

Ventilation/Perfusion Scanning

V̇/Q̇ scanning is indicated when a serious alteration of the normal V̇/Q̇ relationship is suspected. V̇/Q̇ studies are ordered most often to diagnose and follow a suspected pulmonary embolus. V̇/Q̇ scanning is approximately 90% accurate in determining this diagnosis. Comparing the perfusion scan with the results of a clinical examination may improve this percentage.[15]

The V̇/Q̇ scan consists of a ventilation scan and a perfusion scan. The ventilation scan is performed by having the patient inhale a radiolabeled gas and air mixture through a mask. The perfusion scan is performed by giving the patient an intravenous injection of a radioisotope. Scintillation cameras record the gamma radiation images produced by the isotope as it is breathed or perfused into the lung. When an obstruction of the isotope's flow into an area of the lung occurs, the diminished radioactivity is reflected in the camera image of that zone.[2,15]

Because the results are less than 100% accurate in predicting pulmonary emboli, most V̇/Q̇ scans are interpreted in one of four ways. The scan is interpreted as normal when the perfusion scan is normal, and the probability of pulmonary embolism approaches zero. A low probability interpretation is given when there are small V̇/Q̇ mismatches, when there are focal V̇/Q̇ matches with no corresponding radiographic abnormalities, or when the perfusion defects are considerably smaller than the radiographic abnormalities. This finding is associated with

BOX 18.6 Chest Radiograph Interpretation

Step 1
Look at the different densities (black, gray, and white), and answer this question: What is air, fluid, tissue, and bone?

Step 2
Look at the shape or form of each density, and answer this question: What normal anatomic structure is this?

Step 3
Look at the right and left sides, and answer this question: Are the findings the same on both sides, or are there physiologic and pathophysiologic differences?

Step 4
Look at all the structures (bones, mediastinum, diaphragm, pleural space, and lung tissue), and answer this question: Are any abnormalities present?

Step 5
Look for all tubes, wires, and lines, and answer this question: Are the tubes, wires, and lines in the proper place?

a 12% chance of pulmonary embolus.[2,15] An intermediate or indeterminate probability is assigned when there are severe diffuse airflow obstructions; perfusion defects corresponding in size and position to radiographic abnormalities; and a single, moderate V̇/Q̇ mismatch without a corresponding radiographic abnormality. A high probability interpretation is used when the perfusion defects are substantially larger than the radiographic abnormalities or when there is one or more large or two or more moderate V̇/Q̇ mismatches with no corresponding radiographic abnormalities. This finding is seen infrequently but has a highly predictive value.[15]

Chest Radiography

Chest radiography is an important diagnostic procedure for any critically ill patient. Chest x-ray examinations aid in the diagnosis of various disorders and complications and assist in the evaluation of treatment.[16,17] When interpreting a chest radiograph, a systematic method is used for viewing (Box 18.6). Areas of the radiographic film that are assessed include bones, mediastinum, diaphragm, pleural space, and lung tissue. Fig. 18.4 provides an example of a normal chest radiograph.

Bones

The clavicles, ribs, thoracic and cervical spine, and scapulas are assessed. The clavicles should be symmetric, and the ribs should

FIG. 18.4 Normal Chest Radiograph. *1*, trachea; *2*, carina; *3*, right main bronchi; *4*, left main bronchi; *5*, right hilar structure; *6*, left hilar structure; *7*, right horizontal fissure; *8*, right cardiac border formed by the right atrium; *9*, left cardiac border formed by the left ventricle; *10*, aortic knob; *11*, descending thoracic aorta; *12*, right paratracheal line; *13*, right hemidiaphragm; *14*, left hemidiaphragm; *15*, right costophrenic angle; *16*, left costophrenic angle; *17*, gastric air bubble; *18*, gas in the colon. (From Corne J, Kumaran M. *Chest X Ray Made Easy*. 4th ed. London: Elsevier; 2016.)

be an equal distance apart. Intervertebral disk spaces should be evident, indicating an adequately exposed inspiratory film.[16,17] The thoracic and cervical spine should be straight, without signs of curvature. The scapulas usually appear as areas of added density in the upper lung fields. There should be no evidence of fractures, calcification and lesions (increased density), or demineralization (decreased density).[16,17]

Mediastinum

The structures assessed in the mediastinal area are the aortic knob and the trachea. The trachea should be positioned in the midline, with a slight deviation to the right as the trachea approaches the carina.[15] Shifting of the mediastinal structures can occur with atelectasis and removal of all or a portion of a lung (toward the area of involvement), pneumothorax (away from the area of involvement), pleural effusion, and tumors.[16,17]

Diaphragm

The diaphragm should be clearly visible, with sharp costophrenic angles seen where the chest wall and the tapered edges of the diaphragm meet.[17] The level of the diaphragm (on deep inspiration) should appear at the 10th or 11th rib,[17] with the right side 1 to 2 cm higher than the left side.[17] A gastric air bubble may be found under the left side of the diaphragm.[16,17] An elevated diaphragm may be seen in pregnancy, obesity,

conditions that cause air or fluid to accumulate in the peritoneal space, and intestinal obstruction.[17] An elevated hemidiaphragm is associated with several conditions, including phrenic nerve injury, previous chest surgery, subphrenic abscess, trauma, stroke, tumor, pneumonia, and radiation therapy.[17] Flattening of the diaphragm can be a sign of increased air in the lungs, as occurs with chronic COPD or a pleural effusion.[17] Obliteration or "blunting" of the costophrenic angle can occur with pleural effusion, atelectasis, or pneumothorax.[17]

Pleural Space

Identification of the pleural space on a chest radiograph is an abnormal finding. The pleural space is not visible unless air (pneumothorax) or fluid (pleural effusion) enters the space. As fluid accumulates in the pleural space, the fluid surrounds the lung and eventually compresses it. With a pleural effusion, blunting of the costophrenic angle may be evident first, with flattening of the diaphragm and obscuring of the heart borders occurring as the effusion grows.[17] With a pneumothorax, the pleural edges become evident as the examiner looks through and between the images of the ribs on the film. A thin line appears just parallel to the chest wall, indicating where the lung markings have pulled away from the chest wall.[17] The collapsed lung manifests as an area of increased density separated by an area of radiolucency (blackness).

Lung Tissue

The lung tissue is viewed for any areas of increased density or increased radiolucency that may indicate an abnormality. Increased density can be the result of accumulation of fluid in the lungs (water, pus, blood, edema fluid) or collapse of lung tissue (with atelectasis or pneumothorax). Increased radiolucency is caused by increased air in the lungs, as may occur with COPD.[17] In some patients, a fine line may be present on the right side at approximately the level of the sixth rib in the mid-lung field. This is a normal finding and represents the horizontal fissure, which separates the right upper lobe from the right middle lobe.[17]

Tubes, Wires, and Lines

The chest radiograph is assessed for proper placement of all tubes, wires, and lines. When properly positioned, an endotracheal tube is 2 to 3 cm above the carina, and a nasogastric tube runs the length of the esophagus, with the tip in the stomach.[17] The origin of a central venous catheter is observed as a thin, continuous, radiopaque line at the level of the jaw, progressing toward the superior vena cava in an internal jugular approach, whereas a subclavian approach originates in the clavicular area. A pulmonary artery catheter is viewed running through the right atrium and right ventricle into the pulmonary artery.[17] Additional items that may be present include temporary or permanent pacing wires, a permanent pacing generator, an implantable cardioverter defibrillator, a peripherally inserted central catheter, chest tubes (pleural or mediastinal), electrocardiographic electrodes, and surgical markers and clips.[17]

Nursing Management

Nursing management of a patient undergoing a diagnostic procedure involves a variety of interventions, which include preparing the patient psychologically and physically for the procedure, monitoring the patient's responses to the procedure, and assessing the patient after the procedure. Preparing the patient includes teaching the patient about the procedure, answering any questions, and positioning the patient for the procedure. Monitoring the patient's responses to the procedure includes observing the patient for signs of pain, anxiety, or respiratory distress and monitoring vital signs, lung sounds, and oxygen saturation. Assessing the patient after the procedure includes observing for complications of the procedure and medicating the patient for any postprocedural discomfort.

BEDSIDE MONITORING

Capnography

Capnography is the measurement of exhaled carbon dioxide (CO_2) gas and is also known as *end-tidal CO_2* monitoring. Normally, alveolar and arterial carbon dioxide concentrations are equal in the presence of normal $\dot{V}/\dot{Q}$ relationships. In a patient who is hemodynamically stable, the partial pressure of end-tidal CO_2 ($P_{ET}CO_2$) can be used to estimate the $Paco_2$, with $P_{ET}CO_2$ levels 1 to 5 mm Hg less than $Paco_2$ levels. The practitioner must determine first that a normal $\dot{V}/\dot{Q}$ relationship exists before correlation of $P_{ET}CO_2$ and $Paco_2$ can be assumed.[18] Causes of increased $P_{ET}CO_2$ include situations in which carbon dioxide production is increased, such as hyperthermia, sepsis, and seizures, or in which alveolar ventilation is decreased, such as respiratory depression. Causes of decreased $P_{ET}CO_2$ include situations in which carbon dioxide production is decreased, such as hypothermia, cardiac arrest, and pulmonary embolism, or in which alveolar ventilation is increased, such as hyperventilation.[18]

In the critical care area, continuous capnography is used for assessment and monitoring of the patient's ventilatory status in various situations, including weaning from mechanical ventilation and undergoing procedural sedation. Assessment of changes in physiologic dead space can be carried out with $P_{ET}CO_2$ monitoring, based on the degree of difference between $Paco_2$ and $P_{ET}CO_2$. As the severity of pulmonary impairment increases, so does the disparity between $Paco_2$ and $P_{ET}CO_2$, as indicated by an increased gradient. A gradient of greater than 5 mm Hg can be seen with underperfused alveolar-capillary units (dead space–producing situations) and nonperfused alveolar-capillary units (alveolar dead space). Increased dead space ventilation is a result of decreased pulmonary blood flow or cardiac output and lung disease. This leads to an abnormality in the transfer of carbon dioxide from the blood to the lung. The result is a $P_{ET}CO_2$ level that is lower than the $Paco_2$ level because of the mixing of carbon dioxide between perfused and nonperfused units. The end result is an increased or widened $Paco_2/P_{ET}CO_2$ gradient.[18]

The noninvasive measurement of $P_{ET}CO_2$ enables assessment of the adequacy of cardiopulmonary resuscitation and endotracheal tube placement. Decreased pulmonary blood flow is associated with lower $P_{ET}CO_2$ values, reflected clinically by decreased cardiac output, as in the case of cardiopulmonary resuscitation. During endotracheal intubation, a low $P_{ET}CO_2$ reading indicates that the tube is positioned in the stomach because the amount of carbon dioxide in the esophagus is expected to be low.[18]

There are three forms of capnography: mainstream, side-stream, and proximal diverting. All forms can be used in intubated patients, but side-stream and microstream capnography can also be used in nonintubated patients, broadening the application of $P_{ET}CO_2$ monitoring. Mainstream capnography measures the carbon dioxide level directly by a sensor in the exhalation port of the ventilator tubing. During exhalation, gas passes over the sensor, and the information is transferred by an electrical cable to the display unit. The display unit produces a waveform, called a *capnogram* (Fig. 18.5), and a numeric recording ($P_{ET}CO_2$). Disadvantages to this form of capnography include the weight of the sensor on the ventilator tubing and possible obstruction of the sensor by secretions and condensation. In side-stream capnography, the carbon dioxide gas is continuously aspirated through a side port in the ventilator tubing or nasal cannula and is measured and analyzed by a side unit. Disadvantages to this form of capnography include obstruction of the sampling tube with secretions and slow response time. Proximal diverting capnography is a newer and improved version of side-stream capnography that transports gas a short distance from the airway to a site where the sensor is located, reducing the bulkiness at the airway.[18]

Capnography and $P_{ET}CO_2$ analysis have many diverse applications in the critical care area, but the practitioner must never assume that the $P_{ET}CO_2$ values reflect $Paco_2$ values without waveform analysis. Any change in the waveform can indicate a change in the patient's pulmonary status and warrants further evaluation. Loss of the waveform may signal loss of effective respirations.[18]

FIG. 18.5 Capnogram. Normal findings on a capnogram. $A \rightarrow B$ indicates the baseline; $B \rightarrow C$, the expiratory upstroke; $C \rightarrow D$, the alveolar plateau; D, the partial pressure of end-tidal carbon dioxide; and $D \rightarrow E$, the inspiratory downstroke. (From Frakes M. Measuring end-tidal carbon dioxide: clinical applications and usefulness. *Crit Care Nurse.* 2001;21[5]:23.)

Pulse Oximetry

Pulse oximetry is a noninvasive method for monitoring oxygen saturation (Spo_2) and is indicated in any situation in which the patient's oxygenation status requires continuous observation. A pulse oximeter consists of a microprocessor and a probe that attaches to the patient's forehead, finger, ear, toe, or nose. The probe consists of two light-emitting diodes and a photodetector (Fig. 18.6). The diodes transmit red and infrared light wavelengths through the pulsating arterial vascular bed to the photodetector on the other side. The percentage of oxygen saturation is determined by the difference in absorbance of the red and infrared light caused by the difference in color between oxygen-bound (bright red) and oxygen-unbound (dark red) hemoglobin. The photodetector converts the light signals into an electric signal that is sent to the microprocessor, which converts the electric signal into a digital reading. The pulse oximeter is considered very accurate; readings vary less than 4% to 5% at a saturation level greater than 70%. However, several physiologic and technical factors limit the monitoring system.[18]

Physiologic limitations of pulse oximetry include elevated levels of abnormal hemoglobins, the presence of vascular dyes, and poor tissue perfusion. The pulse oximeter cannot differentiate between normal and abnormal hemoglobin. Elevated levels of abnormal hemoglobin falsely elevate the Spo_2. Vascular dyes such as methylene blue, indigo carmine, indocyanine green, and fluorescein interfere with pulse oximetry and can lead to falsely low readings. Poor tissue perfusion to the area with the probe leads to loss of pulsatile flow and signal failure.[18] In a critically ill patient, pulse oximetry is reliable only for monitoring the patient's oxygenation status. Pulse oximetry is an unreliable method for monitoring the patient's ventilatory status. The ability of a pulse oximeter to detect hypoventilation is accurate only when the patient is breathing room air. Because most critically ill patients require some form of oxygen therapy, pulse oximetry is an unreliable method of detecting hypercapnia and should *not* be used for this purpose.[18]

Technical limitations of pulse oximetry include bright lights, excessive motion, and incorrect placement of the probe. Bright lights may interfere with the photodetector and cause inaccurate results. The probe must be covered to limit optical interference. Excessive motion can mimic arterial pulsations and can lead to false readings. Incorrect placement of the probe can lead to inaccurate results because part of the light can reach the photodetector without having passed through blood (optical shunting). Interventions to limit these problems include using

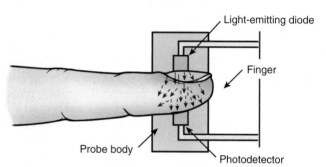

FIG. 18.6 Pulse Oximeter Finger Probe. (From Wilkins RL, Stoller JK, Scanlan CL, eds. *Egan's Fundamentals of Respiratory Care.* 8th ed 8. St. Louis: Mosby; 2006.)

the proper probe in the appropriate spot (not using a finger probe on the ear), applying the probe according to the directions, and ensuring that the area being monitored has adequate perfusion.[18]

SUMMARY

Laboratory Studies

- Interpretation of ABG levels involves looking at the Pao_2 (normal range, 80 to 100 mm Hg), the pH (normal range, 7.35 to 7.45), the $Paco_2$ (normal range, 35 to 45 mm Hg), and HCO_3^- (normal range, 22 to 26 mEq/L).
- The efficiency of oxygenation can be assessed by measuring the degree of intrapulmonary shunting using the classic shunt equation and oxygen tension indices (Pao_2/Fio_2 ratio, Pao_2/Pao_2 ratio, and A-a gradient).
- Sputum specimens are crucial for rapid identification and treatment of pulmonary infections.

Diagnostic Procedures

- Fiberoptic bronchoscopy and thoracentesis are often used as diagnostic and therapeutic procedures.
- PFTs are used for preoperative assessment, evaluating lung mechanics, diagnosing and tracking pulmonary diseases, and monitoring therapy.
- $\dot{V}/\dot{Q}$ scanning is indicated when a serious alteration of the normal $\dot{V}/\dot{Q}$ relationship is suspected, such as with a pulmonary embolus.
- Chest x-ray examination aids in the diagnosis of various pulmonary disorders and assists in the evaluation of treatments.

Bedside Monitoring

- Capnography is a noninvasive method used to monitor a patient's ventilatory status by measurement of exhaled carbon dioxide gas.
- Pulse oximetry is a noninvasive method used to monitor a patient's oxygenation status by measurement of oxygen saturation.

ⓔ Visit the Evolve site for additional study materials.

REFERENCES

1. Cohen Z. Gas exchange and transport. In: Kacmarek RM, Stoller JK, Heuer AJ, eds. *Egan's Fundamentals of Respiratory Care.* ed 11. St. Louis: Elsevier; 2017.
2. Chernecky C, Berger B. *Laboratory Tests and Diagnostic Procedures.* ed 6. St. Louis: Elsevier; 2013.
3. Meiner SE. Theories of aging. In: Meiner SE, ed. *Gerontology Nursing.* ed 5. St. Louis: Elsevier; 2015.
4. Beach W. Acid base balance. In: Kacmarek RM, Stoller JK, Heuer AJ, eds. *Egan's Fundamentals of Respiratory Care.* ed 11. St. Louis: Elservier; 2017.
5. Scanlan CL. Interpretation of blood gases. In: Heuer AJ, Scanlon CL, eds. *Wilkin's Clinical Assessment in Respiratory Care.* ed 7. St. Louis: Elsevier; 2014.
6. Mireles-Cabodevila E, Chatburn RL. Ventilation. In: Kacmarek RM, Stoller JK, Heuer AJ, eds. *Egan's Fundamentals of Respiratory Care.* ed 11. St. Louis: Elsevier; 2017.
7. Fisher DF. Solutions, body fluids and electrolytes. In: Kacmarek RM, Stoller JK, Heuer AJ, eds. *Egan's Fundamentals of Respiratory Care.* ed 11. St. Louis: Elsevier; 2017.
8. American Association for Clinical Chemistry. Lab tests online: Bacterial sputum culture. https://labtestsonline.org/understanding/analytes/sputum-culture/tab/sample/#.Vg1PEsfMrak.gmail. 2014 Accessed October 15, 2016.
9. Kallet R. Interpreting clinical and laboratory data. In: Kacmarek RM, Stoller JK, Heuer AJ, eds. *Egan's Fundamentals of Respiratory Care.* ed 11. St. Louis: Elsevier; 2017.
10. Altobelli N. Airway management. In: Kacmarek RM, Stoller JK, Heuer AJ, eds. *Egan's Fundamentals of Respiratory Care.* ed 11. St. Louis: Elsevier; 2017.
11. American Society of Anesthesiologists. Practice guidelines for preoperative fasting and the use of pharmacologic agents to reduce the risk of pulmonary aspiration: application to healthy patients undergoing elective procedures. *Anesthesiology.* 2011;114(3):495–511.
12. Strange C. Pleural diseases. In: Kacmarek RM, Stoller JK, Heuer AJ, eds. *Egan's Fundamentals of Respiratory Care.* ed 11. St. Louis: Elsevier; 2017.
13. Kasmani R, et al. Re-expansion pulmonary edema following thoracentesis. *CMAJ.* 2000-2002;182(18).
14. Cohen Z. Pulmonary function testing. In: Kacmarek RM, Stoller JK, Heuer AJ, eds. *Egan's Fundamentals of Respiratory Care.* ed 11. St. Louis: Elsevier; 2017.
15. Tonelli AR, Dweik RA. Pulmonary vascular disease. In: Kacmarek RM, Stoller JK, Heuer AJ, eds. *Egan's Fundamentals of Respiratory Care.* ed 11. St. Louis: Elsevier; 2017.
16. Azok JT, Stoller JK. Review of thoracic imaging. In: Kacmarek RM, Stoller JK, Heuer AJ, eds. *Egan's Fundamentals of Respiratory Care.* ed 11. St. Louis: Elsevier; 2017.
17. Corne J, Kumaran M. *Chest X Ray Made Easy.* ed 4. London: Elsevier; 2016.
18. Gentile MA, Heuer AJ, Kallet RH. Analysis and monitoring of gas exchange. In: Kacmarek RM, Stoller JK, Heuer AJ, eds. *Egan's Fundamentals of Respiratory Care.* ed 11. St. Louis: Elsevier; 2017.

19

Pulmonary Disorders

Kathleen M. Stacy

Understanding the pathology of a disease, the areas of assessment on which to focus, and the usual medical management allows the critical care nurse to more accurately anticipate and plan nursing interventions. This chapter focuses on pulmonary disorders commonly seen in the critical care environment.

ACUTE LUNG FAILURE

Description

Acute lung failure (ALF),[1] also known as acute respiratory failure, is a clinical condition in which the pulmonary system fails to maintain adequate gas exchange.[1,2] It is the most common type of organ failure seen in the critical care unit, with approximately 56% of the patients in the critical care unit experiencing it.[1] One-third of patients with ALF requiring mechanical ventilation die in the hospital.[3]

ALF results from a deficiency in the performance of the pulmonary system (Fig. 19.1).[2,4] It usually occurs secondary to another disorder that has altered the normal function of the pulmonary system in such a way as to decrease the ventilatory drive, decrease muscle strength, decrease chest wall elasticity, decrease the lung's capacity for gas exchange, increase airway resistance, or increase metabolic oxygen requirements.[1,5]

ALF can be classified as hypoxemic normocapnic respiratory failure (type I) or hypoxemic hypercapnic respiratory failure (type II), depending on analysis of the patient's arterial blood gases (ABGs). In type I respiratory failure, the patient presents with a low arterial oxygen pressure (PaO_2) and a normal arterial carbon dioxide pressure ($PaCO_2$); in type II respiratory failure, the patient presents with a low PaO_2 and a high $PaCO_2$.[2,4]

Etiology

The causes of ALF may be classified as *extrapulmonary* or *intrapulmonary*, depending on the origin of the patient's primary disorder. Extrapulmonary causes include disorders that affect the brain, the spinal cord, the neuromuscular system, the thorax, the pleura, and the upper airways. Intrapulmonary causes include disorders that affect the lower airways and alveoli, the pulmonary circulation, and the alveolar-capillary membrane.[1,6] Table 19.1 lists the different etiologies of ALF and their associated disorders.

Pathophysiology

Hypoxemia is the result of impaired gas exchange and is the hallmark of ALF. Hypercapnia may be present, depending on the underlying cause of the problem. The main causes of hypoxemia are alveolar hypoventilation, ventilation/perfusion ($\dot{V}/\dot{Q}$) mismatching, and intrapulmonary shunting.[1,2,7] Type I respiratory failure usually results from $\dot{V}/\dot{Q}$ mismatching and intrapulmonary shunting, whereas type II respiratory failure usually results from alveolar hypoventilation, which may or may not be accompanied by $\dot{V}/\dot{Q}$ mismatching and intrapulmonary shunting.[2]

Alveolar Hypoventilation

Alveolar hypoventilation occurs when the amount of oxygen being brought into the alveoli is insufficient to meet the metabolic needs of the body.[6] This can be the result of increasing metabolic oxygen needs or decreasing ventilation.[5] Hypoxemia caused by alveolar hypoventilation is associated with hypercapnia and commonly results from extrapulmonary disorders.[1,2,7]

Ventilation/Perfusion Mismatching

$\dot{V}/\dot{Q}$ mismatching occurs when ventilation and blood flow are mismatched in various regions of the lung in excess of what is normal. Blood passes through alveoli that are underventilated for the given amount of perfusion, leaving these areas with a lower than normal amount of oxygen. $\dot{V}/\dot{Q}$ mismatching is the most common cause of hypoxemia and is usually the result of alveoli that are partially collapsed or partially filled with fluid.[1,2,7]

Intrapulmonary Shunting

Intrapulmonary shunting, the extreme form of $\dot{V}/\dot{Q}$ mismatching, occurs when blood reaches the arterial system without participating in gas exchange. The mixing of unoxygenated (shunted) blood and oxygenated blood lowers the average level of oxygen present in the blood. Intrapulmonary shunting occurs when blood passes through a portion of a lung that is not ventilated. This may be the result of (1) alveolar collapse secondary to atelectasis or (2) alveolar flooding with pus, blood, or fluid.[1,2,7]

If allowed to progress, hypoxemia can result in a deficit of oxygen at the cellular level. As the tissue demands for oxygen continue and the supply diminishes, an oxygen supply/demand imbalance occurs, and tissue hypoxia develops. Decreased oxygen to the cells contributes to impaired tissue perfusion and the development of lactic acidosis and multiple-organ dysfunction syndrome.[8]

Assessment and Diagnosis

A patient with ALF may experience a variety of clinical manifestations, depending on the underlying cause and the extent of tissue hypoxia. The clinical manifestations commonly seen in patients with ALF are usually related to the development of hypoxemia, hypercapnia, and acidosis (Fig. 19.2).[9] Because the clinical symptoms are so varied, they are not considered reliable in predicting the degree of hypoxemia or hypercapnia[5] or the severity of ALF.

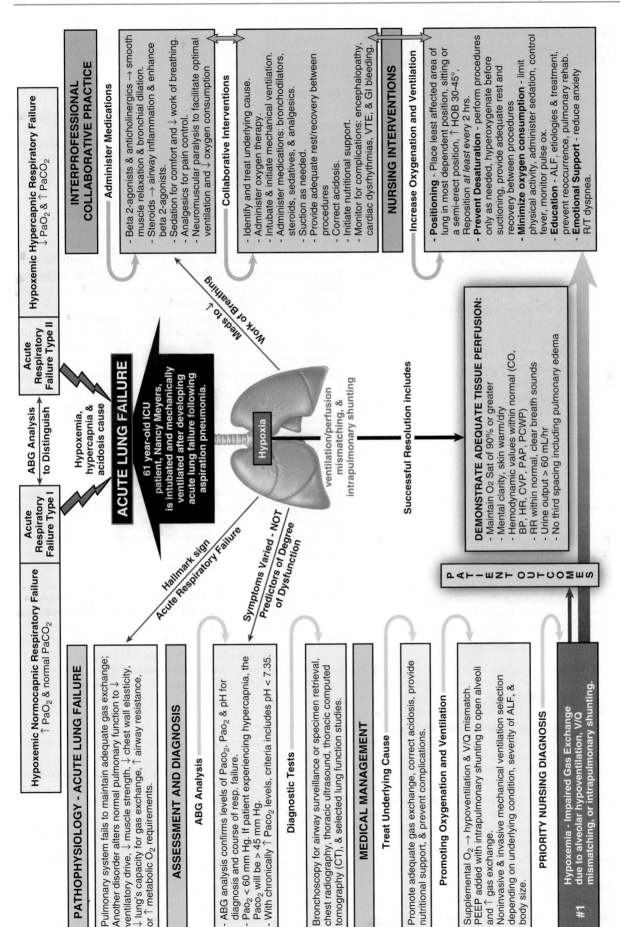

FIG. 19.1 Concept Map for Acute Lung Failure. *O₂,* Oxygen; *ABG,* Arterial Blood Gases; *PaCO₂,* Partial pressure of carbon dioxide in arterial blood; *PaO₂,* Partial pressure of oxygen in arterial blood; *pH,* A measure of the degree to which a solution is acidic or alkaline; *CT,* Computed tomography, *V/Q Mismatch,* Ventilation perfusion mismatch; *PEEP,* Positive End Expiratory Pressure *ALF,* Acute Lung Failure; *O₂ Sat,* Oxygen saturation; *CO,* Cardiac Output; *BP,* Blood Pressure; *HR,* Heart Rate; *CVP,* Central Venous Pressure; *PAP,* Pulmonary Artery Pressure; *PCWP,* Pulmonary Capillary Wedge Pressure; *mL/hr,* milliliters/hour; *VTE,* Venous Thromboembolism; *HOB,* Head of Bed Pulse; *Ox,* Pulse oximetry; *GI,* Gastrointestinal; *Hrs,* Hours; *R/T,* Related

To Concept maps created by © DEANNE A. BLACH, MSN, RN

PATHOPHYSIOLOGY - ACUTE LUNG FAILURE

Pulmonary system fails to maintain adequate gas exchange; Another disorder alters normal pulmonary function to ↓ ventilatory drive, ↓ muscle strength, ↓ chest wall elasticity, ↓ lung's capacity for gas exchange, ↑ airway resistance, or ↑ metabolic O₂ requirements.

Hypoxemic Normocapnic Respiratory Failure
↑ PaO₂ & normal PaCO₂

Acute Respiratory Failure Type I

ABG Analysis to Distinguish

Hypoxemia, hypercapnia & acidosis cause

Acute Respiratory Failure Type II

Hypoxemic Hypercapnic Respiratory Failure
↓ PaO₂ & ↑ PaCO₂

INTERPROFESSIONAL COLLABORATIVE PRACTICE

Administer Medications

- Beta 2-agonists & anticholinergics → smooth muscle relaxation & bronchial dilation.
- Steroids → airway inflammation & enhance beta 2-agonists.
- Sedation for comfort and ↓ work of breathing.
- Analgesics for pain control.
- Neuromuscular paralysis to facilitate optimal ventilation and ↓ oxygen consumption

Collaborative Interventions

- Identify and treat underlying cause.
- Administer oxygen therapy.
- Intubate & initiate mechanical ventilation.
- Administer medications: bronchodilators, steroids, sedatives, & analgesics.
- Suction as needed.
- Provide adequate rest/recovery between procedures
- Correct acidosis.
- Initiate nutritional support.
- Monitor for complications: encephalopathy, cardiac dysrhythmias, VTE, & GI bleeding.

NURSING INTERVENTIONS

Increase Oxygenation and Ventilation

- **Positioning** - Place least affected area of lung in most dependent position, sitting or a semi-erect position, ↑ HOB 30-45°, Reposition *at least* every 2 hrs.
- **Prevent Desaturation** - perform procedures only as needed, hyperoxygenate before suctioning, provide adequate rest and recovery between procedures
- **Minimize oxygen consumption** - limit physical activity, administer sedation, control fever, monitor pulse ox.
- **Education** - ALF, etiologies & treatment, prevent reoccurrence, pulmonary rehab.
- **Emotional Support** - reduce anxiety R/T dyspnea.

ACUTE LUNG FAILURE

61 year-old ICU patient, Nancy Meyers, is intubated and mechanically ventilated after developing acute lung failure following aspiration pneumonia.

Meds to ↑ Work of Breathing

Hypoxia

Hallmark sign
Acute Respiratory Failure

Symptoms Varied - NOT of Degree of Dysfunction

ventilation/perfusion mismatching, & intrapulmonary shunting

Successful Resolution includes

DEMONSTRATE ADEQUATE TISSUE PERFUSION:

- Maintain O₂ Sat of 90% or greater
- Mental clarity, skin warm/dry
- Hemodynamic values within normal (CO, BP, HR, CVP, PAP, PCWP)
- RR within normal, clear breath sounds
- Urine output > 60 mL/hr
- No third spacing including pulmonary edema

PATIENT OUTCOMES

ASSESSMENT AND DIAGNOSIS

ABG Analysis

- ABG analysis confirms levels of PaCO₂, PaO₂ & pH for diagnosis and course of resp. failure.
- PaO₂ < 60 mm Hg. If patient experiencing hypercapnia, the PaCO₂ will be > 45 mm Hg.
- With chronically ↑ PaCO₂ levels, criteria includes pH < 7.35.

Diagnostic Tests

Bronchoscopy for airway surveillance or specimen retrieval, chest radiography, thoracic ultrasound, thoracic computed tomography (CT), & selected lung function studies.

MEDICAL MANAGEMENT

Treat Underlying Cause

Promote adequate gas exchange, correct acidosis, provide nutritional support, & prevent complications.

Promoting Oxygenation and Ventilation

Supplemental O₂ → hypoventilation & V/Q mismatch. PEEP added with intrapulmonary shunting to open alveoli and ↑ gas exchange.
Noninvasive & invasive mechanical ventilation selection depending on underlying condition, severity of ALF, & body size.

PRIORITY NURSING DIAGNOSIS

#1 Hypoxemia - Impaired Gas Exchange due to alveolar hypoventilation, V/Q mismatching, or intrapulmonary shunting.

TABLE 19.1 Etiologies of Acute Lung Failure

Affected Area	Disorders[a]
Extrapulmonary	
Brain	Drug overdose (opioids, sedatives)
	Central alveolar hypoventilation syndrome
	Brain trauma or lesion
	Postoperative general anesthesia depression
Spinal cord	Guillain-Barré syndrome
	Poliomyelitis
	Amyotrophic lateral sclerosis
	Spinal cord trauma or lesion
Neuromuscular system	Myasthenia gravis
	Multiple sclerosis
	Neuromuscular-blocking agents
	Organophosphate poisoning
	Muscular dystrophy
	Critical illness polyneuropathy
Thorax	Massive obesity
	Chest trauma
Pleura	Pleural effusion
	Pneumothorax
	Malignancy
Upper airways	Sleep apnea
	Tracheal obstruction
	Epiglottitis
	Vocal cord paralysis
Intrapulmonary	
Lower airways and alveoli	Chronic obstructive pulmonary disease
	Asthma
	Bronchiolitis
	Cystic fibrosis
	Pneumonia
Pulmonary circulation	Pulmonary emboli
Alveolar-capillary membrane	ARDS
	Inhalation of toxic gases
	Near-drowning

ARDS, acute respiratory distress syndrome.
[a]Not an inclusive list.

Diagnosing and following the course of respiratory failure is best accomplished by ABG analysis. ABG analysis confirms the level of $Paco_2$, Pao_2, and blood pH. ALF is generally accepted as being present when the Pao_2 is less than 60 mm Hg. If the patient is also experiencing hypercapnia, the $Paco_2$ will be greater than 45 mm Hg. In patients with chronically elevated $Paco_2$ levels, these criteria must be broadened to include a pH less than 7.35.[9]

Various additional tests are performed depending on the patient's underlying condition. These include bronchoscopy for airway surveillance or specimen retrieval, chest radiography, thoracic ultrasound, thoracic computed tomography (CT), and selected lung function studies.[10]

Medical Management

Medical management of a patient with ALF is aimed at treating the underlying cause, promoting adequate gas exchange, correcting acidosis, initiating nutrition support, and preventing complications. Medical interventions to promote gas exchange are aimed at improving oxygenation and ventilation.[1]

Oxygenation

Actions to improve oxygenation include supplemental oxygen administration, with either a low-flow system[11] or a high-flow system,[12] and the use of positive pressure ventilation.[7] The purpose of oxygen therapy is to correct hypoxemia; although the absolute level of hypoxemia varies in each patient, most treatment approaches aim to keep the arterial hemoglobin oxygen saturation greater than 90%.[5] The goal is to keep the tissues' needs satisfied but not produce hypoxemia or hyperoxemia.[11] Supplemental oxygen administration is effective in treating hypoxemia related to alveolar hypoventilation and $\dot{V}/\dot{Q}$ mismatching. When intrapulmonary shunting exists, supplemental oxygen alone is ineffective. In this situation, positive pressure is necessary to open collapsed or fluid-filled alveoli and facilitate their participation in gas exchange. Positive pressure is delivered via invasive and noninvasive mechanical ventilation. To avoid intubation, positive pressure is usually administered initially noninvasively via a mask.[13] A recent study comparing low-flow oxygen, high-flow oxygen, and noninvasive ventilation found that high-flow oxygen therapy and noninvasive ventilation were superior to low-flow oxygen therapy in the treatment of hypoxemia. The study also found that high-flow oxygen therapy is better tolerated and more comfortable than noninvasive ventilation.[12] For further information on supplemental oxygen therapy and noninvasive ventilation, see Chapter 20.

Ventilation

Interventions to improve ventilation include the use of noninvasive and invasive mechanical ventilation. Depending on the underlying cause and the severity of the ALF, the patient may be treated initially with noninvasive ventilation.[13] However, one study found that patients with respiratory acidosis and a pH less than 7.25 at initial presentation was more likely to need invasive mechanical ventilation.[14] The selection of ventilatory mode and settings depends on the patient's underlying condition, severity of respiratory failure, and body size. Initially, the patient is started on volume ventilation in the assist/control mode. In a patient with chronic hypercapnia, the settings are adjusted to keep the ABG values within the parameters expected to be maintained by the patient after extubation.[15] For further information on mechanical ventilation, see Chapter 20.

Pharmacology

Medications to facilitate dilation of the airways may also be beneficial in the treatment of ALF. Bronchodilators, such as beta-2 agonists and anticholinergic agents, aid in smooth muscle relaxation and are of particular benefit to patients with airflow limitations. Methylxanthines, such as aminophylline, are no longer recommended because of their negative side effects. Steroids also are often administered to decrease airway inflammation and enhance the effects of the beta-2 agonists. Mucolytics and expectorants are also no longer used because they have been found to be of no benefit in this patient population.[16]

Sedation is necessary in many patients to assist with maintaining adequate ventilation. Sedation can be used to comfort the patient and decrease the work of breathing, particularly if the patient is fighting the ventilator. Analgesics are

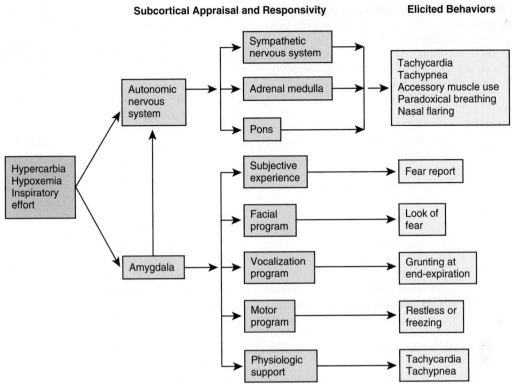

Subcortical Appraisal and Responsivity   **Elicited Behaviors**

FIG. 19.2 Model of Respiratory Distress Behaviors Activated From Subcortical Stimulation. (From Campbell ML. Respiratory distress: a model of responses and behaviors to an asphyxial threat for patients who are unable to self-report. *Heart Lung.* 2008;37[1]:54–60.)

administered for pain control.[17,18] In some patients, sedation does not decrease spontaneous respiratory efforts enough to allow adequate ventilation. Neuromuscular paralysis may be necessary to facilitate optimal ventilation. Paralysis also may be necessary to decrease oxygen consumption in severely compromised patients.[18]

Acidosis

Acidosis may occur in a patient for many reasons. Hypoxemia causes impaired tissue perfusion, which leads to the production of lactic acid and the development of metabolic acidosis. Impaired ventilation leads to the accumulation of carbon dioxide and the development of respiratory acidosis. Once the patient is adequately oxygenated and ventilated, the acidosis should correct itself. The use of sodium bicarbonate to correct metabolic acidosis has been shown to be of minimal benefit to the patient and is no longer recommended as first-line treatment. Bicarbonate therapy shifts the oxygen-hemoglobin dissociation curve to the left and can worsen tissue hypoxia. Sodium bicarbonate may be used if metabolic acidosis is severe (pH less than 7.2), refractory to therapy, and causing dysrhythmias or hemodynamic instability.[19]

Nutrition Support

The initiation of nutrition support is of utmost importance in the management of a patient with ALF. The goals of nutrition support are to meet the overall nutrition needs of the patient while avoiding overfeeding, to prevent nutrition delivery–related complications and to improve patient outcomes.[20] Failure to provide the patient with adequate nutrition support leads to the development of malnutrition. Both malnutrition

and overfeeding can interfere with the performance of the pulmonary system, further perpetuating ALF. Malnutrition decreases the patient's ventilatory drive and muscle strength, whereas overfeeding increases carbon dioxide production, which increases the patient's ventilatory demand, resulting in respiratory muscle fatigue.[21]

The enteral route is the preferred method of nutrition administration. If the patient cannot tolerate enteral feedings or cannot receive enough nutrients enterally, he or she will be started on parenteral nutrition. Because the parenteral route is associated with a higher rate of complications, the goal is to switch to enteral feedings as soon as the patient can tolerate them.[20,21] Nutrition support is initiated before the third day of mechanical ventilation for well-nourished patients and within 24 hours for malnourished patients.[20,21]

Complications

Patients with ALF may experience many complications, including ischemic-anoxic encephalopathy,[22] cardiac dysrhythmias,[23] venous thromboembolism (VTE),[24] and stress ulcers.[25] Ischemic-anoxic encephalopathy results from hypoxemia, hypercapnia, and acidosis.[22] Dysrhythmias are precipitated by hypoxemia, acidosis, electrolyte imbalances, and the administration of beta-2 agonists.[23] Maintaining oxygenation, normalizing electrolytes, and monitoring medication levels facilitate the prevention and treatment of encephalopathy and dysrhythmias.[22,23] VTE is precipitated by venous stasis resulting from immobility and can be prevented through the use of intermittent pneumatic compression devices and low-dose unfractionated heparin or low-molecular-weight heparin (LMWH).[24] Stress ulcers can be prevented through the use of histamine receptor antagonists and proton pump inhibitors. However, the use of stress ulcer prophylaxis has been associated with an increased risk of ventilator-associated pneumonia.[25] In addition, the patient is at risk for the complications associated with the artificial airway, mechanical ventilation, enteral and parenteral nutrition, and vascular access devices.

Nursing Management

The nursing management plan for a patient with ALF incorporates a variety of nursing diagnoses (Box 19.1). Nursing actions are driven by the specific cause of the respiratory failure, although there are some common interventions that are appropriate for all patients with ALF. The nurse has a significant role in optimizing oxygenation and ventilation, providing comfort and emotional support, maintaining surveillance for complications, and educating the patient and family.

Optimize Oxygenation and Ventilation

Nursing interventions to optimize oxygenation and ventilation include positioning, preventing desaturation, and promoting secretion clearance.

Positioning. Positioning of a patient with ALF depends on the type of lung injury and the underlying cause of hypoxemia. For patients with $\dot{V}/\dot{Q}$ mismatching, positioning is used to facilitate better matching of ventilation with perfusion to optimize gas exchange.[26] Because gravity normally facilitates preferential ventilation and perfusion to the dependent areas of the lungs, the best gas exchange would take place in the dependent areas of the lungs.[26] Thus the goal of positioning is to place the least affected area of the patient's lung in the most dependent position. Patients with unilateral lung disease are positioned with the healthy lung in a dependent position.[26,27] Patients with diffuse lung disease may benefit from being positioned with the right lung down because it is larger and more vascular than the left lung.[27,28] For patients with alveolar hypoventilation, the goal of positioning is to facilitate ventilation. These patients benefit from nonrecumbent positions such as sitting or a semierect position.[29] Elevating the head of the bed 30 to 45 degrees has also been shown to decrease the risk of aspiration; however, it also has been shown to increase the risk of pressure ulcers.[30] Frequent repositioning (at least every 2 hours) is beneficial in optimizing the patient's ventilatory pattern and $\dot{V}/\dot{Q}$ matching.[31]

Preventing desaturation. Numerous activities can prevent desaturation from occurring, including performing procedures only as needed, hyperoxygenating the patient before suctioning, providing adequate rest and recovery time between procedures, and minimizing oxygen consumption. Interventions to minimize oxygen consumption include limiting the patient's physical activity, administering sedation to control anxiety, and providing measures to control fever.[29] The patient is continuously monitored with a pulse oximeter to warn of signs of desaturation.

Promoting secretion clearance. Interventions to promote secretion clearance include providing adequate systemic hydration, humidifying supplemental oxygen, coughing, and suctioning. Postural drainage and chest percussion and vibration have been found to be of little benefit in critically ill patients[32,33] and are not discussed here.

To facilitate deep breathing, the patient's thorax is maintained in alignment, and the head of the bed is elevated 30 to 45 degrees. This position best accommodates diaphragmatic descent and intercostal muscle action.

Deep breathing and incentive spirometry are started as soon as possible after the patient is extubated. Deep breathing involves having the patient take a deep breath and holding it for approximately 3 seconds or longer. Incentive spirometry involves having the patient take at least 10 deep, effective breaths per hour using an incentive spirometer. These actions help prevent atelectasis and reexpand any collapsed lung tissue. The chest is auscultated during inflation to ensure that all dependent parts of the lung are well ventilated and to help the patient understand the depth of breath necessary for optimal effect. Coughing is avoided unless secretions are present because it promotes collapse of the smaller airways.

Educate the Patient and Family

Early in the patient's hospital stay, the patient and family are taught about ALF, its causes, and its treatment. Closer to discharge, the patient education plan focuses on the interventions necessary for preventing the reoccurrence of the precipitating disorder (Box 19.2). If the patient smokes, he or she is encouraged to stop smoking and is referred to a smoking cessation program (Box 19.3). In addition, the importance of participating in a pulmonary rehabilitation program is stressed.

Interprofessional collaborative management of a patient with ALF is outlined in Box 19.4.

ACUTE RESPIRATORY DISTRESS SYNDROME

Description

Acute respiratory distress syndrome (ARDS) is a systemic process that is considered to be the pulmonary manifestation of multiple-organ dysfunction syndrome.[34] It is characterized by noncardiac pulmonary edema and disruption of the

---

◎ BOX 19.1   NURSING DIAGNOSES

Acute Lung Failure

- Impaired Gas Exchange related to alveolar hypoventilation, p. 1030
- Impaired Gas Exchange related to ventilation-perfusion mismatching or intrapulmonary shunting, p. 1030
- Ineffective Breathing Pattern related to musculoskeletal fatigue or neuromuscular impairment, p. 1035
- Risk for Aspiration, p. 1040
- Imbalanced Nutrition: Less Than Body Requirements related to lack of exogenous nutrients and increased metabolic demand, p. 1029
- Risk for Infection, p. 1046
- Impaired Spontaneous Ventilation related to respiratory muscle fatigue or metabolic factors, p. 1031
- Acute Confusion related to sensory overload, sensory deprivation, and sleep pattern disturbance, p. 1007
- Anxiety related to threat to biologic, psychologic, social integrity, p. 1012
- Disturbed Body Image related to functional dependence on life-sustaining technology, p. 1022
- Compromised Family Coping related to critically ill family member, p. 1014
- Deficient Knowledge related to lack of previous exposure to information, p. 1020 (See Box 19.2, Patient Education Plan for Acute Lung Failure)

BOX 19.2 PATIENT EDUCATION PLAN

Acute Lung Failure

Before the patient's discharge, the patient should be able to teach back the following topics:

- Pathophysiology of disease
- Specific etiology
- Modification of precipitating factors
- Importance of taking medications
- Breathing techniques (eg, pursed-lip breathing, diaphragmatic breathing)
- Energy conservation techniques
- Measures to prevent pulmonary infections (eg, proper nutrition, handwashing, immunization against *Streptococcus pneumoniae* and influenza viruses)
- Signs and symptoms of pulmonary infections (eg, sputum color change, shortness of breath, fever)
- Cough enhancement techniques (eg, cascade cough, huff cough, end-expiratory cough, augmented cough)

Additional information for the patient can be found at the following websites:

- American Lung Association: http://www.lung.org
- Smokefree.gov: http://smokefree.gov
- Healthfinder—U.S. Department of Health and Human Services: http://healthfinder.gov
- WebMD: http://www.webmd.com
- ARDS Foundation: http://www.ardsusa.org

alveolar-capillary membrane as a result of injury to either the pulmonary vasculature or the airways.[35]

Many different diagnostic criteria have been used to identify ARDS, which has led to confusion, particularly among researchers. In 2012, in an attempt to address the limitations of the existing definition of ARDS, the ARDS Definition Task Force drafted a new definition (known as the Berlin Definition) of ARDS.[36] This definition eliminated the term "acute lung injury" and proposed three distinct categories (mild, moderate, and severe) of ARDS based on the severity of hypoxemia. The Berlin Definition of ARDS is as follows:

- Timing—Within 1 week of known clinical insult or new or worsening respiratory symptoms
- Chest imaging—Bilateral opacities not fully explained by effusions, lobar/lung collapse, or nodules
- Origin of edema—Respiratory failure not fully explained by heart failure or fluid overload; objective assessment needed to exclude hydrostatic edema if no risk factor present
- Oxygenation—Mild (200 mm Hg less than PaO_2/fraction of inspired oxygen [FIO_2] less than or equal to 300 mm Hg with positive end-expiratory airway pressure [PEEP] or continuous positive airway pressure [CPAP] greater than or equal to 5 cm H_2O); moderate (100 mm Hg less than PaO_2/FIO_2 less than or equal to 200 mm Hg with PEEP greater than or equal to 5 cm H_2O); or severe (PaO_2/FIO_2

QSEN BOX 19.3 QSEN: Evidence-Based Practice

Smoking Cessation Guidelines

The following are the key recommendations of the updated guideline Treating Tobacco Use and Dependence, based on the literature review and expert panel opinion:

1. Tobacco dependence is a chronic disease that often requires repeated intervention and multiple attempts to quit. Effective treatments exist, however, that can significantly increase rates of long-term abstinence.
2. It is essential that clinicians and health care delivery systems consistently identify and document tobacco use status and treat every tobacco user seen in a health care setting.
3. Tobacco dependence treatments are effective across a broad range of populations. Clinicians should encourage every patient willing to make a quit attempt to use the counseling treatments and medications recommended in this Guideline.
4. Brief tobacco dependence treatment is effective. Clinicians should offer every patient who uses tobacco at least the brief treatments shown to be effective in this Guideline.
5. Individual, group, and telephone counseling are effective, and their effectiveness increases with treatment intensity. Two components of counseling are especially effective, and clinicians should use these when counseling patients making a quit attempt:
   - Practical counseling (problem solving/skills training)
   - Social support delivered as part of treatment
6. Numerous effective medications are available for tobacco dependence, and clinicians should encourage their use by all patients attempting to quit smoking—except when medically contraindicated or with specific populations for which there is insufficient evidence of effectiveness (eg, pregnant women, smokeless tobacco users, light smokers, and adolescents).
   - Seven first-line medications (five nicotine and two nonnicotine) reliably increase long-term smoking abstinence rates:

- Bupropion SR
- Nicotine gum
- Nicotine inhaler
- Nicotine lozenge
- Nicotine nasal spray
- Nicotine patch
- Varenicline
- Clinicians also should consider the use of certain combinations of medications identified as effective in this Guideline.

7. Counseling and medication are effective when used by themselves for treating tobacco dependence. The combination of counseling and medication, however, is more effective than either alone. Thus, clinicians should encourage all individuals making a quit attempt to use both counseling and medication.
8. Telephone quitline counseling is effective with diverse populations and has broad reach. Therefore clinicians and health care delivery systems should both ensure patient access to quitlines and promote quitline use.
9. If a tobacco user currently is unwilling to make a quit attempt, clinicians should use the motivational treatments shown in this Guideline to be effective in increasing future quit attempts.
10. Tobacco dependence treatments are both clinically effective and highly cost-effective relative to interventions for other clinical disorders. Providing coverage for these treatments increases quit rates. Insurers and purchasers should ensure that all insurance plans include the counseling and medication identified as effective in this Guideline as covered benefits.

From Fiore MC, et al. *Treating Tobacco Use and Dependence: 2008 Update Clinical Practice Guideline.* Rockville, MD: US Department of Health and Human Services Public Health Service; 2008. Available from http://www.ncbi.nlm.nih.gov/books/NBK63952/.

Interprofessional Collaborative Practice: Acute Lung Failure

- Identify and treat underlying cause.
- Administer oxygen therapy.
- Intubate patient.
- Initiate mechanical ventilation.
- Administer medications:
  - Bronchodilators
  - Steroids
  - Sedatives
  - Analgesics
- Position patient to optimize ventilation/perfusion matching.
- Suction as needed.
- Provide adequate rest and recovery time between procedures.
- Correct acidosis.
- Initiate nutrition support.
- Maintain surveillance for complications:
  - Encephalopathy
  - Cardiac dysrhythmias
  - Venous thromboembolism
  - Gastrointestinal bleeding
- Provide comfort and emotional support.

BOX 19.5 Risk Factors for Acute Respiratory Distress Syndrome

Direct Injury
Aspiration
Near-drowning
Toxic inhalation
Pulmonary contusion
Pneumonia
Oxygen toxicity
Transthoracic radiation

Indirect Injury
Sepsis
Nonthoracic trauma
Hypertransfusion
Cardiopulmonary bypass
Severe pancreatitis
Embolism—air, fat, amniotic fluid
Disseminated intravascular coagulation
Shock states

less than or equal to 100 mm Hg with PEEP greater than or equal to 5 cm H_2O).[36]

The mortality rate for ARDS is estimated to be 34% to 58%.[37]

Etiology

A wide variety of clinical conditions is associated with the development of ARDS. These are categorized as *direct* or *indirect*, depending on the primary site of injury (Box 19.5).[35,38] Direct injuries are injuries in which the lung epithelium sustains a direct insult. Indirect injuries are injuries in which the insult occurs elsewhere in the body and mediators are transmitted via the bloodstream to the lungs. Sepsis, aspiration of gastric contents, diffuse pneumonia, and trauma were found to be major risk factors for the development of ARDS.[37]

Pathophysiology

The progression of ARDS can be described in three phases: exudative, fibroproliferative, and resolution. ARDS is initiated with stimulation of the inflammatory-immune system as a result of a direct or indirect injury (Fig. 19.3). Inflammatory mediators are released from the site of injury, resulting in the activation and accumulation of the neutrophils, macrophages, and platelets in the pulmonary capillaries. These cellular mediators initiate the release of humoral mediators that cause damage to the alveolar-capillary membrane.[38]

Exudative Phase

Within the first 72 hours after the initial insult, the exudative phase or acute phase ensues. Once released, the mediators cause injury to the pulmonary capillaries, resulting in increased capillary membrane permeability leading to the leakage of fluid filled with protein, blood cells, fibrin, and activated cellular and humoral mediators into the pulmonary interstitium. Damage to the pulmonary capillaries also causes the development of microthrombi and elevation of pulmonary artery pressures. As fluid enters the pulmonary interstitium, the lymphatics are overwhelmed and unable to drain all the accumulating fluid, resulting in the development of interstitial edema. Fluid is then forced from the interstitial space into the alveoli, resulting in alveolar edema. Pulmonary interstitial edema also causes compression of the alveoli and small airways. Alveolar edema causes swelling of the type I alveolar epithelial cells and flooding of the alveoli. Protein and fibrin in the edema fluid precipitate the formation of hyaline membranes over the alveoli. Eventually, the type II alveolar epithelial cells are also damaged, leading to impaired surfactant production. Injury to the alveolar epithelial cells and the loss of surfactant lead to further alveolar collapse.[38,39]

Hypoxemia occurs as a result of intrapulmonary shunting and $\dot{V}/\dot{Q}$ mismatching secondary to compression, collapse, and flooding of the alveoli and small airways. Increased work of breathing occurs as a result of increased airway resistance, decreased functional residual capacity (FRC), and decreased lung compliance secondary to atelectasis and compression of the small airways. Hypoxemia and the increased work of breathing lead to patient fatigue and the development of alveolar hypoventilation. Pulmonary hypertension occurs as a result of damage to the pulmonary capillaries, microthrombi, and hypoxic vasoconstriction leading to the development of increased alveolar dead space and right ventricular afterload. Hypoxemia worsens as a result of alveolar hypoventilation and increased alveolar dead space. Right ventricular afterload increases and leads to right ventricular dysfunction and a decrease in cardiac output (CO).[38]

Fibroproliferative Phase

The fibroproliferative phase begins as disordered healing and starts in the lungs. Cellular granulation and collagen deposition occur within the alveolar-capillary membrane. The alveoli become enlarged and irregularly shaped (fibrotic), and the pulmonary capillaries become scarred and obliterated. This leads

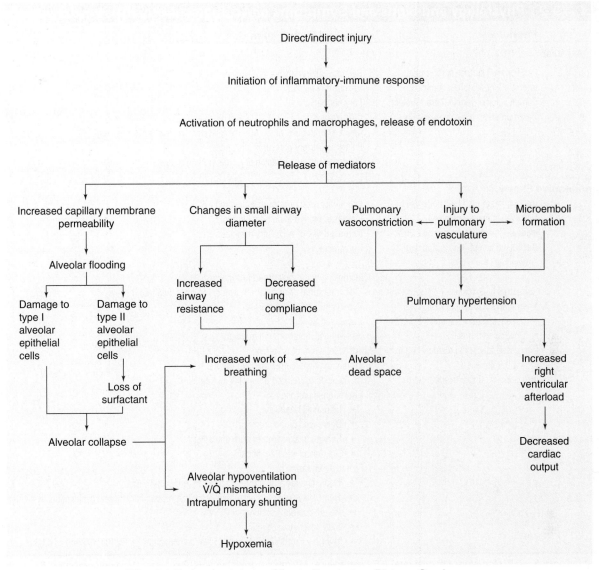

FIG. 19.3 Pathophysiology of Acute Respiratory Distress Syndrome.

to further stiffening of the lungs, increasing pulmonary hypertension, and continued hypoxemia.[38,39]

Resolution Phase

Recovery occurs over several weeks as structural and vascular remodeling take place to reestablish the alveolar-capillary membrane. The hyaline membranes are cleared, and intraalveolar fluid is transported out of the alveolus into the interstitium. The type II alveolar epithelial cells multiply, some of which differentiate to type I alveolar epithelial cells, facilitating the restoration of the alveolus. Alveolar macrophages remove cellular debris.[38,39]

Assessment and Diagnosis

A patient with ARDS initially may be seen with a variety of clinical manifestations, depending on the precipitating event. As the disorder progresses, the patient's signs and symptoms can be associated with the phase of ARDS that he or she is experiencing (Table 19.2). During the exudative phase, the patient presents with tachypnea, restlessness, apprehension, and moderate increase in accessory muscle use. During the fibroproliferative phase, the patient's signs and symptoms progress to agitation, dyspnea, fatigue, excessive accessory muscle use, and fine crackles as respiratory failure develops.[40,41]

ABG analysis shows a low Pao_2, despite increases in supplemental oxygen administration (refractory hypoxemia).[40] The $Paco_2$ initially is low as a result of hyperventilation but eventually increases as the patient fatigues. The pH is high initially but decreases as respiratory acidosis develops.[40,41]

Initially the chest x-ray film may be normal because changes in the lungs do not become evident for up to 24 hours. As the pulmonary edema becomes apparent, diffuse, patchy interstitial and alveolar infiltrates appear. This progresses to multifocal consolidation of the lungs, which appears as a "whiteout" on the chest radiograph.[40]

Medical Management

Medical management of a patient with ARDS involves a multifaceted approach. This strategy includes treating the underlying cause, promoting gas exchange, supporting tissue oxygenation,

TABLE 19.2	Physiology and Signs and Symptoms of Acute Respiratory Distress Syndrome	
Phase	**Physiology**	**Physical Examination**
Exudative Phase		
	Parenchymal surface hemorrhage	Restless, apprehensive, tachypneic
	Interstitial or alveolar edema	Respiratory alkalosis
	Compression of terminal bronchioles	Pao_2 normal
	Destruction of type I alveolar cells	CXR: normal
		Chest examination: moderate use of accessory muscles, lungs clear
		Pulmonary artery pressures: elevated
		Pulmonary artery occlusion pressure: normal or low
Fibroproliferative Phase		
	Destruction of type II alveolar cells	Pulmonary artery pressures: elevated
	Gas exchange compromised	Increased workload on right ventricle
	Increased peak inspiratory pressure	Increased use of accessory muscles
	Decreased compliance (static and dynamic)	Fine crackles
		Increasing agitation related to hypoxia
	Refractory hypoxemia:	CXR: interstitial or alveolar infiltrates; elevated diaphragm
	• Intraalveolar atelectasis	Hyperventilation; hypercarbia
	• Increased shunt fraction	Decreased Svo_2
	• Decreased diffusion	Widening alveolar-arterial gradient
	Decreased functional residual capacity	Increased work of breathing
	Interstitial fibrosis	Worsening hypercarbia and hypoxemia
	Increased dead space ventilation	Lactic acidosis (related to aerobic metabolism)
		Alteration in perfusion:
		• Increased heart rate
		• Decreased blood pressure
		• Change in skin temperature and color
		• Decreased capillary filling
		End-organ dysfunction:
		• Brain: change in mentation, agitation, hallucinations
		• Heart: decreased cardiac output → angina, HF, papillary muscle dysfunction, dysrhythmias, MI
		• Renal: decreased urinary or GFR
		• Skin: mottled, ischemic
		• Liver: elevated SGOT, bilirubin, alkaline phosphatase, PT/PTT; decreased albumin

CXR, chest radiograph; *GFR*, glomerular filtration rate; *HF*, heart failure; *MI*, myocardial infarction; *Pao₂*, arterial oxygen pressure; *PT*, prothrombin time; *PTT*, partial thromboplastin time; *SGOT*, serum glutamate oxaloacetate transaminase; *Svo₂*, venous oxygen saturation.
Modified from Phillips JK: Management of patients with acute respiratory distress syndrome. *Crit Care Nurs Clin North Am.* 1999;11(2):233–247.

and preventing complications. Given the severity of hypoxemia, the patient is intubated and mechanically ventilated to facilitate adequate gas exchange.[38]

Ventilation

Traditionally patients with ARDS were ventilated with a mode of volume ventilation, such as assist/control ventilation or synchronized intermittent mandatory ventilation (SIMV), with tidal volumes adjusted to deliver 10 to 15 mL/kg. Current research indicates that this approach may have actually led to further lung injury. It is now known that repeated opening and closing of the alveoli cause injury to the lung units (atelectrauma) resulting in inhibited surfactant production and increased inflammation (biotrauma) resulting in the release of mediators and an increase in pulmonary capillary membrane permeability. In addition, excessive pressure in the alveoli (barotrauma) or excessive volume in the alveoli (volutrauma) leads to excessive alveolar wall stress and damage to

the alveolar-capillary membrane, resulting in air escaping into the surrounding spaces.[38,42] Thus several different approaches have been developed to facilitate the mechanical ventilation of patients with ARDS.

Low tidal volume. Low tidal volume ventilation uses smaller tidal volumes (6 mL/kg) to ventilate the patient in an attempt to limit the effects of barotrauma and volutrauma. The goal is to provide the maximum tidal volume possible, while maintaining end-inspiratory plateau pressure less than 30 cm H_2O. To allow for adequate carbon dioxide elimination, the respiratory rate is increased to 20 to 30 breaths/min.[42,43]

Permissive hypercapnia. Permissive hypercapnia uses low tidal volume ventilation in conjunction with normal respiratory rates in an attempt to limit the effects of atelectrauma and biotrauma. To maintain normocapnia, the patient's respiratory rate normally would have to be increased to compensate for the small tidal volume. In ARDS, increasing the respiratory rate can lead to worsening alveolar damage. Thus the patient's carbon dioxide level is allowed to increase, and the patient becomes hypercapnic. As a general rule, the patient's $Paco_2$ should not rise faster than 10 mm Hg per hour and overall should not exceed 80 to 100 mm Hg. Because of the negative cardiopulmonary effects of severe acidosis, the arterial pH is generally maintained at 7.20 or greater. To maintain the pH, the patient may be given intravenous sodium bicarbonate, or the respiratory rate, tidal volume, or both are increased. Permissive hypercapnia is contraindicated in patients with increased intracranial pressure, pulmonary hypertension, seizures, and heart failure.[44]

Pressure control ventilation. In pressure control ventilation mode, each breath is delivered or augmented with a preset amount of inspiratory pressure as opposed to tidal volume, which is used in volume ventilation. Thus the actual tidal volume the patient receives varies from breath to breath. Pressure control ventilation is used to limit and control the amount of pressure in the lungs and decrease the incidence of volutrauma. The goal is to keep the patient's plateau pressure (end-inspiratory static pressure) lower than 30 cm H_2O. A known problem with this mode of ventilation is that as the patient's lungs get stiffer, it becomes harder and harder to maintain an adequate tidal volume, and severe hypercapnia can occur.[42,43]

Inverse ratio ventilation. Another alternative ventilatory mode that is used in managing patients with ARDS is inverse ratio ventilation (IRV), either pressure controlled or volume controlled. IRV prolongs the inspiratory time and shortens the expiratory time, thus reversing the normal inspiratory-to-expiratory ratio. The goal of IRV is to maintain a more constant mean airway pressure throughout the ventilatory cycle, which helps keep alveoli open and participating in gas exchange. It also increases FRC and decreases the work of breathing. In addition, as the breath is delivered over a longer period of time, the peak inspiratory pressure in the lungs is decreased. A major disadvantage to IRV is the development of auto-PEEP. As the expiratory phase of ventilation is shortened, air can become trapped in the lower airways, creating unintentional PEEP (or auto-PEEP), which can cause hemodynamic compromise and worsening gas exchange. Patients on IRV usually require heavy sedation with neuromuscular blockade to prevent them from fighting the ventilator.[42,43]

High-frequency oscillatory ventilation. High-frequency oscillatory ventilation is another alternative ventilatory mode that is used in patients who remain severely hypoxemic despite the treatments previously described. The goal of this method of ventilation is similar to that of IRV in that it uses a constant airway pressure to promote alveolar recruitment while avoiding overdistention of the alveoli. High-frequency oscillatory ventilation uses a piston pump to deliver very low tidal volumes (1 to 3 mL/breath) at very high rates or oscillations (300 to 900 breaths/min). Current research has failed to demonstrate that this method of ventilation provides any additional benefit over conventional ventilation.[45]

Oxygen Therapy

Oxygen is administered at the lowest level possible to support tissue oxygenation. Continued exposure to high levels of oxygen can lead to oxygen toxicity, which perpetuates the entire process. The goal of oxygen therapy is to maintain an arterial hemoglobin oxygen saturation of 90% or greater using the lowest level of oxygen—preferably less than 0.50.[11]

Positive end-expiratory pressure. Because the hypoxemia that develops with ARDS is often refractory or unresponsive to oxygen therapy, it is necessary to facilitate oxygenation with PEEP. The purpose of using PEEP in a patient with ARDS is to improve oxygenation while reducing Fio_2 to less toxic levels. PEEP has several positive effects on the lungs, including opening collapsed alveoli, stabilizing flooded alveoli, and increasing FRC. Thus PEEP decreases intrapulmonary shunting and increases compliance. PEEP also has several negative effects, including (1) decreasing CO as a result of decreasing venous return secondary to increased intrathoracic pressure and (2) barotrauma as a result of gas escaping into the surrounding spaces secondary to alveolar rupture. The amount of PEEP a patient requires is determined by evaluating both arterial hemoglobin oxygen saturation and CO. In most cases, a PEEP of 10 to 15 cm H_2O is adequate. If PEEP is too high, it can result in overdistention of the alveoli, which can impede pulmonary capillary blood flow, decrease surfactant production, and worsen intrapulmonary shunting. If PEEP is too low, it allows the alveoli to collapse during expiration, which can result in more damage to alveoli.[42]

Extracorporeal and intracorporeal gas exchange. Extracorporeal and intracorporeal gas exchanges are last-resort techniques used in the treatment of severe ARDS when conventional therapy has failed. These methods allow the lungs to rest by facilitating the removal of carbon dioxide and providing oxygen external to the lungs by means of an "artificial lung," or membrane/fiber oxygenator. Extracorporeal membrane oxygenation (ECMO) and extracorporeal carbon dioxide removal are two techniques that employ this type of technology. ECMO is similar to cardiopulmonary bypass in that blood is removed from the body and pumped through a membrane oxygenator, where CO_2 is removed and O_2 is added, and then returned to the body. Extracorporeal carbon dioxide removal is a variation of ECMO in which the primary focus is removal of CO_2.[46]

Tissue Perfusion

Adequate tissue perfusion depends on an adequate supply of oxygen being transported to the tissues. An adequate CO and hemoglobin level is critical to oxygen transport. CO depends on heart rate, preload, afterload, and contractility. Various fluids and medications are used to manipulate this parameter. Newer approaches to fluid management include maintaining a very low intravascular volume (pulmonary artery occlusion pressure of 5 to 8 mm Hg) with fluid restriction and diuretics, while supporting the CO with vasoactive and inotropic medications. The goal is to decrease the amount of fluid leakage into the lungs.[47]

Nursing Management

The nursing management plan for a patient with ARDS incorporates a variety of nursing diagnoses (Box 19.6). The nurse has a significant role in optimizing oxygenation and ventilation, providing comfort and emotional support, and maintaining surveillance for complications.

Optimize Oxygenation and Ventilation

Nursing interventions to optimize oxygenation and ventilation include positioning, preventing desaturation, and promoting secretion clearance. For further discussion of these interventions, see Nursing Management of Acute Lung Failure earlier in this chapter. One additional nursing intervention that can be used to improve the oxygenation and ventilation of a patient with ARDS is prone positioning.

◎ BOX 19.6 **NURSING DIAGNOSES**
Acute Respiratory Distress Syndrome

- Impaired Gas Exchange related to ventilation/perfusion mismatching or intrapulmonary shunting, p. 1030
- Decreased Cardiac Output related to alterations in preload, p. 1015
- Imbalanced Nutrition: Less Than Body Requirements related to lack of exogenous nutrients or increased metabolic demand, p. 1029
- Risk for Aspiration, p. 1040
- Risk for Infection, p. 1046
- Anxiety related to threat to biologic, psychologic, and/or social integrity, p. 1012
- Disturbed Body Image related to functional dependence on life-sustaining technology, p. 1022
- Compromised Family Coping related to critically ill family member, p. 1014

Prone positioning. Numerous studies have shown that prone positioning of a patient with ARDS results in an improvement in oxygenation. Although many theories propose how prone positioning improves oxygenation, the discovery that with ARDS there is greater damage to the dependent areas of the lungs probably provides the best explanation. It was originally thought that ARDS was a diffuse homogeneous disease that affected all areas of the lungs equally. It is now known that the dependent lung areas are more heavily damaged than the nondependent lung areas. Turning the patient prone improves perfusion to less damaged parts of lungs and improves $\dot{V}/\dot{Q}$ matching and decreases intrapulmonary shunting. Prone positioning appears to be more effective when initiated during the early phases of ARDS.[48] For more information on prone positioning, see Chapter 20.

Interprofessional collaborative management of a patient with ARDS is outlined in Box 19.7.

PNEUMONIA

Description

Pneumonia is an acute inflammation of the lung parenchyma that is caused by an infectious agent that can lead to alveolar consolidation. Pneumonia can be classified as community-acquired pneumonia (CAP), hospital-acquired pneumonia (HAP), or health care–associated pneumonia (HCAP).[49] Pneumonia is referred to as community acquired when it occurs outside of the hospital or within 48 hours of admission to the hospital.[50] Severe CAP requires admission to the critical care unit and accounts for approximately 22% of all patients with pneumonia. The mortality for this patient group is approximately 50%, with increasing age as a major risk factor.[51] Pneumonia is referred to as hospital acquired when it occurs while the patient is in the hospital for at least 48 hours.[49] Ventilator-associated pneumonia (VAP) is a subgrouping of HAP that refers to development of pneumonia after the insertion of an artificial airway.[49] VAP is one of the most common infections acquired in the critical care unit.[52] Pneumonia is referred to as health care associated when it is acquired in health care environments outside of the traditional hospital setting.[49]

Etiology

The spectra of etiologic pathogens of pneumonia vary with the type of pneumonia, as do the risk factors for the disease.

QSEN BOX 19.7 **QSEN: Teamwork and Collaboration**

Interprofessional Collaborative Practice: Acute Respiratory Distress Syndrome

- Administer oxygen therapy.
- Intubate patient.
- Initiate mechanical ventilation:
  - Permissive hypercapnia
  - Pressure control ventilation
  - Inverse ratio ventilation
- Use PEEP.
- Administer medications:
  - Bronchodilators
  - Sedatives
  - Analgesics
  - Neuromuscular blocking agents
- Maximize cardiac output:
  - Preload
  - Afterload
  - Contractility
- Position patient prone.
- Suction as needed.
- Provide adequate rest and recovery time between procedures.
- Initiate nutrition support.
- Maintain surveillance for complications:
  - Encephalopathy
  - Cardiac dysrhythmias
  - Venous thromboembolism
  - Gastrointestinal bleeding
  - Atelectrauma
  - Biotrauma
  - Volutrauma
  - Barotrauma
  - Oxygen toxicity
- Provide comfort and emotional support.

PEEP, positive end expiratory pressure.

Severe Community-Acquired Pneumonia

Pathogens that can cause severe CAP include *Streptococcus pneumoniae, Legionella* species, *Haemophilus influenzae, Moraxella catarrhalis, Staphylococcus aureus, Mycoplasma pneumoniae,* respiratory viruses, *Chlamydia pneumoniae,* and *Pseudomonas aeruginosa.*[50,51] Numerous factors increase the risk for developing CAP, including alcoholism; chronic obstructive pulmonary disease; and comorbid conditions such as diabetes, malignancy, and coronary artery disease. Impaired swallowing and altered mental status also contribute to the development of CAP because they result in an increased exposure to the various pathogens owing to chronic aspiration of oropharyngeal secretions.[51]

Hospital-Acquired Pneumonia

Pathogens that can cause HAP include *Escherichia coli, H. influenzae,* methicillin-sensitive *S. aureus, S. pneumoniae, P. aeruginosa, Acinetobacter baumannii,* methicillin-resistant *S. aureus, Klebsiella* spp., and *Enterobacter* spp. Two of the pathogens most frequently associated with VAP are *S. aureus* and *P. aeruginosa.* Risk factors for HAP can be categorized as host related, treatment related, and infection control related (Box 19.8).[53]

BOX 19.8 Risk Factors for Hospital-Acquired Pneumonia

Host-Related

Advanced age
Altered level of consciousness
Chronic obstructive pulmonary disease
Altered immune system
Severity of illness
Poor nutrition
Hemodynamic compromise
Trauma
Smoking
Dental plaque

Treatment-Related

Mechanical ventilation
Endotracheal intubation
Unintentional extubation
Bronchoscopy
Nasogastric tube
Previous antibiotic therapy
Elevated gastric pH secondary to histamine receptor antagonists, proton pump inhibitors, and enteral feedings
Upper abdominal surgery
Thoracic surgery
Supine position

Infection Control-Related

Poor handwashing practices

TABLE 19.3 Precipitating Conditions of Pneumonia

Condition	Etiologies
Depressed epiglottal and cough reflexes	Unconsciousness, neurologic disease, endotracheal or tracheal tubes, anesthesia, aging
Decreased cilia activity	Smoke inhalation, smoking history, oxygen toxicity, hypoventilation, intubation, viral infections, aging, COPD
Increased secretion	COPD, viral infections, bronchiectasis, general anesthesia, endotracheal intubation, smoking
Atelectasis	Trauma, foreign body obstruction, tumor, splinting, shallow ventilations, general anesthesia
Decreased lymphatic flow	Heart failure, tumor
Fluid in alveoli	Heart failure, aspiration, trauma
Abnormal phagocytosis and humoral activity	Neutropenia, immunocompetent disorders, patients receiving chemotherapy
Impaired alveolar macrophages	Hypoxemia, metabolic acidosis, cigarette smoking history, hypoxia, alcohol use, viral infections, aging

COPD, chronic obstructive pulmonary disease.

Health Care–Associated Pneumonia

Pathogens that can cause HCAP are similar to pathogens causing both CAP and HAP, with *P. aeruginosa* and methicillin-resistant *S. aureus* being the most common in the United States.[54] Risk factors for HCAP include prior hospitalization (hospitalized for 2 or more days within the last 90 days); receiving hemodialysis; receiving intravenous antibiotic therapy, chemotherapy, or wound care within 30 days; residing in a long-term care facility or with a family member with multidrug-resistant infection; and an immunocompromised state. These patients are at a higher risk of developing multidrug-resistant organisms.[55]

Pathophysiology

Development of acute pneumonia implies a defect in host defenses, a particularly virulent organism, or an overwhelming inoculation event. Bacterial invasion of the lower respiratory tract can occur by inhalation of aerosolized infectious particles, aspiration of organisms colonizing the oropharynx, migration of organisms from adjacent sites of colonization, direct inoculation of organisms into the lower airway, spread of infection to the lungs from adjacent structures, spread of infection to the lung through the blood, and reactivation of latent infection (usually in the setting of immunosuppression). The most common mechanism appears to be aspiration of oropharyngeal organisms.[56] Table 19.3 lists the precipitating conditions that can facilitate the development of pneumonia.

Fig. 19.4 depicts the pathophysiology of HAP. Colonization of the patient's oropharynx with infectious organisms is a major contributor to the development of HAP. The oropharynx normally has a stable population of resident flora that may be anaerobic or aerobic. When stress occurs, such as with illness, surgery, or infection, pathogenic organisms replace normal resident flora. Previous antibiotic therapy also affects the resident flora population, making replacement by pathologic organisms more likely. The pathogens are then able to invade the sterile lower respiratory tract.[53]

Disruption of the gag and cough reflexes, altered consciousness, abnormal swallowing, and artificial airways all predispose the patient to aspiration and colonization of the lungs and subsequent infection. Histamine-2 agonists, antacids, and enteral feedings also contribute to this problem because they raise the pH of the stomach and promote bacterial overgrowth. The nasogastric tube then acts as a wick, facilitating the movement of bacteria from the stomach to the pharynx, where the bacteria can be aspirated.[53]

Infection results in pulmonary inflammation with or without significant exudates. Increased capillary permeability occurs, leading to increased interstitial and alveolar fluid. V̇/Q̇ mismatching and intrapulmonary shunting occur, resulting in hypoxemia as lung consolidation progresses. Untreated pneumonia can result in ALF and initiation of the inflammatory-immune response. In addition, the patient may develop a pleural effusion. This is the result of the vascular response to inflammation, whereby capillary permeability is increased, and fluid from the pulmonary capillaries diffuses into the pleural space.[57]

Prevention of VAP is discussed in the mechanical ventilation section of Chapter 20.

Assessment and Diagnosis

The clinical manifestations of pneumonia vary with the offending pathogen. The patient may first be seen with a variety of signs and symptoms including dyspnea, fever, and cough (productive or nonproductive). Coarse crackles on auscultation and dullness to percussion may also be present.[52] Patients with severe CAP may present with confusion and disorientation,

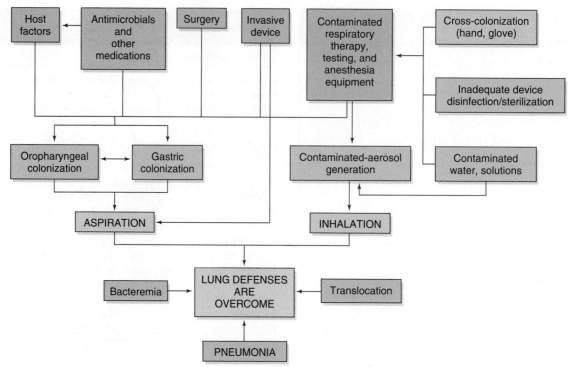

FIG. 19.4 Pathophysiology of Pneumonia. (From Tablan OC, et al. Guideline for prevention of nosocomial pneumonia. The Hospital Infection Control Practices Advisory Committee, Centers for Disease Control and Prevention. *Am J Infect Control.* 1994;22[4]:247–292.)

tachypnea, hypoxemia, uremia, leukopenia, thrombocytopenia, hypothermia, and hypotension.[57]

Chest radiography is used to evaluate a patient with suspected pneumonia. The diagnosis is established by the presence of a new pulmonary infiltrate. The radiographic pattern of the infiltrates varies with the organism.[53] A sputum Gram stain and culture are done to facilitate identification of the infectious pathogen. In 50% of cases, a causative agent is not identified.[53] A diagnostic bronchoscopy may be needed, particularly if the diagnosis is unclear or current therapy is not working.[52] In addition, a complete blood count with differential, chemistry panel, blood cultures, and ABGs is obtained.[53]

Medical Management

Medical management of a patient with pneumonia includes antibiotic therapy, oxygen therapy for hypoxemia, mechanical ventilation if ALF develops, fluid management for hydration, nutrition support, and treatment of associated medical problems and complications. For patients having difficulty mobilizing secretions, a therapeutic bronchoscopy may be necessary.[52]

Antibiotic Therapy

Although bacterium-specific antibiotic therapy is the goal, this may not always be possible because of difficulties in identifying the organism and the seriousness of the patient's condition. The time involved obtaining cultures is balanced against the need to begin some treatment based on the patient's condition. Empiric therapy has become a generally acceptable approach. In this approach, choice of antibiotic treatment is based on the most likely etiologic organism while avoiding toxicity, superinfection, and unnecessary cost. If available, Gram stain results are used to guide choices of antibiotics. Antibiotics that offer broad coverage of the usual pathogens in the hospital or community

are chosen. Failure to respond to such therapy may indicate that the chosen antibiotic regimen does not appropriately cover all the etiologic pathogens or that a new source of infection has developed.[52,53]

At the present time, the Centers for Medicare and Medicaid Services and The Joint Commission standards for managing patients with CAP require that the first dose of antibiotics be administered within 6 hours of arrival to the hospital. This time frame is very controversial and has been the subject of much debate. Individuals in favor of the standard believe that early antibiotic administration leads to improved outcomes, whereas individuals not in favor of the standard believe it leads to the overuse of antibiotics. More research is needed to clarify the issue.[58]

Independent Lung Ventilation

In patients with unilateral pneumonia or severely asymmetric pneumonia, independent lung ventilation, an alternative mode of mechanical ventilation, may be necessary to facilitate oxygenation. As the alveoli in the affected lung become flooded with pus, the lung becomes less compliant and difficult to ventilate. This results in a shifting of ventilation to the good lung without a concomitant shift in perfusion and thus an increase in $\dot{V}/\dot{Q}$ mismatching. Independent lung ventilation allows each lung to be ventilated separately, controlling the amount of flow, volume, and pressure each lung receives. A double-lumen endotracheal tube is inserted, and each lumen is usually attached to a separate mechanical ventilator. The ventilator settings are then customized to the needs of each lung to facilitate optimal oxygenation and ventilation.[59]

Nursing Management

The nursing management plan for a patient with pneumonia incorporates a variety of nursing diagnoses (Box 19.9). The

⊚ BOX 19.9 NURSING DIAGNOSES

Pneumonia

- Ineffective Airway Clearance related to excessive secretions or abnormal viscosity of mucus, p. 1034
- Impaired Gas Exchange related to ventilation/perfusion mismatching or intrapulmonary shunting, p. 1030
- Imbalanced Nutrition: Less Than Body Requirements related to lack of exogenous nutrients or increased metabolic demand, p. 1029
- Risk for Aspiration, p. 1040
- Risk for Infection, p. 1046
- Anxiety related to threat to biologic, psychologic, and/or social integrity, p. 1012
- Powerlessness related to lack of control over current situation or disease progression, p. 1038
- Compromised Family Coping related to critically ill family member, p. 1019

nurse has a significant role in optimizing oxygenation and ventilation, preventing the spread of infection, providing comfort and emotional support, and maintaining surveillance for complications. The patient's response to antibiotic therapy is monitored for adverse effects.

Optimize Oxygenation and Ventilation

Nursing interventions to optimize oxygenation and ventilation include positioning, preventing desaturation, and promoting secretion clearance. For further discussion of these interventions, see Nursing Management of Acute Lung Failure earlier in this chapter.

Prevent Spread of Infection

Prevention is directed at eradicating pathogens from the environment and interrupting the spread of organisms from person to person. Significant progress has been made in removing contaminants from the patient environment through proper disinfection of respiratory equipment and increased use of disposable supplies. Other possible environmental sources of pathogens include suctioning equipment and indwelling lines. These invasive tools must be given proper aseptic care.[60]

Proper hand hygiene is the most important measure available to prevent the spread of bacteria from person to person (Box 19.10). Hand hygiene is performed before and after touching a patient or their surroundings, before a procedure, and after exposure to any body fluids.[61] In addition, meticulous oral care, including suctioning of the secretions pooling above the cuff of the artificial airway, is critical to decreasing the bacterial colonization of the oropharynx.[60] Oral care is discussed further in Chapter 20.

Interprofessional collaborative management of a patient with pneumonia is outlined in Box 19.11.

ASPIRATION PNEUMONITIS

Description

The presence of abnormal substances in the airways and alveoli as a result of aspiration is misleadingly called *aspiration pneumonia*. This term is misleading because the aspiration of toxic substances into the lung may or may not involve an infection. *Aspiration pneumonitis* is a more accurate term because injury to the lung can result from the chemical, mechanical, or bacterial characteristics of the aspirate.[62]

QSEN BOX 19.10 QSEN: Quality Improvement

Hand Hygiene Guidelines

The following are the key recommendations of the Hand Hygiene Task Force, based on the literature review and expert panel opinion:

- Wash hands with soap and water when visibly dirty or contaminated with blood and other body fluids.
- When washing hands with soap and water, wet hands first with water, apply an amount of product recommended by the manufacturer to hands, and rub hands together vigorously for at least 15 seconds, covering all surfaces of the hands and fingers. Rinse hands with water, and dry thoroughly with a disposable towel. Use towel to turn off the faucet. Avoid using hot water because repeated exposure to hot water may increase the risk of dermatitis.
- If hands are not visibly soiled, use an alcohol-based hand rub for routinely decontaminating hands.
- When decontaminating hands with an alcohol-based hand rub, apply product to palm of one hand and rub hands together, covering all surfaces of hands and fingers, until hands are dry (follow the manufacturer's recommendations regarding the volume of product to use).
- Decontaminate hands before and after having direct contact with patients.
- Decontaminate hands before and after donning gloves.
- Wear gloves when contact with blood or other potentially infectious materials, mucous membranes, or nonintact skin could occur.
- Change gloves during patient care if moving from a contaminated body site to a clean body site.
- Remove gloves after caring for a patient. Do not wear the same pair of gloves for the care of more than one patient, and do not wash gloves between uses with different patients.
- Decontaminate hands after contact with inanimate objects (including medical equipment).
- Do not wear artificial fingernails or extenders when having direct contact with patients at high risk (eg, those in critical care units or operating rooms).
- Keep natural nails tips less than ¼-inch long.

From Boyce JM, Pittet D; Healthcare Infection Control Practices Advisory Committee; HICPAC/SHEA/APIC/IDSA Hand Hygiene Task Force. Guideline for hand hygiene in health care settings. Recommendations of Healthcare Infection Control Practices Advisory Committee, and the HICPAC/SHEA/APIC/IDSA Hand Hygiene Task Force. Society for Healthcare Epidemiology of America/Association for Professionals in Infection Control/Infectious Diseases Society of America. *MMWR Recomm Rep.* 2002;51(RR16):1–45.

QSEN BOX 19.11 QSEN: Teamwork and Collaboration

Interprofessional Collaborative Practice: Pneumonia

- Administer oxygen therapy.
- Initiate mechanical ventilation as required.
- Administer medications:
  - Antibiotics
  - Bronchodilators
- Position patient to optimize ventilation/perfusion matching.
- Suction as needed.
- Provide adequate rest and recovery time between procedures.
- Maintain surveillance for complications:
  - Acute lung failure
- Provide comfort and emotional support.

TABLE 19.4   Risk Factors for Aspiration

Risk Factor	Rationale
Decreased LOC, because of either CNS problems or use of sedatives	Decreased ability to protect airway from oropharyngeal secretions and regurgitated gastric contents
	Cough and gag reflexes diminish as LOC diminishes, whether from CNS disorder or sedation
	Slowed gastric emptying
	Decreased tone of lower esophageal sphincter
Supine position	Increases probability of gastroesophageal reflux
Presence of nasogastric tube	Interferes with closure of lower esophageal sphincter
	Biofilm on tube predisposes to aspiration of pathogenic organisms
Vomiting	Sudden and forceful entry of gastric contents into oropharynx predisposes to aspiration
	Predisposes to displacement of feeding tube ports into esophagus
Feeding tube ports positioned in esophagus	Infused feedings reflux into oropharynx
Tracheal intubation	Reduction in upper airway defense related to ineffective cough, desensitization of oropharynx and larynx, disuse atrophy of laryngeal muscles, and esophageal compression by an inflated cuff
Mechanical ventilation	Positive abdominal pressure predisposes to aspiration of gastric contents, probably by increasing gastroesophageal reflux
Accumulation of subglottic secretions above endotracheal cuff	Subglottic secretions can leak around cuff into lower respiratory tract, especially when cuff is deflated
Inadequate cuff inflation of tracheal devices	Persistent low cuff pressure (eg, 20 cm H_2O) predisposes to aspiration of oropharyngeal secretions and refluxed gastric contents
Gastric feeding site when gastric emptying significantly impaired	Accumulation of formula and gastrointestinal secretions predisposes to gastroesophageal reflux and aspiration
High GRVs	High GRVs predispose to gastroesophageal reflux and aspiration
Bolus feedings	Volume of infused formula may exceed tolerance of patients who have poor cough and gag reflexes
Poor oral health	Colonized oropharyngeal secretions may be aspirated into respiratory tract
Advanced age	Older patients tend to have reduced swallowing ability and are more likely to have neurologic disorders that increase aspiration risks
	Strong association between advanced age and probability of developing pneumonia once aspiration has occurred
Hyperglycemia	Mild hyperglycemia can cause delayed gastric emptying by disrupting postprandial antral contractions

CNS, central nervous system; GRVs, gastric residual volumes; LOC, level of consciousness.
From Metheny NA. Strategies to prevent aspiration-related pneumonia in tube-fed patients. Respir Care Clin N Am. 2006;12(4):603–617.

Etiology

Numerous factors have been identified that place the patient at risk for aspiration (Table 19.4). Gastric contents and oropharyngeal bacteria (see Pneumonia earlier in this chapter) are the most common aspirates of critically ill patients.[62-64] The effects of gastric contents on the lungs vary based on the pH of the liquid. If the pH is less than 2.5, the patient will develop a severe chemical pneumonitis resulting in hypoxemia. If the pH is greater than 2.5, the immediate damage to the lungs will be lessened, but the elevated pH may have promoted bacterial overgrowth of the stomach.[62,63] Once the bacteria-laden gastric contents are aspirated into the lungs, overwhelming bacterial pneumonia can develop.[63]

Pathophysiology

The type of lung injury that develops after aspiration is determined by many factors, including the quality of the aspirate and the status of the patient's respiratory defense mechanisms.

Acid Liquid

The aspiration of acid (pH less than 2.5) liquid gastric contents results in the development of bronchospasm and atelectasis almost immediately. Over the next 4 hours, tracheal damage, bronchitis, bronchiolitis, alveolar-capillary breakdown, interstitial edema, and alveolar congestion and hemorrhage occur.[64] Severe hypoxemia develops as a result of intrapulmonary

shunting and $\dot{V}/\dot{Q}$ mismatching. As the disorder progresses, necrotic debris and fibrin fill the alveoli, hyaline membranes form, and hypoxic vasoconstriction occurs, resulting in elevated pulmonary artery pressures.[63,64] The clinical course follows one of three patterns: (1) rapid improvement in 1 week, (2) initial improvement followed by deterioration and development of ARDS or pneumonia, or (3) rapid death from progressive ALF.[64]

Acid Food Particles

The aspiration of acid (pH less than 2.5) nonobstructing food particles can produce the most severe pulmonary reaction because of extensive pulmonary damage. Severe hypoxemia, hypercapnia, and acidosis occur.[63,64]

Nonacid Liquid

The aspiration of nonacid (pH greater than 2.5) liquid gastric contents is similar to acid liquid aspiration initially, but minimal structural damage occurs. Intrapulmonary shunting and $\dot{V}/\dot{Q}$ mismatching usually start to reverse within 4 hours, and hypoxemia clears within 24 hours.[63,64]

Nonacid Food Particles

The aspiration of nonacid (pH greater than 2.5) nonobstructing food particles is similar to acid aspiration initially, with significant edema and hemorrhage occurring within 6 hours. After the initial reaction, the response changes to a foreign body–type reaction with granuloma formation occurring around the food particles within 1 to 5 days.[64] In addition to hypoxemia, hypercapnia and acidosis occur as a result of hypoventilation.[62,63]

Assessment and Diagnosis

Clinically patients present with signs of acute respiratory distress, and gastric contents may be present in the oropharynx. Patients have shortness of breath, coughing, wheezing, cyanosis, and signs of hypoxemia. Tachypnea, tachycardia, hypotension, fever, and crackles also are present. Copious amounts of sputum are produced as alveolar edema develops.[62,63]

ABGs reflect severe hypoxemia. Changes on chest radiography appear 12 to 24 hours after the initial aspiration, with no one pattern being diagnostic of the event. Infiltrates appear in various distribution patterns depending on the position of the patient during aspiration and the volume of the aspirate. If bacterial infection becomes established, leukocytosis and positive sputum cultures occur.[63]

Medical Management

Management of a patient with aspiration lung disorder includes both emergency and follow-up treatment. When aspiration is witnessed, emergency treatment is instituted to secure the airway and minimize pulmonary damage. The patient's head is turned to the side, and the oral cavity and upper airway is suctioned immediately to remove the gastric contents.[63,64] Direct visualization by bronchoscopy is indicated to remove large particulate aspirate or to confirm an unwitnessed aspiration event. Bronchoalveolar lavage is not recommended because this practice disseminates the aspirate in lungs and increases damage.[64]

After airway clearance, attention is given to supporting oxygenation and hemodynamics. Hypoxemia is corrected with supplemental oxygen or mechanical ventilation with PEEP, if necessary.[63,64] Hemodynamic changes result from fluid shifts into the lungs that can occur after massive aspirations. Monitoring intravascular volume is essential, and judicious amounts of replacement fluids are instituted to maintain adequate urinary output and vital signs.[63,64]

Empiric antibiotic therapy is usually not indicated after aspiration of gastric contents. However, antibiotic therapy is considered if VAP is suspected or the aspiration event occurred in the presence of a small bowel obstruction or colonized gastric contents.[64] Corticosteroids have not been demonstrated to be of any benefit in the treatment of aspiration pneumonitis and are not recommended.[63,64]

Nursing Management

The nursing management plan for a patient with aspiration lung disorder incorporates a variety of nursing diagnoses (Box 19.12). The nurse has a significant role in optimizing oxygenation and ventilation, preventing further aspiration events, providing comfort and emotional support, and maintaining surveillance for complications.

Optimize Oxygenation and Ventilation

Nursing interventions to optimize oxygenation and ventilation include positioning, preventing desaturation, and promoting secretion clearance. For further discussion of these

BOX 19.12   NURSING DIAGNOSES

Aspiration Pneumonitis

- Impaired Gas Exchange related to ventilation/perfusion mismatching or intrapulmonary shunting, p. 1030
- Ineffective Airway Clearance related to excessive secretions or abnormal viscosity of mucus, p. 1034
- Risk for Aspiration, p. 1040
- Risk for Infection, p. 1046
- Anxiety related to threat to biologic, psychologic, and/or social integrity, p. 1012
- Ineffective Coping related to situational crisis and personal vulnerability, p. 1036
- Compromised Family Coping related to critically ill family member, p. 1014

interventions, see Nursing Management of Acute Lung Failure earlier in this chapter.

Prevent Aspiration

One of the most important interventions for preventing aspiration is identifying patients at risk for aspiration (Box 19.13). Actions to prevent aspiration include confirming feeding tube placement, checking for signs and symptoms of feeding intolerance, elevating the head of the bed at least 30 to 45 degrees, feeding the patient via a small-bore feeding tube or gastrostomy tube, avoiding the use of a large-bore nasogastric tube, ensuring proper inflation of artificial airway cuffs, and frequent suctioning of the oropharynx of an intubated patient to prevent secretions from pooling above the cuff of the tube. For patients at risk for aspiration or intolerant of gastric feedings, the feeding tube is placed in the small bowel.[65]

Interprofessional collaborative management of a patient with aspiration pneumonitis is outlined in Box 19.14.

ACUTE PULMONARY EMBOLISM

Description

A pulmonary embolism (PE) occurs when a clot (thrombotic embolus) or other matter (nonthrombotic embolus) lodges in the pulmonary arterial system, disrupting the blood flow to a region of the lungs (Fig. 19.5). Most thrombotic emboli arise from the pelvic and deep leg veins,[66] particularly the iliac, femoral, and popliteal veins. Other sources include the right ventricle, the upper extremities, and the pelvic veins. Nonthrombotic emboli arise from fat, tumors, amniotic fluid, air, and foreign bodies. This section focuses on thrombotic emboli.

Etiology

Numerous predisposing factors and precipitating conditions put a patient at risk for developing a PE (Box 19.15). Of the three predisposing factors (ie, hypercoagulability, injury to vascular endothelium, and venous stasis [Virchow triad]), endothelial injury appears to be the most significant.[66]

The American Heart Association has developed a classification schema for an acute PE, which stratifies patients into one of three categories: massive, submassive, or low risk. A massive PE is defined as an acute PE with sustained hypotension (systolic blood pressure less than 90 mm Hg) for more than 15 minutes, the need for inotropes not based on other causes,

BOX 19.13 QSEN: Evidence-Based Practice

Aspiration Prevention Guidelines

The following are the expected practice guidelines from the updated AACN Practice Alert: Preventing Aspiration:

1. Maintain head-of-bed elevation at an angle of 30–45 degrees, unless contraindicated. [Level B]
2. Use sedatives as sparingly as feasible. [Level C]
3. For tube-fed patients, assess placement of the feeding tube at 4-hour intervals. [Level C]
4. For patients receiving gastric tube feedings, assess for gastrointestinal intolerance to the feedings at 4-hour intervals. [Level C]
5. For tube-fed patients, avoid bolus feedings in those at high risk for aspiration. [Level E]
6. Consult with physician about obtaining a swallowing assessment before oral feedings are started for recently extubated patients who have experienced prolonged intubation. [Level C]
7. Maintain endotracheal cuff pressures at an appropriate level, and ensure that secretions are cleared from above the cuff before it is deflated. [Level B]

Levels of Evidence

Level A—Meta-analysis of quantitative studies or metasynthesis of qualitative studies with results that consistently support a specific action, intervention, or treatment

Level B—Well-designed, controlled studies with results that consistently support a specific action, intervention, or treatment

Level C—Qualitative studies, descriptive or correlational studies, integrative reviews, systematic reviews, or randomized controlled trials with inconsistent results

Level D—Peer-reviewed professional and organizational standards with the support of clinical study recommendations

Level E—Multiple case reports, theory-based evidence from expert opinions, or peer-reviewed professional organizational standards without clinical studies to support recommendations

Level M—Manufacturer's recommendations only

Modified from American Association of Critical-Care Nurses: AACN Practice Alert: Preventing Aspiration. http://www.aacn.org/WD/practice/docs/practicealerts/aacn-aspiration-practice-alert.pdf. 2011. Accessed October 2015.

BOX 19.14 QSEN: Teamwork and Collaboration

Interprofessional Collaborative Practice: Aspiration Pneumonitis

- Administer oxygen therapy.
- Secure patient's airway.
- Place patient in slight Trendelenburg position.
- Turn patient to right lateral decubitus position.
- Suction patient's oropharyngeal area.
- Initiate mechanical ventilation as required.
- Maintain surveillance for complications:
  - Pneumonia
  - Acute lung failure
  - Acute respiratory distress syndrome
- Provide comfort and emotional support.

or signs of shock. A submassive PE is defined as an acute PE with evidence of right ventricular dysfunction or myocardial necrosis. A patient with none of these conditions is defined as low risk.[67]

Pathophysiology

A massive PE occurs with the blockage of a lobar or larger artery, resulting in occlusion of the pulmonary vascular bed. Blockage of the pulmonary arterial system has both pulmonary and hemodynamic consequences.[66] The effects on the pulmonary system are increased alveolar dead space, bronchoconstriction, and compensatory shunting.[68] Hemodynamic effects include an increase in pulmonary vascular resistance and right ventricular workload.[69,70]

Increased Dead Space

An increase in alveolar dead space occurs because an area of the lung is receiving ventilation without being perfused. The ventilation to this area is known as *wasted ventilation* because it does not participate in gas exchange. This effect leads to alveolar dead space ventilation and an increase in the work of breathing. To limit the amount of dead space ventilation, localized bronchoconstriction occurs.[70]

Bronchoconstriction

Bronchoconstriction develops as a result of alveolar hypocarbia, hypoxia, and the release of mediators. Alveolar hypocarbia occurs as a consequence of decreased carbon dioxide in the affected area and leads to constriction of the local airways, increased airway resistance, and redistribution of ventilation to perfused areas of the lungs. Various mediators are released from the site of the injury, either from the clot or the surrounding lung tissue, which further causes constriction of the airways. Bronchoconstriction promotes the development of atelectasis.[70]

Compensatory Shunting

Compensatory shunting occurs as a result of the unaffected areas of the lungs having to accommodate the entire CO. A situation results in which perfusion exceeds ventilation and blood is returned to the left side of the heart without participating in gas exchange. This leads to the development of hypoxemia.[70]

Hemodynamic Consequences

The major hemodynamic consequence of a PE is the development of pulmonary hypertension, which is part of the effect of a mechanical obstruction when more than 50% of the vascular bed is occluded. In addition, the mediators released at the injury site and the development of hypoxia cause pulmonary vasoconstriction, which further exacerbates pulmonary hypertension. As the pulmonary vascular resistance increases, so does the workload of the right ventricle, as reflected by an increase in pulmonary artery pressures. Consequently, right ventricular failure occurs, which can lead to decreases in left ventricular preload, CO, and blood pressure and shock.[66,68-70]

Assessment and Diagnosis

A patient with a PE may have numerous presenting signs and symptoms, with the most common being tachycardia and tachypnea. Additional signs and symptoms that may be present

FIG. 19.5 Pathophysiology of Pulmonary Embolism. Thromboemboli travel through the right side of the heart to reach the lungs. LA, left atrium; LV, left ventricle; RA, right atrium; RV, right ventricle.

BOX 19.15 Risk Factors for Pulmonary Thromboembolism

Predisposing Factors

Venous stasis
  Atrial fibrillation
  Decreased cardiac output
  Immobility
Injury to vascular endothelium
  Local vessel injury
  Infection
  Incision
  Atherosclerosis
Hypercoagulability
  Polycythemia

Precipitating Conditions

Previous pulmonary embolus
Cardiovascular disease
  Heart failure
  Right ventricular infarction
  Cardiomyopathy
  Cor pulmonale
Surgery
  Orthopedic
  Vascular
  Abdominal
Cancer
  Ovarian
  Pancreatic
  Stomach
  Extrahepatic bile duct system
Trauma (injury or burns)
  Lower extremities
  Pelvis
  Hips
Gynecologic status
  Pregnancy
  Postpartum
  Birth control pills
  Estrogen replacement therapy

include dyspnea, apprehension, increased pulmonic component of the second heart sound (P_1), fever, crackles, pleuritic chest pain, cough, evidence of deep vein thrombosis (DVT), and hemoptysis.[66] Syncope and hemodynamic instability can occur as a result of right ventricular failure.[69]

Initial laboratory studies and diagnostic procedures that may be done include ABG analysis, D-dimer, electrocardiogram (ECG), chest radiography, and echocardiography. ABGs may show a low Pao_2, indicating hypoxemia; a low $Paco_2$, indicating hypocarbia; and a high pH, indicating a respiratory alkalosis. The hypocarbia with resulting respiratory alkalosis is caused by tachypnea.[68] An elevated D-dimer occurs with a PE and many other disorders. A normal D-dimer does not occur with a PE and can be used to rule out a PE as the diagnosis.[66] The most frequent ECG finding seen in a patient with a PE is sinus tachycardia.[66] The classic ECG pattern associated with a PE—S wave in lead I and Q wave with inverted T wave in lead III—is seen in less than 20% of patients.[66] Other ECG findings associated with a PE include right bundle-branch block, new-onset atrial fibrillation, T-wave inversion in the anterior or inferior leads, and ST-segment changes.[70] Chest x-ray findings vary from normal to abnormal and are of little value in confirming the presence of a PE. Abnormal findings include cardiomegaly, pleural effusion, elevated hemidiaphragm, enlargement of the right descending pulmonary artery (Palla sign), a wedge-shaped density above the diaphragm (Hampton hump), and the presence of atelectasis.[68] Transthoracic or transesophageal echocardiography is also useful in the identification of a PE because it can provide visualization of any embolus in the central pulmonary arteries. In addition, it can be used for assessing the hemodynamic consequences of the PE on the right side of the heart.[70]

Differentiating a PE from other illnesses can be difficult because many clinical manifestations of a PE are found in a variety of other disorders.[67] Therefore various other tests may be necessary, including V̇/Q̇ scintigraphy, pulmonary angiography, and DVT studies.[66,68,70] With the advent of more sophisticated CT scanners, spiral CT is also being used to diagnose a PE.[68-70] A definitive diagnosis of a PE requires confirmation by a high-probability V̇/Q̇ scan, an abnormal pulmonary angiogram or CT scan, or strong clinical

TABLE 19.5 Venous Thromboembolism Prophylaxis

Condition	Prophylaxis
General surgery	Unfractionated heparin 5000 units SC TID *or*
	Enoxaparin 40 mg SC QD *or*
	Dalteparin 2500 or 5000 units SC QD
Orthopedic surgery	Warfarin (target INR 2.0–3.0) *or*
	Enoxaparin 30 mg SC BID *or*
	Enoxaparin 40 mg SC QD *or*
	Dalteparin 2500 or 5000 units SC QD *or*
	Fondaparinux 2.5 mg SC QD
Neurosurgery	Unfractionated heparin 5000 units SC BID *or*
	Enoxaparin 40 mg SC QD *and*
	Graduated compression stockings/intermittent pneumatic compression
	Consider surveillance lower extremity ultrasonography
Oncologic surgery	Enoxaparin 40 mg SC QD
Thoracic surgery	Unfractionated heparin 5000 units SC TID *and*
	Graduated compression stockings/intermittent pneumatic compression
Medical patients	Unfractionated heparin 5000 units SC TID *or*
	Enoxaparin 40 mg SC QD *or*
	Dalteparin 5000 units SC QD *or*
	Fondaparinux 2.5 mg SC QD *or*
	Graduated compression stockings/intermittent pneumatic compression for patients with contraindications to anticoagulation
	Consider combination pharmacologic and mechanical prophylaxis for very high-risk patients
	Consider surveillance lower extremity ultrasonography for intensive care unit patients

BID, twice daily; *INR*, international normalized ratio; *QD*, daily; *SC*, subcutaneous; *TID*, three times daily.
From Piazza G, Goldhaber SZ. Acute pulmonary embolism: part II treatment and prophylaxis. *Circulation.* 2006;114(3):e42–e47.

suspicion coupled with abnormal findings on lower extremity DVT studies.[68]

Medical Management

Medical management of a patient with a PE involves both prevention and treatment strategies. Prevention strategies include the use of prophylactic anticoagulation with low-dose or adjusted-dose heparin, LMWH, or oral anticoagulants (Table 19.5). The use of pneumatic compression has also been demonstrated as an effective method of prophylaxis in low-risk patients.[24]

Treatment strategies include preventing the recurrence of a PE, facilitating clot dissolution, reversing the effects of pulmonary hypertension, promoting gas exchange, and preventing complications. Medical interventions to promote gas exchange include supplemental oxygen administration, intubation, and mechanical ventilation.[66]

Prevention of Recurrence

Interventions to prevent the recurrence of a PE include the administration of unfractionated or LMWH and warfarin (Coumadin).[66,71] Heparin is administered to prevent further clots from forming and has no effect on the existing clot. The heparin dose is adjusted to maintain the activated partial thromboplastin time in the range of two to three times of upper normal.[66,70,71] Warfarin is started at the same time, and when the international normalized ratio (INR) reaches 3.0, the heparin is discontinued. The INR is maintained between 2.0 and 3.0. The patient remains on warfarin for 3 to 12 months, depending on his or her risk for thromboembolic disease.[66,70,72]

Interruption of the inferior vena cava is reserved for patients in whom anticoagulation is contraindicated.[72] The procedure involves placement of a percutaneous venous filter (eg, Greenfield filter) into the vena cava, usually below the renal arteries. The filter prevents further thrombotic emboli from migrating into the lungs.[73]

Clot Dissolution

The administration of fibrinolytic agents in the treatment of PE has had limited success. At the present time, fibrinolytic therapy is reserved for patients with a massive PE and concomitant hemodynamic instability. Either recombinant tissue-type plasminogen activator or streptokinase may be used. The therapeutic window for using fibrinolytic therapy is up to 14 days, although the most benefit is usually obtained when given within 48 hours.[70]

If fibrinolytic therapy is contraindicated, a pulmonary embolectomy may be performed to remove the clot. Generally, pulmonary embolectomy is performed as an open procedure while the patient is on cardiopulmonary bypass. An emerging alternative to surgical embolectomy is catheter embolectomy. It appears to be particularly useful if surgical embolectomy is unavailable or is contraindicated. It appears to be most successful when performed within 5 days of the occurrence of the PE.[72]

Reversal of Pulmonary Hypertension

To reverse the hemodynamic effects of pulmonary hypertension, additional measures may be taken including the administration of inotropic agents and fluid. Fluids are administered to increase right ventricular preload, which would stretch the right ventricle and increase contractility, overcoming the elevated pulmonary arterial pressures. Inotropic agents also can be used to increase contractility to facilitate an increase in CO.[66,70]

Nursing Management

Prevention of PE is a major nursing focus because most critically ill patients are at risk for this disorder. Nursing actions are aimed at preventing the development of DVT (Box 19.16), which is a major complication of immobility and a leading cause of PE. These measures include the use of pneumatic compression devices, active/passive range-of-motion exercises involving foot extension, adequate hydration, and progressive ambulation.[24]

The nursing management plan for a patient with a PE incorporates a variety of nursing diagnoses (Box 19.17). The nurse has a significant role in optimizing oxygenation and ventilation, monitoring for bleeding, providing comfort and emotional support, maintaining surveillance for complications, and educating the patient and family.

Optimize Oxygenation and Ventilation

Nursing interventions to optimize oxygenation and ventilation include positioning, preventing desaturation, and promoting secretion clearance. For further discussion of these

BOX 19.16 QSEN: Evidence-Based Practice

Venous Thromboembolism Prevention Guidelines

The following are the expected practice guidelines from the updated AACN Practice Alert: Venous Thromboembolism Prevention:

1. Assess all patients on admission to the critical care unit for risk factors of VTE and anticipate orders for VTE prophylaxis based on risk assessment. [Level D]
2. Clinical eligibility and regimens for VTE prophylaxis include:
   - Moderate-risk patients (medically ill and postoperative patients): Low-dose unfractionated heparin, LMWH, or fondaparinux [Level B]
   - High-risk patients (major trauma, spinal cord injury, or orthopedic surgery): LMWH, fondaparinux, or oral vitamin K antagonist [Level B]
   - Patients with high risk for bleeding: Mechanical prophylaxis including graduated compression stockings and/or intermittent pneumatic compression devices [Level B]
   - Mechanical prophylaxis may also be anticipated in conjunction with anticoagulant-based prophylaxis regimens
3. Review daily—with the physician and during multidisciplinary rounds—each patient's current VTE risk factors, including clinical status, necessity for CVC, current status of VTE prophylaxis, risk for bleeding, and response to treatment. [Level E]
4. Maximize patient mobility whenever possible, and take measures to reduce amount of time patient is immobile because of the effects of treatment (eg, pain, sedation, neuromuscular blockade, mechanical ventilation). [Level E]
5. Ensure that mechanical prophylaxis devices are fitted properly and in use at all times except when being removed for cleaning and/or inspection of skin. [Level E]

Levels of Evidence

Level A—Meta-analysis of quantitative studies or metasynthesis of qualitative studies with results that consistently support a specific action, intervention, or treatment

Level B—Well-designed, controlled studies with results that consistently support a specific action, intervention, or treatment

Level C—Qualitative studies, descriptive or correlational studies, integrative reviews, systematic reviews, or randomized controlled trials with inconsistent results

Level D—Peer-reviewed professional and organizational standards with the support of clinical study recommendations

Level E—Multiple case reports, theory-based evidence from expert opinions, or peer-reviewed professional organizational standards without clinical studies to support recommendations

Level M—Manufacturer's recommendations only

CVC, central venous catheter; *LMWH*, low-molecular-weight heparin; *VTE*, venous thromboembolism.
Modified from American Association of Critical-Care Nurses. AACN practice alert: venous thromboembolism prevention. http://www.aacn.org/WD/Practice/Docs/PracticeAlerts/VTE%20Prevention%2004-2010%20final.pdf. 2010. Accessed October 2015.

BOX 19.17 NURSING DIAGNOSES

Acute Pulmonary Embolism

- Impaired Gas Exchange related to ventilation/perfusion mismatching or intrapulmonary shunting, p. 1030
- Acute Pain related to transmission and perception of cutaneous, visceral, muscular, or ischemic impulses, p. 1010
- Risk for Aspiration, p. 1040
- Anxiety related to threat to biologic, psychologic, and/or social integrity, p. 1012
- Powerlessness related to lack of control over current situation or disease progression, p. 1038
- Compromised Family Coping related to critically ill family member, p. 1014

BOX 19.18 PATIENT EDUCATION PLAN

Acute Pulmonary Embolism

Before the patient's discharge, the patient should be able to teach back the following topics:
- Pathophysiology of disease
- Specific etiology
- Modification of precipitating factors
- Measures to prevent DVT (eg, avoid tight-fitting clothes, crossing legs, and prolonged sitting or standing; elevate legs when sitting; exercise)
- Signs and symptoms of DVT (eg, redness, swelling, sharp or deep leg pain)
- Importance of taking medications
- Signs and symptoms of anticoagulant complications (eg, excessive bruising, discoloration of skin, changes in color of urine or stools)
- Measures to prevent bleeding (eg, use soft-bristle toothbrush, caution when shaving)

Additional information for the patient can be found at the following websites:
- Vascular Web: http://www.vascularweb.org/vascularhealth/Pages/pulmonary-embolism.aspx
- Healthfinder—US Department of Health and Human Services: http://healthfinder.gov
- WebMD: http://www.webmd.com

DVT, deep vein thrombosis.

---

interventions, see Nursing Management of Acute Lung Failure earlier in this chapter.

Monitor for Bleeding

Patients receiving anticoagulant or fibrinolytic therapy are observed for signs of bleeding. The patient's gums, skin, urine, stool, and emesis are monitored for signs of overt or covert bleeding. In addition, monitoring the patient's INR or activated partial thromboplastin time is critical to managing the anticoagulation therapy.

Educate the Patient and Family

Early in the patient's hospital stay, the patient and family are taught about pulmonary embolus, its causes, and its treatment (Box 19.18). Closer to discharge, the patient's education plan focuses on the interventions necessary for preventing the reoccurrence of DVT and subsequent emboli, signs and symptoms of DVT and anticoagulant complications, and measures to prevent bleeding. If the patient smokes, he or she is encouraged to stop smoking and is referred to a smoking cessation program.

Interprofessional collaborative management of a patient with a pulmonary embolus is outlined Box 19.19.

BOX 19.19   QSEN: Teamwork and Collaboration

Interprofessional Collaborative Practice: Acute Pulmonary Embolism

- Administer oxygen therapy.
- Intubate patient.
- Initiate mechanical ventilation.
- Administer medications:
  - Fibrinolytic therapy
  - Anticoagulants
  - Bronchodilators
  - Inotropic agents
  - Sedatives
  - Analgesics
- Administer fluids.
- Position patient to optimize ventilation/perfusion matching.
- Maintain surveillance for complications:
  - Bleeding
  - Acute respiratory distress syndrome
- Provide comfort and emotional support.

STATUS ASTHMATICUS

Description

Asthma is a chronic obstructive pulmonary disease that is characterized by partially reversible airflow obstruction, airway inflammation, and hyperresponsiveness to a variety of stimuli.[74] Status asthmaticus is a severe asthma attack that fails to respond to conventional therapy with bronchodilators, which may result in ALF.[75,76]

Etiology

The precipitating cause of the attack is usually an upper respiratory infection, allergen exposure, or a decrease in antiinflammatory medications. Other factors that have been implicated include overreliance on bronchodilators, environmental pollutants, lack of access to health care, failure to identify worsening airflow obstruction, and noncompliance with the health care regimen.[75]

Pathophysiology

An asthma attack is initiated when exposure to an irritant or trigger occurs, resulting in the initiation of the inflammatory-immune response in the airways. Bronchospasm occurs along with increased vascular permeability and increased mucus production. Mucosal edema and thick, tenacious mucus further increase airway responsiveness. The combination of bronchospasm, airway inflammation, and hyperresponsiveness results in narrowing of the airways and airflow obstruction. These changes have significant effects on the pulmonary and cardiovascular systems.[75]

Pulmonary Effects

As the diameter of the airways decreases, airway resistance increases, resulting in increased residual volume, hyperinflation of the lungs, increased work of breathing, and abnormal distribution of ventilation. $\dot{V}/\dot{Q}$ mismatching occurs, which results in hypoxemia. Alveolar dead space also increases as hypoxic vasoconstriction occurs, resulting in hypercapnia.[75]

Cardiovascular Effects

Inspiratory muscle force also increases in an attempt to ventilate the hyperinflated lungs. This results in a significant increase in negative intrapleural pressure, leading to an increase in venous return and pooling of blood in the right ventricle. The stretched right ventricle causes the intraventricular septum to shift, impinging on the left ventricle. In addition, the left ventricle has to work harder to pump blood from the markedly negative pressure in the thorax to elevated pressure in systemic circulation. This leads to a decrease in CO and a fall in systolic blood pressure on inspiration (pulsus paradoxus).[75]

Assessment and Diagnosis

The patient may initially present with a cough, wheezing, and dyspnea. As the attack continues, the patient develops tachypnea, tachycardia, diaphoresis, increased accessory muscle use, and pulsus paradoxus greater than 25 mm Hg. Decreased level of consciousness, inability to speak, significantly diminished or absent breath sounds, and inability to lie supine herald the onset of ALF.[74-76]

Initial ABGs indicate hypocapnia and respiratory alkalosis caused by hyperventilation. As the attack continues and the patient starts to fatigue, hypoxemia and hypercapnia develop.[76] Lactic acidosis also may occur as a result of lactate overproduction by the respiratory muscles. The end result is the development of respiratory and metabolic acidosis.

Deterioration of pulmonary function tests despite aggressive bronchodilator therapy is diagnostic of status asthmaticus and indicates the potential need for intubation. A peak expiratory flow rate (PEFR) less than 40% of predicted or forced expiratory volume in 1 second (maximum volume of gas that the patient can exhale in 1 second) less than 20% of predicted indicates severe airflow obstruction, and the need for intubation with mechanical ventilation may be imminent.[77]

Medical Management

Medical management of a patient with status asthmaticus is directed toward supporting oxygenation and ventilation. Bronchodilators, corticosteroids, oxygen therapy, and intubation and mechanical ventilation are the mainstays of therapy.[76]

Bronchodilators

Inhaled beta-2 agonists and anticholinergics are the bronchodilators of choice for status asthmaticus. Beta-2 agonists promote bronchodilation and can be administered by nebulizer or metered-dose inhaler (MDI). Usually larger and more frequent doses are given, and the medication is titrated to the patient's response. Anticholinergics that inhibit bronchoconstriction are not very effective by themselves, but in conjunction with beta-2 agonists, they have a synergistic effect and produce a greater improvement in airflow. The routine use of xanthines is not recommended in the treatment of status asthmaticus because they have been shown to have no therapeutic benefit.[75-77]

Many studies have focused on the bronchodilator abilities of magnesium. Although it has been demonstrated that magnesium is inferior to beta-2 agonists as a bronchodilator, it may be beneficial in patients who are refractory to conventional treatment. A bolus of 1 to 4 g of intravenous magnesium given over 10 to 40 minutes has been reported to produce desirable effects.[75-77]

Many other studies are evaluating the effects of leukotriene inhibitors such as zafirlukast, montelukast, and zileuton in the treatment of status asthmaticus. Leukotrienes are inflammatory mediators known to cause bronchoconstriction and airway inflammation. Research suggests that these agents may be beneficial as bronchodilators in patients who are refractory to beta-2 agonists.[77]

Systemic Corticosteroids

Intravenous or oral corticosteroids also are used in the treatment of status asthmaticus. Their antiinflammatory effects limit mucosal edema, decrease mucus production, and potentiate beta-2 agonists. It usually takes 6 to 8 hours for the effects of the corticosteroids to become evident.[76] The use of inhaled corticosteroids for the treatment of status asthmaticus is undecided at the present time.[75,76] Initial studies indicate they may be beneficial in certain patient populations.[76]

Oxygen Therapy

Initial treatment of hypoxemia is with supplemental oxygen. High-flow oxygen therapy is administered to keep the patient's oxygen saturation greater than 92%.[75] Another therapy currently under investigation is the use of heliox. A mixture of helium and oxygen, heliox has a lower density and higher viscosity than an oxygen and air mixture. Heliox is believed to reduce the work of breathing and improve gas exchange because it flows more easily through constricted areas. Studies have shown that it reduces air trapping and carbon dioxide and helps relieve respiratory acidosis.[75]

Intubation and Mechanical Ventilation

Indications for mechanical ventilation include cardiac or respiratory arrest, disorientation, failure to respond to bronchodilator therapy, and exhaustion.[75-77] A large endotracheal tube (8 mm) is used to decrease airway resistance and to facilitate suctioning of secretions. Ventilating the patient with status asthmaticus can be very difficult. High inflation pressures are avoided because they can result in barotrauma. The use of PEEP is monitored closely because the patient is prone to developing air trapping. Patient-ventilator asynchrony also can be a major problem. Sedation and neuromuscular paralysis may be necessary to allow for adequate ventilation of the patient.[75,77]

Nursing Management

The nursing management plan for a patient with status asthmaticus incorporates a variety of nursing diagnoses (Box 19.20). The nurse has a significant role in optimizing oxygenation and ventilation, providing comfort and emotional support, maintaining surveillance for complications, and educating the patient and family. A systematic review examined the impact of severe asthma on the quality of life and found that the symptoms and activity limitations had a negative impact on the quality of life for these patients.[78]

Optimize Oxygenation and Ventilation

Nursing interventions to optimize oxygenation and ventilation include positioning, preventing desaturation, and promoting secretion clearance. For further discussion of these interventions, see Nursing Management of Acute Lung Failure earlier in this chapter.

Educate the Patient and Family

Early in the patient's hospital stay, the patient and family are taught about asthma, its triggers, and its treatment (Box 19.21).

BOX 19.20 NURSING DIAGNOSES

Status Asthmaticus

- Impaired Gas Exchange related to alveolar hypoventilation, p. 1030
- Impaired Gas Exchange related to ventilation/perfusion mismatching or intrapulmonary shunting, p. 1030
- Ineffective Breathing Pattern related to musculoskeletal fatigue or neuromuscular impairment, p. 1035
- Ineffective Airway Clearance related to excessive secretions or abnormal viscosity of mucus, p. 1034
- Risk for Infection, p. 1046
- Anxiety related to threat to biologic, psychologic, and/or social integrity, p. 1012
- Disturbed Body Image related to actual change in body structures, function, or appearance, p. 1022
- Compromised Family Coping related to critically ill family member, p. 1014

BOX 19.21 PATIENT EDUCATION PLAN

Status Asthmaticus

Before the patient's discharge, the patient should be able to teach back the following topics:
- Pathophysiology of disease
- Specific etiology
- Early warning signs of worsening airflow obstruction (20% decrease in PEFR below predicted or personal best, increase in cough, shortness of breath, chest tightness, wheezing)
- Treatment of attacks
- Importance of taking prescribed medications and avoidance of over-the-counter asthma medications
- Correct use of an inhaler (with and without spacer device)
- Correct use of a peak flowmeter
- Removal or avoidance of environmental triggers (eg, pollen; dust; mold spores; cat and dog dander; cold, dry air; strong odors; household aerosols; tobacco smoke; air pollution)
- Measures to prevent pulmonary infections (eg, proper nutrition and handwashing, immunization against *Streptococcus pneumoniae* and influenza viruses)
- Signs and symptoms of pulmonary infection (eg, sputum color change, shortness of breath, fever)
- Importance of participating in pulmonary rehabilitation program

Additional information for the patient can be found at the following websites:
- Asthma and Allergy Foundation of America: http://www.aafa.org
- American Lung Association: http://www.lung.org
- Healthfinder—US Department of Health and Human Services: http://healthfinder.gov
- WebMD: http://www.webmd.com

PEFR, peak expiratory flow rate.

Closer to discharge, the patient education plan focuses on the interventions necessary for preventing the recurrence of status asthmaticus, early warning signs of worsening airflow obstruction, correct use of an inhaler and a peak flowmeter, measures to prevent pulmonary infections, and signs and symptoms of a pulmonary infection. If the patient smokes, he or she is

QSEN BOX 19.22   QSEN: Teamwork and Collaboration

Interprofessional Collaborative Practice: Status Asthmaticus

- Administer oxygen therapy.
- Intubate patient.
- Initiate mechanical ventilation.
- Administer medications:
  - Bronchodilators
  - Corticosteroids
  - Sedatives
- Maintain surveillance for complications:
  - Acute lung failure
  - Provide comfort and emotional support.

TABLE 19.6   Air Leak Disorders

Type	Description
Pneumothorax	
Spontaneous	
Primary	Disruption of the visceral pleura that allows air from the lung to enter the pleural space; occurs spontaneously in patients *without* underlying lung disease
Secondary	Disruption of the visceral pleura that allows air from the lung to enter the pleural space; occurs spontaneously in patients *with* underlying lung disease
Traumatic	
Open	Laceration in the parietal pleura that allows atmospheric air to enter the pleural space; occurs as a result of penetrating chest trauma
Closed	Laceration in the visceral pleura that allows air from the lung to enter the pleural space; occurs as a result of blunt chest trauma
Iatrogenic	Laceration in the visceral pleura that allows air from the lung to enter the pleural space; occurs as a result of therapeutic or diagnostic procedures, such as central line insertion, thoracentesis, and needle aspiration
Tension	Occurs when air is allowed to enter the pleural space but not to exit it; as pressure increases inside the pleural space, the lung collapses, and the mediastinum shifts to the unaffected side; may result from a spontaneous or traumatic pneumothorax
Barotrauma/Volutrauma	
Pulmonary interstitial emphysema	Air in the pulmonary interstitial space
Subcutaneous emphysema	Air in the subcutaneous tissues
Pneumomediastinum	Air in the mediastinal space
Pneumopericardium	Air in the pericardial space
Pneumoperitoneum	Air in the peritoneal space
Pneumoretroperitoneum	Air in the retroperitoneal space

encouraged to stop smoking and is referred to a smoking cessation program. In addition, the importance of participating in a pulmonary rehabilitation program is stressed.

Interprofessional collaborative management of a patient with status asthmaticus is outlined in Box 19.22.

AIR LEAK DISORDERS

Description

Air leak disorders consist of conditions that result in extraalveolar air accumulation. These disorders are commonly divided into two categories: pneumothorax[79,80] and barotrauma.[81] A pneumothorax occurs with the accumulation of air or other gas in the pleural space.[79,80] Barotrauma is the result of excessive pressure in the alveoli that can lead to extreme alveolar wall stress and damage to the alveolar-capillary membrane, causing air to escape into the surrounding spaces.[81] Individual air leak disorders are described in Table 19.6.

Etiology

The two main causes of air leak disorders are (1) disruption of the parietal or visceral pleura, which allows air to enter the pleural space,[79,80] and (2) rupture of alveoli, which allows air to enter the interstitial space.[81] Disruption of the parietal pleura occurs as the result of penetrating trauma to the chest wall, which allows atmospheric air to enter the pleural space (traumatic open pneumothorax).[79,80] Disruption of the visceral pleura occurs as a result of entry of air into the pleural space from the lung. This may be caused by blunt chest wall trauma (traumatic closed pneumothorax), diagnostic or therapeutic procedures (traumatic iatrogenic pneumothorax), diseases of the pulmonary system (secondary spontaneous pneumothorax), or ruptured subpleural blebs (primary spontaneous pneumothorax).[79,80] Alveolar rupture occurs as a result of a change in the pressure gradient between the alveoli and the surrounding interstitial space. An increase in alveolar pressure or a decrease in interstitial pressure can lead to overdistention of the alveoli, rupture, and air leakage into the interstitial space. One of the most common causes of barotrauma is mechanical ventilation.[81]

Pathophysiology

The pathologic consequences of pneumothorax and of barotrauma or volutrauma are different.

Pneumothorax

Regardless of the cause, the entry of air into the pleural space compresses the affected lung. As the lung collapses, the alveoli become underventilated, causing $\dot{V}/\dot{Q}$ mismatching and intrapulmonary shunting. If the pneumothorax is large, hypoxemia ensues, and ALF quickly develops. Increased pressure within the chest can lead to shifting of the mediastinum, compression of the great vessels, and decreased CO.[79,80]

Barotrauma

After air enters the interstitial space, it travels though the pulmonary interstitium (pulmonary interstitial emphysema); out through the hilum; and into the mediastinum (pneumomediastinum), pleural space (pneumothorax), subcutaneous tissues (subcutaneous emphysema), pericardium (pneumopericardium), peritoneum (pneumoperitoneum), and retroperitoneum (pneumoretroperitoneum).[81] Except for pneumothorax, the resultant disorders are usually benign. Pneumomediastinum has been associated with decreased venous return and upper

FIG. 19.6 Left-Sided Tension Pneumothorax. Notice the shift of the heart and mediastinum to the right. (From Des Jardin T, Burton GC. *Clinical Management and Assessment of Respiratory Disease.* 3rd ed. St. Louis: Mosby; 1995.)

FIG. 19.7 Heimlich Valve. (Courtesy and © Becton, Dickinson and Company.)

FIG. 19.8 Underwater-Seal Drainage System. (Courtesy Atrium Medical Corporation, Hudson, NH.)

airway obstruction,[82] and pneumopericardium has been associated with cardiac tamponade.[83]

Assessment and Diagnosis

The clinical manifestations of a pneumothorax depend on the degree of lung collapse. If the pneumothorax is large, decreased respiratory excursion on the affected side may be noticed, along with bulging intercostal muscles. The trachea may deviate away from the affected side. Percussion reveals hyperresonance with decreased or absent breath sounds over the affected area. ABG analysis demonstrates hypoxemia and hypercapnia.[79,80] A chest radiograph confirms the pneumothorax with increased translucency evident on the affected side (Fig. 19.6).[80,84]

The clinical manifestations of barotrauma are much more subtle. Subcutaneous emphysema is manifested by crepitus, usually around the face, neck, and upper chest.[80] Stabbing substernal pain with position changes and with increased ventilation is the most commonly reported symptom of a pneumomomediastinum.[82] A clicking or crunching sound synchronous with the heart sounds may be heard over the apex of the heart (Hamman sign).[82] A friction rub may be heard with a pneumopericardium.[83] Barotrauma is also confirmed by radiography. Extraalveolar air, as evidenced by increased translucency, is present in the affected area (eg, chest, abdomen).[85]

Medical Management

Medical management of air leak disorders varies depending on the severity of the specific disorder. Usually, only a pneumothorax would require treatment, and that would depend on its size. A pneumothorax of less than 15% usually requires no treatment other than supplemental oxygen administration, unless complications occur or underlying lung disease or injury is present.[79,80]

A pneumothorax greater than 15% requires intervention to evacuate the air from the pleural space and facilitate reexpansion of the collapsed lung.[80,86] Interventions include aspiration of the air with a needle and placement of a small-bore (12 to 20 Fr) or large-bore (24 to 40 Fr) chest tube. Chest tubes are inserted into the pleural space to remove fluid or air, reinstate the negative intrapleural pressure, and reexpand a collapsed lung.[80,86] The trend appears to be toward placement of a small-bore tube, as the smaller tubes are more comfortable for the patient and just as effective as large-bore tubes. Patients on mechanical ventilation with a pneumothorax secondary to barotrauma are best managed with large-bore chest tubes.[87]

Chest tubes are usually inserted in the fourth or fifth intercostal space on the midaxillary line. After the tube is inserted, it is attached to a Heimlich valve or a chest drainage system. The Heimlich valve is a small one-way valve device that allows air to exit from the pleural space but not enter it (Fig. 19.7). It can be used alone or attached to a drainage bag.[80]

A chest drainage system is a disposable plastic unit that has three separate chambers: a water-seal or dry-seal chamber, a suction-control chamber, and a drainage-collection chamber (Fig. 19.8). In a system with a water-seal chamber, the chamber is filled to the 2-cm level. The water-seal chamber acts as a one-way valve, allowing air to escape from the chest but not to enter it. In a system with a dry-seal chamber, a mechanical one-way valve takes the place of the water seal. The suction-control chamber is adjusted to the desired level of suction. After the chest tubes are placed, the suction-control chamber is attached to an external suction regulator, which is adjusted until the desired level of suction is established (usually 20 cm H_2O). Any fluid draining from the chest will be evident in the collection chamber. Connection points of the drainage tubing are sealed with tape, and an occlusive dressing is applied over the chest tube insertion site. After the tubes are inserted and connected to either device, a chest radiograph is obtained to confirm reexpansion of the lung.[80,88]

Surgical intervention may be necessary in patients with a persistent air leak or failure of the lung to expand within 3 to 5 days. The preferred procedure is a video-assisted thoracoscopic surgery.[86] Two conditions that require emergency intervention for immediate relief are a tension pneumothorax and a tension pneumopericardium.

Tension Pneumothorax

A tension pneumothorax develops when air enters the pleural space on inhalation and cannot exit on exhalation. As pressure inside the pleural space increases, it results in collapse of the lung and shifting of the mediastinum and trachea to the unaffected side (see Fig. 19.6). The resultant effect is decreased venous return and compression of the unaffected lung. Clinical signs include diminished breath sounds, hyperresonance to percussion, tachycardia, and hypotension. Treatment comprises administration of supplemental oxygen and insertion of a large-bore needle or catheter into the second intercostal space at the midclavicular line of the affected side. This action relieves the pressure within the chest. The needle remains in place until the patient is stabilized and a chest tube is inserted.[79,86]

Tension Pneumopericardium

A tension pneumopericardium develops when air enters the pericardial space and has no outlet for exiting. As pressure inside the pericardium increases, it results in compression of the heart and the development of cardiac tamponade. A pericardiocentesis is performed immediately to relieve the pressure within the pericardial sac.[83]

Nursing Management

The nursing management plan for a patient with an air leak disorder incorporates a variety of nursing diagnoses (Box 19.23). The nurse has a significant role in optimizing oxygenation and ventilation, maintaining the chest drainage system, providing comfort and emotional support, and maintaining surveillance for complications.

Optimize Oxygenation and Ventilation

Nursing interventions to optimize oxygenation and ventilation include positioning, preventing desaturation, and promoting secretion clearance. For further discussion of these interventions, see Nursing Management of Acute Lung Failure earlier in this chapter.

Maintain Chest Drainage System

Maintaining the chest drainage system involves careful attention to the suction applied and to maintenance of unobstructed drainage tubes. Kinks and large loops of tubing must be avoided because they impede drainage and air evacuation, which may prevent timely lung reexpansion or may result in a tension pneumothorax. Retained drainage also becomes an excellent medium for bacterial growth. The system is routinely observed for air leaks.[88]

If an air leak is present, the source is identified. To determine whether the source is within the system or within the patient, systematic brief clamping of the drainage tube is performed. A padded clamp is placed on the drainage tubing as close to the chest dressing as possible. If the air leak stops, the leak is located between the patient and the clamp. The air leak can be within the patient or at the insertion site. The clamp is then removed, and the chest tube site is exposed. The tube is inspected at the site where it enters the chest to ensure that all the eyelets are within the patient. If an eyelet port is outside the chest, it can be a source of an air leak and must be occluded, which may require the attention of the physician. After the insertion site has been eliminated as a leakage source, the chest dressing is reapplied, securely covering the site. If the air leak does not stop when a clamp is placed on the chest tube, the leak must be located between the clamp and the drainage collector. It can be found by releasing the clamp and moving it down the tubing a few inches at a time until the bubbling stops. After the area of the leak is located, it can be taped to reestablish a seal, or the system can be replaced.[88]

A sterile occlusive dressing and a bottle of sterile water should be available at the patient's bedside at all times. If the chest drainage system is inadvertently interrupted, the chest tube is placed a few centimeters into the bottle of water while the drainage system is reestablished. If the chest tube is inadvertently dislodged at the insertion site, a sterile dressing is placed on the site and taped on three sides. The fourth side should be left open to allow air to escape from the chest to avoid causing a tension pneumothorax. Immediate implementation of these techniques minimizes or prevents the formation of a pneumothorax and avoids greater complications.

Throughout the duration of chest tube placement, the patient is assessed periodically for reexpansion of the lung and for complications associated with the chest drainage system. The thorax and lungs are assessed, paying particular attention to any tracheal deviation, asymmetry of chest movement, presence of subcutaneous emphysema, characteristics of breathing, quality of lung sounds, and presence of tympany or percussion sounds, which are indicative of pneumothorax.

Interprofessional collaborative management of a patient with an air leak disorder is outlined in Box 19.24.

LONG-TERM MECHANICAL VENTILATOR DEPENDENCE

Description

Long-term mechanical ventilator dependence (LTMVD) is a secondary disorder that occurs when a patient requires assisted

BOX 19.24 QSEN: Teamwork and Collaboration

Interprofessional Collaborative Practice: Air Leak Disorders

- Administer oxygen therapy
- Intubate patient as needed
- Initiate mechanical ventilation as needed
- Evacuate air from the pleural space
  - Percutaneous catheter attached to Heimlich valve
  - Chest tube to chest drainage system
- Maintain surveillance for complications
  - Acute lung failure
- Maintain chest drainage system
- Provide comfort and emotional support

BOX 19.25 Physiologic Factors Contributing to Long-Term Mechanical Ventilator Dependence

Decreased gas exchange
  Ventilation/perfusion mismatching
  Intrapulmonary shunting
  Alveolar hypoventilation
  Anemia
  Acute heart failure
Increased ventilatory workload
  Decreased lung compliance
  Increased airway resistance
  Small endotracheal tube
  Decreased ventilatory sensitivity
  Improper positioning
  Abdominal distention
  Dyspnea
Increased ventilatory demand
  Increased pulmonary dead space
  Increased metabolic demands
  Improper ventilator mode/settings
  Metabolic acidosis
  Overfeeding
Decreased ventilatory drive
  Respiratory alkalosis
  Metabolic alkalosis
  Hypothyroidism
  Sedatives
  Malnutrition
Increased respiratory muscle fatigue
  Increased ventilatory workload
  Increased ventilatory demand
  Malnutrition
  Hypokalemia
  Hypomagnesemia
  Hypophosphatemia
  Hypothyroidism
  Critical illness polyneuropathy
  Inadequate muscle rest

ventilation longer than expected given the patient's underlying condition.[89] It is the result of complex medical problems that do not allow the weaning process to take place in a normal and timely manner. Generally, the patient has failed multiple weaning attempts.[90] A review of the literature reveals a great deal of confusion regarding an exact definition of LTMVD, particularly in regard to an actual time frame. In 2005, the National Association for Medical Direction of Respiratory Care Consensus Panel recommended that LTMVD (which they referred to as prolonged mechanical ventilation) be defined as "the need for greater than or equal to 21 consecutive days of mechanical ventilation for greater than or equal to 6 hours per day."[91]

Etiology and Pathophysiology

Approximately 20% of patients requiring mechanical ventilation develop LTMVD.[92] A wide variety of physiologic and psychologic factors contribute to the development of LTMVD. Physiologic factors include conditions that result in decreased gas exchange, increased ventilatory workload, increased ventilatory demand, decreased ventilatory drive, and increased respiratory muscle fatigue (Box 19.25).[90,92] Psychologic factors include conditions that result in loss of breathing pattern control, lack of motivation and confidence, and delirium (Box 19.26).[93] The development of LTMVD also is affected by the severity and duration of the patient's current illness and any underlying chronic health problems.[94]

Medical and Nursing Management

The goal of medical and nursing management of patients with LTMVD is successful weaning. The Third National Study Group on Weaning from Mechanical Ventilation, sponsored by the American Association of Critical-Care Nurses, proposed the Weaning Continuum Model, which divides weaning into three stages: preweaning, weaning process, and weaning outcome.[95] The management of a patient with LTMVD is described within this framework. In addition, the common nursing diagnoses for this patient population are listed in Box 19.27.

Preweaning Stage

For a patient with LTMVD, the preweaning phase consists of resolving the precipitating event that necessitated ventilatory assistance and preventing the physiologic and psychologic factors that can interfere with weaning. Before any attempts

at weaning, the patient is assessed for weaning readiness, an approach is determined, and a method is selected.[93,96]

Weaning preparedness. The patient should be physiologically and psychologically prepared to initiate the weaning process by addressing factors that can interfere with weaning. Aggressive medical management to prevent and treat $\dot{V}/\dot{Q}$ mismatching, intrapulmonary shunting, anemia, heart failure, decreased lung compliance, increased airway resistance, acid–base disturbances, hypothyroidism, abdominal distention, and electrolyte imbalances should be initiated. In addition, interventions to decrease the work of breathing should be implemented, such as replacing a small endotracheal tube with a larger tube or a tracheostomy, suctioning airway secretions, administering bronchodilators, optimizing the ventilator settings and trigger sensitivity, initiating early mobilization, and positioning the patient in straight alignment with the head of the bed elevated at least 30 degrees. Enteral or parenteral nutrition is started, and the patient's nutrition state optimized. Physical therapy is initiated for a patient with critical illness polyneuropathy because increased mobility facilitates weaning. A means

BOX 19.26   Psychologic Factors Contributing to Long-Term Mechanical Ventilator Dependence

Loss of breathing pattern control
  Anxiety
  Fear
  Dyspnea
  Pain
  Ventilator asynchrony
  Lack of confidence in ability to breathe
Lack of motivation and confidence
  Inadequate trust in staff
  Depersonalization
  Hopelessness
  Powerlessness
  Depression
  Inadequate communication
Delirium
  Sensory overload
  Sensory deprivation
  Sleep deprivation
  Pain
  Medications

BOX 19.27   NURSING DIAGNOSES

Long-Term Mechanical Ventilation Dependence

- Dysfunctional Ventilatory Weaning Response related to physical, psychosocial, or situational factors, p. 1024
- Risk for Aspiration, p. 1040
- Imbalanced Nutrition: Less Than Body Requirements related to lack of exogenous nutrients or increased metabolic demand, p. 1029
- Risk for Infection, p. 1046
- Acute Confusion related to sensory overload, sensory deprivation, and sleep pattern disturbance, p. 1007
- Disturbed Body Image related to functional dependence on life-sustaining technology, p. 1022
- Relocation Stress Syndrome related to transfer out of intensive care unit, p. 1039
- Powerlessness related to lack of control over current situation or disease progression, p. 1038
- Compromised Family Coping related to critically ill family member, p. 1014

of communication should be established with the patient. Sedatives can be administered to provide anxiety control, but it is critical to avoid respiratory depression.[96]

Weaning readiness. Although various methods for assessing weaning readiness have been developed, none has proven to be very accurate in predicting weaning success in a patient with LTMVD. One study indicated that the presence of left ventricular dysfunction, fluid imbalance, and nutrition deficiency increased the duration of mechanical ventilation. Another study suggested that the upward trending of the albumin level may be predictive of weaning success. Because so many variables can affect the patient's ability to wean, any assessment of weaning readiness should incorporate these variables. Cardiac function, gas exchange, pulmonary mechanics, nutrition status, electrolyte and fluid balance, and motivation are considered when making the decision to wean. This assessment is ongoing to reflect the dynamic nature of the process.[97]

Weaning approach. Although weaning patients requiring short-term mechanical ventilation is a relatively simple process that can usually be accomplished with a nurse and respiratory therapist, weaning a patient with LTMVD is a much more complex process that usually requires a multidisciplinary team approach. Multidisciplinary weaning teams that use a coordinated and collaborative approach to weaning have demonstrated improved patient outcomes and decreased weaning times. The team ideally consists of a physician, nurse, respiratory therapist, dietitian, physical therapist, social worker or case manager, and clinical nurse specialist. Additional members, if possible, include an occupational therapist, a speech therapist, and a discharge planner. Working together, the team members develop a comprehensive plan of care for the patient that is efficient, consistent, progressive, and cost-effective.[98] Several studies have demonstrated successful weaning through the use of nurse and respiratory therapist–managed protocols.[99]

Weaning method. Various weaning methods are available, and no one method has consistently proven to be superior to the others. These methods include T-tube (T-piece), CPAP, pressure support ventilation (PSV), and SIMV. One multicenter study lends evidence to support the use of PSV for weaning over T-tube or SIMV weaning. Often these weaning methods are used in combination with each other, such as SIMV with PSV, CPAP with PSV, or SIMV with CPAP.[90,94]

Weaning Process Stage

For a patient with LTMVD, the weaning process phase consists of initiating the weaning method selected and minimizing the physiologic and psychologic factors that can interfere with weaning.[92,93] It is imperative that the patient not become exhausted during this phase because this can result in a setback in the weaning process.[96] During this phase, the patient is assessed for weaning progress and signs of weaning intolerance.[94]

Weaning initiation. Ideally weaning is initiated in the morning while the patient is rested. Before starting the weaning process, the patient is given an explanation of how the process works and a description of the sensations to expect and is reassured that he or she will be closely monitored and returned to the original ventilator mode and settings if any difficulty occurs.[94] This information is reinforced with each weaning attempt. One study showed that family presence during the weaning trial was beneficial and that the trials were longer when the family was present.[100]

T-tube and CPAP weaning are accomplished by removing the patient from the ventilator and placing the patient on a T-tube or placing the patient on CPAP mode for a specified duration of time, known as a weaning trial, for a specified number of times per day. When the weaning trial is over, the patient is placed on the assist-control mode or similar mode and allowed to rest to prevent respiratory muscle fatigue. The duration of time spent weaning is gradually increased, as is the frequency, until the patient is able to breathe spontaneously for 24 hours. If PSV is used in conjunction with CPAP, the PSV is initially set to provide the patient with an assisted tidal volume of 10 to 12 mL/kg, and this is gradually weaned until a level of 6 to 8 cm H_2O of pressure support is achieved. Weaning with SIMV and PSV is accomplished by gradually decreasing

TABLE 19.7 Indications of Weaning Intolerance and Interventions

Indicator	Etiology	Intervention
Pulmonary Signs (Emotional)		
Altered breathing pattern	Inadequate understanding of weaning process	Build trust in staff; consistent care providers
Dyspnea intensity		Encouragement; concrete goals for extubation
Change in facial expression	Inability to control breathing pattern	Involve patient in process and planning daily activities
		Efficient communication established
	Environmental factors	Organize care; avoid interruptions during weaning
		Adequate sleep
		Calm, caring presence of nurse; nonsedating anxiolytics
		Measure dyspnea
		Fan; music
		Biofeedback; relaxation; breathing control
		Family involvement; normalizing daily activities
Pulmonary Signs (Physiologic)		
Accessory muscle use	Airway obstruction	Suction/air-mask bag unit ventilation; manually ventilate patient
Prolonged expiration	Secretions/atelectasis	
Asynchronous movements of chest and abdomen	Bronchospasm	Bronchodilators
	Patient position/kinked	Sitting upright in bed or chair or per patient preference
Retractions	ET tube	
Facial expression changes	Increased workload or muscle	
Dyspnea	Fatigue	
Shortened inspiratory time	Caloric intake	Nutrition assessment
Increased breathing frequency, decreased Vt	Electrolyte imbalances	Assess electrolytes; give replacements as necessary
	Inadequate rest	Rest between weaning trials (ie, SIMV frequency rate >5)
	Patient/ventilator interactions	Assess ventilator settings (ie, flow rate, trigger sensitivity)
	Increased Ve requirement	Muscle training if appropriate
	Infection	Check for infection (treat if indicated)
	Overfeeding	Appropriate caloric intake
	Respiratory alkalosis	Baseline ABGs achieved (ventilate according to pH)
	Anxiety	Coaching to regularize breathing pattern; give nonsedating anxiolytics
	Pain	Judicious use of analgesics
CNS Changes		
Restless/irritable	Hypoxemia/hypercarbia	Increase Fio_2
Decreased responsiveness		Return to mechanical ventilation
		Discern etiology and treat
CV Deterioration		
Excessive change in BP or HR	Heart failure	Diuretics as ordered
	Increase venous return	Beta-blockers
Dysrhythmias	Ischemia	Increase Fio_2
Angina		Return to mechanical ventilation
Dyspnea		Discern etiology and treat

ABGs, arterial blood gases; *BP*, blood pressure; *CNS*, central nervous system; *CV*, cardiovascular; *ET*, endotracheal; *Fio₂*, fraction of inspired oxygen; *HR*, heart rate; *SIMV*, synchronized intermittent mandatory ventilation; *Ve*, respiratory minute volume; *Vt*, tidal volume.
Modified from Knebel AR: When weaning from mechanical ventilation fails. *Am J Crit Care*, 1(3):19-29, 1992

the number of breaths or the amount of pressure support the patient receives by a specified amount until the patient is able to breathe spontaneously for 24 hours.[94]

Weaning progress. Weaning progress can be evaluated using various methods. Evaluation of weaning progress when using a weaning method that gradually withdraws ventilatory support, such as SIMV or PSV, can be accomplished by measuring the percentage of the minute ventilation requirement that is provided by the ventilator. If the percentage steadily decreases, weaning is progressing. Evaluation of weaning progress when using a weaning method that removes ventilatory support, such

as T-tube or CPAP, can be accomplished by measuring the amount of time the patient remains free from support. If the time steadily increases, weaning is progressing.[94]

Weaning intolerance. Once the weaning process has begun, the patient is continuously assessed for signs of intolerance. When present, these signs indicate when to place the patient back on the ventilator or to return the patient to the previous ventilator settings. Commonly used indicators include dyspnea; accessory muscle use; restlessness; anxiety; change in facial expression; changes in heart rate and blood pressure; rapid, shallow breathing; and discomfort.[97] Table 19.7 lists the different weaning intolerance indicators and actions that can be taken to control or prevent them.

Facilitative therapies. Additional therapies may be needed to facilitate weaning in a patient who is having difficulty making weaning progress. These therapies include ventilatory muscle training and biofeedback. Inspiratory muscle training is used to enhance the strength and endurance of the respiratory muscles. Biofeedback can be used to promote relaxation and assist in the management of dyspnea and anxiety.[94]

Weaning Outcome Stage

Two outcomes are possible for a patient with LTMVD: weaning completed and incomplete weaning.[94]

Weaning completed. Weaning is deemed successful when a patient is able to breathe spontaneously for 24 hours without ventilatory support. When this occurs, the patient may be extubated or decannulated at any time, although this is not necessary for weaning to be considered successful.[95]

QSEN BOX 19.28 **QSEN: Informatics**

Internet Resources

American Association of Critical-Care Nurses: http://www.aacn.org
Society for Critical Care Medicine: http://www.sccm.org
Respiratory Nursing Society: http://respiratorynursingsociety.org
American Association of Respiratory Care: http://www.aarc.org
American College of Chest Physicians: http://www.chestnet.org/accp
NHLBI ARDS Network: http://www.ardsnet.org
American College of Physicians: http://www.acponline.org
American Lung Association: http://www.lung.org
American Medical Association: http://www.ama-assn.org
American Thoracic Society: http://www.thoracic.org
Centers for Disease Control and Prevention: http://www.cdc.gov
National Institutes for Health: http://www.nih.gov
PubMed Health: http://www.ncbi.nlm.nih.gov/pubmedhealth
American Society for Parenteral and Enteral Nutrition: http://www.nutrition-care.org

---

Incomplete weaning. Weaning is deemed incomplete when a patient has reached a plateau (5 days at the same ventilatory support level without any changes) in the weaning process despite managing the physiologic and psychologic factors that impede weaning. Thus the patient is unable to breathe spontaneously for 24 hours without full or partial ventilatory support. Once this occurs, the patient is placed in a subacute ventilator facility or discharged home on a ventilator with home care nursing follow-up.[95]

SUMMARY

Acute Lung Failure

- ALF is a clinical condition in which the pulmonary system fails to maintain adequate gas exchange; it results from a deficiency in the performance of the pulmonary system.
- Hypoxemia is the hallmark of ALF and is the result of impaired gas exchange as a result of alveolar hypoventilation, $\dot{V}/\dot{Q}$ mismatching, or intrapulmonary shunting.
- Medical management focuses on treatment of the underlying cause, promotion of adequate gas exchange, correction of acidosis, initiation of nutrition support, and prevention of

complications (ie, ischemic-anoxic encephalopathy, cardiac dysrhythmias, VTE, and gastrointestinal bleeding).
- Nursing actions include optimizing oxygenation and ventilation (by positioning, preventing desaturation, and promoting secretion clearance), providing comfort and emotional support, maintaining surveillance for complications, and educating the patient and family.

Acute Respiratory Distress Syndrome

- ARDS is characterized by noncardiac pulmonary edema and disruption of the alveolar-capillary membrane as a result of injury to the pulmonary vasculature or the airways.
- The hallmark of ARDS is refractory hypoxemia.
- Medical management focuses on treatment of the underlying cause, promotion of gas exchange, support of tissue oxygenation, and prevention of complications.
- Nursing actions include optimizing oxygenation and ventilation, providing comfort and emotional support, and maintaining surveillance for complications.

Pneumonia

- Pneumonia is an acute inflammation of the lung parenchyma caused by an infectious agent that can lead to alveolar consolidation and can be classified as community acquired or hospital acquired.
- Medical management focuses on initiation of antibiotic therapy, administration of oxygen and mechanical ventilation, management of fluids and nutrition support, and treatment of complications.
- Nursing actions include optimizing oxygenation and ventilation, preventing the spread of infection, providing comfort and emotional support, and maintaining surveillance for complications.

Aspiration Pneumonitis

- Aspiration pneumonitis is the presence of abnormal toxic substances in the airways and alveoli, resulting in injury to the lungs.
- Medical management focuses on clearance of the toxic substance from the airways, support of oxygenation, and maintenance of hemodynamics.
- Nursing actions include optimizing oxygenation and ventilation, preventing further aspiration events, providing comfort and emotional support, and maintaining surveillance for complications.

Pulmonary Embolism

- A PE occurs when a clot (thrombotic embolus) or other matter (nonthrombotic embolus) lodges in the pulmonary arterial system, disrupting the blood flow to a region of the lungs.
- Medical management focuses on prevention of the recurrence of PE, initiation of clot dissolution, reversal of the effects of pulmonary hypertension, promotion of gas exchange, and prevention of complications.
- Nursing actions include optimizing oxygenation and ventilation, monitoring for bleeding, providing comfort and emotional support, maintaining surveillance for complications, and educating the patient and family.

Status Asthmaticus

- Status asthmaticus is a severe asthma attack that fails to respond to conventional therapy with bronchodilators; it may result in ALF.

- Medical management focuses on support of oxygenation (by bronchodilators, corticosteroids, and oxygen therapy) and ventilation.
- Nursing actions include optimizing oxygenation and ventilation, providing comfort and emotional support, maintaining surveillance for complications, and educating the patient and family.

Air Leak Disorders

- Air leak disorders consist of conditions that result in extraalveolar air accumulation and are classified into two categories: pneumothorax and barotrauma/volutrauma.
- Two conditions that require emergency intervention for immediate relief are a tension pneumothorax and a tension pneumopericardium.
- Nursing actions include optimizing oxygenation and ventilation, maintaining the chest drainage system, providing comfort and emotional support, and maintaining surveillance for complications.

Long-Term Mechanical Ventilation Dependence

- LTMVD is a secondary disorder that occurs when a patient requires assisted ventilation for longer than expected given the patient's underlying condition.
- Weaning can be divided into three stages: preweaning, weaning process, and weaning outcome.
- The preweaning phase consists of resolving the precipitating event that necessitated ventilatory assistance and preventing the physiologic and psychologic factors that can interfere with weaning.
- The weaning process phase consists of initiating the weaning method selected and minimizing the physiologic and psychologic factors that can interfere with weaning.
- Weaning is deemed successful when the patient is able to breathe spontaneously for 24 hours without ventilatory support.
- Ⓔ Visit the Evolve site for additional study materials.

REFERENCES

1. Mac Sweeney R, McAuley DF, Matthay MA. Acute lung failure. *Semin Respir Crit Care Med.* 2011;32(5):607–625.
2. Schneider J, Sweberg T. Acute respiratory failure. *Crit Care Clin.* 2013;29(2):167–183.
3. Wright BJ. Lung-protective ventilation strategies and adjunctive treatments for the emergency medicine patient with acute respiratory failure. *Emerg Med Clin N Am.* 2014;32(4):871–887.
4. Balk R, Bone RC. Classification of acute respiratory failure. *Med Clin North Am.* 1983;67(3):551–556.
5. Markou NK, Myrianthefs PM, Baltopoulos GJ. Respiratory failure: an overview. *Crit Care Nurs Q.* 2004;27(4):353–379.
6. Raju P, Manthous CA. The pathogenesis of respiratory failure: an overview. *Respir Care Clin N Am.* 2000;6(2):195–212.
7. Lee WL, Slutsky AS. Acute hypoxemic respiratory failure and ARDS. In: Broaddus VC, et al., ed. *Murray and Nadel's Textbook of Respiratory Medicine.* 6th ed. Philadelphia: Saunders; 2016.
8. Loiacono LA, Shapiro DS. Detection of hypoxia at the cellular level. *Crit Care Clin.* 2010;26(2):409–421.
9. Hill NS. Acute ventilatory failure. In: Broaddus VC, et al., ed. *Murray and Nadel's Textbook of Respiratory Medicine.* 6th ed. Philadelphia: Saunders; 2016.
10. Dakin J, Griffiths M. The pulmonary physician in critical care 1: pulmonary investigations for acute respiratory failure. *Thorax.* 2002;57(1):79–85.
11. Martin SD, Grocott MPW. Oxygen therapy in critical illness: precise control of arterial oxygenation and permissive hypoxemia. *Crit Care Med.* 2013;41(2):423–432.
12. Frat JP, et al. Sequential application of oxygen therapy via high-flow nasal cannula and noninvasive ventilation in acute respiratory failure: an observational pilot study. *Respir Care.* 2015;60(2):170–178.
13. Gregorett C, et al. Noninvasive ventilation in critically ill patients. *Crit Care Clin.* 2015;31(3):435–457.
14. Soo Hoo GW, Hakimian N, Santiago SM. Hypercapnic respiratory failure in COPD patients: response to therapy. *Chest.* 2000;117(1):169–177.
15. Ward NS, Dushay KM. Clinical concise review: mechanical ventilation of patients with chronic obstructive pulmonary disease. *Crit Care Med.* 2008;36(5):1614–1619.
16. Dodwell RL, Kendall JB. Respiratory system: applied pharmacology. *Anaesth Intensive Care Med.* 2014;15(11):517–521.
17. Barr J, et al. Clinical practice guidelines for the management of pain, agitation, and delirium in adult patients in the intensive care unit. *Crit Care Med.* 2013;41(1):263–306.
18. Greenberg SB, Vender J. The use of neuromuscular blocking agents in the ICU: where are we now? *Crit Care Med.* 2013;41(5):1332–1344.
19. Kraut JA, Madias NE. Lactic acidosis. *N Engl J Med.* 2014;371(24):2309–2319.
20. McClave SA, et al. Guidelines for the provision and assessment of nutrition support therapy in the adult critically ill patient: Society of Critical Care Medicine (SCCM) and American Society for Parenteral and Enteral Nutrition (ASPEN). *J Parenter Enteral Nutr.* 2016;40(2):159–211.
21. Casaer MP, Van den Berghe G. Nutrition in the acute phase of critical illness. *N Engl J Med.* 2014;370(13):1227–1236.
22. Boot R. Delirium: a review of the nurses role in the intensive care unit. *Intensive Crit Care Nurs.* 2012;28(3):185–189.
23. van der Jagt, Miranda DR. Beta-blockers in intensive care medicine: potential benefit in acute brain injury and acute respiratory distress syndrome. *Recent Pat Cardiovasc Drug Discov.* 2012;7(2):141–151.
24. Kahn SR, et al. Prevention of VTE in nonsurgical patients: antithrombotic therapy and prevention of thrombosis, 9th ed: American College of Chest Physicians Evidence-Based Clinical Practice Guidelines. *Chest.* 2012;141(suppl 2):e195S–e226S.
25. Webster B, Newman C. Gastrointestinal dysfunction. *Surgery (Oxford).* 2015;33(10):505–509.
26. Wong WP. Use of body positioning in the mechanically ventilated patient with acute respiratory failure: application of Sackett's rules of evidence. *Physiother Theory Pract.* 1999;15(1):25–41.
27. Johnson KL, Meyenburg T. Physiological rationale and current evidence for therapeutic positioning of critically ill patients. *AACN Adv Crit Care.* 2009;20(3):228–242.
28. Marklew A. Body positioning and its effect on oxygenation—a literature review. *Nurs Crit Care.* 2006;11(1):16–22.
29. Cosenza JJ, Norton LC. Secretion clearance: state-of-the-art from a nursing perspective. *Crit Care Nurse.* 1986;6(4):23–39.
30. Metheny NA, Frantz RA. Head-of-bed elevation in critically ill patients: a review. *Crit Care Nurse.* 2013;33(3):53–66.
31. Krishnagopalan S, et al. Body positioning of intensive care patients: clinical practice versus standards. *Crit Care Med.* 2002;30(11):2588–2592.
32. Stiller K. Physiotherapy in intensive care: an updated systematic review. *Chest.* 2013;144(3):825–847.
33. Stickland SL, et al. AARC clinical practice guideline: effectiveness of nonpharmacologic airway clearance therapies in hospitalized patients. *Respir Care.* 2013;58(12):2187–2193.
34. Del Sorbo L, Slutsky AS. Acute respiratory distress syndrome and multiple organ failure. *Curr Opin Crit Care.* 2011;17(1):1–6.
35. Khan A, Kantrow S, Taylor DE. Acute respiratory distress syndrome. *Hosp Med Clin.* 2015;4(4):500–512.
36. The ARDS Definition Task Force. Acute respiratory distress syndrome: the Berlin Definition. *JAMA.* 2012;307(23):2526–2533.
37. Blank R, Napolitano LM. Epidemiology of ARDS and ALI. *Crit Care Clin.* 2011;27(3):439–458.
38. Dechert RE, Hass CF, Ostwani W. Current knowledge of acute lung injury and acute respiratory distress syndrome. *Crit Care Nurs Clin N Am.* 2012;24(3):377–401.
39. Matthay MA, Zemans RL. The acute respiratory distress syndrome: pathogenesis and treatment. *Annu Rev Pathol.* 2011;6:147–163.

40. Saguil A, Fargo M. Acute respiratory distress syndrome: diagnosis and management. *Am Fam Physician*. 2012;85(4):352–358.

41. Matthay MA, Ware LB, Zimmerman GA. The acute respiratory distress syndrome. *J Clin Invest*. 2012;122(8):2731–2740.

42. Bieh M, Kashiouris MG, Gajic O. Ventilator-induced lung injury: minimizing its impact in patients with or at risk for ARDS. *Respir Care*. 2013;58(3):927–937.

43. Ochiai R. Mechanical ventilation of acute respiratory distress syndrome. *J Intensive Care*. 2015;3(1):25.

44. Contreras M, Masterson C, Laffey JG. Permissive hypercapnia: what to remember. *Curr Opin Anaesthesiol*. 2015;28(1):26–37.

45. Shekar K, et al. To ventilate, oscillate, or cannulate? *J Crit Care*. 2013;28(5):655–662.

46. Abrams D, Brodie D. Extracorporeal circulatory approaches to treat acute respiratory distress syndrome. *Clin Chest Med*. 2014;35(4):765–779.

47. Gattinoni L, Cressoni M, Brazzi L. Fluids in ARDS: from onset through recovery. *Curr Opin Crit Care*. 2014;20(4):373–377.

48. Dirkes S, et al. Prone positioning: is it safe and effective? *Crit Care Nurs Q*. 2012;35(1):64–75.

49. American Thoracic Society. Infectious Diseases Society of America: Guidelines for the management of adults with hospital-acquired, ventilator-associated, and healthcare-associated pneumonia. *Am J Respir Crit Care Med*. 2005;171(4):388–416.

50. Remington LT, Sligi WI. Community-acquired pneumonia. *Curr Opin Pulm Med*. 2014;20(3):215–224.

51. Prina E, Raznzani OT, Torres A. Community-acquired pneumonia. *Lancet*. 2015;386(9998):1097–1108.

52. Ottosen J, Evans H. Pneumonia: challenges in the definition, diagnosis, and management of disease. *Surg Clin North Am*. 2014;95(6):130501317.

53. Nair GB, Niederman MS. Nosocomial pneumonia: lessons learned. *Crit Care Clin*. 2013;29(3):521–546.

54. Labelle A, Kollef MH. Healthcare-associated pneumonia: approach to management. *Clin Chest Med*. 2011;32(3):507–515.

55. Lopez A, Amaro R, Polverion E. Does health care associated pneumonia really exist? *Eur J Intern Med*. 2012;23(5):407–411.

56. Komiya K, Ishii H, Kadota J. Healthcare-associated pneumonia and aspiration pneumonia. *Aging Dis*. 2014;6(1):27–37.

57. Driver C. Pneumonia part 1: pathology, presentation and prevention. *Br J Nurs*. 2012;21(2).

58. Pines JM. Timing of antibiotics for acute, severe infections. *Emerg Med Clin North Am*. 2008;26(2):245–257.

59. Anantham D, Jagadesan R, Tiew PE. Clinical review: independent lung ventilation in critical care. *Crit Care*. 2005;9(6):594–600.

60. Osman MF, Askari R. Infection control in the intensive care unit. *Surg Clin North Am*. 2014;94(6):1175–1194.

61. Kendall A, et al. Point-of-care hand hygiene: preventing infection behind the curtain. *Am J Infect Control*. 2012;40(suppl 1):S3–S10.

62. Paintal HS, Kuschner WG. Aspiration syndromes: 10 clinical pearls every physician should know. *Int J Clin Pract*. 2007;61(5):846–852.

63. Marik PE. Pulmonary aspiration syndrome. *Curr Opin Pulm Med*. 2011;17(3):148–154.

64. Raghavendran K, et al. Aspiration-induced lung injury. *Crit Care Med*. 2011;39(4):818826.

65. Schallom M, et al. Gastroesophageal reflux in critically ill patients. *Dimens Crit Care Nurs*. 2013;32(2):69–77.

66. Truong TTN, Jones SD, Dunn AS. Pulmonary embolism. *Hosp Med Clin*. 2014;3(4).

67. Jaff MR, et al. Management of massive and submassive pulmonary embolism, iliofemoral deep vein thrombosis, and chronic thromboembolic pulmonary hypertension: a scientific statement from the American Heart Association. *Circulation*. 2011;123(16):1788–1830.

68. Tonelli AR, Dweik RA, Arroliga AC. Pulmonary vascular disease. In: Kacmarek RM, Stoller JK, Heuer AJ, eds. *Egan's Fundamentals of Respiratory Care*. 10th ed. St. Louis: Mosby; 2013.

69. Smithburger PL, Campbell S, Kane-Gill SL. Alteplase treatment of acute pulmonary embolism in the intensive care unit. *Crit Care Nurse*. 2013;33(2):17–27.

70. Moorjani N, Price S. Massive pulmonary embolism. *Cardiol Clin*. 2013;31(4):503–518.

71. Kearon C, et al. Antithrombotic therapy for VTE disease: antithrombotic therapy and prevention of thrombosis, 9th ed: American College of Chest Physicians Evidence-Based Clinical Practice Guidelines. *Chest*. 2012;141(suppl 2):419S–e494S.

72. Samoukovic G, Malas T, deVarennes B. The role of pulmonary embolectomy in the treatment of acute pulmonary embolism: a literature review from 1968 to 2008. *Interact Cardiovasc Thorac Surg*. 2010;11(3):265–270.

73. Fairfax LM, Sing RF. Vena cava interruption. *Crit Care Clin*. 2011;27(4):781–804.

74. Fanta CH, Long AA. Difficult asthma: assessment and management, part 2. *Allergy Asthma Proc*. 2012;33(4):313–323.

75. Mannam P, Siegel MD. Analytic review: management of life-threatening asthma in adults. *J Intensive Care Med*. 2010;25(1):3–15.

76. Murata A, Ling PM. Asthma diagnosis and management. *Emerg Med Clin N Am*. 2012;30(2):203–222.

77. Restrepo RD, Peters J. Near-fatal asthma: recognition and management. *Curr Opin Pulm Med*. 2008;14(1):13–23.

78. Likhar N, et al. The impact of severe asthma on the quality of life: a systematic review. *Value in Health*. 2015;18(7):A710.

79. Strange C. Pleural diseases. In: Kacmarek RM, Stoller JK, Heuer AJ, eds. *Egan's Fundamentals of Respiratory Care*. 10th ed. St. Louis: Mosby; 2013.

80. van Berkel V, Kuo E, Meyers BF. Pneumothorax, bullous disease, and emphysema. *Surg Clin N Am*. 2010;90(5):935–953.

81. Flanders S, Gunn S. Pulmonary issues in acute and critical care: pulmonary embolism and ventilator-induced lung injury. *Crit Care Nurs Clin N Am*. 2011;23(4):617–634.

82. Banki F, et al. Pneumomediastinum: etiology and a guide to diagnosis and treatment. *Am J Surg*. 2013;206(6):1001–1006.

83. Xu Y, Xu Z, Wang Y. Cardiac tamponade due to pneumopericardium. *Pak J Med Sci*. 2014;30(4):924–929.

84. Azok JT, Stoller JK. A review of thoracic imaging. In: Kacmarek RM, Stoller JK, Heuer AJ, eds. *Egan's Fundamentals of Respiratory Care*. 11th ed. St. Louis: Elsevier; 2017.

85. Hakim SY, et al. Pneumoperitoneum in a patient with pneumothorax and blunt neck trauma. *Int J Surg Case Rep*. 2014;5(12):1106–1109.

86. Yarmus L, Feller-Kopman D. Pneumothorax in the critically ill patient. *Chest*. 2012;141(4):1098–1105.

87. Cooke DT, David EA. Large-bore and small-bore chest tubes: types, function, and placement. *Thorac Surg Clin*. 2013;23(1):17–24.

88. Kane CJ, York NL. Minton LA: Chest tubes in the critically ill patient. *Dimens Crit Care Nurs*. 2013;32(3):111–117.

89. Knebel AR, et al. Weaning from mechanical ventilation: concept development. *Am J Crit Care*. 1994;3(6):416–420.

90. White AC. Long-term mechanical ventilation: management strategies. *Respir Care*. 2012;57(6):889–897.

91. MacIntyre NR, et al. Management of patients requiring prolonged mechanical ventilation: report of a NAMDRC Consensus Conference. *Chest*. 2005;128(6):3937–3954.

92. Navalesi P, et al. Prolonged weaning: from the intensive care unit to home. *Rev Port Pneumol*. 2014;20(5):264–272.

93. MacIntyre NR. Psychological factors in weaning from mechanical ventilatory support. *Respir Care*. 1995;40(3):277–2781.

94. Burns SM. Weaning from mechanical ventilation. In: Burns SM, ed. *Care of Mechanically Ventilated Patients*. 2nd ed. Sudbury, MD: Jones & Bartlett; 2007.

95. Knebel AR, et al. Weaning from mechanical ventilatory support: refinement of a model. *Am J Crit Care*. 1998;7(2):149–152.

96. El-Khatib MF, Bou-Khalil P. Clinical review: liberation from mechanical ventilation. *Crit Care*. 2008;12(4):221.

97. Cox CE, Carson SS. Prolonged mechanical ventilation. In: MacIntyre NR, Branson RD, eds. *Mechanical Ventilation*. 2nd ed. St. Louis: Saunders; 2009.

98. White V, Curry J, Botti M. Multidisciplinary team developed and implemented protocols to assist mechanical ventilation weaning: a systematic review of literature. *Worldviews Evid Based Nurs*. 2011;8(1):51–59.

99. Hass CF, Loik PS. Ventilator discontinuation protocols. *Respir Care*. 2012;57(10):1649–1662.

100. Happ MB, et al. Family presence and surveillance during weaning from prolonged mechanical ventilation. *Heart Lung*. 2007;36(1):47–57.

20

Pulmonary Therapeutic Management

Kathleen M. Stacy

OXYGEN THERAPY

Normal cellular function depends on the delivery of an adequate supply of oxygen to the cells to meet their metabolic needs. The goal of oxygen therapy is to provide a sufficient concentration of inspired oxygen to permit full use of the oxygen-carrying capacity of the arterial blood; this ensures adequate cellular oxygenation, provided that the cardiac output and hemoglobin concentration are adequate.[1,2]

Principles of Therapy

Oxygen is an atmospheric gas that must also be considered a medication because—similar to most other medications—it has detrimental as well as beneficial effects. Oxygen is one of the most commonly used and misused medications. As a medication, oxygen must be administered for good reason and in a proper, safe manner.[1] Oxygen is usually ordered in liters per minute (L/min), as a concentration of oxygen expressed as a percentage (eg, 40%), or as a fraction of inspired oxygen (FIO_2; eg, 0.4).

The primary indication for oxygen therapy is hypoxemia.[3] The amount of oxygen administered depends on the pathophysiologic mechanisms affecting the patient's oxygenation status. In most cases, the amount required should provide an arterial partial pressure of oxygen (PaO_2) of greater than 60 mm Hg or an arterial hemoglobin saturation (SaO_2) of greater than 90% during rest and exercise.[2] The concentration of oxygen given to an individual patient is a clinical judgment based on the many factors that influence oxygen transport, such as hemoglobin concentration, cardiac output, and arterial oxygen tension.[2]

After oxygen therapy has begun, the patient is continuously assessed for level of oxygenation and the factors affecting it. The patient's oxygenation status is evaluated several times daily until the desired oxygen level has been reached and has stabilized. If the desired response to the amount of oxygen delivered is not achieved, the oxygen supplementation is adjusted, and the patient's condition is reevaluated. It is important to use this dose-response method so that the lowest possible level of oxygen is administered that will still achieve a satisfactory PaO_2 or SaO_2.[2,3]

Methods of Delivery

Oxygen therapy can be delivered by many different devices (Table 20.1). Common problems with these devices include system leaks and obstructions, device displacement, and skin irritation. These devices are classified as low-flow, reservoir, or high-flow systems.[3]

Low-Flow Systems

A low-flow oxygen delivery system provides supplemental oxygen directly into the patient's airway at a flow of 8 L/min or less. Because this flow is insufficient to meet the patient's inspiratory volume requirements, this method of oxygen delivery results in a variable FIO_2 as the supplemental oxygen is mixed with room air. The patient's ventilatory pattern affects the FIO_2 of a low-flow system: As this pattern changes, differing amounts of room air gas are mixed with the constant flow of oxygen. A nasal cannula is an example of a low-flow device.[3]

Reservoir Systems

A reservoir system incorporates some type of device to collect and store oxygen between breaths. When the patient's inspiratory flow exceeds the oxygen flow of the oxygen delivery system, the patient is able to draw from the reservoir of oxygen to meet his or her inspiratory volume needs. Less mixing of the inspired oxygen occurs with room air than in a low-flow system. A reservoir oxygen delivery system can deliver a higher FIO_2 than a low-flow system. Examples of reservoir systems are simple face masks, partial rebreathing masks, and nonrebreathing masks.[3]

High-Flow Systems

With a high-flow system, the oxygen flows out of the device and into the patient's airways in an amount sufficient to meet all inspiratory volume requirements. This type of system is not affected by the patient's ventilatory pattern. A high-flow system uses either an air-entrainment system or a blending system to mix air and oxygen to achieve the desired FIO_2. An air-entrainment mask is an example of a high-flow system that delivers precisely controlled oxygen at the lower FIO_2 range.[3]

One newer high-flow system is the high-flow nasal cannula. With this system, warmed and humidified oxygen is delivered to the patient via a nasal cannula using a blending system. This system has been shown to improve oxygenation and ventilation and decrease the work of breathing in a patient with acute lung failure. A high-flow nasal cannula also is more comfortable and better tolerated than similar therapies.[4]

Complications of Oxygen Therapy

Oxygen, similar to most medications, has adverse effects and complications resulting from its use. The adage, "If a little is good, a lot is better," does not apply to oxygen. The lung is designed to handle a concentration of 21% oxygen, with some adaptability to higher concentrations, but adverse effects and oxygen toxicity can result if a high concentration is administered for too long.[5]

487

TABLE 20.1   Oxygen Therapy Systems

Category	Device	Flow	FIO2 Range (%)	FIO2 Stability	Advantages	Disadvantages	Best Use
Low-flow	Nasal cannula	0.25–8 L/min (adults) ≤2 L/min (infants)	22–45	Variable	Use on adults, children, infants; easy to apply; disposable, low cost; well tolerated	Unstable, easily dislodged; high flows uncomfortable; can cause dryness or bleeding; polyps, deviated septum may block flow	Stable patient needing low FIO2; home care patient requiring long-term therapy
	Nasal catheter	0.25–8 L/min	22–45	Variable	Use on adults, children, infants; good stability; disposable, low cost	Difficult to insert; high flows increase back-pressure; needs regular changing; polyps, deviated septum may block insertion; may provoke gagging, air swallowing, aspiration	Procedures in which cannula is difficult to use (bronchoscopy); long-term care for infants
	Transtracheal catheter	0.25–4 L/min	22–35	Variable	Lower oxygen usage/cost; eliminates nasal/skin irritation; improved compliance; increased exercise tolerance; increased mobility; enhanced image	High cost; surgical complications; infection; mucus plugging; lost tract	Home care or ambulatory patients who need increased mobility or who do not accept nasal oxygen
Reservoir	Reservoir cannula	0.25–4 L/min	22–35	Variable	Lower oxygen usage/cost; increased mobility; less discomfort because of lower flows	Unattractive, cumbersome; poor compliance; must be regularly replaced; breathing pattern affects performance	Home care or ambulatory patients who need increased mobility
	Simple mask	5–12 L/min	35–50	Variable	Use on adults, children, infants; quick, easy to apply; disposable, inexpensive	Uncomfortable; must be removed for eating; prevents radiant heat loss; blocks vomitus in unconscious patients	Emergencies; short-term therapy requiring moderate FIO2
	Partial rebreathing mask	6–10 L/min (prevent bag collapse on inspiration)	35–60	Variable	Same as simple mask; moderate to high FIO2	Same as simple mask; potential suffocation hazard	Emergencies; short-term therapy requiring moderate to high FIO2
	Nonrebreathing mask	6–10 L/min (prevent bag collapse on inspiration)	55–70	Variable	Same as simple mask; high FIO2	Same as simple mask; potential suffocation hazard	Emergencies; short-term therapy requiring high FIO2
	Nonrebreathing circuit (closed)	3 × $\dot{V}_E$ (prevent bag collapse on inspiration)	21–100	Fixed	Full range of FIO2	Potential suffocation hazard; requires 50 psi air or oxygen; blender failure common	Patients requiring precise FIO2 at any level (21%–100%)
High-flow	Air-entrainment mask	Varies; should provide output flow >60 L/min	24–50	Fixed	Easy to apply; disposable, inexpensive; stable, precise FIO2	Limited to adult use; uncomfortable, noisy; must be removed for eating; FIO2 >0.40 not ensured; FIO2 varies with back-pressure	Unstable patients requiring precise low FIO2
	Air-entrainment nebulizer	10–15 L/min input; should provide output flow of at least 60 L/min	28–100	Fixed	Provides temperature control and extra humidification	FIO2 <28% or >0.40 not ensured; FIO2 varies with back-pressure; high infection risk	Patients with artificial airways requiring low to moderate FIO2
	Blending system (open)	Should provide output flow of at least 60 L/min	21–100	Fixed	Full range of FIO2	Requires 50 psi air + oxygen; blender failure or inaccuracy common	Patient with high $\dot{V}_E$ who need high FIO2

TABLE 20.1	Oxygen Therapy Systems—cont'd						
Category	Device	Flow	F_{IO_2} Range (%)	F_{IO_2} Stability	Advantages	Disadvantages	Best Use
	High-flow cannula system	Up to 40 L/min (depending on system)	35–90	Variable or fixed depending on system and input flow	Wide range of F_{IO_2} and relative or absolute humidity; use on adults, children, infants	F_{IO_2} not ensured depending on input flow and patient breathing pattern; infection risk	Patients of all ages with high or variable V_E who need supplemental oxygen, positive pressure, or humidity

F_{IO_2}, fraction of inspired oxygen; V_E, minute volume.
Modified from Heuer AJ: Medical gas therapy. In: Kacmarek RM, Stoller JK, Heuer AJ, eds. *Egan's Fundamentals of Respiratory Care*, 10th ed. St. Louis, 2013, Mosby.

Oxygen Toxicity

The most detrimental effect of breathing a high concentration of oxygen is the development of oxygen toxicity. Oxygen toxicity can occur in any patient who breathes oxygen concentrations of greater than 50% for longer than 24 hours. Oxygen toxicity is most likely to develop in patients who require intubation, mechanical ventilation, and high oxygen concentrations for extended periods.[3]

Hyperoxia, or the administration of higher-than-normal oxygen concentrations, produces an overabundance of oxygen free radicals. These radicals are responsible for the initial damage to the alveolar-capillary membrane. Oxygen free radicals are toxic metabolites of oxygen metabolism. Normally, enzymes neutralize the radicals, preventing any damage from occurring. During the administration of high levels of oxygen, the large number of oxygen free radicals produced exhausts the supply of neutralizing enzymes. Damage to the lung parenchyma and vasculature occurs, resulting in the initiation of acute respiratory distress syndrome (ARDS).[2,5]

Many clinical manifestations are associated with oxygen toxicity. The first symptom is substernal chest pain that is exacerbated by deep breathing. A dry cough and tracheal irritation follow. Eventually, definite pleuritic pain occurs on inhalation, followed by dyspnea. Upper airway changes may include a sensation of nasal stuffiness, sore throat, and increased pressure sensation in the ears. Chest radiographs and pulmonary function tests show no abnormalities until symptoms are severe. Complete, rapid reversal of these symptoms occurs as soon as normal oxygen concentrations are restored.[5]

Carbon Dioxide Retention

In patients with severe chronic obstructive pulmonary disease (COPD), carbon dioxide (CO_2) retention may occur as a result of administration of oxygen in high concentrations. Numerous theories have been proposed for this phenomenon. One states that the normal stimulus to breathe (ie, increasing CO_2 levels) is muted in patients with COPD and that decreasing oxygen levels become the stimulus to breathe. If hypoxemia is corrected by the administration of oxygen, the stimulus to breathe is abolished; hypoventilation develops, resulting in a further increase in the arterial partial pressure of carbon dioxide ($Paco_2$).[2,3] Another theory is that the administration of oxygen abolishes the compensatory response

of hypoxic pulmonary vasoconstriction. This results in an increase in perfusion of underventilated alveoli and the development of dead space, producing ventilation/perfusion ($\dot{V}/\dot{Q}$) mismatch. As alveolar dead space increases, so does CO_2 retention.[2,3] One further theory states that the increase in CO_2 is related to the ratio of deoxygenated to oxygenated hemoglobin (Haldane effect). Deoxygenated hemoglobin carries more CO_2 compared with oxygenated hemoglobin. Administration of oxygen increases the proportion of oxygenated hemoglobin, which causes increased release of CO_2 at the lung level.[5] Because of the risk of CO_2 accumulation, all patients who are chronically hypercapnic require careful low-flow oxygen administration.[3]

Absorption Atelectasis

Another adverse effect of high concentrations of oxygen is absorption atelectasis. Breathing high concentrations of oxygen washes out the nitrogen that normally fills the alveoli and helps hold them open (residual volume). As oxygen replaces the nitrogen in the alveoli, the alveoli start to shrink and collapse. This occurs because oxygen is absorbed into the bloodstream faster than it can be replaced in the alveoli, particularly in areas of the lungs that are minimally ventilated.[2,3]

Nursing Management

Nursing management of a patient receiving oxygen therapy focuses on ensuring the oxygen is being administered as ordered and observing for complications of the therapy. Confirming that the oxygen therapy device is properly positioned and replacing it after removal is important. During meals, an oxygen mask is changed to a nasal cannula if the patient can tolerate one. A patient receiving oxygen therapy is also transported with the oxygen. In addition, oxygen saturation is periodically monitored using a pulse oximeter.

ARTIFICIAL AIRWAYS

Pharyngeal Airways

Pharyngeal airways are used to maintain airway patency by keeping the tongue from obstructing the upper airway. The two types of pharyngeal airways are *oropharyngeal* and *nasopharyngeal airways*. Complications of these airways include trauma to the oral or nasal cavity, obstruction of the airway, laryngospasm, gagging, and vomiting.[6,7]

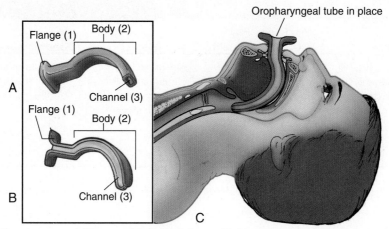

FIG. 20.1 Oropharyngeal Airways. (A) Guedel airway. (B) Berman airway. (C) Airway in place. (From Barnes TA. Emergency cardiovascular life support. In: Kacmarek RM, Stoller JK, Heuer AJ, eds. *Egan's Fundamentals of Respiratory Care*, 10th ed. St. Louis: Mosby; 2013.)

Oropharyngeal Airway

An oropharyngeal airway is made of plastic and is available in various sizes. The proper size is selected by holding the airway against the side of the patient's face and ensuring that it extends from the corner of the mouth to the angle of the jaw. If the airway is improperly sized, it will occlude the airway.[6,7] An oral airway is placed by inserting a tongue depressor into the patient's mouth to displace the tongue downward and then passing the airway into the patient's mouth, slipping it over the patient's tongue (Fig. 20.1).[7] When properly placed, the tip of the airway lies above the epiglottis at the base of the tongue. An oropharyngeal airway is used only in an unconscious patient who has an absent or diminished gag reflex.[6,7]

Nasopharyngeal Airway

A nasopharyngeal airway is usually made of plastic or rubber and is available in various sizes. The proper size is selected by holding the airway against the side of the patient's face and ensuring that the nasopharyngeal airway extends from the tip of the nose to the ear lobe.[6,7] A nasal airway is placed by lubricating the tube and inserting it midline along the floor of the naris into the posterior pharynx.[7] When properly placed, the tip of the airway lies above the epiglottis at the base of the tongue.[6,7]

Endotracheal Tubes

An endotracheal tube (ETT) is the most commonly used artificial airway for providing short-term airway management. Indications for endotracheal intubation include maintenance of airway patency, protection of the airway from aspiration, application of positive pressure ventilation, facilitation of pulmonary toilet, and use of high oxygen concentrations.[8] An ETT may be placed through the orotracheal route via direct laryngoscopy or video laryngoscopy or the nasotracheal route via blind nasal intubation.[9] In most situations involving emergency placement, the orotracheal route is used because this route is simpler and allows the use of a larger diameter ETT. Nasotracheal intubation provides greater patient comfort over time and is preferred in patients with a jaw fracture.[8] The advantages of orotracheal and nasotracheal intubation are presented in Table 20.2.

TABLE 20.2	Advantages of Orotracheal, Nasotracheal, and Tracheostomy Tubes	
Orotracheal Tubes	**Nasotracheal Tubes**	**Tracheostomy Tubes**
Easier access	Easily secured and stabilized	Easily secured and stabilized
Avoids nasal and sinus complications	Reduces risk of unintentional extubation	Reduces risk of unintentional decannulation
Allows for larger diameter tube, which facilitates	Well tolerated by patient	Well tolerated by patient
• Work of breathing • Suctioning • Fiberoptic bronchoscopy	Enables swallowing and oral hygiene	Enables swallowing, speech, and oral hygiene
	Facilitates communication	Avoids upper airway complications
	Avoids need for bite block	Allows for larger diameter tube, which facilitates • Work of breathing • Suctioning • Fiberoptic bronchoscopy

ETTs are available in various sizes, which are based on the inner diameters of the tubes, and have a radiopaque marker that runs the length of the tube. On one end of the tube is a cuff that is inflated with the use of the pilot balloon. Because of the high incidence of cuff-related problems, low-pressure, high-volume cuffs are preferred. On the other end of the tube is a 15-mm adapter that facilitates connection of the tube to a manual resuscitation bag (MRB), T-tube, or ventilator (Fig. 20.2).[10,11]

Rapid Sequence Intubation

Rapid sequence intubation (RSI) is a seven-step process that is often used to intubate a critically ill patient. This method is considered safer for the patient, as it decreases the risk of aspiration.[12,13]

FIG. 20.2 Endotracheal Tube. (Image used by permission from Nellcor Puritan Bennett LLC, Boulder, CO.)

A   B

FIG. 20.3 Insertion of Tube With Laryngoscope in Place. (A) Insert tube with the tip initially against the right buccal mucosa so that a clear view of the vocal cords can be maintained at all times. As it advances, watch the tube pass through the cord. (B) Tube is correctly placed when the tip is 2–3 cm beyond the vocal cords. (From Pfenninger JL, Fowler GC, eds. *Pfenninger and Fowler's Procedures for Primary Care*, 3rd ed. Philadelphia: Elsevier; 2011.)

FIG. 20.4 **Carbon Dioxide Detector.** Disposable colorimetric CO_2 detector for confirming tracheal intubation. (From Altobelli N. Airway management. In: Kacmarek RM, Stoller JK, Heuer AJ, eds. Egan's Fundamentals of Respiratory *Care*, 10th ed. St. Louis: Mosby; 2013.)

Step 1—preparation. Before intubation, the necessary equipment is gathered and organized to facilitate the procedure. Readily available equipment includes a suction system with catheters and tonsil suction, an MRB with a mask connected to 100% oxygen, a laryngoscope handle with assorted blades, ETTs in various sizes, and a stylet. Before the procedure is started, all equipment is inspected to ensure that the equipment is in working order. The patient is prepared for the procedure, if possible, with an intravenous catheter in place and monitored with a pulse oximeter.[12,13]

Step 2—preoxygenation. Once everything is ready, the patient is preoxygenated with 100% oxygen for 3 to 5 minutes via a tight-fitting face mask. If the patient is unable to maintain adequate spontaneous ventilations, assisted ventilations are initiated with an MRB. The goal is to avoid positive pressure ventilation, if possible, as this intervention increases the chances of gastric distention and the risk of aspiration.[12,13]

Step 3—pretreatment. While the patient is being preoxygenated, the patient is pretreated with adjunct medications to decrease the physiologic response to intubation. These medications include lidocaine, fentanyl, and atropine. A very low dose of a paralytic agent may be administered to prevent fasciculations. The use of these medications depends on the patient's underlying condition. If possible, pretreatment occurs 3 minutes before the next step.[12-14]

Step 4—paralysis with induction. A sedative agent and a paralytic agent are administered in "rapid sequence" to achieve induction and paralysis. Various sedative agents, including etomidate, midazolam, ketamine, and propofol, are used to facilitate rapid loss of consciousness. Induction dosages for these medications are usually slightly higher than the typical dosages used for sedation. The two most commonly administered neuromuscular blocking agents used to facilitate skeletal muscle relaxation are succinylcholine and rocuronium.[12-14]

Step 5—protection and positioning. The procedure is initiated by positioning the patient with the neck flexed and head slightly extended in the "sniff" position. The oral cavity and pharynx are suctioned, and any dental devices are removed.

Step 6—placement of endotracheal tube. The ETT is inserted into the trachea (Fig. 20.3), and placement is confirmed.[12,13] Each intubation attempt is limited to 30 seconds to prevent hypoxemia. After the ETT is inserted, the patient is assessed for bilateral breath sounds and chest movement. Absence of breath sounds is indicative of an esophageal intubation, whereas breath sounds heard over only one side of the chest is indicative of a main stem intubation. A disposable end-tidal CO_2 detector (Fig. 20.4) is used to initially verify correct airway placement, after which the cuff of the tube is inflated and the tube is secured. Finally, a chest radiograph is obtained to confirm placement.

The tip of the ETT should be approximately 3 to 4 cm above the carina when the patient's head is in the neutral position.[8]

Step 7—postintubation management. After final adjustment of the ETT position is complete, the level of insertion (marked in centimeters on the side of the tube) at the teeth is noted. The ETT is then secured to patient's face using tape or a commercial tube holder (Fig. 20.5). Securing the tube stabilizes it to prevent movement and potential dislodgment.[8]

Complications

Numerous complications can occur during the intubation procedure, including nasal and oral trauma, pharyngeal and hypopharyngeal trauma, vomiting with aspiration, and cardiac arrest.[15] Tracheal rupture is a rare and often fatal complication that is associated with emergent intubation.[16] Hypoxemia and hypercapnia can also occur, resulting in bradycardia, tachycardia, dysrhythmias, hypertension, and hypotension.[8,15]

Several complications can occur while the ETT is in place, including nasal and oral inflammation and ulceration, sinusitis and otitis, laryngeal and tracheal injuries, and tube

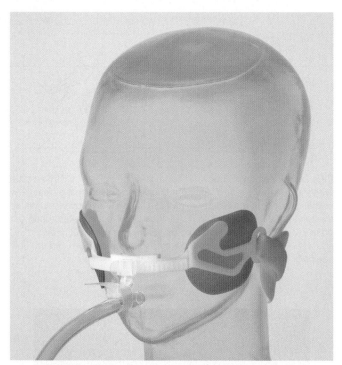

FIG. 20.5 Commercial Tube Holder. Anchor Fast oral ETT fastener. (Courtesy Hollister Incorporated, Libertyville, IL.)

obstruction and displacement. Other complications can occur days to weeks after the ETT is removed, including laryngeal and tracheal stenosis and a cricoid abscess (Table 20.3). Delayed complications usually require some form of surgical intervention.[17,18]

Tracheostomy Tubes

A tracheostomy tube is the preferred method of airway maintenance in a patient who requires long-term intubation. Although no ideal time to perform the procedure has been identified, it is commonly accepted that if a patient has been intubated or is anticipated to be intubated for longer than 7 to 10 days, a tracheostomy should be performed.[19] A tracheostomy is also indicated in several other situations such as the presence of an upper airway obstruction secondary to trauma, tumors, or swelling and the need to facilitate airway clearance secondary to spinal cord injury, neuromuscular disease, or severe debilitation.[20,21]

A tracheostomy tube provides the best route for long-term airway maintenance because this route avoids the oral, nasal, pharyngeal, and laryngeal complications associated with an ETT. The tube is shorter, has a wider diameter, and is less curved than an ETT; the resistance to airflow is less; and breathing is easier. Additional advantages of a tracheostomy tube include ease with secretion removal, increased patient acceptance and comfort, capability of the patient to eat and talk if possible, and easier ventilator weaning.[8,20] See Table 20.2 for a list of the advantages of a tracheostomy tube.

Tracheostomy tubes are made of plastic or metal and may have one or two lumens. Single-lumen tubes consist of the tube; a built-in cuff, which is connected to a pilot balloon for inflation purposes; and an obturator, which is used during tube insertion. Double-lumen tubes consist of the tube with the attached cuff, the obturator, and an inner cannula that can be removed for cleaning and then reinserted or, if disposable, replaced by a new sterile inner cannula. The inner cannula can be removed

quickly if the cannula becomes obstructed, making the system safer for patients with significant secretion problems. Single-lumen tubes provide a larger internal diameter for airflow, so airflow resistance is reduced, and the patient can ventilate through the tube with greater ease. Plastic tracheostomy tubes also have a 15-mm adapter on the end (Fig. 20.6).[20,21]

Tracheostomy Procedure

A tracheostomy tube is inserted by an open procedure or a percutaneous procedure. An open procedure is usually performed in the operating room, whereas a percutaneous procedure can be done at the patient's bedside.[21-23]

Complications

Numerous complications can occur during the tracheostomy procedure, including misplacement of the tracheal tube, hemorrhage, laryngeal nerve injury, pneumothorax, pneumomediastinum, and cardiac arrest.[17,21,22] Several complications can occur while the tracheostomy tube is in place, including stomal infection, hemorrhage, tracheomalacia, tracheoesophageal fistula, tracheoinnominate artery fistula, and tube obstruction and displacement.[21,22] Many complications can occur days to weeks after the tracheostomy tube is removed, including tracheal stenosis and tracheocutaneous fistula (Table 20.4). Delayed complications usually require some form of surgical intervention.[21]

Nursing Management

Nursing management of a patient with an endotracheal or tracheostomy tube requires some additional measures to address the effects associated with tube placement on the respiratory and other body systems. Nursing interventions for a patient with an artificial airway include providing humidification, managing the cuff, suctioning, establishing a method of communication, and providing oral hygiene. Because the tube bypasses the upper airway system, warming and humidifying the air must be performed by external means. Because the cuff of the tube can cause damage to the walls of the trachea, proper cuff inflation and management are imperative. In addition, the normal defense mechanisms are impaired, and secretions may accumulate; thus suctioning may be needed to promote secretion clearance. Because the tube does not allow airflow over the vocal cords, developing a method of communication is also very important. Last, observing the patient to ensure proper placement of the tube and patency of the airway is essential.

Patient safety is of paramount importance when caring for a patient with an artificial airway, as loss of the tube can result in loss of the patient's airway. In the event of unintentional extubation or decannulation, the patient's airway is opened with the head tilt–chin lift maneuver and maintained with an oropharyngeal or nasopharyngeal airway. If the patient is not breathing, he or she is manually ventilated with a manual resuscitation bag and face mask with 100% oxygen. In the case of a tracheostomy, the stoma is covered to prevent air from escaping through it. If the tracheostomy remains open, consideration is given to ventilating the patient through the stoma instead of the mouth.

One study examined patients' perception of ETT-related discomforts. Of the patients, 46% reported remembering having the ETT while in the critical care unit. Most of these patients found the discomfort associated with the ETT and the inability to speak very stressful. In addition, some patients continued to have problems with hoarseness, sore throat, and voice changes days to months later.[24]

TABLE 20.3 Complications of Endotracheal Tubes

Complications	Causes	Prevention and Treatment
Tube obstruction	Patient biting tube	*Prevention:*
	Tube kinking during repositioning	Place bite block.
	Cuff herniation	Sedate patient PRN.
	Dried secretions, blood, or lubricant	Suction PRN.
	Tissue from tumor	Humidify inspired gases.
	Trauma	*Treatment:*
	Foreign body	Replace tube.
Tube displacement	Movement of patient's head	*Prevention:*
	Movement of tube by patient's tongue	Secure tube to upper lip.
	Traction on tube from ventilator tubing	Restrain patient's hands as needed.
		Sedate patient PRN.
	Self-extubation	Ensure that only 2 inches of tube extend beyond lip.
		Support ventilator tubing.
		Treatment:
		Replace tube.
Sinusitis and nasal injury	Obstruction of paranasal sinus drainage	*Prevention:*
	Pressure necrosis of nares	Avoid nasal intubations.
		Cushion nares from tube and tape or ties.
		Treatment:
		Remove all tubes from nasal passages.
		Administer antibiotics.
Tracheoesophageal fistula	Pressure necrosis of posterior tracheal wall, resulting from overinflated cuff and rigid nasogastric tube	*Prevention:*
		Inflate cuff with minimal amount of air necessary.
		Monitor cuff pressures every 8 hours.
		Treatment:
		Position cuff of tube distal to fistula.
		Place gastrostomy tube for enteral feedings.
		Place esophageal tube for secretion clearance proximal to fistula.
Mucosal lesions	Pressure at tube and mucosal interface	*Prevention:*
		Inflate cuff with minimal amount of air necessary.
		Monitor cuff pressures every 8 hours.
		Use appropriate size tube.
		Treatment:
		May resolve spontaneously.
		Perform surgical intervention.
Laryngeal or tracheal stenosis	Injury to area from end of tube or cuff, resulting in scar tissue formation and narrowing of airway	*Prevention:*
		Inflate cuff with minimal amount of air necessary.
		Monitor cuff pressures every 8 hours.
		Suction area above cuff frequently.
		Treatment:
		Perform tracheostomy.
		Place laryngeal stent.
		Perform surgical repair.
Cricoid abscess	Mucosal injury with bacterial invasion	*Prevention:*
		Inflate cuff with minimal amount of air necessary.
		Monitor cuff pressures every 8 hours.
		Suction area above cuff frequently.
		Treatment:
		Perform incision and drainage of area.
		Administer antibiotics.

PRN, as needed.

Humidification

Humidification of air normally is performed by the mucosal layer of the upper respiratory tract. When this area is bypassed, as occurs with ETT and tracheostomy tubes or when supplemental oxygen is used, humidification by external means is necessary. Various humidification devices add water to inhaled gas to prevent drying and irritation of the respiratory tract, to prevent undue loss of body water, and to facilitate secretion removal.[25,26] The humidification device provides inspired gas conditioned (heated) to body temperature and saturated with water vapor.[27]

Valve used for cuff inflation, deflation, and pressure measurement
Face plate
Slots for tube ties
Disposable inner cannula
Fenestrations
Pilot balloon
Outer cannula
Cuff (inflated)
Obturator

Outer cannula
Valve used to inflate and deflate cuff and measure cuff pressure
Pilot balloon
Cuff (inflated)
Face plate
Slots for attachment of tube ties
Obturator
Cuff inflation tube

FIG. 20.6 Tracheostomy Tubes. (A) Dual-lumen cuffed tracheostomy tube with disposable inner cannula. (B) Dual-lumen cuffed fenestrated tracheostomy tube. (C) Single-lumen cannula cuffed tracheostomy tube. (From Rees HC. Care of patients requiring oxygen therapy or tracheostomy. In: Ignatavicius DD, Workman ML, eds. *Medical-Surgical Nursing*, 7th ed. St. Louis: Elsevier; 2013.)

TABLE 20.4	**Complications of Tracheostomy Tubes**	
Complications	**Causes**	**Prevention and Treatment**
Hemorrhage	Vessel opening after surgery Vessel erosion caused by tube	*Prevention:* Use appropriate size tube. Treat local infection. Suction gently. Humidify inspired gases. Position tracheal window not lower than third tracheal ring. *Treatment:* Pack lightly. Perform surgical intervention.
Wound infection	Colonization of stoma with hospital flora	*Prevention:* Perform routine stoma care. *Treatment:* Remove tube, if necessary. Perform aggressive wound care and débridement. Administer antibiotics.

TABLE 20.4 **Complications of Tracheostomy Tubes—cont'd**

Complications	Causes	Prevention and Treatment
Subcutaneous emphysema	Positive pressure ventilation Coughing against tight, occlusive dressing or sutured or packed wound	*Prevention:* Avoid suturing or packing wound closed around tube. *Treatment:* Remove any sutures or packing, if present.
Tube obstruction	Dried blood or secretions False passage into soft tissues Opening of cannula positioned against tracheal wall Foreign body Tissue from tumor	*Prevention:* Suction PRN. Humidify inspired gases. Use tube with removable inner cannula. Position tube so that opening does not press against tracheal wall. *Treatment:* Remove or replace inner cannula. Replace tube.
Tube displacement	Patient movement Coughing Traction on ventilatory tubing	*Prevention:* Use commercial tube holder. Use tubes with adjustable neck plates for patients with short necks. Support ventilatory tubing. Sedate patient PRN. Restrain patient PRN. *Treatment:* Cover stoma and manually ventilate patient by mouth. Replace tube.
Tracheal stenosis	Injury to area from end of tube or cuff, resulting in scar tissue formation and narrowing of airway	*Prevention:* Inflate cuff with minimal amount of air necessary. Monitor cuff pressures every 8 hours. *Treatment:* Perform surgical repair.
Tracheoesophageal fistula	Pressure necrosis of posterior tracheal wall, resulting from overinflated cuff and rigid nasogastric tube	*Prevention:* Inflate cuff with minimal amount of air necessary. Monitor cuff pressures every 8 hours. *Treatment:* Perform surgical repair.
Tracheoinnominate artery fistula	Direct pressure from elbow of cannula against innominate artery Placement of tracheal stoma below fourth tracheal ring High-lying innominate artery	*Prevention:* Position tracheal window not lower than third tracheal ring. *Treatment:* Hyperinflate cuff to control bleeding. Remove tube and replace with ETT, and apply digital pressure through stoma against sternum. Perform surgical repair.
Tracheocutaneous fistula	Failure of stoma to close after removal of tube	*Treatment:* Perform surgical repair.

ETT, endotracheal tube; *PRN,* as needed.

Cuff Management

Because the cuff of the ETT or tracheostomy tube is a major source of the complications associated with artificial airways, proper cuff management is essential. To prevent the complications associated with cuff design, only low-pressure, high-volume cuffed tubes are used in clinical practice.[8,10] Even with these tubes, cuff pressures can be generated that are high enough to lead to tracheal ischemia and injury. Proper cuff inflation techniques and cuff pressure monitoring are critical components of the care of a patient with an artificial airway.[8,10]

Cuff pressure monitoring. Cuff pressures are monitored at a minimum of every shift with a cuff pressure manometer (Fig. 20.7). Cuff pressures are maintained within 20 to 30 mm Hg (27 to 41 cm H_2O) because greater pressures decrease blood flow to the capillaries in the tracheal wall and lesser pressures increase the risk of aspiration. Pressures greater than 30 mm Hg (41 cm H_2O) should be reported to the physician. Cuffs are not routinely deflated because this increases the risk of aspiration.[8]

Foam cuff tracheostomy tubes. One tracheostomy tube on the market has a cuff made of foam that is self-inflating (Fig. 20.8). The cuff is deflated during insertion, after which the pilot

FIG. 20.7 Cuff Pressure Manometer. Aneroid pressure manometer for cuff inflation and measuring cuff pressures. (From Ignatavicius DD, Workman ML, eds. *Medical-Surgical Nursing*, 7th ed. St. Louis: Elsevier; 2013.)

FIG. 20.8 Foam Cuff Tracheostomy Tube. (Courtesy Smiths Medical, Inc., London, United Kingdom.)

port is opened to atmospheric pressure (room air), and the cuff self-inflates. After inflation, the foam cuff conforms to the size and shape of the patient's trachea, reducing the pressure against the tracheal wall. The pilot port can be left open to atmospheric pressure or attached to the mechanical ventilator tubing, allowing the cuff to inflate and deflate with the cycling of the ventilator. Routine maintenance of a foam cuff tracheostomy tube includes aspirating the pilot port every 8 hours to measure cuff volume, to remove any condensation from the cuff area, and to assess the integrity of the cuff. Removal is accomplished by deflating the cuff; this can be complicated if the plastic sheath covering the foam is perforated. If perforation occurs, the foam may not be deflatable because the air cannot be totally aspirated.[21]

Subglottic secretion removal. The cuff has also been implicated in the development of ventilator-associated pneumonia (VAP). Fluids can leak around the cuff into the airway, resulting in microaspiration. Bacteria-laden oral secretions trickle down the larynx and pool above the cuff of the artificial airway. These secretions are referred to as *subglottic secretions.* Subglottic secretions can then leak into

the lower airways around the cuff via the longitudinal folds that form in the cuff as it accommodates to the shape of the airway, when an underinflated cuff fails to form a proper seal in the airway, or in the event of inadvertent movement of the ETT within airway. The use of established cuff inflation techniques, monitoring of cuff pressures, using an appropriate method of tube stabilization, and oral hygiene are important interventions for preventing this problem.[28] Deep oropharyngeal suctioning to remove subglottic secretions is performed at least every 12 hours and before deflating the cuff or moving the tube.[29]

Specialized tubes are available to allow for the continuous removal of subglottic secretions. These tubes have an additional lumen, with an opening above the cuff, which is connected to continuous (-20 to -30 cm H_2O) suction (Fig. 20.9).[10] These tubes are recommended for patients who are expected to be intubated for longer than 48 to 72 hours.[10] One issue with these tubes is that the aspiration lumen can become clogged, and a small amount of air needs to be injected into the aspiration port every few hours.

Suctioning

Suctioning is often required to maintain a patent airway in a patient with an ETT or tracheostomy tube. Suctioning is a sterile procedure that is performed only when the patient needs it and not on a routine schedule.[30,31] Indications for suctioning include the presence of coarse crackles over the trachea on auscultation,[30] coughing, visible secretions in the airway, a sawtooth pattern on the flow-volume loop on the ventilator monitor,[30,31] increased peak airway pressures on the ventilator, decreasing oxygenation saturation, and acute respiratory distress.[31] Complications associated with suctioning include hypoxemia, atelectasis, bronchospasms, dysrhythmias, increased intracranial pressure, and airway trauma.[31]

There are two different methods for suctioning based on the type of catheter. The open suction method requires disconnecting the patient from the ventilator and inserting a single-use, disposable, suction catheter into the artificial airway. The closed suction method requires a sterile, closed tracheal suction system and allows the patient to remain on the ventilator when suctioned. The closed method is preferable, as the evidence suggests that this method appears to limit the hypoxemia associated with suctioning.[13,31]

There are two different techniques for suctioning depending on how deeply the suction catheter is inserted into the trachea: shallow suctioning and deep suctioning. For shallow suctioning, the suction catheter is inserted to the end of the ETT or tracheostomy tube, and then the suction is applied. For deep suctioning, the suction catheter is inserted until resistance is met, the catheter is pulled back approximately 1 cm, and then suction is applied.[13,31] Evidence suggests that shallow suctioning is as effective as deep suctioning for secretion removal and is associated with fewer complications.[13]

Complications. Hypoxemia can result because the oxygen source is disconnected from the patient or the oxygen is removed from the patient's airways when the suction is applied. Atelectasis is thought to occur when the suction catheter is larger than one-half of the diameter of the ETT. Excessive negative pressure occurs when suction is applied, promoting collapse of the distal airways. Bronchospasms are the result of stimulation of the airways with the suction catheter. Cardiac dysrhythmias, particularly bradycardias, are attributed to

FIG. 20.9 Endotracheal and Tracheostomy Tubes With Subglottic Suction Ports. (From Altobelli N. Airway management. In: Kacmarek RM, Stoller JK, Heuer AJ, eds. *Egan's Fundamentals of Respiratory Care*, 10th ed. St. Louis: Mosby; 2013.)

FIG. 20.10 Closed Tracheal Suction System. (Modified from Sills JR. *Entry-Level Respiratory Therapist Exam Guide*. St. Louis: Mosby; 2000.)

vagal stimulation. Airway trauma occurs with impaction of the catheter in the airways and excessive negative pressure applied to the catheter.[8,31]

Suctioning protocol. Many protocols regarding suctioning have been developed. Several practices have been found to be helpful in limiting the complications of suctioning. Hypoxemia can be minimized by hyperoxygenating the patient with 100% oxygen for 30 to 60 seconds before suctioning and for at least 60 seconds after suctioning.[31,32] Atelectasis can be avoided by using a suction catheter with an external diameter of less than one-half of the internal diameter of the ETT.[31,32] Using 120 mm Hg or less of suction decreases the chances of hypoxemia, atelectasis, and airway trauma.[31,32] Limiting the duration of each suction pass to 10 to 15 seconds also helps minimize hypoxemia, airway trauma, and cardiac dysrhythmias.[13,31,32] The process of applying intermittent (instead of continuous) suction has been shown to be of no benefit.[33] The instillation of normal saline to help remove secretions has not been proved to be of any benefit, and it may contribute to the development of hypoxemia as well as lower airway colonization resulting in VAP.[13,31,34]

Closed tracheal suction system. One device to facilitate the suctioning of a patient on a ventilator is the closed tracheal suction system (CTSS) (Fig. 20.10). This device consists of a suction catheter in a plastic sleeve that attaches directly to the ventilator tubing. The CTSS allows the patient to be suctioned while remaining on the ventilator. Advantages of the CTSS include maintenance of oxygenation and PEEP during suctioning, reduction of hypoxemia-related complications, and protection of staff members from the patient's secretions. The CTSS is convenient to use, requiring only one person to perform the procedure.[32]

Concerns related to the CTSS include autocontamination, inadequate removal of secretions, and increased risk of unintentional extubation resulting from the extra weight of the system on the ventilator tubing. Autocontamination has been shown not to be an issue if the catheter is cleaned properly after every use. Inadequate removal of secretions may or may not be a problem, and further investigation is required

to settle this issue.[32] Although recommendations for changing the catheter vary, one study indicated that the catheter could be changed on an as-needed basis without increasing the incidence of VAP.[35] One study found that suctioning with the CTSS caused massive aspiration of fluid around the tracheal tube cuff as a result of a significant decrease in airway pressure.[36]

Communication

Impaired communication is a major stressor for a patient with an artificial airway. This stress is related to the inability to speak, insufficient explanations from staff members, inadequate understanding, fear of being unable to communicate, and difficulty with communication methods.[37] Many interventions can facilitate communication for a patient with an ETT or tracheostomy tube. These include establishing an environment that fosters communication, performing a complete assessment of the patient's ability to communicate, anticipating the patient's needs, teaching the patient and family how to communicate, using a variety of methods to communicate, and facilitating the patient's ability to communicate by providing the patient with his or her eyeglasses or hearing aid.[38]

Methods to facilitate communication in this patient population include the use of verbal and nonverbal language and various devices to assist the patient on short-term and long-term ventilator assistance. Nonverbal communication may include the use of sign language, gestures, lip reading, pointing, facial expressions, or eye blinking. Simple devices include pencil and paper; Magic Slates; magnetic boards with plastic letters; picture, alphabet, or symbol boards; and flash cards. More sophisticated devices include typewriters, computers, talking ETT and tracheostomy tubes, and external handheld vibrators. Regardless of the method selected, the patient must be taught how to use the device.[38]

Passy-muir valve. The Passy-Muir valve is a device used to assist a mechanically ventilated patient with a tracheostomy to speak. This one-way valve opens on inhalation, allowing air to enter the lungs through the tracheostomy tube, and closes on exhalation, forcing air over the vocal cords and out the mouth, permitting the patient to speak (Fig. 20.11). Before the valve can be placed on a tracheostomy tube, the cuff must be deflated to allow air to pass around the tube, and the tidal volume of the ventilator must be increased to compensate for the air leak. In addition to aiding communication, the Passy-Muir valve can assist a ventilator-dependent patient with relearning normal breathing patterns. The valve is contraindicated in patients with laryngeal or pharyngeal dysfunction, excessive secretions, or poor lung compliance.[38]

Oral Hygiene

Patients with artificial airways are extremely susceptible to developing VAP because of microaspiration of subglottic secretions. These secretions are full of microorganisms from the patient's mouth. Because the cuff of the artificial airway does not form a tight seal in the patient's airway, these secretions seep around the cuff into the patient's lungs, promoting the development of VAP.[39] Although bacteria are normally present in a patient's mouth, increased amounts of bacteria and more resistant bacteria are present in critically ill patients. Decreased salivary flow, poor mucosal status, and dental plaque all contribute to this problem.[40]

Proper oral hygiene has been shown to decrease the incidence of VAP.[41,42] However, studies have shown that routine oral care is not a priority intervention for many nurses.[43] No evidence-based protocol exists for oral care at the present time. Research studies are lacking, particularly with regard to frequency and effectiveness of different procedures. However, most experts agree that oral care should consist of brushing the patient's teeth with a soft toothbrush to reduce plaque, brushing the patient's tongue and gums with a foam swab to stimulate the tissue,[40] and performing deep oropharyngeal suctioning to remove any secretions that have pooled above the patient's cuff.[39] In addition, chlorhexidine solution (0.12% to 0.2%) should be applied to the inside of the mouth to decrease the prevalence of oropharyngeal organisms. To be effective, chlorhexidine should be applied with a sponge swab to the teeth, tongue, and inside of the oral cavity. To have the greatest effect, chlorhexidine should be applied four times daily.[44] This procedure has been shown to reduce oral colonization of bacteria and to decrease the incidence of VAP, particularly in patients who have undergone cardiac surgery or trauma.[45] A sample oral care protocol is outlined in Box 20.1.

Extubation and Decannulation

An artificial airway is removed when it is no longer needed. Extubation, the process of removing an ETT, is a simple procedure that can be done at the bedside.[46] Before the cuff of an ETT or tracheostomy tube is deflated in preparation for removal, it is important to ensure that secretions are cleared from above the tube cuff. Complications of extubation include sore throat, stridor, hoarseness, odynophagia, vocal cord immobility, pulmonary aspiration, and cough.[46] Decannulation is the process of

FIG. 20.11 Passy-Muir Valve. (Redrawn from Manzano JL, et al. Verbal communication of ventilator dependent patients. *Crit Care Med.* 1993;21[4]:512–517, 1993; with permission.)

Air movement through vocal cords

Unidirectional valve

BOX 20.1 Sample Oral Care Protocol

Standard of Care

1. The oral cavity is assessed initially and daily by the RN.
2. Unconscious patients and patients with artificial airways (endotracheal or tracheostomy tubes) are provided oral care every 4 hours and as needed.
3. Patients with cuffed artificial airways have oropharyngeal and subglottic secretions suctioned at least every 12 hours and before repositioning of the tube or deflation of the cuff.

Procedure

1. Set up suction equipment.
2. Position patient's head to the side, or place patient in semi-Fowler position.
3. Provide suction, as needed, to patients with an artificial airway to remove any oropharyngeal and subglottic secretions (secretions that migrate down the tube and settle on top of the cuff).
4. Brush teeth using a suction toothbrush and small amounts of water and alcohol-free antiseptic oral rinse.
   - Brush for approximately 1–2 minutes.
   - Exert gentle pressure while moving in short horizontal or circular strokes.
5. Gently brush surface of tongue.
6. Use suction swab to clean the teeth and tongue if brushing causes discomfort or bleeding.
   - Place swab perpendicular to gum line, applying gentle mechanical action for 1–2 minutes.
   - Turn swab in clockwise rotation to remove mucus and debris.
7. Swab mouth (teeth, tongue, and oral cavity) with 15 mL of 0.12% chlorhexidine every 6 hours.
8. Apply mouth moisturizer inside mouth.
9. Apply lip balm, if needed.

removing a tracheostomy tube. This is also a simple process that can be performed at the bedside. After removal of the tracheostomy tube, the stoma is usually covered with a dry dressing with the expectation that it will close within several days.[47,48] Difficulty removing the tracheostomy tube because of a tight stoma is usually the only complication associated with decannulation.[47]

INVASIVE MECHANICAL VENTILATION

Indications

Mechanical ventilation is the process of using an apparatus to facilitate the transport of oxygen and CO_2 between the atmosphere and the alveoli for the purpose of enhancing pulmonary gas exchange. Mechanical ventilation is indicated for physiologic and clinical reasons. Physiologic objectives include supporting cardiopulmonary gas exchange (alveolar ventilation and arterial oxygenation), increasing lung volume (end expiratory lung inflation and functional residual capacity), and reducing the work of breathing. Clinical objectives include reversing hypoxemia and acute respiratory acidosis, relieving respiratory distress, preventing or reversing atelectasis and respiratory muscle fatigue, permitting sedation and neuromuscular blockade, decreasing oxygen consumption, reducing intracranial pressure, and stabilizing the chest wall.[49-52]

Use of Mechanical Ventilators
Types of Ventilators

The two main types of ventilators available at the present time are (1) positive pressure ventilators and (2) negative pressure ventilators. Negative pressure ventilators are applied externally to the patient and decrease the atmospheric pressure surrounding the thorax to initiate inspiration. They generally are not used in the critical care environment. Positive pressure ventilators use a mechanical drive mechanism to force air into the patient's lungs through an ETT or tracheostomy tube.[51]

Ventilator Mechanics

To properly ventilate the patient, the ventilator must complete four phases of ventilation: (1) change from exhalation to inspiration, (2) inspiration, (3) change from inspiration to exhalation, and (4) exhalation. The ventilator uses four different variables to begin, sustain, and terminate each of these phases. These variables are described in terms of *volume*, *pressure*, *flow*, and *time*.[51,53,54]

Trigger. The phase variable that initiates the change from exhalation to inspiration is called the *trigger*. Breaths may be pressure triggered or flow triggered, depending on the sensitivity setting of the ventilator and the patient's inspiratory effort, or they may be time triggered, depending on the rate setting of the ventilator. A breath that is initiated by the patient is known as a *patient-triggered* or *patient-assisted* breath, whereas a breath that is initiated by the ventilator is known as a *machine-triggered* or *machine-controlled* breath.[51,53,54]

A *time-triggered breath* is a machine-controlled breath that is initiated by the ventilator after a preset length of time has elapsed and is controlled by the rate setting on the ventilator (eg, a rate of 10 breaths/min yields 1 breath every 6 seconds). *Flow-triggered* and *pressure-triggered* breaths are patient-assisted breaths that are initiated by decreased flow or pressure, respectively, within the breathing circuit. Flow triggering (also known as *flow-by*) is controlled by adjusting the flow-sensitivity setting of the ventilator, whereas pressure triggering is controlled by adjusting the pressure-sensitivity setting. Many ventilators offer the various types of triggers in combination. For example, a breath may be time triggered and flow triggered, depending on the patient's ability to interact with the ventilator and initiate a breath.[51,53,54]

Limit. The variable that maintains inspiration is called the *limit* or *target*. Inspiration can be pressure limited, flow limited, or volume limited. A *pressure-limited breath* is one in which a preset pressure is attained and maintained during inspiration. A *flow-limited breath* is one in which a preset flow is reached before the end of inspiration. A *volume-limited breath* is one in which a preset volume is delivered during the inspiration. However, the limit variable does not end inspiration; it only sustains it.[51,53,54]

Cycle. The variable that ends inspiration is called the *cycle*. The classification of positive pressure ventilators is based on this variable: volume-cycled, pressure-cycled, flow-cycled, and time-cycled ventilators. *Volume-cycled ventilators* are designed to deliver a breath until a preset volume is delivered. *Pressure-cycled ventilators* deliver a breath until a preset pressure is reached within the patient's airways. *Flow-cycled ventilators* deliver a breath until a preset inspiratory flow rate is achieved. *Time-cycled ventilators* deliver a breath over a preset time interval.[51,53,54]

Baseline. The variable that is controlled during exhalation is called the *baseline*. Pressure is almost always used to adjust this variable. The patient exhales to a certain baseline pressure that is set on the ventilator. The baseline variable may be set at zero (ie, atmospheric pressure) or above atmospheric pressure (ie, PEEP).[51,53,54]

Modes of Ventilation

The term *ventilator mode* refers to how the machine ventilates the patient. Selection of a particular mode of ventilation determines how much the patient will participate in his or her own ventilatory pattern. The choice depends on the patient's situation and the goals of treatment. The mode is determined by the combination of phase variables selected. Many modes are available (Table 20.5), and some may be used in conjunction with others.[49-54] Because brands of ventilators vary in their ability to perform certain functions, not all modes are available on all ventilators.[53-55]

Ventilator Settings

Settings on the ventilator allow the ventilator parameters to be individualized to the patient and allow selection of the desired ventilation mode (Table 20.6). Each ventilator has a patient-monitoring system that allows all aspects of the patient's ventilatory pattern to be assessed, monitored, and displayed.[49,52-54,56]

Complications

Mechanical ventilation is often lifesaving, but, similar to other interventions, it is not without complications. Some complications are preventable, whereas others can be minimized but not eradicated. Physiologic complications associated with mechanical ventilation include ventilator-induced lung injury, cardiovascular compromise, gastrointestinal disturbances, patient-ventilator dyssynchrony, and VAP.

Ventilator-Induced Lung Injury

Mechanical ventilation can cause two different types of injury to the lungs: (1) air leaks and (2) biotrauma.[54,57] Air leaks related to mechanical ventilation are the result of excessive

TABLE 20.5 Modes of Mechanical Ventilation

Mode of Ventilation	Clinical Application	Nursing Implications
Continuous mandatory (volume or pressure) ventilation (CMV), also known as assist/control (AC) ventilation: Delivers gas at preset tidal volume or pressure (depending on selected cycling variable) in response to patient's inspiratory efforts and initiates breath if patient fails to do so within preset time.	Volume-controlled (VC) CMV is used as primary mode of ventilation in spontaneously breathing patients with weak respiratory muscles.	Hyperventilation can occur in patients with increased respiratory rates
	Pressure-controlled (PC) CMV is used in patients with decreased lung compliance or increased airway resistance, particularly when patient is at risk for volutrauma.	Sedation may be necessary to limit number of spontaneous breaths
		Patient on VC-CMV is monitored for volutrauma Patient on PC-CMV is monitored for hypercapnia
Pressure-regulated volume control ventilation (PRVCV): Variation of CMV that combines volume and pressure features; delivers preset tidal volume using lowest possible airway pressure; airway pressure will not exceed preset maximum pressure limit.	PRVCV is used in patients with rapidly changing pulmonary mechanics (airway resistance and lung compliance), limiting potential complications.	
Pressure-controlled inverse ratio ventilation (PC-IRV): PC-CMV mode in which inspiratory-to-expiratory (I:E) time ratio is >1:1.	PC-IRV is used in patients with hypoxemia refractory to PEEP; longer inspiratory time increases functional residual capacity and improves oxygenation by opening collapsed alveoli, and shorter expiratory time induces auto-PEEP that prevents alveoli from recollapsing.	Requires sedation and/or pharmacologic paralysis because of discomfort
		Increased intrathoracic pressure can result in excessive air trapping and decreased cardiac output
Intermittent mandatory (volume or pressure) ventilation (IMV), also known as synchronous intermittent mandatory ventilation (SIMV): Delivers gas at preset tidal volume or pressure (depending on selected cycling variable) and rate, while allowing patient to breathe spontaneously; ventilator breaths are synchronized to patient's respiratory effort.	VC-IMV is used as primary mode of ventilation in many clinical situations and as weaning mode. PC-IMV is used in patients with decreased lung compliance or increased airway resistance when the need to preserve the patient's spontaneous efforts is important.	May increase work of breathing and promote respiratory muscle fatigue
		Patient is monitored for hypercapnia, particularly with PC-IMV
Adaptive support ventilation (ASV): Ventilator automatically adjusts settings to maintain 100 mL/min/kg of minute ventilation; pressure support.	ASV is computerized mode of ventilation that increases or decreases ventilatory support based on patient needs; can be used with any patient requiring volume-controlled ventilation.	Not intended as a weaning mode
		Adapts to changes in patient position
Continuous positive airway pressure (CPAP): Positive pressure applied during spontaneous breaths; patient controls rate, inspiratory flow, and tidal volume.	CPAP is spontaneous breathing mode used in patients to increase functional residual capacity and improve oxygenation by opening collapsed alveoli at end expiration; it is also used for weaning.	Side effects include decreased cardiac output, volutrauma, and increased intracranial pressure
		No ventilator breaths are delivered in PEEP or CPAP mode unless used with CMV or IMV
Airway pressure release ventilation (APRV): Two different levels of CPAP (inspiratory and expiratory) are applied for set periods of time, allowing spontaneous breathing to occur at both levels.	APRV is spontaneous breathing mode used to maintain alveolar recruitment without imposing additional peak inspiratory pressures that could lead to barotrauma.	Patient needs to be monitored for hypercapnia
Pressure support ventilation (PSV): Preset positive pressure used to augment patient's inspiratory efforts; patient controls rate, inspiratory flow, and tidal volume.	PSV is spontaneous breathing mode used as primary mode of ventilation in patients with stable respiratory drive to overcome any imposed mechanical resistance (eg, artificial airway).	Patient is monitored for hypercapnia
	PSV can also be used with IMV to support spontaneous breaths.	Advantages include reduced patient work of breathing and improved patient-ventilator synchrony

TABLE 20.5   Modes of Mechanical Ventilation—cont'd

Mode of Ventilation	Clinical Application	Nursing Implications
Volume-assured pressure support ventilation (VAPSV), also known as pressure augmentation (PA): Variation of PSV with set tidal volume to ensure that patient receives minimum tidal volume with each pressure support breath.	VAPSV is spontaneous breathing mode used to treat acute respiratory illness and to facilitate weaning.	Advantages include increased patient comfort, decreased work of breathing, decreased respiratory muscle fatigue, and promotion of respiratory muscle conditioning
Neurally adjusted ventilatory assist (NAVA): Partial ventilatory support mode that uses electrical activity of diaphragm to control patient ventilator interaction.	NAVA delivers assisted breath in proportion to and in synchrony with patient's respiratory effort.	Requires esophageal catheter (similar to naso-gastric tube) that measures electrical signal to diaphragm
Independent lung ventilation (ILV): Each lung is ventilated separately.	ILV is used in patients with unilateral lung disease, bronchopleural fistulas, or bilateral asymmetric lung disease.	Requires double-lumen ETT, two ventilators, sedation, and pharmacologic paralysis
High-frequency ventilation (HFV): Delivers small volume of gas at rapid rate. • *High-frequency positive- pressure ventilation (HFPPV):* Delivers 60–100 breaths/min • *High-frequency jet ventilation (HFJV):* delivers 100–600 cycles/min • High-frequency oscillation (HFO): delivers 900–3000 cycles/min	HFV is used in situations in which conventional mechanical ventilation compromises hemodynamic stability, in patients with bronchopleural fistulas, during short-term procedures, and with diseases that create risk of volutrauma.	Patients require sedation and/or pharmacologic paralysis Inadequate humidification can compromise airway patency Assessment of breath sounds is difficult

ETT, endotracheal tube; *PEEP,* positive end expiratory pressure.

TABLE 20.6   Ventilator Settings

Parameter	Description	Typical Settings
Respiratory rate or frequency	Number of breaths ventilator delivers per minute	6–20 breaths/min
V_T	Volume of gas delivered to patient during each ventilator breath	6–10 mL/kg 4–8 mL/kg in ARDS
Oxygen concentration (F_{IO_2})	F_{IO_2} delivered to patient	May be set between 21% and 100%; adjusted to maintain Pa_{O_2} level >60 mm Hg or Sp_{O_2} level >92%
PEEP	Positive pressure applied at end of expiration of ventilator breaths	3–5 cm H_2O
PS	Positive pressure used to augment patient's inspiratory efforts	5–10 cm H_2O
Inspiratory flow rate and time	Speed with which V_T is delivered	40–80 L/min Time: 0.8–1.2 seconds
I:E ratio	Ratio of duration of inspiration to duration of expiration	1:2 to 1:1.5 unless inverse ratio ventilation is desired
Sensitivity	Determines amount of effort patient must generate to initiate a ventilator breath; it may be set for pressure triggering or flow triggering	Pressure trigger: 0.5–1.5 cm H_2O below baseline pressure Flow trigger: 1–3 L/min below baseline flow
High pressure limit	Regulates maximal pressure ventilator can generate to deliver V_T; when pressure limit is reached, ventilator terminates breath and spills undelivered volume into atmosphere	10–20 cm H_2O above peak inspiratory pressure

ARDS, acute respiratory distress syndrome; *F_{IO_2},* fraction of inspired oxygen; *I:E,* inspiratory to expiratory; *Pa_{O_2},* arterial oxygen pressure; *PEEP,* positive end expiratory time; *PS,* pressure support; *Sp_{O_2},* oxygen saturation as measured by pulse oximetry; *V_T,* tidal volume.

pressure in the alveoli (barotrauma), excessive volume in the alveoli (volutrauma), or shearing caused by repeated opening and closing of the alveoli (atelectrauma).[54,58] Barotrauma, volutrauma, and atelectrauma can lead to excessive alveolar wall stress and damage to the alveolar-capillary membrane, resulting in air leakage into the surrounding spaces. The air then travels out through the hilum and into the mediastinum (pneumomediastinum), pleural space (pneumothorax), subcutaneous tissues (subcutaneous emphysema), pericardium (pneumopericardium), peritoneum (pneumoperitoneum), and retroperitoneum (pneumoretroperitoneum). The resultant disorders vary from fairly benign to potentially lethal—the most lethal of which is a pneumothorax or pneumopericardium resulting in cardiac tamponade.[54,59]

Barotrauma, volutrauma, and atelectrauma can also cause the release of cellular mediators and initiation of the inflammatory-immune response. This type of ventilator-induced injury is known as *biotrauma.*[54,60] Biotrauma can result in the development of ARDS.[61] To limit ventilator-induced lung injury, the plateau pressure (pressure needed to inflate the alveoli) is kept at less than 32 cm H_2O, PEEP is used to avoid end expiratory collapse and reopening, and the tidal volume is set at 6 to 10 mL/kg.[57,60]

Cardiovascular Compromise

Positive pressure ventilation increases intrathoracic pressure, which decreases venous return to the right side of the heart. Impaired venous return decreases preload, which results in a decrease in cardiac output. As a secondary consequence, hepatic and renal dysfunction may occur. Positive pressure ventilation impairs cerebral venous return. In patients with impaired autoregulation, positive pressure ventilation can result in increased intracranial pressure.[54,62]

Gastrointestinal Disturbances

Gastrointestinal disturbances can occur as a result of positive pressure ventilation. Gastric distention occurs when air leaks around the ETT or tracheostomy tube cuff and overcomes the resistance of the lower esophageal sphincter. Vomiting can occur as a result of pharyngeal stimulation from the artificial airway.[9] These problems can be prevented by inserting a nasogastric tube and ensuring appropriate cuff inflation. Hypomotility and constipation may occur as a result of immobility and the administration of paralytic agents, analgesics, and sedatives.

Patient-Ventilator Dyssynchrony

Because the ventilatory pattern is normally initiated by the establishment of negative pressure within the chest, the application of positive pressure can lead to patient difficulties in breathing while on the ventilator. To achieve optimal ventilatory assistance, the patient should breathe in synchrony with the machine. The selected mode of ventilation, the settings, and the type of ventilatory circuitry used can increase the work of breathing and lead to breathing out of synchrony with the ventilator. Patient-ventilator dyssynchrony can result in decreased effectiveness of mechanical ventilation, the development of auto-PEEP, and psychologic distress. Patients who are not breathing in synchrony with the ventilator appear to be fighting or "bucking" the ventilator. To minimize this problem, the ventilator is adjusted to accommodate the patient's spontaneous breathing pattern and to work with the patient. If this is not possible, the patient may need to be sedated or pharmacologically paralyzed.[63-65]

Ventilator-Associated Pneumonia

VAP is a type of hospital-acquired pneumonia that refers to the development of pneumonia 48 to 72 hours after endotracheal intubation.[66] A great potential for the development of pneumonia exists after placement of an artificial airway because the tube bypasses or impairs many of the normal defense mechanisms of the lung. After an artificial airway has been placed, contamination of the lower airways follows within 24 hours. This results from many factors that directly and indirectly promote airway colonization. The use of respiratory therapy devices (eg, ventilators, nebulizers, intermittent positive pressure breathing machines) also can increase the risk of pneumonia.[53,67] The severity of the patient's illness, increased age, and the presence of ARDS or malnutrition significantly increase the likelihood that an infection will ensue. Therapeutic measures such as nasogastric intubation and gastric alkalization with enteral feedings or medications facilitate the development of pneumonia.

Nasogastric tubes promote aspiration by acting as a wick for stomach contents, whereas enteral feedings, antacids, histamine inhibitors, and proton pump inhibitors increase the pH level of the stomach, promoting the growth of bacteria that can then be aspirated (Fig. 20.12).[68] Additional information on managing a patient with pneumonia is provided in Chapter 19. Prevention of VAP is crucial; strategies to prevent VAP are listed in Box 20.2.

Semirecumbency. Positioning of a patient who requires mechanical ventilation is very important. Semirecumbent positioning (elevation of the head of the bed 30 to 45 degrees) reduces the incidence of gastroesophageal reflux and subsequent aspiration of oropharyngeal secretions and decreases the incidence of VAP. The head of the patient's bed is elevated to 30 to 45 degrees at all times unless contraindicated (eg, hemodynamic instability, presence of intraaortic balloon pump, physician's order to the contrary). However, this intervention increases the risk of skin shear on the coccyx, and extra surveillance is mandatory for prevention of pressure ulcers.[69,70]

Sedation vacation. Many patients receiving mechanical ventilation require sedation to ameliorate symptoms of anxiety and stress associated with critical illness. However, the prolonged use of sedation has been shown to contribute to the development of complications, including oversedation, prolonged mechanical ventilation, and delirium. To decrease the incidence of these complications, the concept of a "sedation vacation" has been developed. A "sedation vacation" is simply the daily interruption of sedation to evaluate the patient and his or her need for continued sedation and mechanical ventilation. Not every patient is a candidate for this procedure. Contraindications include hemodynamic instability, increased intracranial pressure, ongoing agitation, seizures, alcohol withdrawal, and use of neuromuscular blocking agents. If the patient is able to tolerate being off the sedation for more than 4 hours (this number varies depending on the protocol being used), the sedation is discontinued. Signs of intolerance include ongoing agitation, increased respiratory rate, decreasing oxygen saturation, cardiac dysrhythmias, and signs of respiratory distress.[71]

Other measures to reduce incidence of ventilator-associated pneumonia. Studies have shown that use of an ETT with a polyurethane cuff may decrease the incidence of VAP. A traditional ETT has a polyvinyl low-pressure, high-volume cuff. When the cuff is inflated, folds form in the cuff, allowing fluids and air to leak around the cuff and into the lungs; this is why subglottic secretion removal is so important. Polyurethane cuffs are much thinner than the traditional polyvinyl cuffs and do not form folds when they are inflated. No leakage of fluids into the lungs occurs.[67,72,73] In addition, some evidence suggests that the shape of the cuff may also affect this issue. A taper-shaped cuff appears to be better for preventing fluid leakage compared with a cylindrical cuff commonly found on most tubes.[74]

Another meta-analysis found limited evidence to support the use of silver-coated ETTs to reduce the incidence and delay the onset of VAP compared with a regular ETT.[75] The silver-coated tube decreases the incidence of VAP by preventing bacterial colonization and biofilm formation. Biofilm is formed when bacteria cling to the inner lumen of the ETT and then secrete an exopolysaccharide substance. This substance forms a gelatinous matrix that allows bacteria to thrive on a nonbiologic surface.[72,73]

FIG. 20.12 Pathogenesis of Ventilator-Associated Pneumonia. (Redrawn from Sachdev G, Napolitano LM. Postoperative pulmonary complications: pneumonia and acute respiratory failure. *Surg Clin North Am.* 2012;92[2]:321–344.)

QSEN BOX 20.2 QSEN: Evidence-Based Practice

Ventilator-Associated Pneumonia Prevention Strategies

- Use noninvasive positive pressure ventilation when possible.
- Avoid or minimize the use of sedation.
- Conduct a spontaneous awakening trial daily unless contraindicated.
- Conduct a spontaneous breathing trial daily unless contraindicated.
- Initiate early mobilization and exercise.
- Begin intermittent or continuous subglottic secretion removal.
- Elevate the head of the bed 30–45 degrees.
- Change ventilator circuits only when visibly soiled.
- Perform routine oral care with chlorhexidine.
- Consider administration of prophylactic probiotics.
- Consider selective decontamination of the oropharynx and/or the digestive tract.

Modified from Klompas M, et al. Strategies to prevent ventilator-associated pneumonia in acute care hospitals: 2014 update. *Infect Control Hosp Epidemiol.* 2014;35(8):915–936.

Weaning

Weaning is the gradual withdrawal of the mechanical ventilator and the reestablishment of spontaneous breathing. Weaning is begun only after the original process for which ventilator support was required has been corrected and patient stability has been achieved. Other factors to consider when weaning are length of time on ventilator, sleep deprivation, and nutritional status. Major factors that affect the patient's ability to wean include the ability of the lungs to participate in ventilation and respiration, cardiovascular performance, and psychologic readiness.[76] This discussion focuses on weaning of a patient from short-term (3 days or less) mechanical ventilation. Management of weaning in a patient on long-term mechanical ventilation is discussed in Chapter 19.

Readiness to Wean

Patients are screened every day for their readiness to be weaned. The screen includes an evaluation of the patient's level of consciousness, physiologic and hemodynamic stability, adequacy of oxygenation and ventilation, spontaneous breathing capability, and respiratory rate and pattern.[76] Routine parameters that are usually assessed are presented in Table 20.7.

The rapid shallow breathing index (RSBI) can predict weaning success. To calculate an RSBI, the patient's respiratory rate and minute ventilation are measured for 1 minute during spontaneous breathing. The measured respiratory rate is then divided by the tidal volume (expressed in liters). An RSBI of less than 105 is considered predictive of weaning success. If the patient is receiving sedation, the medication is discontinued at least 1 hour before the RSBI is measured. If the patient meets criteria for weaning readiness and has an RSBI of less than 105, a spontaneous breathing trial can be performed.[77] One study showed that implementation of a weaning program that incorporated daily spontaneous breathing trials had a positive impact on extubation rates and no effect on reintubation rates.[78] Fig. 20.13 outlines one approach for a spontaneous breathing trial.

After the patient's readiness to be weaned has been established, the patient is prepared for the weaning trial. The patient is positioned upright to facilitate breathing and suctioned to ensure airway patency. The process is explained to the patient, and the patient is offered reassurance and diversional activities. The patient is assessed immediately before the start of the trial and frequently during the weaning period for signs of weaning intolerance (Box 20.3).[76,77,79,80]

Weaning Methods

Numerous methods can be used to wean a patient from the ventilator. The method selected depends on the patient, his or her pulmonary status, and length of time on the ventilator. The three main methods for weaning are (1) T-tube (T-piece) trials, (2) synchronized intermittent mandatory ventilation (SIMV), and (3) pressure support ventilation (PSV).[76,79,81] Regardless of the method selected, evidence shows that using a standardized approach decreases weaning time and length of stay in the critical care unit.[82]

T-piece trials. T-piece weaning trials consist of alternating periods of ventilatory support (usually assist/control ventilation or continuous mandatory ventilation) with periods of spontaneous breathing. The trial is initiated by removing the patient from the ventilator and having the patient breathe spontaneously on a T-piece oxygen delivery system. After a set amount of time, the patient is placed back on the ventilator. The goal is to progressively increase the duration of time spent off the ventilator. During the weaning process, the patient is observed closely for respiratory muscle fatigue.[76,79,81]

TABLE 20.7	Conventional Weaning Parameters	
Parameters	**Weanable Values**	**Normal Ranges**
NIF (cm H₂O)	<−20	<−50
VC (mL/kg)	>10	>65–75
VT (mL/kg)	<5	>5–7
RR (breaths/min)	<32	12–20
VE (L/min)	>10	>10
RSBI (RR/VT)	<105	<40

NIF, negative inspiratory force; *RR,* respiratory rate; *RSBI,* rapid shallow breathing index; *VC,* vital capacity; *VE,* minute ventilation; *VT,* tidal volume.

From Benjamin IJ, ed. *Andreoli and Carpenter's Cecil Essentials of Medicine,* 9th ed. Philadelphia: Saunders; 2016.

Approach to Discontinuing Ventilation/Extubation

1. Daily assessment: Is patient ready for a spontaneous breathing trial?
   • General: resolving process, patient alert, no continuous sedation
   • Gas exchange: P/F > 200; FIO₂ ≤ 50%
   • Hemodynamics: no vasopressors
   • Respiratory: PEEP ≤ 5-7 cm H₂O

Evaluate and treat reversible causes of failure
• Sedation, fluid status, myocardial ischemia, pain control, bronchodilator need, etc.

Yes

2. Initiate screening for spontaneous breathing trial (SBT):
   • Monitor patient with ECG, oximetry
   • Patient breathes spontaneously on T-piece, or on PSV of 5-7 cm H₂O
   • Monitor physiologic variables (RR, gas exchange, hemodynamics, subjective comfort)

If patient physiologically unstable

Reinstitute ventilation
• Stable, nonfatiguing, comfortable

If patient physiologically stable, continue

Failed criterion

3. Continue SBT for 30-120 minutes:
   Discontinue if any of the following occurs:
   • General: ↑ anxiety or sweating
   • Gas exchange: SpO₂ < 88%; PaCO₂ ↑ by >10 mm Hg
   • Hemodynamics: sustained HR changes of >± 20% OR HR > 140/min; SBP < 90 OR > 180 mm Hg
   • Respiratory: RR > 35/min for >5 min; signs of ↑ WOB (paradoxical breathing, accessory muscles...)

Reintubate

No failure criterion met

Failure

4. Extubate

5. Monitor

FIG. 20.13 Liberation Algorithm. Algorithm for assessing whether a patient is ready to be liberated from mechanical ventilation and extubated. ECG, electrocardiogram; HR, heart rate; PEEP, positive end expiratory pressure; P/F, Pao₂/Fio₂ ratio; PSV, pressure support ventilation; RR, respiratory rate; SBP, systolic blood pressure; SpO₂, oxygen saturation as measured by pulse oximetry; WOB, work of breathing. (From Goldman L, Scharfer AI, editors: *Goldman-Cecil medicine,* ed 25, Philadelphia: Elsevier; 2016.)

Continuous positive airway pressure may be added to prevent atelectasis and improve oxygenation.[79,81]

Synchronized intermittent mandatory ventilation trials. The goal of SIMV weaning is the gradual transition from ventilatory support to spontaneous breathing. SIMV weaning is initiated by placing the ventilator in the SIMV mode and slowly decreasing the rate, usually one to three breaths at a time, until a rate of zero or near-zero is reached. An arterial blood gas (ABG) sample is usually obtained 30 minutes after the trial. This method of weaning can increase the work of breathing, and the patient must be closely monitored for signs of respiratory muscle fatigue.[76,79,81]

Pressure support ventilation trials. PSV weaning consists of placing the patient on the pressure support mode and setting the pressure support at a level that facilitates the patient's achieving a spontaneous tidal volume of 10 to 12 mL/kg. PSV augments the patient's spontaneous breaths with a positive pressure boost during inspiration. During the weaning process, the level of pressure support is gradually decreased in increments of 3 to 6 cm H_2O, while the tidal volume is maintained at 10 to 15 mL/kg until a level of 5 cm H_2O is achieved. If the patient is able to maintain adequate spontaneous respirations at this level, extubation is considered. PSV also can be used with SIMV weaning to help overcome the resistance in the ventilator system.[76,79,81]

Nursing Management

Routine assessment of patients requiring mechanical ventilation includes monitoring for patient-related and ventilator-related complications.

Patient Assessment

Assessment of a patient requiring mechanical ventilation focuses on the pulmonary system, placement of the ETT or tracheostomy tube, and monitoring for the development of subcutaneous emphysema and dyssynchrony with the ventilator. Bedside evaluation of vital capacity, minute ventilation, ABG values, and other pulmonary function tests may be warranted, according to the patient's condition. The use of pulse oximetry can facilitate continuous, noninvasive assessment of oxygenation. The use of capnography may facilitate continuous noninvasive assessment of ventilation. Static and dynamic compliance are also monitored to assess for changes in lung compliance (see Appendix B).[83]

Symptom Management

Patients requiring mechanical ventilation may present with a variety of disturbing symptoms, including anxiety, pain, shortness of breath, confusion and agitation, and sleep disturbances. These symptoms are often managed with sedation and analgesic medications. As discussed earlier, these medications could contribute to prolonged mechanical ventilation and delirium. Nonpharmacologic interventions have been shown to be of benefit to these patients. These interventions include promoting a healing environment, promoting sleep, and interventions to lessen anxiety (eg, music therapy, guided imagery, nursing presence, and animal-assisted therapy). Nursing activities to promote a healing environment include minimizing noise levels, ensuring the patient has access to natural light, establishing a method of communication with the patient, and providing the patient with explanations of what is occurring around them.[84] Referral to a complementary and alternative therapy specialist (if one is available) is also appropriate.

ABCDEF Bundle

Another bundle that has been proposed is the Awakening and Breathing Coordination, Delirium Monitoring, Early Mobility, and Family Engagement and Empowerment (ABCDEF) bundle. This bundle focuses on enhancing communication between team members in the critical care unit, standardizing patient care processes, and decreasing the incidence of delirium and prolonged weakness associated with critical illness.[85] The ABCDEF bundle activities are presented in Box 20.4. To facilitate the implementation of the ABCDEF bundle, the patient must be allowed to sleep. Box 20.5 discusses issues surrounding sleep disturbance in the critically ill patient.

Ventilator Assessment

Assessment of the ventilator includes a review of all the ventilator settings and alarms. A clear understanding of the alarms and their related problems is important (Table 20.8). Peak inspiratory pressure, exhaled tidal volume, and ABGs are also monitored.

Patient Safety

Several measures are required to maintain a trouble-free ventilator system. These include maintaining a functional manual resuscitation bag connected to oxygen at the bedside, ensuring that the ventilator tubing is free of water, positioning the ventilator tubing to avoid kinking, maintaining the patency of ventilator tubing and connections, changing ventilator tubing per hospital policy, and monitoring the temperature of the inspired air. If the ventilator malfunctions, the patient is removed from the ventilator and ventilated manually with a manual resuscitation bag. Alarms should be sufficiently audible with respect to distance and competing noise within the unit. Issues regarding patient transport are addressed in Box 20.6.

NONINVASIVE VENTILATION

Noninvasive ventilation (NIV) is an alternative method of ventilation that uses a mask instead of an ETT to deliver the therapy.

BOX 20.3 Weaning Intolerance Indicators

- Decrease in level of consciousness
- Systolic blood pressure increased or decreased by 20 mm Hg
- Diastolic blood pressure greater than 100 mm Hg
- Heart rate increased by 20 beats/min
- Premature ventricular contractions greater than 6 per minute, couplets, or runs of ventricular tachycardia
- Changes in ST segment (usually elevation)
- Respiratory rate greater than 30 breaths/min or less than 10 breaths/min
- Respiratory rate increased by 10 breaths/min
- Spontaneous tidal volume less than 250 mL
- $Paco_2$ increased by 5–8 mm Hg and/or pH less than 7.30
- Spo_2 less than 90%
- Use of accessory muscles of ventilation
- Complaints of dyspnea, fatigue, or pain
- Paradoxical chest wall motion or chest abdominal asynchrony
- Diaphoresis
- Severe agitation or anxiety unrelieved by reassurance

Paco₂, arterial carbon dioxide pressure; *Spo₂*, oxygen saturation as measured by pulse oximetry.

QSEN BOX 20.4 **QSEN: Patient-Centered Care**

ABCDEF Bundle

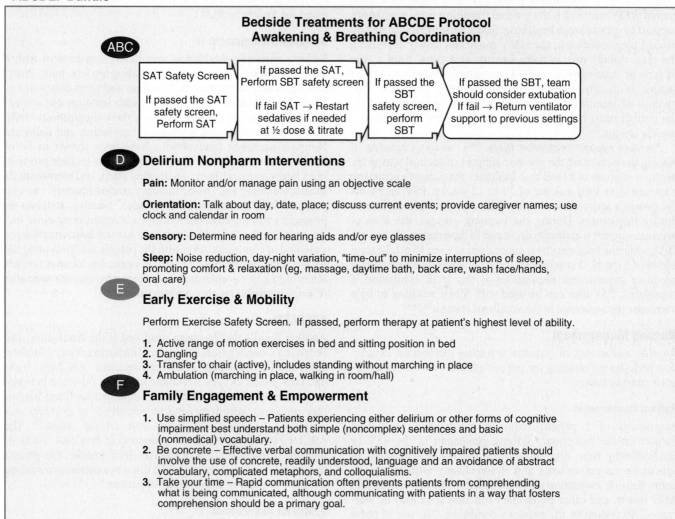

Bedside Treatments for ABCDE Protocol
Awakening & Breathing Coordination

ABC

| SAT Safety Screen

If passed the SAT safety screen, Perform SAT | If passed the SAT, Perform SBT safety screen

If fail SAT → Restart sedatives if needed at ½ dose & titrate | If passed the SBT safety screen, perform SBT | If passed the SBT, team should consider extubation
If fail → Return ventilator support to previous settings |

D Delirium Nonpharm Interventions

Pain: Monitor and/or manage pain using an objective scale

Orientation: Talk about day, date, place; discuss current events; provide caregiver names; use clock and calendar in room

Sensory: Determine need for hearing aids and/or eye glasses

Sleep: Noise reduction, day-night variation, "time-out" to minimize interruptions of sleep, promoting comfort & relaxation (eg, massage, daytime bath, back care, wash face/hands, oral care)

E Early Exercise & Mobility

Perform Exercise Safety Screen. If passed, perform therapy at patient's highest level of ability.

1. Active range of motion exercises in bed and sitting position in bed
2. Dangling
3. Transfer to chair (active), includes standing without marching in place
4. Ambulation (marching in place, walking in room/hall)

F Family Engagement & Empowerment

1. Use simplified speech – Patients experiencing either delirium or other forms of cognitive impairment best understand both simple (noncomplex) sentences and basic (nonmedical) vocabulary.
2. Be concrete – Effective verbal communication with cognitively impaired patients should involve the use of concrete, readily understood, language and an avoidance of abstract vocabulary, complicated metaphors, and colloquialisms.
3. Take your time – Rapid communication often prevents patients from comprehending what is being communicated, although communicating with patients in a way that fosters comprehension should be a primary goal.

SAT, spontaneous awakening trial; *SBT*, spontaneous breathing trial.
Modified from ICU Delirium and Cognitive Impairment Study Group: Bedside Treatments for ABCDE Protocol. http://www.icudelirium.org/docs/AB-CDEF_Pocket_Reference.pdf. Accessed December 9, 2015.

Advantages of this type of ventilation include decreased frequency of hospital-acquired pneumonia; increased comfort; and the noninvasive nature of the procedure, which allows easy application and removal. NIV is indicated in type I and type II acute respiratory failure, cardiogenic pulmonary edema, and other situations in which intubation is not an option. Contraindications to NIV include hemodynamic instability; dysrhythmias; apnea; uncooperativeness; intolerance of the mask; recent upper airway or esophageal surgery; and inability to maintain a patent airway, clear secretions, or properly fit the mask.[86]

NIV can be applied with a full face, nasal, or face mask and ventilator or with a BiPAP machine (Respironics Inc., Murrysville, PA) (Fig. 20.14). One study found that a full face mask is better tolerated than a nasal mask and associated with a diminished incidence of pressure ulcers.[87] This type of ventilation uses a combination of PSV and PEEP supplied by a ventilator or inspiratory and expiratory positive airway pressure supplied by a BiPAP machine to assist the spontaneously breathing patient with ventilation. On inspiration, the patient receives PSV or inspiratory positive airway pressure to increase tidal volume and minute ventilation, resulting in increased alveolar ventilation, a decreased $Paco_2$ level, relief of dyspnea, and reduced accessory muscle use. On expiration, the patient receives PEEP or expiratory positive airway pressure to increase functional residual capacity, resulting in an increased Pao_2 level. Humidified supplemental oxygen is administered to maintain a clinically acceptable Pao_2 level, and timed breaths may be added, if necessary.[88]

Nursing Management

Nursing management of a patient receiving NIV includes many different interventions. Routine assessment of these patients includes monitoring for patient-related and ventilator-related complications. As with invasive mechanical ventilation, the patient must be closely monitored. Respiratory rate, accessory muscle use, and oxygenation status are continually assessed to ensure that the patient is tolerating this method of ventilation. Continuous pulse oximetry is also used.[88,89]

BOX 20.5   QSEN: Patient-Centered Care

Sleep Promotion

Sleep disturbance in critically ill patients stems from various factors including stress associated with critical illness and the critical care environment, pain, and muscular and joint discomfort resulting from bed rest. Bright nocturnal light, excessive noise, and frequent interruptions for care procedures may also disturb sleep in critically ill patients. Because a primary cause of sleep pattern disturbance in patients in the critical care unit is a state of heightened anxiety and discomfort, nursing interventions such as massage that promote relaxation and comfort may be effective. Providing a relaxed, caring environment that encourages confidence in care providers may also assist the patient to relax. Allowing close family members to sit quietly at the bedside while the patient rests may comfort the family and the patient and allow the patient to rest better. Nurses should limit interruptions for care procedures and should coordinate the care among other disciplines to allow patients time for consolidated nocturnal sleep and a daytime nap. Draperies or blinds should be opened during the day to allow patients to receive bright natural light and to help orient them to time of day, lights should be dimmed at night. Noise from staff, squeaky carts, alarms, televisions, slamming doors, and ringing phones should be minimized. Offering the patient earplugs or eye shields may help decrease noise, limit the effects of light, and promote sleep.

The key to ensuring adequate ventilatory support is a properly fitted mask. A nasal mask, face mask, or full-face mask may be used, depending on the patient. A properly fitted mask minimizes air leakage and discomfort for the patient. Transparent dressings placed over the pressure points of the face help minimize air leakage and prevent facial pressure ulcers caused by the mask.[89] The BiPAP machine is able to compensate for air leaks.[88]

The patient is positioned with the head of the bed elevated at 45 degrees to minimize the risk of aspiration and to facilitate breathing. Insufflation of the stomach is a complication of this mode of therapy and places the patient at risk for aspiration. The patient is closely monitored for gastric distention, and a nasogastric tube is placed for decompression, as necessary. Patients are often very anxious and have high levels of dyspnea before the initiation of noninvasive mechanical ventilation. After adequate ventilation has been established, anxiety and dyspnea are usually sufficiently relieved. Heavy sedation is avoided, but if it is needed, it would constitute the need for intubation and invasive mechanical ventilation. It is important to spend 30 minutes with the patient after initiation of NIV because the patient needs reassurance and must learn how to breathe on the machine.[87] The patient who requires NIV with a face mask should never

TABLE 20.8   Troubleshooting Ventilator Alarms

Problem	Causes	Interventions
Low exhaled Vт	Altered settings; any condition that triggers high- or low-pressure alarm; patient stops spontaneous respirations; leak in system preventing Vт from being delivered; cuff insufficiently inflated; leak through chest tube; airway secretions; decreased lung compliance; spirometer disconnected or malfunctioning	Check settings; evaluate patient, check respiratory rate; check all connections for leaks; suction patient's airway; check cuff pressure; calibrate spirometer.
Low inspiratory pressure	Altered settings; unattached tubing or leak around ETT; ETT displaced into pharynx or esophagus; poor cuff inflation or leak; tracheoesophageal fistula; peak flows that are too low; low Vт; decreased airway resistance resulting from decreased secretions or relief of bronchospasm; increased lung compliance resulting from decreased atelectasis; reduction in pulmonary edema; resolution of ARDS; change in position	Reset alarm; reconnect tubing; modify cuff pressures; tighten humidifier; check chest tube; adjust peak flow to meet or exceed patient demand and correct for patient's Vт; reposition or change ETT.
Low exhaled minute volume	Altered settings; leak in system; airway secretions; decreased lung compliance; malfunctioning spirometer; decreased patient-triggered respiratory rate resulting from medications, sleep, hypocapnia, alkalosis, fatigue, change in neurologic status	Check settings; assess patient's respiratory rate, mental status, work of breathing; evaluate system for leaks; suction airway; assess patient for changes in disease state; calibrate spirometer.
Low PEEP/CPAP pressure	Altered settings; increased patient inspirator/flows; leak; decreased expiratory flows from ventilator	Check settings and correct; observe for leaks in system; if unable to correct problem, increase PEEP settings.
High respiratory rate	Increased metabolic demand; medication administration; hypoxia; hypercapnia; acidosis; shock; pain; fear; anxiety	Evaluate ABGs; assess patient; calm and reassure patient.
High-pressure limit	Improper alarm setting; airway obstruction resulting from patient fighting ventilator (holding breath as ventilator delivers Vт); patient circuit collapse; tubing kinked; ETT in right main stem bronchus or against carina; cuff herniation; increased airway resistance resulting from bronchospasm, airway secretions, plugs, and coughing; water from humidifier in ventilator tubing; decreased lung compliance resulting from tension pneumothorax, change in patient position, ARDS, pulmonary edema, atelectasis, pneumonia, or abdominal distention	Reset alarms; clear obstruction from tubing; unkink and reposition patient off of tubing; empty water from tubing; check breath sounds; reassure patient and sedate if necessary; check ABGs for hypoxemia; observe for abdominal distention that would put pressure on diaphragm; check cuff pressures; obtain chest radiograph and evaluate for ETT position, pneumothorax, and pneumonia; reposition ETT; give bronchodilator therapy.
Low-pressure oxygen inlet	Improper oxygen alarm setting; oxygen not connected to ventilator; dirty oxygen intake filter	Correct alarm setting; reconnect or connect oxygen line to 50-psi source; clean or replace oxygen filter.
I:E ratio	Inspiratory time longer than expiratory time; use of an inspiratory phase that is too long with a fast rate; peak flow setting too low, whereas rate too high; machine too sensitive	Change inspiratory time or adjust peak flow; check inspiratory phase, or hold; check machine sensitivity.
Temperature	Sensor malfunction; overheating resulting from too low or no gas flow; sensor picking up outside airflow (from heater, open door or window, air conditioner); improper water levels	Test or replace sensor; check gas flow; protect sensor from outside source that would interfere with readings; check water levels.

ABGs, arterial blood gases; *ARDS,* acute respiratory distress syndrome; *CPAP,* continuous positive airway pressure; *ETT,* endotracheal tube; *I:E,* inspiratory to expiratory; *PEEP,* positive end expiratory pressure; *Vт,* tidal volume.
Modified from Flynn JBM, Bruce NP. *Introduction to Critical Care Nursing Skills.* St. Louis: Mosby; 1993.

Intrahospital Transport of Critically Ill Patients

The following is an excerpt from the "Guidelines for the Interhospital and Intrahospital Transport of Critically Ill Patients":

1. Pretransport Coordination and Communication
   - Confirm receiving unit readiness to receive patient
   - Nurse to nurse handoff (if patient care responsibility is being transferred to a nurse in the receiving area)
   - Notify respiratory therapist and/or other members of the health care team of timing of transport and request equipment support, as needed
   - Mechanical ventilator in receiving unit (for mechanically ventilated patients)
2. Accompanying Personnel
   - A minimum of two people should accompany a critically ill patient (one of whom should be a critical care nurse)
   - Unstable patients should be accompanied by a physician
3. Accompanying Equipment
   - Blood pressure monitor or cuff
   - Pulse oximeter
   - Cardiac monitor with defibrillator
   - Basic resuscitation medications (emergency cart should be readily available in receiving unit)
   - Additional sedatives and narcotic analgesics
   - Additional intravenous fluids and medications
   - Oxygen delivery device attached to oxygen source with at least a 30-minute reserve or manual resuscitation bag and/or transport ventilator (for mechanically ventilated patients)
   - Transport ventilator must have alarms and back up battery
4. Monitoring During Transport
   - Continuous electrocardiographic monitoring
   - Continuous pulse oximetry
   - Periodic measurement of blood pressure, pulse rate, and respiratory rate

From Warren J, et al. Guidelines for the inter- and intrahospital transport of critically ill patients. *Crit Care Med.* 2004;32(1):256–262.

FIG. 20.14 BiPAP via Face Mask. (Courtesy Respironics Inc., Murrysville, PA.)

be restrained. The patient must be able to remove the mask if it becomes displaced or the patient vomits. A displaced mask can force the patient's bottom jaw inward and occlude the patient's airway.

POSITIONING THERAPY

Positioning therapy can help match ventilation and perfusion through the redistribution of oxygen and blood flow in the lungs, which improves gas exchange. On the basis of the concept that preferential blood flow occurs to the gravity-dependent areas of the lungs, positioning therapy is used to place the least damaged portion of the lungs into a dependent position. The least damaged portions of the lungs receive preferential blood flow, resulting in less $\dot{V}/\dot{Q}$ mismatch. Two approaches to position therapy are (1) prone positioning and (2) rotation therapy.

Prone Positioning

Prone positioning is a therapeutic modality that is used to improve oxygenation in patients with ARDS.[90-92] It involves turning the patient completely over onto his or her stomach in the face-down position. Although numerous theories have been proposed to explain how prone positioning improves oxygenation, the discovery that ARDS causes greater damage to the dependent areas of the lungs probably provides the best explanation. It was originally thought that ARDS was a diffuse, homogeneous disease that affected all areas of the lungs equally. It is now known that the dependent lung areas are more heavily damaged than the nondependent lung areas. Turning the patient to the prone position improves perfusion to the less damaged areas of the lungs, improves $\dot{V}/\dot{Q}$ match, and decreases intrapulmonary shunting. Prone positioning can be used to facilitate the mobilization of secretions and provide pressure relief. Prone positioning is contraindicated in patients with increased intracranial pressure, hemodynamic instability, spinal cord injuries, or abdominal surgery. Patients who are unable to tolerate the face-down position are also not appropriate candidates for this type of therapy.[90-92]

No standard has been established for the length of time a patient should remain in the prone position. A review of the research on this subject revealed a wide variation ranging from 12 to 20 hours.[92] The therapy is considered successful if the patient has an improvement in Pao₂ of greater than 10 mm Hg within 30 minutes of being placed in the prone position.[93] The positioning schedule (length of time in the prone position and frequency of turning) is usually based on the patient's tolerance of the procedure, the success of the procedure in improving the patient's Pao₂, and whether the patient is able to sustain improvements in Pao₂ when turned back to the supine position. Prone positioning is discontinued when the patient no longer demonstrates a response to the position change.[93]

The biggest limitation to prone positioning is the actual mechanics of turning the patient. Numerous methods have been discussed in the literature, including manually turning the patient and positioning with pillows to support the patient and use of the RotoProne Therapy System (ArjoHuntleigh, Sweden) (Fig. 20.15).[90] Regardless of the method used, the abdomen must be allowed to hang free to facilitate diaphragmatic descent.

Before the patient is turned to the prone position, his or her eyes are lubricated and taped closed, tubes and drains are secured, and the procedure is explained to the patient and family. A team is organized to implement the turning procedure, and one member is positioned at the head of the bed to maintain the patient's airway. Complications of the procedure include dislodgment or obstruction of tubes and drains,

FIG. 20.15 RotoProne Therapy System. (Courtesy Kinetic Concepts, Inc., San Antonio, TX. RotoProne is a trademark of the ArjoHuntleigh group of companies.)

hemodynamic instability, massive facial edema, pressure ulcers, aspiration, and corneal ulcerations.[90,92]

Rotation Therapy

Automated turning beds to provide rotation therapy are often used in the critical care setting. *Kinetic therapy* and *continuous lateral rotation therapy* (CLRT) are two forms of rotation therapy. The patient is continuously turned from side to side with a rotation of 40 degrees or greater (kinetic therapy) or with a rotation of less than 40 degrees (CLRT).[94] Two types of beds can perform this type of therapy: (1) an oscillation bed, in which the mattress inflates and deflates to provide rotation, and (2) a kinetic bed, in which the entire platform of the bed rotates.[95]

Rotation therapy is thought to improve oxygenation through better matching of ventilation to perfusion and to prevent pulmonary complications associated with bed rest and mechanical ventilation.[96,97] However, to achieve such benefits, rotation must be aggressive, and the patient must be turned at least 40 degrees per side, with a total arc of at least 80 degrees, for at least 18 hours a day.[97,98] CLRT has been shown to be of minimal pulmonary benefit to critically ill patients.[94] Kinetic therapy decreases the incidence of VAP, particularly in patients with neurologic problems and in patients who have undergone surgery.[98] In one study, kinetic therapy decreased the incidence of VAP and lobar atelectasis in medical, surgical, and trauma patients.[97]

Complications of the procedure include dislodgment or obstruction of tubes, drains, and lines; hemodynamic instability; and pressure ulcers. Lateral rotation does not replace manual repositioning to prevent pressure ulcers.[99] Repositioning changes the relationship of the patient's posterior surface to the mattress. This gives the skin a chance to reperfuse and to ventilate. Repositioning shifts weight-bearing points. To prevent pressure ulcers, the patient is positioned 30 degrees from the surface of the mattress regardless of the degree of rotational turn. One study found that patients receiving rotational therapy still developed pressure ulcers of the sacrum, occiput, and heels.[100]

THORACIC SURGERY

The term *thoracic surgery* refers to numerous surgical procedures that involve opening the thoracic cavity (thoracotomy), the organs of respiration, or both. Indications for thoracic surgery range from tumors and abscesses to repair of the esophagus and thoracic vessels.[101] Table 20.9 describes various thoracic surgical procedures and their indications. This discussion focuses only on the surgical procedures that involve the removal of lung tissue.

Preoperative Care

Before surgery, a complete evaluation of the patient is needed to determine the appropriateness of surgery as a treatment and to determine whether lung tissue can be removed without jeopardizing respiratory function. This is especially important when a lobectomy or pneumonectomy is being considered. When resection is being undertaken for tumor treatment, preoperative care includes evaluation of the type and extent of the tumor and the physical condition of the patient.[102]

The evaluation of the patient's physical status focuses on the adequacy of cardiopulmonary function. The preoperative evaluation includes pulmonary function tests to determine the patient's ability to manage with less lung tissue. Cardiac function is also evaluated. Uncontrolled dysrhythmias, acute myocardial infarction, severe chronic heart failure, and unstable angina all are contraindications to surgery.[103,104]

Surgical Considerations

The type and location of surgery dictate the type of surgical approach that is used. The most common approach is the posterolateral thoracotomy, which allows for exposure of both the lung and the mediastinum. Other approaches that are used include anterolateral thoracotomy and median sternotomy.[101]

Special care is taken to avoid drainage of blood or secretions into the unaffected lung during surgery (Fig. 20.16) because such an occurrence could cause hypoxemia and cardiac dysfunction. A double-lumen ETT is used during surgery to protect the unaffected lung from secretions and necrotic tumor fragments. To decrease the incidence of hypoxemia during the procedure, 5 to 10 cm H_2O of PEEP is maintained to the deflated lung. In addition, the deflated lung is intermittently ventilated during the procedure.[105]

Complications and Medical Management

Many complications are associated with a lung resection, including acute respiratory failure, bronchopleural fistula, hemorrhage, cardiovascular disturbances, and mediastinal shift.

Acute Lung Failure

In the postoperative period, acute respiratory failure may result from atelectasis or pneumonia. Atelectasis can occur as a result of anesthesia, the surgical procedure, immobilization, and pain. Treatment is aimed at correcting the underlying problems and supporting gas exchange. Supplemental oxygen and mechanical ventilation with PEEP may be necessary.[106]

Bronchopleural Fistula

Development of a postoperative bronchopleural fistula is a major cause of mortality after a lung resection. A bronchopleural

TABLE 20.9   Thoracic Surgeries

Procedure	Definition	Indications
Pneumonectomy 	Removal of entire lung with or without resection of mediastinal lymph nodes	Malignant lesions Unilateral tuberculosis Extensive unilateral bronchiectasis Multiple lung abscesses Massive hemoptysis Bronchopleural fistula
Lobectomy 	Resection of one or more lobes of lung	Lesions confined to single lobe Pulmonary tuberculosis Bronchiectasis Lung abscesses or cysts Trauma
Segmental resection 	Resection of bronchovascular section of lung lobe	Small peripheral lesions Bronchiectasis Congenital cysts or blebs
Wedge resection 	Removal of small wedge-shaped section of lung tissue	Small, peripheral lesions (without lymph node involvement) Peripheral granulomas Pulmonary blebs
Bronchoplastic reconstruction (also called *sleeve resection*) 	Resection of lung tissue and bronchus with end-to-end reanastomosis of bronchus	Small lesions involving carina or major bronchus without evidence of metastasis May be combined with lobectomy

TABLE 20.9 Thoracic Surgeries—cont'd

Procedure	Definition	Indications
Lung volume reduction surgery	Resection of most damaged portions of lung tissue, allowing more normal chest wall configuration	Severe emphysema
Bullectomy	Resection of large bulla (airspace that is >1 cm in diameter that formed as a result of pulmonary tissue destruction)	Severe emphysema with large bullae compressing surrounding tissue
Open lung biopsy	Resection of small portion of lung for biopsy	Failure of closed lung biopsy Removal of small lesions
Decortication	Removal of fibrous membrane from pleural surface of lung	Fibrothorax resulting from hemothorax or empyema
Drainage of empyema	Drainage of pus in pleural space	Acute and chronic infections
Partial rib resection	Removal of one or more ribs to allow healing of underlying lung tissue	Chronic empyemic infections
VATS	Endoscopic procedure performed through small incisions in chest	Evaluation of pulmonary, pleural, mediastinal, or pericardial conditions Biopsy of lung, pleural, or mediastinal lesions Recurrent spontaneous pneumothorax Evacuation of emphysema, hemothorax, pleural effusion, or pericardial effusion Blebectomy or bullectomy Pleurodesis Sympathectomy Closure of bronchopleural fistula Lysis of adhesions

VATS, video-assisted thoracoscopy.

A   B

FIG. 20.16 Positions for Thoracotomy Incisions. (A) Lateral position for posterolateral incision. (B) Semilateral position for axillary or anterolateral position. (From Rothrock JC, ed. *Alexander's Care of the Patient in Surgery.* 15th ed. St. Louis: Elsevier; 2015.)

fistula develops when the suture line fails to secure occlusion of the bronchial stump, and an opening develops into the pleural space.[107] This can result from an imperfect stump closure, perforation of the stump (eg, with a suction catheter), high pressure within the airways (eg, caused by mechanical ventilation), or infection.[108,109] During surgery, careful attention is given to isolating and closing the bronchus in an attempt to secure a lasting seal with subsequent stump healing.[101] In addition, early extubation is encouraged to eliminate the possibility of perforation of the stump and high airway pressures.[108] Clinical manifestations of a bronchopleural fistula include shortness of breath and coughing up serosanguineous sputum. Immediate surgery is usually necessary to close the stump and prevent flooding of the remaining lung with fluid from the residual space.[109] If this occurs, the patient is placed with the operative side down (remaining lung up), and a chest tube is inserted to drain the residual space.[101]

Hemorrhage

Hemorrhage is an early, life-threatening complication that can occur after a lung resection and can result from bronchial or intercostal artery bleeding or disruption of a suture or clip around a pulmonary vessel.[108] Excessive chest tube drainage can signal the presence of this complication. During the immediate postoperative period, chest tube drainage is measured every 15 minutes; this frequency is decreased as the patient stabilizes. If chest tube drainage is greater than 100 mL/h, fresh blood is noted, or a sudden increase in drainage occurs, hemorrhage should be suspected.

Cardiovascular Disturbances

Cardiovascular complications after thoracic surgery include dysrhythmias and pulmonary edema. Resections of a large lung area or a pneumonectomy may be followed by an increase in central venous pressure. With the loss of one lung, the right ventricle must empty its stroke volume into a vascular bed that has been reduced by 50%. This means a higher pressure system is created, which increases right ventricular workload and precipitates right ventricular failure. Depending on previous heart function, acute decompensation of both ventricles can result. Measures are aimed at supporting cardiac function and avoiding intravascular volume excess. These measures include optimizing preload, afterload, and contractility with vasoactive agents.[108]

Postoperative Nursing Management

Nursing care of a patient who has had thoracic surgery incorporates many nursing diagnoses (Box 20.7). Nursing interventions include optimizing oxygenation and ventilation, preventing atelectasis, monitoring chest tubes, assisting the patient to return to an adequate activity level, providing comfort and emotional support, and maintaining surveillance for complications.

Optimizing Oxygenation and Ventilation

Nursing interventions to optimize oxygenation and ventilation include positioning, preventing desaturation during procedures, and promoting secretion clearance.

Preventing Atelectasis

Nursing interventions to prevent atelectasis include proper patient positioning and early ambulation, deep-breathing exercises, incentive spirometry, and pain management. The goal is to promote maximal lung ventilation and prevent hypoventilation.

Patient positioning and early ambulation. When positioning the patient, the nurse considers the surgical incision site and the type of surgery. After a lobectomy, the patient is turned onto the nonoperative side to promote $\dot{V}/\dot{Q}$ matching. When the good lung is dependent and blood flow is greater to the area with better ventilation, $\dot{V}/\dot{Q}$ matching is better. $\dot{V}/\dot{Q}$ mismatching results when the affected lung is positioned down because of the increase in blood flow to an area with less ventilation. The patient is turned frequently to promote secretion removal but should have the affected lung dependent as little as possible. A patient who has had a pneumonectomy is positioned supine or on the operative side during the initial period. Turning onto the operative side promotes splinting of the incision and facilitates deep-breathing exercises. Tilting the patient slightly toward the unaffected side is possible, but the surgeon should indicate when free side-to-side positioning is safe.[109]

When sitting at the bedside or ambulating, patients must be encouraged to keep the thorax in straight alignment while they breathe deeply. This position best accommodates diaphragmatic descent and intercostal muscle action. The sitting or standing position provides enhanced ventilation to areas of the lung that are dependent in the supine position, accommodating

maximal inflation and promoting gas exchange. Ambulation is essential in restoring lung function and is initiated as soon as possible.

Deep breathing and incentive spirometry. Deep breathing and incentive spirometry are performed regularly by patients who have undergone a thoracotomy. Deep breathing involves having the patient take a deep breath and holding the breath for approximately 3 seconds or longer. Incentive spirometry involves having the patient take at least 10 deep, effective breaths per hour using an incentive spirometer. These activities help reexpand collapsed lung tissue, promoting early resolution of the pneumothorax in patients with partial lung resections. The chest is auscultated during inflation to ensure that all dependent parts of the lung are well ventilated and to help the patient understand the depth of breath necessary for optimal effect. Coughing, which is encouraged only when secretions are present, assists in mobilizing secretions for removal.[110]

Pain management. Pain can be a major problem after thoracic surgery. Pain can increase the workload of the heart, precipitate hypoventilation, and inhibit mobilization of secretions. Clinical manifestations of pain include tachypnea, tachycardia, elevated blood pressure, facial grimacing, splinting of the incision, hypoventilation, moaning, and restlessness. Several alternatives for pain management after thoracic surgery can be used. The two most common methods are systemic narcotic administration and epidural narcotic administration. Opioids can be administered intravenously or via patient-controlled analgesia. In addition, the patient is assisted with splinting the incision with a pillow or blanket when deep breathing and coughing. Splinting stabilizes the area and reduces pain when moving, deep breathing, or coughing.[106]

Maintaining Chest Tube System

Chest tubes are placed after most thoracic surgery procedures to remove air and fluid. The drainage initially appears bloody, becoming serosanguineous and then serous over the first 2 to 3 days postoperatively. Approximately 100 to 300 mL of drainage occurs during the first 2 hours postoperatively, which decreases to less than 50 mL/h over the next several hours. Routine stripping of chest tubes is not recommended because excessive negative pressure can be generated in the chest. If blood clots are present in the drainage tubing or an obstruction is present, the chest tubes may be carefully milked. The chest tube may be placed to suction or water seal.[111]

During auscultation of the lungs, air leaks are evaluated. In the early phase, an air leak is commonly heard over the affected area because the pleura have not yet tightly sealed. As healing occurs, this leak should disappear. An increase in an air leak or the appearance of a new air leak warrants prompt investigation of the chest drainage system to discover whether air is leaking into the system from outside or whether the leak is originating from the incision. Increased air leaks not related to the thoracic drainage system may indicate disruption of sutures.[108]

Assisting Patient to Return to Adequate Activity Level

Within a few days after surgery, range-of-motion exercises for the shoulder on the operative side are performed. The patient frequently splints the operative side and avoids shoulder movement because of pain. If immobility is allowed, stiffening of the shoulder joint can result. This is referred to as *frozen shoulder* and may require physical therapy and rehabilitation to regain satisfactory range of motion of the shoulder joint.[109]

◎ BOX 20.7 NURSING DIAGNOSES

Thoracic Surgery

- Ineffective Breathing Pattern related to decreased lung expansion, p. 1035
- Impaired Gas Exchange related to ventilation-perfusion mismatching or intrapulmonary shunting, p. 1030
- Impaired Gas Exchange related to alveolar hypoventilation, p. 1030
- Acute Pain related to transmission and perception of cutaneous, visceral, muscular, or ischemic impulses, p. 1010
- Anxiety related to threat to biologic, psychologic, or social integrity, p. 1012
- Disturbed Body Image related to actual change in body structures, function, or appearance, p. 1022
- Compromised Family Coping related to critically ill family member, p. 1014

The patient is usually able to sit in a chair the day after surgery. Activity is systematically increased, with attention to the patient's activity tolerance. With adequate pulmonary function before surgery and a surgical approach designed to preserve respiratory function, full return to previous activity levels is possible. This may take 6 months to 1 year, depending on the tissue resected and the patient's general condition.[101]

PHARMACOLOGY

Numerous pharmacologic agents are used in the care of a critically ill patient with pulmonary dysfunction. Table 20.10 reviews these agents and the special considerations necessary for administering them.

Bronchodilators and Adjuncts

Medications to facilitate removal of secretions and dilate airways are of major benefit in the treatment of pulmonary disorders. Mucolytics are administered to help liquefy mucus secretions, which facilitates their removal. Bronchodilators such as beta-2 agonists and anticholinergic agents aid in smooth muscle relaxation and are of particular benefit to patients with airflow limitations. Steroids are often used in conjunction with beta-2 agonists to enhance their effects and to decrease airway inflammation.[112-114]

Neuromuscular Blocking Agents

Sedation is necessary in many patients to assist with maintaining adequate ventilation. Sedation can be used to comfort the patient and to decrease the work of breathing, particularly if the

---

TABLE 20.10 Pharmacologic Management

Pulmonary Disorders

Medication	Dosage	Actions	Special Considerations
NMBAs			
Vecuronium (Norcuron)	Loading dose: 0.08–0.1 mg/kg IV	Used to paralyze patient to decrease oxygen demand and avoid ventilator dyssynchrony	*Boxed Warning From FDA:* Risk of anaphylactic and anaphylactoid type adverse reactions, including fatalities reported in association with use of neuromuscular blockers.
	IV infusion: 0.8–1.2 mcg/kg/min		
Pancuronium (Pavulon)	Loading dose: 0.06–0.1 mg/kg IV		Administer sedative and analgesic agents concurrently because NMBAs have no sedative or analgesic properties.
	IV infusion: 0.02–0.04 mg/kg/h		
Rocuronium (Zemuron)	Loading dose: 0.6–1.2 mg/kg IV		Evaluate level of paralysis q4h using peripheral nerve stimulator.
	IV infusion: 10–12 mcg/kg/min		
Atracurium (Tracrium)	Loading dose: 0.30–0.50 mg/kg IV		Protect patients from environment because they are unable to respond.
	IV infusion: 4-12 mcg/kg/min		
Cisatracurium (Nimbex)	Loading dose: 0.15–0.2 mg/kg IV		Prolonged muscle paralysis may occur after discontinuation of paralytic agent.
	IV infusion: 0.5–10.2 mcg/kg/min		
Mucolytics			
Acetylcysteine (Mucomyst)	Nebulizer, 20% solution: 3–5 mL tid–qid	Used to decrease viscosity and elasticity of mucus by breaking down disulfide bonds within mucus	May be administered with a bronchodilator because medication can cause bronchospasms and inhibit ciliary function.
	Nebulizer, 10% solution: 6–10 mL tid–qid		Treatment considered effective when bronchorrhea develops and coughing occurs.
			Antidote for acetaminophen overdose.
Beta-2 Agonists			
Epinephrine (Adrenalin)	Nebulizer, 1% solution: 2.5–5 mg (0.25–0.5 mL) qid	Used to relax bronchial smooth muscle and dilate airways to prevent bronchospasms	May cause skeletal muscle tremors.
Racemic epinephrine	Nebulizer, 2.25% solution: 5.625–11.25 mg (0.25–0.5 mL) qid		Higher doses may cause tachycardia, palpitations, increased blood pressure, dysrhythmias, and angina.
Isoetharine 1% (Bronkosol)	Nebulizer, 1% solution: 2.5–5 mg (0.25–0.5 mL) qid		May increase serum glucose and decrease serum potassium levels.
Terbutaline	MDI, 340 mcg/puff: 1–2 puffs qid		Treatment considered effective when breath sounds improve and dyspnea is lessened.

Continued

TABLE 20.10   Pharmacologic Management—cont'd

Medication	Dosage	Actions	Special Considerations
Metaproterenol (Alupent, Meta-prel)	MDI, 200 mcg/puff: 2 puffs q4–6h Nebulizer, 5% solution: 15 mg (0.3 mL) tid–qid		Only approximately 10% of administered dose reaches the site of action within the lungs.
Albuterol (Proventil, Ventolin)	MDI, 650 mcg/puff: 2–3 puffs tid–qid Nebulizer, 5% solution: 2.5 mg (0.5 mL) tid–qid		
Levalbuterol (Xopenex)	MDI, 90 mcg/puff: 2 puffs tid–qid Nebulizer: 0.63 mg q6–8h		
Anticholinergic Agents			
Ipratropium (Atrovent)	Nebulizer, 0.02% solution: 0.5 mg (2.5 mL) q6–8h	Used to block constriction of bronchial smooth muscle and reduce mucus production	There are relatively few adverse effects because systemic absorption is poor.
Xanthines			
Theophylline	Loading dose: 4.6 mg/kg IV	Used to dilate bronchial smooth muscle and reverse diaphragmatic muscle fatigue	Administer loading dose over 30 minutes.
	IV infusion: 0.4–0.8 mg/kg/h		Monitor serum blood levels; therapeutic level is 10–20 mg/dL.
Aminophylline	Loading dose: 5.7 mg/kg IV		Administer with caution to patients with cardiac, renal, or hepatic disease.
	IV infusion: 0.5–1 mg/kg/h		Signs of toxicity include central nervous system excitation, seizures, confusion, irritability, hyperglycemia, headache, nausea, hypotension, and dysrhythmias.
Inhaled Corticosteroids			
Beclomethasone (Vanceril, Beclovent)	MDI, 42 mcg/puff: 2 puffs tid–qid	Used to decrease airway inflammation and enhance effectiveness of beta agonists	Suppresses inflammatory response and interferes with ability to fight infection.
Flunisolide (AeroBid)	MDI, 250 mcg/puff: 2 puffs bid		Oral candidiasis is a side effect that can be minimized by having patients rinse their mouths after treatment.
Triamcinolone (Azmacort)	MDI, 100 mcg/puff: 2 puffs tid–qid		

FDA, US Food and Drug Agency; *IV,* intravenous/intravenously; *MDI,* metered-dose inhaler, *NMBAs,* neuromuscular blocking agents; *qid,* four times a day; *tid,* three times a day.
Data from *ClinicalKey Drug Monographs.* https://www.clinicalkey.com/#!/browse/drugs. Accessed December 8, 2015.

patient is fighting the ventilator. More information about sedation is provided in Chapter 9. In some patients, sedation does not decrease spontaneous respiratory efforts enough to allow adequate ventilation, and patient-ventilator dyssynchrony may develop. Neuromuscular paralysis may be necessary to facilitate optimal ventilation. Paralysis also may be necessary to decrease oxygen consumption in a patient who is severely compromised.[115-117]

The nursing management plan for a patient receiving a neuromuscular blocking agent incorporates many additional interventions. Because paralytic agents only halt skeletal muscle movement and do not inhibit pain or awareness, they must be administered with a sedative or anxiolytic agent. Pain medication is administered if the patient has a pain-producing illness or surgery. Providing reorientation and explanations for all procedures is crucial because the patient can still hear but cannot move or see. The patient is also at high risk for developing the complications of immobility, so interventions related to the prevention of skin breakdown, atelectasis, and deep vein thrombosis are also implemented. Patient safety is another concern because the patient cannot react to the environment. Special precautions are taken to protect the patient at all times.[118]

Peripheral Nerve Stimulator

Long-term use of neuromuscular blocking agents can result in prolonged neuromuscular blockade and skeletal muscle weakness. To avoid this complication, the patient's level of paralysis is carefully monitored with the use of a peripheral nerve stimulator (PNS). The PNS delivers an electrical stimulus (single twitch, posttetanic count, double-burst stimulation, or train-of-four [TOF]) to a preselected nerve (ulnar, facial, posterior tibial, or peroneal) by electrodes (needle, ball, or pregelled), and the response is monitored to gauge the level of paralysis.[118]

In most cases, the ulnar nerve is used, with pregelled electrodes being placed 2 to 3 inches proximal to the crease of the wrist (Fig. 20.17). The TOF stimulation test, which delivers four electrical stimuli in a row, is the most common test used. When

FIG. 20.17 Peripheral Nerve Stimulator (PNS). Note placement of electrodes along the ulnar nerve. DBS, double-burst stimulation; TOF, train-of-four.

Path of ulnar nerve

On-off and intensity dial switch

Intensity increases progressively as the dial is turned from setting 1 through 10

the ulnar nerve is stimulated with TOF, the expected response is four twitches (adduction) of the thumb medially across the palm of the hand. The number of twitches correlates with the level of paralysis: four twitches indicates less than 75% blockade; three twitches, approximately 75% blockade; two twitches, approximately 80% blockade; one twitch, approximately 90% blockade; and 0 twitch, 100% blockade. The neuromuscular blocking agent usually is titrated to maintain an 80% blockade (two twitches). The goal is to administer the smallest dose possible of the paralytic agent, to avoid prolonged weakness after the therapy is discontinued.[118]

Use of the PNS for estimating the degree of paralysis is not without problems. Poor skin contact, improper electrode placement, edema in the extremity being monitored, and malfunction of the device can lead to overestimation of the degree of blockade. The patient appears to have a zero-twitch TOF response, but evidence of muscle movement is present. More problematic is underestimation of the degree of blockade. Direct stimulation of the muscle or mistaking finger responses for responses of the thumb can result in a false-positive twitch response. This can result in unnecessary administration of additional doses of the paralytic agent. It is imperative that the patient's twitch response be correlated with clinical observations of patient movement.[118]

CASE STUDY 20.1 Patient With Acute Respiratory Failure

Brief Patient History

Mr. B is a 63-year-old man who is clinically obese. He has a long history of chronic obstructive pulmonary disease (COPD) associated with smoking two packs of cigarettes a day for 40 years. During the past week, Mr. B has experienced a flu-like illness with fever, chills, malaise, anorexia, diarrhea, nausea, vomiting, and a productive cough with thick, brownish, purulent sputum.

Clinical Assessment

Mr. B is admitted to the intermediate care unit from the emergency department with acute respiratory insufficiency. He is sitting up in bed, leaning forward, with his elbows resting on the over-the-bed table. Mr. B is breathing through his mouth, taking rapid shallow breaths, using his accessory muscles

---

to ventilate. On inhalation, his nostrils flare and his accessory muscles retract. During exhalation, Mr. B uses pursed-lip breathing, and his intercostal muscles bulge. He appears anxious and irritable and is able to speak only one or two barely audible words between each breath. Auscultation reveals crackles posteriorly over the right and left lower lung fields.

Diagnostic Procedures

His admission chest radiograph reveals infiltrates in the right lower lobe and left lower lobe. Gram stain of a sputum sample shows numerous gram-positive diplococci. His baseline vital signs are as follows: blood pressure of 110/60 mm Hg, heart rate of 108 beats/min (sinus tachycardia), respiratory rate of 30 breaths/min, and temperature of 101.3°F. His baseline arterial blood gas values on a 28% Venturi face mask are as follows: Pao_2 of 58 mm Hg, $Paco_2$ of 33 mm Hg, pH of 7.52, Hco_3^- level of 28, and oxygen saturation of 88%.

Medical Diagnosis

Mr. B is diagnosed with community-associated pneumococcal pneumonia.

Questions

1. What major outcomes do you expect to achieve for this patient?
2. What problems or risks must be managed to achieve these outcomes?
3. What interventions must be initiated to monitor, prevent, manage, or eliminate the problems and risks identified?
4. What interventions should be initiated to promote optimal functioning, safety, and well-being of the patient?
5. What possible learning needs do you anticipate for this patient?
6. What cultural and age-related factors may have a bearing on the patient's plan of care?

QSEN QSEN: Informatics

Internet Resources

American Association of Critical-Care Nurses: http://www.aacn.org
Society for Critical Care Medicine: http://www.sccm.org
Respiratory Nursing Society: http://respiratorynursingsociety.org
American Holistic Nurses Association: http://www.ahna.org
American Association of Respiratory Care: http://www.aarc.org
American College of Chest Physicians: http://www.chestnet.org/accp
NHLBI ARDS Network: http://www.ardsnet.org
American College of Physicians: http://www.acponline.org
American College of Surgeons: http://www.facs.org
American Lung Association: http://www.lung.org
American Medical Association: http://www.ama-assn.org
American Thoracic Society: http://www.thoracic.org
American Holistic Medical Association: http://www.holisticmedicine.org
ICU Delirium and Cognitive Impairment Study Group: http://www.icudelirium.org/index.html
Centers for Disease Control and Prevention: http://www.cdc.gov
National Institutes for Health: http://www.nih.gov
PubMed Health: http://www.ncbi.nlm.nih.gov/pubmedhealth

SUMMARY

Oxygen Therapy

- Oxygen is a medication, and the primary indication for its use is hypoxemia.
- Oxygen can be delivered by various methods, including low-flow systems, reservoir systems, and high-flow systems.

- Complications of oxygen therapy include oxygen toxicity, CO_2 retention, and absorption atelectasis.

Artificial Airways

- Artificial airways (oropharyngeal and nasopharyngeal) are used to maintain airway patency by keeping the tongue from obstructing the upper airway.
- ETTs (oral and nasal) are used to maintain airway patency, to protect the airway from aspiration, to facilitate access to invasive positive pressure ventilation, and to aid in secretion removal.
- Complications of ETTs include tube obstruction, tube displacement, sinusitis and nasal injury, tracheoesophageal fistula, mucosal lesions, laryngeal or tracheal stenosis, and cricoid abscess.
- Tracheostomy tubes provide the best method of long-term airway maintenance.
- Complications of tracheostomy tubes include hemorrhage, wound infection, subcutaneous emphysema, tube obstruction, tube displacement, tracheal stenosis, tracheoesophageal fistula, tracheoinnominate artery fistula, and tracheocutaneous fistula.
- Cuff pressure is monitored every shift and is maintained at 20 to 25 mm Hg (24 to 30 cm H_2O).
- Humidification is required for all ETTs and tracheostomy tubes.
- Complications associated with suctioning can be minimized if hyperoxygenation is initiated before the start of the procedure, each suction pass is limited to 10 to 15 seconds, and normal saline is not instilled.
- Oral care consists of brushing the patient's teeth with a soft toothbrush to reduce plaque, brushing the patient's tongue and gums with a foam swab to stimulate the tissue, and performing deep oropharyngeal suction to remove any secretions that have pooled above the cuff.
- An artificial airway is removed when it is no longer needed.

Invasive Mechanical Ventilation

- Indications for mechanical ventilation include supporting cardiopulmonary gas exchange (alveolar ventilation and arterial oxygenation), increasing lung volume (end expiratory lung inflation and functional residual capacity), and reducing the work of breathing.
- Complications associated with mechanical ventilation include ventilator-induced lung injury, cardiovascular compromise, gastrointestinal disturbances, patient-ventilator dyssynchrony, and VAP.
- Strategies to prevent VAP ("VAP Bundle") include elevation of the head of the bed, daily "sedation vacations" and assessment of readiness to extubate, peptic ulcer disease prophylaxis, deep vein thrombosis prophylaxis, and daily oral care with chlorhexidine.
- Weaning is the gradual withdrawal of the mechanical ventilator and the reestablishment of spontaneous breathing; weaning begins only after the original process for which ventilator support was required has been corrected and patient stability has been achieved.

Noninvasive Mechanical Ventilation

- Noninvasive mechanical ventilation uses a mask instead of an ETT to administer positive pressure ventilation and is indicated in type I and type II acute respiratory failure, cardiogenic pulmonary edema, and other situations in which intubation is not an option.

- Respiratory rate, accessory muscle use, and oxygenation status are continually assessed to ensure that the patient is tolerating this method of ventilation.

Positioning Therapy

- On the basis of the concept that preferential blood flow occurs to the gravity-dependent areas of the lungs, positioning therapy is used to place the least damaged portion of the lungs into a dependent position.
- Prone positioning involves turning the patient completely over onto his or her stomach in the face-down position; prone positioning is used to improve oxygenation in ARDS.
- Kinetic therapy (continuous turning of a patient from side to side with a 40-degree or greater rotation) and CLRT (continuous turning with a less than 40-degree rotation) are two forms of rotation therapy.
- Rotation therapy is thought to improve oxygenation through better matching of ventilation to perfusion and to prevent pulmonary complications associated with bed rest and mechanical ventilation.

Thoracic Surgery

- The term *thoracic surgery* refers to numerous surgical procedures that involve opening the thoracic cavity (thoracotomy) or the organs of respiration, or both; indications for thoracic surgery range from tumors and abscesses to repair of the esophagus and thoracic vessels.
- Before surgery, a complete evaluation of the patient is needed to determine the appropriateness of surgery as a treatment and whether lung tissue can be removed without jeopardizing respiratory function.
- The most common approach is the posterolateral thoracotomy, which allows for exposure of the lung and the mediastinum.
- Complications of a lung resection include acute respiratory failure, bronchopleural fistula, hemorrhage, cardiovascular disturbances, and mediastinal shift.
- Nursing actions include optimizing oxygenation and ventilation, preventing atelectasis, monitoring chest tubes, assisting the patient to return to an adequate activity level, providing comfort and emotional support, and maintaining surveillance for complications.

Pharmacology

- Mucolytics are administered to help liquefy mucus secretions, which facilitates removal.
- Bronchodilators, such as beta-2 agonists and anticholinergic agents, aid in smooth muscle relaxation and are of particular benefit to patients with airflow limitations.
- Steroids are often used in conjunction with beta-2 agonists to enhance their effects and to decrease airway inflammation.
- Sedation is necessary in many patients to assist with maintaining adequate ventilation; sedation can be used to comfort the patient and to decrease the work of breathing, particularly if the patient is fighting the ventilator.
- Neuromuscular paralysis may be necessary to facilitate optimal ventilation and to decrease oxygen consumption in a severely compromised patient.
- To avoid prolonged neuromuscular blockade, the patient's level of paralysis is carefully monitored by means of a PNS.

ℯ Visit the Evolve site for additional study materials.

REFERENCES

1. Nippers I, Sutton I. Oxygen therapy: professional compliance with national guidelines. *Br J Nurs.* 2014;23(7):382-386.

2. O'Driscoll BR, Howard LS, Davison AG, et al. BTS guideline for emergency oxygen use in adult patients. *Thorax.* 2008;63(suppl 6):vi1-vi68.

3. Heuer AJ. Medical gas therapy. In: Kacmarek RM, Stoller JK, Heuer AJ, eds. *Egan's fundamentals of respiratory care.* 10th ed. St. Louis: Mosby; 2013.

4. Ward JJ. High-flow oxygen administration by nasal cannula for adult and perinatal patients. *Respir Care.* 2013;58(1):98-120.

5. Marin DS, Grocott MPW. Oxygen therapy in critical illness: precise control of arterial oxygenation and permissive hypoxemia. *Crit Care Med.* 2013;41(2):423-432.

6. Barnes TA. Emergency cardiovascular life support. In: Kacmarek RM, Stoller JK, Heuer AJ, eds. *Egan's fundamentals of respiratory care.* 10th ed. St. Louis: Mosby; 2013.

7. Davies JD, Costa BK, Ascuitto AJ. Approaches to manual ventilation. *Respir Care.* 2014;59(6):810-824.

8. Altobelli N. Airway management. In: Kacmarek RM, Stoller JK, Heuer AJ, eds. *Egan's fundamentals of respiratory care.* 10th ed. St. Louis: Mosby; 2013.

9. Mechlin MW, Hurford WE. Emergency tracheal intubation: techniques and outcomes. *Respir Care.* 2014;59(6):881-894.

10. Haas CF, Eakin RM, Konkle MA, et al. Endotracheal tubes: old and new. *Respir Care.* 2014;59(6):933-955.

11. Colice GL. Technical standards for tracheal tubes. *Clin Chest Med.* 1991;12:433.

12. Dalley CB, Tola DH, Kesten KS. Providing safe passage: rapid sequence intubation for advanced practice nursing. *AACN Adv Crit Care.* 2012;23(3):270-283.

13. Overbeck MC. Airway management of respiratory failure. *Emerg Med Clin North Am.* 2016;34(1):97-127.

14. El-Orbany M, Connolly LA. Rapid sequence induction and intubation: current controversy. *Anesth Analg.* 2010;110(5):1318-1325.

15. Kabrhel C, Thomsen TW, Setnick GS, et al. Videos in clinical medicine. Orotracheal intubation. *N Eng J Med.* 2007;356(17):e15.

16. Miñambres E, Burón J, Ballesteros MA, et al. Tracheal rupture after endotracheal intubation: a literature systematic review. *Eur J Cardiothorac Surg.* 2009;35(6):1056-1062.

17. Pacheco-Lopez P, Berkow LC, Hillet AT, et al. Complications of airway management. *Respir Care.* 2014;59(6):1006-1021.

18. Gaissert HA, Burns J. The compromised airway: tumors, strictures, and tracheomalacia. *Surg Clin N Am.* 2010;90(5):1065-1089.

19. Durbin CG. Tracheostomy: why, when, and how? *Respir Care.* 2010;55(8):1056-1068.

20. Cheung NH, Napolitano LM. Tracheotomy: epidemiology, indications, timing, technique, and outcomes. *Respir Care.* 2014;59(6):895-919.

21. Morris LL, Afifi MS. *Tracheostomies: the complete guide.* New York: Springer; 2010.

22. Vallamkondu V, Visvanathan V. Clinical review of adult tracheostomy. *J Perioper Pract.* 2011;21(5):172-176.

23. Cabrini L, Monti G, Landoni G, et al. Percutaneous tracheostomy, a systematic review. *Acta Anaesthesiol Scand.* 2012;56(3):270-281.

24. Samuelson KA. Adult intensive care patients' perception of endotracheal tube-related discomforts: a prospective evaluation. *Heart Lung.* 2011;40(1):49-55.

25. Restrepo RD, Walsh BK. AARC Clinical Practice Guidelines. Humidification during invasive and noninvasive mechanical ventilation: 2012. *Respir Care.* 2012;57(5):782-788.

26. Fink J, Ari A. Humidity and bland aerosol therapy. In: Kacmarek RM, Stoller JK, Heuer AJ, eds. *Egan's fundamentals of respiratory care.* 10th ed. St. Louis: Mosby; 2013.

27. Branson RK, Gomaa D, Rodriquez D. Management of the artificial airway. *Respir Care.* 2014;59(6):974-990.

28. Hamilton VA, Grap MJ. The role of the endotracheal tube cuff in microaspiration. *Heart Lung.* 2012;41(2):167-172.

29. Browne JA, Evans D, Christmas LA, et al. Pursuing excellence: development of an oral hygiene protocol for mechanically ventilated patients. *Crit Care Nurs Q.* 2011;34(1):25-30.

30. Sole ML, Bennett M, Ashworth S. Clinical indicators for endotracheal suctioning in adult patients receiving mechanical ventilation. *Am J Crit Care.* 2015;24(4):318-225.

31. American Association for Respiratory Care. AARC Clinical Practice Guidelines. Endotracheal suctioning of mechanically ventilated patients with artificial airways 2010. *Respir Care.* 2010;55(6):758-764.

32. Pedersen CM, Rosedahl-Nielsen M, Hjermind J, et al. Endotracheal suctioning of the adult intubated patient–what is the evidence. *Intensive Crit Care Nurs.* 2009;25(1):21-30.

33. Czarnik RE, Stone KS, Everhart CC, et al. Differential effects of continuous versus intermittent suction on tracheal tissue. *Heart Lung.* 1991;20(2):144-151.

34. Caparros ACS. Mechanical ventilation and the role of saline instillation in suctioning adult intensive care unit patients. *Dimens Crit Care Nurs.* 2014;33(4):246-253.

35. Jelic S, Cunningham JA, Factor P. Clinical review: airway hygiene in the intensive care unit. *Crit Care.* 2008;12(2):209.

36. Dave MH, Frotzler A, Madjdpour C, et al. Massive aspiration past the tracheal tube cuff caused by closed tracheal suction system. *J Intensive Care Med.* 2011;26(5):326-329.

37. Jenabzadeh NE, Chlan L. A nurse's experience being intubated and receiving mechanical ventilation. *Crit Care Nurse.* 2011;31(6):51-54.

38. Grossbach I, Stranberg S, Chlan L. Promoting effective communication for patients receiving mechanical ventilation. *Crit Care Nurse.* 2011;31(3):46-61.

39. Leasure AR, Stirlen J, Lu SH. Prevention of ventilator-associated pneumonia through aspiration of subglottic secretions: a systematic review and meta-analysis. *Dimens Crit Care Nurs.* 2012;31(2):102-117.

40. Andrews T, Steen C. A review of oral preventative strategies to reduce ventilator-associated pneumonia. *Nurs Crit Care.* 2013;18(3):116-122.

41. Parsons S, Lee C, Strickert D, et al. Oral care and ventilator-associated pneumonia: an integrated review of the literature. *Dimens Crit Care Nurs.* 2013;32(3):138-145.

42. Shi Z, Xie H, Wang P, et al. Oral hygiene care for critically ill patients to prevent ventilator-associated pneumonia. *Cochrane Database Syst Rev.* 2013;13:8. CD008367.

43. Feider LL, Mitchell P, Bridges E. Oral care practices for orally intubated critically ill adults. *Am J Crit Care.* 2010;19(2):175-183.

44. Zukerman LM. Oral chlorhexidine use to prevent ventilator-associated pneumonia in adults. *Dimens Crit Care Nurs.* 2016;35(1):25-36.

45. Hillier B, Wilson C, Chamberlain D, et al. Preventing ventilator-associated pneumonia through oral care, product selection, and application method: a literature review. *AACN Adv Crit Care.* 2013;24(1):38-58.

46. Artime CA, Hagberg CA. Tracheal extubation. *Respir Care.* 2014;59(6):991-1005.

47. O'Connor HH, White AC. Tracheostomy decannulation. *Respir Care.* 2010;55(8):1076-1081.

48. Hess DR, Altobelli NP. Tracheostomy tubes. *Respir Care.* 2014;59(6):956-973.

49. Kracz M, Vitkus A, Papadakos PJ, et al. State-of-the-art mechanical ventilation. *J Cardiothorac Vasc Anesth.* 2012;26(3):486-506.

50. Archambault PM, St-Onge M. Invasive and noninvasive ventilation in the emergency department. *Emeg Med Clin N Am.* 2012;30(2):421-429.

51. Tobias JD. Conventional mechanical ventilation. *Saudi J Anaesth.* 2010;4(2):86-98.

52. Chatburn RL, Volsko TA. Mechanical ventilators. In: Kacmarek RM, Stoller JK, Heuer AJ, eds. *Egan's fundamentals of respiratory care.* 10th ed. St. Louis: Mosby; 2013.

53. Cairo JM. *Pilbeam's mechanical ventilation: physiological and clinical applications.* 6th ed. St. Louis: Elsevier; 2016.

54. MacIntyre NR, Branson RD, eds. *Mechanical ventilation.* 2nd ed. St. Louis: Saunders; 2009.

55. Mireles-Cabodevila E, Hatipoglu U, Chatburn RL. A rationale framework for selecting modes of ventilation. *Respir Care.* 2013;58(2):348-366.

56. Kacmarek RM. Initiating and adjusting invasive ventilatory support. In: Kacmarek RM, Stoller JK, Heuer AJ, eds. *Egan's fundamentals of respiratory care*. 10th ed. St. Louis: Mosby; 2013.

57. Gattinoni L, Protti A, Caironi P, et al. Ventilator-induced lung injury: the anatomical and physiological framework. *Crit Care Med*. 2010;38(suppl 10):S539-S548.

58. Biehl M, Kashiouris MG, Gajic O. Ventilator-induced lung injury: minimizing its impact in patients with or at risk for ARDS. *Respir Care*. 2013;58(6):927-934.

59. Wahla AS, Khan FZ. Development of massive pneumopericardium after intubation and positive pressure ventilation. *J Coll Physicians Surg Pak*. 2012;22(6):401-401.

60. Terragni P, Ranieri VM, Brazzi L. Novel approaches to minimize ventilator-induced lung injury. *Curr Opin Crit Care*. 2015;21(1):20-25.

61. Dreyfuss D, Ricard JD, Gaudry S. Did studies on HFOV fail to improve ARDS survival because they did not decrease VILI? On the potential validity of a physiological concept enounced several decades ago. *Intensive Care Med*. 2015;41(12):2076-2086.

62. Frazier SK. Cardiovascular effects of mechanical ventilation and weaning. *Nurs Clin North Am*. 2008;43(1):1-15.

63. Branson RD, Blakeman TC, Robinson BRH. Asynchrony and dyspnea. *Respir Care*. 2013;58(6):973-986.

64. Haas CF, Bauser KA. Advanced ventilator modes and techniques. *Crit Care Nurs Q*. 2012;35(1):27-38.

65. Grossbach I, Chlan L, Tracy MF. Overview of mechanical ventilator support and management of patient- and ventilator-related responses. *Crit Care Nurse*. 2011;31(3):30-45.

66. Rebmann T, Green LR. Preventing ventilator-associated pneumonia: An executive summary of the Association for Professionals in Infection Control and Epidemiology, Inc, Elimination Guide. *Am J Infect Control*. 2010;38(8):647-649.

67. Mietto C, Pinciroli R, Patel N, et al. Ventilator associated pneumonia: evolving definitions and preventive strategies. *Respir Care*. 2013;58(6):990-1003.

68. Kallet RH. The vexing problem of ventilator-associated pneumonia: observations on pathophysiology, public policy, and clinical science. *Respir Care*. 2015;60(10):1495-1508.

69. Schallom M, Dykeman B, Metheny N, et al. Head-of-bed elevation and early outcomes of gastric reflux, aspiration and pressure ulcers: a feasibility study. *Am J Crit Care*. 2015;24(1):57-66.

70. Burk RS, Grap MJ. Backrest position in prevention of pressure ulcers and ventilator-associated pneumonia: conflicting recommendations. *Heart Lung*. 2012;41(6):536-545.

71. Berry E, Zecca H. Daily interruptions of sedation: a clinical approach to improve outcomes in critically ill patients. *Crit Care Nurse*. 2012;32(1):43-51.

72. Ramirez P, Bassi GL, Torres A. Measures to prevent nosocomial infections during mechanical ventilation. *Curr Opin Crit Care*. 2012;18(1):86-92.

73. Coppadoro A, Bittner E, Berra L. Novel preventive strategies for ventilator-associated pneumonia. *Crit Care*. 2012;16(2):210.

74. Blot S, Rello J, Vogelaers D. What is new in the prevention of ventilator-associated pneumonia? *Curr Opin Pulm Med*. 2011;17(3):155-159.

75. Tokmaji G, Vermeulen H, Muller MC, et al. Silver-coated endotracheal tubes for the prevention of ventilator-associated pneumonia in critically ill patients. *Cochrane Database Syst Rev*. 2015;12:8. CD009201.

76. Kacmarek RM. Discontinuing ventilatory support. In: Kacmarek RM, Stoller JK, Heuer AJ, eds. *Egan's fundamentals of respiratory care*. 10th ed. St. Louis: Mosby; 2013.

77. Penuelas O, Thille AW, Esteban A. Discontinuation of ventilatory support: new solutions to old dilemmas. *Curr Opin Crit Care*. 2015;21(1):74-81.

78. Robertson TE, Sona C, Schallom L, et al. Improved extubation rates and earlier liberation from mechanical ventilation with implementation of a daily spontaneous-breathing trial protocol. *J Am Coll Surg*. 2008;206(3):489-495.

79. Burns SM. Weaning from mechanical ventilation. In: Burns SM, ed. *AACN Protocols for Practice: Care of the mechanically ventilated patient*. 2nd ed. Sudbury, MA: Jones and Bartlett; 2007.

80. McConville JF, Kress JP. Weaning patients from the ventilator. *N Engl J Med*. 2012;367(23):2233-2239.

81. Caroleo S, Agnello F, Abdallah K, et al. Weaning from mechanical ventilation: an open issue. *Minerva Anestesiol*. 2007;73(7-8):417-427.

82. Blackwood B, Burns KE, Cardwell CR, et al. Protocolized versus non-protocolized weaning for reducing the duration of mechanical ventilation in critically ill adult patients. *Cochrane Database Syst Rev*. 2014;11:CD006904.

83. Bekos V, Marini JJ. Monitoring the mechanically ventilated patient. *Crit Care Clin*. 2007;23(3):575-611.

84. Tracy MF, Chlan L. Nonpharmacological interventions to management common symptoms in patient receiving mechanical ventilation. *Crit Care Nurse*. 2011;31(3):19-28.

85. ICU Delirium and Cognitive Impairment Study Group: ABCDEF Bundle. http://www.icudelirium.org/medicalprofessionals.html. Accessed December 9, 2015.

86. Hess DR. Noninvasive ventilation for acute respiratory failure. *Respir Care*. 2013;58(6):950-969.

87. Schallom M, Cracchiolo L, Falker A, et al. Pressure ulcer incidence in patients wearing nasal-oral versus full-face noninvasive ventilation masks. *Am J Crit Care Nurs*. 2015;24(4):349-357.

88. Williams PF. Noninvasive ventilation. In: Kacmarek RM, Stoller JK, Heuer AJ, eds. *Egan's fundamentals of respiratory care*. 10th ed. St. Louis: Mosby; 2013.

89. Visscher MO, White CC, Jones JM. Face masks for noninvasive ventilation: fit, excess skin hydration, and pressure ulcers. *Respir Care*. 2015;60(11):1536-1547.

90. Dirkes S, Dickenson S, Havey R, et al. Prone positioning: is it safe and effective? *Crit Care Nurs Q*. 2012;35:64-75.

91. Kallet RH. A comprehensive review of prone position in ARDS. *Respir Care*. 2015;60(11):1660-1687.

92. Athota KP, Millar D, Branson RD, et al. A practical approach to the use of prone therapy in acute respiratory distress syndrome. *Exper Rev Respir Med*. 2014;8(4):453-463.

93. Wright AD, Flynn M. Using the prone position for ventilated patients with respiratory failure: a review. *Nurs Crit Care*. 2011;16(1):19-27.

94. Goldhill DR, Imhoff M, McLean B, et al. Rotational bed therapy to prevent and treat respiratory complications: a review and meta-analysis. *Am J Crit Care*. 2007;16(1):50-61.

95. Stiller K. Physiotherapy in intensive care: towards an evidence-based practice. *Chest*. 2000;118(6):1801-1813.

96. Staudinger T, Bojic A, Holzinger U, et al. Continuous lateral rotation therapy to prevent ventilator-associated pneumonia. *Crit Care Med*. 2010;38(2):486-490.

97. Ahrens T, Kollef M, Stewart J, et al. Effect of kinetic therapy on pulmonary complications. *Am J Crit Care*. 2004;13(5):376-383.

98. Collard HR, Saint S, Matthay MA. Prevention of ventilator-associated pneumonia: an evidence-based systematic review. *Ann Intern Med*. 2003;138(6):494-501.

99. Powers J, Daniels D. Turning points: implementing kinetic therapy in the ICU. *Nurs Manage*. 2004;35(5):supple 1-7.

100. Wanless S, Aldridge M. Continuous lateral rotation therapy – a review. *Nurs Crit Care*. 2012;17(1):28-35.

101. Lemin MAG. Thoracic surgery. In: Rothrock JC, ed. *Alexander's care of the patient in surgery*. 15th ed. St. Louis: Elsevier; 2015.

102. Keogy BF, Alexander D. Preoperative assessment for thoracic surgery. *Anaesthes Intensive Care Med*. 2014;16(2):59-62.

103. Davies AN, Saravanan P. Tests of pulmonary function before thoracic surgery. *Anaesthes Intensive Care Med*. 2014;15(11):495-498.

104. von Groote-Bidlingmaier F, Koegelenberg CF, Bolliger CT. Functional evaluation before lung resection. *Clin Chest Med*. 2011;32(4):773-787.

105. Senturk M, Slinger P, Cohen E. Intraoperative mechanical ventilation strategies for one-lung ventilation. *Best Pract Res Clin Anaesthesiol*. 2015;29(3):357-369.

106. Sachdev G, Napolitano LM. Postoperative pulmonary complications: pneumonia and acute respiratory failure. *Surg Clin N Am*. 2012;92(2):321-344.

107. Shekar K, Foot C, Fraser J, et al. Bronchopleural fistula: an update for intensivists. *J Crit Care*. 2010;25(1):47-55.

108. Soll C, Hahnloser D, Frauenfelder T. The postpneumonectomy syndrome: clinical presentation and treatment. *Eur J Cardiothorac Surg*. 2009;35(2):319-324.

109. Brenner Z, Addona C. Caring for the pneumonectomy patient: challenges and changes. *Crit Care Nurse*. 1995;15(5):65-72.

110. Hirsch CA. Airway clearance therapy. In: Kacmarek RM, Stoller JK, Heuer AJ, eds. *Egan's fundamentals of respiratory care*. 10th ed. St. Louis: Mosby; 2013.

111. Kane CJ, York NL, Minton LA. Chest tubes in the critically ill patient. *Dimens Crit Care Nurs*. 2013;32(3):111-117.

112. Dodwell RL, Kendall JB. Respiratory system: applied pharmacology. *Anaesthe Intensive Care Med*. 2014;15(11):517-522.

113. Gardenhire DS. Airway pharmacology. In: Kacmarek RM, Stoller JK, Heuer AJ, eds. *Egan's fundamentals of respiratory care*. 10th ed. St. Louis: Mosby; 2013.

114. Meyer KC. COPD 2013: an update on treatment and newly approved medications for pharmacists. *J Am Pharm Assoc* (2003). 2003;53(6):e219-e229.

115. Hraiech S, Dizier S, Papazian L. The use of paralytics in patients with acute respiratory failure. *Clin Chest Med*. 2014;35(4):753-763.

116. Greenberg SB, Vender J. The use of neuromuscular blocking agents in the ICU: where are we now? *Crit Care Med*. 2013;41(5):1332-1344.

117. Price D, Kenyon NJ, Stollenwerk N. A fresh look at paralytics in the critically ill: real promise and real concern. *Ann Intensive Care*. 2012;2(1):43.

118. Lien CA, Kopman AF. Current recommendations for monitoring depth of neuromuscular blockade. *Curr Opin Anaesthesiol*. 2014;27(6):616-622.

21

Neurologic Anatomy and Physiology

Kathleen M. Stacy

The nervous system is the "executive suite" of the human body. It directs all other systems and provides the unique ability for thought, emotion, understanding of complex information, and integration of numerous stimuli. As the recipient of all sensory information for analysis, the nervous system generates intellectual and motor responses aimed at maintaining the integrity of life structures. Critical care nurses must attain a basic understanding of the anatomy and physiology of this complex system because the nervous system serves as the basis for innervation and proper functioning of all other systems. This chapter reviews the anatomic divisions and functions of the central nervous system (CNS), including the cellular microstructure, protective encasement, networked functions, and mechanisms aimed at maintenance of structural and physiologic integrity. The cranial nerves, a component of the peripheral nervous system (PNS), are presented in tabular form.

DIVISIONS OF THE NERVOUS SYSTEM

The nervous system is the most highly organized system of the body, with all its parts functioning as an inseparable unit. This system is usually classified by anatomic function.

Anatomic Divisions

The CNS comprises the brain and the spinal cord. The PNS comprises 12 pairs of cranial nerves, 31 pairs of spinal nerves, and all other nerves serving a variety of functions throughout the body.[1,2]

Physiologic Divisions

The somatic, or voluntary, nervous system is composed of fibers that connect the CNS with structures of the skeletal muscles and the skin. The autonomic, or involuntary, nervous system is composed of fibers that connect the CNS with smooth muscle, cardiac muscle, internal organs, and glands. The autonomic nervous system includes sympathetic and parasympathetic branches.[1,2]

Most activities of the nervous system originate from sensory receptors such as visual, auditory, or tactile receptors. This sensory information is transmitted to the CNS by afferent fibers (sensory fibers). Efferent fibers (motor fibers) transmit the CNS response to the periphery to produce a motor response, such as contraction of skeletal muscles, contraction of the smooth muscles of organs, or secretion by endocrine glands. To better understand the macrostructure and functions of the nervous system, it helps to study the microstructure, or the cellular level.[1-4]

MICROSTRUCTURE OF THE NERVOUS SYSTEM

Two types of cells make up the nervous system: (1) neurons and (2) neuroglia. Neurons are the cells primarily charged with the functional work of the nervous system, including receipt of information, integration, and transmission or conduction of nerve impulses to recipient cells. Neuroglial cells serve as the support infrastructure of the nervous system, providing protection and a structural foundation for neurons and participating in neuronal repair.[1-4]

Neuroglia

In the nervous system, 6 to 10 times more neuroglial cells exist than do neurons. Neuroglial cells consist of four types: (1) *astroglia (astrocytes)*, (2) *oligodendroglia*, (3) *ependyma*, and (4) *microglia* (Fig. 21.1). These cells provide the neuron with structural support, nourishment, and protection (Table 21.1).[1-4] They retain the ability to replicate, but they can replicate abnormally and are the primary source of CNS neoplasms.[3,4]

Neurons

Neurons are the basic functional unit within the CNS, and they are charged with the highly specialized task of data integration and signal transmission. The CNS is made up of more than 10 billion neurons.[1,2] The cellular appearance of neurons varies, but each cell contains three basic components: (1) the cell body, (2) dendrites, and (3) an axon (Fig. 21.2). Neurons are structurally classified as *unipolar*, a cell body with one process that divides into a central branch (one axon) and a peripheral branch (one dendrite); as *bipolar*, a cell body with two processes (one axon and one dendrite); or *multipolar*, a cell body with one axon and several dendrites. The cell body (soma) controls the metabolic activity of the neuron and contains the organelles, such as the nucleus, mitochondria, endoplasmic reticulum, Golgi apparatus, and liposomes, which are necessary for cellular metabolism and maintenance.[1-3] Compared with other body cells, the neuron's protein-embedded membrane with its phospholipid bilayer is unique, consisting of specialized pores

FIG. 21.1 Neuroglial Cells. (A) Astrocytes along the capillary. (B) Oligodendrocytes along the nerves. (C) Microglia (phagocytes). (D) Ependymal cells form a sheet that lines fluid cavities in the brain. (From Black JM, Hawks JH. *Medical-Surgical Nursing: Clinical Management for Positive Outcomes.* 8th ed. Philadelphia: Saunders; 2009.)

TABLE 21.1	Neuroglial Cells
Cell Type	**Function**
Astroglia (astrocyte)	Supplies nutrients to neuron structure and to support framework for neurons and capillaries; forms part of blood–brain barrier
Oligodendroglia	Forms myelin sheath in central nervous system
Ependyma	Lines ventricular system; forms choroid plexus, which produces cerebrospinal fluid
Microglia	Occurs mainly in white matter; phagocytizes waste products from injured neurons

that work as ion-specific channels or pumps to promote passage of ions through an otherwise impermeable plasma membrane.[4]

The neuronal cell body is the life support unit of the neuron. The metabolic demands of these specialized units necessitate uninterrupted perfusion with glucose and oxygen to maintain neuronal life and optimal functioning. Originally, it was believed that CNS neuronal repair was impossible, but research has validated that neurons are more *plastic* than was previously thought, although rates of repair (plasticity) or restoration of neuronal function are driven by factors that remain largely unknown.[5-7] Within the brain and the spinal cord, neuronal cell bodies make up regions of gray matter. Outside the CNS, *ganglia* are cell bodies within the PNS that reside near and work closely with CNS neurons.[1-4]

Dendrites form the receptive component of the neuron; they are branched fibers extending only a short distance from the cell body. Each neuron may have several dendrites, which function as impulse receivers for the cell body. The axon is the part of the neuron concerned with transmission of impulses away from the cell body to other neurons, muscle cells, endocrine glands, or some other effector organ.[8] Neurons contain only one axon, whose length may be microscopic or, in some cases, may extend

up to 4 feet. Some axons are protected by a myelin sheath, a white phospholipid complex laid down by Schwann cells in the PNS and by oligodendroglia in the CNS. The myelin sheath protects neuronal axons and provides insulation for the conduction of nerve impulses.[8,9] Fibers enclosed in the sheath are called *myelinated fibers*; fibers that are not enclosed are called *unmyelinated fibers*. The white matter of the CNS is composed of myelinated fiber tracts.[8]

Myelinated fibers use a process called *saltatory conduction* to support rapid axonal transmission of nerve impulses.[3,4,9] Structurally, axons participating in this form of impulse transmission are laid out with a noncontinuous myelin cover, interrupted with 2-micron bare segments called the *nodes of Ranvier*. These nodes are packed with sodium channels, making them extremely sensitive to membrane depolarization. Because segments of the axon covered by myelin are impervious to sodium influx, impulse transmission is pulled down the length of the axon to the next node of Ranvier. Saltatory conduction increases transmission velocity up to 100-fold, allowing transmission at rates of 120 m/s.[1,4]

Neuronal function is driven by depolarization-repolarization cycles, similar to that described for cardiac physiology (see Chapter 11), but what makes the nervous system so exceptional is its ability to undergo the depolarization-repolarization cycle up to 1000 times per second to ensure optimal receipt, integration, and transmission of information throughout the body.[3] The movement of ions across the neuronal membrane generates electrical action potentials (Fig. 21.3). Neuronal resting membrane potential (RMP) is −65 mV, approximating the equilibrium potential for potassium; on depolarization, sodium channels open, shifting the equilibrium potential in the positive direction.[1,3,4]

Mechanisms for ionic movement involve two types of neuronal channels: (1) *voltage-gated* and (2) *ligand-gated.* Many pharmaceutical and therapeutic agents in use at the present time

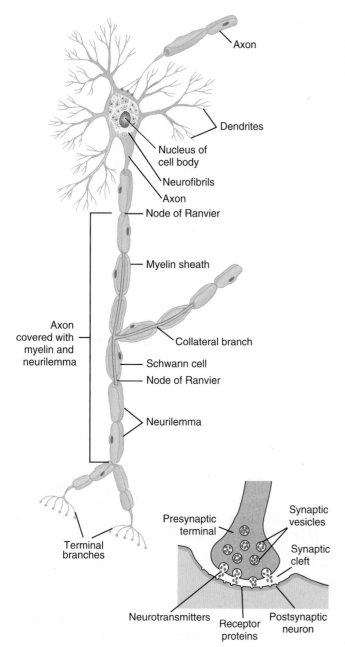

FIG. 21.2 **Neuron.** A neuron (the basic element of the nervous system) and a chemical synapse. (From Black JM, Hawks JH. *Medical-Surgical Nursing: Clinical Management for Positive Outcomes.* 8th ed. Philadelphia: Saunders; 2009.)

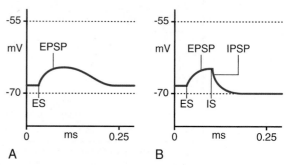

FIG. 21.3 **Transmission.** (A) Transmitter-gated excitatory ionotropic receptor. Binding of the transmitter (*red*, in this example representing glutamate) has opened the pore of a "mixed" Na⁺-K⁺ cation channel. A large influx of sodium ions has depolarized the membrane, as shown by the excitatory postsynaptic potential (EPSP). (B) Transmitter-gated inhibitory ionotropic receptor. Binding of the transmitter (*blue*, representing gamma-aminobutyric acid receptor A) has opened the pore of a chloride channel. Inward chloride conductance has been increased, and the inhibitory postsynaptic potential (IPSP) restores the membrane potential to its resting state: neuronal voltage-gated channel selectivity. (From Fitzgerald MJT, Gruener G, Mtui E. *Clinical Neuroanatomy and Neuroscience.* 6th ed. Philadelphia: Elsevier; 2012.)

or undergoing testing manipulate these ionic transport mechanisms. Voltage-gated channels become activated with changes in transmembrane electrical potential, promoting sodium and calcium influx and potassium efflux. These channels are the primary drivers of cellular action potentials.[1,2] Ligand-gated channels are primarily concerned with mitigating the response of a postsynaptic neuron to synapse and are discussed in more detail later.[1,2]

Action potentials begin with the influx of sodium, producing a focal zone of membrane depolarization at some level between −55 mV and −35 mV. After this critical threshold is reached, numerous sodium channels open, resulting in fast and massive localized depolarization of the plasma membrane. Rapid sodium influx (upstroke phase) increases the membrane

potential to between 70 mV and 90 mV. As the membrane potential changes locally, it stimulates adjoining regions in the neuron to begin depolarization in a self-propagating fashion until depolarization is complete. Within 1 ms of opening, sodium channels close and become inactive.[1-4]

Depolarization causes potassium channels to open, allowing this ion to flow out into the extracellular space, promoting the onset of repolarization. Potassium efflux triggers the cell membrane to return to a potassium equilibrium potential of approximately −75 mV, allowing potassium to reenter the cell but maintaining greater polarity than RMP to hold the cell refractory to another depolarization stimulus. Cellular pumps that depend on a steady supply of adenosine triphosphate are also activated to remove sodium and restore the −65 mV RMP, allowing the cycle to begin anew.[1-4]

After an action potential reaches the axon terminal, the action potential initiates a cascade of events that promote interneuronal communication, or *synapse.* Two types of synapse exist: (1) electrical and (2) chemical. In an electrical synapse, gap junctions made up of narrow (3.5-nm) bridges allow cytoplasm and intracellular metabolites to pass in an essentially continuous fashion between neurons, facilitating impulse conduction from one neuron to the next.[1,2,4] In a chemical synapse, which is involved in most synaptic events, no physical bridge exists between neurons. Instead, a large synaptic cleft of 20 to 40 nm prevents direct action potential transmission from one

Myelin:
1) Multiple sclerosis
2) Guillain-Barré

Cell Body:
1) Trauma
2) Stroke
3) Metabolic disorders - glycogen storage, peroxisomes, etc.

Axons:
1) Diffuse axonal injury (trauma)
2) Axonopathies
3) Tetrodotoxin, saxitoxin - sodium channels
4) Local anesthetics - sodium channels
5) Tetraethylammonium - potassium channels

Pre-synaptic level:
1) Eaton-Lambert myasthenic syndrome
2) Botulinum toxin
3) Tetanus toxin
4) α-latrotoxin
5) Reserpine, guanethidine

Post-synaptic Receptor Level:
1) Organophosphates
2) Neuromuscular blockers - atracurium, succinylcholine
3) Myasthenia gravis
4) Strychnine poisoning
5) Selective serotonin reuptake inhibitors
6) Cocaine / amphetamines
7) Tricyclic antidepressants
8) Curare

FIG. 21.4 Neuronal Pathophysiology. (Modified from Layon AJ, Gabrielli A, Friedman WA. *Textbook of Neurointensive Care.* Philadelphia: Saunders; 2004.)

neuron to another. When the wave of depolarization reaches the presynaptic terminal, it signals the release of neurotransmitters into the synaptic cleft.[1,2]

The two classifications of neurotransmitters are (1) small-molecule transmitters and (2) neuroactive peptides. Examples of small-molecule transmitters include acetylcholine, dopamine, norepinephrine, epinephrine, serotonin, histamine, gamma-aminobutyric acid (GABA), glycine, and glutamate. Neuroactive peptides include pituitary peptides, hypothalamic-releasing hormones, and neurohypophyseal hormones. This chapter is primarily concerned with the small-molecule transmitters, which are stored in vesicles within the axon terminal and released into the synapse through a process called *exocytosis.* Exocytosis is stimulated by arrival of the action potential in the axon terminal and results in release of neurotransmitters into the synaptic cleft, where these molecules rapidly diffuse to interact with postsynaptic receptors.[1,2,4]

Ligand-gated channels are activated by binding of ligand agonists to receptors on the postsynaptic neuron. Ions passing through ligand-gated channels promote an excitatory or inhibitory response within postsynaptic neurons. Examples of excitatory ligand-gated channel receptors include the inotropic glutamate receptors (*N*-methyl-D-aspartate, alpha-amino-3-hydroxyl-5-methyl-4-isoxazolepropionic acid, and kainite), which are primarily concerned with gating sodium, potassium, and calcium ions. Examples of inhibitory ligand-gated channel receptors include GABA receptors, glycine receptors, and nicotinic acetylcholine receptors. Most GABA receptors are found in the brain, where GABA serves as the primary inhibitory neurotransmitter, whereas glycine serves as the primary postsynaptic inhibitory neurotransmitter of the spinal cord. GABA and glycine channels gate chloride ions, which inhibit by promoting repolarization to the chloride equilibrium potential (−60 mV) and by short-circuiting incoming excitatory potentials by gating anions and clamping the membrane shut to excitatory cations (shunting). In other words, when inhibitor neurotransmitters are released, the neuron's internal charge becomes more negative, and the resistance to depolarization is increased.[1]

Metabotropic receptors contribute to impulse transmission, promoting sustained effects of postsynaptic excitation or inhibition. Examples of metabotropic receptors include catecholamine receptors, neuropeptide receptors, and muscarinic receptors.[1,4]

Termination of the synapse reaction is most commonly accomplished through reuptake, in which transporter proteins embedded in neuron and glial cell membranes direct neurotransmitter molecules within the cleft to move back to the intracellular compartment for vesicle repackaging. Neurotransmitters may also go through enzyme degradation, with their component parts taken up for further neurotransmitter synthesis and storage. Ultimately, remaining neurotransmitter diffuses away from the synaptic cleft.[1,2,4]

The response in the postsynaptic neuron to synapse is an excitatory or inhibitory potential. Membrane potentials are not strong enough by themselves to generate a complete action potential within the postsynaptic neuron, but they are instead summarized or integrated by the neuronal cell body in the process of information transmission.[9] When the postsynaptic neuron is bombarded with excitatory potentials, they may combine (*summation*) to become capable of stimulating an action potential.[1-4]

Examples of disease-induced or chemically induced mechanisms that alter neuronal transmission are provided in Fig. 21.4.

CENTRAL NERVOUS SYSTEM

The CNS consists of the brain and the spinal cord. Serving as the control unit for all body systems, the remarkably delicate CNS requires significant protection to preserve normal function. This section addresses the anatomy and physiology of the brain and the spinal cord, supporting the critical care nurse's understanding of pathophysiologic changes that contribute to clinical examination findings.

Cranial Protective Mechanisms

Cranium

The outermost protective measures underneath the integument are the bony structures that encase the CNS. The skull, or cranium, surrounds the brain and is composed of eight flat, irregular bones fused at sutures during early childhood (Fig. 21.5).[1,2] The skull protects the brain from direct force and superficial trauma, although excessive force may fracture the skull, destroying this protective mechanism and driving bony fragments into fragile brain tissue.[10]

If the skull is seen from the inside, the superior surfaces form a smooth inner wall, whereas the basilar skull contains ridges and folds with sharp edges.[1,2] Traumatic impact to the head often results in fracture of the basilar skull as a result of gravitational forces that displace energy in a downward fashion toward the skull base.

The cranium is a solid, nonexpanding bony vault with only one large opening at the base called the *foramen magnum*, through which the brainstem projects and connects to the spinal cord. Several other very small openings in the base of the skull allow entrance and exit of blood vessels and nerve fibers.[1,2]

Meninges

The meninges lie directly beneath the skull, forming another source of protection for the CNS. The meninges consist of three layers: (1) the *dura mater*, (2) the *arachnoid mater*, and (3) the *pia mater* (Fig. 21.6).[1,2,11]

Dura mater. The outermost layer of meninges directly beneath the skull is the dura mater. *Dura* is the Latin term for "tough," and true to its name, this layer is made up of fibrous tissue that is double-folded to support the CNS, nerves, and vascular structures.[1,3] Within the double layers of the dura mater lie venous sinuses that collect blood from intracranial and meningeal veins for drainage into the internal jugular veins.[11]

Four extensions of the dura mater directly support and separate specific areas of the brain: (1) the falx cerebri, (2) the tentorium cerebelli, (3) the falx cerebelli, and (4) the diaphragma sellae. The falx cerebri divides the right and left hemispheres of the brain vertically through the longitudinal fissures extending from the frontal lobe to the occipital lobe. The tentorium cerebelli forms a tent between the occipital lobes and the cerebellum and separates the cerebral hemispheres from the brainstem and the cerebellum. Structures within the brain that are located above the tentorium are often referred to as *supratentorial*, whereas structures located below the tentorium are referred to as *infratentorial* and make up the region of the brain called the *posterior fossa*. The falx cerebelli forms the division between the two lateral lobes of the cerebellum, and the diaphragma sellae forms a roof over the sella turcica, which houses the pituitary gland.[1,2]

The main blood supply for the dura mater is the middle meningeal artery. This artery lies on the surface of the dura in the epidural space and within grooves formed on the inside of the parietal bone. Traumatic disruption of the parietal bone may result in tearing of the middle meningeal artery and development of an epidural hematoma.[12] A potential space exists between the dura mater and the arachnoid mater. This area contains numerous unsupported small veins that may become disrupted and torn when traumatic head injury occurs, leading to development of a subdural hematoma.[12]

Arachnoid mater. The arachnoid membrane is a delicate, fragile membrane that loosely surrounds the brain. Fine threads of elastic tissue called *trabeculae* connect the arachnoid to the pia mater, creating a spongy, web-like structure called the *subarachnoid space*.[11] Cerebrospinal fluid (CSF) circulates freely in the subarachnoid space, which also contains the origins of the brain's large arteries where they enter the skull and differentiate into anterior and posterior circulatory branches.[1,2,13] Rupture of an artery within the subarachnoid space allows for blood to mix with CSF, producing a *subarachnoid hemorrhage*.[12]

At the base of the brain, widened areas of subarachnoid space form cisterns, or spaces, that are filled with CSF. The largest of these cisterns, the cisterna magna, lies between the medulla and the cerebellum, and it communicates with the fourth ventricle.[1,2]

Tufts of arachnoid membrane, called *arachnoid villi*, or granulations, project into the superior sagittal and transverse venous sinuses. Absorption of CSF by arachnoid villi allows its removal by the venous drainage system.[1,2,4] The delicate structure of the arachnoid villi places them at risk for obstruction by blood in subarachnoid hemorrhage, resulting in *obstructive hydrocephalus*.[14]

Pia mater. The pia mater adheres directly to brain tissue. Rich in small blood vessels that supply a large volume of arterial blood to the CNS, this membrane closely follows all folds and convolutions of the brain's surface. Tufts or folds of the pia mater in the lateral, third, and fourth ventricles form a portion of the choroid plexus that is responsible for the production of CSF.[1,3]

Ventricular System

The *ventricular system* consists of four CSF-filled canals lined with ependymal cells, a type of neuroglial cell (Fig. 21.7). This system is made up of two large *lateral ventricles* that each lie within a hemisphere of the cerebral cortex. Extending from the frontal lobes to the occipital lobe, the lateral ventricles consist of a body; an atrium; and frontal, temporal, and occipital horns.[1-3,13] When cannulation of the ventricular system is required for intracranial pressure monitoring, CSF drainage, or placement of a CSF shunt, the frontal horn of the lateral ventricle on the nondominant side of the brain is most often selected.[15,16]

The foramen of Monro connects the two lateral ventricles with a central cavity, the *third ventricle*. Located directly above the midbrain, the walls of the third ventricle are formed by the thalami. The *cerebral aqueduct* (aqueduct of Sylvius) is the canal between the third ventricle and *fourth ventricle*, which lies between the brainstem and the cerebellum. At the base of the fourth ventricle, two openings—the *foramen of Luschka* and the *foramen of Magendie*—open into the subarachnoid space.[1,2] Blockage of CSF flow occurring within the ventricular system obstructs the normal circulation of CSF, causing dilation of the ventricles, a condition called *obstructive hydrocephalus*.[14]

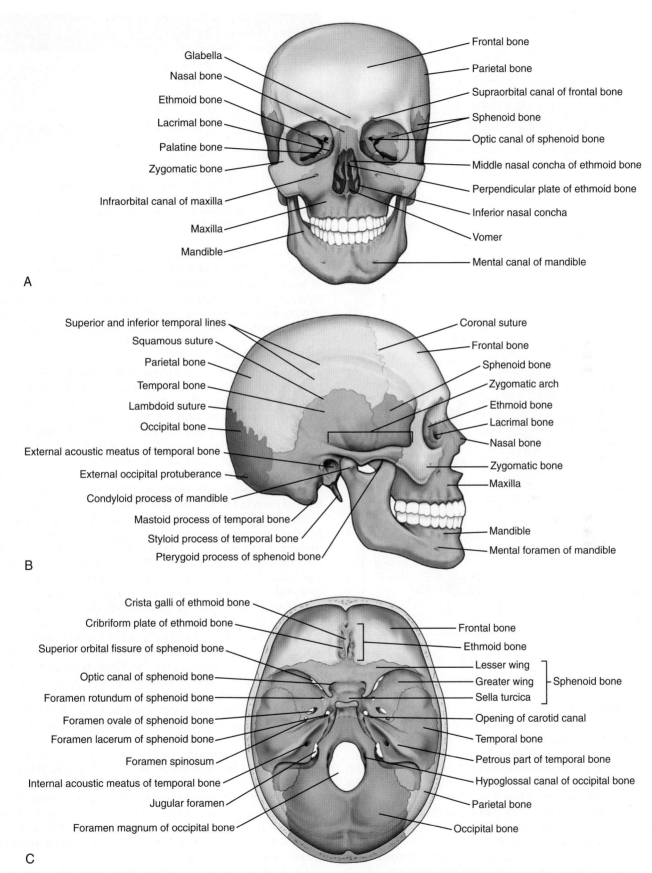

Glabella
Nasal bone
Ethmoid bone
Lacrimal bone
Palatine bone
Zygomatic bone
Infraorbital canal of maxilla
Maxilla
Mandible

Frontal bone
Parietal bone
Supraorbital canal of frontal bone
Sphenoid bone
Optic canal of sphenoid bone
Middle nasal concha of ethmoid bone
Perpendicular plate of ethmoid bone
Inferior nasal concha
Vomer
Mental canal of mandible

A

Superior and inferior temporal lines
Squamous suture
Parietal bone
Temporal bone
Lambdoid suture
Occipital bone
External acoustic meatus of temporal bone
External occipital protuberance
Condyloid process of mandible
Mastoid process of temporal bone
Styloid process of temporal bone
Pterygoid process of sphenoid bone

Coronal suture
Frontal bone
Sphenoid bone
Zygomatic arch
Ethmoid bone
Lacrimal bone
Nasal bone
Zygomatic bone
Maxilla
Mandible
Mental foramen of mandible

B

Crista galli of ethmoid bone
Cribriform plate of ethmoid bone
Superior orbital fissure of sphenoid bone
Optic canal of sphenoid bone
Foramen rotundum of sphenoid bone
Foramen ovale of sphenoid bone
Foramen lacerum of sphenoid bone
Foramen spinosum
Internal acoustic meatus of temporal bone
Jugular foramen
Foramen magnum of occipital bone

Frontal bone
Ethmoid bone
Lesser wing
Greater wing ⎬ Sphenoid bone
Sella turcica
Opening of carotid canal
Temporal bone
Petrous part of temporal bone
Hypoglossal canal of occipital bone
Parietal bone
Occipital bone

C

FIG. 21.5 Skull. (A) Anterior view. (B) Skull viewed from the right side. (C) Floor of the cranial cavity viewed from above. (From Patton KT, Thibodeau GF. *Anatomy and Physiology.* 8th ed. St. Louis: Mosby; 2013.)

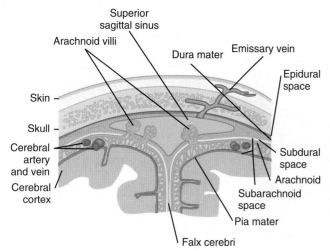

FIG. 21.6 Meninges. Coronal section of the meninges through the superior sagittal sinus. (From Black JM, Hawks JH. *Medical-Surgical Nursing: Clinical Management for Positive Outcomes.* 8th ed. Philadelphia: Saunders; 2009.)

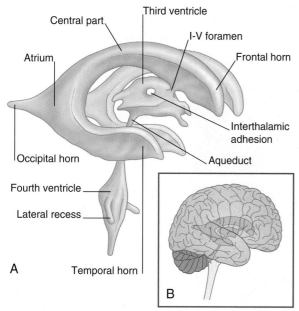

FIG. 21.7 Ventricular System. (A) Isolated cast. (B) Ventricular system in situ. (From Fitzgerald MJT, Gruener G, Mtui E. *Clinical Neuroanatomy and Neuroscience.* 6th ed. Philadelphia: Elsevier; 2012.)

Cerebrospinal Fluid

CSF fills the ventricular system and surrounds the brain and spinal cord in the subarachnoid space. Protection of the CNS is further provided by CSF, which acts as a shock absorber when energy is displaced in traumatic injury. CSF is normally clear, colorless, and odorless. CSF is secreted by the choroid plexuses of the ventricular system, although small amounts are also synthesized by capillaries of the pia mater. Believed to be a filtrate of blood, CSF contains some unique properties that make its synthesis a mystery (Table 21.2).[1,2,13]

The production of CSF occurs at a rate of approximately 20 mL/h, or 500 mL/day. With a circulating volume of 135 to 150 mL, CSF must be regularly resorbed to prevent development of hydrocephalus. Resorption through intact arachnoid villi is favored by increased hydrostatic pressure mechanics that

TABLE 21.2 **Normal Values for Cerebrospinal Fluid**	
Property	**Values**
pH	7.35–7.45
Specific gravity	1.007
Appearance	Clear and colorless
Cells	0 WBCs/mm³; 0 RBCs/mm³; 0–10 lymphocytes/mm³
Glucose	50–75 mg/dL (two-thirds of blood sugar value)
Protein	5–25 mg/dL
Volume	135–150 mL
Pressure	70–200 mm H$_2$O (lumbar puncture); 3–15 mm Hg (ventricular)

RBCs, red blood cells; *WBCs,* white blood cells.

maintain CSF volume within normal limits. The flow of CSF begins in the lateral ventricles, moves through the foramina of Monro into the third ventricle, moves through the cerebral aqueduct into the fourth ventricle, and moves out the foramen of Magendie and the foramina of Luschka into the subarachnoid space of the brain and spinal cord (Fig. 21.8).[1-3,13]

Blood–Brain Barrier

The blood–brain barrier is a physiologic mechanism that helps maintain the delicate metabolic balance in the CNS. The blood–brain barrier regulates the transport of nutrients, ions, water, and waste products through selective permeability.[1,2,17]

Stabilization of the physical and chemical environment surrounding the neurons of the CNS is the task of the blood–brain barrier. Many substances such as metabolites or toxic compounds cannot cross the blood–brain barrier. Other substances such as antibiotics cross slowly, resulting in lower concentrations of them in the brain than in other areas of the body.[17]

The blood–brain barrier operates on the concept of *tight junctions* between adjacent cells and consists of three separate barriers.[1,3] The *vascular endothelial barrier* is formed by tight junctions between the endothelial cells of cerebral blood vessels. The *blood–CSF barrier* consists of tight junctions between the epithelial cells of the choroid plexus. The *arachnoid barrier* is created by tight junctions between the cells that form the outermost layer of the arachnoid mater. The selective permeability of the blood–brain barrier keeps out toxic or harmful compounds and protects neuronal function.[18]

Passage of substances across the blood–brain barrier is a function of particle size, lipid solubility, and protein-binding potential. Most medications or compounds that are lipid soluble and stable at body pH rapidly cross the blood–brain barrier. The blood–brain barrier is also highly permeable to water, oxygen, carbon dioxide, and glucose.[18]

The blood–brain barrier exists only in certain areas of the CNS. The areas in which it does not exist—the pineal region, the basal hypothalamus, and the floor of the fourth ventricle—require contact with plasma to sense changes in concentration of glucose and carbon dioxide and changes in serum osmolality.[1] Initiation of feedback mechanisms by the hypothalamus in response to these changes regulates the internal environment of the remainder of the body.[4]

Of clinical significance, disruption or alteration of blood–brain barrier permeability occurs with injury to brain tissue from trauma, toxic insults, and ischemic injury. Brain irradiation also may alter the permeability of the blood–brain barrier,

FIG. 21.8 Flow of Cerebrospinal Fluid. Fluid produced by filtration of blood by the choroid plexus of each ventricle flows inferiorly through the lateral ventricles, interventricular foramen, third ventricle, cerebral aqueduct, fourth ventricle, and subarachnoid space and to blood. (From Patton KT, Thibodeau GF. *Anatomy and Physiology.* 8th ed. St. Louis: Mosby; 2013.)

although intravenously administered chemotherapeutic agents have been shown to have little effect on blood–brain barrier permeability.[19]

Cerebrum

The cerebrum is the largest portion of the brain, constituting 80% of its weight, and is composed of two cerebral hemispheres (right and left), separated by the longitudinal fissure and connected at the base by the *corpus callosum* (Fig. 21.9B).[1,2,20] The outermost aspect of the cerebrum is called the *cerebral cortex* and is made up of *gray matter*, consisting of neuronal cell bodies. Directly below the cerebral cortex lies *white matter*, consisting of myelinated axons, which communicate impulses from the cerebral cortex to other areas of the brain. White matter tracts consist of three types of fibers: (1) *commissural* (transverse), (2) *projection*, and (3) *association*.[1,2,20] Commissural fibers are tracts that communicate between the two cerebral hemispheres, and the corpus callosum is the largest commissural tract. Projection fibers communicate between the cerebral cortex and the lower regions of the brain and the spinal cord. Association fibers communicate between various regions of the same hemisphere.[1,2,20]

The cerebral hemispheres are divided into the *frontal, parietal, temporal,* and *occipital* lobes (Fig. 21.9A). The *rhinencephalon* is often labeled the fifth lobe of the cerebral cortex. Lying deep inside the cerebrum and anatomically associated with the temporal lobe, the rhinencephalon is sometimes referred to as the *limbic lobe.*[1,2,20]

The primary functions of the cerebral cortex include sensory, motor, and intellectual (cognitive) functions, making this area of the brain vital to normal human functioning and providing capabilities that make humans unique as a species.[3,4,20] Brodmann's classification of cerebral cortical cytoarchitecture identifies more than 100 unique areas and provides a useful way to localize specific cortical functions within the brain (Fig. 21.9C).[3] This section covers the areas within Brodmann's classification that are commonly assessed in relation to the development of specific neurologic pathology.

Frontal Lobe

The frontal lobe lies underneath the frontal bone of the skull and is separated posteriorly from the parietal lobe by the central sulcus (fissure of Rolando) and inferiorly from the temporal lobe by the lateral fissure (sylvian fissure) (see Fig. 21.9A). The major functions of the frontal lobe are voluntary motor function, cognitive function (orientation, memory, insight, judgment, arithmetic, and abstraction), and expressive language (verbal and written).[1,2,20]

The prefrontal areas (see Fig. 21.9C), located just behind the frontal bone's distribution over the forehead, are concerned with cognition.[3,4] These areas work in concert with other areas of the brain to intellectually appraise and respond to environmental information or stimuli. They augment the intellect with socially trained emotional responses learned over the course of childhood and young adulthood, and they participate in triggering autonomic nervous system responses such as tachycardia

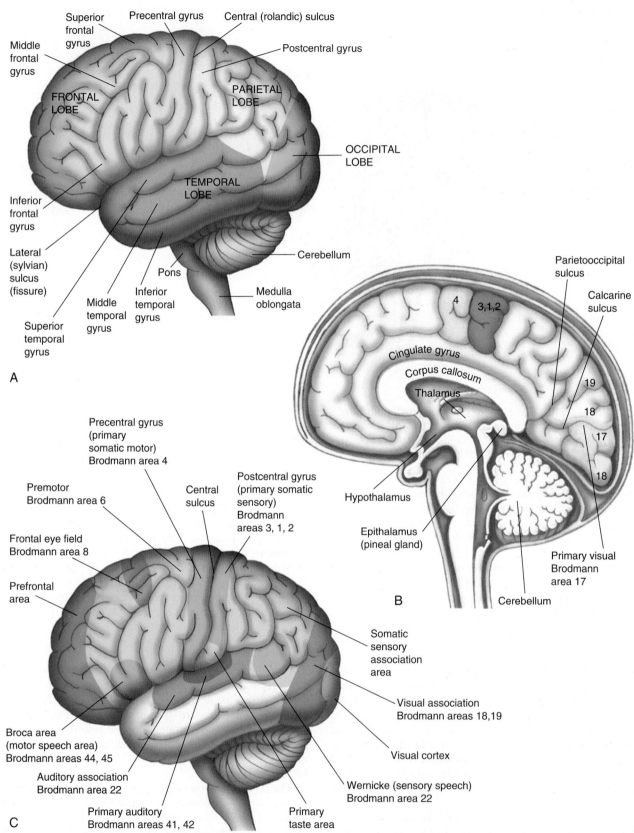

FIG. 21.9 Cerebral Hemispheres. (A) Left hemisphere of cerebrum, lateral view. (B) Functional areas of the cerebral cortex, midsagittal view. (C) Functional areas of the cerebral cortex, lateral view. (From Huether SE, McCance KL: *Understanding Pathophysiology*. 5th ed. St. Louis: Mosby; 2012.)

in relation to situational needs.[3,4] The location of the prefrontal cortex makes it vulnerable to traumatic injury, often resulting in profound changes in cognitive capacity and social responses to environmental stimuli after brain injury.[21]

The motor strip of the frontal cortex is represented by Brodmann area 4 (see Fig. 21.9C) and consists of cell bodies for neurons associated with *voluntary (pyramidal) motor* functions. Because most voluntary motor tracts cross over to the opposite side as they descend through the brainstem, the right motor strip represents voluntary motor function for the left side of the body, and vice versa.[3,4] The motor *homunculus* (Fig. 21.10B) is a graphic representation of the distribution of voluntary motor function throughout area 4. Appearing as an upside-down man, the foot of the homunculus is illustrated on the superior medial aspects of the frontal lobes, with the knees, hips, trunk, and shoulders extending along the lateral surfaces and with the hands, thumb, head, face, and tongue represented in a lateral inferior distribution extending to the sylvian fissure. The homunculus demonstrates larger body part size to denote areas with greater representation because of the amount of dexterity associated with the part's function. The large surface area of the trunk occupies a relatively small part of the motor strip, whereas smaller body areas such as the thumb or tongue, which involve a great deal of dexterity and fine motor movement, occupy a larger area of the motor strip.[3] Damage to the motor strip results in compromise of motor function on the opposite side of the body.[22]

Broca area (Brodmann areas 44 and 45) is located at the inferior frontal gyrus close to the motor strip's facial distribution (see Fig. 21.9C). Most commonly, Broca area is located on the left side of the frontal lobe, although it occasionally is located in the right frontal hemisphere. Broca area is responsible for expressive language and is used in the formation of verbal and written communication.[3,4,23] Damage occurring to this area results in disability ranging from difficulties with word finding to an expressive or nonfluent aphasia, in which verbal and written communication are significantly compromised, although verbal language reception and comprehension may remain intact.[22,23]

Parietal Lobe

The parietal lobe lies directly behind the frontal lobe on the opposite side of the central sulcus. The posterior border of the parietal lobe is the parieto-occipital fissure, which separates the parietal lobe from the occipital lobe (see Fig. 21.9A). The parietal lobes are primarily concerned with sensory functions, including integration of sensory information; awareness of body parts; interpretation of touch, pressure, and pain; and recognition of object size, shape, and texture.[1]

The parietal lobe contains a sensory strip (Brodmann areas 1, 2, and 3) that lies opposite the motor strip of the frontal lobe (see Fig. 21.9C). Similar to the homunculus of the motor strip, a sensory homunculus recreates a caricature of an upside-down man (Fig. 21.10A) representing areas that account for receipt and initial analyses of sensory information from different areas of the body. Areas of the body with greater sensory needs occupy larger areas on the sensory strip, which is concerned with deep or internal sensations and with cutaneous sensations such as touch, pressure, position, and vibration.[1,2] Injury to these areas may result in tactile sensory loss on the opposite side of the body.[22]

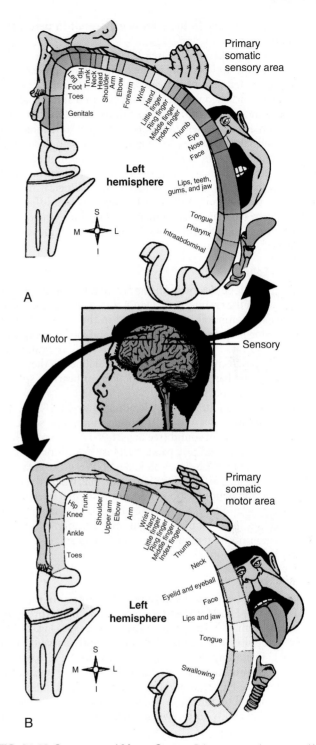

FIG. 21.10 Sensory and Motor Cortex. Primary somatic sensory (A) and motor (B) areas of the cortex. (From Patton KT, Thibodeau GF: *Anatomy and Physiology.* 8th ed. St. Louis: Mosby; 2013.)

The somatic sensory associative area of the parietal lobe (see Fig. 21.9C) facilitates further assessment of sensory stimuli, promoting an ability to determine size, shape, texture, locality of stimuli, temperature, vibration, and precise purpose of familiar objects based solely on tactile discrimination. Interpretive aspects of the response of the parietal lobe to stimuli include awareness of body parts, perceptual orientation in space, and recognition of environmental spatial relationships.[1] Injury to these areas may result in perceptual neglect or inattention.[3]

Wernicke area (Brodmann area 22) is partially located within the parietal lobe and partially in the temporal lobe, most commonly on the left side of the cerebral cortex (see Fig. 21.9C). This area is concerned with reception of written and verbal language and includes many intricate connections to other parts of the brain associated with auditory and visual functions, cognitive appraisal, and expressive language.[1] Injury to this area of the brain may result in disability ranging from minor receptive language dysfunction to *receptive* or *fluent aphasia*, in which expressive language function remains but is illogical in content or a "word salad." When brain injury includes the areas important to language reception and expression, *global aphasia* may result, significantly limiting receipt and expression of language.[23]

Temporal Lobe

The temporal lobe lies beneath the temporal bone in the lateral portion of the cranium (see Fig. 21.9A). The anterior, lower border of the temporal lobe is encased in the sphenoid wing. With a strong blow to the head, the temporal lobe is easily contused and lacerated as it moves against this hard, irregular surface. Separated from the frontal and parietal lobes by the lateral fissure, this lobe has the primary functions of hearing, speech, behavior, and memory.[1,2,20]

The primary auditory areas (Brodmann areas 41 and 42) receive sound impulses and assist in determining the source as well as the meaning of sound (see Fig. 21.9C).[3,4] Injury to these areas may result in auditory perceptual loss.[24] Auditory centers in the temporal lobe are closely linked with Wernicke area.[4]

In the superior portion of the temporal lobe, where the frontal, parietal, and temporal lobes meet, is an essential interpretive area in which auditory, visual, and somatic association areas are integrated into complex thought and memory.[3,4] Seizures in this region of the temporal lobe cause auditory, visual, and sensory hallucinations.[25]

Occipital Lobe

The occipital lobe forms the most posterior aspects of the cerebral cortex (see Fig. 21.9A) and is concerned with interpretation of visual stimuli.[1,2,20] The primary visual cortex (see Fig. 21.9C) receives impulses from projections of the optic nerve (cranial nerve II). These impulses are then referred to the visual associative areas (Brodmann areas 18 and 19) for interpretation and integration (see Fig. 21.9C).[3,4] Injury to the occipital lobes may result in cortical blindness, in which the eye structures remain intact but the ability to receive and interpret visual stimuli is lost.[26]

Limbic Lobe

The rhinencephalon, or limbic lobe, lies medially along the inner aspects of the temporal lobe. The core of the limbic system consists of the hippocampus and the amygdaloid nucleus.[1,2,20] Compared with animals living in the wild, the limbic lobe is poorly developed in humans as a result of the sophisticated cognitive capabilities of the frontal lobe, which mediate many of the protective strategies used by humans in everyday life. The limbic lobe's primary functions are related to self-preservation and include functions such as recall of pleasurable as well as unpleasant or potentially dangerous events, modification of mood and emotional responses in relation to perceived events,

interpretation of smell, and augmentation of visceral processes (eg, heart rate, respiration) associated with emotion.[2] When the injured prefrontal cortex results in cognitive disability, this controversial area of the brain may take on increased control to support self-preservation needs. This may result in significantly aberrant behavior that is frequently judged as socially unacceptable.[27]

Internal Capsule

Fiber tracts from many portions of each half of the cerebrum converge in the area of the brain known as the *internal capsule* as they progress toward the brainstem and the spinal cord. The internal capsule contains afferent and efferent fibers (Fig. 21.11). Afferent (sensory) impulses destined for the cortex travel through the internal capsule in the following succession: brainstem to thalamus to internal capsule to cerebral cortex. Efferent (motor) fibers leaving the cortex also pass through the internal capsule.[1,2] Injury to a portion of the internal capsule may result in pure sensory loss, motor loss, or both on the opposite side of the body with preservation of cortical function.[28]

Basal Ganglia

The basal ganglia participate in regulating extrapyramidal (involuntary) motor function.[1-4] Located deep within the white matter of the cerebral hemispheres, the basal ganglia consist of four nuclei: (1) the corpus striatum (caudate nucleus and putamen), (2) the globus pallidus, (3) the substantia nigra, and (4) the subthalamic nucleus[1,2] (see Fig. 21.11). The basal ganglia are considered a telencephalic, or cerebral, structure, and they are embryologically separate from the thalamus, which is considered a diencephalic structure.[1,2]

Although the basal ganglia play a major role in regulating voluntary motor function, they do not provide direct input to motor tracts through the spinal cord. Instead, input from the

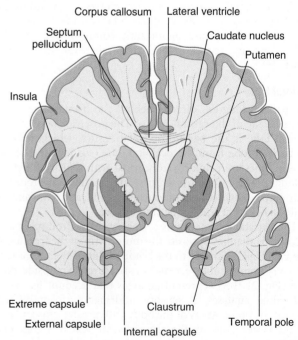

FIG. 21.11 Internal Capsule. Coronal section through the anterior limb of the internal capsule. (From Fitzgerald MJT, Gruener G, Mtui E. *Clinical Neuroanatomy and Neuroscience*. 6th ed. Philadelphia: Elsevier; 2012.)

cerebral cortex stimulates basal ganglia output, which is sent to the brainstem and the thalamus for relay back to the frontal cortex.[4,29] Ultimately, the basal ganglia integrate associated movements and postural adjustments with voluntary motor movement, suppressing skeletal muscle tone as needed to provide fluid, smooth motor function.[4] Dysfunction of the basal ganglia may result in tremor or other involuntary movements; rigid, nonfluid muscle tone; and slowness of movement without paralysis.[29]

Diencephalon

The diencephalon lies below the cerebral cortex and consists of two structures: (1) the thalamus and (2) the hypothalamus (Fig. 21.12).[1,2] Although structurally wedded to the hypothalamus, the pituitary gland is considered an endocrine organ and is not a part of the CNS. Pituitary gland anatomy and physiology are discussed in detail in Chapter 30.

Thalamus

The thalamus consists of two connected ovoid masses of gray matter and forms the lateral walls of the third ventricle (see Fig. 21.12). The two thalami serve as a relay station and gatekeeper for motor and sensory stimuli, preventing or enhancing transmission of impulses based on the behavioral needs of the person. More than 50 nuclei support thalamic function and are divided into specific relay nuclei and nonspecific diffusely projecting nuclei.[1,2] Relay nuclei have a specific relationship or trajectory within the cerebral cortex, whereas diffusely projecting nuclei are thought to mediate cortical arousal.[3,4] Thalamic injury may result in sensory or motor dysfunction, or both, when normal impulse pathways are interrupted.[30]

Hypothalamus

The hypothalamus is located below the thalamus and is connected to the pituitary gland by the hypothalamic or pituitary stalk (see Fig. 21.12).[1,2] Neural control of emotion involves many regions of the brain, including the amygdala and limbic associations with the prefrontal cortex, but to ensure homeostasis, these systems all work through the hypothalamus to coordinate the body's behavioral responses to emotion. The hypothalamus maintains internal homeostasis through its ability to stimulate autonomic nervous system response and endocrine system function in relation to body needs, giving the hypothalamus a role in temperature regulation, regulation of food and water intake, control of pituitary hormone release, and augmentation of overall autonomic nervous system output to a sympathetic or parasympathetic state.[3,4]

Cerebellum

The cerebellum (Fig. 21.13), or hindbrain, is separated from the cerebrum by the dural fold called the *tentorium cerebelli.* Accounting for one-fifth of the brain's size, the cerebellum consists of two lateral hemispheres connected by the *vermis.* The

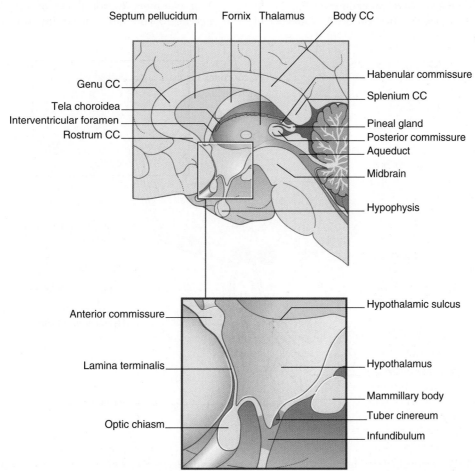

FIG. 21.12 Diencephalon. The diencephalon and its boundaries. CC, corpus callosum. (From Fitzgerald MJT, Gruener G, Mtui E. *Clinical Neuroanatomy and Neuroscience.* 6th ed. Philadelphia: Elsevier; 2012.)

cerebellum is composed of an outer layer of gray matter, or cortex, with a core of white matter tracts lying beneath.[1,2]

Cerebellar impulses are communicated to descending motor pathways to integrate spatial orientation and equilibrium with posture and muscle tone, ensuring synchronized adjustments in movement that maintain overall balance and motor coordination (see Fig. 21.13).[3,4] Cerebellar monitoring and adjustment of motor activity occurs simultaneously with movement, enabling significant control of fine motor function.[3,4,31] The cerebellum is bombarded with information related to the goals of movement and disparities between actual and intended movements. Axons projecting into the cerebellum are 40 times more numerous than the axons leaving the cerebellum to ensure adequate receipt of motor information.[31] Injury to the cerebellum produces *ataxia*, defined as preservation of motor strength with lack of control (coordination) over fine motor function.[32]

Brainstem

The brainstem consists of three major divisions: (1) the midbrain, (2) the pons, and (3) the medulla oblongata. The brainstem is packed with sensory and motor pathways traveling between the spinal cord and the brain and contains numerous centers that regulate vital mechanisms throughout the body.[1,2]

Midbrain

The midbrain forms the junction between the pons and the diencephalon. The cell bodies of cranial nerves III and IV originate in the midbrain (Table 21.3). The midbrain is divided by a sagittal plane into the two cerebral peduncles (Fig. 21.14) and anatomically constitutes the location of the aqueduct of

Sylvius.[1,2] The major function of the midbrain is to relay stimuli to and from the brain through ascending sensory tracts and descending motor pathways.[3,4]

Pons

Located above the medulla, the pons relays information to and from the brain through sensory and motor pathways. The posterior aspects of the pons make up the upper surface of the fourth ventricle (see Fig. 21.14).[1,2] Two respiratory control centers are located in the pons: the apneustic and pneumotaxic centers. The apneustic center controls the length of inspiration and expiration, whereas the pneumotaxic center controls respiratory rate.[3,4]

The cell bodies of cranial nerves V (trigeminal), VI (abducens), VII (facial), and VIII (acoustic) are located in the pons (see Table 21.3).[1,2] The medial longitudinal fasciculus is an important fiber tract in the pons that connects cranial nerves III, IV, and VI with the vestibular portion of the acoustic nerve and pontine paramedian reticular formation, allowing coordinated and appropriate movements of the eyes in response to noise, motion, position, and arousal. The structural integrity of the brainstem may be assessed through clinical stimulation of the medial longitudinal fasciculus in caloric testing.[3,4]

Medulla Oblongata

The medulla oblongata forms the last section of the brainstem, situated between the pons and the spinal cord (see Fig. 21.14). In the pyramids of the medulla, decussation (crossing) of voluntary motor fibers occurs, lending the name *pyramidal* to voluntary motor function (Box 21.1). Below

FIG. 21.13 Principal Cerebellar Efferents. *Arrows* indicate directions of impulse conduction. (From Fitzgerald MJT, Gruener G, Mtui E. *Clinical Neuroanatomy and Neuroscience.* 6th ed. Philadelphia: Elsevier; 2012.)

TABLE 21.3 Cranial Nerves

Cranial Nerve	Origin and Course	Function
I—Olfactory		
Sensory	Found in the mucosa of the nasal cavity; only cranial nerves with cell body are located in peripheral structure (nasal mucosa). It passes through the cribriform plate of the ethmoid bone and goes on to olfactory bulbs at the floor of the frontal lobe. Final interpretation is in the temporal lobe.	Smell. However, the system is more than receptor and interpreter for odors; perception of smell also sensitizes other body systems and responses, such as salivation, peristalsis, and sexual stimulus. Loss of sense of smell is called *anosmia*.
II—Optic		
Sensory	Ganglion cells of the retina converge to the optic disc and form the optic nerve. Nerve fibers pass to the optic chiasm, which is above the pituitary gland. Some fibers decussate; others do not. The two tracts go to the lateral geniculate body near the thalamus and then on to the end station for interpretation in the occipital lobe.	Vision

A-Total blindness of right eye
B-Bitemporal hemianopsia
C-Left nasal hemianopsia
D-Left homonymous hemianopsia
E-Left homonymous hemianopsia inferior quadrant
F-Left homonymous hemianopsia superior quadrant

III—Oculomotor		
Motor	Originates in the midbrain and emerges from the brainstem at the upper pons.	Extraocular movement of eyes
Motor	Motor fibers go to superior, medial, and inferior recti and to the inferior oblique for eye movement and levator muscle of the eyelid.	Raising of eyelid

Continued

TABLE 21.3 Cranial Nerves—cont'd

Cranial Nerve	Origin and Course	Function
Parasympathetic	Parasympathetic fibers go to ciliary muscles and iris of eye.	Constriction of pupil; changing shape of lens

Superior rectus tested by gaze up and out

Inferior oblique tested by gaze up and in

Medial rectus tested by gaze directed in toward nose (medial)

Inferior rectus tested by gaze down and out

G.J.Wassilchenko

A   B   C

IV—Trochlear		
Motor	Midbrain origin near oculomotor nerve, emerges at upper pons near cerebral peduncle; motor fibers go to superior oblique muscle of the eyeball.	Extraocular movement of eyes

Superior oblique tested by gaze down and in

G.J.Wassilchenko

A   B   C

TABLE 21.3   Cranial Nerves—cont'd

Cranial Nerve	Origin and Course	Function
V—Trigeminal		
Sensory	Originates in the fourth ventricle and emerges at lateral parts of the pons; has three branches to face: ophthalmic, maxillary, and mandibular.	*Ophthalmic branch:* Sensation to cornea, ciliary body, iris, lacrimal gland, conjunctiva, nasal mucosal membranes, eyelids, eyebrows, forehead, and nose *Maxillary branch:* Sensation to skin of cheek, lower lid, side of nose and upper jaw, teeth, mucosa of mouth, sphenopalatine-pterygoid region, and maxillary sinus *Mandibular branch:* Sensation to skin of lower lip, chin, ear, mucous membrane, teeth of lower jaw, and tongue
Motor	Goes to temporalis, masseter, pterygoid gland, and anterior part of digastric muscles (all for mastication) and tensor tympani and tensor veli palatine muscles (clench jaw).	Supplies muscles for chewing (mastication) and opening jaw

Ophthalmic branch
Trigeminal nerve
Maxillary branch
Mandibular branches

G.J.Wassilchenko

Cranial Nerve	Origin and Course	Function
VI—Abducens		
Motor	Posterior part of pons goes to lateral rectus muscle for eye movement. Lateral rectus tested by gaze directed outward away from nose (lateral).	Extraocular eye movement; rotates eyeball outward

Lateral rectus tested by gaze directed outward away from nose (lateral)

A   B   C

G.J.Wassilchenko

Continued

TABLE 21.3 Cranial Nerves—cont'd

Cranial Nerve	Origin and Course	Function
VII—Facial		
Sensory	Lower portion of pons goes to anterior two-thirds of tongue and soft palate.	Taste in anterior two-thirds of tongue; sensation to soft palate
Motor	Pons to muscles of forehead, eyelids, checks, lips, ears, nose, and neck.	Movement of facial muscles to produce facial expressions, close eyes
Parasympathetic	Pons to salivary gland and lacrimal glands.	Secretory for salivation and tears
VIII—Acoustic		
Sensory	Nerve has two divisions.	
	Cochlear division originates in spinal ganglia of the cochlea, with peripheral fibers to the organ of Corti in the internal ear. It goes to the pons, and impulses are transmitted to the temporal lobe.	Hearing
	Vestibular division originates in the otolith organs of the semicircular canals in the inner ear and in the vestibular ganglion. It terminates in the pons, with some fibers continuing to cerebellum. It is the only cranial nerve that originates wholly within a bone, the petrous portion of the temporal bone.	Equilibrium
IX—Glossopharyngeal		
Sensory	Posterior one-third of tongue for taste sensation and sensations from soft palate, tonsils, and opening to mouth in back of oral pharynx (fauces). Fibers go to the medulla and then to the temporal lobe for taste and sensory cortex for other sensations.	Taste in posterior one-third of tongue; sensation in back of throat; stimulation elicits gag reflex
Motor	Medulla to constrictor muscles of pharynx and stylopharyngeal muscles.	Voluntary muscles for swallowing and phonation
Parasympathetic	Medulla to parotid salivary gland through the otic ganglia.	Secretory, salivary glands; carotid reflex
X—Vagus		
Sensory	Sensory fibers in back of the ear and posterior wall of the external ear go to the medulla oblongata and on to the sensory cortex.	Sensation behind ear and part of external ear meatus
Motor	Fibers go from the medulla oblongata through the jugular foramen with glossopharyngeal nerve and on to the pharynx, larynx, esophagus, bronchi, lungs, heart, stomach, small intestine, liver, pancreas, and kidneys.	Voluntary muscles for phonation and swallowing; involuntary activity of visceral muscles of heart, lungs, and digestive tract
Parasympathetic	Medulla oblongata to the larynx, trachea, lungs, aorta, esophagus, stomach, small intestines, and gallbladder.	Carotid reflex; autonomic activity of respiratory tract and digestive tract, including peristalsis and secretion from organs
XI—Spinal Accessory		
Motor	The nerve has two roots: cranial and spinal. Cranial portion arises at several rootlets at the side of medulla, runs below the vagus, and is joined by the spinal portion from motor cells in cervical cord. Some fibers go along with vagus nerve to supply motor impulse to pharynx, larynx, uvula, and palate. Major portion goes to the sternomastoid and trapezius muscles, branches to cervical spinal nerves C2-C4.	Some fibers for swallowing and phonation; turning head and shrugging shoulders
XII—Hypoglossal		
Motor	Arises in the medulla oblongata and goes to the muscles of the tongue.	Movement of tongue necessary for swallowing and phonation

the point of decussation, stimuli from the right side of the brain control movement for the left side of the body and vice versa.[1,2]

Centers for control of involuntary functions such as swallowing, vomiting, hiccupping, coughing, heart rate, arterial vasoconstriction, and respiration are located within the medulla oblongata. The medullary respiratory center works in conjunction with the apneustic and pneumotaxic centers in the pons to control respiratory function and is responsible for the rhythm of respiration.[3,4] The cell bodies of cranial nerves IX (glossopharyngeal), X (vagus), XI (spinal accessory), and XII (hypoglossal) are located in the medulla oblongata (see Fig. 21.14 and Table 21.3).[1,2]

Reticular Formation

The reticular formation (RF) of the brainstem is located at the core of the brainstem and is active in modulating sensation, movement, consciousness, reflexive behaviors, and the activities of the cranial nerves arising from the brainstem (III through XII). The RF extends from the upper pons to the diencephalon.[1,2] The ascending RF is referred to as the reticular activating system (RAS) and is responsible for increasing wakefulness, vigilance, and responsiveness of cortical and thalamic neurons to sensory stimuli.[30] In the thalamus, the RAS activates relay

FIG. 21.14 Brainstem and Diencephalon. (A) Anterior aspect. (B) Posterior aspect (shifted slightly to lateral). (From Patton KT, Thibodeau GF. *Anatomy and Physiology*. 8th ed. St. Louis: Mosby; 2013.)

BOX 21.1   Decussation of Voluntary Motor Fibers

FIG. A The Stage Is Set. The subject's right hand is about to click the mouse while the eyes are directed elsewhere. The coronal section identifies key structures.

Continued

BOX 21.1   Decussation of Voluntary Motor Fibers—cont'd

FIG. B Afferents. The left parietal lobe constructs a map of the right hand in relation to the mouse, based on information sent to the left somatic sensory cortex (postcentral gyrus) from the skin and deep tissues. The information is relayed by three successive sets of neurons from the skin and by another set of three neurons from the deep tissues. The first set in each case is composed of first-order or primary afferent neurons. These neurons are called unipolar because each axon emerges from a single point (or pole) of the cell body and divides in a T-shaped manner to provide continuity of impulse conduction from tissue to central nervous system. The primary afferent neurons terminate by forming contacts known as synapses on the multipolar (more or less star-shaped) cells of the second-order (secondary) set. The axons of the second-order neurons project across the midline before turning up to terminate on third-order (tertiary) multipolar neurons projecting to the postcentral gyrus.

Primary afferents activated by contacts with the skin of the hand (S1) terminate in the posterior horn of the gray matter of the spinal cord. Second-order cutaneous afferents (S2) cross the midline in the anterior white commissure and ascend to the thalamus within the spinothalamic tract (STT), to be relayed by third-order neurons to the hand area of the sensory cortex.

The most significant deep tissue sensory organs are neuromuscular spindles (muscle spindles) contained within skeletal muscles. The primary afferents supplying the muscle spindles of the intrinsic muscles of the hand belong to large unipolar neurons whose axons (labeled M1) ascend ipsilaterally (on the same side of the spinal cord) within the posterior funiculus. They synapse in the nucleus cuneatus in the medulla oblongata. The multipolar second-order neurons send their axons across the midline in the sensory decussation. The axons ascend (M2) through pons and midbrain before synapsing on third-order neurons (M3) projecting from thalamus to sensory cortex. *PCML,* posterior column–medial lemniscal pathway; *STT,* spinothalamic tract.

BOX 21.1 Decussation of Voluntary Motor Fibers—cont'd

FIG. C Cerebellar Control. Before the brain sends an instruction to click the mouse, it requires information on the current state of contraction of the muscles. This information is constantly being sent from the muscles to the cerebellar hemisphere on the same side. As indicated in the diagram, M1 neurons are dual-purpose sensory neurons. At their point of entry to the posterior funiculus, they give off a branch, here labeled C1, to a spinocerebellar neuron that projects (C2) to the ipsilateral cerebellum. From here, a cerebellothalamic neuron (C3) is shown projecting across the midbrain to the contralateral thalamus, where a further neuron (C4) relays information to the hand area of the motor cortex in the precentral gyrus.

FIG. D Motor Output. Multipolar neurons in the left motor cortex now fire impulses along the upper motor neurons that constitute the corticospinal tract (CST), which crosses to the opposite side in the motor decussation. The CST synapses on lower motor neurons projecting from the anterior horn of the spinal gray matter to activate flexor muscles of the index finger and local stabilizing muscles.

Note that a copy of the outgoing message is sent to the right cerebellar hemisphere by way of transverse fibers of the pons (TFP) originating in multipolar neurons located on the left side of the pons.

Modified from Fitzgerald MJT, Gruener G, Mtui E. *Clinical Neuroanatomy and Neuroscience.* 6th ed. Philadelphia: Elsevier; 2012.

and diffuse projection nuclei to increase distribution of sensory stimuli throughout the cerebral cortex.[3,4] The RAS also works through activation of the hypothalamus, which results in diffuse cortical stimulation and autonomic stimulation.[1] Damage to the thalamic or hypothalamic RAS pathways results in impaired consciousness.[33]

Arterial Circulation

The brain constitutes 2% of the body's weight but uses 20% of the body's total resting cardiac output, requires approximately 750 mL of blood flow per minute, and can extract 45% of arterial oxygen to meet normal metabolic needs.[4] The brain has no reserve of oxygen or glucose, making reductions of these substances critical to the disruption of normal cellular function.[4] Two pairs of arteries, the internal carotid arteries and the vertebral arteries, provide blood to the brain and are anatomically separated into the anterior and posterior circulations

that connect at the base of the brain to form the circle of Willis (Fig. 21.15).[1,2] Knowledge of the brain's arterial supply as it correlates to neurologic function is an essential aspect of neuroscience critical care nursing, especially in the care of patients who had experienced a stroke.

Anterior Circulation

The anterior circulation of the brain is supplied by the right and left internal carotid arteries and their branches (Fig. 21.16). Originating as the common carotids, the left common carotid takes off from the arch of the aorta, whereas the right common carotid originates from the innominate artery. At the level of the cricothyroid junction, the common carotid splits to form the external and internal carotid arteries. The external carotid feeds the face, the scalp, and the skull and includes the branch called the *middle meningeal artery*, which lies between the skull and the dura mater.[1,2]

The internal carotid artery continues upward through the carotid siphon and enters the base of the skull through an opening in the petrous bone. At the base of the brain, the internal carotid gives off the right and left middle cerebral arteries; the right and left anterior cerebral arteries (ACAs), which are connected by the anterior communicating artery (ACoA); and the two posterior communicating arteries (PCoAs). The anterior circulation provides 80% of the blood flow to the cerebral hemispheres, covering the needs of the frontal lobes and most of the parietal and temporal lobes and supplying the subcortical structures residing above the brainstem. The internal carotid artery gives rise to the ophthalmic artery at the siphon before bifurcating into the anterior cerebral and middle cerebral arteries. The ophthalmic artery supplies blood to the optic nerve and eye and may reverse its course to supplement the arterial blood volume of the anterior circulation in the case of internal carotid artery occlusion.[1,2]

Posterior Circulation

The posterior circulation begins with the two vertebral arteries (Fig. 21.17), which originate from the subclavian arteries and travel posteriorly through small openings in the lateral spinous processes of the cervical spine. They enter the skull through the foramen magnum, and at the level of the pons, the two vertebral arteries fuse to form the basilar artery. The terminal portion of the vertebral arteries gives rise to two important arterial branches before basilar artery fusion: the posterior inferior cerebellar arteries. Two major infratentorial branches of the basilar artery include the anterior inferior cerebellar arteries and the superior cerebellar arteries, which together with the posterior inferior cerebellar arteries supply the cerebellum. The distal basilar artery gives rise to the two posterior cerebral arteries, which emerge in the supratentorial region to supply the posterior aspects of the cerebral cortex.[1,2]

Circle of Willis

The circle of Willis is a vascular supply system unique to the brain's circulation (see Fig. 21.14). Located above the optic chiasm in the subarachnoid space, the circle is fed by branches of the internal carotid and basilar arteries. The anterior circulation is connected between the two ACAs by the ACoA and to the posterior circulation by the two PCoAs.[1,2] Approximately 50% of the population has a complete or "ideal" circle of Willis. In others, atretic (small and nonfunctional or hypoplastic) segments often are found in the first branch of the ACAs, called A1; in the first branch of the posterior cerebral arteries, called P1; and in the PCoAs. When complete, the circle of Willis is capable of supporting some degree of collateral blood flow in the case of arterial occlusion, although a sufficient arterial supply in the face of arterial obstruction is not guaranteed.[34]

Venous Circulation

Venous drainage occurs through venous sinuses, many of which are housed in the double-folded membrane of the dura mater (Fig. 21.18). Capillaries drain into venules, which then flow into cerebral veins, ultimately emptying into sinuses located throughout the cranium. Blood from these sinuses empties into the internal jugular vein, which empties into the superior vena cava (Fig. 21.19). Cerebral veins have thinner walls relative to veins in the general circulation and lack a muscular layer or valves.[1,2]

Spinal Cord

The spinal cord, one division of the CNS, extends from the medulla below the foramen magnum. Similar to the brain, the spinal cord is composed of gray and white matter, although

FIG. 21.15 Cerebral Arteries. View from below the cerebral hemispheres, showing the cortical branches and territories of the three cerebral arteries. *ACA,* anterior cerebral artery; *ICA,* internal carotid artery; *MCA,* middle cerebral artery; *PCA,* posterior cerebral artery. (From Fitzgerald MJT, Gruener G, Mtui E. *Clinical Neuroanatomy and Neuroscience.* 6th ed. Philadelphia: Elsevier; 2012.)

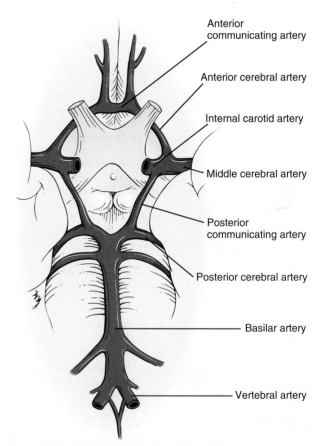

FIG. 21.16 Circle of Willis. (From Swartz MH. *Textbook of Physical Diagnosis: History and Examination.* 7th ed. Philadelphia: Saunders; 2014.)

gray matter in the spinal cord is located internally, and the white matter is on its surface. The distal end of the spinal cord tapers to the *conus medullaris,* which is situated at the level of the first or second lumbar vertebra. Exiting from the spinal cord are 31 pairs of spinal nerves, which exit through intervertebral

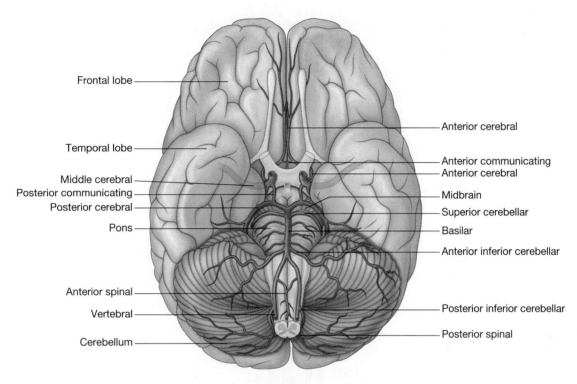

FIG. 21.17 Posterior Arterial Distribution. Arteries at the base of the brain. (From Drake RL, Vogl AW, Mitchell AWM. *Gray's Anatomy for Students*, 3rd ed. Philadelphia: Churchill Livingstone; 2015.)

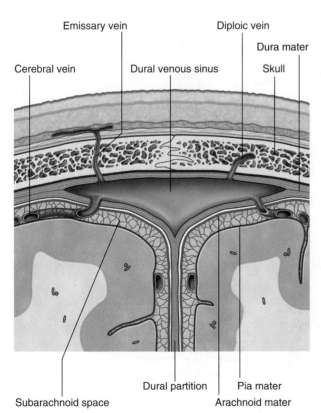

FIG. 21.18 Dural Venous Sinuses. (From Drake RL, Vogl AW, Mitchell AWM. *Gray's Anatomy for Students*, 3rd ed. Philadelphia: Churchill Livingstone; 2015.)

foramina. Because the spinal cord ends at vertebrae L1 and the final nerve roots do not exit until the coccyx, long lengths of nerves, called the *cauda equina*, extend below the conus medullaris toward their associated intervertebral foramina to exit the spinal canal (Fig. 21.20).[1,2]

Spinal Protective Mechanisms

Protective mechanisms similar to those listed for the brain provide protection to the spinal cord.[1,2]

Vertebral Column

The bony structure that encases the spinal cord is the vertebral column. Comprising 33 vertebrae and 24 intervertebral disks, this column is held together by ligaments and tendons. The vertebral column provides support and protection for the spinal cord and the structure and flexibility required for body movement. The vertebrae are divided into sections in relation to their appearance (Fig. 21.21). There are 7 cervical vertebrae, 12 thoracic vertebrae, 5 lumbar vertebrae, 5 sacral vertebrae (fused together as one), and 4 coccygeal vertebrae (fused together as one).[1,2]

Although differences in vertebral appearance exist, the basic structure includes a vertebral body connected by two pedicles to the transverse processes. Two laminae connect the transverse processes to the posterior segment of the vertebra, the spinous process, forming a ring. The center of the spinal foramen is the canal housing the spinal cord.[1,2]

Intervertebral Disks

Vertebral bodies are separated by an intervertebral disk. These fibrocartilaginous structures lie between each vertebral body, extending from the cervical vertebra to the beginning of the sacrum. Intervertebral disks are composed of two layers. The

FIG. 21.19 Venous Circulation.

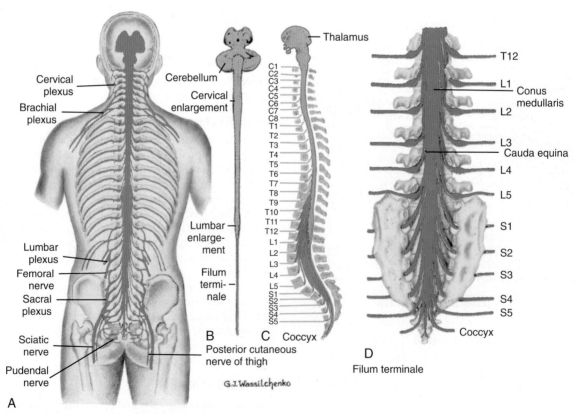

FIG. 21.20 Spinal Cord Within the Vertebral Canal and Exiting Spinal Nerves. (A) Posterior view in situ. (B) Anterior view. (C) Lateral view. (D) Cauda equina.

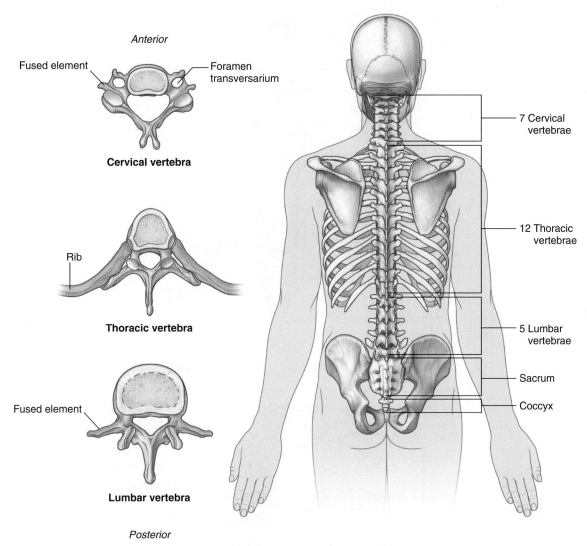

Anterior

Fused element — — Foramen transversarium

Cervical vertebra

Rib

Thoracic vertebra

Fused element

Lumbar vertebra

Posterior

7 Cervical vertebrae

12 Thoracic vertebrae

5 Lumbar vertebrae

Sacrum

Coccyx

FIG. 21.21 Vertebrae. (From Drake RL, Vogl AW, Mitchell AWM. *Gray's Anatomy for Students*, 3rd ed. Philadelphia: Churchill Livingstone; 2015.)

inner core, called the *nucleus pulposus*, is a soft, gelatinous material that assists in shock absorbency. Surrounding the nucleus pulposus is the anulus fibrosus, a thick, tough outer layer.[1,2] The diagnosis of herniated disk refers to dislocation of the normal anatomic position of an intervertebral disk that compromises or puts pressure on a spinal nerve.[35]

Meninges

The meninges of the spinal cord are similar to the meninges in the cranium (Fig. 21.22). The dura mater is a continuation of the intracranial dura mater and encases the cord, the nerve roots, and the spinal nerves until they exit from the vertebral column. The dura extends to the level of the second sacral vertebra, even though the spinal cord itself ends at the L1 or L2 level.[1,2]

The arachnoid mater provides the same web-like, delicate structure as in the cranium, with CSF flow within the subarachnoid space. Because the spinal cord terminates at L2 and the meninges continue to S2, a volume of CSF is contained in the lumbar cistern and constitutes the site targeted for a lumbar puncture. The pia mater of the spinal cord is a thicker, firmer, less vascular membrane than that in the cranium.[1,2]

Spinal Nerves

The 31 pairs of spinal nerves include 8 cervical, 12 thoracic, 5 lumbar, 5 sacral, and 1 coccygeal (see Fig. 21.20). In the cervical region, the first seven pairs of nerves exit the cord above the corresponding vertebrae. The C8 nerve pair exits the spinal cord below the C7 vertebra. From this point on, all thoracic, lumbar, and sacral nerves exit below the corresponding vertebrae.[1,2] In other words, spinal cord segments associated with each spinal nerve and the corresponding vertebra do not directly line up.

The spinal nerve has two roots: (1) the dorsal root and (2) the ventral root. The dorsal root is an afferent pathway that carries sensory impulses from the body into the spinal cord. The ventral root is an efferent pathway that carries motor information from the spinal cord to the body. The dorsal and ventral roots join together as they exit the spinal foramen and become a spinal nerve (see Fig. 21.22).[1,2] Distribution of the sensory components of each spinal nerve are illustrated as dermatomes. Dermatome diagrams facilitate identification of sensory innervation throughout the body (Fig. 21.23).[1]

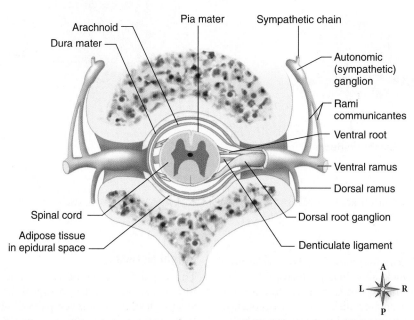

FIG. 21.22 Coverings of the Spinal Cord. The dura mater is shown in purple. Note how it extends to cover the spinal nerve roots and nerves. The arachnoid is highlighted in pink, and the pia mater is highlighted in orange. (From Patton KT, Thibodeau GF. *Anatomy and Physiology.* 8th ed. St. Louis: Mosby; 2013.)

Gray and White Matter

The spinal cord is composed of gray matter and white matter. The central gray matter, which appears in the shape of an "H," consists of cell bodies, small projection fibers, and glial support cells. The gray matter of the spinal cord has been divided into areas based on cell body type and location. The three main divisions are (1) the anterior horn, (2) the lateral horn, and (3) the posterior horn. The anterior horn contains motor neurons and is the final junction for motor information before exiting the CNS. The lateral horn contains preganglionic fibers of the autonomic nervous system: sympathetic fibers T1 to L2 and parasympathetic fibers S2 to S4. The posterior horn contains

sensory neurons and becomes the entry point for afferent impulses to the CNS.[1,2]

The white matter, which surrounds the gray matter, contains the myelinated ascending and descending tracts, which carry information to and from the brain (Fig. 21.24). Spinal tracts are named in such a way that the prefix denotes the origin of the tract, and the suffix is the destination, promoting easy identification of sensory or motor tracts.[1,2] Sensory tracts begin with the prefix *spino-*, and motor tracts end with the suffix *-spinal* (Tables 21.4 and 21.5). The complexity of spinal cord tracts is beyond the scope of this chapter, which is limited to the tracts that are most clinically significant and easily tested.

FIG. 21.23 Dermatome Distribution of Spinal Nerves. (A) The front of the body's surface. (B) The back of the body's surface. (C) The side of the body's surface. The *inset* shows the segments of the spinal cord connected with each of the spinal nerves associated with the sensory dermatomes shown. C, cervical segments and spinal nerves; L, lumbar segments and spinal nerves; S, sacral segments and spinal nerves; T, thoracic segments and spinal nerves. (From Patton KT, Thibodeau GA. *Anatomy and Physiology*. 8th ed. St. Louis: Mosby; 2013.)

FIG. 21.24 Spinal Cord Tracts of the White Matter. (From Patton KT, Thibodeau GF. *Anatomy and Physiology*. 8th ed. St. Louis: Mosby; 2013.)

TABLE 21.4 Major Ascending Tracts of Spinal Cord

Name	Function	Location	Origin*	Termination†
Lateral spinothalamic	Pain, temperature, and crude touch on opposite side	Lateral white columns	Posterior gray column on opposite side	Thalamus
Anterior spinothalamic	Crude touch and pressure	Anterior white columns	Posterior gray column on opposite side	Thalamus
Fasciculi gracilis and cuneatus	Discriminating touch and pressure sensations, including vibration, stereognosis, and two-point discrimination; also conscious kinesthesia	Posterior white columns	Spinal ganglia on same side	Medulla
Anterior and posterior spinoc-erebellar	Unconscious kinesthesia	Lateral white columns	Anterior or posterior gray column	Cerebellum
Spinotectal	Touch related to visual reflexes	Lateral white columns	Posterior gray columns	Superior colliculus (midbrain)

*Location of cell bodies of neurons from which axons of tract arise.
†Structure in which axons of tract terminate.
From Patton KT, Thibodeau GA: *Anatomy and Physiology*. 8th ed. St. Louis: Mosby; 2013.

TABLE 21.5 Major Descending Tracts of Spinal Cord

Name	Function	Location	Origin*	Termination†
Lateral corticospinal (or crossed pyramidal)	Voluntary movement, contraction of individual or small groups of muscles, particularly muscles moving hands, fingers, feet, and toes of opposite side	Lateral white columns	Motor areas or cerebral cortex of opposite side from tract location in cord	Lateral or anterior gray columns
Anterior corticospinal (direct pyramidal)	Same as lateral corticospinal except mainly muscles of same side	Anterior white columns	Motor cortex but on same side as location in cord	Lateral or anterior gray columns
Reticulospinal	Maintain posture during movement	Anterior white columns	Reticular formation (midbrain, pons, medulla)	Anterior gray columns
Rubrospinal	Coordination of body movement and posture	Lateral white columns	Red nucleus (of midbrain)	Anterior gray columns
Tectospinal	Head and neck movement during visual reflexes	Anterior white columns	Superior colliculus (midbrain)	Medulla and anterior gray columns
Vestibulospinal	Coordination of posture or balance	Anterior white columns	Vestibular nucleus (pons, medulla)	Anterior gray columns

*Location of cell bodies of neurons from which axons of tract arise.
†Structure in which axons of tract terminate.

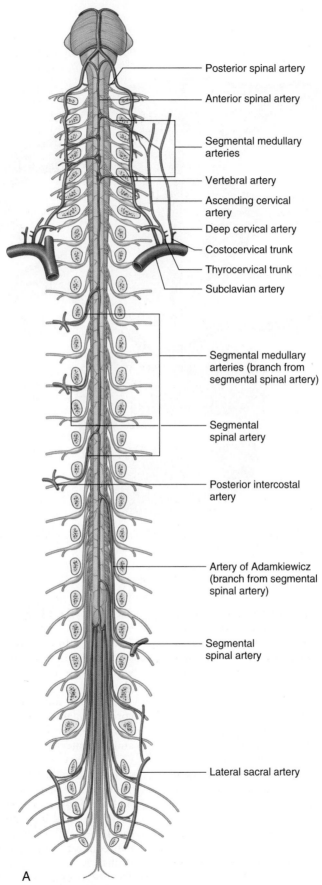

Posterior spinal artery

Anterior spinal artery

Segmental medullary
arteries

Vertebral artery

Ascending cervical
artery

Deep cervical artery

Costocervical trunk

Thyrocervical trunk

Subclavian artery

Segmental medullary
arteries (branch from
segmental spinal artery)

Segmental
spinal artery

Posterior intercostal
artery

Artery of Adamkiewicz
(branch from segmental
spinal artery)

Segmental
spinal artery

Lateral sacral artery

A

FIG. 21.25 Arteries That Supply the Spinal Cord. (A) Anterior view of spinal cord (not all segmental spinal arteries are shown).

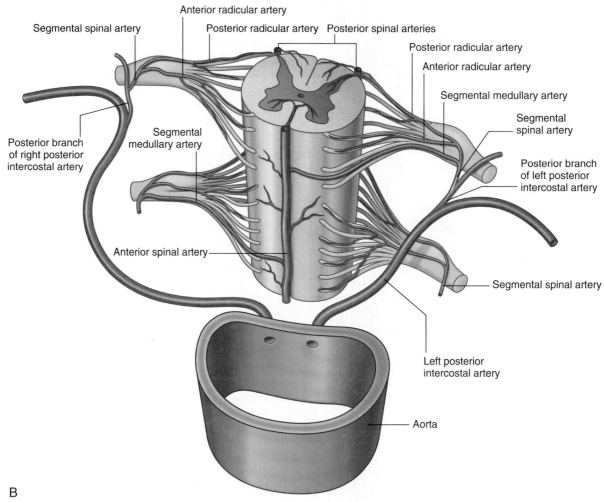

FIG. 21.25, cont'd (B) Segmental supply of spinal cord. (From Drake RL, Vogl AW, Mitchell AWM. *Gray's Anatomy for Students*, 3rd ed. Philadelphia: Churchill Livingstone; 2015.)

Vascular Supply

Arterial blood supply to the spinal cord is provided by branches of the vertebral arteries and small radicular arteries that enter through intervertebral foramina. They combine to form the anterior spinal and two posterior spinal arteries. These three arteries, along with some additional radicular arterial flow from cervical, intercostal, lumbar, and sacral arteries, feed the entire length of the spinal cord (Fig. 21.25).[36]

Arterial supply to the spinal cord is segmented at best, making portions of the spinal cord that receive blood supply from two separate sources vulnerable to low-flow states. The most vulnerable of these areas are C2 to C3, T1 to T4, and L1 to L2. Evidence of this tenuous blood supply is occasionally evident after surgical procedures that involve cross-clamping of the aorta, resulting in spinal cord infarction.[36]

SUMMARY

Anatomy
- Nervous tissue is composed of neurons and neuroglial cells.
- The CNS comprises the brain and spinal cord.

- The somatic nervous system is composed of fibers that connect the CNS with structures of the skeletal muscles and the skin.
- The autonomic nervous system (sympathetic and parasympathetic) is composed of fibers that connect the CNS with smooth muscle, cardiac muscle, internal organs, and glands.
- The brain is contained within the cranial vault, the spinal cord is contained within the vertebral column, and both are surrounded by the meninges (dura mater, arachnoid mater, and pia mater).
- CSF fills the ventricular system and surrounds the brain and spinal cord in the subarachnoid space.
- Two pairs of arteries (internal carotid arteries and vertebral arteries) provide blood to the brain and are anatomically separated into the anterior (right and left ACAs and the ACoA) and posterior (right and left PCoAs) circulations that connect at the base of the brain to form the circle of Willis.
- The PNS comprises the cranial nerves, the spinal nerves, and all other nerves serving a variety of functions throughout the body.

Physiology

- Neurons perform the functional work of the nervous system, including receipt of information, integration, and transmission of nerve impulses to recipient cells.
- Neuroglial cells (astrocytes, oligodendroglia, ependyma, and microglia) serve as the support infrastructure of the nervous system, providing protection, structural support, and neuronal repair.
- Most activities of the nervous system originate from sensory receptors such as visual, auditory, or tactile receptors and are transmitted to the CNS by afferent fibers (sensory fibers).
- Efferent fibers (motor fibers) transmit the CNS response to the periphery to produce a motor response, such as contraction of skeletal muscles, contraction of the smooth muscles of organs, or secretion by endocrine glands.
- The flow of CSF begins in the lateral ventricles, moves through the foramina of Monro into the third ventricle, moves through the cerebral aqueduct into the fourth ventricle, and moves out the foramen of Magendie and the foramina of Luschka into the subarachnoid space of the brain and spinal cord.
- The primary functions of the cerebral cortex include sensory, motor, and cognitive functions.
- The primary functions of the cerebellum include balance and motor coordination.
- The primary function of the brainstem (midbrain, pons, and medulla) is the regulation of vital functions such as breathing.
- Voluntary motor movement is controlled by the motor strip in the frontal cortex, and as the tracts descend through the brainstem, they cross over to the opposite side. The right motor strip controls the left side of the body, and vice versa.
- Broca area is located in the left frontal lobe and is responsible for expression of written and verbal language. Damage to the area can result in expressive aphasia.
- Wernicke area is located in the left parietal lobe and is responsible for reception of written and verbal language. Damage to the area can result in receptive aphasia.
- The circle of Willis provides collateral blood flow to the brain.
- ⓔ Visit the Evolve site for additional study materials.

REFERENCES

1. Patton KT, Thibodeau GA: *Anatomy and Physiology*, ed. 8, St. Louis, 2013, Mosby.
2. FitzGerald MJT, Gruener G, Mtui E, editors: *Clinical Neuroanatomy and Neuroscience*, ed 5, Philadelphia, 2012, Elsevier.
3. Koeppen BM, Stanton BA: *Berne and Levy: Physiology*, ed 6, Philadelphia, 2010, Mosby.
4. Hall JE: *Guyton and Hall Textbook of Medical Physiology*, ed 13, Philadelphia, 2016, Saunders.
5. Liu J, et al.: Neural plasticity after spinal cord injury, *Neural Regen Res* 7(5):386–391, 2012.
6. Warraich Z, Kleim JA: Neural plasticity: the biological substrate for neurorehabilitation, *PM R* 2(12 suppl 2):S208–S219, 2010.
7. Nudo RJ: Neural bases of recovery after brain injury, *J Commun Disord* 44(5):515–520, 2011.
8. Patel DR, Feucht C: Basic concepts in neurotransmission, *Pediatr Clin North Am* 58(1):21–31, 2011.
9. Aggarwal S, Yurlova L, Simon M: Central nervous system myelin: structure, synthesis and assembly, *Trends Cell Biol* 21(10):585–593, 2011.
10. Mohindra S, Singh H, Savardekar A: Importance of an intact dura in management of compound elevated fractures; a short series and literature review, *Brain Inj* 26(2):194–198, 2012.
11. Patel N, Kirmi O: Anatomy and imaging of the normal meninges, *Semin Ultrasound CT MR* 30(6):559–564, 2009.
12. Garq A: Vascular brain pathologies, *Neuroimaging Clin N Am* 21(4):897–926, 2011.
13. Sakka L, Coll G, Chazal J: Anatomy and physiology of cerebrospinal fluid, *Eur Ann Otorhinolaryngol Head Neck Dis* 128(6):309–316, 2011.
14. Toma AK: Hydrocephalus, *Surgery (Oxford)* 33(8):384–389, 2015.
15. Perez-Barcena J, Llompart-Pou JA: Intracranial pressure monitoring and management of intracranial hypertension, *Crit Care Clin* 30(4):735–750, 2014.
16. American Association of Neuroscience Nurses: *Guide to the Care of the Patient Undergoing Intracranial Pressure Monitoring/External Ventricular Drainage or Lumbar Drainage: AANN Clinical Practice Guideline Series*, Glenview, IL, 2011, The Association.
17. Mahringer A, et al.: The ABC of the blood-brain barrier-regulation of drug efflux pumps, *Curr Pharm Des* 17(26):2762–2770, 2011.
18. Bauer HC, et al.: "You shall not pass"—tight junctions of the blood brain barrier, *Front Neurosci* 8:392, 2014.
19. Lawther BK, Kumar S, Krovvidi H: Blood-brain barrier, *Contin Educ Anesth Crit Care Pain* 11(4):128–132, 2011.
20. Rhoton Jr AL: The cerebrum. Anatomy, *Neurosurgery* 61(Suppl 1):37–118, 2007.
21. Lengenfelder J, et al.: Assessing frontal behavioral syndromes and cognitive functions in traumatic brain injury, *Appl Neuropsychol Adult* 22(1):7–15, 2015.
22. Samara A, Tsangaris GT: Brain asymmetry: both sides of the story, *Expert Rev Proteomics* 8(6):693–703, 2011.
23. Change EF, Raygor KP, Berger MS: Contemporary model of language organization: an overview for neurosurgeons, *J Neurosurg* 122(2):250–261, 2015.
24. Gainotti G: What the study of voice recognition in normal subjects and brain-damaged patients tells us about models of familiar people recognition, *Neuropsychologia* 49(9):2273–2282, 2011.
25. Ono T, Galanopoulou AS: Epilepsy and epileptic syndrome, *Adv Exp Med Biol* 724:99–113, 2012.
26. Ricciardi E, Pietrini P: New light from the dark: what blindness can teach us about brain function, *Curr Opin Neurol* 24(4):357–363, 2011.
27. Roxo MR: The limbic system conception and its historical evolution, *ScientificWorldJournal* 11:2428–2441, 2011.
28. Hiraga A: Pure motor monoparesis due to ischemic stroke, *Neurologist* 17(6):301–308, 2011.
29. Helie S, Chakravarthy S, Moustafa AA: Exploring the cognitive and motor functions of the basal ganglia: an integrative review of computational cognitive neuroscience models, *Front Comput Neurosci* 7:174, 2013.
30. Amici S: Thalamic infarcts and hemorrhages, *Front Neurol Neurosci* 30:132–136, 2012.
31. Roostaei T, et al.: The human cerebellum: a review of physiologic neuroanatomy, *Neurol Clin* 32(4):859–869, 2014.
32. Massaquoi SG: Physiology of clinical dysfunction of the cerebellum, *Handb Clin Neurol* 103:37–62, 2012.
33. Brogan ME, Provencio JJ: Spectrum of catastrophic brain injury: coma and related disorders of consciousness, *J Crit Care* 29(4):679–682, 2014.
34. Vrselja Z, et al.: Function of circle of Willis, *J Cereb Blood Flow Metab* 34(4):578–584, 2014.
35. Izzo R, et al.: Spinal pain, *Eur J Radiol* 84(5):746–756, 2015.
36. Melissano G, et al.: An anatomical review of spinal cord blood supply, *J Cardiovasc Surg (Torino)* 56(5):699–706, 2015.

Neurologic Clinical Assessment and Diagnostic Procedures

Darlene M. Burke

Assessment of a critically ill patient with neurologic dysfunction includes a review of the patient's health history, a focused clinical assessment, and an analysis of laboratory data. Numerous invasive and noninvasive diagnostic procedures may also be performed to assist in the identification of the patient's disorder. A thorough assessment of a patient with neurologic dysfunction is imperative for the early identification and treatment of neurologic disorders and serves as source of comparison for ongoing assessments of the patient. The most important finding in any neurologic assessment is change, which should be reported promptly. Early identification of neurologic deterioration is vital to preventing secondary brain injury.[1] Other medical conditions as well as the administration of medications can affect the clinical assessment and should be taken into consideration when the results of the neurologic examination are abnormal.

The completed assessment serves as the foundation for developing the management plan for the patient. The assessment process can be brief or can involve a detailed history and examination, depending on the nature and immediacy of the patient's condition. This chapter focuses on clinical assessments, laboratory studies, and diagnostic procedures for critically ill patients with neurologic dysfunction.

HISTORY

Common to all neurologic assessments is the need to obtain a comprehensive history of events preceding hospitalization. An adequate neurologic history includes information about clinical manifestations, associated complaints, precipitating factors, progression, and familial occurrences (Box 22.1).[2] The ideal historian for recounting this information is someone who is able to provide a detailed description and chronology of events. If the patient is incapable of serving as the historian, family members or significant others who have contact with the patient on a daily basis should be contacted as soon as possible. Through history taking, the caregiver gains valuable information that directs him or her to focus on certain aspects of the patient's clinical assessment.[3]

FOCUSED CLINICAL ASSESSMENT

The clinical assessment helps establish baseline data about the physical dimensions of the patient's condition. The neurologic evaluation of a critically ill patient comprises five major components: (1) level of consciousness, (2) motor function, (3) pupillary function, (4) respiratory function, and (5) vital signs.

A complete neurologic examination requires assessment of all five components.[3,4]

Level of Consciousness

Assessment of the level of consciousness is the most important aspect of the neurologic examination. In most situations, a patient's level of consciousness deteriorates before any other neurologic changes are noticed. These deteriorations often are subtle and must be monitored carefully. Assessment of level of consciousness focuses on two areas: (1) evaluation of arousal or alertness and (2) appraisal of content of consciousness or awareness.[3,5] Different levels of consciousness from full alertness to coma have been defined (Box 22.2).[3] Because these and other terms used to categorize the level of consciousness are frequently used imprecisely, it is often recommended to avoid using them. Instead, a brief description of the applied stimulus and arousal pattern is preferred.[6]

Evaluation of Arousal

Assessment of the arousal component of consciousness is an evaluation of the reticular activating system and its connection to the thalamus and the cerebral cortex. Arousal is the lowest level of consciousness, and observation centers on the patient's ability to respond to verbal or noxious stimuli in an appropriate manner.[5] To stimulate the patient, the nurse begins with verbal stimuli in a normal tone. If the patient does not respond, the nurse increases the stimuli by talking very loudly to the patient. If there is still no response, the nurse further increases the stimuli by gently shaking the patient. If previous attempts to arouse the patient are unsuccessful, noxious stimuli are employed using central stimulation techniques.[6] Central stimulation produces an overall body response and is more reliable than peripheral stimulation.[6] Two common central stimulation techniques are the *sternal rub* and the *trapezius muscle pinch*. A sternal rub is conducted by applying pressure to the center of the sternum with the knuckles of a clenched fist.[3] A trapezius muscle squeeze involves pitching or squeezing the trapezius muscle located at the angle of the shoulder and the neck muscle.[3] The symmetry and pattern of the motor response to noxious stimuli, as well as associated neurologic symptoms, are documented for all patients suspected to have a neurologic disease.[6]

Appraisal of Awareness

Content of consciousness is a higher level function, and appraisal of awareness is concerned with assessment of the patient's orientation to person, place, time, and situation.[5] Assessment of content of consciousness requires the patient to give appropriate answers to various questions. Changes in the patient's

BOX 22.1 DATA COLLECTION

Neurologic History

Common Neurologic Symptoms
- Fainting
- Dizziness
- Blackouts
- Seizures
- Headache
- Memory loss
- Weakness
- Paralysis
- Tremors or other involuntary movements
- Pain
- Numbness
- Tingling
- Speech disturbances
- Vision disturbances

Events Preceding Onset of Symptoms
- Travel
- Animal contact
- Falls
- Infection
- Dental problems or procedures
- Sinus or middle ear infections
- Prodromal symptoms
- Food or drugs ingested

Progression of Symptoms
- Initial onset
- Evolution
- Frequency
- Severity
- Duration
- Associated activities or aggravating factors

Family History
- Stroke (arteriovenous malformation, aneurysm)
- Diabetes mellitus
- Hypertension
- Seizures
- Tumors
- Headaches
- Emotional problems or depression

Medical History

Child
- Birth injuries, congenital defects, encephalitis, meningitis, bedwetting, fainting, seizures, trauma

Adult
- Diabetes; hypertension; cardiovascular, pulmonary, kidney, liver, or endocrine disease; tuberculosis; tropical infection; sinusitis; visual problems; tumors; psychiatric disorders

Surgical History
- Neurologic, ear-nose-throat, dental, eye surgery

Traumatic History
- Motor vehicle accidents; falls; blows to head, neck, or back; being knocked unconscious

Allergies
- Drug, food, environment

Patient Profile
- Personal habits
- Use of alcohol, recreational drugs, over-the-counter medications, smoking, dietary habits, sleeping patterns, elimination patterns, exercise habits
- Recent life changes
- Living conditions
- Working conditions
- Exposure to toxins, chemicals, fumes; occupational duties
- General temperament

Current Medication Use
- Sedatives, tranquilizers
- Anticonvulsants
- Psychotropics
- Anticoagulants
- Antibiotics
- Calcium channel blockers
- Beta-blockers
- Nitrates
- Oral contraceptives

answers that indicate increasing degrees of confusion and disorientation may be the first sign of neurologic deterioration.[2]

Glasgow Coma Scale

The most widely recognized tool for assessing level of consciousness is the Glasgow Coma Scale (GCS).[7] This scored scale is based on evaluation of three categories: (1) eye opening, (2) verbal response, and (3) best motor response (Table 22.1). The highest possible score on the GCS is 15, and the lowest score is 3. A score of 7 or less on the GCS usually indicates coma. Originally, the scoring system was developed to assist in general communication concerning the severity of neurologic injury. However, the usefulness of the GCS has been called into question, particularly because of poor interrater reliability.[8] Several points should be kept in mind when the GCS is used for serial

assessment. The GCS provides data about level of consciousness only and should never be considered a complete neurologic examination. Additionally, the GCS is not a sensitive tool for evaluation of an altered sensorium and does not account for possible aphasia or mechanical intubation. The GCS is also a poor indicator of lateralization of neurologic deterioration.[9] *Lateralization* involves decreasing motor response on one side or unilateral changes in pupillary reaction. To overcome the limitations of the GCS, research into alternative neurologic assessment tools is ongoing. One tool, the Full Outline of UnResponsiveness (FOUR) score, may be a suitable alternative or complementary tool for the GCS.[10] The FOUR score incorporates eye opening and eye movements, brainstem reflexes, respiration patterns, several motor responses, and specific ways to assess comprehension to a command.[11,12]

BOX 22.2 Categories of Consciousness

Alert	Patient responds immediately to minimal external stimuli.
Confused	Patient is disoriented to time or place but usually oriented to person, with impaired judgment and decision making and decreased attention span.
Delirious	Patient is disoriented to time, place, and person, with loss of contact with reality, and often has auditory or visual hallucinations.
Lethargic	Patient displays a state of drowsiness or inaction, in which patient needs an increased stimulus to be awakened.
Obtunded	Patient displays dull indifference to external stimuli, and response is minimally maintained. Questions are answered with a minimal response.
Stuporous	Patient can be aroused only by vigorous and continuous external stimuli. Motor response is often withdrawal or localizing to stimulus.
Comatose	Vigorous stimulation fails to produce any voluntary neural response.

From Barker E. *Neuroscience Nursing: A Spectrum of Care*. 3rd ed. St. Louis: Mosby; 2008.

Motor Function

Assessment of motor function focuses on muscle size and tone and on an estimation of muscle strength. Each side is assessed individually and compared with the other.[9]

Evaluation of Muscle Size and Tone

Initially, muscles are inspected for size and shape. The presence of atrophy is noted. Muscle tone is assessed by evaluating opposition to passive movement. The patient is instructed to relax the extremity while the nurse performs passive range-of-motion movements and evaluates the degree of resistance. Muscle tone is appraised for signs of flaccidity (no resistance), hypotonia (little resistance), hypertonia (increased resistance), spasticity, or rigidity.[13]

Estimation of Muscle Strength

Having the patient perform movements against resistance assesses muscle strength. The strength of the movement is graded on a six-point scale (Box 22.3). The patient is asked to extend both arms with the palms turned upward and to hold that position with the eyes closed. If the patient has a weaker side, that arm will drift downward and pronate. The lower extremities are tested by asking the patient to push and pull the feet against resistance or to elevate the legs.[13]

Abnormal Motor Responses

If the patient is incapable of comprehending and following a simple command, noxious stimuli are necessary to determine motor responses. The stimulus is applied to each extremity separately to allow evaluation of individual extremity function. Peripheral stimulation is used to assess motor function.[3,4] Motor responses elicited by noxious stimuli are interpreted differently from responses elicited by voluntary demonstration.[3] These responses may be classified as shown in Box 22.4.

Abnormal flexion also is known as *decorticate posturing* (Fig. 22.1A). In response to painful stimuli, the upper extremities exhibit flexion of the arm, wrist, and fingers, with adduction

TABLE 22.1 Glasgow Coma Scale

Category	Score	Response
Eye opening	4	Spontaneous: Eyes open spontaneously without stimulation
	3	To speech: Eyes open with verbal stimulation but not necessarily to command
	2	To pain: Eyes open with noxious stimuli
	1	None: No eye opening regardless of stimulation
Verbal response	5	Oriented: Accurate information about person, place, time, reason for hospitalization, and personal data
	4	Confused: Answers not appropriate to question, but use of language is correct
	3	Inappropriate words: Disorganized, random speech, no sustained conversation
	2	Incomprehensible sounds: Moans, groans, and incomprehensible mumbles
	1	None: No verbalization despite stimulation
Best motor response	6	Obeys commands: Performs simple tasks on command; able to repeat performance
	5	Localizes to pain: Organized attempt to localize and remove painful stimuli
	4	Withdraws from pain: Withdraws extremity from source of painful stimuli
	3	Abnormal flexion: Decorticate posturing spontaneously or in response to noxious stimuli
	2	Extension: Decerebrate posturing spontaneously or in response to noxious stimuli
	1	None: No response to noxious stimuli; flaccid

BOX 22.3 Muscle Strength Grading Scale

0/5	No movement or muscle contraction
1/5	Trace contraction
2/5	Active movement with gravity eliminated
3/5	Active movement against gravity
4/5	Active movement with some resistance
5/5	Active movement with full resistance

BOX 22.4 Classification of Abnormal Motor Function

Spontaneous	Occurs without regard to external stimuli and may not occur by request
Localization	Occurs when the extremity opposite the extremity receiving pain crosses midline of body in an attempt to remove the noxious stimulus from the affected limb
Withdrawal	Occurs when the extremity receiving the painful stimulus flexes normally in an attempt to avoid the noxious stimulus
Decortication	Abnormal flexion response that may occur spontaneously or in response to noxious stimuli (see Fig. 22.1A and C)
Decerebration	Abnormal extension response that may occur spontaneously or in response to noxious stimuli (see Fig. 22.1B and C)
Flaccid	No response to painful stimuli

FIG. 22.1 Abnormal Motor Responses. (A) Decorticate posturing. (B) Decerebrate posturing. (C) Decorticate posturing on right side and decerebrate posturing on left side of body.

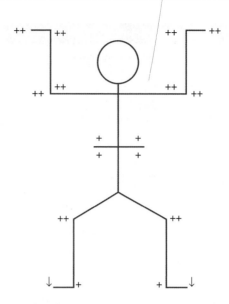

Scoring Deep Tendon Reflexes

Grade	Deep Tendon Reflex Response
0	No response
1+	Sluggish or diminished
2+	Active or expected response
3+	More brisk than expected, slightly hyperactive
4+	Brisk, hyperactive, with intermittent or transient clonus

FIG. 22.2 Reflex Scoring. The patient's reflex scores are recorded by entering the correct scores at the correct location on the stick figure. (From Barker E. *Neuroscience Nursing: A Spectrum of Care.* 3rd ed. St. Louis: Mosby; 2008.)

of the limb. The lower extremity exhibits extension, internal rotation, and plantar flexion. Abnormal flexion occurs with lesions above the midbrain, located in the region of the thalamus or cerebral hemispheres. Abnormal extension also is known as *decerebrate rigidity* or *posturing* (Fig. 22.1B): when the patient is stimulated, the teeth clench, and the arms are stiffly extended, adducted, and hyperpronated. The legs are stiffly extended, with plantar flexion of the feet. Abnormal extension occurs with lesions in the area of the brainstem.[9] Because abnormal flexion and extension appear similar in the lower extremities, the upper extremities are used to determine the presence of these abnormal movements. It is possible for the patient to exhibit abnormal flexion on one side of the body and extension on the other (Fig. 22.1C).[3,4] Outcome studies indicate that abnormal flexion has a less serious prognosis than extension or decerebrate posturing.[9] Onset of posturing or a change from abnormal flexion to abnormal extension requires immediate physician notification.

Evaluation of Reflexes

Deep tendon reflexes (DTRs) are usually evaluated by a physician when a complete neurologic evaluation is performed. DTRs are tested by tapping the appropriate tendon using a reflex or percussion hammer. For reflex testing to be accurate, the muscle needs to be relaxed, and the joint needs to be at midposition.[5] The four reflexes tested are (1) Achilles (ankle jerk), (2) quadriceps (knee jerk), (3) biceps, and (4) triceps. DTRs are graded on a scale from 0 (absent) to 4 (hyperactive). A DTR grade of 2 is normal (Fig. 22.2). Hyperreflexia is associated with upper motor neuron interruption, and areflexia is associated with lesions of the lower motor neurons.[13]

Superficial reflexes are normal if present and abnormal if absent. Superficial reflexes are tested by stimulating cutaneous receptors of the skin, cornea, or mucous membrane. Stroking, scratching, or touching can be used as the stimulus (Table 22.2). The corneal reflex is present if the eyelids quickly close when the cornea is lightly stroked with a wisp of cotton. An alternative approach is to drop a small amount of water or saline onto the cornea.[4,13] The pathway for the corneal reflex is formed by the trigeminal nerve (cranial nerve [CN] V), the facial nerve (CN VII), and the pons. The pharyngeal reflex is present if retching or gagging occurs with stimulation of the back of the pharynx.[4,13]

The presence of pathologic reflexes is an abnormal neurologic finding.[10] The grasp reflex is present when tactile stimulation of the palm of the hand produces a grasp response that is not a conscious voluntary act. The grasp reflex is a primitive reflex that normally disappears with maturational development. Presence of the grasp reflex in an adult indicates cortical damage. Babinski reflex is a pathologic sign in any individual older than 2 years. The presence of this reflex is tested by slow, deliberate stroking of the lateral half of the sole of the foot. Sustained extensor response of the big toe is indicative of a positive Babinski reflex. This response is sometimes accompanied by the fanning out of the other four toes. Flexor response of all the toes in response to the same stimulus is a normal finding and indicates absence of Babinski reflex (Fig. 22.3). Babinski reflex is a significant neurologic finding because it indicates an upper motor neuron lesion in the brain, brainstem, or spinal cord.[14] The disease may be degenerative, neoplastic, inflammatory,

TABLE 22.2   Superficial Reflexes

Reflex	Nerves Involved	Normal Reaction
Corneal	CN V and VII	Prompt closure of both eyelids when cornea touched with wisp of cotton
Pharyngeal	CN IX and X	Gagging response to pharyngeal stimulation
Abdominal	Epigastric (T6-T9); midabdominal (T9-T11); hypogastric (T11-L1)	Contraction of abdominal muscle when stroked, so that a brief, brisk movement of umbilicus toward stimulus occurs
Cremasteric	L1, L2	Elevation of testicle when inner aspect of thigh stroked
Anal		Contraction of anal ring as perineum is stroked or scratched
Bulbocutaneous	S4, S5	
Anocutaneous	S5	
Plantar	L5, S1	Flexion of toes from stimulation of sole of foot

CN, cranial nerve.
From Barker E. *Neuroscience Nursing: A Spectrum of Care*. 3rd ed. St. Louis: Mosby; 2008.

FIG. 22.3 Babinski Reflex. (A) Test maneuver: Using a blunt point, scratch the sole of the foot as shown. (B) Normal response (absence of Babinski response) is plantar flexion of the toes. (C) Abnormal response (presence of Babinski response) is dorsiflexion of the big toe and often a fanning of the other toes. (From Black JM, Hawks JH, eds. *Medical-Surgical Nursing: Clinical Management for Positive Outcomes*. 8th ed. Philadelphia: Saunders; 2009.)

vascular, or posttraumatic. Babinski reflex may also become positive during transtentorial herniation.[3]

Pupillary Function

Assessment of pupillary function focuses on three areas: (1) estimation of pupil size and shape, (2) evaluation of pupillary reaction to light, and (3) assessment of eye movements. Pupillary function is an extension of the autonomic nervous system. Parasympathetic control of the pupil occurs through innervation of the oculomotor nerve (CN III), which exits from the brainstem in the midbrain area. When the parasympathetic fibers are stimulated, the pupil constricts. Sympathetic control originates in the hypothalamus and travels down the entire length of the brainstem. When the sympathetic fibers are stimulated, the pupil dilates. Pupillary changes provide a valuable assessment tool because of pathway locations. The oculomotor nerve lies at the junction of the midbrain and the tentorial notch. Any increase of pressure that exerts force down

through the tentorial notch compresses the oculomotor nerve. Oculomotor nerve compression results in a dilated, nonreactive pupil. Sympathetic pathway disruption occurs with involvement in the brainstem. Loss of sympathetic control leads to pinpoint, nonreactive pupils. Control of eye movements occurs with interaction of three cranial nerves: (1) oculomotor (CN III), (2) trochlear (CN IV), and (3) abducens (CN VI). The pathways for these cranial nerves provide integrated function through the internuclear pathway of the medial longitudinal fasciculus (MLF) located in the brainstem. The MLF provides coordination of eye movements with the vestibular nerve (CN VIII) and the reticular formation.[15]

Estimation of Pupil Size and Shape

Diameter of the pupil is documented in millimeters with the use of a pupillometer to reduce the subjectivity of description. Most people have pupils of equal size, between 2 and 5 mm. A discrepancy up to 1 mm between the two pupils is normal; it is called *anisocoria* and occurs in 16% to 17% of humans.[16] Change or inequality in pupil size, especially in patients who previously have not shown this discrepancy, is a significant neurologic sign. It may indicate impending danger of herniation and should be reported immediately. With the location of CN III at the notch of the tentorium, pupil size and reactivity play a key role in the physical assessment of intracranial pressure (ICP) changes and herniation syndromes. Changes in pupil size occur for other reasons in addition to CN III compression. Large pupils can result from the instillation of cycloplegic agents such as atropine or scopolamine or can indicate extreme stress. Extremely small pupils can indicate opioid overdose, lower brainstem compression, or bilateral damage to the pons.[16,17]

Pupil shape is included in the assessment of pupils. Although the pupil is normally round, an irregularly shaped or oval pupil may be observed in patients who have undergone eye surgery. Initial stages of CN III compression from elevated ICP can cause the pupil to have an oval shape.[3,16]

Evaluation of Pupillary Reaction to Light

The pupillary light reflex depends on optic nerve (CN II) and oculomotor nerve (CN III) function (Fig. 22.4).[12,16] The technique for evaluation of the pupillary light response involves use of a narrow-beamed bright light shined into the pupil from the outer canthus of the eye. If the light is shined directly onto the pupil, glare or reflection of the light may prevent the assessor's proper visualization. Pupillary reaction to light is identified as

Metabolic imbalance

Small, reactive, and regular

Diencephalic dysfunction
Small and reactive

Dysfunction of third cranial nerve
Sluggish, dilated, and fixed

Dysfunction of tectum (roof)
of the midbrain
Large "fixed" hippus

Pontine dysfunction
Pinpoint

Midbrain dysfunction
Midposition and fixed

FIG. 22.4 Abnormal Pupillary Responses.

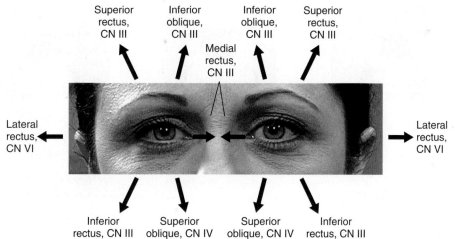

Superior rectus, CN III

Inferior oblique, CN III

Medial rectus, CN III

Inferior oblique, CN III

Superior rectus, CN III

Lateral rectus, CN VI

Lateral rectus, CN VI

Inferior rectus, CN III

Superior oblique, CN IV

Superior oblique, CN IV

Inferior rectus, CN III

FIG. 22.5 Extraocular Eye Movements. (From Ball JW, et al. *Seidel's Guide to Physical Examination.* 7th ed. St. Louis: Mosby; 2015.)

brisk, sluggish, or nonreactive or fixed.[3] Each pupil is evaluated for direct light response and for consensual response. The consensual pupillary response is constriction in response to a light shone into the opposite eye.[3] This reflex occurs as a result of the crossing of nerve fibers at the optic chiasm.[3] Evaluation of consensual response is necessary to rule out optic nerve dysfunction as a cause for lack of a direct light reflex. Because the optic nerve is the afferent pathway for the light reflex, shining a light into a blind eye produces neither a direct light response in that eye nor a consensual response in the opposite eye. A consensual response in a blind eye produced by shining a light into the opposite eye demonstrates an intact oculomotor nerve. Oculomotor compression associated with transtentorial herniation affects the direct light response and the consensual response in the affected pupil.[3,4,15,16]

Assessment of Eye Movement

In a conscious patient, the function of the three cranial nerves of the eye and their MLF innervation can be assessed by asking the patient to follow a finger through the full range of eye motion. If the eyes move together into all six fields, extraocular movements are intact (Fig. 22.5).[3,15]

In an unconscious patient, assessment of ocular function and innervation of the MLF is performed by eliciting the doll's eye reflex. If the patient is unconscious as a result of trauma, the nurse must ascertain the absence of cervical injury before performing this examination. To assess the oculocephalic reflex, the nurse holds the patient's eyelids open and briskly turns the head to one side and observes the eye movement and then briskly turns the head to the other side and observes the eye movement again. If the eye movement deviates to the opposite direction in which the head is turned, the doll's eye reflex is present, and the oculocephalic reflex arc is intact (Fig. 22.6A). If the oculocephalic reflex arc is not intact, the reflex is absent.

This lack of response, in which the eyes remain midline and move with the head, indicates significant brainstem injury (see Fig. 22.6C). The reflex may also be absent in severe metabolic coma. An abnormal oculocephalic reflex is present when the eyes rove or move in opposite directions from each other (see Fig. 22.6B). An abnormal oculocephalic reflex indicates some degree of brainstem injury.[3,4,15]

The oculovestibular reflex is performed by a physician, often as one of the final clinical assessments of brainstem function. After confirmation that the tympanic membrane is intact, the patient's head is raised to a 30-degree angle, and 20 to 100 mL of ice water is injected into the external auditory canal. The

FIG. 22.6 Oculocephalic Reflex (Doll's Eye Reflex). (A) Normal. (B) Abnormal. (C) Absent.

A

B

C

FIG. 22.7 Oculovestibular Reflex (Cold Caloric Test). (A) Normal. (B) Abnormal. (C) Absent.

normal eye movement response is a conjugate, slow, tonic nystagmus, deviating toward the irrigated ear and lasting 30 to 120 seconds. This response indicates brainstem integrity. Rapid nystagmus returns the eye position back to the midline only in a conscious patient with cortical functioning (Fig. 22.7).[3,10] An abnormal response is disconjugate eye movement, which indicates a brainstem lesion, or no response, which indicates little or no brainstem function. The oculovestibular reflex may be temporarily absent in reversible metabolic encephalopathy.[8] This test is an extremely noxious stimulation and may produce a decorticate or decerebrate posturing response in a comatose patient. In a conscious patient, this procedure may produce nausea, vomiting, or dizziness.[3,15,17]

Respiratory Function

Assessment of respiratory function focuses on two areas: (1) observation of respiratory pattern and (2) evaluation of airway status. The activity of respiration is a highly integrated function that receives input from the cerebrum, brainstem, and metabolic mechanisms. In clinical assessment, correlations exist among altered levels of consciousness, the level of brain or brainstem injury, and the patient's respiratory pattern. Under the influence of the cerebral cortex and the diencephalon, three brainstem centers control respirations. The lowest center, the *medullary respiratory center*, sends impulses through the vagus nerve to innervate muscles of inspiration and expiration. The *apneustic* and *pneumotaxic centers of the pons* are responsible for the length of inspiration and expiration and the underlying respiratory rate.[3,4,10]

Observation of Respiratory Pattern

Changes in respiratory patterns assist in identifying the level of brainstem dysfunction or injury (Fig. 22.8 and Table 22.3). Evaluation of the respiratory pattern must include assessment of the effectiveness of gas exchange in maintaining adequate oxygen and carbon dioxide levels. Hypoventilation is common in patients with altered level of consciousness. Alterations in oxygenation or carbon dioxide levels can result in further neurologic dysfunction. ICP increases with hypoxemia or hypercapnia.[3,4,10]

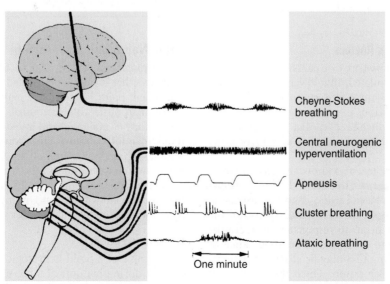

Cheyne-Stokes breathing

Central neurogenic hyperventilation

Apneusis

Cluster breathing

Ataxic breathing

One minute

FIG. 22.8 Abnormal Respiratory Patterns. Abnormal respiratory patterns with corresponding levels of central nervous system activity.

TABLE 22.3   Respiratory Patterns

Pattern of Respiration	Description of Pattern	Significance
Cheyne-Stokes breathing	Rhythmic crescendo and decrescendo of rate and depth of respiration; includes brief periods of apnea	Usually seen with bilateral deep cerebral lesions or some cerebellar lesions
Central neurogenic hyperventilation	Very deep, very rapid respirations with no apneic periods	Usually seen with lesions of midbrain and upper pons
Apneustic breathing	Prolonged inspiratory and/or expiratory pause of 2–3 seconds	Usually seen in lesions of middle to lower pons
Cluster breathing	Clusters of irregular, gasping respirations separated by long periods of apnea	Usually seen in lesions of lower pons or upper medulla
Ataxic respirations	Irregular, random pattern of deep and shallow respirations with irregular apneic periods	Usually seen in lesions of medulla

Evaluation of Airway Status

Evaluation of respiratory function in a patient with a neurologic deficit must include assessment of airway maintenance and secretion control. Cough, gag, and swallow reflexes responsible for protection of the airway may be absent or diminished.[18]

Vital Signs

Assessment of vital signs focuses on two areas: (1) evaluation of blood pressure and (2) observation of heart rate and rhythm. As a result of the brain and brainstem influences on cardiac, respiratory, and body temperature functions, changes in vital signs could be signs of deterioration in neurologic status.[3,4]

Evaluation of Blood Pressure

A common manifestation of intracranial injury is systemic hypertension. Cerebral autoregulation, responsible for the control of cerebral blood flow (CBF), frequently is lost with any type of intracranial injury. After cerebral injury, the body often is in a hyperdynamic state (increased heart rate, blood pressure, and cardiac output) as part of a compensatory response. With the loss of autoregulation as blood pressure increases, CBF and cerebral blood volume increase, and ICP increases. Control of systemic hypertension is necessary to stop this cycle, but caution must be exercised. The mean arterial pressure must be maintained at a level sufficient to produce adequate CBF in the presence of elevated ICP. Attention must also be paid to the pulse pressure because widening of this value may occur in the late stages of intracranial hypertension.[18,19]

Observation of Heart Rate and Rhythm

The medulla and the vagus nerve provide parasympathetic control to the heart. When stimulated, this lower brainstem system produces bradycardia. Sympathetic stimulation increases the rate and contractility. Various intracranial pathologies and abrupt ICP changes can produce bradycardia, premature ventricular contractions, Q–T interval changes, and myocardial damage.[20]

Cushing reflex. Cushing reflex, also known as *Cushing triad* or *Cushing phenomena*, is a set of three clinical manifestations (systolic hypertension, bradycardia, and abnormal respirations) related to pressure on the medullary area of the brainstem. These signs may occur in response to intracranial hypertension or a herniation syndrome. The appearance of Cushing reflex is a late finding that may be absent in patients with severe neurologic deterioration. Once this pattern of vital signs occurs, it may be too late to completely reverse intracranial hypertension.[6]

QSEN BOX 22.5   QSEN: Teamwork and Collaboration

Rapid Neurologic Assessment of the Conscious Patient

The following outline should be used for handoff of a critically ill conscious patient with neurologic dysfunction:

1. *Level of consciousness:* Address the patient and ask a variety of orientation questions; avoid obvious, overused questions about name, date, and place, and focus on questions about recent and past events from the patient's experiences, such as spouse's name, home address, or what was eaten at the previous meal. As examiner, you should be aware of the correct answers to all questions asked.
2. *Facial movements:* During assessment of level of consciousness, observe the patient's facial movements for symmetry, and listen to speech patterns for evidence of slurred speech.
3. *Pupillary function and eye movements:* Perform pupil check, and assess extraocular eye movements.
4. *Motor assessment:* Assess movement and strength in upper and lower extremities.
5. *Sensory:* With a finger, stroke the patient bilaterally on the face and upper aspect of the arm, hand, leg, and foot; ask the patient to identify what is touched and any difference in sensation between the two sides.
6. *Vital signs:* Observe alterations in blood pressure, heart rate or rhythm, respiratory pattern, or temperature.
7. *Change in status:* Ask the patient if he or she feels any differences between this and the previous examination.

Rapid Neurologic Assessment

A neurologic assessment should be organized, thorough, and simple so that it can be performed accurately and easily at each assessment point.[3] A complete neurologic assessment covers all major areas of neurologic control. Any abnormalities identified can be further evaluated and investigated in a more focused and rapid manner. Findings are always evaluated with respect to findings of previous examinations. One critical assessment point is handoff between nurses who are caring for the patient. It is extremely important that the off-going nurse perform a neurologic assessment with the on-coming nurse. This ensures reliability of the assessment and decreases variability between caregivers.

Conscious Patient

An example of a rapid neurologic assessment that can be performed during handoff of a conscious patient with known or potential neurologic deficit is outlined in Box 22.5. This assessment, which usually takes less than 4 minutes, is meant to provide a starting point. If any neurologic deficit is identified that is new or different from the last assessment, more detailed attention must be focused on that abnormality.

Unconscious Patient

In the assessment of an unconscious patient (Box 22.6), initial efforts are directed at achieving maximal arousal of the patient. Calling the patient's name, patting the chest, or shaking a shoulder accomplishes this task. After the patient has been stimulated, the examiner can proceed with the neurologic evaluation. As in the assessment of a conscious patient, if any abnormalities or changes from previous assessment are noticed, further investigation is required. This assessment takes 3 to 4 minutes.

Neurologic Changes Associated With Intracranial Hypertension

Assessment of a patient for signs of increasing ICP is an important responsibility of the critical care nurse. Increasing ICP can be identified by changes in level of consciousness, pupillary reaction, motor response, vital signs, and respiratory patterns (Fig. 22.9).[10,21]

DIAGNOSTIC PROCEDURES

The nursing management of a patient undergoing a neurodiagnostic procedure involves a variety of interventions. Nursing activities are directed toward preparing the patient psychologically and physically for the procedure, monitoring the patient's responses to the procedure, and assessing the patient after the procedure. Preparation includes teaching the patient about the procedure, answering questions, and transporting and positioning the patient for the procedure. During the procedure, the nurse observes the patient for signs of pain, anxiety, or hemorrhage and monitors vital signs. After the procedure, the nurse observes for complications of the procedure and medicates the patient for any postprocedure discomfort. Any evidence of increasing ICP is immediately reported

---

QSEN BOX 22.6   **QSEN: Teamwork and Collaboration**

Rapid Neurologic Assessment of the Unconscious Patient

The following outline should be used for handoff of a critically ill unconscious patient with neurologic dysfunction:

1. *Level of consciousness:* Perform Glasgow Coma Scale assessment.
2. *Pupillary assessment:* Perform pupillary assessment with special attention to size, reactivity, and shape of pupil compared with the opposite eye.
3. *Motor examination:* Assess each extremity individually using a predetermined coding score of motor movement.
4. *Respiratory pattern:* If the patient is not receiving mechanical ventilation, observe respiratory patterns for evidence of deteriorating level of function.
5. *Vital signs:* Include a comparison of preassessment vital signs with vital signs after assessment, paying special attention to arterial blood pressure and intracranial pressure, if these parameters are being monitored.

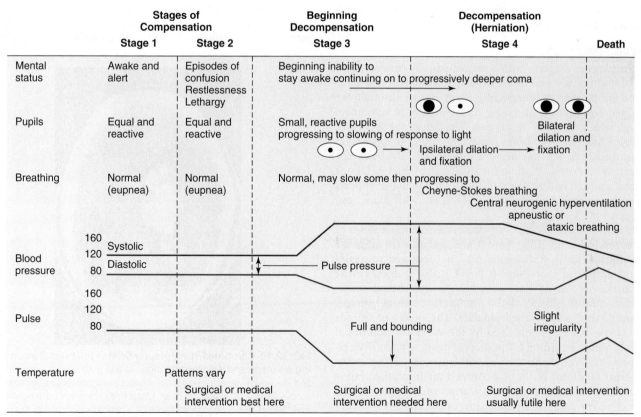

FIG. 22.9 Signs and Symptoms of Intracranial Hypertension. Clinical correlates of compensated and decompensated phases of intracranial hypertension. (From Beare PG, Myers JL, eds. *Principles and Practice of Adult Health Nursing.* 3rd ed. St. Louis: Mosby; 1998.)

to the physician, and emergency measures to maintain circulation must be initiated.

Radiologic Procedures

The following discussion focuses on the more commonly performed radiologic procedures that are used for the diagnosis of a critically ill patient with a neurologic dysfunction.

Skull and Spine Films

The purpose of radiographs of the skull or spine is to identify fractures, anomalies, or possible tumors. The role of skull radiographs in trauma has diminished with the advent of computed tomography (CT). If the patient is to undergo a CT scan during the initial assessment process, a skull radiograph may be unnecessary.[22]

The procedure for obtaining skull and spine radiographs is relatively painless. In many situations, a single lateral view of the skull is adequate, but in some situations, a full skull series is required. A skull series consists of four different views: (1) lateral, (2) posteroanterior, (3) half-axial (Towne), and (4) submentovertical (base) views.[22] A cervical spine series consists of four views: (1) atlas and axial, (2) anteroposterior, (3) lateral, and (4) oblique. A thoracic and lumbar spine series consists of two views: (1) anteroposterior and (2) lateral.[22]

Proper patient positioning is essential, especially for radiographs of the spine. Spinal precautions (eg, cervical collar, strict maintenance of head alignment) must be maintained until lateral radiographs confirm the integrity of the cervical structures. Nursing care involves positioning the patient to obtain adequate radiographs. The cervical spine must be treated as unstable until proved otherwise in any situation in which traumatic injury, especially head injury, is the cause of the patient's admission to the critical care unit.[23]

Computed Tomography

CT provides the clinician with a mathematically reconstructed view of multiple sections of the head and body. This is accomplished by passage of intersecting x-ray beams through the examined area and measurement of the density of substances through which the x-ray beams pass. The denser the substance through which an x-ray beam passes, the whiter it appears on the finished film. The less dense a substance is, the blacker it appears. With normal findings for a CT scan of the head, bone appears white, blood appears off-white, brain tissue appears shaded gray, cerebrospinal fluid (CSF) appears off-black, and air appears black (Fig. 22.10).[24]

CT offers rapid, convenient, noninvasive visualization of structures and is the diagnostic study of choice for an acute head injury. Serial evaluations may be obtained to verify midline shift and increasing ICP.[25] CT also is used in the diagnostic work-up of space-occupying lesions, hemorrhage, vascular abnormalities, skull fractures, cerebral edema, hydrocephalus, and severe headache. The utility of CT for acute stroke has been enhanced by the advent of additional CT techniques including CT perfusion imaging and CT angiography.[26] CT can be performed with and without the use of a contrast medium. Without a contrast medium, the scan is noninvasive, requires no premedication of the patient, and is effective for analysis and location of normal brain structures. The use of an intravenously injected contrast medium enhances the vascular areas and enables detection of vascular lesions or further definition of lesions identified on a non–contrast-enhanced scan. The letter "C" is evident on the radiograph when contrast has been used.[24]

Nursing management of a patient undergoing CT can be divided into two areas of focus: (1) observation of the patient's tolerance of the procedure and (2) observation of the patient's reaction to the dye used in contrast-enhanced scanning. Because of the associated activity and positioning, transporting and scanning of a critically ill patient with known or suspected intracranial hypertension can cause deterioration in the patient's condition. The nurse must always remain with the patient during CT scanning and closely observe the neurologic status, vital signs, and, if monitored, ICP.[23]

If the patient is scheduled to receive a contrast agent for CT scanning, questions about possible sensitivity to iodine-based dye must be asked beforehand, if possible. During infusion of the dye and for 10 to 30 minutes afterward, the patient is observed closely for an anaphylactic reaction. Less than 1% of all patients undergoing contrast-enhanced CT have severe anaphylactic reactions, shock, or cardiac arrest. Another potential complication of the dye is acute kidney failure. Two measures reported to reduce the incidence and severity of renal dysfunction after contrast-enhanced CT are (1) antihistamine administration and (2) adequate hydration before and after the study.[22]

Magnetic Resonance Imaging

Magnetic resonance imaging (MRI) produces images with greater detail than CT and provides views of several planes (sagittal, coronal, axial, and oblique) that cannot be obtained with CT. No ionizing radiation is used. For MRI, the patient is placed in a large magnetic field that stimulates the nuclei of the atoms of the body. Introduction of radiofrequency waves causes resonance of the nuclei, which is emitted as the nuclei relax. A computer constructs an image of the tissue (Fig. 22.11). Intravenous administration of a non–iodine-based contrast

FIG. 22.10 Computed Tomography Scan of the Brain Demonstrating an Intracerebral Hemorrhage. In this patient with hypertension and an acute severe headache, noncontrast computed tomography scan shows a large area of fresh blood in the region of the right thalamus. Blood also is seen in the anterior and posterior horns of the lateral ventricles. Because blood is denser than cerebrospinal fluid, it is layered dependently. (From Mettler FA. *Essentials of Radiology*. 3rd ed. Philadelphia: Saunders; 2014.)

medium enhances the images by influencing the magnetic environment and signal intensity.[22,24]

With MRI, small tumors, whose tissue densities are different from densities of the surrounding cells, can be identified before they could be visualized through any other radiographic test. MRI also can detect areas of cerebral infarct within minutes of stroke as well as identify small hemorrhages deep in the brain that are invisible on CT. Magnetic resonance perfusion and diffusion-weighted imaging may be used in the setting of acute ischemic stroke to establish the presence of brain tissue at risk (penumbra) for dying if ischemia continues.[27] MRI with contrast is the preferred study for detection of infectious and inflammatory processes of the central nervous system (CNS), malignancy, and metastatic lesions; cervical spine imaging; and postoperative evaluation of tumor recurrence. MRI also is the diagnostic study of choice in the evaluation of spinal cord injury.[25]

Nursing management for a patient undergoing MRI is focused on the patient's tolerance of the procedure. Concerns related to transport of the patient with neurologic problems for MRI are identical to the concerns discussed for CT. Teaching

and preparation of the patient are essential for successful performance of MRI. The procedure is lengthy and requires the patient to lie motionless in a tight, enclosed space. Many patients experience anxiety, panic, and an acute sense of claustrophobia. Mild sedation, a blindfold, or both may be necessary. A patient with neurologic impairment may be unable to comprehend the instructions, and sedation, possibly combined with neuromuscular blockade, is required. Removal of all metal from the patient's body and clothing is essential because the basis of MRI is a strong magnetic field. MRI safety is further discussed in Box 22.7.

Cerebral Angiography

The following discussion focuses on more commonly performed angiography procedures that are used for diagnosis in a critically ill patient with a neurologic dysfunction.

Conventional angiography. Conventional angiography involves the injection of radiopaque contrast medium into the intracranial or extracranial vasculature (Fig. 22.12). With the use of serial radiologic filming, an angiogram traces the flow of blood from the arterial circulation through the capillary

FIG. 22.11 Normal Magnetic Resonance Imaging Anatomy of the Brain. (A) Coronal projection. (B) Sagittal projection. (From Mettler FA. *Essentials of Radiology.* 3rd ed. Philadelphia: Saunders; 2014.)

QSEN BOX 22.7 **QSEN: Patient Safety Alert**

Preventing Accidents and Injuries in the MRI Suite

Magnetic resonance imaging (MRI) was applied to health care in the late 1970s to provide never-before-seen two- and three-dimensional views of body tissue and structure. Today, more than 10 million MRI, or MR, scans are done in the United States each year.[1] While the capabilities of the MRI scanner are well-recognized, its inherent dangers may not be as well known. The following types of injury can and have occurred during the MRI scanning process:

1. "Missile effect" or "projectile" injury in which ferromagnetic objects (those having magnetic properties) such as ink pens, wheelchairs, and oxygen canisters are pulled into the MRI scanner at rapid velocity.
2. Injury related to dislodged ferromagnetic implants such as aneurysm clips, pins in joints, and drug infusion devices.
3. Burns from objects that may heat during the MRI process, such as wires (including lead wires for both implants and external devices) and surgical staples, or from the patient's body touching the inside walls (the bore) of the MRI scanner during the scan.[2]
4. Injury or complication related to equipment or device malfunction or failure caused by the magnetic field. For example, battery-powered devices (laryngoscopes, microinfusion pumps, monitors, etc.) can suddenly fail to operate; some programmable infusion pumps may perform erratically;[3] and pacemakers and implantable defibrillators may not behave as programmed.
5. Injury or complication due to failure to attend to patient support systems during the MRI. This is especially true for patient sedation or anesthesia in MRI arenas. For example, oxygen canisters or infusion pumps run out and staff must either leave the MRI area to retrieve a replacement or move the patient to an area where a replacement can be found.
6. Acoustic injury from the loud knocking noise that the MRI scanner makes.
7. Adverse events related to the administration of MRI contrast agents.
8. Adverse events related to cryogen handling, storage, or inadvertent release in superconducting MR imaging system sites.

Five MRI-related cases in the Joint Commission's Sentinel Event database resulted in four deaths and affected four adults and one child. One case was caused by a projectile, three were cardiac events, and one was a misread MRI scan that resulted in delayed treatment.

In 2005, Jason Launders, MSc, a medical physicist with the ECRI Institute, conducted an independent analysis of the FDA's MAUDE (Manufacturer and User Facility Device Experience Database) reporting database over a 10-year time span, which revealed 389 reports of MRI-related events, including nine deaths: three related to pacemaker failure; two to insulin pump failure; and the remaining four events related to implant disturbance, a projectile, and asphyxiation from a cryogenic mishap during installation of an MR imaging system. More than 70 percent of the 389 reports were burns; 10 percent were projectile related; another 10 percent were "other events, including implant disturbance; 4 percent were acoustic injuries; 4 percent were fire related; and 2 percent were internal heating related.

The most common patient injuries in the MRI suite are burns and the most common objects to undergo significant heating are wires and leads. Other objects associated with burns are pulse oximeter sensors and cables, cardiorespiratory monitor cables, safety pins, metal clamps, drug delivery patches (which may contain metallic foil), and tattoos (which may contain iron oxide pigment). Less common injuries involve pacemakers. The American College of Radiology[2] recommends that implanted cardiac pacemakers and implantable cardioverter/defibrillators should be considered a relative contraindication for MRI. Any exception should be considered on a case-by-case basis and only if the site is staffed with individuals with the appropriate radiology and cardiology knowledge and expertise.[2]

While only one missile-effect case has been reported to the Joint Commission, they are more common than is generally recognized. Many people—including

health care workers—are unaware that the magnets in the MRI scanner are always "on" and that turning them "off" (quenching) is an expensive and potentially dangerous undertaking, involving the controlled release of cryogenic gases that can be deadly if released into a contained area. As a result of the magnets, many of the objects pulled into the MRI scanner are cleaning equipment or tools taken into the MRI suite by housekeeping staff or maintenance workers.

Risk reduction strategies

Conventional metal detectors have been used to help identify metal objects in and on patients, but they are not 100 percent accurate and can give false-positives and false-negatives.[4] Furthermore, metal detectors cannot alert personnel to all objects that are subject to heating, malfunction or failure during an MRI scan.[5] However, the recent availability of ferromagnetic detectors may help in screening patients for objects left on their person, according to Dr. Emanuel Kanal, chair of the ACR's Magnetic Resonance Safety Committee. A recent study concludes that ferromagnetic detectors have 99 percent sensitivity.[6]

A report on projectile cylinder accidents in the American Journal of Radiology[7] recommends strategies to prevent missile-effect accidents, including implementing protocols that allow maintenance and housekeeping personnel to enter the MRI suite only after proper safety education and when no patient is in the suite. A number of preventive measures for hazards in the MRI environment are recommended by Dr. Kanal[8] and are supported by the ECRI Institute[9], including:

- Appoint a safety officer who is responsible for implementing and enforcing safety procedures in the MRI suite.
- Implement systems to support safe MRI practice such as written protocols and checklists and periodically review, and assess compliance with your organization's MRI policies, procedures and protocols.
- In general, do not bring any device or equipment into the MRI environment unless it is proven to be MR Safe or MR Conditional. MR Safe items pose no known hazard in all MRI environments, and MR Conditional items have been demonstrated to pose no known hazards in a specified MRI environment with specified conditions of use.[10] The Safety of "MR conditional" items must be verified with the specific scanner and MR environment in which they will be used.

Joint Commission recommendations

The Joint Commission offers the following recommendations and strategies to health care organizations for reducing MRI accidents and injuries:

1. Restrict access to all MRI sites by implementing the four zone concept as defined in the ACR Guidance Document for Safe MR Practices: 2007.[2] The four zone concept provides for progressive restrictions in access to the MRI scanner:
   - Zone I: General public
   - Zone II: Unscreened MRI patients
   - Zone III: Screened MRI patients and personnel
   - Zone IV: Screened MRI patients under constant direct supervision of trained MR personnel
2. Use trained personnel to screen all nonemergent patients twice, providing two separate opportunities for them to answer questions about any metal objects they may have on them, any implanted devices, drug delivery patches, tattoos, and any electrically, magnetically, or mechanically activated devices they may have. If the patient is unconscious or unable to answer questions, question the patient's family member or surrogate decision maker. If this person is unsure, use other means to determine if the patient has implants or other devices that could be negatively affected by the MRI scan (eg, look for scars or deformities, scrutinize the patient's history, use plain-film radiography, use ferromagnetic detectors to assist in the screening process, etc.).[2,8]

QSEN   BOX 22.7   QSEN: Patient Safety Alert—cont'd

Preventing Accidents and Injuries in the MRI Suite

3. Ensure that the MRI technologist has the patient's complete and accurate medical history to ensure that the patient can be safely scanned. All implants should be checked against product labeling or manufacturer literature specific to that implant, or peer-reviewed published data regarding the device or implant in question. Technologists should be provided with ready access to this information.

4. Have a specially trained staff person who is knowledgeable about the MRI environment accompany any patients, visitors and other staff who are not familiar with the MRI environment inside the MRI suite at all times.[2,8]

5. Annually, provide all medical and ancillary staff who may be expected to accompany patients to the MRI suite with safety education about the MRI environment and provide all staff and patients and their families with appropriate materials (eg, guidelines, brochure, poster) that explain the potential for accidents and adverse events in the MRI environment

6. Take precautions to prevent patient burns during scanning, including:
   - Ensure that no items (such as leads) are formed into a loop, since magnetic induction can occur and cause burns.[4]
   - If the patient's body touches the bore of the MRI scanner, use nonconductive foam padding to insulate the patient's skin and tissues.[2]
   - Place a cold compress or ice pack on EKG leads, surgical staples, and tattoos that will be exposed to radiofrequency irradiation during the MR imaging process.[2]

7. Only use equipment (eg, fire extinguishers, oxygen tanks, physiologic monitors, and aneurysm clips) that has been tested and approved for use during MRI scans.[2]

8. Proactively plan for managing critically ill patients who require physiologic monitoring and continuous infusion of life sustaining drugs while in the MRI suite.

9. Provide all MRI patients with hearing protection (ie, ear plugs).

10. Never attempt to run a cardio-pulmonary arrest code or resuscitation within the MR magnet room itself.

Ferromagnetic Objects

buffing machines
chest tube stands
clipboards (patient charts)
gurneys
hairpins
hearing aids
identification badges
insulin pumps
keys
medical gas cylinders
mops
nail clippers and nail files
oxygen cylinders
pulse oximeters
pacemakers
pagers
paper clips
pens and pencils
IV poles
prosthetic limbs
shrapnel
sandbags (with metal filings)
steel shoes
stethoscopes
scissors
staples
tools
vacuum cleaners
watches
wheelchairs

References

1. "Fatal MRI Accident is First of Its Kind", www.webmd.com/content/Article/34/1728_85340.htm.
2. ACR Guidance Document for Safe MR Practices: 2007, *AJR* 188, June 2007. http://www.acr.org/SecondaryMainMenuCategories/quality_safety/MRSafety/safe_mr07.aspx.
3. "Ensuring Safety for Infants Undergoing Magnetic Resonance Imaging," *Medscape*, http://www.medscape.com/viewarticle/499273
4. Radiographic Imaging CEU Source, LLC, Part 6, MRI Safety For Health Care Personnel
5. "What's New in MR Safety", *Health Devices* Vol. 34(No. 10), October 2005. ECRI. Includes a "Starter List of Devices and Equipment for Use in the MR Environment.".
6. Thomas S, Kanal E: Ferromagnetic Detector to Screen Patients for Metallic Foreign Bodies Prior to MR Imaging, *Abstract presented at the American Society of Neuroradiology annual meeting in Toronto*, May 2005. http://www.koppdevelopment.com/articles/abstract.htm.
7. Projectile Cylinder Accidents Resulting from the Presence of Ferromagnetic Nitrous Oxide or Oxygen Tanks in the MR Suite, *AJR* 177, July 2001.
8. Emanuel Kanal MD, Magnetic Resonance Safe Practice Guidelines of the University of Pittsburgh Medical Center, 2001.

9. Hazard Report: Patient Death Illustrates the Importance of Adhering to Safety Precautions in Magnetic Resonance Environments, *Health Devices*(30)8, August 2001, ECRI.
10. American Society of Testing and Materials F 2503-05, *Standard Practice for Marking Medical Devices and Other Items for Safety in the Magnetic Resonance Environment*

VA National Centers for Patient Safety MR Hazard Summary and MR Hazard Summary—August 2001 Update, www.patientsafety.gov/SafetyTopics/mrihazardsummary.html

Burns in MRI Patients Wearing Transdermal Patches, *ISMP Medication Safety Alert!®*, April 8, 2004. www.ismp.org/Newsletters/acutecare/articles/20040408.asp?ptr=y.

"Burns in MRI Patients Wearing Transdermal Patches" video web cast: *FDA Patient Safety News*, U.S. Food and Drug Administration, July 2004. Show #29 www.accessdata.fda.gov/scripts/cdrh/cfdocs/psn/transcript.cfm?show=29.

"Working Together to Improve MRI Safety," *The Joint Commission Perspectives on Patient Safety* Vol. 7(Issue 2), February 2007.

"Evaluating MRI Safety for Specific Populations: Preparing for pediatric, geriatric, and acute patients," *The Joint Commission Perspectives on Patient Safety* Vol. 7(Issue 6), June 2007.

From The Joint Commission: Sentinel Event Alert, no. 38, February 4, 2008. Available at http://www.jointcommission.org/assets/1/18/SEA_38.PDF. Accessed May 12, 2016. For additional MRI Safety Resources, visit the Joint Commission Resources website.

bed to the venous circulation. Cerebral angiography allows visualization of the lumen of vessels to provide information about patency, size (narrowing or dilation), irregularities, or occlusion. Angiography is used in the diagnosis of cerebral aneurysm, vasospasm, arteriovenous malformation, carotid artery disease, and some vascular tumors. Angiography also is used to evaluate cerebral vasculature in patients with stroke. Information obtained from the angiogram guides the surgeon in choosing the operative approach or provides information to make medical management decisions other than surgery.[28]

FIG. 22.12 Cerebral Angiography. (From Ehrlich RA, Daly JA. *Patient Care in Radiography.* 8th ed. St. Louis: Mosby; 2013.)

The procedure involves placement of a catheter in the femoral artery and threading it up the aorta and into the origin of the cerebral circulation. Other injection sites include direct carotid or vertebral artery puncture or placement of a catheter in the brachial, axillary, or subclavian artery. Several views of vessels can be studied by means of angiography. A four-vessel angiogram involves injections into the right and left internal carotid arteries and the right and left vertebral arteries. If the area of suspected disease already has been identified, a single-vessel study may be all that is required. This is particularly true when angiography is used as a follow-up in the evaluation of intracranial vascular surgery. If carotid artery disease is a working diagnosis, the angiographic study may include views of the arch of the aorta and of the external and internal carotid arteries.[22]

After the catheter is appropriately placed, the contrast medium is injected. A rapid succession of radiographs is taken as the contrast medium progresses through the cerebral circulation. Separate injections of contrast medium are administered for each vessel being studied.[26]

Nursing management associated with this invasive procedure is comprehensive. Renal insufficiency, bleeding, and cardiac instability are contraindications to cerebral angiography and must be assessed before the procedure. As with contrast-enhanced CT, the nurse must assess the patient for possible sensitivity to iodine-based contrast dye before angiography. Patient education is essential to patient preparation. The patient's complete understanding of the role this procedure plays in diagnosis as well as the process itself relieves anxiety about the unknown and ensures cooperation in what is commonly an uncomfortable procedure.[23]

Before the procedure, the patient has no oral intake (NPO status) for at least 4 hours. Sedation is administered immediately before the procedure. Discomforts during the procedure include the need to lie still on a cold, hard table and the possibility of pain during preparation and insertion of the groin catheter. The patient often experiences a hot, burning sensation when the contrast medium is injected, especially if it is injected into the external carotid system. Preparation of patients for this burning sensation assures them that it is not an abnormal occurrence.[23]

The patient must be made aware of the postprocedure assessment. After the procedure, adequate hydration is necessary to assist the kidneys in clearing the heavy dye load. Inadequate hydration may lead to renal dysfunction and possibly shutdown. If the patient cannot tolerate oral fluids, an intravenous line is placed before the procedure is begun. Postprocedure assessment involves measurement of vital signs, neurologic evaluation, observation of the puncture site, and assessment of neurovascular integrity distal to the puncture site every 15 minutes for the first hour. Any abnormalities must be reported immediately. The patient is kept on bed rest for 8 to 12 hours.[23]

Complications associated with cerebral angiography include (1) cerebral embolus caused by the catheter dislodging a segment of atherosclerotic plaque in the vessel; (2) hemorrhage or hematoma formation at the insertion site; (3) vasospasm of a vessel caused by the irritation of catheter placement; (4) thrombosis of the extremity distal to the injection site; and (5) allergic or adverse reaction to the contrast medium, including renal impairment.[22]

Digital subtraction angiography. Digital subtraction angiography (DSA) eliminates the shadows and distortions of bone or other material that sometimes block the viewing of the cerebral vessels.[22] Radiographs taken before and after intravenous or intraarterial dye injection are superimposed on each other, and all matching digital images are subtracted by the computer. Only the dye-enhanced cerebral vessels are left for study and evaluation.[29] Intraarterial two-dimensional DSA is particularly useful in detecting ruptured intracranial aneurysms, and three-dimensional DSA offers an even more precise demonstration of the aneurysm anatomy.[29] In addition, an advantage of DSA over conventional arteriography is that significantly less dye is used. The major disadvantage of DSA is that the patient must remain motionless during the entire procedure. Even swallowing interferes significantly with the imaging process. Complications and nursing management for DSA are similar to those described for cerebral angiography.[23]

Magnetic resonance angiography. Magnetic resonance angiography (MRA) offers noninvasive visualization of the cerebrovascular system.[25] It uses MRI technology to evaluate CBF and provide details about cerebral vessels. MRA of the carotid arteries has become an established complement to preoperative ultrasound evaluation. MRA is also used to identify intracranial aneurysms, stroke, arteriovenous malformations, and vasospasm.[25] Contrast-enhanced MRA may be performed to improve image resolution and reduce artifact. The most commonly used agent is gadolinium, a nonnephrotoxic contrast medium that is injected intravenously.[24]

Computed tomography angiography. CT angiography is a technique that uses high-speed helical CT technology with the administration of contrast medium to visualize the cerebrovascular system. With its three-dimensional reconstructions, CT angiography can simultaneously demonstrate the bony skull base and its related vasculature, making it a valuable diagnostic tool for the management of patients with cerebrovascular disease. Use of ionizing radiation and an iodine-based intravascular contrast medium with CT angiography is a disadvantage compared with MRA, but it is quicker and requires less patient cooperation than MRA.[30]

Myelography

Myelography is radiographic examination of the spinal cord and vertebral column after injection of contrast medium into the subarachnoid space through the lumbar region of the

FIG. 22.13 Lumbar Puncture. With the patient in a flexed position to maximize the space between vertebrae, the lumbar puncture needle is inserted between L4 and L5 to gain entry to the subarachnoid space. (From Monahan FD, et al. *Phipps' Medical-Surgical Nursing: Health and Illness Perspectives.* 8th ed. St. Louis: Mosby; 2007.)

spine between L2 and L3 or L3 and L4 or by cisternal puncture. Myelography allows visualization of the spinal canal, the subarachnoid space around the spinal cord, and the spinal nerve roots (Fig. 22.13). MRI has replaced myelography in most cases, but myelography may be necessary in postoperative patients with multiple clips or metallic hardware. Possible risks involved in the use of myelography include injection of the dye outside the subarachnoid space, arachnoiditis as a result of irritation of the arachnoid membranes from a foreign material, and allergic reaction. Other adverse reactions include confusion, hallucinations, headache, grand mal seizure, chest pain, and dysrhythmias.[31] Postprocedure care includes keeping the patient's head elevated 45 degrees for 8 hours, monitoring neurologic status, and encouraging intake of oral fluids.[23]

Cerebral Blood Flow and Metabolism Imaging

Measurement of CBF provides valuable information for clinical management of critical care patients with neurologic problems.[32] The average CBF in a human is 55 mL/100 g of brain per minute, but actual values may vary widely across gray and white matter. The ischemic threshold for CBF is approximately 18 mL/100 g per minute, with 10 mL/100 g per minute often considered the threshold for irreversible injury.[33] CBF is influenced by mean arterial pressure, ICP, and partial pressure of carbon dioxide and oxygen.[34] However, the measurements of CBF and cerebral perfusion pressure (CPP) do not address the brain's metabolic need for oxygen. Neuronal demand for oxygen is governed by the metabolic rate. The rate at which the brain consumes oxygen is known as the cerebral metabolic rate of oxygen ($CMRO_2$), the normal value of which is 3.4 mL/100 g per minute. Measurement of $CMRO_2$ is a valuable tool for assessing brain vitality and function and has been shown to be a better marker of injury severity in hypoxia-ischemia than CBF alone.[35] The following discussion focuses on the more commonly performed imaging studies that assess

CBF and cerebral metabolism in critically ill patients with neurologic dysfunction.

Perfusion Computed Tomography

Perfusion CT allows rapid evaluation of cerebral perfusion. A perfusion CT scan is obtained by passing x-rays through the brain, as in a regular CT scan; however, in addition to revealing the structure of brain tissue, perfusion CT measures CBF, cerebral blood volume, and mean transit time. This is done by scanning the patient several times every few seconds before, during, and after intravenous delivery of an iodine-containing contrast agent that absorbs the x-rays. Perfusion CT has been found to be useful for diagnosis of cerebral ischemia and infarction associated with stroke and for evaluation of cerebral ischemia associated with vasospasm after subarachnoid hemorrhage.[36]

Xenon Computed Tomography

Xenon CT is used to study regional CBF. The scan is a computerized radiographic study of the brain that is performed while the patient breathes a carefully regulated flow of xenon, which is a colorless, odorless gas. It has higher resolution in blood flow measurements than other techniques such as positron emission tomography (PET). Xenon CT has been used in the evaluation of a wide variety of disorders and has been most useful in the evaluation of cerebrovascular disease and brain metabolism. Xenon CT studies are occasionally used to determine brain death.[37]

Perfusion Magnetic Resonance Imaging

Perfusion MRI can provide a relative and absolute measurement of the parameters of cerebral microvascularization: regional blood volume, mean transit time, and regional blood flow. The two most common methods for imaging perfusion are (1) the dynamic susceptibility contrast approach, which detects the first passage of an intravascular contrast agent such as gadolinium, and (2) arterial spin labeling, which uses magnetically labeled arterial blood water as a diffusible flow tracer.[38] The main applications of first-pass perfusion MRI are identification of vascular pathologies (ischemic strokes, vasospasm) and tumoral pathologies. Progress in sequencing and the very magnetic high fields are expected to lead to improvements in the spin labeling technique.[39]

Carotid Ultrasonography

Although ultrasound technology does not provide an absolute measure of CBF, it is a noninvasive technique to provide information about the flow velocity of blood through the carotid vessels. Carotid duplex studies are used as a routine screening procedure for intraluminal narrowing of the common and internal carotid arteries as a result of atherosclerotic plaques. A Doppler probe is placed externally over the vessel, where high-frequency sound waves (ultrasound) are generated, and blood flow velocities are calculated. As the diameter of the vessel changes, the velocity of the flow of blood through the vessel changes; the higher the flow velocity, the narrower is the vessel. Carotid duplex studies are noninvasive, inexpensive, and painless.[23] When changes in flow velocities that may indicate significant occlusion of the vessel are identified, CT angiography or MRA may be used to verify the degree of severity of the narrowed vessel. If necessary, cerebral angiography is performed to confirm ambiguous or equivocal findings.[40]

Emission Tomography Studies

The following discussion focuses on two different nuclear medicine studies that may be used to evaluate critically ill patients with neurologic dysfunction.

Positive Emission Tomography. A PET scan is a nuclear medicine study that uses CT technology to produce a three-dimensional image of detailed biochemical changes in brain tissue as it traces the brain's metabolic activity.[41] Oxygen-15 (^{15}O)–labeled water is injected into the patient, and the PET camera measures the amount of the radiotracer as it flows through the brain, which allows for the measurement of CBF, the fraction of oxygen extracted from the arterial blood by the cerebral tissue, and $CMRO_2$.[42] During the procedure, the patient needs to lie still and may be asked to think, reason, and remember.[23] The amount of radiation the patient is exposed to is very small—about one to three times the normal human annual exposure to background radiation. One consideration with regard to cerebral PET is the long scan time during which a patient's physiologic condition must remain stable.[40]

Single-Photon Emission Computed Tomography. Another nuclear medicine scanning procedure that integrates CT and a radioactive tracer to produce a three-dimensional measurement of regional CBF is single-photon emission computed tomography (SPECT). The test differs from PET in that tracer stays in the bloodstream rather than being absorbed by surrounding tissue, limiting the images to areas where blood flows. SPECT is cheaper and more readily available than higher resolution PET. The major clinical uses of SPECT are to detect cerebrovascular disease, seizures, and tumors.[43]

Electrophysiology Studies

The following discussion focuses on two frequently performed electrophysiology studies that are used in the diagnosis and management of critically ill patients with neurologic dysfunction.

Electroencephalography

Electroencephalography (EEG) records electrical impulses generated by the brain, commonly called *brain waves*. The nurse caring for a patient with a neurologic dysfunction must be aware of the appropriate indications for use and the limitations of this diagnostic procedure. The purpose of EEG is to detect and localize abnormal electrical activity. This abnormal activity can be defined as *slowing*, which occurs in areas of injury or infarct, or as *spikes* and *waves* seen in irritated tissue. Indications for the use of EEG include suspected seizure activity, cerebral infarct, metabolic encephalopathies, altered consciousness, infectious disease, some head injuries, and confirmation of brain death.[23,44]

Noninvasive electrodes are placed on the head, and the electrical impulses detected are transferred to a central recording device that records the information in wave form. Six types of waves or rhythms may be present (Table 22.4). Intermittent slowing with triphasic wave morphology is associated with metabolic encephalopathy. Continuous, generalized slowing in the delta or theta range is associated with anoxic damage. The combination of alpha-waves that do not change with stimulation and a coma state is called *alpha-coma*, and it is associated with a poor prognosis.[45]

Other EEG abnormalities associated with poor prognosis are *burst suppression* (occasional generalized bursts of activity with intervening inactivity or severe voltage depression) and *periodic patterns* (generalized spikes at fixed intervals of one to two per second). Absence of electrical activity on EEG, termed *electrocerebral silence*, can occur transiently in the period immediately after cardiopulmonary resuscitation, severe hypothermia, and CNS depressant overdose. Enduring electrocerebral silence provides evidence for the clinical determination of brain death.[45]

EEG has significant limitations. Only electrical activity involving large areas of cortex is recorded on EEG. The accuracy of EEG depends on the location of electrophysiologic activity. Abnormal EEG findings are not cause specific. Similar EEG changes occur with a variety of conditions. The EEG result can be normal even when significant pathology is present.[44]

In preparing the patient for EEG, the nurse must stress the noninvasive aspects of this procedure. During the procedure, the awake patient may be asked to perform certain simple tasks such as blinking, closing the eye, or swallowing. Occasionally, testing must be performed during sleep or after a period of sleep deprivation.[23]

TABLE 22.4 Types of Electrical Brain Waves

Wave	Duration	Description
Delta	1–4 cycles/s	Normal; seen in stages 3 and 4 of sleep
Alpha	8–13 cycles/s	Normal; relaxed state with eyes closed; often seen in occipital leads
Theta	4–7 cycles/s	Less common in adults than in children; characteristic of coma in brain injury
Beta	12–40 cycles/s	Fast waves indicating mental or physical activity
Sleep spindles	12–14 cycles/s	Seen in stage 2 sleep, not rapid eye movement
Spike and slow waves	Variable	Seen in irritable brain tissue (eg, seizure)

Evoked Potentials

Evoked potentials are cerebral electrical impulses generated in response to a sensory stimulus. Impulses are recorded as they travel through the brainstem and into the cerebral cortex. Measuring evoked potentials is a sophisticated way of observing the status of sensory pathways as they enter the CNS, travel through the brainstem, and reach the cerebral cortex. Evoked potential studies are used in the determination of prognosis in coma and the existence and extent of brainstem or spinal cord injury in a traumatically injured patient. Evaluation of evoked potentials is valuable during therapeutically induced comas such as barbiturate coma inasmuch as these sensory pathways are unaffected by the depressive activity of such medications. Evoked potentials are monitored intraoperatively during spinal surgery and cerebral tumor dissection.[44]

The four types of evoked potential tests are (1) visual evoked responses (VERs), (2) brainstem auditory evoked responses (BAERs), (3) somatosensory evoked responses (SSERs), and (4) motor evoked potentials (MEPs). VERs involve monitoring the visual pathways through the brainstem and cortex in response to the patient's viewing a shifting geometric pattern on a screen or a flashing light stimulus emitted from a mask placed over the eye.[44] BAERs involve monitoring the auditory pathway through the brainstem and cortex in response to a rhythmic clicking sound sent through earphones placed over the patient's ears. BAERs are useful in assessing brainstem integrity in the critical care unit when cranial nerve testing cannot be performed or is inconclusive.[44] SSERs involve monitoring of sensory pathways from the extremities ascending the spinal cord through the brainstem and into the cortex. This is performed by administering a small electrical shock to a nerve root in the periphery such as the ulnar or radial nerve. SSERs can be used to evaluate cortical functioning after cardiac arrest or head trauma. SSERs also are used routinely during spinal surgery.[44] MEPs assess the functional integrity of descending motor pathways. The motor cortex is stimulated by direct high-voltage electrical stimulation through the scalp or use of a magnetic field to induce an electrical current within the brain. Electrical stimulation is a painful procedure and must be reserved for anesthetized patients. Magnetic stimulation is painless.[44]

LABORATORY STUDIES

The major laboratory study performed in a patient with neurologic dysfunction is analysis of CSF obtained by a lumbar puncture or a ventriculostomy.[3,4]

Cerebrospinal Fluid Analysis

The main purpose of a lumbar puncture is to obtain CSF for analysis. CSF opening pressure may also be obtained. CSF samples are evaluated for the presence of subarachnoid blood or infection, or they are sent for laboratory analysis (Table 22.5).[46]

A lumbar puncture involves the introduction of a 20- to 22-gauge hollow needle into the subarachnoid space at L3 to L4 or L4 to L5, below the end of the spinal cord, which usually is at L1 or L2 (see Fig. 22.13). The patient can be placed in the lateral decubitus position, with the knees and head tightly tucked, or in the sitting position, leaning over a bedside table or some other support. Before initiating the procedure, the patient's coagulation profile is checked for abnormalities.[47,48]

Two life-threatening risks associated with lumbar puncture include (1) possible brainstem herniation, if the ICP is elevated, and (2) respiratory arrest associated with neurologic deterioration. During the procedure, the nurse must monitor the patient's neurologic and respiratory status. If the patient is not fully alert and cooperative, the nurse may need to assist the patient in maintaining the position necessary for the lumbar puncture. The long-standing routine of keeping the patient flat in bed for several hours after a lumbar puncture to prevent a headache has been refuted by scientific study.[4]

MULTIMODAL BEDSIDE MONITORING

Monitoring for secondary brain injury is a fundamental aspect of caring for critically ill patients with neurologic dysfunction. By using more than one monitoring technique, the observer is more likely to determine whether a genuine change in cerebral physiology has occurred and what the most appropriate intervention should be.[15,49,50] The following discussion focuses on multimodal techniques to monitor ICP, CPP, brain oxygenation, CBF, cerebral metabolism, and brain function.

Intracranial Pressure Monitoring

ICP monitoring is recommended as a part of protocol-driven care in patients who are at risk of elevated ICP based on clinical or imaging features.[51] In general, indications for ICP monitoring include traumatic brain injury (TBI), intracranial hemorrhage (ICH), subarachnoid hemorrhage (SAH), hydrocephalus, hepatic failure with encephalopathy, acute ischemic stroke with large infarction, and meningitis.[52] A contraindication for ICP monitoring is coagulopathy.[52] The appropriate threshold for ICP has not been defined.[51] However, the normal range for ICP in adults is generally 5 to 15 mm Hg,[49,53] and the threshold for intracranial hypertension is considered to be greater than 20 mm Hg.[51] It is recommended that ICP monitoring be used in conjunction with other intracranial monitoring devices to enhance clinical decision making.[51]

Both noninvasive and invasive methods of monitoring ICP are available.[54] Noninvasive techniques of measuring ICP include transcranial Doppler (TCD), tympanic membrane displacement, optic nerve sheath diameter, CT/MRI, and pupillometry.[53] Noninvasive techniques do not have the complications related to invasive techniques. However, the noninvasive techniques have yet to measure ICP accurately enough to be used as alternatives to invasive measurement.[53] Pupillometry is discussed later in this chapter.

Types of Intracranial Pressure Monitoring Devices

There are several different invasive methods of ICP monitoring. Depending on the location and type of brain injury as well as the monitoring technique, ICP monitoring can be undertaken in different intracranial anatomic locations: intraventricular, intraparenchymal, epidural, subdural, and subarachnoid (Fig. 22.14).[53] The most commonly used ICP monitoring devices use the intraventricular and intraparenchymal locations.

Intraventricular catheter device. The ventricular catheter with external strain gauge transducer is considered the gold standard for ICP monitoring, allowing for accurate and reliable ICP waveform and measurement as well as CSF

TABLE 22.5 Analysis of Cerebrospinal Fluid

Characteristic	Normal Findings	Abnormal Findings	Possible Causes and Comments
Pressure	<200 mm H_2O	<60 mm H_2O	Faulty needle placement
			Dehydration
			Spinal block along subarachnoid space
			Block of foramen magnum
			Hydrocephalus
		>200 mm H_2O	Muscle tension
			Abdominal compression
			Brain tumor
			Subdural hematoma
			Brain abscess
			Brain cyst
			Cerebral edema (any cause)
Color	Clear, colorless	Cloudy or turbid	Cloudy as a result of microorganisms (eg, WBCs)
			Turbid as a result of increased cell count
		Yellow (xanthochromic)	Breakdown of RBCs with RBC pigments, high protein count
		Smoky	RBCs
Blood	None	Red blood cells: Blood tinged	Traumatic tap: Bloody in first sample
		Grossly bloody	Traumatic tap: Bloody in all samples
Volume	150 mL	Increase	Hydrocephalus
Specific gravity	1.007	Increase	Infection, presence of cells or protein
WBCs	0–5 cells/mm³	<500 cells/mm³	Bacterial or viral infections of meninges, neurosyphilis, subarachnoid hemorrhage, infarction, abscess, tuberculous meningitis, metastatic lesions
		>500 cells/mm³	Purulent infection
Glucose	50–75 mg/dL or 60%–70% of blood glucose	<40 mg/dL	Bacterial meningitis, tuberculosis, parasitic, fungal carcinomatous, subarachnoid hemorrhage
		>80 mg/dL	May not be of neurologic significance
Chloride	700–750 mg/dL	Decreased (<625 mg/dL)	Meningeal infection, tuberculosis meningitis, hypochloremia
		Increased (>800 mg/dL)	May not be of neurologic significance; correlated with blood levels of chloride and not routine; done only on request
Culture and sensitivity	No organisms present	*Neisseria* or *Streptococcus*	Identify organisms to begin therapy; Gram stain for some cultures may take several weeks
Serology for syphilis	Negative	Positive	Syphilis
Protein[a]	15–50 mg/dL	Increased (>60 mg/dL)	Bacterial meningitis, brain tumors (benign and malignant), complete spinal block, ALS, Guillain-Barré syndrome, subarachnoid hemorrhage, infarction, CNS trauma, CNS degenerative diseases, herniated disk, DM with polyneuropathy
		Decreased (<10 mg/dL)	May not be of neurologic significance
Osmolality	295 osm/L	Increased	Protein, WBCs, microorganisms, RBCs
Lactate	10–20 mg/dL	Increased	Bacterial, seizure activity, fungal meningitis, CNS trauma, coma related to toxic or metabolic causes

[a]Blood in CSF will increase the protein level.

ALS, amyotrophic lateral sclerosis; *CNS*, central nervous system; *CSF*, cerebrospinal fluid; *DM*, diabetes mellitus; *RBC*, red blood cell; *WBC*, white blood cell.

From Barker E: *Neuroscience Nursing: A Spectrum of Care.* 3rd ed. St. Louis: Mosby; 2008.

drainage.[49,53–55] The ventriculostomy catheter is radiopaque and MRI compatible.[52] The most common method for placement of the catheter is a coronal burr hole approach at Kocher point, with the tip of the device located in the third ventricle. After CSF is obtained, the primed external ventricular drainage system is connected to the catheter and tunneled to exit a few centimeters away from the burr hole.[52] Intraventricular monitoring of ICP can complicated by difficulties with catheter insertion, postoperative hemorrhage, and catheter-associated ventriculitis.[49,55] The risk of infection may be decreased by using an antibiotic-impregnated or silver-coated catheter.[49]

A disadvantage of using an intraventricular catheter device is that repeated zeroing and leveling with the anatomic reference point for the foramen of Monro is required.[55] The external reference for the foramen of Monro varies but is commonly the external auditory meatus.[55] Whichever reference point is used, it must remain consistent for a particular patient and preferably for an institution.[52] Among the most common issues with a ventriculostomy catheter is decreased CSF drainage.[52] An institutional policy will most likely dictate which maneuvers may be performed by critical care nurses to improve drainage.

Intraparenchymal microsensor device. ICP monitors inserted into brain parenchyma work through the use of fiberoptic,

FIG. 22.14 Intracranial Pressure Monitoring Sites. (From Lewis SL, et al. *Medical-Surgical Nursing: Assessment and Management of Clinical Problems.* 9th ed. St. Louis: Elsevier; 2014.)

FIG. 22.15 Normal Intracranial Pressure Waveform. (From Bader MK, Littlejohns LR. *AANN Core Curriculum for Neuroscience Nursing.* 4th ed. St. Louis: Elsevier; 2004.)

FIG. 22.16 Abnormal Intracranial Pressure Waveform. (From Bader MK, Littlejohns LR. *AANN Core Curriculum for Neuroscience Nursing.* 4th ed. St. Louis: Elsevier; 2004.)

strain gauge, or pneumatic technologies. Fiberoptic devices transmit light via a fiberoptic cable toward a displaceable mirror. Changes in ICP move the mirror, and the differences in intensity of the reflected light are translated to an ICP value.[52,53] Another parameter that may be measured with the fiberoptic transducer-tipped catheters is brain temperature.[52] With strain gauge device technology, ICP is calculated when ICP bends the transducer and changes the level of resistance.[53] Pneumatic sensor technology measures ICP by using a small balloon in the distal end of the catheter to register changes in pressure.[53] Pneumatic sensors also allow for quantitative measurement of intracranial compliance.[53]

The accuracy of the devices depends on their placement relative to the site of injury. The catheter can be easily placed via a cranial access device, via a burr hole, or during a craniotomy. However, the device may not be a good gauge of global ICP if pockets of increased ICP arise secondary to focal brain injuries.[54] Additional disadvantages of intraparenchymal microsensor devices are that microtransducer systems can encounter drift when used for more than 5 days, in vivo calibration and CSF drainage are impossible, and transducer-tipped catheters are not MRI compatible.[52,54,56] An error message or loss of waveform on the ICP monitor may indicate a broken catheter or malposition of the catheter.[52,53]

Combination intraventricular/fiberoptic catheter. The intraventricular/fiberoptic catheter combines the capability of external ventricular drainage of CSF with monitoring of ICP. This hybrid device can be used to monitor ICP intermittently or continuously and to drain CSF intermittently or continuously.[55] There are advantages and disadvantages to using the combination catheter. A disadvantage is that the catheter can be zeroed only before insertion. However, because the transducer is in the tip of the fiberoptic catheter, there is no external strain gauge transducer and no repetitive zeroing and leveling of a transducer with the anatomic reference point for the foramen of Monro.55 An advantage of the catheter is that it allows for CSF drainage. However, to prevent underdrainage or overdrainage of CSF, attention must be paid to the level of the reference point of the drip chamber to the anatomic reference point for the foramen of Monro and the setting of the pressure level at the top of the graduated burette (drip chamber).[55] Consequences of CSF underdrainage include headache, neurologic deterioration, hydrocephalus, increased ICP, secondary neuronal injury,

herniation, and death.[55] Consequences of CSF overdrainage include headache, subdural hematoma, pneumocephalus, ventricular collapse, herniation, and death.

Intracranial Pressure Waves

ICP waveform analysis provides information that may identify patients with decreased adaptive capacity who are at risk for increases in ICP and decreases in CPP.[57] ICP pulse waveform is observed on a continuous, real-time pressure display, and it corresponds to each heartbeat.[57] The waveform arises primarily from pulsations of the major intracranial arteries but also receives retrograde venous pulsations.[57] Although a systolic and diastolic component to the ICP waveform is evident, ICP is read as a mean value.[52]

Normal intracranial pressure waveform. The normal ICP wave has three or more defined peaks (Fig. 22.15). The first peak (P1) is called the *percussion wave*. Originating from the pulsations of the choroid plexus, it has a sharp peak and is fairly consistent in its amplitude. The second peak (P2) is called the *tidal wave*. The tidal wave varies more in shape and amplitude, ending on the dicrotic notch. The P2 portion of the pulse waveform has been most directly linked to the state of decreased compliance. When the P2 component is equal to or higher than P1, decreased compliance occurs (Fig. 22.16). Immediately after the dicrotic notch is the third wave (P3), which is called the *dicrotic wave*. After the dicrotic wave, the pressure usually tapers down to the diastolic position unless retrograde venous pulsations add a few more peaks.[57] In performing basic checks of whether the ICP signal is truly representative of the ICP, it is important to ensure that there is an oscillating pressure curve with the progressively decreasing P1, P2, and P3 notches present, indicating propagation of the cardiac pulse pressure signal.[53] Loss of the ICP waveform may indicate blockage, loose system connections, or possibly transducer failure. A numeric value without a corresponding waveform is of no value.[52]

A, B, and C pressure waves are not true waveforms (Fig. 22.17). Rather, they are the graphically displayed trend data of ICP over time. These waves reflect spontaneous alterations in ICP associated with respiration, systemic blood pressure, and deteriorating neurologic status.

FIG. 22.17 Intracranial Pressure Waves. Composite diagram of A-waves (plateau waves), B-waves (sawtooth waves), and C-waves (small rhythmic waves). (From Barker E. *Neuroscience Nursing: A Spectrum of Care.* 3rd ed. St. Louis: Mosby; 2008.)

FIG. 22.18 Pupillometer. (Courtesy Neuroptics, Inc.)

A-Waves. Also called *plateau waves* because of their distinctive shape, A-waves are the most clinically significant of the three types. They usually occur in an already elevated baseline ICP (>20 mm Hg) and are characterized by sharp increases in ICP of 30 to 69 mm Hg, which plateau for 2 to 20 minutes and then return to baseline. The cause of A-waves is unknown, but they may result from vasodilation and increased CBF, decreased venous outflow (and increased cerebral blood volume), fluctuations in arterial partial pressure of carbon dioxide ($Paco_2$) (and changes in cerebral blood volume), or decreased CSF absorption. B-waves often precede A-waves. Plateau waves are considered significant because of the reduced CPP associated with ICP, in the range of 50 to 100 mm Hg. Transient signs of intracranial hypertension, such as a decreased level of consciousness, bradycardia, pupillary changes, or respiratory changes, may accompany these waves. Some research suggests that prolonged increases in ICP associated with plateau waves may result in transient and permanent cell damage from ischemia.[57]

B-Waves. B-waves are sharp, rhythmic oscillations with a sawtooth appearance that occur every 30 seconds to 2 minutes and can increase the ICP from 5 to 70 mm Hg. They are a normal physiologic phenomenon that can occur in any patient, but they are amplified in states of low intracranial compliance. B-waves appear to reflect fluctuations in cerebral blood volume.[57]

C-Waves. C-waves are small, rhythmic waves that occur every 4 to 8 minutes at normal levels of ICP. They are related to normal fluctuations in respiration and systemic arterial pressure.[57]

Pupillometry

Quantitative measurement and classification of pupillary reactivity using a handheld pupillometer (Fig. 22.18) and the Neurological Pupil index (NPi) is a technique to trend increased ICP in patients with severe TBI, aneurysmal SAH, or ICH.[58] The pupillometer is a handheld infrared system that automatically tracks and analyzes pupil dynamics over a 3-second period.[52] A detachable headrest facilitates the correct and consistent placement of the pupillometer in front of the eye. The device has been specifically designed to minimize possible interobserver variability in the pupillary evaluation.[52] The NPi classifies pupil reactivity through the use of an algorithm. An inverse relationship between decreasing pupil reactivity and increasing ICP has been identified with the use of pupillometry and the NPi.[52,58] Additional research is needed to fully determine the usefulness of the pupillometer to detect early change in pupil size related to increased ICP before neurologic deterioration.[52]

Cerebral Perfusion Pressure Monitoring

Measurement of ICP allows for an estimation of CPP.[59] CPP is the blood pressure gradient across the brain, and it is calculated as the difference between the incoming mean arterial pressure (MAP) and the opposing ICP on the arteries: (CPP = MAP − ICP). CPP is related to CBF and is modifiable through its relationship with MAP and ICP.[49] Adequate CPP provides some protection against secondary ischemia; however, to date, the adequate CPP for each patient is unknown. Evidence-based guidelines such as the Brain Trauma Foundation Guidelines for the Management of Severe Traumatic Brain Injury support a CPP range of 50 to 70 mm Hg for adults.[60] However, the CPP threshold may vary from patient to patient, depending on such factors as variation of how the MAP is measured, autoregulatory status, and intracranial compliance.[51] Cerebral autoregulation is the intrinsic ability of the cerebral vessels to constrict and dilate as needed to maintain adequate cerebral perfusion.[55] Intracranial compliance is defined as a change in ICP in relationship to the change in intracranial volume. It is likely that a CPP threshold exists on an individual basis and that optimal CPP can be identified by multimodality monitoring.[49]

Cerebral autoregulation is impaired with brain injury, and the CBF becomes passively dependent on the systemic blood flow.[55] The cerebral blood vessels are no longer able to react to maintain CPP in response to a change in blood pressure.[55] Continuous bedside monitoring of autoregulatory efficiency is possible through online calculation of derived indices such as the pressure reactivity index and may be useful in broad targeting of cerebral perfusion management goals and prognostication in acute brain injury.[49,51]

Cerebral Blood Flow Monitoring

CBF monitoring provides an understanding of the perfusion status of the brain.[50] Tools used in the clinical and research setting for the assessment of CBF are TCD, transcranial color-coded duplex sonography (TCCS), thermal diffusion flowmetry (TDF), and laser Doppler flowmetry (LDF)

Transcranial Doppler

TCD is an established technique for assessing cerebral hemodynamics in real time, measuring relative changes rather than actual CBF. CBF velocity is measured through cranial windows (thinned areas) of the skull. Three areas commonly used are (1) the temporal bone (transtemporal), (2) the eye (transorbital), and (3) the foramen magnum (transoccipital). Depending on the angle of the Doppler probe, flow velocities can be measured in the anterior, middle, or posterior cerebral arteries and the vertebral and basilar arteries.[61]

The noninvasive technique and portability of the equipment allow frequent bedside monitoring of flow velocity and of vascular diameter. Use of serial TCD studies for the detection of cerebral vasospasm greatly reduces the need for cerebral angiograms to verify and follow post-SAH vasospasm.[61] Additional uses of TCD include identification of intracranial lesions in a patient with stroke, evaluation of flow-velocity changes during carotid endarterectomy, and detection of CBF changes associated with increased ICP. TCD has been used to detect cerebral circulatory arrest in brain death determination, but it must be accompanied by clinical evaluation and additional diagnostic tests because intracranial circulation may be preserved in patients who are brain dead.[49,52,61] Current recommendations for TCCS include predicting (1) angiographic vasospasm after aneurysmal SAH, (2) delayed ischemic neurologic deficits caused by vasospasm after aneurysmal SAH, and (3) vasospasm after traumatic SAH.[51]

The limitations of TCD must be understood. Its accuracy is operator dependent. Correct location and angle of the probe are essential. A few patients have temporal bones too thick for ultrasound penetration. A normal TCD study does not completely rule out the presence of vasospasm because vasospasm may not be evident in the particular vessel examined. TCD results are always evaluated in conjunction with clinical assessment findings.[61] During the TCD study, the patient experiences only mild pressure at the transducer site. No pain is involved. The patient must remain still during the study, which lasts 15 to 90 minutes.[61]

Transcranial Color-Coded Duplex Sonography

TCCS is a noninvasive ultrasound study that enables the visualization of the intracranial structures and basal cerebral arteries and the measurement of blood flow velocities through the arteries. The color component of the study provides more reliable data compared with traditional TCD. TCCS can detect narrowing or occlusion of cerebral arteries, screen for vasospasm, and monitor changes in intracranial dynamics.[51] Arteriovenous malformations also can be detected with TCCS.[62] Current recommendations for TCCS include predicting (1) angiographic vasospasm after aneurysmal SAH, (2) delayed ischemic neurologic deficits caused by vasospasm after aneurysmal SAH, and (3) vasospasm after traumatic SAH.[51] TCCS has been found to be superior to TCD in the detection of angiographically proven vasospasm after aneurysmal SAH.[51]

Thermal Diffusion Flowmetry

Although less commonly used in the critical care setting compared with the above-described technologies, direct CBF monitoring may be conducted with TDF.[52] TDF has been used to diagnose delayed cerebral ischemia in patients with SAH. Thermal diffusion therapy allows the quantitative measurement of regional CBF, which is considered an important upstream monitoring parameter indicative of tissue viability.[63] With this method, a thermal diffusion regional CBF microprobe is placed 20 to 25 mm below the cortical surface via a small burr hole and is secured by tightening a metal bolt. When the microprobe is in place, the nurse attaches it to an umbilical cord and monitor to begin calibration.[63] The microprobe includes a heated distal thermistor and a proximal thermistor. The distal thermistor measures blood flow via heat transfer to the capillaries. A microprocessor then converts this information into a measure of CBF in milliliters per 100 g per minute, which is represented as the K-value on the monitor. As a general rule, mean thermal diffusion regional CBF values range from 18 to 25 mL/100 g per minute.[63]

It is important to consider that CBF values measured by thermal diffusion regional CBF vary, depending on the placement of the probe.[63] Another important consideration with the use of TDF is that the monitor provides CBF parameters only within a temperature range of 25°C to 39.5°C.[63] Therefore patient cooling should be considered if the temperature of the brain is greater than 38.5°C.[63] Other considerations with the use of TDF are that the probe can be viewed on CT or with radiography and is not compatible with MRI. Also, because the TDF monitor does not run on battery power, the probe must be disconnected from the umbilical cord and secured to the patient's head dressing before patient transport. Additionally, if the probe is used in conjunction with a microdialysis catheter, the two catheters must be separated by 2 mm for accurate results.[63]

Laser Doppler Flowmetry

LDF provides continuous measurement of red blood cell velocity in the cerebral capillaries to determine cortical CBF.[52] The laser diffusion flowmetry probe may be inserted into the brain parenchyma or placed on the cerebral cortex.[52] In contrast to TDF, laser diffusion flowmetry does not quantify CBF absolutely but provides a measure of relative change in flow in a small brain volume of 1 to 2 mm³.[52] LDF has been used intraoperatively and in severe TBI and aneurysmal SAH vasospasm.[52]

Cerebral Oxygenation and Metabolic Monitoring

Maintenance of adequate brain tissue oxygenation and key brain energy substrates is a critical objective in the management of critically ill patients with neurologic disorders. The following methods may be used in the critical care unit to monitor the patient's cerebral oxygenation status and cerebral metabolic state.

Brain Tissue Oxygen Pressure

Monitoring brain parenchymal oxygen tension ($Pbto_2$) has been shown to be a reliable and sensitive diagnostic method to monitor cerebral oxygenation. $Pbto_2$ uses a device similar to pulse oximetry that allows continuous monitoring of regional tissue oxygenation and, in particular, areas of high ischemic risk.[50,52,64] The device consists of a monitoring probe on the end of a catheter, which is inserted into the brain parenchyma and attached to a bedside monitor (Fig. 22.19). The probe may be inserted into the damaged portion of the brain to measure regional oxygenation or inserted into the undamaged portion of the brain to measure global oxygenation. Placement of the

— Catheter

FIG. 22.19 LICOX Monitor. The LICOX brain tissue oxygen system involves a catheter inserted through an intracranial bolt. The system measures oxygen in the brain, brain tissue temperature, and intracranial pressure. (Modified from Lewis SL, et al. *Medical-Surgical Nursing: Assessment and Management of Clinical Problems*. 9th ed. St. Louis: Elsevier; 2014.)

catheter itself causes some microtrauma, and values obtained in that area may not be valid from 30 minutes up to 2 hours after placement.[52]

Normal $Pbto_2$ is 23 to 35 mm Hg.[51] A $Pbto_2$ threshold of less than 20 mm Hg represents compromised brain oxygen and is a threshold at which to consider intervention. $Pbto_2$ monitoring is safe and provides accurate data for up to 10 days with measured responses to interventions (eg, changes in CPP, ventilator targets, pharmacologic sedation, and transfusion) and can be used to guide therapy.[51] Observational studies suggest a potential benefit when $Pbto_2$-guided therapy is added to a management protocol for severe TBI.[51] However, it is recommended that brain oxygen monitors be used with clinical indicators and other monitoring modalities for accurate prognostication.[51]

Retrograde Jugular Bulb Oxygen Saturation

Oxygen levels in the cerebral venous outflow may inversely correlate with global brain oxygen consumption.[50] Therefore oxygen saturation in the jugular bulb ($Sjvo_2$) may be used for indirect estimation of cerebral oxygen consumption.[50]

To measure $Sjvo_2$, a fiberoptic catheter is placed retrograde through the internal jugular vein into the jugular bulb and attached to a bedside monitor.[64] Normal $Sjvo_2$ is 55% to 70%.[52] $Sjvo_2$ of less than 50% represents global cerebral ischemia, and $Sjvo_2$ of greater than 75% represents an absolute or relative global hyperemia that exceeds the brain's metabolic demand. Both $Sjvo_2$ less than 50% and $Sjvo_2$ greater than 75% have been associated with unfavorable outcomes.[52] Indications for $Sjvo_2$ monitoring include risk for global hypoxia, severe TBI, and aneurysmal SAH.[52]

A limitation of $Sjvo_2$ monitoring is that $Sjvo_2$ readings are affected by the position and movement of the patient's head.[65] Inaccuracies with $Sjvo_2$ monitoring can also occur with catheter misplacement, contamination with extracerebral blood when the catheter abuts the blood vessel wall, or thrombosis occurring around the catheter tip.[51]

Near-Infrared Spectroscopy

Brain oxygenation also can be assessed using transcranial near-infrared spectroscopy (NIRS).[52] A noninvasive monitor of cerebral oxygenation, NIRS quantifies the relative concentrations of oxygenated and deoxygenated hemoglobin through reliance on the transmission and absorption of near-infrared light as it passes through tissue.[49,66] NIRS has many potential advantages over other monitoring techniques: It is a noninvasive technique, has high temporal and spatial resolution, and provides simultaneous measurements over multiple regions of interest.[49] However, no studies demonstrate that data from NIRS use alone can influence outcomes in adult neurocritical care.[51]

Cerebral Microdialysis

Cerebral microdialysis is a neuromonitoring method that measures the concentration of chemicals found in the brain parenchyma, with the goal of detecting neurochemical changes indicative of primary and secondary brain injury.[34] It is used as a bedside monitor to detect impending cerebral ischemia-hypoxia and assess the bioenergetic state of the injured human brain by measuring key brain energy substrates (glucose) and metabolites (lactate and pyruvate).[49]

Cerebral microdialysis involves placement of a small catheter into the brain parenchyma, either during surgery or through a burr hole, which is secured by a cranial bolt. This microdialysis catheter has a 10-mm semipermeable distal membrane.[63] When fluid isotonic to the tissue interstitium is pumped into the catheter, the catheter acts like an artificial blood capillary. It is through diffusion that the metabolic markers glucose, pyruvate, lactate, glutamate, and glycerol are collected from the interstitial fluid and analyzed hourly.[34] Lactate and pyruvate are ischemic metabolites, and the ratio of lactate to pyruvate is currently the best early biomarker of secondary ischemic injury.[63] A lactate-to-pyruvate ratio greater than 40 is indicative of cerebral metabolic crisis.[67] Glycerol, a marker of cell membrane damage, and glutamate, an excitatory amino acid, provide additional evidence of developing brain injury.[68] Monitoring cerebral microdialysis is recommended in patients with or at risk for cerebral ischemia, hypoxia, energy failure, and glucose deprivation.[51]

Continuous Electroencephalography Monitoring

Continuous EEG provides dynamic information about brain function, permitting early detection of changes in neurologic status.[67] This is especially useful when the clinical examination is limited. The primary reason for EEG in the intensive care unit is to detect nonconvulsive status epilepticus.[50] Recurrent seizures may aggravate brain injury; seizures in patients with ICH are associated with ICP surges and midline shifts, which underscore the importance of early detection and management of seizures using continuous EEG monitoring.[50] In 10% to 20% of comatose patients with poor-grade SAH, nonconvulsive seizures may be detected on continuous EEG.[69] Continuous EEG should be considered in patients with poor-grade SAH who fail to improve or who have neurologic deterioration of undetermined etiology.[69] The drawbacks to the use of continuous EEG are that it is an expensive, labor-intensive program that requires expertise for interpretation and is subject to artifact from the intensive care unit environment.[70,71]

▌ S U M M A R Y

History

- A neurologic history includes information about clinical manifestations, associated complaints, precipitating factors, progression of symptoms, familial occurrences, and events preceding the onset of symptoms.
- If the patient's condition permits, additional information is gathered regarding the patient's personal and social status, general health status, and family history.

Focused Clinical Assessment

- The five major components of a neurologic examination are evaluation of (1) level of consciousness, (2) motor function, (3) pupillary function, (4) respiratory function, and (5) vital signs.
- Assessment of the level of consciousness focuses on evaluation of arousal and appraisal of awareness.
- Assessment of motor function focuses on evaluation of muscle size and tone and estimation of muscle strength.
- Assessment of pupillary function focuses on estimation of pupil size and shape, evaluation of pupillary reaction to light, and appraisal of eye movements.
- Assessment of respiratory functions focuses on observation of respiratory pattern and evaluation of airway status.
- Assessment of vital signs focuses on evaluation of blood pressure and observation of heart rate.
- Increasing ICP can be identified by changes in the level of consciousness, pupillary reaction, motor response, vital signs, and respiratory patterns.

Diagnostic Procedures

- Radiologic procedures are often performed to identify abnormalities of the brain, spinal cord, and surrounding bone and tissue. These tests include skull and spine radiography, CT, MRI, cerebral angiography, and myelography.
- Imaging of CBF and metabolism can help to define the cause and extent of brain injury, identify appropriate treatments, and predict the outcome. These tests include perfusion CT, xenon CT, perfusion MRI, carotid duplex sonography, PET, and SPECT.
- Electrophysiology studies are often performed to evaluate the electrical impulses of the brain. These tests include EEG, VERs, BAERs, SSERs, and MEPs.

Laboratory Studies

- CSF analysis is performed (by lumbar puncture or ventriculostomy) to look for the presence of blood or infection in the subarachnoid space.

Multimodal Monitoring

- ICP monitoring is used in patients with suspected intracranial hypertension. Measurement of ICP allows for an estimation of CPP, which is the blood pressure gradient across the brain. ICP and CPP monitoring are recommended as a part of protocol-driven care and should be used in conjunction with other intracranial monitors to guide medical and surgical interventions and detect life-threatening imminent herniation.
- CBF monitoring plays an important role in neurologic care because the brain depends on continuous blood flow to supply glucose and oxygen. TCD, TCCS, TDF, and LDF are techniques to monitor CBF.

- Measurements of brain oxygenation and metabolism provide insight into understanding acute brain injury and ways to manage secondary brain injury. Techniques to monitor brain oxygenation, metabolism, or both include $Pbto_2$, $Sjvo_2$, NIRS, and cerebral microdialysis.
- Continuous EEG is used to detect nonconvulsive seizures.
- Ⓔ Visit the Evolve site for additional study materials.

REFERENCES

1. McGlinsey A, Kirk A: Neurological assessment: early identification of neurological deterioration is vital to preventing secondary brain injury. Available at http://nursing.advanceweb.com/Continuing-Education/CE-Articles/Neurological-Assessment.aspx Accessed November 2, 2015.
2. Daroff RB, et al.: Diagnosis of neurological disease. In Daroff RB, et al.: *Bradley's Neurology in Clinical Practice*, ed 7, Philadelphia, 2016, Elsevier.
3. Barker E: The neurologic assessment. In Barker E, editor: *Neuroscience Nursing: A Spectrum of Care*, ed 3, St. Louis, 2008, Mosby.
4. Bader MK, Littlejohns LR: *AANN Core Curriculum for Neuroscience Nursing*, ed 5, Glenview, IL, 2010, American Association of Neuroscience Nurses.
5. Koita J, et al.: The mental status examination in emergency practice, *Emerg Med Clin North Am* 28(3):439–451, 2010.
6. Restrepro RD, Cohen Z: Neurologic assessment. In Heuer AJ, Scanlan CL, editors: *Wilkin's Clinical Assessment in Respiratory Care*, ed 7, St. Louis, 2014, Elsevier.
7. Teasdale G, Jennett W: Assessment of coma and impaired consciousness—a practical scale, *Lancet* 2(7872):81–84, 1974.
8. Green SM: Cheerio, laddie! Bidding farewell to the Glasgow Coma Scale, *Ann Emerg Med* 58(5):427–430, 2011.
9. Kornbluth J, Bhardwaj A: Evaluation of coma: a critical appraisal of popular scoring systems, *Neurocrit Care* 14(1):134–143, 2011.
10. Berger JR: Stupor and coma. In Daroff RB, et al, editors: *Bradley's Neurology in Clinical Practice*, ed 7, Philadelphia, 2016, Elsevier.
11. Jalali R, Rezaei M: A comparison of the Glasgow Coma Scale Score with Full Outline of Unresponsiveness Scale to predict patients' traumatic brain injury outcomes in intensive care units, *Crit Care Res Pract* 289803:2014, 2014.
12. Kramer AA, et al.: A multicenter prospective study of interobserver agreement using the Full Outline of Unresponsiveness score coma scale in the intensive care unit, *Crit Care Med* 40(9):2671–2676, 2012.
13. Ball JW, et al.: *Seidel's Guide to Physical Examination*, ed 8, St. Louis, 2015, Mosby.
14. McGee S: *Evidence-Based Physical Diagnosis*, ed 3, Philadelphia, 2012, Saunders.
15. Thurtell MJ, Rucker JC: Pupillary and eyelid abnormalities. In Daroff RB, et al, editors: *Bradley's Neurology in Clinical Practice*, ed 7, Philadelphia, 2016, Elsevier.
16. Adoni A, McNett M: The pupillary response in traumatic brain injury: a guide for trauma nurses, *J Trauma Nurs* 14(4):191–196, 2007.
17. Bishop BS: Pathologic papillary signs: self-learning module. Part II, *Crit Care Nurs* 11(7):58–67, 1991.
18. Haddad SH, Arabi YM: Critical care management of severe traumatic brain injury in adults, *Scand J Trauma Resusc Emerg Med* 20:12, 2012.
19. Saiki RL: Current and evolving management of traumatic brain injury, *Crit Care Nurs Clin North Am* 21(4):549–559, 2009.
20. Samuels MA: The brain-heart connection, *Circulation* 116(1):77–84, 2007.
21. Yuh EL, Dillon WP: Intracranial hypotension and intracranial hypertension, *Neuroimaging Clin N Am* 20(4):597–617, 2010.
22. Van Thielen T, et al.: Imaging techniques and anatomy. In Adam A, et al, editors: *Grainger & Allison's Diagnostic Radiology: A Textbook of Medical Imaging*, ed 6, London, 2015, Elsevier Churchill Livingstone.
23. Chernecky CC, Berger BJ: *Laboratory Tests and Diagnostic Procedures*, ed 6, St. Louis, 2013, Elsevier.
24. Cogbill TH, Ziegelbein KJ: Computed tomography, magnetic resonance, and ultrasound imaging: basic principles, glossary of terms, and patient safety, *Surg Clin North Am* 91(1):1–14, 2011.

25. Ajtai B, et al.: Structural imaging using magnetic resonance imaging and computed tomography. In Daroff RB, et al, editors: *Bradley's Neurology in Clinical Practice*, ed 7, Philadelphia, 2016, Elsevier.

26. Crownover BK, Bepko JL: Appropriate and safe use of diagnostic imaging, *Am Fam Physician* 87(7):494–501, 2013.

27. Patkar D, et al.: New advances in MRI, *JIMSA* 26(1):59–64, 2013.

28. McInnis LA, et al.: Angiography: from a patient's perspective, *Crit Care Nurs Clin North Am* 22(1):51–60, 2010.

29. Ahn SS, Kim YD: Three-dimensional digital subtraction angiographic evaluation of aneurysm remnants after clip placement, *J Korean Neurosurg Soc* 47(3):185–190, 2010.

30. National Imaging Associates: NIA Standard Clinical Guidelines. Available at http://www.niahealthcare.com/media/629554/2014-nia-standard-clinical-guidelines.pdf. 2014 Accessed on December 11, 2015.

31. Griffin N, Grant LA: The spine. In Grant LA, Griffin N, editors: *Grainger & Allison's Diagnostic Radiology Essentials*, London, 2013, Churchill Livingstone.

32. Kim N, et al.: Noninvasive measurement of cerebral blood flow and blood oxygenation using near-infrared and diffuse correlation spectroscopies in critically brain-injured adults, *Neurocrit Care* 12(2):173–180, 2010.

33. Noble K: Traumatic brain injury and increased intracranial pressure, *J Perianesth Nurs* 25(4):242–248, 2010.

34. Barazangi N, Hemphill JC: Advanced cerebral monitoring in neurocritical care, *Neurol India* 56(4):405–414, 2008.

35. Jain V, et al.: MRI estimation of global brain oxygen consumption rate, *J Cereb Blood Flow Metab* 30(9):1598–1607, 2010.

36. Wintermark M, et al.: Cerebral perfusion CT: technique and clinical applications, *J Neuroradiol* 35(5):253–260, 2008.

37. Carlson AP, et al.: Xenon-enhanced cerebral blood flow at 28% xenon provides uniquely safe access to quantitative, clinically useful cerebral blood flow information: a multicenter study, *AJNR Am J Neuroradiol* 32(7):1315–1320, 2011.

38. Van Boven RW, et al.: Advances in neuroimaging of traumatic brain injury and posttraumatic stress disorder, *J Rehabil Res Dev* 46(6):717–757, 2009.

39. Hoa D: Brain perfusion imaging. Available at https://www.imaios.com/en/e-Courses/e-MRI/Cerebral-perfusion-imaging Accessed December 11, 2015.

40. Adamczyk P, Liebeskind DS: Vascular imaging: computed tomographic angiography, magnetic resonance angiography, and ultrasound. In Daroff RB, et al, editors: *Bradley's Neurology in Clinical Practice*, ed 7, Philadelphia, 2016, Elsevier.

41. Miletich RS: Positron emission tomography for neurologists, *Neurol Clin* 27(1):61–88, 2009.

42. Meyer PT, et al.: Functional neuroimaging: functional magnetic resonance imaging, positron emission tomography, and single-photon emission computed tomography. In Daroff RB, et al, editors: *Bradley's Neurology in Clinical Practice*, ed 7, Philadelphia, 2016, Elsevier.

43. Zukotynski K, et al.: Central nervous system. In Christain PE, Waterstram-Rich KM, editors: *Nuclear Medicine and PET/CT: Technology and Techniques*, ed 7, St. Louis, 2012, Elsevier.

44. Hahn CD, Emercon RG: Electroencephalography and evoked potentials. In Daroff RB, et al, editors: *Bradley's Neurology in Clinical Practice*, ed 7, Philadelphia, 2016, Elsevier.

45. Andraus ME, Alves-Leon SV: Non-epileptiform EEG abnormalities: an overview, *Arq Neuropsiquiatr* 69(5):829–835, 2011.

46. Welch H, Hasbun R: Lumbar puncture and cerebrospinal fluid analysis, *Handb Clin Neurol* 96:31–49, 2010.

47. Sladky JH, Piwinski SE: Lumbar puncture technique and lumbar drains, *Atlas Oral Maxillofac Surg Clin North Am* 23(2):169–176, 2015.

48. Euerle BD: Spinal puncture and cerebrospinal fluid examination. In Roberts JR, Hedges JR, editors: *Roberts and Hedges' Clinical Procedures in Emergency Medicine*, ed 6, Philadelphia, 2014, Saunders.

49. Kirkman MA, Smith M: Intracranial pressure monitoring, cerebral perfusion pressure estimation, and ICP/CPP-guided therapy: a standard of care or optional extra after brain injury? *Br J Anaesth* 112(1):35–46, 2014.

50. Ko SB: Multimodality monitoring in the neurointensive care unit: a special perspective for patients with stroke, *J Stroke* 15(2):99–108, 2013.

51. Le Roux P, et al.: Consensus summary statement of the International Multidisciplinary Consensus Conference on Multimodality Monitoring in Neurocritical Care: a statement for healthcare professionals from the Neurocritical Care Society and the European Society of Intensive Care Medicine, *Neurocrit Care* 21(Suppl 2):S1–S26, 2014.

52. Blisset PA: Hemodynamic and intracranial monitoring in neurocritical care. In Lough ME, editor: *Hemodynamic Monitoring: Evolving Technologies and Clinical Practice*, St. Louis, 2016, Elsevier.

53. Raboel PH, Barteck J: Intracranial pressure monitoring: invasive versus on-invasive methods—a review, *Crit Care Res Pract* 950393:2012, 2012.

54. Tan KT, Ming HC: Options for managing raised intracranial pressure, *Proceedings of Singapore Healthcare* 24(3):156–164, 2015.

55. Slazinski T: Combination intraventricular/fiberoptic catheter insertion (assist), monitoring, nursing care, troubleshooting, and removal. In Wiegand DLM, editor: *AACN Procedure Manual for Critical Care*, ed 6, St. Louis, 2011, Saunders.

56. Slazinski T: Intracranial bolt and fiberoptic catheter insertion (assist), intracranial pressure monitoring, care, troubleshooting, and removal. In Wiegand DLM, editor: *AACN Procedure Manual for Critical Care*, ed 6, St. Louis, 2011, Saunders.

57. American Association of Neuroscience Nurses: *AANN Clinical Practice Guideline Series. Guide to the Care of the Patient Undergoing Intracranial Pressure Monitoring/External Ventricular Drainage or Lumbar Drainage*, Glenview, IL, 2011, The Association.

58. Chen JW, et al.: Pupillary reactivity as an early indicator of increased intracranial pressure: the introduction of the Neurological Pupil Index, *Surg Neurol Int* 2:82, 2011.

59. Brain Trauma Foundation, American Association of Neurological Surgeons, Congress of Neurological Surgeons, et al.: Guidelines for the management of severe traumatic brain injury. VII. Intracranial pressure monitoring, *J Neurotrauma* 24(Suppl 1):S45–S54, 2007.

60. Brain Trauma Foundation, American Association of Neurological Surgeons, Congress of Neurological Surgeons, et al.: Guidelines for the management of severe traumatic brain injury. IX. Cerebral perfusion thresholds, *J Neurotrauma* 24(Suppl 1):S59–S64, 2007.

61. Bouzat P, et al.: Transcranial Doppler after traumatic brain injury: is there a role? *Curr Opin Crit Care* 20(2):153–160, 2014.

62. Marshall SA, Nyguist P, Ziai WC: The role of transcranial Doppler ultrasonography in the diagnosis and management of vasospasm after aneurysmal subarachnoid hemorrhage, *Neurosurg Clin N Am* 21(2):291–303, 2010.

63. Cecil S, et al.: Traumatic brain injury: advanced multimodal neuromonitoring from theory to practice, *Crit Care Nurse* 31(2):25–36, 2011.

64. Bader MK: Recognizing and treating ischemic insults to the brain: the role of brain tissue oxygen monitoring, *Crit Care Nurs Clin North Am* 18(2):243–256, 2006.

65. Slazinski T: Jugular venous oxygen saturation monitoring: insertion (assist), patient care, troubleshooting, and removal. In Wiegand DLM, editor: *AACN Procedure Manual for Critical Care*, ed 6, St. Louis, 2011, Saunders.

66. Murkin JM, Arango M: Near-infrared spectroscopy as an index of brain and tissue oxygenation, *Br J Anesth* 103(suppl 1):i3–i13, 2009.

67. Vulliemoz S, et al.: Imaging compatible electrodes for continuous electroencephalogram monitoring in the intensive care unit, *J Clin Neurophysiol* 26(4):236–243, 2009.

68. Hemphill JC, et al.: Multimodal monitoring and neurocritical care bioinformatics, *Nat Rev Neurol* 7(8):451–460, 2011.

69. Diringer MN, et al.: Critical care management of patients following aneurysmal subarachnoid hemorrhage: recommendations from the Neurocritical Care Society's multidisciplinary consensus conference, *Neurocrit Care* 15(2):211–240, 2011.

70. Young GB: Continuous EEG monitoring in the ICU: challenges and opportunities, *Can J Neurol Sci* 36(Suppl 2):S89–S91, 2009.

71. Wijdicks E, Rabinstein AA: Critical care neurology: five new things, *Neurol Clin Pract* 1(1):34–40, 2011.

23

Neurologic Disorders and Therapeutic Management

Lourdes Januszewicz

To accurately anticipate and plan nursing interventions for patients with neurologic disorders, the critical care nurse must have an understanding of the disease pathology, determine the areas of focused assessment, and be well acquainted with the medical management of the patient. Despite a wide array of neurologic disorders, only a few disorders routinely require care in the critical care environment.

STROKE

Stroke is a descriptive term for the sudden onset of acute neurologic deficit persisting for more than 24 hours and caused by the interruption of blood flow to the brain. Stroke is the fourth leading cause of death in the United States, preceded by heart disease, cancer, and chronic respiratory disease. Each year, approximately 795,000 people have a stroke; 610,000 of strokes annually are first attacks, and 185,000 are recurrent attacks.[1]

Strokes are classified as ischemic and hemorrhagic (Fig. 23.1). Hemorrhagic strokes can be further categorized as subarachnoid hemorrhages (SAHs) and intracerebral hemorrhages (ICHs). Approximately 87% of all strokes are ischemic, 10% are ICHs, and 3% are SAHs.[1] Although less common, hemorrhagic strokes (ICHs and SAHs) have a higher mortality rate compared with ischemic strokes. Approximately 8% to 12% of ischemic strokes and 37% to 38% of hemorrhagic strokes result in death within 30 days.[1] In 2012, the annual cost for care and loss of productivity was estimated to be $71.6 billion.[1]

The national concern for the incidence and effects of stroke is illustrated by the inclusion of emergent stroke care in the American Heart Association guidelines for basic and advanced life support. Major public education programs, stroke appraisal screening programs, development of stroke centers, and algorithms for stroke management are based on the success that these same approaches have had with coronary artery disease.

Ischemic Stroke
Description
Ischemic stroke results from interruption of blood flow to the brain and accounts for 88% of all strokes.[2] The interruption can be the result of a thrombotic or embolic event. Thrombosis can form in large vessels (large-vessel thrombotic strokes) or small vessels (small-vessel thrombotic strokes). Embolic sources include the heart (cardioembolic strokes) and atherosclerotic plaques in larger vessels (atheroembolic strokes). In 25% of the cases, the underlying cause of the stroke is unknown (cryptogenic strokes).[3]

Strokes are preventable. Most thrombotic strokes are the result of the accumulation of atherosclerotic plaque in the vessel lumen, especially at the bifurcations or curves of the vessel. The pathogenesis of cerebrovascular disease is identical to the pathogenesis of coronary vasculature. The greatest risk factor for ischemic stroke is hypertension.[2] Other risk factors are dyslipidemia, diabetes, smoking, and carotid atherosclerotic disease.[1,4] Common sites of atherosclerotic plaque are the bifurcation of the common carotid artery, the origins of the middle and anterior cerebral arteries, and the origins of the vertebral arteries.[2] Ischemic strokes resulting from vertebral artery dissection have been reported after chiropractic manipulation of the cervical spine.[4]

Etiology
An embolic stroke occurs when an embolus from the heart or lower circulation travels distally and lodges in a small vessel, obstructing the blood supply. At least 20% of ischemic strokes are attributed to a cardioembolic phenomenon.[2] The most common cause of cardiac emboli is atrial fibrillation. It is responsible for approximately 50% of all cardiac emboli.[5] Other sources of cardiac emboli are from mitral stenosis, mechanical valves, atrial myxoma, endocarditis, and recent myocardial infarction.[2] Researchers hypothesize that a patent foramen ovale or atrial septal aneurysms may be the cause of cryptogenic stroke.[3]

Pathophysiology
Ischemic stroke is a cerebral hemodynamic insult. When cerebral blood flow (CBF) is reduced to a level insufficient to maintain neuronal viability, ischemic injury occurs. In focal stroke, an area of hypoperfused tissue, the ischemic penumbra, surrounds a core of ischemic cells. The ischemic penumbra can be salvaged with return of blood flow. However, sustained anoxic insult initiates a chain of biochemical events leading to apoptosis, or cellular death.[6]

The phenomenon of a focal ischemic stroke is identical to myocardial infarction, which is why the term *brain attack* is used in public education strategies. Often, a history of transient ischemic attacks, brief episodes of neurologic symptoms that last less than 24 hours, offers a warning that stroke is likely to occur. Sudden onset indicates embolism as the final insult to flow.[2] The size of the stroke depends on the size and location of the occluded vessel and the availability of collateral blood flow.

COLLABORATIVE CARE INTERVENTIONS

Patient Education Priorities

- Pathophysiology of disease & specific cause.
- Risk factor modification.
- Importance of taking medications.
- Activities of daily living.
- Measures to prevent injuries of impaired limbs.
- Measures to compensate for residual deficits.
- Basic rehabilitation techniques.
- Participating in rehab program or support group.

Treatment with rtPA • *Monitor for Bleeding

- Start treatment within 4.5 hours of the onset.
- Dosage -0.9 mg/kg total, 10% given as IV bolus, followed by continuous IV infusion over 1 hr.
- No anticoagulants during the first 24 hours.
- R/O contraindications: head trauma, prior stroke, recent MI or major surgery, active bleeding or recent noncompressible arterial puncture.
- Systolic BP < 185 mm Hg & diastolic < 110 mm Hg.
- INR 1.7 or < aPTT must be WNL.
- Platelet count at least 100 000 mm³.
- Blood glucose > 40 mg/dL or < 400 mg/dL.
- No seizure with postictal residual impairments.
- No multilobar infarction.

NURSING INTERVENTIONS

Early recognition of neurologic or hemodynamic deterioration

- Perform frequent neurologic assessments.
- Early recognition of neuro & hemodynamic deterioration: closely monitor VS, pulse ox, monitor & treat seizure activity.
- BP control with IV labetalol or nicardipine.
- Protect patient's airway; provide ventilatory assistance, as required.
- Maintain surveillance for complications: cerebral edema, hemorrhage, seizures, impaired swallowing, aspiration, DVD, PE pressure ulcers, neurologic deficits.
- Provide comfort and emotional support.
- Develop an appropriate rehab program.

George Hammond suffers an ischemic stroke from a cardioembolic episode of atrial fibrillation.

Ischemic Stroke

Results in

Acute Neurological Deficit
↓ Cerebral Perfusion

Early identification → treat symptoms early → ↓ mortality.

GOALS OF MEDICAL MANAGEMENT

- Identify and treat the underlying cause.
- Dissolve the clot and reperfuse the ischemic brain.
- Reverse or minimize the effects of stroke.
- Prevent complications.

The patient will demonstrate adequate cerebral perfusion by

- Maintaining vital functions and develop no further neurologic deterioration.
- Maintaining airway and acceptable ABGs.
- Preserving physiologic body functions.

PATIENT OUTCOMES

HISTORY AND PHYSICAL

Risk Factors

Atrial Fibrillation • Hypertension • Dyslipidemia
Diabetes • Smoking • Carotid Artery Disease

Pathophysiology – Cerebral Hemodynamic Insult

Acute neurologic deficit for > 24 hours caused by interruption of cerebral blood flow as a result of a thrombotic or embolic event. Cerebral edema, secondary hemorrhage, and seizures are the major acute complications of ischemic stroke.

Assessment & Diagnosis

- Focal neuro signs persisting > 24 hours.
- Hemiparesis, aphasia, & hemianopia.
- Stupor, coma, confusion, & agitation.
- Seizures can occur within 24 hours of insult.

Assess for Signs of ↑ ICP

- Assess for signs of ↑ ICP: ↓ LOC, Cushing triad, papilledema, posturing, pupil changes, projectile vomiting, altered breathing patterns, & headache.

PRIORITY NURSING DIAGNOSES

- Risk for Ineffective Cerebral Tissue Perfusion.
- Unilateral Neglect, related to perceptual disruption.
- Impaired Verbal Communication R/T cerebral speech center injury.
- Impaired Swallowing R/T neuromuscular impairment, fatigue, and limited awareness.
- Anxiety R/T threat to biologic, psychologic, or social integrity.
- Deficient Knowledge: Discharge Regimen R/T lack of previous exposure to information.

FIG. 23.1 Concept Map for Stroke. *aPTT,* activated partial thromboplastin time; *ICP,* intracranial pressure; *INR,* international normalized ratio; *LOC,* loss of consciousness; *Pulse ox,* pulse oximetry; *R/T,* related to; *rtPA,* recombinant tissue plasminogen activator; *R/O,* rule out; *VS,* vital signs; *WNL,* within normal limits. (Concept maps illustration created by © DEANNE A. BLACH, MSN, RN.)

Global ischemia results when severe hypotension or cardiopulmonary arrest provokes a transient decrease in blood flow to all areas of the brain.[6]

Cerebral edema sufficient to produce clinical deterioration develops in 10% to 20% of patients with ischemic stroke and can result in intracranial hypertension. The edema results from a loss of normal metabolic function of the cells and peaks at 4 days.[2] This process is commonly the cause of death during the first week after a stroke.[7] Secondary hemorrhage at the site of the stroke lesion, known as *hemorrhagic conversion*, and seizures are the two other major acute neurologic complications of ischemic stroke.[7,8]

Assessment and Diagnosis

The characteristic sign of an ischemic stroke is the sudden onset of focal neurologic signs persisting for more than 24 hours.[2] These signs usually occur in combination. Box 23.1 lists common patterns of neurologic symptoms associated with an ischemic stroke. Hemiparesis, aphasia, and hemianopia are common. Changes in the level of consciousness (LOC) usually occur only with brainstem or cerebellar involvement, seizure, hypoxia, hemorrhage, or elevated intracranial pressure (ICP). These changes may be exhibited as stupor, coma, confusion, and agitation.[9] The reported frequency of seizures in patients with ischemic stroke is approximately 11%. If seizures occur, they are usually seen within 24 hours of an insult.[8]

The National Institutes of Health Stroke Scale (NIHSS) is often used as the basis of the focused neurologic examination.[10] The score ranges from 0 to 42 points; the higher the score, the more neurologically impaired the patient is. A change of four points on the scale indicates significant neurologic change. The components of the NIHSS include LOC; LOC questions; LOC commands; gaze; visual fields; face, arm, and leg strength; sensation; limb ataxia; and language function. A copy of the NIHSS with complete instructions is available at http://www.ninds.nih.gov/disorders/stroke/strokescales.htm.

Confirmation of the diagnosis of ischemic stroke is the first step in the emergent evaluation of these patients. Differentiation from intracranial hemorrhage is vital. In most instances, noncontrast computed tomography (CT) scanning is the method of choice for this purpose, and it is considered the most important initial diagnostic study. In addition to excluding intracranial hemorrhage, CT can assist in identifying early neurologic complications and the cause of the insult. Magnetic resonance imaging (MRI) can demonstrate infarction of cerebral tissue earlier than CT and is an appropriate alternative to a noncontrast CT scan for excluding intercereberal hemorrhage.[10]

Because of the strong correlation between acute ischemic stroke and heart disease, 12-lead electrocardiography and continuous cardiac monitoring are suggested to detect a cardiac cause or coexisting condition. A chest radiograph is obtained if lung disease is suspected. However, obtaining these studies should not delay the administration of fibrinolysis.[10] Echocardiography is valuable in identifying a cardioembolic phenomenon when a sufficient index of suspicion warrants its use.[2] Laboratory studies to evaluate hematologic and renal function, coagulation, electrolyte and glucose levels, and troponin are also recommended. Arterial blood gas analysis is performed if hypoxia is suspected. A lumbar puncture may be performed if a SAH is suspected and the CT scan is normal.[10]

Medical Management

Rapid diagnosis of stroke and initiation of treatment are important to maximize recovery, prevent recurrence of stroke, and prevent complications. Fibrinolytic therapy with intravenous recombinant tissue plasminogen activator (rtPA) is recommended within 3 hours of onset of ischemic stroke to facilitate dissolution of the clot.[11] Inclusion and exclusion criteria for patients who should be considered for fibrinolysis are listed in Box 23.2. The time frame for rtPA has been extended to 4.5 hours with some additional exclusions including patients older than 80 years of age, patients taking oral anticoagulants, patients with a baseline NIHSS score greater than 25, patients with evidence of ischemic injury involving more than one-third of the middle cerebral artery territory, and patients with a history of both stroke and diabetes.[11] The diagnosis must be confirmed with CT scan before rtPA administration.[10] The recommended dosage of rtPA is 0.9 mg/kg up to a maximum dosage of 90 mg; 10% of the total dose is administered as an initial intravenous bolus, and the remaining 90% is administered by intravenous infusion over 60 minutes.[10,11]

The desired result of fibrinolytic therapy is to dissolve the clot and reperfuse the ischemic brain. The goal is to reverse or minimize the effects of stroke.[12] Bleeding, especially intracranial hemorrhage, is the major risk and complication of rtPA therapy. In contrast to fibrinolytic protocols for acute myocardial infarction, subsequent therapy with anticoagulant or antiplatelet agents is not recommended after rtPA administration in ischemic stroke. Patients receiving fibrinolytic therapy for stroke should not receive aspirin, heparin, warfarin, ticlopidine, or any other antithrombotic or antiplatelet medications for at least 24 hours after treatment.[10]

BOX 23.1   Neurologic Abnormalities in Acute Ischemic Strokes

Left (Dominant) Hemisphere
Aphasia; right hemiparesis; right-sided sensory loss; right visual field defect; poor right conjugate gaze; dysarthria; difficulty in reading, writing, or calculating

Right (Nondominant) Hemisphere
Neglect of left visual space, left visual field defect, left hemiparesis, left-sided sensory loss, poor left conjugate gaze, extinction of left-sided stimuli, dysarthria, spatial disorientation

Brainstem, Cerebellum, and Posterior Hemisphere
Motor or sensory loss in all four limbs, crossed signs, limb or gait ataxia, dysarthria, dysconjugate gaze, nystagmus, amnesia, bilateral visual field defects

Small Subcortical Hemisphere or Brainstem (Pure Motor Stroke)
Weakness of face and limbs on one side of body without abnormalities of higher brain function, sensation, or vision

Small Subcortical Hemisphere or Brainstem (Pure Sensory Stroke)
Decreased sensation of face and limbs on one side of body without abnormalities of higher brain function, motor function, or vision

From Adams HP, et al. Guidelines for the management of patients with acute ischemic stroke: a statement for healthcare professionals from a special writing group of the Stroke Council, American Heart Association. *Circulation*. 1994;90(3):1588–1601.

BOX 23.2 Inclusion and Exclusion Characteristics of Patients With Ischemic Stroke Who Could Be Treated With Intravenous Recombinant Tissue Plasminogen Activator Within 3 Hours From Symptom Onset

Inclusion Criteria

- Diagnosis of ischemic stroke causing measurable neurologic deficit
- Onset of symptoms <3 h before beginning treatment
- Age ≥18 years

Exclusion Criteria

- Significant head trauma or prior stroke in previous 3 months
- Symptoms suggest subarachnoid hemorrhage
- Arterial puncture at noncompressible site in previous 7 days
- History of previous intracranial hemorrhage
- Intracranial neoplasm, arteriovenous malformation, or aneurysm
- Recent intracranial or intraspinal surgery
- Elevated blood pressure (systolic >185 mm Hg or diastolic >110 mm Hg)
- Active internal bleeding
- Acute bleeding diathesis, including but not limited to
  - Platelet count <100,000/mm^3
  - Heparin received within 48 h, resulting in abnormally elevated aPTT greater than upper limit of normal
  - Current use of anticoagulant with INR >1.7 or PT >15 s
  - Current use of direct thrombin inhibitors or direct factor Xa inhibitors with elevated sensitive laboratory tests (eg, aPTT, INR, platelet count, and ECT; TT; or appropriate factor Xa activity assays)
- Blood glucose concentration <50 mg/dL (2.7 mmol/L)
- CT demonstrates multilobar infarction (hypodensity greater than one-third cerebral hemisphere)

Relative Exclusion Criteria

More recent experience suggests that under some circumstances—with careful consideration and weighing of risk to benefit—patients may receive fibrinolytic therapy despite one or more relative contraindications. Consider risk to benefit of IV rtPA administration carefully if any of the following relative contraindications are present:

- Minor or rapidly improving stroke symptoms (clearing spontaneously)
- Pregnancy
- Seizure at onset with postictal residual neurologic impairments
- Major surgery or serious trauma within previous 14 days
- Recent gastrointestinal or urinary tract hemorrhage (within previous 21 days)
- Recent acute myocardial infarction (within previous 3 months)

Notes

1. The checklist includes some FDA-approved indications and contraindications for administration of IV rtPA for acute ischemic stroke. Recent guideline revisions have modified the original FDA-approved indications. A physician with expertise in acute stroke care may modify this list.
2. Onset time is defined as either the witnessed onset of symptoms or the time last known normal if symptom onset was not witnessed.
3. In patients without recent use of oral anticoagulants or heparin, treatment with IV rtPA can be initiated before availability of coagulation test results but should be discontinued if INR is >1.7 or PT is abnormally elevated by local laboratory standards.
4. In patients without history of thrombocytopenia, treatment with IV rtPA can be initiated before availability of platelet count but should be discontinued if platelet count is <100,000/mm^3.

aPTT, activated partial thromboplastin time; *CT,* computed tomography; *ECT,* ecarin clotting time; *FDA,* US Food and Drug Administration; *INR,* international normalized ratio; *IV,* intravenous; *PT,* partial thromboplastin time; *rtPA,* recombinant tissue plasminogen activator; *TT,* thrombin time. From Jauch EC, et al. Guidelines for the early management of patients with acute ischemic stroke. A guideline for healthcare professionals from the American Heart Association/American Stroke Association. *Stroke.* 2013; 44(3):870–947.

The major barriers to effective application of fibrinolytic therapy for ischemic stroke are prehospital and in-hospital delays.[12,13] To help decrease delays, the public needs to be educated about stroke symptoms and activation of the emergency medical system. Emergency medical system responders need adequate education and training on managing a patient with an acute ischemic stroke, focusing on stabilization and transport of the patient quickly to the emergency department. The receiving hospital should ideally have certification for primary stroke treatment and have expert staff and the infrastructure to care for a patient with complex stroke.[10]

Other emergent care of a patient with ischemic stroke must include airway protection and ventilatory assistance to maintain adequate tissue oxygenation.[10] Hypertension is often present in the early period as a compensatory response, and in most cases, blood pressure must not be lowered (Table 23.1). For patients who have not received fibrinolytic therapy, antihypertensive therapy is considered only if the diastolic blood pressure is greater than 120 mm Hg or the systolic blood pressure is greater than 220 mm Hg.[10] Criteria are different for patients who have received rtPA. Their blood pressure is maintained at less than 180/105 mm Hg to prevent intracranial hemorrhage. Intravenous labetalol or nicardipine is used to achieve blood pressure control. If these agents are ineffective, nitroprusside

should be considered.[10] Body temperature and glucose levels also must be normalized.[10]

Medical management also includes the identification and treatment of acute complications such as cerebral edema or seizure activity. Prophylaxis for these complications is not recommended. However, deep vein thrombosis (DVT) prophylaxis should be initiated to decrease the risk of pulmonary embolism. One study demonstrated that improved outcomes for patients with ischemic stroke can be achieved by managing swallowing issues, initiating DVT prophylaxis, and treating hypoxemia.[14] Surgical decompression is recommended if a large cerebellar infarction compresses the brainstem.[10]

Subarachnoid Hemorrhage
Description

SAH is bleeding into the subarachnoid space, which usually is caused by rupture of a cerebral aneurysm or arteriovenous malformation (AVM).[7] At the time of autopsy, approximately 4% of the population has been found to have one or more aneurysms.[13] With improvements in imaging techniques, an increased number of incidental intracranial aneurysms has been found. CT angiography and magnetic resonance angiography can detect 95% of all aneurysms. Among patients younger than 40 years, more men than women are likely to have SAHs, whereas among patients older than 40 years, more women have

TABLE 23.1 Blood Pressure Management for Stroke According to the American Stroke Association Guidelines

BP[a]	Treatment
Nonthrombolytic Candidates	
DBP >140 mm Hg	Sodium nitroprusside (0.5 mcg/kg/min); aim for 10%–20% reduction in DBP
SBP >220 mm Hg, DBP 121–140 mm Hg, or MAP[b] >130 mm Hg	10–20 mg of labetalol[c] given by IVP over 1–2 min; may repeat or double labetalol every 20 min to maximum dose of 300 mg
SBP <220 mm Hg, DBP = 120 mm Hg, or MAP[b] <130 mm Hg	Emergency antihypertensive therapy is deferred in the absence of aortic dissection, acute myocardial infarction, severe congestive heart failure, or hypertensive encephalopathy
Thrombolytic Candidates	
Pretreatment	
SBP >185 mm Hg or DBP >110 mm Hg	1–2 inches of nitroglycerin paste ("nitro paste") or 1–2 doses of 10–20 mg of labetalol[c] given by IVP; if BP is not reduced and maintained to <185/110 mm Hg, the patient should not be treated with tPA
During and After Treatment	
Monitor BP	BP is monitored every 15 min for 2 h, then every 30 min for 6 h, and then hourly for 16 h
DBP >140 mm Hg	Sodium nitroprusside (0.5 mcg/kg/min)
SBP >230 mm Hg or DBP 121–140 mm Hg	10 mg of labetalol[c] given by IVP over 1–2 min; may repeat or double labetalol every 10 min to a maximum dose of 300 mg or give initial labetalol bolus and then start a labetalol drip at 2–8 mg/min
	If BP not controlled by labetalol, consider sodium nitroprusside
SBP 180–230 mm Hg or DBP 105–120 mm Hg	10 mg of labetalol[c] given by IVP; may repeat or double labetalol every 10–20 min to a maximum dose of 300 mg or give initial labetalol bolus and then start a labetalol drip at 2–8 mg/min

BP, blood pressure; *DBP,* diastolic blood pressure; *IVP,* intravenous push; *MAP,* mean arterial pressure; *SBP,* systolic blood pressure; *tPA,* tissue-type plasminogen activator.

[a]All initial BPs should be verified before treatment by repeating reading in 5 minutes.

[b]As estimated by one-third of the sum of SBP and double DBP.

[c]Labetalol should be avoided in patients with asthma, cardiac failure, or severe abnormalities in cardiac conduction. For refractory hypertension, alternative therapy may be considered with sodium nitroprusside or enalapril.

From Bader MK, Littlejohns LR. *AANN Core Curriculum for Neuroscience Nursing.* 4th ed. St. Louis: Elsevier; 2004.

SAHs. Aneurysmal SAH is associated with a mortality rate of 25% to 50%, with most patients dying on the first day after the insult.[13] Hemorrhage from AVM rupture has a better chance of survival and is associated with an overall mortality rate of 10% to 15%.[14] Known risk factors for SAH include hypertension, smoking, and alcohol or stimulant use.[15]

Etiology

Cerebral aneurysm rupture accounts for approximately 85% of all cases of spontaneous SAH.[1] An aneurysm is an outpouching of the wall of a blood vessel that results from weakening of the wall of the vessel (Table 23.2).[13] Of aneurysms, 90% are congenital—the cause of which is unknown. The other 10% can be the result of traumatic injury (that stretches and tears the muscular middle layer of the arterial vessel) or infectious material (most often from infectious vegetation on valves of the left side of the heart after bacterial endocarditis) that lodges against a vessel wall and erodes the muscular layer, or they are of undetermined cause.[15] Multiple aneurysms occur in approximately 30% of cases and often are bilateral, occurring in the same location on both sides of the cerebral vascular system.[16]

AVM rupture is responsible for approximately 6% of all SAHs.[16] An AVM is a tangled mass of arterial and venous blood vessels that shunt blood directly from the arterial side into the venous side, bypassing the capillary system. AVMs may be small, focal lesions or large, diffuse lesions that occupy almost an entire hemisphere.[15] They are always congenital,

although the exact embryonic cause for these malformations is unknown. They also occur in the spinal cord and the renal, gastrointestinal, and integumentary systems.[16] Small, superficial AVMs are seen as port-wine stains of the skin. In contrast to SAH from an aneurysm in middle-aged patients, SAH from an AVM usually occurs in the second to fourth decades of life.[15,16]

Pathophysiology

The pathophysiologies of the two most common causes of SAH, cerebral aneurysm and AVM, are distinctly different.

Cerebral aneurysm. As an individual with a congenital cerebral aneurysm gets older, blood pressure increases, and more stress is placed on the poorly developed thin vessel wall. Ballooning of the vessel occurs, giving the aneurysm a berry-like appearance. Most cerebral aneurysms are saccular or berry-like, with a stem or neck. Aneurysms are usually small, are 2 to 7 mm in diameter, and often occur at the base of the brain on the circle of Willis.[14] Fig. 23.2 illustrates the usual distribution between the vessels. Most cerebral aneurysms occur at the bifurcation of blood vessels.[15,16]

The aneurysm becomes clinically significant when the vessel wall becomes so thin that it ruptures, sending arterial blood at a high pressure into the subarachnoid space. For a brief moment after the aneurysm ruptures, ICP is thought to approach mean arterial pressure, and cerebral perfusion decreases.[16] In other situations, the unruptured aneurysm expands and places pressure on surrounding structures. This is particularly true with

TABLE 23.2   Classification of Aneurysms

Types of Aneurysms	Characteristics
Berry or saccular	Most common type, usually congenital; appears at a bifurcation in anterior circulation, primarily at the base of the brain or circle of Willis and its branches; grows from the base of the arterial wall with a neck or stem; contains blood; thinned dome is usually the site of rupture
Giant or fusiform	Can have an irregular shape and be >2.5 cm and atherosclerotic; involves mainly the internal carotid or vertebrobasilar artery; rarely ruptures; has no stem; may act like a space-occupying lesion in the brain; difficult to manage
Mycotic	Rare form; usually occurs from septic emboli, usually results from bacterial infection, which weakens the vessel wall, causing dilation involving distal branches of the middle cerebral arteries
Dissecting	May occur during angiography; caused by trauma, syphilis, arteriosclerosis, or when blood is forced between layers of the arterial wall; intima is pulled away from the medial layer, allowing blood to enter
Traumatic	Sometimes called a *pseudoaneurysm*, which may resolve after trauma
Charcot-Bouchard	Small aneurysm that can be seen in the area of the basal ganglia or brainstem in individuals with a history of hypertension; chronic hypertension causes fibrinoid necrosis in the penetrating and subcortical arteries, weakening arterial walls and causing formation of small aneurysmal outpouching

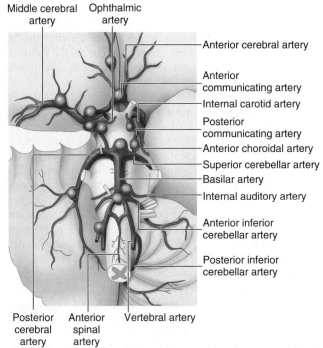

Middle cerebral artery
Ophthalmic artery
Anterior cerebral artery
Anterior communicating artery
Internal carotid artery
Posterior communicating artery
Anterior choroidal artery
Superior cerebellar artery
Basilar artery
Internal auditory artery
Anterior inferior cerebellar artery
Posterior inferior cerebellar artery
Posterior cerebral artery
Anterior spinal artery
Vertebral artery

FIG. 23.2 Common Sites of Berry Aneurysms. The size of the aneurysm in the drawing is proportional to the frequency of occurrence at the various sites. (From Goldman L, Schafer AI, eds. *Goldman-Cecil medicine*, 25th ed. St. Louis: Elsevier; 2016.)

RIGHT   LEFT

FIG. 23.3 Cerebral Angiogram. Cerebral angiography shows the location of an aneurysm *(arrow)* at the posterior communicating artery. (From Tortorici M. *Fundamentals of Angiography*. St. Louis: Mosby; 1982.)

posterior communicating artery aneurysms because they put pressure on the oculomotor nerve (cranial nerve III), causing ipsilateral pupil dilation and ptosis.[16]

Arteriovenous malformation. The pathophysiologic features of an AVM are related to the size and location of the malformation. One or more cerebral arteries, also known as *feeders*, supply an AVM. These feeder arteries tend to enlarge over time and increase the volume of blood shunted through the malformation and increase the overall mass effect. Large, dilated, tortuous draining veins develop as a result of increasing arterial blood flow being delivered at a higher than normal pressure. Normal vascular flow has a mean arterial pressure of 70 to 80 mm Hg, a mean arteriole pressure of 35 to 45 mm Hg, and a mean capillary pressure that decreases from 35 to 10 mm Hg as it connects with the venous side. Lack of this capillary bridge allows blood with a mean pressure of 35 to 45 mm Hg to flow into the venous system. In contrast to arteries, veins have no muscular layer and become extremely engorged and rupture easily. Some patients with AVMs also have cerebral atrophy, which is the result of chronic ischemia secondary to the shunting of blood through the AVM and away from normal cerebral circulation.[16]

Assessment and Diagnosis

A patient with a SAH characteristically has an abrupt onset of pain, described as the "worst headache of my life." A brief loss of consciousness, nausea, vomiting, focal neurologic deficits, and a stiff neck may accompany the headache.[14-18] The SAH may result in coma or death.

The patient's history may reveal one or more incidences of sudden onset of headache with vomiting in the weeks preceding a major SAH. These are small "warning leaks" of an aneurysm in which small amounts of blood ooze from the aneurysm into

the subarachnoid space. The presence of blood is an irritant to the meninges, particularly the arachnoid membrane, and the irritation causes headache, stiff neck, and photophobia. These warning leaks seldom are detected because the condition is not severe enough for the patient to seek medical attention. If a neurologic deficit such as third cranial nerve palsy develops before aneurysm rupture, medical intervention is sought, and the aneurysm may be surgically secured before the devastation of a rupture can occur. Symptoms of unruptured AVM—headaches with dizziness or syncope or fleeting neurologic deficits—also may be found in the history.[18]

Diagnosis of SAH is based on clinical presentation, CT findings, and lumbar puncture results. Noncontrast CT is the cornerstone of definitive SAH diagnosis.[17-19] In 95% of the cases, CT demonstrates blood in the subarachnoid space if performed within 48 hours of the hemorrhage.[13,18] On the basis of the appearance and the location of the SAH, diagnosis of the cause—aneurysm or AVM—may be made from the CT scan. MRI is not routinely used, but it may provide greater sensitivity for detecting the areas of SAH clot and the potential location of the bleed.[17]

If the initial CT finding is negative, a lumbar puncture is performed to obtain cerebrospinal fluid (CSF) for analysis. CSF after SAH appears bloody and has a red blood cell count greater than 1000 cells/mm³. If the lumbar puncture is performed more than 5 days after the SAH, the CSF fluid is xanthochromic (dark amber) because the blood products have broken down.[15] Cloudy CSF usually indicates some type of infectious process such as bacterial meningitis, not SAH.[16]

After the SAH has been documented, cerebral angiography is necessary to identify the exact cause of the hemorrhage (Fig. 23.3). If a cerebral aneurysm rupture is the cause, angiography is essential for identifying the exact location of the aneurysm in preparation for surgery.[17-19] After the aneurysm has been located, it is graded using the Hunt and Hess classification scale. This scale categorizes the patient on the basis of the severity of the neurologic deficits associated with the hemorrhage (Box 23.3).[20] If AVM rupture is the cause, angiography is necessary to identify the feeding arteries and draining veins of the malformation.[15]

Medical Management

SAH is a medical emergency, and time is of the essence. Preservation of neurologic function is the goal, and early diagnosis is crucial. Initial treatment must always support vital functions. Airway management and ventilatory assistance may be necessary.[17] A ventriculostomy is performed to control ICP if the patient's LOC is depressed.[18]

Evidence suggests that only 19% of the deaths attributable to aneurysmal SAH are related to the direct effects of the initial hemorrhage.[21] Rebleeding accounts for 22% of deaths from aneurysmal SAH, cerebral vasospasm accounts for 23%, and nonneurologic medical complications account for 23%.[21] Principal nonneurologic causes of death are systemic inflammatory response syndrome and secondary organ dysfunction.[22] After initial intervention has provided the necessary support for vital physiologic functions, medical management of acute SAH is aimed primarily at prevention and treatment of the complications of SAH, which may produce further neurologic damage and death.[18]

BOX 23.3   Hunt and Hess Classification of Subarachnoid Hemorrhage

- *Grade I:* Asymptomatic or minimal headache and slight nuchal rigidity
- *Grade II:* Moderate to severe headache, nuchal rigidity, but no neurologic deficit other than cranial nerve palsy
- *Grade III:* Drowsiness, confusion, or mild focal deficit
- *Grade IV:* Stupor, moderate to severe hemiparesis, possible early decerebrate rigidity, and vegetative disturbances
- *Grade V:* Deep coma, decerebrate rigidity, moribund appearance

From Hunt WE, Hess RM. Surgical risks as related to time of intervention in the repair of intracranial aneurysms. *J Neurosurg.* 1968; 28:14–20.

Rebleeding. Rebleeding is the occurrence of a second SAH in an unsecured aneurysm or, less commonly, an AVM.[13] The incidence of rebleeding during the first 24 hours after the first bleed is 4%, with a 1% to 2% chance per day in the following month. The mortality rate associated with aneurysmal rebleeding is approximately 70%.[18]

Historically, conservative measures to prevent rebleeding have included blood pressure control and SAH precautions (see "Nursing Management"). An elevation in blood pressure is a normal compensatory response to maintain adequate cerebral perfusion after a neurologic insult. In the belief that hypertension contributes to rebleeding, nitroprusside, metoprolol, or hydralazine has been commonly used to maintain a systolic blood pressure no greater than 140 mm Hg.[18] Individualized guidelines must be determined on the basis of the clinical condition and preexisting values of the patient. Evidence suggests that rebleeding has more to do with variations in blood pressure than it does with absolute values and that blood pressure control does not reduce the incidence of rebleeding.[19]

Surgical clipping of aneurysms. Definitive treatment for the prevention of rebleeding is surgical clipping or endovascular coiling with complete obliteration of the aneurysm.[18,19] Timing of the operation is a key medical management issue. Since the introduction of microsurgery and improved surgical techniques, patients commonly are taken to the operating room within the first 48 hours after rupture.[18] This early surgical intervention to secure the aneurysm eliminates the risk of rebleeding and allows more aggressive therapy to be used in the postoperative period for the treatment of vasospasm.[18,19] Early surgery also allows the neurosurgeon to flush out the excess blood and clots from the basal cisterns (reservoir of CSF around the base of the brain and circle of Willis) to reduce the risk of vasospasm.[22] Careful consideration of the patient's clinical situation is necessary in determining the optimal time for surgery.

The surgical procedure involves a craniotomy to expose and isolate the area of aneurysm. A clip is placed over the neck of the aneurysm to eliminate the area of weakness (Fig. 23.4). This is a technically difficult procedure that requires the skill of an experienced neurosurgeon. It is not uncommon, particularly

FIG. 23.4 Clipping of a Posterior Communicating Artery Aneurysm. (A) *Solid curved line* shows the typical skin incision, and *dashed lines* show the craniotomy location. (B) Application of the clip to the aneurysm.

in early surgery, for the clot to break away from the aneurysm as it is surgically exposed. Extensive hemorrhage into the craniotomy site results, and cessation of the hemorrhage often causes increased neurologic deficits. Deficits also may occur as a result of surgical manipulation to gain access to the site of the aneurysm.[18]

Surgical excision of arteriovenous malformations. Management of AVM has traditionally involved surgical excision or conservative management of symptoms such as seizures and headache. The decision for surgical excision depends on the location and size of the AVM. Some malformations are located so deep in the cerebral structures (thalamus or midbrain) that attempts to remove the AVM would cause severe neurologic deficits. History of a previous hemorrhage and the patient's age and overall condition are also taken into account when making the decision regarding surgical intervention.[18]

Surgical excision of large AVMs includes the risk of reperfusion bleeding. As feeding arteries of the AVM are clamped off, the arterial blood that usually flowed into the AVM is diverted into the surrounding circulation. In many cases, the surrounding tissue has been in a state of chronic ischemia, and the arterial vessels feeding these areas are maximally dilated. As arterial blood begins to flow at a higher volume and pressure into these dilated arteries, blood may seep from the vessels. Evidence of reperfusion bleeding in the operating room is an indication that no more arterial blood can be diverted from the AVM without risk of serious ICH. In the postoperative phase, low blood pressure is maintained to prevent further reperfusion bleeding. For large AVMs, two to four stages of surgery may be required over 6 to 12 months.[18]

Embolization. Embolization is used to secure a cerebral aneurysm or AVM that is surgically inaccessible because of size, location, or medical instability of the patient. Embolization involves several new interventional neuroradiology techniques. All techniques use a percutaneous transfemoral approach in a manner similar to angiography. Under fluoroscopy, the catheter is threaded up to the internal carotid artery. Specially developed microcatheters are then manipulated into the area of the vascular anomaly, and embolic materials are placed endovascularly. Three embolization techniques are used, depending on the underlying pathologic derangement.[17]

The first type of embolization is used for an AVM. Small polymeric silicone (Silastic) beads or glue is slowly introduced into the vessels feeding the AVM. Blood flow carries the material to the site, and embolization is achieved. This procedure may be used in combination with surgery. One to three sessions of embolization of the feeding vessels are performed to reduce the size of the lesion before a craniotomy is performed for total excision. The primary risk of this procedure is lodging of the embolic substance in a vessel that feeds normal tissue, which creates an embolic stroke with the immediate onset of neurologic symptoms.[23]

The second type of embolization involves placement of one or more detachable coils into an aneurysm to produce an endovascular thrombus (Fig. 23.5). The advantage of this technique is that an electrical current creates a positive charge on the coil, which induces electrothrombosis. Complications include embolic stroke, coil migration, overproduction of the clot, subtotal occlusion and intraprocedural rupture of the vasculature, and death.[23]

Cerebral vasospasm. The presence or absence of cerebral vasospasm significantly affects the outcome of aneurysmal SAH. This complication does not occur with SAH resulting from AVM rupture. Cerebral vasospasm is a narrowing of the lumen of the cerebral arteries, possibly in response to subarachnoid blood clots coating the outer surface of the blood vessels. Because aneurysms usually occur at the circle of Willis, the major vessels responsible for feeding the cerebral circulation are affected by vasospasm. Depending on the arterial vessels involved in the vasospasm reaction, decreased arterial flow occurs in large areas of the cerebral hemispheres.[24]

It is estimated that 70% of all patients with SAH develop vasospasm, which can be demonstrated on angiography.[25] Of these patients, 32% develop symptomatic vasospasm, resulting in ischemic stroke or death in up to 23% of patients despite the use of maximal therapy.[25] The onset of vasospasm is usually 7 to 10 days after the initial hemorrhage.[19] The three recommended treatments for the management of vasospasm are hemodynamic augmentation, oral nimodipine, and transluminal cerebral angioplasty.[19,24,25]

Hemodynamic augmentation. Hemodynamic augmentation therapy involves increasing the patient's blood pressure and cardiac output with vasoactive medications. Systolic blood pressure is maintained between 150 mm Hg and 160 mm Hg. The increase in pressure forces blood through the vasospastic area at higher pressures. Many anecdotal reports exist of neurologic deficits of patients improving as systolic pressure increases from 130 mm Hg to between 150 mm Hg and 160 mm Hg.[24] Prior recommendations for the treatment of cerebral vasospasm also included induced hemodilution and hypervolemia; however, these therapies are no longer recommended because they were not supported through research.[19,24] Hypervolemia and hypovolemia should be avoided, and euvolemia should be maintained.[19]

The obvious deterrent to the use of induced hypertension is the risk of rebleeding in an unsecured aneurysm. Surgical clipping of the aneurysm before hemodynamic augmentation therapy is preferred. Cerebral edema, elevated ICP, heart failure, and electrolyte imbalance are also risks of hemodynamic augmentation therapy. Careful monitoring of the patient's neurologic status, hemodynamic parameters, ICP, and serum electrolytes is necessary.[24]

Nimodipine. Nimodipine is strongly recommended to reduce the poor outcomes associated with vasospasm. The exact nature of the effect of nimodipine is unclear, but the use of the medication has demonstrated consistently positive effects on outcome without any demonstrable effect on the incidence or severity of vasospasm.[19,25] A dose of 60 mg of nimodipine is given orally every 4 hours for 21 days.[24] Nimodipine may produce hypotension, especially when administered concurrently with other antihypertensive agents.[25]

Cerebral angioplasty. Cerebral angioplasty is used when pharmacologic management of cerebral vasospasm has failed. It is performed only when CT or MRI provides evidence that infarction has not occurred. An interventional neuroradiologist performs the procedure, and the patient is placed under procedural sedation. The technique of cerebral angioplasty is very similar to the technique used in the coronary vasculature. Risks include intimal perforation or rupture; cerebral artery thrombosis or embolism; recurrence of stenosis; and severe, diffuse vasospasm unresponsive to therapy. Hemorrhage at the femoral site also may occur. This procedure is recommended when conventional therapy is unsuccessful.[19]

Hyponatremia

Hyponatremia develops in up to 50% of patients with SAH as a result of central salt-wasting syndrome. It usually occurs during the same period as vasospasm, several days after the initial hemorrhage.[18] Sodium is replenished with isotonic fluids in patients with SAH; the use of fluid restriction to treat hyponatremia is associated with a poor outcome.[19]

Hydrocephalus

Hydrocephalus is a late complication that occurs in approximately 25% of patients after SAH.[15] Blood that has circulated in the subarachnoid space and has been absorbed by the arachnoid villi may obstruct the villi and reduce the rate of CSF absorption. Over time, increasing volumes of CSF in the intracranial

space produce communicating hydrocephalus. Treatment consists of placing a drain to remove CSF. This can be accomplished temporarily, by inserting a ventriculostomy, or permanently, by placing a ventriculoperitoneal shunt.[18,19]

Intracerebral Hemorrhage
Description

ICH is bleeding directly into cerebral tissue.[26,27] ICH destroys cerebral tissue, causes cerebral edema, and increases ICP. The source of intracerebral bleeding is usually a small artery, but it also can result from rupture of an AVM or aneurysm. The most important cause of spontaneous ICH is hypertension, and this section concentrates on spontaneous hypertensive ICH.[28]

Spontaneous ICH accounts for at least 10% of all stroke admissions.[27] The likelihood of death or disability is higher with ICH than with ischemic stroke or SAH. The mortality rate for hemorrhagic stroke is 50% within 1 month. Only 20% of

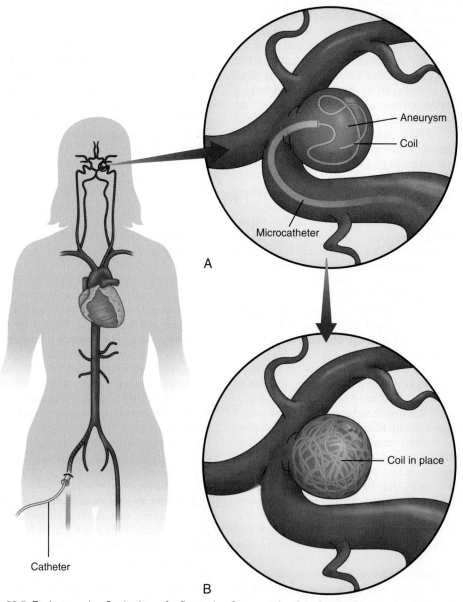

FIG. 23.5 Endovascular Occlusion of a Posterior Communicating Artery Aneurysm. (A) Insertion of the microcatheter into the aneurysm through the right femoral artery, aorta, and left carotid artery. (B) Occlusion of the aneurysm with coils.

patients with ICH return to a functional life at 6 months.[29] The key risk factors for ICH are age-associated cerebral amyloid angiopathy and hypertension.[27]

Etiology

ICH is most often caused by hypertensive rupture of a cerebral vessel, resulting from a long-standing history of hypertension.[27] Other possible causes of spontaneous ICH are anticoagulation or fibrinolytic therapy, coagulation disorders, drug abuse, and hemorrhage into a cerebral infarct or brain tumors.[18,30] Often, on questioning, a patient with a hypertensive hemorrhage admits to having discontinued antihypertensive medication 2 to 3 weeks before the hemorrhage.

Pathophysiology

The pathophysiology of ICH is caused by continued elevated blood pressure exerting force against smaller arterial vessels that have become damaged from arteriosclerotic changes. Eventually, these arteries break, and blood bursts from the vessels into the surrounding cerebral tissue, creating a hematoma. ICP rises precipitously in response to the increase in overall intracranial volume.[30]

Assessment and Diagnosis

Initial assessment usually reveals a critically ill patient who often is unconscious and requires ventilatory support. History from a relative or significant other describes a sudden onset of focal deficit often accompanied by severe headache, nausea, vomiting, and rapid neurologic deterioration. Signs and symptoms vary, depending on the location of the ICH.[30] Approximately 50% of patients sustain early loss of consciousness, a key feature that differentiates ICH from ischemic stroke. More than one-half of patients with ICH present with a smooth progression of neurologic symptoms, an uncommon finding in cases of ischemic stroke or SAH.[31] One-third of patients have maximal symptoms at onset. Assessment of vital signs usually reveals a severely elevated blood pressure (200/100 to 250/150 mm Hg). Signs of increased ICP are often present by the time the patient arrives in the emergency department. Diagnosis is established easily with CT. Angiography is recommended only in patients considered surgical candidates and if a clear cause of hemorrhage is not evident.[27-31]

Medical Management

ICH is a medical emergency. Initial management requires attention to airway, breathing, and circulation. Intubation is usually necessary. Blood pressure management must be based on individual factors. Reduction in blood pressure is usually necessary to decrease ongoing bleeding, but lowering blood pressure too much or too rapidly may compromise cerebral perfusion pressure (CPP), especially in a patient with elevated ICP. National guidelines recommend keeping the *mean* arterial blood pressure less than 130 mm Hg in patients with a history of hypertension by moderate blood pressure reduction to a mean arterial pressure less than 110 mm Hg.[31] Vasopressor therapy after fluid replenishment is recommended if systolic blood pressure is less than 90 mm Hg.[28]

Increased ICP is common with ICH and is a major contributor to mortality. Recommended management includes mannitol, when indicated; hyperventilation; and neuromuscular blockade with sedation. Steroids are avoided. CPP must be maintained at greater than 70 mm Hg.[28,29]

The goal for fluid management is euvolemia, with a recommended pulmonary artery occlusion pressure of 10 to 14 mm Hg. Body temperature is maintained at less than 38.5°C by using acetaminophen or cooling blankets. Euglycemia, a blood glucose level less than 140 mg/dL, is maintained by using insulin therapy, but hypoglycemia should be avoided. Use of short-acting benzodiazepines or propofol is recommended to treat agitation or hyperactivity. Pneumatic compression devices are used to decrease the risk of pulmonary embolism. Prophylactic anticonvulsant therapy is sometimes used.[28,31]

The benefit of surgical treatment for spontaneous ICH is unclear. Recommendations for surgical removal of the clot depend on the size and location of the hematoma, the patient's ICP, and other neurologic symptoms.[31] Medical treatment is recommended if the hemorrhage is small (<10 cm) or neurologic deficit is minimal.[28,31] Likewise, surgery offers no improvement in outcome for patients with a Glasgow Coma Scale (GCS) score of 4 or less. Surgical evacuation of the clot is recommended for patients with cerebellar hemorrhage greater than 3 cm with neurologic deterioration or hydrocephalus with brainstem compression, as well as for young patients with moderate or large lobar hemorrhage with clinical deterioration.[28,31] Numerous techniques are being investigated to lessen the risk of brain damage associated with craniotomy for ICH.

Interprofessional collaborative management of a patient with ICH is outlined in Box 23.4.

Nursing Management

The nursing management plan for a patient with stroke incorporates a variety of nursing diagnoses (Box 23.5). The nurse has a significant role in monitoring for changes in neurologic and hemodynamic status, maintaining surveillance for complications, providing comfort and emotional support, and educating the patient and family.

Monitor for Changes in Neurologic and Hemodynamic Status

The goal of frequent assessments is early recognition of neurologic or hemodynamic deterioration. Close monitoring of the patient's neurologic signs and vital signs is essential and requires almost continuous observation. Automatic noninvasive devices such as a blood pressure cuff and a pulse oximeter are helpful. Seizure activity must be identified and treated immediately. It is essential that all personnel working with the patient be aware of the desired hemodynamic and neurologic parameters set by the physician and that the physician be notified at the first sign of any changes.

Maintain Surveillance for Complications

A patient with stroke should be monitored closely for signs of bleeding, vasospasm, and increased ICP. Other complications of stroke include aspiration, malnutrition, pneumonia, DVT, pulmonary embolism, pressure ulcers, contractures, and joint abnormalities.[16] Nursing measures to prevent these complications are well known.

Additional complications that may be seen in a patient with stroke are related to the area of the brain that has been damaged. Damage to the temporoparietal area can create various disturbances that affect the patient's ability to interpret sensory information. Damage to the dominant hemisphere (usually left) produces problems with speech and

QSEN BOX 23.4   QSEN: Evidence-Based Practice

Spontaneous Intracerebral Hemorrhage Management Guidelines

The following are class 1 recommendations from the American Heart Association and American Stroke Association. Class 1 recommendations are conditions for which evidence and general agreement exist that the procedure or treatment is useful and effective.

- A baseline severity score should be performed as part of the initial evaluation of patients with ICH.
- Rapid neuroimaging with CT or MRI is recommended to distinguish ischemic stroke from ICH.
- Patients with a severe coagulation factor deficiency or severe thrombocytopenia should receive appropriate factor replacement therapy or platelets, respectively.
- Patients with ICH whose INR is elevated because of VKA should have their VKA withheld, should receive therapy to replace vitamin K–dependent factors and correct the INR, and should receive IV vitamin K.
- Patients with ICH should receive intermittent pneumatic compression for prevention of venous thromboembolism beginning the day of hospital admission.
- Initial monitoring and management of patients with ICH should take place in an intensive care unit or a dedicated stroke unit with physician and nursing neuroscience acute care expertise.
- Blood glucose levels should be monitored, and hyperglycemia and hypoglycemia should be avoided.
- Patients with clinical seizures should be treated with antiseizure medications.
- Patients with a change in mental status who are found to have electrographic seizures on EEG should be treated with antiseizure medications.
- A formal screening procedure for dysphagia should be performed in patients before the initiation of oral intake to reduce risk of pneumonia.
- Given the potentially serious nature and complex pattern of evolving disability and the increasing evidence for efficacy, it is recommended that all patients with ICH have access to multidisciplinary rehabilitation.
- Patients with cerebellar hemorrhage who are deteriorating neurologically or who have brainstem compression, hydrocephalus, or both from ventricular obstruction should undergo surgical removal of the hemorrhage as soon as possible.

CT, computed tomography; *EEG*, electroencephalography; *ICH*, intracerebral hemorrhage; *INR*, international normalized ratio; *IV*, intravenous; *MRI*, magnetic resonance imaging; *VKA*, vitamin K antagonists.
Modified from Hemphill JC, et al. Guidelines for the management of spontaneous intracerebral hemorrhage: a guideline for healthcare professionals from the American Heart Association/American Stroke Association. *Stroke.* 2015;46(7):2032–2060.

BOX 23.5   NURSING DIAGNOSES

Stroke

- Risk for Ineffective Cerebral Tissue Perfusion, p. 1042
- Acute Pain related to transmission and perception of cutaneous, visceral, muscular, or ischemic impulses, p. 1010
- Unilateral Neglect related to perceptual disruption, p. 1048
- Impaired Verbal Communication related to cerebral speech center injury, p. 1033
- Impaired Swallowing related to neuromuscular impairment, fatigue, and limited awareness, p. 1032
- Risk for Aspiration, p. 1040
- Risk for Infection, p. 1046
- Anxiety related to threat to biologic, psychologic, or social integrity, p. 1012
- Disturbed Body Image related to actual change in body structure, function, or appearance, p. 1022
- Compromised Family Coping related to critically ill family member, p. 1014

language and abstract and analytic skills. Damage to the nondominant hemisphere (usually right) produces problems with spatial relationships. The resulting deficits include agnosia, apraxia, and visual field defects. Perceptual deficits are not as readily noticeable as motor deficits, but they may be more debilitating and may lead to inability to perform skilled or purposeful tasks. The patient also may experience impaired swallowing.[17,20]

Bleeding and vasospasm. In a patient with a cerebral aneurysm, sudden onset of, or an increase in, headache and nausea and vomiting, increased blood pressure, and changes in respiration herald the onset of rebleeding. The first indication of vasospasm is usually the appearance of new focal or global neurologic deficits.

SAH precautions must be implemented to prevent any stress or straining that could potentially precipitate rebleeding. Precautions include blood pressure control; bed rest; a dark, quiet environment; and stool softeners. Short-acting analgesics and sedatives are used to relieve pain and anxiety. The patient must be kept calm. Limb restraints cause straining and must be avoided. The head of the bed should be elevated to 35 to 45 degrees at all times. The patient is taught to avoid any activities that correspond to performance of the Valsalva maneuver, such as pushing with the legs to move up in bed, straining for a bowel movement, or holding his or her breath during procedures or discomfort. DVT precautions are routinely implemented. Caregivers collaborate with the patient and family to establish a visitation plan to meet patient and family needs. Often, family members at the bedside can assist the patient to remain calm.[17,19,20]

Increased intracranial pressure. Numerous signs and symptoms of increased ICP can be observed. A change in the LOC is the most sensitive indicator. Others include unequal pupil size, decreased pupillary response to light, headache, projectile vomiting, altered breathing patterns, Cushing triad (bradycardia, systolic hypertension, and bradypnea), diminished brainstem reflexes, papilledema, and abnormal extension (decerebrate posturing) or flexion (decorticate posturing).[17,19,20]

Damage to nondominant hemisphere. Patients with pathologic conditions affecting the nondominant hemisphere may exhibit emotional lability, with periods of euphoria, impulsiveness, and inattention. A short attention span, lack of insight, and poor judgment may lead to injuries as the patient attempts to perform activities beyond his or her capabilities. These patients also may experience agnosia, visual field defects, and apraxia.[17,19,20]

Agnosia. Agnosia is a disturbance in the perception of familiar sensory (eg, verbal, tactile, visual) information. Unilateral neglect is a form of agnosia characterized by an unawareness or denial of the affected half of the body. This denial may range from inattention to refusing to acknowledge a paralysis by neglecting the involved side of the body or by denying ownership of the side, attributing the paralyzed arm or leg to someone else. The neglect also may extend to extrapersonal space. This defect most often results from right hemispheric brain damage that causes left hemiplegia.

Other types of agnosia exist in addition to unilateral neglect. Some patients are unable to recognize objects visually (visual object agnosia), whereas others cannot recognize faces (prosopagnosia) and may have to rely on the voice or characteristic mannerisms of a familiar person to identify that person. Tactile agnosia is a perceptual disorder in which a patient is unable to recognize by touch alone an object that has been placed in his or her hand. This may occur even in the presence of an intact sense of touch. If allowed to see or hear the object, the patient usually recognizes it.

Spatial orientation is affected, resulting in interference with the patient's ability to judge position, distance, movement, form, and the relationship of his or her body parts to surrounding objects. Patients may confuse concepts such as "up and down" or "forward and backward." They may have difficulty following a route from one place to another and may get lost in areas that were once familiar. Patients with stroke may also experience reading and writing problems related to visual perception and visuospatial deficits. One type of spatial dyslexia is related to unilateral spatial neglect. The patient may not look at the beginning of a line of written material that appears on the left. Instead, the patient fixes attention on a point to the right of the beginning of the line and reads to the end of the line. If asked to draw a design, the person completes only half of a design or drawing.

Visual field defects. Visual field defects may accompany agnosia, although they do not cause it. A hemispheric lesion can interrupt the visual pathways, with the resulting visual defect dependent on the location and extent of the lesion. At the optic chiasm, nerve fibers coming from the nasal half of each retina cross to the opposite side, whereas fibers coming from the temporal half of each retina do not cross. This partial crossing allows binocular vision. In the optic chiasm, fibers from the nasal half of each retina join the uncrossed fibers from the temporal half of the retina to form the optic tract. Impulses conducted to the right hemisphere by the right optic tract represent the left field of vision, and impulses conducted to the left hemisphere by the left optic tract represent the right field of vision. Optic radiations extend back to the occipital lobes. Visual defects restricted to a single field, right or left, are called *homonymous hemianopsia.*

The nurse may be the first person to notice that the patient has this defect. A patient with hemianopsia may neglect all sensory input from the affected side and initially may appear unresponsive if approached from the affected side. If the nurse approaches the patient from the healthy side, the patient may be quite alert. The patient eating food only from one half of the tray is another clue to hemianopsia. Hemianopsia may recede gradually with time. Many patients can learn to scan their environment visually to compensate for the defect, although in the acute stage of stroke, the patient may be too lethargic to follow instructions in methods of visual scanning. This visual defect can lead to fear and confusion and can present a risk to the patient's safety.

Apraxia. Lesions in the parietal lobe and in other cortical structures can result in apraxia, an inability to perform a learned movement voluntarily. Although a patient may understand the task to be performed and may have intact motor ability, the patient cannot perform the task and often fumbles and makes mistakes. For example, a patient experiencing dressing apraxia may be unable to orient clothing in space, becoming tangled in his or her clothes when attempting to dress.

Damage to dominant hemisphere. Damage to the dominant hemisphere produces problems with speech and language. Impaired communication is a condition that results from a patient's difficulty in expressing and exchanging thoughts, ideas, or desires.[17,19,20] The posterior temporoparietal area contains the receptive speech center known as *Wernicke area.* The center for the perception of written language lies anterior to the visuoreceptive areas. Located at the base of the motor strip of the frontal lobe and slightly anterior to it is *Broca area,* also known as the *motor speech center.* These sensory and motor areas are connected by a large bundle of nerve fibers. Rather than receptive and motor language functions being entirely within discrete areas, it is thought that language is an integrated sensorimotor process, control of which is roughly located in these areas in the dominant cerebral hemisphere. It also is recognized that the elaborately complex functions of speech and language depend on other associative areas of the cerebrum and their thalamic connections. Consequently, much inconsistency exists in the degree of communication impairment among patients with lesions located in the same area of the brain.

Aphasia is a loss of language abilities caused by brain injury, usually to the dominant hemisphere. It involves more than just understanding speech or expressing oneself through verbal means. *Language* is a much broader term, referring to what the individual is attempting to interpret or convey through listening, speaking, reading, writing, and gesturing. Most cases of aphasia are partial rather than complete. The severity of the disorder depends on the area and the extent of the cerebral damage.

Receptive aphasia. Receptive aphasia, also referred to as *sensory, Wernicke,* or *fluent aphasia,* occurs when the connection between the primary auditory cortex in the temporal lobe and the angular gyrus in the parietal lobe is destroyed. The patient's comprehension of speech is impaired, but he or she can still talk if the motor area for speech (Broca area) is intact. The patient may talk excessively, with many errors in the use of words. The patient can hear the examiner but cannot comprehend what is being said and cannot repeat the examiner's words. These patients may talk nonsense, with rambling speech that gives little information. Patients with receptive aphasia also cannot read words, although they can see them.

Expressive aphasia. Expressive aphasia, also known as *motor, Broca,* or *nonfluent aphasia,* is primarily a deficit in language output or speech production. Depending on the size and exact location of the lesion, wide variation in the motor deficit can result. Expressive aphasia can range from a mild dysarthria (imperfect articulation as a result of weakness or lack of coordination of speech musculature) to incorrect intonation and phrasing and, in its most severe form, to complete loss of ability to communicate through verbal and written means. In this severe form of aphasia, the patient also experiences a loss of ability to communicate through conventional gestures such as nodding or shaking the head for "yes" or "no." In most cases of expressive aphasia, the muscles of articulation are intact. If speech is possible at all, the words "yes" and "no" are occasionally uttered, sometimes appropriately. Some patients may sing the words of well-known songs. Other patients, when excited or angered, may utter expletives. Some patients with expressive aphasia struggle or hesitate in trying to express words. They struggle to form words while using motor musculature (*verbal apraxia*), an articulatory disorder that is a feature of some expressive types of aphasia. All these difficulties lead to exasperation and despair in the patient. Most patients with expressive aphasia also have severely impaired writing ability. Although penmanship may be intact, they are unable to express themselves through writing—a deficit called *agraphia*. If the right hand is paralyzed, as is often the case, the patient still cannot write or print with the left hand. In the recovery phase of severe expressive aphasia, patients become able to speak aloud to some degree, although words are uttered slowly and laboriously. However, many patients are able to learn to communicate ideas to some extent.

Global aphasia. Global aphasia results when a massive lesion affects the motor and sensory speech areas. The patient cannot transform sounds into words and cannot comprehend spoken words. All language modalities are affected, and impairment may be so severe that the patient may be unable to communicate on any level. These patients usually have severe hemiplegia and homonymous hemianopsia. Their language function rarely recovers to a significant degree unless the lesion is caused by some transient disorder, such as cerebral edema or a metabolic derangement.

Impaired swallowing. Normal swallowing occurs in four phases that are controlled by the cranial nerves. Damage to the brain, brainstem, or cranial nerves may result in various swallowing deficits that could place the patient at risk for aspiration. A patient with stroke is observed for signs of dysphagia, including drooling; difficulty handling oral secretions; absence of gag, cough, or swallowing reflexes; moist, gurgling voice quality; decreased mouth and tongue movements; and the presence of dysarthria. A speech therapy consultation is initiated if any of these signs are present, and the patient must not be orally fed. In the absence of these warning signs, the patient may be fed, as ordered by the physician, although he or she must be continually monitored for signs of aspiration.[17,19,30]

Educate the Patient and Family

Rehabilitation starts in the critical care area, with a multidisciplinary team designing and implementing an individualized plan for maximizing the patient's potential for neurologic rehabilitation. Early in the patient's hospital stay, the patient and family must be taught about stroke, its causes, and its treatment (Box 23.6). Closer to discharge, teaching focuses on the interventions necessary for preventing the recurrence of the event and on maximizing the patient's rehabilitation potential. The patient's family must be encouraged to participate in the patient's care; learn how to feed, dress, and bathe the patient; and learn some basic rehabilitation techniques. The importance of participating in a neurologic rehabilitation program or a support group, or both, must be stressed.

Interprofessional collaborative management of a patient with stroke is outlined in Box 23.7.

COMA

Description

Normal consciousness requires awareness and arousal. Awareness is the combination of cognition (mental and intellectual) and affect (mood) that can be construed based on the

---

BOX 23.6 PATIENT EDUCATION PLAN

Stroke

Before the patient's discharge, the patient should be able to teach back the following topics:
- Pathophysiology of disease
- Specific cause
- Risk factor modification
- Importance of taking medications
- Activities of daily living
- Measures to prevent injuries of impaired limbs
- Measures to compensate for residual deficits
- Basic rehabilitation techniques
- Importance of participating in neurologic rehabilitation program or support group

Additional information for the patient can be found at the following websites:
- National Stroke Association website (http://www.stroke.org)
- American Stroke Association website (http://www.strokeassociation.org/STROKEORG)

QSEN BOX 23.7 QSEN: Teamwork and Collaboration

Interprofessional Collaborative Practice Management: Stroke

- Distinguish the cause of the stroke:
  - Ischemic
  - Subarachnoid hemorrhage
  - Cerebral aneurysm
  - AVM
  - Intracerebral bleed
- Implement treatment according to cause of bleed:
  - Ischemic
  - Fibrinolytic therapy
  - Blood pressure control
  - Subarachnoid hemorrhage
  - Surgical aneurysm clipping or AVM excision
  - Embolization
  - Intracerebral bleed
  - Blood pressure control
- Protect patient's airway.
- Provide ventilatory assistance, as required.
- Perform frequent neurologic assessments.
- Maintain surveillance for complications:
  - Cerebral edema and intracranial hypertension
  - Cerebral vasospasm and ischemia
  - Rebleeding
  - Impaired swallowing
  - Neurologic deficits
  - Hyponatremia
  - Hydrocephalus
- Provide comfort and emotional support.
- Design and implement appropriate rehabilitation program.
- Educate patient and family.

AVM, arteriovenous malformation.

patient's interaction with the environment.[9] Alterations of consciousness may be the result of deficits in awareness, arousal, or both.[32] The four discrete disorders of consciousness are (1) coma, (2) vegetative state, (3) minimally conscious state, and (4) locked-in syndrome. Coma is characterized by the absence of both wakefulness and awareness, whereas a *vegetative state* is characterized by the presence of wakefulness with the absence of awareness. In a *minimally conscious state*, wakefulness is present, and awareness is severely diminished but not absent. *Locked-in syndrome* is characterized by the presence of wakefulness and awareness, but with quadriplegia and the inability to communicate verbally; thus the patient appears to be unconscious.[33] Box 23.8 lists the disorders of consciousness in descending order of wakefulness.

Coma is the deepest state of unconsciousness; arousal and awareness are lacking.[9,32,33] The patient cannot be aroused and does not demonstrate any purposeful response to the surrounding environment.[32] Coma is a symptom rather than a disease, and it occurs as a result of some underlying process.[9,32] The incidence of coma is difficult to ascertain because a wide variety of conditions can induce coma.[9,32] This state of unconsciousness is commonly encountered in the critical care unit, and it is the focus of the following discussion.

Etiology

The causes of coma can be divided into two general categories: (1) structural or surgical and (2) metabolic or medical. Structural causes of coma include ischemic stroke, ICH, trauma, and brain tumors.[34] Metabolic causes of coma include drug overdose, infectious diseases, endocrine disorders, and poisonings.[34] The three most common causes of nontraumatic coma are stroke, anoxia, and poisonings.[35] Coma demands immediate attention, resulting in a high percentage of admissions to all hospital services.[35] Box 23.9 lists the possible causes of coma.

Pathophysiology

Consciousness involves arousal, or wakefulness, and awareness. Neither of these functions is present in a patient in coma.

Ascending fibers of the reticular activating system (RAS) in the pons, hypothalamus, and thalamus maintain arousal as an autonomic function. Neurons in the cerebral cortex are responsible for awareness. Diffuse dysfunction of both cerebral hemispheres and diffuse or focal dysfunction of the RAS can produce coma.[9,36,37] Structural causes usually produce compression or dysfunction in the area of the ascending RAS, whereas most medical causes lead to general dysfunction of both cerebral hemispheres.[37] Trauma, hemorrhage, and tumor can damage the ascending RAS, leading to coma. Destruction of large regions of bilateral cerebral hemispheres can be the result of seizures or viral agents. Toxic drugs, toxins, or metabolic abnormalities can suppress cerebral function.[34,36,37]

Assessment and Diagnosis

The clinical diagnosis of the comatose state is readily established by assessment of the LOC. However, determining the full nature and cause of coma requires a thorough history and physical examination. A medical history is essential because events immediately preceding the change in the LOC can often provide valuable clues to the origin of the coma. When limited information is available and the coma is profound, the response of the patient to emergent treatment may provide clues to the underlying diagnosis; for example, a patient who becomes responsive with the administration of naloxone can be presumed to have ingested some type of opiate.[36]

Detailed serial neurologic examinations are essential for all patients in coma. Assessment of pupillary size and reaction to light (normal, sluggish, or fixed), extraocular eye movements (normal, asymmetric, or absent), motor response to pain (normal, decorticate, decerebrate, or flaccid), and breathing pattern yields important clues for determining whether the cause of coma is structural or metabolic.[9,36]

The areas of the brainstem that control consciousness and pupillary responses are anatomically adjacent. The sympathetic

---

BOX 23.8 Continuum of Descending States of Consciousness

Consciousness
↓
Wakefulness
↓
Arousal
↓
Drowsiness
↓
Confusion
↓
Inattentiveness
↓
Delirium
↓
Stupor
↓
Vegetative state
↓
Coma

BOX 23.9 Causes of Coma

Structural or Surgical Coma	Metabolic or Medical Coma
Trauma	Infection
Epidural hematoma	Meningitis
Subdural hematoma	Encephalitis
Diffuse axonal injury	Metabolic encephalopathy
Brain contusion	Metabolic conditions
Intracerebral hemorrhage	Hypoglycemia
Subarachnoid hemorrhage	Hyperglycemia
Posterior fossa hemorrhage	Hyperosmolar states
Supratentorial hemorrhage	Uremia
Hydrocephalus	Hepatic encephalopathy
Ischemic stroke	Hypertensive encephalopathy
Tumor	Hypoxic encephalopathy
Other causes	Hyponatremia
	Hypercalcemia
	Myxedema
	Intoxication
	Opioid overdose
	Alcohol
	Poisonings
	Psychogenic causes

and parasympathetic nervous systems control pupillary dilation and constriction, respectively. The anatomic directions of these pathways are known, and changes in pupillary responses can help identify where a lesion may be located (see Fig. 22.4 in Chapter 22). For example, if damage occurs in the midbrain region, pupils will be slightly enlarged and unresponsive to light. Lesions that compress the third nerve result in a fixed and dilated pupil on the same side as the neurologic insult. Pupillary responses are usually preserved when the cause of coma is metabolic in origin. Pupillary light responses are often the key to differentiating between structural and metabolic causes of coma.[9,36-38]

Areas of the brainstem adjacent to areas responsible for consciousness also control oculomotor eye movement. The ability to maintain conjugate gaze requires preservation of the internuclear connections of cranial nerves III, VI, and VIII via the medial longitudinal fasciculus.[39] As with pupillary responses, structural lesions that impinge on these pathways cause oculomotor dysfunction such as a dysconjugate gaze. Deficits in extraocular eye movements usually accompany a structural cause.[9,34,38]

Focal or asymmetric motor deficits usually indicate structural lesions.[9,34] Abnormal motor movements may also help pinpoint the location of a lesion. Decorticate posturing (abnormal flexion) can be seen with damage to the diencephalon. Decerebrate posturing (abnormal extension) can be seen with damage to the midbrain and pons. Flaccid posturing is an ominous sign and can be seen with damage to the medulla.[38]

Abnormal breathing patterns may also assist in differentiating structural from metabolic causes of coma. Cheyne-Stokes respirations are seen in patients with cerebral hemispheric dysfunction or metabolic suppression. Central neurogenic hyperventilation, or Kussmaul breathing, occurs with metabolic acidosis or damage to the midbrain and upper pons. Apneustic breathing may occur with damage to the pons, hypoglycemia, and anoxia. Ataxic breathing occurs with damage to the medulla. Agonal breathing occurs with failure of the respiratory centers in the medulla.[36,38]

In addition to physical assessment, laboratory studies and diagnostic procedures are done. Structural causes of coma are usually readily apparent with CT or MRI.[39,40] Laboratory studies are also used to identify metabolic or endocrine abnormalities.[36] Evoked potentials are useful in facilitating a differential diagnosis between the disorders of consciousness and in evaluating a patient's prognosis. Generally, a patient in coma, with absence of brainstem auditory evoked responses, is considered to have a poor prognosis of recovery.[33] Occasionally, the cause of coma is never clearly determined.

Medical Management

The goal of medical management of a patient in coma is identification and treatment of the underlying cause of the condition. Initial medical management includes emergency measures to support vital functions and prevent further neurologic deterioration. Protection of the airway and ventilatory assistance are often needed. Administration of thiamine (at least 100 mg), glucose, and a opioid antagonist is suggested when the cause of coma is not immediately known.[9,36] Thiamine is administered before glucose because the coma produced by thiamine deficiency, Wernicke encephalopathy, can be precipitated by a glucose load.[9]

A patient who remains in coma after emergent treatment requires supportive measures to maintain physiologic body functions and prevent complications. Intubation for continued airway protection and nutrition support is essential. Fluid and electrolyte management is often complex because of alterations in the neurohormonal system. Anticonvulsant therapy may be necessary to prevent further ischemic damage to the brain.[9,34,36]

The health care team and the patient's family make decisions jointly regarding the level of medical management to be provided. Family members require informational support in terms of the probable cause of coma and the prognosis for recovery of consciousness and function. Prognosis depends on the cause of coma and the length of time unconsciousness persists. Only 15% of patients in nontraumatic coma make a satisfactory recovery.[37] Metabolic coma usually has a better prognosis compared with coma caused by a structural lesion, and traumatic coma usually has a better outcome compared with nontraumatic coma.[34,37]

Much research has been directed toward identifying the prognostic indicators for a patient in coma after a cardiopulmonary arrest. In a meta-analysis, the best predictors of poor outcome after cardiac arrest were lack of corneal or papillary response at 24 hours and lack of motor movement at 72 hours. However, regardless of the cause or duration of coma, outcome for an individual cannot be predicted with 100% accuracy.[41] Research has focused on induced hypothermia in patients after cardiac arrest. The use of hypothermia has demonstrated improved neurologic outcomes and survival rates. When a patient remains comatose after return of spontaneous circulation, the body is cooled to 32°C to 34°C for up to 24 hours.[42,43]

Nursing Management

The nursing management plan for a patient in coma incorporates a variety of nursing diagnoses (Box 23.10) and is directed by the specific cause of coma, although some common interventions are used. The patient in coma totally depends on the health care team. The nurse has a significant role in monitoring for changes in neurologic status and clues to the origin of coma, supporting all body functions, maintaining surveillance for complications, providing comfort and emotional support, and initiating rehabilitation measures.[9] Measures to support body functions include promoting pulmonary hygiene, maintaining skin integrity, initiating range-of-motion exercises, managing bowel and bladder functions, and ensuring adequate nutrition support.

Eye Care

The blink reflex is often diminished or absent in a patient in coma. The eyelids may be flaccid and may depend on body

---

◎ BOX 23.10 NURSING DIAGNOSES

Coma

- Ineffective Airway Clearance related to excessive secretions or abnormal viscosity of mucus, p. 1034
- Ineffective Breathing Pattern related to decreased lung expansion, p. 1035
- Imbalanced Nutrition: Less Than Body Requirements related to lack of exogenous nutrients and increased metabolic demand, p. 1029
- Risk for Aspiration, p. 1040
- Risk for Infection, p. 1046
- Compromised Family Coping related to critically ill family member, p. 1014

positioning to remain in a closed position, and edema may prevent complete closure. Loss of these protective mechanisms results in drying and ulceration of the cornea, which can lead to permanent scarring and blindness.[9]

Two interventions that are commonly used to protect the eyes are instilling saline or methylcellulose lubricating drops and taping the eyelids in the shut position. Evidence suggests that an alternative technique may be more effective in preventing corneal epithelial breakdown. In addition to instilling saline drops every 2 hours, a polyethylene film is taped over the eyes, extending beyond the orbits and eyebrows. The film creates a moisture chamber around the cornea and assists in keeping the eyes moist and in the closed position. This technique also prevents damage to the eyes that results from tape or gauze being placed directly on the delicate skin of the eyelids.[44]

Interprofessional collaborative management of a patient in coma is outlined in Box 23.11.

GUILLAIN-BARRÉ SYNDROME

Description

Guillain-Barré syndrome (GBS), once thought to be a single entity characterized by inflammatory peripheral neuropathy, is a combination of clinical features with various forms of presentation and multiple pathologic processes. A full discussion of this complex condition is beyond the scope of this chapter. Most cases of GBS do not require admission to the critical care unit. However, the prototype of GBS, known as *acute inflammatory demyelinating polyradiculoneuropathy* (AIDP), involves a rapidly progressive, ascending peripheral nerve dysfunction, which leads to paralysis that may produce respiratory failure. Because of the need for ventilatory support, AIDP is one of the few peripheral neurologic diseases that necessitates care in a critical care environment.[45] In this discussion, all references to GBS pertain to the AIDP prototype.

The annual incidence of GBS is 1.8 cases per 100,000 persons.[45] It occurs more often in men and is the most commonly acquired demyelinating neuropathy. Occasionally, clusters of cases are reported, as occurred following the 1977 swine flu vaccinations.[45]

QSEN BOX 23.11 QSEN: Teamwork and Collaboration

Interprofessional Collaborative Practice: Coma

- Identify and treat the underlying cause.
- Protect the airway.
- Provide ventilatory assistance, as required.
- Support circulation, as required.
- Initiate nutrition support.
- Provide eye care.
- Protect skin integrity.
- Initiate range-of-motion exercises.
- Maintain surveillance for complications:
  - Infections
  - Metabolic alterations
  - Cardiac dysrhythmias
  - Temperature alterations
- Provide comfort and emotional support.
- Plan for the rehabilitation program.

Etiology

The precise cause of GBS is unknown, but the syndrome involves an immune-mediated response involving cell-mediated immunity and development of IgG antibodies. Most patients report a viral infection 1 to 3 weeks before the onset of clinical manifestations, usually involving the upper respiratory tract.[45,46]

Numerous antecedent causes, or triggering events, have been associated with GBS. They include viral infections (eg, influenza virus; cytomegalovirus; hepatitis A, B, or C virus; Epstein-Barr virus; human immunodeficiency virus), bacterial infections (eg, gastrointestinal *Campylobacter jejuni*, *Mycoplasma pneumoniae*), vaccines (eg, rabies, tetanus, influenza), lymphoma, surgery, and trauma.[45,46]

Pathophysiology

GBS affects the motor and sensory pathways of the peripheral nervous system and the autonomic nervous system functions of the cranial nerves. The major finding in AIDP-type GBS is a segmental demyelination process of the peripheral nerves. GBS is thought to be an autoimmune response to antibodies formed in response to a recent physiologic event. T cells migrate to the peripheral nerves, resulting in edema and inflammation. Macrophages invade the area and break down the myelin. Inflammation around this demyelinated area causes further dysfunction. Some axonal damage also occurs.[45,46]

The myelin sheath of the peripheral nerves is generated by Schwann cells and acts as an insulator for the peripheral nerve. Myelin promotes rapid conduction of nerve impulses by allowing the impulses to jump along the nerve by means of the nodes of Ranvier. Disruption of the myelin fiber slows and may eventually stop the conduction of impulses along the peripheral nerves. In GBS, the more thickly myelinated fibers of motor pathways and the cranial nerves are more severely affected than the thinly myelinated sensory fibers of cutaneous pain, touch, and temperature.[45,46]

After the temporary inflammatory reaction stops, myelin-producing cells begin the process of reinsulating the demyelinated portions of the peripheral nervous system. When remyelination occurs, normal neurologic function should return. In some instances, the axon may be damaged during the inflammatory process. The degree of axonal damage is responsible for the degree of neurologic dysfunction that persists after recovery.[45,46]

Assessment and Diagnosis

Symptoms of GBS include motor weakness, paresthesias and other sensory changes, cranial nerve dysfunction (especially oculomotor, facial, glossopharyngeal, vagal, spinal accessory, and hypoglossal), and some autonomic dysfunction. The usual course of GBS begins with an abrupt onset of lower extremity weakness that progresses to flaccidity and ascends over hours to days. Motor loss usually is symmetric, bilateral, and ascending. In the most severe cases, complete flaccidity of all peripheral nerves, including spinal and cranial nerves, occurs.[46-48]

The patient is admitted to the hospital when lower extremity weakness prevents mobility. Admission to the critical care unit is necessary when progression of weakness threatens respiratory muscles. As weakness progresses, close observation of the patient is essential. Frequent assessment of the respiratory system, including ventilatory parameters such as inspiratory force and tidal volume, is necessary. The most common cause of death of patients with GBS is respiratory arrest. As the disease progresses and respiratory effort weakens, intubation and mechanical ventilation are necessary. Frequent assessment of neurologic deterioration is continued until the patient reaches the peak of the disease, and a plateau occurs.[46,47]

The diagnosis of GBS is based on clinical findings plus CSF analysis and nerve conduction studies. The diagnostic finding is elevated CSF protein with normal cell count.[46] The increased protein count usually occurs after the first week but does not occur in approximately 10% of cases. Nerve conduction studies that test the velocity at which nerve impulses are conducted show significant reduction, as the demyelinating process of the disease suggests.[47]

Medical Management

With no curative treatment available, the medical management of GBS is limited. The disease must run its course, which is characterized by ascending paralysis that advances over 1 to 3 weeks and then remains at a plateau for 2 to 4 weeks.[46] The plateau stage is followed by descending paralysis and return to normal or near-normal function. The main focus of medical management is the support of bodily functions and the prevention of complications.[47]

Plasmapheresis and intravenous immunoglobulin are used to treat GBS[45,46,49,50] and have been shown to be equally effective.[45] Plasmapheresis involves the removal of venous blood through a catheter, separation of plasma from blood cells, and reinfusion of the cells plus autologous plasma or another replacement solution. Although the number of exchanges may vary, four to six exchanges usually are performed over a 5- to 8-day period.[45] Intravenous immunoglobulin has emerged as the preferred therapy because of convenience and availability. The usual dose is 0.4 mg/kg for 5 days.[47]

Nursing Management

The nursing management plan for a patient with GBS incorporates a variety of nursing diagnoses and interventions (Box 23.12). The goal of nursing management is to support all normal body functions until the patient can do so on his or her own. Although the condition is reversible, patients with GBS require extensive long-term care because recovery can be a long process. The nurse has a significant role in maintaining surveillance for complications, initiating rehabilitation, facilitating nutrition support, providing comfort and emotional support, and educating the patient and family.

Maintain Surveillance for Complications

Continuous assessment of the progressive paralysis associated with GBS is essential to timely intervention and the prevention of respiratory arrest and further neurologic insult. After the patient is intubated and placed on mechanical ventilation, close observation for pulmonary complications such as atelectasis, pneumonia, and pneumothorax is necessary. Autonomic dysfunction (dysautonomia) in a patient with GBS can produce variations in heart rate and blood pressure that can reach extreme values.[46,51] Hypertension and tachycardia may require beta-blocker therapy. All patients with GBS must be observed for this phenomenon.[48]

Initiate Rehabilitation

In patients with GBS, immobility may last for months. The usual course of GBS involves an average of 10 days of symptom

---

BOX 23.12 NURSING DIAGNOSES

Guillain-Barré Syndrome

- Ineffective Breathing Pattern related to musculoskeletal fatigue or neuromuscular impairment, p. 1035
- Acute Pain related to transmission and perception of cutaneous, visceral, muscular, or ischemic impulses, p. 1010
- Activity Intolerance related to prolonged immobility or deconditioning, p. 1006
- Risk for Aspiration, p. 1040
- Imbalanced Nutrition: Less Than Body Requirements related to lack of exogenous nutrients or increased metabolic demand, p. 1029
- Risk for Infection, p. 1046
- Anxiety related to threat to biologic, psychologic, or social integrity, p. 1012
- Powerlessness related to lack to control over current situation or disease progression, p. 1038
- Ineffective Coping related to situational crisis and personal vulnerability, p. 1036
- Compromised Family Coping related to critically ill family member, p. 1014

---

progression and 10 days of maximal level of dysfunction, followed by 2 to 48 weeks of recovery. Although GBS usually is completely reversible, the patient will require physical and occupational rehabilitation because of the problems of long-term immobility. Rehabilitation starts in the critical care area, with a multidisciplinary team designing and implementing an individualized plan for maximizing the patient's potential for rehabilitation.[51]

Facilitate Nutrition Support

Nutrition support is implemented early in the course of the disease. Because recovery from GBS is a long process, adequate nutrition support will remain a problem for an extended period. Nutrition support usually is accomplished through the use of enteral feeding.

Provide Comfort and Emotional Support

Pain control is another important component in the care of a patient with GBS. Although patients may have minimal to no motor function, most sensory functions remain, causing patients considerable muscle ache and pain. Because of the length of this illness, a safe, effective, long-term solution to pain management must be identified.[51] These patients also require extensive psychological support. Although the illness is almost 100% reversible, lack of control over the situation, constant pain or discomfort, and the long-term nature of the disorder create coping difficulties for patients. GBS does not affect the LOC or cerebral function. Interaction and communication with the patient are essential elements of the nursing management plan.

Educate the Patient and Family

Early in the patient's hospital stay, the patient and family must be taught about GBS and its different treatments (Box 23.13). As the patient moves toward discharge, teaching focuses on the interventions to maximize the patient's rehabilitation potential. The patient's family must be encouraged to participate in the patient's care and to learn some basic

BOX 23.13   PATIENT EDUCATION PLAN

Guillain-Barré Syndrome

Before the patient's discharge, the patient should be able to teach back the following topics:

- Pathophysiology of disease
- Importance of taking medications
- Measures to compensate for residual deficits
- Basic rehabilitation techniques
- Importance of participating in neurologic rehabilitation program, if necessary

Additional information for the patient can be found at the following website:

- GBS/CIDP Foundation International website (http://www.gbs-cidp.org)

QSEN   BOX 23.14   QSEN: Teamwork and Collaboration

Interprofessional Collaborative Practice: Guillain-Barré Syndrome

- Support bodily functions:
  - Protect airway
  - Provide ventilatory assistance, as required
- Initiate treatments to limit duration of syndrome:
  - Plasmapheresis
  - Intravenous immunoglobulin
- Initiate nutrition support.
- Maintain surveillance for complications:
  - Infections
  - Cardiac dysrhythmias
  - Blood pressure alterations
  - Temperature alterations
- Provide comfort and emotional support.
- Design and implement appropriate rehabilitation program.
- Educate patient and family.

rehabilitation techniques. The importance of participating in a neurologic rehabilitation program (if necessary) must be stressed.

Interprofessional collaborative management of patients with GBS is outlined in Box 23.14.

CRANIOTOMY

Types of Surgery

A craniotomy is performed to gain access to portions of the central nervous system (CNS) inside the cranium, usually to allow removal of a space-occupying lesion such as a brain tumor (Table 23.3). Common procedures include tumor resection or removal, cerebral decompression, evacuation of hematoma or abscess, and clipping or removal of an aneurysm or AVM. Most patients who undergo craniotomy for tumor resection or removal do not require care in a critical care unit. Patients who do require such care usually need intensive monitoring or are at greater risk for complications because of underlying cardiopulmonary dysfunction or the surgical approach used.[52] Box 23.15 provides definitions of common neurosurgical terms.

Preoperative Care

Protection of the integrity of the CNS is a major priority of care for a patient awaiting a craniotomy. Optimal arterial oxygenation, hemodynamic stability, and cerebral perfusion are essential for maintaining adequate cerebral oxygenation. Management of seizure activity is essential for controlling metabolic needs.

Detailed assessment and documentation of the patient's preoperative neurologic status are imperative for accurate postoperative evaluation. Attention is focused on identifying and describing the nature and extent of any preoperative neurologic deficits. When pituitary surgery is planned, a thorough evaluation of endocrine function is necessary to prevent major intraoperative and postoperative complications.[53]

Trends in health care demand judicious use of routine preoperative studies. Depending on the type of surgery to be performed and the general health of the patient, preoperative screening may include a complete blood cell count; tests for blood urea nitrogen, creatinine, and fasting blood sugar; chest radiography; and electrocardiography. A blood type and crossmatch may also be ordered.[54]

Preoperative teaching is necessary to prepare the patient and family for what to expect in the postoperative period. A description of the intravascular lines and intracranial catheters used during the postoperative period allows the family to focus on the patient and not be overwhelmed by masses of tubing. Some or all of the patient's hair is shaved off in the operating room, and a large, bulky, turban-like craniotomy dressing is applied. Most patients experience some degree of postoperative eye or facial swelling and periorbital ecchymosis. An explanation of these temporary changes in appearance helps alleviate the shock and fear many patients and families experience in the immediate postoperative period.[54]

All patients who undergo craniotomy require instruction to avoid activities known to provoke sudden changes in ICP. These activities include bending, lifting, straining, and the Valsalva maneuver. Patients commonly elicit the Valsalva maneuver during repositioning in bed by holding their breath and straining with a closed epiglottis. This is prevented effectively by teaching the patient to continue to breathe deeply through the mouth during all position changes.[54]

Patients undergoing transsphenoidal surgery require preparation for the sensations associated with nasal packing. Patients often awaken with alarm because of the inability to breathe through the nose. Preoperative instruction in mouth breathing and avoidance of coughing, sneezing, or blowing of the nose facilitates postoperative cooperation.[53]

The psychosocial issues associated with the prospect of neurosurgery cannot be overemphasized. Few procedures are as threatening as procedures involving the brain or spinal cord. For some patients, the fear of permanent neurologic impairment may be as ominous as or more ominous than the fear of death. Steps to meet the needs of the patient and the family include collaboration with religious and social services personnel, patient-controlled visitation, and provision of as much privacy as the patient's condition permits. The patient and family must be provided with the opportunity to express their fears and concerns jointly and apart from each other.[52]

Surgical Considerations

Although the emphasis in the surgical approach for most other types of surgery is to gain adequate exposure of the surgical site,

TABLE 23.3 Types of Brain Tumors Occurring in Adults

Type	Pathology
Gliomas	
Astrocytomas (grades I–III)	Nonencapsulated, tend to infiltrate brain tissue; arise in any part of brain connective tissue; infiltrate primarily cerebral hemisphere tissue; not well outlined, so difficult to excise completely; grow rapidly—most patients live months to years after diagnosis; tumors assigned grade I–IV, with IV being most malignant
Glioblastoma multiforme (also called astrocytoma grade IV)	
Oligodendroglioma (grades I–III)	
Ependymoma (grades I–IV)	
Medulloblastoma	
Tumors From Support Structures	
Meningiomas	Arise from meningeal coverings of brain; usually benign but may undergo malignant changes; usually encapsulated, and surgical cure possible; recurrence possible
Neuromas (acoustic neuroma, schwannoma)	Arise from Schwann cells inside auditory meatus on vestibular portion of cranial nerve VIII; usually benign but may undergo cellular change and become malignant; will regrow if not completely excised; surgical resection often difficult because of location
Pituitary adenoma	Arise from various tissues; surgical approach usually successful; recurrence possible
Developmental (Congenital) Tumors	
Dermoid, epidermoid, craniopharyngioma	Arise from embryonic tissue in various sites in brain; success of surgical resection depends on location and invasiveness
Angiomas	Arise from vascular structures; usually difficult to resect
Metastatic Tumors	
	Cancer cells spreading to brain via circulatory system; surgical resection difficult; even with treatment, prognosis poor; survival beyond 1–2 y uncommon

From Monahan FD, et al, eds. *Phipps' Medical-Surgical Nursing: Health and Illness Perspective.* 8th ed. St. Louis: Mosby; 2007.

BOX 23.15 Operative Terms

- *Burr hole:* Hole made into the cranium using a special drill
- *Craniotomy:* Surgical opening of the skull
- *Craniectomy:* Removal of a portion of the skull without replacing it
- *Cranioplasty:* Plastic repair of the skull
- *Supratentorial:* Above the tentorium, separating the cerebrum from the cerebellum
- *Infratentorial:* Below the tentorium; includes the brainstem and the cerebellum; an infratentorial surgical approach may be used for temporal or occipital lesions
- *Stereotactic:* Minimally invasive surgical intervention that uses a three-dimensional coordinate system to localize a specific area of the brain for ablation, biopsy, dissection, or radiosurgery

the neurosurgeon must select a route that also produces the least amount of disruption to the intracranial contents. Neural tissue is unforgiving. A significant portion of neurologic trauma and postoperative deficits is related to the surgical pathway through the brain tissue, rather than to the procedure performed at the site of pathology. Depending on the location of the lesion and the surgical route chosen, a transcranial or a transsphenoidal approach is used to open the skull.

Transcranial Approach

In the transcranial approach, a scalp incision is made, and a series of burr holes is drilled into the skull to form an outline of the area to be opened (Fig. 23.6). A special saw is used to cut between the holes. In most cases, the bone flap is left attached to the muscle to create a hinge effect. In some cases, the bone flap is removed completely and placed in the abdomen for later retrieval and implantation or discarded and replaced with synthetic material. Next, the dura mater is opened and retracted. After the intracranial procedure, the dura mater and the bone flap are closed, the muscles and scalp are sutured, and a turban-like dressing is applied.[52]

Transsphenoidal Approach

The transsphenoidal approach is the technique of choice for removal of a pituitary tumor without extension into the intracranial vault (Fig. 23.7).[53,54] This approach involves creating a microsurgical entrance into the cranial vault through the nasal cavity. The sphenoid sinus is entered to reach the anterior wall of the sella turcica. The sphenoid bone and the dura mater are then opened to gain intracranial access. After removal of the tumor, the surgical bed is packed with a small section of adipose tissue grafted from the patient's abdomen or thigh. After closure of the intranasal structures, nasal splints and soft packing or nasal tampons impregnated with antibiotic ointment are placed in the nasal cavities. Occasionally, epistaxis balloons are used instead. A nasal drip pad or mustache-type dressing is placed at the base of the nose to catch surgical drainage.[52]

The patient may be placed in the supine, prone, or sitting position for a craniotomy procedure. A skull clamp connected to skull pins is used to position and secure the patient's head throughout the operation. During a transsphenoidal approach or a transcranial approach into the infratentorial area, the patient's head is elevated during surgery. This position places the patient at risk for an air embolism. Air can enter the vascular system through the edges of the dura mater or a venous opening. Continuous monitoring of the patient's heart sounds by Doppler signal allows immediate recognition of this complication. If air embolism occurs, an attempt may be made to withdraw the embolus from the right atrium through a central

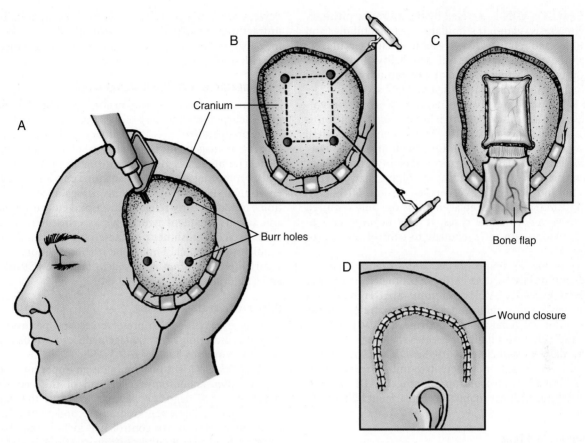

FIG. 23.6 Craniotomy Procedure. (A) Burr holes are drilled into skull. (B) Skull is cut between burr holes with a surgical saw. (C) Bone flap is turned back to expose cranial contents. (D) After surgery, bone flap is replaced, and wound is closed. (From Monahan FD, et al. editors: *Phipps' Medical-Surgical Nursing: Health and Illness Perspective.* 8th ed. St. Louis: Mosby; 2007.)

FIG. 23.7 Transsphenoidal Hypophysectomy.

line. Flooding the surgical field with irrigation fluid and placing a moistened sterile surgical sponge over the surgical site creates an immediate barrier to any further air entrance.[52]

Postoperative Medical Management

Definitive management of a postoperative neurosurgical patient varies, depending on the underlying reason for the craniotomy.

During the initial postoperative period, management is usually directed toward the prevention of complications. Complications associated with a craniotomy include intracranial hypertension, surgical hemorrhage, fluid imbalance, cerebrospinal fluid leak, and DVT.

Intracranial Hypertension

Postoperative cerebral edema is expected to peak 48 to 72 hours after surgery. If the bone flap is not replaced at the time of surgery, intracranial hypertension will produce bulging at the surgical site. Close monitoring of the surgical site is important so that integrity of the incision can be maintained. Management of intracranial hypertension after craniotomy is usually accomplished through CSF drainage, patient positioning, and steroid administration.[54]

Surgical Hemorrhage

Surgical hemorrhage after a transcranial procedure can occur in the intracranial vault and manifests as signs and symptoms of increasing ICP. Hemorrhage after a transsphenoidal craniotomy may be evident from external drainage, the patient's complaint of persistent postnasal drip, or excessive swallowing. Loss of vision after pituitary surgery indicates an evolving hemorrhage. Postoperative hemorrhage requires surgical reexploration.[55]

Fluid Imbalance

Fluid imbalance in a patient after craniotomy usually results from a disturbance in production or secretion of antidiuretic hormone (ADH). ADH is secreted by the posterior pituitary (neurohypophysis) gland. It stimulates the renal tubules and collecting ducts to retain water in response to low circulating blood volume or increased serum osmolality. Inoperative trauma or postoperative edema of the pituitary gland or hypothalamus can result in insufficient ADH secretion. The outcome is unabated renal water loss even when blood volume is low and serum osmolality is high. This condition is known as *diabetes insipidus* (DI). The polyuria associated with DI is often more than 200 mL/h. Urine specific gravity of 1.005 or less and elevated serum osmolality provide evidence of insufficient ADH. The loss of volume may provoke hypotension and inadequate cerebral perfusion. DI is usually self-limiting, and fluid replacement is the only required therapy. However, in some cases, it may be necessary to administer vasopressin intravenously to control the loss of fluid.[56]

The syndrome of inappropriate antidiuretic hormone (SIADH) commonly occurs with neurologic insult and results from excessive ADH secretion. SIADH manifests as inappropriate water retention with hyponatremia in the presence of normal renal function. Urine specific gravity is elevated, and urine osmolality is greater than serum osmolality. The dangers associated with SIADH include circulating volume overload and electrolyte imbalance, both of which may impair neurologic functioning. SIADH is usually self-limiting, with the mainstay of treatment being fluid restriction.[56]

Cerebrospinal Fluid Leak

Leakage of CSF results from an opening in the subarachnoid space, as evidenced by clear fluid draining from the surgical site. When this complication occurs after transsphenoidal surgery, it is evidenced by excessive, clear drainage from the nose or persistent postnasal drip.[57] To differentiate CSF drainage from postoperative serous drainage, a specimen is tested for glucose content. A CSF leak is confirmed by glucose values of 30 mg/dL or greater. Management of a patient with a CSF leak includes bed rest and head elevation. Lumbar puncture or placement of a lumbar subarachnoid catheter may be used to reduce CSF pressure until the dura mater heals. The risk of meningitis associated with CSF leak often necessitates surgical repair to reseal the opening.[58]

Deep Vein Thrombosis

Patients who have undergone neurosurgery are at particularly high risk for development of DVT. Research has demonstrated that these patients have a variety of additional risk factors, including preoperative leg weakness, longer preoperative and postoperative stay in the critical care unit, longer operative procedure time, prone positioning on frames with flexion of the hips or knees, longer time in the postanesthesia care unit, more days on bed rest, lengthy operative procedures, and delay of postoperative mobility and activity.[59,60] Clinical manifestations of DVT include leg or calf pain and erythema, warmth, and swelling of the affected limb. However, a patient with a DVT is often asymptomatic, and the diagnosis is not made until the patient experiences a pulmonary embolus.[61] The primary treatment for DVT is prophylaxis. After neurosurgery, sequential (intermittent) pneumatic compression sleeves are effective in reducing the incidence of DVT. Effectiveness is enhanced when these devices are initiated in the preoperative period. Low-dose unfractionated heparin or low-molecular-weight heparin may also be used prophylactically in high-risk patients when the risk of bleeding has decreased.[62]

Postoperative Nursing Management

The nursing management plan for a patient after neurosurgery incorporates a variety of nursing diagnoses (Box 23.16). As in preoperative care, the primary goal of postcraniotomy nursing management is protection of the integrity of the CNS. The nurse has a significant role in preserving adequate CPP, promoting arterial oxygenation, providing comfort and emotional support, maintaining surveillance for complications, initiating early rehabilitation, and educating the patient and family. Frequent neurologic assessment is necessary to evaluate accomplishment of these objectives and to identify problems and quickly intervene if complications do arise. A ventriculostomy often is placed to facilitate ICP monitoring and CSF drainage.

Preserve Cerebral Perfusion

Nursing interventions to preserve cerebral perfusion include patient positioning, fluid management, and avoidance of postoperative vomiting and fever.

Positioning. Patient positioning is an important component of care after craniotomy. The head of the bed should be elevated 30 to 45 degrees at all times to reduce the incidence of hemorrhage, facilitate venous drainage, and control ICP. Other positioning measures to control ICP include maintaining the patient's head in a neutral position at all times and avoiding neck or hip flexion. These rules of positioning must be followed throughout all nursing activities, including linen changes and transporting the patient for diagnostic evaluation. Most patients after craniotomy can be turned from side to side within these restrictions, using pillows for support, except in some cases of extensive tumor removal, cranioplasty, and when the bone flap is not replaced. Specific orders from the surgeon must be obtained in these instances. A patient with an infratentorial incision may be restricted to only a very small pillow under the head to prevent strain on the incision. Avoidance of anterior or lateral neck flexion also protects the integrity of this type of incision.

Fluid management. Fluid management is another important component of postcraniotomy care. Hourly monitoring of fluid intake and output facilitates early identification of fluid imbalance. Urine specific gravity must be measured if DI is suspected. Fluid restriction may be ordered as a routine measure to lessen the severity of cerebral edema or as

---

⊚ **BOX 23.16   NURSING DIAGNOSES**

Craniotomy

- Decreased Intracranial Adaptive Capacity related to failure of normal intracranial compensatory mechanisms, p. 1018
- Ineffective Cerebral Tissue Perfusion, p 1042
- Acute Pain related to transmission and perception of cutaneous, visceral, muscular, or ischemic impulses, p. 1010
- Disturbed Body Image related to actual change in body structure, function, or appearance, p. 1022

treatment for the fluid and electrolyte imbalances associated with SIADH.[56]

Avoidance of vomiting and fever. Postoperative vomiting must be avoided to prevent sharp spikes in ICP and possibly surgical hemorrhage. Antiemetics are administered as soon as nausea is apparent. Early nutrition in the patient is beneficial. If the patient is unable to eat, enteral hyperalimentation delivered through a feeding tube is the preferred method of nutrition support and can be initiated 24 hours after surgery. Postoperative fever may also adversely affect ICP and increase the metabolic needs of the brain. Acetaminophen is administered orally, rectally, or through a feeding tube. External cooling measures such as a hypothermia blanket may be necessary.

Promote Arterial Oxygenation

Routine pulmonary care is used to maintain airway clearance and prevent pulmonary complications. To prevent dangerous elevations in ICP, this care measure must be performed using proper technique and at time intervals that are adequately spaced from other patient care activities. If pulmonary complications arise, consideration must be given to maintaining adequate oxygenation during repositioning. It may be necessary to restrict turning to only the side that places the good lung down.

Provide Comfort and Emotional Support

Pain management in patients after craniotomy primarily involves control of headache. Small doses of intravenous morphine are used in the critical care setting. Oral analgesics should be started as soon as can be tolerated. Nonopioid medications such as tramadol may be used as an adjunct medication.[63] Because opioid analgesics cause constipation, administration of stool softeners and initiation of a bowel program are important components of postcraniotomy care. Constipation is hazardous because straining to have a bowel movement can create significant elevations in blood pressure and ICP.

Maintain Surveillance for Complications

Following neurosurgery, patients are at risk for infection, corneal abrasions, and injury from falls or seizures.

Infection. After neurosurgery, patients are at risk for a variety of infections, including meningitis, cerebral abscesses, bone flap infections, and subdural empyema.[64] Care of the incision and surgical dressings is specific to the institution and the physician. The rule of thumb for a craniotomy dressing is to reinforce it as needed and change it only on a physician's order. A drain is often left in place to facilitate decompression of the surgical site. If a ventriculostomy is present, it is treated as a component of the surgical site. All drainage devices must be secured to the dressing to prevent unintentional displacement with patient movement. Sterile technique is required to prevent infection. Postoperatively, infection should be suspected if the patient exhibits signs of mental status changes, headache, fever, and purulent drainage and swelling around the incision site.[64]

Corneal abrasions. Routine eye care may be necessary to prevent corneal drying and ulceration. Periorbital edema interferes with normal blinking and eyelid closure, which are essential to adequate corneal lubrication. Saline drops are instilled every 2 hours. If the patient remains in a comatose state, covering the eyes with a polyethylene film extending over the orbits and eyebrows may be beneficial.[13,65]

Injury. After craniotomy, the patient may experience periods of altered mentation. Protection from injury may require the use of restraint devices. The side rails of the bed must be padded to protect the patient from injury. Having a family member stay at the bedside or the use of music therapy is often helpful to keep the patient calm during periods of restlessness. In rare circumstances, continuous sedation with or without neuromuscular blockade may be necessary to control patient activity and metabolic needs on a short-term basis.

Initiate Early Rehabilitation

Increased activity, including ambulation, is begun as soon as tolerated by the patient in the postoperative period. Rehabilitation measures and discharge planning may begin in the critical care unit, but discussion is beyond the scope of this chapter. Transfer to a general care or rehabilitation unit is usually accomplished as soon as the patient is deemed stable and free of complications.

Educate the Patient and Family

Preoperatively, the patient and family should be taught about the precipitating event necessitating the need for the craniotomy and its expected outcome (Box 23.17). The severity of the disease and the need for critical care management postoperatively must be stressed. As the patient moves toward discharge, teaching focuses on medication instructions, incisional care including the signs of infection, and the signs and symptoms of increased ICP. If the patient has neurologic deficits, teaching focuses on the interventions to maximize the patient's rehabilitation potential, and the patient's family members must be encouraged to participate in the patient's care and to learn some basic rehabilitation techniques. The importance of participating in a neurologic rehabilitation program must be stressed.

INTRACRANIAL HYPERTENSION

Pathophysiology

The intracranial space comprises three components: (1) brain substance (80%), (2) CSF (10%), and (3) blood (10%). Under

---

✳ BOX 23.17   PATIENT EDUCATION PLAN

Craniotomy

Before the patient's discharge, the patient should be able to teach back the following topics:

Before Surgery
- Pathophysiology and expected outcome of underlying disease
- Need for intensive care management after surgery
- Routine preoperative surgical care

After Surgery
- Routine postoperative surgical care
- Discharge medications—purpose, dosage, and side effects
- Incisional care
- Signs and symptoms of infection
- Signs and symptoms of increased intracranial pressure
- Measures to compensate for residual deficits
- Basic rehabilitation techniques
- Importance of participating in neurologic rehabilitation program
  Additional information for the patient can be found at the following website:
- National Brain Tumor Society website (www.braintumor.org)

normal physiologic conditions, the mean ICP is maintained at less than 15 mm Hg.[66-68] Essential to understanding the pathophysiology of ICP, the Monro-Kellie hypothesis proposes that an increase in volume of one intracranial component must be compensated by a decrease in one or more of the other components so that total volume remains fixed. This compensation, although limited, includes displacing CSF from the intracranial vault to the lumbar cistern, increasing CSF absorption, and compressing the low-pressure venous system.[67,68] Pathophysiologic alterations that can elevate ICP are outlined in Table 23.4.

Volume-Pressure Curve

When capable of compliance, the brain can tolerate significant increases in intracranial volume without much increase in ICP. However, the amount of intracranial compliance has a limit. After this limit has been reached, a state of decompensation with increased ICP results. As the ICP increases, the relationship between volume and pressure changes and small increases in volume may cause major elevations in ICP (Fig. 23.8).[67] The exact configuration of the volume-pressure curve and the point at which the steep increase in pressure occurs vary among patients. The configuration of this curve is also influenced by the cause and the rate of volume increases within the

intracranial vault; for example, neurologic deterioration occurs more rapidly in a patient with an acute epidural hematoma than in a patient with a meningioma of the same size.[66] Regardless of how fast the pressure increases, intracranial hypertension occurs when ICP is greater than 20 mm Hg.[67]

Cerebral Blood Flow and Autoregulation

CBF corresponds to the metabolic demands of the brain and is normally 50 mL/100 g of brain tissue/min. Although the brain makes up only 2% of body weight, it requires 15% to 20% of the resting cardiac output and 15% of the body's oxygen demands. The normal brain has a complex capacity to maintain constant CBF, despite wide ranges in systemic arterial pressure—an effect known as *autoregulation.* A mean arterial pressure of 50 to 150 mm Hg does not alter CBF when autoregulation is functioning. Outside the limits of this autoregulation, CBF becomes passively dependent on the perfusion pressure.[67]

Factors other than arterial blood pressure that affect CBF are conditions that result in acidosis, alkalosis, and changes in metabolic rate. Conditions that cause acidosis (eg, hypoxia, hypercapnia, ischemia) result in cerebrovascular dilation. Conditions causing alkalosis (eg, hypocapnia) result in cerebrovascular constriction. Normally, a reduction in metabolic rate (eg, from hypothermia or barbiturates) decreases CBF, and increases in metabolic rate (eg, from hyperthermia) increase CBF.[66,69]

Arterial blood gases exert a profound effect on CBF. Carbon dioxide, which affects the pH of the blood, is a potent vasoactive substance. Carbon dioxide retention (hypercapnia) leads to cerebral vasodilation, with increased cerebral blood volume, whereas hypocapnia leads to cerebral vasoconstriction and a reduction in cerebral blood volume. However, prolonged hypocapnia, especially at an arterial partial pressure of carbon dioxide ($Paco_2$) level less than 20 mm Hg, can lead to cerebral ischemia. Low arterial partial pressure of oxygen (Pao_2) levels, especially less than 40 mm Hg, lead to cerebral vasodilation, which increases the intracranial blood volume and can

TABLE 23.4 **Mechanisms of Intracranial Pressure Elevation**	
Pathophysiology	**Examples**
Disorders of CSF	
Overproduction of CSF	Choroid plexus tumors (papilloma or carcinoma)
Communicating hydrocephalus	Obstructed arachnoid villi
	Old subarachnoid hemorrhage
Noncommunicating hydrocephalus	Posterior fossa tumor obstructing aqueduct
	Aqueductal stenosis
Interstitial edema	Any of above
Disorders of Intracranial Blood Flow	
Intracranial hemorrhage	Epidural hematoma
	Subdural hematoma
	Intraparenchymal hematoma
Vasospasm	Subarachnoid hemorrhage
Vasodilation	Elevated $Paco_2$
Increasing cerebral blood volume	Hypoxia
Disorders of Brain Substance	
Expanding mass lesion with local vasogenic edema	Brain tumor
	Abscess
	Brain injury
	Ischemic stroke
Ischemic brain injury with cytotoxic edema	Anoxic brain injury
	Hypoxic encephalopathy
Increased cerebral metabolic rate increasing CBF	Seizures
	Hyperthermia

CBF, cerebral blood flow; *CSF,* cerebrospinal fluid; *Paco₂,* arterial partial pressure of carbon dioxide.

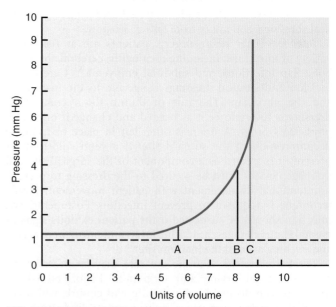

FIG. 23.8 Intracranial Volume-Pressure Curve. (A) Pressure is normal, and increases in intracranial volume are tolerated without increases in intracranial pressure. (B) Increases in volume may cause increases in pressure. (C) Small increases in volume may cause larger increases in pressure.

contribute to increased ICP. High Pao$_2$ levels have not been shown to affect CBF in either direction.[66,69]

Assessment and Diagnosis

The numerous signs and symptoms of increased ICP include decreased LOC, Cushing triad (bradycardia, systolic hypertension, and widening pulse pressure), diminished brainstem reflexes, papilledema, decerebrate posturing (abnormal extension), decorticate posturing (abnormal flexion), unequal pupil size, projectile vomiting, decreased pupillary reaction to light, altered breathing patterns, and headache.[70] Patients may exhibit one or all of these symptoms, depending on the underlying cause of the elevation in ICP. One of the earliest and most important signs of increased ICP is a decrease in the LOC. This change must be reported immediately to the physician.[69,70]

In a patient with suspected intracranial hypertension, a monitoring device may be placed within the cranium to quantify ICP. Under normal physiologic conditions, the mean ICP is maintained at less than 15 mm Hg. The device is used to monitor serial ICPs and assist with the management of intracranial hypertension. An increase in ICP can decrease blood flow to the brain, causing brain damage. The monitoring device can also provide a sterile access for draining excess CSF. The four sites for monitoring ICP are the intraventricular space, the subarachnoid space, the epidural space, and the parenchyma. Each site has advantages and disadvantages for monitoring ICP. The type of monitor chosen depends on the suspected pathologic condition and the physician's preferences.[68-71] Chapter 22 provides a more detailed discussion of ICP monitoring.

Medical and Nursing Management

After intracranial hypertension is documented, therapy must be prompt to prevent secondary insults (Fig. 23.9). Although the exact pressure level denoting intracranial hypertension is uncertain, most current evidence suggests that ICP generally must be treated when it exceeds 20 mm Hg.[66,69] All therapies are directed toward reducing the volume of one or more of the components (eg, blood, brain, CSF) that lie within the intracranial vault. A major goal of therapy is to determine the cause of the elevated pressure and, if possible, to remove the cause.[66,69] In the absence of a surgically treatable mass lesion, intracranial hypertension is treated medically. Nurses play an important role in rapid assessment and implementation of appropriate therapies for reducing ICP.

Positioning and Other Nursing Activities

Positioning of the patient is a significant factor in the prevention and treatment of intracranial hypertension. Head elevation has long been advocated as a conventional nursing intervention to control ICP, presumably by increasing venous return; however, this may decrease CPP. Close monitoring of ICP and CPP should be done with positioning, customizing positioning to maximize CPP and minimize ICP.[68]

Positions that impede venous return from the brain cause elevations in ICP. Obstruction of jugular veins or an increase in intrathoracic or intraabdominal pressure is communicated as increased pressure throughout the open venous system, impeding drainage from the brain and increasing ICP. Positions that decrease venous return from the head (eg, Trendelenburg, prone, extreme flexion of the hips, and angulation of the neck) must be avoided if possible. If changes to positions such as Trendelenburg are necessary to provide adequate pulmonary care, critical care nurses must closely monitor ICP and vital signs.[66]

Some routine nursing activities affect ICP and may be harmful. Use of positive end-expiratory pressures greater than 20 cm H$_2$O, coughing, suctioning, tight tracheostomy tube ties, and Valsalva maneuver have been associated with increases in ICP. Cumulative increases in ICP have been reported when care activities are performed one after another. Conversely, family contact and gentle touch have been associated with decreases in ICP.[66]

Hyperventilation

Controlled hyperventilation has been an important adjunct of therapy for patients with increased ICP. The rationale employed in hyperventilation is that if Paco$_2$ can be reduced from its normal level of 35 to 40 mm Hg to a range of 25 to 30 mm Hg in a patient with intracranial hypertension, vasoconstriction of cerebral arteries, reduction of CBF, and increased venous return will result. This practice is being reexamined. Additional research has indicated that severe or prolonged hyperventilation can reduce cerebral perfusion and lead to cerebral ischemia and infarction.[72] The current trend is to maintain Paco$_2$ levels on the lower side of normal (35 mm Hg ± 2) by carefully monitoring arterial blood gas measurements and by adjusting ventilator settings.[68-71]

Although hypoxemia must be avoided, excessively high levels of oxygen offer no benefits, and increasing inspired oxygen concentrations to greater than 60% may lead to toxic changes in lung tissue. The use of pulse oximetry has led to greater awareness of the circumstances, such as pain and anxiety, which can cause oxygen desaturation and elevate ICP.[66]

Temperature Control

Directly proportional to body temperature, cerebral metabolic rate increases 7% per 1°C of increase in body temperature.[69,70] This fact is significant because as the cerebral metabolic rate increases, blood flow to the brain must increase to meet the tissue demands. To avoid the increase in blood volume associated with an increased cerebral metabolic rate, nurses must prevent hyperthermia in a patient with a brain injury. Antipyretics and cooling devices must be used when appropriate while the source of the fever is being determined.[69,70]

Blood Pressure Control

Maintenance of arterial blood pressure in the high-normal range is essential in patients with brain injury. Inadequate perfusion pressure decreases the supply of nutrients and oxygen requirements for cerebral metabolic needs. However, a blood pressure that is too high increases cerebral blood volume and may increase ICP.[69] Fig. 23.10 shows the relationship between blood pressure and ICP.

Control of systemic hypertension may require nothing more than the administration of a sedative agent. Small, frequent doses may be sufficient to blunt noxious stimuli and prevent them from triggering increases in blood pressure. When sedation proves inadequate in controlling systemic arterial hypertension, antihypertensive agents are used. Care must be taken in choosing these agents because many of the peripheral vasodilators (eg, nitroprusside, nitroglycerin) also are cerebral vasodilators. All antihypertensives are believed to cause some degree

POSTCRANIOTOMY – INTRACRANIAL HTN

Pathophysiology – Increase of Fluid in Brain

Intracranial volume shift displaces CSF from intracranial vault → lumbar cistern → ↑ CSF absorption → compresses low-pressure venous system.

Intracranial HTN → ICP > 20 mm Hg

- Postop cerebral edema peaks 48-72 hours after surgery.
- Without bone flap, intracranial HTN → bulging.

Assessment & Diagnosis

↓ LOC, Cushing triad, ↓ brainstem reflexes, papilledema, decerebrate & decorticate posturing, unequal pupil size, projectile vomiting, ↓ pupillary reaction to light, altered breathing patterns, & headache.

Patient may have one or all - S/S of ↑ ICP

- ↑ ICP: ↓ LOC, Cushing triad, papilledema, posturing, pupil changes, projectile vomiting, altered breathing patterns, & headache.
- Early & significant sign of ↑ ICP is ↓ LOC.

PRIORITY NURSING DIAGNOSES

- Risk for Ineffective Cerebral Tissue Perfusion.
- Impaired Verbal Communication R/T cerebral injury and intubation.
- Impaired Swallowing R/T neuromuscular impairment, fatigue, and limited awareness.
- Anxiety R/T threat to biologic, psychologic, or social integrity.
- Deficient Knowledge: Discharge Regimen R/T lack of previous exposure to information.

Doug Hamad is 48 hours postcraniotomy including removal of a cranial bone flap. Recovering in the Neuro-Intensive Care Unit, his ICP is measured at 23 mm Hg.

Intracranial Hypertension

Results in

↓ Cerebral Perfusion

GOALS OF MEDICAL MANAGEMENT
Early identification → treat symptoms early → ↓ mortality.

- Document intracranial hypertension (ICP > 20 mm Hg).
- Prevent secondary insults.
- ↓ Volume of blood, brain, and/or CSF.
- Determine cause and remove, if possible.
- Prevent complications

The patient will demonstrate adequate cerebral perfusion pressure:

- Maintaining vital functions and develop no further neurologic deterioration.
- Maintaining airway and acceptable ABGs.
- Preserving physiologic body functions.

PATIENT OUTCOMES

COLLABORATIVE CARE INTERVENTIONS

Patient Education Priorities

- Educate about precipitating event, craniotomy, & expected outcomes.
- Critical care management postoperatively.
- Closer to discharge, focus on medications, incisional care, safety, S/S infection & ↑ ICP.
- If neuro deficits present, encourage family to get involved in care and learn basic rehabilitation.
- Participation in support group as indicated for family & patient.

Frequent Neurological Assessments to Identify Problems Early

- Preserve adequate cerebral perfusion pressure.
- Hourly I/O, urine SG if DI suspected, fluid restriction for cerebral edema or to treat SIADH.
- Medicate with antiemetics to avoid vomiting.
- Acetaminophen and/or external cooling for postoperative fever.
- Promote arterial oxygenation.
- Provide comfort and emotional support.
- Maintain surveillance for complications: (infection, corneal abrasions, falls or seizures).
- Initiate early rehabilitation.
- Monitor function of ventriculostomy to facilitate ICP monitoring and sterile access for CSF drainage.

NURSING INTERVENTIONS TO ↓ ICP

Rapid Assessment & Measures to ↓ ICP

- Position patient to achieve maximal ↓ in ICP.
- Reduce environmental stimulation.
- Maintain normothermia.
- Control ventilation to ensure a normal PaCO₂ level (35 ± 2 mm Hg).
- Administer diuretic agents, anticonvulsants, sedation, analgesia, paralytic agents, & vasoactive medications to ensure cerebral perfusion pressure (CPP) > 70 mm Hg.

FIG. 23.9 Concept Map for Intracranial Hypertension. *CPP*, cerebral perfusion pressure; *CSF*, cerebrospinal fluid; *DI*, diabetes insipidus; *HTN*, hypertension; *ICP*, intracranial pressure; *I/O*, intake and output; *LOC*, level of consciousness; *PaCo₂*, partial pressure of carbon dioxide in arterial blood. *R/T*, related to; *S/S*, signs and symptoms; *SG*, specific gravity; *SIADH*, syndrome of inappropriate secretion of antidiuretic hormone. (Concept map illustration created by © DEANNE A. BLACH, MSN, RN.)

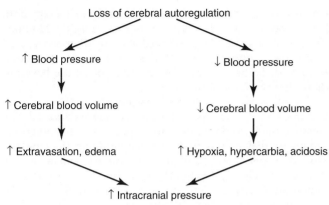

FIG. 23.10 Loss of Pressure Autoregulation.

INTRAVENTRICULAR CATHETER

FIG. 23.11 **Intermittent Drainage System.** Intermittent drainage involves draining cerebrospinal fluid (CSF) through a ventriculostomy when intracranial pressure exceeds the upper pressure parameter set by the physician. Intermittent drainage is achieved by opening the three-way stopcock to allow CSF to flow into the drainage bag for brief periods (30–120 seconds) until the pressure is below the upper pressure parameter. (From Barker E, ed. *Neuroscience Nursing: A Spectrum of Care.* 3rd ed. St. Louis: Mosby; 2008.)

of cerebral vasodilation. To reduce this vasodilating effect, concurrent treatment with beta-blockers (eg, metoprolol, labetalol) may be beneficial.[66,69]

Systemic hypotension should be treated aggressively with fluids to maintain a systolic blood pressure greater than 90 mm Hg. Crystalloids, colloids, and blood products can be used, depending on the patient's condition. Studies have demonstrated a positive effect on ICP and CPP with hypertonic saline.[73] If fluids fail to adequately elevate the patient's blood pressure, the use of inotropic agents may be necessary.[66]

Seizure Control

The incidence of posttraumatic seizures in patients with head injury has been estimated to be 15% to 20%. Because of the risk of a secondary ischemic insult associated with seizures, many physicians prescribe anticonvulsant medications prophylactically. Seizures cause metabolic requirements to increase, which results in elevation of CBF, cerebral blood volume, and ICP, even in paralyzed patients. If blood flow cannot match demand, ischemia develops, cerebral energy stores are depleted, and irreversible neuronal destruction occurs.[69] Phenytoin is the recommended medication for seizure prophylaxis. A loading dose of 15 to 20 mg/kg is administered intravenously over 30 minutes followed by 100 mg intravenously every 8 hours, titrated to therapeutic level, for 7 days.[74,75] Fast-acting, short-duration agents such as lorazepam may be indicated for breakthrough seizures until therapeutic medication levels can be achieved.

Cerebrospinal Fluid Drainage

CSF drainage for intracranial hypertension may be used with other treatment modalities (Figs. 23.11 and 23.12). CSF drainage is accomplished by the insertion of a pliable catheter into the anterior horn of the lateral ventricle (ventriculostomy), preferably on the nondominant side. This drainage can help support the patient through periods of cerebral edema by controlling spikes in ICP. A major advantage of ventriculostomy is its dual role as a monitoring device and a treatment modality.[76] Care should be taken to avoid infection. However, cleansing ointment such as bacitracin or povidone is not recommended. Ventriculitis occurs in 10% to 20% of patients with a ventriculostomy.[77]

Hyperosmolar Therapy

Osmotic diuretics and hypertonic saline have also been used to reduce increased ICP. In the presence of an intact blood–brain barrier, hyperosmolar therapy is used to draw water from brain

FIG. 23.12 **Continuous Drainage System.** Continuous drainage involves placing the drip chamber of the drainage system at a specified level above the foramen of Monro (usually 15 cm). The system is left open to allow continuous drainage of cerebrospinal fluid into the chamber (which drains into a collection bag) against a pressure gradient that prevents excessive drainage and ventricular collapse.

tissue into the intravascular compartment. The direction of flow is from the hypoconcentrated tissue to the hyperconcentrated cerebral vasculature. If the situation becomes reversed and the tissue becomes hyperconcentrated in relation to the cerebral vasculature, a rebound phenomenon may occur. These agents have little direct effect on edematous cerebral tissue situated in an area of a defective blood–brain barrier; instead, they require an intact blood–brain barrier for osmosis to occur.[69,78]

The most widely used osmotic diuretic is mannitol, a large-molecule agent that is retained almost entirely in the extracellular compartment and has little of the rebound effect observed with other osmotic diuretics. Administration of mannitol increases CBF and induces cerebral vasoconstriction as part of the brain's autoregulatory response to keep blood flow constant.[69,78]

Perhaps the most common difficulty associated with the use of osmotic agents is the provocation of electrolyte disturbances. Careful attention must be paid to body weight and fluid and electrolyte stability. Serum osmolality must be kept between 300 and 320 mOsm/L. Hypernatremia and hypokalemia often are associated with repeated administration of osmotic agents. Central venous pressure readings must be monitored to prevent hypovolemia. Smaller doses of mannitol simplify fluid and electrolyte management, and their use is encouraged whenever possible.[78]

Hypertonic saline, given in concentrations ranging from 3% to 23.4%, can also be used to treat increased ICP. Some studies suggest that hypertonic saline is as equally effective as mannitol for reducing increased ICP.[73] Adverse effects include electrolyte abnormalities, hypotension, pulmonary edema, acute renal failure, hemolysis, central pontine myelinolysis, coagulopathy, and dysrhythmias.[78]

Control of Metabolic Demand

Any treatment modality that increases the incidence of noxious stimulation to the patient carries with it the potential for increasing ICP. Noxious stimuli include pain, the presence of an endotracheal tube, coughing, suctioning, repositioning, bathing, and many other routine nursing interventions. Agents used to reduce metabolic demands include the use of benzodiazepines such as midazolam and lorazepam, intravenous sedative-hypnotics such as propofol, opioid narcotics such as fentanyl and morphine, and neuromuscular blocking agents such as vecuronium and atracurium. These agents may be administered separately or in combination via continuous drip or as an intravenous bolus on an as-needed basis.[66,79]

The preferred treatment regimen begins with the administration of benzodiazepines for sedation and narcotics for analgesia. If these agents fail to blunt the patient's response to noxious stimuli, propofol or a neuromuscular blocking agent is added. The use of these medications is recommended only in patients who have an ICP monitor in place because sedatives, opioids, and neuromuscular blocking agents affect the reliability of neurologic assessment. The use of neuromuscular blocking agents without sedation is not recommended because these agents can cause skeletal muscle paralysis and because they have no analgesic effect and do not adequately protect the patient from pain and the physiologic responses that can occur from pain-producing procedures.[69,79] If these agents fail to control ICP, barbiturate therapy is considered.

Barbiturate therapy. Barbiturate therapy is a treatment protocol developed for the management of uncontrolled intracranial hypertension that has not responded to the conventional treatments previously described.[69] The two most commonly used medications in high-dose barbiturate therapy are (1) pentobarbital and (2) thiopental. The goal with either medication is a reduction of ICP to 15 to 20 mm Hg while a mean arterial pressure of 70 to 80 mm Hg is maintained.

Patients are maintained on high-dose barbiturate therapy until ICP has been controlled within the normal range for 24 hours. Barbiturates must never be stopped abruptly; they are tapered slowly over approximately 4 days. Despite the theoretical reasons for barbiturate use, clinical trials of its use have not shown improved outcome.[66,74]

Complications of high-dose barbiturate therapy can be disastrous unless a specific and organized approach is used. The most common complications are hypotension, hypothermia, and myocardial depression. If any complications occur and are allowed to persist unchecked, they may cause secondary insults to an already damaged brain. Hypotension, the most common complication, results from peripheral vasodilation and can be compounded in an already dehydrated patient who has received large doses of an osmotic diuretic in an attempt to control ICP. Careful monitoring of fluid status by central venous pressure or a pulmonary artery catheter can help prevent this complication. Myocardial depression results from cardiac muscle suppression and can be avoided by frequent monitoring of fluid status, cardiac output, and serum drug levels. If an adequate cardiac output cannot be maintained in the presence of normothermia, barbiturates must be reduced, regardless of serum levels.[66,79]

Interprofessional collaborative management of intracranial hypertension in a patient is outlined in Box 23.18.

Herniation Syndromes

The goal of neurologic evaluation, ICP monitoring, and treatment of increased ICP is to prevent herniation. Herniation of intracerebral contents results in the shifting of tissue from one compartment of the brain to another and places pressure on cerebral vessels and vital function centers of the brain. If unchecked, herniation rapidly causes death as a result of the cessation of CBF and respirations.[66]

Supratentorial Herniation

The four types of supratentorial herniation syndrome are (1) uncal; (2) central, or transtentorial; (3) cingulate; and (4) transcalvarial (Fig. 23.13).

Uncal herniation. Uncal herniation is the most common herniation syndrome. In uncal herniation, a unilateral, expanding mass lesion, usually of the temporal lobe, increases ICP, causing lateral displacement of the tip of the temporal lobe (uncus). Lateral displacement pushes the uncus over the edge of the tentorium, puts pressure on the oculomotor nerve (cranial nerve III) and the posterior cerebral artery ipsilateral to

---

QSEN BOX 23.18 **QSEN: Teamwork and Collaboration**

Interprofessional Collaborative Practice: Intracranial Hypertension

- Position patient to achieve maximal ICP reduction.
- Reduce environmental stimulation.
- Maintain normothermia.
- Control ventilation to ensure normal Paco$_2$ level (35 mm Hg ± 2).
- Administer diuretic agents, anticonvulsants, sedation, analgesia, paralytic agents, and vasoactive medications to ensure CPP >70 mm Hg.
- Drain cerebrospinal fluid for ICP >20 mm Hg.

CPP, cerebral perfusion pressure; *ICP,* intracranial pressure; *Paco$_2$,* arterial partial pressure of carbon dioxide.

the lesion, and flattens the midbrain against the opposite side. Clinical manifestations of uncal herniation include ipsilateral pupil dilation, decreased LOC, respiratory pattern changes leading to respiratory arrest, and contralateral hemiplegia leading to abnormal flexion (decorticate) or abnormal extension (decerebrate) posturing. If no intervention occurs, uncal herniation results in fixed and dilated pupils, flaccidity, and respiratory arrest.[66,80]

Central herniation. In central, or transtentorial, herniation, an expanding mass lesion of the midline, frontal, parietal, or occipital lobe results in downward displacement of the hemispheres, basal ganglia, and diencephalon through the tentorial notch. Central herniation often is preceded by uncal and cingulate herniation. Clinical manifestations of central herniation include loss of consciousness; small, reactive pupils progressing to fixed, dilated pupils; respiratory changes leading to respiratory arrest; and abnormal flexion (decorticate)

posturing progressing to flaccidity. In the late stages, uncal and central herniation syndromes affect the brainstem similarly.[66,80]

Cingulate herniation. Cingulate herniation occurs when an expanding lesion of one hemisphere shifts laterally and forces the cingulate gyrus under the falx cerebri. Cingulate herniation occurs often. When a lateral shift is observed on CT scan, cingulate herniation has occurred. Little is known about the effects of cingulate herniation, and no accompanying clinical manifestations exist to assist in its diagnosis. Cingulate herniation is not in itself a life-threatening condition, but if the expanding mass lesion that caused cingulate herniation is not controlled, uncal or central herniation will follow.[66,80]

Transcalvarial herniation. Transcalvarial herniation is the extrusion of cerebral tissue through the cranium. In the presence of severe cerebral edema, transcalvarial herniation occurs through an opening from a skull fracture or craniotomy site.[66]

Infratentorial Herniation

The two infratentorial herniation syndromes are (1) upward transtentorial herniation and (2) downward cerebellar herniation.

Upward transtentorial herniation. Upward transtentorial herniation occurs when an expanding mass lesion of the cerebellum causes protrusion of the vermis (central area) of the cerebellum and the midbrain upward through the tentorial notch. Compression of the third cranial nerve and diencephalon occurs. Blockage of the central aqueduct and distortion of the third ventricle obstruct CSF flow. Deterioration progresses rapidly.[66,80]

Downward cerebellar herniation. Downward cerebellar herniation occurs when an expanding lesion of the cerebellum exerts pressure downward, sending the cerebellar tonsils through the foramen magnum. Compression and displacement of the medulla oblongata occur, rapidly resulting in respiratory and cardiac arrest.[66,79]

PHARMACOLOGIC AGENTS

Many pharmacologic agents are used in the care of patients with neurologic disorders. Table 23.5 reviews the various agents used and any special considerations necessary for administering them.

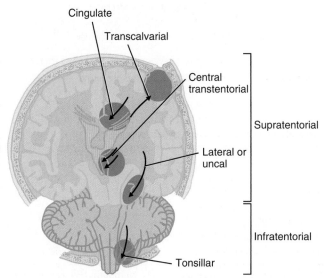

FIG. 23.13 Types of Intracranial Herniation. (From Linton AD, ed. *Introduction to Medical-Surgical Nursing.* 6th ed. St. Louis: Elsevier; 2016.)

TABLE 23.5 Pharmacologic Management

Neurologic Disorders

Medication	Dosage	Action	Special Considerations
Anticonvulsants			
Phenytoin (Dilantin)	Loading dose: 10–20 mg/kg IV	Prevents influx of sodium at cell membrane	Monitor serum levels closely; therapeutic level is 10–20 mg/L (if hypoalbuminuria, monitor free phenytoin serum levels: therapeutic level of 0.1–0.2 mg/L)
	Maintenance dose: 100 mg q6–8h IV		Infuse phenytoin no faster than 50 mg/min; administer with normal saline only because it precipitates with other solutions
Fosphenytoin (Cerebyx)	Loading dose: 15-20 mg/kg IV	Prevents influx of sodium at cell membrane	Monitor serum levels closely; therapeutic level is 10–20 mg/L
	Maintenance dose: 4–6 mg/kg/24 h IV		Dosage, concentration, and infusion rate of fosphenytoin expressed as FE
Barbiturates			
Phenobarbital	Loading dose: 6–8 mg/kg IV	Produces CNS depression and reduces spread of epileptic focus	May depress cardiac and respiratory function
	Maintenance dose: 1–3 mg/kg/24 h IV		Administer phenobarbital at a rate of 60 mg/min; monitor serum level closely; therapeutic level is 15–40 mcg/mL

Continued

TABLE 23.5 Pharmacologic Management—cont'd

Neurologic Disorders

Medication	Dosage	Action	Special Considerations
Pentobarbital	Loading dose: 3–10 mg/kg over 30 min Maintenance dose: 0.5–3 mg/kg/h IV	Induces barbiturate coma	Monitor serum level of pentobarbital closely; therapeutic level for coma is 15–40 mg/L
Osmotic Diuretics			
Mannitol	1–2 g/kg IV	Treats cerebral edema by pulling fluid from extravascular space into intravascular space; requires intact blood–brain barrier	Side effects include hypovolemia and increased serum osmolality
			Monitor serum osmolality and notify physician if >310 mOsm/L
			Warm and shake before administering to ensure crystals are dissolved
Calcium Channel Blockers			
Nimodipine (Nimotop)	60 mg q4h NG or PO for 21 days	Decreases cerebral vasospasm	Side effects include hypotension, palpitations, headache, and dizziness
			Monitor blood pressure frequently when implementing therapy
Local Anesthetics			
Lidocaine	50–100 mg IV or 2 mL of 4% solution	Blunts effects of tracheal stimulation on intracranial pressure	Must be administered not longer than 5 min before suctioning
Thrombolytics			
tPA	0.9 mg/kg total, with 10% of dose administered as IV bolus over 1 min and 90% of dose administered as continuous IV infusion over 1 h	Converts plasminogen to plasmin to dissolve clot	Treatment must start within 4.5 h of onset of symptoms
			Do not exceed 90 mg
			Do not use anticoagulants during the first 24 h
			Monitor patient for bleeding

CNS, central nervous system; *FE*, phenytoin sodium equivalents; *IV*, intravenous/intravenously; *NG*, nasogastric; *PO*, by mouth; *tPA*, tissue-type plasminogen activator.

Data from *ClinicalKey Drug Monographs*. https://www.clinicalkey.com/#!/browse/drugs. Accessed May 12, 2016.

CASE STUDY 23.1   Patient With a Neurologic Problem

Brief Patient History

Mr. P is a 24-year-old man. While he was water skiing, he was hit by a boat. He was rescued from the water by friends. He was immobilized and transported to the hospital by paramedics called to the scene.

Clinical Assessment

Mr. P is admitted to the emergency department with abrasions and bruising to his head and shoulders. He is having difficulty breathing and is unable to move his extremities. He complains of neck pain, and he has a cervical collar in place. He has urinary and fecal incontinence. He does not have motor, sensory, or deep tendon reflexes from the neck to the feet. He is awake and able to talk.

Diagnostic Procedures

Magnetic resonance imaging (MRI) performed on admission showed an incomplete spinal cord transection. Baseline vital signs include the following: blood pressure of 85/60 mm Hg, heart rate of 48 beats/min (sinus bradycardia),

respiratory rate of 8 breaths/min, temperature of 99.3°F, and oxygen saturation of 88%. The Glasgow Coma Scale score was 10.

Medical Diagnosis

Mr. P is diagnosed with an incomplete spinal cord transection and neurogenic shock.

Questions

1. What major outcomes do you expect to achieve for this patient?
2. What problems or risks must be managed to achieve these outcomes?
3. What interventions must be initiated to monitor, prevent, manage, or eliminate the problems and risks identified?
4. What interventions should be initiated to promote optimal functioning, safety, and well-being of the patient?
5. What possible learning needs do you anticipate for this patient?
6. What cultural and age-related factors may have a bearing on the patient's plan of care?

SUMMARY

Stroke

- A stroke is the sudden onset of an acute neurologic deficit persisting for more than 24 hours, and it is caused by the interruption of blood flow to the brain.
- Strokes are classified as ischemic or hemorrhagic. Hemorrhagic strokes can be further categorized as SAHs (cerebral aneurysms and AVMs) and ICHs.
- Nursing interventions focus on monitoring for changes in neurologic status, maintaining surveillance for complications, providing comfort and emotional support, initiating rehabilitation measures, and educating the patient and family.

Ischemic Stroke

- The two main causes of ischemic stroke are thrombosis and embolism, resulting in a neuronal tissue injury from decreased or absent blood flow.
- The characteristic sign of an ischemic stroke is the sudden onset of focal neurologic signs persisting for more than 24 hours. The signs depend on the affected portion of the brain.
- Medical management focuses on preservation of brain tissue through fibrinolytic therapy, management of blood pressure, and treatment of complications.

Subarachnoid Hemorrhage

- SAH is bleeding into the subarachnoid space, and it is usually caused by rupture of a cerebral aneurysm or AVM.
- Medical management focuses on preservation of neurologic function, support of vital functions, and treatment of complications (rebleeding, vasospasm, hyponatremia, and hydrocephalus).

Intracerebral Hemorrhage

- ICH is bleeding directly into cerebral tissue, and it is usually caused by rupture of a small artery in the brain resulting from hypertension.
- Medical management focuses on preservation of neurologic function, control of blood pressure, support of vital functions, and management of intracranial hypertension.

Coma

- The two main causes of coma are structural (eg, ischemic stroke, ICH, trauma, brain tumors) and metabolic (eg, drug overdose, infectious diseases, endocrine disorders, poisonings).
- Coma is the deepest state of unconsciousness; arousal and awareness are lacking as a result of diffuse dysfunction of both cerebral hemispheres or diffuse or focal dysfunction of the RAS.
- Medical management focuses on identification and treatment of the underlying cause of the condition and support of vital functions.
- Nursing interventions focus on supporting all body functions, maintaining surveillance for complications, providing comfort and emotional support, initiating rehabilitation measures, and educating the patient and family.

Guillain-Barré Syndrome

- Guillain-Barré syndrome involves a rapidly progressive, ascending peripheral nerve dysfunction leading to paralysis that may produce respiratory failure.
- Medical management focuses on support of vital functions and the administration of treatments to limit the duration of the syndrome.
- Nursing interventions focus on maintaining surveillance for complications, initiating rehabilitative measures, providing comfort and emotional support, and educating the patient and family about the disorder.

Craniotomy

- A craniotomy is performed to gain access to portions of the CNS inside the cranium for the purposes of tumor resection or removal, cerebral decompression, evacuation of hematoma or abscess, or repair of an aneurysm or AVM.
- Postoperative medical management focuses on preventing complications, including intracranial hypertension, hemorrhage, fluid imbalances, CSF leaks, and DVT.
- Nursing interventions focus on positioning the patient's head in accordance with the physician's orders, monitoring the patient's intake and output, administering medications to control vomiting and fever, promoting postoperative pulmonary care, providing comfort and emotional support, maintaining surveillance for complications, initiating rehabilitative measures, and education of the patient and family.

Intracranial Hypertension

- One of the earliest signs of increased ICP is a decrease in LOC.
- ICP can be measured using an ICP monitor, and it should be treated when it exceeds 20 mm Hg.
- Medical and nursing management is directed toward reducing the volume of one or more of the components (eg, blood, brain, CSF) that lie within the intracranial vault.
- Herniation of intracerebral contents results in the shifting of tissue from one compartment of the brain to another and places pressure on cerebral vessels and vital function centers of the brain. If unchecked, it rapidly causes death.

ⓔ Visit the Evolve site for additional study materials.

REFERENCES

1. Mozaffarian D, et al. Heart disease and stroke statistics—2016 update: a report from the American Heart Association. *Circulation.* 2016;133(4):447–454.
2. Biller J, Ruland S, Schneck MJ. Ischemic cerebrovascular disease. In: Daroff RB, et al., ed. *Bradley's Neurology in Clinical Practice.* 7th ed. Philadelphia: Elsevier; 2016.
3. Fonseca AC, Ferro JM. Cyptogenic stroke. *Eur J Neurol.* 2015;22(4):618–623.
4. Murphy DR. Current understanding of the relationship between cervical manipulation and stroke: what does it mean for the chiropractic profession? *Chiropr Osteopat.* 2010;18:22.
5. Amin H, Nowak RJ, Schindler JL. Cardioembolic stroke: practical considerations for patient risk management. *Postgrad Med.* 2014;126(1):55–65.
6. Boss BJ, Huether SE. Disorders of central and peripheral nervous system and the neuromuscular junction. In: McCance KL, Huether SE, eds. *Pathophysiology: The Biologic Basis for Disease in Adults and Children.* ed 7. St. Louis: Mosby; 2014.
7. Seder DB, Mayer SA. Critical care management of subarachnoid hemorrhage and ischemic stroke. *Clin Chest Med.* 2009;30(1):103–122.
8. Zhang C, et al. Risk factors for post-stroke seizures: a systematic review and meta-analysis. *Epilepsy Res.* 2014;108(10):1806–1810.
9. Barker E. Altered states of consciousness and sleep. In: Barker E, ed. *Neuroscience Nursing: A Spectrum of Care.* ed 3. St. Louis: Mosby; 2008.
10. Jauch EC, et al. Guidelines for the early management of patients with acute ischemic stroke. A guideline for healthcare professionals from the American Heart Association/American Stroke Association. *Stroke.* 2013;44(3):870–947.
11. Damaerschalk BM, et al. Scientific rationale for the inclusion and exclusion criteria for intravenous alteplase in acute ischemic stroke. A statement for health professionals from the American Heart Association/American Stroke Association. *Stroke.* 2016;47(2):581–621.
12. Bravata DM, et al. Processes of care associated with acute stroke outcomes. *Arch Intern Med.* 2010;170(9):804–810.
13. Anderson T. Current and evolving management of subarachnoid hemorrhage. *Crit Care Nurs Clin N Am.* 2009;21(4):529–539.
14. Venti M. Subarachnoid and intraventricular hemorrhage. *Front Neurol Neurosci.* 2012;30:149–153.
15. Pillai P, et al. Management of aneurysms, subarachnoid hemorrhage, and arteriovenous malformations. In: Barker E, ed. *Neuroscience Nursing: A Spectrum of Care.* ed 3. St. Louis: Mosby; 2008.
16. Szeder V, Tateshima S, Duckwiler GR. Intracranial aneurysms and subarachnoid hemorrhage. In: Daroff RB, et al., ed. *Bradley's Neurology in Clinical Practice.* ed 7. Philadelphia: Elsevier; 2016.
17. Raya AK, Diringer MN. Treatment of subarachnoid hemorrhage. *Crit Care Clin.* 2014;30(4):719–733.
18. Alexander S, et al. *Care of the Patient With Aneurysmal Subarachnoid Hemorrhage. AANN Clinical Practice Guidelines Series.* Glenview, IL: American Association of Neuroscience Nurses; 2012.
19. Connolly ES, Rabinstein AA, Carhuapoma JR. Guidelines for the management of aneurysmal subarachnoid hemorrhage: a guideline for healthcare professionals from the American Heart Association/American Stroke Association. *Stroke.* 2012;43(6):1711–1737.
20. Hunt WE, Hess RM. Surgical risks as related to time of intervention in the repair of intracranial aneurysms. *J Neurosurg.* 1968;28(1):14–20.
21. Solenski NJ, et al. Medical complications of aneurysmal subarachnoid hemorrhage: a report of the multicenter, cooperative aneurysm study. Participants of the Multicenter Cooperative Aneurysm Study. *Crit Care Med.* 1995;23(6):1007–1017.
22. Classen J, et al. Effect of acute physiologic derangements on outcome after subarachnoid hemorrhage. *Crit Care Med.* 2004;32(3):832–838.
23. Ellis JA, Lavine SD. Role of embolization for cerebral arteriovenous malformations. *Methodist Debakey Cardiovasc J.* 2014;10(4):234–239.
24. Baggott CD, Aagaard-Kienitz B. Cerebral vasospasm. *Neurosurg Clin N Am.* 2014;25(3):497–528.
25. Keyrouz SG, Diringer MN. Clinical review: prevention and therapy vasospasm in subarachnoid hemorrhage. *Crit Care.* 2007;11(4):220.
26. Treggiari MM. Participants in the International Multi-disciplinary Consensus Conference on the Critical Care Management of Subarachnoid Hemorrhage: hemodynamic management of subarachnoid hemorrhage. *Neurocrit Care.* 2011;15(2):329–335.
27. Rincon F, Mayer SA. Clinical review: critical care management of spontaneous intracerebral hemorrhage. *Crit Care.* 2008;12(6):237.
28. Hsieh PC, et al. Current updates in perioperative management of intracerebral hemorrhage. *Neurol Clin.* 2006;19(3):401–414.
29. Godoy DA, et al. Steps to consider in the approach and management of critically ill patient with spontaneous intracerebral hemorrhage. *World J Crit Care Med.* 2015;4(3):213–229.
30. Mayer SA. Hemorrhagic cerebrovascular disease. In: Goldman L, Schafer AI, eds. *Goldman-Cecil Medicine.* ed 25. St. Louis: Elsevier; 2016.
31. Hemphill JC, et al. Guidelines for the management of spontaneous intracerebral hemorrhage: a guideline for healthcare professionals from the American Heart Association/American Stroke Association. *Stroke.* 2015;46(7):2032–2060.
32. Hoesch RE, Koenig MA, Geocardin RG. Coma after global ischemic brain injury: pathophysiology and emerging therapies. *Crit Care Clin.* 2008;24(1):25–44.
33. Gawryluk JR, et al. Improving the clinical assessment of consciousness with advances in electrophysiological and neuroimaging techniques. *BMC Neurol.* 2010;10:11.
34. Hocker S, Rabinstein AA. Management of the patient with diminished responsiveness. *Neurol Clin.* 2012;30(1):1–9.
35. Horsting MW, et al. The etiology and outcome of non-traumatic coma in critical care: a systematic review. *BMC Anesthesiol.* 2015;15:65.
36. Ropper AH. Coma. In: Kasper D, et al., ed. *Harrison's Principles of Internal Medicine.* ed 19. New York: McGraw-Hill; 2016.
37. Edlow JA, et al. Diagnosis of reversible causes of coma. *Lancet.* 2014;384(9959):2064–2076.
38. Boss BJ, Huether SE. Alteration in cognitive systems, cerebral hemodynamics, and motor function. In: McCance KL, Huether SE, eds. *Pathophysiology: The Biologic Basis for Disease in Adults and Children.* ed 7. St. Louis: Mosby; 2014.
39. Berger JR. Stupor and coma. In: Daroff RB, et al., ed. *Bradley's Neurology in Clinical Practice.* ed 7. Philadelphia: Elsevier; 2016.
40. Rosenberg RN. Consciousness, coma, and brain death 2009. *JAMA.* 2009;201(11):1172–1174.
41. Bruno MA. From unresponsive wakefulness to minimally conscious PLUS and functional locked-in syndromes: recent advances in our understanding of disorders of consciousness. *J Neurol.* 2011;258(7):1373–1384.
42. Weng Y, Sun S. Therapeutic hypothermia after cardiac arrest in adults: mechanism of neuroprotection, phases of hypothermia, and methods of cooling. *Crit Care Clin.* 2012;28(2):231–243.
43. Hessel EA. Therapeutic hypothermia after in-hospital cardiac arrest: a critique. *J Cardiothorac Vasc Anesth.* 2014;28(3):789–799.
44. Cortese D, Capp L, McKinley S. Moisture chamber versus lubrication for the prevention of corneal epithelial breakdown. *Am J Crit Care.* 1995;4(6):425–428.
45. Yuki N, Hartung HP. Guillain-Barré syndrome. *N Engl J Med.* 2012;366(24):2294–2304.
46. van den Berg B, et al. Guillain-Barré syndrome: pathogenesis, diagnosis, treatment and prognosis. *Nat Rev Neurol.* 2014;10(8):469–482.
47. Randall DP. Guillain-Barré syndrome. *Dis Mon.* 2010;56(5):256–261.
48. Shah DN. The spectrum of Guillain-Barré syndrome. *Dis Mon.* 2010;56(5):262–265.
49. Cortese I, et al. Evidence-based guideline update: plasmapheresis in neurologic disorders: report of the Therapeutics and Technology Assessment Subcommittee of the American Academy of Neurology. *Neurology.* 2011;76(3):294–300.
50. Patwa HS, et al. Evidence-based guideline: intravenous immunoglobulin in the treatment of neuromuscular disorders: report of the Therapeutics and Technology Assessment Subcommittee of the American Academy of Neurology. *Neurology.* 2012;78(13):1009–1015.

51. Mullings KR, Alleva JT, Hudgins TH. Rehabilitation of Guillain-Barré syndrome. *Dis Mon*. 2010;56(5):288–292.

52. Krizman Germanovich SJ. Neurosurgery. In: Rothrock JC, ed. *Alexander's Care of the Patient in Surgery*. ed 15. St. Louis: Elsevier; 2015.

53. Miller BA, Loachimescu AG, Oyesiku NM. Contemporary indications for transsphenoidal pituitary surgery. *World Neurosurg*. 2014;82(6 Suppl):S147–S151.

54. Yuan W. Managing the patient with transsphenoidal pituitary tumor resection. *J Neurosurg Nurs*. 2013;45(2):101–107.

55. Fugate JE. Complications of neurosurgery. *Continuum (Minneap Minn)*. 2015;21(5 Neurocritical Care):1425–1444.

56. Hannon MJ, Finucane FM, Sherlock M, et al. Clinical review: disorders of water homeostasis in neurosurgical patients. *J Clin Endocrinol Metab*. 2012;97(5):1423–1433.

57. Ausiello JC, Bruce JN, Freda PU. Postoperative assessment of the patient after transsphenoidal pituitary surgery. *Pituitary*. 2008;11(4):391–401.

58. Daele JJ, Goffart Y, Machiels S. Traumatic, iatrogenic, and spontaneous cerebrospinal fluid (CSF) leak: endoscopic repair. *B-ENT*. 2011;7(Suppl 17):47–60.

59. Collen JF, et al. Prevention of venous thromboembolism in neurosurgery: a metaanalysis. *Chest*. 2008;134(2):237–249.

60. Schneck MJ. Venous thromboembolism in neurologic disease. *Handb Clin Neurol*. 2014;119:298–2304.

61. Anthony M. Nursing assessment of deep vein thrombosis. *Medsurg Nurs*. 2013;22(2):95–98.

62. Gould MK, et al. Prevention of VTE in nonorthopedic surgical patients: antithrombotic therapy and prevention of thrombosis, 9th ed: American College of Chest Physicians evidence-based clinical practice guidelines. *Chest*. 2012;141(Suppl 2):e227S.

63. Hansen MS, et al. Pain treatment after craniotomy: where is the (procedure-specific) evidence? A qualitative systematic review. *Eur J Anaesthesiol*. 2011;28(12):821–829.

64. Dashti SR, et al. Operative intracranial infection following craniotomy. *Neurosurg Focus*. 2008;24(6):E10.

65. Kocacal Guler E, Eser I, Eqrilmez S. Effectiveness of polyethylene covers versus carbomer drops (Viscotears) to prevent dry eye syndrome in the critically ill. *J Clin Nurs*. 2011;20(13-14):1916–1922.

66. Barker E. Intracranial pressure and monitoring. In: Barker E, ed. *Neuroscience Nursing: A Spectrum of Care*. ed 3. St. Louis: Mosby; 2008.

67. Eigsti J, Henke K. Anatomy and physiology of neurological compensatory mechanisms. *Dimens Crit Care Nurs*. 2006;25(5):197–202.

68. Blissitt PA. Hemodynamic and intracranial dynamic monitoring in neurocritical care. In: Lough ME, ed. *Hemodynamic Monitoring: Evolving Technologies and Clinical Practice*. ed 1. St Louis: Elsevier; 2016.

69. Perez-Barcena J, Llompart-Pou JA, O'Phelan KM. Intracranial pressure monitoring and management of intracranial hypertension. *Crit Care Clin*. 2014;30(4):735–750.

70. Latorre JG, Greer DM. Management of acute intracranial hypertension: a review. *Neurologist*. 2009;15(4):193–207.

71. Bhatia A, Gupta AK. Neuromonitoring in the intensive care unit. I. Intracranial pressure and cerebral blood flow monitoring. *Intens Care Med*. 2007;33(7):1263–1271.

72. Curley G, Kavanagh BP, Laffey JG. Hypocapnia and the injured brain: more harm than benefit. *Crit Care Med*. 2010;38(5):1348–1359.

73. Mortazavi MM, et al. Hypertonic saline for treating raised intracranial pressure: literature review with meta-analysis. *Neurosurg*. 2012;116(1):210–221.

74. Saiki RL. Current and evolving management of traumatic brain injury. *Crit Care Nurs Clin N Am*. 2009;21(4):549–559.

75. Haddad SH, Arabi YM. Critical care management of severe traumatic brain injury in adults. *Scand J Trauma Resusc Emerg Med*. 2012;20:12.

76. Leeper B, Lovasik D. Cerebrospinal drainage systems: external ventricular and lumbar drains. In: Littlejohns LR, Bader MK, eds. *AACN-ANNA Protocols for Practice: Monitoring Technologies in Critically Ill Neuroscience Patients*. Sudbury, MA: Jones & Bartlett; 2009.

77. Atkinson RA, et al. Silver-impregnated external-ventricular-drain-related cerebrospinal fluid infections: a meta-analysis. *J Hosp Infect*. 2016;92(3):263–272.

78. Fink ME. Osmotherapy for intracranial hypertension: mannitol versus hypertonic saline. *Continuum (Minneap Minn)*. 2012;18(3):640–654.

79. Stevens RD, et al. Emergency neurological life support: intracranial hypertension and herniation. *Neurocrit Care*. 2012;17(Suppl 1):S60–S65.

80. Fisher CM. Brain herniation: a revision of classic concepts. *Can J Neurol Sci*. 1995;22(2):83–91.

24

Kidney Anatomy and Physiology

Mary E. Lough

The kidneys are complex organs responsible for numerous functions and substances necessary to maintain homeostasis. The primary roles of the kidneys are to remove metabolic wastes, maintain fluid–electrolyte balance, and help achieve acid–base balance. Hormones produced by the kidneys have an important role in blood pressure control, red blood cell production, and bone metabolism. The kidneys are important in maintaining the intracellular and extracellular environment required by all cells to function effectively. When a patient experiences kidney dysfunction, some or all of the functions of the kidneys may be decreased or absent, leading to altered homeostasis.

This chapter provides an overview of the anatomy and physiologic processes of the kidneys. An understanding of normal kidney function is essential to understanding the pathophysiology, symptoms, and therapeutic management of kidney disease and failure.

MACROSCOPIC ANATOMY

The kidneys are paired organs located retroperitoneally, one on each side of the vertebral column between T12 and L3.[1] The right kidney is slightly lower than the left because of the position of the liver. Each kidney is approximately 12 cm long, 6 cm wide, and 2.5 cm thick in an adult. Kidney size and weight vary between men and women: 125 to 170 g in men and 115 to 155 g in women.[1] The kidneys are protected anteriorly and posteriorly by the rib cage and by a tough fibrous capsule that encloses each kidney. Additional protection is provided by a cushion of perirenal fat and the support of the kidney fascia.

Internally, the kidneys are made up of two distinct areas: the cortex and the medulla. The kidney *cortex* is the outer layer and contains the glomeruli, proximal tubules, cortical portions of the loops of Henle, distal tubules, and cortical collecting ducts. The kidney cortex is approximately 1 cm in thickness. The kidney *medulla* is the inner kidney layer, made up of the pyramids, which contain the medullary portions of the loops of Henle, the vasa recta, and the medullary portions of the collecting ducts. Numerous pyramids taper and join to form a minor calyx; several minor calyces join to form a major calyx. The major calyces then join and enter the funnel-shaped *kidney pelvis,* a 5- to 10-mL conduit that directs urine into the ureter (Fig. 24.1).

The kidney system also includes the urinary drainage system—the ureters, bladder, and urethra (Fig. 24.2). The ureters are fibromuscular tubes that exit the central part of the kidney pelvis. The ureters are 28 to 34 cm in length and enter the urinary bladder at an oblique angle. As urine is formed by the kidneys, the urine flows through the ureters by peristalsis. The peristaltic action of the ureters and the angle at which the ureters enter the bladder help prevent reflux of urine from the bladder back up into the kidneys. The bladder is a muscular sac within the pelvis and has a capacity of 280 to 500 mL. Urine leaves the bladder through the urethral orifice and is excreted from the body through the urethra. The male urethra is approximately 20 cm long; the female urethra is 3 to 5 cm long.

VASCULAR ANATOMY

The kidneys are highly vascular and receive up to 20% of the cardiac output—approximately 1 to 1.2 L/min of blood flow.[2] Blood enters the kidneys through the renal arteries, which branch bilaterally from the abdominal aorta. The renal artery divides into arterial branches that become progressively smaller vessels, eventually ending with the afferent arterioles. A single *afferent arteriole* supplies blood to each glomerulus, a tuft of capillaries that is the first structure of the nephron. The nephron is often described as the *functional unit* of the kidneys.[1]

Blood exits the glomerulus by the *efferent arteriole,* which connects with the peritubular capillary network, also known as the *vasa recta* (straight vessels), that parallel the long loops of Henle. The intricate capillary network maintains the intracapillary pressure that allows water and solutes to move between the tubules and the capillaries for urine formation and the concentration and dilution of urine. The capillaries then rejoin and form gradually enlarging venous vessels, until the blood leaves each kidney through the renal vein and returns to the general circulation by the inferior vena cava.[2]

MICROSCOPIC STRUCTURE AND FUNCTION

Each kidney is made up of approximately 1 million nephrons, the functional units of the kidneys. Because of the vast number of nephrons, the kidneys can continue to function even when several thousand nephrons are damaged or destroyed by

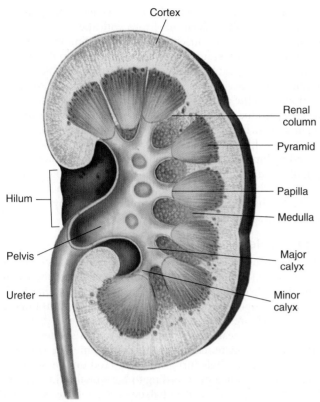

FIG. 24.1 **Cross Section of the Kidney.** (From Thompson JM, et al. *Mosby's Clinical Nursing.* 5th ed. St. Louis: Mosby; 2002.)

FIG. 24.3 **Components of the Nephron.** (From Thompson JM, et al. *Mosby's Clinical Nursing.* 5th ed. St. Louis: Mosby; 2002.)

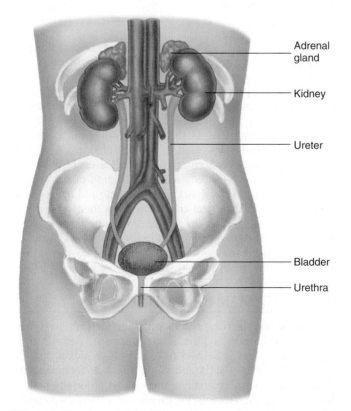

FIG. 24.2 **Structures of the Urinary System.** (From Thompson JM, et al. *Mosby's Clinical Nursing.* 5th ed. St. Louis: Mosby; 2002.)

disease or injury. Each nephron has the ability to perform all the individual functions of the kidneys. The nephron is made up of several distinct structures: glomerulus, Bowman capsule, proximal tubule, loop of Henle, distal tubule, and collecting duct (Fig. 24.3).

Two types of nephrons make up each kidney: the cortical nephrons and the juxtamedullary nephrons. Most are cortical nephrons. These superficial cortical nephrons have glomeruli located in the outer cortex and have short loops of Henle. The midcortical nephrons are located lower in the cortex and have loops of Henle that may be short or long. Both types of cortical nephrons perform excretory and regulatory functions. The remaining nephrons are juxtamedullary nephrons with glomeruli located deep in the cortex and extending into the medullary layer of the kidney. The juxtamedullary nephrons have long loops of Henle that have an important role in the concentration and dilution of urine. The peritubular capillaries, known as the vasa recta, surround the juxtamedullary nephrons maintaining a concentration gradient to concentrate the urine.

Glomerulus

The first structure of each nephron is the glomerulus, a high-pressure capillary bed that serves as the filtering point for the blood. Positive filtration pressure in the glomerulus is achieved as a result of the high arterial pressure as the blood enters the *afferent arteriole* and the resistance created by the smaller *efferent arteriole* as the blood exits the glomerulus. As a result of the positive-pressure gradient, fluid and solutes are filtered through the glomerular capillary walls. The glomerulus has three layers: endothelium, basement membrane, and epithelium. The inner endothelial layer lines the glomerulus and contains numerous pores that allow filtration of fluid and small solutes from the blood. The middle basement membrane layer also controls filtration according to the size, electrical charge, protein-binding capability, and shape of the molecules. This complex is also described as the *glomerular filtration barrier.* It is freely permeable to water and small or midsized molecules, but large molecules such as albumin and red blood cells are prevented from entering the filtrate.[3] The presence of large molecules in the urine is a signal that the glomerular membrane is damaged. The outer epithelium layer contains pores that allow the filtered blood, or filtrate, into the Bowman space.

Bowman Capsule

A filtrate of plasma, usually called the *ultrafiltrate,* enters the Bowman space, which is surrounded by the Bowman capsule, a tough, membranous layer of epithelial cells that completely surrounds the glomerular capillary bed. The Bowman space is located between the capillary walls of the glomerulus and the inner layer of the Bowman capsule and contains the initial filtrate from the blood. Fluid, solutes, and other substances filtered by the glomerulus collect in the space. The Bowman space is a continuous structure that joins the first portion of the nephron's tubular system—the proximal tubule.[1]

Proximal Tubule

The *proximal tubule* is located in the cortex of the kidney and has a large surface area available for solute and fluid transportation. The proximal tubule resorbs (takes back) most of the filtered water and sodium and many of the solutes the body does not routinely excrete in the urine. Solutes that are usually resorbed include all of the glucose; some of the water-soluble vitamins; most of the phosphate and bicarbonate; and much of the potassium, chloride, and calcium that is filtered by the glomerulus. Proteins are resorbed in the proximal tubule by two specialized receptors known as megalin and cubilin that bind albumin and vitamin-binding proteins.[1] Creatinine is minimally resorbed and is excreted in the urine.

In addition to its major role in resorbing water and solutes from the filtrate, the proximal tubule secretes organic anions and cations into the tubular lumen. Ammonia is produced from the metabolism of glutamine in the mitochondria of the proximal tubule cells, where ammonia (NH_3) combines with hydrogen (H^+) to form ammonium (NH_4^+), which is secreted into the proximal tubule lumen.[1]

Because of the large amount of solutes in the glomerular filtrate, the fluid that enters the proximal tubule is hyperosmotic. When the filtrate leaves the proximal tubule and enters the loop of Henle, it is isosmotic (equivalent to plasma) as a result of the resorption of solutes and water.

Loop of Henle

After selective resorption in the proximal tubule, the isosmotic filtrate enters the loop of Henle. The *loop of Henle* consists of a thin descending limb, a thin ascending limb, and a thick ascending limb. There are two types of nephrons: the cortical nephrons with short loops of Henle and the juxtamedullary nephrons with long loops of Henle. The nephrons with short loops of Henle do not have a thin ascending limb. As a result, the cortical nephrons perform excretory and regulatory functions but play only a minor role in the concentration or dilution of urine. The juxtamedullary nephrons have glomeruli that are next to (juxtaposed to) the medulla near where the

cortex and medulla sections of the kidney join and contain a thin ascending limb. These nephrons with the thin ascending limbs are critical for concentrating and diluting the urine by means of the countercurrent mechanism. The thin descending limb is very permeable to water but fairly impermeable to urea, sodium, and other solutes. As a result, water (but not solute) is resorbed into the general circulation, and a more concentrated filtrate is produced. The filtrate then moves up the thin ascending limb, which is impermeable to water but allows movement of sodium, chloride, and urea back into the filtrate. The thick ascending limb is also impermeable to water but allows resorption of sodium, chloride, potassium, calcium, and bicarbonate. Because of the low water and high solute resorption in the loop of Henle, the filtrate leaves the ascending limb hypoosmotic (more dilute than plasma).

Distal Tubule

The hypoosmotic filtrate enters the distal tubule located in the cortex of the kidney. The first portion of the distal tubule contains the cells of the *macula densa,* which are specialized cells that are a component of the juxtaglomerular apparatus important in blood pressure control. The first section of the distal tubule is impermeable to water and transports solutes such as sodium, bicarbonate, calcium, and potassium. The later section of the distal tubule further regulates sodium, bicarbonate, potassium, and calcium according to hormonal influences and the acid–base and electrolyte balance needs of the body. The permeability of the late distal tubule is influenced by antidiuretic hormone (ADH). In the presence of ADH, the late distal tubule is impermeable to water but resorbs some solutes, and the filtrate remains hypoosmotic. In the absence of ADH, the late distal tubule is more permeable to water, and the filtrate may become isosmotic.

Collecting Duct

Several distal tubules join to form a collecting duct that begins in the cortex and extends through the medulla to empty into the papilla. The final composition of the urine occurs in the collecting duct, primarily because of the transport of potassium, sodium, and water. Water permeability is determined by the absence or presence of ADH. In the absence of ADH or with small amounts of ADH, the urine becomes dilute, whereas larger amounts of ADH result in concentrated urine. The filtrate usually is more concentrated when it leaves the collecting duct than it was when it entered. Acidification of the urine is accomplished by the transport of bicarbonate and hydrogen in the collecting duct. Several collecting ducts then combine to form the pyramids. After the urine leaves the collecting ducts, no change in the composition of the filtrate occurs. Box 24.1 summarizes tubular resorption and secretion in the various structures of the nephron.

NERVOUS SYSTEM INNERVATION

The autonomic nervous system provides the primary innervation to the kidneys and the urinary drainage system. Kidney neural innervation is derived from the celiac plexus and the sympathetic plexuses of the abdominal viscera to form the renal plexus. The renal plexus enters the kidneys along the path of the renal arteries. The inferior mesenteric plexus, hypogastric plexus, and pudendal nerve from the sacral region serve the urinary bladder, ureters, and urethra.

BOX 24.1   Tubular Resorption and Secretion

Glomerulus
- Filters fluid and solutes from blood

Proximal Tubule
- Resorbs Na^+, K^+, Cl^-, HCO_3^-, urea, glucose, and amino acids
- Filtrate leaves isosmotic

Loop of Henle
- Resorbs Na^+, K^+, Cl^-
- Blocks resorption of H_2O from ascending limb
- Countercurrent mechanism dilutes or concentrates urine
- Filtrate leaves hypoosmotic

Distal Tubule
- Na^+, K^+, Ca^{2+}, PO_4^{3-} selectively resorbed
- H_2O resorbed in the presence of antidiuretic hormone (ADH)
- Na^+ resorbed in the presence of aldosterone
- Filtrate leaves hypoosmotic

Collecting Duct
- Resorption similar to that in distal tubule
- H_2O resorbed in the presence of ADH
- HCO_3^- and H^+ resorbed or secreted to acidify urine
- Filtrate leaves hyperosmotic or hypoosmotic, depending on body needs

Nervous system control in the urinary tract is reflected in the process of micturition, or the release of urine. Bladder fullness stimulates stretch receptors in the bladder wall and a portion of the urethra. Signals are carried through nerves in the sacral area and return as parasympathetic messages to contract the detrusor muscle of the bladder. With a full bladder, contractions usually are powerful enough to relax the external sphincter. Sympathetic stimulation returns the external sphincter to contraction after the urine is released. The cerebral cortex and brainstem portions of the central nervous system also exert control over the urinary bladder. The central nervous system regulates the micturition reflex, frequency, and external sphincter tone and allows conscious control over release of urine from the bladder.

URINE FORMATION

The nephrons are responsible for removing metabolic substances and waste products from the blood and retaining essential electrolytes and water as needed by the body. The entire blood volume of an individual is filtered by the kidneys 60 to 70 times each day, resulting in approximately 180 L of filtrate. The glomerular filtration rate (GFR), or the amount of filtrate formed in the nephrons, is approximately 125 mL/min. The kidneys must reduce the 180 L of filtrate to an average of 1 to 2 L of urine per day. Although 180 L of filtrate is formed, 99% of it is resorbed, and only 1% is excreted as urine. The three processes necessary for changing the 180 L of filtrate into 1 to 2 L of urine are glomerular filtration, tubular resorption, and tubular secretion.

Glomerular Filtration

The first process in urine formation is glomerular filtration, which depends on glomerular blood flow, pressure in the Bowman space, and plasma oncotic pressure.[2] Glomerular

blood flow is the most important of these three factors and is maintained through an autoregulatory mechanism within the kidneys.[2] The autoregulatory mechanism maintains consistent kidney blood flow and perfusion at a constant level as long as the mean arterial pressure (MAP) remains between 80 mm Hg and 180 mm Hg. The afferent and efferent arterioles of the glomeruli have the ability to increase or decrease the glomerular blood flow rate through selective dilation and constriction. When the MAP is decreased, the afferent arteriole dilates, and the efferent arteriole constricts to maintain a higher pressure in the glomerular capillary bed and maintain the GFR at 125 mL/min. The ability of the kidneys to autoregulate blood flow begins to fail when the MAP is less than 80 mm Hg or greater than 180 mm Hg.

The second factor that influences the GFR is the pressure in the Bowman space. An increase in pressure in this space decreases filtration because the increased pressure resists the movement of solutes and water from the capillaries into the space. For example, if the tubules of the nephrons are blocked by cellular debris, backward pressure is exerted on the Bowman space, the GFR decreases to less than 125 mL/min, and urine output decreases.

The third factor that influences GFR is plasma oncotic pressure. When the oncotic pressure in the blood is decreased (as in disease states that result in low plasma protein levels), pressure in the glomerular capillary bed is decreased. Although the MAP in the glomerulus favors filtration, decreased amounts of fluid and solutes leave the capillaries and enter the Bowman space because the oncotic pressure gradient in the plasma that encourages movement of fluid and solutes out of the plasma is less favorable. Filtration still occurs, but it is decreased from the normal 125 mL/min, resulting in a decrease in the amount of filtrate and urine.

The status of the glomerular filtration system is assessed by measuring the GFR. Creatinine is used as a measure of the GFR because it is a waste product produced at a fairly constant rate by the muscles, is freely filtered by the glomerulus, and is minimally resorbed or secreted by the tubules. Most of the creatinine produced by the body is excreted by the kidneys, making the creatinine clearance a good screening and follow-up test for estimating the GFR. Creatinine clearance usually mirrors the GFR, so that a normal creatinine clearance rate is approximately 125 mL/min. A creatinine clearance rate less than 100 mL/min reflects a GFR of less than 100 mL/min and is a signal of decreased kidney function. A creatinine clearance rate (and GFR) less than 20 mL/min results in symptoms of kidney failure.

Tubular Resorption

The second process in the formation of urine is tubular resorption—the movement of a substance from the tubular lumen (filtrate) into the peritubular capillaries (blood). Tubular resorption allows the 180 L of solutes and water filtered by the glomerulus to be taken back into the circulation, decreasing the 180 L of filtrate to 1 to 2 L of urine per day. Most tubular resorption occurs in the proximal tubule and occurs by passive and active transport processes.

Passive Transport

Passive transport of substances in the tubule depends on changes in concentration gradients and does not require energy. Diffusion and osmosis are the primary passive transport processes in the nephrons. Diffusion is the spontaneous movement of molecules or solutes from an area of higher concentration to an area of lower concentration across a semipermeable membrane (not all substances cross, particularly large molecules). For example, when water is resorbed by the tubules, the concentration of urea in the tubules is increased. Urea then diffuses across the semipermeable membrane of the tubule and reenters the plasma to achieve balance in the concentration gradient.

Osmosis is the movement of water from an area of lower solute concentration to an area of higher solute concentration. Osmosis occurs any time the concentration of solutes on one side of a semipermeable membrane is greater than the concentration of solutes on the other side of the membrane. For example, when the concentration of sodium is greater in the peritubular capillaries than in the tubules, water passively moves from the tubules into the capillaries to balance the concentration gradient.

Active Transport

Active transport of substances into or out of the tubules requires substances to move against an electrochemical gradient, and it takes energy in the form of adenosine triphosphate (ATP). In active transport, the substance combines with a carrier and then diffuses across the semipermeable tubular membrane. Substances that are actively resorbed include glucose, amino acids, calcium, potassium, and sodium. The rate at which substances can be actively resorbed depends on the availability of the carriers, saturation of the carriers, and availability of energy. The transport maximum refers to the maximum rate at which substances can be resorbed and varies according to each substance.

The threshold concentration of a substance is important in active transport. The threshold of a substance is the plasma level of a substance at which none of the substance appears in the urine.[2] When the threshold of a substance in the plasma is exceeded, progressively larger amounts of the substance appear in the urine because the large amounts cannot be resorbed. For example, the serum threshold concentration for glucose is approximately 180 mg/dL. At or below a plasma glucose concentration of 180 mg/dL, all glucose is actively resorbed from the kidney tubules back into the circulation, and none is excreted in the urine. When the plasma glucose concentration is greater than 180 mg/dL, the threshold concentration is exceeded, and some of the glucose cannot be resorbed from the tubules and is excreted in the urine.

Tubular Secretion

The third process in urine formation is tubular secretion, the transport of substances from the peritubular capillaries into the lumen of the tubules. Tubular secretion allows the body to remove excess substances; it occurs by diffusion and by active transport, and it depends on the needs of the body. For example, potassium, hydrogen, medications, or medication metabolites are secreted into the tubules to decrease their concentration in the body. Tubular secretion plays a lesser role than tubular resorption in changing the filtrate into urine.

FUNCTIONS OF THE KIDNEYS

The formation of urine through the processes previously described is a major function of the kidneys. The kidneys are also responsible for other functions essential to maintaining homeostasis, including the elimination of metabolic wastes,

blood pressure regulation, the regulation of erythrocyte production, the activation of vitamin D, prostaglandin synthesis, acid–base balance, and fluid–electrolyte balance.

Elimination of Metabolic Wastes

Metabolic processes in the body produce waste products that are selectively filtered out of the circulation by the kidneys. Urea, uric acid, and creatinine are by-products of protein metabolism that the kidneys filter out of the circulation and excrete in the urine. Metabolic acids, bilirubin, and medication metabolites are also eliminated as waste products.

Urea

Urea and creatinine are the primary waste products that are measured in determining kidney function. Urea is measured as blood urea nitrogen; this is the end product of protein metabolism and results from the breakdown of ammonia in the liver. The level of urea in the blood is influenced by protein breakdown, the amount of protein in the diet, fluid volume, and excretion from the kidneys. The body forms approximately 25 to 28 g of urea per day. More urea is formed if protein intake is high or if the individual is in a catabolic state and is breaking down body protein stores. Urea is primarily excreted in the urine and accumulates if the glomerulus is unable to filter it from the blood.

Creatinine

Creatinine is an end product of protein metabolism produced by the muscles. Creatinine is normally completely filtered and minimally resorbed by the kidneys. As a result, creatinine is excreted in the urine. Similar to urea, creatinine accumulates when the glomerulus is unable to filter it from the blood. The level of creatinine in the blood provides an indicator of kidney function.

Blood Pressure Regulation

The kidneys regulate arterial blood pressure by maintaining the circulating blood volume by means of fluid balance and by altering peripheral vascular resistance through the renin-angiotensin-aldosterone system (RAAS). Regulation by the RAAS occurs in the *juxtaglomerular apparatus* (JGA), a group of specialized cells located around the afferent arteriole where the distal tubule and afferent arteriole make contact (see Fig. 24.3).[4,5] Another group of specialized cells is located near the distal tubule; known as the *macula densa,* these cells control a feedback mechanism from the distal tubule to the afferent arteriole to control blood flow through the afferent arteriole.[4]

An increase in tubular filtrate in the macula densa causes the afferent arteriole to constrict and decrease the GFR and the amount of filtrate produced. Conversely, a decrease in the amount of tubular filtrate results in afferent arteriole dilation, an increased GFR, and an increased amount of filtrate.

The JGA synthesizes, stores, and releases renin.[5] *Renin* is released in response to reduced pressure in the glomerulus, sympathetic stimulation of the kidneys, and a decrease in the amount of sodium in the distal tubule.[5] Renin enters the lumen of the afferent arteriole and is released into the general circulation. Renin is then converted to angiotensin I, which is further converted to angiotensin II as the blood circulates through the lungs. *Angiotensin II* is an active compound that causes afferent and efferent arteriole vasoconstriction, resulting in increased vascular resistance, and it maintains

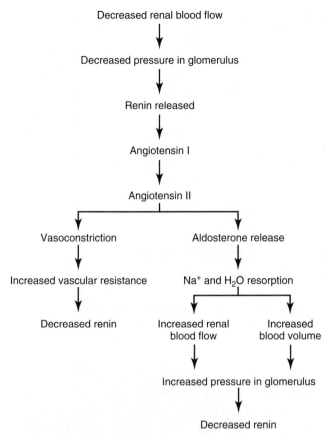

Decreased renal blood flow

↓

Decreased pressure in glomerulus

↓

Renin released

↓

Angiotensin I

↓

Angiotensin II

Vasoconstriction → Increased vascular resistance → Decreased renin

Aldosterone release → Na$^+$ and H$_2$O resorption → Increased renal blood flow / Increased blood volume → Increased pressure in glomerulus → Decreased renin

FIG. 24.4 Renin-Angiotensin-Aldosterone System.

hydrostatic pressure within the kidneys. A powerful vasoconstrictor, angiotensin II also causes increased systemic vascular resistance and increased arterial blood pressure. Intracellular actions of angiotensin II constitute an emerging area of research.[6,7] Angiotensin II also stimulates the release of aldosterone by the adrenal cortex.

Aldosterone acts on the distal tubule to facilitate sodium and water resorption, resulting in an expanded circulating blood volume and increased blood pressure. When the arterial blood pressure increases, the JGA reduces the release of renin, and the RAAS is less active. Fig. 24.4 summarizes the major aspects of the renin-angiotensin-aldosterone mechanism.

Erythrocyte Production

The kidneys secrete erythropoietin, the hormone that controls erythrocyte (red blood cell) production in the bone marrow. Erythropoietin is released in response to a decrease in the amount of oxygen delivered to the kidneys, such as in anemia or prolonged hypoxia. The hormone remains active for approximately 24 hours after release and stimulates the bone marrow to increase the production of erythrocytes. The absence of erythropoietin, which occurs in individuals with kidney failure, results in a profound anemia that is treated by administering synthetic erythropoietin or by blood transfusion therapy.[8,9]

Vitamin D Activation

The kidneys convert vitamin D from food sources into an active form for use by the body. Active vitamin D stimulates the absorption of calcium by the intestine and resorption of calcium

by the tubules so that calcium is available for bone and tooth metabolism and blood clotting functions.[10] When the kidneys fail, the body is unable to convert dietary vitamin D to its active form, calcium is poorly absorbed, and bone disease and other immunologic deficiencies result. Lack of vitamin D may also be responsible for changes in the immune system that increase the risk of infection in patients with chronic kidney disease.[11]

Prostaglandin Synthesis

Prostaglandins are vasoactive substances that dilate or constrict the arteries. The kidney produces two vasodilatory prostaglandins: prostaglandin E$_1$ (PGE$_1$) and prostaglandin I$_2$ (PGI$_2$).[12] The prostaglandins produced by the kidneys have only local blood flow effects with minimal or no systemic effects. The primary prostaglandins produced by the kidneys are the vasodilators PGE$_1$ and PGI$_2$, which act on the afferent arteriole to maintain blood flow and glomerular perfusion and filtration. The vasodilating effects of the prostaglandins also counteract the effects of angiotensin II and the sympathetic nervous system on the kidneys and maintain blood flow to the kidney despite systemic vasoconstriction. Another prostaglandin that may affect kidney function is prostaglandin F$_2$ (PGF$_2$), which contributes to vasoconstriction in times of volume depletion. Box 24.2 lists the effects of prostaglandins.

Acid–Base Balance

The kidneys are actively involved in acid–base regulation by resorbing or excreting acids and bases in the kidney tubules. For example, bicarbonate, the principal blood buffer, is resorbed from the tubules, and hydrogen, a potent organic acid, is secreted into the tubules. However, the tubules do not function as rapidly in altering acid–base concentrations as do the lungs; the kidneys regulate the day-to-day balance rather than coping with emergencies requiring an immediate physiologic response.

FLUID BALANCE

Regulation of the total amount of water in the body is vital for homeostasis, and it is one of the most important functions of the kidneys. In the absence of effective kidney function, fluid volume overload occurs and threatens homeostasis. Similarly, if the kidneys are unable to preserve adequate amounts of fluid, a severe volume deficit occurs that also disrupts homeostasis.

Fluid Compartments

The fluid of the body is present in distinct internal spaces or compartments. The compartments are separated from each other by semipermeable membranes with openings (pores)

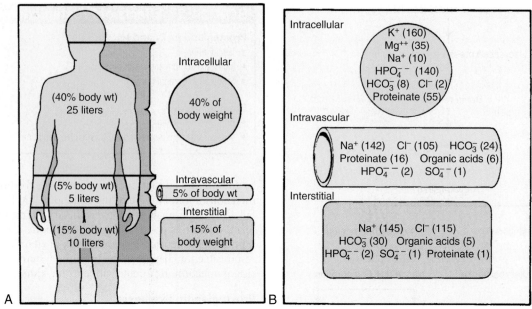

FIG. 24.5 (A) Fluid compartments. (B) Electrolytes by fluid compartment.

that allow molecules of specific size and molecular weight to pass through, while preventing larger, heavier molecules from doing so. As a result of the semipermeable membrane, fluid movement between the compartments is dynamic and constant.

Water makes up 45% to 60% of body weight.[13] The body has two main fluid compartments: intracellular and extracellular. The *intracellular compartment* is the fluid inside each of the body's cells and accounts for 40% of the total body water content.[13] The remaining fluid is outside the body's cells and makes up the *extracellular compartment*. The extracellular compartment is composed of two distinct subcompartments: *intravascular* and *interstitial*. The *intravascular compartment*, referring to the fluid within the blood vessels, accounts for 5% of the body water. The interstitial compartment corresponds to the fluid in the tissue spaces outside of the body cells and the blood vessels and accounts for 15% of body water. Approximate amounts of fluid contained in each compartment are shown in Fig. 24.5A. With an increase in body fat, the body fluid percentage decreases because fat contains a smaller and less significant amount of water than muscle.

Electrolytes

Electrolytes are elements or compounds that, when dissolved in water, dissociate into ions, electrically charged atomic particles. Ions in solution in the fluid allow the fluid to conduct an electrical current. A balance exists between cations (positively charged ions), anions (negatively charged ions), and other substances in the fluid compartments. Maintaining this balance is important to the normal function of all body systems. Electrolytes exist in differing amounts in each of the fluid compartments. The primary electrolytes and other substances of importance in fluid and electrolyte balance are shown by fluid compartment in Fig. 24.5B.

Fluid Physiology

An overall understanding is needed of the structures containing or balancing fluids and electrolytes and the physiologic forces

that govern their movement and balance. Knowledge of factors that inhibit or enhance the transfer of fluids and electrolytes is required.

Tonicity

The terms *isotonic, hypotonic,* and *hypertonic* all refer to tonicity, or the osmolality of body fluids. *Osmolality* is a measure of the number of particles (solute) in a solution, and the value is stated in milliosmoles per kilogram of water. The normal osmolality of body fluids is 275 to 295 mOsm/kg of body weight. Different hospital laboratories may use slightly different numbers, such as 280 to 300 mOsm/kg.[13]

Fig. 24.6 shows the effects of the tonicity (osmolality) of fluid in the body. An isotonic solution has approximately the same concentration of particles as the blood plasma; cells within an isotonic solution maintain consistency and do not lose or gain fluid to their surroundings. A *hypertonic solution* contains a

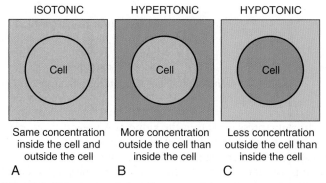

FIG. 24.6 (A) Isotonic solution. The extracellular solute concentration is the same as the intracellular concentration, with no movement of water into or out of the cell. (B) Hypertonic solution. The extracellular solute concentration is greater than the intracellular concentration. Water moves from the cell into the extracellular compartment. (C) Hypotonic solution. The extracellular solute concentration is less than the intracellular concentration. Water moves from the extracellular compartment into the cell.

greater concentration of particles than that inside the cell and causes fluid to be drawn out of the cells. Used inappropriately, too much fluid may be withdrawn, causing a withering of the cell (crenation). A *hypotonic solution* contains a lesser concentration of particles than that inside the cell and causes fluid to be drawn into the cells. If used incorrectly, a hypotonic solution can cause too much fluid to enter the cell, causing the cells to swell and burst (hemolysis).

Hydrostatic Pressure

The force of left ventricular contraction of the heart propels the blood through the circulatory system, causing the blood to exert pressure against the vessel walls. This hydrostatic pressure creates the tendency for fluids and dissolved substances to move into the interstitial spaces by filtration (movement of fluid and substances from an area of high pressure to one of low pressure). Without opposing forces counteracting the hydrostatic pressure, fluid would leave the intravascular space until the space was depleted. Although hydrostatic pressure favors fluid and electrolyte movement out of the intravascular compartment, the colloid osmotic pressure of the plasma holds the fluid and substances in the intravascular space.

Osmotic Pressure

Osmotic pressure is created by solutes and other substances (eg, albumin, globulin, fibrinogen) suspended in fluid. Colloid osmotic pressure is created primarily by the presence of plasma proteins in the intravascular space. Plasma proteins exert a pull on water molecules and produce osmotic pressure, which retains fluid within the intravascular compartment. This force is maintained because proteins are large and cannot move or be transported across the semipermeable membrane unless the permeability of the membrane is changed by disease or other assaults on the body (eg, burns, infections). Similarly, the solute and protein content of the interstitium results in interstitial colloid osmotic pressure. A decrease in serum protein lessens the osmotic pressure in the intravascular space so that the interstitial oncotic pressure is greater than the intravascular pressure and pulls fluid from the vascular space into the interstitial space, causing edema.

Diffusion, Osmosis, and Active Transport

Fluid balance within the compartments is achieved through the processes of diffusion, osmosis, and active transport. Just as in the kidney tubule cells, these three processes are constantly at work in other parts of the body to facilitate the movement of water and solutes to maintain homeostasis between the intracellular and extracellular compartments.

Movement of Water

The combined effects generated by ventricular contraction, colloid osmotic pressure in the intravascular space, solute content of the extracellular fluid (ECF), and solutes in the intracellular fluid (ICF) cause constant movement between the ICF and ECF compartments.[13] Ultimately, a state of equilibrium is established, with a balance of fluid throughout the fluid compartments. An increase in plasma volume results in increased capillary hydrostatic pressure, forcing fluid into the interstitial space and creating edema. A decrease in plasma volume causes the movement of fluid from the interstitium into the vascular space because the interstitial hydrostatic pressure is greater than the capillary hydrostatic pressure.

BOX 24.3   Factors Stimulating Release of Antidiuretic Hormone

- Hyperosmolality of extracellular fluid
- Hypovolemia
- Increased body temperature
- Medications
- Opioids
- Antineoplastics
- Oral hypoglycemics
- Beta-adrenergics
- Severe emotional or physical stress

BOX 24.4   Factors Stimulating Release of Aldosterone

- Hypovolemia
- Hyponatremia
- Hyperkalemia
- Stress—emotional, physical

Factors Controlling Fluid Balance

Antidiuretic Hormone and Aquaporins

ADH, also known as *vasopressin,* is secreted by the posterior pituitary gland and functions as the primary controller of ECF volume.[14] Feedback messages for release of ADH are sent by osmoreceptors (water receptors) located in the hypothalamus. As serum osmolality increases to greater than 285 mOsm/kg (normal range, 275 to 295 mOsm/kg), ADH is released and carried through the circulation to the nephrons. The kidney distal tubules, connecting tubules, and collecting ducts alter their permeability to water by the action of *aquaporins.*[14] ADH action on osmolality in the kidney is predominantly mediated through the aquaporins. The normal range of urinary osmolality is from 500 to 800 mOsm/kg. Box 24.3 identifies several additional mechanisms that stimulate the release of ADH. In addition to the usual stimuli, the presence of severe emotional or physical stress can initiate ADH release through the limbic system that surrounds the hypothalamus.

Aldosterone

Box 24.4 shows several factors that stimulate the release of aldosterone. The relationship between sodium and water plays an important role in the influence of the RAAS on body water regulation (see Fig. 24.4). A reduction in vascular volume stimulates the release of renin. Renin is converted to angiotensin I, which is converted to the powerful vasoconstrictor angiotensin II. Angiotensin II stimulates the adrenal glands to secrete aldosterone, which acts on the distal tubules to resorb sodium from the tubular lumen into the circulation. When sodium is retained, so is water. Angiotensin II also constricts the renal vasculature, reducing kidney blood flow and available glomerular filtrate, sending a signal to the posterior pituitary to release ADH. The two systems intertwine to maintain fluid–electrolyte balance.

Atrial Natriuretic Peptide

An additional influence on fluid and electrolyte regulation comes from the synthesis of atrial natriuretic peptide (ANP). This hormone is secreted from cells in the atria of the heart in

---

BOX 24.5   Factors Stimulating Release of Atrial Natriuretic Peptide

- Hypernatremia
- Hypervolemia
- Vasoconstriction
- Decreased cardiac output
- Increased cardiac preload and afterload
- Increased systemic vascular resistance

BOX 24.6   Functions of Potassium

Normal Serum Value

- 3.5–4.5 mEq/L

Functions

- Transmission of nerve impulses
- Intracellular osmolality
- Enzymatic reactions
- Acid–base balance
- Myocardial, skeletal, and smooth muscle contractility

BOX 24.7   Factors Affecting Resorption and Secretion of Potassium

- Sodium balance: Sodium deficit results in potassium loss
- Acid–base balance: Acidosis moves hydrogen into the cell and potassium out, with potassium being excreted in urine
- Diuretics: Increased loss of potassium in distal tubule
- Gastrointestinal losses: Vomiting, gastric suction may remove potassium
- Insulin: Promotes movement of potassium into the cell
- Epinephrine: Enhances potassium resorption from distal tubule

---

BOX 24.8   Functions of Sodium

Normal Serum Value

- 135–145 mEq/L

Functions

- Body fluid movement and retention
- Extracellular osmolality
- Active transport mechanism (with potassium)
- Neuromuscular activity
- Enzyme activities
- Acid–base balance

---

response to hypernatremia, stimulation of stretch receptors as a result of increased volume, and increased pressure in the heart (Box 24.5). ANP affects sodium and water balance by blocking aldosterone and ADH production, initiating vasodilation, and stimulating increased sodium and water excretion by the collecting ducts of the kidneys. The physiologic effects of ANP include a reduction in fluid overload through diuresis, decreased cardiac workload, and reduction in cardiac preload and afterload.

ELECTROLYTE BALANCE

Potassium

Potassium (K^+) is the primary intracellular electrolyte and is responsible for numerous physiologic functions (Box 24.6). As with many solutes, diffusion and active transport across the cell membrane maintain potassium balance. Potassium leaves the cell by diffusion, moving toward the area of lesser concentration outside the cell, but it must be actively transported back into the cell to maintain cellular stability.[13] One of the most important potassium functions in the body—that of aiding nervous impulse conduction and muscle contraction—is accomplished with the movement of potassium across the cell membrane. The gastrointestinal tract and skin excrete small amounts of potassium, but the major controllers of potassium stores are the kidneys.[13] Potassium is resorbed by the proximal tubules and secreted into the distal tubules as needed to maintain balance. Resorption and secretion of potassium are influenced by many factors (Box 24.7). Of the estimated 60 to 100 mEq/day ingested by an individual, 90% of the potassium is resorbed before arriving at the distal tubule, where the remainder is usually excreted.

Potassium and sodium are in a constant state of competition within the body despite the need for electrolytes and their different functions. Because both electrolytes are cations, one intracellular and one extracellular, potassium and sodium must remain in balance to preserve electrical neutrality at the cell membrane. In the presence of aldosterone, potassium is excreted by the tubules, and sodium is retained. Potassium wasting may occur despite the body's need for potassium. If potassium stores are low within the cell, the other intracellular electrolytes (magnesium and phosphorus) are often similarly depleted.

Sodium

Sodium (Na^+) is the most abundant extracellular electrolyte in the body and is associated with fluid balance and the amount of water retained or excreted by the kidneys.[13] Along the length of the nephron, sodium is resorbed from the filtrate. This is an active metabolic process that is regulated by site-specific sodium transporters.[15] When diuretics are administered, sodium absorption is inhibited, and consequently sodium is eliminated in the urine.[15] Sodium plays an essential role in the transmission of nerve impulses through the sodium pump, or active transport mechanism, at the cellular level. Sodium is key to many physiologic functions (Box 24.8).

The body contains a complex system of safeguards and feedback mechanisms to protect the level of sodium in the ECF. Sodium balance is regulated by the kidneys, adrenal glands (aldosterone secretion), and posterior pituitary gland (ADH secretion). Most sodium resorption occurs in the proximal tubule under the influence of aldosterone. Because of the extremely sensitive mechanism for retaining sodium, ingestion of large amounts of sodium is unnecessary.

Calcium

Calcium (Ca^{2+}) is the electrolyte of greatest quantity in the body, with stores estimated at 1200 g. Of the total body calcium, 99% is contained in the bones.[16] The remaining 1% is contained primarily in the ECF in the vascular space. The calcium contained within bone is in an inactive form that maintains bone strength and is a ready storehouse for mobilization

---

BOX 24.9   Functions of Calcium

Normal Serum Value
- 8.5–10.5 mg/dL

Functions
- Hardness of bone and teeth
- Skeletal muscle contraction
- Blood coagulation
- Cellular permeability
- Heart muscle contraction

BOX 24.10   Functions of Phosphorus

Normal Serum Value
- 2.5–4.5 mg/dL

Functions
- Intracellular energy production (adenosine triphosphate)
- Bone hardness
- Structure of cellular membrane
- Oxygen delivery to tissues
- Enzyme regulation (adenosine triphosphatase)

---

of calcium to the serum in cases of depletion.[16] In addition to bone metabolism, calcium is responsible for numerous other important functions, including myocardial contractility, coagulation, and neuromuscular activity (Box 24.9).

The mobilization of calcium from bone stores is accomplished through the influence of *parathyroid hormone.* The calcium in the intravascular space (plasma calcium) exists in three forms: ionized, protein bound, or complexed. *Ionized calcium* is the active form and functions in cell membrane stability and blood clotting. Protein-bound calcium, which ionizes more quickly than the calcium in the bone, is readily put to use during an immediate crisis. Complexed calcium is combined with other anions such as chloride, citrate, or phosphate and is available for filtration by the glomerulus for potential removal in the urine. Ionized calcium not needed for physiologic functions is returned to the bone under the influence of the hormone *calcitonin.*

In the ionized (active) form, calcium plays an important role in maintaining the internal integrity of the cell. The amount of ionized calcium in the serum depends on changes in serum pH and on the availability of plasma protein, primarily albumin. Because changes in pH and albumin levels occur with relative frequency, the measurement of total serum calcium alone can be deceptive. To accurately determine the ionized calcium, it is necessary to measure it with a laboratory test because the results of calculated values are unreliable. Estimation of ionized calcium levels—calculated from the serum albumin and total serum calcium—have been found to be inaccurate in critically ill patients. The total serum calcium and the ionized calcium values often are measured. Increasingly, the ionized calcium value is the one used to accurately guide calcium management in critically ill patients.

Calcium levels depend on individual dietary intake and on a variety of physiologic mechanisms related to absorption. The uptake of calcium is influenced by the levels of phosphorus, magnesium, vitamin D and its breakdown products, parathyroid hormone, and calcitonin.

Phosphorus

As with calcium and magnesium, the serum values of phosphorus represent a minute portion of the actual body stores. Approximately 80% of the phosphorus is found in the bones.[16] Most of the remaining phosphorus is intracellular, with only a small amount in the ECF. The primary function of phosphorus is the formation of ATP, which provides intracellular energy for active transport mechanisms across the cell membrane. Additional functions of phosphorus include cell membrane structure, acid–base balance, oxygen delivery to the tissues, cellular immunity, and bone strength (Box 24.10).

Absorption of phosphorus occurs in the gastrointestinal tract, and serum phosphorus levels change frequently and dramatically, particularly in response to the ingestion of phosphate-rich foods such as milk, red meats, poultry, and fish. Most excretion occurs in the kidneys. More than 90% of the phosphorus in the plasma is filtered by the glomerulus, and approximately 80% is resorbed by the proximal tubules. Resorption by the kidneys is increased when body stores are low, and it is combined with sodium and excess hydrogen ions to maintain acid–base balance.

Phosphorus abnormalities are evident early in the course of kidney failure.[17] The Third National Health and Nutrition Examination Survey (NHANES III; 1988–1994, which included 14,722 adults) revealed that people with mild or moderate kidney dysfunction—defined as a urinary creatinine clearance rate of 50 to 60 mL/min—already have elevations of serum phosphorus and potassium levels.[17,18] In contrast, serum ionized calcium remains relatively unchanged until the creatinine clearance rate is extremely low (less than 20 mL/min) and kidney failure is advanced.

Magnesium

Magnesium is the second most important and abundant intracellular electrolyte; approximately 60% of it is located in the bone.[13] The ECF contains only approximately 1% of the body's magnesium, and the remaining amount resides in the ICF. The levels of other intracellular electrolytes, such as calcium and potassium, are affected by the level of magnesium. For example, calcium and magnesium compete for absorption in the gastrointestinal tract. If the dietary intake of calcium is higher than intake of magnesium, calcium is preferentially resorbed and vice versa. The most important functions of magnesium are ensuring the transport of sodium and potassium across the cell membrane and as a cofactor in many intracellular enzyme reactions. Depletion of magnesium liberates potassium to the ECF, which causes an increase in the excretion of potassium by the kidney and hypokalemia. Magnesium also plays a role in maintaining neuromuscular activity, protein synthesis, and intracellular energy production (Box 24.11).

Chloride

Chloride (Cl^-) is predominantly found in the ECF. Changes in serum chloride levels usually indicate changes in the other electrolytes or in acid–base balance. Chloride plays a major role in maintaining serum osmolality, water balance, and acid–base balance. Additional functions of chloride are listed in Box 24.12.

Chloride is usually ingested with sodium in the form of salt and is resorbed or excreted in the proximal tubules of the

---

BOX 24.11   Functions of Magnesium

Normal Serum Value
- 1.3–2.1 mEq/L

Functions
- Neuromuscular transmission
- Contraction of heart muscle
- Activation of enzymes for cellular metabolism
- Active transport at cellular level
- Transmission of hereditary information

BOX 24.12   Functions of Chloride

Normal Serum Value
- 97–110 mEq/L

Functions
- Body fluid osmolality (with sodium)
- Body water balance (with sodium)
- Acid–base balance
- Acidity of body fluids, especially gastric secretions
- Red blood cell oxygenation and carbon dioxide transport

---

kidney. Chloride is actively transported out of the tubules into the interstitium with sodium to help maintain the high tubular interstitial osmolality and the mechanism for concentrating the urine.

Bicarbonate

Bicarbonate (HCO_3^-) is an anion in the ECF, and it performs the essential function of maintaining the acid–base balance.[13] Although bicarbonate is not solely responsible for the acid–base balance, it is the major ECF buffer. Bicarbonate levels in the body are in balance with carbonic acid (H_2CO_3) levels. The ratio between the two must remain proportional at 1 mEq of carbonic acid to 20 mEq of bicarbonate; otherwise, acid–base disturbances will result. When the carbonic acid level is elevated, acidosis results. When the bicarbonate level is high, alkalosis results.

The kidneys regulate the amount of bicarbonate available in the ECF. Resorption of bicarbonate occurs primarily from the proximal tubule into the peritubular capillaries. Bicarbonate is also produced in the distal tubule and resorbed into the blood in response to acid–base balance and body requirements. The kidneys resorb or excrete bicarbonate in response to the number of hydrogen ions present as part of the body's buffer system. More bicarbonate is resorbed when a large number of hydrogen ions are present, and more is excreted when few hydrogen ions are present.

Effects of Aging

Kidney function declines gradually with age, but this usually does not affect homeostasis in a healthy older adult unless proteinuria is present.[19,20] Proteinuria is associated with complications in both the kidney and the cardiovascular systems.[19] With aging, the GFR declines by approximately 0.75 mL/min per year.[19] However, despite the gradual decrease in the GFR and the associated reduction in clearance of creatinine, serum creatinine levels may not rise. This occurs because the reduced muscle mass associated with aging produces less creatinine to be excreted by the kidneys, essentially masking the overall effects of aging on the kidneys. As a result, relatively low levels of serum creatinine in older adults may be associated with reductions in the GFR and creatinine clearance. The gradual decline in kidney function that occurs with aging usually is not a threat to homeostasis because the remaining GFR is adequate. The Cockcroft-Gault formula is used to estimate GFR and includes age in the formula (see Chapter 25).[19] However, when older adults become ill, the decline in kidney function can be accelerated, making older adults especially susceptible to acute and chronic kidney dysfunction.

The kidneys carry out many functions. Although fluid balance is perhaps the most obvious function, an understanding of the numerous other roles of the kidneys provides crucial information for the care of any critically ill patient.

SUMMARY

Anatomy
- The kidneys are paired organs located retroperitoneally, one on each side of the vertebral column between T12 and L3.
- The nephron is the functional unit of the kidney; it comprises the glomerulus, proximal tubule, loop of Henle, distal tubule, and collecting ducts.

Physiology
- The kidneys play a major role in maintaining homeostasis.
- Important functions of the kidneys include waste product removal, fluid–electrolyte balance, and acid–base balance.
- Hormone functions of the kidneys support red blood cell production, blood pressure regulation, and bone metabolism.
- Kidney function declines gradually with age, making older adults more susceptible to kidney dysfunction during illness.
- Visit the Evolve site for additional study materials.

REFERENCES

1. Nielsen S, et al. Anatomy of the kidney. In: Taal MW, et al., eds. *Brenner & Rector's The Kidney.* 9th ed. Vol. 1. Philadelphia: Saunders; 2011.
2. Munger KA, et al. The renal circulations and glomerular ultrafiltration. In: Taal MW, et al., eds. *Brenner & Rector's The Kidney.* 9th ed. Vol. 2. Philadelphia: Saunders; 2011.
3. Menon MC, Chuang PY, He CJ. The glomerular filtration barrier: components and crosstalk. *Internat J Nephrol.* 2012. Article ID 749010, 9 pages http://dx.doi.org/10.1155/2012/749010.
4. Kurtz A. Renin release: sites, mechanisms, and control. *Annu Rev Physiol.* 2011;73:377.
5. Perlewitz A, Persson AE, Patzak A. The juxtaglomerular apparatus. *Acta Physiol.* 2012;205(1):6.
6. Velez JC. The importance of the intrarenal renin-angiotensin system. *Nat Clin Pract Nephrol.* 2009;5(2):89.
7. Kumar R, et al. The intracrine renin-angiotensin system. *Clin Sci.* 2012;123(5):273.
8. Moore E, Bellomo R. Erythropoietin (EPO) in acute kidney injury. *Ann Intensive Care.* 2011;1(1):3.
9. Ramanath V, et al. Anemia and chronic kidney disease: making sense of the recent trials. *Rev Recent Clin Trials.* 2012;7(3):187.
10. Kandula P, et al. Vitamin D supplementation in chronic kidney disease: a systematic review and meta-analysis of observational studies and randomized controlled trials. *Clin J Am Soc Nephrol.* 2011;6(1):50.
11. Sterling KA, et al. The immunoregulatory function of vitamin D: implications in chronic kidney disease. *Nat Rev Nephrol.* 2012;8(7):403.

12. Wang H, et al. Prostaglandin E1 for preventing the progression of diabetic kidney disease. *Cochrane Database Syst Rev*. 2010;(5):CD006872.

13. Rhoda KM, Porter MJ, Quintini C. Fluid and electrolyte management: Putting a plan in motion. *JPEN J Parent Enteral Nutr*. 2011;35(6):675.

14. Knepper MA. Systems biology in physiology: the vasopressin signaling network in kidney. *Am J Physiol Cell Physiol*. 2012;303(11):C1115.

15. Bernstein PL, Ellison DH. Diuretics and salt transport along the nephron. *Semin Nephrol*. 2011;31(6):475.

16. Bonjour JP. Calcium and phosphate: a duet of ions playing for bone health. *J Am Coll Nutr*. 2011;30(5 Suppl 1):438S.

17. O'Seaghdha CM, et al. Serum phosphorus predicts incident chronic kidney disease and end-stage renal disease. *Nephrol Dial Transplant*. 2011;26(9):2885.

18. Hsu CY, Chertow GM. Elevations of serum phosphorus and potassium in mild to moderate chronic renal insufficiency. *Nephrol Dial Transplant*. 2002;17(8):1419.

19. Verma V, et al. Proteinuria in the elderly: Avaluation and management. *Int Urol Nephrol*. 2012;44(6):1745.

20. Peters R, et al. Kidney function in the very elderly with hypertension: data from the hypertension in the very elderly (HYVET) trial. *Age Ageing*. 2013;42(2):253.

25

Kidney Clinical Assessment and Diagnostic Procedures

Mary E. Lough

Understanding the anatomic structures and physiologic workings of the kidneys provides the basis for understanding the clinical manifestations that signal kidney or renal vascular dysfunction. The body produces many clinical signs and symptoms that indicate kidney disorders. However, these signs and symptoms are often subtle, and although some symptoms point directly to the kidneys, many are exhibited by other body systems. A detailed history and careful physical examination help focus on the kidneys as the source of symptoms and often uncover the cause of the problem.

HISTORY

The history begins with a description of the chief complaint or primary problem, stated in the patient's own words. A description of the chief complaint includes the onset, location, duration, and factors or strategies that lessen or aggravate the problem.[1] The patient should be encouraged to describe the effects of any treatment for the problem, prescription and nonprescription medications taken to alleviate symptoms, efforts taken to determine the cause of the problem, and procedures performed to improve the problem. A careful history that explores symptoms fully is an essential component of the clinical assessment.

Predisposing factors for acute kidney dysfunction are obtained during the history including the use of over-the-counter medicines, recent infections requiring antibiotic therapy, antihypertensive medicines, and any diagnostic procedures performed using radiopaque contrast dye.[2] Nonsteroidal antiinflammatory medications (eg, ibuprofen), antibiotics (especially aminoglycosides), antihypertensives (especially medicines that block angiotensin),[3] and iodine-based dyes may cause an acute or chronic decline in kidney function. A history of recent onset of nausea and vomiting or appetite loss caused by taste changes (uremia often causes a metallic taste) may provide clues to the rapid onset of kidney problems.[2] Symptoms that indicate rapid fluid volume gains are explored. For example, weight gains of more than 2 lb per day, sleeping on additional pillows, and sitting in a chair to sleep are signals of volume overload and potential cardiac stress related to kidney dysfunction. Fluid volume overload and edema are frequent findings in severe critical illness related to systemic inflammation, fluid loss from capillaries, volume administration, and acute kidney injury (AKI).[4]

In addition to determining the immediate reason for admission to the critical care unit, compiling a complete medical and social history is important. Similar symptoms, problems, or treatment for similar complaints in the past may help establish the cause of the current problem or provide clues

for treatment. For example, a history of obstructive urologic problems, frequent kidney infections, or previous AKI or kidney failure may signal risk factors for current kidney problems. The patient, family member, or significant other should be encouraged to provide as much detail as possible during the history.

The family history may provide important information that suggests the kidneys are the source of the patient's symptoms. For example, the patient may reveal that one or two close family members have always had swelling of the extremities or high blood pressure. These symptoms should lead to questions about a history of kidney problems in the family. Box 25.1 summarizes the information gained from a kidney history.

PHYSICAL EXAMINATION

In the critical care area, nursing assessment does not routinely include a full physical examination of the kidneys and urologic system. However, many of the assessment parameters for the kidneys provide information related to the volume status of the patient and are helpful in numerous patients regardless of kidney function or status. Although not often performed in the depth described in the following sections, the critical care nurse must be aware of how to perform a thorough kidney assessment in stable patients and as needed in patients with kidney dysfunction.

Inspection
Bleeding
Visual inspection related to the kidneys focuses on the patient's flank and abdomen. Kidney trauma is suspected if a purplish discoloration is present on the flank (Grey Turner sign) or near the posterior 11th or 12th ribs. Bruising, abdominal distention, and abdominal guarding may also signal kidney trauma or a hematoma around a kidney. Individuals who have experienced a traumatic injury should be carefully assessed for signs of kidney trauma.[1]

Volume
Inspection is especially helpful in looking for signs of volume depletion or overload that may signal or lead to kidney problems. Fluid volume assessment begins with an inspection of the patient's jugular neck veins. The supine position facilitates normal jugular venous distention. An absence of distention (flat neck veins) indicates hypovolemia. Assessment continues with the head of the bed elevated 45 to 90 degrees.[1] Fluid overload exists when the neck veins remain distended more than 2 cm above the sternal notch when the bed is at 45 degrees.

BOX 25.1   DATA COLLECTION

Kidney History

Common Kidney-Related Symptoms
- Dyspnea
- Peripheral dependent edema
- Nocturia
- Nausea
- Metallic taste in mouth
- Loss of appetite
- Headache
- Rapid weight gain
- Itching
- Dry, scaly skin
- Weakness, fatigue
- Cognitive function changes
- Mental status changes

Patient Profile
- Personal habits
- Use of over-the-counter medications, herbs, vitamins, and dietary supplements
- Illicit drug use
- Change in employment caused by illness
- Financial problems resulting from illness (eg, cost, time off work)
- Sexual function (eg, decreased libido, amenorrhea)

Risk Factors
- Family history
- Hypertension
- Diabetes mellitus
- Prior acute kidney injury

Medical History
Child
- Nephrotic syndrome, streptococcal infection, hypoplastic kidneys, obstructive uropathy

Adult
- Frequent urinary tract infections
- Calculi
- Vasculitis
- Use of iodine-based radiographic contrast media
- Use of nonsteroidal antiinflammatory medications

Family History
- Hypertension
- Diabetes mellitus
- Polycystic kidney disease
- Kidney disease
- Chronically swollen extremities

Current Medication Use
- Nonsteroidal antiinflammatory medications
- Antibiotics
- Antihypertensives
- Diuretics

Past Kidney Studies
- Urinalysis with proteinuria
- Creatinine clearance
- KUB radiograph
- Intravenous pyelogram
- Kidney ultrasound
- Renal arteriography
- Kidney biopsy

KUB, kidney-ureter-bladder.

Inspection of the veins of the hand may be helpful in assessing volume status and is performed by observing for venous distention when the hand is held in the dependent position. Venous filling that takes longer than 5 seconds suggests hypovolemia. When the hand is elevated, the distention should disappear within 5 seconds. If distention does not disappear within 5 seconds after the hand is elevated, fluid overload is suspected.

Assessment of skin turgor provides additional data for identifying fluid-related problems. To assess turgor, the skin over the forearm is picked up and released.[5] Normal elasticity and fluid status allow an almost immediate return to shape after the skin is released. In the presence of fluid volume deficit, the skin remains raised and does not return to its normal position for several seconds.[5] Because of the loss of skin elasticity in older persons, skin turgor assessment may not be an accurate fluid assessment measure for this age group.[6]

Inspection of the oral cavity provides clues to fluid volume status. When a fluid volume deficit exists, the mucous membranes of the mouth become dry. However, mouth breathing and some medicines (eg, antihistamines) can also dry the mucous membranes temporarily. The most accurate way to assess the oral cavity is to inspect the mouth using a tongue blade and light. Dryness of the oral cavity is more indicative of fluid volume deficit than complaints of a dry mouth.

Edema

Edema is the presence of excess fluid in the interstitial space, and it can be a sign of volume overload.[4] In the presence of volume excess, edema may develop in dependent areas of the body, such as the feet and legs of an ambulatory person or the sacrum of an individual confined to bed. However, edema does not always indicate fluid volume overload. A loss of albumin from the vascular space can cause peripheral edema despite hypovolemia or normal fluid states. A critically ill patient may have a low serum albumin level (hypoalbuminemia) because of inadequate nutrition after surgery, a burn, or a head injury and may exhibit edema as a result of the loss of plasma oncotic pressure and not as a result of volume overload. Edema also may signal circulatory difficulties. An individual who is fluid balanced but who has poor venous return may experience pedal edema after prolonged sitting in a chair with the feet dependent. Similarly, an individual with heart failure may experience edema because the left ventricle is unable to pump blood effectively through the vessels. A key

TABLE 25.1 **Pitting Edema Scale**

Rating	Approximate Equivalent
+1	2-mm depth
+2	4-mm depth (lasting up to 15 s)
+3	6-mm depth (lasting up to 60 s)
+4	8-mm depth (lasting longer than 60 s)

BOX 25.2 **Orthostatic Hypotension Assessment**

1. Take blood pressure (BP) and heart rate (HR) with patient lying down.
2. Assist patient to sitting position.
   Monitor patient for complaints of dizziness or imbalance. Take BP and HR immediately and record.
   Take BP and HR after 3 min and record.
3. Assist patient to a standing position (if patient is not dizzy or loses balance). Assess as above.

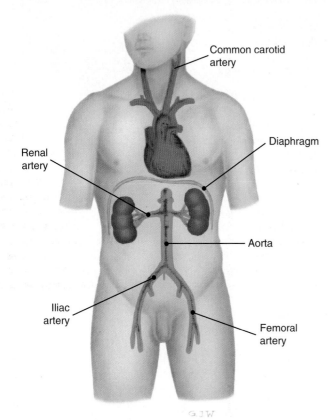

FIG. 25.1 Sites for Auscultation of Bruits.

feature that distinguishes edema resulting from excess volume or hypoalbuminemia from circulatory compromise is that the edema does not reverse with elevation of the extremity.

Edema can be assessed by applying fingertip pressure on the swollen area over a bony prominence, such as the ankles, pretibial areas (shins), and sacrum. If the indentation made by the fingertip does not disappear within 15 seconds, pitting edema exists. Pitting edema indicates increased interstitial volume, and it usually is not evident until significant weight gain has occurred. Edema also may appear in the hands and feet, around the eyes, and in the cheeks. In patients confined to a wheelchair or bed, dependent areas such as the feet and sacrum are the areas most likely to demonstrate edema. One way of measuring the extent of edema is by using a subjective scale of 1 to 4, with 1 indicating only minimal pitting and 4 indicating severe pitting (Table 25.1).[1] Other scales for assessing and measuring edema also can be used (see Table 12.3).

Auscultation

Auscultation of the kidneys yields virtually no useful information. However, the renal arteries are auscultated for a bruit, a blowing or swishing sound that resembles a cardiac murmur

(Fig. 25.1). The examiner listens for bruits above and to the left and right of the umbilicus.[1] A renal artery bruit usually indicates stenosis, which may lead to acute or chronic kidney dysfunction secondary to compromised blood flow to one or both kidneys. A bruit over the upper portion of the abdominal aorta may indicate an aneurysm or a stenotic area that can decrease blood flow to the kidneys.

Auscultation is especially helpful in providing information about extracellular fluid volume status. Listening for specific sounds in the heart and lungs provides information about the presence or absence of increased fluid in the interstitium or vascular space.

Heart

Auscultation of the heart requires assessing the rate and rhythm and listening for extra sounds. Fluid overload is often accompanied by a third or fourth heart sound, which is best heard with the bell of the stethoscope.[1] Increased heart rate alone provides little information about fluid volume, but combined with a low blood pressure, it may indicate hypovolemia.

The heart is auscultated for the presence of a pericardial friction rub. A rub can best be heard at the third intercostal space to the left of the sternal border while the patient leans slightly forward.[1] A pericardial friction rub indicates pericarditis, and it may result from uremia in a patient with kidney failure.

Blood Pressure

Blood pressure and heart rate changes are very useful in assessing fluid volume deficit.[3] In stable critically ill patients or in patients on a telemetry unit, orthostatic vital sign measurements provide clues to blood loss, dehydration, unexplained syncope, and the effects of some antihypertensive medications. A decrease in systolic blood pressure of 20 mm Hg or more, a decrease in diastolic blood pressure of 10 mm Hg or more, or an increase in pulse rate of more than 15 beats/min from lying to sitting or from sitting to standing indicates orthostatic hypotension. Box 25.2 describes how to assess for orthostatic hypotension. The decrease in blood pressure occurs because a sufficient preload is not immediately available when the patient changes position. The heart rate increases in an attempt to maintain cardiac output and circulation. Orthostatic hypotension produces subjective feelings of weakness, dizziness, or faintness. Orthostatic hypotension occurs with hypovolemia, prolonged bed rest, or as a side effect of medications that affect blood volume or blood pressure.

Lungs

Lung assessment is essential in gauging fluid status. Crackles indicate fluid overload. Dyspnea with mild exertion, dyspnea at night that prevents sleeping in a supine position (orthopnea), or dyspnea that awakens the individual from sleep (paroxysmal

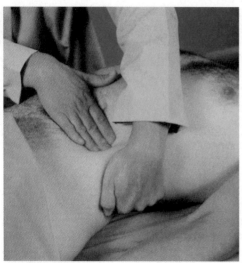

FIG. 25.2 Palpation of the Kidney. (From Barkauskas V, et al. *Health and Physical Assessment*. 3rd ed. St. Louis: Mosby; 2002.)

FIG. 25.3 Test for the Presence of a Fluid Wave. (From Barkauskas V, et al. *Health and Physical Assessment*. 3rd ed. St. Louis: Mosby; 2002.)

nocturnal dyspnea) may indicate pooling of fluid in the lungs. Shallow, gasping breaths with periods of apnea reflect severe acid–base imbalances.

Palpation

Although rarely performed in critically ill patients, palpation of the kidneys in stable patients provides information about the size and shape of the kidneys. Palpation of the kidneys is done through the bimanual capturing approach. Capturing is accomplished by placing one hand posteriorly under the flank of a supine patient with the examiner's fingers pointing to the midline and placing the opposite hand just below the rib cage anteriorly.[1,2] The patient is asked to inhale deeply while pressure is exerted to bring the hands together (Fig. 25.2). As the patient exhales, the examiner may feel the kidney between the hands. After each kidney is palpated in this manner, the two kidneys should be compared for size and shape. Each kidney should be firm and smooth, and the two organs should be of equal size. The examiner is usually unable to palpate a normal left kidney. The right kidney is more easily palpated because of its lower position, caused by downward displacement by the liver. Problems should be suspected if a mass (cancer) or an irregular surface (polycystic kidneys) is palpated, a size difference is detected, the kidney extends significantly lower than the rib cage on either side, or there is evidence of recent blunt trauma.[1]

Percussion

Percussion is performed to detect pain in the area of a kidney or to determine excess accumulation of air, fluid, or solids around the kidneys. Percussion of the kidneys also provides information about kidney location, size, and possible problems. Similar to palpation, percussion of the kidneys is not a routine part of a nursing assessment in critical care. However, the information gained through percussion can provide important patient care data.

Kidneys

Percussion of a kidney is performed with the patient in a side-lying or sitting position, with the examiner's hand placed over the costovertebral angle (lower border of the rib cage on the flank).[1] Striking the back of the hand with the opposite fist produces

a dull thud, which is normal. Pain may indicate infection (eg, urinary tract infection that has extended into the kidneys) or injury resulting from trauma. Traumatic injury to the kidneys should be assessed in the presence of a penetrating abdominal wound, blunt abdominal trauma, or a fractured pelvis or ribs.

Abdomen

Observation and percussion of the abdomen may help in assessing fluid status. Percussing the abdomen with the patient in the supine position generally yields a dull sound (solid bowel contents or fluid) or a hollow sound (gaseous bowel).[1]

Ascites, or excess fluid accumulation and distention of the abdominal cavity, is an important observation in determining fluid overload. Differentiating ascites from distortion caused by solid bowel contents is accomplished by producing a fluid wave. A fluid wave is elicited by exerting pressure to the abdominal midline while one hand is placed on the right or left flank.[1] Tapping the opposite flank produces a wave in the accumulated fluid that can be felt under the hands (Fig. 25.3). Other signs of ascites include a protuberant, rounded abdomen and abdominal striae.[1]

Individuals with kidney failure may have ascites caused by volume overload, which forces fluid into the abdomen as a result of increased capillary hydrostatic pressures. However, ascites may or may not represent fluid volume excess. Severe ascites in patients with compromised liver function may result from decreased plasma proteins. The ascites occurs because the increased vascular pressure associated with liver dysfunction forces fluid and plasma proteins from the vascular space into the interstitial space and abdominal cavity. Although the patient may exhibit marked edema, the intravascular space is volume depleted, and the patient is hypovolemic.

ADDITIONAL ASSESSMENTS

Weight Monitoring

One of the most important assessments of kidney and fluid status is the patient's weight. In the critical care unit, weight is monitored for each patient every day and is an important vital sign measurement. Significant fluctuations in body weight over a 1- to 2-day period indicate fluid gains and losses. Rapid weight gains or losses of more than 2 lb per day usually indicate fluid rather than nutritional factors; 1 L of fluid equals 1 kg, or approximately 2.2 lb.

Whenever possible, the patient is weighed during admission to the critical care unit. It is important to document whether the current weight differs significantly from the weight 1 to 2 weeks before admission to the hospital. The patient is weighed daily for comparison with the previous day's weight. The weight is obtained at the same time each day, with the patient wearing the same amount of clothing and using the same scales. The individual's weight is of critical importance to the dialysis nurse caring for a patient with acute or chronic kidney failure. The differences in weight from day to day are used to calculate the amount of fluid to remove during a dialysis treatment.

Intake and Output Monitoring

Similar to patient weight, intake and output are monitored for all patients in the critical care unit. Intake and output can be compared with the patient's weight to evaluate fluid gains or losses more accurately. Urinary output plus insensible fluid losses (perspiration, stool, and water vapor from the lungs) can vary by 750 to 2400 mL/day. When intake exceeds output (eg, excessive intravenous fluid, decreased urine output), a positive fluid balance exists. With impaired kidney function, the positive fluid balance results in fluid volume overload. Conversely, if output exceeds intake (eg, fever, increased respiration, profuse sweating, vomiting, diarrhea, gastric suction, diuretic therapy), a negative fluid balance exists, and volume deficit results. During a 24-hour period, fever can increase skin and respiratory losses by 75 mL per 1°F increase in temperature.

Individuals with AKI often exhibit a decrease in urine output, or oliguria (less than 0.5 mL/kg per hour in adults; less than 1 mL/kg per hour in infants and young children). However, there may be a normal or only slightly decreased urine output that reflects water removal without solute removal in the early phases of AKI. Although urine output is a sensitive indicator, kidney function cannot be accurately determined by urine output alone. For additional information on AKI, see Chapter 26.

Abnormal output of body fluids creates fluid imbalances and causes electrolyte and acid–base disturbances. For example, gastrointestinal suction or loss by diarrhea can result in fluid deficit, sodium and potassium deficits, and metabolic acidosis from excessive loss of bicarbonate.

In maintaining daily records of intake and output, all gains or losses must be recorded. A standard list of the fluid volume held in various containers (eg, milk cartons, juice containers) expedites this process. Discussions about the importance of accurate recording of intake and output with the patient and family or friends are necessary and can improve the accuracy of assessment of intake and output volumes.

Hemodynamic Monitoring

Body fluid status is accurately reflected in measurements of cardiovascular hemodynamics. Measurements such as central venous pressure (CVP), pulmonary artery occlusion pressure (PAOP), cardiac index (CI), and mean arterial pressure (MAP) provide a clear picture of the increases or decreases in vascular volume returning to and being ejected from the heart.[7] Volume depletion and volume overload are easily detected by the use of

TABLE 25.2 Hemodynamic Assessment of Fluid Status

Measurement	Volume Depletion	Volume Overload
CVP	<2 mm Hg	>5 mm Hg
PAOP	<5 mm Hg	>12 mm Hg
CI	<2.2 L/min/m²	>4 L/min/m²
MAP	Decreased	Increased

CI, cardiac index; CVP, central venous pressure; MAP, mean arterial pressure; PAOP, pulmonary artery occlusion pressure.

central venous or arterial catheters, from which pressure measurements can be obtained (Table 25.2).

A central venous catheter often is inserted to evaluate fluid volume status and to measure the CVP. The CVP represents the filling pressure of the right atrium and is a measurement of right ventricular preload. The CVP changes with fluctuations in volume status. A normal CVP is 2 to 5 mm Hg. In volume depletion, the CVP is less than 2 mm Hg, whereas volume overload is reflected by readings of more than 5 mm Hg (see "Central Venous Pressure Monitoring" in Chapter 13 for more information on CVP interpretation).

If the patient has coexisting cardiopulmonary disease or if more information about hemodynamic function is required, a pulmonary artery catheter may be inserted. This catheter provides information about left ventricular filling pressures and cardiac output. The PAOP represents the left atrial pressure required to fill the left ventricle. When the left ventricle is full at the end of diastole, it represents the volume of blood available for ejection. It is also known as left ventricular preload and is measured by the PAOP. The normal PAOP is 5 to 12 mm Hg. In fluid volume excess, the PAOP increases. In fluid volume deficit, the PAOP is low.[7]

The CI demonstrates the cardiac output, or amount of blood ejected by the left ventricle over 1 minute, standardized for body size. The normal CI is 2.2 to 4 L/min per m². Compensatory mechanisms in early hypovolemic shock maintain the CI at or near normal. With prolonged fluid loss, the CI decreases. Fluid volume overload increases heart rate, which increases cardiac output, but only to a point. Left ventricular failure may result from massive volume overload, such as with acute heart failure resulting from kidney failure, in which case the CI decreases. The most common cause of AKI in which hemodynamic monitoring is indicated is severe sepsis.[7]

MAP is regulated by cardiac output and systemic vascular resistance (SVR) and represents an averaged blood pressure within the arterial system. Changes in cardiac output or SVR inevitably result in corresponding MAP changes. For example, an increase in SVR during the early stages of hypovolemic shock leads to elevation of the MAP. Ongoing fluid losses eventually lead to decreased cardiac output, which leads to a reduction in MAP. The net effect of a decreased MAP on the kidneys is a reduction in effective blood flow, which may lead to AKI.

Other Observations

Kidney system dysfunction often leads to fluid and electrolyte imbalances and the retention of metabolic waste products. Some of the disturbances in fluid, electrolyte, and waste product levels are accompanied by clinical manifestations less observable or measurable than manifestations previously mentioned but that indicate a change from normal function. Box 25.3 summarizes

BOX 25.3 Fluid and Electrolyte Assessment

Fluid Status

- Skin turgor
- Mucous membranes
- Intake and output
- Presence of edema or ascites
- Neck and hand vein engorgement
- Lung crackles (rales)
- Dyspnea
- Central venous pressure <2 mm Hg or >5 mm Hg
- Pulmonary artery occlusive pressure <5 mm Hg or >12 mm Hg
- Tachycardia
- Hypertension, hypotension
- Cardiac index <2.2 L/min/m^2
- S_3, S_4 heart sounds
- Headache
- Blurred vision
- Vertigo on rising
- Papilledema
- Mental changes
- Serum osmolality

Electrolyte and Waste Product Status

- Complete blood cell count
- Serum electrolyte levels
- Nitrogen waste products (blood urea nitrogen [BUN])
- Electrocardiogram tracings (potassium, calcium, magnesium levels)
- Behavioral and mental changes (sodium, BUN levels)
- Chvostek and Trousseau signs (calcium levels)
- Changes in peripheral sensation (numbness, tremor—sodium, potassium, calcium levels)
- Muscle strength (potassium, BUN)
- Gastrointestinal changes (nausea and vomiting—BUN)
- Itching (calcium, phosphorus, BUN)
- Therapies that can alter electrolyte status (gastrointestinal suction, diuretics, antihypertensives, calcium channel blockers)

important aspects to consider during kidney and fluid and electrolyte assessment.

Sudden or slowly developing changes in cognitive function and mental status must be investigated. For example, acidosis often results in disorientation. Lethargy, decreased attention or memory, coma, and confusion may result from sodium, calcium, or magnesium excess or deficit or retained waste products. Apprehension or anxiety may result from sodium deficit, a shift of fluid from the plasma to the interstitium, or respiratory changes caused by fluid volume overload. Apathy and withdrawal may accompany hypovolemic states.

Patients with kidney failure and the accompanying systemic increases in electrolytes, fluids, and nitrogenous waste products may exhibit apathy, restlessness, mental status changes, and withdrawal.[2] The speed of onset depends on how rapidly or slowly the kidney failure progresses and alters homeostasis.

LABORATORY ASSESSMENT

There is no single or ideal laboratory test or marker that detects a decrease in kidney function. Laboratory tests used to detect and diagnose kidney dysfunction have limitations, but when

reviewed daily for changes or trends, they provide valuable information concerning the status of the kidneys.[8] AKI must be identified as early as possible because it is associated with significant mortality in critically ill patients.[9]

Blood Urea Nitrogen

Blood urea nitrogen (BUN) is a by-product of protein and amino acid metabolism. The normal value for BUN is 5 to 20 mg/dL; this value is increased when kidney function deteriorates. With kidney dysfunction, the BUN is elevated because of a decrease in the glomerular filtration rate (GFR) and resulting decrease in urea excretion. Elevations in the BUN can be correlated with the clinical manifestations of uremia; as BUN increases, symptoms of uremia become more pronounced.[2] However, a decrease in the GFR with an increase in the BUN also may be caused by hypovolemia and dehydration, nephrotoxic medications, or a sudden hypotensive episode. In these cases, the increase in BUN is caused by a decreased GFR in the presence of normal kidney function. BUN is also increased by changes in protein metabolism that occur with excessive protein intake and catabolism. A catabolic state may occur with starvation (or chronic poor nutrition in a critically ill patient), severe infection, surgery, or trauma. The BUN level also may be elevated as the result of hematoma resorption, gastrointestinal bleeding, excessive licorice ingestion, or steroid or tetracycline therapy. A decrease in the BUN level may indicate volume overload, liver damage, severe malnutrition (as a result of depleted protein stores), use of phenothiazines, or pregnancy.

Creatinine

Creatinine is a by-product of muscle and normal cell metabolism, and it appears in serum in amounts generally proportional to the body muscle mass. The normal serum creatinine level is approximately 0.5 to 1.2 mg/dL; this value is slightly higher in men than women. Creatinine is freely filtered by the glomerulus, easily excreted by the kidney tubules, and minimally resorbed or secreted in the tubules.[2] Creatinine levels are fairly constant and are affected by fewer factors than BUN levels. As a result, the serum creatinine level is a more sensitive and specific indicator of kidney function than BUN. Creatinine excess occurs most often in patients with kidney failure resulting from impaired excretion. However, the body's production and release of creatinine may vary during muscle wasting in acute illness, leading to a falsely low serum level of creatinine. Elevated levels of creatinine are seen in muscle growth disorders such as acromegaly, with traumatic skeletal muscle injury, and with some medications that decrease creatinine removal (eg, trimethoprim, cimetidine) in the absence of kidney dysfunction. Malnutrition can result in transient increases in creatinine levels, as the rapid muscle catabolism associated with malnutrition releases increased amounts of creatinine into the circulation.

Blood Urea Nitrogen-to-Creatinine Ratio

Another useful diagnostic parameter in kidney disease is the ratio of BUN to creatinine. The usual ratio of BUN to creatinine is 10:1, and a change in the ratio may indicate kidney dysfunction. For example, if BUN and creatinine levels are elevated and maintained at an approximate ratio of 10:1, the disorder is intrarenal, or affecting the tubules of the kidneys. If the ratio of BUN to creatinine levels is greater than 10:1, the cause is most likely prerenal (eg, hypovolemia). In prerenal kidney failure, the creatinine is excreted by functioning tubules, but the urea

BOX 25.4 Creatinine Clearance Calculations[a]

Measured: 24-Hour Urine

(Urine creatinine × Volume of urine) /Serum creatinine

Estimated: Adults—Cockcroft-Gault Formula

[(140 − Age) × Body weight (kg)] / [72 × Plasma creatinine (mg/dL)]

For women, multiply the result by 0.85.

Estimated: Adults—Modification of Diet in Renal Disease Formula

186 × (Plasma creatinine) − 1.154 × (Age in years) − 0.203

For women, multiply the result by 0.742.
For African Americans, multiply the result by 1.210.[b]

Estimated: Children

$\leq$ 10 kg : 0.45 × Height (cm)/Serum creatinine (mg/dL)

> 10 , < 70 kg : 0.55 × Height (cm)/Serum creatinine (mg/dL)

$\geq$ 70 kg : [1.55 × Age (y)] + 0.5 × Height (cm)/Serum creatinine (mg/dL)

[a]Online calculators available from the National Kidney Foundation at http://www.kidney.org/professionals.
[b]Both risk factor assessments apply for African American women. The number would be multiplied by both 0.742 (woman) and 1.210 (African American).

nitrogen is retained because of the poor GFR and hemoconcentration, leading to the increased ratio. In the diagnosis of prerenal kidney failure, the ratio is a more useful indicator of kidney function than the separate tests of BUN and creatinine.[6]

Creatinine Clearance

The urine creatinine clearance is a measure of how well the kidneys remove creatinine. Because of the relatively constant rate at which creatinine is produced and the nearly complete removal of creatinine by normal kidneys, the ability of the kidneys to remove (clear) creatinine from the blood is an indication of how well the glomeruli and tubules are working. Measuring the creatinine clearance—the amount of creatinine in the excreted urine and the amount of creatinine in the blood over 24 hours—provides a reliable and accurate estimate of glomerular filtration and of kidney function.[2] The normal value for creatinine clearance is 110 to 120 mL/min; values less than 50 mL/min indicate significant kidney dysfunction. The creatinine clearance is traditionally measured using a 12-hour or 24-hour urine collection and blood sample. Newer methods use a random, smaller volume urine specimen and blood sample. Creatinine clearance can also be estimated from the serum creatinine level (Box 25.4), a method commonly used in the critical care unit. The estimated or calculated creatinine clearance is widely used to determine changes in medication dosing with kidney dysfunction because of the many medications excreted by the kidneys.

Cystatin C

Although not widely used in practice, cystatin C is another serum marker for kidney function. Cystatin C is a substance synthesized and released by most cells in the body at a constant rate.[10] Similar to creatinine, cystatin C is filtered easily by the glomerulus and not secreted or resorbed by the tubules. The advantage of cystatin C is that it is metabolized by the tubules. In normal kidney function, cystatin C levels are very low because the glomerulus filters it and the tubules metabolize it. In kidney dysfunction, the glomerular filtration of cystatin C is reduced and not provided to the tubules for metabolism. Cystatin C is affected by fewer factors (eg, age, sex, muscle mass) than creatinine, and a change in its level can be detected earlier during AKI than creatinine.[10] Cystatin C and other kidney-related biomarkers may become more widely used as kidney function markers as additional clinical validation studies are completed.[10]

Osmolality

The serum osmolality reflects the concentration or dilution of vascular fluid and measures the dissolved particles in the serum. The normal serum osmolality is 275 to 295 mOsm/L.[3] An elevated osmolality level indicates hemoconcentration or dehydration, and a decreased osmolality level indicates hemodilution or volume overload. When the serum osmolality level increases, antidiuretic hormone (ADH) is released from the posterior pituitary gland and stimulates increased water resorption in the kidney tubules. This expands the vascular space, returns the serum osmolality level back to normal, and results in more concentrated urine and an elevated urine osmolality level. The opposite occurs with a decreased serum osmolality level, which inhibits the production of ADH. The decreased ADH results in increased excretion of water in the tubules, producing dilute urine with a low osmolality, and returns the serum osmolality level back to normal. Sodium accounts for 85% to 95% of the serum osmolality value; doubling the serum sodium level gives an estimate of the serum osmolality level in healthy individuals. Other particles in the serum can increase the osmolality and need to be considered in patients with common comorbid conditions. A more precise estimation of serum osmolality can be calculated from the following formula:

$$2 \times Na \ (mEq/L) + BUN/3 \ (mg/dL) + Glucose/18 \ (mg/dL)$$

The calculated serum osmolality level is a useful tool while awaiting full laboratory results. Measured serum osmolality is a useful parameter in determining fluid balance and fluid replacement therapy for critically ill patients. Serum osmolality is also a useful parameter in determining disorders of ADH secretion that may occur in critically ill patients. A decreased serum osmolality level may indicate syndrome of inappropriate ADH secretion, or too much ADH, whereas an elevation of the serum osmolality level may indicate diabetes insipidus, or too little ADH.

Anion Gap

The *anion gap* is a calculation of the difference between the measurable extracellular plasma cations (sodium and potassium) and the measurable anions (chloride and bicarbonate).[3] In plasma, sodium is the predominant cation, and chloride is the predominant anion. Extracellular potassium concentration in plasma is so small that it is generally ignored, leaving the following equation for calculation of the anion gap:

$$[Na^+] - ([Cl^-] + [HCO_3^-])$$

The normal anion gap is 8 to 16 mEq/L, a range that has been verified in a healthy population of adults.[11] The "gap" represents the unmeasurable ions present in the extracellular fluid (phosphates, sulfates, ketones, lactate). An increased anion gap level usually reflects overproduction or decreased excretion of acid products and indicates metabolic acidosis; a decreased anion gap indicates metabolic alkalosis.

Acute and chronic kidney failure can increase the anion gap because of retention of acids and altered bicarbonate resorption.[12] The anion gap is also increased in diabetic ketoacidosis caused by ketone production. The measurement of the anion gap is a rapid method for identifying acid–base imbalance but cannot be used to pinpoint the source of the acid–base disturbance specifically.

Hemoglobin and Hematocrit

The hemoglobin and hematocrit levels can indicate increases or decreases in intravascular fluid volume. Hemoglobin and hematocrit values vary between sexes; the hemoglobin level in men is normally 13.5 to 17.5 g/dL and in women is 12 to 16 g/dL. The hematocrit level is 40% to 54% in men and 37% to 47% in women. Hematocrit levels are higher in newborns (up to 65%) and decrease to adult ranges between the ages of 4 and 10 years. Hemoglobin transports oxygen and carbon dioxide and is important in maintaining cellular metabolism and acid–base balance.[3]

The hematocrit value is the proportion or concentration of red blood cells (RBCs) in a volume of whole blood and is expressed as a percentage. The hematocrit level is approximately three times the hemoglobin level if the individual is in a normal fluid balance. An increase in the hematocrit value often indicates a fluid volume deficit, which results in hemoconcentration. Although rare, true disorders of RBC production, such as polycythemia, can result in an increased hematocrit level.

Conversely, a decreased hematocrit value can indicate fluid volume excess because of the dilutional effect of the extra fluid load. Decreases also can result from blood loss, liver damage, or hemolytic reactions. A decreased hematocrit level may indicate the anemia of kidney failure or may reflect fluid volume overload. If the hematocrit value is decreasing but the hemoglobin concentration remains constant, the cause is fluid volume overload. Decreased hematocrit values and hemoglobin concentrations indicate a true loss of RBCs. The history and bedside assessment including hemodynamic monitoring data aid in determining whether fluid imbalances or disease states, or both, are responsible for changes in hematocrit levels in a critically ill patient. Anemia is a frequent finding in patients with kidney failure, complicating management in critical illness.[13]

Albumin

Slightly more than 50% of the total plasma protein is serum albumin. It is manufactured in the liver, and a normal blood level is 3.5 to 5 g/dL. Albumin is primarily responsible for the maintenance of colloid osmotic pressure, which functions to hold fluid in the vascular space. The blood vessel walls, because of their impermeability to plasma proteins, prevent albumin from leaving the vascular space. However, in some disease states, such as severe burns (cell membrane destruction) or nephrotic syndrome (increased glomerular capillary permeability to protein and protein loss in the urine), albumin is lost from the vascular space.

Decreased albumin levels in the vascular space result in a fluid shift from the plasma to the interstitium, creating peripheral edema. A decreased albumin level can result from protein-calorie malnutrition, which occurs in many critically ill patients in whom available stores of albumin are depleted. A decrease in the plasma oncotic pressure results, and fluid shifts from the vascular space to the interstitial space. Liver disease or severe injury to the liver also causes a decrease in albumin levels, as the diseased liver fails to synthesize sufficient albumin. Severe portal hypertension can force albumin and other plasma proteins into the abdominal cavity, resulting in ascites.

Increased albumin levels are rare. The body uses a fixed amount of protein for energy and body cell replacement and converts excess protein into stored fat. If all plasma protein levels are elevated, fluid volume deficit (hemoconcentration) is suspected.

Urinalysis

Analysis of the urine provides excellent information about the patient's kidney function and condition relative to fluids and electrolytes. Specific tests and abnormal indications are presented in Table 25.3. In a critically ill patient, a routine urinalysis specimen may be obtained to rule out the presence of urinary protein or glucose. A sterile urine culture may be obtained if a urinary tract infection is suspected.

Urine Appearance

Physical examination of the urine focuses on a general inspection of urine color, clarity, and odor. Normal urine is pale yellow, but it may vary as a result of food intake (carrots, beets, rhubarb), medications (phenytoin, nitrofurantoin, phenazopyridine), or metabolic by-products (bilirubin, methemoglobin). Clarity of the urine may be affected by bacteria, white blood cells (WBCs), or urates. Normal urine has minimal odor; a strong odor may be caused by concentrated urine (as in dehydrated states), infection, medicines (especially vitamins), or foods (broccoli, asparagus).[14]

Urine pH

Urine pH indicates the acidity or alkalinity of the urine. The normal urinary pH is acidic with a range from 4.5 to 8.[14] The kidneys regulate acid–base balance; more hydrogen ions are excreted than bicarbonate ions, causing the acidity of the urine. Changes in metabolic function and kidney function produce changes in urinary pH.

An increase in urinary acidity (decreased pH) indicates retention of sodium and acids by the body, which occurs in intrarenal AKI. A decrease in urinary acidity (increased pH or more alkaline) means the body is retaining bicarbonate. In the presence of normal kidney function, urinary pH levels are greatly affected by diet and medications. Certain food groups such as citrus fruits and vegetables lead to alkaline urine, whereas a diet high in protein can produce acidic urine. In the critical care unit, patients receiving total parenteral nutrition or a high-protein tube-feeding formula may have acidic urine because of high protein intake.

Urine Specific Gravity

Specific gravity measures the density or weight of urine compared with that of distilled water. The normal urinary specific gravity is 1.005 to 1.025.[14] For comparison, the specific gravity of distilled water is 1.000. Because urine is composed of many solutes and substances suspended in water, the specific gravity should always be higher than that of water.

TABLE 25.3   Urinalysis Results

Test	Normal	Possible Causes for Increased Values	Possible Causes for Decreased Values
pH	4.5–8.0	Alkalosis	Acidosis Intrarenal AKI
Specific gravity	1.003–1.030[a]	Volume deficit Glycosuria Proteinuria Prerenal AKI (>1.020)	Volume overload Intrarenal AKI
Osmolality	300–1200 mOsm/kg	Volume deficit Prerenal AKI (urine > serum osmolality)	Volume excess Intrarenal AKI (urine < serum osmolality)
Protein	30–150 mg/24 h[b]	Trauma Infection Intrarenal AKI Transient with exercise Glomerulonephritis	
Sodium	40–220 mEq/24 h	High-sodium diet Intrarenal AKI	Prerenal AKI
Creatinine	1–2 g/24 h		Intrarenal AKI Chronic kidney failure
Urea	6–17 g/24 h		Intrarenal AKI Chronic kidney failure
Myoglobin	Absent	Crush injury Rhabdomyolysis	
RBCs	0–5[c]	Trauma Intrarenal AKI Infection Strenuous exercise Renal artery thrombus	
WBCs	0–5[c]	Infection	
Bacteria	None to few	Infection	
Casts	None to few	RBC: Glomerular disease WBC: Pyelonephritis Glomerular disease Nephrotic syndrome Epithelial: Glomerular disease	

AKI, Acute kidney injury; *RBC,* red blood cell; *WBC,* white blood cell.
[a]Adult value; newborn value is slightly lower at 1.001–1.020.
[b]Higher values usually apply for persons after exercise; lower values apply for persons at rest.
[c]Cells per low-power field.

The specific gravity reflects hydration status and indicates the ability of the kidneys to dilute or concentrate the urine. Decreases in specific gravity reflect the inability of the kidneys to excrete the usual solute load into the urine (less dense with fewer solutes). Increases in specific gravity are caused by dehydration (more concentrated urine) or occur with additional glucose (diabetes) or protein (glomerular dysfunction) that increase urine density.[14] A fixed specific gravity (does not vary with fluid intake) suggests early kidney dysfunction because the kidneys are unable to excrete or resorb water and solutes.

Urine Osmolality

The urine osmolality may be measured in tandem with the serum osmolality. The simultaneous measurement of serum and urine osmolality levels provides an accurate assessment of fluid status. The normal urine osmolality level is 500 to 1200 mOsm/kg and depends on resorption or excretion of water in the kidney tubules. The urine osmolality level increases (and urine output decreases) during fluid volume deficit because of the retention of fluid by the body. The urine osmolality level decreases (and urine output increases) during volume excess because fluid is excreted by the kidneys.

Urine Protein

Protein normally is absent from urine because protein molecules are too large to be filtered across the intact glomerular capillary membrane. Protein amounts greater than 150 mg/day signal compromise of the glomerular membrane and intrinsic kidney damage.[14]

Traditionally, quantitative measurement of the amount of protein in the urine required a 24-hour urine collection.[14] A "spot" or random urine sample can also be used, as the correlation between the two tests is very strong.[14] Both the amount of protein and the amount of creatinine in the urine specimen are measured. A normal *urine protein-to-urine creatinine ratio* is less than 0.2; a protein-to-creatinine ratio of 3.5 indicates that approximately 3.5 g of protein are being excreted per day, indicating severe protein loss by the kidneys.

Urine Glucose

Glycosuria is defined as glucose in the urine. Glucose normally is completely resorbed by the kidney tubules, and the urine should be free of glucose. Urinary glucose should not exceed 130 mg/day.[14] In the presence of acute or chronic kidney failure, glycosuria is an unreliable indicator of the level of hyperglycemia because of the damaged nephrons. In the critical care unit, only the serum glucose level is measured.

Urine Ketones

Ketones in the urine are abnormal and signal hyperglycemia caused by type 1 diabetes or starvation ketosis.[14]

Urine Electrolytes

Levels of electrolytes in the urine are not measured as often as levels in serum, but they can yield information about kidney function. To measure urinary electrolyte levels, a 24-hour urine sample may be needed, although potassium and sodium can be measured in a randomly collected specimen.

Urine Sodium. The most commonly measured electrolyte in urine is sodium. Urinary sodium is a reflection of the action of aldosterone and subsequent retention or excretion of sodium by the kidney tubules to maintain fluid balance. In the presence of hypovolemia, the kidney tubules retain sodium (and water), and the amount of sodium in the urine and the fractional excretion of sodium are very low. The opposite is true with volume overload and with kidney diseases that cause sodium wasting. The amount of sodium in the urine can help in determining the pathology of AKI as long as diuretics have not been administered. In prerenal AKI caused by ineffective circulation reaching the kidneys, the urine sodium level is low. If AKI results from damage to the kidney tubules, the urine sodium level is normal or elevated.

Urine Sediment

The presence of sediment such as epithelial cells and casts in urine aids in identifying problems related to the kidneys.[14] A fresh urine specimen, tested 30 to 60 minutes after collection, is important.[14] Urine becomes more alkaline after it has been collected, resulting in a change in the urine sediment (eg, casts dissolve, cells lyse). The presence or absence of urine sediment can be helpful in identifying the cause of AKI. In prerenal AKI, the kidneys are not injured, and urinary sediment is absent. However, in intrarenal AKI, the kidney glomeruli or tubules are damaged, allowing urinary sediment containing casts and epithelial cells in the urine.[14]

Casts are cylindrical structures composed mainly of mucoprotein (Tamm-Horsfall protein), which is secreted by epithelial cells lining the loops of Henle, the distal tubules, and the collecting ducts. Casts may form in the presence of epithelial cells, RBCs, or WBCs in the tubular lumen. These cells or clumps of cellular breakdown products can adhere to and be surrounded by the fibrillar mucoprotein matrix, and the resulting casts are washed out of the kidney tubular system in the urinary flow. Casts differ in composition and size and correlate with the severity and type of kidney damage. For example, WBC casts indicate pyelonephritis, or they may occur during acute glomerulonephritis. RBC casts indicate glomerulonephritis. Hyaline casts, which consist of Tamm-Horsfall protein, are associated with kidney parenchymal disease and glomerular capillary membrane inflammation. Consistent appearance of epithelial cells shed by the lining of the nephron may indicate nephritis. Although small numbers of epithelial cells normally appear in the urine and an occasional cast may be found, their consistent appearance is abnormal.[14]

Hematuria

Obvious and microscopic hematuria may signal kidney damage. Although a few RBCs in the urine are normal, discernibly bloody urine usually indicates bleeding within the urinary tract or kidney trauma. Microscopic hematuria may occur normally after strenuous exercise or the insertion of a retention catheter; this should disappear within 48 hours.

The presence of myoglobin can make the urine appear red. Microscopic examination of the urine fails to reveal RBCs, with myoglobin being present instead. Myoglobin in the urine may result from skeletal muscle damage (eg, traumatic crush injury) or rhabdomyolysis. Rhabdomyolysis may develop in patients admitted to a critical care unit for many reasons, including traumatic injury, cocaine abuse, status epilepticus, heat prostration, or collapse during intense physical exercise (eg, running a marathon race on a hot day). Damaged muscle cells release myoglobin that blocks the tubules within the kidney to cause intrarenal AKI.

URINE TOXICOLOGY SCREEN

Urine can be screened to detect the presence of alcohol, illegal drugs, prescription and nonprescription medications, and other substances that are excreted via the kidneys.[15] This is often referred to as a urine drug screen.[15] Urine toxicology tests conducted in the emergency department or the critical care unit are considered screening tests and are not diagnostic of a disease state.[15] These analyses are typically undertaken to provide information about causes of an altered level of consciousness rather than to identify kidney-related problems.

IMAGING STUDIES

Although laboratory assessment is used most often in diagnosing kidney problems in critically ill patients, imaging studies can confirm or clarify causes of particular disorders. Imaging assessment includes the use of ultrasound and radiologic techniques. Ultrasound is a noninvasive imaging technique that is available in most hospitals. Kidney ultrasound is especially useful in determining the size, shape, and contour of the kidneys; the presence of masses or cysts; and the presence of renal artery stenosis.[16] Radiologic assessment ranges from basic to more complex (Table 25.4) and provides information about abnormal masses, abnormal fluid collections, obstructions, vascular supply alterations, and other disorders of the kidneys and urinary tract.[16]

Some radiologic studies require the use of a contrast agent or injection of a radiopaque dye. Because many of the dyes used in radiology are potentially nephrotoxic, they must be used carefully in patients with AKI or chronic kidney disease.[17,18] To prevent contrast-induced nephrotoxicity, adequate hydration before and after the test and careful monitoring of kidney function are always indicated.[17,18]

KIDNEY BIOPSY

The increase in kidney imaging has led to an increase in the detection of kidney tumors, some benign and some cancerous.[19,20] Kidney biopsy is the definitive tool for diagnosing

TABLE 25.4 Kidney Imaging Tests

Test	Comments
KUB radiograph	Flat-plate radiograph of abdomen; determines position, size, and structure of kidneys, urinary tract, and pelvis; useful for evaluating the presence of calculi and masses; usually followed by additional tests
IVP	Intravenous injection of contrast agent with radiography; allows visualization of internal kidney tissues
Angiography	Injection of contrast agent into arterial blood perfusing kidneys; allows visualization of renal blood flow; may also visualize stenosis, cysts, clots, trauma, and infarctions
CT	Radioisotope is administered by intravenous route and absorbed by kidneys; scintillation photography is performed in several planes; spiral or helical CT allows rapid imaging; density of image helps evaluate kidney vessels, perfusion, tumors, cysts, stones/calculi, hemorrhage, necrosis, and trauma
Ultrasound	High-frequency sound waves are transmitted to kidneys and urinary tract, and image is viewed on oscilloscope; noninvasive; identifies fluid accumulation or obstruction, cysts, stones/calculi, and masses; useful for evaluating kidney before biopsy
MRI	Scanner produces three-dimensional images in response to application of high-energy radiofrequency waves to tissues; produces clear images; density of image may indicate trauma, cysts, masses, malformation of vessels or tubules, stones/calculi, and necrosis

CT, computed tomography; *IVP,* intravenous pyelogram; *KUB,* kidney-ureter-bladder; *MRI,* magnetic resonance imaging.

disease processes involving the parenchyma of the kidney. Percutaneous needle biopsy involves inserting a needle through the flank to obtain a specimen of cortical and medullary kidney tissue. Some small tumors are amenable to ablation.[19,20] An open biopsy is a surgical procedure and is rarely done in critically ill patients. Biopsy is the last choice for diagnostic assessment in critically ill patients because of the periprocedural risks of bleeding, hematoma, and infection.

SUMMARY

Clinical Assessment

- Predisposing factors for acute kidney dysfunction are obtained during the history including the use of over-the-counter medicines, recent infections requiring antibiotic therapy, antihypertensive medicines, and any diagnostic procedures performed using radiopaque contrast dye.
- Urine output may be decreased or normal, depending on the cause of the kidney dysfunction. Low urine output alone is insufficient to identify AKI.

Laboratory Studies

- BUN is a by-product of protein and amino acid metabolism. BUN is increased when kidney function deteriorates.
- Serum creatinine is used to trend kidney function in critical illness, as creatine is not resorbed by the kidney tubules and increases when kidney function deteriorates.

- Cystatin C is a newer serum biomarker for early identification of AKI.
- Electrolyte derangements are frequent in kidney failure including sodium, potassium, phosphate, calcium, chloride, and bicarbonate.
- Anion gap is increased in kidney failure in association with electrolyte and acid–base changes.
- Urinalysis can provide valuable information about kidney function, but results are unreliable if the patient has recently been given diuretics.

Diagnostic Procedures

- Ultrasound, computed tomography, and magnetic resonance imaging are noninvasive tests used to obtain images of the kidney.
- Kidney biopsy is rarely performed in critically ill patients.
- ⓔ Visit the Evolve site for additional study materials.

REFERENCES

1. Ball JW, et al. *Seidel's Guide to Physical Examination.* 8th ed. St. Louis: Elsevier; 2015.
2. American Association of Nephrology Nurses Association (ANNA). *Core Curriculum for Nephrology Nursing.* 6th ed. Pitman NJ; American Nephrology Nurses Association: 2015.
3. Wadel HM, Textor SC. The role of the kidney in regulating arterial blood pressure. *Nat Rev Nephrol.* 2012;8(10):602.
4. O'Connor ME, Prowle JR. Fluid overload. *Crit Care Clin.* 2015;31(3):803.
5. de Vries Feyens C, de Jager CP. Images in clinical medicine: decreased skin turgor. *N Engl J Med.* 2011;364. e6.
6. Morley JE. Dehydration, hypernatremia, and hyponatremia. *Clin Geriatr Med.* 2015;31:389.
7. Davison DL, Patel K, Chawla LS. Hemodynamic monitoring in the critically ill: spanning the range of kidney function. *Am J Kidney Dis.* 2012;59:715.
8. Singbartl K, Joannidis M. Short-term effects of acute kidney injury. *Crit Care Clin.* 2015;31:751.
9. Vaara ST, et al. The attributable mortality of acute kidney injury: a sequentially matched analysis. *Crit Care Med.* 2014;42(4):878.
10. Weekley CC, Peralta CA. Advances in the use of multimarker panels for renal risk stratification. *Curr Opin Nephrol Hypertens.* 2012;21:301.
11. Farwell WR, Taylor EN. Serum anion gap, bicarbonate and biomarkers of inflammation in healthy individuals in a national survey. *CMAJ.* 2010;182:137.
12. Abramowitz MK, Hostetter TH, Melamed ML. The serum anion gap is altered in early kidney disease and associates with mortality. *Kidney Int.* 2012;82:701.
13. Babitt JL, Lin HY. Mechanisms of anemia in CKD. *J Am Soc Nephrol.* 2012;23:1631.
14. Lerma EV, Rosner MH. Urinalysis. In: Lerna EV, Nisenson AR, eds. *Nephrology Secrets.* 3rd ed. Philadelphia: Elsevier; 2012.
15. Markway EC, Baker SN. A review of the methods, interpretation, and limitations of the urine drug screen. *Orthopedics.* 2011;34:877.
16. Rosen A, Simpson WL. Renal imaging techniques. In: Lerna EV, Nisenson AR, eds. *Nephrology Secrets.* 3rd ed. Philadelphia: Elsevier; 2012.
17. Isaac S. Contrast-induced nephropathy: nursing implications. *Crit Care Nurs.* 2012;32:41.
18. Stacul F, et al. Contrast induced nephropathy: updated ESUR Contrast Media Safety Committee guidelines. *Eur Radiol.* 2011;21:2527.
19. Hu R, et al. Role of percutaneous needle core biopsy in diagnosis and clinical management of renal masses. *Hum Pathol.* 2015;46(4):570.
20. Shin BJ, et al. Contemporary status of percutaneous ablation for the small renal mass. *Curr Urol Rep.* 2016;17:23.

26

Kidney Disorders and Therapeutic Management

Mary E. Lough

ACUTE KIDNEY INJURY

Acute kidney injury (AKI) describes the spectrum of acute-onset kidney disorders that can range from mild impairment of kidney function through acute kidney failure that requires renal replacement therapy (dialysis).[1,2] Severe AKI is characterized by a sudden decline in glomerular filtration rate (GFR), with subsequent retention of products in the blood that are normally excreted by the kidneys; this disrupts electrolyte balance, acid–base homeostasis, and fluid volume equilibrium. A transition to greater use of the word *kidney* rather than *renal* reflects a trend in the nephrology literature that emphasizes the vulnerability of the kidney during critical illness.[1,2]

Critical Illness and Acute Kidney Injury

Critical care patients with AKI have a longer length of hospital stay, more complications, and higher mortality.[1,2] Mortality associated with AKI ranges from 15% to 60%.[2] One reason for poor survival is that critical care patients often have coexisting medical conditions that increase their susceptibility to the development of AKI. High-risk diagnoses include heart failure, shock, respiratory failure, and sepsis.[3] The multinational Acute Kidney Injury–Epidemiologic Prospective Investigation (AKI-EPI) study examined the incidence of AKI in 97 hospitals in 33 countries and reported that AKI occurred in more than half of critically ill patients.[3] The most frequent causes of AKI were sepsis (40%), hypovolemia (34%), drug/medication related (14%), and cardiogenic shock (13%).[3] One-third of patients were mechanically ventilated, and half were on vasopressors at the time of AKI diagnosis.[3] Mortality with a diagnosis of AKI was 24%; in contrast, mortality was 5% for critically ill patients with functional kidneys.[3] A diagnosis of kidney failure dramatically increases risk of death from complications of critical illness.

Typically, a patient is not admitted to the critical care unit with a diagnosis of AKI alone; there is always coexisting hemodynamic, cardiac, pulmonary, or neurologic compromise. Many patients come into the hospital with underlying changes in kidney function, such as an elevated serum creatinine level, although they have no symptoms and are often unaware of their compromised kidney function. The lack of kidney reserve places these patients at increased risk for AKI if complications occur in any other organ systems. As a result, the picture of AKI in the modern critical care unit has changed to encompass patients with kidney injury who also have multisystem dysfunction that complicates their clinical course.

DEFINITIONS OF ACUTE KIDNEY INJURY

One of the challenges of estimating the incidence of AKI in the critical care unit has been the wide variation in definitions that have been used. Measurement of kidney function is indirect, and the diagnosis of AKI is predominantly derived from changes in urine output and elevation of serum creatinine level, with the understanding that changes in these values reflect a decline in the GFR.[1,2] Urine output is sometimes a problematic measure to use because diuretics artificially increase the urine output but may not alter the course of kidney failure. The clinical insult may have direct effects on the kidney, such as the inflammation associated with sepsis, which accounts for almost 50% of AKI seen in critical care units.[1]

RIFLE Criteria

The risk of critically ill patients developing AKI has been classified by a multinational group of nephrologists.[1,2] The classification uses the acronym *RIFLE*—risk, injury, failure, loss, and end-stage kidney disease.[2] The RIFLE system classifies AKI in three categories of increasing severity (R, I, F) and two outcome criteria (L, E) based on GFR status reflected by the change in urine output or loss of kidney function (Table 26.1).[2] If AKI is superimposed on a kidney that is already compromised, the term *chronic* is added to the RIFLE criteria to denote the cause as acute-on-chronic kidney failure.[2]

TABLE 26.1 RIFLE Criteria for Acute Kidney Dysfunction

RIFLE	Serum Creatinine Criteria[a]	Urine Output Criteria
*R*isk	Serum Cr increased 1.5 times above normal *or*	UO <0.5 mL/kg/h for 6 h
	Serum Cr increase ≥0.3 mg/dL	
*I*njury	Serum Cr increased 2 times above normal	UO <0.5 mL/kg/h for 12 h
*F*ailure	Serum Cr increased 3 times above normal *or*	UO <0.3 mL/kg/h for 24 h *or* anuria for 12 h (oliguria)
	Serum Cr ≥4 mg/dL *or*	
	Serum Cr acute rise ≥0.5 mg/dL	
*L*oss	Persistent AKI—complete loss of kidney function for >4 weeks	
*E*SKD	End-stage kidney disease	

[a]All serum creatinine references are based on changes from baseline.
AKI, acute kidney injury; *Cr,* creatinine; *UO,* urine output.
Data from Kellum JA, et al. Definition and classification of acute kidney injury. *Nephron Clin Pract.* 2008;109(4):c182.

BOX 26.1   Acute Kidney Injury Network Criteria for Diagnosis of Acute Kidney Injury

- *Definition:* Acute kidney injury (AKI) is an abrupt (within 48 h) reduction in kidney function defined as
  - An absolute increase in serum creatinine level of more than or equal to 0.3 mg/dL (more than or equal to 26.4 µmol/L)
  - A percentage increase in serum creatinine of more than or equal to 50% (1.5-fold from baseline)
  - A reduction in urine output (documented oliguria of less than 0.5 mL/kg/h for more than 6 h)

Explanatory Notes

- *Serum creatinine:* These criteria include an absolute and a percentage change in creatinine to accommodate variations related to age, sex, and body mass index and to reduce the need for a baseline creatinine level, but they do require at least two serum creatinine values within 48 h.
- *Urine output:* The urine output criterion was included based on the predictive importance of this measure but with the awareness that urine outputs may not be measured routinely in non–critical care unit settings. It is assumed that the diagnosis based on the urine output criterion alone will require exclusion of urinary tract obstructions that reduce urine output or of other easily reversible causes of reduced urine output.
- *Clinical context:* These criteria should be used in the context of the clinical presentation and after adequate fluid resuscitation when applicable. Many acute kidney diseases exist, and some may result in AKI. Because diagnostic criteria are not documented, some cases of AKI may not be diagnosed.
- *Physiologic state:* AKI may be superimposed on or lead to chronic kidney disease.

Data from Mehta RL, et al, for the Acute Kidney Injury Network. Report of an initiative to improve outcomes in acute kidney injury. *Crit Care.* 2007;11(2):R31.

BOX 26.2   Acute Kidney Injury

Prerenal Acute Kidney Injury
- Prolonged hypotension (sepsis, vasodilation)
- Prolonged low cardiac output (heart failure, cardiogenic shock)
- Prolonged volume depletion (dehydration, hemorrhage)
- Renovascular thrombosis (thromboemboli)

Intrarenal Acute Kidney Injury
- Kidney ischemia (advanced stage of prerenal acute kidney injury)
- Endogenous toxins (rhabdomyolysis, tumor lysis syndrome)
- Exogenous toxins (radiocontrast dye, nephrotoxic medications)
- Infection (acute glomerulonephritis, interstitial nephritis)

Postrenal Acute Kidney Injury
- Obstruction (urethra, prostate, or bladder)
- Rare as a cause of acute kidney injury in critical care

Acute Kidney Injury Network Criteria

The Acute Kidney Injury Network criteria are listed in Box 26.1. These criteria are similar to the criteria proposed by the RIFLE group. Both groups make the point that in an acutely ill patient, small changes in the serum creatinine level and urine output may signal important declines in GFR and kidney function.[2]

Types of Acute Kidney Injury

Acute kidney injury may be classified by the location of the insult relative to kidney anatomy: *prerenal* (before), *intrarenal* (within), and *postrenal* (after) (Box 26.2). This remains a useful way to imagine the relationship between anatomy and functional insults to the kidney, although there are often several complications of critical illness that may predispose to development of AKI. An overview of the development and possible outcomes of AKI is presented in Fig. 26.1.

Prerenal Acute Kidney Injury

Any condition that decreases blood flow, blood pressure, or kidney perfusion before arterial blood reaches the renal artery that supplies the kidney may be anatomically described as *prerenal* AKI.[1] When arterial hypoperfusion secondary to low cardiac output, hemorrhage, vasodilation, thrombosis, or other cause reduces the blood flow to the kidney, glomerular filtration decreases, and consequently urine output decreases (see Box 26.2). This is a major reason the critical care nurse monitors urine output on an hourly basis.[4,5] Initially, in prerenal states, the integrity of the kidney's nephron structure and function may be preserved. If normal perfusion and cardiac output are restored quickly, the kidney recovers with no permanent injury. However, if the prerenal insult is not corrected, GFR declines, blood urea nitrogen (BUN) concentration rises (prerenal azotemia),[1] and the patient develops oliguria and is at risk for significant kidney damage. *Oliguria,* defined as urine output less than 400 mL/day, or urine output less than 0.5 mL/kg per hour,[4] with an elevated serum creatinine, is a classic finding in AKI. Prerenal azotemia is associated with a lower mortality rate than other forms of AKI.[6]

Intrarenal Acute Kidney Injury

Any condition that produces an ischemic or toxic insult directly at parenchymal nephron tissue places the patient at risk for development of *intrarenal* AKI (see Box 26.2).[1] Ischemic damage may be caused by prolonged hypotension or low cardiac output. Toxic injury reaction may occur in response to substances that damage the kidney tubular endothelium, such as some antimicrobial medications and the contrast dye used in radiologic diagnostic studies. The insult may involve the glomeruli and the tubular epithelium. When the internal filtering structures are pathologically affected, the condition was previously known as *acute tubular necrosis,* although the newer term of AKI is now used more often.[1]

Postrenal Acute Kidney Injury

Any obstruction that hinders the flow of urine from beyond the kidney through the remainder of the urinary tract may lead to *postrenal* AKI. This is an uncommon cause of kidney failure in critically ill patients.[1] When monitoring of the urine output reveals a sudden decrease in the patient's urine output from the urinary catheter, a blockage may be responsible. Sudden development of *anuria* (urine output less than 100 mL/24 h) should prompt verification that the urinary catheter is not occluded.

Azotemia

The term *azotemia* is used to describe an acute increase in the BUN level often associated with prerenal AKI.[1,6] *Uremia* is another term used to describe an elevated BUN value.

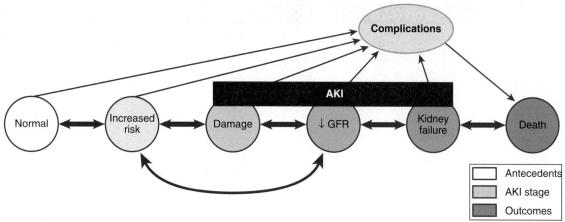

FIG. 26.1 Model of Components of Acute Kidney Injury. (Modified from Acute Kidney Injury Network. AKI Conceptual Model, developed at the Vancouver Summit 2006. http://www.akinet.org.)

TABLE 26.2 Normal Serum Electrolyte Values

Electrolyte	Normal Value
Sodium	135–145 mEq/L
Potassium	3.5–4.5 mEq/L
Chloride	98–108 mEq/L
Calcium	8.5–10.5 mg/dL or 4.5–5.8 mEq/L
Phosphorus	2.7–4.5 mg/dL
Magnesium	1.5–2.5 mEq/L
Bicarbonate	24–28 mEq/L

TABLE 26.3 Initial Urine Laboratory Analysis Findings in Acute Kidney Injury[a]

Assessment	Prerenal[b]	Intrarenal[c]	Postrenal[d]
Urine volume	Normal	Oliguria or nonoliguria	Oliguria to anuria
Urine specific gravity	>1.020	1.010	1.000–1.010
Urine osmolality (mOsm/kg)	>350	<300	300–400
Urine sodium (mEq/L)	<20	>30	20–40
FENa (%)	<1%	>2%–3%	1%–3%
BUN/Cr ratio	20:1	Ischemic: 20:1 Toxic: 10:1	10:1
Urine microscopy (sediment)	Normal	Dark granular casts, hyaline casts, kidney epithelial cells	Normal

[a]Results of urine laboratory tests are valid only in the absence of diuretics.
[b]Urine in prerenal failure is concentrated, with low sodium.
[c]Urine in intrarenal failure shows kidney damage because the nephron cannot concentrate urine or conserve sodium, and evidence of kidney damage (casts) is seen.
[d]Urine test results in postrenal failure vary because findings initially depend on the hydration status of the patient rather than the status of the kidney. Anuria, urine volume less than 100 mL/24 h; *BUN,* blood urea nitrogen; *Cr,* creatinine; *FENa,* fractional excretion of sodium; oliguria, urine volume of 100–400 mL/24 h; polyuria, urine volume excessive over 24 h.

ASSESSMENT AND DIAGNOSIS

Laboratory Assessment

When AKI is suspected, the degree of injury is assessed using blood analysis. Most serum levels of electrolytes become increasingly elevated as AKI develops (Table 26.2). Urinalysis values are also altered by AKI, although these values are not predictive of outcome in critical illness. Consequently, urinary electrolytes are rarely measured (Table 26.3).[1] Clinical findings associated with AKI are listed in Table 26.4. Normal and abnormal urinalysis findings and reasons for their significance are summarized in Chapter 25.

Acidosis

Acidosis (pH less than 7.35) is one of the trademarks of severe acute kidney insult. Metabolic acidosis occurs as a result of the accumulation of unexcreted waste products. The acid waste products consist of strong negative ions (anions), elevated serum phosphorus levels (hyperphosphatemia), and other normally unmeasured ions (eg, sulfate, urate, lactate) that decrease the serum pH. A low serum albumin concentration, which often occurs in AKI, has a slight alkalinizing effect, but it is not enough to offset the metabolic acidosis. Respiratory compensation and mechanical ventilatory support are rarely sufficient to reverse the metabolic acidosis. Acidosis in AKI is complex, as evidenced by the fact that many patients with AKI maintain a normal anion gap; the reasons for this are unknown. Information on acidosis and arterial blood gas interpretation is presented in Chapter 18. Anion gap measurement is discussed in Chapter 25.

Blood Urea Nitrogen

The BUN level is an unreliable indicator of kidney injury as an individual test.[1] The BUN concentration is changed by protein intake, blood in the gastrointestinal tract, and cell catabolism, and it is diluted by fluid administration. A BUN-to-creatinine ratio may be calculated to determine the cause of AKI (see Table 26.3). The BUN-to-creatinine ratio is most useful in diagnosing prerenal AKI (often described as prerenal azotemia), in which the BUN level is greatly elevated relative to the serum creatinine value, although critically ill patients can be developing AKI before changes in this ratio are evident.[6]

Serum Creatinine

Creatinine is a by-product of muscle metabolism that is formed nonenzymatically from creatine in muscles.[7] Creatinine

TABLE 26.4 Serum Electrolytes in Acute Kidney Failure

Electrolyte Disturbance	Serum Value	Clinical Findings	Electrolyte Disturbance	Serum Value	Clinical Findings
Potassium			Hypercalcemia	>10.5 mg/dL or >5.8 mEq/L	Deep bone pain
Hypokalemia	<3.5 mEq/L	Muscular weakness			Excessive thirst
		Cardiac irregularities on ECG			
		Abdominal distention and flatulence			Anorexia
		Paresthesia			Lethargy, weakened muscles
		Decreased reflexes			
		Anorexia	**Magnesium**		
		Dizziness, confusion	Hypomagnesemia	<1.4 mEq/L	Choroid or athetoid muscle activity
		Increased sensitivity to digitalis			Facial tics, spasticity
Hyperkalemia	>4.5 mEq/L	Irritability and restlessness			Cardiac dysrhythmias
		Anxiety	Hypermagnesemia	>2.5 mEq/L	CNS depression
		Nausea and vomiting			Respiratory depression
		Abdominal cramps			Lethargy
		Weakness			Coma
		Numbness and tingling (fingertips and circumoral)			Bradycardia
					Changes on ECG
		Cardiac irregularities on ECG			
			Phosphorus		
Sodium			Hypophosphatemia	<3.0 mg/dL	Hemolytic anemias
Hyponatremia	<135 mEq/L	Disorientation			Depressed white blood cell function
		Muscle twitching			Bleeding (decreased platelet aggregation)
		Nausea, vomiting, abdominal cramps			
		Headaches, dizziness			Nausea, vomiting
		Seizures, postural hypotension			Anorexia
		Cold, clammy skin	Hyperphosphatemia	>4.5 mg/dL	Tachycardia
		Decreased skin turgor			Nausea, diarrhea, abdominal cramps
		Tachycardia			Muscle weakness, flaccid paralysis
		Oliguria			Increased reflexes
Hypernatremia	>145 mEq/L	Extreme thirst			
		Dry, sticky mucous membranes	**Chloride**		
		Altered mentation	Hypochloremia	<98 mEq/L	Hyperirritability
		Seizures (later stages)			Tetany or muscular excitability
					Slow respirations
Calcium			Hyperchloremia	>108 mEq/L	Weakness, lethargy
Hypocalcemia	<8.5 mg/dL or <4.5 mEq/L	Irritability			Deep, rapid breathing
		Muscular tetany, muscle cramps			Possible unconsciousness (later stages)
			Albumin		
		Decreased cardiac output (decreased contractions)	Hypoalbuminemia	<3.8 g/dL	Muscle wasting
		Bleeding (decreased ability to coagulate)			Peripheral edema (fluid shift)
		Changes on ECG			Decreased resistance to infection
		Positive Chvostek or Trousseau signs			Poorly healing wounds

CNS, central nervous system; *ECG,* electrocardiogram.

is completely excreted when kidney function is normal.[7] Consequently, when the kidneys are not working, the serum creatinine level rises. Even small increases in serum creatinine represent a significant decline in GFR.[7] Serum creatinine level is assessed daily to follow the trend of kidney function and to determine whether it is stable, improving, or worsening.

Creatinine Clearance

If the patient is making sufficient urine, urinary creatinine clearance can be measured. A normal urinary creatinine clearance rate is 120 mL/min, but this value decreases with kidney failure. Critical care patients with severe AKI manifest elevated serum

creatinine and may be oliguric. Consequently, the urinary creatinine clearance rate is rarely measured during critical illness.[7]

Fractional Excretion of Sodium

The fractional excretion of sodium (FENa) in the urine can be measured early in the course of AKI to differentiate between prerenal AKI and interrenal AKI (parenchymal). An FENa value less than 1% (in the absence of diuretics) suggests prerenal compromise because *resorption* of almost all of the filtered sodium is an appropriate response to decreased perfusion to the kidneys. If diuretics are administered, the test is meaningless. An FENa value greater than 2% implies that the kidney cannot concentrate the sodium and that the damage is intrarenal (acute tubular necrosis). FENa values do not have any predictive benefit in critical illness and are rarely measured.[1]

Urinary sodium is measured in milliequivalents per liter. Interpretation of results is similar to the FENa. A urinary sodium concentration less than 10 mEq/L (low) suggests a pre-renal condition. A urinary sodium level greater than 40 mEq/L (in the presence of elevated serum creatinine and the absence of a high sodium load) suggests that intrarenal damage has occurred (see Table 26.2). As with other urinalysis tests, the use of diuretics invalidates any results. Because diuretics alter resorption of water and produce dilute urine, the test result does not reflect actual kidney function.

AT-RISK DISEASE STATES AND ACUTE KIDNEY INJURY

Many patients come into the critical care unit with disease states that predispose them to the development of AKI. Many others already have kidney damage but are unaware of this condition (Fig. 26.2).

Underlying Chronic Kidney Disease

The incidence of chronic kidney disease (CKD) in the United States is approximately 10%, or 1 in 10 people.[8] Clinical practice guidelines for the management of end-stage kidney disease categorize kidney dysfunction into five stages. Because of the large numbers of adults with kidney dysfunction (diagnosed or not), kidney function must be assessed on all critically ill patients at risk for fluid and electrolyte imbalance. The GFR associated with each stage and the numeric population estimates for each stage of kidney dysfunction are shown in Table 26.5. Most people in the early stages of kidney disease are unaware of their condition.[9]

Older Age and Acute Kidney Injury

Among adults older than 60 years, the prevalence of CKD in the United States is close to 25%.[8] The number of older adults with CKD is increasing in tandem with the increase in diabetes and hypertension in the US population.[10]

Heart Failure and Acute Kidney Injury

There is a strong association between kidney failure and heart failure.[11] Heart-kidney interactions have been categorized into five subtypes under the term *cardiorenal syndromes*.[12] One feature that is often encountered is a resistance to use of high-potency loop diuretics such as furosemide.

Several risk factors for atherosclerotic cardiovascular disease, notably hypertension and diabetes, are also detrimental to the kidney over the long-term. Maintenance of blood pressure below 130/80 mm Hg and blood glucose within the normal range decreases the risk of developing both CKD and the atherosclerotic cardiac diseases such as coronary artery disease and peripheral artery disease.

Respiratory Failure and Acute Kidney Injury

There is a significant association between kidney failure and respiratory failure.[3] Mechanical ventilation can alter kidney function. Positive-pressure ventilation reduces blood flow to the kidney, lowers the GFR, and decreases urine output. These effects are intensified with the addition of positive end-expiratory pressure. AKI increases inflammation, causes the lung vasculature to become more permeable, and contributes to the development of acute respiratory distress syndrome. Patients with AKI are more likely to require prolonged mechanical ventilatory support.[13,14] Patients with chronic lung conditions such as chronic obstructive pulmonary disease have a 41% increased risk of death if they also have AKI.[15]

Sepsis and Acute Kidney Injury

Sepsis causes almost half of cases of AKI in critically ill patients.[1,3] Sepsis and septic shock create hemodynamic instability and reduce perfusion to the kidney.[16,17] In severely septic patients, inflammation increases vascular permeability, and much of this fluid may move into the third space (interstitial space). In half of patients with septic shock, vasopressors are used after volume resuscitation.[16,17] Vasopressors raise blood pressure and increase systemic vascular resistance, but they also may raise the vascular resistance within the kidney microvasculature.

Trauma and Acute Kidney Injury
Trauma Admissions

Trauma patients have different demographics than other critical care populations. Patients are always emergency admissions, are younger, are more often male, and have fewer coexisting illnesses.[18] A 5-year retrospective study of 9449 trauma admissions to critical care units in Australia and New Zealand used the RIFLE criteria to determine incidence of AKI in the first 24 hours after admission; 18% of trauma patients developed AKI.[18] However, if patients were older or had preexisting comorbid illnesses, their risk of AKI increased to 35%.[18] Although these AKI numbers are high, they likely underestimate the true incidence because the study did not include patients who developed AKI later than 24 hours after admission to the critical care unit.[18]

Rhabdomyolysis

Trauma patients with major crush injuries have an elevated risk of kidney failure because of the release of creatine and myoglobin from damaged muscle cells, a condition called *rhabdomyolysis*.[19] Myoglobin in large quantities is toxic to the kidney. A major goal of treatment is to prevent rhabdomyolysis-induced AKI. The mortality rate is low, provided that adequate crystalloid volume is administered early in the course of treatment.[20] It is important to trend the serum potassium levels. Life-threatening hyperkalemia can occur as cell lysis permits intracellular potassium to be released into the bloodstream.[21]

The level of creatine kinase (CK), a marker of systemic muscle damage, increases in patients with rhabdomyolysis. One trauma service reported that of 2083 critical care trauma admissions, 85% had elevated CK levels, and 10% developed AKI resulting from rhabdomyolysis.[21] A CK level of 5000 units/L was the lowest abnormal value in patients who developed AKI associated with rhabdomyolysis.[21]

Crystalloid volume resuscitation is the primary treatment for preservation of adequate kidney function and prevention of AKI. In many hospitals, intravenous (IV) fluids are alkalinized by the addition of sodium bicarbonate, and urine output is increased by IV administration of the diuretic mannitol. A bicarbonate and mannitol regimen is instituted to prevent acidosis and hyperkalemia because both are frequent complications of rhabdomyolysis. Close attention is paid to hourly urine output that can be dark

FLUIDS & MEDICATIONS - IMPROVE PERFUSION

Crystalloid Volume Resuscitation
- Sodium Bicarbonate added to alkalinize solution.
- Osmotic diuretic mannitol given to ↑ U/O.
- Bicarb and mannitol regimen instituted to prevent acidosis and hyperkalemia.
- Assess urine hourly for amount & color.
- Monitor BUN, serum creatinine, & electrolytes.

Hyperkalemia and hypocalcemia can result in life-threatening cardiac dysrhythmias.

NURSING INTERVENTIONS

- Fluid resuscitation with crystalloids and colloids.
- Hemodynamic monitoring and fluid balance.
- VS, CO, daily weight, I/O, focused physical assessment
- Insert a urinary drainage catheter to accurately record hourly U/O. Remove as soon as clinically feasible to prevent CAUTI.
- Fluid Restriction calculated on U/O & insensible losses.
- Frequent skin care with emollients, discouraging scratching, and administering phosphate-binding medications.
- Monitor ABGs to maintain pH within normal range.
- Prevent blood loss, minimize blood withdrawal.
- Because of risk for GI bleed - stress ulcer prophylaxis and testing for occult blood with stool, NG tube drainage, & emesis.
- Educate patient and family about AKI prognosis, treatment, and possible complications.
- Encourage patient and family to voice concerns, frustrations, or fears, allowing some control over situation.

Prevent complications including ischemic-anoxic encephalopathy cardiac dysrhythmias, venous thromboembolism (VTE),and stress ulcers.[5]

↑ Perfusion

Monitor for life-threatening complications

Responding

ACUTE KIDNEY INJURY

62 year-old ICU patient, Marcus Jones, develops sepsis with sustained hypotension and suffers an acute kidney injury.

Fluid & Electrolyte Balance

Nurse's Role is to
- Expand intravascular volume to achieve & maintain hemodynamic stability.
- Recognize S/S of circulatory overload.
- Prevent clinical manifestations of electrolyte and acid-base imbalances.
- Use measures to remove fluid, solutes, & toxins in the circulation.
- Provide comfort & emotional support.
- Maintain surveillance for complications.

Analysis

DEMONSTRATE ADEQUATE FLUID VOLUME:
- Hemodynamic values within normal (CO, BP, HR, CVP, PAP, PAOP)
- Electrolytes and H/H within normal range
- Maintain O₂ Sat of 90% or greater
- Mental clarity, skin warm/dry,
- Urine output > 60 mL/hr
- RR within normal, clear breath sounds

P A T I E N T   O U T C O M E S

Prerenal AKI

Fluid Status

Life-Threatening Electrolyte Disturbances

PATHOPHYSIOLOGY - ACUTE KIDNEY INJURY

Hemodynamic instability from sepsis induced hypotension → ↓ perfusion to the kidney. Inflammation ↑ vascular permeability → interstitial edema. Edema 2° to fluid retention → inadequate U/O, ↓ serum albumin → ↓ oncotic pressure, inflammation ↑ vascular permeability → fluid movement from vessels into interstitial spaces.

FOCUSED PHYSICAL ASSESSMENT

Assessing Fluid Balance

- Thirst, ↓ skin turgor and lethargy → extracellular fluid depletion.
- Pulmonary congestion, ↑ heart failure, and ↑ BP → intravascular fluid volume overload.
- Patient remains "intravascularly dry" and hemodynamically unstable, because retained fluid is not inside a vascular compartment.
- Assess frequently for pitting edema over bony prominences & dependent areas.

Interpreting Electrolyte Balance

Hyperkalemia
- Monitor ECG: peaked T waves, widening of QRS, ventricular tachycardia or fibrillation.
- IV diuretics (if patient producing urine).
- IV administration of D₅₀ & regular insulin
- K⁺ - binding resins orally, NG tube, or rectally.
- Dialysis

Hypernatremia and Hyponatremia
- Can be ↑ or ↓ depending on fluid volume.

Hypocalcemia and Hyperphosphatemia
- Serum calcium levels ↓ results from multiple factors, including hyperphosphatemia.

Medical Management
Prevention, compensation ↓ kidney function, and regeneration of kidney functional capacity.
Key Treatment - Prevention strategies, fluid balance, anemia, medications, and electrolytes.

PRIORITY NURSING DIAGNOSIS

Excess Fluid Volume related to kidney dysfunction

FIG. 26.2 Concept Map for Acute Kidney Injury. *BP,* blood pressure; *BUN,* blood, urea, creatinine; *CAUTI,* catheter associated urinary tract infection; *CO,* cardiac output; *CVP,* central venous pressure; *ECG,* electrocardiogram; *HR,* heart rate; *I/O,* intake and output; *O₂ Sat,* oxygen saturation; *RR,* respiratory rate; *S/S,* signs and symptoms; *SvO₂,* mixed venous oxygen saturation; *U/O,* urine output; *VS,* vital signs. Concept maps created by © DEANNE A. BLACH, MSN, RN.

TABLE 26.5 Decreased Kidney Function by Stage in Adult US Population

Stage[*]	Population Affected[*]	GFR and Diagnosis[*]	Percentage Who Know They Have Kidney Dysfunction (%)[†]
1	9 million (3.3%)	Normal; persistent albuminuria	40.5
2	5.3 million (3.0%)	60–89; persistent albuminuria	29.3
3	7.6 million (4.3%)	30–59	22.0
4	400,000 (0.2%)	15–29	44.5
5	300,000 (0.2%)	<15: ESKD	100

[*]Data from Coresh J, et al. Prevalence of chronic kidney disease and decreased kidney function in the adult US population: Third National Health and Nutrition Examination Survey. *Am J Kidney Dis.* 2003;41(1):1.
[†]Data from Nickolas TL, et al. Awareness of kidney disease in the US population: Findings from the National Health and Nutrition Examination Survey (NHANES) 1999 to 2000. *Am J Kidney Dis.* 2004;44(2):185.
ESKD, end-stage kidney disease; *GFR,* glomerular filtration rate (mL/min/1.73 m² of body surface area).

brown or tea-colored,[20] CK levels, serum creatinine levels, serum potassium levels, and any signs of compartment syndrome in all patients admitted with this diagnosis.

Contrast-Induced Nephrotoxic Injury and Acute Kidney Injury

More than 1 million radiologic studies or procedures that involve use of IV radiopaque contrast medium are performed every year. Patients most at risk of contrast-induced nephropathy (CIN) are patients with preexisting CKD, an elevated baseline serum creatinine level, and dehydration.[22-24] The clinical definition of CIN is an increase in serum creatinine concentration of 0.5 mg/dL or more, or a 25% increase from the patient's baseline within 3 days of contrast medium exposure, without an alternative clinical explanation for development of AKI.[23] The effects of reversible, contrast-induced AKI may not be limited to the immediate hospitalization; it has been linked to increased mortality in the 5-year period after the reversible AKI compared with similar patients who did not have kidney injury.[22-24]

Radiopaque Contrast Medium

High-molecular-weight contrast medium is a potential cause of nephrotoxicity. A recommended strategy to prevent CIN involves use of a lower quantity of contrast medium per study and use of nonionic, low-osmolar or iso-osmolar (iohexol) contrast media that are less nephrotoxic.[22,23]

Promote Hydration and Avoid Dehydration

The best method of prevention is aggressive hydration with IV normal saline during and after the procedure.[22,23] After some diagnostic intravascular catheterization procedures, an alert patient is asked to drink several liters of water over a 12-hour period to protect the kidney. Avoiding dehydration is vital.

Medications

The addition of sodium bicarbonate, because of its alkalinizing effect, may confer protection to the vulnerable kidney beyond hydration with normal saline only.[23] Other strategies such as adjunctive use of *N*-acetylcysteine or hemofiltration have shown conflicting results in research studies and are not recommended.[23]

Potentially nephrotoxic medications are also stopped before the procedure. Metformin, a medication that decreases insulin resistance in type 2 diabetes, has been associated with lactic acidosis in rare instances.[23] For patients with elevated serum creatinine, metformin is stopped the day before any procedure involving contrast medium and not started again for 48 hours when serum creatinine has returned to baseline.[24]

The mainstay measures to protect the kidney from contrast-induced AKI are to use the smallest dose possible of low-osmolar or iso-osmolar contrast medium, provide vigorous fluid volume expansion, stop all nephrotoxic medications, and avoid repeat contrast media injections within 48 hours.[22]

Catheter-Associated Urinary Tract Infection

Most critically ill patients have a urinary drainage catheter inserted to record hourly urine output accurately.[25] This is an appropriate use of a urinary catheter during critical illness. However, because of the risk of catheter-associated urinary tract infection (CAUTI), the catheter should be removed as soon as clinically feasible.[26-28] Critically ill patients who have a protracted illness have a significant risk of contracting a CAUTI, especially if the catheter is required for several days.[28] Additionally, critically ill patients who have developed a CAUTI have a higher mortality and longer lengths of stay.[29]

The focus on prevention of CAUTI has gained considerable momentum. The US Centers for Medicare and Medicaid Services no longer provides reimbursement for hospital-acquired CAUTI because it is considered a preventable infection. The Joint Commission has identified prevention of CAUTI as a national patient safety goal.[30] Prevention is the best cure, and many critical care units have adopted a "bundle" approach to eliminate CAUTI.[31-34] The essential components of CAUTI prevention are as follows:

1. Avoid unnecessary use of urinary catheters
2. Insert urinary catheters using aseptic technique
3. Adopt evidence-based standards for maintenance of urinary catheters
4. Review the need for the urinary catheter daily and remove the catheter promptly

Interventions to prevent CAUTI are listed in Box 26.3.

Hemodynamic Monitoring and Fluid Balance

Hemodynamic monitoring is important for the analysis of fluid volume status in a critically ill patient with AKI.[35] Hemodynamic monitoring includes surveillance of changes in vital signs including cardiac output. The range of monitoring devices has expanded, and assessment may be continuous or intermittent and be invasive, minimally invasive, or noninvasive as described in Chapter 13.

Daily Weight

A less "high-tech" method but also important is a daily weight. The daily weight, combined with accurate intake and output monitoring, is a powerful indicator of fluid gains or losses over 24 hours. A 1-kg weight gain over 24 hours represents 1000 mL (1 liter) of additional fluid retention.

QSEN BOX 26.3 **QSEN: Patient Safety Alert**

Prevention of Catheter-Associated Urinary Tract Infections

1. Avoid Unnecessary Use of Indwelling Urinary Catheters
Critical Care Indications
Accurate measurements of urinary output
Prolonged immobilization (eg, potentially unstable thoracic or lumbar spine, multiple traumatic injuries such as pelvic fractures)

Perioperative Indications
Urologic or genitourinary tract surgery
Prolonged duration of surgery (catheters inserted for this reason should be removed in the postanesthesia care unit)
Large-volume infusions or diuretics administered during surgery
Intraoperative monitoring of urinary output

Other Indications
Acute urinary retention or bladder outlet obstruction
Assist in healing of open sacral or perineal wounds in incontinent patients
Improve comfort for end-of-life care if needed

2. Insert Urinary Catheters Using Aseptic Technique
Hand Hygiene
Wash hands thoroughly before or after any patient care activity
Use gloves when touching catheter site or meatus

Sterile Technique and Sterile Equipment
Use standard supply kits that contain all necessary items:
- Sterile gloves, drape, sponges, antiseptic solution for cleaning meatus, single-use packet of lubricant jelly for insertion
- Use as small a catheter as possible to minimize urethral trauma
- Single attempt to insert urinary catheter
- Use new catheter if second attempt at catheterization is required

3. Adopt Evidence-Based Standards for Maintenance of Urinary Catheters
Maintenance of Closed Drainage System
Maintain sterile closed drainage system
Maintain unobstructed urine flow (avoid dependent loops)
Keep drainage bag below the level of the bladder at all times

Do not allow drainage bag to touch the floor
Empty collection bag regularly, using a separate container for each patient
Do not allow drainage spigot to touch the collection container
Do not break the system to collect a urine sample. Collect from sampling port in the tubing drainage system, disinfecting the port and aspirating using aseptic technique
Avoid catheter irrigation except in the case of an obstructed catheter; use a bladder ultrasound scan to determine if there is urine in the bladder
Routine scheduled replacement of catheters is not recommended

Catheter Securement and Hygiene
Keep urinary catheter secured to prevent catheter movement and urethral friction
Do not clean periurethral area with antiseptics. Urethral cleaning during a bath is appropriate

4. Review Need for Urinary Catheter Daily and Remove Catheter Promptly
Documentation and Monitoring
Document when catheter was inserted
Nurses and physicians should review the need for the urinary catheter for every patient every day

Hospital Strategies to Ensure Early Removal of Urinary Catheters
Ensure clinicians are aware that longer duration of catheter use increases catheter-associated urinary tract infection (CAUTI) risk. This awareness can be reinforced by
- Alerts in computerized ordering systems
- Automatic stops on catheter orders at 24 h, 48 h, or 72 h, depending on the clinical situation
- Development of standardized nursing protocols that allow nurses to remove urinary catheters if predetermined criteria are met

Know Your Own CAUTI Data
Each critical care unit should ensure that all nurses and physicians are aware of their unit/patient statistics on CAUTI per 1000 catheter days
Publicize strategies used to prevent CAUTI

Based on data from Gould CV, et al. *Guideline for prevention of catheter associated urinary tract infections 2009.* Centers for Disease Control and Prevention. http://www.cdc.gov/hicpac/pdf/cauti/cautiguideline2009final.pdf. 2009. Accessed October 9, 2016.

Physical Assessment

Physical signs and symptoms are used to assess fluid balance. Signs that suggest extracellular fluid depletion include thirst, decreased skin turgor, and lethargy. Signs that imply intravascular fluid volume overload include pulmonary congestion, increasing heart failure, and rising blood pressure. A patient with untreated AKI is edematous. The following factors contribute to this state:

1. Fluid retention is caused by inadequate urine output.
2. Low serum albumin levels create a lower oncotic pressure in the vasculature, and more fluid seeps out into the interstitial spaces to cause peripheral edema.
3. Inflammation associated with AKI or a coexisting nonrenal disease increases vascular permeability, facilitating fluid movement from the vessels into interstitial spaces.

In critical illness, even though there is peripheral edema, and the patient may have gained 8 L of fluid over his or her

"dry-weight" baseline, the patient may remain "intravascularly dry" and hemodynamically unstable because the retained fluid is not inside a vascular compartment and cannot contribute to maintenance of hemodynamic stability. A patient with AKI is assessed frequently for pitting edema over bony prominences and in dependent body areas.

Electrolyte Balance
Potassium

Electrolyte levels require frequent observation, especially in the critical phases of AKI when potassium can quickly reach levels of 6.0 mEq/L or higher (see Table 26.4). Specific electrocardiogram changes are associated with hyperkalemia, including peaked T waves, a widening of the QRS interval, and ultimately ventricular tachycardia or fibrillation.[36] If hyperkalemia is identified, all potassium supplements are stopped. If the patient is producing urine, IV diuretics can be administered. Acute hyperkalemia can be treated temporarily by IV administration of insulin and glucose. An infusion of 50 mL of 50% dextrose accompanied by 10 units of regular insulin forces potassium out of the serum and into the cells.[37]

To treat smaller increases in serum potassium, nonabsorbable potassium-binding resins may be used. The binding resins can be administered orally, through a nasogastric (NG) tube, or rectally to treat hyperkalemia. Cation exchange resins employ either sodium (Kayexalate) or calcium (Sorbisterit, Ca-Resonium, Argamate) and exchange the cation for potassium across the gastrointestinal wall.[37,38] The potassium is contained in the lower gastrointestinal tract and is eliminated with the stool. Potassium-binding resins and dialysis are the only permanent methods of potassium removal to treat hyperkalemia.

Sodium

Alterations in sodium level are an expected finding in kidney failure (see Table 26.4). Both hypernatremia (elevated serum sodium) and hyponatremia (low serum sodium) are associated with increased mortality with kidney failure[39]; this is unrelated to whether or not the patient has a diagnosis of heart failure.[39]

Calcium and Phosphorus

Serum calcium levels are reduced (hypocalcemia) in kidney failure (see Table 26.4). This reduction results from multiple factors, including hyperphosphatemia. Chronically elevated serum phosphorus levels (above 5.5 mg/dL) are associated with higher mortality rates for patients with kidney failure.[40,41] Calcium and phosphorus levels are regulated by a complex physiologic feedback mechanism involving parathyroid hormone and fibroblast growth factor. Normally, parathyroid hormone helps calcium be resorbed back into the bloodstream at the proximal tubule and distal nephron, and it promotes excretion of phosphorus by the kidney to maintain homeostasis. In kidney failure, this mechanism is nonfunctional; the serum phosphorus level rises, and the serum calcium level falls. Consequently, patients with kidney failure must take oral phosphate binder medications to control serum phosphorus.[42]

Calcium Replacement

Most calcium in the bloodstream is bound to protein. Calcium levels can be measured in two ways: total calcium or ionized calcium. Protein-calcium binding confounds the measurement of accurate calcium levels. In the past, calculations were used to estimate the amounts of protein-bound versus unbound calcium, but these calculations have been shown to produce inaccurate results. The metabolically active, non–protein-bound portion is known as *ionized calcium* and is the preferred method of measurement.[43] Without adequate levels of serum calcium, a compensatory mechanism "steals" calcium from the bones, making the patient with kidney failure more vulnerable to fractures. Maintaining adequate calcium stores in the body is important and is achieved by administration of calcium supplements and vitamin D.[41]

Dietary Phosphorus–Binding Medications

A second method used in tandem with calcium supplements to achieve normal calcium levels is to reduce the level of phosphorus in the bloodstream.[42] Phosphorus is present in many foods, especially foods with a high protein content or food additives such as dairy products, processed meats, some carbonated drinks, and nuts.[44] After eating these foods, free phosphorus passes from the gastrointestinal tract into the bloodstream and raises the serum level. Medications that bind dietary phosphorus in the gastrointestinal tract are administered orally or by NG tube. The binding agent must be taken at the same time as a meal. After the dietary phosphorus is bound to the binding substance in the bowel, it is eliminated from the intestine with stool.[40] This lowers the serum phosphorus level.

The types of dietary phosphorus binders used have changed over the years. The original binders were aluminum salts (aluminum hydroxide) that bound dietary phosphorus effectively in the gastrointestinal tract but conferred aluminum toxicity because some of the aluminum metal was also absorbed. For this reason, aluminum binders have largely been abandoned.[40] The second generation dietary phosphorus–binding agents that are widely prescribed use calcium salts including calcium carbonate or calcium acetate (PhosLo) to bind dietary phosphorus in the gastrointestinal tract. Calcium-based medications are safer, but elevated serum calcium levels and calcium deposits in other areas of the body (extraosseous calcification) are a problem.

A third generation of nonabsorbable dietary phosphorus–binding medications is available. These are non–aluminum-based, non–calcium-based medications and include sevelamer hydrochloride (Renagel) and lanthanum carbonate (Fosrenol). These medications have a good safety profile and are frequently prescribed to lower serum phosphorus levels in patients with CKD.[40]

Medical Management
Treatment Goals

Treatment goals for patients with AKI focus on prevention, compensation for the deterioration of kidney function, and regeneration of kidney functional capacity. Key treatment areas include prevention strategies, fluid balance, anemia, medications, and electrolyte imbalance.

Prevention

The only truly effective remedy for AKI is prevention. Effective prevention requires assessment of the patient's risk for AKI. Knowledge of the most frequent causes of AKI in critically ill patients is essential if prevention strategies are to be enacted. The critical care team collaborates closely with the clinical pharmacist to avoid medications with nephrotoxic side effects in patients with AKI or CKD. Nonsteroidal antiinflammatory medications for pain relief are avoided in patients with elevated creatinine levels. The use of intravascular contrast dye is preferably delayed until the patient is fully rehydrated.

Fluid Resuscitation

Prerenal failure is caused by decreased perfusion and flow to the kidney. It is often associated with trauma, hemorrhage, hypotension, and major fluid losses. If contrast dye is used, aggressive fluid resuscitation with normal saline (NaCl) is recommended. The objectives of volume replacement are to replace fluid and electrolyte losses and to prevent ongoing loss. Maintenance IV fluid therapy is initiated when oral fluid intake is inadvisable. Maintenance fluids are calculated with consideration for individual body surface area. Adults require approximately 1500 mL/m^2 per 24 hours; fever, burns, and trauma significantly increase fluid requirements. Other important criteria when calculating fluid volume replacement include baseline metabolism, environmental temperature, and humidity. The rate of replacement depends on cardiopulmonary reserve, adequacy of kidney function, urine output, fluid balance, ongoing loss, and type of fluid replaced.

Crystalloids and colloids. Crystalloids and colloids refer to two different types of IV fluids used for volume management in critically ill patients. These IV solutions are used on all types of patients, not just patients with acute kidney failure. Adequacy of IV fluid replacement depends on strict, ongoing evaluation and frequent adjustment. Frequent monitoring of serum electrolyte levels is required, and strictly regulated intake and output are correlated with daily weight records. In septic shock, hemodynamic readings are frequently undertaken. After a fluid challenge, a merely minimal increase in central venous pressure implies that additional fluid replacement is required. Continued decreases in central venous pressure, pulmonary artery occlusion pressure, and the cardiac index indicate ongoing volume losses.

Which IV fluid to select to successfully resuscitate hemodynamically unstable patients has been a controversial topic in critical care. The debate centers on the differences between crystalloid and colloid solutions.

Crystalloids. Crystalloid solutions, which are balanced salt solutions, are in widespread use for maintenance infusion and replacement therapy. Crystalloid fluids include normal saline solution (0.9 NaCl), half-normal saline solution (0.45 NaCl), and lactated Ringer solution (Table 26.6). Lactated Ringer solution usually is avoided in patients with kidney failure because it contains potassium. A noncrystalloid solution that may be infused is dextrose (5% or 10%) in water (D_5W, $D_{10}W$).

TABLE 26.6 Frequently Used Intravenous Solutions

Solution	Electrolytes	Indications
Crystalloids[a]		
Dextrose in water (D_5W), isotonic	None	Maintain volume Replace mild loss Provide minimal calories
Normal saline solution (0.9% NaCl)	Sodium: 154 mEq/L Chloride: 154 mEq/L Osmolality: 308 mEq/L	Maintain volume Replace mild loss
Half-normal saline solution (0.45% NaCl)	Sodium: 77 mEq/L Chloride: 77 mEq/L	Free water replacement Correct mild hyponatremia Free water and electrolyte replacement (fluid- and electrolyte-restricted conditions)
Lactated Ringer solution	Sodium: 130 mEq/L Potassium: 4 mEq/L Calcium: 2.7 mEq/L Chloride: 107 mEq/L Lactate: 27 mEq/L pH: 6.5	Fluid and electrolyte replacement (contraindicated for patients with kidney or liver disease or in lactic acidosis)
Colloids		
5% Albumin (Albumisol)	Albumin: 50 g/L Sodium: 130–160 mEq/L Potassium: 1 mEq/L Osmolality: 300 mOsm/L Osmotic pressure: 20 mm Hg pH: 6.4–7.4	Volume expansion Moderate protein replacement Achievement of hemodynamic stability in shock states
25% Albumin (salt-poor)	Albumin: 240 g/L Globulins: 10 g/L Sodium: 130–160 mEq/L Osmolality: 1500 mOsm/L pH: 6.4–7.4	Concentrated form of albumin sometimes used with diuretics to move fluid from tissues into vascular space for diuresis
Hetastarch	Sodium: 154 mEq/L Chloride: 154 mEq/L Osmolality: 310 mOsm/L Colloid osmotic pressure: 30–35 mm Hg	Synthetic polymer (6% solution) used for volume expansion Hemodynamic volume replacement after cardiac surgery, burns, sepsis
LMWD	Glucose polysaccharide molecules with average molecular weight of 40,000; no electrolytes	Volume expansion and support (contraindicated for patients with bleeding disorders)
HMWD	Glucose polysaccharide molecules with average molecular weight of 70,000; no electrolytes	Used prophylactically in some cases to prevent platelet aggregation; available in saline and glucose solutions

[a]For crystalloid solutions that contain electrolytes, specific concentrations of electrolytes and pH vary according to the manufacturer.
HMWD, high-molecular-weight dextran; *LMWD,* low-molecular-weight dextran.

Colloids. Colloids are solutions containing oncotically active particles that are used to expand intravascular volume to achieve and maintain hemodynamic stability. Albumin (5% and 25%) and hetastarch are colloid solutions (see Table 26.6). Colloids expand intravascular volume, and the effect can last 24 hours, although the use of colloids in critical care volume resuscitation is discouraged because of increased cost without evidence of increased benefit.[45]

The controversy over whether colloids or crystalloid IV fluids are most effective for volume resuscitation appears to have been put to rest by a series of randomized clinical trials and meta-analytic reviews. The SAFE study (*saline versus albumin fluid evaluation*) was a randomized, prospective, double-blind trial that examined whether the selection of resuscitation fluid in the critical care unit affected survival at 28 days.[45] This was a huge study, with almost 7000 critical care patients randomly assigned to two similar groups. One group received 4% albumin, and the other group received 0.9 normal saline (NaCl) for fluid resuscitation.[45] The patients in both groups were similar in terms of organ dysfunction, mechanical ventilator support (64% of patients), and renal replacement therapy (1% of patients). The SAFE results showed that there was no difference in the mortality rate, time in the critical care unit, ventilator days, or renal replacement therapy days.[45] The researchers concluded that albumin and saline should be considered clinically equivalent treatments for intravascular volume expansion in critically ill patients.[45] The exception was for patients with traumatic brain injury, in which case albumin was associated with a higher mortality rate.[46]

The findings of the SAFE study investigators have been validated by a systematic review of randomized trials of crystalloids versus colloids that reported no difference in mortality rates for critically ill and injured patients based on resuscitation fluid.[47] Consequently, colloids are not favored because of their higher cost, and crystalloids are the recommended fluid to use for resuscitation in critical care.

Fluid restriction. Fluid restriction constitutes a large part of medical treatment for acute kidney failure. Fluid restriction is used to prevent circulatory overload and the development of interstitial edema when the kidneys cannot remove excess volume. The fluid requirements are calculated on the basis of daily urine volumes and insensible losses. Obtaining daily weight measurements and keeping accurate intake and output records is essential. Patients with kidney failure are usually restricted to 1 L of fluid per 24 hours if the urine output is 500 mL or less. Insensible losses range from 500 to 750 mL/day.

Fluid removal. Acute kidney failure results in retention of water, solutes, and potential toxins in the circulation, and prompt measures are needed to decrease their levels. Diuretics are used to stimulate urine output in the early stages of AKI. Renal replacement therapy (hemodialysis or hemofiltration) is another choice, particularly if volume overload exacerbates pulmonary edema or heart failure.

Pharmacologic Management

The first step is to stop all nephrotoxic medications. Second, if medications are eliminated through the kidneys, it is important to decrease the frequency of administration (eg, from every 6 hours to every 12 or 24 hours) or to decrease the dose and to monitor the concentration by measuring serum medication levels.

Diuretics

Diuretics are used to stimulate urinary output in a patient with fluid overload and functioning kidneys. Care must be taken in their use to avoid the creation of secondary electrolyte abnormalities (Table 26.7). Diuretics reduce volume overload and are helpful for symptoms such as pulmonary edema, but they have not been shown to prevent AKI.[48] Diuretics are used in many patients other than those with incipient kidney failure.

Loop diuretics. Loop diuretics include furosemide (Lasix), bumetanide (Bumex), and torsemide.[49] Furosemide is the most frequently used diuretic in critical care patients. It may be administered orally, as an IV bolus, or as a continuous IV infusion. Electrolyte abnormalities are frequently encountered, and close monitoring of serum potassium, magnesium, and sodium is essential. Loop diuretics block the Na-K-2Cl transporter in the nephron on the ascending limb of the loop of Henle, where most sodium is reabsorbed (Fig. 26.3). This diuresis is also a *natriuresis,* as sodium is excreted in the urine. Diuretic resistance can develop over time in patients with chronic heart failure or kidney failure who were taking loop diuretics at home before they were admitted to the hospital.[50] Their higher diuretic medication dosages are a reflection of diuretic resistance.[50]

Thiazide diuretics. Diuretics from different classes may be prescribed in combination. A thiazide diuretic such as chlorothiazide (Diuril) or metolazone (Zaroxolyn) may be administered and followed by a loop diuretic to take advantage of the fact that these medications work on different parts of the nephron (see Fig. 26.3).[51] Creatinine clearance affects the efficacy of thiazide diuretics. Metolazone is a more effective diuretic in kidney failure when the creatinine clearance is less than 30 mL/min. A normal creatinine clearance is 120 mL/min (see Table 26.7). Sometimes a thiazide diuretic is added to a loop diuretic to compensate for the development of loop diuretic resistance.[50]

Osmotic diuretics. Osmotic diuretics, such as mannitol, are prescribed to increase urine output and decrease fluid overload. It is important to use an in-line 5-micron filter when administering this IV medication. Mannitol is frequently administered to patients with brain injury and increased intracranial pressure. More information on the use of mannitol in patients with neurologic disorders can be found in Chapter 23 under hyperosmolar therapy. Mannitol is filtered by the glomerulus, is not absorbed by the nephron, and works in the proximal tubule and the descending section of the loop of Henle via aquaporin water channels (see Fig. 26.3).[49]

Carbonic anhydrase inhibitor diuretics. Only one carbonic anhydrase inhibitor acts as a diuretic, and it is used in very specific clinical circumstances. Acetazolamide (Diamox) acts on the proximal tubule, where it inhibits the carbonic anhydrase enzyme allowing more bicarbonate (HCO_3^-) to be released into the filtrate resulting in an alkaline diuresis (see Fig. 26.3). Acetazolamide is administered to treat the metabolic alkalosis that sometimes occurs after aggressive diuresis with loop diuretics.[52] Acid–base balance and serum bicarbonate levels are frequently monitored when acetazolamide is used to treat metabolic alkalosis (see Table 26.7).

Potassium-sparing diuretics. Spironolactone (Aldactone) is a "potassium-sparing" diuretic. Spironolactone inhibits the aldosterone mineralocorticoid receptor in the late distal tubule and collecting duct of the kidneys causing potassium to be retained and sodium to be excreted (see Fig. 26.3). At

TABLE 26.7 Pharmacologic Management
Kidney-Related Medications

Medication	Dosage	Action	Special Considerations
Diuretics			
Loop Diuretics			
Furosemide (Lasix)	20–80 mg/day	Acts on loop of Henle to inhibit sodium and chloride resorption (natriuresis)	Ototoxicity if administered too rapidly or with other ototoxic medications Caution with sulfa allergy
Bumetanide (Bumex)	0.5–2 mg/day		Monitor intake and output, hydration; monitor for hypotension; Titrate to maintenance, may increase by 20 to 40 mg orally at 6- to 8-hour intervals after the previous dose; this individual dose may be given once or twice daily; MAX 600 mg/day orally Caution with sulfa allergy
Thiazide Diuretics			
Chlorothiazide (Diuril)	500–1000 mg/ once or twice /day PO/IV	Inhibits sodium, chloride resorption in distal tubule	Enhanced with low-sodium diet; 500 to 1000 mg ORALLY once or twice daily; may also give intermittently (alternate days or 3 to 5 days per week). Use IV only when patient cannot take by mouth; caution with sulfa allergy Synergistic effect with loop diuretics
Metolazone (Zaroxolyn)	2.5–10 mg/day PO initial dose May increase to 20 mg/day with edema	Inhibits sodium, chloride resorption in distal tubule	Effective to creatinine clearance of 10 mL/min; caution with sulfa allergy
Osmotic Diuretics			
Mannitol	0.25–1.0 g/kg IV infusion as 15%–20% solution over 30–90 min	Increases urine output because higher plasma osmolality Increases flow of water from tissues, causing increased GFR Increases serum sodium, potassium levels	Often used in head injury to decrease cerebral edema Can be used to promote urinary secretion of toxic substances Mannitol may crystallize at low temperatures, use in-line 5-micron IV filter with >15% (>15 g/100 mL) solutions
Potassium-Sparing Diuretics			
Spironolactone (Aldactone)	100 mg/day for 5 days PO	Exert effects on collecting duct; retains potassium, increases sodium diuresis	Weak diuretic effect Potassium supplements not required; monitor for hyperkalemia Used as an aldosterone blocker to treat heart failure
Vaptans			
Conivaptan (Vaprisol)	Loading dose: 20 mg IV as 30-min infusion Continuous IV infusion: 20 mg over 24 h After first day, can be increased to 40 mg/24 h Maximum infusion is 4 days	Blocks V2 aquaporin channels in collecting tubules	Used only in hyponatremia with hypervolemia Monitor volume status and serum sodium frequently

BP, blood pressure; *ECG*, electrocardiogram; *GFR*, glomerular filtration rate; *GI*, gastrointestinal; *IV*, intravenous/intravenously; *PO*, by mouth.

high dosages, it has a diuretic action, although that is rarely the rationale behind its use today. Spironolactone is most often administered as an *aldosterone antagonist* in the management of heart failure.

Vaptans

A newer class of medications collectively described as *vaptans* inhibit the effect of antidiuretic hormone (vasopressin) on the V2 aquaporin channels in the collecting ducts of the kidney (see Fig. 26.3). Blockage of the aquaporin channels renders the collecting ducts impermeable, resulting in solute-free water excretion or *aquadiuresis*.[53] Vaptans are used to correct symptomatic hypervolemic hyponatremic (dilutional) states. The clinical intent is to eliminate water and retain sodium. These medications must not be administered for hypovolemic hyponatremia or anuria. Conditions that can cause dilutional hyponatremia include *syndrome of inappropriate antidiuretic hormone secretion* described in Chapter 32, liver cirrhosis with ascites, and heart failure. Only two vaptans are approved by the US Food and Drug Administration (FDA) for use in the United States. Conivaptan (Vaprisol), which is administered intravenously, is approved for short-term use in the hospital only (see Table 26.7). Tolvaptan (Samsca) is available only as an oral medication.[53]

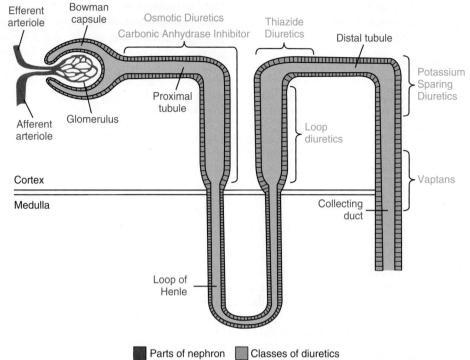

FIG. 26.3 Pharmacologic Site of Action of Diuretics in the Nephron.

Dopamine

Low-dose dopamine (2 to 3 mcg/kg per minute), previously known as renal-dose dopamine, is frequently infused to stimulate blood flow to the kidney. Dopamine is effective in increasing urine output in the short-term, but tolerance of the dopamine renal receptor to the medication is theorized to develop in critically ill patients who are most at risk for AKI. Renal-dose dopamine does not prevent onset of AKI, decrease the need for dialysis, or reduce mortality.[1] At this point, the support for routine use of low-dose dopamine for the prevention of AKI remains anecdotal only. Low-dose dopamine infusions may have other therapeutic uses, such as increasing urine output, in combination with furosemide in patients with heart failure.[54]

Acetylcysteine

Acetylcysteine (Mucomyst, Mucosil) is an *N*-acetyl derivative of the amino acid l-cysteine. It has been used for many years as a mucolytic agent to assist with expectoration of thick pulmonary secretions. It is also frequently prescribed for patients with mildly elevated serum creatinine levels before a radiologic study using contrast dye.[24] In research trials, the addition of acetylcysteine to normal saline hydration did not reduce the incidence of contrast-induced AKI.[23]

Dietary Phosphorus Binders

Many patients with kidney failure are prescribed a dietary phosphorus–binding medication (see earlier section on "Dietary Phosphorus–Binding Medications").[40-42] Many dietary phosphorus binders are available, and some important issues concern all of them. The dietary phosphorus binder must be taken at the time of the meal. If it is taken 2 hours later, it will increase only the level of the binding substance (eg, calcium) in the bloodstream and will not lower the serum phosphorus level. Related issues, such as the quantity of phosphorus in the diet, should be discussed with a clinical nutritionist (dietitian).

Nutrition

Diet or nutritional supplementation for a patient with AKI in the critical care unit is designed to account for the diminished excretory capacity of the kidney. The recommended energy intake is between 20 and 30 kcal/kg per day, with 1.2 to 1.5 g/kg of protein per day to control azotemia (increased BUN level). Oral nutrition is preferred, and if the patient cannot eat, enteral nutrition is recommended over parenteral (IV) nutrition.[55,56] Fluids are limited, and monitoring of blood glucose levels is recommended. The electrolytes potassium, sodium, and phosphorus are strictly limited.

Nursing Management

Nursing management of a patient with AKI involves a variety of nursing diagnoses (Box 26.4). "Prevention is the best cure" is an old saying that captures the role of the critical care nurse, who evaluates all patients for level of kidney function, risk of infection, fluid imbalance, electrolyte disturbances, anemia, readiness to learn, and need for education.

Risk Factors for Acute Kidney Injury

Some individuals are at increased risk for AKI as a complication during hospitalization, and the alert critical care nurse recognizes potential risk factors and acts as a patient advocate. Patients at risk include older patients because their GFR may be decreased, dehydrated patients with kidney hypoperfusion, patients with increased creatinine levels before their hospitalization, and patients undergoing a radiologic procedure involving contrast dye.

Infectious Complications

A critical care patient with infectious complications is at risk for AKI. Signs of infection such as an increased white blood cell count, redness at a wound or IV line site, or increased temperature are always a cause for concern. A urinary catheter may be inserted to facilitate accurate urine measurement. However, any indwelling catheter is a potential source for infection. When the patient no longer makes large quantities of urine and is hemodynamically stable, the catheter must be removed promptly. If the patient cannot void urine spontaneously, a scheduled intermittent urinary catheterization is performed to minimize the risk of infection from an indwelling catheter and drainage system. This method allows the patient's bladder to be emptied, but the catheter does not remain in place.

Fluid Balance

Intravascular fluid balance is often assessed on an hourly basis for a critically ill patient who has hemodynamic lines inserted. Hemodynamic values (heart rate, blood pressure, central venous pressure, pulmonary artery occlusion pressure, cardiac output, and cardiac index) and daily weight measurements are correlated with intake and output. Urine output is measured hourly by means of a urinary catheter and drainage bag throughout all phases of AKI, particularly in response to diuretics. Any fluid removed with dialysis is included in the daily fluid balance. Recognition of the clinical signs and symptoms of fluid overload is important. Excess fluid moves from the vascular system into the peripheral tissues (dependent edema), abdomen (ascites), and lungs (crackles, pulmonary edema, and pulmonary effusions); around the heart (pericardial effusions); and into the brain (increased intracranial swelling).

Electrolyte Imbalance

Hyperkalemia, hypocalcemia, hyponatremia, hyperphosphatemia, and acid–base imbalances occur during AKI (see Table 26.4). Clinical manifestations of these electrolyte imbalances must be prevented, and their associated side effects must be controlled. The more likely imbalances are hyperkalemia and hypocalcemia, which can result in life-threatening cardiac dysrhythmias.[36] Dilutional hyponatremia may develop as fluid overload worsens in patients with oliguria. Monitoring the serum sodium level is important to prevent this complication. Hyperphosphatemia results in severe pruritus. Nursing care is directed at soothing the itching by performing frequent skin care with emollients, discouraging scratching, and administering phosphate-binding medications. The acid–base imbalances that occur with AKI are monitored by arterial blood gas analyses. The goal of treatment is to maintain the pH within the normal range.

Preventing Anemia

Anemia is an expected side effect of kidney failure that occurs because the kidney no longer produces the hormone *erythropoietin*.[57] As a result, the bone marrow is not stimulated to produce erythrocytes (red blood cells). Additionally, the normal erythrocyte survival of 80 to 120 days is decreased in patients with CKD on dialysis to 70 to 80 days, increasing their risk for anemia.[57] Care is taken to prevent blood loss in patients with AKI, and blood withdrawal is minimized as much as possible. Irritation of the gastrointestinal tract from metabolic waste accumulation is expected, and stress ulcer prophylaxis must be prescribed. Gastrointestinal bleeding remains a possibility. Stool, nasogastric tube drainage, and emesis are routinely tested for occult blood.

Erythropoiesis-stimulating medications. Anemia associated with CKD may be treated pharmacologically by the administration of recombinant human erythropoietin. Three medications are approved by the FDA for treatment of CKD-associated anemia in the United States: epoetin alfa (Procrit, Epogen), darbepoetin alfa (Aranesp), and methoxy polyethylene glycol–epoetin beta (Mircera).[57] These agents stimulate erythrocyte production by the bone marrow.[57] Adjunctive treatments include administration of iron supplements, vitamin B_{12}, vitamin B_6, and folate. Erythropoietin has been shown to prevent anemia and reduce blood transfusions before dialysis, but it does not slow the progression of kidney disease.[58]

Patient Education

Accurate and uncomplicated information must be provided to the patient and family about AKI including its prognosis, treatment, and possible complications. Education of the patient can be challenging because elevations of BUN and creatinine levels can negatively affect the level of consciousness. Sleep-rest disorders and emotional upset often occur as complications of AKI and can disrupt short-term memory. Encouraging the patient and family to voice concerns, frustrations, or fears and allowing the patient to control some aspects of the acute care environment and treatment also are essential (Box 26.5).

RENAL REPLACEMENT THERAPY: DIALYSIS

Two types of renal replacement therapy are available for the treatment of AKI: intermittent hemodialysis (IHD) therapy and continuous renal replacement therapy (CRRT).

✳ BOX 26.5 PATIENT EDUCATION PLAN

Acute Kidney Injury

Before discharge, the patient should be able to teach back the following topics:

- Pathophysiology of acute kidney injury as a sudden decline in kidney function that caused an acute buildup of toxins in the blood.
- Explain level of kidney function after discharge from the hospital (if known).
- Explain diet and fluid restrictions.
- Emphasize need for exercise and rest.
- Describe medications and adverse effects.
- Explain need for ongoing follow-up with health care professional.
- Explain purpose of dialysis and importance of regular treatments.

Hemodialysis

Hemodialysis roughly translates as "separating from the blood." Indications and contraindications for hemodialysis are listed in Box 26.6. As a treatment, hemodialysis separates and removes from the blood the excess electrolytes, fluids, and toxins by means of a hemodialyzer (Fig. 26.4). Hemodialysis is efficient in removing solutes. Because levels of electrolytes, toxins, and fluids increase between treatments, hemodialysis occurs on a regular basis. Traditional hemodialysis treatments last 3 to 4 hours. A newer option is the use of *sustained low-efficiency dialysis* (SLED) that is run daily for 8 hours or 12 hours. Sometimes in critical illness this mode is run continuously (C-SLED). In the acute phase of kidney failure, hemodialysis is performed daily. Should the patient's condition progress to chronic kidney failure, the dialysis frequency gradually decreases to three times per week.

Hemodialyzer

Hemodialysis works by circulating blood outside the body through synthetic tubing to a dialyzer, which consists of hollow-fiber tubes. The dialyzer is sometimes described as an artificial kidney (Fig. 26.5). While the blood flows through the membranes, which are semipermeable, a fluid (dialysate bath) bathes the membranes and, through osmosis and diffusion, performs exchanges of fluid, electrolytes, and toxins from the blood to the bath, where toxins and dialysate then pass out of the artificial kidney. The blood and the dialysate bath are shunted in opposite directions (countercurrent flow) through the dialyzer to match the osmotic and chemical gradients at the most efficient level for effective dialysis.

Ultrafiltration

To remove fluid, a positive hydrostatic pressure is applied to the blood, and a negative hydrostatic pressure is applied to the dialysate bath. The two forces together, called *transmembrane pressure,* pull the excess fluid from the blood. The difference between the two values, expressed in millimeters of mercury represents the transmembrane pressure and results in fluid extraction, known as *ultrafiltration,* from the vascular space.

Anticoagulation

Heparin or sodium citrate is added to the system just before the blood enters the dialyzer to anticoagulate the blood within the dialysis tubing.[59] Without an anticoagulant, the blood clots because its passage through the foreign tubular substances of

---

BOX 26.6 Indications and Contraindications for Hemodialysis

Indications
- Blood urea nitrogen level greater than 90 mg/dL
- Serum creatinine level of 9 mg/dL
- Hyperkalemia
- Medication toxicity
- Intravascular and extravascular fluid overload
- Metabolic acidosis
- Symptoms of uremia
- Pericarditis
- Gastrointestinal bleeding
- Changes in mentation
- Contraindications to other forms of dialysis

Contraindications
- Hemodynamic instability
- Inability to anticoagulate
- Lack of access to circulation

FIG. 26.4 Hemodialyzer.

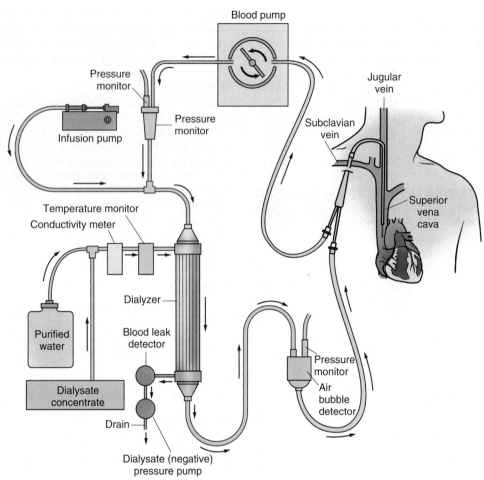

FIG. 26.5 Components of a Hemodialysis System.

the dialysis machine activates the clotting mechanism. Heparin can be administered by bolus injection or intermittent infusion. It has a short half-life, and its effects subside within 2 to 4 hours. If necessary, the effects of heparin are easily reversed with the antidote protamine sulfate. When there is concern about the development of heparin-induced thrombocytopenia, alternative anticoagulants can be used. Citrate can be infused as an anticoagulant by intermittent bolus or continuous infusion.

Vascular Access

Hemodialysis requires access to the bloodstream. Various types of temporary and permanent devices are in clinical use. It is important for patient safety to be able to recognize these different vascular access devices and to care for them properly. This section discusses temporary vascular access catheters used in the acute care hospital environment and permanent methods used for long-term hemodialysis.

Temporary vascular access. Subclavian and *femoral* veins are catheterized when short-term access is required or when a graft or fistula vascular access is nonfunctional in a patient requiring immediate hemodialysis. Subclavian and femoral catheters are routinely inserted at the bedside. Most temporary catheters are venous lines only. Blood flows out toward the dialyzer and flows back to the patient through the same catheterized vein. A dual-lumen venous catheter is most commonly used. It has a central partition running the length of the catheter. The outflow catheter section pulls the blood flow through openings

that are proximal to the inflow openings on the opposite side (Fig. 26.6). This design helps prevent dialyzing the same blood just returned to the area (recirculation), which would severely reduce the efficiency of the procedure. A silicone rubber dual-lumen catheter with a polyester cuff designed to decrease catheter-related infections is also available.

Permanent vascular access. The common denominator in permanent vascular access devices is a conduit connection between the arterial circulation and the venous circulation.

Arteriovenous fistula. The arteriovenous fistula is created by surgically exposing a peripheral artery and vein, creating a side-by-side opening in the artery and the vein to join the two vessels together. The high arterial flow creates a swelling of the vein, or a pseudoaneurysm, at which point (when healed) a large-bore needle can be inserted to obtain arterial outflow to the dialyzer. Inflow is accomplished through a second large-bore needle inserted into a peripheral vein distal to the fistula (Fig. 26.7A). Fistulas are the preferred mode of access because of the durability of blood vessels, relatively few complications, and less need for revision compared with other access methods. An initial disadvantage of a fistula concerns the time required for development of sufficient arterial flow to enlarge the new access. The minimum reported length of time before a fistula can be cannulated for dialysis is 14 days, but the time lag for many patients can be longer. Ideally, the fistula should be established 6 months before the requirement for hemodialysis to ensure it is usable for dialysis when required.[60]

Double Lumen Catheter

FIG. 26.6 Temporary Dialysis Venous Access Catheter.

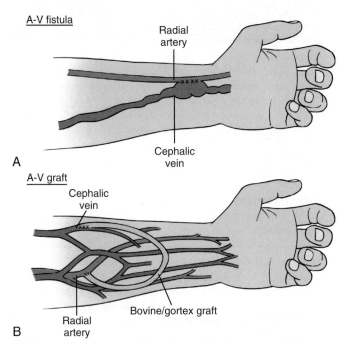

FIG. 26.7 Vascular Access for Hemodialysis. (A) Arteriovenous fistula between the vein and artery. (B) Internal synthetic graft connects the artery and vein.

In caring for a patient with a fistula, there are some important nursing priorities to ensure the ongoing viability of the vascular access and safety of the limb (Table 26.8). The critical care nurse frequently assesses the quality of blood flow through the fistula. A patent fistula has a thrill when palpated gently with the fingers and has a bruit if auscultated with a stethoscope. The extremity should be pink and warm to the touch. No blood pressure measurements, IV infusions, or laboratory phlebotomy procedures are performed on the arm with the fistula.

The arteriovenous fistula is the preferred long-term access for hemodialysis. It provides the most favorable long-term patency for hemodialysis access if patients require long-term hemodialysis.

Arteriovenous grafts. Arteriovenous grafts connect a vein and artery to allow vascular access for dialysis in chronic kidney failure. The graft is a tube made of synthetic material that is surgically implanted inside the limb. The area is surgically opened, and an artery and a vein are located. A tunnel is created in the tissue where the graft is placed. Anastomoses are made

TABLE 26.8 Complications and Nursing Management of Arteriovenous Fistula/Graft

Type	Complications	Nursing Management
Fistula	Thrombosis	Teach patients to avoid wearing constrictive clothing on limbs containing access.
	Infection	Teach patients to avoid sleeping on or bending accessed limb for prolonged periods.
	Pseudoaneurysm	Use aseptic technique when cannulating access.
	Vascular steal syndrome	Avoid repetitious cannulation of one segment of access.
	Venous hypertension	Offer comfort measures, such as warm compresses and ordered analgesics, to lessen pain of vascular steal.
	Carpal tunnel syndrome	
	Inadequate blood flow	Teach patients to develop blood flow in fistulas through exercises (squeezing a rubber ball) while applying mild impedance to flow just distal to the access (at least once per day for 10–15 min).
		Avoid too-early cannulation of new access.
Graft	Bleeding	Teach patients to avoid wearing constrictive clothing on accessed limbs.
	Thrombosis	Avoid repeated cannulation of one segment of access.
	False aneurysm formation	Use aseptic technique when cannulating access.
	Infection	Monitor for changes in arterial or venous pressure while patients are on dialysis.
	Arterial or venous stenosis	Provide comfort measures to reduce pain of vascular steal (eg, warm compresses, analgesics as ordered).
	Vascular steal syndrome	

with the graft ends connected to the artery and vein. The blood is allowed to flow through the graft, and the surgical area is closed. The graft creates a raised area that looks like a large peripheral vein just under the skin (Fig. 26.7B). Two large-bore needles are used for outflow from and inflow to the graft during dialysis. For grafts and fistulas, firm pressure must be applied to stop any bleeding after needle removal at the end of the hemodialysis treatment (see Table 26.8).

TABLE 26.9   Comparison of Continuous Renal Replacement Therapy Modes

Type	Ultrafiltration Rate	Fluid Replacement	Mode of Solute Removal	Indication
SCUF	100–300 mL/h	None	None	Fluid removal
CVVH	500–800 mL/h	Predilution or postdilution, calculating hourly net loss	Convection	Fluid removal, moderate solute removal
CVVHD	500–800 mL/h	Predilution or postdilution, subtracting dialysate, then calculating hourly net loss	Diffusion	Fluid removal, maximum solute removal
CVVHDF		Predilution or postdilution, subtracting dialysate, then calculating hourly net loss	Convection and diffusion	Maximal fluid removal, maximal solute removal

CVVH, continuous venovenous hemofiltration; *CVVHD*, continuous venovenous hemodialysis; *CVVHDF*, continuous venovenous hemodiafiltration; *SCUF*, slow continuous ultrafiltration.

Tunneled catheters. While waiting for the fistula or graft to mature to be ready for access, some patients with CKD may have a tunneled, cuffed catheter placed in either the internal or the external jugular vein. The cuff and tunneling are physical barriers to reduce central venous line infections. Modern catheters are made of silicone or Silastic elastomers making them more pliable than temporary catheters.

Medical Management

Medical management involves the decision to place a vascular access device and then to choose the most appropriate type and location for each patient. Patients in the critical care setting who require vascular access for hemodialysis typically use a temporary hemodialysis catheter. The exact quantity of fluid and solute removal to be achieved by hemodialysis is determined individually for each patient by clinical examination and review of all relevant laboratory results.

Nursing Management

A non–critical care nurse who is specially trained in dialysis manages the IHD. The dialysis nurse typically comes to the patient's bedside with the hemodialysis machine. During the acute phase of treatment, hemodialysis occurs daily. The frequency is reduced to 3 days per week as the patient becomes hemodynamically stable. The essential role of the critical care nurse during dialysis is to monitor the patient's hemodynamic status and ensure the patient remains hemodynamically stable. A patient with AKI on hemodialysis depends on a viable venous access catheter. When not in use, the catheter is "heparin-locked" to preserve patency. The critical care nurse provides education about the disease process and treatment plan to the patient and family.

Continuous Renal Replacement Therapy

CRRT is a newer mode of dialysis that has many similarities to traditional hemodialysis. CRRT is a continuous therapy that is monitored by the critical care nurse, and it may continue over many days. The venous blood is circulated through a highly porous hemofilter. As with traditional hemodialysis, access and return of blood are achieved through a large venous catheter (venovenous).[61] The CRRT system allows the continuous removal of fluid from the plasma. The patient's blood flow is 100 to 200 mL/min, and the dialysate flow ranges from 20 to 30 mL/kg per minute. The fluid removal rate varies depending on the particular CRRT method used and removal of solutes (urea, creatinine, and electrolytes), as listed in Table 26.9. The removed fluid is described as *ultrafiltrate*. In an ideal situation, the hydrostatic pressure exerted by a mean arterial pressure greater than 70 mm Hg would propel a continuous flow of blood through

BOX 26.7   Indications and Contraindications for Continuous Renal Replacement Therapy

Indications
- Need for large fluid volume removal in hemodynamically unstable patient
- Hypervolemic or edematous patients unresponsive to diuretic therapy
- Patients with multiple-organ dysfunction syndrome
- Ease of fluid management in patients requiring large daily fluid volume
- Replacement for oliguria
- Administration of total parenteral nutrition
- Contraindication to hemodialysis and peritoneal dialysis
- Inability to be anticoagulated

Contraindications
- Hematocrit greater than 45%
- Terminal illness

the hemofilter to remove fluid and solute. However, because many critically ill patients are hypotensive and cannot provide adequate flow through the hemofilter, an electric roller pump "milks" the tubing to augment flow. If large amounts of fluid are to be removed, IV replacement solutions are infused. Indications and contraindications for CRRT are listed in Box 26.7.

Controversy exists about when CRRT should be started, the optimal dialysis dose, which patients can derive the greatest benefit, and when CRRT should be discontinued. The debate over the optimal "dose" of dialysis is likely to continue because although clinical trials have not shown a difference in mortality between critically ill patients receiving intensive or nonintensive dialysis regimens,[61] the amount of dialysis in the research studies was greater than that normally achieved in clinical practice.[61] Therefore, the debate continues.

Because controlled removal and replacement of fluid is possible over many hours or days with CRRT, hemodynamic stability is maintained. This makes CRRT highly advantageous for use in hemodynamically unstable patients with multisystem problems. Several modes of CRRT are used in critical care units; a partial list follows:

1. Slow continuous ultrafiltration (SCUF)
2. Continuous venovenous hemofiltration (CVVH)
3. Continuous venovenous hemodialysis (CVVHD)
4. Continuous venovenous hemodiafiltration (CVVHDF)

The decision about which type of therapy to initiate is based on clinical assessment, metabolic status, severity of uremia, whether a particular treatment modality is available at that institution, and other factors.

TABLE 26.10 Size of Molecules Cleared by Continuous Renal Replacement Therapy

Type of Molecule	Size of Molecule	Solutes	Solute Removal Method
Small	<500 daltons	Urea, creatinine	Convection, diffusion
Middle	500–5000 daltons	Vancomycin	Convection better than diffusion
Low-molecular-weight (small) proteins	5000–50,000 daltons	Cytokines, complement	Convection or absorption onto hemofilter
Large proteins	>50,000 daltons	Albumin	Minimal removal

Continuous Renal Replacement Therapy Terminology

In CRRT, solutes are removed from the blood by *diffusion* or *convection*. Both processes remove fluid, and the two methods remove molecules of different sizes.

Diffusion. Diffusion describes the movement of solutes along a *concentration gradient* from a high concentration to a low concentration across a semipermeable membrane. This is the main mechanism used in hemodialysis. Solutes such as creatinine and urea cross the dialysis membrane from the blood to the dialysis fluid compartment.

Convection. Convection occurs when a pressure gradient is set up so that the water is pushed or pumped across the dialysis filter and carries the solutes from the bloodstream with it. This method of solute removal is known as *solvent drag,* and it is commonly employed in CRRT.

Absorption. The filter attracts solute, and molecules attach (adsorb) to the dialysis filter. The size of solute molecules is measured in *daltons.* The different sizes of molecules that can be removed by convection or diffusion methods are shown in Table 26.9. Tiny molecules such as urea and creatinine are removed by diffusion and convection (all methods). As the molecular size increases beyond 500 daltons, convection is the more efficient method (Table 26.10).

Ultrafiltrate volume. The fluid that is removed each hour is not called *urine;* it is known as *ultrafiltrate.*

Replacement fluid. Typically, some of the ultrafiltrate is replaced through the CRRT circuit by a sterile replacement fluid. The replacement fluid can be added before the filter (prefilter dilution) or after the filter (postfilter dilution).[61] The purpose is to increase the volume of fluid passing through the hemofilter and improve convection of solute.

Anticoagulation. Because the blood outside the body is in contact with artificial tubing and filters, the coagulation cascade and complement cascades are activated. To prevent the hemofilter from becoming obstructed by clotting, or clotting off, low-dose anticoagulation must be used.[61] The dose should be low enough to have no effect on the patient's anticoagulation parameters. Systemic anticoagulation is not the goal. Typical anticoagulant choices include unfractionated heparin and sodium citrate.[61] Citrate is an effective prefilter anticoagulant, which has the side effect that it *chelates* (binds to and removes) calcium from the blood. Consequently, ionized calcium levels are verified, and calcium is replaced per protocol when sodium citrate is the anticoagulant.

Modes of Continuous Renal Replacement

Because of the design of the CRRT machine, it is impossible to look at the outside and follow the flow of blood and, if used, dialysate. Each of the CRRT modes is described, and diagrams are employed to clarify the mode of CRRT that is used.

Slow continuous ultrafiltration. SCUF slowly removes fluid (100 to 300 mL/h) through a process of ultrafiltration (Fig. 26.8A). This consists of a movement of fluid across a semipermeable membrane. SCUF has minimal impact on solute removal. However, SCUF is an infrequent clinical choice because it requires both arterial and venous access for effective functioning, and the circuit is more likely to thrombose (clot off) than other CRRT methods that use higher flows. Because small amounts of fluid are gently removed, initially it was hoped that SCUF would be a suitable choice for edematous patients with acute heart failure and diminished perfusion to the kidneys that were unresponsive to diuretics. Currently, intermittent *ultrafiltration* using a peripheral venous catheter is more likely to be used to remove excess volume from patients with acute decompensated heart failure when the kidneys are unresponsive to diuretics.

Continuous venovenous hemofiltration. CVVH is indicated when the patient's clinical condition warrants removal of significant volumes of fluid and solutes. Fluid is removed by ultrafiltration in volumes of 5 to 20 mL/min or up to 7 to 30 L/24 h. Removal of solutes such as urea, creatinine, and other small non–protein-bound toxins is accomplished by convection. The replacement fluid rate of flow through the CRRT circuit can be altered to achieve desired fluid and solute removal without causing hemodynamic instability. Replacement fluid can be added via a prehemofilter replacement fluid (Fig. 26.8B) or posthemofilter replacement fluid.

As with other CRRT systems, the blood outside the body is anticoagulated, and the ultrafiltrate is drained off by gravity or by the addition of negative-pressure suction into a large drainage bag. Because large volumes of fluid may be removed in CVVH, some of the removed ultrafiltrate volume must be replaced hourly with a continuous infusion (replacement fluid) to avoid intravascular dehydration. Replacement fluids may consist of standard solutions of bicarbonate, potassium-free lactated Ringer solution, acetate, or dextrose. Electrolytes such as potassium, sodium, calcium chloride, magnesium sulfate, and sodium bicarbonate may be added. The formula used to calculate the volume removed from the patient follows along with an example:

$$\text{Ultrafiltrate in bag} + \text{Other output} - (\text{CWH replacement fluid} + \text{IV/oral/NG intake}) = \text{Output}$$
$$1000 \text{ mL} - 800 \text{ mL} = 200 \text{ mL/h output}$$

Continuous Venovenous Hemodialysis

CVVHD is technically similar to traditional hemodialysis, and it removes solute by diffusion because of a slow (15 to 30 mL/min) countercurrent drainage flow on the membrane side of the hemofilter (Fig. 26.8C). Blood and fluid move by countercurrent flow through the hemofilter. *Countercurrent* means the blood flows in one direction, and the dialysate flows in the opposite direction. As with other types of CRRT and hemodialysis, although arterial access is always possible, venovenous vascular access is the most common choice.

CVVHD is indicated for patients who require large-volume removal for severe uremia or critical acid–base imbalances or for patients who are resistant to diuretics. A mean arterial pressure of at least 70 mm Hg is desirable for effective volume removal and dialysis, and it is most effective when used over days, not hours. The use of replacement fluid is optional and depends on the patient's clinical condition and plan of care. The critical care nurse is responsible for calculating the hourly intake and output, identifying fluid trends, and replacing excessive losses. This therapy is ideal for hemodynamically unstable patients in the critical care setting because they do not experience the abrupt

fluid and solute changes that can accompany standard hemodialysis treatments.

Continuous venovenous hemodiafiltration. Another CRRT option is CVVHDF, which combines two of the previously described methods (CVVH and CVVHD) to achieve maximal fluid and solute removal. A strong transmembrane pressure is applied to the hemofilter to push water across the filter, and a negative pressure is applied at the other side to pull fluid across the membrane and produce large volumes of ultrafiltrate and

FIG. 26.8 Continuous Renal Replacement Therapy (CRRT) Systems. (A) Slow continuous ultrafiltration. (B) Continuous venovenous hemofiltration.

to create a "solvent drag" (CVVH method). The blood and the dialysate are circulated in a countercurrent flow pattern to remove fluid and solutes by diffusion (hemodialysis method). CVVHDF can remove large volumes of fluid and solute because it employs diffusion gradients and convection.

Complications

Potential problems associated with CRRT and appropriate nursing interventions are listed in Table 26.11. Complications are often related to the rate of flow through the system. If the patient becomes hypotensive or the access lines remain kinked, the ultrafiltration rate decreases. This can lead to increased clot formation within the hemofilter. As the surface of the hemofilter becomes more clotted, it does not provide effective fluid or solute clearance, and CRRT is stopped; a new CRRT circuit must then be set up. The most common reasons for interruption in CRRT are clotting and patient clinical issues.

FIG. 26.8, cont'd (C) Continuous venovenous hemofiltration dialysis. (D) Continuous venovenous hemodiafiltration.

The critical care nurse monitors the pressures displayed on the CRRT machine screen to monitor the positive pressure of fluid going into the hemofilter (inflow) and the pressures coming out of the hemofilter to ensure that resistance to the negative-pressure pull of the fluid across the hemofilter membrane has not developed. Other patient-related complications include fluid and electrolyte alterations, bleeding because of anticoagulation, or problems with the access site such as dislodgment or infection.

Medical Management

The choice of the method of blood purification to use to treat AKI is a medical decision. There is no clinical or research consensus about whether IHD or CRRT is the most beneficial, and no difference in outcomes has been shown in clinical research trials.[61,62] Age, sex, and preexisting chronic conditions are of little help in determining whether to select IHD or CRRT. Often the acute clinical diagnosis, physician's preference, availability of the CRRT machine, and knowledgeable nurses and physicians at the hospital are the deciding factors.

The current trend is to start IHD or CRRT earlier rather than later in the course of AKI, especially for hemodynamically unstable patients.[61-63] There is no definitive number at which renal replacement therapy is initiated. The threshold to begin treatment is based on an increasing serum creatinine and the patient's illness, especially organ failure. If the patient has severe electrolyte imbalance or fluid overload, even earlier intervention may be required.[63]

Nursing Management

Critical care nurses play a vital role in monitoring patients receiving CRRT. In many critical care units, the CRRT system is set up by the dialysis staff but is run on a 24-hour basis by

TABLE 26.11 Complications Associated With Continuous Renal Replacement Therapy

Problem	Cause	Clinical Manifestations	Nursing Management
Decreased ultrafiltration rate	Hypotension	Ultrafiltration rate decreased	Observe filter and arteriovenous system
	Dehydration	Minimal flow through blood lines	Control blood flow
	Kinked lines		Control coagulation time
	Bending of catheters		Position patient on back
	Clotting of filter		Lower height of collection container
Filter clotting	Obstruction	Ultrafiltration rate decreased, despite height of collection container being lower	Control anticoagulation (heparin/citrate)
	Insufficient heparinization		Maintain continuous system anticoagulation
			Call physician
			Remove system
			Prime catheters with anticoagulated solution
			Prime new system; connect it
			Start predilution with 1000 mL saline 0.9% solution/h
			Do not use three-way stopcocks
Hypotension	Increased ultrafiltration rate	Bleeding	Control amount of ultrafiltration
	Blood leak	Call physician	Control access sites
	Disconnection of one of lines		Clamp lines
Fluid and electrolyte changes	Too much or too little removal of fluid	Changes in mentation	Observe for
	Inappropriate replacement of electrolytes	↑ or ↓ CVP	Changes in CVP or PAOP
	Inappropriate dialysate	↑ or ↓ PAOP	Changes in vital signs
		ECG changes	ECG change resulting from electrolyte abnormalities
		↑ or ↓ BP and heart rate	Monitor output values every hour
		Abnormal electrolyte levels	Control ultrafiltration
Bleeding	System disconnection	Oozing from catheter insertion site or connection	Monitor ACT no less than once every hour (heparin)
	↑ Heparin dose		Adjust heparin dose within specifications to maintain ACT
			Monitor serum calcium if using citrate as an anticoagulant
			Observe dressing on vascular access for blood loss
			Observe for blood in filtrate (filter leak)
Access dislodgment or infection	Catheter or connections not secured	Bleeding from catheter site or connections	Observe access site at least once every 2 h
	Break in sterile technique	Inappropriate flow or infusion	Ensure that clamps are available within easy reach at all times
	Excessive patient movement	Fever	Observe strict sterile technique when dressing vascular access
		Drainage at catheter site	

ACT, activated coagulation time; *BP,* blood pressure; *CRRT,* continuous renal replacement therapy; *CVP,* central venous pressure; *ECG,* electrocardiogram; *PAOP,* pulmonary artery occlusion pressure; ↑, increased; ↓, decreased.

critical care nurses with additional training. Complications may be related to the CRRT circuit, the CRRT pump, or the patient (Box 26.8). The critical care nurse monitors fluid intake and output, prevents or detects potential complications (eg, bleeding, hypotension), identifies trends in electrolyte laboratory values, supervises safe operation of the CRRT equipment, and provides patient and family education about the patient's condition and the use of CRRT.

Peritoneal Dialysis

Peritoneal dialysis (PD) is a less "high-tech" modality used in patients with CKD.[64,65] When a PD-dependent patient is admitted to the critical care unit with a nonrenal acute illness, PD may be continued, but the patient is more often converted to hemodialysis or CRRT because of the critical illness. PD involves the introduction of sterile dialyzing fluid through an implanted catheter into the abdominal cavity. The dialysate bathes the peritoneal membrane, which covers the abdominal organs and overlies the capillary beds that support the organs. By the processes of osmosis, diffusion, and active transport, excess fluid and solutes travel from the peritoneal capillary fluid through the capillary walls, through the peritoneal membrane, and into the dialyzing fluid. After a selected period, the fluid is drained out of the abdomen by gravity (Fig. 26.9). The process is then repeated at regular, prescribed intervals. At home, patients generally have four peritoneal dialysate exchanges per day or use an automated PD exchange overnight when sleeping.[64,65]

The structure of the peritoneal membrane and capillary blood flow to the peritoneum account for the relatively slow nature of PD. The small capillary pores, the capillary membrane, the interstitium, the mesothelium of the peritoneum, and the fluid film layers in the capillary and the peritoneal cavity provide formidable barriers to fluid and solute passage. The volume of dialysate instilled into the abdomen affects the clearance. Normally, PD-dependent patients are well versed in the amount, type, and frequency of dialysate to be infused into the abdomen, with subsequent drainage by gravity into a waste bag. The primary nursing consideration is to avoid contamination of the access point and monitor the patient's vital signs during this process. The dialysate should be instilled at body temperature to be comfortable, provide some vasodilation, and provide increased solute transport in the peritoneum. The length of time the solution remains in the peritoneal cavity, called the *dwell time*, and the solution composition affect the outcome. The dwell time affects the amount of fluid removed from the peritoneal capillaries, although a longer dwell time does not remove proportionately more fluid because of osmotic equilibration across the membranes. The various glucose concentrations of the dialysate provide different rates of fluid removal.[64,65]

Catheter Placement

Most catheters have four segments: an external segment outside the abdomen, a tunnel segment that passes through subcutaneous tissue and muscle, a cuff for stabilization at the peritoneal membrane, and an internal segment with numerous holes for fast delivery and drainage of dialysate (Fig. 26.9). The infusion and removal of the dialysate fluid are sterile procedures.

Infection

The most significant infection risk to the patient with the use of PD is development of peritonitis and sepsis from catheter contamination. Serious infection is also a reason for admitting a patient who uses PD to the hospital.[64,65] Clinicians must remain vigilant for signs of localized catheter or abdominal infection manifested by catheter site redness, site swelling, cloudy dialysis effluent after the dwell time, and abdominal tenderness or pain. Assessment for signs and symptoms of systemic infection, such as a sudden increase in the white blood cell count, increased temperature, and malaise, is also required.

Nursing Management

Nursing management of a patient receiving PD is complex. Nurses are vigilant about prevention and detection of complications related to PD (Table 26.12). The critical care nurse observes for signs and symptoms of infection, monitors fluid volume status, infuses the dialysate fluid, observes drainage of the ultrafiltrate fluid, prevents complications associated with the PD catheter, and provides patient and family education. Patients who use PD are knowledgeable partners in the maintenance of their health because of the huge commitment they make in daily management of their PD care.[64-66]

BOX 26.8   Complications of Continuous Renal Replacement Therapy

Circuit
- Air embolism
- Clotted hemofilter
- Poor ultrafiltration
- Blood leaks
- Broken filter
- Recirculation or disconnection
- Access failure
- Catheter dislodgment

Pump
- Circuit pressure alarm
- Decreased inflow pressure
- Decreased outflow pressure
- Increased outflow resistance
- Air bubble detector alarm
- Power failure
- Mechanical dysfunction

Patient
- Code or emergency situation
- Dehydration
- Hypotension
- Electrolyte imbalances
- Acid–base imbalances
- Blood loss or hemorrhage
- Hypothermia
- Infection

FIG. 26.9 Peritoneal Dialysis. (A) Inflow. (B) Outflow (drains by gravity). (From Thompson JM, et al. *Mosby's Clinical Nursing.* 5th ed. St. Louis: Mosby; 2002.)

TABLE 26.12 Complications Associated With Peritoneal Dialysis

Complication	Nursing Management	Complication	Nursing Management
Peritonitis	Assess for signs and symptoms: cloudy effluent, abdominal pain, rebound tenderness, nausea and vomiting, fever. Obtain effluent sample for culture. Administer antibiotics as ordered. Teach patient and family about signs and symptoms and prevention.	Rectal pain	Ensure a sufficient reservoir of fluid. Use a slow infusion rate.
		Shoulder pain	Ensure that all air is primed from infusion tubing. Attempt draining effluent with the patient in a knee-chest position. Administer mild analgesics as ordered.
Exit site infection	Monitor site daily for signs and symptoms of infection: induration, erythema, purulence, hyperthermia. Increase daily cleaning of site. Apply topical antibiotics as ordered (controversial). Teach patient and family to avoid creams and lotions around exit site.	Hernia	Monitor for increase in size of or pain in the area of the hernia. Dialyze with patient in the supine position. Use abdominal binder or support for the hernia (as long as not binding on catheter exit site).
Catheter tunnel infection	Assess for signs and symptoms of infection: pain along tunnel, induration for several centimeters away from catheter, erythema leading away from exit site, drainage at exit site or as tunnel is "milked" toward exit site. Teach patient and family about signs and symptoms of infection. Teach patient and family to avoid pulling on PD catheter to avoid trauma to exit site. Emphasize need to maintain the cleansing regimen at exit site.	Fluid overload	Increase use of hypertonic solutions. Decrease oral fluid intake. Shorten dwell times. Weigh patients daily and before and after PD. Monitor lung sounds and peripheral edema.
		Dehydration	Assess patients for decreased skin turgor, muscle cramps, hypotension, tachycardia, and dizziness. Discontinue hypertonic solutions. Increase oral fluid intake. Lengthen dwell times.
Fluid obstruction	Change position of the patient (standing, lying, side-lying, knee-chest). Relieve the patient's constipation. Irrigate the catheter. Ensure that sufficient fluid is in the abdomen (sometimes requires a residual reservoir of approximately 50 mL).	Blood-tinged effluent	Monitor for change in effluent color (clear yellow to pink or rust). Administer heparin, as ordered, to prevent fibrin formation. Obtain a patient history about catheter trauma and patient activity before appearance of complication.

PD, peritoneal dialysis.

CASE STUDY 26.1   Patient With a Kidney Problem

Brief Patient History

Ms. L is a 32-year-old woman who is found in the street near the hospital. She is awake but confused. She is unable to give any medical history and has no idea how long she has been in the street.

Clinical Assessment

Ms. L is admitted to the critical care unit with muscle pain and minimal dark urine output. She continues to be confused, but her neurologic examination results are otherwise normal. She repeatedly tells the nurses that she is tired, has pain everywhere, and just wants to sleep. She is able to move all her extremities and has no signs of injury on skin examination.

Diagnostic Procedures

Laboratory tests show the following results: creatinine phosphokinase level of 40,400 units/L, serum myoglobin level of 2.5 mg/L, urinary myoglobin level of 300 mg/L, and serum potassium level of 4.8 mEq/dL. Baseline vital signs are as follows: blood pressure of 85/60 mm Hg, heart rate of 128 beats/min (sinus tachycardia), respiratory rate of 18 breaths/min, temperature of 101.3°F, and oxygen saturation of 98%.

The toxicology screen shows that the patient tested positive for cocaine. The Glasgow Coma Scale score is 14.

Medical Diagnosis

Ms. L is diagnosed with rhabdomyolysis.

Questions

1. What major outcomes do you expect to achieve for this patient?
2. What problems or risks must be managed to achieve these outcomes?
3. What interventions must be initiated to monitor, prevent, manage, or eliminate the problems and risks identified?
4. What interventions should be initiated to promote optimal functioning, safety, and well-being of the patient?
5. What possible learning needs do you anticipate for this patient?
6. What cultural and age-related factors may have a bearing on the patient's plan of care?

QSEN BOX 26.9   QSEN: Informatics

Internet Resources

National Kidney Foundation: https://www.kidney.org
National Kidney Foundation: Professional Resources:
    https://www.kidney.org/professionals/links
National Kidney Foundation: Patient and Family Resources:
    https://www.kidney.org/patients/resources

SUMMARY

Acute Kidney Injury

- Risk factors for development of AKI include sepsis, cardiac surgery, and diabetes.
- Many critically ill patients have AKI as a complication of their illness. The initial reason for admission to the critical care unit might have been sepsis, hypovolemic shock, trauma, or major surgery. If AKI develops, mortality and morbidity rates increase.
- Vigorous hydration with normal saline is the most effective intervention to prevent CIN and AKI.

Catheter-Associated Urinary Tract Infection

- CAUTI is a significant risk in critical illness. Prevention strategies include avoiding unnecessary use of urinary catheters; insertion of urinary catheters using aseptic technique; adoption of evidence-based standards for maintenance of urinary catheters; and daily clinical review of the need for the urinary catheter and, if not needed, prompt removal.

Diuretics and Renal Replacement Therapies

- Diuretics increase urine output but do not protect against the development of kidney failure. Diuretics are categorized into different groups based on their pharmacology and site of action in the nephron. The most frequently used diuretics are loop diuretics, thiazide diuretics, and osmotic diuretics. Two diuretics from different classes can act synergistically to increase urine output when the pharmacologic action of each diuretic is on a different part of the nephron.
- Acute care renal replacement therapies include IHD and CRRT. Both are valuable in acute kidney failure, and one method is not superior to the other in terms of mortality outcomes or recovery of kidney function.
- PD is a home-based method of dialysis. If a patient with PD is admitted to the hospital with a noncritical illness unrelated to the abdominal cavity, the patient may continue the PD regimen. However, this modality is not suitable for patients with critical illness. The biggest risk faction is peritoneal infection and sepsis.

ⓔ Visit the Evolve site for additional study materials.

REFERENCES

1. Bellomo R. Acute renal failure. *Semin Respir Crit Care Med.* 2011;32(5):639.
2. Singbartl K, Kellum JA. AKI in the ICU: Definition, epidemiology, risk stratification, and outcomes. *Kidney Int.* 2012;81(9):819.
3. Hoste EAJ, et al. Epidemiology of acute kidney injury in critically ill patients—the multinational AKI-EPI study. *Intensive Care Med.* 2015;41(8):1411.
4. Prowle JR, et al. Oliguria as predictive biomarker of acute kidney injury in critically ill patients. *Crit Care.* 2011;15(4):R172.
5. Macedo E, et al. Defining urine output criterion for acute kidney injury in critically ill patients. *Nephrol Dial Transplant.* 2011;26(2):509.
6. Morley JE. Dehydration hypernatremia and hyponatremia. *Clin Geriatr Med.* 2015;31:389.
7. Endre ZH, Pickering JW, Walker RJ. Clearance and beyond: the complementary roles of GFR measurement and injury biomarkers in acute kidney injury (AKI). *Am J Physiol Renal Physiol.* 2011;301(4):F697.
8. National Kidney and Urologic Diseases Information Clearinghouse (NKUDIC). http://kidney.niddk.nih.gov/kudiseases/pubs/kustats/. Accessed March 23, 2016.
9. Hoerger TJ, et al. The future burden of CKD in the United States: A simulation model for the CDC CKD Initiative. *Am J Kidney Dis.* 2015;65(3):403.
10. Grams ME, et al. Lifetime incidence of CKD stages 3-5 in the United States. *Am J Kidney Dis.* 2013;62(2):245.
11. Jentzer JC, Chawla LS. A clinical approach to the acute cardiorenal syndrome. *Crit Care Clin.* 2015;31:685.
12. Ronco C, et al. Cardio-renal syndromes: Report from the consensus conference of the acute dialysis quality initiative. *Eur Heart J.* 2010;31(6):703.
13. Vieira Jr JM, et al. Effect of acute kidney injury on weaning from mechanical ventilation in critically ill patients. *Crit Care Med.* 2007;35(1):184.
14. Pan SW, et al. Acute kidney injury on ventilator initiation day independently predicts prolonged mechanical ventilation in intensive care unit patients. *J Crit Care.* 2011;26(6):586.

15. Navaneethan SD, et al. Mortality outcomes of patients with chronic kidney disease and chronic obstructive pulmonary disease. *Am J Nephrol.* 2016;43:39.

16. Singer M, et al. The third international consensus definitions for sepsis and septic shock. *JAMA.* 2016;315(8):801.

17. Shankar-Hari M, et al. Developing a new definition and assessing new clinical criteria for septic shock: for the Third International Consensus Definitions for Sepsis and Septic Shock (Sepsis-3). *JAMA.* 2016;315(8):775.

18. Bagshaw SM, et al. A multi-center evaluation of early acute kidney injury in critically ill trauma patients. *Ren Fail.* 2008;30(6):581.

19. Delaney KA, Givens ML, Vohra RB. Use of RIFLE criteria to predict the severity and prognosis of acute kidney injury in emergency department patients with rhabdomyolysis. *J Emerg Med.* 2012;42(5):521.

20. Shapiro ML, Baldea A, Luchette FA. Rhabdomyolysis in the intensive care unit. *J Intensive Care Med.* 2011;27(6):335.

21. Parekh R, Care DA, Tainter CR. Rhabdomyolysis: Advances in diagnosis and treatment. *Emerg Med Pract.* 2012;14(3):1.

22. Weisbord SD, Palevsky PM. Contrast associated acute kidney injury. *Crit Care Clin.* 2015;31:725.

23. Stacul F, et al. Contrast induced nephropathy: Updated ESUR Contrast Media Safety Committee guidelines. *Eur Radiol.* 2011;21(12):2527.

24. Isaac S. Contrast-induced nephropathy: nursing implications. *Crit Care Nurse.* 2012;32(3):41.

25. Hartley SE, Valley SC. Prevention of catheter-associated urinary tract infections in the hospital. *Hosp Med Clin.* 2015:258.

26. Institute for Healthcare Improvement. Getting started kit: prevent catheter-associated urinary tract infections how-to guide. http://www.bestcare.org.za/file/view/CAUTI-IHI-howtoguide.pdf. Accessed March 16, 2016.

27. Urinary tract infection (catheter-associated urinary tract infection [CAUTI] and non-catheter-associated urinary tract infection [UTI]) and other urinary system infection [USI]) events 2016. http://www.cdc.gov/n-hsn/pdfs/pscmanual/7psccautincurrent.pdf. Accessed March 16, 2016.

28. Burton DC, et al. Trends in catheter-associated urinary tract infections in adult intensive care units—United States, 1990-2007. *Infect Control Hosp Epidemiol.* 2011;32(8):748.

29. Chant C, et al. Relationship of catheter-associated urinary tract infection to mortality and length of stay in critically ill patients: a systematic review and meta-analysis of observational studies. *Crit Care Med.* 2011;39(5):1167.

30. The Joint Commission. National Patient Safety Goals 2016. https://www.jointcommission.org/assets/1/6/2016_NPSG_HAP.pdf. Accessed September 11, 2016.

31. Rosenthal VD, et al. International Nosocomial Infection Control Consortium (INICC) report, data summary of 36 countries, for 2004-2009. *Am J Infect Control.* 2012;40(5):396.

32. Conway LJ, et al. Adoption of policies to prevent catheter-associated urinary tract infections in United States intensive care units. *Am J Infect Control.* 2012;40(8):705.

33. Saint S, et al. Introducing a catheter-associated urinary tract infection (CAUTI) prevention guide to patient safety (GPS). *Am J Infect Control.* 2014;42:584.

34. Gould C. Catheter-associated urinary tract infection (CAUTI) toolkit. http://www.cdc.gov/HAI/pdfs/toolkits/CAUTItoolkit_3_10.pdf. Accessed March 16, 2016.

35. Davison DL, Patel K, Chawla LS. Hemodynamic monitoring in the critically ill: Spanning the range of kidney function. *Am J Kidney Dis.* 2012;59(5):715.

36. McDonald TJ. Investigating hyperkalemia in adults. *BMJ.* 2015;351: h4762.

37. Sterns RH, et al. Treatment of hyperkalemia: something old, something new. *Kidney Int.* 2016;89:546.

38. McCullough PA. Acute and chronic cardiovascular effects of hyperkalemia: New insights into prevention and clinical management. *Rev Cardiovasc Med.* 2014;15(1):11.

39. Kovesdy CP, et al. Hyponatremia, hypernatremia, and mortality in patients with chronic kidney disease with and without congestive heart failure. *Circulation.* 2012;125(5):677.

40. Hutchison AJ, Smith CP, Brenchley PE. Pharmacology, efficacy and safety of oral phosphate binders. *Nat Rev Nephrol.* 2011;7(10):578.

41. Molony DA, Stephens BW. Derangements in phosphate metabolism in chronic kidney diseases/endstage renal disease: Therapeutic considerations. *Adv Chronic Kidney Dis.* 2011;18(2):120.

42. Gutekunst H. An update on phosphate binders—a dietitian's perspective. *J Ren Nutr.* 2016;26(4): 209.

43. Aberegget SK. Ionized calcium in the ICU: should it be measured and corrected? *Chest.* 2016;149(3):846.

44. Kalantar-Zadeh K, et al. Understanding sources of dietary phosphorus in the treatment of patients with chronic kidney disease. *Clin J Am Soc Nephrol.* 2010;5(3):519.

45. Finfer S, et al. A comparison of albumin and saline for fluid resuscitation in the intensive care unit. *N Engl J Med.* 2004;350(22):2247.

46. SAFE Study Investigators, et al. Saline or albumin for fluid resuscitation in patients with traumatic brain injury. *N Engl J Med.* 2007;357(9):874.

47. Perel P, Roberts I. Colloids versus crystalloids for fluid resuscitation in critically ill patients. *Cochrane Database Syst Rev.* 2007;(4): CD000567.

48. Nigwekar SU, Waikar SS. Diuretics in acute kidney injury. *Semin Nephrol.* 2011;31(6):523.

49. Wile D. Diuretics: a review. *Ann Clin Biochem.* 2012;49(5):419.

50. Felker GM. Loop diuretics in heart failure. *Heart Fail Rev.* 2012;17(2):305.

51. Asare K. Management of loop diuretic resistance in the intensive care unit. *Am J Health Syst Pharm.* 2009;66(18):1635.

52. Kassamali R, Sica DA. Acetazolamide: a forgotten diuretic agent. *Cardiol Rev.* 2011;19(6):276.

53. Lehrich RW, Greenberg A. Hyponatremia and the use of vasopressin receptor antagonists in critically ill patients. *J Intensive Care Med.* 2012;27(4):207.

54. Giamouzis G, et al. Impact of dopamine infusion on renal function in hospitalized heart failure patients: results of the Dopamine in Acute Decompensated Heart Failure (DAD-HF) Trial. *J Card Fail.* 2010;16(12):922.

55. McCarthy MS, Phipps SC. Special nutrition challenges—current approach to acute kidney injury. *Nutr Clin Pract.* 2014;29(1):56.

56. Gervasio JM, Garmon WP, Holowatyj M. Nutrition support in acute kidney injury. *Nutr Clin Pract.* 2011;26(4):374.

57. Ramanath V, et al. Anemia and chronic kidney disease: Making sense of the recent trials. *Rev Recent Clin Trials.* 2012;7(3):187.

58. Cody JD, Hodson EM. Recombinant human erythropoietin versus placebo or no treatment for the anaemia of chronic kidney disease in people not requiring dialysis. *Cochrane Database Syst Rev.* 2016;(1):CD003266.

59. Oudemans-van Straaten HM, Kellum JA, Bellomo R. Clinical review: Anticoagulation for continuous renal replacement therapy—heparin or citrate? *Crit Care.* 2011;15(1):202.

60. Kimball TA, et al. Efficiency of the kidney disease outcomes quality initiative guidelines for preemptive vascular access in an academic setting. *J Vasc Surg.* 2011;54(3):760.

61. Ronco C, et al. Renal replacement therapy in acute kidney injury: controversy and consensus. *Crit Care.* 2015;19:146.

62. Villa G, et al. Renal replacement therapy. *Crit Care Clin.* 2015;31:839.

63. Palevsky P. Renal replacement therapy in acute kidney injury. *Adv Chronic Kidney Dis.* 2013;20(1):236.

64. Catley C. Use if peritoneal dialysis in kidney disease. *Nursing Times.* 2015;48:12–14.

65. Catley C. Peritoneal dialysis: a guide for non-renal nurses. *Nursing Times.* 2015;49/50:18–19.

66. Schaepe C, Bergjan M. Educational interventions in peritoneal dialysis—a narrative review of the literature. *Int J Nurs Stud.* 2015;52(4):882.

27

Gastrointestinal Anatomy and Physiology

Kathleen M. Stacy

The major function of the gastrointestinal (GI) tract is digestion, which is the conversion of ingested nutrients into simpler forms that can be transported from the lumen of the GI tract to the portal circulation and then used in metabolic processes. The GI system also plays a vital role in the detoxification and elimination of bacteria, viruses, chemical toxins, and drugs. Disturbances of the GI system itself or of the complex hormonal and neural controls that regulate the GI tract can severely upset homeostasis and compromise the overall nutritional status of the patient. Any circumvention of the normal feeding mechanism can alter digestive processes or contribute to malabsorption.

A critical care nurse must have a comprehensive knowledge of the anatomy and normal function of the GI tract to facilitate assessment, diagnosis, and intervention in patients with GI dysfunction. The GI tract consists of the mouth, esophagus, stomach, small intestine, and large intestine (Fig. 27.1).

MOUTH

The mouth and accessory organs, which include the lips, cheeks, gums, tongue, palate, and salivary glands, perform the initial phases of digestion, which are ingestion, mastication, and salivation.[1]

Ingestion and Mastication

The mouth is the beginning of the alimentary canal (see Fig. 27.1) and is the means for ingestion and entry of nutrients. The teeth cut, grind, and mix food, transforming it into a form suitable for swallowing and increasing the surface area of food available to mix with salivary secretions. Healthy dentition is vital for this process. Mucous glands located behind the tip of the tongue and serous glands located at the back of the tongue aid in the lubrication of food and in its distribution over the taste buds.[2]

Salivation

Salivation has an important role in the first stage of digestion because saliva lubricates the mouth, facilitates the movement of the lips and the tongue during swallowing, and washes away bacteria. Saliva consists of approximately 99.5% water,[3] which contains a large amount of ions such as potassium, chloride, bicarbonate,[1] thiocyanate, and hydrogen[3]; immunoglobulin

A, which is vital for destroying oral bacteria[1]; and mucus. Approximately 1000 to 1500 mL of saliva is produced each day by three pairs of major salivary glands: (1) the submandibular glands, (2) the sublingual glands, and (3) the parotid glands. Parotid gland secretions are enzymatic, containing amylase (ptyalin), which begins the chemical breakdown of large polysaccharides into dextrins and sugars. The mouth and pharynx also are lined with minor salivary glands that provide additional lubrication.[3]

The salivary glands are regulated by the autonomic nervous system, with parasympathetic effects being predominant. Increased parasympathetic stimulation results in profuse secretions of watery saliva, whereas decreased parasympathetic stimulation results in inhibition of salivation.[1,3]

ESOPHAGUS

The esophagus is a hollow muscular tube that lacks cartilage. In adults, the esophagus is 23 to 25 cm (9 to 10 inches) long and 2 to 3 cm (1 inch) wide. The esophagus is the narrowest part of the digestive tube and lies posterior to the trachea and the heart, with attachments at the hypopharynx and at the cardiac portion of the stomach below the diaphragm. The esophagus begins at the level of the C6 to T1 vertebrae and extends vertically through the mediastinum and diaphragm to the level of T11.[4]

The esophagus has two sphincters: (1) the upper esophageal sphincter (also known as *hypopharyngeal sphincter*) and (2) the lower esophageal sphincter (also known as *cardioesophageal* or *gastroesophageal sphincter*).[4] The upper esophageal sphincter inhibits air from entering the esophagus during respiration. The lower esophageal sphincter controls the passage of food into the stomach and prevents reflux of gastric contents.[1]

Swallowing

The functions of the esophagus are to accept a bolus of food from the oropharynx, transport the bolus through the esophageal body by gravity and peristalsis, and release the bolus into the stomach through the lower esophageal sphincter. This process is known as *swallowing*.[5] Peristalsis consists of waves of circular muscle contractions and relaxations. Peristalsis that is initiated by swallowing is known as *primary peristalsis*, whereas peristalsis that is initiated by esophageal distention is known as

657

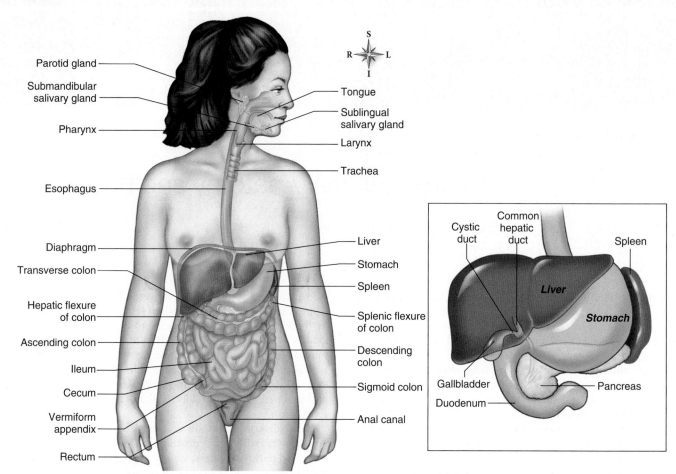

FIG. 27.1 Gastrointestinal System. Overall anatomy of the gastrointestinal system. (From Patton KT, Thibodeau GA. *Anatomy and Physiology.* 8th ed. St. Louis; Elsevier; 2013.)

secondary peristalsis. Peristaltic waves begin in the pharynx and move distally at a rate of 2 to 6 cm/s.[1]

STOMACH

The stomach is an elongated pouch that is approximately 25 to 30 cm (10 to 12 inches) long and 10 to 15 cm (4 to 6 inches) wide at the maximal transverse diameter (Fig. 27.2). The stomach lies obliquely beneath the cardiac sphincter at the esophagogastric junction and above the pyloric sphincter, next to the small intestine. The anatomic divisions of the stomach are the cardia (proximal end), the fundus (portion above and to the left of the cardiac sphincter), the body (middle portion), the antrum (elongated, constricted portion), and the pylorus (distal end connecting the antrum to the duodenum) (Fig. 27.3). The greater curvature, which begins at the cardiac orifice and arches backward and upward around the fundus, is in contact with the transverse colon and the pancreas at the posterior edge. The lesser curvature extends from the cardia to the pylorus. Two sphincters control the rate of food passage: (1) the lower esophageal sphincter at the esophagogastric junction and (2) the pyloric sphincter at the gastroduodenal junction.[6]

The stomach wall has four layers (Fig. 27.4). The outermost layer, the *serous layer (serosa)*, consists of squamous epithelial tissue and continues as a double fold from the lower edge of the stomach to cover the intestine. The second layer, the *muscular layer (muscularis)*, extends from the fundus to the antrum

and consists of three smooth muscle layers: the longitudinal layer, the circular layer, and the oblique layer. The third layer, the *submucous layer (submucosa)*, consists of connective tissue that contains blood vessels, lymphatics, and nerve plexuses. The innermost layer, the *mucous layer (mucosa)*, consists of a muscular layer that is arranged in longitudinal folds, or rugae, that can expand as the stomach fills.[6] This layer also contains glands that secrete approximately 1500 mL/day of gastric juice.[7]

The celiac artery provides the blood supply required for the motor and secretory activities of the stomach. The splenic vein provides venous drainage for the right side of the stomach, and the gastric vein provides venous drainage for the left side.[1] Numerous lymphatic channels arise in the submucosa and terminate in the thoracic duct. The stomach is innervated by the autonomic nervous system. Sympathetic fibers arise from the celiac plexus, and parasympathetic fibers arise from the gastric branch of the vagus nerve.[6]

The epithelial cells of the gastric mucosa are packed very close together and serve as a protective barrier, preventing diffusion of hydrogen ions into the mucosa. The surface epithelial cells produce alkaline mucus and secrete a bicarbonate-laden fluid. The mucus further protects the gastric mucosa by delaying back diffusion of hydrogen ions and trapping them for neutralization by the secreted bicarbonate.[7] The gastric mucosal cells can compensate for cell destruction. Epithelial cells are in a constant state of growth, migration, and desquamation, and they are shed at a rate of 0.5 million cells/min. The gastric mucosa also has the

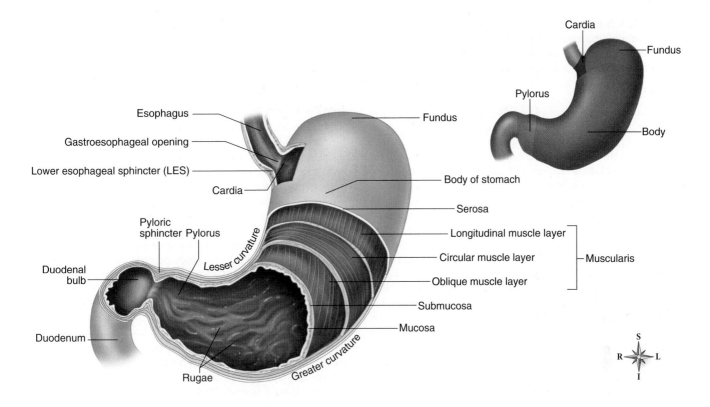

FIG. 27.2 Stomach. The gross anatomy of the stomach. (From Patton KT, Thibodeau GA. *Anatomy and Physiology.* 8th ed. St. Louis; Elsevier; 2013.)

FIG. 27.3 Endoscopic View of the Stomach. (From Soybel DI. Anatomy and physiology of the stomach. *Surg Clin North Am.* 2005;85(5):875–894.)

FIG. 27.4 Gastric Mucosa. The structure of the gastric mucosa. (From Patton KT, Thibodeau GA. *Anatomy and Physiology.* 8th ed. St. Louis; Elsevier; 2013.)

ability to increase blood flow, providing an additional buffer for acid neutralization and aiding in the removal of toxic metabolites and chloride ions from injured mucosa. The gastric mucosal cells synthesize a family of unsaturated fatty acids known as *prostaglandins*. Prostaglandins facilitate mucosal bicarbonate secretion and inhibit acid secretion by preventing the activation of parietal cells by histamine (a local biochemical mediator). Certain lipid-soluble substances such as alcohol, aspirin and other non-steroidal antiinflammatory drugs, regurgitated bile, and uremic toxins can break through the mucosal barrier and penetrate the cells, causing their destruction, edema, and eventual bleeding.[7]

Gastric Secretion

The stomach has two types of glands—*oxyntic* (also known as *gastric glands*), and *pyloric*—that contain cells of various types that secrete 1500 to 2400 mL/day of gastric juice into the lumen, depending on the diet and other stimuli.[7] Gastric juice is composed of hydrochloric acid, pepsin (necessary for the breakdown of protein), mucus, intrinsic factor (necessary for vitamin B_{12} absorption), sodium, and potassium. Pepsinogen, secreted by the chief cells of the stomach lining, is converted to its active form, pepsin, in the acidic environment of the stomach.[1] The cardiac glands secrete mucus and pepsinogen. The oxyntic glands contain parietal cells, which secrete hydrochloric acid and intrinsic factor, and chief cells, which secrete pepsinogen. Pyloric glands contain mucous cells, which secrete mucus and pepsinogen, and G cells, which secrete gastrin (Table 27.1).[6] Gastric glands are stimulated by the parasympathetic stimulation and gastrin and inhibited by gastric inhibitory peptide and enterogastrone. Histamine and entero-oxyntin also stimulate the parietal cells to produce acid, and secretin stimulates the chief cells to produce pepsinogen.[1]

The pH of gastric juice is 1.0, but when mixed with food, the pH rises to 2.0 to 3.0. Gastric juice dissolves soluble foods and has bacteriostatic action against swallowed microorganisms. The composition of gastric secretions depends on a variety of factors, including flow rate, volume, and the time of day. Pain, fear, or rage can inhibit gastric secretion, whereas aggression or hostility can stimulate gastric secretion.[1]

Gastric Motility

The functions of the stomach include food storage, digestion, and emptying. The stomach receives food through the lower esophageal sphincter, stores it for a period, and then mixes the food with gastric secretions. The food is then ground into a semifluid consistency called *chyme*, which is delivered through the pylorus to the duodenum. Gastric motility is regulated by the autonomic nervous system, digestive hormones, and neural reflexes. Gastrin, motilin (see Table 27.1), and parasympathetic stimulation increase gastric motility, whereas secretin, cholecystokinin, enterogastrone, gastric inhibitory peptide (see Table 27.1), and sympathetic stimulation decrease gastric motility. The ileogastric reflex inhibits gastric motility when the ileum is distended.[8]

SMALL INTESTINE

The small intestine, a coiled, folded tube that is approximately 7 m (22 to 23 feet) long, extends from the pyloric sphincter to the cecum and fills most of the abdominal cavity. The small intestine has three anatomic divisions: (1) the duodenum, (2) the

---

TABLE 27.1   Digestive Hormones[a]

Source	Hormone	Stimulus for Secretion	Action
Mucosa of stomach	Gastrin	Presence of partially digested proteins in stomach	Stimulates gastric glands to secrete hydrochloric acid and pepsinogen; growth of gastric mucosa; promotes gastric motility
	Histamine	Acid in stomach	Stimulates acid secretion
	Somatostatin	Acid in stomach	Inhibits acid and pepsinogen secretion and release of gastrin
	Acetylcholine	Vagus and local nerves in stomach	Stimulates release of pepsinogen and acid secretion
	Gastrin-releasing peptide (bombesin)	Vagus and local nerves in stomach	Stimulates gastrin and release of pepsinogen and acid secretion
Mucosa of small intestines	Motilin	Presence of acid and fat in duodenum	Increases GI motility
	Secretion	Presence of chyme (acid, partially digested proteins, and fats) in duodenum	Stimulates pancreas to secrete alkaline pancreatic juice and liver to secrete bile; decreases GI motility; inhibits gastrin and gastric acid secretion
	Cholecystokinin	Presence of chyme (acid, partially digested proteins, and fats) in duodenum	Stimulates gallbladder to eject bile and pancreas to secrete alkaline fluid; decreases gastric motility; constricts pyloric sphincter; inhibits gastrin; delays gastric emptying
	Enteroglucagon	Intraluminal fats and carbohydrates	Weakly inhibits gastric and pancreatic secretion and enhances insulin release, lipolysis, ketogenesis, and glycogenolysis; delays gastric emptying
	Gastric inhibitory peptide	Fat and glucose in small intestine	Inhibits gastric secretion and gastric emptying; stimulates insulin release
	Peptide YY	Intraluminal fat and bile acids	Inhibits postprandial gastric acid and pancreatic secretion; delays gastric and small bowel emptying
	Pancreatic polypeptide	Protein, fat, and glucose in small intestine	Decreases pancreatic bicarbonate
	Vasoactive intestinal peptide	Intestinal mucosa and muscle	Relaxes intestinal smooth muscle; increases blood flow

[a]The digestive hormones are not secreted into the GI lumen but rather into the bloodstream, in which they travel to target tissues. There are >30 peptide hormone genes expressed in the GI tract and >100 hormonally active peptides.
GI, gastrointestinal.
Modified from Johnson LR. *Gastrointestinal Physiology.* 7th ed. St. Louis: Mosby; 2007. Data from Schubert ML, Peura DA. Control of gastric acid secretion in health and disease. *Gastroenterology.* 2008;134(7):1842–1860; and Wren AM, Bloom SR. Gut hormones and appetite control. *Gastroenterology.* 2007;132(6):2116–2130.

jejunum, and (3) the ileum. The duodenum, shaped like the letter "C," begins at the pyloric sphincter of the stomach and ends at the ligament of Treitz. The duodenum is 30 cm (12 inches) long and 4 cm (1 to 1.5 inches) wide.[9] The jejunum, which is 250 cm (8 to 9 feet) long and 4 cm (1 to 1.5 inches) wide, lies in the left iliac and umbilical regions. The ileum, which is 375 cm (12 feet) long and 2.5 cm (1 inch) wide, lies in the hypogastric, right iliac, and pelvic regions. Although the demarcating line between the jejunum and the ileum is arbitrary, the ileum is narrower than the jejunum. The ileocecal valve, located at the terminal end of the ileum at the junction of the cecum and colon, controls the flow of small bowel contents into the large intestine and prevents reflux (Fig. 27.5).[1]

The small intestine has four layers (Fig. 27.6). The outermost layer, the *serous layer (serosa)*, is a continuation of the serous coat surrounding the stomach. The second layer, the *muscular layer (muscularis)*, consists of two smooth muscle layers called the *longitudinal* and *circular layers*. The third layer, the *submucous layer (submucosa)*, consists of connective tissue that contains blood vessels, lymphatics, glands, and nerve plexuses. The innermost layer, the *mucous layer (mucosa)*, consists of simple columnar epithelium.[5] The mucosa and submucosa are arranged in circular folds (plicae circulares),[5] which are largest and most numerous in the jejunum and upper ileum.[1] These folds are covered by a second series of projectile-like folds called *villi*, which are in constant motion—constricting, lengthening,

and shortening (villous movement). The 4 to 5 million villi (see Fig. 27.5) give the intestine a velvety appearance; they are more numerous and larger in the jejunum than in the ileum. Villi contain a network of capillaries and blind lymphatic vessels called *lacteals*. The outer layer of the villus is composed of microvilli. The circular folds of the small intestine, along with the villi and microvilli, increase the digestive-absorptive surface of the small intestine 600 times.[9,10]

The gastroduodenal artery provides the blood supply for the duodenum, and branches of the superior mesenteric artery provide for the jejunum and the ileum. The superior mesenteric vein provides for venous drainage of the small intestine.[11] Numerous lymphatic channels arise in the submucosa and terminate in the thoracic duct. The small intestine is extrinsically innervated by the autonomic nervous system. Sympathetic fibers arise from the celiac plexus, whereas parasympathetic fibers arise from the gastric branch of the vagus nerve. Intrinsic innervation, which initiates motor functions, is provided by Auerbach plexus and Meissner plexus, which are located in the intestinal wall.[1]

Intestinal Secretion

The small intestine has two major types of glands: (1) Brunner glands and (2) intestinal glands. Brunner glands lie in the mucosa of the duodenum and secrete mucus, an alkaline fluid (pH of 9) that neutralizes chyme and protects the mucosa.[10] Intestinal

FIG. 27.5 Small Intestine. The clinical anatomy of the small intestine. (From Thompson JM, et al. *Mosby's clinical nursing.* 5th ed. St. Louis: Mosby; 2002.)

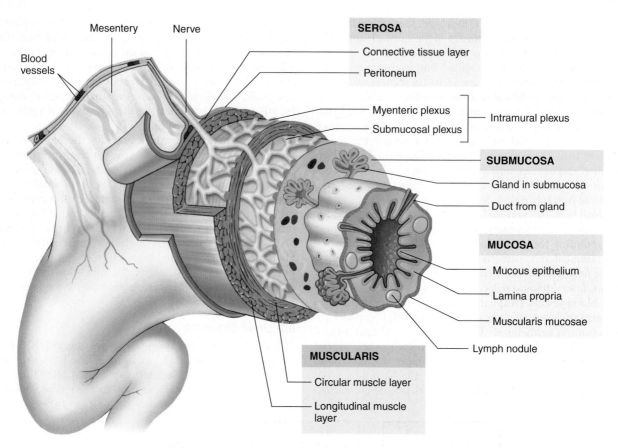

FIG. 27.6 Gastrointestinal wall. Cross section of the gastrointestinal wall. (From Patton KT, Thibodeau GA. *Anatomy and Physiology.* 8th ed. St. Louis; Elsevier; 2013.)

glands are found in pits of the submucosa and are called the *crypts of Lieberkühn*. These crypts secrete 2 to 3 L/day of yellow fluid containing enzymes that assist in nutrient digestion.[7]

Intestinal Motility

Intestinal motility consists of two separate motions: (1) peristalsis and (2) haustral segmentation. Peristalsis is sequential contraction and relaxation of short segments of the small intestine that facilitate digestion and absorption. Haustral segmentation is rhythmic contractions that facilitate the mixing and forward movement of chyme. Haustral segmentation is controlled by Auerbach plexus. Intestinal motility is also affected by neural reflexes located along the length of the small intestine. Motility is inhibited by the intestinointestinal reflex, which is activated by distention of the small intestine, and is stimulated by the gastroileal reflex, which is initiated by an increase in gastric motility.[12]

Digestion and Absorption

The functions of the small intestine include digestion and absorption. Digestion, which involves breaking down large molecules into small ones, is essential for nutrient absorption from the small intestine (Fig. 27.7). Maintenance of pH and osmolality is crucial for digestion in the small intestine. The entry of chyme into the duodenum stimulates the production of secretin, which stimulates the pancreas to secrete a highly alkaline fluid into the duodenum. In the small intestine, chyme mixes with pancreatic enzymes, intestinal enzymes, and bile from the liver and gallbladder and is reduced to absorbable elements of proteins, fats, and

carbohydrates. The nutrients are absorbed through the villi and transported to the liver by the portal system for further processing. The small intestine absorbs up to 8 L/day of fluid, passing only a small part of this fluid into the large intestine. In addition to the nutrients, electrolytes, water, components of saliva, gastric juice, and bile, intestinal and pancreatic secretions are absorbed.[1]

LARGE INTESTINE

The large intestine, which extends from the ileocecal valve to the anus, is approximately 90 to 150 cm (4 to 5 feet) long and 4 to 6 cm (2 inches) in diameter. The large intestine is divided into the ascending colon, hepatic flexure, transverse colon, splenic flexure, descending colon, sigmoid colon, rectum, and anal canal (Fig. 27.8).[10]

The colon has four layers. The outermost layer, the *serous layer (serosa)*, is formed from the visceral peritoneum and covers most of the large intestine, with the exclusion of the sigmoid colon. The second layer, the *muscular layer (muscularis)*, consists of two smooth muscle layers: the *longitudinal* and the *circular* muscles. These muscles work together to propel fecal matter through the colon and to "knead" the stool into a compact bolus. The longitudinal muscle consists of three muscular bands that stretch from the cecum to the distal sigmoid colon. These muscular bands create sacculations of haustra, important clinical features that normally are apparent on a barium enema radiograph. Haustra aid segmentation so that absorption of fluid from the fecal bolus is achieved. The third layer,

FIG. 27.7 Digestion and Absorption of Foodstuffs. (From McCance KL, et al, eds. *Pathophysiology: The Biologic Basis for Disease in Adults and Children.* 7th ed. St. Louis: Elsevier; 2014.)

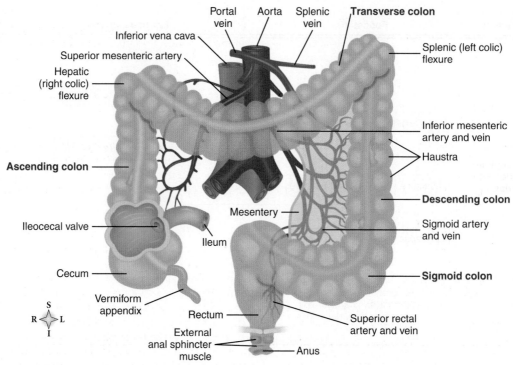

FIG. 27.8 Large Intestine. (Modified from Patton KT, Thibodeau GA. *Anatomy and Physiology.* 8th ed. St. Louis: Elsevier; 2013.)

the *submucous layer (submucosa)*, consists of connective tissue that contains blood vessels, lymphatics, glands, and nerve plexuses. The innermost layer, the *mucous layer (mucosa)*, is lined with simple columnar epithelial cells and contains deep crypts of Lieberkühn that are lined with mucus-producing goblet cells. The mucus eases the passage of the fecal material and protects the mucosal surface from trauma.[10]

The rectum begins at the midsacrum, is 12 to 15 cm (5 inches) long, and is quite angulated. These angles, also known as *Houston valves*, are important in the defecation process because they tend to slow the passage of fecal material in the rectal vault, assisting the continence mechanism.

Arterial blood is supplied to the colon from branches of the superior and inferior mesenteric arteries. Venous drainage occurs through the branches of the superior and inferior mesenteric veins into the portal system. The colon is intrinsically innervated by Auerbach plexus, which controls secretion and motility and is extrinsically innervated by the autonomic nervous system. The sympathetic and parasympathetic branches of the autonomic system innervate the colon, regulating motility. Sympathetic stimulation inhibits colonic activity and constricts the anal sphincters, whereas parasympathetic stimulation increases colonic activity and secretion and relaxes the anal sphincters.[9]

Colonic Motility

Colonic motility consists of haustral shuttling and peristalsis. Haustral shuttling, a variation of haustral segmentation, consists of the contraction and relaxation of the circular muscle. Haustral shuttling moves the contents of the colon back and forth to facilitate the grinding of food masses and fluid absorption. Peristalsis is produced primarily by the longitudinal muscles and propels the fecal bolus forward. Mass peristalsis is a strong, slow contraction in which the distal left colon contracts en masse to move the fecal bolus into the rectum.[13]

Resorption

The major functions of the colon are resorption of water, sodium, chloride, glucose, and urea; dehydration of undigested residue; putrefaction of contents by bacteria; movement of the fecal bolus through the colon; and elimination of the fecal mass. The colon receives approximately 1000 to 2000 mL/day of chyme, and all but 50 to 250 mL is absorbed in the ascending and transverse colon.[5]

The colon contains billions of anaerobic bacteria that putrefy remaining proteins and indigestible residue; synthesize folic acid, vitamin K, nicotinic acid, riboflavin, and some B vitamins; and convert urea salts to ammonium salts and ammonia for absorption into the portal circulation.[1] Common colonic bacteria include *Bacteroides*, *Lactobacillus*, and *Clostridium*.[14]

ACCESSORY ORGANS

The accessory organs of digestion are the liver, biliary system, and pancreas (Fig. 27.9).

Liver

The liver is the largest internal organ in the body. Weighing 1200 to 1600 g (3 to 4 lb), the liver is friable and dark red in color and has a soft-solid consistency. Located in the right upper abdominal quadrant, the liver fits snugly against the right interior diaphragm. The liver is surrounded by connective tissue known as *Glisson capsule*, which is covered by serosa and contains blood vessels and lymphatics. The peritoneum covering the liver forms the falciform ligament, which attaches the liver to the anterior portion of the abdomen between the diaphragm and umbilicus and divides the liver into two main lobes, right and left (see Fig. 27.8). The right lobe, which is six times larger than the left, has three sections: the right lobe

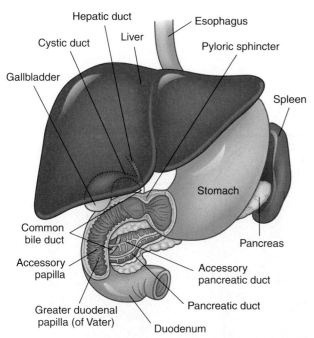

Hepatic duct
Cystic duct
Liver
Esophagus
Pyloric sphincter
Gallbladder
Spleen
Stomach
Common bile duct
Pancreas
Accessory papilla
Accessory pancreatic duct
Greater duodenal papilla (of Vater)
Pancreatic duct
Duodenum

FIG. 27.9 Liver, Gallbladder, and Pancreas. (From McCance KL, et al, eds. *Pathophysiology: The Biologic Basis for Disease in Adults and Children.* 7th ed. St. Louis: Elsevier; 2014.)

proper, the caudate lobe, and the quadrate lobe. The left lobe is divided into two sections. Each lobe is divided into numerous lobules.[10,15]

The liver receives one-third of the total cardiac output from two major sources: (1) the hepatic artery, which provides oxygenated blood, and (2) the portal vein, which is supplied with nutrient-rich blood from the gut, pancreas, spleen, and stomach (Fig. 27.10). The portal vein, which accounts for 75% of the total liver blood flow, branches into sinusoids to transport blood to each lobule. In contrast to capillaries, sinusoids lack a definite cell wall but contain a lining of phagocytic (Kupffer) cells and some nonphagocytic cells of modified epithelium. Sinusoids empty blood into an intralobular vein in the center of the lobule. Intralobular veins empty into larger veins and then into the hepatic vein, which empties on the posterior surface of the liver and eventually into the vena cava. The hepatic artery also divides and subdivides between the lobules, supplying sinusoids with oxygenated blood before emptying into the hepatic vein. Lymphatic spaces are located between liver cells. Lymph drains into lymphatic vessels that surround the hepatic vein and bile ducts.[15]

Nutrient Metabolism

The liver plays a key role in metabolizing and storing carbohydrates, fats, proteins, and vitamins. Glycogen, the stored form of glucose, can be synthesized from glucose or from protein, fat, or lactic acid. Glycogen is broken down to glucose by the liver to maintain normal blood glucose levels. The liver also has a vital role in amino acid metabolism and can synthesize amino acids from metabolites of carbohydrates and fats or can deaminate amino acids to produce ketoacids and ammonia, from which urea is formed. In fat metabolism, the liver hydrolyzes triglycerides to glycerol and fatty acids in the process of ketogenesis and synthesizes phospholipids, cholesterol, and lipoproteins.[10,15]

Hematologic Function

The liver synthesizes plasma proteins such as globulins and albumin, which are important in maintaining the normal osmotic balance of blood. The liver also synthesizes many clotting factors, including fibrinogen and prothrombin. Kupffer cells destroy worn red blood cells, and hepatocytes conjugate bilirubin (by-product of red cell destruction) for excretion.[10,15]

Detoxification and Storage

Steroid hormones are conjugated and polypeptide hormones are inactivated by the liver. The liver stores fat-soluble vitamins, vitamin B_{12}, and the minerals iron and copper. Detoxification of drugs and toxins occurs in Kupffer cells.[10,15]

Bile

The production of bile makes the liver a vital organ in digestion and absorption. The major components of bile are bile pigments, bile salts, cholesterol, neutral fats, phospholipids, inorganic salts, fatty acids, mucin, conjugated bilirubin, lecithin, and water. Traces of albumin, gamma globulin, urea, nitrogen, and glucose are also present in bile. The principal electrolytes of bile are sodium, chloride, and bicarbonate.[15]

Bile emulsifies fat globules and absorbs fat-soluble vitamins. Bile salts also serve as an excretion route for bilirubin, cholesterol, and various hormones. Approximately 80% of bile salts are actively resorbed in the distal ileum and are recycled to the liver through the enterohepatic circulation; only 20% are lost in feces.[1]

Bilirubin

The primary bile pigment, bilirubin, is formed from the heme portion of hemoglobin during the degradation of red blood cells by Kupffer cells. When released into the bloodstream, bilirubin binds to albumin as fat-soluble, unconjugated bilirubin. Taken up by liver hepatocytes, unconjugated bilirubin is conjugated with glucuronic acid to form water-soluble, conjugated bilirubin, which is excreted through hepatic ducts into the large intestine. If the amount of bilirubin sent to the liver is in excess, the ability of the liver to conjugate the bilirubin may be taxed; free, unconjugated or indirect bilirubin appears in the blood. High levels of unconjugated bilirubin in the blood suggest hepatocellular dysfunction, whereas high levels of conjugated bilirubin suggest biliary tract obstruction.[1]

Biliary System

The biliary system (Fig. 27.11) consists of the gallbladder and its related ductal system, including the hepatic, cystic, and common bile ducts. The hepatic duct, from the liver, joins the cystic duct, from the gallbladder, to form the common bile duct, which empties into the duodenum. The common bile duct is surrounded by Oddi sphincter, which pierces the wall of the duodenum and controls the flow of bile into the duodenum. The gallbladder is a pear-shaped organ that is 7 to 10 cm (3 to 4 inches) long and 2.5 to 3.5 cm (approximately 1 inch) wide, lying on the underside of the liver (see Fig. 27.9). The gallbladder is attached to the liver by connective tissue, peritoneum, and blood vessels.[10,16]

Bile

The main functions of the gallbladder are to collect, concentrate, acidify, and store bile. Bile is continuously formed in the liver and excreted into the hepatic duct for transport to the gallbladder through the cystic duct. The gallbladder can store 90 mL of bile and concentrate it approximately 15 to 29 times by removing

FIG. 27.10 Microscopic Structure of the Liver. (A) Diagram shows the location of liver lobules relative to the overall circulatory scheme of the liver. (B and C) Enlarged views of several lobules show how blood from the hepatic portal veins and hepatic arteries flows through sinusoids and past plates of hepatic cells toward a central vein in each lobule *(black arrows)*. Hepatic cells form bile, which flows through bile canaliculi toward hepatic ducts that eventually drain the bile from the liver *(yellow arrows)*. (From Patton KT, Thibodeau GA. *Anatomy and Physiology*. 8th ed. St. Louis: Elsevier; 2013.)

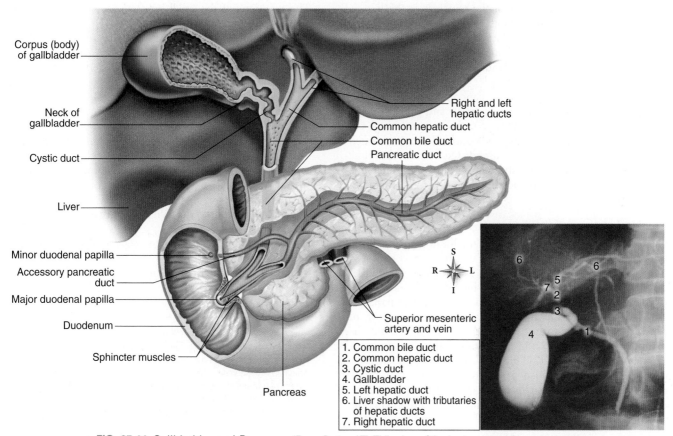

FIG. 27.11 Gallbladder and Pancreas. (From Patton KT, Thibodeau GA. *Anatomy and Physiology.* 8th ed. St. Louis: Elsevier; 2013.)

Labels on figure:
- Corpus (body) of gallbladder
- Neck of gallbladder
- Cystic duct
- Liver
- Minor duodenal papilla
- Accessory pancreatic duct
- Major duodenal papilla
- Duodenum
- Sphincter muscles
- Pancreas
- Right and left hepatic ducts
- Common hepatic duct
- Common bile duct
- Pancreatic duct
- Superior mesenteric artery and vein

1. Common bile duct
2. Common hepatic duct
3. Cystic duct
4. Gallbladder
5. Left hepatic duct
6. Liver shadow with tributaries of hepatic ducts
7. Right hepatic duct

approximately 90% of the water. Cholesterol and pigment are likewise concentrated. Bile, which is golden or orange-yellow in the liver, becomes dark brown when concentrated in the gallbladder. By altering its shape and volume, the gallbladder regulates pressure within the biliary system. Relaxation of the sphincter of Oddi is coordinated with gallbladder contraction through the regulatory action of cholecystokinin. Such factors as sight, smell, and taste can stimulate gallbladder contraction, whereas fear or excitement can decrease contraction. After a meal, the amount of bile entering the duodenum increases as a result of enhanced liver secretion and gallbladder contraction. Intestinal secretion of cholecystokinin and secretin, high levels of bile salts in the blood, and vagal stimulation increase biliary secretion.[15]

Box 27.1 summarizes all the functions of the liver.

Pancreas

The pancreas is a soft, lobulated, fish-shaped gland (see Fig. 27.11) lying beneath the duodenum and the spleen (see Fig. 27.9). The pinkish yellow organ is 15 to 20 cm (6 to 8 inches) long and 5 cm (1 to 1.5 inches) wide. Its anatomic divisions include the *head*, which lies in the C-shaped curve of the duodenum to which the pancreas is attached; the *body*, the main part of the gland, which extends horizontally across the abdomen and is largely hidden behind the stomach; and the *tail*, a thin, narrow portion in contact with the spleen. The main pancreatic duct, called the *duct of Wirsung*, traverses the entire length of the organ. The duct of Wirsung empties exocrine secretions into the ampulla of Vater, which is the same lumen draining the common bile duct, at the entrance to the duodenum.[10]

BOX 27.1   Functions of the Liver

- Secretion of bilirubin, bile salts, cholesterol, fatty acids, calcium, and other electrolytes into bile
- Storage of amino acids, glucose, vitamins, minerals (copper, iron), and blood
- Conversion of complex sugars to simple sugars
- Conversion of carbohydrates to fats
- Conversion of stored glucose (glycogen) to glucose (glycogenolysis)
- Conversion of amino acids and fats to glucose (gluconeogenesis)
- Conversion of amino acids to fatty acids and triglycerides
- Formation of phospholipids and cholesterol
- Formation of lipoproteins from triglycerides and peptides
- Conversion of amino acids to plasma proteins (eg, albumin, fibrinogen, globulins)
- Phagocytosis of old red blood cells
- Formation of clotting factors and heparin
- Conversion of ammonia to urea
- Conversion of creatine to creatinine
- Conversion of vitamin D_3 to 25-hydroxycholecalciferol
- Detoxification of bacteria
- Biotransformation of drugs to active and/or inactive metabolites
- Deactivation of certain hormones

Modified from Dennison RD. *Pass CCRN!* 4th ed. St. Louis: Mosby; 2013.

The internal structural unit of the pancreas is the lobule, consisting of numerous small ducts with secretory cells called *tubuloacinar* cells. Each acinus has a small duct that empties into lobular ducts. Lobules are joined by connective tissue into lobes, which unite to form the gland. The ducts from each lobule empty into the duct of Wirsung.[10]

Arterial blood supply to the pancreas is provided by branches of the superior mesenteric artery and celiac arteries. Venous drainage of the head of the pancreas occurs through the portal vein, and drainage of the body and tail occurs through the splenic vein. The pancreas is innervated by the autonomic nervous system. Sympathetic stimulation decreases pancreatic secretion, and parasympathetic stimulation increases pancreatic secretion.[10]

Exocrine Functions

Exocrine functions of the pancreas are limited to digestion. Acinar cells secrete pancreatic juice, which consists of water, sodium bicarbonate, and electrolytes at a highly alkaline pH. Enzymes produced in the pancreas include trypsin, chymotrypsin, carboxypeptidase, amylase, and lipase. The pancreas also produces a trypsin inhibitor that prevents activation of trypsinogen (inactive form of trypsin), which inhibits autodigestion. Autodigestion is the underlying cause of acute pancreatitis. Pancreatic exocrine function is regulated by digestive hormones. Signals provided primarily by the intestinal hormones *secretin* and *cholecystokinin* stimulate the pancreas to secrete pancreatic juice. The two hormones potentiate the effects of each other on the pancreas.[17]

Endocrine Functions

Endocrine tissue in the pancreas consists of spherical islets called *islets of Langerhans*, which are embedded within the lobules of acinar tissue throughout the pancreas, especially in the distal body and tail. Endocrine products include *insulin*, which is produced in beta cells; *glucagon*, which is produced in alpha cells; and *gastrin*. All of these hormones are secreted directly into the bloodstream.[17]

■ SUMMARY

Anatomy

- The GI tract consists of the mouth (lips, cheeks, gums, tongue, palate, and salivary glands), esophagus, stomach, small intestine, and large intestine.
- The accessory organs of digestion are the liver, biliary system, and pancreas.

Physiology

- The major function of the GI tract is digestion.
- Digestion is the conversion of ingested nutrients into simpler forms that can be transported from the lumen of the GI tract to the portal circulation and then used in metabolic processes.
- The mouth and accessory organs perform the initial phases of digestion, which are ingestion, mastication, and salivation.
- The functions of the stomach include food storage, digestion, and emptying.
- Gastric motility is regulated by the autonomic nervous system, digestive hormones, and neural reflexes.

- The functions of the small intestine include digestion and absorption.
- Intestinal motility consists of peristalsis and haustral segmentation.
- The major functions of the colon include resorption of water, sodium, chloride, glucose, and urea; dehydration of undigested residue; putrefaction of contents by bacteria; movement of the fecal bolus through the colon; and elimination of the fecal mass.
- Colonic motility consists of haustral shuttling and peristalsis.
- The functions of the liver include metabolism and storage of carbohydrates, fats, proteins, and vitamins; synthesis of plasma proteins; detoxification of drugs and toxins; and production of bile.
- The main functions of the gallbladder are to collect, concentrate, acidify, and store bile.
- The main functions of the pancreas are digestion and glucose regulation.

ⓔ Visit the Evolve site for additional study materials.

REFERENCES

1. Huether SE. Structure and function of the digestive system. In: McCance KL, et al., ed. *Pathophysiology: The Biologic Basis for Disease in Adults and Children*. ed 7. St. Louis: Mosby; 2014.
2. Madani FM, Kuperstein AS. Normal variations of oral anatomy and common oral soft tissue lesions: evaluation and management. *Med Clin North Am*. 2014;98(6):1281–1298.
3. Mandel L. Salivary gland disorders. *Med Clin North Am*. 2014;98(6):1407–1449.
4. Oezcelik A, DeMeester SR. General anatomy of the esophagus. *Thorac Surg Clin*. 2011;21(2):289–297.
5. Matsuo K, Palmer JB. Anatomy and physiology of feeding and swallowing: normal and abnormal. *Phys Med Rehabil Clin North Am*. 2008;19(4):691–707.
6. Soybel DI. Anatomy and physiology of the stomach. *Surg Clin North Am*. 2005;85(5):875–894.
7. Hall JE. *Guyton and Hall Textbook of Medical Physiology*. ed 13. Philadelphia: Saunders; 2016.
8. Rostas JW, Mai TT, Richards WO. Gastric motility physiology and surgical intervention. *Surg Clin North Am*. 2011;91(5):983–999.
9. Androulakis J, et al. Embryologic and anatomic basis of duodenal surgery. *Surg Clin North Am*. 2000;80(1):171–199.
10. SGNA. *Gastroenterology Nursing: A Core Curriculum*. ed 5. St. Louis: Society of Gastroenterology Nurses and Associates; 2013.
11. Lin PH, Chaikof EL. Embryology, anatomy, and surgical exposure of the great abdominal vessels. *Surg Clin North Am*. 2000;80(1):417–433.
12. Smout A, Fox M. Weak and absent peristalsis. *Neurogastroenterol Motil*. 2012;24(suppl 1):40–47.
13. Gras B, et al. Motility disorders of the colon and rectum. *Curr Opin Gastroenterol*. 2013;29(1):66–71.
14. Macfarlane GT, Macfarlane SL. Bacteria, colonic fermentation, and gastrointestinal health. *J AOAC Int*. 2012;95(1):50–60.
15. Misdraji J. Embryology, anatomy, histology, and developmental anomalies of the liver. In: Feldman M, Friedman LS, Brandt LJ, eds. *Sleisenger & Fordtran's Gastrointestinal and Liver Disease: Pathophysiology, Diagnosis, and Management*. ed 10. Philadelphia: Saunders; 2016.
16. Adkins RB, Chapman WC, Reddy VS. Embryology, anatomy, and surgical applications of the extrahepatic biliary system. *Surg Clin North Am*. 2000;80(1):363–379.
17. Chen N, et al. The complex exocrine-endocrine relationship and secondary diabetes in exocrine pancreatic disorders. *J Clin Gastroenterol*. 2011;45(10):850–861.

Gastrointestinal Clinical Assessment and Diagnostic Procedures

Jacqueline Fitzgerald Close

Assessment of a critically ill patient with gastrointestinal (GI) dysfunction includes a review of the patient's history, a focused clinical assessment, and analysis of the patient's laboratory data. Numerous invasive and noninvasive diagnostic procedures may also be performed to identify the disorder. A thorough assessment of a patient with GI dysfunction is imperative for early identification and treatment of GI disorders. The completed assessment serves as the foundation for developing the management plan for the patient. Depending on the nature and immediacy of the patient's condition, the assessment process can be brief or can involve a detailed history and examination.[1,2]

HISTORY

Taking a thorough and accurate history is extremely important to the assessment process. The patient's history provides the foundation and direction for the rest of the assessment. The overall goal of the patient interview is to expose key clinical manifestations that will facilitate the identification of the underlying cause of the illness. This information can assist in the development of an appropriate management plan.

The initial presentation of the patient determines the rapidity and direction of the interview. For a patient in acute distress, the history should be curtailed to a few questions about the patient's chief complaint and the precipitating events. For a patient in no obvious distress, the history should focus on current symptoms, the patient's medical history, and the family history. Specific items regarding each of these areas are outlined in Box 28.1, Data Collection.[3,4]

FOCUSED CLINICAL ASSESSMENT

The clinical assessment helps establish baseline data about the physical dimensions of the patient's situation.[3] The abdomen is divided into four quadrants (left upper, right upper, left lower, and right lower) with the umbilicus as the middle point, to specify the location of examination findings (Fig. 28.1 and Box 28.2). Have the patient empty his or her bladder before the examination, as a full bladder could distort the accuracy of the examination.[5] The assessment should proceed when the patient is as comfortable as possible and in the supine position; however, the position may need readjustment if it elicits pain. To prevent stimulation of GI activity, the order for the assessment should be changed to inspection, auscultation, percussion, and palpation.[4]

Inspection

Inspection should be performed in a warm, well-lit environment, and the patient should be in a comfortable position, with the abdomen exposed. Although assessment of the GI system classically begins with inspection of the abdomen, the patient's oral cavity also must be inspected to determine any unusual findings. Abnormal findings of the mouth include temporomandibular joint tenderness, inflammation of gums, missing teeth, dental caries, ill-fitting dentures, and mouth odor.

Observe the skin for pigmentation, lesions, striae, scars, petechiae, signs of dehydration, and venous pattern. Pigmentation may vary considerably and still be within normal limits because of race and ethnic background, although the abdomen usually is of a lighter color than other exposed areas of the skin. Abnormal findings include jaundice, skin lesions, and a tense and glistening appearance of the skin. A deviated umbilicus may be caused by a mass, hernia, fluid, or old scar tissue. An everted umbilicus is apparent with distention.[5] Old striae (stretch marks) usually are silver, whereas pinkish purple striae may indicate Cushing syndrome.[4] A bluish discoloration of the umbilicus (Cullen sign) and of the flank (Grey Turner sign) indicates retroperitoneal bleeding.[1]

Observe the abdomen for contour, noting whether it is flat, slightly concave, or slightly round; observe for symmetry and for movement. Marked distention is an abnormal finding. In particular, ascites may cause generalized distention and bulging flanks. Asymmetric distention may indicate organ enlargement, large masses, hernia, or bowel obstruction.[5] Peristaltic waves should not be visible except in very thin patients. In the case of intestinal obstruction, hyperactive peristaltic waves may be observed. Pulsation in the epigastric area is often a normal finding, but increased pulsation may indicate an aortic aneurysm. Symmetric movement of the abdomen with respirations is usually seen in men.[4,6]

Auscultation

Auscultation of the abdomen provides clinical data regarding the status of bowel motility. Initially, listen with the diaphragm of the stethoscope below and to the right of the umbilicus. The examination proceeds methodically through all four quadrants, lifting and then replacing the diaphragm of the stethoscope lightly against the abdomen (see Fig. 28.1). Normal bowel sounds include high-pitched, gurgling sounds that occur approximately every 5 to 15 seconds or at a rate of 5 to 34 times per minute. Colonic sounds are low-pitched

BOX 28.1   DATA COLLECTION

Gastrointestinal History

Common Gastrointestinal Symptoms
- Oral lesions
- Digestion or indigestion (heartburn)
- Dysphagia
- Nausea
- Vomiting
- Hematemesis
- Change in stool color or contents (eg, clay-colored, tarry, fresh blood, mucus, undigested food)
- Constipation
- Diarrhea
- Abdominal pain
- Jaundice
- Anal discomfort
- Fecal incontinence

Patient Lifestyle
- Usual height and weight
- Dietary habits
  - Usual number of meals or snacks per day
  - Usual fluid intake per day
- Nutrient intake
  - Types of food usually eaten at each meal or snack
  - Food likes and dislikes
  - Religious or medical food restrictions
  - Food intolerances
  - Patient's perceptions and concerns about adequacy of diet and appropriateness of weight
  - Effects of lifestyle on food intake, weight gain or loss
  - Vitamins or nutritional supplements (eg, type, amount, frequency)
- Bowel elimination
  - Usual frequency of bowel movements
  - Usual consistency and color of stool
  - Ability to control elimination of gas and stool
  - Any changes in bowel elimination patterns
  - Use of enemas or laxatives (eg, reason for use, frequency, type, response)
- Alcohol intake (eg, frequency, usual amounts)
- Exercise patterns

Medical History
- Chronic illnesses
- Previous weight gain or loss
- Tooth extractions or orthodontic work
- GI disorders (eg, peptic ulcer, inflammatory bowel disease, polyps, cholelithiasis, diverticular disease, pancreatitis, intestinal obstruction)
- Hepatitis or cirrhosis
- Abdominal surgery
- Abdominal trauma
- Cancer affecting GI system
- Spinal cord injury
- Women: episiotomy or fourth-degree laceration during delivery
- Exposure to infectious agents (eg, foreign travel, water source)

Family History
- Investigate for history of following disorders, and document (+ or −) responses
  - Hirschsprung disease
  - Obesity
  - Metabolic disorders
  - Inflammatory disorders
  - Malabsorption syndromes
  - Familial Mediterranean fever
  - Rectal polyps
  - Polyposis syndromes
  - Cancer of GI tract

Current Medication Use
- Laxatives
- Stool softeners
- Antiemetics
- Antidiarrheals
- Antacids
- Aspirin
- Acetaminophen
- Nonsteroidal antiinflammatory drugs
- Corticosteroids

FIG. 28.1 Abdominal Four Quadrants. (A) Anatomic mapping of the four quadrants of the abdomen. (B) Auscultation for bowel sounds. (From Barkauskas V, Baumann L, Darling-Fisher C. *Health and Physical Assessment.* 3rd ed. St. Louis: Mosby; 2002.)

BOX 28.2 Anatomic Correlates of the Four Quadrants of the Abdomen

Right Upper Quadrant
- Liver and gallbladder
- Pylorus
- Duodenum
- Head of pancreas
- Right adrenal gland
- Portion of right kidney
- Hepatic flexure of colon
- Portion of ascending and transverse colon

Right Lower Quadrant
- Lower pole of right kidney
- Cecum and appendix
- Portion of ascending colon
- Bladder (if distended)
- Ovary and salpinx
- Uterus (if enlarged)
- Right spermatic cord
- Right ureter

Left Upper Quadrant
- Left lobe of liver
- Spleen
- Stomach
- Body of pancreas
- Left adrenal gland
- Portion of left kidney
- Splenic flexure of colon
- Portions of transverse and descending colon

Left Lower Quadrant
- Lower pole of left kidney
- Sigmoid colon
- Portion of descending colon
- Bladder (if distended)
- Ovary and salpinx
- Uterus (if distended)
- Left spermatic cord
- Left ureter

From Barkauskas V, Baumann L, Darling-Fisher C. *Health and Physical Assessment*. 3rd ed. St. Louis: Mosby; 2002.

TABLE 28.1 Abnormal Abdominal Sounds

Sound	Cause
Hyperactive bowel sounds (borborygmi), loud and prolonged	Hunger, gastroenteritis, or early intestinal obstruction
High-pitched, tinkling sounds	Intestinal air and fluid under pressure; characteristic of early intestinal obstruction
Decreased (hypoactive) bowel sounds	Possible peritonitis or ileus
Infrequent and abnormally faint sounds	
Absence of bowel sounds (confirmed only after auscultation of all four quadrants and continuous auscultation for 5 min)	Temporary loss of intestinal motility, as occurs with complete ileus
Friction rubs	Pathologic conditions such as tumors or infection that cause inflammation of peritoneal covering of organ
High-pitched sounds heard over liver and spleen (RUQ and LUQ), synchronous with respiration	
Bruits	Abnormality of blood flow (requires additional evaluation to determine specific disorder)
Audible swishing sounds that may be heard over aortic, iliac, renal, and femoral arteries	
Venous hum	Increased collateral circulation between portal and systemic venous systems
Low-pitched, continuous sound	

LUQ, left upper quadrant; *RUQ*, right upper quadrant.
From Doughty DB, Jackson DB. *Gastrointestinal Disorders*. St. Louis: Mosby; 1993.

sounds with a rumbling quality. A venous hum may be audible sometimes.[7] Table 28.1 lists abnormal abdominal sounds.

Abnormal findings include the absence of bowel sounds throughout a 5-minute period; extremely soft, widely separated sounds; and increased sounds with a high-pitched, loud rushing sound (peristaltic rush). Hyperactive bowel sounds that are tinkling may indicate increased motility related to an early bowel obstruction, diarrhea, or gastroenteritis. Hypoactive bowel sounds may indicate paralytic ileus after surgery, which is very common; peritoneal irritation; or bowel obstruction.[5] Absent bowel sounds may result from inflammation; ileus; electrolyte disturbances; and ischemia, which requires immediate attention. The abdomen should be auscultated for the presence of bruits using the bell of the stethoscope (Fig. 28.2). Bruits are created by turbulent flow over a partially obstructed artery and are always considered an abnormal finding. The aorta,

the right and left renal arteries, and the iliac arteries should be auscultated.[6,7]

Percussion

Percussion is used to elicit information about deep organs such as the liver, spleen, and pancreas (Fig. 28.3). Because the abdomen is a sensitive area, muscle tension may interfere with this part of the assessment. Percussion often helps relax tense muscles, and it is performed before palpation. Percussion in the absence of disease helps delineate the position and size of the liver and spleen, and it assists in the detection of fluid, gaseous distention, and masses in the abdomen.[6]

Percussion should proceed systematically and lightly in all four quadrants. Normal findings include tympany over the empty stomach, tympany or hyperresonance over the intestine, and dullness over the liver and spleen. Abnormal areas of dullness may indicate

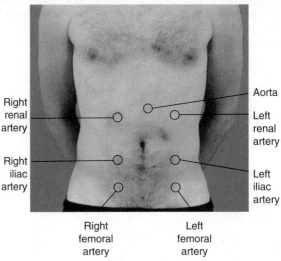

FIG. 28.2 Auscultation for Bruits. The correct placement of the stethoscope is shown on the left. (From Barkauskas V, Baumann L, Darling-Fisher C. *Health and Physical Assessment*. 3rd ed. St. Louis: Mosby; 2002.)

FIG. 28.3 Percussion of the Abdomen. (From Barkauskas V, Baumann L, Darling-Fisher C. *Health and Physical Assessment*. 3rd ed. St. Louis: Mosby; 2002.)

an underlying mass. Tenderness over the liver may indicate inflammation or infection.[5] Solid masses, enlarged organs, and a distended bladder also produce areas of dullness. Dullness over both flanks may indicate ascites and necessitates further assessment.[7]

Palpation

Palpation is the assessment technique most useful in detecting abdominal pathologic conditions. Light and deep palpation of each organ and quadrant should be completed. Light palpation, which has a palpation depth of approximately 1 cm, assesses to the depth of the skin and fascia (Fig. 28.4A). Deep palpation assesses the rectus abdominis muscle and is performed bimanually to a depth of 4 to 5 cm (Fig. 28.4B). Deep palpation is most helpful in detecting abdominal masses. Areas in which the patient complains of tenderness should be palpated last.[7]

Normal findings include no areas of tenderness or pain, no masses, and no hardened areas. Persistent involuntary guarding may indicate peritoneal inflammation, particularly if it continues after relaxation techniques are used. Rebound tenderness, in which pain increases with quick release of a palpated area, indicates an inflamed peritoneum.[4]

Assessment Findings for Common Disorders

Table 28.2 list various common GI disorders and their associated assessment findings.

LABORATORY STUDIES

The value of various laboratory studies used to diagnose and treat diseases of the GI system has been emphasized often. However, no single study provides an overall picture of the functional state of the various organs, and no single value is predictive by itself. Laboratory studies used in the assessment of GI function, liver function, and pancreatic function are presented in Tables 28.3, 28.4, and 28.5.

Diagnostic Procedures

To complete the assessment of a critically ill patient with GI dysfunction, the patient's diagnostic tests are reviewed. Although many procedures exist for diagnosing GI disease, their application in a critically ill patient is limited. Only procedures that are currently used in the critical care setting are presented here.

The nursing management of a patient undergoing a diagnostic procedure involves a variety of interventions. Nursing actions include preparing the patient psychologically and physically for the procedure, monitoring the patient's responses to the procedure, and assessing the patient after the procedure. Preparing the patient includes teaching the patient about the procedure, answering any questions, and transporting and positioning the patient for the procedure. Monitoring the patient's responses to the procedure includes observing the patient for signs of pain, anxiety, or hemorrhage and monitoring vital signs. Assessing the patient after the procedure includes observing for complications of the procedure and

FIG. 28.4 Palpation of the Abdomen. (A) Light palpation. (B) Deep palpation. (From Barkauskas V, Baumann L, Darling-Fisher C. *Health and Physical Assessment.* 3rd ed. St. Louis: Mosby; 2002.)

TABLE 28.2	Assessment Findings of Common Gastrointestinal Disorders		
Condition	**History**	**Symptoms**	**Signs**
RLQ of Abdomen			
Appendicitis	Children (except infants) and young adults	Anorexia	Signs may be absent early
		Nausea	Vomiting
		Early vague epigastric, periumbilical, or generalized pain after 12–24 h; RLQ at McBurney point	Localized RLQ guarding and tenderness after 12–24 h
			Rovsing sign: pain in RLQ with application of pressure, iliopsoas sign
			Obturator sign
			White blood cell count of 10,000/mm³ or shift to left
			Low-grade fever
			Cutaneous hyperesthesia in RLQ
			Signs highly variable
Perforated duodenal ulcer	Prior history	Abrupt-onset pain in epigastric area or RLQ	Tenderness in epigastric area or RLQ
			Signs of peritoneal irritation
			Heme-positive stool
			Increased white blood cell count
Cecal volvulus	Seen most often in older adults	Abrupt severe abdominal pain	Distention
			Localized tenderness
			Tympany
Strangulated hernia	Any age	Severe localized pain	If bowel obstructed, distention
	Women: femoral	If bowel obstructed, generalized pain	
	Men: inguinal		
RUQ of Abdomen			
Liver hepatitis	Any age, often young blood product user	Fatigue	Hepatic tenderness
		Malaise	Hepatomegaly
	Drug addict	Anorexia	Bilirubin elevated
		Pain in RUQ	Jaundice
		Low-grade fever	Lymphocytosis in one-third of cases
		May have severe fulminating disease with liver failure	Liver enzymes elevated
			Hepatitis A or B or antibodies to viruses may be found
Acute hepatic congestion	Usually older adults with acute heart failure	Symptoms of acute heart failure	Hepatomegaly
	Pericardial disease		Acute heart failure
	Pulmonary embolism		
Biliary stones, colic	"Fair, fat, forty" (90%) but can be 30–80 years old	Anorexia	Tenderness in RUQ
		Nausea	Jaundice
		Pain severe in RUQ or epigastric area	
		Episodes lasting 15 min to hours	

Continued

TABLE 28.2   Assessment Findings of Common Gastrointestinal Disorders—cont'd

Condition	History	Symptoms	Signs
Acute cholecystitis	"Fair, fat, forty" (90%) but can be 30–80 years old	Severe RUQ or epigastric pain	Vomiting
		Episodes prolonged up to 6 h	Tenderness in RUQ
			Peritoneal irritation signs
			Increased white blood cell count
Perforated peptic ulcer	Any age	Abrupt RUQ pain	Tenderness in epigastrium, right quadrant, or both
			Peritoneal irritation signs
			Free air in abdomen
LUQ of Abdomen			
Splenic trauma	Blunt trauma to LUQ of abdomen	Pain: LUQ pain of abdomen often referred to left shoulder (Kehr sign)	Hypotension
			Syncope
			Increased dyspnea
			Radiographic studies show enlarged spleen
Pancreatitis	Alcohol abuse	Pain in LUQ or epigastric region radiating to back or chest	Fever
	Pancreatic duct obstruction		Rigidity
			Rebound tenderness
	Infection		Nausea
	Cholecystitis		Vomiting
			Jaundice
			Cullen sign
			Turner sign
			Abdominal distention
			Diminished bowel sounds
Pyloric obstruction	Duodenal ulcer	Weight loss	Increasing dullness in LUQ
		Gastric upset	Visible peristaltic waves in epigastric region
		Vomiting	
LLQ of Abdomen			
Ulcerative colitis	Family history	Chronic, watery diarrhea with bloody mucus	Fever
	Jewish ancestry		
	Cachexia		
		Anorexia	Anemia
		Weight loss	Leukocytosis
		Fatigue	
Colonic diverticulitis	Older than 39 years	Pain that recurs in LUQ	Fever
	Low-residue diet		Vomiting
			Chills
			Diarrhea
			Tenderness over descending colon

LLQ, left lower quadrant; *LUQ*, left upper quadrant; *RLQ*, right lower quadrant; *RUQ*, right upper quadrant.
Modified from Barkauskas V, Baumann L, Darling-Fisher C. *Health and Physical Assessment*. 3rd ed. St. Louis: Mosby; 2002.

medicating the patient for any postprocedural discomfort. Any evidence of GI bleeding should be immediately reported to the physician, and emergency measures to maintain circulation must be initiated.

Endoscopy

Available in several forms, fiberoptic endoscopy is a diagnostic procedure for the direct visualization and evaluation of the GI tract. Endoscopy can provide information about lesions, mucosal changes, obstructions, and motility dysfunction, and a biopsy or removal of foreign objects may be performed during the procedure. The main difference between the various diagnostic forms is the length of the anatomic area that can

be examined. Esophagogastroduodenoscopy permits viewing of the upper GI tract from the esophagus to the upper duodenum, and it is used to evaluate sources of upper GI bleeding (Fig. 28.5). Colonoscopy permits viewing of the lower GI tract from the rectum to the distal ileum, and it is used to evaluate sources of lower GI bleeding. Enteroscopy permits viewing of the small bowel beyond the ligament of Treitz, and it is used to evaluate sources of GI bleeding that have not been identified previously with esophagogastroduodenoscopy or colonoscopy. Endoscopic retrograde cholangiopancreatography enables viewing of the biliary and pancreatic ducts, and it is used in the evaluation of pancreatitis. During this procedure, contrast medium is injected into the ducts through the

TABLE 28.3 Selected Laboratory Studies of Gastrointestinal Function

Test	Normal Findings	Clinical Significance of Abnormal Findings
Stool studies	Resident microorganisms: clostridia, enterococci, *Pseudomonas*, a few yeasts	Detection of *Salmonella typhi* (typhoid fever), *Shigella* (dysentery), *Vibrio cholerae* (cholera), *Yersinia* (enterocolitis), *Escherichia coli* (gastroenteritis), *Staphylococcus aureus* (food poisoning), *Clostridium botulinum* (food poisoning), *Clostridium perfringens* (food poisoning), *Aeromonas* (gastroenteritis)
	Fat: 2–6 g/24 h	Steatorrhea (increased values) resulting from intestinal malabsorption or pancreatic insufficiency
	Pus: none	Large amounts of pus associated with chronic ulcerative colitis, abscesses, and anorectal fistula
	Occult blood: none (ortho-toluidine or guaiac test)	Positive test results associated with bleeding
	Ova and parasites: none	Detection of *Entamoeba histolytica* (amebiasis), *Giardia lamblia* (giardiasis), and worms
D-Xylose absorption	5-h urinary excretion: 4.5 g/L Peak blood level: >30 mg/dL	Differentiation of pancreatic steatorrhea (normal D-xylose absorption) from intestinal steatorrhea (impaired D-xylose absorption)
Gastric acid stimulation	11–20 mEq/h after stimulation	Detection of duodenal ulcers, Zollinger-Ellison syndrome (increased values), gastric atrophy, gastric carcinoma (decreased values)
Manometry[a]	Values vary at different levels of intestine	Inadequate swallowing, motility, sphincter function
Culture and sensitivity of duodenal contents	No pathogens	Detection of *S. typhi* (typhoid fever)
Breath tests		
Glucose or D-xylose breath test	Negative for hydrogen or carbon dioxide	May indicate intestinal bacterial overgrowth
Urea breath test	Negative for isotopically labeled carbon dioxide	Presence of *Helicobacter pylori* infection
Lactose breath test	Negative for exhaled hydrogen	Lactose intolerance

[a]Use of water-filled catheters connected to pressure transducers passed into the esophagus, stomach, colon, or rectum to evaluate contractility.
From McCance KL, et al, eds. *Pathophysiology: The Biologic Basis for Disease in Adults and Children.* 7th ed. St. Louis: Elsevier; 2014.

TABLE 28.4 Common Laboratory Studies of Liver Function

Test	Normal Value	Interpretation
Serum Enzymes		
Alkaline phosphatase	13–39 U/L Male, 12–39 U/L Female, 9–31 U/L	Increases with biliary obstruction and cholestatic hepatitis
Aspartate aminotransferase (AST)[a]	5–40 U/L	Increases with hepatocellular injury (and injury in other tissues, eg skeletal and cardiac muscle)
Alanine aminotransferase (ALT)[b]	5–35 U/L	Increases with hepatocellular injury and necrosis
Lactate dehydrogenase (LDH)	0–250 U/L	Isoenzyme lactate dehydrogenase (LD_5) is elevated with hypoxic and primary liver injury
5′-Nucleotidase	2–11 U/L	Increases with increase in alkaline phosphatase and cholestatic disorders
Bilirubin Metabolism		
Serum bilirubin		
Indirect (unconjugated)	0–1.0 mg/dL	Increases with hemolysis (lysis of red blood cells)
Direct (conjugated)	0–0.3 mg/dL	Increases with hepatocellular injury or obstruction
Total	0–1.0 mg/dL	Increases with biliary obstruction
Urine bilirubin	0.2–1.3 mg/dL	Increases with biliary obstruction
Urine urobilinogen	0.3–2.1 mg/2 h (male) 0.1–1.1 mg/2 h (female)	Increases with hemolysis or shunting or portal blood flow
Serum Proteins		
Albumin	4.0–6.0 g/dL	Decreases with hepatocellular injury
Globulin	2.0–4.0 g/dL	Increases with hepatitis
Total	6–8 g/dL	
Albumin-to-globulin (A/G) ratio	1.5–2.5:1	Ratio reverses with chronic hepatitis or other chronic liver disease
Transferrin	250–300 mcg/dL	Liver damage with decreased values, iron deficiency with increased values
Alpha-fetoprotein	<10 ng/dL	Elevated values in primary hepatocellular carcinoma
Blood Clotting Functions		
Prothrombin time	10–14 s or 90% of control	Increases with chronic liver disease (cirrhosis) or vitamin K deficiency
International normalized ratio (INR)	0.9–1.3	Increased values indicate high chance of bleeding; useful for monitoring effects of drugs such as warfarin
Partial thromboplastin time (PTT)	25–40 s	Increases with severe liver disease or heparin therapy
Bromsulphalein (BSP) excretion	<6% retention in 45 min	Increased retention with hepatocellular injury

[a]Previously serum glutamate oxaloacetate transaminase (SGOT).
[b]Previously serum glutamate pyruvate transaminase (SGPT).
From McCance KL, et al, eds. *Pathophysiology: The Biologic Basis for Disease in Adults and Children.* 7th ed. St. Louis: Elsevier; 2014.

endoscope, and radiographs are obtained.[8] Endoscopy also provides therapeutic benefits for various conditions, including GI bleeding.[9]

Nursing Management

The patient should take nothing by mouth (NPO) for 6 to 12 hours before endoscopy of the upper GI tract. The patient should receive a bowel preparation before endoscopy of the lower GI tract.[8] In some cases, the procedure is performed at the patient's bedside, particularly if the patient is actively bleeding and too unstable to be moved to the GI suite. Fiberoptic endoscopy may present risks for the patient. Although rare, potential complications include perforation of the GI tract, hemorrhage, aspiration, vasovagal stimulation, and oversedation.[8] Signs of perforation include abdominal pain and distention, GI bleeding, and fever.[10]

TABLE 28.5   Common Laboratory Studies of Pancreatic Function

Test	Normal Value	Clinical Significance
Serum amylase	60–180 Somogyi units/mL	Elevated levels with pancreatic inflammation
Serum lipase	1.5 Somogyi units/mL	Elevated levels with pancreatic inflammation (may be elevated with other conditions; differentiates with amylase, isoenzyme study)
Urine amylase	35–260 Somogyi units/h	Elevated levels with pancreatic inflammation
Secretin test	Volume 1.8 mL/kg/h, Bicarbonate concentration: >80 mEq/L, Bicarbonate output: >10 mEq/L/30 s	Decreased volume with pancreatic disease because secretin stimulates pancreatic secretion
Stool fat	2–5 g/25 h	Measures fatty acids: decreased pancreatic lipase increases stool fat

From McCance KL, et al, eds. *Pathophysiology: The Biologic Basis for Disease in Adults and Children.* 7th ed. St. Louis: Elsevier; 2014.

Angiography

Angiography is used as a diagnostic and a therapeutic procedure. Diagnostically, it is used to evaluate the status of the GI circulation (Fig. 28.6).[8] Therapeutically, it is used to achieve transcatheter control of GI bleeding.[11] Angiography may be used for lower GI bleeding and as a way to isolate the bleeding source before surgery. Angiography is used in the diagnosis of upper GI bleeding only when endoscopy fails, and it is used to treat patients (approximately 15%) whose GI bleeding is not stopped with medical measures or endoscopic treatment.[11] Angiography also is used to evaluate cirrhosis, portal hypertension, intestinal ischemia, and other vascular abnormalities.[8]

The radiologist cannulates the femoral artery with a needle and passes a guidewire through it into the aorta. The needle is removed, and an angiographic catheter is inserted over the guidewire. The catheter is advanced into the vessel supplying the portion of the GI tract that is being studied. After the catheter is in place, contrast medium is injected, and serial radiographs are obtained. If the procedure is undertaken to control bleeding, vasopressin (Pitressin Synthetic) or embolic material (Gelfoam) is injected after the site of the bleeding is located.[11]

Nursing Management

Complications include overt and covert bleeding at the femoral puncture site, neurovascular compromise of the affected leg, and sensitivity to the contrast medium. Before the procedure, the patient should be asked about any sensitivity to contrast medium. Assessment after the procedure involves monitoring vital signs, observing the injection site for bleeding, and assessing neurovascular integrity distal to the injection site every 15 minutes for the first 1 to 2 hours. Depending on how the puncture site is stabilized after the procedure, the patient may have to remain flat in bed for a specified length of time. Any evidence

FIG. 28.5 Endoscopic Appearance of a Mallory-Weiss Tear With Mild Oozing. The tear starts at the gastroesophageal junction *(large arrow)* and extends distally into the hiatal hernia *(small arrow).* (From Feldman M, et al. *Sleisenger and Fordtran's Gastrointestinal and Liver Disease.* 10th ed. Philadelphia: Elsevier; 2016.)

FIG. 28.6 Arteriogram of Superior Mesenteric Artery Shows Diverticular Bleeding. Note the area of contrast extravasation. (From Doughty DB, Jackson DB. *Gastrointestinal Disorders.* St. Louis: Mosby; 1993.)

of bleeding or neurovascular impairment must be immediately reported to the physician.[12]

Plain Abdominal Series

Although numerous radiologic studies are available to investigate GI dysfunction further, many of these studies are not performed on critically ill patients because of hemodynamic instability. The radiologic study that is performed most often is the plain abdominal series (Fig. 28.7). An abdominal radiograph is useful in the diagnosis of bowel obstruction and perforation.[13]

Air in the bowel serves as a contrast medium to aid in the visualization of the bowel. Gas patterns (the presence of gas inside or outside the bowel lumen and the distribution of gas in dilated and nondilated bowel) are best revealed by plain radiographs. Common radiologic signs of free air in the abdomen include the presence of air on both sides of the bowel wall and the presence of air in the right upper quadrant anterior to the liver.[13] Free air in the abdomen suggests a perforated bowel, and the need for surgery is paramount. Table 28.6 lists common radiologic findings. Abdominal radiographs are used to verify nasogastric or feeding tube placement.

Nursing Management

An abdominal radiographic series can be obtained at the patient's bedside using a portable x-ray machine. The series includes two views of the abdomen: one in the supine position and one in the upright position. For patients unable to sit upright, a lateral decubitus radiograph may be obtained with the patient's left side down. No special interventions are required before or after the procedure.[12]

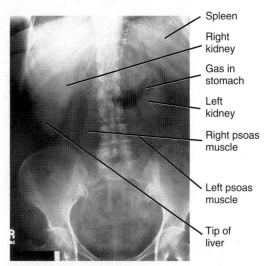

FIG. 28.7 Abdominal Flat Plate Radiograph. Note the air in the patient's stomach. (From Mettler FA. *Essentials of Radiology*. 3rd ed. Philadelphia: Elsevier; 2014.)

TABLE 28.6   Plain Film Findings

Finding	Appearance	Associations
Pneumoperitoneum	Air seen under diaphragm on upright chest or overlying right lobe of liver on left lateral decubitus films	Most commonly associated with bowel perforation, although other causes exist
Peritoneal fluid	Medial displacement of colon separated from flank stripes by fluid density on flat plate	Ascites or hemorrhage
Adynamic ileus	Dilatation of entire intestinal tract, including stomach	Many causes, including trauma, infection (intraabdominal and extraabdominal), metabolic disease, and medications (eg, narcotics)
Sentinel loop	Single distended loop of small bowel containing air-fluid level	Represents localized ileus associated with localized inflammatory process such as cholecystitis, appendicitis, or pancreatitis
Small bowel obstruction	Dilated loops of small bowel (distinguished by valvulae conniventes, thin, transverse linear densities that extend completely across diameter of bowel) with air-fluid levels	Can be associated with other serious pathology such as incarcerated hernia, appendicitis, or mesenteric ischemia
Large bowel obstruction	Dilated loops, usually more peripheral in abdomen (distinguished by haustra—short, thick indentations that do not completely cross bowel and are less frequently spaced than valvulae conniventes)	Can be associated with diverticulitis and malignancy
Cecal volvulus	Usually found in middle or upper abdomen to the left; often kidney-shaped	
Sigmoid volvulus	Dilated loop of colon arising from left side of pelvis and projecting obliquely upward toward right side of abdomen	
Early ischemic bowel findings	May resemble mechanical obstruction with dilated loops and air-fluid levels	
Later ischemic bowel findings	May resemble adynamic ileus; thumbprinting (edema of bowel wall with convex indentations of lumen) and pneumatosis intestinalis (linear or mottled gas pattern in bowel wall)	
Gallbladder emergency findings	Ring of air outlining gallbladder	Emphysematous cholecystitis
	Air in biliary tree combined with signs of small bowel obstruction, possibly with visible calculus in pelvis	Gallstone ileus
AAA	Usually appears left of midline on supine film and anterior to spine in lateral projection; calcification in wall of aneurysm is variable	Ruptured or leaking AAA may reveal loss of psoas shadows or large soft tissue mass

AAA, abdominal aortic aneurysm.
From Hendrickson M, Naparst TR. Abdominal surgical emergencies in the elderly. *Emerg Med Clin North Am.* 2003;21(4):937–969.

FIG. 28.8 Abdominal CT. Abdominal CT scan in a patient with abundant (A) and little (B) intraabdominal fat. *1,* pancreas; *2,* gallbladder; *3,* crus of the diaphragm; *4,* aorta; *5,* superior mesenteric artery; *6,* inferior vena cava with left renal vein; *7,* left kidney; *8,* right kidney; *9,* liver; *10,* bowel; *11,* splenoportal confluence. (From Seeram E. *Computed Tomography: Physical Principles, Clinical Applications, and Quality Control.* 3rd ed. St. Louis: Saunders; 2009.)

Abdominal Ultrasound

Abdominal ultrasound is useful in evaluating the status of the gallbladder and biliary system, the liver, the spleen, and the pancreas. It plays a key role in the diagnosis of many acute abdominal conditions such as acute cholecystitis and biliary obstructions because it is sensitive in detecting obstructive lesions and ascites. Ultrasound is used to identify gallstones and hepatic abscesses, candidiasis, and hematomas. Intestinal gas, ascites, and extreme obesity can interfere with transmission of the sound waves and limit the usefulness of the procedure.[14]

The procedure uses sound waves to produce echoes that are converted into electrical energy and transferred to a screen for viewing. A transducer, which emits and receives sound waves, is moved slowly over the area of the abdomen being studied. Tissues with various densities produce different echoes, which translate into the different structures on the viewing screen.[15]

Nursing Management

An ultrasound scan can be obtained at the patient's bedside using a portable scanning unit. Ultrasound is easily performed, noninvasive, and well tolerated even by critically ill patients. The procedure requires only that the patient lie still for 20 to 30 minutes. No special interventions are required before or after the procedure.[12]

Computed Tomography of the Abdomen

Computed tomography (CT) is a radiographic examination that provides cross-sectional images of internal anatomy (Fig. 28.8).

It may be used to evaluate abdominal vasculature and identify focal points found on nuclear scans as solid, cystic, inflammatory, or vascular.[15] CT detects mass lesions greater than 2 cm in diameter and allows visualization and evaluation of many different aspects of GI disease. It is particularly useful in identifying pancreatic pseudocysts, abdominal abscesses, appendicitis, biliary obstructions, and various GI neoplastic lesions.[16]

The procedure involves taking the patient to the CT scanner, placing the patient on the table, and inserting the area to be studied into the opening of the scanner. Multiple scans are obtained at various angles, and a computer synthesizes images of the structures being studied. Intravenous or GI contrast medium may be used to facilitate imaging of the blood vessels or the GI tract, respectively.[15]

Nursing Management

Before the procedure, the patient should be asked about any sensitivity to contrast medium. The procedure usually takes 30 minutes without contrast medium and 60 minutes with contrast medium, during which time the patient must lie still. No special interventions are required before or after the procedure.[11]

Hepatobiliary Scintigraphy

A hepatobiliary scan is a nuclear scan that is used to assess the status of the liver and the biliary system. It is valuable in detecting GI abnormalities such as acute and chronic cholecystitis, biliary obstruction, and bile leaks, and it yields additional information about organ size.[16]

The scan involves injecting an intravenous technetium-99m (^{99m}Tc)–labeled iminodiacetic agent (radiotracer), such as disofenin (^{99m}Tc DISIDA) or mebrofenin (^{99m}Tc TMBIDA). Serial images are obtained using a gamma (scintillation) camera. The liver cells take up 80% to 90% of the radiotracer, which is then secreted into the bile and transported throughout the biliary system, allowing visualization of the biliary tract, the gallbladder, and the duodenum.[17] Pooling of the iminodiacetic agent around the liver indicates poor uptake and hepatocellular dysfunction.[16]

Nursing Management

The hepatobiliary scan is relatively noninvasive and safe, although the patient must be transported to the nuclear medicine department. The patient may need to maintain NPO status for 2 to 4 hours before the procedure. Sedation is usually not required, but the patient must be able to lie flat and remain still for 60 minutes during the scanning procedure. No special interventions are required after the procedure.[11]

Gastrointestinal Bleeding Scan

A GI bleeding scan is used to evaluate the presence of an active bleed, to identify the site of the bleed, and to assess the need for an arteriogram.[18] The GI bleeding scan is sensitive to low rates of bleeding (0.1 mL/min), but it is reliable only when the patient is actively bleeding and may need to be repeated in 1 to 2 days.[8,18]

The scan is usually performed with intravenous ^{99m}Tc-labeled sulfur colloid or ^{99m}Tc-labeled red blood cells (radiotracers). To tag the red blood cells, a blood sample is taken from the patient. The red blood cells are separated, tagged with ^{99m}Tc, and returned to the patient. Serial images are obtained using a gamma (scintillation) camera. Extravasation and accumulation or pooling of radiotracers in the bowel lumen indicates active bleeding is occurring and facilitates identification of the site.[8,18]

Nursing Management

The GI bleeding scan is relatively noninvasive and safe, although the patient must be transported to the nuclear medicine department. Sedation usually is not required, but the patient must be able to lie flat and remain still for 60 minutes or longer during the scanning procedure. No special interventions are required after the procedure.[12]

Magnetic Resonance Imaging

Magnetic resonance imaging (MRI) is used to identify tumors, abscesses, hemorrhages, and vascular abnormalities. Small tumors, whose tissue densities are different from those of the surrounding cells, can be identified before they would be visible on any other radiographic test.[8] Magnetic resonance angiography is a form of MRI that is used to assess blood vessels and blood flow.[15] Magnetic resonance cholangiopancreatography is a form of MRI used to evaluate the biliary and pancreatic ducts.[19]

During MRI, the patient is placed in a large magnetic field that stimulates the protons of the body. Introduction of radiofrequency waves causes resonance of these protons, which then emit an image that a computer is able to reconstruct for viewing. Intravenous administration of a non–iodine-based contrast medium enhances the image by influencing the magnetic environment and signal intensity.[15]

Nursing Management

The MRI procedure is lengthy and requires that the patient be transported to the scanner. The patient must lie motionless in a tight, enclosed space (if a closed MRI scanner is used), and sedation may be necessary. Removal of all metal from the patient's body is essential because the basis of MRI is a magnetic field. Patients with implanted metal objects are not candidates for the procedure. No special interventions are required after the procedure.[12]

Percutaneous Liver Biopsy

Liver biopsy is a diagnostic procedure that is used to evaluate liver disease. Morphologic, biochemical, bacteriologic, and immunologic studies are performed on the tissue sample to diagnose liver disorders such as cirrhosis, hepatitis, infections, or cancer. A biopsy can also yield information about the progression of the patient's disease and response to therapy.[8,20]

Percutaneous liver biopsy can be performed at the bedside or in the imaging department and involves the use of an imaging-guided needle.[21] Before the test, the patient should maintain NPO status for 6 hours and have blood drawn for coagulation studies. The procedure is performed by anesthetizing the pericapsular tissue, inserting a coring or suction needle between the eighth and ninth intercostal space into the liver while the patient holds his or her breath on exhalation, withdrawing the needle with the sample, and applying pressure to stop the bleeding.[8]

Nursing Management

During liver biopsy, the patient may experience a deep pressure sensation or dull pain that radiates to the right shoulder. After the procedure, the patient is positioned on the right side for 2 hours and kept on complete bed rest for the next 6 to 8 hours.[8,20] Hemorrhage is the major complication associated with liver biopsy, although it occurs in less than 1% of patients. Other complications include damage to neighboring organs (eg, kidney, lung, colon, gallbladder), bile peritonitis, hemothorax, and infection at the needle site. Puncturing of the gallbladder can cause leakage of bile into the abdominal cavity, resulting in peritonitis.[20]

SUMMARY

History

- A review of the patient's current illness and symptoms, including the presence or absence of bleeding, abdominal pain, and dysphagia, is an important part of obtaining the patient's history.
- If the patient's condition permits, additional information regarding the patient's personal and social status; general health status, including nutritional intake, oral hygiene, and bowel elimination; and family history should be obtained.

Focused Clinical Assessment

- To prevent stimulation of GI activity, the order for the assessment should be changed to inspection, auscultation, percussion, and palpation.
- Inspection should focus on the oral cavity, skin, and abdomen.
- Auscultation provides clinical data on the status of bowel motility.
- Normal bowel sounds are high-pitched, gurgling sounds that occur approximately every 5 to 15 seconds, and colonic sounds are low-pitched sounds with a rumbling quality.

- Percussion is used to elicit information about deep organs, such as liver, spleen, and pancreas.
- Light and deep palpation methods are used to detect pathologic conditions of the abdomen.

Laboratory Studies

- No single laboratory study provides an overall picture of the functional state of the various organs.

Diagnostic Procedures

- Fiberoptic endoscopy is a diagnostic procedure for direct visualization and evaluation of the GI tract.
- Angiography is used diagnostically to evaluate the status of GI circulation and therapeutically to achieve control of GI bleeding.
- An abdominal radiograph is useful in the diagnosis of a bowel obstruction and perforation.
- Abdominal ultrasound is used to evaluate the status of the gallbladder and biliary system, the liver, the spleen, and the pancreas.
- CT provides cross-sectional images of the internal anatomy of the abdomen and is used to evaluate abdominal vasculature and identify focal points found on nuclear scans as solid, cystic, inflammatory, or vascular.
- A hepatobiliary scan is a nuclear scan that is used to assess the status of the liver and biliary system.
- A GI bleeding scan is used to evaluate the presence of an active GI bleed, to identify the site of the bleed, and to assess the need for arteriography.
- MRI is used to identify tumors, abscesses, hemorrhages, and vascular abnormalities.
- Liver biopsy is a diagnostic procedure that is used to evaluate liver disease.

ⓔ Visit the Evolve site for additional study materials.

REFERENCES

1. O'Toole MT. Advanced assessment of the abdomen and gastrointestinal problems. *Nurs Clin North Am.* 1990;25(4):771-779.
2. Baid H. The process of conducting a physical assessment: a nursing perspective. *Br J Nurs.* 2006;15(13):710-714.
3. Ball JW, et al. *Seidels's Guide to Physical Examination.* ed 8. St. Louis: Mosby; 2015.
4. Barkauskas V, Baumann L, Darling-Fisher C. *Health and Physical Assessment.* ed 3. St. Louis: Mosby; 2002.
5. Webber JR, Kelley JH. *Health Assessment in Nursing.* ed 5. Philadelphia: Lippincott; 2014.
6. Thompson JM, McFarland GK. *Mosby's Clinical Nursing.* ed 5. St. Louis: Mosby; 2002.
7. O'Hanlon-Nicholas T. Basic assessment series: gastrointestinal system. *Am J Nurs.* 1998;98(4):48-53.
8. Society of Gastroenterology Nurses and Associates. *Gastroenterology Nursing: A Core Curriculum.* ed 4. St. Louis: Society of Gastroenterology Nurses and Associates; 2008.
9. Hwang JH, et al. The role of endoscopy in the management of acute non-variceal upper GI bleeding. *Gastrointest Endosc.* 2012;75(6):1135-1138.
10. Ginzburg L, Greenwald D, Cohen J. Complications of endoscopy. *Gastrointest Endosc Clin North Am.* 2007;17(2):405-432.
11. Walker TG, Salazar GM, Waltman AC. Angiographic evaluation and management of acute gastrointestinal hemorrhage. *World J Gastroenterol.* 2012;18(11):1191-1201.
12. Pangana KD, Pangana TJ, Pagana TN. *Mosby's Diagnostic and Laboratory Test Reference.* ed 12. St. Louis: Mosby; 2015.
13. Iaselli F, et al. Bowel and mesenteric injuries from blunt abdominal trauma: a review. *Radiol Med.* 2015;120(1):21-32.
14. Godfrey EM, Rushbrook SM, Carrol NR. Endoscopic ultrasound: a review of current diagnostic and therapeutic applications. *Postgrad Med J.* 2010;86(1016):346-353.
15. Cogbill TH, Ziegelbein KJ. Computed tomography, magnetic resonance and ultrasound imaging: basic principles, glossary of terms and patient safety. *Surg Clin North Am.* 2011;91(1):1-14.
16. McSweeney SE, O'Donoghue PM, Jhaveri K. Current and emerging techniques in gastrointestinal imaging. *J Postgrad Med.* 2010;56(2):109-116.
17. Lambie H, et al. Tc99m-hepatobiliary iminodiacetic acid (HIDA) scintigraphy in clinical practice. *Clin Radiol.* 2011;66(11):1094-1105.
18. Mellinger JD, et al. Imaging of gastrointestinal bleeding. *Surg Clin North Am.* 2011;91(1):93-108.
19. Grand DF, Beland M, Harris A. Magnetic resonance enterography. *Radiol Clin North Am.* 2013;51(1):99-112.
20. Sargent S, Farrington E. Percutaneous liver biopsy: an overview. *Gastrointest Nurs.* 2011;9(5):35-40.
21. Lipnik AJ, Brown DB. Image-guided percutaneous abdominal mass biopsy. *Radiol Clin North Am.* 2015;53(5):1049-1059.

Gastrointestinal Disorders and Therapeutic Management

Jacqueline Fitzgerald Close

Understanding the pathology of a disease, the areas of assessment on which to focus, and the usual medical management allows the critical care nurse to accurately anticipate and plan nursing interventions. This chapter focuses on gastrointestinal (GI) disorders commonly seen in the critical care environment.

ACUTE GASTROINTESTINAL HEMORRHAGE

Description

GI hemorrhage is a potentially life-threatening emergency and a common complication of critical illness; it results in more than 300,000 hospital admissions yearly.[1] Despite advances in medical knowledge and nursing care, the mortality rate for patients with acute GI bleeding remains at 10% per annum in the United States.[1]

Etiology

GI hemorrhage occurs from bleeding in the upper or lower GI tract. The ligament of Treitz is the anatomic division used to differentiate between the two areas. Bleeding proximal to the ligament is considered to be from the upper GI tract, and bleeding distal to the ligament is considered to be from the lower GI tract.[1-3] The various causes of acute GI hemorrhage are listed in Box 29.1.[4] Only the three main causes of GI hemorrhage commonly seen in the critical care unit are discussed further.

Peptic Ulcer Disease

Peptic ulcer disease (ie, gastric and duodenal ulcers), which results from the breakdown of the gastromucosal lining, is the leading cause of upper GI hemorrhage, accounting for approximately 40% of cases.[5,6] Normally, protection of the gastric mucosa from the digestive effects of gastric secretions is accomplished in several ways. First, the gastroduodenal mucosa is coated by a glycoprotein mucous barrier that protects the surface of the epithelium from hydrogen ions and other noxious substances present in the gut lumen.[6-8] Adequate gastric mucosal blood flow is necessary to maintain this mucosal barrier function. Second, gastroduodenal epithelial cells are protected structurally against damage from acid and pepsin because they are connected by tight junctions that help prevent acid penetration. Third, prostaglandins and nitric oxide protect the mucosal barrier by stimulating the secretion of mucus and bicarbonate and inhibiting the secretion of acid.[6-8]

Peptic ulceration occurs when these protective mechanisms cease to function, allowing gastroduodenal mucosal breakdown. After the mucosal lining is penetrated, gastric secretions autodigest the layers of the stomach or duodenum, leading to injury of the mucosal and submucosal layers. This results in damaged blood vessels and subsequent hemorrhage. The two main causes of disruption of gastroduodenal mucosal resistance are the bacterial action of *Helicobacter pylori* and nonsteroidal antiinflammatory drugs.[9]

Stress-Related Mucosal Disease

Stress-related mucosal disease (SRMD) is an acute erosive gastritis that covers both types of mucosal lesions that are often found in critically ill patients: stress-related injury and discrete stress ulcers.[10-12] Additional terms used to describe this condition include *stress ulcers, stress erosions, stress gastritis, hemorrhagic gastritis,* and *erosive gastritis.* These abnormalities develop within hours of admission and range from superficial mucosal erosions to deep focal lesions and usually affect the upper GI tract.[11] SRMD occurs by means of the same pathophysiologic mechanisms as peptic ulcer disease, but the main cause of disruption of gastric mucosal resistance is increased acid production and decreased mucosal blood flow, resulting in ischemia and degeneration of the mucosal lining.[11] Patients at risk include patients in situations of high physiologic stress, as occurs with mechanical ventilation, extensive burns, severe trauma, major surgery, shock, sepsis, coagulopathy, or acute neurologic disease.[13] SRMD is decreasing in incidence because of advances in therapeutic techniques and prevention of hypoperfusion of the mucosa.[14]

Esophagogastric Varices

Esophagogastric varices are engorged and distended blood vessels of the esophagus and proximal stomach that develop as a result of portal hypertension caused by hepatic cirrhosis, a

---

BOX 29.1	Causes of Acute Gastrointestinal Hemorrhage	
Upper Gastrointestinal Tract	**Lower Gastrointestinal Tract**
Peptic ulcer disease	Diverticulosis
Stress-related erosive syndrome	Angiodysplasia
Esophagogastric varices	Neoplasm
Mallory-Weiss tear	Inflammatory bowel disease
Esophagitis	Trauma
Neoplasm	Infectious colitis
Aortoenteric fistula	Radiation colitis
Angiodysplasia	Ischemia
	Aortoenteric fistula
	Hemorrhoids

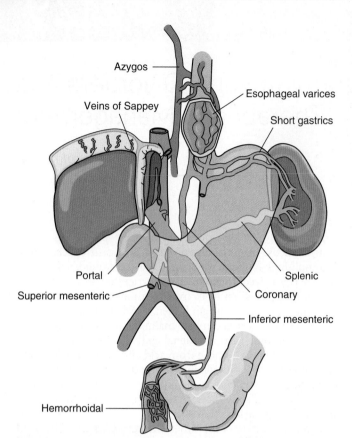

Azygos

Veins of Sappey

Esophageal varices

Short gastrics

Portal

Superior mesenteric

Splenic

Coronary

Inferior mesenteric

Hemorrhoidal

FIG. 29.1 Varices Related to Portal Hypertension. Portal vein, its major tributaries, and the most important shunts (collateral veins) between the portal and caval systems. (From Monahan FD, et al. *Phipps' Medical-Surgical Nursing: Concepts and Clinical Practice.* 8th ed. St. Louis: Mosby; 2007.)

chronic disease of the liver that results in damage to the liver sinusoids (Fig. 29.1). Without adequate sinusoid function, resistance to portal blood flow is increased, and pressures within the liver are elevated. This leads to increased portal venous pressure (portal hypertension), causing collateral circulation to divert portal blood from areas of high pressure within the liver to adjacent areas of low pressure outside the liver, such as into the veins of the esophagus, spleen, intestines, and stomach. The tiny, thin-walled vessels of the esophagus and proximal stomach that receive this diverted blood lack sturdy mucosal protection. The vessels become engorged and dilated, forming esophago-gastric varices that are vulnerable to damage from gastric secretions and that may result in subsequent rupture and massive hemorrhage.[15] The risk of variceal bleeding increases with disease severity and variceal size, but overall, bleeding occurs in 25% to 30% of patients within 2 years of diagnosis, with 20% to 30% mortality from each bleeding episode.[16,17]

Pathophysiology

GI hemorrhage is a life-threatening disorder that is characterized by acute, massive bleeding. Regardless of the cause, acute GI hemorrhage results in hypovolemic shock, initiation of the shock response, and development of multiple organ dysfunction syndrome if left untreated (see Concept Map, Fig. 29.2).[7] However, the most common cause of death in cases of GI hemorrhage is exacerbation of the underlying disease, not intractable hypovolemic shock.

Assessment and Diagnosis

The initial clinical presentation of a patient with acute GI hemorrhage is that of a patient in hypovolemic shock, and the clinical presentation depends on the amount of blood lost (Table 29.1).[2] Hematemesis (bright red or brown, "coffee grounds" emesis), hematochezia (bright red stools), and melena (black, tarry, or dark red stools) are the hallmarks of GI hemorrhage.[2,18]

Hematemesis

A patient who is vomiting blood is usually bleeding from a source above the duodenojejunal junction; reverse peristalsis is seldom sufficient to cause hematemesis if the bleeding point is below this area. The hematemesis may be bright red or look like coffee grounds, depending on the amount of gastric contents at the time of bleeding and the length of time the blood has been in contact with gastric secretions. Gastric acid converts bright red hemoglobin to brown hematin, accounting for the "coffee grounds" appearance of the emesis. Bright red emesis results from profuse bleeding with little contact with gastric secretions.[19]

Hematochezia and Melena

The presence of blood in the GI tract results in increased peristalsis and diarrhea. Hematochezia occurs from massive lower GI hemorrhage and, if rapid enough, upper GI hemorrhage. Melena occurs from digestion of blood from an upper GI hemorrhage and may take several days to clear after the bleeding has stopped.

Laboratory Studies

Laboratory tests can help determine the extent of bleeding, although the patient's hemoglobin level and hematocrit are poor indicators of the severity of blood loss if the bleeding is acute. As whole blood is lost, plasma and red blood cells are lost in the same proportion; if the patient's hematocrit is 45% before a bleeding episode, it will be 45% several hours later.[7] It may take 24 to 72 hours for the redistribution of plasma from the extravascular space to the intravascular space to occur and cause the patient's hemoglobin level and hematocrit value to decrease.[19]

Diagnostic Procedures

To isolate and treat the source of bleeding, an urgent fiber-optic endoscopy is usually undertaken.[20] Before endoscopy, the patient must be hemodynamically stabilized.[21] Tagged red blood cell scanning, angiography, or both may be done to assist with localizing and treating a bleeding lesion in the GI tract when it is impossible to clearly view the GI tract because of continued active bleeding.[19]

Medical Management

Management of a patient at risk for GI hemorrhage may include prophylactic administration of pharmacologic agents for neutralization or suppression of gastric acids. These agents include histamine-2 (H_2) antagonists and proton-pump inhibitors (PPIs).[5,22] However, pharmacologic management to prevent stress ulcers is not without risks. Acid suppressive therapy is associated with increased bacterial colonization of the upper GI tract and increased risk of developing ventilator-associated pneumonia.[10] A meta-analysis suggested that patients who are receiving enteral feedings may not require stress ulcer prophylaxis.[10] Priorities in the medical management of a patient with

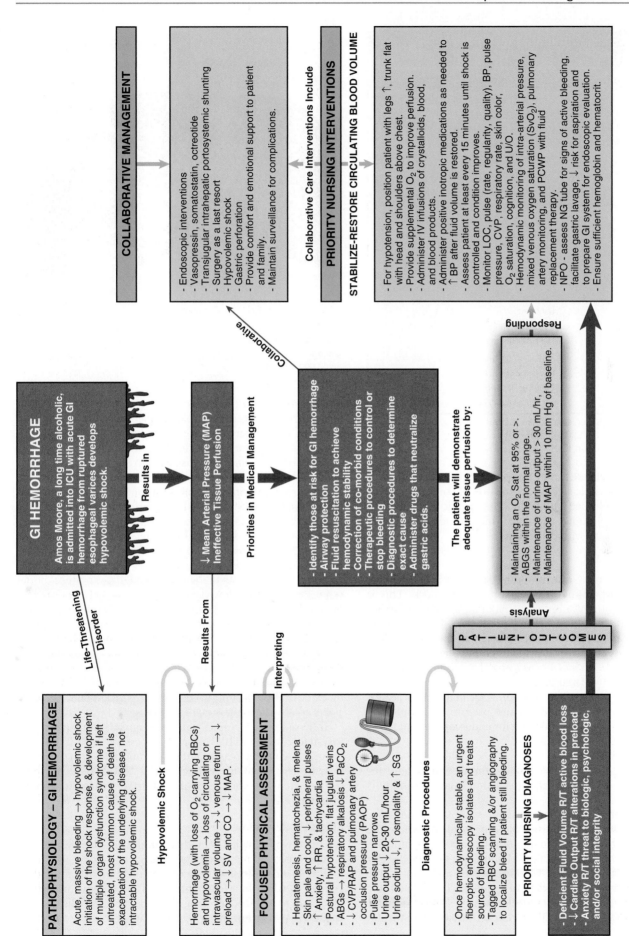

COLLABORATIVE MANAGEMENT

- Endoscopic interventions
- Vasopressin, somatostatin, octreotide
- Transjugular intrahepatic portosystemic shunting
- Surgery as a last resort
- Hypovolemic shock
- Gastric perforation
- Provide comfort and emotional support to patient and family.
- Maintain surveillance for complications.

Collaborative Care Interventions Include

PRIORITY NURSING INTERVENTIONS

STABILIZE-RESTORE CIRCULATING BLOOD VOLUME

- For hypotension, position patient with legs ↑, trunk flat with head and shoulders above chest.
- Provide supplemental O_2 to improve perfusion.
- Administer IV infusions of crystalloids, blood, and blood products.
- Administer positive inotropic medications as needed to ↑ BP after fluid volume is restored.
- Assess patient at least every 15 minutes until shock is controlled and condition improves.
- Monitor LOC, pulse (rate, regularity, quality), BP, pulse pressure, CVP, respiratory rate, skin color, O_2 saturation, cognition, and U/O.
- Hemodynamic monitoring of intra-arterial pressure, mixed venous oxygen saturation (SvO_2), pulmonary artery monitoring, and PCWP with fluid replacement therapy.
- NPO - assess NG tube for signs of active bleeding, facilitate gastric lavage, ↓ risk for aspiration and to prepare GI system for endoscopic evaluation.
- Ensure sufficient hemoglobin and hematocrit.

Responding

GI HEMORRHAGE

Amos Moore, a long time alcoholic, is admitted into ICU with acute GI hemorrhage from ruptured esophageal varices develops hypovolemic shock.

Results in

↓ Mean Arterial Pressure (MAP) Ineffective Tissue Perfusion

Priorities in Medical Management

- Identify those at risk for GI hemorrhage
- Airway protection
- Fluid resuscitation to achieve hemodynamic stability
- Correction of co-morbid conditions
- Therapeutic procedures to control or stop bleeding
- Diagnostic procedures to determine exact cause
- Administer drugs that neutralize gastric acids.

The patient will demonstrate adequate tissue perfusion by:

- Maintaining an O_2 Sat at 95% or >.
- ABGS within the normal range.
- Maintenance of urine output > 30 mL/hr,
- Maintenance of MAP within 10 mm Hg of baseline.

Analysis

Collaborative

P A T I E N T   O U T C O M E S

PATHOPHYSIOLOGY – GI HEMORRHAGE

Acute, massive bleeding → hypovolemic shock, initiation of the shock response, & development of multiple organ dysfunction syndrome if left untreated, most common cause of death is exacerbation of the underlying disease, not intractable hypovolemic shock.

Life-Threatening Disorder

Hypovolemic Shock

Hemorrhage (with loss of O_2 carrying RBCs) and hypovolemia → loss of circulating or intravascular volume → ↓ venous return → ↓ preload → ↓ SV and CO → ↓ MAP.

Results From

Interpreting

FOCUSED PHYSICAL ASSESSMENT

- Hematemesis, hematochezia, & melena
- Skin pale and cool, ↓ peripheral pulses
- ↑ Anxiety, ↑ RR, & tachycardia
- Postural hypotension, flat jugular veins
- ABGs → respiratory alkalosis ↓ $PaCO_2$
- ↓ CVP/RAP and pulmonary artery occlusion pressure (PAOP)
- Pulse pressure narrows
- Urine output ↓ 20-30 mL/hour
- Urine sodium ↓, ↑ osmolality & ↑ SG

Diagnostic Procedures

- Once hemodynamically stable, an urgent fiberoptic endoscopy isolates and treats source of bleeding.
- Tagged RBC scanning &/or angiography to localize bleed if patient still bleeding.

PRIORITY NURSING DIAGNOSES

- Deficient Fluid Volume R/T active blood loss
- ↓ Cardiac Output R/T alterations in preload
- Anxiety R/T threat to biologic, psychologic, and/or social integrity

FIG. 29.2 Concept Map for Gastrointestinal Hemorrhage. (Illustrated by Deanne A. Blach, RN MSN.)

TABLE 29.1 Clinical Classification of Hemorrhage

Class	Blood Loss (%)	Clinical Signs and Symptoms
1	≤15	Pulse rate: normal or <100 beats/min (supine) Capillary refill <3 s Urine output: adequate (30–35 mL/h) Orthostatic hypotension Apprehensive
2	15–30	Pulse rate: increased (>100 beats/min) Capillary refill: sluggish Pulse pressure: decreased Blood pressure: normal (supine) Tachypnea Urine output: low (25–30 mL/h)
3	30–40	Pulse rate: ≥120 beats/min (supine) Hypotension Skin: cool, pale Confused Hyperventilating Urine output: low (5–15 mL/h)
4	≥40	Profoundly hypotensive Pulse rate: ≥140 beats/min Confused, lethargic Urine output minimal

From Klein DG. Physiologic response to traumatic shock. *AACN Clin Issues Crit Care Nurs.* 1990;1(3):505–521.

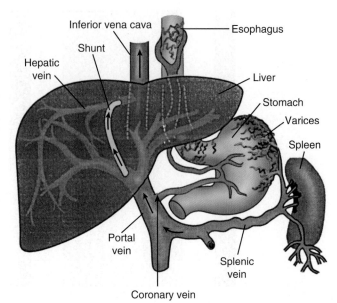

FIG. 29.3 Transjugular Intrahepatic Portosystemic Shunt (TIPS). Anatomic location of TIPS. (From Vargas HE, Gerber D, Abu-Elmagd K. Management of portal hypertension-related bleeding. *Surg Clin North Am.* 1999;79(1):1–22.)

GI hemorrhage include airway protection; fluid resuscitation to achieve hemodynamic stability; correction of comorbid conditions, if possible (eg, coagulopathy); therapeutic procedures to control or stop bleeding; and diagnostic procedures to determine the exact cause of the bleeding.[5,21]

Stabilization

The initial treatment priority is the restoration of adequate circulating blood volume to treat or prevent shock. This is accomplished with the administration of intravenous infusions of crystalloids, blood, and blood products.[22] Hemodynamic monitoring can help guide fluid replacement therapy, particularly in patients at risk for heart failure.[7] Supplemental oxygen therapy is initiated to increase oxygen delivery and improve tissue perfusion.[7,22] A large nasogastric tube may be inserted to confirm the diagnosis of active bleeding; facilitate gastric lavage; decrease the risk for aspiration; and prepare the esophagus, stomach, and proximal duodenum for endoscopic evaluation.[4]

Controlling Bleeding

Interventions to control bleeding are the second priority for a patient with GI hemorrhage after hemodynamic stability is achieved.

Peptic ulcer disease. In a patient with GI hemorrhage related to peptic ulcer disease, bleeding hemostasis may be accomplished by endoscopic injection therapy in conjunction with thermal or hemostatic clips.[20] Endoscopic thermal therapy uses heat to cauterize the bleeding vessel, and endoscopic injection therapy uses a variety of agents such as hypertonic saline, epinephrine, ethanol, and sclerosants to induce localized vasoconstriction of the bleeding vessel.[6] Intraarterial infusion

of vasopressin into the gastric artery or intraarterial injection of an embolizing agent (eg, Gelfoam pledgets, polyvinyl alcohol particles, coils) can be performed during arteriography to control bleeding after the site has been identified.[19]

Stress-related mucosal disease. In a patient with GI hemorrhage caused by SRMD, bleeding hemostasis may be accomplished by intraarterial infusion of vasopressin and intraarterial embolization. Endoscopic therapies provide minimal benefit because of the diffuse nature of the disease.[19]

Esophagogastric varices. In acute variceal hemorrhage, control of bleeding may be initially accomplished through the use of pharmacologic agents and endoscopic therapies. Intravenous vasopressin, somatostatin, and octreotide can reduce portal venous pressure and slow variceal hemorrhaging by constricting the splanchnic arteriolar bed.[16] Two commonly used endoscopic therapies are endoscopic injection sclerotherapy and endoscopic variceal ligation (EVL).[23] Endoscopic injection sclerotherapy controls bleeding by injection of a sclerosing agent in or around the varices. This creates an inflammatory reaction that induces vasoconstriction and results in the formation of a venous thrombosis. During EVL, bands are placed around the varices to create an obstruction to stop the bleeding.[24]

If these initial therapies fail, transjugular intrahepatic portosystemic shunt (TIPS) may be necessary. In a TIPS procedure, a channel between the systemic and portal venous systems is created to redirect portal blood, reducing portal hypertension and decompressing the varices to control bleeding (Fig. 29.3).[23,24]

Surgical Intervention

A patient who remains hemodynamically unstable despite volume replacement may need urgent surgery.

Peptic ulcer disease. Surgical intervention is required to control bleeding in a few patients.[25] The operative procedure of choice to control bleeding from peptic ulcer disease is a vagotomy and pyloroplasty. During this procedure, the vagus

FIG. 29.4 Portosystemic Shunt Operative Procedures. (From Copstead LC, Banasik JL. *Pathophysiology*. 5th ed. St. Louis: Elsevier; 2013.)

nerve to the stomach is severed, eliminating the autonomic stimulus to the gastric cells and reducing hydrochloric acid production. Because the vagus nerve also stimulates motility, a pyloroplasty is performed to provide for gastric emptying.[26]

Stress-related mucosal disease. In the past, several operative procedures were used to control bleeding from SRMD. Because of the advent of stress ulcer prophylaxis, the incidence of hemorrhage from SRMD is markedly decreased.[22]

Esophagogastric varices. If medical treatment is unsuccessful and angiographic interventional TIPS procedure is not available, operative procedures to control bleeding gastroesophageal varices may be undertaken. Although rarely performed, operative interventions focus on some form of shunting (Fig 29.4).[25] These shunt procedures are also referred to as *decompression procedures* because they result in the diversion of portal blood flow away from the liver and decompression of the portal system. The portacaval shunt procedure has two variations: (1) an *end-to-side portacaval shunt procedure*, which involves the ligation of the hepatic end of the portal vein with subsequent anastomosis to the vena cava, and (2) a *side-to-side portacaval shunt procedure*, during which the side of the portal vein is anastomosed to the side of the vena cava. A *mesocaval shunt procedure* involves the insertion of a graft between the superior mesenteric artery and the vena cava. During a *distal splenorenal shunt procedure*, the splenic vein

is detached from the portal vein and anastomosed to the left renal vein.[27]

Nursing Management

All critically ill patients should be considered at risk for stress ulcers and GI hemorrhage. Routine assessment of gastric fluid pH monitoring is controversial.[12,28] Maintaining the pH between 3.5 and 4.5 is a goal of prophylactic therapy. Gastric pH measurements made with litmus paper or direct nasogastric tube probes may be used to assess gastric fluid pH and the effectiveness or need for prophylactic agents.[28] Patients at risk also should be assessed for the presence of bright red or coffee grounds emesis; bloody nasogastric aspirate; and bright red, black, or dark red stools.[4] Any signs of bleeding should be promptly reported to the physician.

The nursing management plan for a patient experiencing acute GI hemorrhage incorporates a variety of nursing diagnoses (Box 29.2). The nurse plays a significant role in administering volume replacement, initiating gastric lavage, providing comfort and emotional support to the patient and the family, maintaining surveillance for complications, and educating the patient and family.

Administer Volume Replacement

Measures to facilitate volume replacement include obtaining intravenous access and administering prescribed fluids and

Acute Gastrointestinal Hemorrhage

- Deficient Fluid Volume related to absolute loss, p. 1019
- Decreased Cardiac Output related to alterations in preload, p. 1015
- Risk for Aspiration, p. 1040
- Imbalanced Nutrition: Less Than Body Requirements related to lack of exogenous nutrients and increased metabolic demand, p. 1029
- Risk for Infection, p. 1046
- Powerlessness, p. 1038
- Compromised Family Coping critically ill family member, p. 1014
- Deficient Knowledge related to lack of previous exposure to information, p. 1020 (see Patient Education Plan, Box 29.3)

blood products. Two large-diameter peripheral intravenous catheters should be inserted to facilitate the rapid administration of prescribed fluids.[1]

Initiate Gastric Lavage

One measure to prepare the patient for endoscopy is the initiation of gastric lavage. It is used to evacuate blood from the stomach and improve visualization during endoscopy. Gastric lavage is performed by inserting a large-bore nasogastric tube into the stomach and irrigating it with normal saline until the returned solution is clear. It is important to keep accurate records of the amount of fluid instilled and aspirated to ascertain the true amount of bleeding.[1] However, this practice has been called into question as unnecessary and is no longer routinely recommended.[29]

Maintain Surveillance for Complications

The patient should be continuously observed for signs of gastric perforation. Although a rare complication, gastric perforation constitutes a surgical emergency. Signs and symptoms include sudden, severe, generalized abdominal pain with significant rebound tenderness and rigidity. Perforation should be suspected when fever, leukocytosis, and tachycardia persist despite adequate volume replacement.[30]

Educate the Patient and Family

Early in the hospital stay, the patient and family should be taught about acute GI hemorrhage and its causes and treatments. Closer to discharge, teaching should focus on the interventions necessary for preventing the recurrence of the precipitating disorder and steps to take if another bleed should occur. If the patient abuses alcohol, the patient should be encouraged to stop drinking and be referred to an alcohol cessation program (Box 29.3).

Interprofessional collaborative management of the patient with acute GI hemorrhage is outlined in Box 29.4.

ACUTE PANCREATITIS

Description

Acute pancreatitis is an inflammation of the pancreas that produces exocrine and endocrine dysfunction that may also involve surrounding tissues, remote organ systems, or both. The clinical course can range from a mild, self-limiting disease to a systemic process characterized by organ failure,

Acute Gastrointestinal Hemorrhage

Before the patient's discharge, the patient should be able to teach back the following topics:
- Gastrointestinal hemorrhage
- Specific cause
- Precipitating factor modification
- Interventions to reduce further bleeding episodes
- Importance of taking medications
- Lifestyle changes
- Stress management
- Diet modifications
- Alcohol cessation
- Smoking cessation

Additional information for the patient can be found at the following websites:
- Alcoholics Anonymous: http://www.aa.org
- International Foundation for Functional Gastrointestinal Disorders: http://www.iffgd.org
- Healthfinder—US Department of Health and Human Services: http://healthfinder.gov
- Web MD: http://www.webmd.com

Interprofessional Collaborative Practice: Acute Gastrointestinal Hemorrhage

- Initiate fluid resuscitation to achieve hemodynamic stability.
  - Crystalloids
  - Colloids
  - Blood and blood products
- Determine the cause of bleeding.
  - Gastric lavage
- Control bleeding.
  - Endoscopic interventions
  - Vasopressin, somatostatin, octreotide
  - Transjugular intrahepatic portosystemic shunt
  - Surgery (last resort)
- Provide comfort and emotional support.
- Maintain surveillance for complications.
  - Hypovolemic shock
  - Gastric perforation

sepsis, and death. In approximately 80% of patients, it takes the milder form of *edematous interstitial pancreatitis*; the remaining 20% of patients develop severe *acute necrotizing pancreatitis*.[31] Reported mortality rates for acute pancreatitis range from 2% to 15% overall, with a steadily increasing rate of approximately 20,000 deaths per year in the United States.[32,33] Several prognostic scoring systems have been developed to predict the severity of acute pancreatitis. One of the most commonly used is Ranson criteria (Box 29.5).[34] If the patient has 0 to 2 factors present, the predicted mortality rate is 2%; with 3 to 4 factors, the rate is 15%; with 5 to 6 factors, the rate is 40%; and with 7 to 8 factors, the rate is 100%.[34-36]

BOX 29.5 Ranson Criteria

At Admission

- Age >55 years
- Hypotension
- Abnormal pulmonary findings
- Abdominal mass
- Hemorrhagic or discolored peritoneal fluid
- Increased serum LDH levels (>350 U/L)
- AST >250 U/L
- Leukocytosis (>16,000/mm³)
- Hyperglycemia (>200 mg/dL; no diabetes history)
- Neurologic deficit (confusion, localizing signs)

During Initial 48 Hours of Hospitalization

- Fall in hematocrit >10% with hydration or hematocrit <30%
- Necessity for massive fluid and colloid replacement
- Hypocalcemia (<8 mg/dL)
- Arterial P_{O_2} <60 mm Hg with or without acute respiratory distress syndrome
- Hypoalbuminemia (<3.2 mg/dL)
- Base deficit >4 mEq/L
- Azotemia

AST, aspartate aminotransferase; *LDH*, lactate dehydrogenase; P_{O_2}, partial pressure of oxygen.
From Latifi R, McIntosh JK, Dudrick SJ. Nutritional management of acute and chronic pancreatitis. *Surg Clin North Am.* 1991;71(3):579–595.

BOX 29.6 Causes of Acute Pancreatitis

- Biliary disease (stones, sludge, common bile duct obstruction)
- Toxins (ethyl alcohol, methyl alcohol, scorpion, venom, parathion)
- Smoking
- Medications
- Hypercalcemia (hyperparathyroidism)
- Hyperlipidemia
- Tumors
- Infections (bacterial, viral, parasitic)
- Trauma (abdominal, surgical, endoscopic)
- Hypoperfusion
- Vasculitis
- Pregnancy
- Hypothermia
- Sphincter of Oddi dysfunction
- Autoimmune diseases
- Ampullary stenosis
- Idiopathic cause

Etiology

The two most common causes of acute pancreatitis are gallstone migration and alcoholism.[36] Together, they account for approximately 80% of cases.[19] Less common causes are quite diverse and include surgical trauma, hypercalcemia, various toxins, ischemia, infections, and the use of certain medications (Box 29.6). In 20% of patients with acute pancreatitis, no etiologic factor can be determined.[19,31]

Pathophysiology

In acute pancreatitis, the normally inactive digestive enzymes become prematurely activated within the pancreas itself, leading to autodigestion of pancreatic tissue. The enzymes become

BOX 29.7 Clinical Manifestations of Acute Pancreatitis

- Pain
- Vomiting
- Nausea
- Fever
- Abdominal distention
- Abdominal guarding
- Abdominal tympany
- Hypoactive or absent bowel sounds
- Severe disease
- Peritoneal signs
- Ascites
- Jaundice
- Palpable abdominal mass
- Grey Turner sign
- Cullen sign
- Signs of hypovolemic shock

From Krumberger JM. Acute pancreatitis. *Crit Care Nurs Clin North Am.* 1993;5(1):185–202.

activated through various mechanisms, including obstruction of or damage to the pancreatic duct system, alterations in the secretory processes of the acinar cells, infection, ischemia, and other unknown factors.[7,36]

Trypsin is the enzyme that becomes activated first. It initiates the autodigestion process by triggering the secretion of proteolytic enzymes, such as kallikrein, chymotrypsin and elastase, phospholipase A, and lipase. Release of kallikrein and chymotrypsin results in increased capillary membrane permeability, leading to leakage of fluid into the interstitium and the development of edema and relative hypovolemia. Elastase is the most harmful enzyme in terms of direct cell damage. It dissolves the elastic fibers of blood vessels and ducts, leading to hemorrhage. Phospholipase A, in the presence of bile, destroys the phospholipids of cell membranes, causing severe pancreatic and adipose tissue necrosis. Lipase flows into the damaged tissue and is absorbed into the systemic circulation, resulting in fat necrosis of the pancreas and surrounding tissues.[7,37]

The extent of injury to the pancreatic cells determines the type of acute pancreatitis that develops. If injury to the pancreatic cells is mild and without necrosis, edematous pancreatitis develops. The acinar cells appear structurally intact, and blood flow is maintained through small capillaries and venules. This form of acute pancreatitis is self-limiting. If injury to the pancreatic cells is severe, acute necrotizing pancreatitis develops.[32,37] Cellular destruction in pancreatic injury results in the release of toxic enzymes and inflammatory mediators into the systemic circulation and causes injury to vessels and other organs distant from the pancreas; this may result in systemic inflammatory response syndrome, multiorgan failure, and death.[19,36] Local tissue injury results in infection, abscess and pseudocyst formation, disruption of the pancreatic duct, and severe hemorrhage and shock.[19]

Assessment and Diagnosis

The clinical manifestations of acute pancreatitis range from mild to severe and often mimic the manifestations of other disorders (Box 29.7). Acute onset of abdominal pain, nausea, and vomiting are hallmark symptoms.[19,32,37] Epigastric to peri-umbilical pain may vary from mild and tolerable to severe and incapacitating. Many patients report a twisting or knife-like sensation that radiates to the low dorsal region of the back. The patient may obtain some comfort by leaning forward or assuming a semifetal position. Other clinical findings include fever, diaphoresis, weakness, tachypnea, hypotension, and tachycardia. Depending on the extent of fluid loss and hemorrhage, the patient may exhibit signs of hypovolemic shock.[19,37]

Physical Examination

The results of physical assessment usually reveal hypoactive bowel sounds and abdominal tenderness, guarding, distention, and tympany. Findings that may indicate pancreatic hemorrhage include Grey Turner sign (gray-blue discoloration of the flanks) and Cullen sign (discoloration of the umbilical region); however, these signs are rare and usually seen several days into the illness.[19] A palpable abdominal mass indicates the presence of a pseudocyst or abscess.[19]

Laboratory Studies

Assessment of laboratory data usually demonstrates elevated levels of serum amylase and lipase. Serum lipase is more pancreas specific than amylase and a more accurate marker for acute pancreatitis. Amylase is present in other body tissues, and other disorders (eg, intraabdominal emergencies, renal insufficiency, salivary gland trauma, liver disease) may contribute to an elevated level. In contrast to other serum enzymes, amylase is excreted in urine, and this clearance increases with acute pancreatitis. Measurement of urinary versus serum amylase should be considered in light of the patient's creatinine clearance. The serum amylase level may be elevated for only 3 to 5 days; if the patient delays seeking treatment, a normal level (false-negative result) may be detected. A marker of severity may be determined with a serum cross-reactive (C-reactive) protein level.[19,38] Leukocytosis, hypocalcemia, hyperglycemia, hyperbilirubinemia, and hypoalbuminemia may also be present (Table 29.2).[19,36,38]

Diagnostic Procedures

An abdominal ultrasound scan is obtained as part of the diagnostic evaluation to determine the presence of biliary stones. Contrast-enhanced computed tomography (CT) is considered the gold standard for diagnosing pancreatitis and for ascertaining the overall degree of pancreatic inflammation and necrosis.[19,32]

Medical Management

Initial management of a patient with severe acute pancreatitis includes ensuring adequate pain management, fluid and electrolyte replacement, providing nutrition support, and correcting metabolic alterations.[35] Careful monitoring for systemic and local complications is critical. Current evidence-based guidelines for the management of a patient with acute pancreatitis are presented in Box 29.8.

Fluid Management

Because pancreatitis is often associated with massive fluid shifts, intravenous crystalloids and colloids are administered immediately to prevent hypovolemic shock and maintain hemodynamic stability. Electrolytes are monitored closely, and abnormalities

TABLE 29.2   Laboratory Tests and Diagnostic Procedures for Acute Pancreatitis

Study	Finding In Pancreatitis
Laboratory Studies	
Serum amylase	Elevated
Serum isoamylase	Elevated
Urine amylase	Elevated
Serum lipase (if available)	Elevated
Serum triglycerides	Elevated
Cross-reactive protein	Elevated
Glucose	Elevated
Calcium	Decreased
Magnesium	Decreased
Potassium	Decreased
Albumin	Decreased or increased
White blood cell count	Elevated
Bilirubin	May be elevated
Liver enzymes	May be elevated
Prothrombin time	Prolonged
Arterial blood gases	Hypoxemia, metabolic acidosis

Diagnostic Procedures
- Abdominal ultrasonography
- Computed tomography scan
- Magnetic resonance imaging
- Endoscopic retrograde cholangiopancreatography
- Abdominal radiographs (flat plate and upright or decubitus)
- Chest radiographs (posteroanterior and lateral)

Modified from Krumberger JM. Acute pancreatitis. *Crit Care Nurs Clin North Am.* 1993;5(1):185–202.

such as hypocalcemia, hypokalemia, and hypomagnesemia are corrected.[37] If hyperglycemia develops, exogenous insulin may be required.

Nutrition Support

Over the past 3 decades, nutrition support has shifted. Previously, conventional nutrition management was to place the patient on a nothing by mouth (NPO) regimen and institute intravenous hydration. The rationale was to rest the inflamed pancreas and prevent enzyme release. Enteral or parenteral support should be initiated if oral intake is withheld more than 5 to 7 days.[39] Randomized clinical trials have demonstrated that enteral feeding (gastric or jejunal) is safe and cost-effective and is associated with fewer septic and metabolic complications than other methods.[40-42] Enteral feeding enhances immune modulation and maintenance of the intestinal barrier, and it avoids complications associated with parenteral nutrition. Early initiation of enteral feeding is preferred over total parenteral nutrition.[39] However, total parenteral nutrition still has a role for critically ill patients with acute pancreatitis who do not tolerate enteral feeding or when nutrition goals are not reached within 2 days.[37,41,42] In the past, nasogastric suction was also recommended, but this intervention has not been shown to be beneficial and should be instituted only if the patient has persistent vomiting, obstruction, or gastric distention.[37]

QSEN BOX 29.8   QSEN: Evidence-Based Practice

Acute Pancreatitis Management Guidelines

A. Diagnosis of Acute Pancreatitis and Etiology

1. The definition of acute pancreatitis is based on the fulfillment of "2 out of 3" of the following criteria: clinical (upper abdominal pain), laboratory (serum amylase or lipase >3× upper limit of normal), or imaging (CT, MRI, ultrasonography) criteria. (GRADE 1B, strong agreement)

2. On admission, the etiology of acute pancreatitis should be determined using detailed personal (ie, previous acute pancreatitis, known gallstone disease, alcohol intake, medication and drug intake, known hyperlipidemia, trauma, recent invasive procedures such as ERCP) and family history of pancreatic disease, physical examination, laboratory serum tests (ie, liver enzymes, calcium, triglycerides), and imaging (ie, right upper quadrant ultrasonography). (GRADE 1B, strong agreement)

3. In patients considered to have idiopathic acute pancreatitis, after negative routine work-up for biliary etiology, EUS is recommended as the first step to assess for occult microlithiasis, neoplasms, and chronic pancreatitis. If EUS is negative, (secretin-stimulated) MRCP is advised as a second step to identify rare morphologic abnormalities. CT of the abdomen should be performed. If etiology remains unidentified, especially after a second attack of idiopathic pancreatitis, genetic counseling (not necessarily genetic testing) should be considered. (GRADE 2C, weak agreement)

B. Prognostication/Prediction of Severity

4. SIRS is advised to predict severe acute pancreatitis at admission and persistent SIRS at 48 hours. (GRADE 2B, weak agreement)

5. During admission, a three-dimension approach is advised to predict outcome of acute pancreatitis combining host risk factors (eg, age, comorbidity, body mass index), clinical risk stratification (eg, persistent SIRS), and monitoring response to initial therapy (eg, persistent SIRS, blood urea nitrogen, creatinine). (GRADE 2B, strong agreement)

C. Imaging

6. The indication for initial CT assessment in acute pancreatitis can be (1) diagnostic uncertainty, (2) confirmation of severity based on clinical predictors of severe acute pancreatitis, or (3) failure to respond to conservative treatment or in the setting of clinical deterioration. Optimal timing for initial CT assessment is at least 72–96 hours after onset of symptoms. (GRADE 1C, strong agreement)

7. Follow-up CT or MRI in acute pancreatitis is indicated when there is a lack of clinical improvement, when there is clinical deterioration, or especially when invasive intervention is considered. (GRADE 1C, strong agreement)

8. It is recommended to perform multidetector CT with thin collimation and slice thickness (ie, 5 mm or less), 100–150 mL of nonionic intravenous contrast material at a rate of 3 mL/s, during the pancreatic and/or portal venous phase (ie, 50–70 s delay). During follow-up, only a portal venous phase (monophasic) is generally sufficient. For MRI, the recommendation is to perform axial fat-saturated T2 and fat-saturated T1 scanning before and after intravenous gadolinium contrast administration. (GRADE 1C, strong agreement)

D. Fluid Therapy

9. Ringer lactate is recommended for initial fluid resuscitation in acute pancreatitis. (GRADE 1B, strong agreement)

10a. Goal-directed intravenous fluid therapy with 5–10 mL/kg/h should be used initially until resuscitation goals (see 10b) are reached. (GRADE 1B, weak agreement)

10b. The preferred approach to assessing the response to fluid resuscitation should be based on one or more of the following: (1) noninvasive clinical targets of heart rate <120 beats/min, mean arterial pressure 65–85 mm Hg (8.7–11.3 kPa), and urinary output >0.5–1 mL/kg/h; (2) invasive clinical targets of stroke volume variation and intrathoracic blood volume determination; and (3) biochemical targets of hematocrit 35%–44%. (GRADE 2B, weak agreement)

E. Intensive Care Management

11. Intensive care management is recommended for patients diagnosed with acute pancreatitis and one or more of the parameters identified at admission as defined by the guidelines of the Society of Critical Care Medicine. Furthermore, patients with severe acute pancreatitis as defined by the revised Atlanta Classification (ie, persistent organ failure) should be treated in an intensive care setting. (GRADE 1C, strong agreement)

12. Management in, or referral to, a specialist center is necessary for patients with severe acute pancreatitis and for those who may need interventional radiologic, endoscopic, or surgical intervention. (GRADE 1C, strong agreement)

13. A specialist center in the management of acute pancreatitis is defined as a high-volume center with up-to-date intensive care facilities including options for organ replacement therapy and with daily (ie, 7 days per week) access to interventional radiology, interventional endoscopy with EUS and ERCP assistance, and surgical expertise in managing necrotizing pancreatitis. Patients should be enrolled in prospective audits for quality control issues and into clinical trials whenever possible. (GRADE 2C, weak agreement)

14. Early fluid resuscitation within the first 24 hours of admission for acute pancreatitis is associated with decreased rates of persistent SIRS and organ failure. (GRADE 1C, strong agreement)

15. Abdominal compartment syndrome (ACS) is defined as a sustained intraabdominal pressure >20 mm Hg that is associated with new-onset organ failure. (GRADE 2B, strong agreement)

16. Medical treatment of ACS should target (1) hollow viscera volume, (2) intravascular/extravascular fluid, and (3) abdominal wall expansion. Invasive treatment should be used only after multidisciplinary discussion in patients with a sustained intraabdominal pressure >25 mm Hg with new-onset organ failure refractory to medical therapy and nasogastric/rectal decompression. Invasive treatment options include percutaneous catheter drainage of ascites, midline laparostomy, bilateral subcostal laparostomy, or subcutaneous linea alba fasciotomy. In case of surgical decompression, the retroperitoneal cavity and the omental bursa should be left intact to reduce the risk of infecting peripancreatic and pancreatic necrosis. (GRADE 2C, strong agreement)

F. Preventing Infectious Complications

17. Intravenous antibiotic prophylaxis is not recommended for the prevention of infectious complications in acute pancreatitis. (GRADE 1B, strong agreement)

18. Selective gut decontamination has shown some benefits in preventing infectious complications in acute pancreatitis, but further studies are needed. (GRADE 2B, weak agreement)

19. Probiotic prophylaxis is not recommended for the prevention of infectious complications in acute pancreatitis. (GRADE 1B, strong agreement)

G. Nutrition Support

20. Oral feeding in predicted mild pancreatitis can be restarted once abdominal pain is decreasing and inflammatory markers are improving. (GRADE 2B, strong agreement)

21. Enteral tube feeding should be the primary therapy in patients with predicted severe acute pancreatitis who require nutrition support. (GRADE 1B, strong agreement)

22. Either elemental or polymeric enteral nutrition formulations can be used in acute pancreatitis. (GRADE 2B, strong agreement)

23. Enteral nutrition in acute pancreatitis can be administered via either the nasojejunal or the nasogastric route. (GRADE 2A, strong agreement)

Continued

QSEN BOX 29.8   QSEN: Evidence-Based Practice—cont'd

Acute Pancreatitis Management Guidelines

24. Parenteral nutrition can be administered in acute pancreatitis as second-line therapy if nasojejunal tube feeding is not tolerated and nutrition support is required. (GRADE 2C, strong agreement)

H. Biliary Tract Management

25. ERCP is not indicated in predicted mild biliary pancreatitis without cholangitis. (GRADE 1A, strong agreement) ERCP is probably not indicated in predicted severe biliary pancreatitis without cholangitis. (GRADE 1B, strong agreement) ERCP is probably indicated in biliary pancreatitis with common bile duct obstruction. (GRADE 1C, strong agreement) ERCP is indicated in patients with biliary pancreatitis and cholangitis. (GRADE 1B, strong agreement)

26. Urgent ERCP (<24 h) is required in patients with acute cholangitis. Currently, there is no evidence regarding the optimal timing of ERCP in patients with biliary pancreatitis without cholangitis. (GRADE 2C, strong agreement)

27. MRCP and EUS may prevent a proportion of ERCPs that would otherwise be performed for suspected common bile duct stones in patients with biliary pancreatitis who do not have cholangitis, without influencing the clinical course. EUS is superior to MRCP in excluding the presence of small (<5 mm) gallstones. MRCP is less invasive, less operator-dependent, and probably more widely available than EUS. Therefore, in clinical practice there is no clear superiority for either MRCP or EUS. (GRADE 2C, strong agreement)

I. Indications for Intervention in Necrotizing Pancreatitis

28. Common indications for intervention (radiologic, endoscopic, or surgical) in necrotizing pancreatitis are (1) clinical suspicion of or documented infected necrotizing pancreatitis with clinical deterioration, preferably when the necrosis has become "walled-off," and (2) in the absence of documented infected necrotizing pancreatitis, ongoing organ failure for several weeks after the onset of acute pancreatitis, preferably when the necrosis has become walled-off. (GRADE 1C, strong agreement)

29. Routine percutaneous FNA of peripancreatic collections to detect bacteria is not indicated because clinical signs (ie, persistent fever, increasing inflammatory markers) and imaging signs (ie, gas in peripancreatic collections) are accurate predictors of infected necrosis in the majority of patients. Although the diagnosis of infection can be confirmed by FNA, there is a risk of false-negative results. (GRADE 1C, strong agreement)

30. Indications for intervention (radiologic, endoscopic, or surgical) in sterile necrotizing pancreatitis are (1) ongoing gastric outlet, intestinal, or biliary obstruction due to mass effect of walled-off necrosis (ie, arbitrarily >4–8 weeks after onset of acute pancreatitis); (2) persistent symptoms (eg, pain, "persistent unwellness") in patients with walled-off necrosis without signs of infection (ie, arbitrarily >8 weeks after onset of acute pancreatitis); and (3) disconnected duct syndrome (ie, full transection of the pancreatic duct in the presence of pancreatic necrosis) with persisting symptomatic (eg, pain, obstruction) collections with necrosis without signs of infection (ie, arbitrarily >8 weeks after onset of acute pancreatitis). (GRADE 2C, strong agreement)

J. Timing of Intervention in Necrotizing Pancreatitis

31. For patients with proven or suspected infected necrotizing pancreatitis, invasive intervention (ie, percutaneous catheter drainage, endoscopic transluminal drainage/necrosectomy, minimally invasive or open necrosectomy) should be delayed where possible until at least 4 weeks after initial presentation to allow the collection to become walled-off. (GRADE 1C, strong agreement)

32. The best available evidence suggests that surgical necrosectomy should ideally be delayed until collections have become walled-off, typically 4 weeks after the onset of pancreatitis, in all patients with complications of necrosis. No subgroups have been identified that might benefit from earlier or delayed intervention. (GRADE 1C, strong agreement)

K. Intervention Strategies in Necrotizing Pancreatitis

33. The optimal interventional strategy for patients with suspected or confirmed infected necrotizing pancreatitis is initial image-guided percutaneous (retroperitoneal) catheter drainage or endoscopic transluminal drainage, followed, if necessary, by endoscopic or surgical necrosectomy. (GRADE 1A, strong agreement)

34. Percutaneous catheter or endoscopic transmural drainage should be the first step in the treatment of patients with suspected or confirmed (walled-off) infected necrotizing pancreatitis. (GRADE 1A, strong agreement)

35. There are insufficient data to define subgroups of patients with suspected or confirmed infected necrotizing pancreatitis who would benefit from a different treatment strategy. (GRADE 2C, strong agreement)

L. Timing of Cholecystectomy (or Endoscopic Sphincterotomy)

36. Cholecystectomy during index admission for mild biliary pancreatitis appears safe and is recommended. Interval cholecystectomy after mild biliary pancreatitis is associated with a substantial risk of readmission for recurrent biliary events, especially recurrent biliary pancreatitis. (GRADE 1C, strong agreement)

37. Cholecystectomy should be delayed in patients with peripancreatic collections until the collections either resolve or persist beyond 6 weeks, at which time cholecystectomy can be performed safely. (GRADE 2C, strong agreement)

38. In patients with biliary pancreatitis who have undergone sphincterotomy and are fit for surgery, cholecystectomy is advised because ERCP and sphincterotomy prevent recurrence of biliary pancreatitis but not gallstone-related gallbladder disease (ie, biliary colic and cholecystitis). (GRADE 2B, strong agreement)

CT, computed tomography; *ERCP*, endoscopic retrograde cholangiopancreatography; *EUS*, endoscopic ultrasonography; *FNA*, fine-needle aspiration; *MRCP*, magnetic resonance cholangiopancreatography; *MRI*, magnetic resonance imaging; *SCCM*, Society of Critical Care Medicine; *SIRS*, systemic inflammatory response syndrome.
From Working Group IAP/APA Acute Pancreatitis Guidelines: IAP/APA evidence-based guidelines for the management of acute pancreatitis. *Pancreatology.* 2013;13(4 Suppl 2):e1–e15.

Systemic Complications

Acute pancreatitis can affect every organ system, and recognition and treatment of systemic complications are crucial to management of the patient (Box 29.9). The most serious complications are hypovolemic shock, acute respiratory distress syndrome (ARDS), acute kidney injury (AKI), and GI hemorrhage. Hypovolemic shock is the result of relative hypovolemia resulting from third spacing of intravascular volume and vasodilation caused by the release of inflammatory immune mediators. Fluid accumulates in the abdominal cavity resulting in intraabdominal hypertension and abdominal compartment syndrome.[43] Inflammatory mediators also contribute to the development of ARDS and AKI. Other possible pulmonary complications include pleural effusions, atelectasis, and pneumonia.[37]

BOX 29.9   Complications of Acute Pancreatitis

Respiratory
- Early hypoxemia
- Pleural effusion
- Atelectasis
- Pulmonary infiltration
- Acute respiratory distress syndrome
- Mediastinal abscess

Cardiovascular
- Hypotension and shock
- Pericardial effusion
- ST-T changes

Renal
- Acute tubular necrosis
- Oliguria
- Renal artery or vein thrombosis

Hematologic
- Disseminated intravascular coagulation
- Thrombocytosis
- Hyperfibrinogenemia

Endocrine
- Hypocalcemia
- Hypertriglyceridemia
- Hyperglycemia

Neurologic
- Fat emboli
- Psychosis
- Encephalopathy and coma

Ophthalmic
- Purtscher retinopathy (sudden blindness)

Dermatologic
- Subcutaneous fat necrosis

Gastrointestinal or Hepatic
- Intraabdominal hypertension/abdominal compartment syndrome
- Hepatic dysfunction
- Obstructive jaundice
- Stress ulceration
- Erosive gastritis
- Paralytic ileus
- Duodenal obstruction
- Pancreatic
  - Pseudocyst
  - Phlegmon
  - Abscess
  - Ascites
- Bowel infarction
- Massive intraperitoneal bleed
- Perforation
  - Stomach
  - Duodenum
  - Small bowel
  - Colon

◎ BOX 29.10   NURSING DIAGNOSES
Acute Pancreatitis

- Acute Pain related to transmission and perception of cutaneous, visceral, muscular, or ischemia impulses, p. 1010
- Deficient Fluid Volume related to relative fluid loss, p. 1019
- Decreased Cardiac Output related to alterations in preload, p. 1019
- Ineffective Breathing Pattern related to decreased lung expansion, p. 1035
- Imbalanced Nutrition: Less Than Body Requirements related to lack of exogenous nutrients or increased metabolic demand, p. 1029
- Anxiety related to threat to biologic, psychologic, or social integrity, p. 1012
- Compromised Family Coping related to critically ill family member, p. 1014
- Deficient Knowledge related to lack of previous exposure to information, p. 1020 (see Patient Education Plan, Box 29.11)

Local Complications

Local complications include the development of infected pancreatic necrosis and pancreatic pseudocyst.[19,32,38] The necrotic areas of the pancreas can lead to development of a widespread pancreatic infection (infected pancreatic necrosis), which significantly increases the risk of death.

Prophylactic antibiotics may not reduce mortality in patients suspected to have necrotizing pancreatitis.[44] Intravenous antibiotics should not be used prophylactically, but if sepsis, abscess, or biliary calculi are evident, they are indicated.[37] When the patient develops infected necrosis, surgical intervention is necessary.[36] The procedure of choice is a minimally invasive necrosectomy, which entails careful débridement of the necrotic tissue in and around the pancreas. A pancreatic pseudocyst is a collection of pancreatic fluid enclosed by a nonepithelialized wall. Cyst formation may result from liquefaction of a pancreatic fluid collection or from direct obstruction in the main pancreatic duct.[37] A pancreatic pseudocyst may (1) resolve spontaneously; (2) rupture, resulting in peritonitis; (3) erode a major blood vessel, resulting in hemorrhage; (4) become infected, resulting in abscess; or (5) invade surrounding structures, resulting in obstruction. Treatment involves drainage of the pseudocyst surgically, endoscopically, or percutaneously.[36,37,43]

Nursing Management

The nursing management plan for a patient with pancreatitis incorporates a variety of nursing diagnoses (Box 29.10). The nurse plays a significant role in providing comfort and emotional support, maintaining surveillance for complications, and educating the patient and family.

Provide Comfort and Emotional Support

Pain management is a major priority in acute pancreatitis. Administration of around-the-clock analgesics to achieve pain relief is essential. Morphine, fentanyl, and hydromorphone are the commonly used narcotics for pain control.[37] Relaxation techniques and the knee-chest position can also assist in pain control.

Maintain Surveillance for Complications

The patient is routinely monitored for signs of local or systemic complications (see Box 29.9). Intensive monitoring of each of the organ systems is imperative because organ failure is a major indicator of the severity of the disease.[19] Intraabdominal

BOX 29.11   PATIENT EDUCATION PLAN

Acute Pancreatitis

Before the patient's discharge, the patient should be able to teach back the following topics:

- Pancreatitis
- Specific cause
- Precipitating factor modification
- Interventions to reduce further episodes
- Importance of taking medications
- Lifestyle changes
- Diet modification
- Stress management
- Alcohol cessation
- Diabetes management, if needed

Additional information for the patient can be found at the following websites:

- The Pancreatitis Association, Inc.: http://pancassociation.org

Alcoholics Anonymous: http://www.aa.org

- International Foundation for Functional Gastrointestinal Disorders: http://www.iffgd.org
- Healthfinder—U.S. Department of Health and Human Services: http://healthfinder.gov
- Web MD: http://www.webmd.com

BOX 29.12   Signs and Symptoms of Pancreatic Infection

Symptoms

- Persistent abdominal pain
- Abdominal tenderness

Signs

- Prolonged fever
- Abdominal distention
- Palpable abdominal mass
- Vomiting

Diagnostics

- Laboratory findings
- Increased white blood cell count
- Persistent elevation of serum amylase
- Hyperbilirubinemia
- Elevated alkaline phosphatase level
- Positive culture and Gram stain
- Radiography or computed tomography findings
- Pancreatic inflammation or enlargement
- Necrosis
- Cystic or mass lesions
- Fluid accumulations
- Pseudocyst abscess

Modified from Krumberger JM. Acute pancreatitis. *Crit Care Nurs Clin North Am.* 1993;5(1):185–202.

QSEN   BOX 29.13   QSEN: Teamwork and Collaboration

Interprofessional Collaborative Practice: Acute Pancreatitis

- Ensure adequate circulating volume.
- Provide nutrition support.
- Correct metabolic alterations.
- Minimize pancreatic stimulation.
- Provide comfort and emotional support.
- Maintain surveillance for complications.
- Pancreatic pseudocyst
- Infected pancreatic necrosis
- Pancreatic abscess
- Intraabdominal compartment syndrome
- Acute respiratory distress syndrome
- Multiple organ dysfunction syndrome

---

pressure monitoring is initiated if intraabdominal hypertension is suspected. The patient is closely monitored for signs and symptoms of pancreatic infection, which include increased abdominal pain and tenderness, fever, and increased white blood cell count (Box 29.11).[19]

Educate the Patient and Family

Early in the patient's hospital stay, the patient and family should be taught about acute pancreatitis and its causes and treatment. Closer to discharge, teaching should focus on the interventions necessary for preventing the recurrence of the precipitating disorder. If sustained, permanent damage to the pancreas has occurred, the patient will require teaching specific to diet modification and supplemental pancreatic enzymes. Diabetes education may also be necessary. If the patient abuses alcohol, the patient should be encouraged to stop drinking and be referred to an alcohol cessation program (Box 29.12).

Interprofessional collaborative management of the patient with pancreatitis is outlined in Box 29.13.

ACUTE LIVER FAILURE

Description

Acute liver failure (ALF) is a life-threatening condition characterized by severe and sudden liver cell dysfunction, coagulopathy, and hepatic encephalopathy.[45] Although uncommon, ALF is associated with a mortality rate of 40%, and it usually occurs in patients without preexisting liver disease.[45] Because liver transplantation is one of the few definitive treatments, a patient with ALF should be transferred to a critical care unit and strongly considered for referral to a major medical center where transplantation services are available.[45]

Etiology

The causes of ALF include infections, medications, toxins, hypoperfusion, metabolic disorders, and surgery (see Box 29.13); however, viral hepatitis and medication-induced liver damage are the predominant causes in North America. Patients are usually healthy before the onset of symptoms because ALF tends to occur in patients with no known liver history. A thorough medication and health history is imperative to determine a possible cause. The patient should be questioned about exposure to environmental toxins, hepatitis, intravenous drug use, sexual history, viral hepatitis, medication toxicity, and poisoning.

Additional vascular causes such as thrombosis; ischemia; Budd-Chiari syndrome (blocked venous outflow from small hepatic veins to inferior vena cava from thrombosis)[46]; and metabolic disorders such as Reye syndrome (acute, often fatal liver disease),[47] Wilson disease (disease of defective copper metabolism that damages liver and brain),[48] galactosemia (rare disease in infants in which they cannot metabolize galactose resulting in hepatocellular damage),[49] and fructose intolerance should be considered.[45]

Pathophysiology

ALF develops over 1 to 3 weeks, followed by the development of hepatic encephalopathy within 8 weeks, in a patient with a previously healthy liver. The interval between the failure of the liver and the onset of hepatic encephalopathy usually is less than 2 weeks. The underlying cause is massive necrosis of the hepatocytes.[50]

ALF results in numerous derangements, including impaired bilirubin conjugation, decreased production of clotting factors, depressed glucose synthesis, and decreased lactate clearance. This results in jaundice, coagulopathies, hypoglycemia, and metabolic acidosis. Other effects of ALF include increased risk of infection and altered carbohydrate, protein, and glucose metabolism. Hypoalbuminemia, fluid and electrolyte imbalances, and acute portal hypertension contribute to the development of ascites.[45] Hepatic encephalopathy is thought to result from failure of the liver to detoxify various substances in the bloodstream, and it may be worsened by metabolic and electrolyte imbalances.[50]

The patient may experience various other complications, including cerebral edema, cardiac dysrhythmias, acute respiratory failure, sepsis, and AKI. Cerebral edema and increased intracranial pressure (ICP) develop as a result of breakdown of the blood–brain barrier and astrocyte swelling. Circulatory failure that mimics sepsis is common in ALF and may exacerbate low cerebral perfusion pressure.[51] Hypoxemia, acidosis, electrolyte imbalances, and cerebral edema can precipitate the development of cardiac dysrhythmias. Acute respiratory failure, progressing to ARDS, intrapulmonary shunting, ventilation-perfusion mismatch, sepsis, and aspiration may contribute to the universal arterial hypoxemia.[51]

Assessment and Diagnosis

Early recognition of ALF is essential. The diagnosis should include potentially reversible conditions (eg, autoimmune hepatitis) and should differentiate ALF from decompensating chronic liver disease. Prognostic indicators such as coma grade, serum bilirubin, prothrombin time, coagulation factors, and pH should be assessed, and potential causes should be investigated.[45]

Signs and symptoms of ALF include headache, hyperventilation, jaundice, mental status changes, palmar erythema, spider nevi, bruises, and edema. The patient should be evaluated for the presence of asterixis, or "liver flap," which is best described as the inability to voluntarily sustain a fixed position of the extremities. Asterixis is best recognized by downward flapping of the hands when the patient extends the arms and dorsiflexes the wrists. Hepatic encephalopathy is assessed by using a grading system that stages the encephalopathy according to the patient's clinical manifestations (Box 29.14). Diagnostic findings include prolonged prothrombin times; elevated levels

BOX 29.14 Causes of Acute Liver Failure

Infections
- Hepatitis A, B, C, D, E, non-A, non-B, non-C
- Herpes simplex virus (types 1 and 2)
- Epstein-Barr virus
- Varicella zoster
- Dengue fever virus
- Rift Valley fever virus

Medications or Toxins
- Industrial substances (chlorinated hydrocarbons, phosphorus)
- *Amanita phalloides* (mushrooms)
- Aflatoxin (a toxic metabolite of fungus)
- Medications (isoniazid, rifampin, halothane, methyldopa, tetracycline, valproic acid, monoamine oxidase inhibitors, phenytoin, nicotinic acid, tricyclic antidepressants, isoflurane, ketoconazole, trimethoprim-sulfamethoxazole, sulfasalazine, pyrimethamine, octreotide)
- Acetaminophen toxicity
- Cocaine

Hypoperfusion
- Venous obstructions
- Budd-Chiari syndrome
- Veno-occlusive disease
- Ischemia

Metabolic Disorders
- Wilson disease
- Tyrosinemia
- Heat stroke
- Galactosemia

Surgery
- Jejunoileal bypass
- Partial hepatectomy
- Liver transplantation failure

Other Causes
- Reye syndrome
- Acute fatty liver of pregnancy
- Massive malignant infiltration
- Autoimmune hepatitis

of serum bilirubin, aspartate aminotransferase, alkaline phosphatase, and serum ammonia; and decreased levels of serum albumin.[50] Arterial blood gases reveal respiratory alkalosis, metabolic acidosis, or both. Hypoglycemia, hypokalemia, and hyponatremia also may be present.[50,51]

Factors I (fibrinogen), II (prothrombin), V, VII, IX, and X are produced exclusively by the liver. Prothrombin time may be the most useful of these in the evaluation of acute ALF because levels may be 40 to 80 seconds above control values. Test results show decreased levels of plasmin and plasminogen and increased levels of fibrin and fibrin-split products. Platelet counts may be less than 100,000/mm^3.[50]

Medical Management

Medical interventions are directed toward management of the multiple system impact of ALF.

Ammonia Levels

Antibiotics such as neomycin, metronidazole, and rifaximin and lactulose, which is the gold standard, are administered to remove or decrease production of nitrogenous wastes in the large intestine. Antibiotics reduce bacterial flora of the colon; this aids in decreasing ammonia formation by decreasing bacterial action on the protein in feces. Side effects include renal toxicity and hearing impairment. Lactulose, a synthetic ketoanalogue of lactose split into lactic acid and acetic acid in the intestine, is given orally through a nasogastric tube or as a retention enema. The result is the creation of an acidic environment that results in ammonia being drawn out of the portal circulation. Lactulose has a laxative effect that promotes expulsion.[50,51]

Complications

Bleeding is best controlled through prevention. If an invasive procedure (eg, central line placement, ICP monitor) will be performed or the patient develops active bleeding, vitamin K, fresh frozen plasma (to maintain a reasonable prothrombin time), and platelet transfusions are necessary.[25] Metabolic disturbances such as hypoglycemia, metabolic acidosis, hypokalemia, and hyponatremia should be monitored and treated appropriately. Prophylactic antibiotic administration may be initiated because the patient is at high risk for an infection.[25] The development of cerebral edema necessitates ICP monitoring. Treatment with mannitol has been shown to be beneficial in managing ICP in a patient with ALF, but it must be used with caution in patients with renal failure to avoid hyperosmolarity.[51] Other interventions to control ICP include elevating the head of the bed to 30 degrees, treating fever and hypertension, minimizing noxious stimulation, and correcting hypercapnia and hypoxemia.[25] Renal failure develops in 70% of patients with ALF; continuous renal replacement therapy provides renal support.[25] Hemodynamic instability is a common complication necessitating fluid administration and vasoactive medications to prevent prolonged episodes of hypotension. A pulmonary artery catheter may be used to guide clinical management.[50]

If ALF continues and the patient shows no immediate signs of improvement or reversal, the patient should be considered for a liver transplantation. Prompt referral to a transplantation center should be a high priority for patients experiencing ALF.[25,45]

Nursing Management

The nursing management plan for a patient with ALF incorporates a variety of nursing diagnoses (Box 29.15). The nurse plays a significant role in protecting the patient from injury, providing comfort and emotional support, maintaining surveillance for complications, and educating the patient and family.

Protect the Patient from Injury

Use of benzodiazepines and other sedatives is discouraged in a patient with ALF because pertinent neurologic changes may be masked and hepatic encephalopathy may be exacerbated.[51] These patients are often very difficult to manage because they may be extremely agitated and combative. Physical restraint may be necessary to prevent injury to the patient; however, all other nursing interventions must be tried before restraints are considered.

Maintain Surveillance for Complications

As the neurologic condition worsens, respiratory depression and arrest can occur quickly. Continuous pulse oximetry monitoring and arterial blood gas analysis are helpful in assessing adequacy of respiratory efforts. A thorough neurologic assessment should be performed at least every hour, with changes reported immediately.

Educate the Patient and Family

Early in the patient's hospital stay, the patient and family should be taught about ALF and its causes and treatment. Closer to discharge, teaching should focus on the interventions necessary for preventing the recurrence of the precipitating cause. If the patient is considered a candidate for liver transplantation, the patient and family will need specific information regarding the procedure and care. Evaluation for liver transplantation may include screening for medical contraindications, human immunodeficiency virus serology, anticipated compliance, and assessment of the social support system. Psychiatric and other specialty team consultations are necessary for a thorough evaluation of the patient's suitability for a liver transplantation (Box 29.16).

Interprofessional collaborative management of the patient with ALF is outlined in Box 29.17.

BOX 29.15   Staging of Hepatic Encephalopathy

I. Euphoria or depression, mild confusion, slurred speech, disordered sleep rhythm; slight asterixis and normal EEG

II. Lethargy, moderate confusion; marked asterixis and abnormal EEG

III. Marked confusion, incoherent speech, sleeping but arousable; asterixis present and abnormal EEG

IV. Coma; initially responsive to noxious stimuli, later unresponsive; asterixis absent and abnormal EEG

EEG, electroencephalogram.

BOX 29.16   NURSING DIAGNOSES

Acute Liver Failure

- Ineffective Breathing Pattern related to decreased lung expansion, p. 1035
- Impaired Gas Exchange related to ventilation-perfusion mismatching or intrapulmonary shunting, p. 1030
- Decreased Cardiac Output related to alterations in preload, p. 1019
- Decreased Cardiac Output related to alterations in heart rate, p. 1016
- Decreased Intracranial Adaptive Capacity related to failure of normal compensatory mechanisms, p. 1018
- Risk for Infection, p. 1046
- Imbalanced Nutrition: Less Than Body Requirements related to lack of exogenous nutrients or increased metabolic demand, p. 1029
- Disturbed Body Image related to actual change in body structure, function, or appearance, p. 1022
- Compromised Family Coping related to critically ill family member, p. 1014
- Deficient Knowledge related to lack of previous exposure to information, p. 1020 (see Patient Education Plan, Box 29.17)

GASTROINTESTINAL SURGERY

Types of Surgery

GI surgery refers to a wide variety of surgical procedures that involve the esophagus, stomach, intestine, liver, pancreas, or biliary tract. Indications for GI surgery are numerous and include bleeding or perforation from peptic ulcer disease, obstruction, trauma, inflammatory bowel disease, and malignancy. Patients may be admitted to the critical care unit for monitoring after GI surgery as a result of their underlying medical condition; however, this section focuses only on several surgical procedures that commonly require postoperative critical care.

✳ BOX 29.17 **PATIENT EDUCATION PLAN**

Acute Liver Failure

Before the patient's discharge, the patient should be able to teach back the following topics:
- Specific cause
- Precipitating factor modification
- Interventions to reduce further episodes
- Importance of taking medications
- Lifestyle changes
- Diet modification
- Alcohol cessation

Additional information for the patient can be found at the following websites:
- American Liver Foundation: http://www.liverfoundation.org
- National Liver Foundation: http://www.nlfindia.com
- Alcoholics Anonymous: http://www.aa.org
- International Foundation for Functional Gastrointestinal Disorders: http://www.iffgd.org
- Healthfinder—U.S. Department of Health and Human Services: http://healthfinder.gov
- Web MD: http://www.webmd.com

Esophagectomy

Esophagectomy is usually performed for cancer of the distal esophagus and gastroesophageal junction. The technically difficult procedure involves the removal of part or all of the esophagus, part of the stomach, and lymph nodes in the surrounding area. The stomach is then pulled up into the chest and connected to the remaining part of the esophagus. If the entire esophagus and stomach must be removed, part of the bowel may be used to form the esophageal replacement (Figs. 29.5 and 29.6).[52]

Two approaches may be used for esophageal resection: *transhiatal* or *transthoracic* (see Figs. 29.5 and 29.6). In both approaches, the stomach is mobilized through an abdominal incision and then transposed into the chest. The anastomosis of the stomach to the esophagus is performed in the chest (transthoracic) or in the neck (transhiatal). The approach selected depends on the location of the tumor, the patient's overall health and pulmonary function, and the experience of the surgeon. After surgery, the patient has a nasogastric tube in place, and it should not be manipulated because of the potential to damage the anastomosis. Patients who undergo transthoracic esophagectomy have chest tubes.[52]

Pancreaticoduodenectomy

The standard operation for pancreatic cancer is a pancreaticoduodenectomy, also called the *Whipple procedure.* In the Whipple procedure, the pancreatic head, the duodenum, part of the jejunum, the common bile duct, the gallbladder, and part of the stomach are removed. The continuity of the GI tract is restored by anastomosing the remaining portion of the pancreas, the bile duct, and the stomach to the jejunum (Fig. 29.7).[52]

Bariatric Surgery

Bariatric surgery refers to surgical procedures of the GI tract that are performed to induce weight loss. Bariatric procedures

FIG. 29.5 Overview of Transhiatal Esophagectomy. (A) Transhiatal esophagectomy with (B) gastric mobilization and (C) gastric pull-up for cervical esophagogastric anastomosis. (Modified from Ellis FH. Esophagogastrectomy for carcinoma: technical considerations based on anatomic location of lesion. *Surg Clin North Am.* 1980;60(2):265–279.)

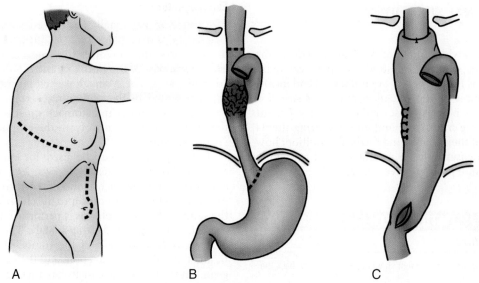

FIG. 29.6 Overview of Transthoracic Esophagectomy. Transthoracic esophagectomy with (A) esophageal resection, (B) gastric mobilization, and (C) intrathoracic anastomosis for a midesophageal tumor. (Modified from Ellis FH. Esophagogastrectomy for carcinoma: technical considerations based on anatomic location of lesion. *Surg Clin North Am.* 1980;60(2):265–279.)

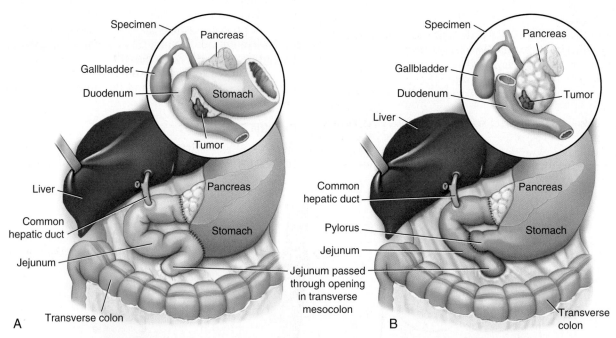

FIG. 29.7 Standard and Pylorus-Preserving Whipple Procedures. (A) The standard Whipple procedure involves resection of the gastric antrum, head of pancreas, distal bile duct, and entire duodenum with reconstruction as shown. (B) The pylorus-preserving Whipple procedure does not include resection of the distal stomach, pylorus, or proximal duodenum.

are divided into three broad types: (1) restrictive, (2) malabsorptive, and (3) combined restrictive and malabsorptive.[53] Restrictive procedures such as vertical banded gastroplasty (Fig. 29.8A) and gastric banding (Fig. 29.8B) reduce the capacity of the stomach and limit the amount of food that can be consumed. Malabsorptive procedures such as biliopancreatic diversion (Fig. 29.8C) alter the GI tract to limit the digestion and absorption of food. The Roux-en-Y gastric bypass (Fig. 29.8D) combines both strategies by creating a small gastric

pouch and anastomosing the jejunum to the pouch (Fig 29.8E). Food then bypasses the lower stomach and duodenum, resulting in decreased absorption of digestive materials.[53]

Most bariatric procedures can be performed using an open or laparoscopic surgical technique. Although laparoscopic approaches are more technically difficult to perform, they have largely replaced open procedures because they are associated with decreased pulmonary complications, less postoperative pain, reduced length of hospital stay, fewer wound

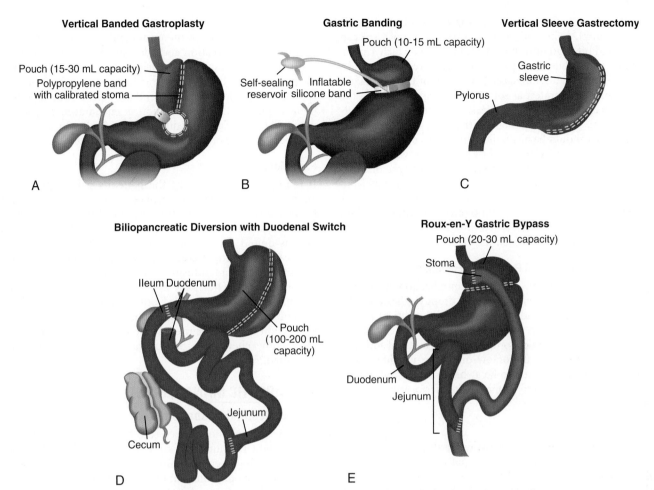

FIG. 29.8 Bariatric Surgical Procedures. (A) Vertical banded gastroplasty involves creating a small gastric pouch. (B) Adjustable gastric banding uses a band to create a gastric pouch. (C) Vertical sleeve gastrectomy involves creating a sleeve-shaped stomach by removing approximately 80% of the stomach. (D) Biliopancreatic diversion with duodenal switch procedure creates an anastomosis between the stomach and intestine. (E) Roux-en-Y gastric bypass procedure involves constructing a gastric pouch whose outlet is a Y-shaped limb of small intestine. (From Lewis SL, et al. *Medical-Surgical Nursing: Assessment and Management of Clinical Problems.* 9th ed. St. Louis: Elsevier; 2014.)

complications (eg, infections, incisional hernia), and an earlier return to full activity.[52,53] Open procedures are performed on patients who have had prior upper abdominal surgery, who are morbidly obese, or who may be unable to tolerate the increased abdominal pressure associated with laparoscopic procedures.[52]

Preoperative Care

A thorough preoperative evaluation should be conducted to evaluate the patient's physical and mental status and identify risk factors that may affect the postoperative course. Because obesity is associated with a higher incidence of comorbidities such as cardiovascular disease, hypertension, diabetes, gastroesophageal reflux, obstructive sleep apnea, and heart failure, an extensive work-up may be required for the patient who will undergo bariatric surgery.[52,54]

Complications and Medical Management

Several complications are associated with GI surgery, including respiratory failure, atelectasis, pneumonia, anastomotic leak, deep vein thrombosis, pulmonary embolus, and bleeding.

Morbidly obese patients are at even greater risk for many postoperative complications.[53]

Pulmonary Complications

The risk for pulmonary complications is substantial after GI surgery, and adverse respiratory events such as atelectasis and pneumonia are twice as likely to occur in an obese patient.[54] Aggressive pulmonary exercise should be initiated in the immediate postoperative period. Early ambulation and adequate pain control assist in reducing the risk of developing atelectasis. Suctioning, chest physiotherapy, or bronchodilators may be needed to optimize pulmonary function. Patients should be closely monitored for the development of oxygenation problems. Treatment should be aimed at supporting adequate ventilation and gas exchange. Mechanical ventilation may be required in the event of respiratory failure.

Anastomotic Leak

An anastomotic leak is a severe complication of GI surgery. It occurs when there is a breakdown of the suture line in a surgical anastomosis and results in leakage of gastric or intestinal contents into the abdomen or mediastinum (transthoracic esophagectomy).[54] The clinical signs and symptoms of a leak can be subtle and often go unrecognized. They include tachycardia, tachypnea, fever, abdominal pain, anxiety, and restlessness.[54] In a patient who had an esophagectomy, a leak of the esophageal anastomosis may manifest as subcutaneous emphysema in the chest and neck.[48] If undetected, a leak can result in sepsis, multiorgan failure, and death. Patients with progressive tachycardia and tachypnea should have a radiologic study (upper GI study with a contrast agent [Gastrografin] or CT scan with contrast medium) to rule out an anastomotic leak.[54] The type of treatment depends on the severity of the leak. If the leak is small and well contained, it may be managed conservatively by maintaining NPO status, administering antibiotics, and draining fluid percutaneously. If the patient is deteriorating rapidly, an urgent laparotomy is indicated to repair the defect.[52,54]

Deep Vein Thrombosis and Pulmonary Embolism

Pulmonary embolism is a very serious complication of any surgical procedure. Deep vein thrombosis prophylaxis should be initiated before surgery and continued until the patient is fully ambulatory to reduce the risk of clot development. Typically, a combination of sequential compression devices and subcutaneous unfractionated heparin or low-molecular-weight heparin is used. Patients determined to be at high risk for pulmonary embolism may benefit from prophylactic inferior vena cava filter placement.[52]

Bleeding

Upper GI bleeding is an uncommon but life-threatening complication of GI surgery. Early bleeding usually occurs at the site of the anastomosis and can usually be treated through endoscopic intervention. Surgical revision may be needed for persistent, uncontrolled bleeding. Late bleeding is usually a result of ulcer development. Medical therapy is aimed at the prevention of this complication through administration of H_2 antagonists or PPIs.[5]

Postoperative Nursing Management

The nursing management plan for the patient who has had GI surgery incorporates a variety of nursing diagnoses (Box 29.18). The nurse plays a significant role in optimizing oxygenation and ventilation, preventing atelectasis, promoting ambulation, providing comfort and emotional support, and maintaining surveillance for complications.

Pulmonary Management

Nursing interventions in the postoperative period are focused on promoting ventilation and adequate oxygenation and preventing complications such as atelectasis and pneumonia. After the patient is extubated, deep-breathing exercises and incentive spirometry should be initiated, and the patient should perform them regularly. Early ambulation is encouraged to promote maximal lung inflation, reducing the risk of pulmonary complications and the potential for pulmonary embolus.

Pain Management

It is imperative to manage the patient's pain appropriately after GI surgery. Adequate analgesia is necessary to promote the mobility of the patient and decrease pulmonary complications. Initial pain management may be accomplished by intravenous opioid (morphine, hydromorphone) administration by means of a patient-controlled analgesia pump or through continuous epidural infusion of an opioid and local anesthetic (bupivacaine).[52] Oral pain medications can be started after an anastomosis leak is ruled out. Nonpharmacologic interventions such as positioning, application of heat or cold, and distraction may also be used. If the patient's pain is not being sufficiently relieved, the pain management service should be consulted.[52,54]

THERAPEUTIC MANAGEMENT

Gastrointestinal Intubation

Because GI intubation is used so often in critical care units, it is important for nurses to know the clinical indications and responsibilities inherent in tube use. The three categories of GI tubes are based on function: (1) nasogastric suction tubes, (2) long intestinal tubes, and (3) feeding tubes (Box 29.19). Feeding tubes are discussed in Chapter 7.

Nasogastric Suction Tubes

Nasogastric tubes remove fluid regurgitated into the stomach, prevent accumulation of swallowed air, may partially decompress the bowel, and reduce the patient's risk for aspiration. Nasogastric tubes also can be used for collecting specimens, assessing the presence of blood, and administering tube feedings. The most common nasogastric tubes are the single-lumen Levin tube and the double-lumen Salem sump. The Salem sump has one lumen that is used for suction and drainage and another that allows air to enter the patient's stomach and prevents the tube from adhering to the gastric wall and damaging

---

QSEN BOX 29.18 QSEN: Teamwork and Collaboration

Interprofessional Collaborative Practice: Acute Liver Failure

- Decrease ammonia levels.
- Control bleeding.
- Correct metabolic alterations.
- Prevent infection.
- Prepare patient for liver transplantation, if necessary.
- Protect patient from injury.
- Provide comfort and emotional support.
- Maintain surveillance for complications:
  - Cerebral edema
  - Renal failure

BOX 29.19 NURSING DIAGNOSES

Gastrointestinal Surgery

- Ineffective Breathing Pattern related to decreased lung expansion, p. 1035
- Impaired Gas Exchange related to alveolar hypoventilation, p. 1030
- Decreased Cardiac Output related to alterations in preload, p. 1015
- Acute Pain related to transmission and perception of cutaneous, visceral, muscular, or ischemic impulses, p. 1010
- Anxiety related to threat to biologic, psychologic, or social integrity, p. 1012
- Disturbed Body Image related to actual change in body structure, function, or appearance, p. 1022
- Deficient Knowledge related to lack of previous exposure to information, p. 1020

the mucosa. The tube is passed through the nose or mouth into the nasopharynx and then down through the pharynx into the esophagus and stomach. The length of time the nasogastric tube remains in place depends on its use. The tube is then placed to gravity, low intermittent suction, or low continuous suction, and in rare instances, it is clamped.[55]

Nursing management focuses on preventing complications common to this therapy, such as ulceration and necrosis of the nares, esophageal reflux, esophagitis, esophageal erosion and stricture, gastric erosion, and dry mouth and parotitis from mouth breathing. Interference with ventilation and coughing, aspiration, and loss of fluid and electrolytes can be critical problems. Interventions include irrigating the tube every 4 hours with normal saline, ensuring the blue air vent of the Salem sump is patent and maintained above the level of the patient's stomach, and providing frequent mouth and nares care (Box 29.20).[55]

Long Intestinal Tubes

Miller-Abbott, Cantor, and Andersen tubes are examples of long, weighted-tip intestinal tubes that are placed preoperatively or intraoperatively. Their considerable length allows removal of the contents of the intestine to treat an obstruction that cannot be managed by a nasogastric tube. These tubes can decompress the small bowel and can splint the small bowel intraoperatively or postoperatively. Because progression of the tubes depends on bowel peristalsis, their use is contraindicated in patients with paralytic ileus and severe mechanical bowel obstructions.

Interventions used in the care of a patient with a long intestinal tube are similar to interventions used with a nasogastric tube. The patient should be observed for (1) gaseous distention of the balloon section, which makes removal difficult; (2) rupture of the balloon; (3) overinflation of the balloon, which can lead to intestinal rupture; and (4) reverse intussusception if

the tube is removed rapidly. Intestinal tubes should be removed slowly; usually 6 inches of the tube is withdrawn every hour.[55]

Endoscopic Injection Therapy

Endoscopic injection therapy is used to control bleeding of ulcers. It may be performed emergently, electively, or prophylactically. An endoscope is introduced through the patient's mouth, and endoscopy of the esophagus and stomach is performed to identify the bleeding varices or ulcers. An injector with a retractable 23- to 25-gauge needle is introduced through the biopsy channel of the endoscope. The needle is then inserted in or around the varices or into the area around the ulcer, and a liquid agent is injected (Fig. 29.9). The most commonly used agent is epinephrine, which results in localized vasoconstriction and enhanced platelet aggregation. Sclerosing agents such as ethanolamine, alcohol, and polidocanol also may be used. These agents cause an inflammatory reaction in the vessel that results in thrombosis and eventually produces a fibrous band. Repeated sclerotherapy results in the development of supportive scar tissue around the varices. Other embolic agents are used, including fibrinogen and thrombin, which when injected together react to form an active fibrin clot, and "glues" (N-butyl cyanoacrylate), which are used as a sealant to stop the bleeding.[20,24,56]

Endoscopic Variceal Ligation

EVL involves applying bands or metal clips around the circumference of the bleeding varices to induce venous obstruction and control bleeding. EVL has replaced endoscopic sclerotherapy of variceal hemorrhage (Fig. 29.10). One or 2 days after the procedure, necrosis and scar formation promote band and tissue sloughing. Fibrinous deposits within the healing ulcer potentiate vessel obliteration. Band ligation is accomplished through endoscopy, with multiple bands placed per session.[16] The procedure may be repeated on an inpatient or outpatient basis every 1 or 2 weeks until all the varices are obliterated.[56] EVL controls bleeding in approximately 80% to 90% of cases.[56] The most common complication of EVL is the development of superficial mucosal ulcers. Varices may reoccur, as local banding does not affect portal pressure.[16,57]

FIG. 29.9 Endoscopic Sclerosis of Varices. (From Copstead LC, Banasik JL. *Pathophysiology.* 5th ed. St. Louis: Elsevier; 2013.)

| Site of bleeding identified | Contact made between ligator and varix | Suction applied to draw varix into ligator lumen | O ring released around neck of varix | Hemostasis achieved |

FIG. 29.10 Endoscopic Band Ligation. (From Copstead LC, Banasik JL. *Pathophysiology.* 5th ed. St. Louis: Elsevier; 2013.)

Transjugular Intrahepatic Portosystemic Shunt

TIPS is an angiographic interventional procedure for decreasing portal hypertension. TIPS is advocated for (1) patients with portal hypertension who are also experiencing active bleeding or have poor liver reserve, (2) transplant recipients, and (3) patients with other operative risks.[25,57] The TIPS procedure is usually performed by a gastroenterologist, vascular surgeon, or interventional radiologist.

Portal hypertension is confirmed by direct measurement of the pressure in the portal vein (gradient greater than 10 mm Hg). Cannulation is achieved through the internal jugular vein, and an angiographic catheter is advanced into the middle or right hepatic vein. The midhepatic vein is then catheterized, and a new route is created connecting the portal and hepatic veins using a needle and guidewire with a dilating balloon. A polytetrafluoroethylene-coated stent is then placed in the liver parenchyma to maintain that connection (Fig. 29.11). The increased resistance in the liver is bypassed.[25,58] TIPS may be performed in patients with bleeding varices, with refractory bleeding varices, or as a bridge to liver transplantation if the candidate becomes hemodynamically unstable. Postprocedural care should include observation for overt (cannulation site) or covert (intrahepatic site) bleeding, hepatic or portal vein laceration (resulting in rapid loss of blood volume), and inadvertent puncture of surrounding organs. Other complications include hepatic encephalopathy, liver failure, bacteremia, and stent stenosis.[25,58]

PHARMACOLOGIC AGENTS

Many pharmacologic agents are used in the care of patients with GI disorders. Table 29.3 reviews the various agents and any special considerations necessary for administering them.

Antiulcer Agents

Many different antiulcer agents are commonly used in the critical care setting, including H$_2$ antagonists, gastric PPIs, and gastric mucosal agents.[59] There is no clear evidence as to which method provides the best outcome for the patient.

H$_2$ antagonists are used to decrease the volume and concentration of gastric secretions and control gastric pH, decreasing the incidence of stress-related upper GI bleeding. These agents work by blocking histamine stimulation of the H$_2$ receptors on the gastric parietal cells, reducing acid production.[60] Although these medications may be administered orally, intramuscularly, or intravenously, they usually are given intravenously in the critical care setting.

PPIs decrease gastric acid secretion by binding to the proton pump, blocking the release of acid from the gastric parietal cells.[60] PPIs are potent acid inhibitors and have greater suppressive ability than H$_2$ antagonists; however, they are also associated with an increased risk of ventilator-associated pneumonia and *Clostridium difficile* infections (see Box 29.20).[61] Esomeprazole, pantoprazole, and lansoprazole are available for intravenous administration. Oral PPIs are formulated as enteric-coated tablets or as delayed-release capsules containing enteric-coated granules. Absorption occurs in an alkaline environment and begins only after the granules leave the stomach and enter the duodenum.

In contrast to H$_2$ antagonists or PPIs, sucralfate does not affect gastric acid concentration but rather exerts its action locally. Sucralfate reacts with hydrochloric acid to form a sticky, paste-like substance that adheres to the surface of the ulcer and shields it from pepsin, acid, and bile. Sucralfate predominantly binds to damaged GI mucosa, with minimal adherence to normal tissue.[62] It is administered orally or through a gastric tube. Sucralfate should not be crushed but may be dissolved in 10 mL of water to form a slurry. It is also available as a suspension. If given with enteral feedings, the feeding should be held 1 hour before administration and 1 hour after administration.

Vasopressin

Vasopressin is used to control gastric ulcer and variceal bleeding. It is administered intraarterially, through a catheter inserted

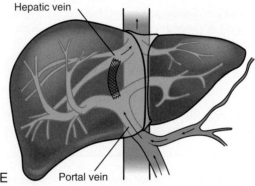

FIG. 29.11 Transjugular Intrahepatic Portosystemic Shunt (TIPS). (A) Needle directed through liver parenchyma to portal vein. (B) Needle and guidewire passed down to midportal vein. (C) Balloon dilation. (D) Deployment of stent. (E) Intrahepatic shunt from portal to hepatic vein. (From Urden LD, Stacy KM, Lough ME. *Priorities in Critical Care Nursing.* 7th ed. St. Louis: Mosby; 2016.)

into the right or left gastric artery (through the femoral artery, aorta, and celiac trunk) or intravenously. It causes splanchnic and systemic vasoconstriction, subsequently reducing portal blood flow and pressure.[24,63-65]

A major side effect of the medication is systemic vasoconstriction, which can result in cardiac ischemia, chest pain, hypertension, acute heart failure, dysrhythmias, phlebitis, bowel ischemia, and cerebrovascular accident. These side effects can be offset with concurrent administration of nitroglycerin.[24,63,64] Other complications include bradycardia and fluid retention. Nursing responsibilities associated with the use of this therapy include maintenance of a patent infusion line and continuous monitoring for vasoconstrictive complications of therapy. Because of the known adverse effects, vasopressin is not the first choice of treatment.[63,64]

Octreotide

Octreotide, a long-acting synthetic analogue of somatostatin, is a peptide that is administered parenterally in a patient with acute bleeding and cirrhosis. It reduces splanchnic vasodilation and portal pressure through the inhibition of secretion of various vasodilator hormones, and it is as effective as vasopressin in treating variceal bleeding with minimal side effects. Combined with endoscopic therapy, octreotide is the preferred treatment for achieving hemostasis.[16]

TABLE 29.3 Pharmacologic Management
Gastrointestinal Disorders

Medication	Dosage	Actions	Special Considerations
Antacids	30–90 mL q1–2h PO or NG; possibly titrated to NG pH	Used to buffer stomach acid and raise gastric pH	Can cause diarrhea or constipation and electrolyte disturbances
			Irrigate NG tube with water after administration because antacids can clog tube
Histamine-2 (H$_2$) Antagonists			
Cimetidine (Tagamet)	300 mg q6h IV or PO	Used to reduce volume and concentration of gastric secretions	Side effects include CNS toxicity (confusion or delirium) and thrombocytopenia
Ranitidine (Zantac)	150–300 mg q12h PO or 50 mg q8h IV		Separate administration of antacids and PO histamine blocking agents by 1 h
Famotidine (Pepcid)	40 mg daily PO or 20 mg q12h IV		Dosage adjustments recommended for patients with moderate (creatinine clearance <50 mL/min) or severe (creatinine clearance <10 mL/min) renal insufficiency
Nizatidine (Axid)	150 mg q12h PO or 300 mg q24h		
Gastric Mucosal Agents			
Sucralfate (Carafate)	1 g q6h NG or PO, given 1 h before meals and at bedtime	Forms an ulcer-adherent complex with proteinaceous exudates	Requires an acid medium for activation; do not administer within 30 min of antacid
		Covers ulcer and protects against acid, pepsin, and bile salts	May cause severe constipation
			May cause decreased absorption of certain medications
Gastric Proton-Pump Inhibitors			
Omeprazole (Prilosec)	20–40 mg q12h PO	Inactivates acid, or hydrogen, acid pump, blocking secretion of hydrochloric acid by gastric parietal cells	Capsules should be swallowed intact
Lansoprazole (Prevacid)	15–30 mg q24h PO		May increase levels of phenytoin, diazepam, warfarin
	30 mg over 30 min q24h IV		May be administered concomitantly with antacids
Rabeprazole (Aciphex)	20–40 mg q24h PO		Associated with higher incidence of *Clostridium difficile* infection and ventilator-associated pneumonia
Esomeprazole (Nexium)	40 mg q12–24h PO		
	20–40 mg q24h IV		
Pantoprazole (Protonix)	20–80 mg q24h PO		
	80 mg q8–12h IV		
Vasopressin			
(Pitressin Synthetic)	Loading dose of 20 U over 20 min IV, followed by 0.2–0.4 U/min IV infusion	Decreases splanchnic blood flow, reducing portal pressure	Side effects include coronary, mesenteric, and peripheral vasoconstriction
	Doses can be increased to 0.9 U/min, if necessary		May be administered concurrently with nitroglycerin to minimize side effects
Somatostatin			
Octreotide (Sandostatin)	Bolus dose of 25–50 mcg followed by IV infusion of 25–50 mcg/h for 48 h	Decreases splanchnic blood flow, reducing portal pressure	May cause hyperglycemia or hypoglycemia when initiating drip and changing dosages

CNS, central nervous system; *IV*, intravenous/intravenously; *NG*, nasogastric; *PO*, by mouth.
Data from *ClinicalKey Drug Monographs*. https://www.clinicalkey.com/#!/browse/drugs. Accessed December 18, 2015.

CASE STUDY 29.1 Patient With Gastrointestinal Issues

Brief Patient History
Mrs. S is a 70-year-old woman with a long history of chronic back pain. She has been taking nonsteroidal antiinflammatory drugs for several years. She was recently started on warfarin for atrial fibrillation.

Clinical Assessment
Mrs. S is admitted to the critical care unit because she is vomiting bright red blood. She is pale and diaphoretic and complains of epigastric pain.

Diagnostic Procedures
Vital signs include the following: blood pressure of 70/40 mm Hg, heart rate of 130 beats/min (sinus tachycardia), respiratory rate of 30 breaths/min, and temperature of 101.3°F. Her urine output is 15 mL/h, hemoglobin level is 9 g/dL, and international normalized ratio (INR) is 5.3.

Medical Diagnosis
Mrs. S is diagnosed with upper gastrointestinal bleeding.

Questions
1. What major outcomes do you expect to achieve for this patient?
2. What problems or risks must be managed to achieve these outcomes?
3. What interventions must be initiated to monitor, prevent, manage, or eliminate the problems and risks identified?
4. What interventions should be initiated to promote optimal functioning, safety, and well-being of the patient?
5. What possible learning needs do you anticipate for this patient?
6. What cultural and age-related factors may have a bearing on the patient's plan of care?

SUMMARY

Acute Gastrointestinal Hemorrhage

- Acute GI hemorrhage can be caused by peptic ulcer disease or stress-related erosive syndrome, and it can result in hypovolemic shock.
- Medical management focuses on restoration of hemodynamic stability and control of bleeding. Nursing actions include administering volume replacement, controlling bleeding, and maintaining surveillance for complications.

Acute Pancreatitis

- Acute pancreatitis can be caused by gallstones and alcoholism, and it can result in autodigestion of the pancreas.
- Medical management focuses on fluid management, nutrition support, and control of systemic and local complications.
- Nursing actions include providing comfort and emotional support and maintaining surveillance for complications.

Acute Liver Failure

- ALF is a life-threatening condition characterized by severe and sudden liver cell dysfunction, coagulopathy, and hepatic encephalopathy.
- Medical management focuses on treatment of elevated ammonia levels and control of complications such as bleeding, metabolic disturbances, and cerebral edema.
- Nursing actions include protecting the patient from injury and maintaining surveillance for complications.

Gastrointestinal Surgery

- Complications of GI surgery include atelectasis, pneumonia, anastomosis leak, deep vein thrombosis, and bleeding.
- Postoperative nursing actions include managing pain and preventing complications.

Therapeutic Management

- Nasogastric suction tubes and long intestinal tubes are often used in the management of GI disorders.

- Endoscopic procedures to control bleeding include endoscopic injection therapy and EVL.
- TIPS is an angiographic interventional procedure for decreasing portal hypertension.
- Common pharmacologic agents used in the management of GI disorders include H_2 antagonists, gastric mucosal agents, PPIs, vasopressin, and octreotide.

Ⓔ Visit the Evolve site for additional study materials.

REFERENCES

1. Khamaysi I, Gralnek IM. Acute upper gastrointestinal bleeding (UGIB)—initial evaluation and management. *Best Pract Res Clin Gastroenterol.* 2013;27(5):633-638.
2. Prasad KM, Tokar JL. Acute gastrointestinal bleeding. *Ann Intern Med.* 2013;159(3):ITC2-1-ITC15.
3. Acosta RD, Wong RKH. Differential diagnosis of upper gastrointestinal bleeding proximal to the ligament of Treitz. *Gastrointest Endosc Clin North Am.* 2011;21(4):555-566.
4. Kumar R, Mills AM. Gastrointestinal bleeding. *Emerg Med Clin North Am.* 2011;29(2):239-252.
5. Ghassemi KA, Kovacs TO, Jensen DM. Gastric acid inhibition in the treatment of peptic ulcer hemorrhage. *Curr Gastroenterol Rep.* 2009;11(6):462-469.
6. Schubert ML. Gastric secretion. *Curr Opin Gastroenterol.* 2014;30(6):578-582.
7. Doig AK, Huether SE. Alterations of digestive function. In: McCance KL, Huether SE, eds. *Pathophysiology: The Biologic Basis for Disease in Adults and Children.* ed 7. St. Louis: Elsevier; 2014.
8. Schubert ML, Peura DA. Control of gastric acid secretion in health and disease. *Gastroenterology.* 2008;134(7):1842-1860.
9. Ferri FF. *Ferri's Clinical Advisor 2016.* Philadelphia: Elsevier; 2016.
10. Marik P, et al. Stress ulcer prophylaxis in the new millennium: a systematic review and meta-analysis. *Crit Care Med.* 2010;38(11):2222-2228.
11. Bardou M, Quenot JP, Barkun A. Stress-related mucosal disease in the critically ill patient. *Nat Rev Gastroenterol Hepatol.* 2015;12(5):98-107.
12. Ali T, Harty RF. Stress-induced ulcer bleeding in critically ill patients. *Gastroenterol Clin North Am.* 2009;38(2):245-265.
13. Pilkington KB, Wagstaff MJ, Greenwood JE. Prevention of gastrointestinal bleeding due to stress ulceration: a review of current literature. *Anaesth Intensive Care.* 2012;40(2):253-259.
14. Tulassay Z, Herszenyi L. Gastric mucosal defense and cytoprotection. *Best Pract Res Clin Gastroenterol.* 2010;24(2):99-108.
15. Stevens A, Path JL, Scott I. *Core Pathology.* ed 3. St. Louis: Elsevier; 2009.
16. Cat TB, Liu-DeRyke X. Medical management of variceal hemorrhage. *Crit Care Nurs Clin North Am.* 2010;22(3):381-393.
17. Bambha K, et al. Predictors of early re-bleeding and mortality after acute variceal haemorrhage in patients with cirrhosis. *Gut.* 2008;57(6):814-820.
18. Jessee MA. Stool studies: tried, true, and new. *Crit Care Nurs Clin Am.* 2010;22(1):129-145.
19. Goldman L, Schafer A. *Goldman-Cecil Medicine.* ed 25. Philadelphia: Elsevier; 2016.
20. Huang JH, et al. The role of endoscopy in acute non-variceal upper GI bleeding. *Gastrointest Endosc.* 2012;60(4):497-504.
21. Sudheendra D, et al. Radiologic techniques and effectiveness of angiography to diagnose and treat acute upper gastrointestinal bleeding. *Gastrointest Endosc Clin North Am.* 2011;21(4):697-705.
22. Klein A, Gralnek IM. Acute, nonvariceal upper gastrointestinal bleeding. *Curr Opin Crit Care.* 2015;21(2):154-162.
23. Yoshida H, et al. Treatment modalities for bleeding esophagogastric varices. *J Nihon Med Sch.* 2012;79(1):19-30.
24. Opio CK, Garcia-Tsao G. Managing varices: drugs, bands, and shunts. *Gastroenterol Clin North Am.* 2011;40(3):561-579.
25. Garcia-Tsao G, Bosch J. Management of varices and variceal hemorrhage in cirrhosis. *N Engl J Med.* 2010;362(9):823-832.
26. Lundell L. Acid secretion and gastric surgery. *Dig Dis.* 2011;29(5):487-490.

27. Costa G, Cruz RJ Jr, Abu-Elmagd KM. Surgical shunt versus TIPS for treatment of variceal hemorrhage in the current era of liver and multivisceral transplantation. *Surg Clin North Am.* 2010;90(4):891-905.

28. Ghosh T, et al. Review article: methods of measuring gastric acid secretion. *Aliment Pharmacol Ther.* 2011;33(7):768-781.

29. Simon TG, Travis AC, Saltzman JR. Initial assessment and resuscitation in nonvariceal upper gastrointestinal bleeding. *Gastrointest Endosc Clin N Am.* 2015;25(3):429-442.

30. Milosavljevic T, et al. Complications of peptic ulcer disease. *Dig Dis.* 2011;29(5):491-493.

31. Khan AS, Latif SU, Eloubeidi MA. Controversies in the etiologies of acute pancreatitis. *JOP.* 2010;11(6):545-552.

32. Lankisch PG, Apte M, Banks PA. Acute pancreatitis. *Lancet.* 2015;386(9988):85-96.

33. Singla A, et al. National hospital volume in acute pancreatitis: analysis of the Nationwide Inpatient Sample 1998-2006. *HPB (Oxford).* 2009;11(5):391-387.

34. Ranson JH, et al. Prognostic signs and the role of operative management in acute pancreatitis. *Surg Gynecol Obstet.* 1974;139(1):69-81.

35. Munsell MA, Buscaglia JM. Acute pancreatitis. *J Hosp Med.* 2010;5(4):241-250.

36. Lerch MM, Gorelick FS. Models of acute and chronic pancreatitis. *Gastroentoerology.* 2013;144(6):1180-1193.

37. Muniraj T, et al. Acute pancreatitis. *Dis Mon.* 2012;58(3):98-144.

38. Chernecky CC, Berger BJ. *Laboratory tests and diagnostic procedures.* ed 6. St. Louis: Saunders; 2013.

39. American Society for Parenteral and Enteral Nutrition (ASPEN) Board of Directors. Clinical guidelines for the use of parenteral and enteral nutrition in adult and pediatric patients. *JPEN J Parenter Enteral Nutr.* 2009;33(1):255-259.

40. Quan H, Wang X, Guo C. A meta-analysis of enteral nutrition and total parenteral nutrition in patient with acute pancreatitis. *Gastroenterol Res Pract.* 2011;698248:2011.

41. Al-Omran M, et al. Enteral versus parenteral nutrition for nutrition for acute pancreatitis. *Cochrane Database Syst Rev.* 2010;(1):CD002837.

42. Moraes JM, et al. A full solid diet as the initial meal in mild acute pancreatitis is safe and results in a shorter length of hospitalization: results from a prospective, randomized, controlled, double-blind clinical trial. *J Clin Gastroenterol.* 2010;44(7):517-522.

43. Working Group IAP/APA Acute Pancreatitis Guidelines. IAP/APA evidence-based guidelines for the management of acute pancreatitis. *Pancreatology.* 2013;13(4 Suppl 2):e1-e15.

44. Villatoro E, Mulla M, Larvin M. Antibiotic therapy for prophylaxis against infection of pancreatic necrosis in acute pancreatitis. *Cochrane Database Syst Rev.* 2010;(5):CD002941.

45. Foston TP, Carpentar D. Acute liver failure. *Crit Care Nurs Clin North Am.* 2010;22(3):395-402.

46. Cheng D, et al. Clinical features and etiology of Budd-Chiari syndrome in Chinese patients: a single-center study. *J Gastroenterol Hepatol.* 2013;28(6):1061-1067.

47. Lopez AM, Hendrickson RG. Toxin-induced hepatic injury. *Emerg Med Clin North Am.* 2014;32(1):103-125.

48. Rahu K, et al. Wilson's disease: a clinical autopsy case report with review of the literature. *J Nat Sci Biol Med.* 2015;6(1):248-252.

49. Bosch AM. Classic galactosemia: dietary dilemmas. *J Inherit Metab Dis.* 2011;34(2):257-260.

50. Mahajan A, Lat I. Correction of coagulopathy in the setting of acute liver failure. *Crit Care Nurs Clin North Am.* 2010;22(3):315-321.

51. Ginès P, et al. Management of critically-ill cirrhotic patients. *J Hepatol.* 2012;56(Suppl 1):S13-S24.

52. Jackson D. Gastrointestinal surgery. In: Rothrock JC, ed. *Alexander's Care of the Patient in Surgery.* ed 15. St. Louis: Elsevier; 2015.

53. Apau D, Whiteing N. Pre- and post-operative nursing considerations of bariatric surgery. *Gastrointest Nurs.* 2011;9(3):44-48.

54. Cannon-Diehl R. Emerging issues for the postbariatric surgical patient. *Crit Care Nurs Q.* 2010;33(4):361-370.

55. Noble KA. Name that tube. *Nursing.* 2003;33(3):56-62.

56. Holster IL, Kuipers EJ. Update on the endoscopic management of peptic ulcer bleeding. *Curr Gastroenterol Rep.* 2011;13(6):525-531.

57. Cárdenas A. Management of acute variceal bleeding: emphasis on endoscopic therapy. *Clin Liver Dis.* 2010;14(2):251-262.

58. Siramolpiwat S. Transjugular intrahepatic postosystemic shunts and portal hypertension-related complications. *World J Gastroenterol.* 2014;20(45):16996-17010.

59. Farrell C, Mercogliano G, Kuntz CL. Overuse of stress ulcer prophylaxis in the critical care setting and beyond. *J Crit Care.* 2010;25(2):214-220.

60. MacLaren R, et al. Proton pump inhibitors and histamine-2 receptor antagonists in the intensive care setting: focus on therapeutic and adverse events. *Expert Opin Drug Saf.* 2015;14(2):269-280.

61. MacLaren R, Reynolds PM, Allen RR. Histamine-2 receptor antagonists vs proton pump inhibitors on gastrointestinal tract hemorrhage and infectious complications in the intensive care unit. *JAMA Intern Med.* 2014;174(4):564-574.

62. Szabo S. "Gastric cytoprotection" is still relevant. *J Gastroenterol Hepatol.* 2014;29(Suppl 4):124-132.

63. Foster KJ, Lin S, Turck CJ. Current and emerging strategies for treating hepatic encephalopathy. *Crit Care Nurs Clin North Am.* 2010;22(3):341-350.

64. Walker TG, Salazar GM, Waltman AC. Angiographic evaluation and management of acute gastrointestinal hemorrhage. *World J Gastroenterol.* 2012;18(11):1191-1201.

65. Miñano C, Garcia-Tsao G. Clinical pharmacology of portal hypertension. *Gastroenterol Clin North Am.* 2010;39(3):681-695.

Endocrine Anatomy and Physiology

Mary E. Lough

Maintaining dynamic equilibrium among the various cells, tissues, organs, and systems of the human body is a highly complex and specialized process. Two systems regulate these critical relationships: the nervous system and the endocrine system. The nervous system communicates by nerve impulses that control skeletal muscle, smooth muscle tissue, and cardiac muscle tissue. The endocrine system controls and communicates by distributing potent hormones throughout the body. Fig. 30.1 lists the endocrine glands and their hormones, target tissues, and actions. When stimulated, the endocrine glands secrete hormones into surrounding body fluids. In the circulation, these hormones travel to specific target tissues, where they exert a pronounced effect. Receptors found on or within these specialized target tissue cells are equipped with molecules that recognize the hormone and bind it to the cell, producing a specific response.

PANCREAS

Anatomy

The pancreas is a long, triangular organ. It is clinically described as consisting of a *head, neck, body,* and *tail.* The head of the organ lies in the C-shaped curvature of the duodenum, and the tail extends behind and below the stomach toward the spleen. The pancreas is approximately 15 cm (6 inches) long and 4 cm (1.5 inches) wide.

Pancreas Blood Supply

The pancreas receives arterial blood supply from many sources. The head of the pancreas receives its blood supply from both *pancreaticoduodenal arteries:* the superior pancreaticoduodenal artery, which is a branch of the common hepatic artery (which comes from the celiac trunk), and the inferior pancreaticoduodenal artery, which branches from the superior mesenteric artery. These two blood supplies anastomose. The neck, body, and tail of the pancreas receive their blood supply from multiple branches of the splenic artery (another branch of the celiac trunk). Venous drainage occurs through the veins that correspond to the arteries and that ultimately empty into the portal vein. The pancreas has two major functions: *digestive* and *hormonal.*

Exocrine Cells

Specialized exocrine cells within the pancreas secrete digestive enzymes into a duct that is 3 mm wide and traverses the length of the pancreas. The pancreatic duct joins with the cystic duct, carrying bile from the liver and gallbladder, before it empties into the duodenum at the major duodenal papilla. This common ductal exit for the two organs raises the danger of a gallstone lodging at the duodenal papilla and blocking the outflow of pancreatic enzymes. Pancreas exocrine anatomy is illustrated in Fig. 27.9 in Chapter 27, and pancreatic digestive juices are discussed as part of the physiology of the gastrointestinal (GI) system. Most pancreatic tissue is devoted to production of exocrine digestive juices.

Endocrine Cells

The pancreas contains specialized endocrine cells that secrete hormones directly into the bloodstream. The endocrine tissue is less than 5% of the total volume of the pancreas. The function of the endocrine hormones is the focus of the following discussion.

Physiology

The physiology of glucose metabolism has traditionally focused exclusively on the pancreas. With increases in knowledge, glucose metabolism physiology has expanded to include cellular glucose transport proteins, known as *glucose transporters (GLUTs),* and incretin proteins from the GI system.

In the pancreas, clusters of cells that appear to form tiny islands among the exocrine cells accomplish the pancreatic endocrine functions. These clusters are known as the *islets of Langerhans* and are composed of four distinct cell types: *alpha, beta, delta,* and *PP.* The locations of the cells that produce these hormones are shown in Fig. 30.2. Alpha cells secrete *glucagon,* beta cells secrete *insulin,* delta cells secrete *somatostatin,* and PP cells secrete *pancreatic polypeptide hormone.*[1] Most cells that make up the islets of Langerhans are glucagon-secreting alpha cells and insulin-secreting beta cells.[1] Glucagon, insulin, somatostatin, and polypeptide hormones are released into the surrounding capillaries to empty into the portal vein, where they are distributed to target cells in the liver. The hormones then travel into general circulation to reach other target cells.

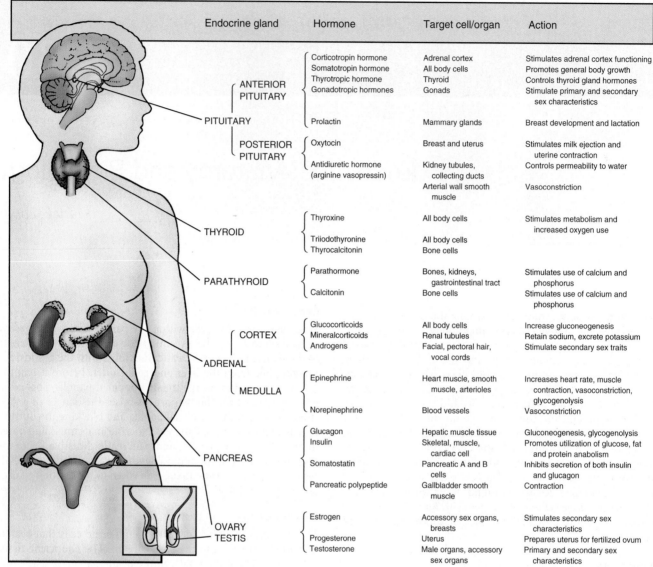

Endocrine gland	Hormone	Target cell/organ	Action
ANTERIOR PITUITARY	Corticotropin hormone	Adrenal cortex	Stimulates adrenal cortex functioning
	Somatotropin hormone	All body cells	Promotes general body growth
	Thyrotropic hormone	Thyroid	Controls thyroid gland hormones
	Gonadotropic hormones	Gonads	Stimulate primary and secondary sex characteristics
PITUITARY	Prolactin	Mammary glands	Breast development and lactation
POSTERIOR PITUITARY	Oxytocin	Breast and uterus	Stimulates milk ejection and uterine contraction
	Antidiuretic hormone (arginine vasopressin)	Kidney tubules, collecting ducts	Controls permeability to water
		Arterial wall smooth muscle	Vasoconstriction
THYROID	Thyroxine	All body cells	Stimulates metabolism and increased oxygen use
	Triiodothyronine	All body cells	
	Thyrocalcitonin	Bone cells	
PARATHYROID	Parathormone	Bones, kidneys, gastrointestinal tract	Stimulates use of calcium and phosphorus
	Calcitonin	Bone cells	Stimulates use of calcium and phosphorus
ADRENAL — CORTEX	Glucocorticoids	All body cells	Increase gluconeogenesis
	Mineralcorticoids	Renal tubules	Retain sodium, excrete potassium
	Androgens	Facial, pectoral hair, vocal cords	Stimulate secondary sex traits
ADRENAL — MEDULLA	Epinephrine	Heart muscle, smooth muscle, arterioles	Increases heart rate, muscle contraction, vasoconstriction, glycogenolysis
	Norepinephrine	Blood vessels	Vasoconstriction
PANCREAS	Glucagon	Hepatic muscle tissue	Gluconeogenesis, glycogenolysis
	Insulin	Skeletal, muscle, cardiac cell	Promotes utilization of glucose, fat and protein anabolism
	Somatostatin	Pancreatic A and B cells	Inhibits secretion of both insulin and glucagon
	Pancreatic polypeptide	Gallbladder smooth muscle	Contraction
OVARY / TESTIS	Estrogen	Accessory sex organs, breasts	Stimulates secondary sex characteristics
	Progesterone	Uterus	Prepares uterus for fertilized ovum
	Testosterone	Male organs, accessory sex organs	Primary and secondary sex characteristics

FIG. 30.1 Location of Endocrine Glands With the Hormones They Produce, Target Cells or Organs, and Hormonal Actions.

Insulin

Insulin is a potent anabolic hormone produced by the beta cells of the pancreas. Elevated levels of blood glucose stimulate insulin production. Insulin is the only hormone produced in the body that directly lowers blood glucose levels. Insulin is responsible for the storage of carbohydrate, protein, and fat nutrients. Insulin also augments the transport of potassium into the cells, decreases the mobilization of fats, and stimulates protein synthesis (Table 30.1). Box 30.1 defines the terms commonly used when discussing glucose and insulin balance. The major stimulant for insulin secretion is an elevation of serum glucose. The greater the increase in blood glucose, the more insulin the normal pancreas produces. Other hormones inhibit the release of insulin (Table 30.2).

Blood Glucose

Blood glucose is reported in millimoles per liter, which is the International System of Units (SI) unit of measurement used throughout the world. In the United States, blood glucose is measured in milligrams per deciliter. The normal blood glucose range is 70 to 100 mg/dL (3.9 to 5.6 mmol/L). To convert mmol/L of glucose to mg/dL, multiply the mmol/L value by 18. To convert mg/dL of glucose to mmol/L, divide the mg/dL value by 18.

In patients who have symptoms of diabetes, pancreatic beta cell destruction has already occurred. With a diagnosis of type 1 diabetes, all the beta cells are nonfunctional. In type 2 diabetes, about half of the beta cells are already destroyed by the time the patient exhibits signs and symptoms of diabetes.[2] The destruction of the beta cells disrupts the homeostatic ability to regulate blood glucose.

Carbohydrate anabolism. Glucose is admitted to the skeletal, cardiac, and adipose cells for use as energy in the presence of effective insulin facilitated by the glucose transporter 4 (GLUT4), as described subsequently. The movement of glucose from the circulation into the intracellular compartment reduces the concentration of glucose in the bloodstream and helps preserve osmolality of the blood. Simultaneously, glucose is available to the cell as its main energy source. Excess glucose in the form of *glycogen* is stored in the hepatic and muscle cells for use as fuel at a later time. In skeletal muscle, 90% of the glucose in the cell is

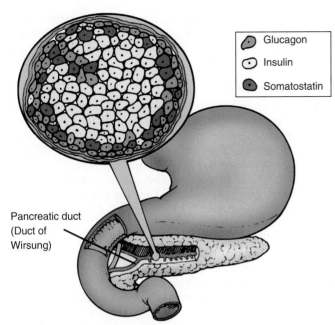

Glucagon
Insulin
Somatostatin

Pancreatic duct
(Duct of
Wirsung)

FIG. 30.2 Macroscopic and Microscopic Structures of the Pancreas and Islets of Langerhans.

TABLE 30.1 Pancreatic Endocrine Cells: Target Tissue and Physiologic Response

Cell	Hormone	Stimulant Release Factor	Target Tissue	Physiologic Response
Alpha	Glucagon	↓ Glucose	Hepatocyte	↑ Glucose in bloodstream
		Exercise	Myocyte	↑ Gluconeogenesis
		↑ Amino acids		↑ Glycogenolysis
		SNS stimulation		↑ Fat mobilization
				↑ Protein mobilization
Beta	Insulin	Glucose	Skeletal cells	↓ Blood glucose
			Muscle cells	↓ Fat mobilization
			Cardiac cells	↑ Fat storage
				↓ Protein mobilization
				↑ Protein synthesis
				↑ Glucogenesis
Delta	Somatostatin	Hyperglycemia	Alpha cells	↓ Blood glucose
			Beta cells	↓ Glycogen secretion
				↓ Insulin secretion
PP	Pancreatic polypeptide	Acute hypoglycemia	Gallbladder	↑ Gallbladder contraction
			Smooth muscle	↓ Pancreatic enzyme

SNS, sympathetic nervous system; ↑, increases; ↓, decreases.

converted to *glycogen* for longer term storage. Glycogen release protects against the effects of hypoglycemia.[3] However, with a diagnosis of type 1 diabetes, glycogen is too abundant after a meal (postprandial hyperglycemia) and insufficient in hypoglycemic states.[3] Newer research suggests that dysregulation of both beta and alpha cells is present in diabetes.[3]

BOX 30.1 Terms Used for Insulin and Glucose Imbalance

- **Anabolism**—constructive phase of metabolism in which the body converts simple substances into more complex compounds in the presence of energy
- **Catabolism**—destructive phase of metabolism in which the body breaks down complex substances to form simpler substances in the presence of energy
- **Gluconeogenesis**—formation of glucose from noncarbohydrate nutrients (eg, fats, protein), which occurs in the liver
- **Glycogen**—storage form of glucose in liver and muscles
- **Glycogenesis**—formation of glycogen from glucose and adenosine triphosphate after a meal when both are plentiful
- **Glycogenolysis**—conversion of glycogen stored in the liver and muscles into usable glucose
- **Osmolality**—measurement of the number of particles in a solution or the concentration of a solution

TABLE 30.2 Insulin Release and Inhibition

Insulin Release (Major Stimulus: High Blood Glucose)	Insulin Inhibition (Major Inhibitor: Low Blood Glucose)
Hormones	
Glucagon	Somatostatin
Corticotropic hormone	Norepinephrine
Thyrotropin	Epinephrine
Somatotropin	
Glucocorticoids	
Incretins	
Medications	
Beta-adrenergic stimulators	Beta-adrenergic blocking agents
Sulfonylurea	Diazoxide
Theophylline	Phenytoin
Acetylcholine	Thiazide or sulfonamide diuretics

Fat anabolism. Adequate, effective insulin levels are important for normal metabolism of lipids. Type 2 diabetes is strongly associated with dyslipidemias and increased risk of atherogenic cardiovascular disease. Type 2 diabetes is characterized by overproduction of large, triglyceride-rich, *very-low-density lipoproteins* and decreased levels of *high-density lipoproteins*.[4] Disorders of carbohydrate and fat metabolism are also associated with metabolic syndrome, a precursor to diabetes and cardiovascular disease.

Protein conservation. Insulin and the GLUTs (see later on) together facilitate the transfer of glucose across the cell wall. By having glucose (carbohydrate) available as the body's fuel source, protein is spared from use as energy. Protein is then available for critical protein synthesis and for amino acid transport into the cells. Protein metabolism also benefits from an adequate insulin supply. The body uses protein for energy sources only in acute hyperglycemia of diabetic ketoacidosis or in starvation states.

Glucagon

Glucagon, synthesized by alpha cells in the pancreas, has the opposite effect of insulin. Glucagon is released during hypoglycemia to induce hepatic glucose output.[3] Because glucagon counterregulates insulin levels and raises blood glucose levels, it is a potent *gluconeogenic hormone.* By means of *gluconeogenesis,* glucagon can form glucose from noncarbohydrate sources such as fat and protein when required. Glucagon release from the pancreas is stimulated by low blood glucose levels, starvation, exercise, or stimulation of the sympathetic nervous system (SNS).[5] Glucagon release protects the brain from the consequences of hypoglycemia.[5]

To meet short-term energy requirements, glucagon stimulates the release of *glycogen* stores from liver and muscle cells. Through a process called *glycogenolysis,* the glycogen stored in the liver is converted into a glucose form that can be used by the cells.[5]

For long-term energy needs, glucagon stimulates glucose release through the more complex process of *gluconeogenesis.* In gluconeogenesis, fat and protein nutrients are rapidly broken down into end products that are then changed into glucose.[5]

A normal blood glucose level is maintained in the healthy body by the *insulin-to-glucagon ratio* (Box 30.2). When the blood glucose level is high, insulin is released, and glucagon is inhibited. When blood glucose levels are low, glucagon rather than insulin is released to raise the blood glucose level. The brain has a very limited supply of glucose, and glucagon release is essential to protect the brain from the effects of hypoglycemia.[6]

Somatostatin

Somatostatin is a hormone that is produced in the pancreatic delta cells. Somatostatin decreases glucagon secretion; in high quantities, it decreases insulin release (see Table 30.1). Hyperglycemia stimulates the activity of the delta cells. It is theorized that the release of insulin enables somatostatin to control beta cell activity. Somatostatin may be involved in the regulation of the postprandial influx of glucose into cells.

Pancreatic Polypeptide

The PP cells within the islets of Langerhans synthesize pancreatic polypeptide hormone.[1] This hormone is released after a meal and remains elevated for several hours suggestive of a role in digestion. Pancreatic polypeptide hormone influences GI motility and gallbladder function. Other functions are not yet understood.

Glucose Transporters

Human cells take up glucose by means of facultative glucose transport proteins. These proteins are specialized by tissue distribution and function as described in Table 30.3.[7] At the cellular level, glucose crosses the cell plasma membrane through *aqueous pores* formed by GLUT transporters. There have been 14 GLUTs identified so far.[8] The GLUT number indicates the order in which the molecular sequence and GLUT tissue locations were identified.[8] The functions of key GLUTs are described in more detail next.

GLUT1 and GLUT3. The central nervous system (CNS) is freely permeable to glucose transported by GLUT1 and GLUT3.[6] The CNS does not rely on insulin for transport of glucose across the neural cell membrane. The brain and other CNS cells require a constant source of glucose because they retain minimal glucose and glycogen stores.

GLUT2. The GLUT2 proteins are associated with glucose sensing and facilitate rapid entry of glucose into specialized cells such as the pancreatic beta cells and into the glucose-sensing cells in the hepatoportal vein area.[8,9] In the intestine, in the presence of a high-glucose meal, GLUT2 proteins may translocate to the apical cell surface to increase glucose absorption from the gut to the bloodstream.[8]

GLUT4. The insulin-responsive GLUT4 protein plays a pivotal role in the way glucose moves from the bloodstream into the cell.[9,10] After a meal, the levels of sugars and amino acids in the bloodstream rise. This increase signals pancreatic

---

BOX 30.2 Insulin-to-Glucagon Ratio: Effects on Carbohydrate, Fat, and Protein Metabolism

Balanced Insulin and Glucagon	Decreased Insulin and Increased Glucagon
↑ Use of glucose by cells	↓ Use of glucose by cells
↑ Movement of potassium intracellularly	↓ Movement of potassium intracellularly
↑ Carbohydrate metabolism	↑ Blood glucose
↓ Gluconeogenesis	↑ Gluconeogenesis
↑ Glycogen storage	↓ Glycogen storage
↓ Glycogenolysis	↑ Glycogenolysis
↓ Lipolysis	↑ Lipolysis
↓ Fat mobilization	↑ Fat mobilization
↑ Fat storage	↓ Fat stores
↓ Protein mobilization	↑ Hepatic metabolism fats
↑ Protein synthesis	↑ Ketogenesis
	↑ Mobilization of protein
	↑ Proteolysis
	↑ Lipoprotein

TABLE 30.3 Glucose Transporter Functions

Glucose Transporter (GLUT)	Anatomic Locations	Function
GLUT1	Erythrocytes, endothelial cells of brain Transport across blood–brain barrier	Basal glucose uptake
GLUT2	Pancreatic beta bells, liver, kidney, small intestine	High-capacity glucose transporter Can transport fructose
GLUT3	Brain cells, nerve cells (axons and dendrites)	Transports glucose into brain and neural tissue
GLUT4	Striated muscle and adipose tissue	Insulin-regulated transport in muscle and fat
GLUT5	Intestine, kidney, testis	Transports fructose
GLUT6	Spleen, leukocytes, brain	
GLUT7	Small intestine, colon, testis	Transports fructose
GLUT8	Testis, brain, muscle, adipocytes	Fuel supply of mature spermatozoa
GLUT9	Liver, kidney	
GLUT10	Liver, pancreas	Muscle-specific fructose transporter
GLUT11	Heart, muscle	
GLUT12	Heart, prostate, mammary gland	
GLUT13	Brain	

beta cells to release insulin into the bloodstream. As the insulin circulates in the vascular system, it activates an insulin receptor on the plasma membrane of cells, primarily peripheral muscle and adipose cells. This receptor initiates signaling cascades inside the cell to activate GLUT4, which resides in intracellular vesicles (storage areas within the cell) until needed. GLUT4 travels from intracellular storage sites to the plasma membrane in response to the signal from the insulin receptor.[10,11] At the cell surface, GLUT4 facilitates the passive transport of glucose along a concentration gradient into striated muscle and fat cells. This increases glucose transport into fat cells by a factor of 20- to 30-fold in healthy individuals.[9] Glucose transport into skeletal muscle accounts for 85% to 90% of postprandial glucose removal from the bloodstream.[9]

In the baseline state (between meals with normal blood glucose), only 4% to 10% of GLUT4 is on the cell surface, whereas 90% is within the cell storage sites.[9] Within 10 to 15 minutes of insulin stimulation of muscle cells, GLUT4 levels at the cell surface double as rapid translocation from the interior to the cell surface occurs. Between meals, the liver normally provides sufficient glucose output to maintain constant circulating blood glucose levels within the normal range.

GLUT5. Fructose absorption is the target for GLUT5 proteins, which are found on the apical membrane of intestinal cells.[8] GLUT5 is of interest because of the high levels of fructose in many modern processed foods and the link between high-fructose foods and obesity.

Incretins

Incretins, which are hormones that are released from the GI tract after a meal, increase the production of insulin from the pancreatic beta cells.[12] Two incretins are of particular clinical importance: (1) *glucagon-like peptide 1 (GLP-1)* and (2) *glucose-dependent insulinotropic polypeptide (GIP).*[12] The physiology of the incretins has been used to develop new medicines that reduce postprandial blood glucose levels in type 2 diabetes (see Table 32.3 in Chapter 32). More insulin is released after oral glucose ingestion than in response to the same amount of intravenous glucose because of release of the gut incretins.[12-14] The increase in insulin secretion caused by stimulation from the

incretins may make up 70% of the insulin response, depending on the size of the meal.[13,14] This incretin effect is impaired in patients with type 2 diabetes.[13,14] The physiologic effects of GIP and GLP-1 are listed in Table 30.4.

Glucose-dependent insulinotropic polypeptide. GIP is an incretin and is described as a "gut hormone"[15] that is synthesized and predominantly released from the K cells of the duodenum and proximal jejunum.[12,15] GIP acts directly on pancreatic beta cells to increase insulin secretion.[15]

Glucagon-like peptide 1. GLP-1 is an incretin that is also described as a "gut hormone."[15] GLP-1 is synthesized and released from the enteroendocrine L cells of the ileum and colon.[13,15] When blood glucose levels are elevated, GLP-1 stimulates insulin release from the pancreas and inhibits glucagon release from the liver. GLP-1 has a short half-life of less than 2 minutes because it is rapidly broken down by the enzyme *dipeptidyl peptidase-4* (DPP-4).[16] *Gliptins* are medicines that have been developed to inhibit the DPP-4 enzyme and slow the inactivation of endogenous GLP-1 to reduce postprandial glucose elevation after a meal.

GLP-1 exerts other beneficial effects, including decreased gastric emptying and the feeling of satiety (feeling of being full) after a meal. When blood glucose levels are within normal range, GLP-1 inhibits the release of somatostatin from the pancreatic delta cells and glucagon from the liver.[14,15]

PITUITARY GLAND AND HYPOTHALAMUS

Anatomy

The hypothalamus is linked to the pituitary gland in two distinct ways: (1) a vascular network connects the anterior portion of the pituitary with the hypothalamus, and (2) a separate pathway of nerve fibers connects the posterior pituitary with the hypothalamus. Understanding the proximity of the hypothalamus and the pituitary gland to each other is necessary to appreciate the correlation that exists between these organs.

The hypothalamus lies in the base of the brain, superior to the pituitary gland. It is composed of specialized nervous tissue responsible for the integrated functioning of the nervous system and endocrine system, which is called *neuroendocrine*

TABLE 30.4 Incretins Impact on Metabolism

Target Organs and Tissues	GIP	GLP-1
Pancreas	Stimulates insulin synthesis and release from pancreatic beta cells after a meal when blood glucose is elevated	Stimulates insulin synthesis and release from pancreatic beta cells after a meal when blood glucose is elevated
	Maintains beta cell mass and function	Maintains beta cell mass and function
	Decreases beta cell death (apoptosis)	Decreases beta cell death (apoptosis)
	Increases GLUT2 expression in the pancreas	Increases GLUT2 expression in pancreas
		Increases somatostatin release from pancreatic delta cells
		Decreases glucagon release from the pancreas
Liver		Decreases release of glucose from the liver
GI system		Delays gastric emptying
CNS		Decreases appetite, sense of satiety after a meal
Muscle		Increases glucose uptake in muscle
Adipose tissue		Increases glucose uptake and free fatty acid synthesis to triglycerides
Bone	Increases bone formation	Increases bone formation
	Decreases bone resorption	Decreases bone resorption

CNS, central nervous system; *GI,* gastrointestinal; *GIP,* glucose-dependent insulinotropic polypeptide; *GLP-1,* glucagon-like peptide 1; *GLUT2,* glucose transporter 2.

control. The hypothalamus weighs approximately 4 g and forms the walls and lower portion of the third ventricle of the brain. The area comprising the floor of the ventricle thickens in the center and elongates. The pituitary gland is suspended from this funnel-shaped portion, called the *infundibulum* or *infundibular stalk,* as illustrated in Fig. 30.3. The infundibular stalk contains a rich vascular supply and a network of communicating neurons that travel from the hypothalamus to the pituitary. The vascular network and neural pathways transport chemical and neural signals and maintain constant communication between the nervous system and the endocrine system.

The pituitary gland is also called the *hypophysis.* It is attached below the hypothalamus and is found recessed in the base of the cranial cavity in a hollow depression of the sphenoid bone known as the *sella turcica.*[17] Secured in such a protected environment, the pituitary is one of the most inaccessible endocrine glands in humans. However, because of this location, the pituitary gland is susceptible to injury from surgical and accidental trauma to the face and head.[18] The pituitary is composed of the anterior lobe and the posterior lobe (see Fig. 30.3). Each component within the pituitary has its own origin, morphology, and function.

Anterior Pituitary

The anterior lobe of the pituitary, also called the *adenohypophysis,* is the largest portion of the gland. It communicates with the hypothalamus by means of a vascular network. The glandular tissue of the anterior pituitary produces several hormones, including adrenocorticotropic hormone (ACTH), thyroid-stimulating hormone (TSH), follicle-stimulating hormone, luteinizing hormone, growth hormone, and prolactin.[17] Information about all the hormones, their target tissues, and their actions is found in Fig. 30.1.

Posterior Pituitary

The posterior lobe of the pituitary gland is also known as the *neurohypophysis.* It retains its continuity with the hypothalamus by means of neural fibers running through the infundibular stalk. The neurohypophysis has no glandular properties but functions as an extension of the hypothalamus. It collects, stores, and later releases hormones that are produced in the hypothalamus. Oxytocin and antidiuretic hormone (ADH) are manufactured in the hypothalamus and stored in the posterior pituitary.[17]

Physiology

The hypothalamus gland is known as the "master gland" because of the influence it has over all areas of body functioning. The hypothalamus controls pituitary gland action and response by secreting substances called *release-inhibiting factors.* These factors control the release or inhibition of hormones. Thyrotropin-releasing hormone (TRH) is an example of a release-inhibiting factor.[17] Virtually every function necessary to maintaining the human body in a state of dynamic equilibrium is regulated in this manner. One of the most important hormones to understand in caring for a critically ill patient is ADH.

Antidiuretic Hormone

ADH, known also as *arginine vasopressin,* is an important hormone responsible for regulating fluid balance within the body.[18,19] ADH acts through specialized vasopressin receptors (V receptors) in specific target tissue:

V_1 receptors in arterial walls
V_2 receptors in kidney collecting ducts
V_3 receptors in pituitary tissue

ADH has two functions: (1) By means of the V_1 receptors, it constricts smooth muscles within the arterial wall, and (2) through V_2 receptors, it regulates fluid balance by altering the permeability of the kidney tubule to water.[19] ADH also contributes to control of the sodium level in the extracellular fluid by control of plasma osmolality. The sodium ion concentration in the plasma largely determines plasma osmolality. Osmoreceptors, located in the hypothalamus, are sensitive to changes in the circulating plasma osmolality.[19]

Disorders of water metabolism are divided into *hyperosmolar* and *hypo-osmolar* states.[19] Hyperosmolar disorders have a deficit of body water relative to body solute. Hypo-osmolar disorders have an excess of body water relative to total body solute.

Sodium and water metabolism are regulated by different but complementary systems within the body. Sodium metabolism is predominately regulated by the renin-angiotensin-aldosterone system (RAAS), and water metabolism is primarily controlled by arginine vasopressin (ADH).

A low sodium level is associated with a low serum osmolality (hypo-osmolar state). When sodium levels rise, plasma osmolality increases (hyperosmolar state). ADH is then released to stimulate water resorption at the nephron to maintain sodium balance. This process decreases water loss from the body and subsequently concentrates and reduces urine volume. Fluid conserved in this manner is returned to the circulating plasma, where it dilutes the concentration (osmolality) of plasma, as shown in Fig. 30.4.

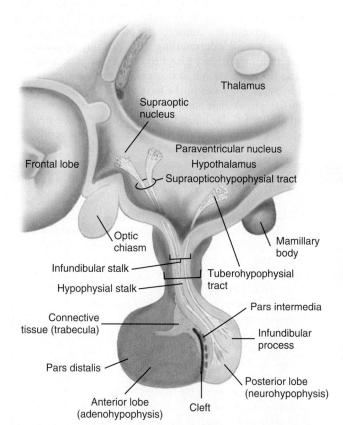

FIG. 30.3 Anatomy of the Hypothalamus and Pituitary Gland and Their Locations in the Skull. (From Thompson JM, et al. *Mosby's Clinical Nursing.* 5th ed. St. Louis: Mosby; 2002.)

The release of ADH increases with hypovolemia.[19] Plasma osmotic pressure and the volume of circulating blood regulate the release of ADH. Stretch receptors located in the left atrium are sensitive to volume changes in the plasma that may be caused by vomiting, diarrhea, or blood loss. Hemorrhage that is sufficient to lower the blood pressure or emesis that is sufficient to reduce fluid volume stimulates the release of ADH. Other factors capable of influencing ADH secretion are pain, stress, malignant disease, surgical intervention, alcohol, and some medications. Table 30.5 lists additional factors that affect ADH levels.

THYROID GLAND

Anatomy

The thyroid gland weighs 15 to 25 g in an adult.[20] The size of the adult gland varies according to the availability of dietary iodine in different geographic regions. The gland partially encases the trachea, is wrapped around the second to fourth tracheal rings anteriorly and laterally, and is located at the level of the sixth and seventh cervical vertebrae posteriorly. The thyroid gland lies inferior to the thyroid cartilage and the articulating surface of the *cricoid cartilage*. This bow-tie–shaped gland has two lateral lobes that are partially covered by the sternohyoid and sternothyroid muscles. The thyroid isthmus, the band of narrow thyroid tissue that connects the lateral lobes, lies directly inferior to the cricoid cartilage, as shown in Fig. 30.5.

Two important nerves associated with speech and swallowing pass close to the thyroid gland. The *recurrent laryngeal nerve* and *superior laryngeal nerve* are branches of the *vagus nerve*. The considerable anatomic variety in the location of these nerves increases the risk of injury during surgical procedures such as thyroidectomy.[20]

The thyroid gland has a rich blood supply from the superior and inferior thyroid arteries. The superior thyroid artery is the first branch of the external carotid artery.[20] Venous drainage is from the superior, middle, and inferior thyroid veins. Lymphatic drainage follows the route of the thyroid veins.[20] The functional units of the thyroid gland are spherical cells called *follicles*. Follicles are filled with the protein *thyroglobulin*.[21]

The parathyroid glands (usually four) are intimately associated with the posterior surface of the thyroid gland. The parathyroid glands derive their name from their anatomic proximity to the thyroid, although they have a completely different function. The parathyroid glands maintain calcium homeostasis.

Physiology

Functioning of the thyroid gland depends on many factors that respond to a delicate hormonal interplay. The hypothalamus, anterior pituitary, dietary intake of iodine, and circulating protein bodies in the blood all affect thyroid gland function.

Pituitary Gland and Thyroid-Stimulating Hormone

The anterior lobe of the pituitary gland secretes TSH, also known as *thyrotropin*. TSH then stimulates the thyroid gland to produce thyroid hormones.

Iodine and Iodide

In the United States, dietary ingestion of iodine ranges from 200 to 500 mcg per person/day. Iodine is added to table salt to ensure adequate amounts in the population. Through a complex process, dietary iodine is absorbed and concentrated in the thyroid follicles. The iodine is oxidized to iodide by the enzyme *thyroid peroxidase*. Through active transport, the amino acid tyrosine binds the iodide to thyroglobulin, eventually yielding triiodothyronine (T_3) and thyroxine (T_4). Most T_3 and T_4 are circulated in the bloodstream bound to proteins. Free thyroid hormone that is not protein bound is responsible for activating thyroid responses throughout the body and is described as free T_3 and free T_4.

Antidiuretic Hormone RELEASE

Hemoconcentration, hypovolemia

↑ Osmoreceptors   ↑ Baroreceptors stimulation — Atria / Aorta / Carotid artery

↓

↑ Release of antidiuretic hormone

↓

↑ Permeability of renal tubule

↓

↑ Water reabsorption/conservation

↓

↓ Serum osmolality   ↓ Urine volume   ↑ Urine osmolality

Antidiuretic Hormone RESTRICTION

Hemodilution, hypervolemia

↑ Hypothalamic osmoreceptors   ↑ Stretch receptors left atrium

↓

↓ Release of antidiuretic hormone

↓

↓ Permeability of renal tubule

↓

↓ Water reabsorption/promote diuresis

↓

↑ Serum osmolality   ↑ Urine output   ↓ Urine osmolality

FIG. 30.4 Physiology of the Release and Restriction of Antidiuretic Hormone.

TABLE 30.5   Antidiuretic Hormone Functions

Antidiuretic Hormone Stimulation	Antidiuretic Hormone Restriction
Increased serum osmolality	Decreased serum osmolality
Emesis	Hypervolemia
Hypovolemia	Water intoxication
Hemorrhage	Cold
Pain	Congenital defect
	Carbon dioxide inhalation

Hypothalamic-Pituitary System Damage

Accidental trauma	Accidental trauma
Surgical trauma	Surgical trauma
Pathologic trauma	Pathologic trauma
Stress: Physical and emotional	
Acute infections	
Malignancies	
Nonmalignant pulmonary disorders	
Stimulated pulmonary baroreceptors	
Nocturnal sleep	

Medications

Nicotine	Phenytoin
Barbiturates	Chlorpromazine
Oxytocin	Reserpine
Glucocorticoids	Norepinephrine
Anesthetics	Ethanol
Acetaminophen	Opioids
Amitriptyline	Lithium
Carbamazepine	Demeclocycline
Cyclophosphamide	Tolazamide
Chlorpropamide	
Potassium-depleting diuretics	
Vincristine	
Isoproterenol	

Thyroglobulin

Thyroglobulin is a key precursor in the biosynthesis of thyroid hormone. Thyroglobulin is stored in the thyroid follicles until needed. TSH release stimulates thyroglobulin secretion into the bloodstream.[21]

Triiodothyronine and Thyroxine

TSH prompts the thyroid cells to produce thyroid hormones (T_3 and T_4) in the presence of iodine in the thyroid follicles. In the normal thyroid gland, 90% of the thyroid hormone that is produced is in the form of T_4, and 10% is T_3. These hormones are named according to the number of iodine atoms in their structure; T_3 has three iodine atoms, and T_4 has four iodine atoms.[21]

Most T_4 is subsequently converted into the more biologically active T_3. Most T_3 in the bloodstream is the result of the conversion of T_4 to T_3 in the peripheral tissues, liver, and kidneys. T_3 acts more rapidly on target tissues compared with T_4, and it is more actively potent. Both thyroid hormones affect the rate at which oxygen is used in the body and thus affect all metabolic processes in the body.

Calcitonin

The thyroid gland produces a third hormone, *thyrocalcitonin,* also called *calcitonin.* This hormone is produced by the parafollicular cells, or C cells, that are found scattered among the thyroid follicular cells. Calcitonin acts in concert with parathyroid hormone to maintain normal calcium blood levels. Calcitonin lowers calcium levels in the blood through urinary excretion and by promoting calcium absorption in the bone. In contrast, parathyroid hormone limits urinary loss and stimulates bones to release calcium. Throughout the remainder of this discussion, thyroid hormone refers collectively to T_3 and T_4, not calcitonin.

Hypothalamic-Pituitary-Thyroid Axis Feedback Loop

The hypothalamic-pituitary-thyroid axis regulates the mechanism for the synthesis and secretion of thyroid hormone. The production and secretion of thyroid hormone are regulated by a feedback mechanism that limits the amount of hormone circulating to the cellular need at that time, as illustrated in Fig. 30.6.

In response to decreased circulating levels of T_3 and T_4, the hypothalamus releases TRH. TRH activates TSH in the anterior pituitary, and TSH stimulates the thyroid gland to manufacture and release the thyroid hormones T_3 and T_4 in the presence of iodine.[21] When serum blood levels of T_3 and T_4 become high, the pituitary inhibits the production of additional TSH. When levels of T_3 and T_4 become too low, the pituitary is stimulated to secrete additional TSH.

T_4 prompts the activation of beta-adrenergic receptors in widespread areas of the body. These receptors trigger an SNS response and release norepinephrine at sympathetic nerve endings.[22] The effect is stimulation of the cardiac tissue, nervous tissue, and smooth muscle tissue as well as an increase in metabolism and thermogenesis (increased body heat). Box 30.3 lists the major actins of thyroid hormones in more detail.

ADRENAL GLAND

Anatomy

The adrenal glands, also called *suprarenal glands,* are small, yellowish, bilateral, pyramidal or semilunar-shaped organs located at the superior pole of the kidney. As a neighbor to the kidney, they are retroperitoneal and embedded in the fat pad of the kidney. The normal adrenal gland is 3 to 4 cm in its longest axis and weighs approximately 5 g in adults (Fig. 30.7). Functionally and histologically, two glands exist within the suprarenal gland: (1) the outer cortex and (2) the inner medulla. Both regions secrete hormones that are integral to the body's response to stress.

Adrenal Cortex

The adrenal cortex is the thicker outer region, and it makes up 85% of the gland. The cortex is composed of three different layers of cells, each with a specific endocrine function: (1) zona glomerulosa, (2) zona fasciculata, and (3) zona reticularis. The cortex secretes cortisol, it regulates fluid homeostasis by means of aldosterone, and it secretes androgens.

Adrenal Medulla

The inner region is called the *adrenal medulla.* The inner medulla is a part of the SNS, and it resembles a cluster of neurons more

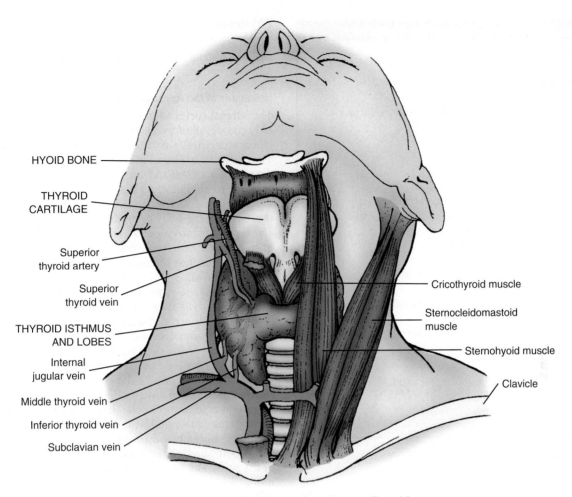

FIG. 30.5 Gross Anatomy of the Human Thyroid.

FIG. 30.6 Hypothalamus-Pituitary-Thyroid Axis Feedback Loop.

than an endocrine gland. The adrenal medulla contains clusters of specialized *chromaffin cells,* which are modified preganglionic sympathetic neurons.[23] Different sets of chromaffin cells contain chromaffin granules that are specific for each of the catecholamines epinephrine or norepinephrine. The granules for each catecholamine appear in different sets of cells within the adrenal medulla. A chromaffin cell usually contains granules only for one catecholamine or the other.

The adrenal medulla is stimulated by the SNS by preganglionic bundles of sympathetic nerve fibers that originate in the spinal cord.[22] The role of the chromaffin cells is to secrete the catecholamines epinephrine and norepinephrine. Under physiologic stress, these hormones produce a widespread excitatory effect described as a "surge of adrenaline" or as the "fight-or-flight response."[23]

Adrenal Blood Supply

The rich arterial blood supply comes to the adrenal gland from three sources (see Fig. 30.7): (1) The superior suprarenal artery is a branch of the inferior phrenic artery, (2) the middle suprarenal artery branches directly off of the aorta, and (3) the inferior suprarenal artery branches off the renal artery. Venous drainage is usually achieved through a single vein from each adrenal gland. The vein from the right adrenal gland drains into the inferior vena cava, and the vein from the left adrenal gland empties into the left renal vein.

BOX 30.3 Thyroid Hormone Functions

- Interact with growth hormone
- Maturation of skeletal system
- Development of central nervous system
- Stimulate carbohydrate metabolism
- Increase rate of glucose absorption from the gastrointestinal tract
- Increase rate of glucose use by the cells
- Accelerate the rate of fat metabolism
- Increase cholesterol degradation in the liver
- Decrease serum cholesterol levels
- Increase protein anabolism and catabolism
- Mobilize protein and release amino acids into circulation
- Increase energy from protein nutrients through gluconeogenesis
- Increase the body's demand for vitamins
- Increase oxygen consumption and use
- Increase basal metabolic rate
- Have marked chronotropic and inotropic effects on the heart
- Increase cardiac output
- Stimulate contractility and excitability of myocardium
- Increase blood volume
- Expand respiratory rate and depth necessary for normal hypoxic and hypercapnic drive
- Promote sympathetic overactivity
- Boost erythropoiesis
- Increase metabolism and clearance of various hormones and pharmacologic agents
- Stimulate bone resorption

Cortex   Medulla

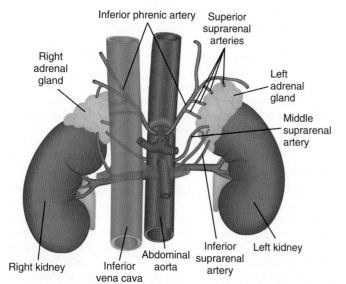

FIG. 30.7 Adrenal Gland. (A) Cross section of the adrenal gland showing the outer cortex and inner medulla. (B) Anatomic relationship of the adrenal glands to the kidneys.

Physiology

The adrenal cortex and the adrenal medulla secrete important and very different hormones. Each part of the gland is functionally independent.

Hormones of the Adrenal Cortex

The adrenal cortex (outer layer) secretes three different classes of hormone, all of which are lipid-based steroid hormones: (1) glucocorticoid, (2) corticosteroid, and (3) mineralocorticoid. The *glucocorticoid* hormone cortisol is secreted from the cells of the zona fasciculata and zona reticularis. Cortisol is released in response to physiologic stress caused by infection, trauma, and the fasting state. In hypoglycemia, the release of cortisol triggers other cells in the body to produce energy from fats and amino acids (proteins) to ensure that the brain receives a steady supply of glucose. Pharmacologic doses (high doses) of glucocorticoids are used to depress the inflammatory response and inhibit the immune system.

Pharmacologic *corticosteroids* are administered to prevent rejection of newly transplanted solid organs (see Chapter 36). Corticosteroids are also used to treat inflammatory disorders, and they are administered when the adrenal gland is cortisol deficient.

The principal *mineralocorticoid* hormone aldosterone is secreted from the cells of the zona glomerulosa. Secretion of aldosterone is the final step in the RAAS. Aldosterone is secreted in response to intravascular hypovolemia, and its target of action is the distal tubules of the kidneys to retain more sodium and water in the bloodstream. In the healthy person, aldosterone contributes to the equilibrium of water and potassium in the body. Fig. 14.18 in Chapter 14 illustrates the neurohormonal role of the RAAS in heart failure. In patients with heart failure, medications to block the effect of aldosterone on the kidneys often are prescribed. The most frequently used medication is spironolactone (Aldactone) (see "Neurohormonal Compensatory Mechanisms in Heart Failure" in Chapter 14). Some androgen hormones such as dehydroepiandrosterone (DHEA) are also secreted from the zona reticularis in the cortex. The function of DHEA is not fully understood.

Hormones of the Adrenal Medulla

The adrenal medulla (inner region) secretes two important catecholamines: *epinephrine,* also known as *adrenaline,* and *norepinephrine,* also known as *noradrenaline.* The adrenal medulla acts as a functional extension of the SNS. With stimulation of the SNS, the chromaffin cells in the adrenal medulla are stimulated to secrete predominantly epinephrine and some norepinephrine into the bloodstream. This results in an epinephrine surge described as the fight-or-flight response. In the critical care unit, intravenous infusions of epinephrine and norepinephrine are used in shock states to raise the blood pressure. The pharmacologic effects of these catecholamines are described in Table 15.18 in Chapter 15.

Hypothalamic-Pituitary-Adrenal Axis

The adrenal glands are physiologically linked to the hypothalamus and the pituitary gland. When the brain perceives a stressful or threatening situation, the hypothalamus releases corticotropin-releasing hormone, which acts on the anterior pituitary to release ACTH, which circulates in the bloodstream to reach the adrenal cortex and stimulate glucocorticoid hormone release. Under stress-free conditions, cortisol is secreted in a diurnal pattern, and levels are highest in the early morning and lowest in the late evening.[24] Illness or trauma disrupts this normal physiology with resultant loss of the diurnal pattern. There is also an association with adrenal insufficiency during critical illness.[25]

SUMMARY

Pancreas

- The pancreas is a long, triangular organ approximately 15 cm long and 4 cm wide. It is situated in the C-shaped curvature of the duodenum and extends behind and below the stomach toward the spleen.
- Insulin is released by the beta cells of the pancreas. An elevated blood glucose level is the stimulus for insulin secretion from the pancreas. The higher the blood glucose, the more insulin the normal pancreas produces.
- Glucagon is synthesized from the alpha cells in the pancreas. Its effect is the opposite of the effect of insulin. Glucagon release is stimulated by hypoglycemia, and it stimulates glucose output from the liver.
- In addition to insulin, human cells take up glucose by means of facultative glucose transport proteins known as GLUTs.
- Incretins are hormones released from the GI tract after a meal that increase the production of insulin from the pancreatic beta cells.

Pituitary

- The pituitary gland is attached below the hypothalamus and recessed in the base of the skull in a hollow depression known as the sella turcica.
- The anterior pituitary gland secretes ACTH, TSH, and other hormones.
- The posterior pituitary gland secretes ADH, also known also as arginine vasopressin.
- Sodium and water metabolism are regulated by two complementary systems within the body: sodium metabolism by the RAAS and water metabolism by arginine vasopressin (ADH).

Thyroid

- The thyroid gland has a "bow-tie" shape. It is wrapped around the trachea anteriorly and laterally at the level of the sixth and seventh cervical vertebrae. The thyroid isthmus, the band of narrow thyroid tissue that connects the lateral lobes, lies directly below the cricoid cartilage.
- The thyroid hormones are T_4 and T_3. Most T_4 is converted to the more potent and biologically active T_3 in the peripheral tissues, liver, and kidneys.
- The thyroid gland produces a third hormone, thyrocalcitonin (calcitonin), which acts in concert with parathyroid hormone to maintain normal calcium blood levels.

Adrenal

- The adrenal glands are small, pyramid-shaped organs located at the superior pole of the kidneys.
- The adrenal gland contains a cortex and medulla that represent two functionally different endocrine zones. The adrenal cortex secretes cortisol and aldosterone. The adrenal medulla secretes epinephrine and norepinephrine.

ⓔ Visit the Evolve site for additional study materials.

REFERENCES

1. Barbieus C, et al. Asymmetrical distribution of delta and PP cells in human pancreatic islets. *J Endocrinol.* 2016;229(2):123.
2. Russo GT, et al. Factors associated with beta-cell dysfunction in type 2 diabetes—the BETADECLINE Study. *PLoS One.* 2014;9(10):e109702.
3. Farhy LS, McCall AL. Glucagon—the new "insulin" in the pathophysiology of diabetes. *Curr Opin Clin Nutr Metab Care.* 2015;18(4):407.
4. Vergès B. Pathophysiology of diabetic dyslipidaemia: Where are we? *Diabetologia.* 2015;58(5):886.
5. Cryer PE. Minireview: glucagon in the pathogenesis of hypoglycemia and hyperglycemia in diabetes. *Endocrinology.* 2012;153(3):1039.
6. Thorens B. Brain glucose sensing and neural regulation of insulin and glucagon secretion. *Diabetes Obes Metab.* 2011;13(suppl 1):82.
7. Thorens B. Sensing of glucose in the brain. *Handb Exp Pharmacol.* 2012;(209):277.
8. Thorens B, Mueckler M. Glucose transporters in the 21st century. *Am J Physiol Endocrinol Metabol.* 2010;298(2):E141.
9. Stringer DM, Zahradka P, Taylor CG. Glucose transporters: cellular links to hyperglycemia in insulin resistance and diabetes. *Nutr Rev.* 2015;73(3):140.
10. Rowland AF, Fazakerley DJ, James DE. Mapping insulin/GLUT4 circuitry. *Traffic.* 2011;12(6):672.
11. Leto D, Saltiel AR. Regulation of glucose transport by insulin: traffic control of GLUT4. *Nat Rev Mol Cell Biol.* 2012;13(6):383.
12. Pais R, Gribble FM, Reimann F. Stimulation of incretin secreting cells. *Ther Adv Endocrinol Metab.* 2016;7(1):24.
13. Ahrén B, Carr RD, Deacon CF. Incretin hormone secretion over the day. *Vitam Horm.* 2010;84:203.
14. Phillips LK, Prins JB. Update on incretin hormones. *Ann N Y Acad Sci.* 2011;1243:E55.
15. Campbell JE, Drucker DJ. Pharmacology, physiology, and mechanisms of incretin hormone action. *Cell Metab.* 2013;17(6):819.
16. Campbell RK. Clarifying the role of incretin-based therapies in the treatment of type 2 diabetes mellitus. *Clin Ther.* 2011;33(5):511.
17. Musumeci G, et al. A journey through the pituitary gland: development, structure and function, with emphasis on embryo-foetal and later development. *Acta Histochem.* 2015;117(4-5):355.
18. Kleindienst A, et al. Hyponatremia in neurotrauma: the role of vasopressin. *J Neurotrauma.* 2015;33(7):615.
19. Knepper MA, Kwon TH, Nielsen S. Molecular physiology of water balance. *N Engl J Med.* 2015;372(14):1349.
20. Mohebati A, Shaha AR. Anatomy of thyroid and parathyroid glands and neurovascular relations. *Clin Anat.* 2012;25(1):19.
21. Stathatos N. Thyroid physiology. *Med Clin North Am.* 2012;96(2):165.
22. Gordan R, Gwathmey JK, Xie LH. Autonomic and endocrine control of cardiovascular function. *World J Cardiol.* 2015;7(4):204.
23. Pérez-Alvarez A, Hernández-Vivanco A, Albillos A. Past, present and future of human chromaffin cells: role in physiology and therapeutics. *Cell Mol Neurobiol.* 2010;30(8):1407.
24. Gibbison B, et al. Dynamic pituitary-adrenal interactions in response to cardiac surgery. *Crit Care Med.* 2015;43(4):791.
25. Boonen E, et al. Reduced nocturnal ACTH-driven cortisol secretion during critical illness. *Am J Physiol Endocrinol Metab.* 2014;306(8):E883.

31

Endocrine Clinical Assessment and Diagnostic Procedures

Mary E. Lough

Assessment of a patient with endocrine dysfunction is a systematic process that incorporates history taking and physical examination. Most of the endocrine glands are deeply encased in the human body. Although the placement of the glands provides security for the glandular functions, their resulting inaccessibility limits clinical examination. Nevertheless, the endocrine glands may be assessed indirectly. The critical care nurse who understands the metabolic actions of the hormones produced by endocrine glands assesses the physiology of a gland by monitoring the target tissue of the gland as listed in Fig. 30.1 in Chapter 30. This chapter describes clinical and diagnostic evaluation of the pancreas, the posterior pituitary, and the thyroid gland.

HISTORY

The initial presentation of the patient determines the rapidity and direction of the history. For a patient in acute distress, the history is curtailed to only a few questions about the patient's chief complaint and precipitating events. For a patient without obvious distress, the endocrine history focuses on four areas: (1) current health status, (2) description of the current illness, (3) medical history and general endocrine status, and (4) family history. Data collection in the endocrine history for diabetes complications is outlined in Box 31.1.

PANCREAS

Physical Assessment

Insulin, which is produced by the pancreas, is responsible for glucose metabolism. The clinical assessment provides information about pancreatic functioning. Clinical manifestations of abnormal glucose metabolism often include hyperglycemia, which is the initial assessment priority for a patient with pancreatic dysfunction.[1,2] Patients with hyperglycemia may be prediabetic, may be hyperglycemic in association with a severe critical illness, or may ultimately be diagnosed with type 1 or type 2 diabetes. All these conditions have specific identifying features. More information on the specific pathophysiology and management of each condition is provided in Chapter 32.

Hyperglycemia

Because severe hyperglycemia affects a variety of body systems, all systems are assessed. The patient may complain of blurred vision, headache, weakness, fatigue, drowsiness, anorexia, nausea, and abdominal pain. On *inspection,* the patient has flushed skin, polyuria, polydipsia, vomiting, and evidence of dehydration. Progressive deterioration in the level of consciousness, from alert to lethargic or comatose, is observed as the hyperglycemia exacerbates. If ketoacidosis occurs, the patient's breathing becomes deep and rapid (Kussmaul respirations), and the breath may have a fruity odor. *Auscultation* of the abdomen may reveal hypoactive bowel sounds. *Palpation* elicits abdominal tenderness. *Percussion* may reveal diminished deep tendon reflexes. Because hyperglycemia results in osmotic diuresis, the patient's fluid volume status is assessed. Signs of dehydration include tachycardia, orthostatic hypotension, and poor skin turgor. The key laboratory tests that assist in assessment are discussed next.

Laboratory Studies

Pertinent laboratory tests for pancreatic function measure short-term and long-term blood glucose levels, which can identify and diagnose diabetes (Table 31.1).

Blood Glucose

The fasting plasma glucose (FPG) level is assessed by a simple blood test after the patient has not eaten for 8 hours (see Table 31.1).[3] A normal FPG level is between 70 and 100 mg/dL.[3] An FPG level between 100 and 125 mg/dL identifies a person who has *prediabetes.*[3] Individuals with prediabetes are at increased risk for complications of diabetes, such as coronary heart disease and stroke. An FPG level of 126 mg/dL (7 mmol/L) or higher is diagnostic of diabetes (see Table 31.1).[3] After a meal, the concentration of glucose increases in the bloodstream. Postprandial blood glucose levels should be less than180 mg/dL (10 mmol/L) (Table 31.2).[3]

All critically ill patients must have blood glucose levels monitored frequently while in the hospital. Clinical practice guidelines from the American Association of Clinical Endocrinologists and the American Diabetes Association recommend instituting insulin therapy when the blood glucose level is greater than 180 mg/dL in a critically ill patient.[4] A target blood glucose range of 140 to 180 mg/dL is recommended.[3,4] During administration of a continuous insulin infusion, point-of-care blood glucose testing is performed hourly or according to hospital protocol to achieve and maintain the blood glucose within the target range.[4,5]

Hypoglycemia is defined as a blood glucose level less than 70 mg/dL (3.9 mmol/L).[3] A complication of intensive glucose control is that hypoglycemic episodes may occur more frequently both in the hospital and with self-management of glucose levels in diabetes.[4,5]

BOX 31.1 DATA COLLECTION: COMPLICATIONS OF DIABETES

Current Health Status

- The body may be unable to adjust to increased insulin needs resulting from sudden physiologic changes such as infection, injury, or surgery. The nurse assesses whether the patient has a severe infection, surgical wound, or traumatic injury.
- Recent or current signs and symptoms
  - Unexplained changes in weight, thirst, hunger
  - Headache, blurred vision
  - Long-standing, unhealed infection
  - Vaginitis, pruritus
  - Leg pain, numbness
- Unexplained change in urinary patterns (eg, daytime and nighttime, frequency, volume)
- Energy or stamina changes
- Endurance level
- Weakness
- Unexplained, excessive fatigue
- Behavior or mental changes (also ask family member or significant other for input)
  - Memory loss
  - Orientation

Assessment of Current Illness: Onset, Characteristics, and Course

- Chronic illness: Physiologic or psychological stress may increase endogenous glucose.

- Recent treatments that could be a source of exogenous glucose
  - Hyperalimentation
  - Peritoneal dialysis
  - Hemodialysis
- Medications, including prescription and over-the-counter preparations: Pharmacologic agents may alter pancreatic function by increasing or decreasing the release of endocrine hormones. Medications also may interfere with hormonal action at the receptor site on the target cell.

Medical History: Questions

- Have you had prior pancreatic surgery?
- Have you ever been told that any of the following applied to you?
  - Too much sugar in the urine
  - Too much sugar in the blood
  - Will probably develop too much sugar later in life
- If you answered yes to any of these questions, what treatment, if any, was prescribed?
- Are you currently following such a treatment?

Family History: Questions

- Has a family member ever been diagnosed with diabetes or "sugar in the blood"?
- If so, how was the condition treated?

TABLE 31.1 Blood Glucose Levels

Patient Status	Fasting BG (mg/dL)	Fasting BG (mmol/L)
Hypoglycemia	<70	<3.9
Normal	70–100	>3.9–5.6
Prediabetes	100–125	5.6–6.9
Diabetes	≥126	≥7.0

BG, blood glucose.
Data from American Diabetes Association. Glycemic targets. *Diabetes Care.* 2016;39(suppl 1):S39.

TABLE 31.2 Blood Glucose Targets Before and After Meals[a]

Blood Test	mg/dL	nmol/L
Preprandial plasma glucose	80–130	4.4–7.2
Postprandial plasma glucose	<180	10.0

[a]These preprandial and postprandial values apply only to nonpregnant adults.
Data from American Diabetes Association. Glycemic targets. *Diabetes Care.* 2016;39(suppl 1):S39.

Before discharge to home, patients with diabetes should be taught to monitor their blood glucose levels. Maintaining blood glucose within the normal range is associated with fewer long-term diabetes-related complications.[1] Laboratory blood tests and point-of-care or self-monitoring of blood glucose represent the standard of care for management of diabetes. However, home monitoring of blood glucose is not the norm despite research evidence that maintaining blood glucose levels as close to normal as possible prolongs life and reduces complications.

Urine Glucose

Testing the urine for glucose is not recommended for patients with diabetes because too much variation exists in the threshold for glucose when diabetes-related kidney damage has occurred. Urine glucose measurements are affected by variation in fluid intake; reflect an average glucose level, not a specific point in time; and are altered by some medications. Urine glucose testing does not offer any help in the identification of hypoglycemia. For all these reasons, urine glucose testing should never be used.

Glycated Hemoglobin

Blood testing of glucose is useful for daily management of diabetes. However, a different blood test is used to achieve an objective measure of blood glucose over an extended period. The *glycated hemoglobin (HbA₁c)* provides information about the average amount of glucose that has been present in the patient's bloodstream over the previous 3 to 4 months. During the 120-day life span of red blood cells (erythrocytes), the hemoglobin within each cell binds to the available blood glucose through a process known as *glycosylation*. Typically, 4% to 6% of hemoglobin contains the glucose group HbA_{1c}. A normal HbA_{1c} value is less than 5.4%, with an acceptable target level of less than 6.5% for diabetic patients.[2] The HbA_{1c} value correlates with specific blood glucose levels as shown in Table 31.3.[3] The American Diabetes Association recommends use of the HbA_{1c} value both during initial assessment of diabetes mellitus and for follow-up to monitor treatment effectiveness.[2]

TABLE 31.3 Correlation Between Hemoglobin A$_{1c}$ Concentration and Plasma Glucose Level

HbA$_{1c}$ (%)	Mean Plasma Glucose Level (mg/dL)	Mean Plasma Glucose Level (mmol/L)
6	126	7.0
7	154	8.6
8	183	10.2
9	212	11.8
10	240	13.4
11	269	14.9
12	298	16.5

HbA$_{1c}$, Glycosylated hemoglobin.
Data from American Diabetes Association. Standards of medical care in diabetes—2016: glycemic targets. *Diabetes Care.* 2016;39(suppl 1):S39.

Blood Ketones

Ketone bodies are a by-product of rapid fat breakdown. Ketone blood levels rise in acute illness, in fasting states, and with sustained elevation of blood glucose in type 1 diabetes in the absence of insulin. In diabetic ketoacidosis, fat breakdown (*lipolysis*) occurs so rapidly that fat metabolism is incomplete, and the ketone bodies (acetone, beta-hydroxybutyric acid, and acetoacetic acid) accumulate in the blood (*ketonemia*) and are excreted in the urine (*ketonuria*). It is recommended that all patients with diabetes perform self-testing or have their blood or urine tested for the presence of ketones during any alteration in level of consciousness or acute illness with an elevated blood glucose level.[6] A blood test that measures *beta-hydroxybutyrate*, the primary metabolite of ketoacidosis, provides the most accurate measurement.[6,7] Self-test meters to measure blood ketones from a fingerstick are now available.[6]

Elevated levels of ketones (ketonemia) may be detected by a fruity, sweet-smelling odor on the exhaled breath. This distinctive breath odor derives from the elimination of acetone as part of the compensatory response to maintain a normal pH.

Urine Ketones

Ketones are eliminated in the urine, and urine may be tested for ketones. Ketonuria is retrospective and indicates that blood ketones were or are elevated.[6,7] Ketonuria may also occur in fasting and starvation states.

PITUITARY GLAND

The pituitary gland, recessed in the base of the cranium, is not accessible to physical assessment. Therefore, the critical care nurse must be aware of the systemic effects of a normally functioning pituitary to be able to identify dysfunction. One essential hormone formed in the hypothalamus but secreted through the posterior pituitary gland is *antidiuretic hormone* (ADH), also known as *vasopressin*.

Physical Assessment

ADH controls the amount of fluid lost and retained within the body. Acute dysfunction of the posterior pituitary or the hypothalamus may result in insufficient or excessive ADH production. The clinical signs of posterior pituitary dysfunction often manifest as fluid volume deficit (insufficient ADH production) or fluid volume excess (excessive ADH production).

Hydration Status

One method to determine the effectiveness of ADH production is to conduct a hydration assessment. This includes observations of skin integrity, skin turgor, and buccal membrane moisture. Moist, shiny buccal membranes indicate satisfactory fluid balance. Skin turgor that is resilient and returns to its original position in less than 3 seconds after being pinched or lifted indicates adequate skin elasticity. The skin over the forehead is the most reliable for testing tissue turgor because this area of skin is less affected by aging.[8] The skin in the groin and axilla is slightly moist to touch in a well-hydrated patient. In older patients, these typical assessment findings may be absent.

Other indicators that the patient's hydration status is adequate for metabolic demands include a balanced intake and output and absence of thirst. However, absence of thirst is an unreliable indicator of dehydration in patients with decreased thirst mechanisms such as older patients and critically ill patients. Absence of abrupt changes in mental status may also indicate normal hydration. Other indicators of normal hydration include absence of edema, stable weight, and urine specific gravity within the normal range (1.005 to 1.030).

Vital Signs

Changes in heart rate, blood pressure, and central venous pressure (when available) are useful to determine fluid volume status. Blood pressure and pulse are monitored frequently. Decreased blood pressure with increased pulse is characteristic of hypovolemia, whereas elevated blood pressure and a rapid, bounding pulse may indicate hypervolemia. Orthostatic hypotension, which occurs when intravascular fluid volume decreases, is identified by a drop in systolic blood pressure of 20 mm Hg or a drop in diastolic blood pressure of 10 mm Hg when the patient changes position from lying to standing.[9]

Weight Changes and Intake and Output

Daily weight changes coincide with fluid retention and fluid loss. Sudden changes in weight can result from a change in fluid balance; 1 L of fluid lost or retained is equal to approximately 2.2 lb, or 1 kg, of weight gained or lost. To use weight as a true determinant of fluid balance, all extraneous variables must be eliminated; this means the same scale is used at the same time each day. Precise measurement and notation of intake and output are used as criteria for fluid replacement therapy.

Laboratory Assessment

No single diagnostic test identifies dysfunction of the posterior pituitary gland. A diagnosis usually is made through the patient's clinical presentation and history. Although serum measurement of ADH is available, it is rarely obtained in critically ill patients.

Serum Antidiuretic Hormone

The normal serum ADH range is approximately 1 to 5 pg/mL, although this range may vary slightly according to the clinical laboratory doing the test. Before ADH measurement, all medications that may alter the release of ADH are withheld for a minimum of 8 hours. Common medications that affect ADH levels include morphine sulfate, lithium carbonate, chlorothiazide, carbamazepine, oxytocin, and selective serotonin reuptake inhibitors. Nicotine, alcohol, positive-pressure and negative-pressure ventilation, and emotional stress also influence ADH.

Serum ADH levels are compared with blood and urine osmolality to differentiate *syndrome of inappropriate antidiuretic hormone (SIADH)* from central *diabetes insipidus (DI)*.[10] Increased ADH levels in the bloodstream compared with a low serum osmolality and elevated urine osmolality confirms the diagnosis of SIADH.[10] Reduced levels of serum ADH in a patient with high serum osmolality, hypernatremia, and reduced urine concentration indicate central DI. Typically, this diagnosis is based on urine output, serum sodium, and serum osmolality rather than serum ADH level.[10] Chapter 32 provides more information about SIADH and DI.

Serum and Urine Osmolality

Values for serum osmolality in the bloodstream range from 275 to 295 mOsm/kg H_2O; there are variations in this range based on the clinical laboratory standard values. *Osmolality* measurements determine the concentration of dissolved particles in a solution. In a healthy person, a change in the concentration of solutes triggers a chain of events to maintain adequate serum dilution. The most accurate measures of the body's fluid balance are obtained when urine and blood samples are collected simultaneously.

Increased serum osmolality stimulates the release of ADH, which reduces the amount of water lost through the kidney. Body fluid is retained at the kidney tubules and collecting ducts to dilute the particle concentration in the bloodstream. According to one clinical guideline, the hypothalamic vasopressin (ADH) osmoreceptors are maximally inhibited at levels less than 280 mOsm/kg H_2O to eliminate water via the kidney. In contrast, at levels greater than 290 mOsm/kg H_2O, the sensation of thirst and hypothalamic vasopressin (ADH) osmoreceptors are maximally stimulated to conserve water.[10] This is a narrow clinical range that is often disrupted in pituitary disease and critical illness.

Decreased serum osmolality inhibits the release of ADH. The kidney tubules increase their permeability, and fluid is eliminated from the body in an attempt to regain normal concentration of particles in the bloodstream. Urine osmolality in a person with normal kidneys depends on fluid intake. With high fluid intake, particle dilution is low, but it increases if fluids are restricted. Therefore, the expected range for urine osmolality is wide, ranging from 50 to 1400 mOsm/kg.

Antidiuretic Hormone Test

The ADH test is used to differentiate *neurogenic* DI (central) from *nephrogenic* (kidney) DI. The patient is challenged with 0.05 to 1.0 mL of intranasally administered ADH in the form of desmopressin (1-deamino-8-D-arginine vasopressin, commonly abbreviated as DDAVP). An intravenous line is inserted before ADH administration, and urine volume and osmolality are measured every 30 minutes for 2 hours before and after the ADH challenge. A patient with normal posterior pituitary function responds to the exogenous ADH by resorbing water at the kidney tubule, raising the urine osmolality slightly. In cases of severe central DI, in which the pituitary is affected, the urine osmolality shows a significant increase (becomes more concentrated), which indicates that the cell receptor sites on the kidney tubules are responsive to vasopressin. Test results in which urine osmolality remains unchanged indicate nephrogenic DI,

suggesting kidney dysfunction because the kidneys are no longer responsive to ADH. This test is rarely performed in the critical care unit because of the unstable hemodynamic and volume status of most patients.

Diagnostic Procedures

In addition to laboratory tests, radiographic examination, computed tomography (CT), and magnetic resonance imaging (MRI) are used to diagnose structural lesions such as cranial bone fractures, tumors, or blood clots in the region of the pituitary.[11,12] Although these procedures do not diagnose DI or SIADH, they are useful in uncovering the likely underlying cause.

Radiographic Examination

A basic radiographic examination of the inferior skull views the *sella turcica* and surrounding bone formation. Bone fractures or tissue swelling at the base of the brain, which are apparent on a radiograph, suggest interference with the vascular supply and nerve impulses to the hypothalamic-pituitary system. Dysfunction may occur if the hypothalamus, infundibular stalk, or pituitary gland is impaired.

Computed Tomography

CT of the base of the skull identifies pituitary tumors, blood clots, cysts, nodules, or other soft tissue masses. This rapid procedure causes no discomfort except that it requires the patient to lie perfectly still. CT studies can be performed with or without radiopaque contrast medium. The contrast dye is given intravenously to highlight the hypothalamus, infundibular stalk, and pituitary gland. This dye may cause allergic reactions in iodine-sensitive individuals, and the patient must be asked about iodine allergy before the test. The size and shape of the sella turcica and the position of the hypothalamus, infundibular stalk, and pituitary are identified.[12]

Magnetic Resonance Imaging

MRI enables the radiologist to visualize internal organs and cellular characteristics of specific tissues. MRI uses a magnetic field rather than radiation to produce high-resolution, cross-sectional images. The soft brain tissue and surrounding cerebrospinal fluid make the brain especially suited to assessment with MRI.[12]

THYROID GLAND

Clinical Assessment

History

The history of any patient in a critical care unit should be as detailed as possible. Information regarding the clinical manifestations of hypothyroidism or hyperthyroidism must be obtained from the patient, family, or others with knowledge of the health history. Sample questions considered pertinent to detection of thyroid disease are provided in Box 31.2.

Physical Examination

The thyroid is palpated for tenderness, nodules, and enlargement and is auscultated for bruits. The normal-size thyroid gland usually is neither visible nor palpable in the anterior neck. Palpation may be done from an anterior or posterior approach. Auscultation of the thyroid is accomplished by use of the bell portion of the stethoscope to identify a bruit or blowing noise

BOX 31.2 DATA COLLECTION: HYPERTHYROIDISM AND HYPOTHYROIDISM

The patient is the best source for the following information. If the patient is unable to respond, the following questions can be directed to family, friends, a significant other, or persons involved in admission of the patient to the critical care unit.

- Have you ever been diagnosed with overactive thyroid, increased metabolism, or hyperthyroidism? What about underactive thyroid, slowed metabolism, or hypothyroidism?
- Have you ever been treated for hyperthyroidism or hypothyroidism?
- Have you ever had an operation for thyroid disease?
- Have you ever received radioactive iodine for thyroid disease?
- Are you taking any medicine for thyroid disease? If so, what is the name of the medicine, and what is the prescribed dose and frequency?
- When did you first notice the constant restlessness or extreme fatigue?
- Has your weight been the same or changed over the past year?
- Has your appetite changed over the past 6 months?
- Have you lost weight even though your appetite has increased (may indicate hyperthyroidism)?
- Have you gained weight or stayed at the same weight even though you have not felt like eating over the past 6 months (may indicate hypothyroidism)?
- Do you always feel warm (may indicate hyperthyroidism)?
- Do you open windows in the house even in winter months?
- Do you wear lightweight clothing even when others are wearing layers of heavier clothing?
- Do you always feel cold (may indicate hypothyroidism)?
- Do you wear multiple layers of clothing despite warm weather or the use of a heater or furnace?
- Do you use several blankets and keep windows closed even in warm weather?
- Do you complain about never being able to "warm up"?
- Over the past 6 months to 1 year, have you developed any of the following?

Hypothyroidism Indicators	Hyperthyroidism Indicators
Loss of coarse, dry scalp hair and outer edge of eyebrow	Hair thinning
Sleepiness, lethargy, depression	Swelling (face, eyes, legs)
Weight gain despite decreased appetite	Insomnia, nervousness, anxiety
Severe constipation	Weight loss despite increased appetite
Muscle and joint pain (hands, wrists, feet)	Diarrhea
Dry, itchy skin	Muscle weakness or wasting; tremors
Increased sensitivity to cold	Warm, moist skin
Bradycardia	Heat intolerance, sweating
Menstruation changes; impaired fertility	Tachycardia, atrial fibrillation
	Menstruation changes; impaired fertility

TABLE 31.4 Thyroid Hormone Blood Tests

Name of Test	Abbreviation	Reference Value (SI)	Reference Value[a]
Thyroid-stimulating hormone (thyrotropin)	TSH	0.4–4.5 mIU/L	
Total serum thyroxine	TT$_4$	581–154 nmol/L	4.0–12.0 mcg/dL
Free thyroxine	FT$_4$	9–23 pmol/L	0.7–1.8 ng/dL
Total serum triiodothyronine	TT$_3$	1.2–2.7 nmol/L	100–200 ng/dL
Free triiodothyronine	FT$_3$	3.2–9.2 pmol/L	208–596 pg/dL
Thyroglobulin[b]	Tg	3.0–40 mcg/L	

SI, International Units.

[a]Some tests are reported with more than one reference value because clinical laboratories use various reference ranges depending on the specifics of the clinical test.

[b]Thyroglobulin (Tg) reference values should be determined locally because serum thyroglobulin concentrations are influenced by local iodide intake. Reference values from Demers LM, et al. Thyroid disease: Pathophysiology and diagnosis. *Clin Lab Med*. 2004;24(1):19.

from the circulation through the thyroid gland. The presence of a bruit indicates enlargement of the thyroid, as evidenced by increased blood flow through the glandular tissue.

Laboratory Studies

Controversy exists about routine measurement of thyroid function in adults without clinical symptoms. The US Preventive Services Task Force 2015 review found the research evidence insufficient to recommend routine screening for thyroid disease in asymptomatic adults.[13] However, thyroid hormone blood test screening is recommended for adults 60 years old and older and for individuals with symptoms of thyroid dysfunction (hypofunction or hyperfunction).[13] There are no recommendations about thyroid hormone screening for critically ill patients.

Thyroid hormone blood tests measure the levels of circulating thyroid hormone and assess the integrity of the hormonal negative feedback response within the hypothalamic-pituitary-thyroid axis. Laboratory diagnosis is based on the simultaneous measurement of thyroid-stimulating hormone (TSH) and free thyroxine (FT$_4$). An inverse linear relationship exists between TSH and FT$_4$.[14] When the hypothalamic-pituitary-thyroid axis is normal, TSH production is inhibited by the presence of free thyroid hormone in the bloodstream (FT$_4$), and the TSH value is normal.[14]

- Hypothyroidism: High TSH and low FT$_4$
- Hyperthyroidism: Low TSH, high FT$_4$, and an increased FT$_3$-to-FT$_4$ ratio

Thyroid-Stimulating Hormone

Over the past decade, laboratory tests developed to analyze TSH have become much more sensitive, allowing more accurate measurement of low levels of thyroid hormone. Thyroid hormone reference ranges in adults are listed in Table 31.4.[14] Because serum values vary slightly between laboratory methods, it is imperative to know the normal reference values used by the hospital clinical laboratory.

The upper limit of normal for some of these values is under scrutiny. A US national survey found the average level of TSH in the population in all ages to be only 1.49 mIU/L, considerably lower than most cited laboratory norms.[14] The serum level of TSH increases as a person grows older, which may signal declining thyroid function, as greater stimulation of the thyroid gland by TSH is required.[14] The average TSH level varies by age, as follows[14]:

1.60 mIU/L after age 50 years
1.79 mIU/L after age 60 years
1.98 mIU/L after age 70 years
2.08 mIU/L after age 80 years

Because this age-adjusted increase is predictable, it is not recommended that laboratories use age-adjusted reference values when assessing thyroid function.[14]

Thyroid Tests in Critically Ill Patients

The incidence of thyroid disease in hospitalized patients is low, estimated at 1% and 2% of all inpatients. In critically ill patients, TSH measurement is usually the first thyroid-related laboratory test that is obtained. Most experts recommend obtaining both TSH and FT$_4$ hormone levels.[15]

Medications and Thyroid Testing

Additional measurement difficulties involve concomitant use of certain medications that interfere with thyroid function and lower serum levels.[16]

TSH secretion is affected by several medications routinely administered in critical care units. Glucocorticoids in large doses may lower the serum level of FT$_3$ and inhibit TSH secretion.[14] Dopamine infusions at greater than 1 mcg/kg per minute directly block TSH release.[16] Amiodarone, an antidysrhythmic medication, is an iodine-rich compound that is structurally similar to T$_3$ and T$_4$.[17] At usual doses, amiodarone contains 35 to 140 times the iodine recommended daily allowance of 150 mcg/day.[17]

Several medications increase the serum level of FT$_4$ by displacing protein-bound T$_4$.[16] Medications that displace protein-bound T$_4$ cause an increase in serum FT$_4$ levels.[16] Salicylates (aspirin), furosemide (Lasix), and unfractionated and low-molecular-weight heparins all raise FT$_4$ serum levels by this mechanism.[16] A more complete list of medications that alter thyroid hormone serum levels is provided in Table 31.5. It is unclear whether it is necessary to adjust pharmacologic management of critically ill patients in response to these medication-laboratory interactions.

Diagnostic Procedures

Diagnostic tests often begin with ultrasonography to visualize a thyroid nodule or tumor.[18] To diagnose hypothyroidism, a nuclear medicine scan using an oral iodine radioactive isotope may be requested.[19] The thyroid-scanning procedure may also detect the presence of ectopic thyroid tissue, thyroid carcinomas, and the amount of viable thyroid glandular tissue after therapeutic irradiation.

ADRENAL GLAND

Primary Adrenal Disorders

Admission to the critical care unit with a primary adrenal disorder is rare. The term *primary* indicates that the principal problem lies within the adrenal gland. Secondary adrenal dysfunction is caused by dysfunction in another gland or by a clinical condition such as sepsis.

TABLE 31.5 Medications That Influence Diagnostic Thyroid Levels

FT$_3$

Increase	Decrease
Methadone	Anabolic steroid
Estrogens	Androgens
Progestins	Salicylates
Amiodarone	Phenytoin
	Lithium
	Reserpine
	Propranolol
	Sulfonamides
	Propylthiouracil
	Methylthiouracil

FT$_4$

Increase	Decrease
Oral contraceptives	Phenytoin
Heparin	Steroids
Aspirin	Diphenylhydantoin
Furosemide	Chlorpromazine
Clofibrate	Lithium
Phenylbutazone	Sulfonylurea
Some NSAIDs	Sulfonamides
Propranolol	Reserpine
Corticosteroids	Chlordiazepoxide
Amiodarone	

TSH

Increase TSH	Decrease TSH and TSH Response to TRH
Metoclopramide	Glucocorticoids
Iodides	Dopamine
Lithium	Heparin
Potassium iodide	Aspirin
Morphine sulfate	Carbamazepine

TBG

Increase	Decrease
Opiates	Androgen therapy
Oral contraceptives	Asparaginase
Estrogens	
Clofibrate	
5-FU	
Perphenazine	

5-FU, 5-fluorouracil; *FT$_3$*, free triiodothyronine; *FT$_4$*, free thyroxine; *NSAIDs*, nonsteroidal anti-inflammatory drugs; *TBG*, thyroxine-binding globulin; *TRH*, Thyrotropin-releasing hormone; *TSH*, thyroid-stimulating hormone.

The adrenal gland is actually two glands in one, as described in Chapter 30, and this may make the history and presentation complex. The adrenal cortex (outer layer) secretes two classes of hormones, and if deficient or released in excess, they may cause clinical symptoms. Two hormones relevant to care of critically ill patients are (1) the glucocorticoid hormone cortisol and (2) the mineralocorticoid hormone aldosterone. *Cortisol* is secreted in response to physiologic stress as a result of infection, trauma, and hypoglycemia. *Aldosterone* is secreted in response to intravascular hypovolemia. It is the final step in the renin-angiotensin-aldosterone system (RAAS) pathway.

The adrenal medulla (inner layer) also secretes two hormones that cause clinical symptoms if they are deficient or released in excess: *epinephrine* and *norepinephrine*. Epinephrine, also known as *adrenaline*, and norepinephrine, also known as *noradrenaline*, are both secreted from the adrenal gland in response to stress.

Clinical Assessment
History
A detailed history may help to identify conditions or medications that may affect adrenal gland function. Primary endocrine disorders are rare, but a history of uncontrolled hypertension despite three or more oral medications may indicate whether endocrine-related hypertension should be investigated. The medication history may help determine whether the patient takes glucocorticoid tablets, and the patient or family should be asked about using steroid creams for dermatologic conditions and about using steroid-based inhalers for chronic obstructive lung disease.

Physical Examination
The physical examination is related to the effects of adrenal dysfunction, and the signs depend on the hormone involved and whether the problem is related to excess or deficiency. This means that the signs and symptoms are very diverse. A methodical approach to assessing all signs and symptoms is important because adrenal disease is often missed or misdiagnosed.

Adrenal Cortex
Primary cushing syndrome. Cushing syndrome is caused by excess release of the glucocorticoid hormone *cortisol*.[20-22] Excess cortisol produces the classic signs and symptoms listed in Box 31.3. Primary Cushing disease is rare, but if a patient is not taking exogenous steroids, it becomes a diagnosis of exclusion when the relevant constellation of signs and symptoms is present.[20-22] The first step is to obtain a serum adrenocorticotropic hormone (ACTH) level in a patient with overt signs of Cushing syndrome. A serum ACTH level less than 2.2 pmol/L (10 pg/mL) is considered diagnostic.[22] Imaging of the pituitary gland to search for a tumor or other injury is performed after the low ACTH value has confirmed Cushing syndrome as the cause of the condition.[22]

Secondary cushing syndrome. Symptoms identical to the symptoms of primary Cushing syndrome (see Box 31.3) occur in patients with the secondary form who are on long-term glucocorticoid therapy with pharmacologic doses, such as transplant recipients who take steroids to prevent solid-organ rejection, patients with chronic obstructive lung disease, or patients with chronic inflammatory conditions. When patients are admitted to the critical care unit, it is important to ascertain whether they are steroid dependent to avoid the deleterious effects of abrupt steroid withdrawal.[22]

Primary Aldosteronism
In patients with primary aldosteronism, the adrenal cortex secretes excess mineralocorticoid (aldosterone) unrelated to the RAAS.[23] In other words, the aldosterone secretion is untethered from the normal RAAS feedback loop (see Fig. 14.18 in Chapter 14). Primary aldosteronism occurs in up to 10% of individuals with medication-resistant hypertension, and approximately one-third also have hypokalemia.[23] This rare condition may cause the patient to present emergently with severe hypertension

---

BOX 31.3   Causes of Cushing Syndrome

Primary Cushing Syndrome
Cushing syndrome is divided into adrenocorticotropin-dependent and adrenocorticotropin-independent types. Adrenocorticotropin is also known as *adrenocorticotropic hormone (ACTH)* or *corticotropin*.

ACTH-Dependent Cushing Syndrome
Most cases (80%) result from a pituitary adenoma that causes the pituitary gland to produce excess ACTH. Excess secretion of ACTH stimulates the adrenal cortex to release excess amounts of *cortisol* into the bloodstream, circumventing the normal inhibitory feedback loop.

The other 20% of cases are caused by ectopic ACTH secretion from small cell cancers of the lung, metastases, and endocrine tumors.

ACTH-Independent Cushing Syndrome
Cases are usually caused by a unilateral adrenal tumor: adrenal adenoma (60%) or adrenal carcinoma (40%).

Secondary or Iatrogenic Cushing Syndrome
The patient takes pharmacologic doses of glucocorticoids, which may be prescribed to prevent rejection after solid-organ transplantation or to treat chronic inflammatory conditions.

Clinical Signs and Symptoms of Cushing Syndrome
- Emotional lability (can range from depression to psychosis)
- Hyperglycemia and poorly controlled type 2 diabetes
- Obesity or weight gain in abdomen
- Rounded face
- Acne
- Thin skin, bruises easily, poor wound healing
- Hypertension
- Hirsutism (excess hair growth)
- Dorsocervical fat pad ("buffalo hump")
- Decreased libido
- Fatigue, weakness

---

and a critically low serum potassium (hypokalemia), which can be lethal if not identified and effectively treated. The diagnostic laboratory test that is recommended is an aldosterone-to-renin ratio.[23] A CT scan of the adrenal-kidney structures is obtained to visualize tumors that may be secreting the excess aldosterone.[23,24] An invasive diagnostic test is adrenal venous sampling of cortisol and aldosterone levels, obtained by an interventional radiologist, to determine if the condition affects one or both adrenal glands.[23,25] Surgical removal of an aldosterone-secreting tumor may be required.

Adrenal Insufficiency
Adrenal insufficiency is a rare disorder of the adrenal cortex that involves hyposecretion of glucocorticoids (cortisol), sometimes occurring with hyposecretion of mineralocorticoids (aldosterone). It is also known as *Addison disease* after Thomas Addison who first described the condition.[26,27] Physiologically, adrenal insufficiency may be envisioned as the inverse of conditions with excess hormone secretion. The laboratory diagnosis involves simultaneous measurements of the serum ACTH level with a cortisol serum level.[27] A low (or normal) serum cortisol in the presence of an elevated ACTH is diagnostic.[27] A serum cortisol value below 100 nmol/L at 9:00 am is also considered diagnostic.[27]

BOX 31.4 **Pheochromocytoma: Signs and Symptoms**^a

BOX 31.4 Pheochromocytoma: Signs and Symptoms[a]

Signs	Symptoms
Hypertension	Headaches
Tachycardia	Dizziness or faintness
Tachypnea	Palpitations, chest pain
Pallor or flushing	Anxiety and nervousness
Hyperglycemia or poorly controlled type 2 diabetes	Excessive sweating
Decreased gastrointestinal motility	Weakness, fatigue
	Weight loss
	Constipation

[a]Not all patients have all signs and symptoms.

Adrenal Crisis

An *adrenal crisis,* also called an *addisonian crisis,* is a life-threatening condition in which the adrenal gland is almost nonfunctional, usually because of destruction of adrenal tissue.[26] The patient presents acutely with critical hypotension, an elevated serum potassium level (hyperkalemia), a low serum sodium level (hyponatremia), and hypoglycemia.

Critical Illness–Related Corticosteroid Insufficiency

The adrenal gland is designed to respond to acute physiologic stress by increasing stress hormones via the hypothalamic-pituitary-adrenal axis.[28] Early in critical illness, a rise in cortisol levels can be documented. However, over time, the adrenal gland may be unable to secrete adequate amounts of stress hormones, especially when critical illness is prolonged. Whether to administer corticosteroids or not remains a subject of fierce debate. Clinicians are awaiting the results of the ADRENAL (*AD*junctive *Co*Rticosteroid Tr*E*atment i*N* Critic*A*lly Il*L* Patients with Septic Shock) study, a major study to help decide this question. The study is expected to randomly assign 3800 mechanically ventilated patients with vasopressor-dependent septic shock to receive either hydrocortisone (200 mg/day) or placebo for 7 days.[29]

Adrenal Medulla

Pheochromocytoma. Pheochromocytomas are rare tumors that arise from the catecholamine-producing *chromaffin cells* of the adrenal medulla.[30] Most produce norepinephrine, but some produce both norepinephrine and epinephrine. These tumors produce a far greater quantity of catecholamines than normal adrenal medullary tissue. The concentrations of catecholamines can be so high within the tumor that it has have been likened to a volcano that is ready to erupt. When huge amounts of norepinephrine or epinephrine are released into the bloodstream, it creates a *catecholamine storm* and a *hypertensive crisis* that can be life-threatening. The body responds to the catecholamine surge as if to a severe fight-or-flight threat by hypertension, tachycardia, increased respiratory rate, and hyperglycemia. The patient may describe symptoms of headache, dizziness, palpitations, chest pain, anxiety, nervousness, and fatigue (Box 31.4).[30] Because the body perceives the catecholamine onslaught as a signal to be ready to escape a threatening situation, it slows down the gastrointestinal tract, and constipation is another symptom. Patients at greatest risk are patients who are admitted to a critical care unit or who

undergo surgery and experience a hypertensive crisis during anesthesia.[30]

The recommended laboratory diagnosis of pheochromocytoma is by measurement of plasma and urine fractionated metanephrines.[30,31] Catecholamines are metabolized into metanephrines. Pheochromocytoma-secreted catecholamine levels fluctuate, making blood levels variable, but catecholamine metabolism into metanephrines is constant, which is the reason this test is preferred.[30] Before the metanephrine blood level is drawn, the patient should be supine and resting for 30 minutes.[30,31] A 24-hour urine collection of excreted catecholamines may be obtained.[30] Finally, genetic testing of the patient and immediate relatives may be requested.[31]

Diagnostic Imaging Procedures

CT is the most widely used test to image the adrenal glands.[24] Percutaneous adrenal biopsy is rarely performed in all cases and is unlikely to be performed in critically ill patients.

SUMMARY

- Assessment of a patient with endocrine dysfunction is a systematic process that incorporates the medical and family history, physical examination, and laboratory test results.

Pancreas
- Normal fasting blood glucose is between 70 and 100 mg/dL. A fasting blood glucose between 110 and 126 mg/dL identifies prediabetes. A blood glucose level greater than 126 mg/dL is diagnostic of diabetes. Hyperglycemia is a frequent finding in critically ill patients.

Pituitary
- Normal range of serum ADH is 1 to 5 pg/mL. All medications that may alter ADH release are withheld for a minimum of 8 hours before ADH measurement.
- Serum osmolality ranges from 275 to 295 mOsm/kg H_2O. Urine osmolality ranges from 50 to 1400 mOsm/kg.
- Serum ADH levels are compared with blood and urine osmolality to differentiate SIADH from central DI.

Thyroid
- Hypothyroidism is identified by high TSH and low FT_4 values.
- Hyperthyroidism is identified by low TSH and high FT_4 values.

Adrenal
- The adrenal gland is designed to respond to acute physiologic stress. In prolonged critical illness and in septic shock, the adrenal gland may not secrete adequate amounts of cortisol. Other rare adrenal conditions that require specific diagnostic tests include Cushing syndrome, primary aldosteronism, adrenal insufficiency, and pheochromocytoma.
- ⓔ Visit the Evolve site for additional study materials.

REFERENCES

1. American Diabetes Association. Standards of medical care in diabetes—2016. *Diabetes Care.* 2016;39(suppl 1):S4.
2. American Diabetes Association. Classification and diagnosis of diabetes. *Diabetes Care.* 2016;39(suppl 1):S13.
3. American Diabetes Association. Glycemic targets. *Diabetes Care.* 2016;39(suppl 1):S39.

4. Moghissi ES, et al. American Association of Clinical Endocrinologists and American Diabetes Association consensus statement on inpatient glycemic control. *Diabetes Care.* 2009;32(6):1119.

5. Jacobi J, et al. Guidelines for the use of an insulin infusion for the management of hyperglycemia in critically ill patients. *Crit Care Med.* 2012;40(12):3251.

6. Kitabchi AE, et al. Hyperglycemic crises in adult patients with diabetes. *Diabetes Care.* 2009;32(7):1335.

7. Arora S, et al. Diagnostic accuracy of point-of-care testing for diabetic ketoacidosis at emergency-department triage: β-Hydroxybutyrate versus the urine dipstick. *Diabetes Care.* 2011;34(4):852.

8. Morley JE. Dehydration, hypernatremia, and hyponatremia. *Clin Geriatr Med.* 2015;31:389.

9. Jones P, Shaw BH, Satish RR. Orthostatic hypotension: Managing a difficult problem. *Expert Rev Cardiovasc Ther.* 2015;13(11):1263.

10. Lamas C, et al. Clinical guidelines for management of diabetes insipidus and syndrome of inappropriate antidiuretic hormone secretion after pituitary surgery. *Endocrinol Nutr.* 2014;61(4):e15.

11. Bresson D, et al. Sellar lesions/pathology. *Otolaryngol Clin North Am.* 2016;49:63.

12. Nunes RH, et al. Imaging in endoscopic cranial skull base and pituitary surgery. *Otolaryngol Clin North Am.* 2016;49:33.

13. LeFevre ML, on behalf of the U.S. Preventive Services Task Force. Screening for thyroid dysfunction: U.S. Preventive Services Task Force Recommendation Statement. *Ann Intern Med.* 2015;162:641.

14. Demers LM. Thyroid disease: Pathophysiology and diagnosis. *Clin Lab Med.* 2004;24(1):19.

15. Merchant NB, Mirza FS. Interpretation of thyroid function tests in hospitalized patients. *Hosp Clin Med.* 2015;4(2):243.

16. Kundra P, Burman KD. The effect of medications on thyroid function tests. *Med Clin North Am.* 2012;96(2):283.

17. Cohen-Lehman J, et al. Effects of amiodarone therapy on thyroid function. *Nat Rev Endocrinol.* 2010;6(1):34.

18. Xie C, et al. Ultrasonography of thyroid nodules: a pictorial review. *Insights Imaging.* 2016;7:77.

19. Hoang JK, et al. Imaging thyroid disease. *Radiol Clin North Am.* 2015;53:145.

20. Nieman LK, et al. The diagnosis of Cushing's syndrome: an Endocrine Society Clinical Practice Guideline. *J Clin Endocrinol Metab.* 2008;93(5):1526.

21. Nieman LK, et al. Cushing's syndrome. The Diagnosis of Cushing's Syndrome—An Endocrine Society Clinical Practice Guideline. *J Clin Endocrinol Metab.* 2015;100(8):2807.

22. Lacroix A, et al. Cushing's syndrome. *Lancet.* 2015;386:913.

23. Funder JW, et al. Case detection, diagnosis, and treatment of patients with primary aldosteronism: an Endocrine Society Clinical Practice Guideline. *J Clin Endocrinol Metabol.* 2008;93(9):3266.

24. Allen BC, Francis IR. Adrenal imaging and intervention. *Radiol Clin North Am.* 2015;53(5):1021.

25. Rossi GP, et al. An expert consensus statement on use of adrenal vein sampling for the subtyping of primary aldosteronism. *Hypertension.* 2014;63:151.

26. Bornstein SR, et al. Diagnosis and treatment of primary adrenal insufficiency: an Endocrine Society Clinical Practice Guideline. *J Clin Endocrinol Metab.* 2016;101(2):364.

27. Brooke AM, Monson JP. Addison's disease. *Medicine.* 2013;41(9):522.

28. Langouche L, Van den Berghe G. Hypothalamic-pituitary hormones during critical illness: a dynamic neuroendocrine response. *Handb Clin Neurol.* 2014;124:115.

29. Venkatesh B, et al. The ADRENAL study protocol: adjunctive corticosteroid treatment in critically ill patients with septic shock. *Crit Care Resusc.* 2013;15(2):83.

30. Thomas RM, et al. Endocrine hypertension: an overview on the current etiopathogenesis and management options. *World J Hypertens.* 2015;5(2):14.

31. Lenders JW, et al. Pheochromocytoma and paraganglioma: an Endocrine Society Clinical Practice Guideline. *J Clin Endocrinol Metab.* 2014;99(6):1915.

32

Endocrine Disorders and Therapeutic Management

Mary E. Lough

The endocrine system is almost invisible when it functions well, but it causes widespread disruption when an organ is suppressed, hyperstimulated, or under physiologic stress. A wide spectrum of possible disorders can result; some are rare, and others are frequently encountered in the critical care unit. This chapter focuses on the neuroendocrine stress associated with critical illness and on disorders of three major endocrine glands: pancreas, posterior pituitary gland, and thyroid gland.

NEUROENDOCRINOLOGY OF STRESS AND CRITICAL ILLNESS

Major neurologic and endocrine changes occur when an individual is confronted with physiologic stress caused by any critical illness, sepsis, trauma, major surgery, or underlying cardiovascular disease.[1] The normal "fight or flight" response that is initiated in times of physiologic or psychological stress is exacerbated in critical illness through activation of the neuroendocrine system, specifically the hypothalamic-pituitary-adrenal (HPA) axis.[2] All endocrine organs are affected by acute critical illness, as shown in Table 32.1.

Acute Neuroendocrine Response to Critical Illness

The fight or flight acute response to physiologic threat is a rapid discharge of the catecholamines *norepinephrine* and *epinephrine* into the bloodstream.[2] Norepinephrine is released from the nerve endings of the sympathetic nervous system. Epinephrine is released from the adrenal glands.

Hypothalamic-Pituitary-Adrenal Axis in Critical Illness

The pituitary gland has two parts (anterior and posterior) that function under control of the hypothalamus (see Figs. 30.1 and 30.3 in Chapter 30). The *posterior pituitary gland* releases antidiuretic hormone (ADH), also known as *vasopressin*, as a component of the physiologic stress response. This hormone is an antidiuretic with a powerful vasoconstrictive effect on blood vessels. The synergistic combination of vasopressin and epinephrine released from the adrenal glands quickly raises blood pressure (BP).

The *anterior pituitary gland* produces several hormones including *corticotropin* (also called adrenocorticotropic hormone), which stimulates release of *cortisol* from the adrenal cortex. Cortisol release is an important protective response to stress. Increased cortisol levels alter carbohydrate, fat, and protein metabolism so that energy is immediately and selectively available to vital organs. However, if critical illness is prolonged, the HPA axis may be unable to respond adequately to prolonged physiologic stress, and adrenal insufficiency may result.[3]

The *adrenal gland* produces cortisol from the cortex and epinephrine from the medulla (see Fig. 30.7 in Chapter 30). Diminished adrenal gland function may result from various causes during critical illness, as follows:

- *Primary hypoadrenalism* describes an intrinsic failure of the adrenal gland to produce normal endogenous glucocorticosteroid hormones (eg, cortisol) and mineralocorticosteroid hormones (eg, aldosterone). In critical illness, failure of the adrenal gland to respond to extended pathologic stress has been documented.[3] Primary adrenal failure outside critical illness is rare.[4]
- *Secondary Cushing syndrome* is a cluster of signs and symptoms that occur after taking high-dose corticosteroids for a period of time. In response to exogenous corticosteroids, the adrenal glands stop production of intrinsic hormones.[5,6] Patients who have been taking steroids before their admission to the hospital need their dosage increased during illness to avoid hypoadrenalism. Primary Cushing syndrome, unrelated to steroid administration, is rare.[7]

Hyperglycemia in Critical Illness

Many factors contribute to hyperglycemia in critical illness, including release of the powerful *counterregulatory hormones:* glucagon, cortisol, and epinephrine.[8] In response to physiologic stress, *glucagon* is released by the pancreatic alpha cells and stimulates the liver to pour glucose into the bloodstream. In healthy individuals, blood insulin levels control glucagon release. When blood glucose levels are less than 80 mg/dL, the stimulus to release insulin from the pancreatic beta cells is suppressed, and the alpha cells are stimulated to release glucagon. The physiologic purpose of glucagon is to prevent hypoglycemia by stimulating the liver to release additional glucose into the bloodstream. However, in diabetes and during critical illness, the normal feedback loop is disrupted. Circulating glucagon can be increased five times the normal value—unrelated to insulin levels—causing hyperglycemia in critical illness.[8] Physiologic stress stimulates release of cortisol and epinephrine from the adrenal glands. These counterregulatory hormones further stimulate glucagon and subsequent release of glucose from the liver.[8]

Under normal physiologic conditions, hyperglycemia and insulin secretion inhibit glucagon release. However, in the acute phase of critical illness, normal physiology is disrupted, and insulin secretion is decreased.[8] This causes a relative insulin deficiency compared with physiologic need. Later in the course of the illness, peripheral tissues may become *insulin resistant,* meaning the tissues are unable to use the available insulin to transport glucose inside the cells.[8]

TABLE 32.1	**Endocrine Responses to Stress**	
Gland or Organ	**Hormone**	**Response or Physical Examination**
Adrenal cortex	Cortisol	↑ Insulin resistance → ↑ glycogenolysis → ↑ glucose circulation
		↑ Hepatic gluconeogenesis → ↑ glucose available
		↑ Lipolysis
		↑ Protein catabolism
		↑ Sodium → ↑ water retention to maintain plasma osmolality by movement of extravascular fluid into the intravascular space
	Glucocorticoid	↓ Connective tissue fibroblasts → poor wound healing
		↓ Histamine release → suppression of immune system
		↓ Lymphocytes, monocytes, eosinophils, basophils
		↑ Polymorphonuclear leukocytes → ↑ infection risk
		↑ Glucose
		↓ Gastric acid secretion
	Mineralocorticoids	↑ Aldosterone → ↓ sodium excretion → ↓ water excretion → ↑ intravascular volume
		↑ Potassium excretion → hypokalemia
		↑ Hydrogen ion excretion → metabolic acidosis
Adrenal medulla	Epinephrine	↑ Endorphins → ↓ pain
	Norepinephrine, epinephrine	↑ Metabolic rate to accommodate stress response
		↑ Live glycogenolysis → ↑ glucose
		↑ Insulin (cells are insulin resistant)
		↑ Cardiac contractility
		↑ Cardiac output
		↑ Dilation of coronary arteries
		↑ Blood pressure
		↑ Heart rate
		↑ Bronchodilation → ↑ respirations
		↑ Perfusion to heart, brain, lungs, liver, and muscle
		↓ Perfusion to periphery of body
		↓ Peristalsis
	Norepinephrine	↑ Peripheral vasoconstriction
		↑ Blood pressure
		↑ Sodium retention
		↑ Potassium excretion
Pituitary	All hormones	↑ Endogenous opioids → ↓ pain
Anterior pituitary	Corticotropin	↑ Aldosterone → ↓ sodium excretion → ↓ water excretion → ↑ intravascular volume
		↑ Cortisol → ↑ blood volume
	Growth hormones	↑ Protein anabolism of amino acids to protein
		↑ Lipolysis → ↑ gluconeogenesis
Posterior pituitary	Antidiuretic hormone	↑ Vasoconstriction
		↑ Water retention → restoration of circulating blood volume
		↓ Urine output
		↑ Hypo-osmolality
Pancreas	Insulin	↑ Insulin resistance → hyperglycemia
	Glucagon	↑ Glycolysis (directly opposes action of insulin)
		↑ Glucose for fuel
		↑ Glycogenolysis
		↑ Gluconeogenesis
		↑ Lipolysis
Thyroid	Thyroxine	↓ Routine metabolic demands during stress
Gonads	Sex hormones	Energy and oxygen supply diverted to brain, heart, muscles, and liver

↑, increased; →, causes; ↓, decreased.

There is a second physiologic system to transport glucose into cells using facilitative *glucose transporters* (GLUTs) (see Table 30.3 in Chapter 30). The normal physiologic stimulus for insulin release from the pancreas is an increase in blood glucose after a meal or hyperglycemia. GLUT2 receptors are located on the surface of the beta cells and transport circulating glucose inside the cell, stimulating insulin release from the beta cell. GLUT2 receptor actions do not depend on insulin. The insulin-independent GLUTs (GLUT1, GLUT2, and GLUT3) are active during physiologic stress but may be unable to keep up with the massive increase in glucose production by the liver.

Managing glucagon release in critical illness is not yet feasible and remains a future goal. Hyperglycemia management is focused on continuous infusion of insulin to maintain blood glucose levels within a safe, near-normal range to reduce morbidity and mortality.[9]

Hyperglycemia Management in Critical Illness

Normal fasting blood glucose levels are between 70 and 100 mg/dL in a healthy person. Critically ill patients frequently have much higher blood glucose levels, and several retrospective analyses have reported that hyperglycemic patients have a higher mortality rate than patients with normal blood glucose values.[8] In 2001, a landmark prospective, randomized study showed a significant reduction in morbidity and mortality among critically ill surgical patients whose blood glucose concentration was maintained between 80 and 110 mg/dL with a continuous insulin infusion compared with patients whose blood glucose was treated only if it was greater than 180 mg/dL.[10,11] These initial studies were greeted with tremendous enthusiasm, and many critical care units adopted stringent glucose control standards to reduce hyperglycemia-associated morbidity and mortality. However, reproducibility of such tight glucose control outside of a research trial was impossible, as shown by the results of follow-up clinical studies.[10,11] The most important trial was the NICE-SUGAR trial.[12] This was a prospective randomized trial of 6014 critically ill patients that compared continuous insulin infusion to achieve tight glucose control (target 81 to 108 mg/dL) with a conventional glucose control range (target below 180 mg/dL). In the tight glucose control group, 6.8% had episodes of severe hypoglycemia (less than 40 mg/dL); in the conventional control group, only 0.5% experienced severe hypoglycemia.[12] There was a 2.6% higher risk of death in the intensive glucose control group (27.5% died) compared with the conventional control group (24.9% died).[12]

Clinical Practice Guidelines for Blood Glucose Management in Critically Ill Patients

As a result of the studies just described, clinical practice guidelines were developed by the American Association of Clinical Endocrinologists and the American Diabetes Association (ADA) that recommend the use of continuous insulin infusions to maintain blood glucose in critical care patients between 140 and 180 mg/dL, with hourly monitoring of blood glucose.[9] The range of 140 to 180 mg/dL was selected to minimize the risk of hypoglycemia while avoiding extreme hyperglycemia. Other glucose control guidelines relevant to critical illness have also been published. The Society of Critical Care Medicine recommends initiating glycemic control when blood glucose rises above 150 mg/dL.[1] Insulin management must be initiated if the blood glucose level is greater than 180 mg/dL.[1] Stress hyperglycemia (greater than 180 mg/dL) occurs in almost one-third of critically ill patients.[8]

Insulin Management in Critically Ill Patients

As a result of the research that has highlighted the deleterious effects of hyperglycemia in critically ill patients, most hospitals have developed an institution-specific glucose-insulin algorithm to lower blood glucose into the targeted range. The vigilance of the critical care nurse is pivotal to the success of any intervention to lower blood glucose using a continuous insulin infusion. As discussed earlier, many glucose control protocols are using less restrictive ranges (140 to 180 mg/dL) because of concerns about iatrogenic hypoglycemia.[1,9]

Frequent Blood Glucose Monitoring

Monitoring the blood glucose with a point of care glucometer is the basis of targeted glucose control. As part of the comprehensive initial assessment, blood sugar is measured by a standard laboratory sample or by a fingerstick capillary blood sample. In many institutions, if blood sugar is greater than 180 mg/dL, the patient is started on a continuous intravenous (IV) insulin infusion. While the glucose is elevated, blood sample measurements are usually obtained hourly, to allow titration of the insulin drip to lower blood glucose.[1] After the patient is stable, blood glucose measurements can be spaced approximately every 2 hours, based on individual hospital protocols.

Several different blood sampling methods are available. A capillary fingerstick is perhaps the easiest initial option, although the fingers can become noticeably marked if there are numerous sticks over several days. Trauma to the fingers is also exacerbated if peripheral perfusion is diminished. If a central venous catheter or an arterial line with a blood conservation system attached is in place, this can be a highly efficient system for sampling because there is no blood wastage. If a blood conservation setup is not attached, use of the venous or arterial catheter for access is unacceptable because of the quantity of "waste" blood that would be discarded.

Point of care testing for blood glucose in critical illness. Point of care testing with a handheld glucometer is frequently used to allow hourly rapid assessment of the blood glucose and titration of a continuous glucose infusion. The point of care tests assay whole blood. However, this has caused some controversy because these devices were typically developed for at-home use and were not developed for use with critically ill patients.[13] For this reason, it is important to verify very high blood glucose values and any low blood glucose values with a blood sample sent to the clinical laboratory for plasma glucose verification. The US Food and Drug Administration (FDA) requires that blood glucose testing devices that are used in the hospital meet standards specific to the inpatient setting.[13,14]

Continuous Insulin Infusion

Many hospitals use insulin infusion protocols for management of stress-induced hyperglycemia. These protocols are implemented and managed by the critical care nurse.[1,9] Effective glucose protocols gauge the insulin infusion rate based on two parameters: (1) the immediate blood glucose result and (2) the rate of change in the blood glucose level since the last hourly measurement. Protocols vary by hospital, but the underlying concepts are similar. The following three examples illustrate blood glucose management strategies:

- Patient A receives 3 units of continuous IV regular insulin per hour and has a blood glucose measurement of 110 mg/dL, but 1 hour ago it was 190 mg/dL; the insulin rate must be decreased to avoid sudden hypoglycemia.
- Patient B receives 3 units of continuous IV regular insulin per hour and has a blood glucose measurement of 110 mg/dL, but 1 hour ago it was 112 mg/dL; in this situation, no change is made in the insulin infusion rate.
- Patient C receives 3 units of continuous IV regular insulin per hour and has a blood glucose measurement of 190 mg/dL, and 1 hour ago it was 197 mg/dL; the insulin rate must be increased to move the patient's blood sugar more rapidly toward the targeted glucose range (ie, 140 to 180 mg/dL, although this range varies by individual hospital protocol).

The important point to emphasize is that the *rate of change* of blood glucose is as important as the *most recent* blood glucose measurement. Each of the patients described in the examples may have the same insulin infusion rate, depending on their catabolic state, but individualization among patients with different diagnoses can be safely achieved as long as the rate of change is also considered.

A person's insulin requirement often fluctuates over the course of an illness. This fluctuation occurs in response to changes in the clinical condition such as development of an infection, caloric alterations caused by stopping or starting enteral or parenteral nutrition, administration of therapeutic steroids, or because the person is less catabolic. A method to allow for corrective incremental changes (up or down) to adapt to the reality of clinical developments and maintain the glucose within the target range is essential. Some protocols alter only the infusion rate, whereas others incorporate bolus insulin doses if the glucose concentration is greater than a preestablished threshold (eg, 180 mg/dL). Typically, after the blood glucose level has remained within the target range for a number of hours (varies according to the hospital protocol), the time interval between measurements for blood glucose monitoring may be extended to every 2 hours.

Transition From Continuous to Intermittent Insulin Coverage

The transition from a continuous insulin infusion to intermittent insulin coverage must be handled with care to avoid large fluctuations in blood glucose levels. Before the conversion, the regular insulin infusion should be at a stable and preferably low rate, and the patient's blood glucose level should be maintained consistently within the target range. The transition from IV to subcutaneous insulin administration depends on numerous factors, including whether the patient is able to eat a consistent amount of dietary carbohydrate.[15]

Clinicians use various methods to calculate the quantity of insulin to prescribe during the transition from IV to subcutaneous insulin to maintain stable blood glucose levels. Fig. 32.1 depicts hypothetical examples of how a combination of basal and bolus insulin regimens (prandial insulin) can work in clinical practice. The application of one calculation method is described for a 67-year-old patient, Alice Smith, who is recovering from critical illness and has recently been weaned from mechanical ventilation and extubated.

1. Ms. Smith is in stable condition on a regular insulin drip at 1 unit/h. She is ready to be transitioned to subcutaneous insulin and will be taking food and liquids by mouth. Her total insulin requirement over the previous 24 hours was 32 units. Ms. Smith will now require basal coverage (provided by subcutaneous intermediate or long-acting insulin) and *prandial* coverage for mealtimes (provided by short-acting subcutaneous insulin).

2. The 30 units of insulin infused during the previous 24 hours is Ms. Smith's required daily insulin dose. To transition to subcutaneous insulin, a proportion of this amount (ie, 75% to 80%) will be divided between basal and prandial components.[9] In this situation, 75% of the 32 units = 24 units. Half of this amount (12 units) will be administered subcutaneously as intermediate or long-acting insulin; the other half will be administered as short-acting insulin to coincide with meals (ie, 4 units with each of three meals).

3. The options for insulin administration for Ms. Smith are as follows:
   Basal insulin: 12 units of glargine once daily *or* 6 units twice daily of neutral protamine Hagedorn (NPH) administered subcutaneously
   Prandial insulin: 4 units of regular insulin given subcutaneously before each meal (short-acting) *or* 4 units of lispro or aspart given subcutaneously with each meal (ultra–short-acting insulin); verify current blood glucose level

Many types of insulin are available for use. These include ultra–short-acting, short-acting, intermediate-acting, long-acting, and combination insulin replacement options as listed in Table 32.2. After the transition to subcutaneous insulin is completed, blood glucose is monitored frequently to maintain blood glucose within the target range and detect hyperglycemia or hypoglycemia.[16]

Corrective Insulin Coverage

A patient may be prescribed supplemental or corrective doses of insulin in addition to the basal/prandial insulin combination. The use of the trio of basal, prandial, and corrective insulin is designed to eliminate the use of the traditional sliding scale. Criticisms of the sliding scale method are that the dosages are rarely reevaluated or adjusted once established and that the scales treat hyperglycemia only after it has occurred; they are not proactive in the manner of the basal/bolus/corrective insulin method. The ADA does not recommend solo use of the sliding scale in hospitalized patients.[17]

Supplemental corrective insulin. A supplemental correction scale can be used to cover any episodes of hyperglycemia above the target range. The corrective insulin amount can be combined with scheduled blood glucose measurements and scheduled insulin administration.

After the transition to subcutaneous insulin, it is important to recheck the blood glucose level. The insulin dosage is adjusted based on the patient's *insulin sensitivity* or, stated another way, according to how much insulin is needed to metabolize each 15 g of carbohydrate intake. Patients who are *insulin resistant* require more insulin than patients who are *insulin sensitive.*

Hypoglycemia Management

It is important to have a protocol for the management of hypoglycemia. The major drawback to use of intensive insulin protocols, as described earlier, is the potential for hypoglycemia.[16] Whenever hypoglycemia is detected, it is important to *stop* any continuous infusion of insulin. An example of one protocol to reverse hypoglycemia follows:

- Blood glucose level less than 40 mg/dL (severe hypoglycemia): Administer 50 mL of dextrose (25 g dextrose) in water ($D_{50}W$) as an IV bolus.
- Blood glucose level between 40 and 70 mg/dL (hypoglycemia): Administer 25 mL of $D_{50}W$ as an IV bolus.

In all cases of hypoglycemia, the blood glucose concentration is monitored every 15 minutes until the blood glucose level has increased to greater than 70 mg/dL.

Nursing Management

Nursing management of a patient with neuroendocrine stress resulting from critical illness incorporates a variety of nursing diagnoses (Box 32.1). The goals of nursing management are to monitor the hyperglycemic side effects of vasopressor therapy, administer

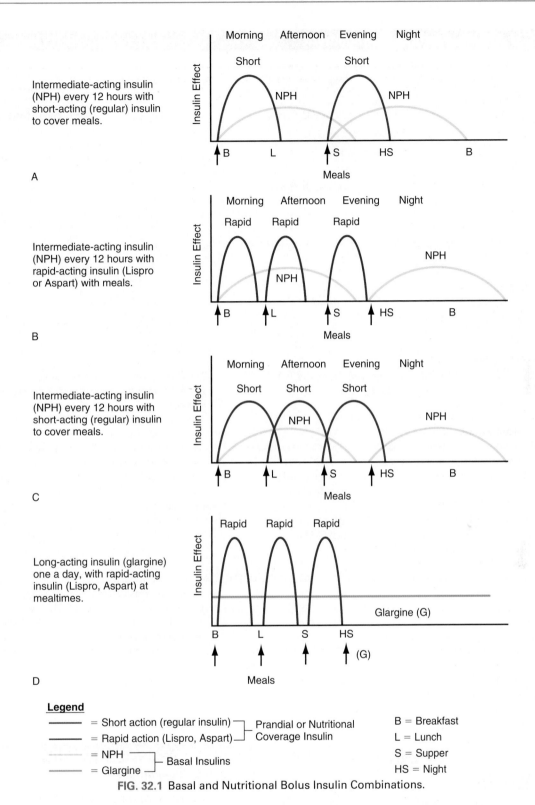

FIG. 32.1 Basal and Nutritional Bolus Insulin Combinations.

prescribed corticosteroids, monitor blood glucose and insulin effectiveness, avoid hypoglycemia, provide nutrition, and provide education to the patient's family and supportive others (Box 32.2).

Monitor Hyperglycemic Side Effects of Vasopressor Therapy

Two vasopressors frequently used as continuous infusions to counteract hypotension also raise blood glucose. Epinephrine and norepinephrine stimulate gluconeogenesis (creation of new glucose), increase liver glycogenolysis (glucose production), increase lipolysis (fat breakdown), suppress insulin secretion, and increase peripheral insulin resistance. All these actions increase blood glucose.

Administer Prescribed Corticosteroids

Critically ill patients with below-normal cortisol levels may be prescribed IV hydrocortisone. Therapeutic steroids increase

TABLE 32.2   Pharmacologic Management
Insulin[a]

Insulin	Route[b]	Action	Onset/Peak/Duration	Special Considerations
Ultra–Short-Acting Insulins				
Aspart (NovoLog)	SC	Insulin replacement, rapid onset	5–15 min/30–90 min/<5 h	Insulin analogue almost *immediately* absorbed; must be taken with food.
				Insulin appearance should be clear.
				Must be used in combination with intermediate-acting or long-acting basal insulin regimen. See Fig. 32.1.
Lispro (Humalog)	SC	Insulin replacement, rapid onset	5–15 min/30–90 min/<5 h	Insulin analogue; almost *immediately* absorbed; must be taken with food.
				Shorter duration of action than regular insulin; should be used with basal longer acting insulin. See Fig. 32.1.
Glulisine (Apidra)	SC	Insulin replacement, rapid onset	5–15 min/30–90 min/<5 h	Insulin analogue.
Short-Acting Insulin				
Regular	IV or SC	Insulin replacement therapy	IV: <15 min SC: 30–60 min/2–3 h/5–8 h	Only type of insulin suitable for IV continuous infusion or IV bolus administration.
Intermediate-Acting Basal Insulin				
Neutral protamine Hagedorn (NPH)	SC	Insulin replacement, intermediate action	2–4 h/4–10 h/10–16 h	NPH is not recommended for SC basal insulin because it has a peak with a less predictable time course than the long-acting insulin analogues
Long-Acting Basal Insulins				
Glargine (Lantus)	SC	Long-acting basal insulin analogue	2–4 h until steady state/no peak Concentration relatively constant over 20–24 h	Synthetic insulin (analogue); differs from human insulin by three amino acids, slow release over 24 h; no peak. Decrease dosage by 20% if switching from NPH to glargine. Must not be diluted or mixed with other insulins. See Fig. 32.1.
Detemir (Levemir)	SC	Long-acting basal insulin analogue	3–8 h until steady state/no peak/5–23 h	
Combination (Premixed) Insulins				
Various	SC	Rapid plus intermediate or long-acting insulin combination	Varies according to combination used	Many combinations exist; examples (long-acting component/short-acting component) include 70/30 regular (70% NPH with 30% regular), NovoLog mix 70/30 (70% aspart-protamine suspension with 30% aspart), and Humalog mix 75/25 (75% lispro-protamine suspension with 25% lispro).

IV, intravenous; *SC*, subcutaneous.
*Dosages are individualized according to patient's age and size.
†Only regular insulin is suitable for IV use.

◎ BOX 32.1   NURSING DIAGNOSES
Stress of Critical Illness

- Deficient Fluid Volume related to absolute loss, p. 1019
- Imbalanced Nutrition: Less Than Body Requirements related to exogenous nutrients and increased metabolic demand, p. 1029
- Risk for Infection, p. 1046
- Risk for Ineffective Peripheral Tissue Perfusion, p. 1044
- Compromised Family Coping related to critically ill family member, p. 1014

✷ BOX 32.2   PATIENT EDUCATION PLAN
Stress of Critical Illness

- Even if the patient is unresponsive because of the underlying critical illness or because of sedation and analgesic medications, brief explanations of procedures are quietly and simply given before interventions.
- During the period of acute illness, questions are answered and information is provided to the family and significant others.
- After recovery, additional information is provided to the patient concerning the illness.

blood glucose levels and can make glycemic control more difficult. Frequent monitoring of the blood glucose concentration is necessary to guide treatment of hyperglycemia in patients receiving IV corticosteroids. Ongoing monitoring for the presence of new infection is mandatory.

Monitor Blood Glucose and Insulin Effectiveness and Avoid Hypoglycemia

The critical care nurse is responsible for the hourly monitoring of blood glucose and titration of the insulin infusion according to the hospital's protocol while the patient is hyperglycemic. The use of standardized protocols makes a systematic approach to the control of blood glucose possible. It is essential and recommended that nurses receive effective and ongoing education about the anabolic impact of insulin therapy in critical illness.[9] Hospital protocols to minimize development of hypoglycemia such as using the target range of 140 to 180 mg/dL[9] and rapid reversal of any occurrence of severe hypoglycemia (below 40 mg/dL) by provision of IV dextrose ($D_{50}W$) are essential.[1]

Provide Nutrition

Whenever an insulin infusion is initiated to lower blood glucose, enteral nutritional support should be considered.[18] Critical illness is associated with significant catabolism of skeletal muscle. The catabolic response to inflammation is much more significant than fasting in a healthy individual because of inflammation, immobility, and the endocrine stress response.[10,18] Enteral nutrition via feeding tube is preferred to IV total parenteral nutrition. Enteral nutrition is associated with better outcomes in critical illness.[1,18] Enteral nutritional formulas have higher carbohydrate content than total parenteral nutrition making it easier to manage fluctuations in blood glucose. If enteral nutrition is stopped or slowed, it is vital that the insulin infusion rate is also decreased to avoid hypoglycemia.

Patient Education

While the patient is acutely ill, most of the educational interventions are directed to the family at the bedside. Numerous explications are required to describe the IV medications, nutritional needs, purpose of insulin, role of corticosteroids (if applicable), ongoing nursing care, prevention of complications, and management of the underlying disease process. Educational topics to discuss are listed in Box 32.2.

Collaborative Management

Standardized protocols designed to manage the complications of critical illness result in lower morbidity and mortality for patients.[1,19] Optimally, all disciplines concerned with the endocrine status of the patient will have participated in the hospital's guidelines related to targeted glucose control.[1,19,20] Guidelines for blood glucose monitoring in critical illness are described in Box 32.3.[1,9,17]

DIABETES MELLITUS

Diabetes mellitus is a progressive endocrinopathy associated with carbohydrate intolerance and insulin dysregulation.

Diagnosis of Diabetes

Diabetes mellitus is diagnosed by measurement of the fasting plasma glucose (FPG) or by a *glycated hemoglobin* greater than 6.5%.[21] The blood glucose may also be called a fasting blood glucose. The benchmarks for a normal blood glucose value have

---

Hyperglycemia Management in Critical Illness

A summary is provided of evidence and evidence-based recommendations for controlling hyperglycemic symptoms related to physiologic stress of critical illness.

Strong Evidence to Support

- Initiate insulin therapy for persistent hyperglycemia greater than 180 mg/dL.
- Once a continuous insulin infusion is initiated, maintain target blood glucose level between 140 and 180 mg/dL.
- Perform frequent blood glucose monitoring to avoid hypoglycemia (hypoglycemia is defined as blood glucose level less than 70 mg/dL; severe hypoglycemia is less than 40 mg/dL).
- For patients who are eating, maintain preprandial blood glucose below 130 mg/dL; maintain 2-h postprandial blood glucose below 180 mg/dL.
- A multidisciplinary team approach to implement institutional guidelines, protocols, and standardized order sets results in fewer hypoglycemic and hyperglycemic events.

References

American Diabetes Association. Standards of medical care in diabetes—2016. *Diabetes Care.* 2016;35(Suppl 1):S11.

Jacobi J, et al. Guidelines for the use of an insulin infusion for the management of hyperglycemia in critically ill patients. *Crit Care Med.* 2012;40(12):3251.

Moghissi ES, et al. American Association of Clinical Endocrinologists and American Diabetes Association consensus statement on inpatient glycemic control. *Endocr Pract.* 2009;15(4):1.

---

been progressively lowered as more knowledge has been gained about the benefits of maintaining the plasma glucose level as close to normal as possible.

Blood glucose values endorsed by the ADA are as follows[21]:
- FPG level 70 to 100 mg/dL (5.6 mmol/L) is a normal fasting glucose.
- FPG level between 100 and 125 mg/dL (5.6 and 6.9 mmol/L) denotes impaired fasting glucose.
- FPG level greater than 126 mg/dL (7 mmol/L) is diagnostic of diabetes (result is verified by testing more than once).

The benefit and importance of maintaining blood glucose at levels as close to normal as possible have been conclusively demonstrated in patients with type 1 and type 2 diabetes. The Diabetes Control and Complications Trial on type 1 diabetes and the United Kingdom Prospective Diabetes Study on type 2 diabetes demonstrated that lifestyle changes and use of medications that lead to consistently normal glucose levels reduce microvascular diabetes-related complications and decrease mortality.

Types of Diabetes

Two distinct types of diabetes are discussed in this chapter:
- Type 1 diabetes results from beta cell destruction, usually leading to absolute insulin deficiency.[21]
- Type 2 diabetes results from a progressive loss of insulin secretion defect in addition to insulin resistance.[21]

The two diseases are different in nature, cause, treatment, and prognosis. A further category of *prediabetes* describes patients with impaired fasting glucose (FPG between 100 and 125 mg/dL) who are likely to develop diabetes in the future and who are at increased risk for coronary artery disease and stroke.[21] Other conditions, such as gestational diabetes, are not discussed in this chapter.

Glycated Hemoglobin

For individuals with diabetes, maintenance of blood glucose within a tight normal range is fundamental to avoid the development of microvascular and neuropathic secondary conditions. Although the plasma glucose value produces a snapshot of the blood glucose concentration at a single point in time, *glycated hemoglobin* (HbA$_{1c}$) measures the percentage of glucose the red blood cells have absorbed from the plasma over the previous 3-month period. The optimal target for patients with diabetes is an HbA$_{1c}$ value less than 6.5%.[21]

Type 1 Diabetes

Type 1 diabetes mellitus accounts for 5% to 10% of all patients with diabetes.[21] It is an autoimmune disease that causes progressive destruction of the beta cells of the islets of Langerhans in the pancreas. Autoantibodies that falsely identify self as a foreign invader to be destroyed can now be identified by laboratory analysis. Autoantibodies that contribute to pancreatic destruction include autoantibodies to the islet cell, to insulin, to glutamic acid decarboxylase (GAD$_{65}$), and to the tyrosine phosphatases IA-2 and IA-2β.[21] One or more of these autoantibodies are present in most patients with type 1 diabetes.[21] Over time, the autoantibodies render the pancreatic beta cells incapable of secreting insulin and regulating intracellular glucose. In type 1 diabetes, the rate of beta cell destruction is highly variable. It occurs rapidly in some patients (mainly children) and more slowly in others (mainly adults).[21] Some patients, particularly children and adolescents, may have ketoacidosis as the first manifestation of their disease.

Genetic predisposition and unknown environmental factors are also believed to play an important role. Patients with type 1 diabetes are prone to development of other autoimmune disorders such as Graves disease (hyperthyroidism), Hashimoto thyroiditis, Addison disease, autoimmune hepatitis, myasthenia gravis, and pernicious anemia.[21] Lack of insulin impairs carbohydrate, protein, and fat metabolism.

Management of Type 1 Diabetes

Patients with type 1 diabetes must receive IV or subcutaneous insulin therapy. Treatment with exogenous insulin replacement restores normal entry of glucose into the cells. The range of insulin replacements available is expanding, and it is essential that critical care nurses be knowledgeable about the different classes of insulin (see Table 32.2). Without insulin, the rapid breakdown of noncarbohydrate substrate, particularly fat, leads to ketonemia, ketonuria, and diabetic ketoacidosis (DKA), a life-threatening complication associated with type 1 diabetes (see later discussion).

Type 2 Diabetes

Type 2 diabetes accounts for 90% to 95% of diabetes.[21] Type 2 diabetes is identified by decreased insulin secretion and *insulin resistance,* with a relative, versus absolute, insulin deficiency. Many patients with type 2 diabetes are obese, with excess adipose tissue concentrated in the abdominal area. The onset of hyperglycemia occurs gradually, and many people are unaware that they have diabetes. Initially, type 2 diabetes is managed by oral medications (noninsulin therapies) because the pancreatic beta cells remain functional. As progressive beta cell dysfunction occurs, a basal long-acting insulin is added to oral noninsulin medications.[22]

Insulin resistance describes a complex metabolic situation in which organ and tissue cells deny entry to insulin and glucose. This creates the clinical paradox in which elevated serum insulin levels and hyperglycemia are present at the same time. Insulin resistance has a strong association with obesity.

Lifestyle Management for Type 2 Diabetes

For most patients with type 2 diabetes, a program comprising weight reduction, increased physical exercise, and a change in diet pattern is the essential first step.[23] The diet should contain less than 30% of calories from fat, with an increased quantity of whole grains, vegetables, and fruits. Crash diets are discouraged, and a gradual program of weight loss is recommended. The exercise program is tailored to the individual but might start with 30 minutes of brisk walking each day if the person was previously sedentary.

Type 2 diabetes increases risk of contracting a wide range of cardiovascular and kidney complications that increase morbidity and mortality. In addition to taking medications to control blood glucose, patients often require medications to lower their BP, lower their cholesterol and triglyceride levels, treat ischemic heart disease, and manage symptoms of heart failure.[23,24]

Pharmacologic Management of Type 2 Diabetes

If lifestyle changes are unsuccessful in reversing the pattern of type 2 diabetes, oral noninsulin antihyperglycemic medications are prescribed as recommended by the ADA (Table 32.3 and Box 32.4). These medications are not oral forms of insulin and have many varied actions as described in Table 32.4.

Metformin. Metformin is an *insulin sensitizer.* This oral medication increases insulin sensitivity in the liver, increasing the ability of insulin to suppress hepatic glucose production. Metformin also increases insulin sensitivity at the peripheral cellular level for fat and muscle, to increase glucose uptake. Metformin is first-line therapy for patients with type 2 diabetes.[22,25] Metformin may be used as monotherapy or be combined with other oral medications that lower blood glucose or combined with basal insulin (see Table 32.3).[24] Metformin is associated with a rare risk of metabolic acidosis. Gastrointestinal side effects are common with metformin.[22]

Sulfonylureas. The *sulfonylureas* (glyburide, glipizide, glimepiride, gliclazide) are oral medications that stimulate secretion of insulin from the pancreatic beta cells (see Table 32.3). They are in a category known as *insulin secretagogues.* Sulfonylureas reduce HbA$_{1c}$ by 1 to 2 percentage points and have a long duration of action. Side effects include hypoglycemia and weight gain. The *meglitinides* (repaglinide and nateglinide) also increase insulin secretion (see Table 32.4) and may be prescribed in place of sulfonylureas if needed.[25]

Thiazolidinediones. The *thiazolidinediones,* also known as *glitazones* (pioglitazone and rosiglitazone), are oral medications that belong to a class of medications called *peroxisome proliferator activated receptor gamma modulators.* These medications increase the sensitivity of muscle, fat, and liver cells to insulin. For this reason, thiazolidinediones are known as *insulin sensitizers.*[26] Side effects such as fluid retention and edema limit use of thiazolidinediones.[26] These medications should be avoided in patients with heart failure.[22,27] Bone loss is also a side effect.[22]

Dipeptidyl peptidase-4 receptor inhibitors. Dipeptidyl peptidase-4 (DPP-4) inhibitors are a newer class of oral antihyperglycemic medications also known as *incretin enhancers* (sitagliptin, vildagliptin, saxagliptin, linagliptin). These medications slow down the degradation of the *glucagon-like peptide-1 (GLP-1)* hormone by the enzyme DPP-4, prolonging the glucose-lowering activity of GLP-1. DPP-4 inhibitors are considered a second-line therapy in type 2 diabetes (see Table

TABLE 32.3 Antihyperglycemic Medications for Management of Type 2 Diabetes

Mono Therapy	Metformin	Metformin	Metformin	Metformin	Metformin	Metformin
Dual Therapy Medications	Metformin + Sulfonylurea	Metformin + Thiazolidinedione	Metformin + DPP-4 Inhibitor	Metformin + SGLT2 Inhibitor	Metformin + GLP-1 Receptor Agonist	Metformin + Insulin
Triple Therapy Medications	Metformin + Sulfonylurea or Thiazolidinedione or DPP-4 Inhibitor or SGLT2 Inhibitor or GLP-1 Receptor Agonist or Insulin	Metformin + Thiazolidinedione or Sulfonylurea or DPP-4 Inhibitor or SGLT2 Inhibitor or GLP-1 Receptor Agonist or Insulin	Metformin + DPP-4 Inhibitor or Sulfonylurea or Thiazolidinedione or SGLT2 Inhibitor or Insulin	Metformin + SGLT2 Inhibitor or Sulfonylurea or Thiazolidinedione or DPP-4 Inhibitor or Insulin	Metformin + GLP-1 Receptor Agonist or Sulfonylurea or Thiazolidinedione or Insulin	Metformin + Insulin or DPP-4 Inhibitor or SGLT2 Inhibitor or GLP-1 Receptor Agonist
Combination Oral + Injectable	Metformin + Basal Insulin + Mealtime Insulin **or** GLP-1 Receptor Agonist					

Data from American Diabetes Association: Approaches to glycemic treatment. *Diabetes Care.* 2016;39(suppl 1):S52-59.

BOX 32.4 Oral Antihyperglycemic Medication Actions

Medications that Sensitize the Body to Insulin (Insulin Sensitizers)
- Biguanides
- Thiazolidinediones

Medications that Stimulate the Pancreas to Make More Insulin (Insulin Secretagogues)
- Sulfonylureas
- Glinides

Medications that Delay Carbohydrate Absorption From Small Intestine
- Alpha-glucosidase inhibitors

Medications that Augment Gut Incretin Hormone Effects
- Incretin mimetics
- Incretin enhancers

Medications that Increase Excretion of Glucose in the Urine
- sodium-glucose cotransporter2 (SGLT2) inhibitors

32.3). These agents have only a modest impact on HbA_{1c} reduction and are rarely associated with hypoglycemia.

DPP-4 inhibitors act on the gastric *incretin* hormones. The main therapeutic target is the incretin hormone GLP-1, which is secreted from the gastric mucosa in response to food ingestion. GLP-1 stimulates the pancreatic beta cells to produce insulin. See Table 30.4 in Chapter 30 for a description of the physiologic effects of incretin hormones.[28]

Sodium-glucose cotransporter 2 inhibitors. The most recently FDA approved medications are *sodium-glucose cotransporter 2 (SGLT2) inhibitors* (see Table 32.3). These oral medications, also known as *glifozins*, inhibit the reabsorption of glucose in the nephron by inhibiting the action of the renal transporter SGLT2.

This results in more glucose being excreted in the urine, and blood glucose is reduced as a result.[29] SGLT2 inhibitors lower HbA_{1c} by approximately 0.5% to 1%.[30] The SGLT2 inhibitors (dapagliflozin, canagliflozin) are used in combination with other antihyperglycemic medications as second-line or third-line treatment.[29] Side effects include genitourinary yeast and urinary tract infections, related to the increased glucose excreted in the urine.[22]

GLP-1 receptor agonists. GLP-1 receptor agonists are known as *incretin mimetics* because they augment activity of GLP-1. These medications (exenatide, liraglutide, albiglutide, dulaglutide) increase insulin secretion from the pancreatic beta cells, lower elevated glucagon levels, and delay gastric emptying. They are approved by the FDA for treatment of type 2 diabetes. The medications in this class are administered by subcutaneous injection. GLP-1 receptor agonists are not a replacement for insulin.

Alpha-glucosidase inhibitors. Alpha-glucosidase inhibitors (acarbose, migitol) are used to reduce postprandial hyperglycemia in type 2 diabetes. Alpha-glucosidase is an enzyme that splits complex carbohydrates into simple sugars in the gastrointestinal tract. These oral medications are taken at the beginning of a meal to inhibit enzyme action and delay gastric absorption of carbohydrates (ie, bread, corn, pasta, beans) into the bloodstream. These medications lower HbA_{1c} by approximately 0.5% to 0.8%.

Polypharmacy in Diabetes

The availability of varied pharmacologic approaches to reduce blood glucose and manage type 2 diabetes can reduce many long-term complications related to hyperglycemia. Often patients may be taking two or three medications for diabetes (see Table 32.3) as well as taking additional medications for coexisting medical conditions. One of the unintended consequences of having so many medications is *polypharmacy* and risk of medication interactions and hypoglycemia; this is recognized as a particular problem for older adults.[31]

TABLE 32.4 Pharmacologic Management
Medications for Type 2 Diabetes

Medication[a]	Dosage	Action	Onset/Peak/Duration	Special Considerations
Metformin				
Metformin (Glucophage)	*Initial dosage:* 500 mg bid or 850 mg in morning; *maximum dosage:* 2550 mg tid	Reduces glucose output from liver	For uo 1–3 h/24 h/24–48 h	Temporarily withhold for up to 48 hours post-procedure if patient has received contrast radiography.
		Increases insulin action by decreasing peripheral insulin resistance		Adverse effects: Lactic acidosis (rare); GI upset.
				Contraindicated in male patients with S.Cr of 1.5 mg/dL or greater and female patients with S.Cr of 1.4 mg/dL or greater.
Sulfonylureas				
Glipizide (Glucotrol)	*Initial dosage:* Immediate-release tablet 5 mg once/day; *maximum dosage:* 40 mg bid	Stimulates insulin release	1 h/1–3 h/12–24 h	Administer with breakfast or after first main meal.
				Also available in extended-release formulation (Glucotrol XL); do not cut, crush, or chew.
				Extended release: *initial dosage:* 5 mg, once daily; *maximum dosage:* 20 mg/day.
				Adjust dosage if creatinine clearance <50 mL/min.
Glyburide (DiaBeta; Micronase)	*Initial dosage:* 2.5 mg once/day; *maintenance dosage:* 1.5–20 mg/day	Stimulates insulin release	1 h/4 h/18–24 h	Administer with breakfast or first main meal.
Glimepiride (Amaryl)	*Initial dosage:* 1–2 mg once/day; *maximum dosage:* 8 mg once/day	Stimulates insulin release	Duration 24 h	Administer with breakfast or first main meal of day.
				Initial dosage is lower in patients with kidney dysfunction (1 mg once/day).
Meglitinides				
Nateglinide (Starlix)	*Initial dosage:* 120 mg tid; *maximum dosage:* 120 mg tid	Stimulates insulin release	Peak <1 h	Administer 15-30 min before meals.
				Cut dosage in half (ie, 60 mg tid) for frail older patients and patients near their HA$_{1c}$ target.
Repaglinide (Prandin)	*Initial dosage:* 1–2 mg tid; *maximum dosage:* 16 mg/day	Stimulates insulin release		Administer 15–30 min before meals.
				Cut dosage in half (ie, 0.5 mg tid) for frail older patients.
Thiazolidinediones				
Pioglitazone (Actos)	*Initial dosage:* 15–30 mg bid; *maximum dosage:* 45 mg once/daily	Increases peripheral insulin sensitivity	Peak 2–3 h	Associated with weight gain, edema, heart failure, bone fractures. Extreme caution if used for patients with heart failure – avoid if possible.
Rosiglitazone (Avandia)	*Initial dosage:* 4 mg once/day or 2 mg bid; *maximum dosage:* 8 mg once/day or 4 mg bid	Increases peripheral insulin sensitivity		Associated with weight gain, edema, heart failure, LDL cholesterol increase, bone fractures.
				Extreme caution in patients with heart failure – avoid if possible.
				FDA warnings on cardiovascular safety.
DPP-4 Receptor Inhibitors				
Sitagliptin	100 mg oral once/day	Inhibits DPP-4 hormone activity		Pancreatitis has occurred.
Saxagliptin	2.5–5 mg oral once/day	Prolongs survival of endogenously released incretin hormones		Reduce dosage for sitagliptin and saxagliptin with kidney dysfunction.
Linagliptin	5 mg oral once/day			No dosage adjustment for kidney dysfunction needed with linagliptin.

TABLE 32.4   Pharmacologic Management—cont'd

Medication[a]	Dosage	Action	Onset/Peak/ Duration	Special Considerations
SGLT2 Inhibitors				
Dapagliflozin	*Initial dosage:* 5 mg once/day; *maximum dosage:* 10 mg once/day.	Increases glucose excretion by blocking SGLT2 glucose uptake in nephron		Decrease dosage per GFR indicating kidney failure.
Canagliflozin	*Initial dosage:* 100 mg/day; *maximum dosage:* 300 mg/day			Avoid with liver failure.
				FDA advisory of increased risk of ketoacidosis. Increased UTI incidence.
GLP-1 Receptor Agonists				
Exenatide (Byetta)	*Initial dosage (immediate release):* 5 mg SC bid; after 1 month may increase to 10 mg bid	Activates GLP-1 receptors in pancreatic beta cells		Avoid if creatinine clearance <30 mL/min.
Exenatide extended release (Bydureon)	*Extended release:* 2 mg once/ week			GI side effects (nausea, vomiting diarrhea).
				Pancreatitis has occurred.
Liraglutide (Victoza)	• *Initial dosage:* 0.6 mg SC once/day (regardless of meals) for 7 days, then increase to 1.2 mg once/day. May increase to 1.8 mg/day if needed; MAX 1.8 mg/day.	Same as above.		Pancreatitis has occurred.
Alpha-Glucosidase Inhibitors				
Acarbose (Precose)	*Initial dosage:* 25 mg tid; *maximum dosage:* 100 mg tid	Delays carbohydrate digestion by blocking absorption of complete carbohydrates in small intestine	Peak 2–3 h	Administer with first bite of each meal.
				GI side effects (flatulence, abdominal pain, diarrhea). Not recommended with severe kidney dysfunction.
Miglitol (Glyset)	*Initial dosage:* 25 mg tid; *maximum dosage:* 100 mg tid		Peak 2–3 h	Administer with first bite of each meal.

bid, twice daily; *DPP-4,* dipeptidyl peptidase-4; *FDA,* US Food and Drug Administration; *GFR,* glomerular filtration rate; *GI,* gastrointestinal; *GLP-1,* glucagon-like peptide-1; *LDL,* low-density lipoprotein; *SC,* subcutaneous; *S. Creat,* Serum Creatine; *SGLT2,* sodium-glucose cotransporter 2; *tid,* three times daily; *UTI,* urinary tract infection.
[a]Combination medications are too numerous to include in this table.

DIABETIC KETOACIDOSIS

Epidemiology and Etiology

DKA is a life-threatening complication of diabetes mellitus. Individuals with type 1 diabetes who are dependent on insulin are typically affected. The diagnostic criteria for DKA are as follows[32]:

- Blood glucose greater than 250 mg/dL
- pH less than 7.3
- Serum bicarbonate less than 18 mEq/L
- Moderate or severe ketonemia or ketonuria

DKA is categorized as mild, moderate, or severe depending on the severity of the metabolic acidosis (assessed by blood pH, bicarbonate, ketones) and by the presence of altered mental status (Table 32.5 and Table 32.6).[32] Hospitalizations for DKA are increasing.[32] DKA accounts for more than 500,000 hospital days per year, with hospital costs that exceed $2.4 billion per year.[32] Infection is the most common precipitating cause of DKA.[32] Symptoms of fatigue and polyuria may precede full-blown DKA, which can develop in less than 24 hours in a patient with type 1 diabetes. In a patient with undiagnosed diabetes, it is unknown how long it may take for DKA to develop as the pancreatic beta cells gradually fail. Hospital admission is generally required for DKA related to new-onset type 1 diabetes. With management by experienced clinicians, the mortality rate from DKA in type 1 diabetics is less than 1%.[32]

Changes in the type of insulin, change in dosage, or increased metabolic demand can precipitate DKA in patients with type 1 diabetes.[32] Life cycle changes, such as growth spurts in an adolescent, require an increase in insulin intake, as do surgery, infection, and trauma. In young patients with diabetes, psychological problems combined with eating disorders are a contributing factor in up to 20% of cases of recurrent ketoacidosis.[32]

Ketoacidosis also occurs with acute pancreatitis. In addition to elevated glucose and acidosis, serum amylase and lipase are

TABLE 32.5   Diagnostic Criteria for Diabetic Ketoacidosis and Hyperglycemic Hyperosmolar Syndrome

	DKA			HHS
	Mild (Plasma Glucose >250 mg/dL)	Moderate (Plasma Glucose >250 mg/dL)	Severe (Plasma Glucose >250 mg/dL)	Plasma Glucose >600 mg/dL
Arterial pH	7.25–7.30	7.00 to <7.24	<7.00	>7.30
Serum bicarbonate (mEq/L)	15–18	10 to <15	<10	>18
Urine ketone[a]	Positive	Positive	Positive	Small
Serum ketone[a]	Positive	Positive	Positive	Small
Effective serum osmolality[b]	Variable	Variable	Variable	>320 mOsm/kg
Anion gap[c]	>10	>12	>12	Variable
Mental status	Alert	Alert/drowsy	Stupor/coma	Stupor/coma

[a]Nitroprusside reaction method.
[b]Effective serum osmolality: 2[measured Na$^+$ (mEq/L)] + glucose (mg/dL)18.
[c]Anion gap: (Na$^+$) − (Cl$^-$ + HCO$_3^-$) (mEq/L).
DKA, diabetic ketoacidosis; *HHS*, hyperglycemic hyperosmolar syndrome.
Data from Kitabchi AE, et al. Hyperglycemic crises in adult patients with diabetes: A consensus statement from the American Diabetes Association. *Diabetes Care.* 2009;32(7):1335.

TABLE 32.6   Comparison of Diabetic Ketoacidosis and Hyperglycemic Hyperosmolar State

Characteristics and Laboratory Tests	DKA	HHS
Cause	Insufficient exogenous glucose for glucose needs	Insufficient exogenous/endogenous insulin for glucose needs
Onset	Sudden (hours)	Slow, insidious (days, weeks)
Precipitating factors	Noncompliance with type 1 diabetes therapy, illness, surgery, decreased activity	Recent acute illness in older patient; therapeutic procedures
Mortality (%)	9–14	10–50
Patients affected	Patients with type 1 diabetes	Patients with type 2 diabetes
Clinical manifestations	Dry mouth, polydipsia, polyuria, polyphagia, dehydration, dry skin, hypotension, weakness	Mental confusion, tachycardia, changes in level of consciousness
	Ketoacidosis, air hunger, acetone breath odor, respirations deep and rapid, nausea, vomiting	No ketosis, no breath odor, respirations rapid and shallow, usually mild nausea/vomiting
Laboratory tests		
Glucose (mg/dL)	300–800	600–2000
Ketones	Strongly positive	Normal or mildly elevated
pH	<7.3	Normal[a]
Osmolality (mOsm/L)	<350	>350
Sodium	Normal or low	Normal or elevated
Potassium (K$^+$)	Normal, low, or elevated (total body K$^+$ depleted)	Low, normal, or elevated
Bicarbonate	<15 mEq/L	Normal
Phosphorus	Low, normal, or elevated (may decrease after insulin therapy)	Low, normal, or elevated (may decrease after insulin therapy)
Urine acetone	Strong	Absent or mild

[a]Exception: In severe HHS, lactic acidosis may develop as a result of dehydration and severe tissue hypoperfusion and ischemia.
DKA, diabetic ketoacidosis; *HHS*, hyperglycemic hyperosmolar state.

abnormally high, which helps to establish pancreatitis as a separate diagnosis from type 1 diabetes. Other nondiabetic causes of ketoacidosis are starvation ketosis and alcoholic ketoacidosis. These cases are distinguished from classic DKA by clinical history and usually by a plasma glucose less than 200 mg/dL.[32]

Pathophysiology

Insulin Deficiency

Insulin is the metabolic key to the transfer of glucose from the bloodstream into the cell, where it can be used immediately for energy or stored for use at a later time. Without insulin, glucose remains in the bloodstream, and cells are deprived of their energy source. A complex pathophysiologic chain of events follows (Fig. 32.2). The release of glucagon from the liver is stimulated when insulin is ineffective in providing the cells with glucose for energy. Glucagon increases the amount of glucose in the bloodstream by breaking down stored glucose (glycogenolysis). Noncarbohydrates (fat and protein) are converted into glucose (gluconeogenesis). Plasma glucose levels for a patient with DKA typically are greater than 250 mg/dL. Elevated serum glucose levels alone do not define DKA; the other crucial determining factor is the presence of ketoacidosis as listed in Table 32.5.[32] Approximately 10% of patients with DKA present to the hospital with a plasma glucose less with 250 mg/dL.[32]

DIABETIC KETOACIDOSIS

Jill Jackson, a 49 year old patient with type 1 diabetes for over 30 years, has developed a wound infection on the bottom of her foot and subsequently developed DKA.

Glucose levels alone do not define DKA

Slow onset 4-10 hours

Aggressive Clinical Management includes

Prevention of progressive decompensation; reverse dehydration, replace insulin, reverse ketoacidosis, & replenish electrolytes.

Successful

Diagnostic Criteria

Life-threatening complication of diabetes

- Blood glucose > 250 mg/dL
- pH < 7.3
- Serum bicarbonate < 18 mEq/L
- Moderate or severe ketonemia or ketonuria

Categories

Depending on the severity of the metabolic acidosis

Categorized as mild, moderate, or severe - assessed by blood pH, bicarbonate, ketones and by the presence of altered mental status.

Pathophysiology

Insulin Deficiency → glucagon release → glycogenolysis. Fat & protein converted into glucose.
Hyperglycemia - ↑ plasma osmolality → dehydration → ↑ catecholamine production → glycogenolysis, lipolysis, & gluconeogenesis.
Fluid Volume Deficit - Polyuria & glycosuria → ↑ osmotic particle load of DKA. ↑ water, sodium, potassium, & phosphorus excreted in urine.
Ketoacidosis - Fat converted into glucose (gluconeogenesis). Ketoacidosis → free fatty acids metabolized into ketones. Acetone → excreted in lungs → characteristic fruity odor of breath.
Acid—Base Balance - ↑ Ketones & ↓ bicarbonate → ↓ serum pH. Kussmaul respirations → release carbonic acid. Acetone exhaled → breath fruity.
Gluconeogenesis - Leaves no reserve protein. Nitrogen accumulates as protein metabolized to urea → ↑ osmotic diuresis & ↑ dehydration.

NURSING DIAGNOSES

- ↓ Cardiac Output R/T alterations in preload.
- ↓ Fluid Volume R/T absolute loss.
- Anxiety R/T threat to biologic, psychologic, & social integrity.
- Disturbed Body Image R/T functional dependence on life-sustaining technology.
- Ineffective Coping R/T situational crisis & personal vulnerability.
- Powerlessness R/T lack of control over current situation or disease progression.
- ↓ Knowledge R/T lack of previous exposure to information.

COLLABORATIVE CARE

Fluids, Insulin, & Electrolytes

- Rapid normal saline infusion using a pump.
- Continuous IV insulin until ketoacidosis subsides.
- Hourly monitoring of BG, K⁺, & ABGs.
- NPO until hyperglycemia under control.
- Goal - ↓ serum glucose 50 - 70 mg/dL/hour.
- When BG < 200 mg/dL, administer D₅W with 0.45% NaCl along with ↓ insulin dose.
- SC insulin given once pt stabilizes & is eating.
- Monitor for hyper/hypoglycemia.
- Accurate I&O, hourly U/O & hourly BG checks.
- Frequent evaluation of VS especially HR, hemodynamic values, & BP.
- Assess respirations frequently (rate, depth, odor).
- Evaluate serum osmolality & sodium, BUN, & creatinine.
- Monitor for FVE, hypoglycemia, hypo/hyperkalemia, hyponatremia, cerebral edema, & infection.
- Monitor for signs of FVE: JVD, DOE: ↓ rate & volume of infusion, ↑ HOB, O₂, & hourly U/O.
- Hypoglycemia - ↑ risk when frequency of BG testing ↑ to 2- to 4-hour intervals.
- Continuous cardiac monitoring - potential for ventricular dysrhythmias.
- Monitor for signs of hyponatremia: abdominal cramping, postural hypotension, & unexpected behavioral changes.
- Frequent neuroassessments - cerebral edema.
- Infection and skin breakdown - meticulous skin and mouth care with sterile technique for all invasive procedures.

NURSING MANAGEMENT GOALS

- Administer fluids, insulin, & electrolytes.
- Monitor response to therapy.
- Maintain surveillance for complications.
- Provide patient education.

PATIENT OUTCOMES

DEMONSTRATE ADEQUATE FLUID REPLACEMENT AND ELECTROLYTE BALANCE:
- ↓ HR, normal BP and normalizing blood glucose levels.
- Absence of ketones in blood and urine.
- Electrolytes within normal range.
- ABGs within normal range.
- Maintain O₂ Saturation of 90% or greater.
- Mental clarity, skin warm/dry.

FIG. 32.2 Concept Map for Diabetic Ketoacidosis. *ABGs*, Arterial blood gases; *BG*, blood glucose; *BP*, blood pressure; *BUN*, blood urea nitrogen; *DKA*, diabetic ketoacidosis; *DOE*, dyspnea on exertion; *FVE*, fluid volume excess; *HOB*, head of bed; *HR*, heart rate; *IV*, intravenous; *I & O*, intake and output; *JVD*, jugular vein distention; *K⁺*, potassium; *NaCl*, sodium chloride; *NPO*, nothing by mouth; *O₂*, oxygen; *pH*, a measure of the degree to which a solution is acidic or alkaline; *R/T*, related to; *SC*, subcutaneous; *U/O*, urine output Concept maps created by © DEANNE A. BLACH, MSN, RN

Hyperglycemia

Hyperglycemia increases plasma osmolality, and the blood becomes hyperosmolar. Cellular dehydration occurs as the hyperosmolar extracellular fluid draws the more dilute intracellular and interstitial fluid into the vascular space in an attempt to return the plasma osmolality to normal. Dehydration stimulates catecholamine production in an effort to provide emergency support. Catecholamine output stimulates further glycogenolysis, lipolysis, and gluconeogenesis, pouring glucose into the bloodstream.

Fluid Volume Deficit

Polyuria (excessive urination) and *glycosuria* (sugar in the urine) occur as a result of the osmotic particle load that occurs with DKA. The excess glucose, filtered at the glomeruli, cannot be resorbed at the kidney tubule and spills into the urine. The unresorbed solute exerts its own osmotic pull in the renal tubules, and less water is returned to circulation through the collecting ducts. As a result, large volumes of water, along with sodium, potassium, and phosphorus, are excreted in the urine, causing a fluid volume deficit. The serum sodium concentration may be decreased because of the movement of water from the intracellular to the extracellular (vascular) space.[32]

Ketoacidosis

In a healthy individual, the presence of insulin in the bloodstream suppresses the manufacture of ketones. In insulin deficiency states, fat is rapidly converted into glucose (gluconeogenesis). *Ketoacidosis* occurs when free fatty acids are metabolized into ketones: Acetoacetate, β-hydroxybutyrate, and acetone are the three ketone bodies that are produced. During normal metabolism, the ratio of β-hydroxybutyrate to acetoacetate is 1:1, with acetone present in only small amounts. In insulin deficiency, the quantities of all three ketone bodies increase substantially, and the ratio of β-hydroxybutyrate to acetoacetate can increase to 10:1. β-Hydroxybutyrate and acetoacetate are the ketones responsible for acidosis in DKA. Acetone does not cause acidosis and is safely excreted in the lungs, causing the characteristic fruity odor.

Ketones are measurable in the bloodstream (ketonemia). Blood tests that measure the quantity of β-hydroxybutyric acid, the predominant ketone body in the blood, are the most useful.[32] Because ketones are excreted by the kidney, they are also measurable in the urine (*ketonuria*). Ketone blood tests are preferred over urine tests for diagnosis and monitoring of DKA in critical care. When the blood and urine become clear of ketones, DKA is resolved.

Acid–Base Balance

The acid–base balance varies depending on the severity of DKA. A patient with mild DKA typically has a pH between 7.25 and 7.30. In severe DKA, the pH can drop below 7.00 (see Table 32.5).[32] Acid ketones dissociate and yield hydrogen ions (H^+), which accumulate and precipitate a fall in serum pH. The level of serum bicarbonate also decreases, consistent with a diagnosis of metabolic acidosis. Breathing becomes deep and rapid (Kussmaul respirations) to release carbonic acid in the form of carbon dioxide (CO_2). Acetone is exhaled, giving the breath its characteristic fruity odor.

Gluconeogenesis

Gluconeogenesis is the process of breaking down fat or protein to make new glucose. Fat is metabolized to ketones, as described earlier. Protein used for gluconeogenesis leaves no reserve protein available for synthesis and repair of vital body tissues. Nitrogen accumulates as protein is metabolized to urea. Urea, added to the bloodstream, increases the osmotic diuresis and accentuates dehydration.

Assessment and Diagnosis
Clinical Manifestations

DKA has a predictable clinical presentation. It is usually preceded by patient complaints of malaise, headache, polyuria (excessive urination), polydipsia (excessive thirst), and polyphagia (excessive hunger). Nausea, vomiting, extreme fatigue, dehydration, and weight loss follow. Central nervous system (CNS) depression, with changes in the level of consciousness, can lead quickly to coma.[32]

A patient with DKA may be stuporous or unresponsive, depending on the degree of fluid-balance disturbance. Physical examination reveals evidence of dehydration, including flushed dry skin, dry buccal membranes, and skin turgor that takes longer than 3 seconds to return to its original position after the skin has been lifted. A dehydrated "sunken eyeball" effect, resulting from lack of fluid in the interstitium of the eyeball, may be observed. Tachycardia and hypotension may signal profound fluid losses. Kussmaul respirations are present, and the fruity odor of acetone may be detected.

Laboratory Studies

Considering the complexity and potential seriousness of DKA, the laboratory diagnosis is straightforward. When the patient has established type 1 diabetes, the presence of hyperglycemia and ketones provides rapid diagnostic confirmation of DKA. Many patients have ketone testing point of care devices at home A blood gas sample can confirm acid–base imbalance. Other clues may be gleaned from the venous blood chemistry panel. CO_2, if measured, is low in the presence of uncompensated metabolic acidosis, and the anion gap is elevated. Serum sodium may be low as a result of the movement of water from the intracellular space into the extracellular (vascular) space.[32] The serum potassium level is often normal; a low serum potassium level in DKA suggests that a significant potassium deficiency may be present.[32]

Medical Management

Diagnosis of DKA is based on the combination of presenting symptoms, patient history, medical history (type 1 diabetes), precipitating factors (if known), and results of serum glucose and urine ketone testing. After diagnosis, DKA requires aggressive clinical management to prevent progressive decompensation. The goals of treatment are to reverse dehydration, replace insulin, reverse ketoacidosis, and replenish electrolytes.

Reversing Dehydration

A patient with DKA is dehydrated and may have lost 5% to 10% of body weight in fluids. Aggressive IV fluid replacement is provided to rehydrate the intracellular and extracellular compartments and prevent circulatory collapse (Fig. 32.3).[32] Assessment of hydration is an important first step in the treatment of DKA.

IV isotonic normal saline (0.9% sodium chloride [NaCl]) is infused to replenish the vascular deficit and to reverse hypotension. For a severely dehydrated patient, 1 L of normal saline is infused immediately. Laboratory assessment of serum osmolality and the serum sodium concentration can help guide subsequent interventions. If the serum osmolality is elevated and serum sodium is high (hypernatremia), infusions of hypotonic

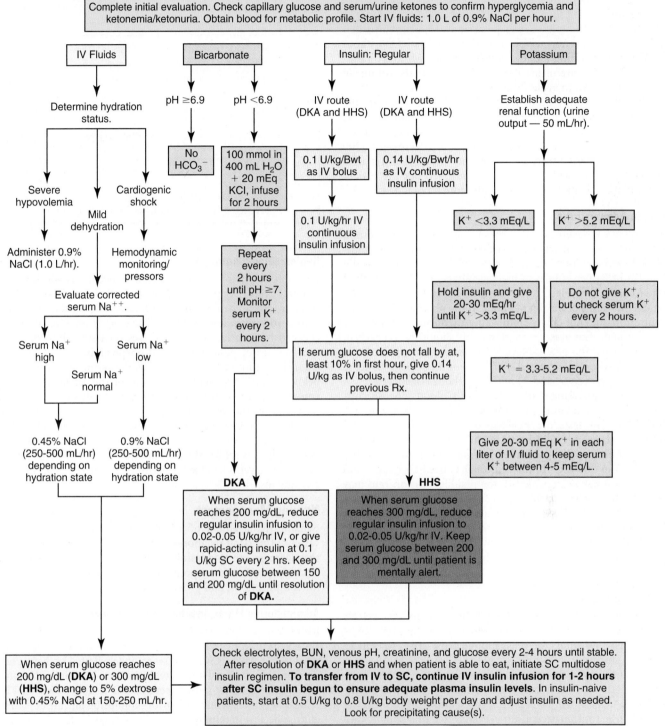

FIG. 32.3 Protocol for Management of Diabetic Ketoacidosis (DKA) and Hyperglycemic Hyperosmolar State (HHS). *ABGs,* Arterial blood gases; *BG,* blood glucose; *BP,* blood pressure; *BUN,* blood, urea, nitrogen; *CV,* cardiovascular; *CVP,* central venous pressure; *DKA,* diabetic ketoacidosis; *DOE,* dyspnea on exertion; *FVE,* fluid volume excess; *HOB,* head of bed; *HR,* heart rate; *I & O,* intake and output; *JVD,* jugular vein distention; *K⁺,* potassium; *UTI,* urinary tract infection; *LOC,* level of consciousness; *MI,* myocardial infarction; *NPO,* nothing by mouth; *O₂ Sat,* oxygen saturation; *SubQ,* subcutaneous; *U/O,* urine output (From Kitabchi AE, et al. Hyperglycemic crises in adult patients with diabetes: A consensus statement from the American Diabetes Association. *Diabetes Care.* 2009;32[7]:1335.)

NaCl (0.45) follow the initial saline replacement. The replacement infusion typically includes 20 to 30 mEq of potassium per liter to restore the intracellular potassium debt, provided that kidney function is normal (see Fig. 32.3).[32] In patients without normally functioning kidneys and in patients with cardiopulmonary disease, careful attention must be paid to the volume of fluid replacement to avoid fluid overload.

After the serum glucose level decreases to 200 mg/dL, the infusing solution is changed to a 50/50 mix of hypotonic saline and 5% dextrose. Dextrose is added to replenish depleted cellular glucose as the circulating serum glucose decreases to 200 mg/dL.[32] Dextrose infusion also prevents unexpected hypoglycemia when the insulin infusion is continued but the patient cannot take in sufficient carbohydrate from an oral diet.

Insulin Administration

In moderate to severe DKA, an initial IV bolus of regular insulin at 0.1 unit for each kilogram of body weight may be administered. Subsequently, a continuous infusion of regular insulin at 0.1 unit/kg per hour is infused simultaneously with IV fluid replacement (see Fig. 32.3).[32] In a 70-kg adult, the infusion would be 7 units of insulin per hour. If the plasma glucose concentration does not fall by 50 to 70 mg/dL during the first hour of treatment, the glucose measurement should be rechecked. When the plasma glucose level is decreasing as expected, the insulin infusion is increased each hour until a steady glucose decline of between 50 and 70 mg/dL per hour is achieved.[32]

Frequent assessment of the patient's blood glucose concentration is mandatory in moderate to severe DKA. Initially, blood glucose tests are performed hourly. The frequency decreases to every 2 to 4 hours as the patient's blood glucose level stabilizes and approaches normal. After the level has decreased to 200 mg/dL, the acidosis has been corrected, and rehydration has been achieved, the insulin infusion rate may be decreased to 0.05 to 0.1 unit/kg per hour. This usually represents 3 to 6 units per hour in an adult receiving a continuous IV insulin infusion. It is important to verify that the serum potassium concentration is not lower than 3.3 mEq/L and to replace potassium if necessary before administering the initial insulin bolus.[32]

Reversing Ketoacidosis

Replacement of fluid volume and insulin interrupts the ketotic cycle and reverses the metabolic acidosis. In the presence of insulin, glucose enters the cells, and the body ceases to convert fats into glucose.

Adequate hydration and insulin replacement usually correct acidosis, and this treatment is sufficient for many patients with DKA. As shown in Fig. 32.3, replacement of bicarbonate is no longer routine except for a severely acidotic patient with a serum pH value lower than 7.0.[32] An indwelling arterial line provides access for hourly sampling of arterial blood gases to evaluate pH, bicarbonate, and other laboratory values in a patient with severe DKA.

Hyperglycemia usually resolves before ketoacidemia does.[32] Patients with type 1 diabetes and DKA may require 6 to 9 L of IV fluid replacement.[33] Volume resuscitation occurs over 24 to 36 hours with most IV crystalloid administered in the first 8 hours.[33] Patients with a new diagnosis of type 1 diabetes take longer to clear urine ketones and require more insulin to achieve normal glycemic control. This is because the blood glucose is typically very elevated on the initial admission.

BOX 32.5 NURSING DIAGNOSES

Diabetic Ketoacidosis

- Decreased Cardiac Output related to alterations in preload, p. 1015
- Deficient Fluid Volume related to absolute loss, p. 1019
- Anxiety related to threat to biologic, psychologic, and social integrity, p. 1012
- Disturbed Body Image related to functional dependence on life-sustaining technology, p. 1022
- Ineffective Coping related to situational crisis and personal vulnerability, p. 1036
- Powerlessness related to lack of control over current situation or disease progression, p. 1038
- Deficient Knowledge related to lack of previous exposure to information, p. 1020 (see Box 32.9, Patient Education Plan for Diabetic Ketoacidosis)

Replenishing Electrolytes

Low serum potassium (hypokalemia) occurs as insulin promotes the return of potassium into the cell and metabolic acidosis is reversed. The potassium level must be 3.3 mEq or greater before administering insulin.[33] The potassium level must be checked frequently, as insulin drives potassium into the cells and the serum potassium can drop precipitously. Potassium chloride is administered as soon as the serum potassium falls below normal. Frequent verification of the serum potassium concentration is required for a patient with DKA receiving fluid resuscitation and insulin therapy.

The serum phosphate level is sometimes low (hypophosphatemia) in DKA. Insulin treatment may make this more obvious as phosphate is returned to the interior of the cell. If the serum phosphate level is less than 1 mg/dL, phosphate replacement is recommended.[32]

Nursing Management

Nursing management of a patient with DKA incorporates a variety of nursing diagnoses (Box 32.5). The goals of nursing management are to administer prescribed fluids, insulin, and electrolytes; monitor response to therapy; maintain surveillance for complications; and provide patient education.

Administering Fluids, Insulin, and Electrolytes

Rapid IV fluid replacement requires the use of a volumetric pump. To ensure effective absorption, insulin is administered intravenously to patients who are severely dehydrated or have poor peripheral perfusion. Patients with DKA are kept on NPO status (nothing by mouth) until hyperglycemia is under control. The critical care nurse is responsible for monitoring the rate of plasma glucose decline in response to insulin. The goal is to achieve a fall in glucose levels of approximately 50 to 70 mg/dL each hour.[32] The coordination involved in monitoring blood glucose, potassium, and often blood gases on an hourly basis is considerable.

When the blood glucose level falls to 200 mg/dL, a 5% dextrose solution (D_5W) with 0.45% NaCl solution is infused to prevent hypoglycemia.[32] At this time, it is likely that the insulin dose per hour will also be decreased. The regular insulin drip is not discontinued until the ketoacidosis subsides, as identified by absence of ketones, by closure of the anion gap, and by a normal pH.[32,33]

Insulin is given subcutaneously after glucose levels, dehydration, hypotension, and acid–base balance are normalized, when the patient is in stable condition and taking an oral diet.

BOX 32.6   Hydration Assessment

- Hourly intake
- Blood pressure changes
  - Orthostatic hypotension
  - Pulse pressure
  - Pulse rate, character, rhythm
- Neck vein filling
- Skin turgor
- Skin moisture
- Body weight
- Central venous pressure
- Hourly output
- Complaints of thirst

Monitoring Response to Therapy

Accurate intake and output (I&O) measurements must be maintained to monitor reversal of dehydration. Hourly urine output is an indicator of kidney function and provides information to prevent overhydration or insufficient hydration. Vital signs, especially heart rate (HR), hemodynamic values, and BP, are continuously monitored to assess response to fluid replacement. Evidence that fluid replacement is effective includes decreased HR, normal BP, and normalizing blood glucose levels. Box 32.6 lists the standard features to be included in an assessment of hydration status. More invasive hemodynamic monitoring, such as a pulmonary artery catheter, is rarely needed. Further evidence of hydration improvement includes a change from a previously weak and rapid pulse to one that is strong and full and a change from hypotension to a gradual elevation of systolic BP. Respirations are assessed frequently for changes in rate, depth, and presence of the fruity acetone odor.

Blood glucose is measured each hour in the initial period. Sometimes potassium is measured just as frequently. The serum osmolality and serum sodium concentration are evaluated, and blood urea nitrogen and creatinine levels are assessed for possible kidney impairment related to decreased organ perfusion. The purpose of these frequent assessments is to determine that the patient's clinical status is improving.

Transition to subcutaneous insulin. When the clinical laboratory indicators are stable and the patient is awake and alert, the transition to subcutaneous insulin and an oral diet can be made.[33] Hyperglycemia is a risk if the subcutaneous insulin dosage is inadequate to maintain a normal blood glucose. In this situation, the anion gap may open up again. Hypoglycemia is also a risk during the transition period. For example, in anticipation of discontinuing the insulin and IV dextrose infusion, a patient receives a subcutaneous dose of insulin and is expected to eat a meal. However, if the patient is then unable to eat an adequate amount, hypoglycemia results from the administration of subcutaneous insulin without adequate carbohydrate.

Surveillance for Complications

A patient with DKA can experience various complications including fluid volume overload, hypoglycemia, hypokalemia or hyperkalemia, hyponatremia, cerebral edema, and infection.

Fluid volume overload. Fluid overload from rapid volume infusion is a serious complication that can occur in a patient with a compromised cardiopulmonary system or kidneys. Neck vein engorgement, dyspnea without exertion, and pulmonary crackles on auscultation signal circulatory overload. Reduction in the rate and volume of infusion, elevation of the head of the bed, and provision of oxygen may be required to manage increased intravascular volume. Hourly urine measurement is mandatory to assess kidney function and adequacy of fluid replacement.

Hypoglycemia. Hypoglycemia is defined as a serum glucose level lower than 70 mg/dL.[32] Most acute care hospitals have specific procedures for management of hypoglycemia (Box 32.7). For example, if hypoglycemia is detected by fingerstick point of care testing at the bedside, a blood sample is sent to the laboratory for verification; the physician is notified immediately; and replacement glucose is given intravenously or orally, depending on the patient's clinical condition, diagnosis, and level of consciousness.

Unexpected behavior change or decreased level of consciousness, diaphoresis, and tremors are physical warning signs that the patient has become hypoglycemic. These symptoms are especially important to recognize if the frequency of blood glucose testing has lengthened to 2- to 4-hour intervals. Up to 30% of individuals who have type 1 diabetes have impaired awareness of their low blood glucose, greatly increasing their risk of severe hypoglycemia (Box 32.7). The physical symptoms associated with hypoglycemia and hyperglycemia are listed in Box 32.8.

Hypokalemia and hyperkalemia. Hypokalemia can occur within the first hours of rehydration and insulin treatment. Continuous cardiac monitoring is required because low serum potassium (hypokalemia) can cause ventricular dysrhythmias.

Hyperkalemia occurs with acidosis or with overaggressive administration of potassium replacement in patients with kidney disease. Severe hyperkalemia is demonstrated on the cardiac monitor by a large, peaked T wave; flattened P wave; and widened QRS complex (see Fig. 13.84 in Chapter 13). Ventricular fibrillation can follow.

Hyponatremia. Elimination of sodium from the body results from the osmotic diuresis and is compounded by the vomiting and diarrhea that can occur during DKA. Clinical manifestations of hyponatremia include abdominal cramping, postural hypotension, and unexpected behavioral changes. NaCl is infused as the initial IV solution. Maintenance of the saline infusion depends on clinical manifestations of sodium imbalance and serum laboratory values.

Risk for cerebral edema. Changes in the patient's neurologic status may be insidious. Alterations in level of consciousness, pupil reaction, and motor function may be the result of fluctuating glucose levels and cerebral fluid shifts. Confusion and sudden complaints of headache are ominous signs that may signal cerebral edema. These observations require immediate action to prevent neurologic damage. Neurologic assessments are performed every hour or as needed during the acute phase of hyperglycemia and rehydration. Assessment of level of consciousness serves as the index of the patient's cerebral response to rehydration therapy.

Risk for infection. Skin care takes on new dimensions for patients with DKA. Dehydration, hypovolemia, and hypophosphatemia interfere with oxygen delivery at the cell site and contribute to inadequate perfusion and tissue breakdown. Patients must be repositioned frequently to relieve capillary pressure and promote adequate perfusion to body tissues. A typical patient with type 1 diabetes is of normal weight or underweight. Bony prominences must be assessed for tissue breakdown, and the patient's body weight must be repositioned every 1 to 2 hours. Irritation of skin from adhesive tape,

BOX 32.7 Hypoglycemia Management

Hypoglycemia Prevention and Management

- Definition: Plasma blood glucose level below 70 mg/dL (3.9 mmol/L).
  - The American Diabetes Association recommends 70 mg/dL plasma blood glucose as the alert threshold for hypoglycemia. Most patients with diabetes do not have symptoms with this blood glucose and this value provides some time to raise the blood glucose and avoid clinical symptoms.
  - Bedside POC glucometers results vary in accuracy. A POC blood glucose less than 70 mg/dL must be double-checked by sending a blood sample to the clinical laboratory *stat*, to measure the plasma blood glucose.
- Hypoglycemia Prevention
  - Close monitoring of blood glucose for all hospitalized patients who receive insulin. Use the laboratory threshold alert of 70 mg/dL, and do not wait for clinical symptoms.
  - Approximately 10% of patients with diabetes admitted to critical care units experience at least one hypoglycemic episode (below 70 mg/dL).
  - Blood glucose testing to detect hypoglycemia is vital because many patients with diabetes do not experience symptoms. This is called *hypoglycemia unawareness*. In patients with diabetes who experience frequent episodes of hypoglycemia, the autonomic nervous system becomes less responsive. This is known as *hypoglycemia-associated autonomic failure*.
  - Patient education before hospital discharge is essential to teach patients how blood glucose monitoring and dietary interventions are used to prevent hypoglycemia.

- Clinical Signs and Symptoms of Acute Hypoglycemia
  - Sedated and intubated patients may not have signs and symptoms
  - Confusion
  - Neurologic changes
  - Seizures
  - Death
- Hypoglycemia Management
  - Stop insulin infusion (if running).
  - Administer 25 grams of hypertonic dextrose (D50) IV immediately.
  - If blood glucose is dangerously low (below 40 mg/dL), some hospital protocols recommend 50 grams D50 IV.
  - Repeat blood glucose value in 15 minutes, and ongoing until blood glucose is greater than 70 mg/dL.
  - Evaluate insulin regimen.
  - Evaluate IV dextrose and carbohydrate nutrition regimen.
  - If the patient can safely swallow, provide 25 grams of carbohydrate orally and recheck blood glucose.
  - Hold subcutaneous insulin. Recheck blood glucose level if subcutaneous insulin has been recently administered, and continue to check blood glucose level based upon the duration of action of the subcutaneous insulin previously administered.

Data from: Seaquist ER et al: Hypoglycemia and Diabetes: A Report of a Workgroup of the American Diabetes Association and The Endocrine Society. Diabetes Care 2013;36:1384–1395.
D50, 50% Dextrose; *IV*, intravenous; *POC*, Point of Care.

BOX 32.8 Clinical Manifestations of Hypoglycemia and Hyperglycemia

Hypoglycemia	Hyperglycemia
Restlessness	Excessive thirst
Apprehension	Excessive urination
Irritability	Hunger
Trembling	Weakness
Weakness	Listlessness
Diaphoresis	Mental fatigue
Pallor	Flushed, dry skin
Paresthesia	Itching
Pallor	Headache
Headache	Nausea
Hunger	Vomiting
Difficulty thinking	Abdominal cramps
Loss of coordination	Dehydration
Difficulty walking	Weak, rapid pulse
Difficulty talking	Postural hypotension
Visual disturbances	Hypotension
Blurred vision	Acetone breath odor
Double vision	Kussmaul respirations
Tachycardia	Rapid breathing
Shallow respirations	Changes in level of consciousness
Hypertension	Stupor
Changes in level of consciousness	Coma
Seizures	
Coma	

shearing force, and detergents should be avoided. Maintenance of skin integrity prevents unwanted portals of entry for microorganisms.

Oral care, including toothbrushing and use of lip balm, helps keep lips supple and prevents cracking. Prepared sponge sticks or moist gauze pads can be used to moisten oral membranes of unconscious patients. Swabbing the mouth moistens the tissue and displaces the bacteria that collect when saliva, which has a bacteriostatic action, is curtailed by dehydration. Conscious patients must be provided the means to self-remove oral bacteria by toothbrushing and frequent oral rinsing.

Strict sterile technique is used to maintain all IV systems. All venipuncture sites are checked every 4 hours for signs of inflammation, phlebitis, or infiltration. Strict surgical asepsis is used for all invasive procedures. Sterile technique is used if urinary catheterization is necessary to obtain urine samples for testing. Urinary catheter care is provided every 8 hours.

Patient Education

It is important to be aware of the knowledge level and adherence history of patients with previously diagnosed diabetes to formulate an appropriate teaching plan. Learning objectives include a discussion of target glucose levels, definition of hyperglycemia and its causes, harmful effects, symptoms, and how to manage insulin and diet when one is unwell and unable to eat. Additional objectives include a definition of DKA and its causes, symptoms, and harmful consequences. The patient and family are also expected to learn the principles of diabetes management. Universal precautions must be emphasized for all family caregivers. The patient and family must also learn the

---

✳ BOX 32.9   PATIENT EDUCATION PLAN
Diabetic Ketoacidosis

Acute Phase
- Explain rationale for critical care unit admission.
- Reduce anxiety associated with critical care unit.

Predischarge
The patient should be able to teach back the following:
- Target glucose levels
- Signs and symptoms of diabetic ketoacidosis
- Self-care monitoring of blood glucose level
- Self-care monitoring of blood ketones
- Insulin regimen
- Sick-day management
- Signs and symptoms to report to health care practitioner

---

warning signs of DKA to report to a health care practitioner. Knowledge-based, independent self-management of blood glucose level and avoidance of diabetes-related complications are the ultimate goals of education of the patient, family, or other support persons using the teach back method (Box 32.9).

Collaborative Management

In all aspects of patient care management, health care professionals work as a team with the major collaborative goal of providing the best possible outcome for each patient. Current guidelines related to collaborative management of patients with DKA are listed in Box 32.10.

HYPERGLYCEMIC HYPEROSMOLAR STATE

Epidemiology and Etiology

Hyperglycemic hyperosmolar state (HHS) is a potentially lethal complication of type 2 diabetes. The hallmarks of HHS are extremely high levels of plasma glucose with resultant elevation in serum osmolality causing osmotic diuresis. Ketosis is absent or mild. Inability to replace fluids lost through diuresis leads to profound dehydration and changes in level of consciousness. The overall mortality rate from HHS ranges from 5% to 20%.[32] Because patients with HHS have type 2 diabetes as an underlying disorder, they are generally older adults with cardiovascular comorbidities.

The diagnostic criteria for HHS are as follows and as shown in Table 32.5[32]:
- Blood glucose greater than 600 mg/dL
- Arterial pH greater than 7.3
- Serum bicarbonate greater than 18 mEq/L
- Serum osmolality greater than 320 mOsm/kg H_2O (320 mmol/kg)
- Absent or mild ketonuria

Most patients with this level of metabolic disruption experience visual changes, mental status changes, and potentially hypovolemic shock.

HHS occurs when the pancreas produces a relatively insufficient amount of insulin for the high levels of glucose that flood the bloodstream. Older adults with type 2 diabetes and cardiovascular conditions are at highest risk. Infection is the usual trigger for development of HHS; the most common infections are pneumonia and urinary tract infections. Other precipitating causes of HHS include stroke, myocardial infarction, trauma, major surgery, and the physiologic stress of critical illness.

QSEN   BOX 32.10   QSEN: Evidence-Based Practice
Diabetic Ketoacidosis

A summary is provided of evidence and evidence-based recommendations for controlling symptoms related to diabetic ketoacidosis.

Strong Evidence to Support
Regular insulin by continuous infusion is recommended.
Replace serum potassium if level is lower than 3.3 mEq/L.
Replace serum phosphate if level is lower than 1.0 mg/dL.

Very Little Evidence to Support
No support for use of routine bicarbonate to correct low serum pH; use may be considered if pH is below 7.0.

Reference
Kitabchi AE, et al. Hyperglycemic crises in adult patients with diabetes: A consensus statement from the American Diabetes Association. *Diabetes Care.* 2009;32(7):1335.

Differences Between Hyperglycemic Hyperosmolar State and Diabetic Ketoacidosis

Clinically, HHS is distinguished from DKA by the presence of extremely elevated serum glucose, more profound dehydration, and minimal or absent ketosis (see Tables 32.5 and 32.6). Another major difference is that protein and fats are not used to create new supplies of glucose in HHS as they are in DKA; as a result, the ketotic cycle is never started or does not occur until the glucose level is extremely elevated.

Pathophysiology

HHS represents a deficit of insulin and an excess of glucagon (Fig. 32.4). Reduced insulin levels prevent the movement of glucose into the cells, allowing glucose to accumulate in the plasma. The decreased insulin triggers glucagon release from the liver, and hepatic glucose is poured into the circulation. As the number of glucose particles increases in the blood, serum hyperosmolality increases. In an effort to decrease the serum osmolality, fluid is drawn from the intracellular compartment (inside the cells) into the vascular bed. Profound intracellular volume depletion occurs if the patient's thirst sensation is absent or decreased. HHS may evolve over days or weeks.[32]

Hemoconcentration persists despite removal of large amounts of glucose in the urine (glycosuria). The glomerular filtration and elimination of glucose by the kidney tubules is ineffective in reducing the serum glucose level sufficiently to maintain normal glucose levels. The hyperosmolality and reduced blood volume stimulate release of ADH to increase the tubular resorption of water. However, ADH is powerless to overcome the osmotic pull exerted by the glucose load. Excessive fluid volume is lost at the kidney tubule, with simultaneous loss of potassium, sodium, and phosphate in the urine. This chain of events results in progressively worsening hypovolemia.

Hypovolemia reduces perfusion to the kidney, and oliguria develops. Although this process conserves water and preserves the blood volume, it prevents further glucose loss, and hyperosmolality increases. Ketosis is absent or mild in HHS.[32]

COLLABORATIVE CARE

Fluids, Insulin, & Electrolytes

Aggressive Clinical Management Includes

- Rapid normal saline infusion using a pump.
- Continuous IV insulin until ketoacidosis subsides.
- Hourly monitoring of BG, K$^+$, & ABGs.
- NPO until hyperglycemia under control.
- Goal - ↓ serum glucose 50 - 70 mg/dL/hour.
- When BG < 200 mg/dL, administer D$_5$W with 0.45% NaCl along with ↓ insulin dose.
- Subcutaneous insulin given once his BG stabilizes & he is eating.
- Monitor for hyper/hypoglycemia.
- Accurate I&O, hourly U/O & hourly BG checks.
- Frequent evaluation of VS especially HR, hemodynamic values, & BP.
- Assess respirations frequently (rate, depth, odor).
- Evaluate serum osmolality & sodium, BUN, & creatinine.

Surveillance for Complications

- Monitor for FVE, hypoglycemia, hypo/hyperkalemia, hyponatremia, cerebral edema, & infection.
- Monitor for signs of FVE: JVD, DOE: ↓ rate & volume of infusion, ↑HOB, O$_2$, & hourly U/O.
- Hypoglycemia - ↑ risk when frequency of BG testing ↑ to 2- to 4-hour intervals.
- Continuous cardiac monitoring - potential for ventricular dysrhythmias.
- Monitor for signs of hyponatremia: abdominal cramping, postural hypotension, & unexpected behavioral changes.
- Frequent neuro assessments - cerebral edema.
- Infection and skin breakdown - meticulous skin and mouth care with sterile technique for all invasive procedures.

NURSING MANAGEMENT GOALS

- Administer fluids, insulin, & electrolytes.
- Monitor response to therapy.
- Maintain surveillance for complications.
- Provide patient education.

HYPERGLYCEMIC HYPEROSMOLAR STATE (HHS)

Assessment of clinical signs of dehydration

65 year old, David Brown, has Type 2 diabetes with underlying cardiovascular disease. He presents to the ED with a UTI, a blood glucose of 660 mg/dL with profound dehydration and lethargy.

Risk — Hypovolemic Shock!

Risk Factors

Medical Management

Same Basic Principles to Treat DKA & HHS

Rapid rehydration, insulin replacement, & K$^+$ replacement. Discover and treat the cause of HHS.

PATIENT OUTCOMES

DEMONSTRATE ADEQUATE FLUID REPLACEMENT AND ELECTROLYTE BALANCE:

- ↓ HR, normal BP and normalizing blood glucose levels.
- Absence of ketones in blood and urine.
- Electrolytes within normal range.
- ABGs within normal range.
- Maintain O$_2$ Saturation of 90% or greater.
- Mental clarity, skin warm/dry.

Diagnostic Criteria

Life-threatening complication of Type 2

- Blood glucose > 600 mg/dL
- pH > 7.3
- Serum bicarbonate > 18 mEq/L
- Absent ketonuria
- Serum bicarbonate > 18 mEq/L
- Serum osmolality > 320 mOsm/kg H$_2$O

↑ Glucose → ↑ serum osmolality → osmotic diuresis. Inability to replace fluids lost through diuresis → profound dehydration & changes in LOC. Insufficient amount of insulin for ↑ serum glucose.

- High risk: older adults with type 2 diabetes & CV conditions.
- Triggers include infection (pneumonia & UTI). Other: stroke, MI, trauma, surgery, & illness.

- Initially, symptoms nonspecific – then malaise, blurred vision, polyuria, polydipsia, weight loss, ↑ weakness.
- Progressive dehydration → mental confusion, convulsions, & coma.
- Profound dehydration → wrinkles in tongue, ↓ salivation, ↓ CVP, ↑ HR, rapid respirations.
- Neurologic status is affected as glucose ↑, especially at levels > 1500 mg/dL. Without intervention, ↓ LOC & coma.

Distinguished from DKA

- Extremely ↑ serum glucose level.
- More profound dehydration than DKA.
- No ketosis.
- No Kussmaul respirations.

- ↓ Cardiac Output R/T alterations in preload.
- ↓ Fluid Volume R/T absolute loss.
- Anxiety R/T threat to biologic, psychologic, & social integrity.
- Disturbed Body Image R/T functional dependence on life-sustaining technology.
- Ineffective Coping R/T vulnerability.
- Powerlessness R/T lack of control.
- ↓ Knowledge R/T lack of previous exposure to info.

Slow Onset over Several Days

Clinical Manifestations

NURSING DIAGNOSES

FIG. 32.4 Concept Map for Hyperglycemic Hyperosmolar.

The sympathetic nervous system reacts to the body's stress response to try to restore homeostasis. Epinephrine, a potent stimulus for gluconeogenesis, is released, and additional glucose is added to the bloodstream. Unless the glycemic diuresis cycle is broken with aggressive fluid replacement and insulin administration, intracellular dehydration negatively affects fluid and oxygen transport to the brain cells. Neurological dysfunction and coma may result. Hemoconcentration increases the blood viscosity, which may result in clot formation; thromboemboli; and cerebral, cardiac, and pleural infarcts.

Assessment and Diagnosis
Clinical Manifestations

HHS has a slow, subtle onset and develops over several days. Initially, the symptoms may be nonspecific and may be ignored or attributed to the patient's concurrent disease processes. History reveals malaise, blurred vision, polyuria, polydipsia (depending on the patient's thirst sensation), weight loss, and increasing weakness. Progressive dehydration follows and leads to mental confusion, convulsions, and eventually coma, especially in older patients.

The physical examination may reveal a profound fluid deficit. Signs of severe dehydration include longitudinal wrinkles in the tongue, decreased salivation, and decreased central venous pressure (CVP), with increases in HR and rapid respirations (Kussmaul air hunger does not occur). In older patients, assessment of clinical signs of dehydration is challenging. Neurologic status is affected as the serum glucose increases, especially at levels greater than 1500 mg/dL. Without intervention, changes in level of conscious and coma occur.

Laboratory Studies

Laboratory studies are used to establish a definitive diagnosis of HHS. Plasma glucose levels are strikingly elevated (greater than 600 mg/dL). Serum osmolality is greater than 320 mOsm/kg. Acidosis is absent (arterial pH greater than 7.3), and the serum bicarbonate concentration is greater than 18 mEq/L. Ketonuria is absent or mild.[32] The patient may have an elevated hematocrit and depleted potassium and phosphorus levels.

Point of care fingerstick or arterial line testing of glucose at the bedside is the usual method for frequent monitoring of the serum blood glucose. Insulin replacement is prescribed according to the blood glucose result. Some electrolytes also can be tested at the bedside (potassium, sodium, ionized calcium), but usually an arterial line is required for frequent blood access. If point of care testing is unavailable, traditional serial laboratory tests keep the critical care team apprised of the fluctuating serum electrolyte levels and provide the basis for electrolyte replacement. Intracellular potassium and phosphate levels usually are depleted as a result of prior osmotic diuresis.[32]

Elevated blood urea nitrogen and creatinine levels suggest kidney impairment as a result of the severe reduction in renal circulation. Metabolic acidosis usually is absent at lower glucose levels. Acidosis may result from starvation ketosis or from an increase in lactic acid production caused by poor tissue perfusion.

Medical Management

The goals of medical management are rapid rehydration, insulin replacement, and correction of electrolyte abnormalities, specifically potassium replacement. The underlying stimulus of HHS must be discovered and treated. The same basic principles used to treat DKA are used for patients with HHS.

Rapid Rehydration

The primary intervention for HHS is rapid rehydration to restore the intravascular volume. The fluid deficit may 150 mL/kg of body weight. The average 150-lb adult can lose more than 7 to 10 L of fluid. Physiologic saline solution (0.9%) is infused at 1 L/h, especially for a patient in hypovolemic shock if there is no cardiovascular contraindication. Several liters of volume replacement may be required to achieve a BP and CVP within normal range. Infusion volumes are adjusted according to the patient's hydration state and sodium level.[32]

Serum sodium concentration is the parameter that is monitored to determine whether to change from isotonic (0.9%) to hypotonic (0.45%) saline. For example, patients with sodium levels equal to or less than 140 mEq/L may be given 0.9% normal saline solution, whereas patients with levels greater than 140 mEq/L are given 0.45% saline solution (see Fig. 32.3).[32] It is difficult to assess the serum sodium level in the presence of hemoconcentration. Another recommendation is to calculate a *corrected sodium value*. This involves adding 1.6 mEq to the sodium laboratory value for each 100 mg/dL plasma glucose above normal.[32] Sodium input should not exceed the amount required to replace the losses. Careful monitoring of the serum sodium level is recommended to avoid a sodium-water imbalance and hemolysis as the hemoconcentration is reduced.

To prevent hypoglycemia in HHS, when the serum glucose decreases to 300 mg/dL, the hydrating solution is changed to D_5W with 0.45% NaCl at 150 to 250 mL/h.[32]

Insulin Administration

Volume resuscitation lowers the serum glucose level and improves symptoms even without insulin administration. However, insulin replacement is recommended in the treatment of HHS because acidosis can develop if insulin is withheld, and insulin facilitates the cellular use of glucose.

Methods to lower the blood glucose level vary in HHS. One method is to administer an IV bolus of regular insulin (0.15 unit/kg of body weight) initially, followed by a continuous insulin drip. Regular insulin, infusing at an initial rate calculated as 0.1 unit/kg hourly (eg, 7 units/h for a person weighing 70 kg) should lower the plasma glucose concentration by 50 to 70 mg/dL during the first hour of treatment. If the measured glucose level does not decrease by this amount, the insulin infusion rate may be doubled until the blood glucose is declining at a rate of 50 to 70 mg/dL per hour.[32]

Insulin resistance. Type 2 diabetes in manifested not only by hyperglycemia but also by insulin resistance. HHS often develops secondary to an illness such as pneumonia or sepsis. In HHS, circulating counterregulatory hormones, also known as *stress hormones* (cortisol, glucagon, epinephrine), increase blood glucose. Patients with HHS often require high doses of insulin initially to overcome the hyperglycemia and insulin resistance. Hourly serial monitoring of the blood glucose level permits safe glycemic management and avoids the most common complication, which is hypoglycemia caused by overzealous insulin administration.[32] After the patient has recovered from the hyperglycemic crisis and insulin has been discontinued, oral medications designed to decrease insulin resistance are individualized to the patient with type 2 diabetes (see Tables 32.3 and 32.4).

Electrolyte Replacement

Increasing the circulating levels of insulin with therapeutic doses of IV insulin promotes the rapid return of potassium and phosphorus into the cell. Serial laboratory tests keep the clinician apprised of the serum electrolyte levels and provide the basis for electrolyte replacement. Potassium typically is added to the IV infusion (see Fig. 32.3). If the serum potassium concentration is lower than 3.3 mEq/L, it is essential to replenish the serum potassium before giving insulin.[32] Many hospitals have potassium replacement algorithms that are used to treat hypokalemia. Serum phosphate levels are carefully monitored, and phosphate is replaced if the level is lower than 1.0 mg/dL.[32]

Nursing Management

Nursing management of a patient with HHS incorporates a variety of nursing diagnoses (Box 32.11). Nursing management goals are similar to the goals outlined for DKA. The critical care nurse administers prescribed fluids, insulin, and electrolytes; monitors the response to therapy; maintains surveillance for complications; and provides patient education.

 BOX 32.11   NURSING DIAGNOSES

Hyperglycemic Hyperosmolar State

- Decreased Cardiac Output related to alterations in preload, p. 1015
- Deficient Fluid Volume related to absolute loss, p. 1019
- Anxiety related to threat to biologic, psychologic, and social integrity, p. 1012
- Deficient Knowledge related to previous lack of exposure to information, p. 1020 (see Box 32.13, Patient Education Plan for Hyperglycemic Hyperosmolar State)

Administering Fluids, Insulin, and Electrolytes

Rigorous fluid replacement and continuous IV insulin replacement must be controlled with an electronic volumetric pump. Accurate I&O measurements are maintained to monitor fluid balance including the total of all fluids administered minus hourly losses, such as urine output and emesis. If the patient is alert, the fluid and electrolytes are replenished orally and via a peripheral IV line. If the patient manifests signs of hypovolemic shock, hemodynamic monitoring may include use of an arterial line and CVP measurements. Arterial line access is very helpful in monitoring serial blood glucose and electrolyte values. The use of a blood conservation system on the arterial line is essential to avoid iatrogenic exsanguination of the patient. Most critical care units have developed protocols or guidelines to ensure that patients in hyperglycemic crisis are managed safely (see Fig. 32.3). The major responsibility for delivery of insulin, hourly monitoring of blood glucose, and infusion of appropriate crystalloid solutions lies with the critical care nurse (Box 32.12). Many hospitals mandate a double-check procedure for medications such as insulin that have the potential to cause harm if wrongly administered.

Monitoring Response to Therapy

BP and HR are monitored to evaluate the degree of dehydration, the effectiveness of hydration therapy, and the patient's fluid tolerance. Because patients with HHS have underlying type 2 diabetes and, if older, are also likely to have preexisting illnesses such as heart failure and kidney failure, it is important to monitor for symptoms of circulatory overload. Symptoms to anticipate include elevated CVP, tachycardia, bounding pulse, dyspnea, tachypnea, lung crackles, and engorged neck veins. The astute critical care nurse is aware of the clinical manifestations of fluid overload and observes for potential complications when rehydrating a patient with HHS and cardiac, pulmonary, or renal disease.

The serum glucose level should decrease by 50 to 70 mg/dL per hour with insulin administration.[32] This decrease is

---

BOX 32.12   Hyperglycemia Prevention and Management

Hyperglycemia Definition: Plasma blood glucose above 180 mg/dL.
- Two serial blood glucose values above 180 mg/dL are evidence of hyperglycemia in critical care.
- Blood glucose target in critical care is between 150-180 mg/dL.

Hyperglycemia Prevention
- In a patient with hyperglycemia, without a pre-existing history of diabetes, the likely causes are hyperglycemia associated with critical illness, or undiagnosed pre-diabetes.
- Type 1 diabetes: A preexisting diagnosis of type 1 diabetes means the patient can never be without insulin coverage. IV or SC insulin must always be provided and blood glucose checked frequently.
- Type 2 diabetes: A preexisting diagnosis of type 2 diabetes means the patient will have an elevated blood glucose when oral medications are stopped. Some patients with type 2 diabetes also have subcutaneous insulin. Hyperglycemia is prevented by use of subcutaneous or IV insulin.
- Use normal saline in IV infusions.
- Monitor blood glucose per hospital protocol.

Hyperglycemia: Clinical Signs and Symptoms
- Hyperglycemia with a history of Type 1 diabetes is generally caused by lack of insulin leading to DKA. Symptoms associated with alteration in level of consciousness range from confusion to coma, with dehydration, and ketoacidosis.
- Hyperglycemia with a history of Type 2 diabetes is often associated with infection leading to HHS, that may takes days to weeks to develop. HHS s associated with alteration in level of consciousness and extreme dehydration. Acidosis can develop in HHS when blood glucose levels are extremely high.

Hyperglycemia Management
- Identify the reason for the hyperglycemia (critical illness stress induced, DKA, HHS). Management varies according to the cause. It is essential to also treat the underlying medical /surgical cause of admission to critical care.
- Administer IV insulin according to hospital protocol. Hourly monitoring of blood glucose during the acute phase of hyperglycemia.
- Rehydrate according to hospital protocol and laboratory values
- Replenish electrolytes according to hospital protocol and laboratory values

Data from: Jacobi J, et al. Guidelines for the use of an insulin infusion for the management of hyperglycemia in critically ill patients. *Crit Care Med.* 2012;40(12):3251-3276.
Kitabchi AE, Umpierrez GE, Miles JM, Fisher JN. Hyperglycemic crises in adult patients with diabetes. *Diabetes Care.* 2009;32(7):1335.
DKA, Diabetic Ketoacidosis, *HHS,* Hyperglycemic, Hyperosmolar Syndrome. *IV,* intravenous; *SC,* subcutaneous.

monitored by hourly blood glucose determinations. Based on the result, the critical care nurse can alter the infusion of insulin according to hospital protocol (see Fig. 32.4).

Surveillance for Complications

The potential complications of HHS are similar to the complications described for DKA and include hypoglycemia, hypokalemia or hyperkalemia, and infection. A patient with HHS is at risk for other complications specific to associated disease entities. A history of cardiovascular, pulmonary, or kidney disease, whether known or latent, places the patient with HHS at high risk for complications.

Patient Education

As the patient's condition improves and the patient demonstrates readiness to learn, education about type 2 diabetes and avoiding a recurrence of HHS becomes a priority (Box 32.13). Most teaching occurs after the patient has left the critical care unit. Teaching topics include a description of type 2 diabetes and how it relates to HHS, dietary restrictions, exercise requirements, medication protocols, home testing of blood glucose, signs and symptoms of hyperglycemia and hypoglycemia, foot care, and lifestyle modifications.[24]

Collaborative Management

Because HHS is an acute condition superimposed on the chronic health problem of type 2 diabetes, many health professionals provide care and work collaboratively to restore homeostasis for each patient (Box 32.14).[34]

DIABETES INSIPIDUS

Diabetes insipidus (DI) is recognized by the vast quantities of very dilute urine that are produced in susceptible patients. In a critically ill patient, the extreme diuresis is most likely to be caused by a lack of ADH (vasopressin). Any patient who has sustained a head trauma or had resection of a pituitary tumor has an increased risk of developing DI. Normally, ADH is produced in the hypothalamus and stored in the posterior pituitary gland (see Chapter 30). Physiologically, ADH is released primarily in response to even small elevations in serum osmolality and secondarily in reaction to hypovolemia or hypotension. DI can occur if (1) the hypothalamus produces insufficient ADH, (2) the posterior pituitary fails to release ADH, or (3) the kidney nephron is resistant (unresponsive) to ADH.[35]

Etiology

DI is divided into three types according to cause: central, nephrogenic, and dipsogenic (Box 32.15). Only central DI, also known as neurogenic DI because of its association with the brain, is encountered with any frequency in the critical care unit.

✳ **BOX 32.13 PATIENT EDUCATION PLAN**

Hyperglycemic Hyperosmolar State

Acute Phase
- Explain rationale for critical care unit admission.

Predischarge
The patient should be able to teach back the following:
- Causes of hyperglycemic hyperosmotic state
- Self-care for diabetes
- Signs and symptoms to report to health care practitioner

QSEN **BOX 32.14 QSEN: Evidence-Based Practice**

Hyperglycemic Hyperosmolar State

A summary is provided of evidence and evidence-based recommendations for controlling symptoms related to hyperglycemic hyperosmolar state.

Strong Evidence to Support
Regular insulin by continuous infusion is recommended to normalize blood glucose.
Replace serum potassium if the level is less than 3.3 mEq/L.
Replace serum phosphate if the level is less than 1 mg/dL.
A multidisciplinary team approach reduces length of stay and improves clinical outcomes.
Close follow-up after discharge is recommended to maintain glycated hemoglobin (A_{1c}) at less than 6.5% and to prevent diabetes-related complications.

Weak Evidence to Support
Use of a sliding insulin scale alone does not represent best practice, because it is associated with both hyperglycemia and hypoglycemia in hospitalized patients.

Reference
Kitabchi AE, et al. Hyperglycemic crises in adult patients with diabetes: A consensus statement from the American Diabetes Association. *Diabetes Care*. 2009;32(7):1335.

BOX 32.15 Causes of Diabetes Insipidus

Central Diabetes Insipidus
Primary Diabetes Insipidus (Rare in Critical Care)
- Antidiuretic hormone (ADH) deficiency caused by hypothalamic-hypophyseal malformation
- Congenital defect
- Idiopathic

Secondary Diabetes Insipidus (Most Common in Critical Care)
- ADH deficiency caused by damage to hypothalamic-hypophyseal system
- Trauma
- Infection
- Surgery
- Primary neoplasms
- Metastatic malignancies

Nephrogenic Diabetes Insipidus
- Inability of kidney tubules to respond to circulating ADH
- Decrease or absence of ADH receptors
- Cellular damage to nephron, especially loop of Henle
- Kidney damage (eg, hydronephrosis, pyelonephritis, polycystic kidney)
- Untoward response to medication therapy (eg, lithium carbonate, demeclocycline)

Dipsogenic Diabetes Insipidus
- Rare form of water intoxication
- Compulsive water drinking

Central Diabetes Insipidus

In central DI, there is an inability to secrete an adequate amount of ADH (arginine vasopressin) in response to an osmotic or nonosmotic stimuli, resulting in inappropriately dilute urine. The synthesis of ADH is incomplete in the hypothalamus, or the release of ADH from the pituitary is interrupted. Central DI can be congenital or acquired.[36] In critical care, the most likely acute cause of central DI is neurosurgery, traumatic head injury, tumors, increased intracranial pressure (ICP), brain death, and infections such as encephalitis or meningitis. Among patients undergoing surgery on the pituitary gland, transient DI occurs in approximately 20% to 30%; permanent DI occurs in 2% to 10% of patients.[36] The degree of hormone replacement required after surgery depends on the quantity of pituitary tissue that has been surgically or endoscopically removed.

Nephrogenic Diabetes Insipidus

Nephrogenic DI is a rare congenital or an acquired disorder that occurs when the vasopressin V_2 receptors on the kidney tubule become nonresponsive to the action of ADH.[37] Some medications cause nephrogenic DI by decreasing the responsiveness of the kidney tubules to ADH. Long-term use of lithium carbonate, prescribed for bipolar disorder, was a frequent culprit in the past.[36]

Dipsogenic Diabetes Insipidus

Dipsogenic DI, also known as *primary polydipsia,* is a rare condition associated with compulsive drinking of more than 5 L of water of fluids daily.[35] Long-standing dipsogenic DI closely mimics nephrogenic DI because the kidney tubules become less responsive to ADH as a result of prolonged conditioning to hypotonic urine.[36,37]

Pathophysiology

The purpose of ADH is to maintain normal serum osmolality and circulating blood volume. Normally, ADH binds to the V_2 receptors on the kidney collecting tubules, causing insertion of water channels, known as *aquaporins,* along the luminal surface. Even small increases in plasma osmolality are sufficient to stimulate ADH release.[38,39] Although there are several types of DI, this discussion focuses on neurogenic (central) DI, the condition encountered in the critical care unit after neurosurgery or head injury (Fig. 32.5).

In DI, as free water is eliminated, the urine osmolality and specific gravity decrease (dilute urine). At the same time, in the bloodstream, the serum sodium concentration and serum osmolality increase. Normally, an increase in the serum osmolality to greater than 290 mOsm/kg H_2O (290 mmol/L) triggers synthesis and release of ADH. If the thirst mechanism is intact, thirst sensors are activated in the hypothalamus causing an acute sensation of thirst that leads the person to drink lots of fluids.[38,39] In central DI, no ADH is released, or the ADH released is insufficient. Without ADH, the kidney collecting tubules are incapable of concentrating urine and retaining water.

As extracellular dehydration ensues, hypotension and hypovolemic shock can occur. If the patient is alert, extreme thirst will lead the patient to replace lost fluids by drinking lots of water. This excessive intake of water reduces the serum osmolality to a more normal level and prevents dehydration. In a patient with decreased level of consciousness, the polyuria leads to severe hypernatremia, dehydration, decreased cerebral perfusion, seizures, loss of consciousness, and death.

Assessment and Diagnosis
Clinical Manifestations

The clinical diagnosis is based on the clinical increase in dilute urine output occurring in the absence of diuretics, a fluid challenge, or hyperglycemia. Central DI is anticipated in conditions in which the underlying disease process is likely to disrupt pituitary function. Central DI that occurs because of increasing ICP is life-threatening. It is imperative that the underlying condition that caused the elevation in ICP be recognized and treated quickly.

Laboratory Studies

The core diagnostic tests used to establish the presence of DI and that evaluate the body's ability to balance fluid and electrolytes are not specific to the endocrine system. The most common tests are serum sodium concentration, serum osmolality, and urine osmolality (Table 32.7). The combination of an obvious clinical picture with high volumes of hypotonic urine, in the presence of the following laboratory criteria, is sufficient to diagnose central DI.[36]
- Serum sodium level greater than 145 mEq/L
- Serum osmolality greater than 295 mOsm/kg H_2O (greater than 295 mmol/L)
- Urine osmolality less than 300 mOsm/kg H_2O (less than 200 mmol/L)
- Urine specific gravity less than 1.005

Serum sodium. The normal serum sodium concentration is 140 mEq/L (range, 135 to 145 mEq/L). In central DI, the serum sodium level can rise precipitously because of the loss of free water. Hypernatremia is usually associated with serum hyperosmolality.

Serum osmolality. Serum osmolality has a range of 275 to 295 mOsm/kg H_2O. Severe DI can increase serum osmolality to greater than 320 mOsm/kg H_2O. Normal values vary slightly between clinical laboratories (eg, 280 to 295 mOsm/ kg H_2O).[39]

Urine osmolality. Urine osmolality is less than 300 mOsm/ kg H_2O (300 mmol/L) in patients with central DI.[36] For greatest accuracy, the urine sample should be collected and tested simultaneously with the blood sample. This test is rarely performed in the critical care unit.

Measurement of antidiuretic hormone. Measurement of the baseline serum ADH level is an additional diagnostic step. This is not typically performed in critical care if the clinical circumstances (eg, head injury with increased ICP) make further testing unnecessary. Normal ADH levels range from 1 to 5 pg/mL. With normal hydration, the normal morning fasting serum level is less than 4 pg/mL. When serum ADH levels are severely depressed (less than 0.5 pg/mL), the osmolality in the urine falls (dilute urine) to less than 100 mOsm/kg H_2O and urine output dramatically increases to 800 to 1000 mL/h.[39]

Medical Management

Immediate management of DI requires an aggressive approach. Treatment goals include restoration of circulating fluid volume, pharmacologic ADH replacement, and treatment of the underlying condition.

COLLABORATIVE MANAGEMENT

Restore Hemodynamic Balance with Fluid Replacement

- Patients able to drink are given voluminous amounts of fluid PO.
- For those unable to drink, hypotonic IV solutions are infused and carefully monitored

Medications—ADH Replacement

- ADH replacement therapy with ADH (vasopressin) or desmopressin (DDAVP).
- DDAVP given IV, SC, or as nasal spray with dosage titrated to antidiuretic response.
- Closely monitor urine output.
- To avoid a medication error, be aware DDAVP is used to manage other conditions including hemorrhage caused by platelet disorders with different dosage ranges.

PRIORITY NURSING INTERVENTIONS

For Patient Unable to Regulate Fluid Needs and Losses

- Critical assessment and management of fluid.
- Rapid IV fluid replacement using a pump. Initially, hypotonic IV solution to replace fluids lost and ↓ serum hyperosmolality.
- Monitor for signs of cardiovascular impairment → fluid intake restricted until urine SG is < 1.015 & normal U/O resumes.
- Monitor HR, BP, CVP, and PAP for indication of response to fluid volume replacement.
- I&O, condition of buccal membranes, skin turgor, daily weights, presence of thirst, & temperature.
- Urinary catheter to monitor U/O.
- Simultaneous urine and blood specimens for determination of osmolality, serum sodium and serum potassium are obtained, and the results are relayed to the physician as necessary.
- Evaluation of response to therapy.
- Surveillance for complications.
- Provision of patient education.

DIABETES INSIPIDUS

Andy Bernalillo, suffered a traumatic brain injury, is admitted into the critical care unit with central diabetes insipidus losing a massive amount of urine.

Patients are unable to synthesize ADH

Results in

Circulatory Collapse

Priorities in Medical Management

- Immediate management requires an aggressive approach.
- Restore circulating fluid volume.
- Pharmacologic ADH replacement.
- Treatment of the underlying condition.

The patient will demonstrate cardiac output and fluid balance by:

- Hemodynamic status is stable - HR, BP, CVP, & PAP indicate adequate fluid status.
- Normal urine output resumes.
- No evidence of dehydration.
- Laboratory values return to normal range (serum sodium, serum osmolality, urine osmolality, & urine specific gravity.

Responding

Analysis

PATIENT OUTCOMES

PATHOPHYSIOLOGY - PITUITARY

Life - Threatening

- Most likely acute causes: neurosurgery, traumatic head injury, tumors, ↑ICP, brain death, encephalitis, or meningitis.
- As free water eliminated → urine osmolality & specific gravity ↓ (dilute urine) → serum sodium ↑ & osmolality ↑. With little or no ADH, kidneys incapable of concentrating urine & retaining water → extracellular dehydration ensues → hypotension and hypovolemic shock occur. In person with ↓ LOC polyuria → severe hypernatremia, dehydration, ↓ cerebral perfusion, seizures, loss of consciousness, & death can occur.

ASSESSMENT & DIAGNOSIS

Clinical Manifestations

- ↑ dilute urine output occurs in absence of diuretics, a fluid challenge, or hyperglycemia.
- Anticipated in conditions with underlying disease disrupting pituitary function.
- Central DI due to ↑ICP is life threatening - underlying condition must be recognized & treated quickly.

Diagnostic Laboratory Tests

The combination of clinical picture with high volumes of hypotonic urine, in the presence of:
- Serum sodium > 145 mEq/L.
- Serum osmolality > 295 mOsm/kg H_2O.
- Urine osmolality < 300 mOsm/kg H_2O.
- Urine specific gravity < 1.005.

Nursing Diagnoses

- ↓ Cardiac Output R/T alterations in preload.
- Deficient Fluid Volume R/T absolute fluid loss.
- Deficient Knowledge R/T lack of previous exposure to information.

FIG. 32.5 Concept Map for Diabetes Insipidus. *BP,* Blood pressure; *CVP,* central venous pressure; *DDAVP,* desmopressin acetate (synthetic analogue of vasopressin); *DI,* diabetes insipidus; *HR,* heart rate; *ICP,* intracranial pressure; *LOC,* level of consciousness; *PAP,* pulmonary artery pressure; *PO,* by mouth; *R/T,* related to; *U/O,* urine output; *SG,* Specific Gravity; *ADH,* Antidiuretic Hormone Concept maps created by © DEANNE A. BLACH, MSN, RN

TABLE 32.7 Laboratory Values for Patients With Diabetes Insipidus and Syndrome of Inappropriate Antidiuretic Hormone

Value	Normal	DI	SIADH
Serum ADH	1–5 pg/mL	Decreased in central DI	Elevated
Serum osmolality (mOsm/L)	275–295	>295	<270
Serum sodium (mEq/L)	135–145	>145	<120
Urine osmolality (mOsm/L)	300–1400	<300	Increased
Urine specific gravity	1.005–1.030	<1.005	>1.030
Urine output	1.0–1.5 L/day	1.0–1.5 L/h	Below normal

ADH, antidiuretic hormone; *DI,* diabetes insipidus; *SIADH,* syndrome of inappropriate antidiuretic hormone.

Volume Restoration

Fluid replacement is provided in the initial phase of treatment to prevent circulatory collapse. Patients who are able to drink are given voluminous amounts of fluid orally to balance output. For patients who are unable to take sufficient fluids orally, hypotonic IV solutions are infused and carefully monitored to restore the hemodynamic balance.

Medications

Central DI requires immediate pharmacologic management. Table 32.8 presents the medications most frequently prescribed to treat central DI and replace ADH.

Medications used for central diabetes insipidus. Patients with central DI who are unable to synthesize ADH require replacement with ADH (vasopressin) or an ADH analogue. The most commonly prescribed medication is the synthetic analogue of ADH, *desmopressin* (DDAVP). DDAVP can be given intravenously, subcutaneously, or as a nasal spray with dosage titrated according to the patient's antidiuretic response. Close monitoring of urine output is advised. To avoid a medication error, it is important to be aware that DDAVP is also used to manage other conditions including hemorrhage caused by platelet disorders and that the dose ranges for these conditions are different. Other medications to treat central DI are available (see Table 32.8) but are rarely used in critical care. DDAVP is used only for central DI. It has no therapeutic value in nephrogenic or dipsogenic DI.

Medications used for nephrogenic diabetes insipidus. Nephrogenic DI is not a diagnosis typically encountered in critical care unless the patient is admitted with this condition in addition to the primary diagnosis. The mainstay of therapy for nephrogenic DI is to stop any medications that are inducing the ADH resistance. Nephrogenic DI is treated with thiazide diuretics.[37]

Nursing Management

Nursing management of a patient with DI incorporates a variety of nursing diagnoses (Box 32.16). Nursing management is directed toward administration of prescribed fluids and medications, evaluation of response to therapy, surveillance for complications, and provision of patient education.

Administration of Fluids

Rapid IV fluid replacement requires the use of a volumetric pump. Initially, a hypotonic IV solution is used to replace fluids lost and reduce the serum hyperosmolality. With any signs of cardiovascular impairment, fluid intake is restricted until urine specific gravity is less than 1.015 and a normal urine output resumes.

Critical assessment and management of fluid status are the most important initial concerns for patients with DI.

Monitoring of HR, BP, CVP, and pulmonary artery pressures (if a pulmonary artery catheter is in place) provides early indications of response to fluid volume replacement. I&O measurement, condition of buccal membranes, skin turgor, daily weight measurements, presence of thirst, and temperature provide a basic assessment list that is vital for the patient who is unable to regulate fluid needs and losses. Placement of a urinary catheter is essential to monitor the urinary output accurately. Simultaneous urine and blood specimens for determination of osmolality, serum sodium, and serum potassium are obtained, and the results are relayed to the physician as necessary. A patient who is unable to satisfy sensations of thirst or to complete any task or self-care activity without the need to urinate may be confused and frightened. For patients who are able to verbalize their fears, having a caring nurse who is interested and nonjudgmental helps to reduce the emotional turmoil associated with their condition.

Administration of Medications

DDAVP by nasal administration is the usual replacement for ADH in critical care. The urine output is recorded hourly to evaluate the response to the medication.

Surveillance for Complications

The most dangerous potential complication of ADH replacement is hypertension and vasospasm of cardiac, cerebral, or mesenteric arterial vessels in response to ADH replacement. In most cases, DDAVP is selected for ADH replacement to minimize this risk. A less serious complication of DI is constipation due to fluid loss; it is treated with dietary fiber, stool softeners, or both.

Patient Education

Educating the patient and the family about the disease process and how it affects thirst, urination, and fluid balance encourages patients to participate in their care and reduces the feelings of hopelessness (Box 32.17). For most critical care patients, central DI is a temporary condition that resolves as the underlying medical condition (eg, brain injury) improves. Patients who are discharged with DI are taught, along with their families, the signs and symptoms of dehydration and overhydration and procedures for accurate daily weight and urine specific gravity measurements. Printed information pertaining to medication actions, side effects, dosages, and timetable is provided as well as an outline of factors that must be reported to the physician.

Collaborative Management

Central DI is a life-threatening condition. The collaborative assessment and clinical skills of all health care professionals and

TABLE 32.8 Pharmacologic Management

Diabetes Insipidus

Medication	Dosage	Actions	Special Considerations
Central Diabetes Insipidus			
DDAVP (available as IV injection, as nasal spray, Rhinal Tube, Rhinyle Drops, Stimate)	Nasal: 10–40 mcg before bed or in divided doses	Central DI	Few side effects.
	Parenteral[a]: 2–4 mcg twice daily	Antidiuretic	Observe for nasal congestion, upper respiratory infection, allergic rhinitis.
		Increases water resorption in nephron	Monitor intake and output, urine osmolality, serum sodium level.
		Prevents and controls polydipsia, polyuria	
Vasopressin (Pitressin)	IV, IM, subcutaneous	Central DI antidiuretic	Monitor fluid volume often, especially in older patients.
	Topical: nasal mucosa	Promotes resorption of water at kidney tubule	Assess cardiac status.
		Decreases urine output	May precipitate angina, hypertension, or myocardial infarction if increased dosage is given to patient with cardiac history.
		Increases urine osmolality	Parenteral extravasation can cause skin necrosis
		Diagnostic aid	
		Increases gastrointestinal peristalsis	
Lypressin (Diapid)	Intranasal: 1–2 sprays (7–14 mcg) in each nostril 4 times daily	Central DI	Proper instillation is important for absorption and action.
		Synthetic ADH	Patient sits upright while holding bottle upright for administration.
		Increases resorption of sodium and water in nephron	Repeat sprays (>2–3) are ineffective and wasteful; if dosage is increased to 2–3 sprays, shorten time between dosing.
			Cough, chest tightness, shortness of breath
Nephrogenic Diabetes Insipidus			
Thiazide diuretics	Varies according to diuretic chosen, patient's size, and age	Nephrogenic DI	Varies according to diuretic chosen.
		Leads to mild fluid depletion	
		Increases resorption of water and sodium in proximal nephron; less fluid travels to distal nephron, excreting less water	
Dipsogenic Diabetes Insipidus			
Anticompulsive disorder medications, anxiolytics, psychopharmacologic agents	Dosage varies	Dipsogenic DI	Varies according to medication chosen.

ADH, antidiuretic hormone; *DDAVP*, desmopressin acetate; *DI*, diabetes insipidus; *IM*, intramuscular; *IV*, intravenous.
[a]IV or subcutaneous administration.

◎ BOX 32.16 NURSING DIAGNOSES

Diabetes Insipidus

- Decreased Cardiac Output related to alterations in preload, p. 1015
- Deficient Fluid Volume related to absolute loss, p. 1019
- Deficient Knowledge related to lack of previous exposure to information, p. 1020 (see Box 32.17, Patient Education Plan for Diabetes Insipidus)

use of a clear plan of care are essential to achieve optimal outcomes for each patient.

SYNDROME OF INAPPROPRIATE SECRETION OF ANTIDIURETIC HORMONE

The opposing syndrome to DI is the *syndrome of inappropriate secretion of antidiuretic hormone* (SIADH), which manifests as a dilutional hyponatremia.[39] A patient with SIADH has an excess of ADH secreted into the bloodstream, more than the amount needed to maintain normal blood volume and serum osmolality. Excessive water is resorbed at the kidney tubule, leading to dilutional hyponatremia.[39]

BOX 32.17 **PATIENT EDUCATION PLAN**

Diabetes Insipidus

Acute Phase
- Explain rationale for critical care unit admission.

Predischarge
- Assess knowledge base
- Measurement of fluid intake and output
- Urine specific gravity
- Causes of diabetes insipidus
- Disease process of diabetes insipidus
- Nutritional information to prevent constipation and diarrhea
- Medications: Explain purpose, side effects, dosage, and how often to use
- Signs and symptoms to report to health care professional

Etiology

Numerous causes of SIADH are observed in patients who are critically ill (Box 32.18). CNS injury, tumors, and diseases that interfere with the normal functioning of the hypothalamic-pituitary system can cause SIADH. A common cause is malignant bronchogenic small cell carcinoma.[39] This type of malignant cell is capable of synthesizing and releasing ADH regardless of the body's needs. With much less frequency, other cancers that involve the brain, head and neck, gastrointestinal system, gynecologic system, and hematologic system are capable of autonomous production of ADH.

Pathophysiology

ADH is a powerful, complex polypeptide compound. When released into the circulation by the posterior pituitary gland, ADH regulates water and electrolyte balance in the body. In SIADH, profound fluid and electrolyte disturbances result from the unsolicited, continuous release of the hormone into the bloodstream (Fig. 32.6). Excessive ADH stimulates the kidney

---

BOX 32.18 **Causes of Syndrome of Inappropriate Secretion of Antidiuretic Hormone**

Malignant Disease Associated With Autonomous Production of Antidiuretic Hormone
- Bronchogenic small cell carcinoma
- Pancreatic adenocarcinoma
- Duodenal, bladder, ureter, and prostatic carcinomas
- Lymphosarcoma, Ewing sarcoma
- Acute leukemia, Hodgkin disease
- Cerebral neoplasm, thymoma

Central Nervous System Diseases That Interfere With Hypothalamic-Hypophyseal System and Increase Production or Release of Antidiuretic Hormone
- Head injury
- Brain abscess
- Hydrocephalus
- Pituitary adenoma
- Subdural hematoma
- Subarachnoid hemorrhage
- Cerebral atrophy
- Guillain-Barré syndrome

Neurogenic Stimuli Capable of Increasing Antidiuretic Hormone
- Decreased glomerular filtration rate
- Physical or emotional stress
- Pain
- Fear
- Trauma
- Surgery
- Myocardial infarction
- Acute infection
- Hypotension
- Hemorrhage
- Hypovolemia

Pulmonary Diseases Believed to Stimulate Baroreceptors and Increase Antidiuretic Hormone
- Pulmonary tuberculosis
- Viral and bacterial pneumonia
- Empyema

- Lung abscess
- Chronic obstructive lung disease
- Status asthmaticus
- Cystic fibrosis

Endocrine Disturbances That Hormonally Influence Antidiuretic Hormone
- Myxedema
- Hypothyroidism
- Hypopituitarism
- Adrenal insufficiency—Addison disease

Medications That Mimic, Increase Release of, or Potentiate Antidiuretic Hormone
- Hypoglycemics
  - Insulin
  - Tolbutamide
  - Chlorpropamide
- Potassium-depleting thiazide diuretics
- Tricyclic antidepressants
  - Imipramine
  - Amitriptyline
- Phenothiazine
  - Fluphenazine
  - Thioridazine
- Thioxanthenes
  - Thiothixene
  - Chlorprothixene
- Chemotherapeutic agents
  - Vincristine
  - Cyclophosphamide
- Opiates
- Carbamazepine
- Clofibrate
- Acetaminophen
- Nicotine
- Oxytocin
- Vasopressin
- Anesthetics

PATHOPHYSIOLOGY

The Opposing Syndrome to Diabetes Insipidus

- Presents as a dilutional hyponatremia.
- Excess ADH secreted into the bloodstream.
- Excessive water resorbed at the kidney tubule, → dilutional hyponatremia.
- Because minimal sodium is present in this fluid, edema usually does not result.
- Without ADH and aldosterone, water is retained, → U/O, ↑ sodium excreted in urine.
- ↑ urine osmolality → ↓ water excretion.
- Malignant bronchogenic small cell carcinoma causes production and release of ADH regardless of the body's needs.

Jerry Kitz is admitted to the critical care unit with SIADH secondary to malignant bronchogenic small cell carcinoma.

SIADH
Syndrome of Inappropriate Secretion of Antidiuretic Hormone

Results in

Dilutional Hyponatremia
↑ Blood Volume
↓ Serum Osmolality

ASSESSMENT & DIAGNOSIS

Clinical Manifestations

- Early clinical manifestations of dilutional hyponatremia include lethargy, anorexia, & N/V.
- Edema usually not present, slight weight gain from ↑ fluid.
- Severe neurologic symptoms usually occur when serum sodium < 120 mEq/L.
- S/S of severe hyponatremia → inability to concentrate, mental confusion, apprehension, seizures, ↓ LOC, coma, & death.

Early recognition of neurologic or hemodynamic deterioration

Laboratory Values

- ↓ Plasma osmolality
- ↑ Urine osmolality
- ↓ Serum sodium
- ↑ Urine sodium
- Measurement of serum ADH levels not recommended for diagnosis.

NURSING DIAGNOSES

- ↓ Cardiac Output R/T alterations in preload.
- ↓ Fluid Volume R/T absolute loss.
- Anxiety R/T threat to biologic, psychologic, & social integrity.
- ↓ Knowledge R/T previous lack of exposure to information.

MEDICATIONS TO CORRECT SIADH

When Water Restriction is Ineffective - Medications

- Indicated for SIADH secondary to a small cell lung carcinoma, the vasopressin receptor antagonists "vaptans" will ↑ water excretion while conserving sodium (aquadiuresis).
- Administer IV infusion of Conivaptan (Vaprisol) or Tolvaptan (Samsca) administered orally.
- Monitor serum sodium levels carefully.
- Monitor for hypotension.
- Astute clinical judgment warranted when using these medications.

NURSING INTERVENTIONS

Patient & Family Health Education

- Show sensitivity to family's fears by using words indicating empathy.
- Teach about SIADH & its effect on water balance, & reasons for fluid restrictions.
- Provide time for the patient & family to ask questions & express their concerns.

Frequent Assessment of Patient's Hydration Status

- Fluids restricted to 500 - 1000 mL per day.
- Slow infusion of 3% saline to replenish sodium without adding extra volume.
- Slowly ↑ serum sodium (10 mEq/L in 24 hrs).
- Evaluate sodium at least every 4 hours during acute phase of sodium replacement.
- Extreme caution is warranted when infusing hypertonic saline solution.
- Calculation of hourly sodium amount and over 24 hours.
- Serial measurements of urine output, serum sodium levels, & serum osmolality.
- Frequent mouth care.
- Daily weight.

GOALS OF MEDICAL MANAGEMENT

RESTORE FLUID AND SODIUM BALANCE

The patient will demonstrate adequate fluid and sodium balance by

Nursing Care Includes

PATIENT OUTCOMES

- Hemodynamic values within normal (CO, BP, HR, CVP, PAP, PAOP)
- Sodium within normal range
- Maintain O₂ Saturation of 90% or greater
- Mental clarity, skin warm/dry
- Urine output ~ 60 mL/hr.
- RR within normal, clear breath sounds

FIG. 32.6 Concept Map for Syndrome of Inappropriate Secretion of Antidiuretic Hormone. *BP,* Blood pressure; *CO,* cardiac output; *CVP,* central venous pressure; *HR,* heart rate; *LOC,* level of consciousness; *N/V,* nausea and vomiting; *O₂,* oxygen; *PAP,* pulmonary artery pressure; *PCWP,* pulmonary capillary wedge pressure; *R/T,* related to; *RR,* respiratory rate; *SIADH,* Syndrome of inappropriate secretion of antidiuretic hormone; *S/S,* signs and symptoms; *U/O,* urine output; Concept maps created by © DEANNE A. BLACH, MSN, RN tubules to retain fluid regardless of need. This results in severe overhydration.

Excessive ADH dramatically alters the sodium balance in the extracellular vascular compartment. The overhydration causes a dilutional hyponatremia and reduces the sodium concentration to critically low levels. In a healthy adult, hyponatremia inhibits the release of ADH. However, in SIADH, increased levels of circulating ADH are unrelated to the serum sodium concentration. Aldosterone production from the adrenal glands is also suppressed. Serum hypo-osmolality leads to a shift of fluid from the extracellular fluid space into the intracellular fluid compartment (inside the cells) in an attempt to equalize osmotic pressure. Because minimal sodium is present in this fluid, edema usually does not result. Without ADH and aldosterone, water is retained, urine output is diminished, and further sodium is excreted in the urine. The urine has an increased osmolality from the decreased water excretion. Urinary concentration is also elevated by excess sodium in the urine. It is believed that, despite the serum hyponatremia, the increased release of ADH promotes sodium loss through the kidneys into the urine.

Assessment and Diagnosis
Clinical Manifestations
The clinical manifestations of SIADH relate to the excess fluids in the extracellular compartment and the proportionate dilution of the circulating sodium. Edema usually is not present, although slight weight gain may occur from the expanded extracellular fluid volume. Early clinical manifestations of dilutional hyponatremia include lethargy, anorexia, nausea, and vomiting. Severe neurologic symptoms usually do not develop until the serum sodium concentration decreases to less than 120 mEq/L. Progressively deteriorating neurologic signs of hyponatremia then predominate, and the patient is admitted to the critical care unit. Symptoms of severe hyponatremia include inability to concentrate, mental confusion, apprehension, seizures, decreased level of consciousness, coma, and death.

Laboratory Values
Patients with SIADH present with very dilute serum, hyponatremia, and concentrated urine. Laboratory values confirm this clinical picture. In SIADH, there is decreased plasma osmolality (less than 275 mOsm/kg H_2O)[40] with increased urine osmolality (greater than 100 mOsm/kg H_2O).[40,41] The low serum sodium (less than 125 mEq/L) is associated with increasingly severe neurologic symptoms. The urine sodium concentration is elevated (greater than 40 mEq/L), congruent with the concentrated urine output of SIADH.[41] Use of diuretics negates the reliability of the urine sodium and urine osmolality levels.[41] See Table 32.7 for the typical laboratory values associated with SIADH and with DI. Measurement of serum ADH levels is not recommended for the diagnosis of SIADH.[40]

Medical Management
In the critical care unit, SIADH often occurs as a secondary disease. Ideally, recognition and treatment of the primary disease will reduce the production of ADH. If the patient is receiving any of the medications suspected to cause SIADH, discontinuing that medication may return ADH levels to normal. Some medications that alter ADH levels are listed in Box 32.18. The goals of medical management are to restore fluid and sodium balance.

Fluid Restriction
Fluid restriction is a cornerstone of the treatment plan for SIADH.[40] Fluids are restricted to 500 to 1000 mL/day.[38]

Sodium Replacement
Patients with severe hyponatremia (less than 125 mEq/L serum sodium) experience severe neurologic symptoms including seizures. Too-rapid serum sodium correction must be avoided to reduce the risk of *osmotic demyelination,* which occurs in the white matter of the brain. Severe neurologic damage or death can result. The demyelination complication can be avoided by increasing the serum sodium slowly, by 8 mEq/L in 24 hours.[40] Serum sodium levels must be evaluated at least every 4 hours during the acute phase of sodium replacement. The serum sodium should not be increased more than 10 mEq/L in 24 hours.[40]

In SIADH, a slow infusion of 3% saline (hypertonic saline) may be used to replenish the serum sodium without adding extra volume.[40] Hypertonic saline solution (3% or greater) can be dangerous if administered too quickly, as described earlier. Calculation of the quantity of sodium that will be administered each hour and over 24 hours is advised.

Medications
Medications are prescribed when water restriction is ineffective in correcting the SIADH. One pharmacologic option is to increase the action of ADH on the V_2 kidney tubule receptors so that more water is excreted.[38,39] This class of medications (described subsequently) is known as vaptans.

Vasopressin receptor antagonists. Vasopressin receptor antagonists are used to treat euvolemic hyponatremia such as SIADH. Medications in this class are also called *vaptans.* Conivaptan (Vaprisol) is approved for use only in hospitalized patients. These medications excrete water while conserving sodium, known as *aquadiuresis.* There is an initial 20-mg IV loading dose over 30 minutes, followed by a 20 mg/day continuous infusion for up to 4 days.[42] If the sodium correction is inadequate, the infusion dose can be increased to 40 mg/day.[42] Conivaptan is a nonselective vasopressin receptor antagonist, which means that it blocks V_1 receptors in the vasculature and V_2 receptors in the kidney. The patient must be observed carefully to avoid hypotension (caused by V_1 receptor blockade). Hypovolemia is a contraindication. Tolvaptan (Samsca) is an oral medication in the same class. This medication may be initiated in the hospital, where serum sodium levels can be monitored to avoid a too-rapid increase in serum sodium after aquadiuresis.

European guidelines for treatment of hyponatremia[40] do not include vaptans for management of SIADH. This omission has caused some controversy and highlighted different ways in which SIADH is managed in different countries.[38] It has also highlighted the importance of clinical judgment when using these medications. It is important to identify if the hyponatremia is transient, related to a medical condition such as pneumonia (vaptans not required), or related to SIADH secondary to a small cell carcinoma in the lung that secretes ADH (vaptans helpful).[38]

Nursing Management
Nursing management of a patient with SIADH incorporates a variety of nursing diagnoses (Box 32.19). Nursing management is directed toward restriction of fluids, surveillance for complications, and provision of patient education.

BOX 32.19 NURSING DIAGNOSES

Syndrome of Inappropriate Secretion of Antidiuretic Hormone

- Deficient Fluid Volume related to decreased secretion of antidiuretic hormone, p. 1019
- Anxiety related to threat to biologic, psychologic, or social integrity, p. 1012

BOX 32.20 PATIENT EDUCATION PLAN

Syndrome of Inappropriate Secretion of Antidiuretic Hormone

Acute Phase
- Explain reasons for admission to the critical care unit.
- Explain reasons for neurologic changes in inappropriate secretion of antidiuretic hormone (SIADH).

Predischarge
The patient should be able to teach back the following:
- Patient-specific cause of SIADH
- How to measure intake and output
- How to measure urine specific gravity (if indicated)
- Signs and symptoms to report to health care professional

Restriction of Fluids

Thorough, astute nursing assessments are required for care of a patient with SIADH while an attempt is made to correct the fluid and sodium imbalance; the systemic effects of hyponatremia occur rapidly and can be lethal. Fluids are restricted to between 500 and 100 mL/day.[39] Accurate measurement of I&O is required. Frequent assessment of the patient's hydration status is accomplished with serial measurements of urine output, serum sodium levels, and serum osmolality. Frequent mouth care (moistening of the buccal membrane) may give comfort during the period of fluid restriction. The patient is weighed daily to gauge fluid retention or loss. Weight gain signifies continual fluid retention, whereas weight loss indicates loss of body fluid.

Patient Education

Rapidly occurring changes in the patient's neurologic status may worry visiting family members. Sensitivity to the family's fears can be shown by words that express empathy and by providing time for the patient and family to ask questions and express their concerns. Patient and family education about SIADH, its effect on water balance, and the reasons for fluid restrictions should be done using the teach back method (Box 32.20).

Collaborative Management

SIADH is a complex condition that requires clinical judgment and a team approach to manage the fluid and electrolyte disruption.[38-40] Effective clinical management requires the skills of many health care professionals working as a team, with goals that are clearly communicated to all team members.

BOX 32.21 Conditions Associated With Hyperthyroidism

- Iodine-induced hyperthyroidism (eg, related to amiodarone therapy)
- Excessive pituitary production of thyroid-stimulating hormone or trophoblastic disease
- Excessive ingestion of thyroid hormone
- Toxic diffuse goiter (Graves disease)
- Toxic adenoma
- Toxic multinodular goiter (Plummer disease)
- Painful subacute thyroiditis
- Silent thyroiditis, including lymphocytic and postpartum variations

THYROID STORM

Description

Thyroid storm always occurs as a complication of preexisting hyperthyroidism.[43] Hyperthyroidism, also called *thyrotoxicosis*, occurs when the thyroid gland produces thyroid hormone in excess of the body's need.[44] The primary cause of hyperthyroidism is *Graves disease*, an autoimmune condition that affects 3% of women and 0.5% of men in the United States.[44] Graves disease is caused by circulating immunoglobulin G antibodies that attack the thyroid-stimulating hormone (TSH) receptor cells on the gland causing release of thyroid hormone unrelated to the normal physiologic feedback mechanisms. The hypothalamus-pituitary-thyroid axis feedback loop is illustrated in Fig. 30.6 in Chapter 30). The antidysrhythmic medication amiodarone causes thyroid dysfunction in 10% to 20% of patients treated with amiodarone.[45,46] Conditions associated with hyperthyroidism are described in Box 32.21.

Thyroid storm, also called *thyroid crisis*, is a rare and life-threatening exacerbation of hyperthyroidism. The pathophysiology underlying the transition from hyperthyroidism to thyroid storm is not fully understood, as thyroid hormone levels are not necessarily different from patients with hyperthyroidism. Activation of the sympathetic nervous system and enhanced sensitivity to the effects of thyroid hormone are apparent. Stopping antithyroid medications and major stressors such as infection, surgery, trauma, pregnancy, or critical illness can precipitate thyroid storm in any patient with preexisting hyperthyroidism. Mortality from thyroid storm is 10%.[47]

Etiology

In thyroid storm, excessive endogenous thyroid hormone increases metabolic activity and stimulates the beta-adrenergic receptors resulting in a heightened sympathetic nervous system response. There is hyperactivity of cardiac tissue, nervous tissue, and smooth muscle tissue and tremendous heat production with an elevated temperature. The biochemical stimulus that precipitates the transition of hyperthyroidism into thyroid storm is unknown.[47] Typically, an added external stressor such as surgery, pregnancy, or infection precipitates thyroid storm.[47]

Pathophysiology

Thyroid hormone increases cellular oxygen consumption in almost all metabolically active cells. Excess metabolism generates heat and critically high fever. Cellular oxygen demands are dramatically increased with increased cardiac output to meet tissue demands. The oxygen demands in the hypermetabolic state are so great that the cardiac system cannot compensate adequately. Hypertension and tachycardia follow.

Gastrointestinal peristalsis increases, resulting in diarrhea, nausea, and vomiting. These symptoms all lead to dehydration and compound the problem of malnutrition and weight loss. Muscular weakness occurs and is compounded by the excessive protein breakdown. Metabolic acidosis is a potential problem.

Hypersensitivity to the increased adrenergic-binding sites potentiates the cardiovascular and nervous system responses to the hypermetabolic state. Atrial fibrillation is a common dysrhythmia in patients with hyperthyroidism, and tachydysrhythmias should be anticipated in thyroid storm, especially in patients with underlying heart disease.[47,48] Pulmonary edema and acute heart failure also can occur. Increased beta-adrenergic activity manifests as emotional lability, fine muscular tremors, agitation, and delirium. Clinical manifestations of thyroid storm are listed in Box 32.22.

Assessment and Diagnosis

The clinical presentation of thyroid storm is characterized by various organ systems, as follows:

1. Thermoregulation: Fever
2. Heart: Atrial fibrillation, supraventricular tachycardia, acute heart failure
3. CNS: Agitation, restlessness, delirium
4. Gastrointestinal: Nausea, vomiting, diarrhea, unexplained jaundice, stupor, coma

Early manifestations may be insidious or missed, creating a paradoxically abrupt presentation of apparently unrelated signs and symptoms. Use of a preestablished thyroid storm scoring system is one method to systematically diagnose thyroid storm (Table 32.9).[43] A score greater than 45 is indicative of thyroid storm.

Laboratory findings are used to confirm the suspicion raised by the clinical signs. The TSH value is extremely low and thyroid hormones (triiodothyronine [T_3] and thyroxine [T_4]) are high compared with normal values (see Table 31.4 in Chapter 31 for normal reference values). These results, in combination with the clinical picture, provide the diagnosis.

No laboratory test is available to differentiate thyroid storm from its predecessor, thyrotoxicosis, for which the laboratory values may be similar. Thyroid storm is identified by a combination of the patient's medical history and exacerbation of clinical manifestations.

Medical Management

The goal of acute medical management of thyroid storm is to reduce the clinical effects of thyroid hormone as rapidly as possible. This includes preventing cardiac decompensation, reducing hyperthermia, and reversing dehydration caused by fever or gastrointestinal losses. In severe cases, *therapeutic plasmaphoresis* (plasma exchange) is used to rapidly reduce circulating thyroid hormone levels.[47]

Prevent Cardiovascular Collapse

The body's heightened sensitivity to the increased adrenergic and catecholamine receptors must be suppressed. Atrial dysrhythmias need to be controlled, and progression of heart failure must be halted. Beta-blockers are the mainstay of therapy for cardiac protection.[43]

BOX 32.22 Clinical Manifestations of Thyroid Storm

Cardiovascular System
Prompted by Increased Affinity of Beta-Adrenergic Receptors in Heart
- Tachycardia
- Systolic murmur
- Increased stroke volume
- Increased cardiac output
- Increased systolic blood pressure (BP)
- Decreased diastolic BP
- Extra systoles
- Paroxysmal atrial tachycardia
- Premature ventricular contraction
- Palpitations
- Chest pain
- Increased cardiac contractility
- Acute heart failure
- Pulmonary edema
- Cardiogenic shock

Central Nervous System
Resulting From Increased Catecholamine Response
- Hyperkinesis
- Nervousness
- Muscle weakness
- Confusion
- Convulsions
- Heat intolerance
- Fine tremor
- Emotional lability
- Frank psychosis
- Apathy
- Stupor
- Diaphoresis

Gastrointestinal System
- Nausea
- Vomiting
- Diarrhea
- Liver enlargement
- Abdominal pain
- Weight loss
- Increased appetite

Integumentary System
- Pruritus
- Hyperpigmentation of skin
- Fine, straight hair
- Alopecia

Thermoregulatory System
- Hyperthermia
- Heat dissipation
- Diaphoresis

Serum or Urine
- Hypercalcemia
- Hyperglycemia
- Hypoalbuminemia
- Hypoprothrombinemia
- Hypocholesterolemia
- Creatinuria

TABLE 32.9 Thyroid Storm Diagnostic Criteria

Criteria	Points
Thermoregulatory Dysfunction	
Temperature (°F)	
99.0–99.9	5
100.0–100.9	10
101.0–101.9	15
102.0–102.9	20
103.0–103.9	25
≥104.0	30
Cardiovascular	
Tachycardia (beats/min)	
100–109	5
110–119	10
120–129	15
130–139	20
≥140	25
Atrial fibrillation	
Absent	0
Present	10
Acute heart failure	
Absent	0
Mild	5
Moderate	10
Severe	20
Gastrointestinal-Hepatic Dysfunction	
Manifestation	
Absent	0
Moderate (diarrhea, abdominal pain, nausea/vomiting)	10
Severe (jaundice)	20
Central Nervous System Disturbance	
Manifestation	
Absent	0
Mild (agitation)	10
Moderate (delirium, psychosis, extreme lethargy)	20
Severe (seizure, coma)	30
Precipitant History	
Status	
Positive	0
Negative	10
Scores Totaled	
>45 Thyroid storm	
25–44 Impending storm	
<25 Storm unlikely	

Modified from Burch and Wartofsky. Life-threatening thyrotoxicosis: thyroid storm. *Endocrinol Metal Clin North Am.* 1993;22:263. In Bahn RS, et al. Hyperthyroidism and other causes of thyrotoxicosis: management guidelines of the American Thyroid Association and American Association of Clinical Endocrinologists. *Endocr Pract.* 2011;17(3):456.

Reduce Hyperthermia

Reduction in body temperature is achieved by use of a cooling blanket and the antipyretic agent acetaminophen.[43] Salicylates (aspirin) are contraindicated because they inhibit protein binding of T_3 to T_4, increasing the level of free, metabolically active thyroid hormone.[47]

Reverse Dehydration

Vigorous fluid replacement must be instituted to treat or prevent dehydration. Antibiotic therapy may be warranted in the presence of systemic infection. Dehydration is treated with large volumes of glucose and isotonic sodium solutions to replace circulating fluid and sodium losses from hypermetabolism.

Pharmacologic Management

Pharmacologic treatment is essential in treatment of thyroid storm.[43] A multimodal medication approach is recommended with monitoring in a critical care unit during the acute phase.[43] Beta-blockers are administered to decrease the peripheral cellular sensitivity to catecholamines, and antithyroid medications are administered to block the synthesis and release of thyroid hormone into the circulation and to inhibit peripheral conversion of T_4 to T_3. Medications used to treat thyroid storm are listed in Table 32.10.

Medications That Block Catecholamine Effect

Beta-adrenergic blocking agents are used to decrease the catecholamine effects of excessive thyroid hormone. Propranolol is the most frequently used medication (see Table 32.10). Beta-blockers have no effect on thyroid hormone but reduce the exaggerated myocardial stimulation and slow the atrioventricular conduction rate. Therapeutic doses vary from patient to patient, but higher doses are typically required for effective control of symptoms. Esmolol, a short-acting IV beta-blocker, may also be used.[43] Nondihydropyridine calcium channel blockers may be effective in controlling HR in patients for whom beta-blockers are contraindicated.[43]

Medications That Block Thyroid Synthesis

The synthesis of new thyroid hormone is blocked by the administration of antithyroid medications. Two agents are frequently used: propylthiouracil (PTU) and methimazole (see Table 32.10).[43] These medications are administered by mouth or via a feeding tube. PTU is especially therapeutic because it blocks thyroid synthesis and blocks conversion of T_4 to T_3. Methimazole has a slower rate of action but is more potent than PTU. Both medications act within 1 to 2 hours after absorption from the gastrointestinal tract. These medications have no impact on previously released thyroid hormone.

Medications That Block Release of Thyroid Hormone

Administration of inorganic iodine blocks the release of any preformed thyroxine that is already in the thyroid gland but not yet released.[43] It is essential that iodine therapy not be administered until adequate inhibition of new hormone synthesis has occurred, as described in Table 32.10.[43] The iodide preparations are rapid acting and have a short duration. They are given approximately 1 hour after administration of the antithyroid medications (described in the previous section) to prevent the iodide from being used for thyroid hormone production and possible worsening of the clinical state.

Some patients with thyroid storm have concomitant adrenal insufficiency and may be prescribed hydrocortisone or dexamethasone during the initial stages of thyroid storm management. See Table 32.10 for a list of the most commonly used medications and their nursing implications for a patient with thyroid storm.

TABLE 32.10 Pharmacologic Management

Thyroid Storm

Medication	Dosage	Actions	Special Considerations
Antithyroid Medications			
Propylthiouracil	Loading dose: 500–1000 mg	Blocks synthesis of thyroid hormone	May cause rash, nausea, vomiting, agranulocytosis, skin hyperpigmentation.
	Maintenance dosage: 250 mg every 4 h	Blocks conversion of T_3 to T_4	Administer with meals to reduce GI effects.
Methimazole	60–80 mg/day	Blocks new hormone synthesis	Monitor signs listed for propylthiouracil. May cause rash, agranulocytosis.
Iodine (saturated solution of potassium iodide)	5 drops (0.25 mL or 250 mg) orally every 6 h	Blocks new hormone synthesis	Do not start until 1 h after antithyroid medications have been administered.
Hydrocortisone	Loading dose: 300 mg IV Maintenance dosage: 100 mg every 8 h	May block conversion of T_4 to T_3	Prophylaxis against adrenal insufficiency. Dexamethasone is alternative medication.
Beta-Blockers			
Propranolol	60–80 mg every 4 h orally. IV initial for rapid effect, 0.5 to 1 mg IV with continuous cardiac monitoring; subsequent doses of 2 to 3 mg IV over 15 minutes, repeated every several hours until effects from oral administration are observed.	Beta-adrenergic blockade	Monitor HR and BP response to beta-blockade.
Esmolol	50–100 mcg/kg/min IV pump	Beta-adrenergic blockade	Monitor HR and BP response to beta-blockade in critical care unit.

BP, blood pressure; *GI*, gastrointestinal; *HR*, heart rate; *IV*, intravenous/intravenously; T_3, triiodothyronine; T_4, thyroxine.
Based on data from Bahn RS, et al. Hyperthyroidism and other causes of thyrotoxicosis: Management guidelines of the American Thyroid Association and American Association of Clinical Endocrinologists. *Endocr Pract.* 2011;17(3):456.

BOX 32.23 NURSING DIAGNOSES

Thyroid Storm

- Hyperthermia related to increased metabolic rate, p. 1026
- Imbalanced Nutrition: Less Than Body Requirements related to lack of exogenous nutrients and increased metabolic demand, p. 1029
- Decreased Cardiac Output related to alterations in heart rate or rhythm, p. 1016
- Anxiety related to threat to biologic, psychologic, and social integrity, p. 1012
- Disturbed Sleep Pattern related to fragmented sleep, p. 1023
- Deficient Knowledge related to lack of previous exposure to information, p. 1020 (see Box 32.24, Patient Education Plan for Thyroid Storm)

Nursing Management

Nursing management of a patient with thyroid storm incorporates a variety of nursing diagnoses (Box 32.23). Nursing interventions are directed toward safe administration and monitoring of the effects of prescribed medications, normalizing body temperature, rehydration with correction of other metabolic derangements, and provision of patient education.

Medication Administration

The timely and ordered sequence of medication administration is essential in the management of thyroid storm (see previous sections on "Pharmacologic Management"). The patient in thyroid storm is agitated, anxious, and unable to rest and benefits from a calm environment. The effects of the antithyroid medications, iodides, and beta-adrenergic blocking agents gradually decrease the neurologic symptoms related to catecholamine sensitivity. HR should decrease with beta-blockade.

The patient and family need to be reassured that this extreme agitation is the result of the disease process and that the medications will help control the nonstop fidgeting and tremors. Frequent reassurance and clear, simple explanations of the patient's condition help decrease the fear brought on by the onset of thyroid storm.

Normalize Body Temperature

In thyroid storm, the patient has hyperthermia related to a hypermetabolic state, as evidenced by a critically high body temperature; diaphoresis; hot, flushed skin; intolerance to heat; tachycardia; and tachypnea. Temperature is assessed frequently until normal body temperature is attained. Nursing measures to provide comfort while the patient is intolerant to heat include a room with a cool environment and a fan to circulate air and comfortable, nonrestrictive bedclothes. A tepid sponge bath helps to reduce heat by evaporation, and cold-pack applications to the groin and axilla increase heat loss at major blood vessels. If antipyretic medications are required, acetaminophen is the agent of choice, and salicylates are avoided.[47]

Rehydration and Correction of Metabolic Derangements

Hyperthermia, tachypnea, diaphoresis, vomiting, and diarrhea predispose the patient to a fluid volume deficit. Fluids and electrolytes are as vigorously replaced as the decompensated cardiovascular system can tolerate. Glucose solutions are given to replace glycogen stores, which are depleted. Insulin is administered to treat the hyperglycemia that results from mobilization of nutrients and glucocorticoids. Hyponatremia from active loss (eg, vomiting) is monitored by means of laboratory serum values. Hyponatremia can be prevented or

BOX 32.24 PATIENT EDUCATION PLAN

Thyroid Storm

Acute Phase
- Explain reasons for critical care unit admission.
- Explain reasons for extreme hypermetabolism.

Predischarge

The patient should be able to teach back the following:
- Patient-specific cause of thyrotoxic crisis
- Medications: Purpose, dosage, how often to use, and side effects
- Signs and symptoms to report to health care professional

treated with isotonic IV fluid replacement. Additional nursing measures focus on frequent hydration assessments (see Box 32.6).

Patient Education

During the critical events surrounding the thyroid storm, the patient and family are given information according to their emotional state and cognitive level of understanding. The cause of the high fever, anxiety, and cardiac dysrhythmias is explained in understandable terms (Box 32.24). The patient and family often are relieved to know that the agitation and nervousness result from circulating hormones that may be decreased by taking daily medications.

Side effects of the specific medication therapy are taught before discharge. Patients treated with beta-blockers are taught to report signs of bradycardia, unexplained fatigue, and orthostatic hypotension, among other untoward effects. Patients discharged with antithyroid medications are alerted to the potential side effect of agranulocytosis (see Table 32.10). Symptoms of *agranulocytosis* include sudden cough, fever, rash, and inflammation. For management or elevated temperature, patients are instructed to use acetaminophen rather than salicylates because salicylates increase the amount of free thyroid hormone in circulation.

Collaborative Management

Management of patients with thyroid storm is derived from the 2011 guidelines issued by the American Thyroid Association and American Association of Clinical Endocrinologists.[43] A patient with thyroid storm requires interventions by many health care professionals, with clearly communicated goals to facilitate rapid recovery.

MYXEDEMA COMA

Description

A severe deficiency of thyroid hormone produces hypothyroidism.[49] There is a spectrum of hypothyroidism, as defined by laboratory tests and clinical symptoms, that ranges from mild to severe. Mild hypothyroidism has subtle symptoms and is treated in the outpatient setting. Severe hypothyroidism is associated with respiratory depression, cardiogenic shock, hypothermia, and coma and is often fatal.[50] Mortality is reported as 25% to 60%.[51,52] The term *myxedema coma* is traditionally used for severe hypothyroidism, although many patients present with decreased levels of consciousness, not necessarily in coma.[50]

Etiology

Myxedema coma is a rare condition, and a high index of suspicion is required to correctly recognize the signs and symptoms. A person may be admitted with myxedema coma after a prolonged period of unrecognized or poorly controlled hypothyroidism.[53] The precipitating event is generally an infection, severe sepsis or other acute illness such as a stroke or acute myocardial infarction, or a reaction to certain medications.[53] For example, the antidysrhythmic medication amiodarone can cause both hyperthyroidism and hypothyroidism.[52]

The following features have been proposed as hallmarks of myxedema coma: Precipitating illness; altered mental status; hypothermia; bradycardia; and abnormal thyroid blood levels,[51] specifically increased TSH and low free T_4 and low free T_3.[51] See Table 31.4 in Chapter 31 for normal values of TSH, FT_3, and FT_4. The TSH level may be higher than 30 mU/L in myxedema coma.[51]

Hypothyroidism affects all body cells and organs and slows the metabolic rate in every system. Hypothyroidism can be caused by damage to the thyroid gland (primary) or can be secondary to pituitary or hypothalamic dysfunction.[54]

Pathophysiology

The effects of hypothyroidism are widespread and varied. When the basal metabolic rate of oxygen consumption is reduced, cells are unable to maintain the processes necessary to sustain life. Without thyroid hormone, protein synthesis is severely curtailed, and amino acid production and repair of tissues are halted. Metabolism of carbohydrate and fat is incomplete, and gluconeogenesis cannot supply additional sources of glucose. Lipolysis is ineffective, and cholesterol collects in the bloodstream. Hypothermia occurs. All systems are affected.

Skin

The composition of the skin changes as deposits of *hyaluronic acid* (a gel-like substance capable of holding large amounts of fluid) accumulate in the interstitial spaces, giving rise to a full appearance of face, hands, and feet. The skin has an overall yellowish appearance resulting from increased carotene deposits. The nails and hair are thin and brittle. Absence of thyroid hormone also leads to decreased or absent sweat production. The hyaluronic acid deposits are evident in heart muscle; skeletal muscles; and muscles of the tongue, pharynx, and proximal esophagus. These striated muscular changes of the tongue, pharynx, and esophagus probably contribute to the hoarse, husky voice and lack of facial expression in patients with hypothyroidism.

Cardiopulmonary System

Interstitial edema impairs cardiac myocytes, resulting in bradycardia and low cardiac output.[51] Serous fluid accumulation in the pericardial sac can cause cardiac tamponade.[55] A decreased sensitivity to catecholamines is present even though serum catecholamine levels are elevated. Resting HR and stroke volume are reduced. The force of myocardial contraction is weakened. There is a decrease in systolic BP and an increase in diastolic BP, causing a narrowed pulse pressure. Electrocardiogram (ECG) typically reveals low-voltage QRS complexes and low-voltage, flattened, or inverted T waves and prolonged Q–T interval.[55]

Pulmonary System

Pleural effusions and muscular changes affect gas exchange. The basal rate of oxygen consumption decreases, with a resulting insensitivity to CO_2. Hypoventilation increases the CO_2 serum content, which increases cerebral hypoxia. Hypoxic and hypercapnic ventilatory drives are severely impaired. Respiratory acidosis can occur. Pleural effusion, reduced vital capacity, and shallow respirations occur with any exertion. Respiratory muscle weakness, sleep apnea, and upper airway obstruction may be present.

Patients with myxedema are in a high-risk category for any surgical procedure or critical care admission because of their limited ventilatory capacity. Respiratory failure and requirement for mechanical ventilation is often the reason for admission to the critical care unit.

Kidneys and Fluid and Electrolyte Balance

Blood flow to the kidney is reduced, and the glomerular filtration rate, urine specific gravity, and urine osmolality are decreased. Elimination of medications by the kidneys is severely slowed in hypothyroidism. Coexisting adrenal insufficiency should also be considered.

Nutrition and Elimination

Decreased gastric motility or ileus is an expected complication for a patient with severe hypothyroidism. Food utilization and nutrient mobilization decrease with insufficient thyroid hormone. Intestinal hypomotility occurs, and serum cholesterol increases. Abdominal distention, decreased intestinal peristalsis, and eventual paralytic ileus lead to extreme constipation. These findings make the provision of enteral nutrition a challenge. In more alert patients, a lack of appetite and inability to eat coexist.

Thermoregulation

Heat production decreases as a result of insufficient energy to maintain the base metabolic rate within the cells. The ability to maintain body heat is further restricted by hypoglycemia. Hypothermia occurs.

Anemia

Anemia is present in many patients with hypothyroidism. Symptoms of fatigue and depression are associated. Erythropoiesis (red blood cell production) is impaired. Coagulation abnormalities may coexist.[55]

Assessment and Diagnosis

The diagnosis of myxedema coma is based on the clinical manifestations of end-stage hypothyroidism. Severe hyperthyroidism (thyroid storm) and severe hypothyroidism (myxedema) are compared in Box 32.25.

Clinical Presentation

The diagnosis of end-stage hypothyroidism is based on the clinical presentation. Increasing signs of somnolence, depression, and diminished mental acuity signal diminished cellular function. Interstitial edema collects in almost all tissues. Organs become infiltrated with the mucoid-rich mucopolysaccharides, compromising organ function. Patients present with cardiovascular collapse, hypothermia, decreased kidney function, fluid excess, hypoventilation, and severe metabolic disorders.

Weight gain is attributed to the collection of mucopolysaccharides in the interstitium, the increase in fluid

---

BOX 32.25 Clinical Manifestations of Hyperthyroidism Compared With Hypothyroidism

Hyperthyroidism (Thyrotoxicosis, Thyroid Storm)	Hypothyroidism (Myxedema, Myxedema Coma)
Elevated T_4, T_3	Decreased T_4, T_3
Decreased TSH	Elevated TSH
Hypercalcemia	Hyponatremia
Hyperglycemia	Hypoglycemia
Metabolic acidosis	Respiratory acidosis, metabolic acidosis
Tachycardia, palpitations, atrial fibrillation	Hypercholesterolemia
Angina	Anemia
ST segment wave changes	Bradycardia
Shortened Q–T interval	Peripheral vasoconstriction
Hypertension	Flattened, inverted T waves
AV block, acute heart failure	Prolonged Q–T and P–R intervals
Hypovolemia	Decreased stroke volume, decreased cardiac output
Shortness of breath, tachypnea	Enlarged heart, pericardial effusion
Hypermetabolism	Increased total body fluid with decreased effective arterial blood volume
Polyphagia	
Weight loss	
Nausea, vomiting, increased peristalsis	Hypoventilation, possible CO_2 retention
Tremor	Depressed metabolism
Extreme restlessness, insomnia, uneasiness, anxiety	Decreased lipolysis, increased cholesterol
Emotional instability, despondency	Weight gain
Diaphoresis	Constipation
Heat intolerance	Seizures
Increased DTRs	Slowness, depression
Muscle weakness or muscle wasting	Impaired short-term memory
Oligomenorrhea	Slow, deliberate speech
	Thickened tongue
	Coarse, dry, scaly, edematous skin
	Hypothermia
	Delirium (myxedema madness)
	Lethargy → stupor → coma (myxedema coma)
	Diminished DTRs
	Paresthesia of hands
	Menorrhagia

AV, atrioventricular; *CO_2*, carbon dioxide; *DTRs*, deep tendon reflexes; *T_3*, triiodothyronine; *T_4*, thyroxine; *TSH*, thyroid-stimulating hormone.

---

retention, and the decrease in metabolism. Paresthesias of hands and feet are caused by hyaluronic acid accumulation in the synovial sacs, which leads to compression of nerves and carpal tunnel syndrome. Compression of nerves interferes with the simplest hand grasp and the ability to raise one's hands. Reflexes contract briskly but take extended seconds to relax.

Hypothermia is a very distressing symptom. Most cases of myxedema are diagnosed in the winter months. A myxedematous patient has hypotension, reduced total blood volume, decreased cardiac output, and bradycardia—all related to a decrease in beta-adrenergic stimulation. Neuropsychiatric symptoms of depression and decreased mental acuity may occur.

BOX 32.26 NURSING DIAGNOSES

Myxedema Coma

- Hypothermia related to decreased metabolic rate, p. 1028
- Impaired Spontaneous Ventilation related to respiratory muscle fatigue or metabolic factors, p. 1031
- Activity Intolerance related to prolonged immobility or deconditioning, p. 1006
- Disturbed Body Image related to functional dependence on life-sustaining technology, p. 1022
- Deficient Knowledge related to lack of previous exposure to information, p. 1020 (see Box 32.27, Patient Education Plan for Myxedema Coma)

Laboratory Studies

Laboratory test results do not differentiate between hypothyroidism and myxedema coma. The blood test results simply confirm the clinical picture. TSH is the first test to order if hypothyroidism is suspected.[50] Typically, patients with myxedema have primary hypothyroidism with a high TSH level and a low T_4 level.[55] If the TSH level is normal or low, other nonthyroid causes must be investigated. TSH is released by the pituitary gland; see Table 31.4 in Chapter 31 for normal reference values. Endocrine studies to evaluate pituitary function should be undertaken.

Medical Management

The patient's primary admitting diagnosis may mask an underlying hypothyroidism. However, clinical manifestations can trigger the alert clinician to suspect a hypofunctioning thyroid. The primary disease condition and the myxedema coma must be treated immediately to improve the patient's chances for recovery. Myxedema coma often necessitates ventilator support, correction of fluid and electrolyte imbalance, correction of other multisystem abnormalities, corticosteroid supplementation, and thyroid hormone replacement.[50]

Pharmacologic Management

Thyroid hormone replacement including type and dosage to treat end-stage hypothyroidism (myxedema coma) is controversial.[56] One method is to replete T_4 levels with an initial dose of levothyroxine (300 to 400 mcg administered intravenously) to saturate the previously empty T_4 binding sites, followed by daily administration of 50 to 100 mcg of levothyroxine.[50]

A serum cortisol level is obtained to evaluate adrenal gland function. Glucocorticoids may be necessary to assist the patient to respond to the stress state of hypothyroidism until a coexisting adrenal insufficiency is ruled out.[56]

Nursing Management

Nursing care of a patient with myxedema coma focuses on management of the precipitating disease and on the severe impact of hypothyroidism on multiple organ systems. Nursing diagnoses associated with management of myxedema coma are listed in Box 32.26.

Pulmonary Care

A patient with myxedema coma who is admitted to the critical care unit may require intubation and mechanical ventilatory support. Individuals who are not intubated are monitored for development of respiratory failure. Arterial blood gas measurements are evaluated to monitor for CO_2 retention and respiratory acidosis.

Cardiac Concerns

Dysrhythmias are common in patients with myxedema and can quickly be identified by continuous ECG monitoring. Expected signs of myxedema, such as flattened or inverted T waves or prolonged Q–T and P–R intervals, resolve in a positive response to thyroxine replacement therapy.

Thermoregulation

Hypothermia gradually improves as the patient is treated with thyroid hormone. Several warm blankets comfortably wrapped around a patient with mild hypothermia may be sufficient to help raise the body temperature to normal. Active warming devices are also used. Continuous assessments are important to avoid too-rapid heating and vasodilation. Electronic devices that can measure accurately at the extreme lower range of body temperatures are used.

Thyroid Replacement Therapy

Older patients and patients with a cardiac history receive IV thyroid hormone replacement with due precautions. Thyroxine can precipitate angina and dysrhythmias. Improvements in the patient's cardiopulmonary and neurologic status, together with changes in T_4 and TSH laboratory values, are used to gauge the success of thyroid hormone replacement therapy.

Skin Care

Patients with myxedema coma have rough, dry skin. Measures are taken to avoid skin breakdown related to decreased circulation and widespread edema. An emollient for skin hydration follows nonsoap baths. Frequent repositioning minimizes pressure against capillary beds over bony prominences.

Elimination

Constipation is managed on a daily basis to avoid impaction. Use of fiber-enriched enteral nutrition may be helpful in an alert patient. Fluids are encouraged as the hypovolemia is corrected and BP stabilizes. Increased fiber is preferable to use of enemas.

Patient Education

Patients with myxedema coma have decreased comprehension and mental acuity. All instructions, procedures, and activities are explained slowly and provided in written form. The patient and family members may experience myriad emotions with one constant—fear of the unknown. Before any teaching, the nurse evaluates the family's ability to accept the patient's slowed thinking and slowed response time.

All instructions given to the patient or family are given verbally and in writing. A written copy of all schedules is given as a reference for home care before discharge. The nurse discusses the medication schedule and the frequency of the medication doses with the patient and family. Side effects of each medication are described. The patient and family need to know the side effects of medications including over-the-counter medications so that they can manage the medications at home. Also, the nurse discusses which signs and symptoms to report to the health care provider (Box 32.27).

Collaborative Management

There are no published guidelines that discuss acute collaborative care management of patients with myxedema coma. Collaborative management is required to decrease mortality in myxedema coma. Early recognition of symptoms and a willingness to request laboratory tests to confirm the diagnosis allow therapy to be instituted as early as possible.

✳ BOX 32.27   PATIENT EDUCATION PLAN
Myxedema Coma

Acute Phase
- Explain reasons for critical care unit admission.
- Explain reasons for extreme hypermetabolism.

Predischarge
The patient should be able to teach back the following:
- Patient-specific cause of thyrotoxic crisis
- Medications: Purpose, dosage, how often to use, and side effects
- Signs and symptoms to report to health care professional

▮ S U M M A R Y

CASE STUDY 32.1   Patient With an Endocrine Disorder

Brief Patient History

Ms. S is a 72-year-old woman with a history of hypertension treated with an angiotensin-converting enzyme inhibitor and thiazide diuretics. She has a past 100-pack/year history of tobacco abuse but quit smoking 2 years ago. She lives independently in a senior apartment. She was brought to the hospital by friends because of a fall. Ms. S states that she has a severe headache but cannot recall whether she hit her head during the fall. She is also having difficulty recalling recent events.

Clinical Assessment

Ms. S is admitted to the critical care unit from the emergency department because of nonspecific electrocardiogram (ECG) changes suggestive of inferior wall ischemia and electrolyte abnormalities. She is awake; alert; and oriented to person, time, and place; she is unable to recall the events leading to her hospitalization. She states that her headache is severe and feels like someone is hitting her head with a hammer. Her skin is warm and dry. Her gait is visibly unsteady.

Diagnostic Procedures

Ms. S's vital signs include the following: blood pressure of 180/92 mm Hg, heart rate of 100 beats/min (sinus rhythm), respiratory rate of 24 breaths/min, and temperature of 98.8°F.

Ms. S reports that her headache is a 10 on the Pain Rating Scale. Laboratory findings include the following: sodium level of 116 mmol/L, potassium level of 3.3 mmol/L, chloride level of 88 mmol/L, carbon dioxide level of 22 mEq/L, magnesium level of 1.8 mg/dL, urinary sodium level of 30 mmol/L, and urine osmolality value of 118 mOsm/L. The test result for troponin I on admission is negative. ECG testing shows a normal sinus rhythm; T wave inversion in leads II, III, and AVF; and a change from prior ECG findings suggestive of inferior wall ischemia. Chest radiography identifies a mass in the right upper lobe that strongly suggests a neoplasm.

Medical Diagnosis

Ms. S is diagnosed with syndrome of inappropriate diuretic hormone.

Questions
1. What major outcomes do you expect to achieve for this patient?
2. What problems or risks must be managed to achieve these outcomes?
3. What interventions must be initiated to monitor, prevent, manage, or eliminate the problems and risks identified?
4. What interventions should be initiated to promote optimal functioning, safety, and well-being of the patient?
5. What possible learning needs do you anticipate for this patient?
6. What cultural and age-related factors may have a bearing on the patient's plan of care?

Stress of Critical Illness
- The endocrine system is complex, and assessment relies heavily on laboratory tests for confirmation of disease processes. To fully participate in the care of patients with these complex conditions, the critical care nurse must be aware of the intricacies of the endocrine system.
- Physiologic stress associated with critical illness causes increased secretion of stress hormones by the HPA pathway, resulting in secretion of cortisol, stimulation of the sympathetic nervous system, and release of norepinephrine and epinephrine to mobilize glucose. If critical illness is prolonged beyond 7 to 10 days, profound suppression of pituitary, thyroid, and adrenal gland function occurs.

Pancreas: Diabetic Ketoacidosis and Hyperglycemic Hyperosmolar State
- Diagnostic criteria for DKA include blood glucose concentration greater than 250 mg/dL, arterial pH value less than 7.3, serum bicarbonate level less than 18 mEq/L, and moderate or severe ketonemia or ketonuria.
- Diagnostic criteria for HHS include blood glucose concentration greater than 600 mg/dL, arterial pH value higher than 7.3, serum bicarbonate level greater than 18 mEq/L, serum osmolality greater than 320 mOsm/kg H_2O (320 mmol/kg H_2O), and absent or mild ketonuria.

Pituitary: Diabetes Insipidus and Syndrome of Inappropriate Secretion of Antidiuretic Hormone
- Central DI occurs when ADH (vasopressin) is not released from the posterior pituitary gland. The excretion of large quantities of hypotonic urine creates the following alterations in serum and urinary laboratory values: serum sodium greater than 145 mEq/L, serum osmolality greater than 295 mOsm/kg H_2O (295 mmol/L), urine osmolality less than 200 mOsm/kg H_2O (200 mmol/L), and urine specific gravity less than 1.005.
- SIADH occurs when excess ADH (vasopressin) is released from the posterior pituitary gland. This stimulates the kidney tubules to retain water, resulting in fluid overload and hyponatremia manifested by the following alterations in serum and urinary laboratory values: decreased plasma osmolality (less than 275 mOsm/kg H_2O) with increased urine osmolality (greater than 100 mOsm/kg H_2O), low serum sodium (less than 125 mEq/L), and elevated urinary sodium (greater than 40 mEq/L).

Thyroid: Thyroid Storm and Myxedema Coma
- Thyroid storm is identified by clinical signs such as high fever, tachycardia, hypertension, and tremor as evidence of the rapid metabolic rate. Laboratory values are similar to values seen in hyperthyroidism: low TSH and high T_4 levels.
- Myxedema coma is characterized by a precipitating illness, hypothermia, hypoventilation, bradycardia, decreased mental acuity, high TSH, and low T_4 levels.

ⓔ Visit the Evolve site for additional study materials.

REFERENCES

1. Jacobi J, et al. Guidelines for the use of an insulin infusion for the management of hyperglycemia in critically ill patients. *Crit Care Med.* 2012;40(12):3251.
2. Gibbison B, Angelini GD, Lightman SL. Dynamic output and control of the hypothalamic-pituitary-adrenal axis in critical illness and major surgery. *Br J Anaesth.* 2013;111(3):347.

3. Boonen E, Bornstein SR, Van den Berghe G. New insights into the controversy of adrenal function during critical illness. *Lancet Diabetes Endocrinol.* 2015;3(10):805.

4. Bornstein SR, et al. Diagnosis and Treatment of Primary Adrenal Insufficiency: an Endocrine Society Clinical Practice Guideline. *J Clin Endocrinol Metab.* 2016;101(2):364.

5. Nieman LK, et al. The diagnosis of Cushing's syndrome: an Endocrine Society Clinical Practice Guideline. *J Clin Endocrinol Metab.* 2008;93(5):1526.

6. Nieman LK, et al. Treatment of Cushing's Syndrome: an Endocrine Society Clinical Practice Guideline. *J Clin Endocrinol Metab.* 2015;100(8):2807.

7. Raff H, Sharma ST, Nieman LK. Physiological basis for the etiology, diagnosis, and treatment of adrenal disorders: cushing's syndrome, adrenal insufficiency, and congenital adrenal hyperplasia. *Compr Physiol.* 2014;4(2):739.

8. Harp JB, Yancopoulos GD, Gromada J. Glucagon Orchestrates Stress-induced Hyperglycemia. *Diabetes Obes Metab.* 2016;18(7):648.

9. Moghissi ES, et al. American Association of Clinical Endocrinologists and American Diabetes Association consensus statement on inpatient glycemic control. *Diabetes Care.* 2009;32(6):1119.

10. Honiden S, Inzucchi SE. Metabolic Management during Critical Illness: Glycemic Control in the ICU. *Semin Respir Crit Care Med.* 2015;36(6):859.

11. Clain J, Ramar K, Surani SR. Glucose control in critical care. *World J Diabetes.* 2015;6(9):1082.

12. NICE-SUGAR Study Investigators, et al. Intensive versus conventional glucose control in critically ill patients. *N Engl J Med.* 2009;360(13):1283.

13. Inoue S, Egi M, Kotani J, Morita K. Accuracy of blood-glucose measurements using glucose meters and arterial blood gas analyzers in critically ill adult patients: systematic review. *Crit Care.* 2013;17(2):R48.

14. Klonoff DC. Point-of-Care Blood Glucose Meter Accuracy in the Hospital Setting. *Diabetes Spectr.* 2014;27(3):174.

15. Dombrowski NC, Karounos DG. Pathophysiology and management strategies for hyperglycemia for patients with acute illness during and following a hospital stay. *Metabolism.* 2013;62(3):326.

16. Frier BM. Hypoglycaemia in diabetes mellitus: epidemiology and clinical implications. *Nat Rev Endocrinol.* 2014;10(12):711.

17. American Diabetes Association. Diabetes Care in the Hospital. *Diabetes Care.* 2016;39(Suppl 1):S99.

18. Casaer MP, Van den Berghe G. Nutrition in the acute phase of critical illness. *N Engl J Med.* 2014;370(13):1227.

19. Rodriguez A, et al. Best Practices for Interdisciplinary Care Management by Hospital Glycemic Teams: Results of a Society of Hospital Medicine Survey Among 19 U.S. Hospitals. *Diabetes Spectr.* 2014;27(3):197.

20. Handelsman Y, et al. American association of clinical endocrinologists and american college of endocrinology - clinical practice guidelines for developing a diabetes mellitus comprehensive care plan - 2015. *Endocr Pract.* 2015;21(Suppl 1):1–87.

21. American Diabetes Association. Classification and Diagnosis of Diabetes. *Diabetes Care.* 2016;39(Suppl 1):S13.

22. Nathan DM. Diabetes: Advances in Diagnosis and Treatment. *JAMA.* 2015;314(10):1052.

23. Fox CS, et al. Update on Prevention of Cardiovascular Disease in Adults With Type 2 Diabetes Mellitus in Light of Recent Evidence: a Scientific Statement From the American Heart Association and the American Diabetes Association. *Diabetes Care.* 2015;38(9):1777.

24. Inzucchi SE, et al. Management of hyperglycemia in type 2 diabetes, 2015: a patient-centered approach: update to a position statement of the American Diabetes Association and the European Association for the Study of Diabetes. *Diabetes Care.* 2015;38(1):140.

25. American Diabetes Association. Approaches to Glycemic Treatment. *Diabetes Care.* 2016;39(Suppl 1):S52.

26. Ahmadian M, et al. PPARγ signaling and metabolism: the good, the bad and the future. *Nat Med.* 2013;19(5):557.

27. Soccio RE, Chen ER, Lazar MA. Thiazolidinediones and the promise of insulin sensitization in type 2 diabetes. *Cell Metab.* 2014;20(4):573.

28. Campbell JE, Drucker DJ. Pharmacology, physiology, and mechanisms of incretin hormone action. *Cell Metab.* 2013;17(6):819.

29. Scheen AJ. Pharmacodynamics, efficacy and safety of sodium-glucose co-transporter type 2 (SGLT2) inhibitors for the treatment of type 2 diabetes mellitus. *Drugs.* 2015;75(1):33.

30. Whalen K, Miller S, Onge ES. The Role of Sodium-Glucose Co-Transporter 2 Inhibitors in the Treatment of Type 2 Diabetes. *Clin Ther.* 2015;37(6):1150.

31. Lipska KJ, Krumholz H, Soones T, Lee SJ. Polypharmacy in the Aging Patient: a Review of Glycemic Control in Older Adults With Type 2 Diabetes. *JAMA.* 2016;315(10):1034.

32. Kitabchi AE, Umpierrez GE, Miles JM, Fisher JN. Hyperglycemic crises in adult patients with diabetes. *Diabetes Care.* 2009;32(7):1335.

33. Gosmanov AR, Gosmanova EO, Dillard-Cannon E. Management of adult diabetic ketoacidosis. *Diabetes Metab Syndr Obes.* 2014;7:255.

34. Garber AJ, et al. Consensus Statement by the American Association of Clinical Endocrinologists and American College of Endocrinology on the Comprehensive Type 2 Diabetes Management Algorithm - 2016 Executive Summary. *Endocr Pract.* 2016;22(1):84.

35. Ball S. Diabetes insipidus. *Medicine.* 2013;41(9):519.

36. Fenske W, Allolio B. Current state and future perspectives in the diagnosis of diabetes insipidus: a clinical review. *Journal Clin Endocrinol Metab.* 2012;97(10):3426.

37. Bockenhauer D, Bichet DG. Pathophysiology, diagnosis and management of nephrogenic diabetes insipidus. *Nat Rev Nephrol.* 2015;11(10):576.

38. Verbalis JG, Grossman A, Hoybye C, Runkle I. Review and analysis of differing regulatory indications and expert panel guidelines for the treatment of hyponatremia. *Curr Med Res Opin.* 2014;30(7):1201.

39. Verbalis JG. Disorders of water metabolism: diabetes insipidus and the syndrome of inappropriate antidiuretic hormone secretion. *Handb Clin Neurol.* 2014;124:37.

40. Spasovski G, et al. Clinical practice guideline on diagnosis and treatment of hyponatraemia. *Intensive Care Med.* 2014;40(3):320.

41. Esposito P, et al. The syndrome of inappropriate antidiuresis: pathophysiology, clinical management and new therapeutic options. *Nephron Clin Pract.* 2011;119(1):c62.

42. Verbalis JG, et al. Hyponatremia treatment guidelines 2007: expert panel recommendations. *American J Med.* 2007;120(11 Suppl 1):S1.

43. Bahn RS, et al. Hyperthyroidism and other causes of thyrotoxicosis: management guidelines of the American Thyroid Association and American Association of Clinical Endocrinologists. *Endocr Pract.* 2011;17(3):456.

44. Burch HB, Cooper DS. Management of Graves Disease: a Review. *JAMA.* 2015;314(23):2544.

45. Bogazzi F, et al. Amiodarone and the thyroid: a 2012 update. *J Endocrinol Invest.* 2012;35(3):340.

46. Cohen-Lehman J, Dahl P, Danzi S, Klein I. Effects of amiodarone therapy on thyroid function. *Nat Review Endocrinol.* 2010;6(1):34.

47. Chiha M, Samarasinghe S, Kabaker AS. Thyroid storm: an updated review. *J Intensive Care Med.* 2015;30(3):131.

48. Collet TH, et al. Subclinical hyperthyroidism and the risk of coronary heart disease and mortality. *Arch Internal Med.* 2012;172(10):799.

49. Garber JR, et al. Clinical practice guidelines for hypothyroidism in adults: cosponsored by the American Association of Clinical Endocrinologists and the American Thyroid Association. *Thyroid.* 2012;22(12):1200.

50. Mathew V, et al. Myxedema coma: a new look into an old crisis. *J Thyroid Res.* 2011;493462.

51. Chiong YV, Bammerlin E, Mariash CN. Development of an objective tool for the diagnosis of myxedema coma. *Transl Res.* 2015;166(3):233.

52. Agarwal V, Parikh V, Otterbeck PE, Lafferty J. Myxedema coma induced by short-term amiodarone therapy. *Am J Med Sci.* 2014;347(3):258.

53. Popoveniuc G, et al. A Diagnostic Scoring System for Myxedema Coma. *Endocrine Practice.* 2014;20(8):808.

54. Dubbs SB, Spangler R. Hypothyroidism: causes, killers, and life-saving treatments. *Emerg Med Clin North Am.* 2014;32(2):303.

55. Klubo-Gwiezdzinska J, Wartofsky L. Thyroid emergencies. *Med Clin North Am.* 2012;96(2):385.

56. Khandelwal D, Tandon N. Overt and subclinical hypothyroidism: who to treat and how. *Drugs.* 2012;72(1):17.

33

Trauma

Eugene E. Mondor

Trauma is the leading cause of death for all individuals age 1 to 44 years.[1] Each year, injury costs the United States hundreds of billions of dollars. It is one of the most demanding health care issues in the United States today, but the impact of trauma in terms of an individual's physical injury, psychological adjustment, lost time from work, disability, and costs to society remains largely underappreciated.

Trauma occurs in many forms. Motor vehicle collisions (MVCs) are the leading cause of death due to injury worldwide with more than 1.25 million deaths reported annually.[2] Sports-related injury, falls, work-related mishaps, and intentional self-harm all produce physical injury. Many trauma patients have underlying alcohol or substance abuse issues. Domestic violence and issues related to alcohol and substance abuse are priority areas with which all health care providers must be actively involved with both public education and injury prevention.

DOMESTIC VIOLENCE AND TRAUMA

Domestic violence constitutes a major public health issue in the United States. It has been reported that approximately 5.3 million episodes of domestic violence among women and 3.2 million episodes among men occur each year in the United States.[3] More than 2 million injuries are reported as a result of domestic violence, with almost one-third of individuals seeking care in the emergency department.[3]

Intimate partner violence (IPV) is a leading cause of injury and death to women; in the United States, it is estimated that 4.8 million women and 2.9 million men are physically assaulted or raped each year.[4] IPV can occur in all age groups and cultures and in heterosexual and same-sex relationships. Many health care facilities and emergency departments routinely screen patients for IPV. Key interventions for victims of IPV are listed in Box 33.1.

ALCOHOL AND SUBSTANCE ABUSE AND TRAUMA

Both alcohol and substance abuse have been implicated in traumatic injury. In 2013, 2.3 million injuries occurred as a result of MVCs, with 32,000 deaths.[5] Of injuries reported, approximately 31% involved alcohol.[5] Alcohol can alter consciousness, affect behavior, and impair judgment and concentration. Alcohol screening has been recommended as a routine component of trauma care.[6]

A strong correlation exists between substance abuse and alcohol use, IPV, and violence-related injuries.[7] Any substance is capable of being abused including alcohol; prescription medications; and illegal drugs such as cocaine, heroin, and crystal methamphetamine. Substance abuse embodies the potential to impair judgment and enhance impulsivity. Emergency and critical care teams screen trauma patients on admission for the presence of alcohol and illicit substances by obtaining blood and urine samples. The Alcohol Use Disorders Identification Test (Table 33.1) is an inexpensive and rapid test that can be used to screen for problem drinking.

MECHANISM OF INJURY

Trauma occurs when an external force of energy impacts the body and causes structural or physiologic alterations, or *injury*. External forces can be radiation, electrical, thermal, chemical, or mechanical forms of energy. Trauma that occurs from high-velocity impact (mechanical energy) is most common. Mechanical energy can produce blunt or penetrating traumatic injuries. Understanding the mechanism of injury helps health care providers predict potential injuries and anticipate the associated care that may be required.

Blunt Trauma

Blunt trauma is seen most often with MVCs, falls, contact sports, or blunt force injuries (eg, trauma caused by a baseball bat). Blunt injury may be difficult to diagnose, as injuries are not always obvious or readily apparent. Blunt injury occurs because of the forces sustained during a rapid change in velocity (deceleration). For example, to estimate the amount of force sustained in an MVC, multiply the person's weight by the miles per hour (speed) the vehicle was traveling. A 130-lb woman in a vehicle traveling at 60 miles/h that hits a brick wall would sustain 7800 lb of force within milliseconds. As the body stops suddenly, tissues and internal organs continue to move forward. This sudden change in velocity can cause significant external and internal injury.

BOX 33.1 Interventions With Victims of Intimate Partner Violence

Provide Validation
- Listen nonjudgmentally.
- "I am concerned for your safety (and the safety of your children)."
- "You are not alone and help is available."
- "You don't deserve the abuse and it is not your fault."
- "Stopping the abuse is the responsibility of your partner not you."

Provide Information
- "Domestic violence is common and happens in all kinds of relationships."
- "Violence tends to continue and often becomes more frequent and severe."

- "Abuse can impact your health in many ways."
- "You are not to blame, but exposure to violence in the home can emotionally and physically hurt your children or other dependent loved ones."

Respond to Safety Issues
- Offer a brochure about safety planning and explain contents to the patient.
- May need to involve assistance of social worker; alert law enforcement agencies when child abuse may be suspected.

From Futures Without Violence (formerly The Family Violence Prevention Fund). *National Consensus Guidelines on Identifying and Responding to Domestic Violence Victimization in Healthcare Settings.* http://www.futureswithoutviolence.org/section/our_work/health/_health_material/_jcaho. Accessed November 26, 2012.

TABLE 33.1 AUDIT Alcohol Screening Questionnaire

Question	Score[a]
How often do you have a drink containing alcohol?	Never
	Monthly or less
	2–4 times per month
	2–3 times per week
	4 or more times per week
How many standard drinks containing alcohol do you have on a typical day when drinking?	1 or 2
	3 or 4
	5 or 6
	7–9
	10 or more
How often do you have 6 or more drinks on one occasion?	
During the past year, how often have you found that you were not able to stop drinking once you had started?	Never
During the past year, how often have you failed to do what was normally expected of you because of drinking?	Less than monthly
	Monthly
During the past year, how often have you needed a drink in the morning to get yourself going after a heavy drinking session?	Weekly
	Daily or almost daily
During the past year, how often have you had a feeling of guilt or remorse after drinking?	
During the past year, have you been unable to remember what happened the night before because you had been drinking?	
Have you or someone else been injured as a result of your drinking?	No
Has a relative or friend or doctor or other health worker been concerned about your drinking or suggested you cut down?	Yes, but not in the past year
	Yes, during the past year

[a]Scores for each question range from 0 to 4, with the first response for each question (never) scoring 0, the second (less than monthly) scoring 1, the third (monthly) scoring 2, the fourth (weekly) scoring 3, and the fifth response (daily or almost daily) scoring 4. For the last two questions, which only have three responses, the scoring is 0, 2, and 4. A score of 8 or more is associated with harmful or hazardous drinking, and a score of 13 or more by women or 15 or more by men is likely to indicate alcohol dependence.
AUDIT, Alcohol Use Disorders Identification Test.

Penetrating Trauma

Penetrating injuries—injuries that puncture the body and result in damage to internal structures—occur with stabbings, firearms, or impalement. Damage is created along the path of penetration. Penetrating injuries can be misleading because the appearance of the external wound may not accurately reflect the extent of internal injury. For instance, bullets can create internal cavitation several times larger than the diameter of the bullet.[8]

Several factors determine the extent of damage sustained as a result of penetrating trauma. Different weapons cause different types of injuries. The severity of a gunshot wound depends on the type of gun, type of ammunition used, and the distance and angle from which the gun was fired. Pellets from a shotgun blast expand on impact and cause multiple injuries to internal structures. Handgun bullets usually damage what is directly in the bullet's path. Inside the body, the bullet can ricochet off bone and create further damage. With penetrating stab wounds, factors that determine the extent of injury include the type and length of object used and the angle of insertion.

PHASES OF TRAUMA CARE

Care of trauma victims during wartime has enhanced knowledge about trauma, triage, and the importance of rapid transport of injured individuals to medical facilities. Military experience has demonstrated that decreasing the time from injury to definitive care can save more lives. Care of critically injured individuals as a result of war has provided insight and knowledge that has helped improve civilian trauma care.

Historically, statistics demonstrated that deaths as a result of trauma occurred in a trimodal distribution.[9] However, at the present time, with advances in trauma resuscitation, most deaths occur in a bimodal distribution (Fig. 33.1).[10,11] The first peak occurs within the first 48 hours after initial injury, and the second peak occurs within days to weeks after injury. Development of the advanced trauma life support (ATLS) guidelines by the American College of Surgeons, enhanced assessment skills of prehospital care providers, expedited transport of injured patients, the presence of designated trauma care centers, creation of evidence-based protocols for injured patients, advancements in critical care, and a focus on injury prevention all have affected the timing of death after trauma.[10,11] In the first peak, death often occurs as a result of severe traumatic brain injury (TBI) or hemorrhage. During the second peak, death frequently

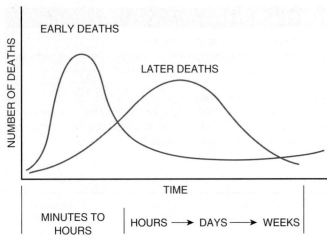

FIG. 33.1 Bimodal Distribution of Trauma Deaths.

occurs in the critical care unit as a result of complications from the initial injury, such as infection or multiple-organ dysfunction syndrome (MODS).

The "golden hour" of trauma resuscitation is frequently looked on as a time frame in which the injured patient will die unless he or she receives definitive care. However, the golden hour should not be considered a time frame, but rather a guideline for all trauma care providers. Components of the golden hour incorporate activation of emergency medical services, stabilization and transport, triage, initial resuscitation, early surgical consultation, and provision of critical care. For a critically injured patient, the primary goal is to minimize the time from injury to definitive care. There is no evidence to suggest that survival rates decrease in trauma patients after 60 minutes.

Major advances have been made in the management of patients with traumatic injuries in the prehospital, emergency department, and critical care settings. Patients with complex, multisystem trauma are frequently admitted to critical care units, and these patients require complex nursing care. Nursing management of a patient with traumatic injuries begins the moment a call for help is received and continues until the patient's death or return to the community. Care of a trauma patient is seen as a continuum that includes multiple phases and locations: prehospital care, emergency department, damage control resuscitation, critical care, intermediate care, and rehabilitation.

Prehospital Care

The goal of prehospital care is immediate identification of life-threatening injuries and transport (ground or air) to the closest appropriate medical facility. Airway maintenance, recognition and control of external bleeding and shock, and immobilization of the patient are essential priorities. Initiation of a peripheral intravenous (IV) line, splinting of fractures, and pain management are also vital components. Prehospital personnel should communicate information needed for triage before arrival at the hospital. Advanced planning for multiply-injured patients by trauma teams is essential.

Emergency Department

The ATLS guidelines assist health care providers with the essential actions necessary for rapid assessment, immediate identification of life-threatening injuries, and initial resuscitation of trauma patients in the emergency department.[9] These guiding principles delineate a systematic approach to initial assessment and care of a trauma patient that includes a rapid primary survey, resuscitation of vital functions, a more detailed secondary survey, and initiation of the most appropriate care. Initially developed for physicians, these guidelines have been adopted worldwide by prehospital care providers and trauma teams, including emergency and critical care nurses, and provides the framework for the ABCDEs of trauma care.

Primary Survey

On arrival of the trauma patient in the emergency department, the primary survey is initiated. The purpose of this initial assessment is to identify and treat any life-threatening injuries that, if left untreated, could potentially cause the patient's death. The five steps in the ATLS primary survey are performed in *ABCDE* sequence (Table 33.2):

A: Airway maintenance with cervical spine protection
B: Breathing and ventilation
C: Circulation with hemorrhage control
D: Disability: Neurologic status
E: Exposure or environmental control

Although many trauma centers use this approach, there is ever-present awareness that many trauma patients die as a result of hemorrhage. Consequently, many trauma facilities have informally adopted the military's *C-ABCDE* approach, where "C" stands for catastrophic hemorrhage.[12] This slight modification to the ABCDE approach of ATLS is intended to emphasize the importance of the immediate assessment, identification, and implementation of measures to control hemorrhage in a trauma patient, without becoming overly preoccupied with other components of the primary survey.

Airway. The patient's airway is assessed for patency and possible airway obstruction. Trauma patients are at risk for ineffective airway clearance, especially in the presence of altered consciousness, effects of drugs and alcohol, and maxillofacial or thoracic injuries. Airway obstruction can be caused by foreign bodies, blood clots, or broken teeth. Airway patency is assessed by inspecting the oropharynx for foreign body obstruction and listening for air movement at the nose and mouth. If the patient can verbally communicate, it is likely that the airway is patent. Patients who have a Glasgow Coma Scale (GCS) score of 8 or less or are unable to protect their own airway usually require the placement of a definitive airway.[9] Airway placement must incorporate cervical spine immobilization. The patient's head should not be rotated, hyperflexed, or hyperextended. The cervical spine must be immobilized at all times in all trauma patients until a cervical spinal cord injury (SCI) has been ruled out.

Breathing. The patient is assessed for signs of visible chest movement. An open, clear airway does not always ensure adequate ventilation and gas exchange. Assessment includes a visual inspection of chest wall integrity and respiratory rate, depth, and symmetry. Auscultation is performed to assess the presence or absence of breath sounds. Decreased or absent breath sounds or alteration in chest wall integrity may necessitate chest tube placement. Supplemental oxygen is administered to all injured patients.[9] Endotracheal intubation may be required for patients who have compromised airways caused by mechanical factors, who are unconscious, or who have ventilatory problems.[9]

Circulation. The next step is to assess for the presence of a palpable pulse, assess any evidence of external or internal hemorrhage, and, if possible, obtain a baseline measurement of the patient's vital signs. Rapid evaluation of circulatory status includes assessment of level of consciousness, skin color, and pulse.[9] The level of consciousness provides data on cerebral perfusion. Ashen, gray facial skin color or white, pale extremities

TABLE 33.2 Primary Survey of Trauma Patient

Survey Component	Trauma Team Assessment	Immediate Care

A—Airway	Immediately assess patient's ability to speak
	Look
	   Are there obvious signs of airway trauma, tachypnea, accessory muscle use?
	Listen
	   Can you hear the patient breathing?
	Feel
	   For air exchange through the mouth
	   For tracheal deviation
		Immobilize spine
		Nondefinitive airway management
		   Oropharyngeal (unconscious patient)
		   Nasopharyngeal (conscious patient)
		When in doubt, secure the airway
		   Endotracheal intubation
		   Emergency cricothyrotomy

B—Breathing	Is the patient breathing?
	Look
	
	   Is the patient's chest rising and falling?
	   Respiratory rate, rhythm, symmetry
	   Is there any evidence of thoracic trauma?
	Listen
	   Quickly auscultate air entry
	   Is there air entry in all lobes?
	Feel
	   Chest wall integrity
		Administer supplemental oxygen
		For life-threatening conditions (eg, tension pneumothorax), insert chest tubes
		Full-support mechanical ventilation (as required)

C—Circulation	Assess pulse quality and rate
	Assess for life-threatening conditions
	   (eg, uncontrolled bleeding, shock)
	Examine and feel patient's skin
	   Warm and dry
	   Cool, pale, and clammy
		Signs and symptoms of poor tissue perfusion
		   Initiate IV access
		   Administer 1–2 L of isotonic IV fluid, then reassess
		If no pulse, begin CPR

D—Disability	Neurologic assessment
	   GCS score
	   Pupils: Size and reactivity?
	   Is patient moving all 4 limbs to command?
	   Any evidence of posturing?
		Consider early neurosurgical consultation
		   Consider early CT scan

E—Exposure	All clothing removed to inspect all body regions
	   Any lacerations, abrasions, bruises?
	   Stab wounds: Entrance?
	   Gunshot wounds: Entrance? Exit?
		Prevent hypothermia
		   Warm blankets
		   Warm IV fluids
		   Increase room temperature

CPR, cardiopulmonary resuscitation; *CT,* computed tomography; *GCS,* Glasgow Coma Scale; *IV,* intravenous.

may be ominous signs of hypovolemia.[9] Central pulses (femoral or carotid artery) are assessed bilaterally for rate, regularity, and quality. If a pulse is not present, cardiopulmonary resuscitation must be initiated immediately.

All trauma patients are considered to be in shock. Trauma patients may or may not exhibit significant deterioration in hemodynamic stability. Measurement and trending of systolic and diastolic blood pressure, mean arterial pressure (MAP), and oxygen saturation on pulse oximetry (Spo_2) readings are more important than individual values. Hypotension in trauma should be attributed to hypovolemia until proven otherwise. Trauma teams are aware that vital signs can initially remain stable even in the face of hemorrhage. External exsanguination is identified and controlled by direct manual pressure on the wound.

Disability. A rapid neurologic assessment is performed. During this important step, the patient's baseline level of consciousness and pupil size and reaction are assessed and documented. The *AVPU* method can be used to quickly describe the patient's level of consciousness:

A: **A**lert
V: Responds to **V**erbal stimuli
P: Responds to **P**ainful stimuli
U: **U**nresponsive

The GCS score can also be used (see Table 22.1 in Chapter 22).

Exposure. In the final step of the primary survey, all of the patient's clothing is removed to facilitate a thorough examination of all body surfaces for the presence of injury. The patient is turned (logrolled) while full spinal precautions are maintained. The spine is carefully palpated for obvious deformity. The occipital lobe, neck, back, buttocks, and extremities are quickly examined for wounds, impaled objects, and bleeding. After clothing is removed, the patient must be protected from hypothermia. This can be accomplished through warm blankets, increasing room temperature, and warmed IV fluids.

Secondary Survey

The secondary survey begins when the primary survey is completed, potentially life-threatening injuries have been identified, and resuscitation has been initiated. In reality, the primary and secondary surveys may seem to occur almost simultaneously. However, the secondary survey is a more detailed, in-depth physical examination of the trauma patient. During the secondary survey, a head-to-toe approach is used to thoroughly examine each body region.

During the secondary survey, the nurse ensures the completion of all necessary procedures, such as an electrocardiogram, radiographic studies (chest, cervical spine, thorax, and pelvis), ultrasonography, and insertion of gastric and urinary catheters. Throughout this survey, the nurse continuously monitors the patient's vital signs (heart rate, blood pressure, MAP, and Spo$_2$) and response to medical therapies. Emotional support to the patient and family also is imperative.

The patient history is also an important aspect of the secondary survey. The patient's pertinent past history can be assessed by use of the mnemonic *AMPLE:*

A: Allergies
M: Medications currently used
P: Past medical illnesses/Pregnancy
L: Last meal
E: Events/Environment related to the injury

Head injury, shock, or the use of drugs or alcohol may preclude obtaining information from the patient. Prehospital care providers (paramedics, emergency medical technicians), family members, or sometimes bystanders can be excellent sources of information. Specific information that must be elicited pertaining to the mechanism of injury is summarized in Box 33.2.

Hemorrhagic shock in trauma. Hypovolemic shock as a result of hemorrhage is the most common type of shock that occurs in trauma patients.[9] The traditional signs and symptoms of hemorrhagic

hypovolemic shock may not appear until approximately 30% to 40% of circulating blood volume is lost.[9] Hemorrhage in trauma must be identified and treated rapidly. Two large-bore (14-gauge to 16-gauge) peripheral IV catheters, the intraosseous device, or central venous catheter is inserted. Blood samples are drawn during the initiation of IV lines (Box 33.3).

The ideal IV fluid for trauma resuscitation has not been established. Current ATLS guidelines suggest an initial infusion of 1 to 2 L of 0.9% normal saline or lactated Ringer solution.[9] Both crystalloid solutions are physiologically isotonic, provide volume to the volume-depleted patient, and are often readily available.

When IV fluid is administered, trauma patients may be categorized as *responders, transient responders,* or *nonresponders.*[9] *Responders* are patients whose hemodynamics steadily improve with the administration of IV fluid. *Transient responders* may exhibit temporary stabilization of vital signs, followed by a decline in patient condition. *Nonresponders* are the most worrisome. These patients do not respond to IV fluid, which often indicates that internal bleeding may be present. Overaggressive volume resuscitation with IV fluids must be avoided to prevent unnecessary complications such as pulmonary edema or exacerbation of hemorrhage.

Damage control resuscitation. Resuscitation in trauma begins during prehospital care and continues simultaneously during the primary and secondary surveys. Damage control resuscitation is an evidence-based strategy employed in trauma centers worldwide to control and assist in stabilization of the trauma patient in hemorrhagic shock.[13] Components of damage control resuscitation include permissive hypotension, massive transfusion protocols, and damage control surgery.[14] Damage control resuscitation begins in the field and continues through the emergency department, operating room, and critical care unit.

Permissive hypotension. Permissive hypotension is employed by most trauma providers. Permissive hypotension involves low-volume IV fluid resuscitation.[15] The goal is to maintain the blood pressure low enough to prevent worsening of hemorrhage but high enough to maintain perfusion of vital organs including the brain. In adult trauma patients, some authors suggest targeting a systolic blood pressure of 80 to 90 mm Hg, and MAP of 50 mm Hg,[13] but these targets are not universally adopted. Aggressively infusing IV fluid into a trauma patient may dilute clotting factors, disrupt any clots that have formed, and exacerbate hemorrhage.[16] Permissive hypotension is contraindicated in TBI.

Massive transfusion protocols. Given the emphasis on use of blood products over crystalloids and correction of trauma-induced coagulopathy, many trauma centers have developed massive transfusion protocols.[17] Approximately 1% to 3% of all trauma patients require activation of the massive transfusion protocol. Having a defined protocol serves as a system-based strategy to facilitate early, timely release of blood products in what can be an often chaotic situation. The massive transfusion protocol outlines the ratio of packed red blood cells, fresh frozen plasma, platelets, and cryoprecipitate to be administered.[18] This is referred to as *hemostatic resuscitation,* where blood components are administered in a ratio that resembles whole blood.

Tranexamic acid is an antifibrinolytic agent used to prevent bleeding in trauma patients. *Thromboelastography* is a newer technique whereby real-time point of care testing of the coagulation profile can be done at the bedside of the trauma patient.[16] The optimal ratio of blood components to be administered to bleeding trauma patients is a major focus in trauma research.[19]

Damage control surgery. Trauma is sometimes referred to as a "surgical disease" because the nature and extent of injuries

---

BOX 33.2 History of Mechanism of Injury

Blunt Trauma

- Height of fall
- Motor vehicle crash extrication time
- Ejection
- Steering wheel deformation
- Location in automobile (passenger, driver, front seat, back seat)
- Restraint status (lap belt, shoulder harness, or combination; unrestrained)
- Speed of automobiles, direction of impact
- Occupants (number and morbidity status)

Penetrating Trauma

- Weapon used (handgun, shotgun, rifle, knife)
- Caliber of weapon
- Number of shots fired
- Sex of assailant
- Position of victim and assailant when injury occurred

BOX 33.3 Blood Samples to Obtain With Intravenous Placement

- Complete blood cell (CBC) count
- Electrolyte profile (Na$^+$, K$^+$, Cl$^-$, carbon dioxide, glucose, blood urea nitrogen, creatinine)
- Coagulation parameters: Prothrombin time, partial thromboplastin time
- Type and screen (ABO compatibility)
- Amylase
- Toxicology screens
- Liver function studies
- Pregnancy test (for women of childbearing age)
- Lactate

usually require operative management. Damage control surgery is a well-established concept in trauma care. Damage control surgery is a strategy of providing essential surgical interventions to control hemorrhage and limit contamination.[20] The goal is to optimize physiology of the actively bleeding patient, not complete definitive repair. Permissive hypotension and massive transfusion protocols are often employed simultaneously during damage control surgery.[20] Reconstruction and formal closure of wounds are often not completed until after resuscitation and stabilization of the patient in the critical care unit have occurred.

BOX 33.4 Nursing Report From Referring Area Using SBAR Method

S: Situation
- Age
- Sex
- Mechanism of injury/injuries sustained
- Admission diagnosis/chief complaint; any loss of consciousness and its duration with current Glasgow Coma Scale score
- Diagnostic tests and procedures completed
- Diagnostic test results and laboratory results
- Medications administered (opiates, sedatives)
- Current issues, including derangements in any physical assessments requiring acute interventions

B: Background
- Significant medical and surgical history
- Home medications

A: Assessments
- Current assessment findings including vital signs, level of consciousness, established airway, and mechanical ventilation settings
- Family members present and assessment of their coping and current knowledge of nature and extent of injuries and treatment plan

R: Recommendations
- Description of plan including fluid volume and blood products

TABLE 33.3 Effects of Trauma Resuscitation

Aspect of Injury or Resuscitation	Impact on Critical Care Management
Prolonged extrication time	Loss of perfusion to vital organs; Severity of shock state
Respiratory and/or cardiac arrest	Effects of loss of perfusion to brain (anoxic injury), kidneys, and other vital organs
Time on backboard	Potentiates risk of skin breakdown to occipital lobe, scapulae, sacrum, coccyx, and heels
Number of units of blood; whether any were not fully crossmatched; packed cells vs whole blood used	Potentiates risk of ARDS, MODS
Prolonged transportation to definitive trauma facility	Worsening of patient condition during transport (eg, hypotension, ongoing bleeding, acid–base imbalance, oxygenation and/or ventilation issues); New-onset bleeding or rebleeding decreases perfusion to vital organs

ARDS, acute respiratory distress syndrome; *MODS,* multiple-organ dysfunction syndrome.

Critical Care Phase

Critically injured trauma patients are frequently admitted to the critical care unit as direct transfers from the emergency department, diagnostic imaging, or operating room. Information the critical care nurse must obtain from prehospital, emergency department, or operating room personnel is summarized using the **SBAR** method: **S**ituation, **B**ackground, **A**ssessment, and **R**ecommendations (Box 33.4). This information is ideally obtained before the patient's admission to the critical care unit to ensure availability of needed personnel, equipment, and supplies, but this may not always be possible. Table 33.3 summarizes the prehospital, emergency department, and operating room resuscitative measures that can affect management of the trauma patient in the critical care unit.

Immediately after the patient's arrival in the critical care unit, the nurse repeats the primary and secondary surveys in accordance with ATLS guidelines to reassess the trauma patient's status. It is essential that the critical care team be aware of all resuscitation strategies that have been initiated up until admission to the critical care unit. Priority nursing care during the critical care phase includes ongoing repeated physical assessments, monitoring laboratory and diagnostic test results, and observing trends in the patient's response to treatment. The nurse is continually aware that the second peak of the bimodal distribution of trauma deaths occurs in the critical care setting as a result of complications including prolonged shock states, acute respiratory distress syndrome (ARDS), sepsis, and MODS. Ongoing nursing assessments are imperative for early detection and treatment of complications.

One of the most important nursing roles is ongoing assessment of the balance between oxygen delivery (supply) and oxygen demand (consumption). Oxygen delivery must be optimized to prevent further system damage. The trauma patient is at high risk for impaired oxygenation as a result of various factors (Table 33.4). Risk factors must be promptly identified and treated to prevent life-threatening sequelae. Prevention and treatment of hypoxemia depend on accurate assessment of the adequacy of pulmonary gas exchange (arterial blood gas), oxygen supply (fraction of inspired oxygen), and oxygen consumption (assessment of level of consciousness, tissue perfusion, capillary refill, urinary output).

Acidosis (pH less than 7.2), hypothermia (temperature less than 35°C), and clinical coagulopathy are often present in trauma

TABLE 33.4 Factors Predisposing Trauma Patients to Impaired Oxygenation

Factor	Impairment
Impaired ventilation	Injury to airway structures, loss of central nervous system regulation of breathing, impaired level of consciousness
Impaired pulmonary gas diffusion	Pneumothorax, hemothorax, aspiration of gastric contents; Shifts to the left of oxyhemoglobin dissociation curve (can result from infusion of large volumes of banked blood, hypocarbia or alkalosis, or hypothermia)
Decreased oxygen supply	Reduced hemoglobin (from hemorrhage); Reduced cardiac output (cardiovascular injury, decreased preload from hemorrhage)

patients. This combination of factors is known as the *lethal triad of death.*[21] For example, hypothermia induced by an open visceral cavity in conjunction with massive blood transfusion can lead to coagulopathy and continued bleeding, which results in shock and metabolic acidosis. The triad of hypothermia, coagulopathy, and acidosis creates a self-propagating cycle that can eventually lead to an irreversible physiologic insult.[21] The goal of the critical care nurse is to continue resuscitation and assist in correcting hypothermia, coagulopathy, and acidosis. Coagulation factors and platelets may be administered to correct coagulopathies. Monitoring arterial blood gases (ABGs) aids in determining acid–base balance. Rewarming techniques are described in Table 33.5.

End Points in Trauma Resuscitation

During resuscitation, all attempts are made to improve cellular oxygenation. Resuscitation is aimed at ensuring adequate perfusion of tissues with fluid, oxygen, and nutrients to support cellular function.[16] No single resuscitation end point is sufficient. Resuscitation end points (variables or parameters) must be viewed across the continuum of trauma resuscitation.

During resuscitation from traumatic hemorrhagic shock, normalization of standard clinical parameters such as blood pressure, heart rate, and urine output is inadequate.[12] Resuscitation end points can be grouped into two major categories: hemodynamic variables and tissue perfusion variables.[22] Base deficit and lactic acid (lactate) values have been well studied to determine the adequacy of cellular oxygenation during trauma resuscitation.[12,22] Optimal resuscitation end points in different types of trauma are ongoing areas of research in trauma care.

Frequent and thorough nursing assessments of all body systems are the cornerstone of medical and nursing management of critically injured trauma patients in critical care. The nurse can detect subtle changes and facilitate the implementation of timely therapeutic interventions to prevent complications often associated with trauma. The nurse must be knowledgeable about specific organ injuries and their associated sequelae. The focus of this chapter is nursing management of adult patients with traumatic injuries in the critical care setting.

SPECIFIC TRAUMA INJURIES

Traumatic Brain Injuries

More than 2.5 million TBIs occur annually; approximately 50,000 Americans die each year of TBI with 280,000 hospitalized as a result of their injury.[23] Adults 65 years old and older are most likely to sustain a TBI and require hospitalization and have the highest percentage of TBI-related deaths.[24] TBI can be caused by both blunt and penetrating trauma. The leading causes of TBI include falls (40%), struck by or against objects (15%), MVCs (14%), and assaults (10%).[16]

Pathophysiology

The pathophysiology of TBI can be divided into two main categories: primary brain injury and secondary brain injury. It is important that the nurse understand these two distinct phases of TBI, as critical care interventions are often directed at limiting the effects of and reducing morbidity and mortality from primary, and more importantly, secondary brain injury.

Primary injury. Primary TBI occurs at the moment of impact as a result of mechanical forces to the head. The extent of and recovery from injury are often related to whether the primary injury was localized (limited to a specific area) or diffuse (widespread) throughout the brain. Primary injuries include injuries that directly damage the brain parenchyma. Examples of primary TBIs include contusion, laceration, shearing injuries, and hemorrhage. Hemorrhage may significantly compress nearby structures. Primary injury may be mild, with little or no neurologic damage, or severe, with major brain and tissue damage. Immediately after the injury, a cascade of neural and vascular processes is activated.

Secondary injury. Secondary injury is the biochemical and cellular response to the initial trauma that can exacerbate the primary injury and cause additional damage and impairment in brain recovery. Secondary injury can be caused by ischemia, hypotension, hypercapnia, cerebral edema, or metabolic derangements.[25] Hypoxia and hypotension, the best-known culprits for secondary injury,[26] typically are the result of extracranial trauma. A self-perpetuating cycle develops that may cause worsening of the primary injury as a result of uncontrolled secondary factors.

Ischemia. Tissue ischemia occurs in areas of poor cerebral perfusion as a result of hypotension or hypoxia. The cells in ischemic areas become edematous. Extreme vasodilation of the cerebral vasculature occurs in TBI in an attempt to supply oxygen and nutrients to the cerebral tissue. This sudden increase in blood volume increases intracranial volume and raises intracranial pressure (ICP).

Hypotension. Initial hypertension in a patient with severe TBI is common. With loss of autoregulation, an increase in blood pressure occurs, which results in increased intracranial blood volume and elevates ICP. Hypertension, observed most frequently after initial TBI, is the body's attempt to perfuse the brain when cerebral circulation is compromised.[27]

Significant hypotension causes inadequate perfusion to neural tissue. Hypotension rarely is associated with TBI, unless terminal medullary failure has occurred. If a trauma patient is unconscious and hypotensive, a detailed assessment of the chest, abdomen, and pelvis must be performed to rule out internal injuries.

TABLE 33.5 Interventions for Rewarming Trauma Patients

Intervention	External Rewarming Procedures	Internal Rewarming Procedures
Passive	Maintain warm room temperature. Remove all wet clothing and linen. Cover patient with blankets. Avoid bathing patient until normothermia is achieved.	Administer warmed, humidified oxygen. Administer warmed IV fluids.
Active	Use radiant heat lamps, heating blankets or pads, and hot water bottles.	Perform gastrointestinal irrigation with warmed solutions. Perform extracorporeal rewarming for profound hypothermia. Use esophageal rewarming tubes.

IV, intravenous.
Adapted from Flarity K. Environmental emergencies. In: Kunz Howard P, Steinmann R, eds. *Sheehy's Emergency Nursing: Principles and Practice.* 6th ed. St. Louis: Mosby; 2010.

Hypercapnia. Hypercapnia is a powerful vasodilator of cerebral vessels. Most often caused by hypoventilation in an unconscious patient, hypercapnia results in cerebral vasodilation, increased cerebral blood flow (volume), and increased ICP.

Cerebral edema. Cerebral edema occurs as a result of the changes in the cellular environment caused by contusion, loss of autoregulation, and increased permeability of the blood–brain barrier. As pressure increases (inside the cranial vault) in an attempt to perfuse the brain, cerebral perfusion decreases, which further compromises brain function. Cerebral edema can be localized around the area of contusion or diffuse as a result of hypotension or hypoxia. The combined effects of increasing pressure and decreasing perfusion precipitate a downward spiral of events. The extent of cerebral edema can sometimes be minimized by managing aspects of secondary injury, such as oxygenation, ventilation, and perfusion.

Classification of Brain Injuries

Injuries of the brain are described by the functional changes or losses that occur. Some of the most common functional abnormalities seen in neurologic trauma are described here.

Skull fracture. Skull fractures are common, but they do not by themselves cause neurologic deficits. Skull fractures can be classified as open (dura mater is torn) or closed (dura mater is not torn), or they can be classified as fractures of the vault or fractures of the base. Common vault fractures occur in the frontal and parietal regions. Basilar skull fractures usually are not visible on conventional skull x-rays; a computed tomography (CT) scan is typically required. Assessment findings may include cerebrospinal fluid (CSF) leakage—described as rhinorrhea (from nose) or otorrhea (from ear), Battle sign (ecchymosis overlying the mastoid process behind the ear), "raccoon eyes" (subconjunctival and periorbital ecchymosis), or palsy of the seventh cranial nerve.

The significance of a skull fracture is that it identifies a patient with a higher probability of having or developing an intracranial hematoma. A significant amount of force is required to fracture the skull. This external force is evident in Fig. 33.2A, which shows a CT scan of a depressed skull fracture with brain tissue injury. In the same patient, the fragmentation of bone in the skull fracture is even more obvious in the *bone window scan* shown in Fig. 33.2B. Bone window views are helpful in

identifying bone tumors, and in trauma a bone window scan provides an enhanced view of cranial abnormalities.

Open skull fractures require surgical intervention to remove bony fragments and close the dura mater. Major complications of basilar skull fractures are cranial nerve injury and leakage of CSF. CSF leakage may result in a fistula, which increases the possibility of bacterial contamination and resultant meningitis.

Concussion. A concussion is a brain injury accompanied by a brief loss of neurologic function, in particular, loss of consciousness. When loss of consciousness occurs, it may last for a few seconds to an hour. Neurologic dysfunctions include confusion, disorientation, and sometimes a period of anterograde or retrograde amnesia. Other clinical manifestations that occur after concussion are headache, dizziness, nausea, irritability, inability to concentrate, impaired memory, and fatigue. The diagnosis of concussion is based primarily on patient history.

Contusion. Contusion, or "bruising" of the brain, is frequently associated with acceleration-deceleration injuries, which result in hemorrhage into the superficial parenchyma. Frontal or temporal lobe contusions are most common and can be seen in a *coup-contrecoup mechanism of injury* (Fig. 33.3A). Coup injury affects the cerebral tissue directly under the point of impact. Contrecoup injury occurs in a line directly opposite the point of impact (Fig. 33.3B). The brain contusions caused by the coup and contrecoup impact is visible on a CT scan (Fig 33.3C).

Clinical manifestations of a contusion are related to the location of the injury, the degree of contusion, and the presence of associated lesions. Contusions can be small, in which localized areas of dysfunction result in a focal neurologic deficit. Larger contusions can evolve over 2 to 3 days after injury as a result of edema and further hemorrhaging. A large contusion can produce a mass effect that can cause a significant increase in ICP. Contusions may lead to the development of intracerebral hematomas.[9]

Contusions of the tips of the temporal lobe are a common occurrence and are of particular concern. Because the inner aspects of the temporal lobe surround the opening in the tentorium (where the midbrain enters the cerebrum), edema in this area can cause rapid deterioration in level of consciousness and can lead to herniation. Because of the location, this deterioration can occur with little or no warning.

Diagnosis of contusion is made by CT scan. If contusions are small, focal, or multiple, they are treated medically with

FIG. 33.2 (A) CT scan of depressed skull fracture shows both brain tissue injury and bone injury. (B) Bone Window scan of the same depressed skull fracture more clearly shows the displaced fragments of bone. CT, Computer Tomography.

FIG. 33.3 Coup and Contrecoup Head Injury After Blunt Trauma. (A) Coup injury: Impact against an object, showing the site of impact and direct trauma to the brain *(a)*, shearing of subdural veins *(b)*, and trauma to the base of the brain *(c)*. (B) Contrecoup injury: Impact within the skull, showing the site of impact from the brain hitting the opposite side of the skull *(a)* and shearing forces throughout the brain *(b)*. These injuries occur in one continuous motion; the head strikes the wall (coup) and then rebounds (contrecoup). (C) CT scan of a Coup and Contracoup Head Injury. The primary injury is located in the right parietal region, with the Contracoup injury in the left frontal/temporal area. Note that a CT scan is always shown as if the reader is looking in a mirror, so that right (R) and left (L) are reversed. CT, Computed Tomography.

serial neurologic assessments. Larger contusions that produce considerable mass effect may require surgical intervention to reduce edema and elevations in ICP. The nurse must pay specific attention to neurologic assessment findings and look for subtle changes in pupillary signs or vital signs, which may indicate potential worsening of the patient's condition. The outcome of cerebral contusion varies.

Cerebral hematoma. Extravasation of blood creates a space-occupying lesion within the cranial vault that can lead to increased ICP. Three types of hematomas are discussed here and illustrated in Fig. 33.4. The first two, epidural hematoma (EDH) and subdural hematoma (SDH), are extraparenchymal (outside of brain tissue) and produce injury by pressure and displacement of intracranial contents. The third type is intraparenchymal, occurring within the brain tissue. Traumatic intracerebral hemorrhage directly damages neural tissue and can produce further injury as a result of pressure and displacement of intracranial contents.

Epidural hematoma. EDH is a collection of blood between the inner skull and the outermost layer of the dura mater (see Fig. 33.4A). Epidural hemorrhage or EDH occurs as a result of trauma to the skull and meninges as seen in the CT scan in Fig 33.5A. On a CT scan, brain tissue appears dark-gray and any collection of blood appears as light-gray. EDHs are most often associated with skull fractures and middle meningeal artery lacerations (two-thirds of patients) or skull fractures with venous bleeding.[28] A blow to the head that causes a linear skull fracture on the lateral surface of the head may tear the middle meningeal artery. As the artery bleeds, it pulls the dura mater away from the skull, creating a pouch that expands into the intracranial space.

The incidence of EDH is relatively low. EDH can occur as a result of low-impact injuries (eg, falls) or high-impact injuries (eg, MVCs). The classic clinical manifestations of EDH include brief loss of consciousness followed by a period of lucidity. Rapid deterioration in the level of consciousness should be

FIG. 33.4 Intracranial Hematomas. (A) Epidural hematoma. (B) Subdural hematoma. (C) Intracerebral hematoma.

FIG. 33.5 Intracranial Hematomas – CT Scans (A) CT scan of an epidural hematoma in the right temporal/parietal area. (B) CT scan of a subdural hematoma in the left frontal/temporal area. Note that a CT scan is always shown as if the reader is looking in a mirror, so that right (R) and left (L) are reversed. CT, Computed Tomography.

anticipated because arterial bleeding into the epidural space can occur quickly. The patient may complain of a severe, localized headache and may be sleepy. A dilated and fixed pupil on the same side as the impact area is a hallmark of EDH.[28] Diagnosis is based on clinical symptoms and evidence of a collection of epidural blood identified on CT scan. Treatment of EDH requires urgent surgical intervention to remove the blood and to cauterize the bleeding vessels.

Subdural hematoma. SDH, which is the accumulation of blood between the dura mater and underlying arachnoid membrane, is most often related to a rupture in the bridging veins between the cerebral cortex and the dura mater (Fig. 33.4B). SDH accounts for approximately 30% of severe head injuries. Acceleration-deceleration and rotational forces are major causes of SDH, which often is associated with cerebral contusions and intracerebral hemorrhage. The three types of SDH—acute, subacute, and chronic—are based on the time frame from injury, and clinical symptoms.

Acute subdural hematoma. Acute SDHs are hematomas that occur after a severe blow to the head. The clinical presentation of acute SDH is determined by the severity of injury to the underlying brain parenchyma at the time of impact and the rate of blood accumulation in the subdural space. The patient often has a decreased level of consciousness on admission; in other situations, the patient has a lucid period before deterioration. Careful observation for deterioration in the level of consciousness or lateralizing signs such as inequality of pupils or motor movements is essential. Rapid surgical intervention, including craniectomy, craniotomy, or burr hole evacuation, can reduce mortality.

Subacute subdural hematoma. Subacute SDHs are hematomas that develop 4 days to 3 weeks after trauma.[29] An SDH occurs within the meninges in the subdural space (Fig 33.4B). SDH is diagnosed by alteration in neurologic symptoms and by CT scan (Fig 33.5B). In subacute subdural bleeding, the expansion of the hematoma occurs at a rate slower than that observed in acute SDH and slower than an epidural bleed. Clinical deterioration of a patient with a subacute SDH is also usually slower than deterioration with an acute SDH, but treatment by surgical intervention, when appropriate, is the same.

Chronic subdural hematoma. Chronic SDH is diagnosed when symptoms appear 21 days or more after injury. Most patients with chronic SDH are in late middle age or are elderly. Individuals at risk for chronic SDH include patients with coordination or balance disturbances and patients receiving anticoagulation therapy. Clinical manifestations of chronic SDH are insidious. The patient may report a variety of symptoms such as lethargy, absent-mindedness, headache, vomiting, stiff neck, and photophobia and may show signs of transient ischemic attack, seizures, pupillary changes, or hemiparesis. Because a history of trauma is often not significant enough to be recalled, chronic SDH seldom is seen as an initial diagnosis. CT evaluation can confirm the diagnosis.

If surgical intervention is required, evacuation of chronic SDH may be accomplished by craniotomy, burr holes, or catheter drainage. Outcome after chronic SDH evacuation varies. Return of neurologic status often depends on the degree of neurologic dysfunction before removal. Because this condition is most common in older or debilitated patients, recovery may be slow.

Intracerebral hematoma. Intracerebral hemorrhage (ICH) results when bleeding occurs deep within cerebral tissue.[28] Traumatic causes of ICH include depressed skull fractures, penetrating injuries (bullet, knife), or sudden acceleration-deceleration motion. The ICH can act as a rapidly expanding space-occupying lesion; late ICH into the necrotic center of a contused area also is possible (Fig. 33.4C). Sudden clinical deterioration of a patient 6 to 10 days after trauma may be the result of ICH.

Medical management of ICH may include surgical or non-surgical approaches. Hemorrhages that are minimal or localized and do not cause significant neurologic or other problems are treated without surgery. Over time, the blood may be reabsorbed. If significant problems with neurologic status occur as a result of the ICH producing a mass effect, surgical removal is necessary. The outcome of a patient with an ICH depends on the location of the hemorrhage. Size, mass effect, and displacement of other intracranial structures also affect the outcome.

Missile injuries. Missile injuries are caused by objects that penetrate the skull to produce significant focal damage but little acceleration-deceleration or rotational injury. The injury may be depressed, penetrating, or perforating (Fig. 33.6). Depressed injuries are caused by fractures of the skull, with penetration of bone into cerebral tissue. Penetrating injury is caused by a missile that enters the cranial cavity but does not exit. A low-velocity penetrating injury (knife) may involve only focal damage and no loss of consciousness. A high-velocity missile (bullet) can produce shock waves that are transmitted throughout the brain in addition to the injury caused by the bullet. Perforating injuries are missile injuries that enter and then exit the brain. Perforating injuries have much less ricochet effect but are still responsible for significant injury.

Risk of infection and cerebral abscess is a concern in cases of missile injuries. If fragments of the missile are embedded within the brain, surgery may be required. Careful consideration of the location and risk of increasing neurologic deficit is weighed against the risk of abscess, infection, or permanent disability. The outcome after missile injury is based on the degree of penetration, the location of the injury, and the velocity of the missile.

Diffuse Axonal Injury. Diffuse axonal injury (DAI) is a term used to describe prolonged posttraumatic coma that is not caused by a mass lesion, although DAI with mass lesions has been reported. DAI covers a wide range of brain dysfunction typically caused by acceleration-deceleration and rotational forces. DAI occurs as a result of damage to the axons or disruption of axonal transmission of the neural impulses.

The pathophysiology of DAI is related to the stretching, shearing, and tearing of axons as a result of movement of the brain inside the cranium at the time of impact. The stretching and tearing of axons result in microscopic lesions throughout the brain, but especially deep within cerebral tissue and the base of the cerebrum. Disruption of axonal transmission of impulses results in loss of consciousness. Unless surrounding tissue areas are significantly injured, causing small hemorrhages, DAI may not be visible on CT or magnetic resonance imaging (MRI).

DAI can be classified as mild, moderate, or severe based on the extent of lesions. A patient with mild DAI may be in a coma for 24 hours and may exhibit periods of decorticate and decerebrate posturing. Patients with moderate DAI may be in a coma for longer than 24 hours and exhibit periods of decorticate and decerebrate posturing. Severe DAI usually manifests as a prolonged, deep coma with periods of hypertension, hyperthermia, and excessive diaphoresis. Treatment of DAI includes support of vital functions. The outcome after severe DAI is often poor because of the extensive physiologic dysfunction of cerebral pathways.

Neurologic Assessment of Traumatic Brain Injury

Neurologic assessment is the most important tool for evaluating a patient with a severe TBI because it can provide information about the severity of injury, offer prognostic information,

and dictate the speed with which further evaluation and treatment must proceed.[25] The cornerstone of neurologic assessment is the GCS score, although assessment of the GCS score is not a complete neurologic examination. Pupillary and motor strength assessment must be incorporated into early and ongoing assessments. After specific injuries are identified, a more thorough, focused neurologic assessment, such as examination of the cranial nerves, is warranted. To assist with the initial assessment, TBIs are divided into three descriptive categories—mild, moderate, or severe—on the basis of the patient's GCS score and duration of the unconscious state.

Degree of injury

Mild brain injury. Mild TBI is described as a GCS score of 13 to 15, with a loss of consciousness that lasts up to 15 minutes. Patients with mild injury often are seen in the emergency department and discharged home with a family member who is instructed to evaluate the patient routinely and to bring the patient back to the hospital if any further neurologic symptoms appear.

Moderate brain injury. Moderate TBI is described as a GCS score of 9 to 12, with a loss of consciousness for up to 6 hours. Patients with this type of TBI usually are hospitalized. They are at high risk for deterioration from increasing cerebral edema and ICP, and serial clinical assessments are important. Hemodynamic and ICP monitoring and ventilatory support are usually not required for these patients unless other systemic injuries make them necessary. A CT scan is obtained on admission. Repeat CT scans are indicated if the patient's neurologic status deteriorates.

Severe brain injury. Patients with a GCS score of 8 or less after resuscitation or patients who deteriorate to that level within 48 hours of admission have a severe TBI. Loss of consciousness may be 6 hours or longer. Patients with severe TBI often receive mechanical ventilation, ICP, and hemodynamic monitoring. A CT scan is performed to rule out any bleeding or mass lesions that can be surgically ameliorated. Patients are admitted to the critical care unit for continual assessment, monitoring, and management.

Nursing assessment of a patient with traumatic brain injury. As in all traumatic injuries, evaluation of a critically injured patient with TBI follows the ABCDE approach of ATLS. Immediate assessments of airway, breathing, and circulation (ABCs) are the first steps in patient assessment. Patients with

G.J.Wassilchenko

FIG. 33.6 Bullet Wounds of the Head. Bullet wounds or other penetrating missile wounds cause an open (compound) skull fracture and damage to brain tissue. Shock wave effects are transmitted throughout the brain. (A) Perforating injury. (B) Penetrating injury.

moderate to severe TBI may require endotracheal intubation with mechanical ventilation to reduce the risk of hypoxia and hypercapnia. After stabilization of the ABCs, a neurologic assessment is performed.

Level of consciousness, motor movements, pupillary response, respiratory function, and vital signs all are part of a complete neurologic assessment of a patient with TBI. Level of consciousness is a patient's degree of arousal and awareness. Consciousness is assessed by obtaining the patient's response to verbal and painful stimuli. Determination of orientation to person, place, and time assesses mental alertness. Pupils are assessed for size, shape, equality, and reactivity. Asymmetry must be reported immediately. Pupils are also assessed for constriction to a light source (parasympathetic innervation) or dilation (sympathetic innervation). Because parasympathetic fibers are present in the brainstem, pupils that are slow to react to light may indicate a brainstem injury. A "blown" pupil can be caused by compression of the third cranial nerve or transtentorial herniation. Bilateral fixed pupils can indicate midbrain involvement.

Neurologic assessments are continuous throughout the patient's stay in the critical care unit as part of the ongoing assessments to detect subtle changes in the patient's condition. Serial assessments include changes in level of consciousness, GCS score, pupils, and hemodynamic status. The use of analgesia, sedation, and muscle relaxants for patients may mask neurologic signs in a patient with a severe head injury. In these situations, careful clinical observation of trends in the patient's condition is essential. When sedation of the patient is required, newer shorter acting sedatives with a very short half-life, such as IV propofol, can be used and turned off, and within minutes, a neurologic examination can be performed.

Diagnostic procedures. The cornerstone of diagnostic procedures for evaluation of TBI is the CT scan.[25] CT is a rapid, noninvasive procedure that can provide invaluable information about the presence of mass lesions (including hemorrhage) and cerebral edema. Serial CT scans may be obtained over a period of several days to assess areas of contusion and ischemia and to detect delayed hematomas. The critical care nurse must always remain with a patient with a TBI during a CT scan and during transport to and from the scanner to provide continuous observation and monitoring. Transporting the patient, moving the patient from the bed to the CT table, and positioning the head flat during the CT scan all are stressful events and can cause severe increases in ICP and decreases in cerebral perfusion pressure (CPP).

Medical Management

Surgical management. If a lesion identified on CT scan is causing a shift of intracranial contents or increasing ICP, surgical intervention is necessary. A craniotomy is performed to remove the EDH, SDH, or large ICH. Patients may also undergo a *decompressive craniectomy* specifically for elevated ICP. This procedure involves removal of the overlying bone flap to allow the underlying brain tissue to expand and swell. This surgical strategy has demonstrated some benefits but remains controversial.[30]

Nonsurgical management. Management of TBI frequently occurs initially in the critical care unit. Nonsurgical management includes management of ICP, maintenance of adequate CPP, ensuring adequate oxygenation, and treatment of any complications (eg, pneumonia, infection). The decision of when to initiate ICP monitoring is critical. ICP monitoring may be required for patients with a GCS score less than 8 and

abnormal findings on a head CT scan.[31] Brain tissue oxygen monitoring may also be used.

Nursing Management

Nursing diagnoses for a patient with TBI are listed in Box 33.5. Priority nursing goals include reduction of increased ICP, limiting or preventing secondary brain injury, and stabilization of vital signs. Ongoing nursing assessments are the foundation of care for patients with TBI. Assessments are the primary mechanism for determining improvement or worsening of the patient's condition. If secondary injury is to be prevented, the critical care nurse (in collaboration with the physicians), must respond immediately to events that increase ICP, reduce MAP, and reduce CPP.

All aspects of care, including hemodynamic management, control of ICP, IV fluid therapy, pulmonary care, acid–base balance, maintenance of body temperature, and control of the environment, can impact outcome after TBI.[25,32] In patients with TBI, changes in cardiovascular function and circulating catecholamines may contribute to hemodynamic instability. Heart rate and blood pressure are continually monitored, with the goal of achieving MAP greater than 60 mm Hg (minimum) to ensure adequate perfusion to the brain. Isotonic IV fluids (eg, 0.9% normal saline) and vasopressors may be required if target MAP is not achieved. Arterial blood pressure should also be continually monitored because hypotension in a patient with TBI is rare and may indicate additional injuries.

Ongoing monitoring of ICP may be necessary in some patients with TBI, and insertion of an external ventricular drain may be required. When an external ventricular drain is in situ, appropriate targets include maintaining ICP less than 15 mm Hg (normal, 0 to 15 mm Hg), and CPP should be maintained at a minimum of 60 mm Hg.[25] In the absence of cerebral ischemia, aggressive attempts to maintain CPP greater than 70 mm Hg have not been supported in the literature and should be avoided secondary to the risk of ARDS.[25]

Initially, the patient is often intubated, mechanically ventilated, and placed on a full support mode of mechanical ventilation (eg, assist control). *Capnography* (monitoring of exhaled carbon dioxide levels) is suggested to monitor for prevention of inadvertent hypercapnia. ABGs are frequently monitored, with particular attention to arterial partial pressure of carbon

---

◎ BOX 33.5 NURSING DIAGNOSES

Traumatic Brain Injury

- Ineffective Breathing Pattern related to neuromuscular impairment, p. 1035
- Impaired Gas Exchange, p. 1030
- Risk for Aspiration related to decreased level of consciousness, impaired laryngeal sensation or reflex; impaired pharyngeal peristalsis or tongue function; impaired laryngeal closure or elevation; increased gastric volume; decreased lower esophageal sphincter pressure, p. 1040
- Risk for Ineffective Cerebral Tissue Perfusion related to cerebral swelling, loss of autoregulation, increased intracranial pressure, hypercapnia, hyperthermia, mechanical ventilation, suctioning, p. 1042
- Imbalanced Nutrition: Less Than Body Requirements related to lack of exogenous nutrients and increased metabolic demand, p. 1029
- Powerlessness related to lack of control over current situation, p. 1038
- Decreased Intracranial Adaptive Capacity related to failure of normal compensatory mechanisms, p. 1018

dioxide (Paco$_2$). Most facilities caring for patients with TBI aim to keep the Paco$_2$ level at 35 to 40 mm Hg, as any increase in Paco$_2$ would increase cerebral blood flow and worsen ICP. When Paco$_2$ levels increase, the tidal volume or minute volume need to be increased on the ventilator. Although pulmonary care must be instituted, endotracheal suctioning can elevate ICP. Techniques to counter elevation in ICP with suctioning are outlined in Box 33.6.

Cerebral oxygen consumption is increased during periods of increased body temperature. As a result, the goal is to achieve normothermia (36°C to 37°C). Monitoring of the patient's temperature, use of antipyretics, cooling blankets, and early identification and work-up for infection are essential. A tremendous catecholamine surge after TBI has been associated with infectious complications and potentially preventable mortality.[33] The use of beta-blockers to suppress this catecholamine surge in patients with TBI has been shown to decrease mortality.[33]

In the early postinjury phase, the patient's environment must be controlled. Stimuli that produce pain, agitation, or discomfort can increase ICP. Nursing interventions should not be clustered; care should be evenly distributed throughout the shift. Explanations can be provided to patients in a calm, soft-spoken manner. Families and significant others are informed about the importance of maintaining a quiet environment. Analgesics and sedatives should be administered as ordered by the physician but should not be routinely used as first-line agents when ICP increases. Patients should be provided several rest periods during hospitalization.

Newer pharmacologic agents have demonstrated promise in the treatment of patients awakening from head trauma. Amantadine has been prescribed to facilitate awakening. Although its full mechanism is only partially understood, it appears to act as an N-methyl-D-aspartate antagonist and indirect dopamine agonist.[34] It has been shown to help patients who are undergoing active rehabilitation to awaken faster.[34]

Spinal Cord Injuries

Approximately 12,000 new SCIs occur annually. Since the 1970s, the median age at injury has increased from 28 years to the current median age of 41 years.[35] The type of primary injury sustained depends on the mechanism of injury. The greatest cause of SCI is MVCs (38%), followed by falls (30%), violence (14.6%), and sports (9%).[35] The diagnosis of SCI begins with a detailed history of events surrounding the incident, precise evaluation of sensory and motor function, and radiographic studies of the spine.

BOX 33.6   Recommendations for Suctioning Patients With Traumatic Brain Injury

- Hyperoxygenate the patient on 100% fraction of inspired oxygen before each passage of suction catheter.
- Apply suction on removal of catheter for no longer than 10 s.
- Limit number of suction catheter passes, preferably to no more than two passes per suctioning episode.
- Minimize airway stimulation (eg, stabilize endotracheal tube, avoid passing suction catheter all the way to carina).

From McQuillan KA, Thurman P. Traumatic brain injuries. In: McQuillan K, et al, eds. *Trauma: From Resuscitation Through Rehabilitation*. St. Louis: Elsevier; 2009.

Pathophysiology

SCIs are the result of a mechanical force that disrupts neurologic tissue or its vascular supply or both. Similar to the pathophysiology of TBI, injury to the spinal cord occurs through both primary and secondary injury mechanisms. Primary injury is the neurologic and vascular damage that occurs at the moment of impact.[36] Secondary injury, which occurs within minutes of injury, refers to the complex biochemical processes affecting cellular function that occur from edema and vascular injury.[36]

Several events occur immediately after SCI that may lead to spinal cord ischemia and loss of neurologic function. A cascade of events includes systemic and local vascular changes, electrolyte and biochemical changes, neurotransmitter accumulation, and local edema (Box 33.7). Collectively, these pathophysiologic events result in exacerbation of the injury, potentially

BOX 33.7   Primary and Secondary Mechanisms of Acute Spinal Cord Injury

Primary Injury Mechanisms
- Acute compression
- Impact
- Missile
- Distraction
- Laceration
- Shear

Secondary Injury Mechanisms
- Systemic effects
- Heart rate: Brief increase, then prolonged bradycardia
- Blood pressure: Brief hypertension, then prolonged hypotension
- Decreased peripheral resistance
- Decreased cardiac output
- Increased (then decreased) levels of circulating catecholamines
- Hypoxia
- Hyperthermia
- Movement of unstable spine leading to worsening compression
- Local vascular changes
- Loss of autoregulation
- Systemic hypotension (neurogenic shock)
- Hemorrhage
- Loss of microcirculation
- Reduction in blood flow
- Vasospasm
- Thrombosis
- Possible electrolyte and acid–base imbalances

Biochemical Changes
- Neurotransmitter accumulation
- Catecholamines (eg, norepinephrine, dopamine)
- Excitotoxicity (eg, increased intracellular glutamate)
- Arachidonic acid release
- Free radical production
- Inflammatory cytokines
- Edema
- Loss of energy metabolism
- Decreased adenosine triphosphate production
- Apoptosis

Adapted from Sekhon LHS, Fehlings MG. Epidemiology, demographics, and pathophysiology of acute spinal cord injury. *Spine*. 2001;26(24S):S2.

extending the level of functional deficit and worsening long-term outcome. Knowledge of the pathophysiology of secondary processes has led to the development of newer therapies, which aim to target cellular changes contributing to injury. Despite ongoing research efforts at repairing primary SCI, minimizing damage by reducing secondary injury has shown the most promise.

How the Spinal Cord Is Injured

Hyperflexion, hyperextension, rotation, and axial loading are four distinct forces by which the spinal cord may be injured. The spinal cord may also be injured by penetrating trauma.

Hyperflexion. Hyperflexion injury is most often seen in the cervical area, especially at the level of C5-C6 because this is the most mobile portion of the cervical spine. This type of injury most often is caused by sudden deceleration motion, as in head-on collisions. Injury occurs from compression of the cord as a result of fracture fragments or dislocation of the vertebral bodies. Instability of the spinal column occurs because of rupture or tearing of the posterior muscles and ligaments.

Hyperextension. Hyperextension injuries involve backward and downward motion of the head. With this injury, often seen in rear-end collisions or MVCs, the spinal cord is stretched and distorted. Neurologic deficits associated with this injury are often caused by contusion and ischemia of the cord without significant bony involvement. *Whiplash* injury is a mild form of hyperextension.

Rotation. Rotation injuries often occur in conjunction with a flexion or extension injury. This may occur in cervical, thoracic, or lumbar sections of the cord. Severe rotation of the neck or body results in tearing of the posterior ligaments and displacement (rotation) of the spinal column.

Axial loading. Axial loading, or compression injury, occurs from vertical force along the spinal cord. This most commonly is seen in a fall from a height in which the person lands on the feet or buttocks. Compression injuries may cause *burst fractures* of the vertebral body that often send bony fragments into the spinal canal or directly into the spinal cord (Fig. 33.7).

Penetrating injuries. Penetrating injury to the spinal cord can be caused by a bullet, knife, or any other object that penetrates the cord. These types of injuries often cause permanent damage by anatomically transecting the spinal cord.

Functional Injury of the Spinal Cord

Functional injury of the spinal cord refers to the degree of disruption of normal spinal cord function. This depends on what specific sensory and motor structures within the cord are damaged. SCIs are classified as complete or incomplete. The most frequent diagnosis at discharge has been incomplete tetraplegia (45%) followed by complete paraplegia (21%).[35] SCI cannot be classified until spinal shock has resolved.

Complete injury. Complete SCI results in a total loss of sensory and motor function below the level of injury. Regardless of the mechanism of injury, the result is a complete dissection of the spinal cord and its neurochemical pathways, resulting in one of two conditions: tetraplegia or paraplegia.

Tetraplegia. With tetraplegia, the injury occurs between the C1-T1 level. Residual muscle function depends on the specific cervical segments involved. The potential functional status resulting from different neurologic levels of injury is described in Table 33.6.

Paraplegia. With paraplegia, the injury occurs in the thoracolumbar region (T2-L1). Patients with injuries in this area may have limited or full use of the arms, and all require a wheelchair. In rare circumstances, a few patients may have limited ability to ambulate short distances with crutches and orthoses. Thoracic L1 and L2 injuries produce paraplegia with variable innervation to intercostal and abdominal muscles.

Incomplete injury. Incomplete SCI results in a mixed loss of voluntary motor activity and sensation below the level of the lesion. Incomplete SCI exists if any function remains below the level of injury. Incomplete injuries can result in a variety

FIG. 33.7 Spinal Cord Compression Burst Fracture. Compression injuries cause burst fractures of the vertebral body that often send bony fragments into the spinal canal or directly into the spinal cord. Mechanisms of injury include hyperflexion, hyperextension, rotation, axial loading (vertical compression), and missile or penetrating injuries.

TABLE 33.6 Quadriplegia Functional Status	
Neurologic Level (Vertebrae) of Complete Injury	**Functional Ability**
C1-C4	Requires electric wheelchair with breath, head, or shoulder controls
C5	Needs electric wheelchair with hand control and/or manual wheelchair with rim projections; may require adaptive devices to assist with ADL
C6	Independent in manual wheelchair on level surface; may need hand controls; adaptive devices may be needed for ADL
C7	Requires manual wheelchair on most surfaces
C8-T1	May need adaptive devices

ADL, activities of daily living.

TABLE 33.7	**Muscle Strength Scale**
5 =	Active movement against maximal resistance
4 =	Active movement through ROM against resistance
3 =	Active movement through ROM against gravity
2 =	Active movement through ROM with gravity eliminated
1 =	Flicker or trace of contraction
0 =	No contraction; total paralysis

ROM, range of motion.

of syndromes, which are classified according to the degree of motor and sensory loss below the level of injury. Some of the more common incomplete injury syndromes are described here.

Brown-séquard syndrome. Brown-Séquard syndrome is associated with damage to only one side of the cord. This produces loss of voluntary motor movement on the same side as the injury, with loss of pain, temperature, and sensation on the opposite side. Functionally, the side of the body with the best motor control has little or no sensation, whereas the side of the body with sensation has little or no motor control.

Central cord syndrome. Central cord syndrome is associated with cervical hyperextension-hyperflexion injury and hematoma formation in the central areas of the cervical cord. This injury produces a motor and sensory deficit more pronounced in the upper extremities than in the lower extremities. Various degrees of bowel and bladder dysfunction may be present.

Anterior cord syndrome. Anterior cord syndrome is associated with injury to the anterior gray horn cells (motor), spinothalamic tracts (pain), anterior spinothalamic tract (light touch), and corticospinal tracts (temperature). The result is a loss of motor function and loss of the sensations of pain and temperature below the level of injury. However, below the level of injury, position sense and sensations of pressure and vibrations remain intact. Anterior cord syndrome is commonly caused by flexion injuries or acute herniation of an intervertebral disk.

Posterior cord syndrome. Posterior cord syndrome is associated with cervical hyperextension injury with damage to the posterior column. This results in the loss of position sense, pressure, and vibration below the level of injury. Motor function and sensation of pain and temperature remain intact. These patients may be unable to ambulate because the loss of position sense impairs spontaneous movement.

Nursing assessment for spinal cord injury. Screening of the spinal cord for injury is an integral part of the assessment for all trauma patients. However, the initial neurologic assessment may not be an accurate indication of eventual motor and sensory loss. The first assessment focuses on the rapid and accurate identification of present, absent, or impaired functioning of the motor, sensory, and reflex systems that coordinate and regulate vital functions. A detailed motor and sensory examination includes the assessment of all 32 spinal nerves for evidence of dysfunction. Carefully mapped pathways for the sensory portion of the spinal nerves, called *dermatomes,* can assist in localizing the functional sensory level of injury. The American Spinal Injury Association suggests that motor function may be graded on a 6-point scale (Table 33.7). Initial evaluation must be performed correctly, and findings must be thoroughly documented in detail so that subsequent serial assessments can rapidly identify deterioration. The American Spinal Injury Association has developed a form that outlines the required

assessments for initial and ongoing classification of SCIs (Fig. 33.8). Ongoing spinal cord assessments must be documented during the critical care phase.

Nursing assessment of a patient with spinal cord injury. On admission to the critical care unit, similar to patients with TBI and all other trauma patients, attention to the ABCs of the ATLS approach is imperative in a patient with known or suspected SCI. Ensuring a patent airway is of primary concern. Assessment of breathing patterns and gas exchange is done after the airway has been secured. The level of SCI often dictates the degree of altered breathing patterns that exists (Table 33.8). Because complete injuries above the C3 level result in paralysis of the diaphragm, patients with these injuries require intubation and mechanical ventilation.

Stabilization of the spinal cord is mandatory to prevent further injury, and spinal precautions are maintained until otherwise ordered. This includes stabilization of the head and neck with manual (handheld) traction during the initial assessment, intubation, and establishment of ventilatory support. Stabilization includes bed rest, a hard collar, and use of logrolling maneuvers until definitive stabilization is achieved.

Maintenance of hemodynamic stability, ensuring adequate tissue perfusion, is a necessary prerequisite to promote recovery of injured spinal cord tissue. Maintaining MAP greater than 85 to 90 mm Hg for the first 5 to 7 days helps maintain perfusion to the injured cord.[37] A patient with SCI is at high risk for or may exhibit alterations in cardiovascular stability, including dysrhythmias. In patients with SCI, it is imperative that the critical care nurse be able to distinguish the difference between hypovolemic shock, spinal shock, and neurogenic shock.

As discussed earlier, hypovolemic shock in trauma occurs in response to fluid volume deficit, often related to hemorrhage. *Spinal shock* is a condition that occurs shortly after traumatic injury to the spinal cord. Spinal shock is complete loss of all muscle tone and normal reflex activity below the level of injury,[9] including loss of rectal tone. In other words, spinal shock is a "concussion" of the spinal cord. Patients with spinal shock may appear completely without function below the area of injury, although not all of the area may be destroyed. It may occur 30 to 60 minutes after injury and may last 3 months.[38]

Neurogenic shock results from injury to the descending sympathetic pathways in the spinal cord. This injury results in loss of vasomotor tone and sympathetic innervation to the heart. Patients with SCI at T6 or above may have profound neurogenic shock as a result of interruption of the sympathetic nervous system and loss of vasoconstrictor response below the level of the injury. Hypotension, bradycardia, and peripheral vasodilation are hallmark signs and symptoms of neurogenic shock. Blood pressure support may be required with the use of sympathomimetic medications. The duration of this shock state can persist for 1 month after injury.

The mechanism of injury often assists trauma teams in distinguishing between these three types of shock. In hypovolemic shock, the patient is often tachycardic. In neurogenic shock, the patient is generally bradycardic. In spinal shock, priapism may be present.

Diagnostic procedures. Radiographic evaluations can identify the severity of damage to the spinal cord. On admission to the emergency department or critical care unit, initial evaluation should include anteroposterior and lateral x-ray views of all areas of the spinal cord. In many medical centers, CT scan has

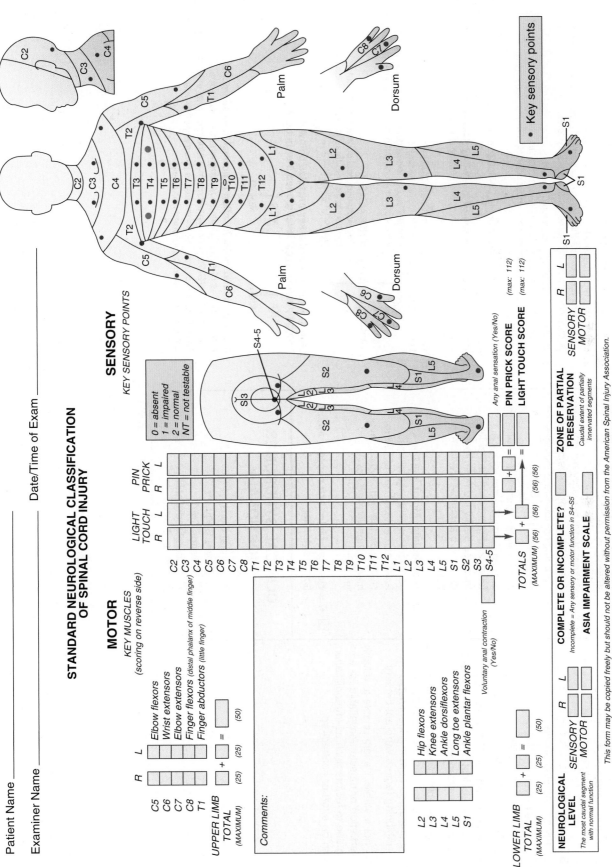

FIG. 33.8 American Spinal Injury Association Classification of Spinal Cord Injuries.

MUSCLE GRADING

0 total paralysis

1 palpable or visible contraction

2 active movement, full range of motion, gravity eliminated

3 active movement, full range of motion, against gravity

4 active movement, full range of motion, against gravity and provides some resistance

5 active movement, full range of motion, against gravity and provides normal resistance

5* muscle able to exert, in examiner's judgment, sufficient resistance to be considered normal if identifiable inhibiting factors were not present

NT not testable. Patient unable to reliably exert effort or muscle unavailable for testing due to factors such as immobilization, pain on effort or contracture.

ASIA IMPAIRMENT SCALE

☐ **A = Complete**: No motor or sensory function is preserved in the sacral segments S4-S5.

☐ **B = Incomplete**: Sensory but not motor function is preserved below the neurological level and includes the sacral segments S4-S5.

☐ **C = Incomplete**: Motor function is preserved below the neurological level, and more than half of key muscles below the neurological level have a muscle grade less than 3.

☐ **D = Incomplete**: Motor function is preserved below the neurological level, and at least half of key muscles below the neurological level have a muscle grade of 3 or more.

☐ **E = Normal**: Motor and sensory function are normal.

CLINICAL SYNDROMES (OPTIONAL)

☐ Central Cord
☐ Brown-Sequard
☐ Anterior Cord
☐ Conus Medullaris
☐ Cauda Equina

STEPS IN CLASSIFICATION

The following order is recommended in determining the classification of individuals with SCI.

1. Determine sensory levels for right and left sides.

2. Determine motor levels for right and left sides.
   Note: in regions where there is no myotome to test, the motor level is presumed to be the same as the sensory level.

3. Determine the single neurological level.
   This is the lowest segment where motor and sensory function is normal on both sides, and is the most cephalad of the sensory and motor levels determined in steps 1 and 2.

4. Determine whether the injury is Complete or Incomplete (sacral sparing).
   If voluntary anal contraction = **No** AND all S4-5 sensory scores = **0** AND any anal sensation = **No**, then injury is COMPLETE. Otherwise injury is incomplete.

5. Determine ASIA Impairment Scale (AIS) Grade:
   Is injury Complete?   If **YES**, AIS=A Record ZPP
   (For ZPP record lowest dermatome or myotome on each side with some (non-zero score) preservation)

   NO →

   Is injury motor incomplete? If **NO**, AIS=B
   (Yes=voluntary anal contraction OR motor function more than three levels below the motor level on a given side.)

   YES →

   Are at least half of the key muscles below the (single) neurological level graded 3 or better?

   NO → AIS=C   YES → AIS=D

If sensation and motor function is normal in all segments, AIS=E
Note: AIS E is used in follow up testing when an individual with a documented SCI has recovered normal function. If at initial testing no deficits are found, the individual is neurologically intact; the ASIA Impairment Scale does not apply.

FIG. 33.8 cont'd

TABLE 33.8 Effects of Spinal Cord Injury on Ventilatory Functions

Neurologic Level (Vertebrae) of Complete Injury	Respiratory Function	Comment
C1-C2	Paralysis of diaphragm	Ventilator dependent
C3-C5	Various degrees of diaphragm paralysis	Some diaphragm control; may need ventilatory support; weaning depends on preinjury pulmonary status
C6-T11	Various degrees of impaired intercostal muscles and abdominal muscles	Compromised respiratory function; reduced inspiratory ability; paradoxical breathing patterns; ineffective cough, sneeze

TABLE 33.9 EAST Guidelines for Cervical Spine Clearance

Trauma Patient Population	Recommendation
Trauma patients who are awake, alert, not intoxicated, neurologically normal, no complaints of neck pain or tenderness with full range of motion of cervical spine	Neck is palpated in all directions for tenderness or pain. If physical examination is negative for pain or tenderness, CT of cervical spine is not required, and cervical collar may be removed.
All other trauma patients with suspected cervical injury must be radiologically evaluated, including patients with neck pain or tenderness, whether alert or with altered mental status/neurologic deficit, or distracting injury	Obtain axial CT from occiput to T1 with sagittal and coronal reconstructions. If CT is positive for injury, continue cervical collar, obtain spine consultation, and obtain MRI. In neurologically intact awake patient with neck pain, if CT is negative (no injury seen), MRI is negative, and adequate flexion/extension radiographs are negative, discontinue cervical collar.
Trauma patients who are obtunded with gross motor function of extremities	Obtain axial CT from occiput to T1 with sagittal and coronal reconstructions. If CT is negative (no injury seen), risk/benefit of additional MRI must be determined in each hospital. Options A. Continue cervical collar until clinical examination can be performed. B. Remove cervical collar on the basis of negative CT alone. C. Obtain MRI. If MRI is negative, collar can be safely removed. Flexion/extension radiographs should not be performed.

CT, computed tomography; *EAST*, Eastern Association of Surgeons in Trauma; *MRI*, magnetic resonance imaging.
Modified from Como JJ, et al. Practice management guidelines for identification of cervical spine injuries following trauma: Update from the Eastern Association for the Surgery of Trauma Practice Management Guidelines Committee. *J Trauma*. 2009;67(3):651.

replaced plain radiography as the principal modality for cervical spine assessment after trauma.[38,39] CT scan of all seven cervical vertebrae and the top of T1 must be obtained to rule out cervicothoracic injury. Flexion and extension views can identify subtle ligament injuries. MRI may also be used for definitive diagnosis of SCI.

The assessment and authorization to remove the cervical collar, known as *clearance of the cervical spine* is challenging in a patient with SCI in the critical care unit. Clearance of the cervical spine is made difficult by alteration in mentation as a result of coexisting injury, analgesia, and sedation; intubation and mechanical ventilation; surgical procedures; and a focus on other, more distracting injuries. The Eastern Association of Surgeons in Trauma developed guidelines for clearance of the cervical spine (Table 33.9).[40]

Medical Management

After assessment and diagnosis of SCI, medical management begins. The primary treatment goal is to preserve remaining neurologic function with either surgical or nonsurgical interventions.

Surgical management. Surgical intervention provides spinal column stability in the presence of an unstable injury. Unstable injuries include disrupted ligaments and tendons and a vertebral column that cannot maintain normal alignment. Identification and immobilization of unstable injuries are particularly important for a patient with incomplete neurologic deficit. Without adequate stabilization, movement and dislocation of the vertebral column may cause a complete neurologic deficit. Various surgical procedures may be performed to achieve decompression (relief of pressure on spinal nerves) and stabilization.

Laminectomy. In the laminectomy procedure, the lamina of the vertebral ring is removed to allow decompression and removal of bony fragments or material from the spinal canal.

Spinal fusion. Spinal fusion involves surgical fusion of two to six vertebral bodies to provide stability and to prevent motion. This may be accomplished by an anterior or posterior surgical approach. Fusion is accomplished through the use of bone chips taken from the iliac crest, bone bank, or artificial bone substitute and by use of wires, pins, or rods.

Other Spinal Cord Surgical Options. Pedicle screw fixation has become the treatment of choice for thoracic and lumbar fracture fixation.[41] This procedure helps stabilize fractured thoracic and lumbar segments of the spinal column. Vertebral plates and bone grafting are also used.

Nonsurgical Management. If the injury to the spinal cord is stable, nonsurgical management is the treatment of choice. Nonsurgical management for cervical and thoracolumbar injuries is discussed in this section.

Cervical Injury. Management of cervical injuries involves the immobilization of the fracture and realignment of any dislocation. This is accomplished through skeletal traction that involves the use of two-point tongs, which are inserted into the skull through shallow burr holes and are connected to weights. Several types of cervical tongs are used. Gardner-Wells and Crutchfield tongs are the most common. These tongs can be applied at the bedside by experienced personnel with the use of a local anesthetic. Weights are applied gradually, with frequent neurologic and radiographic evaluations, until the fracture is reduced (realigned).

After the procedure, the patient must be immobilized on a kinetic therapy bed or a regular bed. The kinetic therapy bed is preferred for cervical immobilization because it maintains alignment of the spinal column, while providing a constant turning motion to reduce pulmonary complications and incidence of skin breakdown.[42] Use of cervical skeletal traction on a regular bed is possible, but it is more difficult to provide adequate care to the pulmonary and integumentary systems because of the extensive degree of immobility.

Halo traction braces are also used for patients with a cervical spine injury. The halo vest consists of a metal ring secured to the skull with two occipital and two temporal screws. The metal ring is attached to steel bars that anchor to the plastic vest to provide cervical immobilization (Fig. 33.9). The halo traction brace immobilizes the cervical spine but allows the patient to ambulate and participate in self-care.

Thoracolumbar Injury. Nonsurgical management of a patient with a thoracolumbar injury is undertaken in the absence of neurologic injury. Generally, this approach frequently involves immobilization. Immobilization is accomplished by bed rest (with the bed flat) or the use of a plastic or fiberglass jacket, a body cast, or a brace, which facilitates early mobility. There is no consensus on the optimal treatment.[41]

Nursing Management

Nursing diagnoses and management for the patient with SCI are summarized in Box 33.8. The goal during the critical care phase is to maintain hemodynamic stability and prevent potentially life-threatening complications, while maximizing the function of all organ systems. Nursing interventions are aimed at preventing secondary damage to the spinal cord and managing the complications of the neurologic deficit. Because almost all body systems are affected by SCI, nursing management must include interventions that promote optimal functioning of each system. Moreover, patients with SCIs have complex psychosocial needs that require a great deal of emotional support from the critical care nurse.

FIG. 33.9 Halo Vest. The halo traction brace immobilizes the cervical spine, which allows the patient to ambulate and participate in self-care.

Neurologic care. Assessment, monitoring, and trending of the patient's GCS score and sensory and motor function are important aspects of nursing the SCI patient in critical care. The use of methylprednisolone as a neuroprotective agent in SCI is controversial.[37] There is no clear consensus on the efficacy of this drug or any other drug in enhancing recovery of cord function after injury.[39] When methylprednisolone is given, the risks of gastrointestinal hemorrhage and wound infection must be considered carefully.

Cardiovascular care. Management of acute cervical SCI involves close hemodynamic monitoring. Current guidelines for the management of acute cervical SCI cite that hypotension (systolic blood pressure less than 90 mm Hg) should be avoided or corrected as soon as possible after acute SCI.[39] It is also considered an option to maintain the MAP at 85 to 90 mm Hg for the first 5 to 7 days after acute SCI to improve spinal cord perfusion.[37,43]

The risk for cardiovascular instability is profound in patients with SCI at the C3-C5 levels, although cardiovascular alterations occur with most injuries above T6. Symptomatic bradyarrhythmias may be treated with an inotropic medication such as isoproterenol or anticholinergic medication such as atropine. Both medications increase heart rate but also increase myocardial oxygen consumption. Another option may be a temporary transcutaneous or transvenous pacemaker.

Alteration in tissue perfusion because of hypotension may require administration of IV fluids. After the fluid volume status has been optimized, inotropic or vasopressor support, or both, may be implemented if systolic blood pressure or MAP remains low. Accurate assessment of fluid volume status is required because pulmonary edema is a threat to patients with SCI.

As with any immobilized patient, the risk for development of deep vein thrombosis (DVT) is high. However, detection of DVT is difficult because pain and tenderness are not applicable to a patient with SCI. Prevention of DVT is imperative and may include a combination of therapies such as low-dose heparin, low-molecular-weight heparin, sequential compression devices, and embolic hose.

Pulmonary care. Pulmonary complications are the most common cause of mortality in patients with SCI.[44] Initial and ongoing nursing assessments of respiratory status are vital for identifying actual or potential impairment in ventilation. Evaluations include observation of respiratory rate and rhythm, observation of symmetry of chest expansion and use

---

◎ **BOX 33.8   NURSING DIAGNOSES**

Spinal Cord Injury

- Impaired Gas Exchange related to alveolar hypoventilation, p. 1030
- Ineffective Breathing Pattern related to decreased lung expansion, p. 1035
- Ineffective Breathing Pattern related to musculoskeletal fatigue or neuromuscular impairment, p. 1035
- Decreased Cardiac Output related to sympathetic blockade, p. 1017
- Autonomic Dysreflexia related to excessive autonomic response to noxious stimuli, p. 1013
- Disturbed Body Image related to actual change in body structure, function, or appearance, p. 1022
- Ineffective Coping related to situational crisis and personal vulnerability, p. 1036

of accessory muscles, inspection of quantity and character of secretions, and auscultation of breath sounds. Serial ABG values provide information on the adequacy of gas exchange.

Intubation and mechanical ventilation are frequently required in acute SCI. The critical care nurse must be aware that the neuromuscular blocking agent *succinylcholine* (suxamethonium) should not be administered to patients with SCI. Use of this depolarizing agent in a patient with SCI not only may aggravate existing injury as a result of fasciculation during induction but also may produce hyperkalemic cardiac arrest.

Patients with lesions at C3 to C5 may eventually be able to be weaned from the ventilator. Some patients with C3 injuries may require mechanical ventilation only at night. Weaning can be a complex process because of the physiologic demands placed on the diaphragm and the psychological effects of fear of the inability to breathe. Various weaning methods are available, and a well-coordinated approach by the nurse, physician, respiratory therapist, and patient is essential. Weaning difficulties are common, and reintubation may be required.

Ineffective airway clearance and impaired gas exchange is a particular problem for a patient with SCI as a result of hypoventilation (paralysis of respiratory muscles), increased bronchial secretions, and atelectasis secondary to decreased cough. Nursing interventions are directed at improving and maintaining adequate gas exchange.

Frequent suctioning of the airway is required. Caution must be used with vigorous suctioning because stimulation of the vagus nerve (which runs alongside the trachea) can cause profound bradycardia. Hyperoxygenation with 100% oxygen before suctioning is recommended.

Chest percussion and repositioning facilitate removal of secretions. Kinetic therapy beds, which can rotate up to 60 degrees on each side, may provide continual postural drainage and mobilization of secretions. To further aid in mobilizing secretions in the presence of an ineffective cough, a technique of cough assistance can be used (Fig. 33.10). This procedure is similar to abdominal thrusts (formerly known as the Heimlich maneuver). Exact hand placement may vary, and it is important to assess which placement works best for the patient. Cough assist machines are also commercially available.

Gastrointestinal and genitourinary care. Initially after SCI, bowel and bladder tone are flaccid. Abdominal distention, constipation, and fecal impaction are major problems

encountered in care of patients with SCI. Innervation between the brain and defecation center in the sacral cord has been disrupted. A bowel program to prevent fecal impaction and encourage normal, regular bowel function may be initiated in the critical care phase. The patient should not go longer than 3 to 4 days without a bowel movement. Laxatives and stool softeners may be needed, especially if the patient is receiving opiates. Aspects of a successful bowel program include consistent timing of evacuation, proper positioning, physical activity, appropriate fluid intake, a high-fiber diet, and reflex stimulation for patients with upper motor neuron injuries.[38,44] Bowel retraining is a major focus of the intermediate care and rehabilitation phase of treatment.

The degree of bladder and urinary sphincter dysfunction depends on the location and completeness of the injury. A Foley catheter is placed on admission, but it should be removed 3 to 4 days later (if possible), at which time the patient is placed on an intermittent catheterization schedule of every 4 to 6 hours. It is not unusual for male patients with an upper motor neuron injury to experience a reflexogenic erection when being catheterized. An overdistended bladder in a patient with an injury at T6 or above may trigger autonomic dysreflexia.

Autonomic dysreflexia is a life-threatening complication that occurs most commonly in the first year after SCI. This condition is caused by a massive sympathetic response to a noxious stimuli (eg, full bladder, fecal impaction) that results in severe hypertension, bradycardia, facial flushing, and pounding headache.[38] Immediate intervention is needed to prevent cerebral hemorrhage and seizures. Treatment is aimed at alleviating the noxious stimuli. Suggestions for treatment of autonomic dysreflexia are provided in Box 33.9.

Integumentary and musculoskeletal care. Patients with SCI are at extremely high risk for pressure ulcers because of the lack of motor control and sensation. Prevention is the best treatment. Diligent assessments, meticulous skin care, and frequent position changes are required. Any evidence of skin breakdown or pressure ulcer development should be assessed, documented, and reported immediately to the most appropriate provider. Specialty surfaces or low-air-loss beds may be necessary for the prevention of pressure ulcers in patients with SCI.

FIG. 33.10 Cough Assistance. One hand or both hands are placed over the upper diaphragm. After the patient inhales, pressure is directed inward and upward as the patient attempts to cough.

BOX 33.9 Autonomic Dysreflexia

- If patient is supine, immediately sit the patient up.
- Begin frequent vital sign monitoring including blood pressure every 5 min.
- Loosen clothing and constrictive devices.
- Immediately begin assessment for underlying cause.
- If indwelling catheter is not placed, catheterize the patient.
- If indwelling catheter is present, do the following:
  - Check system for kinks and obstructions to flow.
  - Irrigate the bladder with small sterile amount of fluid, using strict aseptic technique.
  - If not draining, remove the catheter and replace.
- If acute symptoms persist, suspect fecal impaction:
  - Perform digital examination to check for presence of stool; if present, gently remove.
  - If no stool is found and the abdomen is distended, consider administration of laxative.
- If systolic blood pressure is greater than 150 mm Hg, consider rapid-onset, short-duration antihypertensive agent.
- Do not hesitate to call for immediate medical assistance.

Immobilized patients are at high risk for contractures. When a muscle is denervated, as in the case of SCI, muscle fibers shorten and produce a contracture. Irreversible contractures may result in skin breakdown, inability to perform activities of daily living, poor wheelchair posture, and inability to use adaptive devices. Physical therapy and occupational therapy personnel should be consulted early in the patient's hospitalization. Range-of-motion exercises are initiated as soon as the spine has been stabilized. Footdrop splints should be applied on admission to prevent contractures and prevent skin breakdown of the heels. Hand splints should be applied for quadriplegics. Hand and foot splints should be removed every 2 hours, and the extremities should be examined for evidence of skin breakdown. Nursing management of a patient in skull traction or halo vest includes inspection of pins and traction for security, correct positioning, and maintenance of skin integrity. Traction bars of the halo vest must never be used to lift or reposition the patient, and a wrench must be secured on the front of the vest at all times in case of cardiac arrest.

Another consequence of sympathetic nervous system dysfunction is loss of thermoregulation (*poikilothermy*), in which body temperature is regulated by the external environment. Use of heat or cold for therapeutic or comfort measures may be required but must be used cautiously. Profound changes in body temperature must be avoided. Before antipyretics are given for hyperthermia, a cooling blanket is typically used. Hypothermia can produce bradyarrhythmias and sinus arrest and may impair wound healing.

Maximizing psychosocial adaptation. Nursing management of the patient with SCI must include the provision of dedicated emotional support. In the critical care unit, the patient, family, and significant others often experience anxiety, grief, denial, anger, frustration, and hopelessness because of the nature of the injury, profound and immediate changes required in lifestyle, and the fact that long-term neurologic deficits may remain unknown.

Appropriate nursing interventions include promotion of support systems, which often involve family and friends, and use of coping mechanisms and adaptive skills. Simple, accurate, and consistent information can alleviate fear and anxiety. Feelings of powerlessness may be reduced by including the patient and family in patient care and decision making. Further psychosocial support can be provided by social workers, occupational therapists, psychiatric nurses, and members of the clergy.

Maxillofacial Injuries

Trauma to the face may result in complex physiologic and psychological sequelae. Vital functions that depend on facial integrity include mastication, deglutination, perception of the environment (eg, vision, hearing, speech, olfaction), and respiration. The face represents a direct link to self and to expression by playing a major role in personal identity, appearance, and communication. Consequently, maxillofacial trauma has the potential to produce long-term adverse effects, with varying degrees of sensory, emotional, and psychosocial consequences.

Maxillofacial injury results from blunt or penetrating trauma. Blunt trauma for this injury is exemplified by the unbelted driver or passenger who is thrown into the dashboard or windshield. Associated injuries may include concussion, skull fracture, rhinorrhea, SCI, and fractures of other bones. The facial skeleton serves as an energy-absorbing shield to protect the brain, spinal cord, eyes, and pharynx. Nasal bones, the zygoma, and the mandibular condyle are the most susceptible to fracture. Bullet wounds can be life-threatening injuries because of hemorrhage and airway obstruction. Maxillofacial trauma can result in soft tissue injury ranging from abrasions to destruction of most of the face with accompanying maxillofacial skeletal fractures.

Maxillofacial skeletal injuries. Fractures of the maxilla are diagnosed according to the *Le Fort classification.* Le Fort fractures are classified in three broad categories, depending on the level of the fracture (Fig. 33.11). The most common, Le Fort I, consists of horizontal fractures in which the entire palate moves separately from the lower maxilla (floating palate). Le Fort II fractures are an extension of Le Fort I fractures and resemble a pyramidal fracture. They involve the orbit, ethmoid, and nasal bones (floating maxilla). In a Le Fort III fracture, there is complete craniofacial disruption (floating face). Often associated with severe skull and brain injuries, CSF frequently leaks with Le Fort II and III fractures because there is usually communication between the cranial base and the cribriform

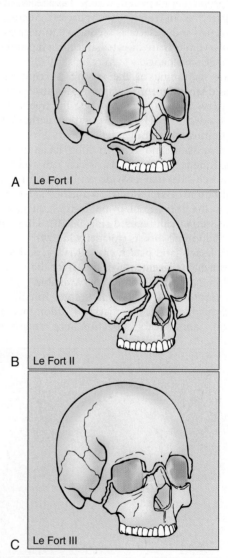

FIG. 33.11 Le Fort Classification. Fractures of the maxillae are diagnosed according to the Le Fort classification, which consists of three broad categories based on the level of the fracture. (A) Le Fort I. (B) Le Fort II. (C) Le Fort III.

plate. A combination of Le Fort fractures is often observed in patients with multisystem trauma.[45]

Physical Assessment and Diagnostic Procedures

Life-threatening complications associated with maxillofacial trauma include airway obstruction and head and cervical spine injuries. Major or minor facial deformities should not distract the trauma team from the standardized ABCDE approach of ATLS primary and secondary surveys.

Patients with maxillofacial trauma are at high risk for ineffective airway clearance. The tongue, edema, hemorrhage, foreign objects, vomit, broken teeth, or bone fragments can obstruct the airway. The "look, listen, and feel" methods (see Table 33.2) should be used to assess airway obstruction. An artificial airway may be required. An oral endotracheal tube may be used unless there is a laryngeal fracture. Nasotracheal or nasogastric intubation is contraindicated in the presence of unstable facial fractures because a fracture of the cribriform plate may exist, and the tube could be inadvertently placed through the fractured base of the cranium and into the brain.[9] In severe maxillofacial trauma, a surgical airway (tracheostomy) may be the best choice for patients with hypopharynx swelling or hemorrhage.[46]

Patients with maxillofacial trauma are also at risk for fluid volume deficit related to hemorrhage as a result of bleeding from the ethmoid or maxillary sinuses. Profuse bleeding through the nares may occur with nasal fractures, maxillary fractures, or cranial base fractures. Control of bleeding with nasal packing, ligation, or arterial embolization may be required.[46] IV fluids are administered to correct deficient fluid volume status.

During the secondary survey, a comprehensive examination of facial structures is begun as part of the head-to-toe assessment. Assessment of the face involves careful inspection and palpation of the orbit and soft tissues. A small abrasion or contusion of the face may seem unobtrusive, but the impact to the underlying structures might have disrupted facial bone integrity, the parotid gland, or facial nerve. The mouth is inspected for traumatic tooth dislodgment, recognizing that some teeth may intrude into the underlying alveolar bone. The ear canal is inspected for occult lacerations of the tympanic membrane.

Maxillofacial trauma often is associated with TBI and cervical SCI. An altered level of consciousness in the presence of maxillofacial fractures strongly suggests neurotrauma. Fractures involving the cranium and tearing of dura mater may enable oral bacterial flora to enter the CSF, placing the patient at risk for meningitis. Nasal and auditory canals must be inspected for discharge. The presence of rhinorrhea or otorrhea should be immediately reported to the physician, and a sample should be tested for glucose to help confirm the drainage is CSF.

CT scan determines the location and displacement of fractures.[9] MRI is also valuable in assessing associated head, neck, and vascular structures for injury and extent of trauma.

Medical Management

Treatment of Le Fort fractures includes direct visualization and reduction of the fragments and stabilization with wires, plates, and screws.

Nursing Management

Nursing diagnoses for the patient with maxillofacial trauma are listed in Box 33.10. Nursing interventions are aimed at maintaining and protecting the airway by reducing the risk of emesis and aspiration. Proper orogastric tube functioning must

be ensured. Antiemetics may be administered. Unless contraindicated, the head of the bed is elevated 30 degrees. If vomiting occurs, the patient is immediately placed in a side-lying or forward position and oral or nasal suctioning is used. If the mandible has been wired postoperatively, wire cutters must be available at the bedside in case of vomiting. Although seldom necessary, the intention in cutting the wires is to prevent aspiration.

Thoracic Injuries

Thoracic injuries involve trauma to the chest wall, lungs, heart, great vessels, and esophagus. Blunt thoracic trauma to the chest most often is caused by MVCs or falls. Second only to head injury or SCI, thoracic injuries account for 25% of trauma deaths.[47] Various mechanisms of blunt trauma are associated with specific injury patterns. In penetrating thoracic injury, the object involved determines the degree of damage sustained to underlying structures. Low-velocity weapons (eg, .22-caliber gun, knife) usually damage only what is in the direct path of the weapon. However, stab wounds that involve the anterior chest wall between the midclavicular lines, the angle of Louis, and the epigastric region are of particular concern because of the proximity of the heart and great vessels.

Specific Thoracic Traumatic Injuries

Chest wall injuries

Rib fractures. Fractures of the ribs can be serious and life-threatening, particularly when there are three or more rib fractures, when preexisting disease (especially cardiopulmonary disease) is present, or when the patient is elderly. Fractures of the first and second ribs are frequently associated with intrathoracic vascular injuries (eg, brachial plexus, great vessels), and because they are protected by the scapula, clavicle, humerus, and muscles, they signify a very high degree of force applied to the thorax.[9] Fractures to the middle ribs may be associated with lung injury, including pulmonary contusion and pneumothorax. Fractures to the lower ribs (7th to 12th) may be associated with abdominal injury, such as spleen and liver injuries.

Localized pain that increases with respiration or that is elicited by rib compression may indicate rib fractures. The pain associated with rib fractures can be aggravated by respiratory excursion. The patient often splints the fractured ribs, takes shallow breaths, and may refuse to cough. This can result in atelectasis and pneumonia. Definitive diagnosis of rib fractures can be made with a chest x-ray.

Interventions include pain control to improve chest expansion and facilitate gas exchange, chest physiotherapy, and early mobilization. The primary goal of pain management in patients

---

◎ BOX 33.10 NURSING DIAGNOSES

Maxillofacial Trauma

- Risk for Aspiration risk factors impaired pharyngeal peristalsis or tongue function; impaired laryngeal sensation or reflex; impaired laryngeal closure or elevation, p. 1040
- Potential for deficient Fluid Volume related to hemorrhage, p. 1019
- Acute Pain related to transmission and perception of cutaneous, visceral, muscular, or ischemic impulses, p. 1010
- Imbalanced Nutrition: Less Than Body Requirements related to lack of exogenous nutrients and increased metabolic demands, p. 1029

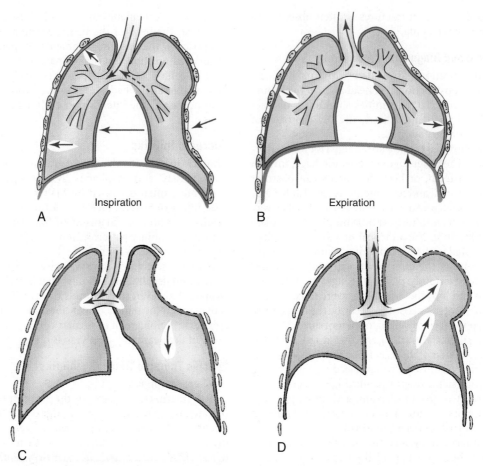

FIG. 33.12 Flail Chest. (A) Normal inspiration. (B) Normal expiration. (C) The area of the lung underlying the unstable chest wall sucks in on inspiration. (D) The same area balloons out on expiration. Notice the movement of the mediastinum toward the opposite lung on inspiration.

with rib fractures is patient comfort and prevention of pulmonary complications. Pain management interventions must be tailored to the individual patient and response to therapy. Nonsteroidal antiinflammatory drugs, intercostal nerve blocks, thoracic epidural analgesia, and opiates may be considered.[48] External splints are not recommended because they may further limit chest wall expansion and add to atelectasis. Surgical plating of fractured ribs is controversial.[49]

Flail chest. Flail chest, caused by blunt trauma, disrupts the continuity of chest wall structures. Typically, a flail segment occurs when two or more ribs are fractured in two or more places and are no longer attached to the thoracic cage, producing a free-floating segment of the chest wall. A flail chest is a clinical diagnosis wherein the so-called flail segment (or floating segment) moves paradoxically compared with the rest of the chest wall (Fig. 33.12).[28] During inspiration, the intact portion of the chest wall expands while the injured part is sucked in. During expiration, the chest wall moves in, and the flail segment moves out. Although the flail segment increases the work of breathing, the main cause of hypoxemia is often underlying pulmonary contusions.[50] The physiologic effects of impaired chest wall motion of a flail chest include decreased tidal volume and vital capacity and impaired cough, which lead to hypoventilation and atelectasis.

Inspection of the thorax reveals paradoxical chest movement. Palpation of the chest may indicate crepitus and tenderness near fractured ribs. A chest x-ray reveals multiple rib fractures. Evidence of hypoxemia may be demonstrated by ABGs, but this does not aid in the diagnosis. Interventions focus on ensuring adequate oxygenation and analgesia to improve ventilation.[48] Intubation and mechanical ventilation may be required.

Ruptured diaphragm. Diagnosis of a diaphragmatic rupture is often missed in trauma patients initially because of the subtle and nonspecific symptoms of this injury. The mechanism of injury appears to be a rapid rise in intraabdominal pressure (IAP) as a result of blunt force applied to the lower part of the chest or upper region of the abdomen.[51] This injury can occur when a person is thrown forward over the edge of the steering wheel in a high-speed MVC. The diaphragm, which offers little resistance to the force, can rupture or tear as a result of high-velocity impact or fractured ribs. Abdominal viscera can gradually enter the thoracic cavity. Massive herniation of abdominal contents into the thoracic cavity can compress the lungs and mediastinum, which decreases venous return, decreases cardiac output, and impairs tissue perfusion. Herniated bowel can become strangulated and perforate. Diaphragmatic rupture can be life-threatening.

Diaphragmatic rupture can produce nonspecific findings, making diagnosis difficult in a busy trauma room. The patient may complain of shoulder pain, shortness of breath, or abdominal tenderness. Auscultation of bowel sounds in the chest or unilateral breath sounds may indicate a ruptured diaphragm.

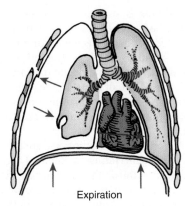

Inspiration   Expiration

FIG. 33.13 Tension Pneumothorax. Tension pneumothorax usually is caused by an injury that perforates the chest wall or pleural space. Air flows into the pleural space with inspiration and becomes trapped. As pressure in the pleural space increases, the lung on the injured side collapses and causes the mediastinum to shift to the opposite side. (From Marx J, et al. Rosen's Emergency Medicine: Concepts and Clinical Practice. 5th ed. St. Louis: Mosby; 2002.)

There may or may not be significant compromise and changes in respiratory effort. A high index of clinical suspicion is required to assist with diagnosis. A chest radiograph may reveal the tip of a nasogastric tube above the diaphragm, a unilaterally elevated hemidiaphragm, a hollow or solid mass above the diaphragm, and a shift of the mediastinum away from the affected side. CT scan and MRI are useful for the evaluation of diaphragmatic injuries in stable trauma patients. Treatment of a ruptured diaphragm includes surgical repair.

Pulmonary injuries

Pulmonary contusion. A pulmonary contusion is a bruise of the lung. Pulmonary contusion is often associated with blunt trauma and other chest injuries, such as rib fractures and flail chest. Pulmonary contusions can occur unilaterally or bilaterally. A contusion manifests initially as a hemorrhage, followed by alveolar and interstitial edema. The edema can remain localized in the contused part or can spread to other areas of the lung. Inflammation negatively affects gas exchange across the alveolar-capillary membrane. As inflammation and edema increase, a decrease in respiratory compliance, increased resistance, and decreased pulmonary blood flow may occur. These processes cause a ventilation-perfusion imbalance that results in progressive hypoxemia and poor ventilation.

Clinical manifestations of pulmonary contusion may take 72 hours after injury to develop.[50] Inspection of the chest wall may reveal ecchymosis at the site of impact. Diminished breath sounds and coarse crackles may be auscultated over the contused lung. The patient may have a cough and blood-tinged sputum. Abnormal lung function can manifest as arterial hypoxemia. Diagnosis is made primarily by imaging studies consistent with pulmonary infiltrates corresponding to the area of external chest impact that manifest within 12 to 24 hours of injury. Pulmonary contusions tend to worsen over 24 to 72 hours after injury and then slowly resolve unless complications occur (eg, infection, ARDS).

Aggressive respiratory care is the cornerstone of care for non-intubated patients with pulmonary contusion. Interventions may include deep-breathing exercises, incentive spirometry, early mobilization, or noninvasive positive pressure ventilation.[48] Chest physiotherapy may not be tolerated if there are coexisting rib fractures. Adequate pain control is achieved with administration of nonsteroidal antiinflammatory drugs,

opiates, intercostal nerve blocks, or thoracic epidural analgesia. Removal of airway secretions is important to avoid infection and to improve ventilation. Patients with unilateral contusions are placed with the injured side up and uninjured side down ("good lung down"). This positioning helps correct the existing ventilation-perfusion mismatch.[50]

Patients with severe contusions may continue to show decompensation, such as respiratory acidosis and increased work of breathing, despite aggressive nursing management. Endotracheal intubation and mechanical ventilation with *positive end-expiratory pressure* (PEEP) may be required. Complications resulting from pulmonary contusions include pneumonia, ARDS, lung abscesses, and pulmonary embolism.

Pneumothoraces in trauma. Pleural damage is common in trauma. These conditions include *pneumothorax* (air in the pleural space), *hemothorax* (blood in the pleural space), or *hemopneumothorax* (air and blood in the pleural space). Pneumothoraces may be managed with chest tubes, analgesia, and surgical consultation, depending on the size of the pneumothorax, hemodynamic stability of the patient, and effects on oxygenation and ventilation. *Tension pneumothorax, open pneumothorax,* and *massive hemothorax,* three additional and potentially life-threatening respiratory problems in trauma, warrant special consideration.

Tension pneumothorax. A tension pneumothorax is caused by an injury that perforates the chest wall or pleural space. Air flows into the pleural space with inspiration and becomes trapped. As pressure in the pleural space increases, the lung on the injured side collapses and causes the mediastinum to shift to the opposite side (Fig. 33.13). As pressure continues to build, the shift exerts pressure on the heart and thoracic aorta, which results in decreased venous return and decreased cardiac output. Tissue perfusion is further hindered because the collapsed lung does not participate in gas exchange.

Clinical manifestations of a tension pneumothorax include dyspnea; tachycardia; hypotension; and sudden chest pain extending to the back, neck, or shoulders. Tracheal deviation (a late sign in tension pneumothorax) can be observed as the trachea shifts away from the injured side. On the injured side, breath sounds may be decreased or absent. Percussion of the chest reveals a hyperresonant sound over the affected side. Diagnosis of tension pneumothorax is made by clinical assessment.

When a tension pneumothorax is suspected in a trauma patient, there is no time for a chest x-ray because this potentially lethal condition must be treated at once.[9] Needle decompression, in which a large-bore (14-gauge) needle is inserted over the second rib on the affected side, is the immediate treatment of choice. This procedure allows release of air from the pleural space. A hissing sound is heard as the tension pneumothorax is converted to a simple pneumothorax. A chest tube is inserted after needle decompression.

Open pneumothorax. An open pneumothorax ("sucking chest wound") is caused by penetrating trauma. Large thoracic wounds (greater than two-thirds the diameter of the trachea) open communication between the atmosphere and intrathoracic cavity.[9] As air moves in and out of the hole in the chest, a sucking sound can be heard on inspiration. Respiratory mechanics become impaired. An open pneumothorax produces the same symptoms as a tension pneumothorax. Subcutaneous emphysema may be palpated around the wound.

Initial management of an open pneumothorax is accomplished by promptly inserting a chest tube. If a chest tube is not immediately available, covering the wound at end expiration with a sterile occlusive dressing, taped securely on three sides and large enough to overlap the edges of the wound, should be used.[9] As the patient breathes in, the dressing gets sucked in to occlude the wound and prevent air from entering the thoracic cavity. On expiration, the dressing moves out permitting the patient to exhale. Surgical intervention may be required to close the wound.

Hemothorax. Blunt or penetrating thoracic trauma can cause bleeding into the pleural space, resulting in a hemothorax (Fig. 33.14). A massive hemothorax results from the accumulation of more than 1500 mL of blood in the thoracic cavity.[28] The source of bleeding may be the intercostal or internal mammary arteries, lungs, heart, or great vessels. Lacerations to the lung parenchyma are low-pressure bleeds and typically stop bleeding spontaneously. Arterial bleeding from hilar vessels usually requires immediate surgical intervention. Increasing vascular blood loss into the pleural space causes decreased venous return and decreased cardiac output.

For patients with massive hemothorax, assessment findings reveal diminished or absent breath sounds over the affected lung and collapsed neck veins. Massive hemothorax can be diagnosed on the basis of clinical manifestations of hypotension associated with the absence of breath sounds or dullness to percussion on one side of the chest.[9,28] Hypovolemic shock may be present.

This potentially life-threatening condition must be treated immediately. Resuscitation with IV fluids is initiated to treat the hypovolemic shock. A chest tube is placed on the affected side to allow drainage of blood. An autotransfusion device can be attached to the chest tube collection chamber. Thoracotomy may be necessary for patients who require persistent blood transfusions or who have significant bleeding (200 mL/h for 2 to 4 hours or more than 1500 mL on initial tube insertion) or when there are accompanying injuries to major cardiovascular structures.[9]

Cardiac and vascular injuries. Cardiac and vascular injuries can result from either blunt or penetrating trauma. The most common causes of blunt cardiac trauma include high-speed MVCs, direct blows to the chest, and falls. Because of its mobility and its location between the sternum and thoracic vertebrae, the heart is susceptible to blunt traumatic injury. Sudden acceleration (as from contact with a steering wheel) can cause the heart to be thrown against the sternum (Fig. 33.15). Sudden deceleration can cause the heart to be thrown against the thoracic vertebrae by a direct blow to the chest, such as blows caused by a baseball, animal kick, or fall.

Penetrating cardiac trauma can occur from mechanical injuries as a result of bullets, knives, or impalements. The chest wall offers little protection to the heart from penetrating trauma. The most common site of injury is the right ventricle because of its anterior position in the mediastinum. Mortality rates from penetrating trauma to the heart are high. Prehospital mortality rates for penetrating cardiac injuries are also high, as most deaths occur within minutes after injury as a result of exsanguination or tamponade.

Specific cardiac and vascular thoracic injuries

Cardiac tamponade. Cardiac tamponade is the progressive accumulation of blood in the pericardial sac (Fig. 33.16). With cardiac tamponade, the accumulation of 120 to 150 mL of blood increases intracardiac pressure and compresses the atria and ventricles. As intracardiac pressure continues to increase, this leads to decreased venous return and decreased preload, which leads to decreased cardiac output.[29] Myocardial hypoxia, heart failure, and cardiogenic shock may occur.

Classic assessment findings associated with cardiac tamponade include the presence of elevated central venous

Hemothorax

FIG. 33.14 Blunt or penetrating thoracic trauma can cause bleeding into the pleural space to form a hemothorax.

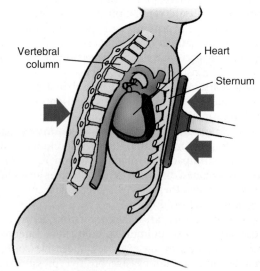

FIG. 33.15 Blunt Cardiac Trauma. Sudden acceleration (as from contact with the steering wheel) can cause the heart to be thrown against the sternum.

pressure with neck vein distention, muffled heart sounds, and hypotension. This is known as *Beck's triad*. These signs are almost universally absent in the case of a traumatic cardiac tamponade.[9] Pulseless electrical activity in the absence of hypovolemia and tension pneumothorax strongly suggests cardiac tamponade.[9] Ultrasonography in the emergency setting may be used in cases of penetrating cardiac injuries to identify a hemopericardium.[52]

Immediate treatment is required to remove the accumulated fluid in the pericardial sac. Pericardiocentesis involves aspiration of fluid from the pericardium by use of a large-bore needle. The inherent risk in this procedure is potential laceration of the coronary artery.

Blunt cardiac injury. *Blunt cardiac injury* (BCI), formerly called *myocardial contusion*, covers a wide spectrum of possible cardiac issues in trauma patients including myocardial contusion, concussion, and rupture. The chambers most often injured are the right atrium and right ventricle because of their anterior position in the chest.[53]

Few clinical signs and symptoms are specific for BCI. Evidence of external chest trauma, such as steering wheel imprint or sternal fractures, should raise suspicion for BCI. However, the presence of a sternal fracture does not predict the incidence of BCI. The patient may complain of chest pain that is similar to anginal pain, but it is not typically relieved with nitroglycerin. Chest pain is usually caused by associated injuries. Guidelines for screening of BCI from the Eastern Association of Surgeons in Trauma are listed in Box 33.11. The patient should be monitored for new onset of dysrhythmias, which, if present, should raise suspicion for BCI.[53] A 12-lead electrocardiogram may reveal dysrhythmias, ST segment changes, bundle branch block, or unexplained sinus tachycardia. Echocardiography and CT scan may reveal possible wall motion abnormalities,

FIG. 33.16 Cardiac tamponade is the progressive accumulation of blood in the pericardial sac.

BOX 33.11   EAST Guidelines for Screening of Blunt Cardiac Injury

- Obtain an admission electrocardiogram (ECG) for all patients in whom there is suspected blunt cardiac injury (BCI).
- If ECG is abnormal, the patient should be admitted for continuous ECG monitoring for 24 to 48 h.
- If the patient is hemodynamically unstable, an echocardiogram may be performed.
- Cardiac biomarkers such as cardiac troponin T values are not useful in predicting which patients will have complications related to BCI.

EAST, Eastern Association for the Surgery of Trauma.

---

pericardial fluid, or valve tearing or rupture. Biomarkers, such as troponin, are of very little diagnostic help for BCI.[53]

Medical management is aimed at preventing and treating complications. This approach includes hemodynamic monitoring in a critical care unit and possible administration of antidysrhythmic medications. Surgical consultation may be required for ruptured valves and pericardial fluid accumulation.

Aortic injury. Blunt traumatic aortic injury is one of the most lethal thoracic injuries and the second most common cause of death in trauma patients.[54] Of patients with blunt traumatic aortic injury, 80% die before reaching hospital.[54] Associated injuries include a first or second rib fracture, high sternal fracture, left clavicular fracture at the level of the sternal margin, and massive hemothorax.

Blunt traumatic aortic injury should be suspected in all trauma patients with a rapid deceleration or acceleration mechanism of injury. The thoracic aorta is relatively mobile and may tear at fixed anatomic points within the thorax. Most partial ruptures of the aorta occur at the ligamentum arteriosum.[55] A complete rupture of the aorta causes death by hemorrhage.

The nurse assesses blood pressure in both arms because a tear in the aortic arch may create a pressure gradient resulting in blood pressure changes between upper extremities. Additional clinical assessment findings include a pulse deficit at any site, unexplained hypotension, sternal pain, precordial systolic murmur, hoarseness, dyspnea, and lower extremity sensory deficits.

An initial chest radiograph is obtained in the upright position after it is considered safe to do so. Radiographic findings suggesting aortic injury include widened mediastinum, obscured aortic knob, and deviation of the left main stem bronchus.[48] CT scan is considered the gold standard for diagnosis of blunt traumatic aortic injury. In indeterminate cases, definitive diagnosis can also be made by aortography. The critical care nurse anticipates early consultation and urgent surgical (open) or endovascular repair.[54]

During the resuscitation phase for a patient with blunt traumatic aortic injury, blood pressure management is the primary goal to minimize injury. Minimizing stress on the vessel is achieved by maintaining the heart rate less than 100 beats/min, ideally using a beta-blocker.[56] The aim is to keep systolic blood pressure less than 100 mm Hg by using antihypertensive agents such as IV nitroglycerin or sodium nitroprusside.[56]

Postoperative care is also directed toward blood pressure stabilization, with the goal of minimizing vessel stress while maintaining tissue perfusion, which typically is accomplished with the use of sodium nitroprusside. Careful assessment for postoperative paraplegia is needed because lack of blood flow to the spinal column might have occurred perioperatively. Paraplegia is closely related to the duration of aortic cross-clamping time intraoperatively. The critical care nurse monitors for signs of bowel ischemia (eg, tube feeding intolerance, lactic acidosis) and acute kidney injury (eg, poor urinary output, rising serum creatinine) because blood flow to the mesentery and kidney may have been compromised as a result of the injury or surgery.

Abdominal Injuries

Abdominal injuries are frequently associated with multisystem trauma. Abdominal injuries are the third leading cause of death secondary to trauma. Injuries to the abdomen may be the result of blunt or penetrating trauma.

Blunt abdominal injuries occur most often from MVCs, falls, and assaults. Blunt trauma to the abdomen can produce injuries to the liver, spleen, and diaphragm. Deceleration and direct forces can produce retroperitoneal hematomas. Penetrating abdominal trauma is caused most often by knives or bullets. Commonly injured organs from knife wounds are the colon, liver, spleen, and diaphragm. Gunshot wounds to the abdomen usually are more serious than stab wounds. Inside the abdomen, a bullet can travel in erratic paths and ricochet off bone. Death from penetrating injuries depends on the injury to major vascular structures and resultant intraabdominal hemorrhage.

Two major life-threatening conditions that can occur after abdominal trauma are hemorrhage and hollow viscus perforation with associated peritonitis. The critical care nurse must pay particular attention to the abdomen after injury for immediate recognition of problems and prevention of complications.

Physical Assessment

Initial assessment of the trauma patient, whether in the emergency department or critical care unit, follows the primary and secondary survey techniques as outlined by ATLS guidelines.[9] The initial physical assessment of the abdomen may be nonspecific or unreliable, given the confounding influences of alcohol, illicit drugs, analgesics, or an altered level of consciousness. The critical care nurse must be aware of specific assessment findings associated with abdominal trauma.

A distended abdomen may indicate the accumulation of blood, fluid, or gas resulting from a perforated organ or ruptured blood vessel. Purplish discoloration of the flanks or umbilicus (Cullen sign) may signify blood in the abdominal wall. Ecchymosis in the flank area (Grey Turner sign) may indicate retroperitoneal bleeding or a pancreatic injury. A hematoma in the flank area suggests kidney injury. Auscultation may reveal normal or absent bowel sounds. The abdomen is assessed for rebound tenderness and rigidity, indicative of peritoneal inflammation. Referred pain to the left shoulder (Kehr sign) may indicate a ruptured spleen or irritation of the diaphragm from bile or other material in the peritoneum. The locations of entry and exit sites associated with penetrating trauma are assessed and documented.

Diagnostic Procedures

Physical examination of the abdomen alone is unreliable in a patient suspected to have abdominal trauma. Insertion of a nasogastric tube serves as a useful diagnostic and therapeutic aid. A nasogastric tube can decompress the stomach, and the contents can be checked for blood.

Laboratory test results may be nonspecific for patients with abdominal trauma. Because of hemoconcentration, hemoglobin and hematocrit results may not reflect actual values. Serial measurements are helpful in diagnosing abdominal injuries. An increasing lactate level is highly suggestive of hypoperfusion.[28]

Diagnostic imaging may occur simultaneously during the ATLS secondary survey. Noninvasive tests include the *focused assessment with sonography for trauma* (FAST) scan, CT, and chest and abdominal x-rays. Diagnostic peritoneal lavage, an invasive technique in which a small catheter is inserted into the abdominal cavity and the abdomen is assessed for the presence of blood, is performed less frequently in many trauma centers. Bedside ultrasound and CT scan have largely replaced diagnostic peritoneal lavage as a diagnostic tool in abdominal trauma.

The FAST examination is performed at most trauma centers to evaluate for the presence of intraabdominal blood.[9] Bedside ultrasonography is used widely in the United States and Canada for the detection of free fluid in the abdomen and hemoperitoneum after injury. FAST is a quick and noninvasive means of

FIG. 33.17 Focused Assessment with Sonography for Trauma (FAST). Quadrants are examined for the presence of free fluid. (From Moore FA, Moore EE. Initial management of life-threatening trauma. In: Ashley SW, editorial chair. *ACS Surgery: Principles and Practice.* Hamilton, Ontario, Canada: Decker Publishing; 2012.)

rapid assessment, but success depends on the skill level of the operator.[9]

Typically, four areas of the abdomen are examined for injury—the subxiphoid area (pericardial effusion and left lobe liver injury), the right upper quadrant (right liver, right kidney, Morrison pouch), the left upper quadrant (left kidney and spleen), and the suprapubic area (bladder and pouch of Douglas) (Fig. 33.17).[57] An extended FAST examination may be completed in some centers to check for pneumothoraces.[57] Although FAST has good sensitivity and specificity, it is not intended to replace the CT scan. Patients with abdominal obesity and patients with ascites may have erroneous results, and further work-up for these patients is warranted. FAST is limited in its ability to diagnose diaphragmatic, intestinal, or pancreatic injuries. FAST is also unable to distinguish between blood and free intraperitoneal fluid.[9] Hemodynamically unstable patients with a positive FAST examination generally undergo emergency surgery to achieve hemostasis.

An initial negative FAST result does not preclude abdominal injury and may be followed by abdominal x-ray, CT scan, or MRI. CT is the mainstay of diagnostic evaluation in a hemodynamically stable patient with abdominal trauma.[58] Abdominal CT provides information about specific organ injury, pelvic injury, and retroperitoneal hemorrhage.

Abdominal Compartment Syndrome

Abdominal compartment syndrome is defined as end-organ dysfunction caused by intraabdominal hypertension (IAH).[59] Increased pressure can be caused by bleeding, ileus, visceral edema, or a noncompliant abdominal wall. Increased pressure within the abdominal cavity can impinge on diaphragmatic excursion and can affect ventilation.

Clinical manifestations of abdominal compartment syndrome include decreased cardiac output, decreased tidal volumes, increased peak pulmonary pressures, decreased urine output, and hypoxia.[59] IAP can be measured through various commercially available devices or a simple pressurized tubing setup. In both instances, the urinary bladder acts as a transducer to estimate the degree of IAP after the injection of 25 mL of sterile saline.[59] IAH is defined as an IAP greater than or equal to 12 mm Hg (normal 5 to 7 mm Hg).[60] IAH may be graded as follows:

IAH grade I (12 to 15 mm Hg)

IAH grade II (16 to 20 mm Hg)

IAH grade III (21 to 25 mm Hg)

IAH grade IV (greater than 25 mm Hg)[60]

The abdominal perfusion pressure is calculated as MAP − IAP (normal value is greater than 60 mm Hg).

Surgical decompression of the abdomen may be required for abdominal pressures greater than 20 to 25 mm Hg accompanied by a taut, tense abdomen and signs of organ dysfunction such as deteriorating heart, lung, and kidney status. After surgical decompression is completed and the pressure is relieved, the patient may return to the critical care unit with an "open abdomen"; in the critical care unit, the abdomen is temporarily closed with a sterile perforated plastic sheet, clips, vacuum-assisted device, or other option, and the skin and abdominal fascia are left open. The wound is closed permanently in the days or weeks following the surgery or, depending on its size, may be allowed to heal by secondary intention and eventual skin grafting.

Specific Abdominal Organ Injuries

Physical assessment findings and abdominal x-ray or CT scan aid in making the diagnosis of abdominal organ injury. Medical and nursing management vary according to specific organ injuries. Liver, spleen, and bowel injuries, which are seen most frequently in patients with multisystem trauma, are discussed here.

Liver injuries. The liver is the second most commonly injured abdominal organ.[61] Trauma to the liver is a significant cause for hemorrhage after trauma.[62] Abdominal CT is considered to be the most reliable diagnostic tool to identify and assess the severity of injury to the liver.[61] The severity of liver injuries is graded to provide a mechanism for determining the amount of trauma sustained, the care needed, and possible outcomes (Table 33.10). Nonoperative management is considered the standard of care for hemodynamically stable patients with liver injury.[61] Patients with liver trauma admitted to the critical care unit are monitored for signs of hemorrhage. Serial serum hematocrit and hemoglobin levels and vital signs are monitored over several days.

Patients with blunt or penetrating liver trauma who are hemodynamically unstable may require surgical intervention to achieve hemostasis. Resection of the devitalized tissue is required for massive injuries. Hemorrhage is common with liver injuries, and ligation of the hepatic arteries or veins may be required. Packing the liver is considered the gold standard in traumatic liver injury.[58] Drains may be placed intraoperatively to prevent hematoma development.

Care of trauma patients with severe liver injuries can be challenging for critical care nurses. Hemodynamic instability can result from hemorrhage and hypovolemic shock, leading to fluid volume deficit, impaired cardiac output, and decreased

TABLE 33.10 Liver Injury Scale

Grade[a]		Injury Description
I	Hematoma	Subcapsular, <10% surface area
	Laceration	Capsular tear, <1 cm parenchymal depth
II	Hematoma	Subcapsular, 10%–50% surface area; intraparenchymal <10 cm in diameter
	Laceration	Capsular tear, 1–3 cm parenchymal depth, <10 cm long
III	Hematoma	Subcapsular, >50% surface area or expanding; ruptured subcapsular or parenchymal hematoma; intraparenchymal hematoma >10 cm or expanding
	Laceration	>3 cm parenchymal depth
IV	Laceration	Parenchymal disruption involving 25%–75% of hepatic lobe or 1–3 Couinaud segments within a single lobe
V	Laceration	Parenchymal disruption involving >75% of hepatic lobe or >3 Couinaud segments within a single lobe
	Vascular	Juxtahepatic venous injuries (retrohepatic vena cava, central major hepatic veins)
VI	Vascular	Hepatic avulsion

[a]Advance one grade for multiple injuries up to grade II.

Modified from Trunkey DD. Hepatic trauma: Contemporary management. *Surg Clin North Am.* 2004;84:437.

TABLE 33.11 Spleen Injury Scale

Grade[a]		Injury Description
I	Hematoma	Subcapsular, <10% surface area
	Laceration	Capsular tear, <1 cm, parenchymal depth
II	Hematoma	Subcapsular, 10%–50% surface area; intraparenchymal <5 cm in diameter
	Laceration	Capsular tear: 1–3 cm parenchymal depth, which does not involve a trabecular vessel
III	Hematoma	Subcapsular, >50% surface area or expanding; ruptured subcapsular or parenchymal hematoma; intraparenchymal hematoma >5 cm or expanding
IV	Laceration	>3 cm parenchymal depth or involving trabecular vessels
	Laceration	Laceration involving segmental or hilar vessels producing major devascularization (>25% of spleen)
V	Laceration	Completely shattered spleen
	Vascular	Hilar vascular injury that devascularizes spleen

[a]Advance one grade for multiple injuries up to grade II.

tissue perfusion. Continued hemodynamic instability (eg, hypotension, decreased cardiac output) despite aggressive medical intervention may indicate continued hemorrhage, in which case an exploratory laparotomy may be required to determine and correct the source of bleeding. A massive transfusion protocol may be implemented to restore blood volume and correct coagulopathies. The patient's postoperative course may be complicated by coagulopathy, acidosis, and hypothermia. Jaundice may occur as a sign of liver dysfunction, but it may also be caused by reabsorption of hematomas or breakdown of transfused red blood cells. A fundamental nursing responsibility is to evaluate the patient's response to medical therapies.

Spleen injuries. The spleen is the organ most commonly injured by blunt abdominal trauma and is second to the liver as a source of life-threatening hemorrhage. Splenic injuries, similar to liver injuries, are graded for the purpose of determining the amount of trauma sustained, the care required, and possible outcomes (Table 33.11). Hemodynamically stable patients may be monitored in the critical care unit, trending serial hematocrit and hemoglobin values and vital signs. The current trend favors nonoperative management.[61,62]

Embolization therapy is a possible option in all grades of spleen injury to help decrease blood loss from the spleen.[63] Patients with splenic injury who exhibit hemodynamic instability and progressive deterioration may require immediate operative intervention with laparotomy.[28] The spleen plays a major role in preventing infection against different organisms, including *Streptococcus, Escherichia,* and *Klebsiella.*[62] Patients who have had a splenectomy are at risk for the development of postsplenectomy sepsis with streptococcal pneumonia. These patients require the polyvalent pneumococcal vaccine (Pneumovax) to help promote immunity against pneumococcal bacteria. Patients should also receive hemophilus B and meningococcal vaccines within 2 weeks of splenectomy.[63] Complications after splenic trauma include wound infection; sepsis; subdiaphragmatic abscess; and fistulas of the colon, pancreas, and stomach.

Hollow viscus injuries. The term *hollow viscus* refers to the hollow organs in the abdomen, such as the stomach, small intestine, and large intestine. Hollow viscus injuries can result from blunt or penetrating trauma. The diagnosis of a hollow viscus injury is challenging, as these injuries may not be readily identifiable during clinical assessment or initially appear on CT scan or ultrasound. A delay in the time to diagnosis contributes to complications.[58] Regardless of the mechanism of injury, intestinal contents (eg, bile, stool, enzymes, bacteria) can leak into the peritoneum and cause peritonitis. Surgical resection and repair is almost always required. The patient's postoperative course is affected by the amount of spillage of intestinal contents. The patient is observed for signs of sepsis and for abscess or fistula formation.

Genitourinary Injuries

Trauma to the genitourinary tract seldom occurs as an isolated injury. A genitourinary injury must be suspected in any patient with pelvic fracture; blunt trauma to the lower chest or flank; contusions, hematoma, or tenderness over the flank, lower abdomen, or perineum; genital swelling or discoloration; blood at the urethral meatus; hematuria after Foley catheter placement; or difficulty with micturition.[9] Similar to all other traumatic injuries, genitourinary injuries can result from blunt or penetrating trauma.

Physical Assessment

Evaluation of genitourinary trauma begins after the ATLS primary survey has been completed. Specific assessment findings may heighten suspicion for genitourinary trauma. A conscious patient may complain of flank pain or colic pain. Rebound tenderness can be elicited if intraperitoneal extravasation of urine has occurred. Inspection may reveal blood at the urethral meatus. Bluish discoloration of the flanks may indicate retroperitoneal bleeding, whereas perineal discoloration may indicate a pelvic fracture and possible bladder or urethral injury. Hematuria is common assessment finding with genitourinary trauma[61]; however, the absence of gross or microscopic hematuria does not exclude a urinary tract injury.[9]

Specific Genitourinary Injuries

Kidney trauma. The kidney is the third most injured organ in blunt abdominal trauma.[61] Contusions or lacerations without urinary extravasation may occur. Injury to the kidney may be reflected by flank ecchymosis and fracture of inferior ribs

or spinous processes. Gross or microscopic hematuria may be present; however, the extent of kidney damage is often inconsistent with the degree of hematuria. Gross hematuria can exist with minor injuries and usually clears within a few hours.

Kidney injury is graded I through V to assist trauma teams in determining the extent of injury.[28] Grade I reflects small contusion and hematoma; and grade V identifies devascularization and avulsion injury.[61] CT is the most accurate modality available for diagnosing kidney injury because it can assess the extent of parenchymal laceration, urine extravasation, surrounding hemorrhage, and the presence of vascular injury.[61]

Contusions and minor lacerations usually can be treated with observation in hemodynamically stable patients. Angiographic embolization is used when possible. Operative interventions may be required in patients with kidney injuries who are hemodynamically unstable with a devascularized segment of the kidney. Postoperative and postinjury complications following kidney trauma include infection, hemorrhage, infarction, extravasation, calcification, and acute kidney injury.

Bladder trauma. A large percentage of bladder injuries result from pelvic fractures.[28] Physical findings may include lower abdominal bruising, distention, and pain. More definitive findings include difficulty in voiding or incomplete recovery of irrigation fluids from catheterized patients. Bladder injuries are classified as extraperitoneal ruptures (60%), intraperitoneal ruptures (30%), or combined injuries (10%).[64] The type of injury depends on the location and strength of blunt force and volume of urine in the bladder at the time of injury. Extraperitoneal rupture of the bladder may be managed conservatively with catheterization and antibiotics for 7 to 10 days.[64] Unresolved extravasation from intraperitoneal rupture requires surgical intervention.

Nursing Management

Nursing management of kidney and bladder trauma is similar to nursing management of genitourinary surgery. Diagnoses that are applicable in caring for a patient with genitourinary trauma include deficient fluid volume, risk for infection, and risk for acute kidney injury.

After admission to the critical care unit, assessment of the patient is done according to ATLS guidelines. Primary nursing interventions for genitourinary trauma include assessment for hemorrhage, maintenance of fluid and electrolyte balance, and maintaining patency of drains and tubes. Measurement of urinary output includes drainage from the urinary catheter, nephrostomy, or suprapubic tubes. Urinary output should be at least 0.5 mL/kg/h.[9] Urine output is measured hourly until bloody drainage and clots have cleared. Gentle irrigation of drainage tubes may be required to clear clots and maintain patency. It is important to monitor the patient's hemoglobin, potassium, creatinine, and urea. Urology consultation, if not already completed, may be necessary. The ideal treatment for bladder injury is unknown.[65]

Musculoskeletal Injuries

Fractures of the hands, feet, and extremities are common in trauma; although painful, such fractures are often not life-threatening. However, the pelvis, when injured, poses potentially life-threatening consequences for a trauma patient.

Pelvic Fractures

The pelvis is a ring-shaped structure composed of the hip bones (ilium, ischium, pubis), sacrum, and coccyx. The pelvis protects the lower urinary tract and major blood vessels and nerves of the lower extremities. Pelvic trauma can result in urologic and neurologic dysfunction and severe, life-threatening hemorrhage.

Blunt trauma to the pelvis can be caused by MVCs, falls, or a crush injury. When the pelvic ring is disrupted, the radius increases, increasing blood volume capacity. Pelvic injuries may be associated with damage to underlying arterial and venous vessels. There is also loss of the tamponade effect of the retroperitoneal tissues and intrapelvic organs, contributing to further bleeding.[66] Because the pelvic area is a highly vascular compartment, it can sequester a large volume of blood. The mortality rate from pelvic trauma ranges from 5% to 50%.[9] Death within 24 hours of injury is most often due to hemorrhagic shock.[9]

Physical Assessment and Diagnostic Procedures

Signs of pelvic fracture include swelling, tenderness, and bruising around the pubis, iliac bones, hips, or sacrum. Perianal ecchymosis (scrotum or vulva), indicating extravasation of urine or blood, may be present. Pain or crepitus on palpation, or "rocking" of the iliac crests, suggests a fractured pelvis, but it is not conclusive.[67] Lower extremity rotation or leg shortening is also suspicious for a pelvic injury. Other possible assessment findings are lower limb paresis; swollen testicles; and vaginal, rectal, or urethral bleeding, which may or may not be accompanied by hematuria. Patients with a suspected pelvic injury should have a rectal examination to assess for SCI or presence of occult or obvious rectal bleeding.

The diagnosis of pelvic fracture is made by an anteroposterior pelvic x-ray with the patient in the supine position or CT scan of the pelvis. Additional radiographs may be required for definitive treatment, but the necessity of obtaining additional films depends on the patient's hemodynamic stability.

Classification of Pelvic Fractures

Pelvic fractures constitute a spectrum of complexity ranging from a single nondisplaced fracture to a life-threatening condition in which there are multiple fractures and crush injuries associated with significant hemorrhage and internal injuries. There is no universally agreed-on classification system for pelvic fractures. Pelvic fractures may be *stable* (intact pelvic ring) or *unstable* (nonintact pelvic ring).[28] Pelvic fractures may be open (continuity with vagina, rectum, or external body surface) or closed. The Young-Burgess system is most frequently used by trauma teams and classifies pelvic fractures based on mechanism of injury.[68]

Anteroposterior compression pelvic injury. When force is applied in the anteroposterior direction, the pelvic diameter widens. In this case, the injury can be completely ligamentous, which manifests as an open sacroiliac joint or open pubic symphysis. This type of injury is commonly associated with vascular injury. Anteroposterior compression pelvic fractures are classified according to severity of injury as follows:
- *Type I anteroposterior injury* includes disruption of the pubic symphysis with less than 2.5 cm of diastasis and with insignificant posterior pelvic involvement.
- *Type II anteroposterior injury* includes disruption of the pubic symphysis of more than 2.5 cm with tearing of associated ligaments.
- *Type III anteroposterior injury* is complete disruption of the pubic symphysis, posterior ligament complexes, and hemipelvic involvement. This is known as the "open book" pelvic fracture.

Lateral compression pelvic injury. Lateral compression forces produce a shortening of the pelvic diameter and typically do not involve ligamentous injury. The pelvic volume is reduced in this type of injury, so hemorrhage is not as common, but localized bleeding may occur.[9] Lateral compression fractures are classified according to severity of injury as follows:
- *Type I lateral compression injury* includes posterior compression of the sacroiliac joint without ligament disruption or an oblique pubic ramus fracture.
- *Type II lateral compression injury* includes rupture of the posterior sacroiliac ligament or internal rotation of the hemipelvis with a crush injury of the sacrum and an oblique pubic ramus fracture.
- *Type III lateral compression injury* includes the findings of type II lateral compression injury with additional evidence of anteroposterior compression to the contralateral hemipelvis.

Vertical shear. A vertical shear pelvic injury occurs when force is applied in a perpendicular plane across the anterior and posterior aspects of the ring. Complete disruption of the hemipelvis associated with major hemipelvic displacement and instability occurs. This type of injury typically occurs in people who fall from a great height and land on one extremity.

Combined pelvic injuries. Combined pelvic injuries are a combination of injury types that do not fit into any one single category.

Medical Management

The priority of medical management of pelvic fractures is to prevent or control life-threatening hemorrhage. Current guidelines suggest that patients with pelvic fractures and hemodynamic instability or signs of ongoing bleeding after nonpelvic sources of blood loss have been ruled out should be considered for angiography with contrast enhancement and embolization. Additionally, patients who have evidence of arterial extravasation on pelvic CT scan may require angiography and embolization independent of hemodynamic status.[68]

Temporary pelvic binders may be applied initially at the scene to help reduce the pelvic ring size and limit the extent of bleeding.[67] Application of pelvic binders may also be accomplished by wrapping the pelvis with a bed sheet or commercially available binder between the greater trochanter and the iliac crests. Advantages of this technique are that it is quick, does not involve specialized training, allows continued access to the patient during trauma resuscitation, and does not require specialized equipment. Although these binders may limit hemorrhage, improvement in mortality has not been demonstrated.[67]

Patients who are hemodynamically stable and have stable pelvic fractures may be treated conservatively with ongoing monitoring of vital signs and collaboration with surgeons for progressive mobility and physical therapy. For unstable polytrauma patients with ongoing hemorrhage and pelvic instability, *damage control orthopedics*—nondefinitive surgical repair of the orthopedic injury—is undertaken.[69] This time-limited approach may involve pelvic packing or application of a pelvic external fixator.[68] Once the patient has stabilized, and generally after several days, definitive management of pelvic fractures may be done with internal screws, nails, or plates to create stability, prevent or correct deformity, and facilitate early mobilization.

Nursing Management

Initial assessment of a trauma patient with a pelvic fracture on admission to the critical care unit proceeds according to ATLS guidelines. Before the patient is moved, the nurse should know whether the physician has classified the pelvic fracture as *stable* or *unstable*. A stable pelvic injury implies that no further pathologic displacement of the pelvis can occur with turning or moving. An unstable pelvic fracture means that further pathologic displacement of the pelvis can occur with turning or moving.

IV fluid resuscitation and hemorrhage control are mainstays of pelvic fracture management. Massive blood loss contributes to alterations in tissue perfusion. On admission, the patient may exhibit hemodynamic instability with abnormal coagulation factors. Interventions include IV fluids and blood products, with recognition that a massive transfusion protocol may be required. The nurse must ensure that an appropriate amount of blood, plasma, and platelets is crossmatched and available if needed.

Essential nursing care includes neurovascular assessment of the lower extremities. Neurologic injury as a result of pelvic fracture may be transient and temporary. Any sudden change in sensation or movement requires prompt notification of the physician. Open pelvic fractures may necessitate complex, time-consuming, and sometimes painful dressing changes. Pain management strategies are essential during dressing changes. Nursing management of external fixation devices is aimed at monitoring for and preventing infection. Most institutions have protocols for pin site care.

Patients with pelvic fractures may have a prolonged critical care course with various degrees of complications. A patient with a pelvic fracture often has other associated injuries, complicating recovery and rehabilitation after injury. The patient is at high risk for several different complications, including development of venous thromboembolism (VTE), ARDS, wound infection, and sepsis.

COMPLICATIONS OF TRAUMA

As a result of vast improvements in prehospital and emergency department care of trauma patients, these patients are surviving their initial multisystem injuries, transport to hospital, and damage control operative procedures. Within the critical care unit, after resuscitation, stabilization, and damage control or definitive surgery, this is often a period of significant vulnerability for trauma patients. Ongoing nursing assessments are imperative for early detection of complications associated with traumatic injuries. Complications increase critical care and hospital length of stay, increase costs, and are associated with increased morbidity and mortality. Some of the most important complications in care of critically injured patients in the critical care, intermediate care, and rehabilitation phases are identified in this section.

Central Nervous System Complications
Pain

Pain may come from many sources, including surgery, procedures, and the injuries themselves. Relief of pain is a major component in the care of trauma patients. Several different strategies of pain management may be used with the trauma patient, including continuous IV infusions, thoracic and lumbar epidural infusions, and intercostal nerve blocks. Pain relief measures are individualized for each patient, based on injuries; contraindications; allergies; and patient, physician, and institutional preferences or protocols.

One issue that often complicates pain management in critical care is the high incidence of substance abuse among patients who sustain traumatic injury. Trauma patients, regardless of any prior substance use history, may require multimodal acute pain management approaches.

Cardiovascular Complications
Compartment Syndrome

Compartment syndrome is a condition in which increased pressure within a limited space compromises circulation, resulting in ischemia and necrosis of tissues within that space. Among patients at high risk for the development of compartment syndrome are patients with upper and lower extremity trauma, including fractures, vascular ruptures, massive tissue injuries, or venous obstruction.

Clinical manifestations of compartment syndrome include obvious swelling and tightness of a limb, paresthesia, and extreme pain in the affected extremity.[9] Diminished pulses and decreased capillary refill do not reliably identify compartment syndrome because they may be intact until after irreversible damage has occurred. Elevated intracompartmental pressures confirm the diagnosis. Treatment can consist of simple interventions such as removing an occlusive dressing or bivalving (cutting) a cast or more complex interventions, including a surgical decompressive fasciotomy.

Venous Thromboembolism

VTE, which includes both DVT and pulmonary emboli, is an important cause of morbidity and mortality in a trauma patient with multiple injuries. Patients with major trauma are at very high risk for VTE.[70] Factors that form the basis of VTE pathophysiology are the same factors that place trauma patients at risk, including endothelial injury (as a result of trauma), hypercoagulopathy (as a result of trauma-induced coagulopathy), and blood stasis (as a result of immobility).

Trauma patients are at the greatest risk for developing VTE early in their hospitalization. Prevention is key. Routine thromboprophylaxis for a high-risk trauma patient includes use of low-molecular-weight heparin (starting as soon as it is considered safe to do so) and use of a mechanical method of prophylaxis such as sequential compression devices.[71] Early mobilization, ensuring the comfort and safety of the patient, and taking into consideration known injuries can also help prevent development of VTE.

Pulmonary Complications
Acute Respiratory Distress Syndrome

Posttraumatic respiratory failure is often due to the development of ARDS.[70] ARDS can be caused by direct or indirect injury to the lungs (see "Acute Respiratory Distress Syndrome" in Chapter 19). Direct injuries in trauma patients include aspiration, inhalation, and pulmonary contusion.[72] Indirect injuries include sepsis, massive transfusion, fat emboli, and missed injury.[72] When ARDS in trauma occurs, it generally develops 24 to 72 hours after the initial injury. Intubation, mechanical ventilation, low-tidal-volume ventilation, and use of PEEP are the mainstays of ARDS treatment.[70,72] In severe cases of ARDS, the trauma patient may need to be placed in a prone position.

Gastrointestinal and Genitourinary Complications
Hypermetabolism

Within 24 to 48 hours after traumatic injury, a predictable hypermetabolic response occurs. The metabolic response to injury mobilizes amino acids and accelerates protein synthesis to support wound healing and the immunologic response to invading organisms. Stress hypermetabolism also occurs after major injury and is characterized by increases in metabolic rate and oxygen consumption. Energy requirements increase to promote immune function and tissue repair. The goal of early nutrition is to maintain host defenses by supporting this hypermetabolism and to preserve lean body mass.[73]

Nutrition support is an essential component in the care of critically ill trauma patients. Most nutrition experts advocate beginning enteral nutrition as early as possible. Current guidelines recommend enteral feedings be initiated, unless otherwise ordered, within 48 hours for all trauma patients.[73] Enteral feeding sites include the gastric route and any site beyond the pylorus of the stomach including the duodenum and jejunum.

Prompt feeding tube placement by the critical care nurse is a priority. Diminished or absent bowel sounds are not a contraindication to initiation of tube feeds. Small bowel function and the ability to absorb nutrients remain intact, despite the presence of gastroparesis and absent bowel sounds. Patients at risk for pulmonary aspiration as a result of gastric retention or gastroesophageal reflux should receive enteral feedings into the jejunum.[74] If enteral feeding is unsuccessful, parenteral nutrition should be initiated.

Acute Kidney Injury

Assessment and ongoing monitoring of kidney function is critical to the survival of the trauma patient. The cause of posttraumatic acute kidney injury is complex and, besides the initial injury, may involve a variety of factors (Box 33.12).

Prevention of kidney failure is the best treatment, and it begins with ensuring sufficient IV fluid volume to provide adequate renal perfusion. Serial assessments of blood urea nitrogen and creatinine levels are commonly used to evaluate kidney function. Progressive deterioration in kidney function requires prompt diagnosis and treatment (see "Acute Kidney Injury" in Chapter 26).

BOX 33.12   Etiologic Factors in Posttraumatic Acute Kidney Injury

- Preexisting disease
  - Hypertension
  - Heart failure
  - Diabetes
  - Chronic kidney disease
  - Chronic liver disease
- Prolonged shock states
- Profound acidosis
- Systemic inflammatory response syndrome or reperfusion injury
- Abdominal compartment syndrome
- Muscle ischemia; myoglobinuria
- Microemboli
- Nephrotoxic medications
- Radiocontrast dye

Rhabdomyolysis and Myoglobinuria

Patients with muscle trauma and crush injuries are susceptible to the development of rhabdomyolysis and, if left untreated, subsequent secondary kidney failure. Crush injuries can compromise blood flow. Decreased arterial blood flow results in the loss of oxygen transport and ischemia. This initiates a cascade of cellular events, including depletion of adenosine triphosphate and failure of the adenosine triphosphatase pumps, which leads to the necrosis of skeletal muscle cells.[75] As cells die, intracellular contents—particularly potassium and myoglobin—are released. Myoglobin, a muscular pigment, is a large molecule that gets lodged in the glomerulus, resulting in myoglobinuria (myoglobin in the urine). Circulating myoglobin can lead to the development of kidney failure by three mechanisms: decreased renal perfusion, cast formation with tubular obstruction, and direct toxic effects of myoglobin in the kidney tubules.[75]

Dark tea-colored urine suggests myoglobinuria. Testing for myoglobin in the urine can be done but may take some time. The most rapid screening test is a serum creatine kinase level. Increased creatine kinase levels are associated with muscle damage and renal failure.[16] Urine output and serial creatine kinase levels should be monitored.

Rhabdomyolysis should be suspected in all patients who experience crush injuries in which blood flow to the muscle is interrupted for a prolonged time. When rhabdomyolysis is diagnosed, treatment is aimed at prevention of subsequent kidney failure. Prevention of kidney dysfunction is paramount through the aggressive administration of IV fluids.[75] IV fluids increase renal blood flow and decrease the concentration of nephrotoxic pigments. Alkalinization of the urine and administration of diuretics have been studied, but their roles in the prevention or management of rhabdomyolysis are not firmly established.[16] Nursing management is directed toward maintaining urinary output, achieving fluid and electrolyte balance, and optimizing hemodynamics to prevent deterioration in kidney function.

Integumentary and Musculoskeletal Complications
Fat Embolism Syndrome

Fat embolism syndrome can occur as a complication of orthopedic trauma. The clinical onset of fat embolism syndrome ranges from 12 hours to 2 weeks after injury.[28] Fat embolism syndrome appears to develop as a result of fat droplets that leak from fractured bone with embolization of the fat droplets to the lungs. These droplets are broken down into free fatty acids that are toxic to the pulmonary microvascular membranes. Pulmonary fat emboli alter pulmonary hemodynamics and pulmonary vascular permeability. The lung becomes highly edematous and hemorrhagic. This may lead to the development of ARDS.[9]

Signs and symptoms may be subtle and nonspecific. The patient may become restless and slightly confused. Hypoxemia, neurologic impairment, and a petechial rash are classic signs and symptoms. The patient may or may not exhibit tachypnea with some degree of respiratory distress.[9] A chest x-ray may reveal patchy infiltrates; a CT scan is often performed to rule out pulmonary embolism. Diagnosis is often clinical and based on patient history, which often involves orthopedic injury.[76] Nursing care is supportive.

Other Complications in Adult Trauma Patients
Infection

Infection is a major source of mortality and morbidity in critical care units. Trauma patients are at risk for infection because of contaminated wounds, intubation and mechanical ventilation, invasive catheters, host susceptibility (including preexisting medical conditions), adverse effect of trauma on the immune system, and the critical care environment. Nursing management must include interventions to decrease and eliminate the patient's risk of infection.

Wound contamination poses a major infection risk for trauma patients, especially with injuries resulting from deep or penetrating trauma. Exogenous bacteria (from the external environment) can enter through open wounds. Exogenous bacteria can be dirt, grass, or debris inoculated into the wound at the time of injury or microorganisms introduced by personnel during wound care. Endogenous bacteria (from the internal environment) can be released as a result of gastrointestinal or genitourinary perforation.

Meticulous wound care is essential. The goals of wound care include removing dead and devitalized tissue, allowing for wound drainage, and promoting wound epithelialization and contraction. Wound healing is accomplished through interventions that promote tissue perfusion including administration of oxygen, IV fluids, and ensuring adequate nutrition support.

Standard interventions for the prevention of ventilator-associated pneumonia, catheter-associated urinary tract infections, and central line–associated bloodstream infection apply to trauma patients. Strict medical aseptic technique for all invasive procedures; sterile technique for invasive catheter care and dressing changes; prompt removal of unnecessary lines, tubes, and drains; and proper hand hygiene are paramount to optimal patient outcome.

Sepsis

A patient with multiple injuries is at risk for development of sepsis and septic shock. In one large-scale study, predictors of sepsis in trauma patients with moderate injuries in critical care included age (increased risk as age increased), male sex, African American ethnicity, hypotension on admission to the emergency department, and MVC as the primary mechanism of injury.[77] Of 373,370 patients in this study, more than 5200 patients developed sepsis (1.41%), and mortality was 18.9% among the patients who developed sepsis.[77]

Possible sources of sepsis in adult trauma patients are contaminated wounds, the presence of invasive catheters, and severe damage to internal organs and structures. The source of the septic nidus must be promptly investigated. Gram stain and cultures of blood, urine, sputum, invasive catheters, and wounds are obtained. Broad-spectrum antibiotic therapy may be initiated before receiving definitive positive culture results, based on the patient's current condition, nature of traumatic injury, hemodynamic stability, and possible severity of infection.

Transfusion-Related Complications

A patient receiving multiple blood products, particularly fresh frozen plasma, must be monitored for *transfusion-related acute lung injury* (TRALI). Signs of TRALI are similar to signs of ARDS, although there is a temporal relationship between the new onset of respiratory distress and the transfusion of blood products.[78] TRALI may occur 6 hours after a transfusion, as evidenced by hypoxemia and bilateral infiltrates on chest x-ray.[78] Treatment consists of lung-protective strategies, which include low-tidal-volume ventilation and PEEP and, if possible, avoidance of subsequent transfusions.[16]

Missed Injury

Posttrauma, once the patient's condition has stabilized, nursing assessment of a patient with multiple injuries may reveal missed injuries. Missed injuries have a reported incidence of approximately 10% in critical care.[79] Missed injuries, which are often orthopedic, may be a cause of morbidity and mortality.[80]

Several factors in critical care contribute to missed injury. Patient factors include patients with head injuries and a GCS score of 8 or less, patients with intoxication at time of admission, patients with greater injury severity scores, and patients receiving analgesia and sedation.[79] Clinician factors may include lack of experience, error in radiologic interpretation, failure to engage other services, or responsibility for multiple patients with competing demands.[79]

In the critical care unit, a missed injury may be suspected if the patient fails to show appropriate response to medical or surgical intervention. Hypotension and a falling hematocrit level despite fluid administration may indicate new-onset or continued bleeding. Change in the character of drainage from wounds or catheters may represent biliary or duodenal injuries. The physician must be notified immediately because potential complications of hemorrhage and infection may be life-threatening. In intermediate care units and rehabilitation facilities, small bone fractures and sprains may manifest as the patient begins to mobilize. Nurses and other health care team members play key roles in identifying missed injuries, particularly when patients regain consciousness and begin to increase their activity.

Multiple Organ Dysfunction Syndrome

Trauma patients are at high risk for MODS, a clinical syndrome of progressive dysfunction of organ systems. It has been estimated that 20% to 50% of MODS in critical care occurs in patients with multiple injuries.[81] MODS can appear 3 to 4 days after admission. Mortality rates for trauma patients with MODS are estimated to be 31% to 80%.[82]

Trauma patients may experience primary and secondary MODS. Organ dysfunction as a result of primary MODS is caused by direct traumatic injury, as may occur with acute lung dysfunction because of pulmonary contusion. Secondary MODS, which occurs later in hospitalization, results from uncontrolled systemic inflammation with resultant organ dysfunction. Treatment is aimed at controlling or eliminating the source of inflammation, maintenance of oxygen delivery and consumption, and nutrition and metabolic support for individual organs.

SPECIAL CONSIDERATIONS

Trauma in Older Patients

Trauma affects people of all ages. Older patients are predisposed to traumatic injuries because of the inevitable consequences of aging. The ability to react to or avoid environmental hazards is impaired because of age-related deterioration of the senses and changes in motor strength, postural stability, balance, and coordination.

Older people are most at risk for falls; these injuries are likely to occur from wet or uneven surfaces, inadequate lighting, or lack of proper footwear.[28] Factors that predispose older people to falls are summarized in Box 33.13. Because falls may be caused by an underlying medical condition (eg, syncope, dysrhythmias, hypotension), management of an older patient who has experienced injury must include an evaluation of events and conditions immediately preceding the fall.

BOX 33.13 Risk Factors for Falls in Older Adults

Acute Illness
- Cerebrovascular accidents
- Dysrhythmias
- Syncope
- Diabetes

Cognitive Impairment
- Dementia

Neuromuscular Disorders
- Arthritis
- Lower extremity weakness
- Unstable gait

Medications
- Antidepressants
- Benzodiazepines
- Diuretics
- Phenothiazines

BOX 33.14 Factors That Predispose Older Adults to Motor Vehicle Crashes

- Alterations in visual and auditory acuity
- Deterioration in strength and slower reaction times
- Diminution of cerebral skills
- Diminution of motor skills
- Exacerbation of acute or chronic medical conditions
- Medications that may interfere with safe driving

Involvement of older adults in MVCs is a consequence of increasing age of the general population and the growing number of older drivers and occupants of motor vehicles. Factors that predispose older adults to MVCs are summarized in Box 33.14. Physiologic deterioration of cerebral and motor skills and alterations in visual and auditory acuity may contribute to causing both older drivers and pedestrians to misjudge or be unable avoid oncoming vehicles.

Trauma in older adults is associated with higher mortality rates, even when the injuries are less severe. Adults 65 years old and older have a higher complication rate and a higher mortality rate because of preexisting medical conditions, decreased physiologic reserve, and decreased ability to compensate for severe injury.[83] Older patients who do survive traumatic injury are often faced with changes in functional status after injury. Relatively minor trauma can be the event that changes the lifestyle of an older person from one of relative independence to one that requires prolonged rehabilitation or skilled nursing care. Discharge planning may begin in the critical care or intermediate care unit.

The concept of *limited physiologic reserve* in an older trauma patient highlights the key difference between the average younger trauma patient with normal physiologic reserve and the older patient with underlying physiologic derangements. Age-related changes that occur in virtually every organ system may not produce evidence of organ dysfunction in the resting state. However, the ability of organs to augment function in response to traumatic stress may be greatly compromised.

Fluid resuscitation is an integral part of trauma resuscitation. Patients on long-term diuretic therapy may require additional volume and enhanced potassium supplementation as a result of chronic volume and potassium depletion. At the same time, these patients may be less likely to tolerate aggressive fluid resuscitation, owing to preexisting cardiac or pulmonary issues. The assessment and management of hypovolemic shock is more complex in older trauma patients. Older adults have limited ability to increase their heart rate in response to blood loss (sometimes because of beta-blocker or calcium channel blocker medication), obscuring one of the earliest signs of hypovolemia—tachycardia.[9] Loss of physiologic reserve and underlying comorbidities are likely to produce further confusing hemodynamic data. Because of lack of physiologic reserve in an older patient, it is imperative that nutrition support is initiated early.

Many older adults take daily anticoagulants or antiplatelet medications or both to prevent thrombotic or embolic complications from preexisting medical conditions. Traumatic injury in conjunction with a prolonged international normalized ratio greatly increases the risk of major hemorrhage. Systemic anticoagulation must be corrected as soon as possible after admission, and when head injury is suspected, a CT scan of the head is urgently obtained.

Trauma protocols are well established for the management of young patients after injury. Clinicians are increasingly recognizing that these protocols must be individualized for older trauma patients.[83] The best outcomes for this patient population have been achieved through early, appropriate, aggressive trauma care, with admission to a trauma center with resources and protocols to provide excellent care to injured adults regardless of age.

Meeting Needs of Family Members and Significant Others

The impact of traumatic injury can be devastating for patients, family members, and significant others. Trauma can precipitate a crisis within the family. The family is faced with an unexpected situation for which the members have had little time to prepare. Family members may exhibit physical and sociocultural reactions and a combination of emotional reactions including anger, fear, powerlessness, confusion, and mistrust. Recovery from traumatic injury can be long and frustrating for families. There may be many peaks and valleys, good days and bad days. During this time, the family may exhaust social and financial support systems. Critical care nurses need to be able to assess, recognize, and address the impact of stressors on families of trauma patients.

A trend has evolved to move away from a paternalistic model of care to one that incorporates the family into all aspects of care. Many family members wish to remain close to their loved ones during these times. Although it may be challenging, family members should be encouraged, to the extent that they are able and wish to do so and maintaining the comfort and safety of the patient, participate in patient care. Bathing, brushing teeth, combing hair, and reading to the patient are excellent strategies to involve families in patient care.

Another valuable intervention is to bring families of trauma patients together in support groups. Trauma family support groups can offer sharing of experiences, expression of emotions, mutual support, sharing of coping strategies, and education about hospital and community resources and services.

CASE STUDY 33.1 Patient With Trauma

Brief Patient History

Mr. G is a 21-year-old man. He was a pedestrian crossing the street in a marked crosswalk when he was hit by a pickup truck traveling at approximately 40 miles/h (64 km/h). He was ejected onto the side of the road. There is visible external damage to the front passenger panel of the truck. On arrival, emergency medical services personnel determined the patient was awake, not following commands, restless, and agitated. His respiratory rate was 22 breaths/min, and breathing was shallow and unlabored. His oxygen saturation on pulse oximetry (SpO_2) was 92%. There was blood oozing from the right side of his head and obvious deformity to his right leg. He was placed in a hard collar, immobilized, and given oxygen via a 15-L nonrebreather mask. He was immediately transported to the hospital.

Clinical Assessment

Mr. G is admitted to the emergency department. The advanced trauma life support primary survey is completed, and the following assessment findings are identified:

- Airway: Moaning incomprehensibly
- Breathing: 24 breaths/min, shallow; obvious right-sided deformity (flail chest)
- Circulation: Pale, cool; palpable carotid and femoral pulses
- Disability: Glasgow Coma Scale score 13 (motor, 5; verbal, 3; eyes, 4); moving all four limbs but not to command
- Exposure: Right scalp laceration; several abrasions; lacerations over face, back, and legs

Diagnostic Procedures

Admission x-ray shows fractured right femur. Computed tomography (CT) scan shows a small subdural hematoma and liver laceration.

Medical Diagnosis

Mr. G is diagnosed with subdural hematoma (secondary to trauma), flail chest, fractured ribs, fractured right femur, and liver laceration.

Admission to Critical Care Unit

On admission to the adult critical care unit after the CT scan, reassessment of the patient is done with the following assessment findings: Heart rate, 142 beats/min (sinus tachycardia); respiratory rate, 30 breaths/min, short, shallow, and labored; blood pressure, 85/46 mm Hg; SpO_2, 86%; temperature, 96.3°F (35.7°C); Glasgow Coma Scale score 7. The patient is difficult to arouse.

Questions

1. What are your immediate priorities for this patient?
2. What care do you anticipate Mr. G will require in the next hour? What care will he require in the next 4 hours?
3. Do you anticipate that Mr. G will require surgery? Explain your rationale.
4. What problems might you anticipate Mr. G may experience as a result of his injuries?
5. What interventions must be initiated to prevent and manage any possible problems?
6. What type of questions might you anticipate the family will ask you? How will you respond?
7. What possible learning needs would you anticipate for this patient?

SUMMARY

- Trauma is costly in terms of disability, health care dollars, and lives lost.
- Traumatic injuries are most frequently caused by high-velocity impact (eg, MVCs) and may be caused by blunt or penetrating mechanisms.

Phases of Trauma Care

- Assessment of the trauma patient is performed in a systematic fashion.
- The initial primary survey focuses on airway, breathing, circulation, disability, and exposure.
- The more detailed secondary survey is an in-depth, head-to-toe physical assessment.
- Resuscitation of the trauma patient involves hemostasis to control hemorrhage, goal-directed volume support to restore cellular oxygenation, maintenance of normothermia, and prevention and correction of acidosis and coagulopathy.
- Assessment and reassessment of the trauma patient in the critical care unit is essential.

Specific Trauma Injuries

- Management of severe TBIs and SCIs in critical care focuses on the prevention of secondary injury by maintaining oxygen delivery to the brain and spinal cord and avoiding complications of prolonged bed rest and immobility.
- Airway compromise is a major focus of care for a patient who has sustained maxillofacial injuries.
- Chest wall and pulmonary injuries require pain management and frequent reassessment of oxygenation and ventilation status.
- Pneumothoraces are often treated with insertion of chest tubes.
- BCI is associated with increased risk of dysrhythmias.
- Abdominal trauma often has nonspecific signs and symptoms; the critical care nurse must maintain increased awareness for abdominal complications.
- Liver and spleen injuries are associated with increased risk of hemorrhage.
- Kidney and bladder injuries are often managed nonoperatively.
- Pelvic fractures may result in tremendous volume loss, and the nurse must remain alert for signs of hemorrhagic shock.
- Complications of trauma may include VTE, infection, sepsis, missed injury, and MODS.
- Ⓔ Visit the Evolve site for additional study materials.

REFERENCES

1. Centers for Disease Control and Prevention. Injury Prevention and Control: Data and Statistics: Ten Leading Causes of Death. http://www.cdc.gov/injury/wisqars/leadingcauses.html; 2013. Accessed February 1, 2016.
2. World Health Organization. Road Traffic Injuries—Fact Sheet No. 358. http://www.who.int/mediacentre/factsheets/fs358/en/; 2015. Accessed February 1, 2016.
3. Burnett LB. Domestic Violence. http://emedicine.medscape.com/article/805546-overview; 2015 Accessed February 1, 2016.
4. Centers for Disease Control and Prevention. Sexual Violence: Prevention Strategies. http://www.cdc.gov/violenceprevention/sexualviolence/prevention.html; 2015. Accessed February 1, 2016.
5. Schroeter K. Trauma nurses making a difference. *J Trauma Nurs*. 2015;22(3):120–121.
6. American College of Surgeons Committee on Trauma. Alcohol Screening and Brief Intervention (SBI) for Trauma Patients: COT Quick Guide. Chicago: American College of Surgeons. https://www.facs.org/~/media/files/quality%20programs/trauma/publications/sbirtguide.ashx; 2007. Accessed September 25, 2016.
7. Clarke SL. Substance use disorders. In: Domino FJ, ed. *The 5-Minute Clinical Consult 2014*. 22nd ed. Philadelphia: Wolters Kluwer; 2014.
8. Stephanopoulos PK, et al. Gunshot wounds: a review of ballistics related to penetrating trauma. *J Acute Dis*. 2014;3(3):178–185.

9. American College of Surgeons. *Advanced Trauma Life Support*. 9th ed. Chicago: American College of Surgeons; 2012.

10. Lansink KWW, Gunning AC, Leenen LPH. Cause of death and time of death distribution of trauma patients in a level I trauma centre in the Netherlands. *Eur J Trauma Emerg Surg*. 2013;39(4):375–383.

11. Sobrino J, Shafi S. Timing and causes of death after injury. *Proc (Bayl Univ Med Cent)*. 2013;26(2):120–123.

12. Kaczynski J. Prevention of tissue hypoperfusion in the trauma patient: Initial management. *Br J Hosp Med*. 2013;74(2):81–84.

13. Kaafarani HMA, Velmahos GC. Damage control resuscitation in trauma. *Scand J Surg*. 2014;103:81–88.

14. Pohlman TH, et al. Damage control resuscitation. *Blood Rev*. 2015;29(4):251–262.

15. Gourgiotis S, et al. Permissive hypotension in bleeding trauma patients: helpful or not and when? *Crit Care Nurse*. 2013;33(6):18–25.

16. Shere-Wolfe RF, Galvagno SM, Grissom TE. (2012). Critical care considerations in the management of the trauma patient following initial resuscitation. *Scand J Trauma Resusc Emerg Med*. 2012;20:68. http://www.sjtrem.com/content/20/1/68. Accessed February 1, 2016.

17. Campion EM, Mackersie RC. Recent developments in the assessment of the multiply injured patient. *Curr Opin Crit Care*. 2014;20(6):620–625.

18. Miller TE. New evidence in trauma resuscitation—is 1:1:1 the answer? *Perioper Med (Lond)*. 2013;2(1):13. http://www.perioperativemedicine-journal.com/content/pdf/2047-0525-2-13.pdf. Accessed February 3, 2016.

19. Holcomb JB, et al. Transfusion of plasma, platelets, and red blood cells in a 1:1:1 vs a 1:1:2 ratio and mortality in patients with severe trauma. *JAMA*. 2015;313(5):471–482.

20. Lamb CM, et al. Damage control surgery in the era of damage control resuscitation. *Br J Anaesth*. 2014;113(2):242–249.

21. Crossan L, Cole E. Nursing challenges with a severely injured patient in critical care. *Nurs Crit Care*. 2013;8(5):236–244.

22. Cestero RF, Dent DL. Endpoints of resuscitation. *Surg Clin North Am*. 2015;95(2):319–336.

23. Centers for Disease Control and Prevention. *Traumatic Brain Injury in the United States: Fact Sheet*; 2015. http://www.cdc.gov/traumaticbraininjury/get_the_facts.html. Accessed February 3, 2016.

24. Centers for Disease Control and Prevention. Severe Traumatic Brain Injury. http://www.cdc.gov/traumaticbraininjury/severe.html; 2014. Accessed February 3, 2016.

25. Dinsmore J. Traumatic brain injury: An evidence-based review of management. *Contin Educ Anaesth Crit Care Pain*. 2013;13(6):189–195.

26. Tran LV. Understanding the pathophysiology of traumatic brain injury and the mechanism of action of neuroprotective interventions. *J Trauma Nurs*. 2014;21(1):30–35.

27. Chowdhury T, et al. Pre-hospital and initial management of head injury patients: an update. *Saudi J Anaesth*. 2014;8(1):114–120.

28. Emergency Nurses Association. *TNCC: Trauma Nursing Core Course* (7th ed.). Des Plaines, IL: Emergency Nurses Association.

29. Meagher RJ. Subdural Hematoma. http://emedicine.medscape.com/article/1137207-overview; 2015. Accessed February 3, 2016.

30. Honeybul S, Ho KM, Lind CR. What can be learned from the DECRA study? *World Neurosurg*. 2013;79(1):159–161.

31. Tang A, et al. Intracranial pressure monitor in patients with traumatic brain injury. *J Surg Res*. 2015;194(2):565–570.

32. Chowdhury T, et al. General intensive care for patients with traumatic brain injury. *Saudi J Anaesth*. 2014;8(2):256–263.

33. Alali AS, et al. Beta blockers for acute traumatic brain injury: A systematic review and meta-analysis. *Neurocrit Care*. 2014;20(3):514–523.

34. Giacino JT, et al. Placebo-controlled trial of amantadine for severe traumatic brain injury. *N Engl J Med*. 2012;366(9):819–826.

35. National Spinal Cord Injury Statistical Center. Spinal cord injury facts and figures at a glance. https://www.nscisc.uab.edu/Public/Facts%202015%20Aug.pdf; 2015. Accessed February 3, 2016.

36. Sarhan F, Saif D, Saif A. An overview of traumatic spinal cord injury: part 1. Aetiology and pathophysiology. *Br J Neurosci Nurs*. 2012;8(6):319–325.

37. Wilson JR, Forgione N, Fehlings MG. (2013). Emerging therapies for acute spinal cord injury. *Can Med Assoc J*. 2013;185(5):485–492.

38. Colangelo J. Care considerations for patients with spinal cord injuries. *Radiol Technol*. 2014;86(1):33–58.

39. Sarhan F, Saif D, Saif A. An overview of traumatic spinal cord injury: part 2. Acute management. *Br J Neurosci Nurs*. 2013;9(3):138–144.

40. Como JJ, Diaz JJ, Dunham CM. Cervical spine injuries following trauma. *J Trauma*. 2009;67(3):651–659.

41. Rajasekaran S, Kanna RM, Shetty AP. Management of thoracolumbar trauma: an overview. *Indian J Orthop*. 2015;49(1):72–82.

42. Prasam ML, et al. Is it safe to use a kinetic therapy bed for care of patients with cervical spine injuries? *Injury*. 2014;46(2):388–391.

43. Ryken TC, et al. The acute cardiopulmonary management of patients with cervical spinal cord injuries. *Neurosurgery*. 2013;72(Suppl 2):84–92.

44. Sarhan F, Saif D, Saif A. An overview of traumatic spinal cord injury: part 3. Rehabilitation. *Br J Neurosci Nurs*. 2012;9(4):187–194.

45. Zilinskiene L, Idle MR, Colley S. Emergency radiology: maxillofacial and skull base trauma. *Trauma*. 2014;16(4):243–255.

46. Barak M, et al. Airway management of the patient with maxillofacial trauma: review of the literature and suggested clinical approach. *Biomed Res Int*. 2015;2015:724032. http://dx.doi.org/10.1155/2015/724032. Accessed February 6, 2016.

47. Mancini MC. Blunt chest trauma. http://emedicine.medscape.com/article/428723-overview; 2014. Accessed February 6, 2016.

48. Stewart DJ. Blunt chest trauma. *J Trauma Nurs*. 2014;21(6):282–286.

49. Muhm M, et al. Severe trauma of the chest wall: surgical rib stabilisation versus non-operative treatment. *Eur J Trauma Emerg Surg*. 2013;39(3):257–265.

50. Battle C, Hutchings H, Evans PA. Blunt chest wall trauma: a review. *Trauma*. 2013;15(2):156–175.

51. Ampatzidou FC, et al. Delayed presentation of diaphragmatic rupture. An unusual case of dyspnea. *Respir Care*. 2015;60(2):e38–e40.

52. Sofia S. Bedside US imaging in multiple trauma patients. Part 1: US findings and techniques. *J Ultrasound*. 2013;16(4):147–159.

53. El-Menyar A, et al. Understanding blunt cardiac injury. *Ann Card Anaesth*. 2012;15(4):287–295.

54. Fox N, et al. Evaluation and management of blunt traumatic aortic injury. *J Trauma Nurs*. 2015;22(2):99–110.

55. Weiser TG. Aortic disruption (traumatic). Merck Manual Professional Version. http://www.merckmanuals.com/professional/injuries-poisoning/thoracic-trauma/aortic-disruption-traumatic; 2015. Accessed February 6, 2016.

56. Neschis DG. *Blunt thoracic aortic injury*. http://www.uptodate.com/contents/blunt-thoracic-aortic-injury; 2015. Accessed February 6, 2016.

57. Knipe H, Bickle I. *Focussed assessment with sonography for trauma*; 2015. http://radiopaedia.org/articles/focussed-assessment-with-sonography-for-trauma-fast-scan. Accessed February 6, 2016.

58. Prachalias AA, Kontis E. Isolated abdominal trauma: diagnosis and clinical management considerations. *Curr Opin Crit Care*. 2014;20(2):218–225.

59. Hunt L, et al. Management of intra-abdominal hypertension and abdominal compartment syndrome: a review. *J Trauma Manag Outcomes*. 2014;8:2. http://www.traumamanagement.org/content/8/1/2. Accessed February 7, 2016.

60. Kirkpatrick AW, et al. Intra-abdominal hypertension and the abdominal compartment syndrome: Updated consensus definitions and clinical practice guidelines from the world society of abdominal compartment syndrome. *Intensive Care Med*. 2013;39(1):1190–1206.

61. Kokabi N, et al. Intra-abdominal solid organ injuries: an enhanced management algorithm. *Can Assoc Radiol J*. 2014;65(4):301–309.

62. Sawhney C, et al. Critical care issues in solid organ injury: review and experience in a tertiary trauma center. *Saudi J Anaesth*. 2014;8(5):29–35.

63. Williamson JML. Splenic injury: diagnosis and management. *Br J Hosp Med*. 2015;76(4):204–229.

64. American Urological Association. Urotrauma: AUA guideline. https://www.auanet.org/common/pdf/education/clinical-guidance/Urotrauma.pdf; 2014. Accessed February 7, 2016.

65. Krader CG. Ideal bladder injury treatment modality unclear. *Urology Times*. 2014;4:22–23.

66. Eastern Association for the Surgery of Trauma. Pelvic fracture hemorrhage—update and systematic review. *J Trauma*. 2011;71(6):1850–1868.

67. Gerecht R. Critical management of deadly pelvic injuries. *J Emerg Med Serv*. 2014;39(12):28–35.

68. Nicola R. Early total care versus damage control: current concepts in orthopaedic care of polytrauma patients. *Int Sch Res Notices Orthop*. 2013. http://dx.doi.org/10.1155/2013/329452. Accessed February 7, 2016.

69. D'Alleyrand JCD, O'Toole RV. The evolution of damage control orthopedics: Current evidence and practical applications of early appropriate care. *Orthop Clin North Am*. 2013;44(4):499–507.

70. Weinacker A. Update on inpatient management of polytrauma patients. *Bangkok Med J*. 2013;6:104–108.

71. DeMuro JP, Hanna AF. Prophylaxis of deep vein thrombosis in trauma patients. *J Blood Disord Transfus*. 2013;4:4. http://dx.doi.org/10.4172/2155-9864.1000151. Accessed February 7, 2016.

72. Bakowitz M, Bruns B, McCunns M. Acute lung injury and the acute respiratory distress syndrome in the injured patient. *Scand J Trauma Resusc Emerg Med*. 2013;20:54. http://www.ncbi.nlm.nih.gov/pmc/articles/pmc3518173/. Accessed February 7, 2016.

73. Bicudo-Salomao A, et al. (2013). Early nutritional therapy in trauma: after A, B,C, D,E, the importance of F (feed). *J Braz Coll Surg*. 2013;40(4):342–346.

74. Preiser J-C, van Zanten ARH, Berger MM. Metabolic and nutritional support of critically ill patients: Consensus and controversies. *Crit Care*. 2015;19:35. http://www.ccforum.com/content/pdf/s13054-015-0737-8.pdf. Accessed February 8, 2016.

75. Williams J, Thorpe C. Rhabdomyolysis. *Contin Educ Anaesth Crit Care Pain*. 2013;6(4):141–143.

76. Weinhouse GL. Fat embolism syndrome. http://www.uptodate.com/contents/fat-embolism-syndrome; 2013. Accessed February 8, 2016.

77. Kisat M, Villegas CV, Onguti S. (2013). Predictors of sepsis in moderately severely injured patients: an analysis of the national trauma data bank. *Surg Infect (Larchmt)*. 2013;14(1):62–68.

78. Alijanpour E, Jabbari A, Hoseini F. Transfusion related acute lung injury in multiple traumatized patients. *Caspian J Intern Med*. 2012;3(3):500–503.

79. Tisherman SA, Forsythe RM. *Trauma Intensive Care*. New York: Oxford University Press; 2013.

80. Roche CD, et al. Missed orthopaedic injuries in adult trauma patients at a major trauma centre. *Trauma*. 2015;17(2):123–127.

81. Siritep U, Thosingha O, Chayaput P. Predictors of multiple organ dysfunction syndrome in patients with major trauma. *Siriraj Med J*. 2013;65(5):137–140.

82. Van Wessem KJP, Leenen LPH. The effect of evolving trauma care on the development of multiple organ dysfunction syndrome. *Eur Trauma Emerg Surg*. 2014;40(2):127–134.

83. Eastern Association for the Surgery of Trauma. Geriatric trauma, evaluation and management of. *J Trauma*. 2012;73(5):S345–S350.

Shock, Sepsis, and Multiple Organ Dysfunction Syndrome

Beverly Carlson and Lorraine Fitzsimmons

Shock is an acute, widespread process of impaired tissue perfusion that results in cellular, metabolic, and hemodynamic alterations. Ineffective tissue perfusion occurs when an imbalance develops between cellular oxygen supply and cellular oxygen demand. This imbalance can occur for a variety of reasons and eventually results in cellular dysfunction and death. This chapter presents an overview of the general shock response, or shock syndrome, followed by a discussion of the various shock states. Information is also provided regarding the pathogenesis and clinical management of systemic inflammatory response syndrome (SIRS) and multiple organ dysfunction syndrome (MODS).

SHOCK SYNDROME

Description

Shock is a complex pathophysiologic process that often results in MODS and death. All types of shock involve ineffective tissue perfusion and acute circulatory failure. The shock syndrome is a pathway involving a variety of pathologic processes that may be categorized in four stages: initial, compensatory, progressive, and refractory. Progression through each stage varies with the patient's prior condition, duration of initiating event, response to therapy, and correction of underlying cause (Fig. 34.1).

Etiology

Shock can be classified as hypovolemic, cardiogenic, or distributive, depending on the pathophysiologic cause and hemodynamic profile. Hypovolemic shock results from a loss of circulating or intravascular volume. Cardiogenic shock results from the impaired ability of the heart to pump. Distributive shock results from maldistribution of circulating blood volume and can be further classified as septic, anaphylactic, or neurogenic. Septic shock is the result of microorganisms entering the body. Anaphylactic shock is the result of a severe antibody-antigen reaction. Neurogenic shock is the result of the loss of sympathetic tone.

Pathophysiology

During the initial stage, cardiac output (CO) is decreased, and tissue perfusion is threatened. Almost immediately, the compensatory stage begins as the body's homeostatic mechanisms attempt to maintain CO, blood pressure, and tissue perfusion. The compensatory mechanisms are mediated by the sympathetic nervous system (SNS) and consist of neural, hormonal, and chemical responses. The neural response includes an increase in heart rate and contractility, arterial and venous vasoconstriction, and shunting of blood to the vital organs. Hormonal compensation includes activation of the renin response and stimulation of the anterior pituitary and adrenal medulla. Activation of the renin response results in the production of angiotensin II, which causes vasoconstriction and the release of aldosterone and antidiuretic hormone, leading to sodium and water retention. Stimulation of the anterior pituitary results in the secretion of adrenocorticotropic hormone (ACTH), which stimulates the adrenal cortex to produce glucocorticoids, causing an increase in blood glucose levels. Stimulation of the adrenal medulla causes the release of epinephrine and norepinephrine, which further enhance the compensatory mechanisms.

During the progressive stage, the compensatory mechanisms begin failing to meet tissue metabolic needs, and the shock cycle is perpetuated. As tissue perfusion becomes ineffective, the cells switch from aerobic to anaerobic metabolism to produce energy. Anaerobic metabolism produces small amounts of energy but large amounts of lactic acid, producing lactic acidemia. Vasodilation and increased vascular permeability from endothelial and epithelial hypoxia and inflammatory mediators results in intravascular hypovolemia, tissue edema, and further decline in tissue perfusion.[1-3] A systemic release of inflammatory mediators in response to tissue hypoxia, especially in gut tissue, produces microcirculatory impairment and derangement of cellular metabolism, facilitating progression of the shock cycle.[1-5] The patient is experiencing SIRS, and irreversible damage begins to occur. Some cells die as a result of apoptosis, an injury-activated, preprogrammed cellular suicide. Others die as the sodium-potassium pump in the cell membrane fails, causing the cell and its organelles to swell. Cellular energy production comes to a complete halt as the mitochondria swell and rupture. At this point, the problem becomes one of oxygen use instead of oxygen delivery. Even if the cell were to receive more oxygen, it would be unable to use it because of damage to the mitochondria. The cell's digestive organelles swell and leak destructive enzymes into the cell, accelerating cell death.[4]

Every system in the body is affected by this process (Box 34.1). Cardiac dysfunction develops as a result of the release of myocardial depressant cytokines.[1-3] Ventricular failure eventually occurs, further perpetuating the entire process. Central nervous system dysfunction develops as a result of cerebral hypoperfusion, leading to failure of the SNS, cardiac and respiratory depression, and thermoregulatory failure. Endothelial injury from hypoxia and inflammatory cytokines and impaired blood flow result in microvascular thrombosis. Hematologic

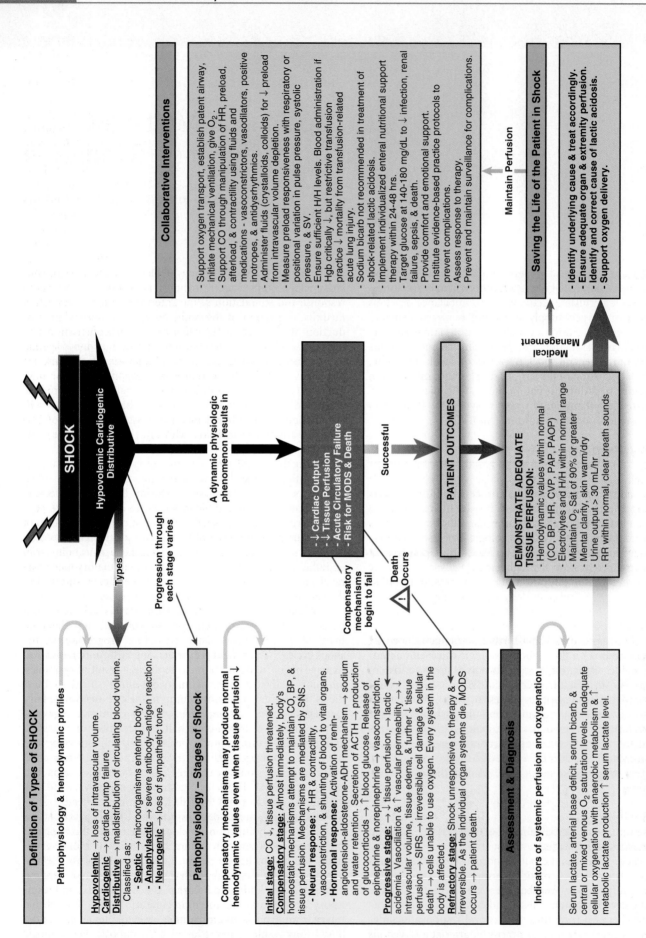

Definition of Types of SHOCK

Pathophysiology & hemodynamic profiles

Hypovolemic → loss of intravascular volume.
Cardiogenic → cardiac pump failure.
Distributive → maldistribution of circulating blood volume.
Classified as:
- **Septic** → microorganisms entering body.
- **Anaphylactic** → severe antibody–antigen reaction.
- **Neurogenic** → loss of sympathetic tone.

Pathophysiology – Stages of Shock

Compensatory mechanisms may produce normal hemodynamic values even when tissue perfusion ↓

Initial stage: CO ↓, tissue perfusion threatened.
Compensatory stage: Almost immediately, body's homeostatic mechanisms attempt to maintain CO, BP, & tissue perfusion. Mechanisms are mediated by SNS.
- **Neural response:** ↑ HR & contractility, vasoconstriction, & shunting of blood to vital organs.
- **Hormonal response:** Activation of renin-angiotension-aldosterone-ADH mechanism → sodium and water retention. Secretion of ACTH → production of glucocorticoids → ↑ blood glucose. Release of epinephrine → norepinephrine → vasoconstriction.
Progressive stage: → ↓ tissue perfusion, → lactic acidemia. Vasodilation & ↑ vascular permeability → ↓ intravascular volume, tissue edema, & further ↓ tissue perfusion → SIRS → irreversible cell damage & cellular death → cells unable to use oxygen. Every system in the body is affected.
Refractory stage: Shock unresponsive to therapy & irreversible. As the individual organ systems die, MODS occurs → patient death.

Assessment & Diagnosis

Indicators of systemic perfusion and oxygenation

Serum lactate, arterial base deficit, serum bicarb, & central or mixed venous O₂ saturation levels. Inadequate cellular oxygenation with anaerobic metabolism & ↑ metabolic lactate production ↑ serum lactate level.

SHOCK

Hypovolemic Cardiogenic Distributive

Types

Progression through each stage varies

A dynamic physiologic phenomenon results in

- ↓ Cardiac Output
- ↓ Tissue Perfusion
- Acute Circulatory Failure
- Risk for MODS & Death

Compensatory mechanisms begin to fail

Death Occurs

Successful

PATIENT OUTCOMES

DEMONSTRATE ADEQUATE TISSUE PERFUSION:
- Hemodynamic values within normal (CO, BP, HR, CVP, PAP, PAOP)
- Electrolytes and H/H within normal range
- Maintain O₂ Sat of 90% or greater
- Mental clarity, skin warm/dry
- Urine output > 30 mL/hr
- RR within normal, clear breath sounds

Medical Management

Collaborative Interventions

- Support oxygen transport, establish patent airway, initiate mechanical ventilation, give O₂.
- Support CO through manipulation of HR, preload, afterload, & contractility using fluids and medications - vasoconstrictors, vasodilators, positive inotropes, & antidysrhythmics.
- Administer fluids (crystalloids, colloids) for ↓ preload from intravascular volume depletion.
- Measure preload responsiveness with respiratory or positional variation in pulse pressure, systolic pressure, & SV.
- Ensure sufficient H/H levels. Blood administration if Hgb critically ↓, but restrictive transfusion practice ↓ mortality from transfusion-related acute lung injury.
- Sodium bicarb not recommended in treatment of shock-related lactic acidosis.
- Implement individualized enteral nutritional support therapy within 24-48 hrs.
- Target glucose at 140-180 mg/dL to ↓ infection, renal failure, sepsis, & death.
- Provide comfort and emotional support.
- Institute evidence-based practice protocols to prevent complications.
- Assess response to therapy.
- Prevent and maintain surveillance for complications.

Maintain Perfusion

Saving the Life of the Patient in Shock

- **Identify underlying cause & treat accordingly.**
- **Ensure adequate organ & extremity perfusion.**
- **Identify and correct cause of lactic acidosis.**
- **Support oxygen delivery.**

FIG. 34.1 Concept Map for Shock. CO – Cardiac Output; BP – Blood Pressure; HR – Heart Rate; O2 Sat – Oxygen saturation; CVP – Central Venous Pressure; PAP – Pulmonary Artery Pressure, PAOP – Pulmonary Artery Occlusion Pressure; SV – Stroke Volume; H/H – Hemoglobin and Hematocrit

BOX 34.1 Consequences of Shock

Cardiovascular
- Ventricular failure
- Microvascular thrombosis

Neurologic
- Sympathetic nervous system dysfunction
- Cardiac and respiratory depression
- Thermoregulatory failure
- Coma

Pulmonary
- Acute lung failure
- Acute respiratory distress syndrome

Renal
- Acute kidney injury

Hematologic
- Disseminated intravascular coagulation

Gastrointestinal
- Gastrointestinal tract failure
- Liver failure
- Pancreatic failure

dysfunction occurs as a result of consumption of clotting factors, release of inflammatory cytokines, and dilutional thrombocytopenia. Disseminated intravascular coagulation (DIC) eventually may develop. Pulmonary dysfunction occurs as a result of increased pulmonary capillary membrane permeability, pulmonary microemboli, and pulmonary vasoconstriction. Ventilatory failure and acute respiratory distress syndrome (ARDS) develop. Renal dysfunction develops secondary to renal vasoconstriction and renal hypoperfusion, leading to acute kidney injury (AKI). Gastrointestinal (GI) dysfunction occurs as a result of splanchnic vasoconstriction and hypoperfusion and leads to failure of the gut organs. Disruption of the intestinal mucosal barrier releases proinflammatory substances into the systemic circulation that further perpetuate the entire shock syndrome.[5]

During the refractory stage, shock becomes unresponsive to therapy and is considered irreversible. As the individual organ systems die, MODS—defined as failure of two or more body systems—occurs. Death is the final outcome. Regardless of the etiologic factors, death occurs from ineffective tissue perfusion because of the failure of the circulation to meet the oxygen needs of the cell.[4]

Assessment and Diagnosis

A patient with a mean arterial blood pressure (MAP) less than 60 mm Hg or with evidence of global tissue hypoperfusion is considered to be in a shock state.[1,3] Because shock is a dynamic physiologic phenomenon, hypotension may occur late in the process or may normalize even when tissue perfusion is still inadequate.[6-9] Clinical manifestations vary according to the underlying cause of shock, the stage of the shock, and the patient's response to shock.

Compensatory mechanisms may produce normal hemodynamic values even when tissue perfusion is compromised.[3,8,10,11] Global indicators of systemic perfusion and oxygenation include serum lactate, arterial base deficit, serum bicarbonate, and central or mixed venous oxygen saturation levels. Inadequate cellular oxygenation with anaerobic metabolism and increased metabolic lactate production increase the serum lactate level.[8,12] The level and duration of this hyperlactatemia are predictive of morbidity and mortality,[7,10-12] and management guided by lactate levels has been effective in improving outcomes.[13,14] The base deficit derived from arterial blood gas (ABG) values also reflects global tissue acidosis and is useful to assess the severity of shock.[6,9-11] Serum bicarbonate is a measure of metabolic acidosis and has been found to correlate well with arterial base deficit.[15] The use of mixed venous oxygen saturation (Svo_2) measured with a pulmonary artery catheter or central venous oxygen saturation ($Scvo_2$) measured with a central venous catheter allows assessment of the balance of oxygen delivery and oxygen consumption and the ratio of oxygen extraction.[3,16-19] As $Scvo_2$ monitoring does not require placement of a pulmonary artery catheter, it is now the preferred method, and its use alone and in conjunction with other measures, particularly serum lactate, has been examined and recommended to assess global oxygenation balance in a variety of critically ill patients.[16-21] Noninvasive indicators of regional tissue perfusion or oxygenation such as sublingual capnometry and subcutaneous or skeletal muscle tissue oxygen saturation measured with near-infrared spectroscopy are also being evaluated.[3,8,18] The sections on different types of shock discuss clinical assessment and diagnosis of the patient in shock.

Medical Management

The major focus of treatment of shock is the improvement and preservation of tissue perfusion. Adequate tissue perfusion depends on an adequate supply of oxygen being transported to the tissues and the cell's ability to use it. Oxygen transport is influenced by pulmonary gas exchange, CO, and hemoglobin level. Oxygen use is influenced by the internal metabolic environment and mitochondrial function. Management of a patient in shock focuses on supporting oxygen delivery.[1,3]

Adequate pulmonary gas exchange is critical to oxygen transport. Establishing and maintaining an adequate airway are the first steps in ensuring adequate oxygenation. After the airway is patent, emphasis is placed on improving ventilation and oxygenation. Therapies include administration of supplemental oxygen and mechanical ventilatory support.

An adequate CO and hemoglobin level are crucial to oxygen transport. CO depends on heart rate, preload, afterload, and contractility. Various fluids and medications are used to manipulate these parameters. The types of fluids used include crystalloids and colloids. The categories of medications used include vasoconstrictors, vasodilators, positive inotropes, and antidysrhythmics.

Fluid administration is indicated for decreased preload related to intravascular volume depletion, and it can be accomplished by use of a crystalloid or colloid solution, or both. Crystalloids are balanced electrolyte solutions that may be hypotonic, isotonic, or hypertonic. Examples of crystalloid solutions used in shock situations are normal saline and lactated Ringer solution. Colloids are protein-containing or starch-containing solutions. Examples of colloid solutions are blood and blood components, such as albumin, and pharmaceutical plasma expanders, such as dextran and mannitol.

The quantity and type of fluid are a subject of debate and depend on the situation.[3,22-27] Excessive volume expansion, more than what increases preload and stroke volume (SV), worsens organ function and may produce coagulopathy, cytokine activation, and abdominal compartment syndrome.[3,24] Methods to measure preload responsiveness include respiratory or positional variations in pulse pressure, systolic pressure, and SV and are more accurate than central venous pressure (CVP).[3] Noninvasive ultrasound is also used to evaluate hemodynamic response to fluid augmentation, although it requires physician interpretation. Fluid resuscitation with normal saline or with albumin produces similar outcomes regardless of baseline serum albumin level.[26,28] Crystalloid solutions are inexpensive and effective. Advantages of colloids include faster restoration of intravascular volume and use of smaller amounts. Colloids are believed to stay in the intravascular space, in contrast to crystalloids, which readily leak into the extravascular space. Disadvantages include expense, allergic reactions, and difficulties in typing and crossmatching blood. Colloids also can leak out of damaged capillaries and cause a variety of additional problems, particularly in the lungs. Hypertonic or hyperoncotic fluids offer no additional benefit over isotonic crystalloids and are not recommended.[3,22,27,29,30]

Blood should be considered to augment oxygen transport if the patient's hemoglobin level is critically low, although what threshold value should be used for a patient in shock or with acute cardiac disease is still undetermined.[3,31] Transfusion of stored red blood cells (RBCs) does not substantially increase oxygen consumption and has been associated with immunosuppression, infection, impairment of microcirculatory flow, increased pulmonary vascular resistance, coagulopathy, and increased mortality. Restrictive transfusion practice has demonstrated lower mortality in a wide variety of patients, including critically ill patients.[3,5,16,31,32] Transfusion-related acute lung injury resulting from immune and nonimmune neutrophil activation has become the leading cause of transfusion-related death and may occur with transfusion of any plasma-containing blood or blood product.[33-35]

Vasoconstrictor agents are used to increase afterload by increasing the systemic vascular resistance (SVR) and improving the patient's blood pressure level. Vasodilator agents are used to decrease preload or afterload, or both, by decreasing venous return and SVR. Positive inotropic agents are used to increase contractility. Antidysrhythmic agents are used to influence heart rate. Box 34.2 lists examples of each of these agents.

Sodium bicarbonate is not recommended in the treatment of shock-related lactic acidosis.[16,36,37] No overall benefit has been found, and the risks associated with its use are significant. These risks include shifting of the oxyhemoglobin dissociation curve to the left, rebound increase in lactic acid production, development of hyperosmolar state, fluid overload resulting from excessive sodium, and rapid cellular electrolyte shifts.[36,37]

A critically ill patient should be started on enteral nutrition support therapy within 24 to 48 hours.[38] The type of nutrition supplementation initiated varies according to the cause of shock, and it should be tailored to the individual patient's needs, as indicated by the underlying condition, laboratory data, and treatment. When enteral feeding is contraindicated, parenteral nutrition should be considered, although a delay of 7 days is recommended for better outcomes.[38-41] Supplementation of enteral feeding with parenteral nutrition to increase caloric intake is a subject of debate but has not been shown to improve patient outcomes.[38,41,42] A delay of 1 week is recommended before consideration of this strategy.[38]

BOX 34.2   Agents Used in the Treatment of Shock

Vasoconstrictors
- Epinephrine (Adrenalin)
- Norepinephrine (Levophed)
- Alpha-range dopamine (Intropin)
- Phenylephrine (Neo-Synephrine)
- Vasopressin (Pitressin)

Vasodilators
- Nitroprusside (Nipride, Nitropress)
- Nitroglycerin (Nitrol, Tridil)
- Hydralazine (Apresoline)
- Labetalol (Normodyne, Trandate)

Inotropes
- Beta-range dopamine (Intropin)
- Dobutamine (Dobutrex)
- Epinephrine (Adrenalin)
- Norepinephrine (Levophed)
- Milrinone (Primacor)

Antidysrhythmics
- Amiodarone (Cordarone)
- Adenosine (Adenocard)
- Procainamide (Pronestyl)
- Labetalol (Normodyne, Trandate)
- Verapamil (Calan, Isoptin)
- Esmolol (Brevibloc)
- Diltiazem (Cardizem)
- Lidocaine (Xylocaine)

Glucose control to a target level of 140 to 180 mg/dL is recommended for all critically ill patients.[43,44] Benefits of glucose control in critically ill patients include lower incidences of infection, renal failure, sepsis, and death.[43-46]

Nursing Management

The nursing management for the patient in shock is a complex and challenging responsibility. It requires an in-depth understanding of the pathophysiology of the disease and the anticipated effects of each intervention as well as a solid understanding of the nursing process. Later sections discuss specific interventions for patients in shock.

The psychosocial needs of the patient and family dealing with shock are extremely important. These needs are based on situational, familial, and patient-centered variables. Nursing interventions for the psychosocial stress of critical illness include providing information on patient status, explaining procedures and routines, supporting the family, encouraging the expression of feelings, facilitating problem solving and shared decision making, individualizing visitation schedules, involving the family in the patient's care, and establishing contacts with necessary resources.[47] The consensus of all relevant professional organizations is that patients and families should be given the option of family presence during invasive procedures and resuscitation.[47-50] Interprofessional collaborative management of a patient with shock is outlined in Box 34.3.

Interprofessional Collaborative Practice: Shock

Support oxygen transport.
- Establish a patent airway.
- Initiate mechanical ventilation.
- Administer oxygen.
- Administer fluids (crystalloids, colloids, blood, and other blood products).
- Administer vasoactive medications.
- Administer positive inotropic medications.
- Ensure sufficient hemoglobin and hematocrit.

Support oxygen use.
- Identify and correct cause of lactic acidosis.
- Ensure adequate organ and extremity perfusion.
- Initiate nutrition support therapy.

Identify underlying cause of shock and treat accordingly.

Provide comfort and emotional support.

Institute evidence-based practice protocols to prevent complications.

Assess response to therapy.

Prevent and maintain surveillance for complications.

HYPOVOLEMIC SHOCK

Description

Hypovolemic shock occurs from inadequate fluid volume in the intravascular space. The lack of adequate circulating volume leads to decreased tissue perfusion and initiation of the general shock response. Hypovolemic shock is the most commonly occurring form of shock (Fig. 34.2).

Etiology

Hypovolemic shock can result from absolute or relative hypovolemia. Absolute hypovolemia occurs when there is a loss of fluid from the intravascular space. This can result from an external loss of fluid from the body or from internal shifting of fluid from the intravascular space to the extravascular space. Fluid shifts can be due to a loss of intravascular integrity, increased capillary membrane permeability, or decreased colloidal osmotic pressure. Relative hypovolemia occurs when vasodilation produces an increase in vascular capacitance relative to circulating volume (Box 34.4).

Pathophysiology

Hypovolemia results in a loss of circulating fluid volume. A decrease in circulating volume leads to a decrease in venous return, which results in a decrease in end-diastolic volume or preload. Preload is a major determinant of SV and CO. A decrease in preload results in a decrease in SV and CO. The decrease in CO leads to inadequate cellular oxygen supply and ineffective tissue perfusion.

Assessment and Diagnosis

The clinical manifestations of hypovolemic shock depend on the severity of fluid loss and the patient's ability to compensate for it. A clinical classification developed by the American College of Surgeons to describe the levels of severity of hypovolemic shock in the trauma setting has been widely accepted, but a test of the validity of this classification suggests that modifications are necessary.[51]

A simpler approach of classifying hypovolemic shock as mild, moderate, or severe is also commonly used. Class I, or mild shock, indicates a fluid volume loss up to 15% to 20% or an actual volume loss up to approximately 750 mL. Compensatory mechanisms maintain CO, and the patient appears free of symptoms other than possibly slight anxiety.[1] As volume loss worsens, the patient may develop cool extremities and increased capillary refill time in response to peripheral vasoconstriction. Class II and class III hypovolemia is consistent with moderate shock.[1] Class II hypovolemia occurs with a fluid volume loss of approximately 15% to 30% or an actual volume loss of 750 to 1500 mL. Falling CO activates more intense compensatory responses. Anxiety increases.[1] The heart rate may increase to more than 100 beats/min in response to increased SNS stimulation unless blocked by preexisting beta-blocker therapy. The pulse pressure narrows as the diastolic blood pressure increases because of vasoconstriction. Postural hypotension develops.[1] The respiratory rate increases as blood loss worsens, and ABG specimens drawn during this phase may reveal respiratory alkalosis, as evidenced by a low partial pressure of carbon dioxide ($Paco_2$). Urine output starts to decline to 20 to 30 mL/h as renal perfusion decreases. The urine sodium level decreases, whereas urinary osmolality and specific gravity increase as the kidneys start to conserve sodium and water. The patient's skin becomes pale and cool with delayed capillary refill because of peripheral vasoconstriction. Jugular veins appear flat as a result of decreased venous return.[1]

Class III hypovolemic shock occurs with a fluid volume loss of 30% to 40% or an actual volume loss of 1500 to 2000 mL. This level of severity may produce the progressive stage of shock as compensatory mechanisms become overwhelmed and ineffective tissue perfusion develops. Blood pressure decreases, but often after tissue hypoperfusion is already significant.[6,9] The heart rate may increase to more than 120 beats/min, and dysrhythmias may develop as myocardial ischemia ensues. During this phase, serum lactate levels increase, and ABG values reveal metabolic acidosis as evidenced by a low bicarbonate (HCO_3^-) and elevated base deficit. Decreased renal perfusion results in the development of oliguria. Blood urea nitrogen and serum creatinine levels start to rise as the kidneys begin to fail. The patient's skin becomes ashen, cold, and clammy, with marked delayed capillary refill. The patient may appear confused as cerebral perfusion decreases.[1]

Class IV hypovolemic shock is severe shock and usually refractory in nature. It occurs with a fluid volume loss of greater than 40% or an actual volume loss of greater than 2000 mL. As the compensatory mechanisms of the body become insufficient, tachycardia and hemodynamic instability worsen, and hypotension ensues. Severe lactic acidosis is present. Peripheral pulses and capillary refill become absent because of marked peripheral vasoconstriction. The skin may appear cyanotic, mottled, and extremely diaphoretic. Organ failure occurs. Urine output ceases. The patient may be confused and agitated, eventually becoming unresponsive. Various clinical manifestations associated with failure of the different body systems develop.[1]

Assessment of the hemodynamic parameters of a patient in hypovolemic shock varies by stage but commonly reveals a decreased CO and cardiac index (CI). Loss of circulating volume leads to a decrease in venous return to the heart, which results in a decrease in the preload of the right and left ventricles.

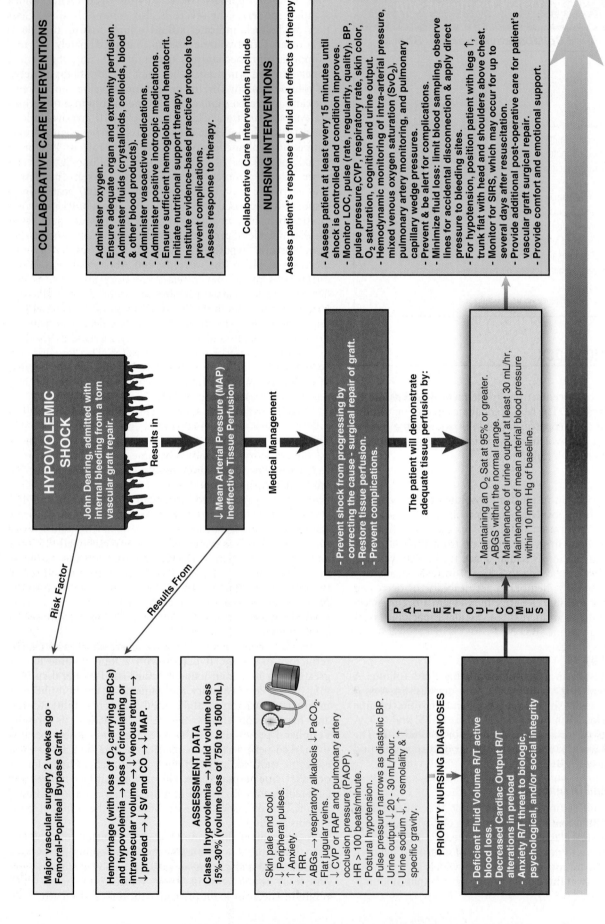

COLLABORATIVE CARE INTERVENTIONS

- Administer oxygen.
- Ensure adequate organ and extremity perfusion.
- Administer fluids (crystalloids, colloids, blood & other blood products).
- Administer vasoactive medications.
- Administer positive inotropic medications.
- Ensure sufficient hemoglobin and hematocrit.
- Initiate nutritional support therapy.
- Institute evidence-based practice protocols to prevent complications.
- Assess response to therapy.

NURSING INTERVENTIONS

Collaborative Care Interventions Include

Assess patient's response to fluid and effects of therapy

- Assess patient at least every 15 minutes until shock is controlled and condition improves.
- Monitor LOC, pulse (rate, regularity, quality), BP, pulse pressure, CVP, respiratory rate, skin color, O₂ saturation, cognition and urine output.
- Hemodynamic monitoring of intra-arterial pressure, mixed venous oxygen saturation (SvO₂), pulmonary artery monitoring, and pulmonary capillary wedge pressures.
- Prevent & be alert for complications.
- Minimize fluid loss: limit blood sampling, observe lines for accidental disconnection & apply direct pressure to bleeding sites.
- For hypotension, position patient with legs ↑, trunk flat with head and shoulders above chest.
- Monitor for SIRS, which may occur for up to several days after resuscitation.
- Provide additional post-operative care for patient's vascular graft surgical repair.
- Provide comfort and emotional support.

HYPOVOLEMIC SHOCK

John Dearing, admitted with internal bleeding from a torn vascular graft repair.

Results in

↓ Mean Arterial Pressure (MAP) Ineffective Tissue Perfusion

Medical Management

- Prevent shock from progressing by correcting the cause - surgical repair of graft.
- Restore tissue perfusion.
- Prevent complications.

The patient will demonstrate adequate tissue perfusion by:

- Maintaining an O₂ Sat at 95% or greater.
- ABGS within the normal range.
- Maintenance of urine output at least 30 mL/hr.
- Maintenance of mean arterial blood pressure within 10 mm Hg of baseline.

P
A
T
I
E
N
T
O
U
T
C
O
M
E
S

Risk Factor

Major vascular surgery 2 weeks ago - Femoral-Popliteal Bypass Graft.

Results From

Hemorrhage (with loss of O₂ carrying RBCs) and hypovolemia → loss of circulating or intravascular volume → ↓ venous return → ↓ preload → ↓ SV and CO → ↓ MAP.

ASSESSMENT DATA
Class II hypovolemia → fluid volume loss 15%-30% (volume loss of 750 to 1500 mL)

- Skin pale and cool.
- ↓ Peripheral pulses.
- ↑ Anxiety.
- ↑ RR.
- ABGs → respiratory alkalosis ↓ PaCO₂.
- Flat jugular veins.
- ↓ CVP or RAP and pulmonary artery occlusion pressure (PAOP).
- HR > 100 beats/minute.
- Postural hypotension.
- Pulse pressure narrows as diastolic BP.
- Urine output ↓ 20 - 30 mL/hour.
- Urine sodium ↓, ↑ osmolality & ↑ specific gravity.

PRIORITY NURSING DIAGNOSES

- Deficient Fluid Volume R/T active blood loss.
- Decreased Cardiac Output R/T alterations in preload
- Anxiety R/T threat to biologic, psychological, and/or social integrity

FIG. 34.2 Concept Map for Hypovolemic Shock. *ABG,* Arterial blood gases; *ABGs,* arterial blood gases; *BP,* blood pressure; *CO,* cardiac output; *CVP,* central venous pressure; *LOC,* level of consciousness; *MAP,* mean arterial pressure; *O₂,* oxygen; *O₂ sat,* oxygen saturation; *PaCO₂,* partial pressure of carbon dioxide in arterial blood. *PaO₂,* partial pressure of oxygen in arterial blood; *R/T,* related to; *SV,* stroke volume; *SvO₂,* mixed venous oxygen saturation; *SIRS,* systemic inflammatory response syndrome.

BOX 34.4 Etiologic Factors in Hypovolemic Shock

Absolute Factors
- Loss of whole blood
  - Trauma or surgery
  - Gastrointestinal bleeding
- Loss of plasma
  - Thermal injuries
  - Large lesions
- Loss of other body fluids
  - Severe vomiting or diarrhea
  - Massive diuresis
  - Loss of intravascular integrity
  - Ruptured spleen
  - Long bone or pelvic fractures
  - Hemorrhagic pancreatitis
  - Hemothorax or hemoperitoneum
  - Arterial dissection or rupture

Relative Factors
- Vasodilation
  - SIRS/sepsis
  - Anaphylaxis
  - Loss of sympathetic stimulation
- Increased capillary membrane permeability
  - SIRS/sepsis
  - Anaphylaxis
  - Thermal injuries
- Decreased colloidal osmotic pressure
  - Severe sodium depletion
  - Hypopituitarism
  - Cirrhosis
  - Intestinal obstruction

SIRS, systemic inflammatory response syndrome.

BOX 34.5 NURSING DIAGNOSES

Hypovolemic Shock

- Deficient Fluid Volume active blood loss, p. 1019
- Deficient Fluid Volume interstitial fluid shift, is on p. 1019
- Decreased Cardiac Output related to alterations in preload, p. 1015
- Imbalanced Nutrition: Less Than Body Requirements related to lack of exogenous nutrients and increased metabolic demand, p. 1029
- Risk for Infection, p. 1046
- Anxiety related to threat to biologic, psychologic, or social integrity, p. 1012
- Compromised Family Coping related to a critically ill family member, p. 1014

is postulated to lessen bleeding and improve survival[22,52-54] and has been demonstrated in a meta-analysis.[53] The type and amount of solutions used for fluid resuscitation and the rate of administration influence immune function; inflammatory mediator release; coagulation; and the incidence of cardiac, pulmonary, renal, and GI complications.[3,22,24,25,27] Consensus on the optimal resuscitative strategy for hypovolemic shock is lacking and is likely situation specific, especially in the case of traumatic hemorrhage.[17,22,24,52,54]

Nursing Management

Prevention of hypovolemic shock is one of the primary responsibilities of the nurse in the critical care unit. Preventive measures include the identification of patients at risk and frequent assessment of the patient's fluid balance. Accurate monitoring of intake and output and daily weights are essential components of preventive nursing care. Early identification and treatment result in decreased mortality.

The nursing management plan for a patient in hypovolemic shock may include numerous nursing diagnoses, depending on the progression of the process (Box 34.5). A patient in hypovolemic shock requires continuous evaluation of intravascular volume, tissue perfusion, and response to therapy. Nursing interventions include minimizing fluid loss, administering volume replacement and vasopressor agents (if needed), assessing response to therapy, providing comfort and emotional support, and preventing and maintaining surveillance for complications.

Measures to minimize fluid loss include limiting blood sampling, observing lines for accidental disconnection, and applying direct pressure to bleeding sites. Measures to facilitate the administration of volume replacement include insertion of large-bore peripheral intravenous catheters and rapid administration of prescribed fluids. Monitoring the patient for adequate tissue perfusion and for clinical manifestations of fluid overload or complications related to fluid and blood product administration is essential for preventing further problems. It is also essential to monitor the patient for SIRS and organ failure, which may occur for up to several days after resuscitation.[55]

CARDIOGENIC SHOCK

Description

Cardiogenic shock is due to failure of the heart to effectively pump blood forward. It can occur with dysfunction of the right or the left ventricle, or both. The lack of adequate pumping function leads to decreased tissue perfusion and circulatory failure (Fig. 34.3). It occurs in approximately 5% to 8% of the

This is evidenced by a decline in the CVP or right atrial pressure (RAP) and pulmonary artery occlusion pressure (PAOP). Vasoconstriction of the arterial system results in an increase in the afterload of the heart, as evidenced by an increase in the SVR. This vasoconstriction may produce inaccurate systolic and diastolic blood pressure values when measured by arterial catheter or noninvasive oscillometry. MAP is more accurate in this low-flow state.[17]

Medical Management

The major goals of therapy for a patient in hypovolemic shock are to correct the cause of the hypovolemia, restore tissue perfusion, and prevent complications. This approach includes identifying and stopping the source of fluid loss, administering fluid to replace circulating volume, and administering vasopressor therapy to maintain tissue perfusion until volume is restored. Fluid administration can be accomplished with use of a crystalloid solution, a colloid solution, blood products, or a combination of fluids. The type of solution used depends on the type of fluid lost, the degree of hypovolemia, the severity of hypoperfusion, and the cause of hypovolemia.

Aggressive fluid resuscitation in trauma and surgical patients is a subject of great debate. Limited or hypotensive (systolic blood pressure 60 to 80 mm Hg or MAP 40 to 60 mm Hg) volume resuscitation in patients with uncontrolled hemorrhage

COLLABORATIVE CARE INTERVENTIONS

- Administer oxygen.
- Ensure adequate organ and extremity perfusion.
- Administer fluids (crystalloids, colloids, blood & other blood products).
- Administer vasoactive medications.
- Administer positive inotropic medications.
- Ensure sufficient hemoglobin and hematocrit.
- Initiate nutritional support therapy.
- Institute evidence-based practice protocols to prevent complications.
- Assess response to therapy.

Collaborative Care Interventions Include

NURSING INTERVENTIONS

- Decrease O_2 demand by providing analgesics & sedatives, position for comfort, limit activities & provide quiet surroundings.
- Close assessment and management of respiratory function to maintain adequate oxygenation including providing supplemental O_2 to maintain adequate ABGs.
- Precise monitoring and management of heart rate, preload, afterload, and contractility.
- Accurate measurement of hemodynamics, controlled administration of fluids and inotropic vasoactive agents.
- Prevent & be alert for complications of drug therapy.
- Immediately recognize & treat dysrhythmias.
- Continuous observation for complications of cardiac mechanical-assist devices: infection, bleeding, thrombocytopenia, hemolysis, embolus, stroke, device malfunction, circulatory compromise of a cannulated extremity, SIRS, and sepsis.
- Provide comfort and emotional support.

Caused by ──── Cardiogenic Shock

Cary Nelson, admitted with anterior MI develops cardiogenic shock 24 hours after admission.

Cardiogenic Shock

Left Anterior Wall MI ST-segment elevation

Results In

- $\rightarrow SV \rightarrow \downarrow CO \rightarrow \downarrow O_2$ to tissues
- $\downarrow LVEDV \rightarrow$ blood flow goes backwards into lungs & causing pulmonary edema.

Impaired Ability of Ventricle to Pump Blood Forward

Blood goes backwards into lungs causing

Pulmonary Edema → Impaired Gas Exchange ↓ Tissue Perfusion

Assessment - early S/S reflect ↓ CO

- Systolic BP < 90 mm Hg
- $\downarrow$ Sensorium; cool, pale, moist skin
- UO < 30 mL/hour
- Chest pain; tachycardia; weak, thready pulse
- $\downarrow S_1$ and S_2 heart sounds
- RR$\uparrow$
- ABGs → respiratory alkalosis ($\downarrow PaCO_2$)
- UA → $\downarrow$ sodium, $\uparrow$ osmolality, $\uparrow$ SG
- $\uparrow$ Serum B-type natriuretic peptide (BNP)

As the LV fails → pulmonary edema results in

- Crackles and rhonchi
- ABGs → Hypoxemia (PaO₂ & SaO₂)
- Development of S_3 and S_4
- JVD indicating right-sided failure
- Dysrhythmias

Death due to cardiogenic shock results from

Cardiopulmonary collapse or multiple organ failure

PRIORITY NURSING DIAGNOSES

- Ineffective Cardiopulmonary Tissue Perfusion R/T acute myocardial ischemia.
- Decreased Cardiac Output R/T alterations in contractility and heart rate.
- Disturbed Body Image related to functional dependence on life-sustaining technology.
- Compromised Family Coping R/T critically ill family member.

AGGRESSIVE MEDICAL MANAGEMENT

- Treat underlying cause.
- Enhance the effectiveness of the pump.
- Improve tissue perfusion.

The patient will demonstrate adequate tissue perfusion by:

- Maintaining an O_2 Sat at 95% or greater.
- ABGS within the normal range.
- Maintenance of urine output at least 30 mL/hr.
- Maintenance of mean arterial blood pressure within 10 mm Hg of baseline.

P A T I E N T   O U T C O M E S

FIG. 34.3 Concept Map for Cardiogenic Shock. *ABGs,* Arterial blood gases; *BP,* blood pressure; *BNP,* b-type natriuretic peptide; *CO,* cardiac output; *LVEDV,* left ventricular end diastolic volume; *O₂,* oxygen; *PaO₂,* partial pressure of oxygen in arterial blood; *RR,* respiratory rate; *R/T,* related to; *SaO₂,* saturation of oxygen; *SG,* specific gravity; *SIRS,* systemic inflammatory response syndrome; *SV,* stroke volume; *UA,* urinary analysis; *UO, urine output.*

patients with an ST segment myocardial infarction (MI), and it is the leading cause of death of patients hospitalized with MI.[56] The mortality rate for cardiogenic shock has decreased with the advent of early revascularization therapy and is currently approximately 40% to 65%.[56-59]

Etiology

Cardiogenic shock can result from problems affecting the muscular function or the mechanical function of the heart or the cardiac rhythm.[57,60] The most common cause is acute MI resulting in the loss of 40% or more of the functional myocardium. It can occur with ST segment elevation or non–ST segment elevation MI.[57] The damage to the myocardium may occur after one massive MI (usually of the anterior wall), or it may be cumulative as a result of several smaller MIs or a small MI in a patient with preexisting ventricular dysfunction.[56] Cardiomyopathy may cause cardiogenic shock as left ventricular function becomes unable to maintain adequate CO. Examples of problems affecting the mechanical function of the heart to fill and eject adequately include severe valvular disease; acute papillary muscle, chordal, or septal rupture; cardiac tamponade; and massive pulmonary embolus (Box 34.6).[57,60]

Pathophysiology

Cardiogenic shock results from the impaired ability of the ventricle to pump blood forward, which leads to a decrease in SV

and an increase in the blood left in the ventricle at the end of systole. The decrease in SV results in a decrease in CO, which leads to decreased cellular oxygen supply and ineffective tissue perfusion. Typically, myocardial performance spirals downward as compensatory vasoconstriction increases myocardial afterload and low blood pressure worsens myocardial ischemia. As left ventricular contractility declines and ventricular compliance decreases, an increase in end-systolic volume results in blood backing up into the pulmonary system and the subsequent development of pulmonary edema. Pulmonary edema causes impaired gas exchange and decreased oxygenation of the arterial blood, which further impair tissue perfusion. In a substantial number of patients, the pathophysiology may follow a different course secondary to activation of inflammatory cytokines. A SIRS response results with systemic vasodilation and, possibly, normalization of the CO.[61] Whether this process contributes to the genesis or the outcome of cardiogenic shock is uncertain, but it is thought to be activated by acute MI and to facilitate development of sepsis.[61] Death caused by cardiogenic shock results from cardiopulmonary collapse or multiple-organ failure.[57]

Assessment and Diagnosis

Various clinical manifestations occur in patients in cardiogenic shock depending on etiologic factors, the patient's underlying medical status, and the severity of the shock state. Although some clinical manifestations are caused by failure of the heart as a pump, many are related to the overall shock response (Box 34.7).

Initially, clinical manifestations reflect the decline in CO. These signs and symptoms include systolic blood pressure less than 90 mm Hg, mean arterial pressure less than 65 mm Hg, or an acute drop in systolic or mean blood pressure of 30 mm Hg or more; decreased sensorium; cool, pale, moist skin; and urine output of less than 30 mL/h.[57,58] The patient also may complain of chest pain. Tachycardia develops to compensate for the decrease in CO. A weak, thready pulse develops, and diminished S_1 and S_2 heart sounds may occur as a result of the decreased contractility. The respiratory rate increases to improve oxygenation. ABG values at this point indicate respiratory alkalosis, as

---

BOX 34.6 **Etiologic Factors in Cardiogenic Shock**

Muscular
- Ischemic injury
  - Acute myocardial infarction
  - Cardiopulmonary arrest
- Acute decompensated heart failure
- Cardiomyopathy
- Acute myocarditis
- Myocardial contusion
- Prolonged cardiopulmonary bypass
- Septic shock
- Hemorrhagic shock
- Medications (beta-adrenergic blockers, calcium channel antagonists, cytotoxic agents)

Mechanical
- Valvular dysfunction
- Papillary muscle dysfunction or rupture
- Septal wall rupture
- Free wall rupture
- Ventricular aneurysm
- Obstructive hypertrophic cardiomyopathy
- Intracardiac tumor
- Pulmonary embolus
- Atrial thrombus
- Cardiac tamponade
- Massive pulmonary embolus
- Constrictive pericarditis

Rhythmic
- Bradydysrhythmias
- Tachydysrhythmias

BOX 34.7 **Clinical Manifestations of Cardiogenic Shock**

- Systolic blood pressure <90 mm Hg
- Acute drop in blood pressure >30 mm Hg
- Heart rate >100 beats/min
- Weak, thready pulse
- Diminished heart sounds
- Change in sensorium
- Cool, pale, moist skin
- Urine output <30 mL/h
- Chest pain
- Dysrhythmias
- Tachypnea
- Crackles
- Decreased cardiac output
- Cardiac index <2.2 L/min/m²
- Increased pulmonary artery occlusion pressure
- Increased right atrial pressure
- Variable systemic vascular resistance

evidenced by a decrease in $Paco_2$. Urinalysis findings demonstrate a decrease in urine sodium level and an increase in urine osmolality and specific gravity as the kidneys start to conserve sodium and water. Serum B-type natriuretic peptide levels are likely to be elevated.

As the left ventricle fails, auscultation of the lungs may disclose crackles and rhonchi, indicating the development of pulmonary edema. Hypoxemia occurs, as evidenced by a fall in Pao_2 and Sao_2 as measured by ABG values. S_3 and S_4 heart sounds may occur. Jugular venous distention is evident with right-sided failure. The patient also may experience dysrhythmias in response to tissue hypoxia, the underlying problem, and drug therapy.[57]

Assessment of the hemodynamic parameters of a patient in cardiogenic shock reveals decreased CO with CI less than 2.2 L/min/m^2 in the presence of an elevated PAOP.[57,58] A proportional pulse pressure (systolic blood pressure/pulse pressure) less than 25% is indicative of left ventricular failure and CI less than 2.2 L/min/m^2 and may be useful when direct measurement of CI is unavailable.[62] Increased filling pressures are necessary to rule out hypovolemia as the cause of circulatory failure. The increase in PAOP reflects an increase in the left ventricular end-diastolic pressure and left ventricular end-diastolic volume resulting from decreased SV. With right ventricular failure, the RAP also increases. Compensatory vasoconstriction typically results in an increase in the afterload of the heart, as evidenced by an increase in the SVR, unless SIRS produces vasodilation and a normal or decreased SVR. Echocardiography confirms the diagnosis of cardiogenic shock, provides noninvasive estimates of PAOP and ejection fraction, and often clarifies etiologic factors.[57,58]

As compensatory mechanisms fail and ineffective tissue perfusion develops, other clinical manifestations appear. Myocardial ischemia progresses, as evidenced by continued increases in heart rate, dysrhythmias, and chest pain. Pulmonary function deteriorates, which leads to respiratory distress. ABG values during this phase reveal respiratory and metabolic acidosis and hypoxemia, as indicated by a high $Paco_2$, low HCO_3^-, and low Pao_2. Renal failure occurs, as exhibited by the development of anuria and increases in blood urea nitrogen and serum creatinine levels. Cerebral hypoperfusion manifests as a decreasing level of consciousness.

Medical Management

Treatment of a patient in cardiogenic shock requires an aggressive approach. The major goals of therapy are to treat the underlying cause, enhance the effectiveness of the pump, and improve tissue perfusion. This approach includes identifying and treating the etiologic factors of heart failure and administering pharmacologic agents or using mechanical devices to enhance CO. Inotropic agents are used to increase contractility and maintain adequate blood pressure and tissue perfusion. Dobutamine is the inotrope of choice.[58] A vasopressor, preferably norepinephrine, may be necessary to maintain blood pressure when hypotension is severe.[57-59] As both of these therapies increase myocardial oxygen demand, the lowest possible doses should be used.[57,58] Diuretics may be used for preload reduction. Vasodilating agents are used for preload and afterload reduction only in specific situations in conjunction with an inotrope or when the patient is no longer in shock. Antidysrhythmic agents should be used to suppress or control dysrhythmias that can affect CO. Intubation and mechanical ventilation are usually necessary to support oxygenation.

The cause of pump failure should be identified as quickly as possible so that measures can be taken to correct the problem if possible. In the setting of acute MI, emergent revascularization by percutaneous coronary intervention or coronary artery bypass graft surgery provides significant survival benefit and is recommended by national guidelines.[57,58,63] Fibrinolytic agents may be used in select patients. Procedural or surgical intervention may be necessary to remedy mechanical etiology.

Mechanical circulatory assist devices are used if adequate tissue perfusion cannot be immediately restored. Options include an intraaortic balloon pump (IABP), percutaneous ventricular assist device (VAD), or extracorporeal membrane oxygenator. The IABP is used to decrease myocardial workload by improving myocardial supply and decreasing myocardial demand. It achieves this goal by improving coronary artery perfusion and reducing left ventricular afterload. However, IABP therapy is no longer recommended for cardiogenic shock associated with acute MI because results of several more recent studies have confirmed a lack of short-term and long-term survival benefit in these patients.[58,59,64] The other mechanical assist devices provide a means to sustain effective organ perfusion, allowing time for effective intervention, healing, permanent placement of a VAD, or cardiac transplantation. Chapter 15 provides more information about these therapies.

Nursing Management

Prevention of cardiogenic shock is one of the primary responsibilities of the nurse in the critical care unit. Preventive measures include the identification of patients at risk, facilitation of early reperfusion therapy for acute MI, and frequent assessment and management of the patient's cardiopulmonary status.

The nursing management plan for a patient in cardiogenic shock may include numerous nursing diagnoses, depending on the progression of the process (Box 34.8). Nursing interventions include limiting myocardial oxygen demand, enhancing myocardial oxygen supply, maintaining adequate tissue perfusion, providing comfort and emotional support, and preventing and maintaining surveillance for complications. Measures to limit myocardial oxygen demand include administering analgesics, sedatives, and agents to control afterload and dysrhythmias; positioning the patient for comfort; limiting activities; providing a calm and quiet environment and offering support to reduce anxiety; and teaching the patient about the condition. Measures to enhance myocardial oxygen supply include administering supplemental oxygen, monitoring the patient's respiratory status, administering prescribed medications, and managing device therapy.

Effective nursing management of cardiogenic shock requires precise monitoring and management of heart rate, preload,

---

BOX 34.8   NURSING DIAGNOSES
Cardiogenic Shock

- Decreased Cardiac Output related to alterations in contractility, p. 1016
- Decreased Cardiac Output related to alterations in heart rate, p. 1016
- Imbalanced Nutrition: Less Than Body Requirements related to lack of exogenous nutrients and increased metabolic demand, p. 1029
- Risk for Infection, p. 1046
- Disturbed Body Image related to functional dependence on life-sustaining technology, p. 1022
- Compromised Family Coping related to a critically ill family member, p. 1014

afterload, and contractility. This is accomplished through accurate measurement of hemodynamic variables and controlled administration of fluids and inotropic and vasoactive agents. Close assessment and management of respiratory function is also essential to maintain adequate oxygenation. Dysrhythmias are common and require immediate recognition and treatment.

Patients who require mechanical device therapy (IABP, VAD, or extracorporeal membrane oxygenator) need to be observed frequently for complications. Complications of mechanical circulatory assist devices include infection, bleeding, thrombocytopenia, hemolysis, embolus, stroke, device malfunction, circulatory compromise of a cannulated extremity, SIRS, and sepsis.

ANAPHYLACTIC SHOCK

Description

Anaphylactic shock, a type of distributive shock, is the result of an immediate hypersensitivity reaction. It is a life-threatening event that requires prompt intervention. The severe and systemic response leads to decreased tissue perfusion and initiation of the general shock response (Fig. 34.4).

Etiology

Anaphylaxis is a systemic reaction caused by an immunologic antibody-antigen response or nonimmunologic activation of mast cells and basophils.[65-69] Numerous triggers have been identified that, when introduced by injection or ingestion or through the skin or respiratory tract, can cause a reaction. This list includes foods, food additives, diagnostic agents, biologic agents, environmental agents, medications, and venoms (Box 34.9).[65,67-69] Anaphylaxis can also be triggered by physical factors and can be idiopathic in nature with no known trigger.[65,67,68] In the hospital environment, latex was once an extremely problematic antigen for patients and health care providers, but efforts to limit and prevent exposure have been highly successful.[68]

Immunologic anaphylactic reactions can be IgE-mediated or non–IgE-mediated responses. IgE is an antibody that is formed as part of the immune response. The first time an antigen enters the body, an antibody IgE, specific for the antigen, is formed. The antigen-specific IgE antibody is then stored by attachment to mast cells and basophils. This initial contact with the antigen is known as a *primary immune response.* The next time the antigen enters the body, the preformed IgE antibody reacts with it, and a secondary immune response occurs. This reaction triggers the release of biochemical mediators from the mast cells and basophils and initiates the cascade of events that precipitates anaphylactic shock.[65,66,68] Some immunologic anaphylactic reactions are non–IgE-mediated. These can be IgG mediated, occur as a result of direct activation of the mast cells, or be mediated by activation of the complement system.[68]

Nonimmunologic direct activation of the mast cells and basophils may occur with exercise or exposure to cold, heat, sunlight, ethanol, or medications. In some cases, multiple mechanisms contribute to the anaphylactic response.[68] The term *anaphylactoid reaction* was formerly used to denote all non–IgE-mediated reactions, but it is no longer recommended because there is no clinical distinction between the various mechanisms.[67-69]

Pathophysiology

Both immunologic and nonimmunologic activation of the mast cells and basophils results in the release of biochemical mediators. These mediators include histamine; tryptase; chymase; carboxypeptidase A3; platelet-activating factor (PAF); heparin; leukotrienes; prostaglandins; and cytokines such as interleukin (IL)-6, IL-33, and tumor necrosis factor (TNF)-alpha, among others.[65,68,69] The activation of the biochemical mediators causes vasodilation; increased capillary permeability; laryngeal edema; bronchoconstriction; excessive mucus secretion; coronary vasoconstriction; inflammation; cutaneous reactions; and constriction of the smooth muscle in the intestinal wall, bladder, and uterus. Coronary vasoconstriction causes severe myocardial depression. Cutaneous reactions cause stimulation of nerve endings, followed by itching and pain.[68]

Peripheral vasodilation results in relative hypovolemia and decreased venous return. Increased capillary membrane permeability results in the loss of intravascular volume into the interstitial space, as much as 35% within 10 minutes, worsening the hypovolemic state.[67] Decreased venous return results in decreased end-diastolic volume and SV. The decline in SV leads to decreased CO and ineffective tissue perfusion. Death may result from airway obstruction or cardiovascular collapse, or both.[65-71]

Assessment and Diagnosis

Anaphylactic shock is a severe systemic reaction that can affect multiple organ systems. Various clinical manifestations occur in a patient in anaphylactic shock, depending on the extent of multisystem involvement. The symptoms usually start to appear within minutes of exposure to the antigen, but they may not occur for hours (Box 34.10).[66,68,71] Symptoms may also reappear after a 1- to 72-hour window of resolution in what is termed a *biphasic reaction.*[68,71,72] These late-phase reactions may be similar to the initial anaphylactic response, milder, or more severe.[72] In *protracted anaphylaxis,* symptoms may last 32 hours.[67]

The cutaneous effects may appear first and include pruritus, generalized erythema, urticaria, and angioedema. Commonly seen on the face and in the oral cavity and lower pharynx, angioedema develops as a result of fluid leaking into the interstitial space. The patient may appear restless, uneasy, apprehensive, and anxious and may complain of being warm. Respiratory effects include the development of laryngeal edema, bronchoconstriction, and mucous plugs. Clinical manifestations of laryngeal edema include inspiratory stridor, hoarseness, a sensation of fullness or a lump in the throat, and dysphagia. Bronchoconstriction causes dyspnea, wheezing, and chest tightness.[68,70,71] GI and genitourinary manifestations, which may develop as a result of smooth muscle contraction, include vomiting, diarrhea, cramping, and abdominal pain.[71]

Hypotension and reflex tachycardia may develop quickly in response to massive vasodilation and rapid loss of circulating volume. Jugular veins appear flat as right ventricular end-diastolic volume is decreased. The eventual outcome is circulatory failure and ineffective tissue perfusion.[68,70,71] The patient's level of consciousness may deteriorate to unresponsiveness.

Assessment of the hemodynamic parameters of a patient in anaphylactic shock reveals a decreased CO and CI. Venous vasodilation and massive volume loss lead to a decrease in preload, which results in a decline in the RAP and PAOP. Vasodilation of the arterial system results in a decrease in the afterload of the

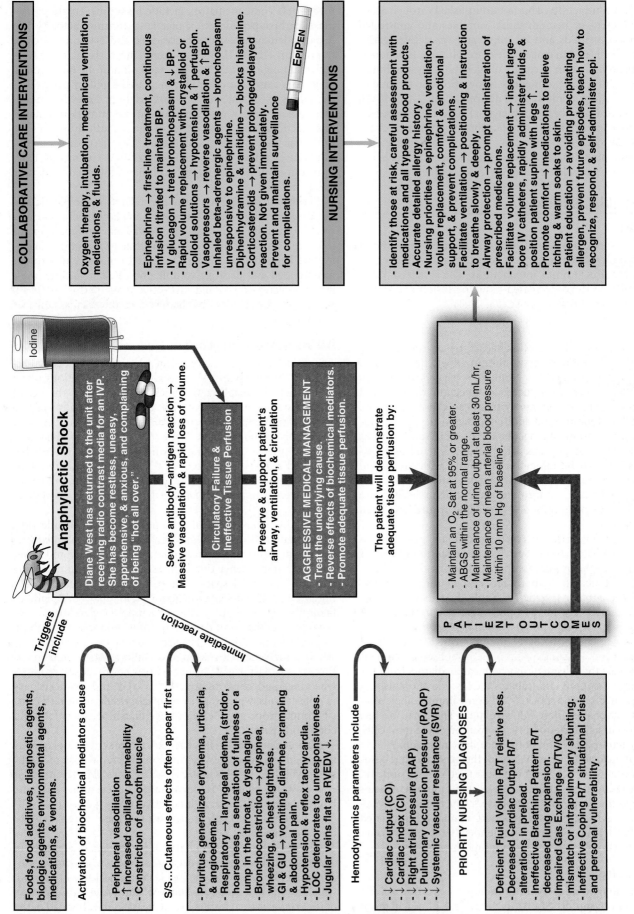

FIG. 34.4 Concept Map for Anaphylactic Shock. *ABGs*, Arterial blood gases; *BP*, blood pressure; *CI*, cardiac index; *CO*, cardiac output; *GI*, gastrointestinal; *GU*, genitourinary; *O₂ Sat*, oxygen saturation; *PAOP*, pulmonary occlusion pressure; *RAP*, right atrial pressure; *R/T*, related to; *RVEDV*, right ventricular end diastolic volume; *S/S*, signs and symptoms; *SVR*, systemic vascular resistance; *V/Q*, ventilation perfusion.

COLLABORATIVE CARE INTERVENTIONS

Oxygen therapy, intubation, mechanical ventilation, medications, & fluids.

- Epinephrine → first-line treatment, continuous infusion titrated to maintain BP.
- IV glucagon → treat bronchospasm & ↓ BP.
- Rapid volume replacement with crystalloid or colloid solutions → hypotension & ↑ perfusion.
- Vasopressors → reverse vasodilation & ↑ BP.
- Inhaled beta-adrenergic agents → bronchospasm unresponsive to epinephrine.
- Diphenhydramine & ranitidine → blocks histamine.
- Corticosteroids → prevent prolonged/delayed reaction. Not given immediately.
- Prevent and maintain surveillance for complications.

NURSING INTERVENTIONS

- Identify those at risk, careful assessment with medications and all types of blood products.
- Accurate detailed allergy history.
- Nursing priorities → epinephrine, ventilation, volume replacement, comfort & emotional support, & prevent complications.
- Facilitate ventilation → positioning & instruction to breathe slowly & deeply.
- Airway protection → prompt administration of prescribed medications.
- Facilitate volume replacement → insert large-bore IV catheters, rapidly administer fluids, & position patient supine with legs ↑.
- Promote comfort → medications to relieve itching & warm soaks to skin.
- Patient education → avoiding precipitating allergen, prevent future episodes, teach how to recognize, respond, & self-administer epi.

Anaphylactic Shock

Diane West has returned to the unit after receiving radio contrast media for an IVP. She has become restless, uneasy, apprehensive, & anxious, and complaining of being "hot all over."

Triggers include

Foods, food additives, diagnostic agents, biologic agents, environmental agents, medications, & venoms.

Activation of biochemical mediators cause

- Peripheral vasodilation
- ↑ Increased capillary permeability
- Constriction of smooth muscle

Immediate reaction

S/S...Cutaneous effects often appear first

- Pruritus, generalized erythema, urticaria, & angioedema.
- Respiratory → laryngeal edema, (stridor, hoarseness, a sensation of fullness or a lump in the throat, & dysphagia).
- Bronchoconstriction → dyspnea, wheezing, & chest tightness.
- GI & GU → vomiting, diarrhea, cramping & abdominal pain.
- Hypotension & reflex tachycardia.
- LOC deteriorates to unresponsiveness.
- Jugular veins flat as RVEDV ↓.

Severe antibody–antigen reaction → Massive vasodilation & rapid loss of volume.

Circulatory Failure & Ineffective Tissue Perfusion

Preserve & support patient's airway, ventilation, & circulation

AGGRESSIVE MEDICAL MANAGEMENT
- Treat the underlying cause.
- Reverse effects of biochemical mediators.
- Promote adequate tissue perfusion.

Hemodynamics parameters include
→ - Cardiac output (CO)
→ - Cardiac index (CI)
→ - Right atrial pressure (RAP)
→ - Pulmonary occlusion pressure (PAOP)
→ - Systemic vascular resistance (SVR)

PRIORITY NURSING DIAGNOSES

- Deficient Fluid Volume R/T relative loss.
- Decreased Cardiac Output R/T alterations in preload.
- Ineffective Breathing Pattern R/T decreased lung expansion.
- Impaired Gas Exchange R/T V/Q mismatch or intrapulmonary shunting.
- Ineffective Coping R/T situational crisis and personal vulnerability.

The patient will demonstrate adequate tissue perfusion by:

- Maintain an O₂ Sat at 95% or greater.
- ABGS within the normal range.
- Maintenance of urine output at least 30 mL/hr,
- Maintenance of mean arterial blood pressure within 10 mm Hg of baseline.

PATIENT OUTCOMES

BOX 34.9   Etiologic Factors in Anaphylactic Shock

Foods
- Eggs and milk
- Fish and shellfish
- Nuts and seeds
- Legumes and cereals
- Soy
- Wheat
- Strawberries
- Avocados
- Any

Food Additives
- Food coloring
- Preservatives

Diagnostic Agents
- Radiocontrast media
- Dehydrocholic acid (Decholin)
- Iopanoic acid (Telepaque)

Biologic Agents
- Blood and blood components
- Insulin and other hormones
- Gammaglobulin
- Seminal fluid
- Vaccines and antitoxins

Environmental Agents
- Pollens, molds, and spores
- Sunlight
- Cold or heat
- Animal dander
- Latex

Drugs
- Antibiotics
- Aspirin
- Nonsteroidal antiinflammatory drugs
- Opioids
- Dextran
- Vitamins
- Muscle relaxants
- Neuromuscular blocking agents
- Barbiturates
- Nonbarbiturate hypnotics
- Protamine
- Infliximab (Remicade)
- Ethanol
- Other

Venoms
- Bees, hornets, yellow jackets, and wasps
- Snakes, jellyfish
- Deer flies
- Fire ants

Physical
- Exercise

BOX 34.10   Clinical Manifestations of Anaphylactic Shock

Cardiovascular
- Hypotension
- Tachycardia
- Bradycardia
- Chest pain

Respiratory
- Lump in throat
- Cough
- Dyspnea
- Dysphagia
- Hoarseness
- Stridor
- Wheezing
- Rhinitis
- Chest tightness

Cutaneous
- Pruritus
- Erythema
- Urticaria
- Angioedema
- Sense of warmth

Neurologic
- Restlessness
- Uneasiness
- Apprehension
- Anxiety
- Dizziness
- Headache
- Sense of impending doom
- Confusion
- Syncope or near syncope

Gastrointestinal
- Nausea
- Vomiting
- Diarrhea
- Cramping abdominal pain

Genitourinary
- Incontinence

Hemodynamic Parameters
- Decreased cardiac output
- Decreased cardiac index
- Decreased right atrial pressure
- Decreased pulmonary occlusion pressure
- Decreased systemic vascular resistance

heart, as evidenced by a decrease in the SVR. Box 34.11 outlines the clinical criteria for diagnosing anaphylaxis.

Medical Management

Treatment of anaphylactic shock requires an immediate and direct approach to prevent death. The goals of therapy are to remove the offending antigen, reverse the effects of the biochemical mediators, and promote adequate tissue perfusion. When the hypersensitivity reaction occurs as a result of administration of medications, dye, blood, or blood products, the infusion should be immediately discontinued. It is often impossible to remove the antigen because it is unknown or has already entered the patient's system.

Reversal of the effects of the biochemical mediators involves the preservation and support of the patient's airway, ventilation, and circulation. This is accomplished through oxygen therapy, intubation, mechanical ventilation, and administration of medications and fluids.

Epinephrine is the first-line treatment of choice for anaphylaxis and should be administered when initial signs and symptoms occur.[67,69,71] It promotes bronchodilation, vasoconstriction, and increased myocardial contractility and inhibits further release of biochemical mediators. In mild cases of anaphylaxis, 0.2 to 0.5 mg (0.3 to 0.5 mL) of a 1:1000 dilution of epinephrine is administered by intramuscular injection into the anterolateral thigh and repeated every 5 to 15 minutes until anaphylaxis is resolved.[65-68,70,71] Subcutaneous injection is no longer recommended.[71] For anaphylactic shock with hypotension, epinephrine is administered intravenously. The intravenous dose is 0.05 to 0.1 mg (1 mL) of a 1:10,000 dilution administered over 5 minutes.[70,71] If hypotension persists, a continuous infusion of epinephrine is recommended, administered at 1 to 4 mcg/min with titration up to 10 mcg/min as needed.[67,70,71] Patients receiving beta-blockers may have a limited response to epinephrine. Intravenous glucagon administered as a 20- to 30-mcg/kg bolus over 5 minutes followed by continuous infusion at 5 to 15 mcg/min is recommended to treat bronchospasm and hypotension in these patients.[66,67,71]

Rapid volume replacement with crystalloid or colloid solutions is also used for patients with hypotension.[66,67,71] Administration of up to 1 L in 5 to 10 minutes is suggested if needed to restore perfusion.[68,71] Vasopressors may be necessary to reverse the vasodilation and increase blood pressure.[66,68,71]

Several medications are used as second-line or third-line adjunctive therapy but are not to be used as substitutes for epinephrine. Inhaled beta-adrenergic agents are used to treat bronchospasm unresponsive to epinephrine.[67,68,70,71] Diphenhydramine (Benadryl), 1 to 2 mg/kg (25 to 50 mg) given by a slow intravenous push, is used to block histamine response.[67,69,71] Ranitidine or cimetidine given in conjunction with diphenhydramine has been found helpful to control cutaneous reactions.[67,71] Corticosteroids are not effective in the immediate treatment of acute anaphylaxis[67,71,73] but may be given with the goal of preventing a prolonged or delayed reaction.[66,69,70]

Nursing Management

Prevention of anaphylactic shock is one of the primary responsibilities of the nurse in the critical care unit. Preventive measures include the identification of patients at risk and cautious assessment of the patient's response to the administration of medications, blood, and blood products. A complete and accurate history of the patient's allergies is an essential component of preventive nursing care. In addition to a list of the allergies, a detailed description of the type of response for each allergy should be obtained.

The nursing management plan for a patient in anaphylactic shock may include numerous nursing diagnoses, depending on the progression of the process (Box 34.12). Nursing interventions include administering epinephrine, facilitating ventilation, administering volume replacement, providing comfort and emotional support, maintaining surveillance for recurrent reactions, and preventing and maintaining surveillance for complications.

Measures to facilitate ventilation include positioning the patient to assist with breathing and instructing the patient to breathe slowly and deeply. Airway protection through prompt administration of prescribed medications is essential. Measures to facilitate the administration of volume replacement include inserting large-bore peripheral intravenous catheters and rapidly administering prescribed fluids. Measures to promote comfort include administering medications to relieve itching and applying warm soaks to skin. Observing the patient for clinical manifestations of a delayed or recurrent reaction is critical. Patient education about how to avoid the precipitating allergen is essential for preventing future episodes of anaphylaxis. Education about how to recognize and respond to a future episode including self-administration of epinephrine is essential to prevent a future life-threatening event.

NEUROGENIC SHOCK

Description

Neurogenic shock, another type of distributive shock, is the result of the loss or suppression of sympathetic tone. The lack of sympathetic tone leads to decreased tissue perfusion and initiation of the general shock response (Fig. 34.5). Neurogenic shock is the most uncommon form of shock.

Etiology

Neurogenic shock can be caused by anything that disrupts the SNS. The problem can occur as the result of interrupted impulse transmission or blockage of sympathetic outflow from the vasomotor center in the brain.[1,74,75] The most common cause is spinal cord injury (SCI). Neurogenic shock may mistakenly be referred to as *spinal shock*. The latter condition refers to loss of neurologic activity below the level of SCI, but it does not necessarily involve ineffective tissue perfusion.[74,75]

Pathophysiology

Loss of sympathetic tone results in massive peripheral vasodilation, inhibition of the baroreceptor response, and impaired thermoregulation. Arterial vasodilation leads to a decrease in SVR and a fall in blood pressure. Venous vasodilation leads to relative hypovolemia and pooling of blood in the venous circuit. The decreased venous return results in a decrease in end-diastolic volume or preload, causing a decrease in SV and CO. The fall in blood pressure and CO leads to inadequate or ineffective tissue perfusion. Loss of sympathetic tone and inhibition of the baroreceptor response result in bradycardia.[74-78] The slow heart rate worsens CO, which further compromises tissue perfusion. Impaired thermoregulation occurs because of loss of vasomotor tone in the cutaneous blood vessels that dilate and constrict to maintain body temperature. The patient becomes poikilothermic, or dependent on the environment for temperature regulation.

Assessment and Diagnosis

A patient in neurogenic shock characteristically presents with hypotension, bradycardia, and warm, dry skin.[74,75,78,79] The decreased blood pressure results from massive peripheral vasodilation. The decreased heart rate is caused by inhibition of the baroreceptor response and unopposed parasympathetic control of the heart.[74,75,78] Consensus on the specific blood pressure and heart rate thresholds for the diagnosis of neurogenic shock has not been established.[74,75] Hypothermia develops from uncontrolled peripheral heat loss. The warm, dry skin occurs as a consequence of pooling of blood in the extremities and loss of vasomotor control in surface vessels of the skin that control heat loss.

Assessment of the hemodynamic parameters of a patient in neurogenic shock reveals a decreased CO and CI. Venous vasodilation leads to a decrease in preload, which results in a decline

in RAP and PAOP. Vasodilation of the arterial system causes a decrease in the afterload of the heart, as evidenced by a decrease in the SVR.[75,78]

Medical Management

Treatment of neurogenic shock requires a careful approach. The goals of therapy are to treat or remove the cause, prevent cardiovascular instability, and promote optimal tissue perfusion. Cardiovascular instability can result from hypovolemia, bradycardia, and hypothermia. Specific treatments are aimed at preventing or correcting these problems as they occur.

Hypovolemia is treated with careful fluid resuscitation. The minimal amount of fluid is administered to ensure adequate tissue perfusion. Volume replacement is initiated for systolic blood pressure less than 90 mm Hg or evidence of inadequate tissue perfusion. Base deficit or lactate levels are recommended to guide fluid resuscitation in patients with SCI.[77] The patient is carefully observed for evidence of fluid overload. Vasopressors are used as necessary to maintain blood pressure and organ perfusion.[1,74,76-79] Higher than typical MAPs are commonly needed for patients with acute SCI to prevent cord ischemia, but optimal pressures have not been determined.[74,77] Bradycardia associated with neurogenic shock rarely requires specific treatment, but atropine, intravenous infusion of a beta-adrenergic agent, or electrical pacing can be used when necessary.[78,80] Hypothermia is treated with warming measures and environmental temperature regulation.

Nursing Management

Prevention of neurogenic shock is one of the primary responsibilities of the nurse in the critical care unit. This includes the identification of patients at risk and constant assessment of the neurologic status. Vigilant immobilization of SCIs and slight elevation of the head of the patient's bed after spinal anesthesia are essential components of preventive nursing care. Early identification allows for early treatment and decreased mortality.

The nursing management plan for a patient in neurogenic shock may include numerous nursing diagnoses, depending on the progression of the process (Box 34.13). Nursing interventions include treating hypovolemia and maintaining tissue perfusion, maintaining normothermia, monitoring for and treating dysrhythmias, providing comfort and emotional support, and preventing and maintaining surveillance for complications.

Venous pooling in the lower extremities promotes the formation of deep vein thrombosis (DVT), which can result in a pulmonary embolism. All patients at risk for DVT should be started on prophylaxis therapy. Prophylactic measures include monitoring of passive range-of-motion exercises, application of sequential pneumatic stockings, and administration of prescribed anticoagulation therapy.

SEPSIS AND SEPTIC SHOCK

Description

Sepsis occurs when microorganisms invade the body and initiate a systemic inflammatory response. This host response often results in perfusion abnormalities with organ dysfunction (sepsis) and eventually circulatory and cellular abnormalities (septic shock). The primary mechanism of this type of shock is maldistribution of blood flow to the tissues (Fig. 34.6).[1,4] Sepsis is estimated to result in more than 700,000 hospitalizations annually

Pathophysiology

Spinal cord injury results in a loss of sympathetic tone → massive peripheral vasodilation, inhibition of baroreceptor response, & impaired thermoregulation.

Assessment & Diagnosis

- ↓ BP → massive peripheral vasodilation.
- ↓ HR → inhibition of baroreceptor response & unopposed parasympathetic control of heart.
- Hypothermia → uncontrolled peripheral heat loss.
- Warm, dry skin → blood pooling in extremities & loss of vasomotor control in surface vessels of the skin that control heat loss.
- ↓ Peripheral pulses
- ↑ Anxiety
- ↑ RR
- ABGs → respiratory alkalosis ↓ $PaCO_2$
- Flat jugular veins.
- Pulse pressure narrows as diastolic BP
- Urine output ↓ 20 - 30 mL/hour

Hemodynamic Parameters

- ↓ CO and CI
- Venous vasodilation → ↓ preload, → ↓ RAP & ↓ PAOP
- Arterial vasodilation → ↓ afterload as evidenced by ↓ SVR

PRIORITY NURSING DIAGNOSES

- Deficient Fluid Volume R/T relative loss.
- Decreased Cardiac Output R/T sympathetic blockade.
- Hypothermia R/T exposure to cold environment, trauma, or damage to the hypothalamus.
- Anxiety R/T threat to biologic, psychological, or social integrity.

24 hours after Jon Walker suffered a T-4 spinal cord injury, he develops hypotension, bradycardia, and warm, dry skin.

Neurogenic Shock

Results in

Sympathetic Blockade Circulatory Failure ↓ Tissue Perfusion

GOALS OF MEDICAL MANAGEMENT

- No further deterioration of neuro functioning.
- Prevent cardiovascular instability.
- Promote optimal tissue perfusion.
- Normalize temperature.

The patient will demonstrate adequate tissue perfusion by

PATIENT OUTCOMES

- Maintaining an O_2 Sat at 95% or greater.
- ABGS within the normal range.
- Maintaining urine output at least 30 mL/hr
- Maintenance of mean arterial blood pressure within 10 mm Hg of baseline or as determined to maintain perfusion to spinal cord.

COLLABORATIVE CARE INTERVENTIONS

- Neurogenic shock is considered an emergency

- Hypovolemia treated with minimal amount of fluid to ensure adequate tissue perfusion.
- Observe for evidence of fluid overload.
- Volume replacement for SBP < 90 mm Hg or evidence of inadequate tissue perfusion.
- Use base deficit or lactate level to guide fluid resuscitation.
- Vasopressors → maintain BP & organ perfusion.
- Higher than typical MAPs often needed to prevent spinal cord ischemia.
- If needed, atropine, an IV beta-blocker, or pacemaker to treat bradycardia.
- Hypothermia treated with warming measures & environmental temperature regulation.

NURSING INTERVENTIONS

- Early identification → treat symptoms early → ↓ mortality.

- Prevention of neurogenic shock → Identify risk, constant neuro assessment, vigilant immobilization of SCI, & slight ↑ HOB after spinal anesthesia to prevent occurrence.
- Treat the symptoms to restore fluids to vascular space.
- Priorities → early identification, treating hypovolemia & maintaining tissue perfusion, maintaining normothermia, monitoring & treating dysrhythmias, providing comfort and emotional support, preventing & maintaining surveillance for complications.
- DVT-prophylactic measures → monitoring passive ROM exercises, application of sequential pneumatic stockings, & administration of prescribed anticoagulation therapy.

FIG. 34.5 Concept Map for Neurogenic Shock. *ABGs,* Arterial blood gases; *BP,* blood pressure; *CI,* cardiac index; *CO,* cardiac output; *DVT,* deep vein thrombosis; *HOB,* head of bed; *HR,* heart rate; *MAP$_s$,* mean arterial pressures; *O$_2$ Sat,* oxygen saturation; *PaCo$_2$,* partial pressure of carbon dioxide in arterial blood; *PAOP,* pulmonary artery occlusion pressure; *RAP,* right atrial pressure; *RR,* respiratory rate; *R/T,* related to; *SBP,* systolic blood pressure; *SCI,* spinal cord injury; *SVR,* systemic vascular resistance.

BOX 34.13   NURSING DIAGNOSES
Neurogenic Shock

- Deficient Fluid Volume related to relative loss, p. 1019
- Decreased Cardiac Output related to sympathetic blockade, p. 1017
- Hypothermia related to exposure to cold environment, trauma, or damage to the hypothalamus, p. 1028
- Imbalanced Nutrition: Less Than Body Requirements related to lack of exogenous nutrients and increased metabolic demand, p. 1029
- Risk for Infection, p. 1046
- Anxiety related to threat to biologic, psychologic, or social integrity, p. 1012
- Compromised Family Coping related to a critically ill family member, p. 1014

in the United States, with an estimated hospital mortality rate of 23% to 50%.[81-84] It is the leading cause of in-hospital death and the 11th leading cause of all deaths in the United States.[82,85] The Third International Consensus Definitions for Sepsis and Septic Shock (Sepsis-3) from the European Society of Intensive Care Medicine and the Society of Critical Care Medicine were published more recently (Box 34.14).[86]

Etiology

Sepsis is caused by a wide variety of microorganisms, including gram-negative and gram-positive aerobes, anaerobes, fungi, and viruses. The source of these microorganisms varies. The respiratory system is the most common site of infection producing sepsis and septic shock, followed by the genitourinary and GI systems.[82,83] Gram-positive bacteria are the predominant cause of sepsis.[83,87] Sepsis and septic shock are associated with a wide variety of intrinsic and extrinsic precipitating factors (Box 34.15). All these factors interfere directly or indirectly with the body's anatomic and physiologic defense mechanisms. Several of the intrinsic factors are not modifiable or are very difficult to control. Several of the extrinsic factors may be required for diagnosis and management. Therefore, all critically ill patients are at risk for septic shock.

Pathophysiology

The syndrome encompassing sepsis and septic shock is a complex systemic response that is initiated when a microorganism enters the body and stimulates the inflammatory/immune system. In a host-pathogen interaction, both the invading organism and the injured tissue release intracellular proteins activating neutrophils, monocytes, lymphocytes, macrophages, mast cells, and platelets as well as numerous plasma enzyme cascades (complement, kinin/kallikrein, coagulation, and fibrinolytic factors). When this reaction is localized, infection is contained and eradicated. However, when the magnitude of the infectious insult is great or the patient is physiologically unable to generate an effective host response, containment fails.[88] The result is a systemic release of the pathogen, activated cells, and mediators, including cytokines, which initiate a chain of complex interactions leading to an uncontrolled SIRS.[88-91]

With systemic activation, various physiologic and pathophysiologic events occur that affect clotting, the distribution of blood flow to the tissues and organs, capillary membrane permeability, and the metabolic state of the body. Subsequently, a systemic imbalance between cellular oxygen supply and demand develops that results in cellular hypoxia, damage, hibernation, and death.[89,91]

Hallmarks of sepsis are endothelial damage and coagulation dysfunction.[91-94] Tissue factor is released from endothelial cells and monocytes in response to stimulation by inflammatory cytokines.[89,92,95,96] Release of tissue factor initiates the coagulation cascade, producing widespread microvascular thrombosis and further stimulation of the systemic inflammatory pathways.[89,90,92,95,96] Diffuse endothelial damage impairs endogenous anticlotting mechanisms.[89,90,92,96] Mediator-induced suppression of fibrinolysis slows clot breakdown. The result is DIC with eventual consumption of coagulation factors, bleeding, and hemorrhage.[90,95,96]

Significant alterations in cardiovascular hemodynamics are caused by the activation of inflammatory cytokines and endothelial damage.[88-90] Ventricular contractility is impaired.[89,90,93] Massive peripheral vasodilation results in the development of relative hypovolemia. Increased capillary permeability produces a loss of intravascular volume to the interstitium, which accentuates the reduction in preload and CO. These changes in global hemodynamics coupled with complex microvascular alterations and thrombosis produce maldistribution of circulating blood volume, decreased tissue perfusion, and inadequate oxygen delivery to the cells. Microcirculatory failure is a key feature of this distributive shock.[89,96] Even if global hemodynamics are restored, occult hypoperfusion secondary to microcirculatory impairment may persist.[96]

Activation of the central nervous system and endocrine system also occurs as part of the response to invading microorganisms. This activation leads to stimulation of the SNS and the release of ACTH. These events trigger the release of epinephrine, norepinephrine, glucocorticoids, aldosterone, glucagon, renin, and growth hormone, resulting in the development of a hypermetabolic state and contributing to vasoconstriction of the renal, pulmonary, and splanchnic beds. Selective vasoconstriction in the splanchnic bed may contribute to hypoperfusion of the GI mucosal barrier, an area particularly vulnerable to the effects of inflammatory cytokines.[90,94] The resulting gut injury propagates the inflammatory response.[2,5,94]

Several metabolic alterations occur as a result of central nervous system, endocrine system, and cytokine activation. The hypermetabolic state increases energy expenditure and oxygen demand, and it contributes to cellular hypoxia. Lactic acid is produced as a result of increased metabolic lactate production and hypoxic anaerobic metabolism. Glucocorticoids, ACTH, epinephrine, glucagon, and growth hormone all are catabolic hormones that are released as part of this response. In conjunction with the inflammatory cytokines, these hormones stimulate catabolism of protein stores in the visceral organs and skeletal muscles to fuel glucose production in the liver, hyperglycemia, and insulin resistance.[91,97] The cytokines also stimulate the use of fats for energy production (lipolysis).[91,97,98]

Metabolic derangements in sepsis and septic shock include an inability of the cells to use oxygen even if blood flow is adequate. Mitochondrial dysfunction is thought to be the underlying mechanism.[89,91,98,99] This bioenergetic failure plays an important role in the development of tissue ischemia and multiple-organ dysfunction.[89,91,98,99] These complex and interrelated pathophysiologic changes produce a pathologic imbalance between cellular oxygen demand and cellular oxygen supply and consumption.

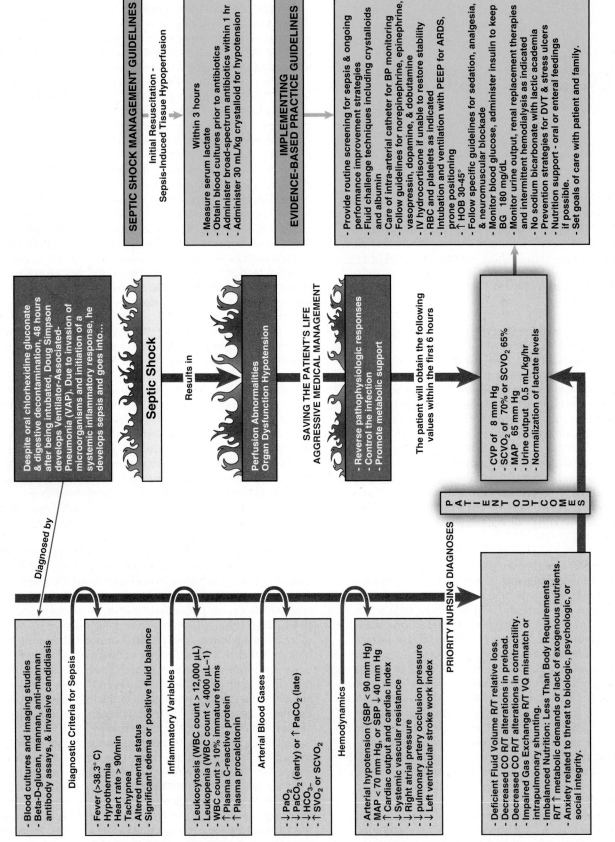

FIG. 34.6 Concept Map for Septic Shock. PaCo2 – Partial pressure of carbon dioxide in arterial blood.PaO2 – Partial pressure of oxygen in arterial blood HCO3 – Sodium Bicarbonate SvO2 Mixed Venous Oxygen Saturation SCVO2 - Mixed Venous Oxygen Saturation MAP – Mean Arterial Pressure SBP – Systolic Blood Pressure R/T – Related To VQ – Ventilation Perfusion: CVP – Central Venous Pressure BP – Blood Pressure: HOB – Head of Bed DVT – Deep Vein Thrombosis

SEPTIC SHOCK MANAGEMENT GUIDELINES

Initial Resuscitation -
Sepsis-Induced Tissue Hypoperfusion

Within 3 hours
- Measure serum lactate
- Obtain blood cultures prior to antibiotics
- Administer broad-spectrum antibiotics within 1 hr
- Administer 30 mL/kg crystalloid for hypotension

IMPLEMENTING EVIDENCE-BASED PRACTICE GUIDELINES

- Provide routine screening for sepsis & ongoing performance improvement strategies
- Fluid challenge techniques including crystalloids and albumin
- Care of intra-arterial catheter for BP monitoring
- Follow guidelines for norepinephrine, epinephrine, vasopressin, dopamine, & dobutamine
- IV hydrocortisone if unable to restore stability
- RBC and platelets as indicated
- Intubation and ventilation with PEEP for ARDS, prone positioning ↑ HOB 30-45°
- Follow specific guidelines for sedation, analgesia, & neuromuscular blockade
- Monitor blood glucose, administer insulin to keep BG 180 mg/dL
- Monitor urine output, renal replacement therapies and intermittent hemodialysis as indicated
- No sodium bicarbonate with lactic academia
- Prevention strategies for DVT & stress ulcers
- Nutrition support - oral or enteral feedings if possible.
- Set goals of care with patient and family.

Despite oral chlorhexidine gluconate & digestive decontamination, 48 hours after being intubated, Doug Simpson develops Ventilator-Associated-Pneumonia (VAP). Due to invasion of microorganisms and initiation of a systemic inflammatory response, he develops sepsis and goes into....

Septic Shock

Results in

Perfusion Abnormalities
Organ Dysfunction Hypotension

SAVING THE PATIENT'S LIFE AGGRESSIVE MEDICAL MANAGEMENT

- Reverse pathophysiologic responses
- Control the infection
- Promote metabolic support

The patient will obtain the following values within the first 6 hours

- CVP of 8 mm Hg
- SCVO₂ of 70% or SCVO₂ 65%
- MAP 65 mm Hg
- Urine output 0.5 mL/kg/hr
- Normalization of lactate levels

Diagnosed by

- Blood cultures and imaging studies
- Beta-D-glucan, mannan, anti-mannan antibody assays, & invasive candidiasis

Diagnostic Criteria for Sepsis

- Fever (>38.3° C)
- Hypothermia
- Heart rate > 90/min
- Tachypnea
- Altered mental status
- Significant edema or positive fluid balance

Inflammatory Variables

- Leukocytosis (WBC count > 12,000 µL)
- Leukopenia (WBC count < 4000 µL–1)
- WBC count > 10% immature forms
- ↑ Plasma C-reactive protein
- ↑ Plasma procalcitonin

Arterial Blood Gases

- ↓ PaO₂
- ↓ PaCO₂ (early) or ↑ PaCO₂ (late)
- ↓ ↑ HCO₃⁻
- ↓ ↑ SVO₂ or SCVO₂

Hemodynamics

- Arterial hypotension (SBP < 90 mm Hg)
  MAP < 70 mm Hg, or SBP ↓40 mm Hg
- ↓ Cardiac output and cardiac index
- ↑ Systemic vascular resistance
- ↓ Right atrial pressure
- ↓ pulmonary artery occlusion pressure
- ↓ Left ventricular stroke work index

PRIORITY NURSING DIAGNOSES

PATIENT OUTCOMES

- Deficient Fluid Volume R/T relative loss.
- Decreased CO R/T alterations in preload.
- Decreased CO R/T alterations in contractility.
- Impaired Gas Exchange R/T VQ mismatch or intrapulmonary shunting.
- Imbalanced Nutrition: Less Than Body Requirements R/T ↑ metabolic demands or lack of exogenous nutrients.
- Anxiety related to threat to biologic, psychologic, or social integrity.

BOX 34.14 New Definitions for Sepsis and Organ Failure

- Sepsis is defined as life-threatening organ dysfunction caused by a dysregulated host response to infection.
- Organ dysfunction can be identified as an acute change in total Sequential [Sepsis-related] Organ Failure Assessment (SOFA) score ≥2 points consequent to the infection.
- The baseline SOFA score (see Fig. 34.7) can be assumed to be zero in patients not known to have preexisting organ dysfunction.
- SOFA score ≥2 reflects an overall mortality risk of approximately 10% in a general hospital population with suspected infection. Patients presenting with modest dysfunction can deteriorate further, emphasizing the seriousness of this condition and the need for prompt and appropriate intervention, if not already being instituted.
- In lay terms, sepsis is a life-threatening condition that arises when the body's response to an infection results in injury to tissues and organs.
- Patients with suspected infection who are likely to have a prolonged intensive care unit stay or to die in the hospital can be promptly identified at the bedside with quick SOFA (qSOFA):
  - Alteration in mental status
  - Systolic blood pressure ≤100 mm Hg
  - Respiratory rate ≥22/min
- Septic shock is a subset of sepsis in which underlying circulatory and cellular/metabolic abnormalities are profound enough to substantially increase mortality.
- Patients with septic shock can be identified with a clinical construct of sepsis with persisting hypotension requiring vasopressors to maintain mean arterial pressure ≥65 mm Hg and having a serum lactate level >2 mmol/L (18 mg/dL) despite adequate volume resuscitation. With these criteria, hospital mortality is >40%.

Modified from Singer M, Deutschman CS, Seymour CW. The third international consensus definitions for sepsis and septic shock. *JAMA.* 2016;315:801.

BOX 34.15 Precipitating Factors Associated With Septic Shock

Intrinsic Factors
- Extreme of age
- Coexisting diseases
  - Malignancies
  - Burns
  - Acquired immunodeficiency syndrome
  - Diabetes
  - Substance abuse
  - Dysfunction of one or more of the major body systems
- Malnutrition

Extrinsic Factors
- Invasive devices
- Medication therapy
- Fluid therapy
- Surgical and traumatic wounds
- Surgical and invasive diagnostic procedures
- Immunosuppressive therapy

The exaggerated systemic inflammatory response associated with sepsis and septic shock results in cell death via both ischemic necrosis and, to a large degree, apoptosis. Apoptosis is a programmed cell death or cellular suicide mediated by caspase-3, a cysteine protease, and affecting endothelial, GI epithelial, and immune cells in particular.[89-91,95] Apoptosis of immune cells results in immunosuppression and secondary infection as well as release of immune cell toxins. Ischemic necrosis and apoptosis stimulate further inflammation, propagating an ongoing cycle of infection, tissue injury, and SIRS.[88,95] If unabated, this situation ultimately results in MODS and death.

Assessment and Diagnosis

Effective treatment of sepsis and septic shock depends on timely recognition. Sepsis-3 advocates the use of the Sequential [Sepsis-related] Organ Failure Assessment (SOFA) score (Fig. 34.7) to facilitate early identification of patients.[86] However, the SOFA score has only more recently been introduced and is not yet fully integrated into practice. Fig. 34.8 outlines how to use the SOFA scoring system in the identification of patient with sepsis and septic shock.

Signs of individual organ dysfunction are discussed later in the chapter. The two most common organs to demonstrate dysfunction in sepsis are the cardiovascular system and the lungs. A patient with persistent hypotension requiring vasopressor therapy despite adequate volume resuscitation is demonstrating cardiovascular dysfunction. Pulmonary dysfunction is manifested by a Pao_2/fraction of inspired oxygen (Fio_2) ratio of less than 300, indicating ARDS.[16,100] Signs indicating septic shock are hypotension despite adequate fluid resuscitation and the presence of perfusion abnormalities such as lactic acidosis, oliguria, or acute change in mentation.

A patient in sepsis or septic shock may present with a variety of clinical manifestations that may change dynamically as the condition progresses (Box 34.16). During the initial stage, massive vasodilation occurs in the venous and arterial beds. Dilation of the venous system leads to a decrease in venous return to the heart, which results in a decrease in the preload of the right and left ventricles. This is evidenced by a decline in RAP and PAOP. Dilation of the arterial system results in a decrease in the afterload of the heart, as evidenced by a decrease in the SVR. The patient's skin becomes pink, warm, and flushed as a result of the massive vasodilation. Myocardial contractility is decreased, as evidenced by a decline in the left ventricular stroke work index and ejection fraction.

The heart rate increases in response to increased SNS, metabolic, and adrenal gland stimulation. If circulating volume and preload are adequate, this results in a normal-to-high CO and CI despite impaired contractility. The pulse pressure widens as the diastolic blood pressure decreases because of the vasodilation, and the systolic blood pressure increases because of the elevated CO. A full, bounding pulse develops. The net result of these changes is a relatively normal blood pressure in sepsis. However, as the reduction in preload and afterload becomes overwhelming and contractility fails, hypotension ensues, resulting in septic shock.

In the lungs, ventilation-perfusion mismatching develops as a result of pulmonary vasoconstriction and the formation of pulmonary microemboli. Hypoxemia occurs, and the respiratory rate increases to compensate for the lack of oxygen. Crackles develop as increased pulmonary capillary membrane permeability leads to pulmonary edema.[100]

Table 1. Sequential [Sepsis-Related] Organ Failure Assessment Score[a]

System	Score 0	1	2	3	4
Respiration					
PaO₂/FiO₂, mm Hg (kPa)	$\geq$400 (53.3)	<400 (53.3)	<300 (40)	<200 (26.7) with respiratory support	<100 (13.3) with respiratory support
Coagulation					
Platelets, ×10³/μL	$\geq$150	<150	<100	<50	<20
Liver					
Bilirubin, mg/dL (μmol/L)	<1.2 (20)	1.2–1.9 (20–32)	2.0–5.9 (33–101)	6.0–11.9 (102–204)	>12.0 (204)
Cardiovascular	MAP $\geq$70 mm Hg	MAP <70 mm Hg	Dopamine <5 or dobutamine (any dose)[b]	Dopamine 5.1–15 or epinephrine $\leq$0.1 or norepinephrine $\leq$0.1[b]	Dopamine >15 or epinephrine >0.1 or norepinephrine >0.1[b]
Central nervous system					
Glasgow Coma Scale score[c]	15	13–14	10–12	6–9	<6
Renal					
Creatinine, mg/dL (μmol/L)	<1.2 (110)	1.2–1.9 (110–170)	2.0–3.4 (171–299)	3.5–4.9 (300–440)	>5.0 (440)
Urine output, mL/d				<500	<200

Abbreviations: FiO₂, fraction of inspired oxygen; MAP, mean arterial pressure; PaO₂, partial pressure of oxygen.

[a]Adapted from Vincent et al.[27]

[b]Catecholamine doses are given as μg/kg/min for at least 1 hour.

[c]Glasgow Coma Scale scores range from 3–15; higher score indicates better neurological function.

FIG. 34.7 Sequential Organ Failure Assessment Score. (From Singer M, Deutschman CS, Seymour CW. The third international consensus definitions for sepsis and septic shock. *JAMA.* 2016;315:801.)

FIG. 34.8 Identifying Patients With Sepsis and Septic Shock. (From Singer M, Deutschman CS, Seymour CW. The third international consensus definitions for sepsis and septic shock. *JAMA.* 2016;315:801.)

The level of consciousness starts to change as a result of decreased cerebral perfusion, immune mediator activation, hyperthermia, and lactic acidosis. This septic encephalopathy is demonstrated by acute onset of impaired cognitive functioning, or delirium, which may fluctuate during its course.[101]

The patient may appear disoriented, confused, combative, or lethargic.

ABG values initially reveal hypocarbia, hypoxemia, and metabolic acidosis. This is demonstrated by low PaO₂ (hypocarbia), low PaCO₂ (hypoxemia), and low HCO₃⁻ (metabolic acidosis)

BOX 34.16 Clinical Manifestations of Septic Shock

- Increased heart rate
- Decreased blood pressure
- Wide pulse pressure
- Full, bounding pulse
- Pink, warm, flushed skin
- Increased respiratory rate (early) or decreased respiratory rate (late)
- Crackles
- Change in sensorium
- Decreased urine output
- Increased temperature
- Increased cardiac output and cardiac index
- Decreased systemic vascular resistance
- Decreased right atrial pressure
- Decreased pulmonary artery occlusion pressure
- Decreased left ventricular stroke work index
- Decreased PaO_2
- Decreased $PaCO_2$ (early) or increased $PaCO_2$ (late)
- Decreased HCO_3^-
- Increased SvO_2 or $ScvO_2$

HCO_3-, bicarbonate; $PaCO_2$, partial pressure of carbon dioxide; PaO_2, partial pressure of oxygen; $ScvO_2$, central venous oxygen saturation; SvO_2, mixed venous oxygen saturation.

QSEN BOX 34.17 QSEN: Evidence-Based Practice

Surviving Sepsis Campaign Bundles

To Be Completed Within 3 Hours of Time of Presentation[a]
1. Measure lactate level.
2. Obtain blood cultures before administration of antibiotics.
3. Administer broad-spectrum antibiotics.
4. Administer 30 mL/kg crystalloid for hypotension or lactate ≥4 mmol/L.

To Be Completed Within 6 Hours of Time of Presentation
5. Apply vasopressors (for hypotension that does not respond to initial fluid resuscitation) to maintain mean arterial pressure (MAP) ≥65 mm Hg.
6. In the event of persistent hypotension after initial fluid administration (MAP <65 mm Hg) or if initial lactate was ≥4 mmol/L, reassess volume status and tissue perfusion, and document findings according to Table 1.
7. Remeasure lactate if initial lactate elevated.

Table 1. Document Reassessment of Volume Status and Tissue Perfusion With

Either
- Repeat focused examination (after initial fluid resuscitation) including vital signs, cardiopulmonary, capillary refill, pulse, and skin findings.

Or two of the following
- Measure central venous pressure.
- Measure $ScvO_2$.
- Perform bedside cardiovascular ultrasound.
- Perform dynamic assessment of fluid responsiveness with passive leg raise or fluid challenge.

[a]"Time of presentation" is defined as the time of triage in the emergency department or, if presenting from another care venue, from the earliest chart annotation consistent with all elements of severe sepsis or septic shock ascertained through chart review.
$ScvO_2$, central venous oxygen saturation.

Modified from Surviving Sepsis Campaign. http://www.survivingsepsis.org/SiteCollectionDocuments/SSC_Bundle.pdf. Retrieved February 2, 2016.

levels. The respiratory alkalosis is caused by the patient's increased respiratory rate. As pathologic pulmonary changes progress and the patient becomes fatigued, the effectiveness of respirations decreases, and $PaCO_2$ increases, resulting in respiratory acidosis. The metabolic acidosis is the result of a lack of oxygen to the cells and the development of lactic acidemia. Serum lactate levels increase above 2 mmol/L because of anaerobic metabolism. SvO_2 may increase because of microcirculatory shunting or decrease because of inadequate oxygen delivery.[89] The white blood cell (WBC) count is elevated as part of the immune response to the invading microorganisms. The WBC differential count reveals an increase in immature neutrophils (shift to the left). This increase occurs because the body has to mobilize increasing numbers of WBCs to fight the infection. An elevated procalcitonin level is a valuable biomarker of significant bacterial infection, and procalcitonin levels have been used in clinical trials to guide antibiotic therapy with positive outcomes.[89,102] Serum glucose levels increase as part of the hypermetabolic response and the development of insulin resistance. The patient's temperature is elevated in response to pyrogens released from the invading microorganisms, immune mediator activation, and increased metabolic activity. Urine output decreases because of decreased perfusion of the kidneys. As impaired tissue perfusion develops, other clinical manifestations appear that indicate the development of MODS.

Medical Management

Treatment of a patient in sepsis or septic shock requires a multifaceted approach. The goals of treatment are to reverse the pathophysiologic responses, control the infection, and promote metabolic support. This approach includes supporting the cardiovascular system and enhancing tissue perfusion, identifying and treating the infection, limiting the systemic inflammatory response, restoring metabolic balance, and initiating nutrition therapy. Dysfunction of the individual organ systems must be prevented. Early treatment reduces mortality.[16,103] Guidelines for the management of sepsis and septic shock have been developed and updated under the auspices of the Surviving Sepsis Campaign (SSC), an international effort of more than 11 organizations to improve patient outcomes.[16] From these guidelines, two groups ("bundles") of selected interventions were identified as having the most impact on patient outcomes (Box 34.17). One bundle lists interventions that need to be implemented within the first 3 hours of presentation, and the other bundle lists interventions that need to be implemented within the first 6 hours. More information regarding these interventions is available at the SSC website (http://www.survivingsepsis.org).

A patient in sepsis or septic shock requires immediate resuscitation of the hypoperfused state. Specific interventions have been aimed at increasing cellular oxygen supply and decreasing cellular oxygen demand. These treatments include administration of fluids, vasopressors, and possibly positive inotropic agents, initially given in the form of a protocolized, quantitative resuscitation to be implemented during the first 6 hours of treatment.[16] This therapy includes aggressive fluid resuscitation to augment intravascular volume and increase preload until a CVP of 8 to 12 mm Hg (12 to 15 mm Hg in mechanically ventilated patients) is achieved. Crystalloids are the initial fluid of choice.[16] A fluid challenge for hypovolemia should be initiated with at least 1000 mL of crystalloids or 300 to 500 mL of colloids over 30 minutes. Vasopressors should be administered as necessary to maintain a MAP of at least 65 mm Hg. These agents reverse the massive peripheral vasodilation and increase SVR. Norepinephrine is recommended as the first-choice agent because of evidence of its superiority in reducing mortality rates and a higher risk of dysrhythmias when dopamine is used.[104,105] When indicated, norepinephrine should be initiated quickly, as delay in starting this therapy has been found to significantly worsen survival.[103] Epinephrine is recommended as an alternative agent if response to norepinephrine is poor.[16] Arterial line placement is recommended for any patient requiring vasopressor therapy. Serum lactate values are used to evaluate the effectiveness of these interventions to restore adequate tissue oxygenation. Intermittent or continuous Scvo$_2$ or Svo$_2$ monitoring has also been used extensively in patients with septic shock as a measure of the effectiveness of oxygen delivery. Current SSC guidelines state that if the Scvo$_2$ is less than 70% or the Svo$_2$ is less than 65% after the CVP goal is achieved, administration of packed RBCs to achieve a hematocrit of at least 30% and inotropic stimulation with dobutamine (administered to a maximum of 20 mcg/kg per minute) to counteract myocardial depression and maintain adequate CO are options to obtain this goal.[16] However, the need for CVP monitoring and for Scvo$_2$ or Svo$_2$ monitoring to guide therapy has been refuted by the results of three major trials and a meta-analysis.[106-109] As a result, the Surviving Sepsis Bundles were modified to include alternative approaches to assess the adequacy of volume resuscitation and restoration of tissue perfusion. Regardless of the method used to assess and document circulatory restoration, the recommended fluid and vasopressor therapies remain the same.

Intubation and mechanical ventilatory support are usually required to optimize oxygenation and ventilation for a patient in sepsis or septic shock. Ventilation with lower than traditional tidal volumes (6 mL/kg vs 12 mL/kg) in patients with ARDS decreases mortality.[110] SSC guidelines recommend the goals of 6 mL/kg of predicted body weight and plateau pressures no more than 30 cm H$_2$O for patients with sepsis or septic shock with ARDS.[16] Increased Paco$_2$ may result from this therapy and is acceptable if tolerated as evidenced by hemodynamic stability. Ventilator settings should include positive end-expiratory pressure (PEEP) and be adjusted to provide the patient with a Pao$_2$ greater than 70 mm Hg. Patients receiving mechanical ventilation should be maintained in a semirecumbent position with the head of the bed raised to 45 degrees to decrease the incidence of ventilator-associated pneumonia.[16] Prone positioning should be considered in a septic patient with ARDS requiring high levels of oxygen.[16] Sedation protocols using intermittent bolus or continuous infusion using a standardized sedation scale and specific goals are recommended for all patients requiring mechanical ventilation. Daily interruption of sedative infusions to allow wakefulness and reevaluation of sedation needs reduces duration of mechanical ventilation and is recommended.[16] Neuromuscular blocking agents should be avoided, if possible, to prevent prolonged blockade after discontinuation.[16]

A key measure in the treatment of septic shock is the initiation of appropriate antibiotic therapy to eradicate the cause of the infection. Antibiotic therapy should be started within 1 hour of recognition of sepsis without delay for cultures.[16] If it can be accomplished with less than a 45-minute delay in antibiotic administration, at least two blood cultures plus urine, sputum, and wound cultures should be obtained to find the location of the infection before such therapy is initiated.[16] Each hour of delay in initial antibiotic administration is associated with a substantial decrease in the survival rate.[111] If the microorganism is unknown, antiinfective therapy with one or more agents known to be effective against likely pathogens should be initiated, with daily reassessment of the regimen. Combination therapy is recommended for known or suspected *Pseudomonas* infection and for neutropenic patients but should be limited to fewer than 3 to 5 days.[16] A specific source of infection should be established within 6 hours of presentation.[16] Surgical intervention to débride infected or necrotic tissue or to drain abscesses may be necessary to facilitate removal of the septic source.[16] Intravascular devices that may be the source of the infection should be removed after establishment of alternative vascular access.

Only one medication was on the market specifically for the treatment of sepsis and septic shock, recombinant human activated protein C, marketed as drotrecogin alfa (Xigris). However, following its implementation in clinical practice, further investigation demonstrated no survival benefit, and the drug was voluntarily withdrawn from the market by the manufacturer.[112-114] Studies of numerous other medications thought to block or alter the effects of immune mediators have failed to demonstrate effectiveness or have been associated with unacceptable adverse effects.[88,93] However, the use of beta-blocker therapy to modulate cardiovascular alterations is currently being evaluated with promising results.[115]

Intravenous hydrocortisone *only* for the patient in septic shock who remains hypotensive despite adequate fluid resuscitation and vasopressor therapy is recommended in the current SSC guidelines.[16] Steroid therapy is to be weaned when vasopressors are no longer required. High doses of steroids of 300 mg/day or more may be harmful and should *not* be used.[16] In a meta-analysis, no support for the use of steroids at any dose was found.[116]

Continuous infusion of intravenous insulin is recommended by SSC guidelines when blood glucose level exceeds 180 mg/dL with a goal blood glucose level of approximately 150 mg/dL.[16,117] Glucose levels should be monitored every 1 to 2 hours until stable and then every 4 hours. Low glucose levels measured by capillary testing may be inaccurate in this population.[16] Platelets should be administered when counts are less than 5000/mm^3, and RBC transfusions are recommended when the hemoglobin level is less than 7 g/dL to obtain a target value of 7 to 9 g/dL.[16] Stress ulcer prophylaxis using H$_2$-receptor antagonists or proton-pump inhibitors and DVT prophylaxis are recommended for all patients with sepsis or septic shock. The Society of Critical Care Medicine guidelines recommend against the use of sodium bicarbonate for lactic acidemia if the pH is equal to or greater than 7.15.[16] Low-dose dopamine infusion for renal protection is not beneficial and should not be used.[16]

The initiation of nutrition therapy is critical in the management of a patient in sepsis or septic shock. The goal is to improve the patient's overall nutrition status, enhance immune function, and promote wound healing. A daily caloric intake of 20 to 30 kcal/kg of usual body weight is recommended for critically ill patients. The enteral route is strongly preferred. Compared with enteral nutrition, parenteral nutrition or a combination of both methods has been associated with higher risk for secondary infection and higher mortality in patients with sepsis or septic shock.[117,118]

Sufficient protein needs to be provided because of the metabolic derangements that develop in the hypermetabolic state. A range of 1.2 to 2.0 g/kg actual body weight per day is recommended for patients with a body mass index less than 30, with progressively larger amounts for patients with higher body mass index.[38] Specific nutrition therapies to reduce the inflammatory and hypermetabolic responses associated with sepsis, such as antioxidant supplementation and feeding with long-chain n-3 polyunsaturated fatty acids, are the source of much debate and evaluation.[100,119] Glutamine is considered by some to be an essential amino acid in critically ill patients and has the most empiric support,[91,119] but others may actually worsen outcomes. Current recommendations stress caution with any immune-modulating formulations in patients with sepsis.[38]

Nursing Management

Nursing management of the patient with sepsis focuses on infection prevention and transmission, early recognition and treatment of sepsis and septic shock, and supportive nursing care.[120] Prevention of sepsis and septic shock is one of the primary responsibilities of the nurse in the critical care unit. These measures include identification of patients at risk and reduction of their risk factors, including exposure to invading microorganisms. Handwashing, aseptic technique, and an understanding of evidence-based practice to reduce nosocomial infection in critically ill patients are essential components of preventive nursing care. Early identification allows for early treatment and decreases mortality. Fig. 34.9 is a simple screening tool that is used to identify patients with sepsis. However, this may change with the introduction of the new sepsis definitions and SOFA score. Subsequent continual observation to detect subtle changes that indicate the progression of the septic process is vitally important, as is evidence-based practice to prevent further infection. Immunosuppression is common as sepsis progresses,[94] and more recent research has found that a resurgence in opportunistic infection in patients with sepsis and septic shock occurs in the later stages, more than 2 weeks after initial diagnosis and treatment.[121] Evidence-based practice to prevent complications of critical illness and prolonged bed rest are essential to prevent further compromise and negative short-term and long-term outcomes. For survivors of sepsis, ongoing mortality and impaired quality of life persist in the months and years after hospital discharge.[122]

The nursing management plan for a patient in septic shock may include numerous nursing diagnoses, depending on the progression of the process (Box 34.18). Nursing interventions include early identification of sepsis syndrome; administering prescribed fluids, medications, and nutrition; providing comfort and emotional support; and preventing and maintaining surveillance for complications. Interprofessional collaborative management of a patient with sepsis or septic shock is outlined in Box 34.19.

MULTIPLE ORGAN DYSFUNCTION SYNDROME

Description

Over the past 2 decades, critical care professionals have witnessed the emergence of MODS, a new clinical syndrome in critically ill patients. MODS results from progressive physiologic failure of two or more separate organ systems in an acutely ill patient such that homeostasis cannot be maintained without intervention.[86] MODS is the major cause of death in patients in critical care units. Mortality is closely linked to the number of organ systems involved. Dysfunction or failure of two or more organ systems is associated with an estimated mortality rate of 54%, which increases to 100% when five organ systems fail.[123] Survivors of MODS may develop generalized polyneuropathy and a chronic form of pulmonary disease from ARDS, complicating recovery. These patients often require prolonged, expensive rehabilitation.[124]

Trauma patients are particularly vulnerable to developing MODS because they often experience ischemia-reperfusion events resulting from hemorrhage, blunt trauma, or SNS-induced vasoconstriction.[125] Other high-risk patients include patients who have experienced infection, a shock episode, various ischemia-reperfusion events, acute pancreatitis, sepsis, burns, aspiration, multiple blood transfusions, or surgical complications.[87] Patients 65 years old or older are at increased risk because of their decreased organ reserve and comorbidities.[126]

Etiology

Organ dysfunction may be the direct consequence of an initial insult (primary MODS) or can manifest latently and involve organs not directly affected in the initial insult (secondary MODS). Patients can experience both primary and secondary MODS (Fig. 34.10). Primary MODS results from a well-defined insult in which organ dysfunction occurs early and is directly attributed to the insult itself. Direct insults initially cause localized inflammatory responses. Primary MODS accounts for only a small percentage of MODS cases. Examples of primary MODS include the immediate consequences of posttraumatic pulmonary failure, thermal injuries, AKI, or invasive infections.[88] These cellular or microcirculatory insults may lead to a loss of critical organ function induced by failure of delivery of oxygen and substrates, coupled with the inability to remove end products of metabolism. The inflammatory response in primary MODS has a less apparent presentation and may resolve without long-term implications. However, primary MODS may "prime" physiologic systems for a more sustained exaggerated inflammatory response that leads to secondary MODS.

Secondary MODS is a consequence of widespread sustained systemic inflammation that results in dysfunction of organs not involved in the initial insult. Secondary MODS develops latently after an initial insult.[88] The early impairment of organs normally involved in immunoregulatory function, such as the liver and the GI tract, intensifies the host response to the insult.[5,127] The initial insult may prime the inflammatory system in such a way that even a mild second insult (hit) may perpetuate a sustained hyperinflammatory response. This "two-hit hypothesis" has been increasingly recognized as an important contributor to morbidity and mortality in patients with secondary MODS.[128]

SIRS and sepsis are common initiating events in the development of secondary MODS. The systemic inflammatory response is an intense host response characterized by sustained generalized inflammation in organs remote from the initial insult. SIRS is widespread inflammation or clinical responses to inflammation that occur in patients with various insults. Clinical conditions and manifestations associated with SIRS are listed in Box 34.20. These insults produce similar or identical systemic inflammatory responses, even in the absence of infection. Manifestations of SIRS must represent an acute alteration from the patient's normal baseline and must not be related to other causes (eg, neutropenia from chemotherapy). Organ dysfunction such as ARDS, AKI, and MODS is a complication

Evaluation for Severe Sepsis Screening Tool

Instructions: Use this optional tool to screen patients for severe sepsis in the emergency department, on the wards, or in the ICU.

1. **Is the patient's history suggestive of a new infection?**

    ❑ Pneumonia, empyema
    ❑ Urinary tract infection
    ❑ Acute abdominal infection
    ❑ Meningitis
    ❑ Skin/soft tissue infection

    ❑ Bone/joint infection
    ❑ Wound infection
    ❑ Bloodstream catheter infection
    ❑ Endocarditis

    ❑ Implantable device infection
    ❑ Other _____

    ___ Yes ___ No

2. **Are any two of the following signs & symptoms of infection both present and new to the patient? Note:** laboratory values may have been obtained for inpatients but may not be available for outpatients.

    ❑ Hyperthermia > 38.3 °C (101.0 °F)
    ❑ Hypothermia < 36 °C (96.8 °F)
    ❑ Tachycardia > 90 bpm

    ❑ Tachypnea > 20 bpm
    ❑ Acutely altered mental status
    ❑ Leukocytosis (WBC count >12,000 mcg-1)

    ❑ Leukopenia (WBC count < 4000 mcg-1)
    ❑ Hyperglycemia (plasma glucose >120 mg/dL) in the absence of diabetes

    ___ Yes ___ No

    If the answer is yes to both either question 1 and 2, *suspicion of infection* is present:

    ✓ Obtain: **lactic acid, blood cultures,** CBC with differential, basic chemistry labs, bilirubin.
    ✓ At the physician's discretion obtain: UA, chest x-ray, amylase, lipase, ABG, CRP, CT scan.

3. **Are any of the following organ dysfunction criteria present at a site remote from the site of the infection that are not considered to be chronic conditions? Note: the remote site stipulation is waived in the case of bilateral pulmonary infiltrates.**

    ❑ SBP < 90 mmHg or MAP < 65 mmHg
    ❑ SBP decrease > 40 mm Hg from baseline
    ❑ Bilateral pulmonary infiltrates with a new (or increased) oxygen requirement to maintain SpO_2 > 90%
    ❑ Bilateral pulmonary infiltrates with PaO2/FiO2 ratio < 300
    ❑ Creatinine > 2.0 mg/dl (176.8 mmol/L) or Urine Output < 0.5 ml/kg/hour for > 2 hours
    ❑ Bilirubin > 2 mg/dl (34.2 mmol/L)
    ❑ Platelet count < 100,000
    ❑ Coagulopathy (INR > 1.5 or aPTT > 60 secs)
    ❑ Lactate > 2 mmol/L (18.0 mg/dl)

    ___ Yes ___ No

If *suspicion of infection* is present AND *organ dysfunction* is present, the patient meets the criteria for SEVERE SEPSIS and should be entered into the severe sepsis protocol.

Date: ___/___/___ (circle: dd/mm/yy or mm/dd/yy)   Time: ___:___ (24 hr. clock)

Version 7.12.2005   © 2005 Surviving Sepsis Campaign and the Institute for Healthcare Improvement

FIG. 34.9 Evaluation for Sepsis Screening Tool. (Redrawn from the Institute for Healthcare Improvement, Cambridge, MA. Copyright 2005 Surviving Sepsis Campaign and the Institute for Healthcare Improvement.)

of SIRS.[123] In epidemiologic studies, SIRS was found to occur in one-third of all hospitalized patients, in 50% to 93% of all patients in critical care units, and in approximately 80% of all patients in surgical critical care units.[129,130]

When SIRS is a result of infection, the term *sepsis* is used. SIRS, sepsis, and septic shock represent a hierarchical continuum of the inflammatory response to infection.[16] Infection and shock are the most common precipitating factors; however, any disease that induces a major inflammatory response can initiate the events that lead to MODS.

When inflammation is not contained locally, consequences occur systemically that lead to organ dysfunction, including intense, uncontrolled activation of inflammatory cells; direct damage of vascular endothelium; disruption of immune cell function; persistent hypermetabolism; and maldistribution of circulatory volume to organ systems. Inflammation becomes a systemic, self-perpetuating process that is inadequately controlled and results in organ dysfunction.[123]

During hypermetabolism, changes occur in cellular anabolic and catabolic function, resulting in autocatabolism. Autocatabolism

BOX 34.18 NURSING DIAGNOSES
Septic Shock

- Deficient Fluid Volume related to relative loss, p. 1019
- Decreased Cardiac Output related to alterations in preload, p. 1015
- Decreased Cardiac Output related to alterations in afterload, p. 1015
- Decreased Cardiac Output related to alteratiasis in contractility, p. 1016
- Impaired Gas Exchange related to ventilation-perfusion mismatching or intrapulmonary shunting, p. 1030
- Imbalanced Nutrition: Less Than Body Requirements related to lack of exogenous nutrients and increased metabolic demand, p. 1029
- Risk for Infection, p. 1046
- Anxiety related to threat to biologic, psychologic, or social integrity, p. 1012
- Compromised Family Coping related to a critically ill family member, p. 1014

manifests as a severe decrease in lean body mass, severe weight loss, anergy, and increased CO and oxygen consumption (Vo_2) resulting from profound alterations in carbohydrate, protein, and fat metabolism.[123] Concurrently, GI, hepatic, and immunologic dysfunction may occur, which intensifies systemic inflammation.[131] Clinical consequences may affect gut function, wound healing, muscle wasting, host response, respiratory function, and continued promotion of the hypermetabolic response.

Not all patients develop MODS from SIRS. The development of MODS appears to be associated with failure to control the source of inflammation or infection, persistent hypoperfusion, flow-dependent Vo_2, or the continued presence of necrotic tissue.[125]

Pathophysiology

Secondary MODS results from altered regulation of the patient's acute immune and inflammatory responses. Dysregulation, or

QSEN BOX 34.19 QSEN: Evidence-Based Practice
Severe Sepsis and Septic Shock Management Guidelines

A. Initial Resuscitation

1. Protocolized, quantitative resuscitation of patients with sepsis-induced tissue hypoperfusion. Goals during first 6 h of resuscitation:
   a. Central venous pressure 8–12 mm Hg.
   b. Mean arterial pressure (MAP) ≥65 mm Hg.
   c. Urine output ≥0.5 mL/kg/h.
   d. Central venous (superior vena cava) or mixed venous oxygen saturation 70% or 65%, respectively (grade 1C).
2. In patients with elevated lactate levels, targeting resuscitation to normalize lactate (grade 2C).

B. Screening for Sepsis and Performance Improvement

1. Routine screening of potentially infected seriously ill patients for severe sepsis to allow earlier implementation of therapy (grade 1C).
2. Hospital-based performance improvement efforts in severe sepsis (ungraded).

C. Diagnosis

1. Cultures before antimicrobial therapy if delay in the start of antimicrobial therapy is <45 min (grade 1C). Two or more sets of blood cultures (aerobic and anaerobic) with at least one drawn percutaneously and one drawn through each vascular access device, unless the device was inserted <48 h ago (grade 1C).
2. 1,3-Beta-D-glucan assay (grade 2B) and mannan and antimannan antibody assays (2C) if available and invasive candidiasis is in differential diagnosis.
3. Imaging studies to confirm potential source of infection (ungraded).

D. Antimicrobial Therapy

1. Goal: Intravenous (IV) antimicrobial therapy within first hour of septic shock (grade 1B) and severe sepsis without septic shock (grade 1C).
2a. Initial empiric antiinfective therapy with drugs active against all likely pathogens and that penetrate adequately into sepsis source tissues (grade 1B).
2b. Antimicrobial regimen reassessed daily for potential deescalation (grade 1B).
3. Low procalcitonin levels or similar biomarkers assist clinicians in discontinuation of therapy in patients who initially appeared septic but have no subsequent evidence of infection (grade 2C).
4a. Combination therapy for neutropenic patients with severe sepsis (grade 2B) and for patients with difficult-to-treat, multidrug-resistant bacterial pathogens (grade 2B). For patients with severe infections associated with

respiratory failure and septic shock, combination therapy with an extended-spectrum beta-lactam and either an aminoglycoside or a fluoroquinolone (for *Pseudomonas aeruginosa* bacteremia) (grade 2B). Combination of beta-lactam and macrolide for patients with septic shock from bacteremic *Streptococcus pneumoniae* infections (grade 2B).

4b. Combination therapy should not be administered for >3–5 days. Deescalation to most appropriate single therapy should be performed as soon as susceptibility profile is known (grade 2B).

5. Duration of therapy typically 7–10 days; longer courses may be appropriate in patients who have a slow clinical response, undrainable foci of infection, bacteremia with *Staphylococcus aureus,* and some fungal and viral infections or immunologic deficiencies (grade 2C).

6. Antiviral therapy initiated as early as possible in patients with severe sepsis or septic shock of viral origin (grade 2C).

7. Antimicrobial agents should not be used in patients with severe inflammatory states determined to be of noninfectious cause (ungraded).

E. Source Control

1. Specific anatomic diagnosis and emergent source control should be diagnosed or excluded as rapidly as possible; source control intervention should be undertaken <12 h after diagnosis, if feasible (grade 1C).
2. When source is potentially infected peripancreatic necrosis, definitive intervention is best delayed until after adequate demarcation of viable tissues (grade 2B).
3. For source control in severely septic patients, effective interventions associated with the least physiologic insult should be used (ungraded).
4. If IV access devices are possible sources, they should be removed promptly after other vascular access has been established (ungraded).

F. Infection Prevention

1a. Selective oral and digestive decontamination should be considered to reduce the incidence of ventilator-associated pneumonia; this can be instituted in settings where it is effective (grade 2B).
1b. Oral chlorhexidine gluconate used to reduce risk of ventilator-associated pneumonia in patients in the intensive care unit (ICU) with severe sepsis (grade 2B).

G. Fluid Therapy of Severe Sepsis

1. Crystalloids initially in resuscitation of severe sepsis and septic shock (grade 1B).

QSEN BOX 34.19 **QSEN: Evidence-Based Practice—cont'd**

Severe Sepsis and Septic Shock Management Guidelines

2. Against hydroxyethyl starches for resuscitation of severe sepsis and septic shock (grade 1B).
3. Albumin in resuscitation of severe sepsis and septic shock when patients require substantial crystalloids (grade 2C).
4. Initial fluid challenge (to minimum of 30 mL/kg of crystalloids) in patients with sepsis-induced tissue hypoperfusion with suspicion of hypovolemia. More rapid administration and greater amounts may be needed in some (grade 1C).
5. Fluid challenge technique applied wherein fluid administration is continued if there is hemodynamic improvement based on dynamic or static variables (ungraded).

H. Vasopressors

1. Vasopressor therapy initially to target MAP of 65 mm Hg (grade 1C).
2. Norepinephrine (NE) as first-choice vasopressor (grade 1B).
3. Epinephrine (added to and potentially substituted for NE) when additional agent is needed to maintain adequate blood pressure (grade 2B).
4. Vasopressin 0.03 units/min can be added to NE to increase MAP or decrease NE dosage (ungraded).
5. Low-dose vasopressin not recommended as single initial vasopressor for treatment of sepsis-induced hypotension. Vasopressin doses >0.03–0.04 units/min should be reserved for salvage therapy (ungraded).
6. Dopamine as an alternative to NE only in highly selected patients (grade 2C).
7. Phenylephrine not recommended in treatment of septic shock except (a) when NE is associated with serious arrhythmias, (b) when cardiac output is high and blood pressure is persistently low, or (c) as salvage therapy when combined inotrope/vasopressor drugs and low-dose vasopressin have failed to achieve MAP target (grade 1C).
8. Low-dose dopamine should not be used for renal protection (grade 1A).
9. All patients requiring vasopressors have an arterial catheter placed as soon as practical (ungraded).

I. Inotropic Therapy

1. A trial of dobutamine infusion up to 20 mcg/kg/min administered or added to vasopressor (if in use) in the presence of (a) myocardial dysfunction or (b) ongoing signs of hypoperfusion, despite adequate intravascular volume and adequate MAP (grade 1C).
2. Not using a strategy to increase cardiac index to predetermined supranormal levels (grade 1B).

J. Corticosteroids

1. Do not use IV hydrocortisone to treat adults if adequate fluid resuscitation and vasopressor therapy are able to restore hemodynamic stability. Otherwise, IV hydrocortisone alone at a dose of 200 mg/day (grade 2C) is suggested.
2. Do not use adrenocorticotropic hormone stimulation test to identify adults who should receive hydrocortisone (grade 2B).
3. If used, hydrocortisone tapered when vasopressors no longer required (grade 2D).
4. Do not use corticosteroids for treatment of sepsis without shock (grade 1D).
5. When hydrocortisone is given, use continuous flow (grade 2D).

K. Blood Product Administration

1. When tissue hypoperfusion has resolved (in absence of extenuating circumstances), red blood cell transfusion is recommended only when hemoglobin decreases to <7.0 g/dL to target hemoglobin concentration of 7.0–9.0 g/dL in adults (grade 1B).
2. Do not use erythropoietin to treat anemia associated with severe sepsis (grade 1B).
3. Do not use fresh frozen plasma to correct laboratory clotting abnormalities in the absence of bleeding or planned invasive procedures (grade 2D).

4. Do not use antithrombin for treatment of severe sepsis and septic shock (grade 1B).
5. In patients with severe sepsis, administer platelets prophylactically when <10,000/mm^3 (10×10^9/L) in absence of apparent bleeding. Prophylactic platelet transfusion suggested when <20,000/mm^3 (20×10^9/L) if patient has significant risk of bleeding. Higher platelet counts ($\geq$50,000/mm^3 [50×10^9/L]) advised for active bleeding, surgery, or invasive procedures (grade 2D).

L. Immunoglobulins

1. Do not use IV immunoglobulins in adults with severe sepsis or septic shock (grade 2B).

M. Selenium

1. Do not use IV selenium for treatment of severe sepsis (grade 2C).

N. Mechanical Ventilation of Sepsis-Induced Acute Respiratory Distress Syndrome

1. Target tidal volume of 6 mL/kg predicted body weight in patients with sepsis-induced acute respiratory distress syndrome (ARDS) (grade 1A vs 12 mL/kg).
2. Measure plateau pressures in patients with ARDS. Initial upper limit goal in a passively inflated lung is $\leq$30 cm H_2O (grade 1B).
3. Apply positive end-expiratory pressure (PEEP) to avoid alveolar collapse at end-expiration (grade 1B).
4. Use strategies based on higher levels of PEEP for patients with sepsis-induced moderate or severe ARDS (grade 2C).
5. Use recruitment maneuvers in patients with sepsis and severe refractory hypoxemia (grade 2C).
6. Use prone positioning in patients with sepsis-induced ARDS and Pao$_2$/Fio$_2$ ratio $\leq$100 mm Hg (grade 2B).
7. Maintain mechanically ventilated sepsis patients with head of bed elevated 30–45 degrees to limit aspiration risk and prevent development of ventilator-associated pneumonia (grade 1B).
8. Use noninvasive mask ventilation (NIV) in patients with sepsis-induced ARDS in whom the benefits of NIV have been carefully considered (grade 2B).
9. Put a weaning protocol in place. Mechanically ventilated patients with severe sepsis should undergo spontaneous breathing trials regularly to evaluate ability to discontinue mechanical ventilation when they (a) are arousable, (b) are hemodynamically stable (without vasopressor agents), (c) have no new potentially serious conditions, (d) have low ventilator and end-expiratory pressure requirements, and (e) have low Fio$_2$ requirements that can be met with a face mask or nasal cannula. If spontaneous breathing trial is successful, consider extubation (grade 1A).
10. Do not routinely use a pulmonary artery catheter for patients with sepsis-induced ARDS (grade 1A).
11. Use a conservative fluid strategy for patients with established sepsis-induced ARDS who do not have evidence of tissue hypoperfusion (grade 1C).
12. In the absence of specific indications, do not use beta-2 agonists for treatment of sepsis-induced ARDS (grade 1B).

O. Sedation, Analgesia, and Neuromuscular Blockade in Sepsis

1. Continuous or intermittent sedation should be minimized in mechanically ventilated patients with sepsis, targeting specific titration end points (grade 1B).
2. Avoid neuromuscular blocking agents (NMBAs) if possible in septic patients *without ARDS* because of risk of prolonged neuromuscular blockade after discontinuation. If NMBAs must be maintained, use either intermittent bolus as required or continuous infusion with train-of-four monitoring (grade 1C).
3. Use a short course of NMBA $\leq$48 h for patients *with* early sepsis-induced ARDS and Pao$_2$/Fio$_2$ <150 mm Hg (grade 2C).

Continued

Severe Sepsis and Septic Shock Management Guidelines

P. Glucose Control

1. A protocolized approach to management in ICU patients with severe sepsis beginning insulin dosing when two consecutive blood glucose levels are >180 mg/dL. Approach should target an upper blood glucose ≤180 mg/dL (grade 1A).
2. Blood glucose values should be monitored every 1–2 h until glucose values and insulin infusion rates stabilize and every 4 h thereafter (grade 1C).
3. Glucose levels obtained with point-of-care testing of capillary blood should be interpreted with caution (ungraded).

Q. Renal Replacement Therapy

1. Continuous renal replacement therapies and intermittent hemodialysis are equivalent in severe sepsis and acute renal failure (grade 2B).
2. Use continuous therapies to facilitate management of fluid balance in hemodynamically unstable septic patients (grade 2D).

R. Bicarbonate Therapy

1. Do not use sodium bicarbonate therapy for improving hemodynamics or reducing vasopressor requirements in patients with hypoperfusion-induced lactic acidemia with pH ≥7.15 (grade 2B).

S. Deep Vein Thrombosis Prophylaxis

1. Patients with severe sepsis should receive daily pharmacoprophylaxis against venous thromboembolism (grade 1B). Accomplish with daily subcutaneous low-molecular-weight heparin (LMWH) (grade 1B vs twice-daily unfractionated heparin [UFH], grade 2C vs three-times-daily UFH). If creatinine clearance <30 mL/min, use dalteparin (grade 1A) or another form of LMWH that has a low degree of renal metabolism (grade 2C) or UFH (grade 1A).
2. Treat patients with severe sepsis with combination of pharmacologic therapy and intermittent pneumatic compression devices if possible (grade 2C).

3. Do not use pharmacoprophylaxis in septic patients who have a contraindication for heparin use (grade 1B). Use mechanical prophylactic treatment (grade 2C), unless contraindicated. When risk decreases, start pharmacoprophylaxis (grade 2C).

T. Stress Ulcer Prophylaxis

1. Give stress ulcer prophylaxis using H_2 blocker or proton-pump inhibitor to patients with severe sepsis or septic shock who have bleeding risk factors (grade 1B).
2. If used, proton-pump inhibitors preferred over H_2 receptor antagonists (grade 2D).
3. Patients without risk factors do not receive prophylaxis (grade 2B).

U. Nutrition

1. Administer oral or enteral feedings rather than either complete fasting or provision of only IV glucose within first 48 h after diagnosis of severe sepsis or septic shock (grade 2C).
2. Avoid mandatory full caloric feeding in first week. Suggest low-dose feeding, advancing only as tolerated (grade 2B).
3. Use IV glucose and enteral nutrition rather than total parenteral nutrition alone or parenteral nutrition in conjunction with enteral feeding in first 7 days after diagnosis of severe sepsis or septic shock (grade 2B).
4. Use nutrition with no specific immunomodulating supplementation in patients with severe sepsis (grade 2C).

V. Setting Goals of Care

1. Discuss goals and prognosis with patients and families (grade 1B).
2. Incorporate goals into treatment and end-of-life care planning (grade 1B).
3. Address goals as early as feasible, but no later than within 72 h of ICU admission (grade 2C).

Fio_2, fraction of inspired oxygen; Pao_2, partial pressure of oxygen.
Data from Dellinger RP, et al. Surviving Sepsis Campaign: International guidelines for management of severe sepsis and septic shock: 2012. *Crit Care Med.* 2014;41:580.

failure to control the host inflammatory response, leads to the excessive production of inflammatory cells and biochemical mediators that cause widespread damage to vascular endothelium and organ damage.[123,132] The compromised immune state of a critically ill patient also fosters an environment conducive to organ failure.

The definitive clinical course of secondary MODS has not been completely identified. Organ dysfunction may occur in a sequential or progressive pattern. Organ dysfunction may begin in the lungs, the most commonly affected major organ, and progress to the liver, gut, and kidneys. Cardiac and bone marrow dysfunction may follow. Neurologic and autonomic system impairment may occur and propagate the progression of organ failure and is associated with illness severity and mortality.[133] Organs may fail simultaneously; for example, kidney dysfunction may occur concurrently with hepatic dysfunction. After the initial insult and resuscitation, patients develop persistent hypermetabolism, a metabolic consequence of sustained systemic inflammation and physiologic stress, followed closely by pulmonary dysfunction, manifested as ARDS.

Certain cellular and biochemical activity evokes the inflammatory and immune responses implicated in SIRS and MODS. The mediators associated with SIRS and MODS can be classified as inflammatory cells, biochemical mediators, or plasma protein systems (Box 34.21). Activation of one mediator often leads to activation of another. The biologic activity of inflammatory cells, biochemical mediators, and plasma protein systems and how they work in concert to cause SIRS and MODS have not been totally determined.

Inflammatory Cells

Neutrophils, macrophages, monocytes, mast cells, platelets, and endothelial cells are inflammatory cells that mediate SIRS through their production of cytokines (biochemical mediators). Along with proinflammatory biochemicals released from damaged or necrotic tissue and circulating catecholamines (stress response), these inflammatory cells create a hypermetabolic state, cause maldistribution of circulatory volume, and alter inflammatory and immune functions.[132]

Neutrophils. During SIRS and MODS, neutrophils are activated systemically and damage normal cells in addition to killing bacteria. Neutrophils adhere to vascular endothelium and release cytotoxic biochemicals, including PAF, TNF-alpha, arachidonic acid (AA) metabolites, and toxic oxygen metabolites.[123,132] These substances cause tissue damage, vascular injury, edema, thrombosis, and hemorrhage in multiple organ systems. During

FIG. 34.10 Pathogenesis of Multiple Organ Dysfunction Syndrome. GI, gastrointestinal; MDF, myocardial depressant factor; MODS, multiple organ dysfunction syndrome; PAF, platelet-activating factor; WBCs, white blood cells. (From McCance KL, Huether SE, ed. Pathophysiology: The Biological Basis for Disease in Adults and Children, ed 7. St. Louis: Elsevier; 2014.)

SIRS or sepsis, neutrophilic function is modulated by other circulating mediators that intensify its inflammatory response, particularly in the liver and the lungs.[100,132]

Monocytes and macrophages. Monocytes and macrophages normally perform three major functions relative to inflammation: antigen processing and presentation, bacterial phagocytosis, and mediator production. Monocytes and macrophages detect, process, and present antigen to lymphocytes for initiation of the humoral and cellular components of the lymphocytic immune response. Macrophages play a significant role in organ injury by producing oxygen metabolites, initiating procoagulant activity, and releasing IL-1 and TNF-alpha.[123] TNF-alpha and IL-1 stimulate neutrophils and lymphocytes to activate the AA cascade. AA metabolites are vasoactive and cause vascular instability and altered organ blood flow. In the lungs, alveolar macrophages produce toxic oxygen metabolites and proteolytic enzymes that destroy alveolar epithelial cells. The role of

macrophages and monocytes in organ dysfunction is linked to their production of TNF-alpha and IL-1.[123,132]

Mast cells. Mast cells are found in all body tissues, especially tissues adjacent to blood vessels. Physical injury, chemical agents, and immunologic or infectious causes activate mast cells and produce mediators through mast cell degranulation and new synthesis that have systemic and local effects. Mast cell–regulated mediators from either process include histamine, TNF-alpha, interleukins, prostaglandins, and various other AA metabolites.[132]

Lymphocytes. Lymphocytes adhere to and are sequestered in the microvascular endothelium. Stimulated T and B lymphocytes produce cytokines such as IL-1 and IL-2, which activate other inflammatory cells.[100,123]

Endothelial cells. The endothelium is a unicellular layer that lines the vascular system. Normally, little interaction occurs between the endothelium and leukocytes. However, during SIRS and MODS, endothelial cells become targets for leukocyte-derived mediators, and they become dysfunctional and release prothrombotic, proinflammatory, and vasoactive mediators. Endothelial damage results in the production of procoagulants such as tissue factor, plasminogen-activating inhibitor, and prostacyclin (prostaglandin I_2), leading to the introduction of thrombin in the microvasculature. Endothelial cells manufacture chemotactic agents that attract neutrophils to areas of inflammation and endothelial injury. Collectively, these processes cause widespread endothelial destruction, intravascular coagulation, vascular instability, and permeability, which are key elements in SIRS and sepsis.[132,134]

Inflammatory mediators that cause endothelial damage include endotoxin, TNF-alpha, IL-1, and PAF. These mediators also recruit and activate neutrophils, activate complement, and perpetuate destruction of the endothelium. Endothelial cells produce and maintain a physiologic equilibrium between endothelin (the most potent vasoconstrictor known) and endothelial cell-derived relaxant factor (nitric oxide), a vasodilator.[132] An alteration in this balance leads to vascular instability, vasodilation, and the perfusion abnormalities commonly seen in patients with SIRS and MODS.[127,132,134]

Biochemical Mediators

Multiple biochemical inflammatory mediators play a role in SIRS and MODS, including proteases, TNF-alpha, interleukins, PAF, AA metabolites, and oxygen metabolites. TNF-alpha,

---

BOX 34.20 Clinical Conditions and Manifestations Associated With Systemic Inflammatory Response Syndrome

Clinical Conditions

- Infection
- Infection of vascular structures (heart and lungs)
- Pancreatitis
- Tissue ischemia or hypoxia
- Multiple trauma with massive tissue injury
- Hemorrhagic shock
- Immune-mediated organ injury
- Exogenous administration of tumor necrosis factor or other cytokines
- Aspiration of gastric contents
- Massive transfusion
- Host defense abnormalities

Clinical Manifestations

- Temperature >38°C or <36°C
- Heart rate >90 beats/min
- Respiratory rate >20 breaths/min or $Paco_2$ <32 mm Hg
- WBC count >12,000 cells/mm³ or <4000 cells/mm³ or >10% immature (band) forms

$Paco_2$, arterial partial pressure of carbon dioxide; *WBC,* white blood cell.

BOX 34.21 Inflammatory Mediators Associated With Systemic Inflammatory Response Syndrome and Multiple-Organ Dysfunction Syndrome

Inflammatory Cells

- Neutrophils
- Macrophages or monocytes
- Mast lymphocytes
- Endothelial

Biochemical Mediators

- Reactive oxygen species
  - Superoxide radical
  - Hydroxyl radical
  - Hydrogen peroxide
- Tumor necrosis factor

- Interleukins
- Platelet-activating factor
- Arachidonic acid metabolites
  - Prostaglandins
  - Leukotrienes
  - Thromboxanes
- Proteases

Plasma Protein Systems

- Complement
- Kinin
- Coagulation

IL-1, and IL-6 appear to be the most important cytokines associated with SIRS and MODS.[135,136]

Reactive oxygen species. Reactive oxygen species are produced in excessive amounts during critical illness and have been implicated in MODS.[137] Oxygen metabolites are normally produced as the result of many physiologic processes. However, the body has numerous antioxidant and enzyme systems to convert free oxygen radicals to nontoxic substances to prevent tissue injury. Excessive oxygen metabolites cause lipid peroxidation and damage to the cell membrane, activate the complement and coagulation cascades, and cause DNA damage. Inflammatory neutrophils cause tissue injury by producing excessive numbers of reactive oxygen metabolites. Reperfusion organ injury is partially attributed to excessive oxygen metabolites. During reperfusion, severe tissue injury follows the massive production of oxygen free radicals. The organs most susceptible to injury include the small intestines, liver, lungs, heart, brain, stomach, muscle, and skin.[138]

Tumor necrosis factor-alpha. TNF-alpha is a polypeptide that is released from macrophages and lymphocytes in response to endotoxin, tissue injury, viral agents, and interleukins. When present in excessive amounts, TNF-alpha causes widespread destruction in most organ systems and is responsible for the pathophysiologic changes in SIRS and septic shock, including fever, hypotension, decreased organ perfusion, and increased capillary permeability.[139] TNF-alpha may precipitate organ injury by causing generalized endothelial injury, fibrin deposition, and a procoagulant state. TNF-alpha causes DIC; interstitial pneumonitis; AKI; and necrosis of the GI tract, liver, and adrenal glands. TNF-alpha stimulates AA metabolism, the clotting cascade, and the production of PAF. Metabolically, excessive TNF-alpha causes hyperglycemia that progresses to hypoglycemia and hypertriglyceridemia. The destructive effects of TNF-alpha are exacerbated by AA metabolites and stress hormones.

Interleukins. Produced mainly by macrophages and lymphocytes, the interleukins are a class of cytokines that have biologic responses similar to TNF-alpha. More than 30 interleukins have been identified. Macrophages secrete substantial amounts of IL-1. IL-1 causes vascular congestion, capillary leakage, and increased coagulation, all of which are associated with SIRS and sepsis. IL-1 has profound vascular endothelial effects, stimulates the production of procoagulants by endothelial cells, increases catabolism of muscle tissue, and causes neutrophilia.[123,132]

Platelet-activating factor. PAF, a potent proinflammatory phospholipid, is released from inflammatory and immune cells in response to a multitude of factors or stimuli. PAF is released by platelets, mast cells, monocytes, macrophages, neutrophils, and endothelial cells. PAF has widespread effects on the heart, the vascular system, procoagulation, platelets, and the lungs. Effects of PAF include platelet aggregation, with resultant microvascular stasis and ischemia in the microvascular bed; platelet release of serotonin, which increases vascular permeability; and increased vasoconstriction from increased production of thromboxane A_2, an AA metabolite.[123]

Arachidonic acid metabolites. AA is a highly metabolic fatty acid that is a precursor of many biologically active substances known as *eicosanoids*. Lipid peroxidation of neutrophil cell membranes induces release of these metabolites.[123] Select eicosanoids are implicated in the pathogenesis of SIRS and MODS. Eicosanoids contribute to organ failure by altering vascular reactivity and permeability and by fostering the accumulation and activation of inflammatory cells. Activation of the AA cascade by hypoxia, ischemia, endotoxin, catecholamines, and tissue injury produces metabolites from the cyclooxygenase and lipoxygenase pathways. AA metabolites produced through the cyclooxygenase pathway are called *prostaglandins* and *thromboxanes*, and AA metabolites from the lipoxygenase pathway are called *leukotrienes* (LTs). AA metabolites have profound effects on vasculature and cause vascular instability and maldistribution of blood flow. Some eicosanoids (eg, prostaglandin H_2, thromboxane A_2, leukotriene D_4) are vasoconstrictors, and others (eg, prostaglandin E_2, prostaglandin I_2) have potent vasodilatory properties. All leukotrienes and thromboxane A_2 enhance capillary membrane permeability and increase vascular leakage. Thromboxane A_2, prostaglandin H_2, and prostaglandin F_2 are potent platelet aggregators.[123]

Proteases. Proteases are proteolytic (protein-digesting) enzymes released from neutrophils. Proteases damage endothelium and contribute to vascular permeability and organ dysfunction.[123] One such protease, neutrophil elastase, damages lung tissue by inducing IL-8 production, attracting additional neutrophils, and stimulating mucus secretion.

Multiple clinical trials have been conducted in an attempt to stop or neutralize the sustained inflammatory response that causes organ dysfunction. These trials have included the use of corticosteroid therapy, antiendotoxin antibodies, anti–tumor necrosis factor monoclonal antibodies, IL-1 receptor antagonists, bradykinin antagonists, PAF antagonists, PAF receptor antagonists, phospholipase A_2 inhibition, nitric oxide synthase inhibition, and antithrombin III. None of trials have demonstrated improved clinical outcomes in patients with sepsis and SIRS.[88]

Assessment and Diagnosis

Secondary MODS is a systemic disease with organ-specific manifestations. Organ dysfunction is influenced by numerous factors, including organ host defense function, response time to the injury, metabolic requirements, organ vasculature response to vasoactive medications, organ sensitivity to damage, and physiologic reserve. The responses of the GI, hepatobiliary, cardiovascular, pulmonary, renal, and hematologic systems are discussed in the following paragraphs. Clinical manifestations of organ dysfunction are outlined in Box 34.22.

Gastrointestinal Dysfunction

The GI tract plays an important role in MODS. GI organs normally have immunoregulatory functions, and the GI tract contains approximately 70% to 80% of the immunologic tissue of the entire body. A normally functioning GI tract prevents bacteria from entering the systemic circulation.[123] Normal gut flora and gut environment are altered in patients with severe SIRS. Healthy probiotics (eg, *Bifidobacterium*, *Lactobacillus*) are decreased in a SIRS state, and pathogenic organisms (eg, *Staphylococcus*, *Pseudomonas*) proliferate.[131]

With microcirculatory failure to the GI tract, the gut's barrier function may be lost, which leads to bacterial translocation, sustained inflammation, endogenous endotoxemia, and MODS.[123,132] Hypoperfusion and shock-like states damage the

BOX 34.22   Clinical Manifestations of Organ Dysfunction

Gastrointestinal
- Abdominal distention and ascites
- Intolerance to enteral feedings
- Paralytic ileus
- Upper or lower gastrointestinal bleeding
- Diarrhea
- Ischemic colitis
- Mucosal ulceration
- Decreased bowel sounds
- Bacterial overgrowth in stool

Liver
- Jaundice
- Hepatomegaly
- Increased serum bilirubin (hyperbilirubinemia)
- Increased liver enzymes
- Increased serum ammonia
- Decreased serum albumin
- Decreased serum transferrin

Gallbladder
- Right upper quadrant tenderness or pain
- Abdominal distention
- Unexplained fever
- Decreased bowel sounds

Metabolic and Nutrition
- Decreased lean body mass
- Muscle wasting
- Severe weight loss
- Negative nitrogen balance
- Hyperglycemia
- Hypertriglyceridemia
- Increased serum lactate
- Decreased serum albumin, serum transferrin, prealbumin
- Decreased retinol-binding protein

Immune
- Infection
- Decreased lymphocyte count
- Anergy

Pulmonary
- Tachypnea
- Acute lung injury pattern of respiratory failure (dyspnea, patchy infiltrates, refractory hypoxemia, respiratory acidosis, abnormal oxygen indices)
- Pulmonary hypertension

Kidney
- Decreased glomerular filtration rate/creatinine clearance
- Increased serum creatinine, blood urea nitrogen levels
- Oliguria, anuria, or polyuria consistent with prerenal azotemia or acute kidney injury
- Urinary indices consistent with prerenal azotemia or acute kidney injury
- Electrolyte imbalance

Cardiovascular
Hyperdynamic
- Decreased pulmonary capillary occlusion pressure
- Decreased systemic vascular resistance
- Decreased right atrial pressure
- Decreased left ventricular stroke work index
- Increased oxygen consumption
- Increased cardiac output, cardiac index, heart rate

Hypodynamic
- Increased systemic vascular resistance
- Increased right atrial pressure
- Increased left ventricular stroke work index
- Decreased oxygen delivery and consumption
- Decreased cardiac output and cardiac index

Central Nervous System
- Lethargy
- Altered level of consciousness
- Fever
- Hepatic encephalopathy

Coagulation or Hematologic
- Thrombocytopenia
- Disseminated intravascular coagulation

Modified from McCance KL, Huether SE, ed. *Pathophysiology: The Biologic Basis for Disease in Adults and Children.* 7th ed. St. Louis: Elsevier; 2014.

normal GI mucosa barrier by decreasing mesenteric blood flow, leading to hypoperfusion of the villi, mucosal edema, ischemic necrosis, sloughing of the mucosa, and malabsorption. The GI tract is extremely vulnerable to oxygen metabolite–induced reperfusion injury. Endothelial injury and GI lesions occur in response to mediator-induced tissue damage. Ischemic events and the absence of feedings can disrupt the normal metabolism of the gastric or intestinal lumen and the normal protective function of the gut barrier.[119,127]

The translocation of GI bacteria through a "leaky gut" into the systemic circulation initiates and perpetuates an inflammatory focus in a critically ill patient.[127] The GI tract harbors organisms that present an inflammatory focus when carried from the gut via the intestinal lymphatics. After hemorrhagic shock, trauma, or a major burn injury, gut-released proinflammatory and tissue injurious factors may lead to acute lung injury, bone marrow failure, myocardial dysfunction, neutrophil activation, RBC injury, and endothelial cell activation and injury. These factors, released from the gut and carried in the mesenteric lymphatics, are capable of causing a septic state and secondary MODS. The "gut-lymph hypothesis" proposes that gut ischemia-reperfusion injury leads to loss of a gut protective barrier, bacterial translocation, and a gut inflammatory response. Gut-derived inflammatory factors are carried in the mesenteric lymph leading to a septic state and distant organ failure and MODS.[2]

Lastly, the oropharynx of a critically ill patient also becomes colonized with potentially pathogenic organisms from the GI tract. Pulmonary aspiration of colonized secretions presents an inflammatory focus that can contribute to concomitant pulmonary dysfunction.[140]

Hepatobiliary Dysfunction

The liver plays a vital role in host homeostasis related to the acute inflammatory response. The liver responds to sustained inflammation by selectively altering carbohydrate, fat, and protein metabolism. Consequently, hepatic dysfunction threatens the patient's survival. The liver normally controls the inflammatory response by several mechanisms. Kupffer cells, which are hepatic macrophages, detoxify substances that may normally induce systemic inflammation and vasoactive substances that cause hemodynamic instability. Failure to detoxify gram-negative bacteria causes endotoxemia, perpetuates SIRS, and may lead to MODS. The liver also produces proteins and antiproteases to control the inflammatory response; however, hepatic dysfunction limits this response.

Common causes of liver failure in critically ill patients are infection-related cholestasis and hepatocellular injury in response to toxins and toxins themselves. In infection-related cholestasis, bacterial toxins and released cytokines affect the uptake and excretion of bilirubin leading to jaundice. In hepatocellular injury, endotoxins and bacteria are phagocytized by Kupffer cells that release hepatotoxic substances that cause cellular damage. Hepatic dysfunction may also occur with organ hypoperfusion, hemolysis, and hepatotoxic medications. Measurements of liver enzymes, bilirubin, ammonia, and liver-produced proteins should be carefully monitored.[140]

The liver and gallbladder are extremely vulnerable to ischemic injury from organ hypoperfusion. Ischemic hepatitis occurs after a prolonged period of physiologic shock and is associated with centrilobular hepatocellular necrosis. The degree of hepatic damage is related directly to the severity and duration of the shock episode. Anoxic and reperfusion injuries damage hepatocytes and the vascular endothelium. Patients at high risk for ischemic hepatitis after a hypotensive event include patients with a history of heart failure or cardiac dysrhythmias. Clinical manifestations of hepatic insufficiency are evident 1 to 2 days after the insult. Jaundice and transient elevations in serum transaminase and bilirubin levels occur. Hyperbilirubinemia results from hepatocyte anoxic injury and an increased production of bilirubin from hemoglobin catabolism. Ischemic hepatitis may resolve spontaneously or progress to acute liver failure. Although ischemic hepatitis is not a life-threatening complication, it can contribute to morbidity and mortality as a component of MODS. Acute liver failure is discussed further in Chapter 29.

Acalculous cholecystitis manifests 3 to 4 weeks after an insult. Its pathogenesis is unclear, but it may be related to ischemic reperfusion injury, PEEP greater than 5 cm H_2O, volume depletion, total parenteral nutrition, opioids, and cystic duct obstruction as a result of hyperviscous bile.[141] Visceral hypotension and vasoactive medication use may decrease perfusion of the gallbladder mucosa contributing to ischemia. Bacterial invasion may stimulate activation of factor XII and initiate the coagulation pathway.[141] Clinical manifestations of acalculous cholecystitis may mimic acute cholecystitis with gallstones. However, patients may demonstrate vague symptoms, including right upper quadrant pain and tenderness. Critical to the detection of acalculous cholecystitis is the recognition of abdominal distention, unexplained fever, loss of bowel sounds, and sudden deterioration in the patient's condition. Approximately 50% of patients with acalculous cholecystitis have gallbladder gangrene, and 10% have gallbladder perforation requiring a cholecystectomy.[141]

Pulmonary Dysfunction

The lungs are frequent and early target organs for mediator-induced injury and are usually the first organs affected in the progression of SIRS to MODS.[142] ARDS is the pulmonary manifestation of MODS. Patients who develop MODS usually have pulmonary symptoms; however, not all patients with ARDS develop secondary MODS. Patients with ARDS who develop SIRS or sepsis concurrently with acute respiratory failure are at the greatest risk for MODS.[143]

ARDS associated with MODS usually occurs 24 to 72 hours after the initial insult. Patients initially exhibit a low-grade fever, tachycardia, dyspnea, and mental confusion. With progression of ARDS dyspnea, hypoxemia, and the work of breathing increase requiring intubation and mechanical ventilation. ARDS results in refractory hypoxemia caused by intrapulmonary shunting, decreased pulmonary compliance, and altered airway mechanics; there usually is radiographic evidence of noncardiogenic pulmonary edema.[144]

Mediators associated with ARDS include inflammatory cells such as polymorphonuclear cells, macrophages, monocytes, endothelial cells, and mast cells and biochemical mediators such as AA metabolites, toxic oxygen metabolites, proteases, TNF, PAF, and interleukins. Intense mediator activity damages the pulmonary vascular endothelium and the alveolar epithelium, resulting in surfactant deficiency, mild pulmonary hypertension, and increased pulmonary capillary permeability leading to increased lung water (noncardiogenic pulmonary edema).[100,144] ARDS is discussed further in Chapter 19.

Kidney Dysfunction

AKI is a common manifestation of MODS. The kidney is highly vulnerable to hypoperfusion and reperfusion injury. Consequently, kidney ischemia-reperfusion injury may be a major cause of kidney dysfunction in MODS. Mechanisms of cellular death may differ in sepsis-induced AKI versus non–sepsis-induced AKI. Acute tubular apoptosis may occur in septic AKI, whereas nonseptic AKI may be associated with necrosis.[145]

A patient with AKI may demonstrate oliguria or anuria resulting from decreased renal perfusion and relative hypovolemia. Early oliguria is likely caused by decreases in renal perfusion related to shock-like states; late oliguria is typically a sign of evolving kidney injury and ischemia. Renal function may become refractory to diuretics, fluid challenges, and vasoactive medications. Prerenal oliguria may progress to AKI, necessitating continuous renal replacement therapies. The frequent use of nephrotoxic medications also intensifies the risk of AKI.

Early recognition of AKI is imperative. However, the lack of early and reliable biomarkers for AKI leads to a delay in initiating treatment. The instability of kidney function in a critically ill patient decreases the validity of measures that are based on creatinine assessment. An elevated serum creatinine level is usually a late sign, but it is typically accepted as the index for renal dysfunction. However, serum creatinine concentrations can vary for reasons other than renal function in patients with organ failure and are rarely at a steady state.[145] It may be preferable to use 8-hour, 12-hour, or 24-hour urinary creatinine clearance values to estimate glomerular filtration rate in critically ill patients, especially when determining medication dosages.[141] Additional signs of kidney impairment include decreased erythropoietin-induced anemia, vitamin D malabsorption, and altered fluid and electrolyte balance. AKI is discussed further in Chapter 26.

Cardiovascular and Hematologic System Dysfunction

The initial cardiovascular response in SIRS or sepsis is myocardial depression; decreased RAP and SVR; and increased venous capacitance, CO, and heart rate. Despite an increased CO, myocardial depression occurs and is accompanied by decreased SVR, increased heart rate, and ventricular dilation. These compensatory mechanisms help maintain CO during the early phase of SIRS or sepsis. An inability to increase CO in response to a low SVR may indicate myocardial failure or inadequate fluid resuscitation, and it is associated with increased mortality. Vo_2 may be twice the normal value and may be flow dependent.[146]

As MODS progresses, heart failure develops. Cardiac dysfunction is characterized by ventricular dilation, decreased diastolic compliance, and decreased systolic contractile function. Cardiovascular function becomes vasopressor dependent. Heart failure may be caused by immune mediators, TNF-alpha, acidosis, or myocardial depressant factor, a substance secreted by the pancreas. Myocardial depression is exacerbated by myocardial hypoperfusion from a low CO state and persistent lactic acidosis. Cardiogenic shock and biventricular failure occur and lead to death.[146] Heart failure is discussed further in Chapter 14, and more information on cardiogenic shock can be found earlier in this chapter.

The most common manifestations of hematologic dysfunction in sepsis or MODS are thrombocytopenia, coagulation abnormalities, and anemia.[147] The most severe is coagulation system dysfunction manifesting as DIC. DIC is a complex, consumptive coagulopathy that occurs in patients with a variety of disorders, including sepsis, tissue injury, and shock; it is overstimulation of the normal coagulation process. DIC results simultaneously in microvascular clotting and hemorrhage in organ systems, leading to thrombosis and fibrinolysis in life-threatening proportions. Clotting factor derangement leads to further inflammation and further thrombosis. Microvascular damage leads to further organ injury. Cell injury and damage to the endothelium activate the intrinsic or extrinsic coagulation pathways.[96,134] Low platelet counts and elevated D-dimer concentrations and fibrinogen degradation products are clinical indicators of DIC. DIC is discussed further in Chapter 37.

Medical Management

A patient with MODS requires multidisciplinary collaboration in clinical management including fluid resuscitation and hemodynamic support (when appropriate), prevention and treatment of infection, maintenance of tissue oxygenation, nutrition and metabolic support, comfort and emotional support, and support for individual organ function. The use of investigational therapies may be part of the patient's clinical management.

Identification and Treatment of Infection

Identification and treatment of the underlying source of inflammation or infection are important ways to reduce mortality. Medical and surgical intervention to remove sources of infection or contamination may limit the inflammatory response and improve chances of recovery. Surgical procedures such as early fracture stabilization, removal of infected organs or tissue, and burn excision are helpful. Appropriate antibiotics are needed if the cause cannot be removed by surgical débridement or incision and draining.[142]

Antibiotic management in septic patients with MODS is a challenge.[148] Ulldemonlins et al provided antibiotic dosing recommendations for critically ill patients with MODS. They purported that tissue hypoperfusion during the early phases of sepsis or septic shock may lead to decreased antibiotic tissue concentrations. Therefore, "higher-than-standard" front-loading doses of *hydrophilic* antibiotics may be considered in the initial course of treatment because their volume of distribution will be significantly increased with tissue hypoperfusion. Hydrophilic antibiotics include beta-lactams, aminoglycosides, and glycopeptides. Hydrophilic antibiotics are cleared mostly by glomerular filtration and tubular secretion. Patients with renal dysfunction require maintenance dose reductions or extended dosing intervals to prevent nephrotoxicity resulting from decreased drug elimination.[148]

Commonly administered *lipophilic* antibiotics include fluoroquinolones, lincosamides, and nitroimidazoles. As these antibiotics are cleared by the liver or kidney, or by both organs, attention to renal and hepatic function for initial and maintenance dosing is needed. In addition, total body weight, especially with obese patients, should be considered with front-loading administration of fluoroquinolones and lincosamides. Macrolides are *lipophilic* antibiotics and allow normal initial and maintenance dosing.

Underdosing of antibiotics may occur with tissue hypoperfusion and with decreased protein binding of highly bound antibiotics in patients with hepatic dysfunction. Overdosing may occur in patients with renal dysfunction secondary to decreased elimination of *hydrophilic* antibiotics and in patients with hepatic dysfunction secondary to decreased metabolism of *lipophilic* antibiotics.

Other timely interventions, such as prevention of skin ulceration and early nutrition support, may improve outcomes. Regardless of the identification of potential risk factors, clinical markers, bacterial contaminants, and investigative approaches for detection and prevention, treatment remains largely supportive, and little improvement in the mortality rate has been appreciated.[88]

Maintenance of Tissue Oxygenation

Normally under steady-state conditions, Vo_2 is relatively constant and independent of oxygen delivery (Do_2) unless delivery becomes severely impaired. The relationship is called *supply-independent oxygen consumption*. Consequently a percentage of oxygen is not used (physiologic reserve). Patients with SIRS or MODS often develop supply-dependent oxygen consumption in which Vo_2 becomes dependent on Do_2, rather than demand, at a normal or high Do_2. When Vo_2 does not equal demand, a tissue oxygen debt develops, subjecting organs to failure.[142]

Hypoperfusion and resultant organ hypoxemia often occur in patients at high risk for MODS, subjecting essential organs to failure. Effective fluid resuscitation and early recognition of flow-dependent Vo_2 is essential, and patients at risk for MODS require hemodynamic monitoring, frequent measurements or surrogate measurements of Do_2 and Vo_2, and serum lactate levels to guide therapy. Serum lactate levels provide information regarding the severity of impaired perfusion and the presence of lactic acidosis and differ significantly in survivors of MODS and nonsurvivors. Failure to maintain adequate oxygenation to vital organs results in organ dysfunction. Despite adequate Do_2, Vo_2 may not meet the needs of the body during MODS.

Patients with ARDS, MODS, or SIRS frequently manifest supply-dependent oxygen consumption and are unable to use oxygen appropriately despite normal delivery.[142] Interventions that decrease oxygen demand and increase oxygen delivery are essential. Sedation, mechanical ventilation, rest, and temperature and pain control may be able to decrease oxygen demand.[133] Oxygen delivery may be increased by maintaining normal hematocrit and Pao₂ levels, using PEEP, increasing preload or myocardial contractility to enhance CO, or reducing afterload to increase CO. Various methods of kinetic or prone therapies are available and may enhance alveolar recruitment, improve oxygenation delivery, and decrease other potential complications.

Nutrition and Metabolic Support

Hypermetabolism in SIRS or MODS results in profound weight loss, cachexia, and loss of organ function. The goal of nutrition support is the preservation of organ structure and function. Although nutrition support may not definitely alter the course of organ dysfunction, it prevents generalized nutrition deficiencies and preserves gut integrity. Enteral nutrition may exert a physiologic effect that downregulates the systemic immune response and reduces oxidative stress.[149] The enteral route is preferable to parenteral support.[38] Enteral feedings are given distal to the pylorus to reduce the risk of pulmonary aspiration. Enteral feedings may limit bacterial translocation. In addition to early nutrition support, the pharmacologic properties of enteral feeding formulas may limit SIRS for selected critical care populations. Supplementation of enteral feedings with glutamine may be beneficial.[89,119] However, the optimal formulation of nutrition support and the use of immune-modulating supplements to improve outcomes in patients with or at risk for MODS continues to be the subject of much debate and study.[38,91,119] Nutrition support is discussed further in Chapter 7.

Nursing Management

Preventive measures include a multitude of assessment strategies to detect early organ manifestations of this syndrome. Patients who continue to experience sites of inflammation, septic foci, and inadequate tissue perfusion may be at higher risk. Handwashing, aseptic technique, and an understanding of how microorganisms can invade the body are essential components of preventive nursing care.

The nursing management plan for a patient with MODS incorporates a variety of nursing diagnoses (Box 34.23). Nursing interventions include preventing development of infection, facilitating oxygen delivery and limiting tissue oxygen demand, facilitating nutrition support, providing comfort and emotional support, and preventing and maintaining surveillance for complications.

Patients are assessed closely for inflammation and infection. Subtle expressions of infection warrant investigation. Nursing measures include strict adherence to standards of practice to prevent infection. Practices related to infection control with invasive hemodynamic monitoring, urinary catheters, endotracheal tubes, intracranial pressure monitoring devices, total parenteral nutrition, and wound care must be stringent to prevent further infection. Prevention of concomitant ventilator-associated pneumonia or aspiration pneumonia is a priority.[16,150]

Measures to limit tissue oxygen consumption include administering analgesics and sedatives, positioning the patient for comfort, limiting activities, offering support to reduce anxiety, providing a calm and quiet environment, and educating the patient and family about the condition. Measures to enhance tissue oxygen supply include administering supplemental oxygen, monitoring the patient's respiratory status, and administering prescribed fluids and medications. Interprofessional collaborative management of a patient with MODS is outlined in Box 34.24.

BOX 34.24   QSEN: Teamwork and Collaboration

Interprofessional Collaborative Practice: Multiple Organ Dysfunction Syndrome

- Support oxygen transport:
  - Establish a patent airway.
  - Initiate mechanical ventilation.
  - Administer oxygen.
  - Administer fluids (crystalloids, colloids, blood, and other blood products).
  - Administer vasoactive medications.
  - Administer positive inotropic medications.
  - Administer antidysrhythmic medications.
  - Ensure sufficient hemoglobin and hematocrit.
- Support oxygen use:
  - Identify and correct cause of lactic acidosis.
  - Ensure adequate organ and extremity perfusion.
- Decrease oxygen demand:
  - Administer sedation or paralytics.
  - Administer antipyretics and external cooling measures.
  - Administer pain medications.
- Identify underlying cause of inflammation and treat accordingly:
  - Remove infected organs or tissue.
  - Administer antibiotics.
  - Initiate nutrition support.
- Treat individual organ dysfunction:
  - Gastrointestinal
  - Hepatobiliary
  - Pulmonary
  - Renal
  - Cardiovascular
  - Coagulation system
- Prevent and maintain surveillance for complications, particularly infection.
- Provide comfort and emotional support.

BOX 34.23   NURSING DIAGNOSES

Multiple Organ Dysfunction Syndrome

- Decreased Cardiac Output related to alterations in preload, p. 1015
- Decreased Cardiac Output related to alterations in afterload, p. 1015
- Decreased Cardiac Output related to alterations in contractility, p. 1016
- Impaired Gas Exchange related to ventilation-perfusion mismatching or intrapulmonary shunting, p. 1030
- Imbalanced Nutrition: Less Than Body Requirements related to lack of exogenous nutrients and increased metabolic demand, p. 1029
- Risk for Infection, p. 1046
- Acute Pain related to transmission and perception of cutaneous, visceral, muscular, or ischemic impulses, p. 1010
- Acute Confusion related to sensory overload, sensory deprivation, and sleep pattern disturbance, p. 1007
- Anxiety related to threat to biologic, psychologic, or social integrity, p. 1012
- Compromised Family Coping related to a critically ill family member, p. 1014

SUMMARY

Shock

- Shock is an acute, widespread process of impaired tissue perfusion that occurs when an imbalance develops between cellular oxygen supply and cellular oxygen demand.
- Shock can be classified as hypovolemic, cardiogenic, or distributive (anaphylactic, neurogenic, and septic), depending on the pathophysiologic cause and hemodynamic profile.
- Shock evolves through four stages—initial, compensatory, progressive, and refractory.
- A patient with a MAP less than 60 mm Hg or with evidence of global tissue hypoperfusion is considered to be in a shock state.
- Management of a patient in shock focuses on supporting oxygen delivery.
- Prevention of shock is one of the primary responsibilities of nurses in the critical care unit.

CASE STUDY 34.1 Patient With Systemic Inflammatory Response Syndrome

Brief Patient History

Mr. Z is a 38-year-old Hispanic construction worker who sustained a liver laceration after falling from a roof. He required an exploratory laparotomy for splenectomy and repair of the liver laceration 4 days earlier. His medical history reveals no chronic health problems, although he smokes 20 packs of cigarettes per year.

Clinical Assessment

Mr. Z is admitted to the medical intensive care unit from the telemetry unit with acute respiratory insufficiency and hypotension. He is using his accessory muscles to breathe. He is speaking Spanish. His abdomen is distended, and there are no bowel sounds. Small amounts of dark green drainage are visible in the nasogastric tube. There is no sign of redness or drainage around the surgical wound.

Diagnostic Procedures

Vital signs are as follows: blood pressure of 78/55 mm Hg, heart rate of 142 beats/min (sinus tachycardia), respiratory rate of 35 breaths/min, temperature of 103.1°F, and urine output of 20 mL over the past 8 hours. Arterial blood gas values on a 100% nonrebreather mask are as follows: pH of 7.22, arterial partial pressure of oxygen of 54 mm Hg, arterial partial pressure of carbon dioxide of 69 mm Hg, bicarbonate level of 18 mEq/L, and oxygen saturation of 88%. The chest radiograph reveals infiltrates in the right lower lobe. Laboratory data reveal a hemoglobin level of 9.8 g/dL, hematocrit of 25%, and white blood cell count of 18,000/mm^3.

Medical Diagnosis

Mr. Z is diagnosed with severe sepsis.

Questions

1. What major outcomes do you expect to achieve for this patient?
2. What problems or risks must be managed to achieve these outcomes?
3. What interventions must be initiated to monitor, prevent, manage, or eliminate the problems and risks identified?
4. What interventions should be initiated to promote optimal functioning, safety, and well-being of the patient?
5. What possible learning needs do you anticipate for this patient?
6. What cultural and age-related factors may have a bearing on the patient's plan of care?

QSEN BOX 34.25 QSEN: Informatics

Internet Resources

American Association of Critical-Care Nurses: http://www.aacn.org/
Society of Critical Care Medicine: http://www.sccm.org/
theheart.org: http://www.theheart.org/
Trauma.org: http://www.trauma.org/
The Food Allergy & Anaphylaxis Network: http://www.foodallergy.org/
Anaphylaxis Campaign: http://www.anaphylaxis.org.uk/
Neurogenic Shock Resource Blog: http://www.neurogenicshock.net/
Surviving Sepsis Campaign: http://www.survivingsepsis.org
Advances in Sepsis: http://www.advancesinsepsis.com/
European Society of Intensive Care Medicine: http://www.esicm.org/
International Sepsis Forum: http://sepsisforum.org/
Survive Sepsis: http://www.survivingsepsis.org/
Sepsis Know From Day 1: http://www.sepsisknowfromday1.com
American College of Physicians: http://www.acponline.org/
American College of Surgeons: http://www.facs.org/
American Medical Association: http://www.ama-assn.org/
National Digestive Diseases Information Clearinghouse: http://digestive.niddk.nih.gov/
National Institutes for Health: http://www.nih.gov/
PubMed Health: http://www.ncbi.nlm.nih.gov/pubmedhealth/
American Society for Parenteral and Enteral Nutrition: http://www.nutrition-care.org/

Hypovolemic Shock

- Hypovolemic shock results from a loss of circulating or intravascular volume as a result of an absolute or relative fluid loss.
- Initial hemodynamic parameters include a decreased CO or CI, decreased CVP or PAOP, and increased SVR.
- Medical management focuses on identifying and stopping the source of fluid loss and administering fluid to replace circulating volume.
- Nursing interventions include minimizing fluid loss, administering volume replacement, assessing response to therapy, providing comfort and emotional support, and preventing and maintaining surveillance for complications.

Cardiogenic Shock

- Cardiogenic shock results from the impaired ability of the heart to pump because of problems affecting the muscular or mechanical function of the heart or dysrhythmias.
- Initial hemodynamic parameters include a decreased CO or CI, increased PAOP or CVP (or both), and increased SVR.
- Medical management focuses on identifying the etiologic factors of pump failure and administering pharmacologic agents to enhance CO.
- Nursing interventions include limiting myocardial oxygen demand, enhancing myocardial oxygen supply, maintaining tissue perfusion, providing comfort and emotional support, and preventing and maintaining surveillance for complications.

Anaphylactic Shock

- Anaphylactic shock results from an immunologic antibody-antigen activation or nonimmunologic activation of mast cells and basophils and the release of biochemical mediators.
- Hemodynamic parameters include decreased CO or CI, decreased RAP or PAOP, and decreased SVR.

- Medical management focuses on removing the offending antigen, reversing the effects of the biochemical mediators, and promoting adequate tissue perfusion.
- Nursing interventions include administering epinephrine, facilitating ventilation, administering volume replacement, providing comfort and emotional support, and preventing and maintaining surveillance for recurrent reactions and complications.

Neurogenic Shock

- Neurogenic shock results from the loss of sympathetic tone as a result of interrupted impulse transmission or blockage of sympathetic outflow from the vasomotor center in the brain.
- Hemodynamic parameters include decreased CO or CI, decreased RAP or PAOP, decreased SVR, and decreased heart rate.
- Medical management focuses on preventing cardiovascular stability and promoting tissue perfusion.
- Nursing interventions include treating hypovolemia and maintaining tissue perfusion, maintaining normothermia, monitoring for and treating dysrhythmias, promoting comfort and emotional support, and preventing and maintaining surveillance for complications.

Sepsis and Septic Shock

- Septic shock results from the initiation of the systemic inflammatory response secondary to microorganisms entering the body.
- Hemodynamic parameters include decreased CO or CI, decreased RAP or PAOP, decreased SVR, and increased heart rate.
- Medical management focuses on reversing the pathophysiologic responses, controlling the infection, and promoting metabolic support.
- Nursing interventions include early identification of the sepsis syndrome; administering prescribed fluids, medications, and nutrition; promoting comfort and emotional support; and preventing and maintaining surveillance for complications.

Systemic Inflammatory Response

- The systemic inflammatory response is an intense host response characterized by generalized inflammation in organs remote from the initial insult.
- Consequences include uncontrolled activation of inflammatory cells, damage of vascular endothelium, disruption of immune cell function, hypermetabolism, and maldistribution of circulatory volume.

Multiple Organ Dysfunction Syndrome

- MODS results from progressive physiologic failure of two or more separate organ systems.
- Organ dysfunction is influenced by numerous factors, including organ host defense function, response time to the injury, metabolic requirements, organ vasculature response to vasoactive medications, and organ sensitivity to damage and physiologic reserve.
- Collaborative management focuses on fluid resuscitation and hemodynamic support, prevention and treatment of infection, maintenance of tissue oxygenation, nutrition and metabolic support, comfort and emotional support, and preservation of individual organ function.

ⓔ Visit the Evolve site for additional study materials.

REFERENCES

1. Maier RV. Approach to the patient with shock. In: Kasper DL, et al., ed. *Harrison's Internal Medicine.* 19th ed. New York: McGraw-Hill; 2015.
2. Deitch EA, Xu D, Kaise VL. Role of the gut in the development of injury and shock induced SIRS and MODS: the gut-lymph hypothesis, a review. *Front Biosci.* 2006;11:520-528.
3. Pieracci FM, Biffl WL, Moore EE. Current concepts in resuscitation. *J Intensive Care Med.* 2012;27(2):79-96.
4. Wilmot LA. Shock: early recognition and management. *J Emerg Nurs.* 2010;36(2):134-139.
5. Yi J, et al. A "clean case" of systemic injury: mesenteric lymph after hemorrhagic shock elicits a sterile inflammatory response. *Shock.* 2015;44(4):336-340.
6. Parks JK, et al. Systemic hypotension is a late marker of shock after trauma: a validation study of Advanced Trauma Life Support principles in a large national sample. *Am J Surg.* 2006;192(6):727-731.
7. Barbee RW, Reynolds PS, Ward KR. Assessing shock resuscitation strategies by oxygen debt repayment. *Shock.* 2010;33(2):113-122.
8. Holley A, et al. Review article: part two: Goal-directed resuscitation—which goals? Perfusion targets. *Emerg Med Australas.* 2012;24(2):127-135.
9. Martin JT, et al. Normal vital signs belie occult hypoperfusion in geriatric trauma patients. *Am Surg.* 2010;76(1):65-69.
10. Neville AL, et al. Mortality risk stratification in elderly trauma patients based on initial arterial lactate and base deficit levels. *Am Surg.* 2011;77(10):1337-1341.
11. Vandromme MJ, et al. Lactate is a better predictor than systolic blood pressure for determining blood requirement and mortality: could prehospital measures improve trauma triage? *J Am Coll Surg.* 2010;210(5):861-869.
12. Jansen TC, van Bommel J, Bakker J. Blood lactate monitoring in critically ill patients: a systematic health technology assessment. *Crit Care Med.* 2009;37(10):2827-2839.
13. Jansen TC, et al. Early lactate-guided therapy in intensive care unit patients: a multicenter, open-label, randomized controlled trial. *Am J Respir Crit Care Med.* 2010;182(6):752-761.
14. Jones AE, et al. Lactate clearance vs central venous oxygen saturation as goals of early sepsis therapy: a randomized clinical trial. *JAMA.* 2010;303(8):739-746.
15. Surbatovic M, et al. Predictive value of sodium bicarbonate, arterial base deficit/excess and SAPS III score in critically ill patients. *Gen Physiol Biophys.* 2009;28(Spec No):271-276.
16. Dellinger RP, et al. Surviving sepsis campaign: international guidelines for management of severe sepsis and septic shock: 2012. *Crit Care Med.* 2013;41(2):580-637.
17. Holley A, et al. Review article: part one: goal-directed resuscitation—which goals? Haemodynamic targets. *Emerg Med Australas.* 2012;24(1):14-22.
18. Nebout S, Pirracchio R. Should we monitor ScVO$_2$ in critically ill patients. *Cardiol Res Pract.* 2012;2012:370697.
19. Joshi R, de Witt B, Mosier JM. Optimizing oxygen delivery in the critically ill: the utility of lactate and central venous oxygen saturation (SCVO2) as a roadmap of resuscitation in shock. *J Emerg Med.* 2014;47(4):493-500.
20. Boyle MS, et al. Central venous oxygen saturation during high-risk general surgical procedures—relationship to complications and clinical outcomes. *Anaesth Intensive Care.* 2014;42(1):28-36.
21. He H, et al. Clinical classification of tissue perfusion based on the central venous oxygen saturation and the peripheral perfusion index. *Crit Care.* 2015;19:330.
22. Alam HB: Advances in resuscitation strategies, *Int J Surg* 9(1):5-12.
23. Bunn F, Trivedi D. Colloid solutions for fluid resuscitation. *Cochrane Database Syst Rev.* 2012;7:CD001319.
24. Cotton BA, et al. The cellular, metabolic, and systemic consequences of aggressive fluid resuscitation strategies. *Shock.* 2006;26(2):115-121.
25. Niemi TT, Miyashita R, Yamakage M. Colloid solutions: a clinical update. *J Anesth.* 2010;24(6):913-925.

26. Perel P, Roberts I, Ker K. Colloids versus crystalloids for fluid resuscitation in critically ill patients. *Cochrane Database Syst Rev.* 2013;2:CD000567.

27. Reinhart K, et al. Consensus statement of the ESICM task force on colloid volume therapy in critically ill patients. *Intensive Care Med.* 2012;38(3):368-383.

28. Study Investigators SAFE, et al. Effect of baseline serum albumin concentration on outcome of resuscitation with albumin or saline in patients in intensive care units: analysis of data from the saline versus albumin fluid evaluation (SAFE) study. *BMJ.* 2006;333 (7577):1044.

29. Bulger EM, et al. Out-of-hospital hypertonic resuscitation after traumatic hypovolemic shock. *Ann Surg.* 2011;253(3):431-441.

30. Patanwala AE, Amini A, Erstad BL. Use of hypertonic saline injection in trauma. *Am J Health Syst Pharm.* 2010;67(22):1920-1928.

31. Carson JL, Carless PA, Hebert PC. Transfusion thresholds and other strategies for guiding allogenic red blood cell transfusion. *Cochrane Database Syst Rev.* 2012;4:CD002042.

32. Collins TA. Packed red blood cell transfusions in critically ill patients. *Crit Care Nurse.* 2011;31(1):25-33.

33. Dennison CA. Transfusion-related acute lung injury: a clinical challenge. *Dimens Crit Care Nurs.* 2008;27(1):1-7.

34. Kopko PM. Transfusion-related acute lung injury. *J Infus Nurs.* 2010;33(1):32-37.

35. Murad MH, et al. The effect of plasma transfusion on morbidity and mortality: a systematic review and meta-analysis. *Transfusion.* 2010;50(6):1370-1383.

36. Kimmoun A, et al. Hemodynamic consequences of severe lactic acidosis in shock states: from bench to bedside. *Crit Care.* 2015;19:175.

37. Rachoin JS, Weisberg LS, McFadden CB. Treatment of lactic acidosis: Appropriate confusion. *J Hosp Med.* 2010;5(4):E1-E7.

38. Taylor BE, et al. Guidelines for the provision and assessment of nutrition support therapy in the adult critically ill patient: society of Critical Care Medicine (SCCM) and American Society for Parenteral and Enteral Nutrition (ASPEN). *Crit Care Med.* 2016;44(2):390-438.

39. Cahill NE, et al. When early enteral feeding is not possible in critically ill patients: results of a multicenter observational study. *J Parenter Enteral Nutr.* 2011;35(2):160-168.

40. Casaer MP, et al. Early versus late parenteral nutrition in critically ill adults. *N Engl J Med.* 2011;365(6):506-517.

41. Wenerman J. Combined enteral and parenteral nutrition. *Curr Opin Clin Nutr Metab Care.* 2012;15(2):161-165.

42. Bost RB, Tjan DH, van Zanten AR. Timing of (supplemental) parenteral nutrition in critically ill patients: a systematic review. *Ann Intensive Care.* 2014;4:31.

43. American Diabetes Association. Diabetes care in the hospital, nursing home, and skilled nursing facility. *Diabetes Care.* 2015;38(suppl 1): S80-S85.

44. Moghissi ES, et al. American Association of Clinical Endocrinologists and American Diabetes Association consensus statement on inpatient glycemic control. *Endocr Pract.* 2009;15(4):353-369.

45. Azevedo JR, et al. Impact of glycemic control on the incidence of acute kidney injury in critically ill patients: a comparison of two strategies using the RIFLE criteria. *Clinics (Sao Paulo).* 2010;65(8):769-773.

46. Wiener RS, Wiener DC, Larson RJ. Benefits and risks of tight glucose control in critically ill adults: a meta-analysis. *JAMA.* 2008;300(8):933-944.

47. American Association of Critical-Care Nurses. AACN Practice Alert: family presence during resuscitation and invasive procedures; 2016. http://www.aacn.org/wd/practice/docs/practicealerts/family-presence-during-resusitation-and-invasive-procedures-pa-2015.pdf. Accessed December 6, 2015.

48. Davidson JE, et al. Clinical practice guidelines for support of the family in the patient-centered intensive care unit: American College of Critical Care Medicine Task Force 2004-2005. *Crit Care Med.* 2007;35(2):605-622.

49. Egging D, et al. Emergency nursing resource: family presence during invasive procedures and resuscitation in the emergency department. *J Emerg Nurs.* 2011;37(5):469-473.

50. Mancini ME, et al. Part 3: ethical Issues: 2015 American Heart Association Guidelines for cardiopulmonary resuscitation and emergency cardiovascular care. *Circulation.* 2015;132(18 suppl 2):S383-S396.

51. Mutschler M, et al. A critical reappraisal of the ATLS classification of hypovolaemic shock: does it really reflect clinical reality? *Resuscitation.* 2011;82:556.

52. Kwan I, et al. Timing and volume of fluid administration for patients with bleeding. *Cochrane Database Syst Rev.* 2014;3:CD002245.

53. Duan C, Li T, Liu L. Efficacy of limited fluid resuscitation in patients with hemorrhagic shock: a meta-analysis. *Int J Clin Exp Med.* 2015;8(7):11645-11656.

54. Bougle A, Harrois A, Duranteau J. Resuscitative strategies in traumatic hemorrhagic shock. *Ann Intensive Care.* 2013;3(1):1.

55. Szopinski J, Kusza K, Semionow M. Microcirculatory responses to hypovolemic shock. *J Trauma.* 2011;71(6):1779-1788.

56. Goldberg RJ, et al. Thirty-year trends (1975 to 2005) trends in the magnitude of, management of, and hospital death rates associated with cardiogenic shock in patients with acute myocardial infarction. *Circulation.* 2009;119(9):1211-1219.

57. Buerke M, et al. Pathophysiology, diagnosis, and treatment of infarction-related cardiogenic shock. *Herz.* 2011;36(2):73-83.

58. Levy B, et al. Experts' recommendations for the management of adult patients with cardiogenic shock. *Ann Intensive Care.* 2015;5(1):52.

59. Thiele H, et al. Intraaortic balloon pump counterpulsation in acute myocardial infarction complicated by cardiogenic shock (IABP-SHOCK II): final 12 months results of a randomized, open-label trial. *Lancet.* 2013;382(9905):1638-1645.

60. Chatterjee K, et al. Analytic reviews: cardiogenic shock with preserved systolic function: a reminder. *J Intensive Care Med.* 2008;23(6):355-366.

61. Shpektor A. Cardiogenic shock: the role of inflammation. *Acute Card Care.* 2010;12(4):115-118.

62. Stevenson LW, Perloff JK. The limited reliability of physical signs for estimating hemodynamics in chronic heart failure. *JAMA.* 1989;261(6):884-888.

63. American College of Emergency Physicians, et al. 2013 ACCF/AHA guideline for the management of ST-elevation myocardial infarction: a report of the American College of Cardiology Foundation/American Heart Association Task Force on Practice Guidelines. *J Am Coll Cardiol.* 2013;61(4):e78-e140.

64. Ahmad Y, et al. Intra-aortic balloon pump therapy for acute myocardial infarction: a meta-analysis. *JAMA Intern Med.* 2015;175(6):931-939.

65. Fineman SM. Optimal treatment of anaphylaxis: antihistamine versus epinephrine. *Postgrad Med.* 2014;126(4):73-81.

66. Kim H, Fischer D. Anaphylaxis. *Allergy Asthma Clin Immunol.* 2011;7(suppl 1):S6.

67. Lieberman P, et al. The diagnosis and management of anaphylaxis practice parameter: 2010 update. *J Allergy Clin Immunol.* 2010;126:477-480.

68. Simons FE, Sheikh A. Anaphylaxis: The acute episode and beyond. *BMJ.* 2013;346:f602.

69. Simons FE, et al. 2015 update of the evidence base: world Allergy Organization anaphylaxis guidelines. *World Allergy Organ J.* 2015;8(1):32.

70. Vander Hoek TL, et al. Part 12: Cardiac arrest in special situations: 2010 American Heart Association Guidelines for cardiopulmonary resuscitation and emergency cardiovascular care. *Circulation.* 2010;122(suppl 3):S829-S861.

71. Campbell RL, et al. Emergency department diagnosis and treatment of anaphylaxis: a practice parameter. *Ann Allergy Asthma Immunol.* 2014;113(6):599-608.

72. Tole JW, Lieberman P. Biphasic anaphylaxis: review of incidence, clinical predictors, and observation recommendations. *Immunol Allergy Clin North Am.* 2007;27(2):309-326.

73. Choo KJ, Simons FE, Sheikh A. Glucocorticoids for the treatment of anaphylaxis. *Cochrane Database Syst Rev.* 2012;4:CD007596.

74. Weaver LC, et al. Disordered cardiovascular control after spinal cord injury. *Handb Clin Neurol.* 2012;109:213-233.

75. Guly HR, et al. The incidence of neurogenic shock in patients with isolated spinal cord injury in the emergency department. *Resuscitation.* 2008;76(1):57-62.

76. Casha S, Christie S. A systematic review of intensive cardiopulmonary management after spinal cord injury. *J Neurotrauma*. 2011;28(8):1479-1495.

77. *Consortium for Spinal Cord Medicine: clinical Practice Guidelines. Early Acute Management in Adults With Spinal Cord Injury: a Clinical Practice Guideline for Health-Care Professionals*. Washington, DC: Paralyzed Veterans of America; 2008.

78. Popa C, et al. Vascular dysfunctions following spinal cord injury. *J Med Life*. 2010;3(3):275-285.

79. Young WF. Shock. In: Stone CK, Humphries RL, eds. *Current Diagnosis and Treatment: emergency Medicine*. 7th ed. New York: McGraw-Hill; 2011.

80. Link MS, et al. Part 7: Adult advanced cardiovascular life support: 2015 American Heart Association guidelines update for cardiopulmonary resuscitation and emergency cardiovascular care. *Circulation*. 2015;132(18 suppl 2):S444-S464.

81. Beale R, et al. Promoting global research excellence in severe sepsis (PROGRESS): lessons from an international sepsis registry. *Infection*. 2009;37(3):222-232.

82. Lagu T, et al. Hospitalizations, costs, and outcomes of severe sepsis in the United States 2003 to 2007. *Crit Care Med*. 2012;40(3):754-761.

83. Mann EA, et al. Comparison of mortality associated with sepsis in the burn, trauma, and general intensive care unit patient: a systematic review of the literature. *Shock*. 2012;37(1):4-16.

84. Sivayoham N, et al. Outcomes from implementing early goal-directed therapy for severe sepsis and septic shock: a 4-year observational cohort study. *Eur J Emerg Med*. 2012;19(4):235-240.

85. Murphy SL, et al. *Deaths: Final data for 2012. National Vital Statistics Reports 63(9)*. Hyattsville, MD: national Center for Health Statistics; 2015. http://www.cdc.gov/nchs/data/nvsr/nvsr63/nvsr63_09.pdf. Accessed December 6, 2015.

86. Singer M, Deutschman CS, Seymour CW. The third international consensus definitions for sepsis and septic shock. *JAMA*. 2016;315(8):801-810.

87. Seymour CW, et al. Marital status and the epidemiology and outcomes of sepsis. *Chest*. 2010;137(6):1289-1296.

88. Fry DE. Sepsis, systemic inflammatory response, and multiple organ dysfunction: the mystery continues. *Am Surg*. 2012;78(1):1-8.

89. Cinel I, Dellinger RP. Advances in pathogenesis and management of sepsis. *Curr Opin Infect Dis*. 2007;20(4):345-352.

90. Nduka OO, Parrillo JE. The pathophysiology of septic shock. *Crit Care Nurs Clin North Am*. 2011;23(1):41-66.

91. Singer M. Mitochondrial function in sepsis: acute phase versus multiple organ failure. *Crit Care Med*. 2007;35(suppl 9):S441-S448.

92. Levi M, van der Poll T, Schultz M. Systemic versus localized coagulation activation contributing to organ failure in critically ill patients. *Semin Immunopathol*. 2012;34(1):167-179.

93. Ait-Oufella H, et al. Microcirculatory disorders during septic shock. *Curr Opin Crit Care*. 2015;21(4):271-275.

94. Vollmar B, Menger MD. Intestinal ischemia/reperfusion: microcirculatory pathology and functional consequences. *Langenbecks Arch Surg*. 2011;396(1):13-29.

95. Stearns-Kurosawa DJ, et al. The pathogenesis of sepsis. *Annu Rev Pathol*. 2011;6:19-48.

96. Semeraro N, et al. Sepsis, thrombosis and organ dysfunction. *Thromb Res*. 2012;129(3):290-295.

97. Tappy L, Chiolero R. Substrate utilization in sepsis and multiple organ failure. *Crit Care Med*. 2007;35(9 suppl):S531-S534.

98. Baumgart K, et al. Pathophysiology of tissue acidosis in septic shock: blocked microcirculation or impaired cellular respiration? *Crit Care Med*. 2008;36(2):640-642.

99. Garrabou G, et al. The effects of sepsis on mitochondria. *J Infect Dis*. 2012;205(3):392-400.

100. Perl M, et al. Pathogenesis of indirect (secondary) acute lung injury. *Expert Rev Respir Med*. 2011;5(1):115-126.

101. Jacob A, Brorson JR, Alexander JJ. Septic encephalopathy: inflammation in man and mouse. *Neurochem Int*. 2011;58(4):472-476.

102. Jensen JU, et al. Procalcitonin-guided interventions against infections to increase early appropriate antibiotics and improve survival in the intensive care unit: a randomized trial. *Crit Care Med*. 2011;39(9):2048-2058.

103. Bai X, et al. Early versus delayed administration of norepinephrine in patients with septic shock. *Crit Care*. 2014;18(5):532.

104. De Backer D, et al. Dopamine versus norepinephrine in the treatment of septic shock: a meta-analysis. *Crit Care Med*. 2012;40(3):725-730.

105. Vasu TS, et al. Norepinephrine or dopamine for septic shock: a systematic review of randomized clinical trials. *J Intensive Care Med*. 2012;27(3):172-178.

106. Angus DC, et al. A systematic review and meta-analysis of early goal-directed therapy for septic shock: The ARISE, ProCESS and ProMISE investigators. *Intensive Care Med*. 2015;41(9):1549-1560.

107. Mouncey PR, et al. Trial of early goal-directed resuscitation for septic shock. *N Engl J Med*. 2015;372(14):1301-1311.

108. ARISE Investigators, et al. Goal-directed resuscitation for patients with early septic shock. *N Engl J Med*. 2014;371(16):1496-1506.

109. The ProCESS Investigators, et al. A randomized trial of protocol-based care for early septic shock. *N Engl J Med*. 2014;370(18):1683-1693.

110. The Acute Respiratory Distress System Network: ventilation with lower tidal volumes as compared with traditional tidal volumes for acute lung injury and the acute respiratory distress syndrome. *N Engl J Med*. 2000;342(18):1301-1308.

111. Kumar A, et al. Duration of hypotension before initiation of effective antimicrobial therapy is the critical determinant of survival in human septic shock. *Crit Care Med*. 2006;34(6):1589-1596.

112. Marti-Carvajal AJ, et al. Human recombinant activated protein C for severe sepsis. *Cochrane Database Syst Rev*. 2012;3:CD004388.

113. Mullard A. Drug withdrawal sends critical care specialists back to basics. *Lancet*. 2011;78(9805):1769.

114. FDA. FDA Drug Safety Communication. Voluntary market withdrawal of Xigris [drotrecogin alfa (activated)] due to failure to show a survival benefit. http://www.fda.gov/Drugs/DrugSafety/ucm277114.htm Accessed February 8, 2016.

115. Sanfilippo F, et al. Beta-blocker use in severe sepsis and septic shock: a systematic review. *Curr Med Res Opin*. 2015;31(10):1817-1825.

116. Volbeda M, et al. Glucocorticosteroids for sepsis: systematic review with meta-analysis and trial sequential analysis. *Intensive Care Med*. 2015;41(7):1220-1234.

117. Elke G, et al. Enteral nutrition is associated with improved outcome in patients with severe sepsis: a secondary analysis of the VISEP trial. *Med Klin Intensivmed Notfmed*. 2013;108(3):223-233.

118. Elke G, et al. Current practice in nutritional support and its association with mortality in septic patients—results from a national, prospective, multicenter study. *Crit Care Med*. 2008;36(6):1762-1767.

119. Beale RJ, et al. Early enteral supplementation with key pharmaconutrients improves Sequential Organ Failure Assessment score in critically ill patients with sepsis: outcome of a randomized, controlled, double-blind trial. *Crit Care Med*. 2008;36(1):131-144.

120. Aitken LM, et al. Nursing considerations to complement the surviving sepsis campaign guidelines. *Crit Care Med*. 2011;39(7):1800-1818.

121. Otto GP, et al. The late phase of sepsis is characterized by an increased microbiological burden and death rate. *Crit Care*. 2011;15(4):R183.

122. Winters BD, et al. Long-term mortality and quality of life in sepsis: a systematic review. *Crit Care Med*. 2010;38(5):1276-1283.

123. Martin LL, Cheek DJ, Morris SD. Shock, multiple organ dysfunction syndrome, and burns in adults. In: McCance KL, Heuther SE, eds. *Pathophysiology: the Biologic Basis for Disease in Adults and Children*. 7th ed. St Louis: Elsevier; 2014.

124. Garnacho-Martin J, et al. Effect of critical illness polyneuropathy on withdrawal from mechanical ventilation and length of stay in septic patients. *Crit Care Med*. 2005;33(2):349-354.

125. Cohn SM, et al. Tissue oxygen saturation predicts the development of organ dysfunction during traumatic shock resuscitation. *J Trauma*. 2007;62(1):44-54.

126. Epstein CD, et al. Oxygen transport and organ dysfunction in the older trauma patient. *Heart Lung*. 2002;31(5):315-326.

127. Mittal R, Coopersmith CM. Redefining the gut as the motor of critical illness. *Trends Mol Med*. 2014;20(4):214-223.

128. Tschoeke SK, et al. The early second hit in trauma management augments the proinflammatory immune response to multiple injuries. *J Trauma*. 2007;62(6):1396-1403.

129. Dulhunty JM, et al. Does severe non-infectious SIRS differ from severe sepsis? Results from a multi-centre Australian and New Zealand intensive care unit study. *Intensive Care Med.* 2008;34(9):1654-1661.

130. Sankoff J, et al. Validation of the Mortality in Emergency Department Sepsis (MEDS) score in patients with the systemic inflammatory response syndrome (SIRS). *Crit Care Med.* 2008;36(2):421-426.

131. Shimizu K, et al. Altered gut flora and environment in patients with severe SIRS. *J Trauma.* 2006;60(1):126-133.

132. Rote NS, Huether SE, McCance KL. Innate immunity: inflammation. In: McCance KL, Heuther SE, eds. *Pathophysiology: the Biologic Basis for Disease in Adults and Children.* 7th ed. St Louis: Elsevier; 2014.

133. Schmidt H, et al. The alteration of autonomic function in multiple organ dysfunction syndrome. *Crit Care Clin.* 2008;24(1):149-163.

134. Gando S. Microvascular thrombosis and multiple organ dysfunction syndrome. *Crit Care Med.* 2010;38(2 suppl):S35-S42.

135. Shapiro NI, Zimmer GD, Barkin AZ. Sepsis syndromes. In: Marx J, ed. *Rosen's Emergency Medicine: concepts and Clinical Practice.* 8th ed. Philadelphia: Elsevier; 2014.

136. Bengmark S. Bioecologic control of inflammation and infection in critical illness. *Anesthesiol Clin.* 2006;24(2):299-323.

137. Abraham E, Singer M. Mechanisms of sepsis-induced organ dysfunction. *Crit Care Med.* 2007;35(10):2408-2416.

138. Biesalski HK, McGregor GP. Antioxidant therapy in critical care—is the microcirculation the primary target? *Crit Care Med.* 2007;35(9 suppl):S577-S583.

139. Teuffle O, et al. Association between tumor necrosis factor-alpha promoter-308A/G polymorphism and susceptibility to sepsis and sepsis mortality: a systematic review and meta-analysis. *Crit Care Med.* 2010;38(1):276-282.

140. Marshall JC, Christou NV, Meakins JL. The gastrointestinal tract. The "undrained abscess" of multiple organ failure. *Ann Surg.* 1993;218(2):111-119.

141. Barie PS, Eachempati SR. Acute acalculous cholecystitis. *Gastroenterol Clin North Am.* 2010;39(2):343-357.

142. Krau SD. Making sense of multiple organ dysfunction syndrome. *Crit Care Nurs Clin North Am.* 2007;19(1):87-97.

143. Bakowitz M, Bruns B, McCunn M. Acute lung injury and the acute respiratory distress syndrome in the injured patient. *Scand J Trauma Resusc Emerg Med.* 2014;20:54.

144. Crouser ED, Exline MC, Fahy RJ. Acute lung injury, pulmonary edema, and multiple system organ failure. In: Kacmarek RM, Stoller JK, Heuer AJ, eds. *Egan's Fundamentals of Respiratory Care.* 10th ed. St. Louis: Elsevier; 2013.

145. Honore PM, et al. Septic AKI in ICU patients, diagnosis, pathophysiology, and treatment type, dosing, and timing: a comprehensive review of recent and future developments. *Ann Intensive Care.* 2011;1(1):32.

146. Zanotti-Cavazzoni SL, Hollenberg SM. Cardiac dysfunction in severe sepsis and septic shock. *Curr Opin Crit Care.* 2009;15(5):392-397.

147. Dhainaut JF, et al. Dynamic evolution of coagulopathy in the first day of severe sepsis: relationship with mortality and organ failure. *Crit Care Med.* 2005;33(2):341-348.

148. Ulldemolins M, et al. Antibiotic dosing in multiple organ dysfunction syndrome. *Chest.* 2011;139(5):1210-1220.

149. McClave SA, Heyland DK. The physiologic response and associated clinical benefits from provision of early enteral nutrition. *Nutr Clin Pract.* 2009;24(3):305-315.

150. Klompas M. Potential strategies to prevent ventilator-associated events. *Am J Respir Crit Care Med.* 2015;192(12):1420-1430.

35

Burns

Jennifer Seigel, Carrie M. Wilson, and Robyn Myers

Since the late 1980s, trends of burn incidence, hospitalization, and mortality all have decreased with advancements in surgical and critical care management and more specialized burn centers.[1,2] These decreases are attributed to fire and burn prevention education, management of burn patients in specialized burn centers, regulation of consumer products, and implementation of occupational safety standards. Many programs and organizations are dedicated to the prevention of burn injury. Societal changes including decreased smoking and alcohol abuse, changes in home cooking practices, and reduced industrial employment also have contributed to the decline in burn incidence. However, despite a decline in overall burn incidence, because of an increase in child maltreatment (3.5 million referrals in 2013), burn injury as a result of physical abuse remains a differential diagnosis in burn patients.[3]

Burn injuries that require medical treatment annually number 450,000 per year.[2] Burn injuries requiring hospitalization total approximately 40,000 per year, and 60% of these patients are admitted to one of the 128 specialized burn centers in the United States.[2]

Great advances have been made in the care of burn patients. In the mid-20th century, many patients died as a result of burn shock. If shock did not cause death, infection or respiratory insufficiency did. With improvements in fluid resuscitation, better critical care management, and the trend toward early excision and grafting, mortality rates have decreased. Focusing management on early eschar excision and grafting leads to earlier resolution of the inflammatory response, better functional outcome, and reduced lengths of hospital stay.[4]

To provide comprehensive, holistic care to burn patients, close collaboration is required among members of the multidisciplinary team. The burn team comprises nurses, physicians, physical therapists, occupational therapists, recreational therapists, nutritionists, psychologists, social workers, family members, and spiritual support staff members. The burn patient is characterized as the universal trauma model. The patient's response to a major burn injury is dramatic and involves multisystem alterations. Knowledge of local and systemic changes associated with patient needs is essential in providing care, which places extraordinary demands on a nurse in a burn practice, who must be both a specialist and a broad-based generalist. The purpose of this chapter is to provide a basic understanding of the complexities of burn care and the patient's response to burn injury.

ANATOMY AND FUNCTIONS OF THE SKIN

The skin is the largest organ of the human body, ranging from 0.2 m^2 in a newborn to more than 2 m^2 in an adult. The integumentary system consists of two major layers: (1) epidermis and (2) dermis (Fig. 35.1).

The outermost layer of the epidermis is 0.07 to 0.12 mm thick, with the deepest layer found on the soles of the feet and the palms of the hands. The epidermis is composed of dead, cornified cells that act as a tough protective barrier against the environment. It serves as a barrier to bacteria and moisture loss.[5] From the surface inward, its five layers are (1) stratum corneum, (2) stratum lucidum, (3) stratum granulosum, (4) stratum spinosum, and (5) stratum germinativum. The deepest layer of the epidermis contains fibronectin, which adheres the epidermis to the basement membrane. The epidermis regenerates every 2 to 3 weeks. The second, thicker layer, the dermis, is 1 to 2 mm thick and lies below the epidermis and regenerates continuously. The dermis is composed of two layers: (1) the more superficial, papillary layer next to the stratum germinativum and (2) the deeper, reticular layer. The dermis, composed primarily of connective tissue and collagenous fiber bundles made from fibroblasts, provides nutrition support to the epidermis. The dermis contains blood vessels; sweat and sebaceous glands; hair follicles; nerves to the skin and capillaries that nourish the avascular epidermis; and sensory fibers that detect pain, touch, and temperature. Mast cells in the connective tissue perform the functions of secretion, phagocytosis, and production of fibroblasts. The hypodermis is beneath the dermis and contains fat, smooth muscle, and areolar tissues. The hypodermis acts as a heat insulator, shock absorber, and nutrition depot.[5]

The skin provides functions crucial to human survival including maintenance of body temperature; a barrier to evaporative water loss; metabolic activity (vitamin D production); immunologic protection by preventing microbes from entering the body; protection against the environment through the sensations of touch, pressure, and pain; and overall cosmetic appearance.

PATHOPHYSIOLOGY AND ETIOLOGY OF BURN INJURY

A burn injury results in tissue loss or damage. Injury to tissue can be caused by exposure to thermal, electrical, chemical, or radiation sources. The temperature or causticity of the burning agent and duration of tissue contact with the source determine the extent of tissue injury. Tissue damage can occur at various temperatures, usually between 40°C (104°F) and 44°C (111.2°F). The burn wound itself is responsible for the local and systemic effects seen in the burn patient. Tissue damage is caused by enzyme malfunction and denaturation of proteins. Prolonged exposure or higher temperatures can lead to cell

FIG. 35.1 Anatomy of the Skin. (From Dains JE. Integumentary system. In: Thompson JM, et al, eds: *Mosby's Clinical Nursing*. 5th ed. St. Louis: Mosby; 2002.)

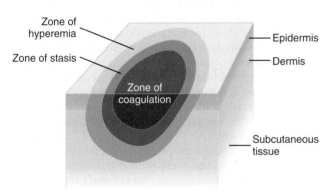

FIG. 35.2 Zones of Burn Injury.

necrosis and a process known as *protein coagulation.* The areas extending outward from this central area of injury sustain various degrees of damage and are identified by zones of injury.[6,7]

Zones of Injury

Three concentric zones are present in burn injury: (1) *zone of coagulation,* (2) *zone of stasis,* and (3) *zone of hyperemia* (Fig. 35.2). The central zone, or zone of coagulation, is the site of most severe damage, and the peripheral zone is the site of least severe damage. The central zone is usually the site of greatest heat transfer, leading to irreversible skin death. This area is surrounded by the zone of stasis, which is characterized by impaired circulation that can lead to cessation of blood flow caused by a pronounced inflammatory reaction. This area is potentially salvageable; however, local or systemic factors can convert it into a full-thickness injury. Some factors that can lead to deeper wound conversion are toxic mediators of the

inflammatory process, infection, inappropriate volume resuscitation, malnutrition, chronic illness, or the local wound care provided. It may take 48 to 72 hours to determine the full extent of injury in this area. The outermost area, the zone of hyperemia, has vasodilation and increased blood flow but minimal cell involvement. Early spontaneous recovery can occur in this area.[7]

CLASSIFICATION OF BURN INJURY

Burns are classified primarily according to the size and depth of injury. However, the type and location of the burn and the patient's age and medical history are also significant considerations. Recognition of the magnitude of burn injury, which is based on the above-mentioned factors, is crucial in the overall plan of care and in decisions concerning patient management and appropriate referral to a burn center (Box 35.1).[2] The patient's age, burn size, and inhalation injury are the cardinal determinants of survival. A study of a large number of burn patients found the biggest predictors of patient mortality to be age, percent total body surface area (TBSA) burned, and inhalation injury.[8]

Size of Injury

Several different methods can be used to estimate the size of the burn area. A quick and easy method is the *rule of nines* (or *Berkow formula*), which often is used in the prehospital setting for initial triage of a burn patient (Fig. 35.3). In this method, the adult body is divided into different surface areas of 9% per area. This method is modified for assessing infants and very small children and accounts for proportionate growth. For example, the head of a 1-year-old child is proportionately larger than the

BOX 35.1   Burn Center Referral

Patients with the following burn injuries are best treated in a certified burn center:

- Partial-thickness burns of 10% or more of total body surface area
- Full-thickness (third-degree) burns in any age group
- Burns of face, hands, feet, genitalia, perineum, or major joints that may result in cosmetic or functional disability
- Electrical burns, including lightning injury
- Inhalation injury
- Chemical burns
- Burns in patients with preexisting medical disorders (eg, diabetes mellitus, symptomatic cardiopulmonary disease) that could complicate management, prolong recovery, or affect mortality
- Burn injury with concomitant trauma (eg, fractures) in which the burn injury poses the greatest risk of morbidity or mortality[a]
- Burns in children in hospitals without qualified personnel or equipment for the care of children
- Burn injury in patients who will require special social, emotional, or long-term rehabilitative intervention

[a]In such cases, if the trauma poses a greater immediate risk, the patient's condition may be stabilized initially in a trauma center before transfer to a burn center. Physician judgment is necessary in these situations.
Modified from American Burn Association. *Burn center referral criteria. Guidelines for the operation of burn centers.* http://www.ameriburn.org Accessed March 26, 2016.

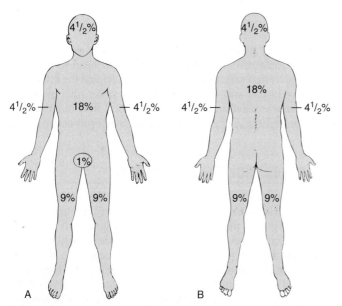

FIG. 35.3 Estimation of Adult Burn Injury: Rule of Nines. (A) Anterior view. (B) Posterior view. (From Marx J, et al. Rosen's Emergency Medicine Concepts and Clinical Practice. 5th ed. St. Louis: Mosby; 2002.)

rest of the body, in contrast to in adults, so the child's head would account for 19% of his or her TBSA, whereas the head of an adult would account for 7% of TBSA.[5] Designated burn centers have access to Berkow formula charts, but local hospitals may not have these charts.

Another method uses the measure of the palmar surface of the victim's hand as a gauge for estimating burn area. The palmar surface (fingertip to wrist), which represents 1% of the TBSA, also can be useful in making burn estimates in the

prehospital setting or for estimating the percentage of involvement in small and scattered areas of burn. Some studies have shown the adult hand's TBSA is calculated to be closer to 0.8% versus 1% for a child.[5]

In the hospital setting, the Lund and Browder method (Fig. 35.4) is the most accurate and accepted method for determining the percentage of burn. Surface area measurements are assigned to each body part in terms of the age of the patient. This method is highly recommended for use with children younger than 10 years because it corrects for smaller surface areas of the lower extremities. It is also recommended for adult burn victims because of its accuracy.

Depth of Burn Injury

Traditionally, burn depth has been classified in degrees of injury based on the amount of injured epidermis, dermis, or both: first-degree, second-degree, third-degree, or fourth-degree burns. However, these terms are not descriptive of the burn surface. The depth of the burn is defined by how much of the skin's two layers are destroyed by the heat source.[5]

Burns are classified as *superficial, partial-thickness, deep-dermal partial-thickness,* or *full-thickness burns.* These descriptions are based on the surface appearance of the wound. Superficial burns include first-degree burns. Partial-thickness burns include various stages of second-degree burns, and full-thickness burns include third-degree burns. Fourth-degree burns extend through all skin layers and extend into muscle, tendon, and bone.[5] Some authorities further separate partial-thickness burns as *superficial* or *deep-dermal partial-thickness burns.* Wound assessment involves recognition of the depth of injury and the size of burn, and it can be challenging even for experienced caregivers. Because the management of burn wounds is closely tied to the correct assessment of wound severity, some newer strategies other than observation are being investigated. Some of these techniques have taken into account the presence of denatured collagen, wound edema, and altered blood flow. One such technique is noncontact laser Doppler imaging, which can give a color perfusion map of the burn wound.[9] Other techniques of assessing burn depth include use of current optical techniques to complement clinical examination, but these optical techniques are based on the premise that functioning blood vessels are retained in viable tissue.[10] Clinical examination is approximately 75% accurate in assessing burn wound depth, but current optical techniques (ie, conventional histology/light microscopy, indocyanine green videoangiography, near-infrared spectroscopy and spectral imaging, in vivo capillary microscopy, orthogonal polarization spectral imaging, reflectance-mode confocal microscopy, laser speckle imaging, spatial frequency domain imaging, photoacoustic microscopy, and polarization-sensitive optical coherence tomography) have both advantages and disadvantages.[10] Research with these techniques is ongoing, but they are limited at the present time by their clinical usefulness at the bedside.

A *superficial (first-degree) burn* involves only the first two or three of the five layers of the epidermis. Erythema and mild discomfort characterize superficial partial-thickness wounds. Pain, the chief symptom, usually resolves in 48 to 72 hours. Common examples of these burn injuries are sunburns and minor steam burns such as may occur while cooking. These wounds usually heal in 2 to 7 days and do not require medical intervention aside from pain relief, management of pruritus (itching), and

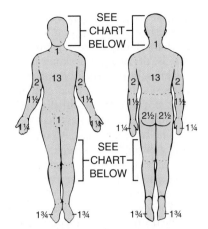

AGE: _____
SEX: _____
WEIGHT: _____
HEIGHT: _____

AREA	Inf.	1-4	5-9	10-14	15	Adult	Part.	Full	Total	Donor areas
HEAD	19	17	13	11	9	7				
NECK	2	2	2	2	2	2				
ANT. TRUNK	13	13	13	13	13	13				
POST. TRUNK	13	13	13	13	13	13				
R. BUTTOCK	2½	2½	2½	2½	2½	2½				
L. BUTTOCK	2½	2½	2½	2½	2½	2½				
GENITALIA	1	1	1	1	1	1				
R.U. ARM	4	4	4	4	4	4				
L.U. ARM	4	4	4	4	4	4				
R.L. ARM	3	3	3	3	3	3				
L.L. ARM	3	3	3	3	3	3				
R. HAND	2½	2½	2½	2½	2½	2½				
L. HAND	2½	2½	2½	2½	2½	2½				
R. THIGH	5½	6½	8	8½	9	9½				
L. THIGH	5½	6½	8	8½	9	9½				
R. LEG	5	5	5½	6	6½	7				
L. LEG	5	5	5½	6	6½	7				
R. FOOT	3½	3½	3½	3½	3½	3½				
L. FOOT	3½	3½	3½	3½	3½	3½				
						TOTAL				

FIG. 35.4 Lund and Browder Burn Estimate Diagram. (Modified from Cardona VD. *Trauma Nursing From Resuscitation Through Rehabilitation.* Philadelphia: Mosby; 1995.)

oral fluids. Swelling can be a common complication that may require intervention. Superficial burns are not included in the calculation of percent burn.

A *partial-thickness (second-degree) burn* involves all the epidermis and part of the underlying dermis.[5] These burns usually are caused by brief contact with flames, hot liquid, or exposure to dilute chemicals (Fig. 35.5). A light to bright red or mottled appearance characterizes superficial second-degree burns. These wounds may appear wet and weeping, may contain bullae, and are extremely painful and sensitive to air currents. These burns blanch painfully.[5] The microvessels that perfuse this area are injured, and permeability is increased resulting in leakage of large amounts of plasma into the interstitium. This fluid lifts off the thin, damaged epidermis, causing blister formation. Despite the loss of the entire basal layer of the epidermis, a burn of this depth heals in 7 to 21 days. Minimal scarring can be expected. Mid-dermal partial-thickness wounds commonly take 4 to 6 weeks to heal.

FIG. 35.5 Partial-Thickness Burn to Left Thigh.

Deep-dermal partial-thickness (second-degree) burns involve the entire epidermal layer and deeper layers of the dermis.[5] These burns often result from contact with hot liquids or solids or with intense radiant energy. A deep-dermal partial-thickness burn usually is not characterized by blister formation. Only a modest plasma surface leakage occurs because of severe impairment in blood supply. The wound surface usually is red with patchy white areas that blanch with pressure. The appearance of the deep-dermal wound changes over time. Dermal necrosis and surface coagulated protein turn the wound from white to yellow (Fig. 35.6). These wounds have a prolonged healing time. They can heal spontaneously as the epidermal elements germinate and migrate until the epidermal surface is restored, or they may require a skin substitute or surgical excision and grafting for wound closure. This process of healing by epithelialization can take up to 6 weeks. Left untreated, these wounds can heal primarily with unstable epithelium, late hypertrophic scarring, and marked contracture formation.[5] Partial-thickness injuries can become full-thickness injuries if they become infected, if blood supply is diminished, or if further trauma occurs to the site. The treatment of choice is surgical excision and skin grafting.

A *full-thickness (third-degree) burn* involves destruction of all the layers of the skin down to and including the subcutaneous fat (Fig. 35.7).[5] The subcutaneous tissue is composed of

FIG. 35.6 Deep-Dermal Partial-Thickness Burn to Thigh.

FIG. 35.7 Full-Thickness Burn to Back of Hand.

adipose tissue, includes the hair follicles and sweat glands, and is poorly vascularized. A full-thickness burn appears pale white or charred, red or brown, and leathery. The surface of the burn may be dry, and if the skin is broken, fat may be exposed. Full-thickness burns usually are painless and insensitive to palpation. Because all the epithelial elements are destroyed, the wound does not heal by reepithelialization. Wound closure of small full-thickness burns (less than 4 cm² area) can be achieved with healing by contraction. All other full-thickness wounds require skin grafting for closure. Extensive full-thickness wounds leave the patient extremely susceptible to infections, fluid and electrolyte imbalances, alterations in thermoregulation, and metabolic disturbances.

The exact depth of many burn wounds cannot be clearly defined on the first inspection, and many burn wounds may contain superficial, mid-dermal, and deep-dermal wounds. A major difficulty is distinguishing deep-dermal partial-thickness from full-thickness injury. It is important to identify the depth of injury for appropriate treatment. Deep-dermal partial-thickness wounds that do not heal within a relatively short time are treated with wound excision and grafting. Burn wounds can evolve over time, and they require frequent reassessment. Special consideration must always be given to very young patients and older patients because of their thin dermal layer. Older adults may also have reduced sensation and blood supply, causing them to be more susceptible to a full-thickness injury. Depressed organ reserves in older adults at the time of burn injury can lead to higher mortality in this age group.[1] Burn injuries in these two age groups may be more severe than they initially appear.

The TBSA of the burn is calculated at the same time that assessment for wound depth occurs. This calculation provides the basis for determining the amount of fluid required for treatment. All burn wound surface area percentages except for superficial burns are used to calculate the patient's fluid requirements.

Types of Injury
Thermal Burns
The most common type of burn is a thermal burn caused by steam, scalds, contact with heat, and fire injuries. Approximately 80% of burns in children are caused by scalds (ie, contact with hot objects or liquids).[5] Toddlers are most often affected by scalding burns. Contact burns are also common. The length of time the hot object is in contact with the skin determines the depth of injury. Flame injuries are often associated with other trauma to the patient. The highest incidence of flame injuries are more common in patients older than 6 years of age.[5] Experimentation with lighters, lighter fluid, fire, firecrackers, and gasoline is more common in children 6 to 16 years old.[5] Contact and flame burns tend to be deep-dermal or full-thickness injuries.

Electrical Burns
Electrical and lightning injuries result in 1500 deaths per year in the United States. Electrical injuries account for 4% of patient admissions to burn centers.[2] Low-voltage (alternating) current (60 to 1000 V) or high-voltage (alternating or direct) current (greater than 1000 V) can cause electrical burns.[11] Children have the highest incidence of electrical injury. These accidents occur as a result of insertion of an object into an outlet or by biting or sucking on an electrical cord. Electrical burns occur

most often in the home; in adults, electrical injuries occur most often in the workplace.[11] Common situations that may increase the risk for electrical injuries include occupational exposure and accidents involving household current.

Chemical Burns

Acid and alkali agents cause chemical burns. Alkali burns commonly result in more severe injuries compared with acid burns. Acid and alkali agents are found in many household and industrial substances such as liquid concrete. Chemical burns most commonly occur in the domestic setting as a result of nonintentional exposure to household chemicals in children younger than age 10 and are preventable.[12] Chemical burns occur most often as a result of deliberate harm in children older than age 10.[12] The concentration of the chemical agent and the duration of exposure are the key factors that determine the extent and depth of damage. Progression of injury from chemical burns to their complete depth may be delayed, and the full extent of the injury may not be apparent until 48 hours after injury. Time must not be wasted in looking for a specific neutralizing agent because the injury is related directly to the concentration of the chemical and the duration of the exposure, and the heat of neutralization can extend the injury.

Radiation Burns

Burns associated with radiation exposure are uncommon. Radiation burns usually are localized and indicate high radiation doses to the affected area. Radiation burns may appear identical to thermal burns.[13] The major difference is the time between exposure and clinical manifestation; it can be days to weeks, depending on the level of the radiation dose. Radiation injury can occur with exposure to industrial equipment such as accelerators and cyclotrons and to equipment used for medical treatment.

Location of Injury

Location of injury can be a determining factor in differentiating the level of care required. According to triage criteria from the American College of Surgeons, burns on the face, hands, feet, genitalia, major joints, and perineum are best treated in a burn center. These burns involve functional areas of the body and often require specialized intervention (Fig. 35.8). Injuries to these areas can result in significant long-term morbidity from impaired function and altered appearance.

Patient Age and History

Patient age and history are significant determinants of survival. Patients considered most at risk are children younger than 2 years and adults older than 60 years. Inhalation injury, electrical burns, and all burns complicated by trauma and fractures (considered major injuries) significantly increase the risk for death. Obtaining the patient's medical history is important, in particular, a history related to cardiac, pulmonary, or kidney dysfunction; diabetes; and central nervous system (CNS) disorders. It is essential to obtain a thorough history, especially for nonverbal patients. Attention should be paid to the description of the burn event to rule out nonaccidental trauma (Fig. 35.9). Social services such as child protective services and the police should be consulted if abuse or neglect is suspected.

Child Abuse

According to the US Department of Health and Human Services Child Maltreatment 2012 report, 3.4 million referrals were made for child maltreatment, and of those, 678,810 were investigated and substantiated for abuse.[3] According to this report, 1640 children died as a result of abuse and neglect. Child abuse or maltreatment should be a differential diagnosis when caring for children with burn injury, as greater than 15% of children who are maltreated sustain physical abuse.[3] Burns account for approximately 6% to 20% of all abuse cases, and severe burns are reported in an estimated 10% of all children who are physically abused.[14] Most often burns in children are accidental but are related to failure of the caregiver or parent to provide adequate supervision. However, the developmental age and size of the child are of key importance in ruling out accidental and nonaccidental burn injuries. The patterns of burns—that is, inflicted burns consistent with immersion or dunking or contact—can be diagnostic of child abuse regardless of history.[15] A delay in seeking treatment or isolated scald or contact burns to the hands, feet, genitalia, or buttocks without a clearly defined mechanism should prompt further investigation for nonaccidental trauma.[4]

FIG. 35.9 Partial-Thickness Iron Burn to Right Buttock From Nonaccidental Trauma.

FIG. 35.8 Partial-Thickness Contact Burn to Palm.

INITIAL EMERGENCY BURN MANAGEMENT

The goals of acute care of a patient with thermal injuries are to save life, minimize disability, and prepare the patient for definitive care. The burn injury may involve multiple organ systems, and the approach to the injured patient should be expeditious and methodical in identifying problems and establishing priorities of care.

The resuscitation phase begins immediately after the burn insult has occurred; therefore, the nurse is concerned with patient management at the scene until admission to an appropriate medical facility. As with any major trauma, the first hour after injury is crucial; however, the first 24 to 36 hours after injury also are important in management of burn patients. Management during this period has a major impact on the patient's survival and ultimate rehabilitation.

Obtaining a history regarding the nature of the injury is important in management of a burn patient. Explosion of a water heater, propane gas, or grain elevator and other types of explosions often throw the patient some distance and may result in concomitant orthopedic, neurologic, and internal trauma. If the burns are chemical, it is valuable to know the specific agents involved. It also helps to know what substance was burned or inhaled and how long the patient was exposed to smoke or superheated air. A detailed patient history should include the mechanism of injury, patient's age, location and size of burn, type and amount of fluid already administered, known allergies, status of tetanus immunization, and significant medical history.

All rings, watches, and jewelry are removed from injured limbs to avoid a tourniquet effect when edema occurs as a result of fluid shifts and fluid resuscitation.

Airway Management

The first priority of emergency burn care is to secure and protect the airway. If there is any possibility of underlying cervical instability, cervical precautions must be initiated. In patients with facial burns, exposure to fire in an enclosed space, or both, inhalation injury should be suspected. Carbon monoxide poisoning is associated with high mortality rates. Carboxyhemoglobin (HbCO) levels are obtained, and oxygen therapy is initiated. Patients with HbCO level elevated greater than 10% and arterial partial pressure of oxygen (Pao_2)/fraction of inspired oxygen (Fio_2) ratio less than 200 have a high probability of needing respiratory support.[4] All patients with major burns or suspected inhalation injury are initially administered 100% oxygen. The nurse should continue to observe the patient for clinical manifestations of impaired oxygenation such as tachypnea, agitation, anxiety, and upper airway obstruction (eg, hoarseness, stridor, wheezing). Early intubation may be lifesaving in a patient who has an inhalation injury because it may be impossible to perform this procedure later, when edema has obstructed the larynx. The need for frequent blood sampling and the benefit of continuous blood pressure monitoring may necessitate placement of an arterial line.

Respiratory Management

Circumferential, full-thickness burns to the chest wall can lead to restriction of chest wall expansion and decreased compliance. Decreased compliance requires higher ventilatory pressures to provide the patient with adequate tidal volumes. In a patient who has not undergone intubation, clinical manifestations of chest wall restriction include rapid, shallow respirations; poor chest wall excursion; and severe agitation. Arterial blood gas analysis reveals a decrease in oxygen tension and an increasing arterial partial pressure of carbon dioxide ($Paco_2$) level. Patients receiving mechanical ventilation have increasing peak airway pressure values.

Escharotomies (burn eschar incisions) may be needed immediately to increase compliance and for improved ventilation.[4] These incisions usually are made bilaterally along the anterior axillary lines and are connected by a transverse incision at the costal margin (Fig. 35.10).

Circulatory Management

The extent and depth of the burn are assessed. The extent of TBSA of the burn is calculated for estimation of fluid resuscitation requirements (Table 35.1); the Parkland formula is the most widely used method of calculation (see Box 35.5, Case Study: Patient With Burns, at the end of the chapter).[6] Burn shock is caused by loss of fluid from the vascular compartment into the area of injury resulting in hypovolemia. The larger the percentage of burn area, the greater is the potential for development of shock. Lactated Ringer solution is infused through a large-bore cannula in a peripheral vein.[6] Lactated Ringer solution, an isotonic crystalloid, is the resuscitation fluid used most often. Given in large amounts, it can restore cardiac output to normal in most patients. It is preferred over normal saline because it most closely matches extracellular fluid. Because isotonic salt solutions generate no difference in osmotic pressure

FIG. 35.10 Preferred Sites of Escharotomy Incisions. (From Carrougher GJ. *Burn Care and Therapy*. St. Louis: Mosby; 1998.)

between plasma and the interstitial space, the entire extracellular space must be expanded to replace intravascular losses. Diuretics should not be given during the resuscitative phase of burn care.

According to the Parkland formula (see Table 35.1), 50% of the calculated amount of fluid is administered to the patient in the first 8 hours after injury; 25% is given in the second 8 hours, and 25% is given in the third 8 hours. Calculated fluid requirements are guidelines. Fluid resuscitation is a dynamic process. The rate of fluid administration is adjusted according to the individual's response, which is determined by monitoring urine output, heart rate, blood pressure, and level of consciousness. Meticulous attention to the patient's intake and output is imperative to ensure that he or she is appropriately resuscitated. Underresuscitation may result in inadequate cardiac output, leading to inadequate organ perfusion and the potential for wound conversion from a partial-thickness to full-thickness injury.[6] Overresuscitation may lead to moderate to severe pulmonary edema, to excessive wound edema causing a decrease in perfusion of unburned tissue in the distal portions of the extremities, or to edema inhibiting perfusion of the zone of stasis resulting in wound conversion. Fluid requirements may be much higher than estimated by using the Parkland formula. The recommendations for these situations are included later in this chapter. For pediatric patients, dextrose-containing intravenous fluid is added at a maintenance rate along with Parkland resuscitation fluid. Pediatric patients need continuous dextrose infusions for vital organs.

Continuous monitoring with electrocardiograms (ECGs) should be used in patients with serious thermal burn injury and in the presence of electrical burns, inhalation injury, or associated traumatic injury. ECG lead placement may present a challenge with extensive burns, and nontraditional locations on nonburned skin should be selected instead.

Pathophysiology of Burn Shock

Burn injuries greater than 20% of TBSA can result in burn shock.[6] *Shock* is defined as inadequate cellular perfusion. Significant burn injury results in hypovolemic shock and tissue trauma. Both cause the production and release of several local and systemic mediators. Burn shock can occur even when hypovolemia is corrected.

The first component of burn shock is hypovolemic shock. At the cellular level, the burning agent produces dilation of the capillaries and small vessels, increasing the capillary permeability. Plasma seeps out into the surrounding tissue, producing blisters and edema. The type, duration, and intensity of the burn all affect the amount and extent of fluid loss. This progressive fluid loss in extensive burns results in significant intravascular fluid volume deficit. Edema occurs locally in the burn wound and systemically in unburned tissues. Edema formation is unique to thermal injury.

Burn edema has been attributed to several factors. Barrier property changes of the capillary wall occur by direct injury and indirect mediator-modulated changes. Increases in permeability of protein and water occur, resulting in edema. In most forms of shock, capillary pressure decreases as a result of arteriolar vasoconstriction. However, an increase in capillary pressure has been found in burned tissue in the first minutes to hours after burn injury, causing capillary leak for the first 24 hours.[4] Coupled with this increase in capillary pressure is a negative interstitial hydrostatic pressure that occurs in the dermis layer of burned skin after thermal injury. This negative interstitial hydrostatic pressure represents an edema-generating mechanism that occurs for approximately 2 hours after injury. Plasma colloid osmotic pressure is decreased as a result of protein leakage into the extravascular space. Plasma is then further diluted with fluid resuscitation. The osmotic pressure is decreased, and further fluid extravasation can occur.

In addition to leaking capillaries, local and systemic mediators cause edema and the cardiovascular problems seen in burn patients. These mediators include histamine, prostaglandins, kinins, and oxygen radicals, and they increase arteriolar vasodilation.[4] Manipulation of these mediators to stop the cascade of burn edema and burn shock is being researched.

The intravascular fluid changes combined with the action of inflammatory mediators and vasoconstricting mediators result in hemodynamic consequences in burn patients.[4] The hemodynamic alterations include decreased myocardial contractility and cardiac output despite adequate volume resuscitation, increased systemic vascular resistance (SVR), and increased pulmonary vascular resistance (PVR). Increased PVR can lead to pulmonary edema. Large but judicious volumes of resuscitation fluids are required to maintain the vascular volume during the first few hours after a large burn injury to provide optimal resuscitation. Early and full fluid resuscitation can prevent the complications of acute kidney injury (AKI), cardiovascular

TABLE 35.1   Formulas for Fluid Replacement or Resuscitation in First 24 Hours

Fluid and Dose Rate	ABA Consensus	Parkland	Modified Brooke	Brooke	Hypertonic
Electrolyte solution	Ringer lactate	Ringer lactate	Ringer lactate	Ringer lactate	Hypertonic lactated saline (sodium, 250 mEq/L)
Dose: mL/kg/% burned[a]	2–4	4	2	1.5	Rate based on urine output of 30–50 mL/h
	50% of fluid over first 8 h; 50% of fluid over next 16 h				
Examples using ABA consensus formula: An 85-kg patient with 35% TBSA burn					
2 mL × 85 kg × 35% = 5950 mL in first 24 h	3 mL × 85 × 35% = 8925 mL	4 mL × 85 × 35% = 11,900 mL			
2975 mL in first 8 h = 372 mL/h	4462 mL in first 8 h = 558 mL/h	5950 mL in first 8 h = 744 mL/h			
2975 mL in next 16 h = 186 mL/h	4462 mL in next 16 h = 279 mL/h	5950 mL in next 16 h = 372 mL/h			

ABA, American Burn Association; *TBSA,* total body surface area.
[a]Adjust these rates to maintain urine output >30 mL/h in adults or 1 mL/kg/h in children.

collapse, and death from shock. However, overresuscitation increases edema formation, which can further impair tissue oxygen diffusion. The nurse must assess the patient's fluid status and response to resuscitation to obtain the optimal response.

Kidney Management

If fluid resuscitation is inadequate, AKI may occur. In the emergency department, an indwelling urinary catheter should be placed for burns greater than 20% of TBSA to monitor urine output and the effectiveness of fluid resuscitation.[6] A catheter may be necessary if the burn extends into the perineal area because of the presence or development of edema. Urinary catheters with temperature probes should be used whenever possible. The nurse measures urine output hourly. Adequate urine output for adults is 0.5 to 1 mL/kg per hour, or 30 to 50 mL/h; in children, it is 1 to 2 mL/kg per hour.[6]

Gastrointestinal System Management

Patients with burns of greater than 20% of TBSA are prone to gastric dilation as a result of paralytic ileus. Nasogastric or orogastric tubes are placed in these patients to prevent abdominal distention, emesis, and potential aspiration. This decrease in gastrointestinal (GI) function is caused by the effects of hypovolemia and the neurologic and endocrine response to injury. GI activity usually returns in 24 to 48 hours. Prophylaxis with histamine blockers or sucralfate is initiated because burn patients are prone to ileus. These acute ulcerations of the duodenum are caused by sloughing of the gastric mucosa resulting from loss of plasma volume after severe burns. Enteral nutrition has been shown to be protective of gastric mucosal integrity and to improve intestinal flow, gastric motility, and intestinal blood flow in burn patients.[16] Enteral nutrition should be started as soon as possible. Patients with severe burns can be safely fed in the duodenum or jejunum within 6 hours of burn injury.[16] Care should be taken to start enteral feeds for burn patients via nasoduodenal or nasojejunal tube promptly.

Extremity Pulse Assessment

Edema formation may cause neurovascular compromise to the extremities; frequent assessments are necessary to evaluate pulses, skin color, capillary refill, and sensation. Arterial circulation is at greatest risk with circumferential burns. If not corrected, reduced arterial flow causes ischemia and necrosis. The Doppler flow probe is one of the best ways to evaluate arterial pulses. An escharotomy may be required to restore arterial circulation and to allow for further swelling. The escharotomy can be performed at the bedside with a sterile field and scalpel. Care must be taken to avoid major nerves, vessels, and tendons. The incision extends through the length of the eschar, over joints, and down to the subcutaneous fat. The incision is placed laterally or medially on the extremity. If a single incision does not restore circulation, bilateral incisions are required (see Fig. 35.8). If escharotomy is required before the patient is transferred to a burn center, consultation with the receiving physician is advised.

Laboratory Assessment

Initial laboratory studies are performed including complete blood count, electrolytes, blood urea nitrogen (BUN), creatinine, urinalysis, glucose, and blood screening. Special situations such as inhalation injury warrant arterial blood gas measurements, HbCO level determination, cultures, alcohol and drug screens, and cyanide levels. A baseline assessment of nutrition status, including albumin and prealbumin, is helpful in monitoring future nutrition needs. Also, creatine kinase, urinalysis, and urine myoglobin, are good indicators of rhabdomyolysis seen in the setting of electrical burn injuries.[6] An ECG is obtained for all patients with electrical burns or preexisting heart disease. Serum lactate is also another good inflammatory marker indicating burn severity.[6]

Wound Care

After wounds have been assessed, topical antimicrobial therapy is not a priority during emergency care. However, the wounds must be covered with clean, dry dressings or sheets. Every attempt must be made to keep the patient warm because of the high risk of hypothermia. The administration of tetanus prophylaxis is recommended for all burns covering more than 10% of the TBSA and for patients with an unknown immunization history.

Burn Center Referral

After initial treatment and stabilization at an emergency department, referral to a burn center is considered (see Box 35.1). A burn center must be able to deliver all therapy required including rehabilitation and must perform personnel training and burn research. Patients meeting the criteria for referral need the expertise of a multidisciplinary team. Referring hospitals must always contact the burn center in their region.[2] Providers in the field should cover the burns with clean, dry cloth until arrival at the burn center. Early communication between the initial provider and the burn center is encouraged by the American Burn Association.[2]

SPECIAL MANAGEMENT CONSIDERATIONS

Inhalation Injury

Inhalation injury can occur in the presence or absence of cutaneous injury. Inhalation injuries are strongly associated with burns sustained in a closed or confined space, and they are associated with increased mortality.[6] Inhalation injury appears in three basic forms, alone or in combination: carbon monoxide poisoning, direct heat injury, and chemical damage. The three types of inhalation injury are carbon monoxide poisoning, upper airway injury, and lower airway injury.

Immediate lifesaving measures in burn patients include management of the airway. The burn patient may exhibit few or no signs of airway distress; however, thermal injury to the airway must be anticipated if facial burns, singed eyebrows and nasal hair, carbon deposits in the oropharynx, and carbonaceous sputum are present or if the history suggests confinement in a burning environment. Any of these findings indicates acute inhalation injury and requires immediate and definitive care. To prevent the necessity of tracheostomy or cricothyrotomy, the use of early intubation and respiratory support must be considered before tracheal edema occurs. Inhalation injury increases the patient's risk of developing pneumonia and acute respiratory distress syndrome (ARDS).[6] Management of ARDS necessitates mechanical ventilatory support and, in extreme cases, high-frequency oscillatory ventilation or extracorporeal membrane oxygenation. The occurrence of inhalation injury with cutaneous burns increases the fluid requirements during resuscitation to a higher level than would be predicted by the cutaneous burn alone.

Carbon Monoxide Poisoning

Carbon monoxide poisoning is the cause of death in persons found dead at the scene of a fire who have few or no cutaneous thermal injuries. Carbon monoxide is a colorless, odorless, and tasteless gas. Inhalation of carbon monoxide, a by-product of the incomplete combustion of carbon, results in its bonding to available hemoglobin, producing HbCO, which effectively decreases oxygen saturation of hemoglobin. The affinity of hemoglobin molecules for carbon monoxide is approximately 200 to 250 times greater than that for oxygen.[17] HbCO binds poorly with oxygen, reducing the oxygen-carrying capacity of blood and causing hypoxemia. The shortage of oxygen at the tissue level is worsened by a shift to the left of the oxyhemoglobin dissociation curve, reflecting the fact that the oxygen in the hemoglobin is not readily given up to the cells.

Measurement of arterial oxygen saturation is of limited value because oxygen saturation may be quite high despite dangerously low levels of oxygen content. Because the pulse oximeter cannot distinguish between oxyhemoglobin and HbCO, it is an unreliable predictor of tissue oxygenation during the initial stages of carbon monoxide poisoning.[17] Arterial blood gas determinations and oxygen saturation are used to accurately assess the hemoglobin oxygen saturation level. A serum HbCO level is obtained at diagnosis. Normal HbCO levels are less than 2%. HbCO levels of 40% to 60% often produce unresponsiveness or obtundation; levels of 15% to 40% may result in various degrees of CNS dysfunction. Levels of 10% to 15%, which can be found in cigarette smokers, rarely produce serious symptoms but may cause a headache.

The major clinical manifestations of severe carbon monoxide poisoning are related to the CNS and the heart. Symptoms associated with carbon monoxide poisoning include headache, dizziness, nausea, vomiting, dyspnea, and confusion.[17] In severe cases, carbon monoxide poisoning may lead to myocardial ischemia and CNS complications caused by reduced oxygen delivery and the already compromised circulatory system. Early signs of carbon monoxide poisoning may include tachycardia, tachypnea, confusion, and lightheadedness. As the carbon monoxide level rises, patients exhibit a decreased level of responsiveness, which may progress to unresponsiveness and respiratory failure.

The treatment of choice for carbon monoxide poisoning is high-flow oxygen administered at 100% through a tight-fitting nonrebreathing mask or endotracheal intubation. The half-life of carbon monoxide in the body is 4 hours at room air (21% oxygen), 2 hours at 40% oxygen, and 40 to 60 minutes at 100% oxygen.[17] The half-life of carbon monoxide is 30 minutes in a hyperbaric oxygen chamber at three times atmospheric pressure. The use of hyperbaric oxygen in the care of burn patients is controversial. Because of the rapid removal of carbon monoxide with the administration of 100% oxygen, the time required to transport a patient who has received oxygen in the field should always be considered to avoid possible underestimation of inhalation injury.

Upper Airway Injury

Burns of the upper respiratory tract include burns involving the pharynx, larynx, glottis, trachea, and larger bronchi. Injuries are caused by direct heat or by chemical inflammation and necrosis. Respiratory injury is most often confined to the upper airway. The heat exchange capability is so efficient that most heat absorption and damage occur in the pharynx and larynx above the true vocal cords.

Heat damage may be severe enough to cause upper airway obstruction at any time, beginning from the moment of injury through the resuscitation period. Caution is needed for patients with severe hypovolemia because supraglottic edema may be delayed until fluid resuscitation is underway and third spacing occurs. Patients must be monitored for hoarseness, stridor, audible airflow turbulence, and the production of carbonaceous sputum. Maximal edema occurs 24 hours after injury with upper airway injuries, and these patients should be observed in the critical care unit for a minimum of 24 hours.[18]

The prediction of an upper airway obstruction is based on consideration of several variables: extent of injury to the face and neck, presence of blisters on or redness of the posterior pharynx, signs of singed nasal hair, increased HbCO levels, increased rate and decreased depth of breathing, hoarseness and stridor (which indicates a significant decrease in the diameter of the airway), increased amount of sputum, and circumstances of the burn event (whether it occurred in an enclosed space or involved superheated gases or steam). Steam has a heat-carrying capacity many times that of dry air, and it is capable of overwhelming the extremely efficient heat-dissipating capabilities of the upper airway.

Intubation is recommended whenever airway patency is questionable, rather than delaying intubation until airway obstruction is so severe that intubation becomes a challenge. After the airway is secure, priority is given to minimizing airway edema, maintaining pulmonary hygiene, and treating bronchospasm. Elevating the head of the bed to 30 degrees or higher decreases airway edema. Therapeutic deep breathing and coughing, early mobility, suctioning, and bronchodilators assist in mobilizing and removing secretions. Fiberoptic bronchoscopy may be required to remove secretions in some patients. Mechanical ventilatory support is necessary when respiratory fatigue or failure occurs. Precautions to prevent ventilator-associated pneumonia should be implemented to avoid secondary infection.

Lower Airway Injury

Heated air rarely causes lower airway injury. If it does, it usually is associated with death at the scene. Lower airway injuries are typically caused by chemical damage to mucosal surfaces. Tracheobronchitis with severe spasm and wheezing may occur in the first minutes to hours after injury. Historically, the most accurate method of documenting lower airway injury is the xenon ventilation-perfusion lung scan. Prolonged retention or symmetry of washout of the radioisotope indicates pulmonary parenchymal injury on the side of the retained emissions. The onset of symptoms is unpredictable after smoke inhalation, and patients at risk must be closely monitored for at least 24 to 48 hours after injury.[17]

Patients with inhalation injuries are at risk for developing pneumonia, acute lung injury, and ARDS. Ventilator management strategies for hypoxia and ARDS in burn patients can be challenging. Lung protective ventilation with low tidal volumes, higher levels of positive end-expiratory pressure, and permissive hypercarbia have shown optimal outcomes and minimized ventilator-induced lung injury.[19] Intrabronchial surfactant and inhaled nitric oxide are other last resorts for treating burn patients with inhalation injuries that have not responded to other means of ventilator support.[17] Treatment of lower airway injury is largely symptomatic. As with upper airway injury management, aggressive pulmonary hygiene, removal of secretions, ventilatory support, and careful fluid resuscitation so as to avoid exacerbating pulmonary edema and ARDS are indicated when caring for burn patients with lower airway inhalation injuries.[18]

Nonthermal Burns
Chemical Burns

Chemical burns can be caused by a variety of products. Acids, alkalis, and organic and inorganic compounds cause chemical burns. The acid or base quality determines the injurious nature of a product. The injury is caused by the pH of the product or by the concentration of the product. In the past, irrigation with neutralizing solutions was recommended to limit the extent and depth of chemical burns. This practice is no longer advocated because neutralizing agents may cause reactions that are exothermic (produce heat), increasing the extent and depth of the burn. It also is possible that the neutralizing agent is neither immediately known nor available. Instead, large amounts of water should be used to flush the area. Clothing and shoes should be removed if they have been in contact with the chemical. Alkali burns of the eyes require continuous irrigation for many hours after the injury. Removal of contact lenses is necessary before irrigation. Litmus paper may be used to assess for neutrality or if further irrigation is needed.[6]

Treatments for chemical burns vary. Phenol burns are first diluted, and then the skin is wiped quickly with polyethylene glycol or vegetable oil to decrease the severity of the burn. Areas exposed to hydrofluoric acid must be copiously irrigated with water; the burned area then can be treated with 2.5% calcium gluconate gel. The patient may need calcium gluconate supplements because the fluoride ion precipitates serum calcium, causing hypocalcemia. White phosphorus can ignite if kept dry, and these wounds must be covered with a moist dressing. After a tar or asphalt injury, the removal of tar or asphalt is best accomplished with the use of petroleum-containing distillates. One such product is Detachol Adhesive Remover (Ferndale Laboratories, Inc., Ferndale, MI). The solution can be placed directly on the wound and gently wiped off. Routine débridement of loose skin is initiated after tar removal. Topical antimicrobial therapy is then provided.

Electrical Burns

In electrical burns, the type and voltage of the circuit, resistance, pathway of transmission through the body, and duration of contact are considered in determining the amount of damage sustained. In these situations, the rescuer also may be injured if he or she becomes part of the electrical circuit. The rescuer must disconnect the electrical source to break the circuit or must know how to avoid becoming part of the circuit. The use of appropriately insulated equipment that diverts the circuit elsewhere is essential. Extreme caution must be used in the rescue of victims.

Electricity always travels toward the ground. The body conducts electrical current as a whole, as opposed to the earlier belief that it traveled most quickly through the nerves and circulatory system. Electrical burns are caused by the thermal conversion of electricity into heat within the tissues, which can cause the skin to only be minimally affected; however, there may be extensive damage to the underlying tissues.[6]

The electrical burn process can result in a profound alteration in acid–base balance and rhabdomyolysis resulting in myoglobinuria, which poses a serious threat to kidney function. Myoglobin is a normal constituent of muscle. With extensive muscle destruction, it is released into the circulatory system and filtered by the kidneys. It can be highly toxic and can lead to AKI. Fluid resuscitation for a patient with an electrical burn does not correlate with the Parkland formula, and the fluid is adjusted according to the patient's urine output. If myoglobin is present in the urine, a urine output greater than 200 mL/h in adults is established until the urine is clear of all myoglobin pigment.[20]

If hemoglobinuria is identified, the clinician should assume that the patient has myoglobinuria and acidosis. Sodium bicarbonate may be administered to bring the pH level into the normal range, to correct a documented acidosis, or to alkalize urine to promote myoglobin excretion. Diuretics such as mannitol also may be administered to increase renal blood flow and glomerular filtration rate to facilitate myoglobin clearance.[20] Sodium bicarbonate infusions and diuretic therapy are called *forced alkaline diuresis*. A baseline ECG and myocardial biomarker levels are obtained while the patient is in the emergency department. The following criteria are used for monitoring the cardiac status of burn patients:

- A history of loss of consciousness or cardiac arrest
- Documentation of cardiac dysrhythmia at the scene of the accident or in the emergency department
- Abnormal ECG findings on admission
- TBSA burns of greater than 20%
- Very young age or advanced age
- Prior history of heart disease

Other burn patients may be admitted to nonmonitored settings and observed closely. Cardiac dysrhythmias must be treated promptly, and a protocol to rule out myocardial infarction must be followed.

BURN NURSING DIAGNOSES AND MANAGEMENT

The clinical course of a burn injury has three phases: (1) resuscitative, (2) acute care, and (3) rehabilitative. Each phase has a unique set of actual and potential problems. The resuscitative phase begins with initial hemodynamic response to the injury and lasts until capillary integrity is restored and the repletion of plasma volume by fluid replacement occurs. Spontaneous diuresis demonstrates that capillaries have regained their integrity. The acute phase begins with the onset of diuresis of fluid mobilized from the interstitial space and ends with the closure of the burn wound. The major focus of the acute phase is wound healing, wound closure, and prevention of infection. The rehabilitative phase begins when the patient is admitted to the hospital, with correction of functional deficits and scar management being major considerations. The rehabilitative phase may last months to years, depending on the severity of injury. The rehabilitation phase should focus on adequate wound healing, preventing scarring and contractures, and psychosocial support of the patient and the family.

Resuscitation Phase

Life-threatening airway and breathing problems, cardiopulmonary instability, and hypovolemia characterize the resuscitation phase, or shock phase. Burn injury affects the structure and function of almost every organ.[21] The magnitude of this pathophysiologic response is proportional to the extent of cutaneous injury. The goal of the resuscitation phase is to maintain vital organ function and perfusion. Emergent interventions for inhalation injury, airway management, and hypovolemia are concurrently addressed.

Oxygenation Alterations

Inhalation injuries have emerged as the most common cause of death in burn patients, whereas 40 to 50 years ago, burn shock followed by burn sepsis accounted for most burn-related deaths. Early diagnosis of inhalation injury is essential to minimize complications and to decrease the mortality rate. Three oxygenation complications are associated with smoke inhalation during the resuscitation phase: (1) *carbon monoxide poisoning,* (2) *upper airway obstruction,* and (3) *chemical pneumonitis.* Evaluation of a patient for inhalation injury includes physical assessment (eg, singed facial hairs, mucosal burns of nose or mouth, carbonaceous sputum), arterial blood gas analysis, HbCO levels, chest radiography, flexible fiberoptic bronchoscopy, xenon-133 lung scan, and pulmonary function tests. Critical care nursing management includes the following:

- Assess breath sounds and the rate and quality of respirations.
- Administer oxygen, as prescribed.
- Monitor HbCO levels.
- Elevate the head of the bed, and implement ventilator-associated pneumonia precautions.
- Assess and assist with pulmonary secretion suctioning.
- Observe for signs of airway obstruction (eg, increased respiratory rate and heart rate, increased work of breathing, use of accessory muscles, stridor, wheezing, hoarseness, crackles).
- Prepare for endotracheal intubation and mechanical ventilation.
- Maintain accurate and timely documentation.

Impaired gas exchange. The most common pulmonary burn complication is carbon monoxide poisoning. High-flow oxygen should be administered at 100% through a nonrebreathing mask or endotracheal intubation until the HbCO level is less than 10% to 15%.

Chemical pneumonitis is caused by inhalation of the by-products of combustion of substances such as cotton, aldehydes, oxides of sulfur, and nitrogen. Burning polyvinyl chloride yields at least 75 potentially toxic compounds, including hydrochloric acid and carbon monoxide. Within days after a burn, ARDS commonly develops in patients with chemical pneumonitis. The primary clinical manifestation of ARDS is hypoxemia that is refractory to oxygen therapy. Early signs include increased pH, decreased $Paco_2$, and increased respiratory rate. Ventilatory support with the use of positive end-expiratory pressure is the treatment of choice.

Ineffective airway clearance. Laryngeal swelling and upper airway obstruction may occur at any time during the first 24 hours after a burn injury. Endotracheal intubation must be accomplished early because this simple procedure can become extremely difficult in the presence of laryngeal edema. Enough time is usually available to intervene after obtaining the history and transporting the patient to the primary hospital. Consequent edema may not manifest for up to 48 hours after the burn incident.[14] A patient who has not initially undergone intubation must be carefully monitored during this critical period. When prolonged ventilatory failure is expected as a result of severe inhalation, a tracheostomy is performed.

Extubation is done only if the patient can meet extubation criteria: level of consciousness assessed as *awake,* intact cough and gag reflexes, inspiratory effort greater than −25 cm H_2O in adults, vital capacity of 10 mL/kg, and decreased volume and tenacity of sputum. Resolution of airway edema can be assessed by deflating the endotracheal cuff and observing the patient's ability to breathe around the endotracheal tube.

Although uncommon, laryngospasm must be addressed. Laryngospasm usually is brought on by airway irritation from inhalation of noxious agents.

Fluid Resuscitation

Current resuscitation protocols emphasize fluid delivery rates based on the extent of burn injury and the patient's weight. The patient's weight measured in kilograms must be obtained on admission to the hospital. The extent of the burn is calculated by using one of the methods previously described. Several formulas are available to guide fluid resuscitation and should be used to assist in the management of fluid replacement (see Table 35.1). The formulas differ primarily in terms of administration, volume, and sodium content. The actual amount of fluid given to any patient must be based on that individual's response.

The type of fluid used in resuscitation and at what point a switch should be made to a colloid solution are controversial topics. No clear-cut guidelines for resuscitation exist. The administration of crystalloid fluid (lactated Ringer solution) for the first 24 to 36 hours after the burn is the most common practice. Lactated Ringer solution is the crystalloid solution of choice because of its physiologic similarity to the composition of extracellular fluid. The addition of lactated Ringer solution with 5% dextrose should be considered as maintenance fluid, especially in the first 24 hours. Assessment for secondary injuries that would affect the choice of fluid should be performed. Ideally, the capillary leak seals approximately 24 hours after the injury, making it possible to give colloid without leakage of protein into the interstitium. Colloid deficits are replaced in the next 24 hours with salt-free albumin or dextran at 0.3 to 1 mL/kg per % TBSA burn. In addition to colloid, maintenance fluids are given to replace evaporative losses, and the amount is adjusted according to the patient's serum electrolyte levels, urine output, weight, volume status, and clinical assessment.

Deficient fluid volume. Physiologic effects of the burn complicate the tissue damage that occurs after the burn insult. Coagulation factors are affected, protein is denatured, and cellular content is ionized. These factors, coupled with dilation of capillaries and small vessels, lead to increased capillary permeability and fluid shifts from the intravascular space to the interstitial space. The lymphatic system, which normally carries away the increased interstitial fluid, may be damaged or overloaded and unable to function to its normal capacity.

In addition to the protein and electrolyte shift, an increased insensible water loss occurs. In a healthy adult, this loss is estimated to be 35 to 50 mL/h. Insensible water loss in a burn patient may be 300 to 3000 mL/day. This increase may be related to temperature elevation, tracheostomy, and the size of the burn.

Burn shock is proportional to the extent and depth of injury. The loss of plasma begins almost immediately after the injury and reaches its peak within the first 48 hours. Desired clinical responses to fluid resuscitation include urinary output of 0.5 to 1 mL/kg per hour, heart rate less than 120 beats/min, blood pressure in the normal to high range, central venous pressure

(CVP) less than 12 cm H_2O or pulmonary artery occlusion pressure less than 18 mm Hg, clear lung sounds, clear sensorium, and absence of intestinal events such as nausea and paralytic ileus. Heart rate, blood pressure, and CVP values are not always accurate or reliable predictors of successful fluid resuscitation.

Potassium and sodium, the two electrolytes of concern during the resuscitation period, must be monitored carefully. *Hyperkalemia* can occur during this phase because of (1) the release of potassium from damaged cells; (2) metabolic acidosis; and (3) impaired kidney function caused by hemoglobinuria, myoglobinuria, or decreased renal perfusion. The patient must be assessed for clinical manifestations of hyperkalemia. Treatment includes correction of acidosis. During the resuscitation phase, using cation-exchange resins or intravenously administered insulin and hypertonic dextrose to transport potassium back into the cell is not recommended because of the unpredictable nature of fluid shifts that occur.

Hypokalemia can occur during the resuscitation phase because of the massive loss of fluids and electrolytes through the burn wounds or because of hemodilution. During the acute phase, it may be related to hemodilution; inadequate replacement; loss associated with diuresis, diarrhea, vomiting, nasogastric drainage, and long hydrotherapy sessions; or the shift of potassium from the intravascular space to the cell after the acidosis has been corrected. Nursing interventions include treating nausea and vomiting, limiting immersive hydrotherapy sessions to less than 30 minutes, preventing fluid volume excess, and judicious replacement of potassium.

Hyponatremia is common during the resuscitation phase because of the loss of sodium through the burn wound, the shift of fluid into the interstitial space, vomiting, nasogastric drainage, diarrhea, and the use of hypotonic salt solutions during the early phase of resuscitation. During this phase, it may be necessary to monitor serum sodium levels every 4 to 8 hours. Hyponatremia also may occur during the acute phase because of hemodilution and loss through the wound, lengthy hydrotherapy sessions, and excessive diuresis resulting from the fluid shift back into the intravascular space. Interventions are followed for treating nausea and vomiting, hydrotherapy sessions are limited, and intravenous replacement of sodium is considered. During diuresis, which occurs during the acute phase, restricting free water intake usually is the only required intervention to increase the serum sodium level.

Risk for Infection

Preventing infection in burn patients is challenging and involves complex decision making. Considerable debate has been ongoing about the infection control precautions to use with burn patients. The burn wound is the most common source of infection in the burn patient. The loss of the protective mechanism of the skin and contamination from the patient's own bacterial flora can lead to bloodstream infections. Some centers advocate routine wound surveillance cultures and wound biopsy to identify infection early. Frequent wound inspection is needed to assess for changes in appearance such as an increase in exudate, odor, or color to minimize the risk of bacteremia. Patients should not be treated with antibiotics prophylactically; rather, treatment should be tailored to positive culture results.[18]

Cross-contamination by direct contact is a significant source of infection and a subsequent cause of sepsis. Effective handwashing technique cannot be overemphasized. Nurses must wash their hands and change gloves when moving from area to area on the same patient. For example, after changing the chest dressing, which may be contaminated with sputum from the tracheostomy, hands must be washed and gloves changed before the nurse moves to the legs. Gowns, gloves, and masks should be worn whenever contact with body fluids occurs. These garments also must be changed and hands washed before caring for a different patient. Maintaining patient-specific dressings and topical agents is recommended. Equipment such as thermometers, intravenous pumps, and stethoscopes should be designated for each patient or, when shared, should be cleaned with appropriate bactericidal cleansers between patients.

Whichever precautions are used, everyone coming in contact with the patient including the patient's family and visitors must be knowledgeable about the standard for infection control. These precautions should be strictly followed by all.

Tissue Perfusion
Ineffective Kidney Tissue Perfusion

Urinalysis to determine the myoglobin level may be performed soon after burn injury. Myoglobinuria can be detected grossly by the dark, port-wine color of the urine. Myoglobin is extremely toxic to the kidneys and can cause massive tubular destruction. It is best treated with rapid fluid administration and forced diuresis with diuretics such as mannitol, an osmotic diuretic. The goal is an hourly urine output that is at least double the general recommendations to flush the kidney tubules. All other diuretics are avoided because they would deplete the already compromised intravascular volume. Sodium bicarbonate is sometimes given intravenously to alkalinize the urine and assist in the elimination of heme pigments.

Maintaining and monitoring the renal system is vital in management of burn patients. Impairment of the renal system may be related to hemoglobinuria, myoglobinuria, hypoperfusion, and hypovolemia. Urinary output must be monitored every hour for the first 48 to 72 hours, and specific gravity values can be used to determine the adequacy of hydration status and renal competency. The urine glucose concentration is monitored, as are urine sodium, creatinine, and BUN levels. Use of an indwelling urinary catheter is appropriate for the first 48 to 72 hours. Because of the tremendous risk of infection related to indwelling catheters, they are removed as soon as possible. However, leaving the catheter in place may be necessary if perineal burns are involved. Oliguria is usually related to inadequate fluid resuscitation but may be associated with AKI. Other signs of kidney failure include increasing creatinine, BUN, phosphorus, and potassium levels; excessive fluid-weight gain; excessive edema; elevated blood pressure; lethargy; and confusion.

The presence of glucose in the urine causes osmotic diuresis. In this clinical situation, urine output is an unreliable estimate of volume status. Because of the increased loss of fluid through the kidneys, glucosuria may suggest the need for additional fluid beyond the original estimates.

Ineffective Cerebral Tissue Perfusion

The patient's neurologic status is assessed frequently during the first few days. Changes may be related to an associated head injury that occurred at the time of burn injury, hypoperfusion related to hypovolemia, hypoxemia associated with inadequate ventilation, carbon monoxide poisoning, or electrolyte imbalances. Patients with electrical burns or major thermal burns may have peripheral neurologic injuries, which may not become evident for several days after the injury. The neurologic assessment includes use of the Glasgow Coma Scale. It is not unusual for the patient to be agitated, restless, and extremely anxious during the resuscitation phase of burn injury as a result of hypovolemia, pain, and fear of disfigurement or death. However, the possibility of neurologic involvement must not be overlooked. Maintaining an adequate mean arterial pressure is essential to ensure adequate cerebral perfusion pressure.

Ineffective Peripheral Tissue Perfusion

Ineffective peripheral tissue perfusion results from third spacing of fluid during the resuscitation phase, which restricts blood flow to extremities. As hypovolemia ensues, vasoconstriction increases, which can be potentiated by the loss of body temperature. Peripheral tissue perfusion must be monitored carefully in all burn patients. Burned as well as unburned areas are carefully assessed for warmth, color, and peripheral pulses. Capillary refill time should be less than 3 seconds in unburned areas. Any clinical manifestation of diminished systemic tissue perfusion must be reported immediately. Nursing actions are taken to minimize any compromise of peripheral circulation. Close monitoring of appropriate fluid resuscitation and careful positioning of the patient are necessary to prevent compromised blood flow. Crossed legs, dependent positions, and pillows under the patient's knees should be avoided. Specialty mattresses and beds may be helpful to prevent secondary skin breakdown and assist with positioning and pulmonary toilet. The limbs should be elevated above the heart to decrease peripheral edema and enhance venous return. Assisted range-of-motion exercises can help to decrease edema.

Monitoring the peripheral circulation is crucial in a burn patient with circumferential, full-thickness burns of the extremities. The resulting edema may severely compromise the venous system and then the arterial system. Neurovascular integrity of extremities with circumferential burns must be assessed every hour for the first 24 to 48 hours using the six "P's": *pulselessness, pallor, pain, paresthesia, paralysis,* and *poikilothermy.* Careful, ongoing assessment is necessary, especially for patients who are intubated and may be unable to communicate pain or paresthesia. The use of a Doppler flowmeter may be necessary. Loss of pulses is a late sign of compromised vascular flow. If any changes are observed, the physician must be notified immediately. Numbness and paresthesia may occur only 30 minutes before loss of pulses. Irreversible nerve ischemia resulting in loss of function may begin after 12 to 24 hours. An escharotomy may become necessary to allow the underlying tissue to expand. In deeper wounds, a fasciotomy, which involves incision into the fascia, may be necessary.

Ineffective Gastrointestinal Tissue Perfusion

Paralytic ileus is a common GI complication that can occur during resuscitation or when sepsis develops. The abdomen and bowel sounds should be assessed every 2 hours during the initial phase and every 4 hours thereafter. If clinical manifestations of a paralytic ileus occur, oral intake is withheld, and a nasogastric tube may be inserted and placed on low suction. Paralytic ileus can be related to hypokalemia, the sympathetic response to severe trauma, or decreased tissue perfusion related to hypovolemia.

A stress ulcer may develop as a result of decreased tissue perfusion to the GI tract, a change in the quantity or quality of mucus (which has a pH of 1), or an increase in gastric acid secretion resulting from the stress response. Gastric acid should be maintained above a pH of 5 through the administration of antacids, histamine blockers, or proton-pump inhibitors to prevent the development of these ulcers. The patient should be carefully monitored for GI bleeding. All stools and gastric content are tested for occult blood. The patient should be observed for epigastric discomfort or fullness, decreased blood pressure, or increased pulse.

Invasive monitoring. The decision to use invasive monitoring techniques requires careful consideration of the potential risk factors and how the data collected will influence the course of treatment. Invasive monitoring should be considered if treatment seems ineffective or if complicating factors such as severe respiratory involvement, major life-threatening injuries, head injuries, or pneumothorax occur. Patients with preexisting medical conditions such as chronic obstructive pulmonary disease, acute heart failure, and kidney failure also may require invasive monitoring.

Invasive monitoring includes direct measurement of CVP, pulmonary artery pressure, arterial pressure, core temperature, cardiac output, SVR, and PVR. The use of an arterial line is considered if serial and frequent arterial blood gas values are required for respiratory management or for hemodynamic instability requiring the titration of vasoactive drugs. Central venous catheters can be helpful in the early stages of fluid resuscitation to deliver the massive amount of fluids required. The physician selects the catheter insertion site based on burn location and the purpose of the catheter. It is preferable not to insert catheters through burned skin. It may be appropriate to use a multilumen catheter that can serve as a route for fluid resuscitation, maintenance fluids, antibiotic therapy, and vasoactive drugs. The risks involved include the increased chance of infection, potential for pneumothorax, and difficulty with insertion if hypovolemia is present.

Pulmonary artery catheters are placed only when necessary for optimal care. They may be essential to the survival of a septic patient despite the risks involved. Pulmonary artery catheters can provide data about pulmonary artery occlusion pressure, cardiac output, stroke volume, SVR and PVR, core temperature, and mixed venous oxygen saturation levels.

Centrally placed intravascular catheters require meticulous care. Strict guidelines should be established and monitored. Catheters are inserted under sterile conditions, and the dressings are changed under the same conditions. Because infection is such a major concern, all invasive catheters should be removed as early as possible.

Hypothermia. Maintenance of thermoregulation is a nursing challenge. A patient with extensive burn injury is at high risk for hypothermia. Hypothermia is especially problematic during initial treatment, during hydrotherapy, during dressing changes, and immediately after surgery. Heat is lost through open burn wounds by means of evaporation and radiation. The patient's core temperature should be maintained between 37.6°C (99.6°F) and 38.3°C (101°F).

Laboratory assessment. Laboratory assessment is another important aspect of burn care. Because of the invasive nature of drawing blood, it is done only if absolutely indicated. Consideration should be given to the age of the patient, the size of the burn, the time since injury, and any underlying disease process.

White blood cell counts usually are monitored for elevation, a sign of sepsis. However, it is not unusual for the white blood cell count to fall to less than 5000/mm^3 within 48 hours after injury. The value may decrease even more—1500/mm^3 to 2000/mm^3—with the use of silver sulfadiazine (SSD). Hemoglobin and hematocrit data can be useful in the resuscitative phase to guide fluid administration. If surgical débridement is required, monitoring blood counts in the postoperative period is important. Serum chemistry information is helpful for ongoing assessment of kidney function and electrolyte balance. The myriad tests available should be used appropriately and as indicated by individual patient needs.

Acute Care Phase

The acute care phase of burn management begins after resuscitation and lasts until complete wound closure is achieved. The early postresuscitation phase is a period of transition from the shock phase to the hypermetabolic phase. Major cardiopulmonary and wound changes occur that substantially alter the manner of patient care from that given during resuscitation. Cardiopulmonary stability is optimal during this period because wound inflammation and infection have not developed. Hypermetabolic changes can be complicated with the onset of wound infection and sepsis. Early wound excision and skin grafting procedures, local wound care, nutrition support, and infection control characterize this phase.

Nurses play a major role in promoting the healing process. As skilled clinicians of the burn team, nurses provide daily wound assessment, hydrotherapy, débridement, preoperative and postoperative management, and pain management.

Immediately after injury, the body responds by initiating a series of physiologic changes to restore skin integrity. These physiologic changes include the inflammatory phase, proliferative phase, and maturation phase.

Inflammatory Phase

The inflammatory phase begins immediately after injury. Vascular changes and cellular activity characterize this period. Changes in the severed vessels occur in an attempt to wall off the wound from the external environment. Platelets, activated as a result of vessel wall injury, aggregate; blood coagulation is initiated; and in larger vessels, smooth muscle tissue contraction occurs, resulting in a reduction in the diameter of the vessel lumen. These brief but important compensatory mechanisms protect the patient from excessive blood loss and increased exposure to bacterial contamination. As vasodilation occurs, blood supply to the wound site increases and is observed as erythema and exudates.[22] Granulocytes invade the wound within 24 hours and initiate the phagocytosis of necrotic tissue and bacteria. Fibroblasts migrate to the wound and multiply, producing a bed of collagen.

Proliferative Phase

The proliferative phase of healing occurs approximately 4 to 20 days after injury. Formation of granulation tissue is key in this phase.[22] The key cell in this phase of healing, the fibroblast, rapidly synthesizes collagen. Collagen synthesis provides the needed strength for a healing wound. Epithelial cells migrate across the wound bed. After these cells contact each other, the wound is covered. This process is known as *epithelialization.* The wound contraction process occurs when specialized fibroblasts known as *myofibroblasts* pull down the wound edges in an effort to close the wound.

Maturation Phase

The maturation phase, or remodeling phase, of healing occurs approximately 21 days after injury. During this period, the wound develops tensile strength, and the collagen becomes increasingly more organized.[22] Regardless of how well collagen realigns itself, the tissue of the wound will never regain the degree of strength or intactness inherent in uninjured tissue.

Impaired Tissue Integrity

Management of the burn wound is the top priority after the resuscitation phase. The depth of the burn wound is the principal determinant of wound management. Expedient closure of the wounds decreases the potential for many complications such as fluid and electrolyte imbalances, loss of proteins and nitrogen, and infection. The major goal of burn wound care is wound closure. Initial débridement is done by removal of blisters and loose skin. The assessment of wound depth by the clinician guides the treatment based on whether the wound will close in a reasonable time with dressings or will require surgical débridement. The assessment of wound depth can be a difficult challenge. There are many alternative dressing regimens for wound closure that are temporary, semipermanent, or permanent. The following objectives must be met for optimal wound closure: control of infection through meticulous cleansing and débridement, promotion of reepithelialization, and preparation of the wound for grafting and closure. Other goals are reduction of scarring and contracture formation and providing patient comfort with appropriate psychological support and pharmacologic intervention.

Factors Affecting Healing of the Burn Wound

Sources of contamination include the patient's endogenous flora found on the skin, the upper respiratory tract, and the GI tract. Exogenous flora found in the patient care setting include bacteria carried by staff members and present in the environment. Patient-specific factors that predispose the patient to infection include age, diabetes, steroid therapy, extreme obesity, severe malnutrition, and infections in remote sites. Because wound healing and clinical infection are inflammatory responses, it is essential to differentiate between normal wound inflammation in the presence of colonization of microorganisms and that of invading organisms. In diagnosing infection, the importance of microbiologic results must be evaluated in conjunction with clinical findings such as excessive erythema, edema, pain, and purulence. Multidrug-resistant pathogens are increasing; therefore, the appropriate diagnosis and choice of antimicrobial treatment should be guided by the intensity of colonization with these organisms as indicated by cultures from various sites.[23] Clinical findings in conjunction with burn wound biopsy or culture results determine the diagnosis of wound infection. A burn wound infection can delay healing and increase scarring, and invasive infection can result in death of the patient.[24] Other factors that affect wound healing are tissue hypoxia from low blood flow to the burn wound, presence of eschar that requires débridement, exudate on the wound that can be harmful to the granulating wound or consume oxygen in the wound, and trauma to the wound from daily dressing changes or lack of protection from the outside environment.

Wound Cleansing

A variety of equally appropriate methods can be used to cleanse burn wounds (eg, sterile normal saline at the bedside, tap water in a hydrotherapy room). At some centers, a mild antimicrobial cleansing agent may be used. Wounds are gently cleaned with a gauze dressing or washcloth and patted dry before application of topical agents. Hydrotherapy facilitates the removal of debris and loose eschar. The prevalence of immersion hydrotherapy has been decreasing as more centers incorporate showering measures.[25] Frequent cleansing and inspection of the wound and unburned skin are performed to assess for signs of healing and local infection. Wound care exposure is limited as much as feasible to prevent hypothermia and decrease exposure to bacteria. Measures to reduce pain and hypothermia are used. Patients must receive adequate premedication with analgesics, opiates, and sedatives.

Wound Care

Although many options for burn wound care are available, the basic principle of maintaining a moist wound environment while preventing wound infection is the standard of care. Benefits include preventing wound desiccation, optimal function of local wound growth factors and proteolytic enzymes to remove dead tissue, increased reepithelialization and collagen synthesis, and decreased wound fluid loss. The most common regimen for burn wound care involves the application of a topical antimicrobial agent, followed by a primary nonstick dressing. An outer layer is applied to provide increased absorption, compression, and occlusion.

Another method consists of covering the wound with a thin layer of gauze or nonadherent dressing that can be impregnated with a petroleum product, with or without a topical antimicrobial. This method is useful for less severe wounds when the amount of drainage has decreased and wound closure has almost been achieved.

Topical Antibiotic Therapy

Burn injuries destroy the function of the skin's protective mechanism, including the function of sebaceous glands. Sebaceous glands normally secrete sebum, which contains fatty acids, including oleic acid. In addition to lubricating the skin, sebum is believed to help destroy some microorganisms, such as streptococci and some strains of staphylococci. Serum is lost from damaged capillaries, providing a rich nutrition medium for bacterial colonization. Topical antibiotic agents are used to control this colonization. Burn infection continues to be a concern during treatment, and topical use of antimicrobial agents plays an important role in the control of burn wound infection.[26] Effective antibacterial agents should control colonization so that specimens for wound biopsy reveal less than 10^5 microorganisms per gram of tissue. With more than 10^5 microorganisms per gram of tissue, control of wound sepsis with topical antibiotics is questionable, and oral or intravenous therapy may then be considered. The topical antibiotics selected must meet several criteria: Side effects must be minimal, resistant strains must not develop with use, application must be easy and rapid, and use must be relatively economical. The most commonly used topical antibiotics are SSD (Silvadene cream), mafenide acetate cream (Sulfamylon), bacitracin ointment, and silver impregnated into the primary dressing (Table 35.2). With multidrug-resistant pathogens increasing, deciding on the appropriate topical treatment is important.

SSD is a broad-spectrum antimicrobial agent with bactericidal action against many gram-negative and gram-positive bacteria associated with burn wound infection. SSD is indicated for use with partial-thickness and full-thickness wounds. It is a white cream that is applied once or twice daily to the burn wound. Moisture provided by the wound exudate may give the SSD cream layer a yellow-gray pseudoeschar. A common side effect of SSD is leukopenia resulting from bone marrow

TABLE 35.2   Pharmacologic Management
Topical Antimicrobial Agents

Agent	Advantages	Disadvantages	Implications
SSD	Painless application	May produce transient leukopenia by bone marrow suppression	Monitor WBC count
	Broad spectrum	Minimal eschar penetration	Observe wounds for tunneling and subeschar infection
	Easy application	Some gram-negative resistance	Monitor culture reports
	Rare sensitivities		
Mafenide acetate cream	Broad spectrum (especially *Pseudomonas* coverage)	Painful application	Provide adequate analgesia
	Easy application	Rare acid–base imbalance	Monitor arterial blood gases
	Penetrates eschar	Frequent sensitivities	Observe for hyperventilation Observe for rashes
Bacitracin	Painless application	No eschar penetration	
	Nonirritating	No gram-negative or fungal coverage	
	Transparent		
	Nontoxic		
Pure silver	Painless application	Keep moist with sterile water, not saline	Maintain dry linens
	Broad spectrum, including fungus and resistant organisms		No reported side effects
	Rare sensitivity		
	Less frequent dressing changes		

SSD, silver sulfadiazine; *WBC*, white blood cell.

suppression, which may develop 24 to 72 hours after application. Rebound to normal leukocyte levels follows onset within 2 to 3 days, and it is not necessary to discontinue SSD use.[26]

Mafenide acetate cream penetrates through burn eschar and is bacteriostatic against many gram-negative and gram-positive organisms.[26] Its use is limited because the application is uncomfortable for the patient, as it creates a burning sensation, and it is rapidly absorbed, requiring dressing changes two or three times daily. It is used routinely for coverage of small wounds involving anatomic areas that contain cartilage such as the ears and nose. Metabolic acidosis can result from the use of mafenide acetate. The patient must be observed closely for hyperventilation (see Table 35.2).

Bacitracin ointment is a topical agent applied to superficial burns and facial burns. Bacitracin is effective against gram-positive organisms but not against gram-negative organisms or fungal organisms. Bacitracin is applied to the wound one or two times daily and covered with a nonstick dressing. The ease of use, cost, and accessibility make it a common treatment in burn wounds. A yeast rash is commonly associated with repeated bacitracin usage.[26]

Silver has long been used for the treatment of wounds because of its broad-spectrum bacteriostatic properties against gram-negative and gram-positive bacteria.[27] Silver has minimal side effects and minimal bacterial resistance. The wound moisture activates the silver and releases it into the wound. An advantage of silver dressings is that the dressing does not need to be changed daily because of the sustained release of silver. Several silver-impregnated dressings are available from different manufacturers. These dressings are a popular choice by patients and providers because they decrease dressing change frequency.

Wound Débridement

Eschar is the nonviable tissue that forms after a burn injury. This tissue has no blood supply, and polymorphonuclear leukocytes, antibodies, and systemic antibodies cannot reach these areas. Eschar provides an excellent medium for bacterial growth, and it is vital that loose eschar is débrided as necessary. Débridement has two major aims: (1) removal of tissue contaminated by foreign bodies and bacteria to protect patients from invasive infection and (2) removal of devitalized tissue. The three types of débridement are mechanical, enzymatic, and surgical.

Mechanical débridement. Mechanical débridement involves the use of scissors and forceps to gently lift and trim loose, necrotic tissue (Fig. 35.11). Only experienced nurses and physicians perform this procedure. Sterile gauze may be used in the form of a wet-to-dry or wet-to-wet dressing to further débride the wound bed.

Enzymatic débridement. Enzymatic débridement involves the topical application of proteolytic substances to the wound bed. These agents are useful in softening eschar and dissolving devitalized tissue. They promote the separation of eschar, which can lead to earlier wound closure.

Surgical débridement. An experienced surgeon performs surgical débridement in the operating room. The goal of débridement is to remove nonviable tissue down to bleeding viable tissue with an electric dermatome or surgical knife.

Skin Substitutes

To assist in wound closure, many temporary and permanent skin substitute dressings have gained popularity in the United

States. A wide variety of products are available. Each dressing has specific indications for use. Temporary substitutes are designed for placement on partial-thickness or clean, excised wounds, and permanent substitutes provide a permanent skin replacement.

Skin substitutes must possess properties that mimic the native epidermis and dermis. They are made from various synthetic materials such as nylon, polyurethane, or solid silicone polymers. Skin barrier substitutes must possess several properties to accomplish their desired effect as a temporary wound covering to protect the granulating tissue and to preserve a clean, viable wound surface for future autografting (Box 35.2). The most important property of these materials is adherence so that the skin substitute can simulate the function of the skin. Adherence must be uniform to prevent fluid accumulation

FIG. 35.11 Anterior Trunk and Bilateral Arm Burn. (A) Before mechanical débridement. (B) After mechanical débridement.

BOX 35.2 Ideal Properties of Skin Substitutes

- Adherence
- Decreased pain
- Easy application and removal
- Intact bacterial barrier
- Shelf storage capability
- Inexpensive in relation to alternatives
- Nonantigenic
- Similar to normal skin in transport of water vapor
- Elastic and durable
- Hemostatic
- Decreased protein and electrolyte loss
- Enhanced natural healing processes

beneath the surface of the substitute, which can lead to bacterial proliferation.

For application of skin substitutes, the wound must be clean and ideally should have a bacterial count of less than 10^5 organisms per gram of tissue. The burn wound must be free from eschar, and hemostasis must exist. Eschar and blood provide an excellent medium for bacterial proliferation, and the presence of blood may interfere with adherence. The surface is cleaned and rinsed with saline solution, and the skin barrier substitutes must be applied according to established procedures using sterile techniques.

Definitive Burn Wound Closure

The primary goal of burn wound management is wound closure during the acute phase. Early excision and grafting of full-thickness (third-degree) burns is the gold standard in burn centers.[26] Some deep-dermal partial-thickness burns that have a prolonged healing time may also benefit from excision and grafting. Early excision should be undertaken to improve functional and cosmetic results, decrease infection risk, decrease in-hospital time, and reduce the cost of burn care. Surgical débridement may begin 3 to 5 days after the burn insult, as soon as hemodynamic stability has been achieved. Some physicians operate within 24 hours of admission if the patient is hemodynamically stable. To minimize contraction, burn wounds over joint surfaces should be excised and grafted as soon as possible. Typically, excision procedures are limited to 20% of the body surface or 2 hours of operating time. In patients with massive burns, excision procedures are commonly staged, requiring the patient to return to the operating room every 2 to 3 days until all wounds have been excised. Table 35.3 summarizes advantages and disadvantages of different graft types.

Autograft

An autograft is a skin graft harvested from a healthy, uninjured donor site on the burn patient and then placed over the patient's burn wound to provide permanent coverage of the wound. Autografts are the only grafts that provide permanent wound coverage. Preferred sites for obtaining these grafts are the thighs, back, and abdomen; however, grafts can be harvested from almost anywhere on the body. Autografting with the patient's own skin from a donor site is the preferred choice for wound closure. However, with large TBSA burns, availability of donor sites can be problematic. When an autograft is unavailable, many alternative methods are used to achieve this goal. Skin substitutes can be used until the patient's own skin is available for harvesting. Previously used and healed donor sites can be used again on later return visits to the operating room.

Surgical excision is performed to mechanically remove necrotic tissue from the burn wound; it may be performed tangentially or fascially. Tangential excision involves sequentially excising the eschar down to bleeding, viable tissue and then placing a split-thickness skin graft over the wound. Fascial excision is used when the wounds are deep and the fat does not appear viable. Sheets of the patient's epidermis and a partial layer of the dermis are harvested with use of a dermatome. These grafts are referred to as *split-thickness skin grafts* and can be applied to the wound bed as a sheet or in meshed form (Fig. 35.12). The size of the mesh is based on the areas requiring grafting and the availability of donor skin. This meshing prevents serum accumulation under the graft and permits coverage of a surface area larger than its original surface.[28] Sheet grafts are placed on the face, neck, lower portions of the arms, and hands when possible. Mesh grafts can cover more area but may not produce the cosmetic appearance desired; therefore, they are usually placed on areas covered by clothing.

The grafts can be secured with sutures, fibrin glue, or staples. The choice of dressing that is placed over the graft varies widely based on physician and institution preference. One choice is fine mesh gauze impregnated with an emollient. It is placed over the graft, covered with a heavy gauze dressing, and secured to the patient with or without a splint, depending on the anatomic area of the graft. A vacuum-assisted closure (VAC) device provides a safe and effective method for securing split-thickness skin grafts, and it is associated with improved graft survival.[29] Negative wound pressure therapy can be used to secure the graft in place. The VAC is reliable and should also be considered when the wound bed and grafting conditions are suboptimal. VAC-trained nursing professionals or physicians remove the dressings on postoperative day 3 to 5 for assessment of adherence and graft survival. Nurses, in collaboration with the multidisciplinary team, provide proper positioning, splinting, and pain management in the postoperative period. Great care must be taken not to disturb the graft. Mobilization of the graft area usually occurs around the first dressing change on postoperative day 3 to 5, according to the surgeon's preference.

TABLE 35.3	**Types of Grafts**		
Graft	**Use**	**Advantages**	**Disadvantages**
Autograft	Provides permanent coverage of burn wounds	Permanent coverage	Lack of available donor sites, which may delay wound coverage
	Used in sheets or meshed form	Nonantigenic	Donor sites are painful partial-thickness wounds
		Least expensive	Must be done in surgical suite
		Meshing allows small amount of tissue to cover large area	
Homograft (allograft)	Temporary wound coverage	Can be placed at bedside or in operating room	Possibility of disease transmission
		Allows for vascularization over deep wound	Antigenic; body rejects in approximately 2 weeks
		Provides better control over bacterial growth than xenograft	Not readily available to all burn centers
			Expensive
			Requires rigorous quality controls

FIG. 35.12 (A) Split-thickness skin graft. (B) Sheet graft to left buttock.

Care of the donor site is equally important because it represents a wound similar to that of a partial-thickness injury. Donor sites can be covered with many different types of dressings. These dressings should not be removed forcibly because this would interfere with the reepithelialization process and cause considerable pain.

Biosynthetic Skin Substitutes

Skin substitutes include homografts (allografts) and heterografts (xenografts). *Homograft skin* can be obtained from living donors or deceased donors (cadaver skin). With advances in cryopreservation, a homograft harvested from cadaver skin can be frozen and stored in a tissue bank. Because it is possible to transmit disease through the application of a homograft, tissue banks must adhere to strict guidelines. Before application, homograft skin is tested for various transmissible diseases including human immunodeficiency virus and hepatitis B surface antigens. Homograft skin can be applied as a biologic dressing for débridement at the bedside or as temporary wound coverage on excised burn wounds. Vascular ingrowth occurs, and the homograft seals the wound and protects it from bacterial invasion; however, it is rejected approximately 2 weeks after its application. Disadvantages include the homograft antigenicity, lack of accessibility, difficulties with storage and quality control, expense of procurement, and possibility of disease transmission from the donor. Homografts are harvested during

the first 4 hours after death, and they are taken from the abdomen, thighs, and back. Homografts usually are available only in centers in which the rigorous processing procedure can be achieved. These centers usually have skin and tissue bank facilities. Procurement of the allograft is much the same as for any other donated organ.

A *xenograft* (heterograft) is a graft transferred between two different species to provide temporary wound coverage. The most common and widely accepted xenograft is pigskin (porcine skin). Pigskin is available in frozen and shelf forms, with each type having a much longer storage life than an allograft. The pigskin is packaged in a variety of ways and in various sizes. It can be meshed or nonmeshed. Pigskin can be used for temporary coverage of full-thickness and partial-thickness wounds, burn wounds, and donor sites. It meets many of the ideal skin substitute properties mentioned previously. It has two disadvantages: (1) It is antigenic, and (2) it has the potential for being digested by the wound collagenase, possibly leading to infection.

After the pigskin is in place, it may be dressed with antibacterial-impregnated dressings or other forms of dressings. Pigskin usually is removed or dissolves because of lack of blood supply in 5 to 7 days. If sloughing or purulent drainage occurs, the xenograft is removed (see Table 35.3).

Synthetic Skin

The lack of available donor sites for major burn injury often delays wound closure. In an effort to minimize infection and to promote healing, many attempts have been made to develop skin substitutes that seal the wound in a functional and cosmetically acceptable fashion. Integra has become a very popular dermal substitute with its ultrathin layer of epidermal autograft used successfully.[30] Integra is intended to be placed on freshly excised, full-thickness burns, and the outer silicone membrane is replaced with an ultrathin epithelial autograft 2 to 3 weeks later. Integra can also lead to more superficial donor sites. A technique that involves the growth and subsequent graft placement of cultured epithelial autograft (CEA) has also become an adjunct to the treatment of burn wounds. A complex process that allows for separation of keratinocytes is performed. The CEA is grown over 2 to 3 weeks to achieve a graft size of 25 cm². This represents an expansion of 50 to 70 times the original specimen. These confluent sheets of cultured epithelial cells are attached to a gauze backing and placed on the wound. Published results reveal that graft acceptance is unpredictable because the CEA lacks dermis. Even when grafts take initially, graft loss can occur later. Compared with other methods, the CEA also is more fragile, and the technique is costly. This therapy is being recommended as an adjunct for traditional split-thickness skin graft, and it continues to be investigated and combined with newer dermal skin substitutes.

Imbalanced Nutrition: Less Than Body Requirements

The basal metabolic rate of a burn patient may be elevated 40% to 100% above the normal rate, depending on the amount of TBSA involved. The metabolic rate is influenced by the amount of protein and albumin lost through the wounds; the catabolic response associated with stress, injuries, fluid loss, fever, infection, and immobility; gender; and height and weight of the patient before the injury. A 10% loss of total body mass leads to immune dysfunction; 20% leads to decreased wound healing; 30% leads to severe infections; a 40% loss leads to death.

Severely burned, catabolic patients can lose 25% of total body mass after acute severe burn injury.[16]

The goal in nutrition management of a burn patient is to provide adequate calories to enhance wound healing. To achieve this goal, nutrition support and a reduction of energy demand are imperative. Every effort should be made to reduce the release of catecholamines, which increase metabolic rate. Pain, fear, anxiety, and cold stimulate release of catecholamine stores. Appropriate interventions for each of these stimuli must be performed. Examples of nonpharmacologic interventions include early excision and burn wound closure; elevation of the environmental temperature to thermal neutrality (31.5°C ± 0.7°C); and high-carbohydrate, high-protein feeds.

Because of the increased nutrition needs of burn patients, oral feedings are usually inadequate, and supplemental enteral feedings are necessary. Caloric requirements are calculated on the basis of the size of the burn; the age, height, and weight of the patient; and stress factors. Protein and caloric requirements for the burn patient are elevated by a negative nitrogen balance. The daily protein requirement may increase to two to four times the normal 0.8 g/kg of body weight. Carbohydrates and fat are used for energy and to spare proteins required for wound healing. Daily caloric intake can be 2 to 20 times higher than normal. Vitamins and minerals usually are given in doses higher than normal. Serum albumin, prealbumin, iron, zinc, calcium, phosphate, and potassium values are monitored, and supplements are given as needed.[16]

Pain Management

Burn injuries are very painful. Pain management must be addressed early and frequently reassessed. Pain is an individualized and subjective phenomenon, and it has physiologic and psychological components. Pain results from the acute burn injury and occurs throughout the phases of healing. Background pain is related to the physiologic changes associated with the burn injury and includes the damage or exposure of the nerve endings within partial-thickness burns and donor sites. Range of motion of the affected limbs and routine activities contribute to background pain. Breakthrough pain is described as episodes of pain more severe than background pain; breakthrough pain is not relieved by routine pain medications. Procedural pain includes pain caused by interventions such as daily wound care, arterial punctures, physical and occupational therapy, and the use of splints.

Initially after burn injury, narcotics are administered intravenously in small doses and titrated to effect. The constant background pain may be addressed with the use of a patient-controlled analgesia device. After hemodynamic stability has occurred and GI function has returned, oral narcotics can be useful. Intramuscular or subcutaneous injections must not be administered because absorption by these routes is unpredictable owing to the fluid shifts that occur with burn injury. Additional premedication and analgesics are necessary during therapeutic procedures. Acetaminophen and nonsteroidal antiinflammatory drugs can be useful in patients who are not at risk for bleeding. Anxiolytics and antidepressants also should be considered and used appropriately. The nurse must be flexible with dosing and should assess the effectiveness of medication by using a numerical or visual analog scale. The nurse should assure the patient that pain control issues will be continually addressed.[31]

Pain continues even after healing; some patients describe the itching, tingling, and paresthesias as being as uncomfortable as the initial injury. Paresthesias are abnormal neurologic sensations of numbness, tingling, or burning that can last 1 year or longer after injury. Inadequate pain management is an issue in many burn units because of the fear of opioid side effects and opioid addiction and the lack of pain evaluation or treatment protocols.

Loss of control, forced dependence, loneliness, and separation from home and family can contribute to anxiety, which heightens the patient's perception of pain. The patient's fears abound in thoughts of disfigurement and loss of love, function, and job. The psychological experience or subjective component may be related to past experiences, anxiety, and altered coping mechanisms. Attention to the psychological component of the patient's pain may lead to useful strategies that decrease perceived pain. If possible, past experiences with pain, hospitalization, and successful coping strategies should be explored. Pain is a psychological and physical experience that accumulates over time and becomes part of the individual's deepest psychology.

Nonpharmacologic techniques such as imagery, hypnosis, and distraction can be effective in reducing anxiety and the pain experience. Giving the patient some control over pain management also can reduce anxiety and the perception of pain. The perception of pain often is increased in a patient who is anxious and lacks control of the situation.

Treatment strategies need to be individualized. Failure to adequately treat pain can increase burn hypermetabolism, result in loss of confidence between the burn team and patient, and lead to the development of psychiatric disorders. The nurse should assess and discuss on a regular basis the patient's psychological status and avoid using psychotropics for analgesia and narcotics for anxiety and depression.

Rehabilitation Phase

The rehabilitation phase is one of recuperation and healing physically and emotionally. This phase can last several years. Psychological rehabilitation is equal in importance to physical rehabilitation in burn patients. The patient may require extensive reconstructive surgery. Psychologically, the patient focuses on attaining specific personal goals related to achieving as much preburn function as possible. A person's preburn level of physical and emotional functioning can greatly affect the course of recovery. Minor and major accomplishments must be praised. This phase is characterized by scar management techniques and by physical and occupational therapies.

The burn team and the patient prepare for the transition to the outside world. Group therapy is a valuable tool used at many burn centers. Patients, family members, and health care providers express ideas and feelings. Burn patients often establish priorities and make realistic decisions about their lives. Staff intervention during this phase is primarily of a supportive nature.

Impaired Physical Mobility

Tremendous advances have been made in the physical care of burn patients. As more patients with larger and deeper burns survive, the challenge to maintain their optimal mobility and cosmetic appearance has been met with increased success. Despite advances in other areas of burn care, contractures still

FIG. 35.13 Severe Contracture to Bilateral Lower Extremities.

develop after a burn injury. A contracture is the shortening of a scar over a joint surface and is the primary cause of functional deficits in burn patients (Fig. 35.13). Contractures develop as a result of various factors including the extent, depth, location, and configuration of the burn; the position of comfort the patient most frequently assumes; the relative underlying muscle strength; and the patient's motivation and compliance. The affected body parts should be positioned to prevent long-term deformity. Frequent change of position also is important and may need to be performed as often as every hour. Burn patients are at greater risk for pressure sores than the general hospital population.

Splints can be used to prevent or correct contracture or to immobilize joints after grafting. If splints are used, they must be checked daily for proper fit and effectiveness. Splints that are used to immobilize body parts after grafting must be left on at all times except to assess the graft site for pressure points during every shift. Splints to correct severe contracture may be off for 2 hours per shift to allow burn care and range-of-motion exercises.

Active exercise is encouraged and is preferred, although active-assisted or gentle-passive exercises also may be an important part of the rehabilitation program. Active exercise maintains muscle mass, aids in restoring protein structures within the muscle tissue, aids in venous and lymphatic return, and reduces the risk of pulmonary embolus and deep vein thrombosis. The patient's tolerance must be carefully evaluated. The number of repetitions of an exercise is proportional to the degree of anticipated contracture and the patient's tolerance. Anticipation of the patient's pain also must be carefully considered. Before range-of-motion exercises and activities of daily living are performed, the need for pain medication must be assessed. Nursing diagnoses for the burn patient are summarized in Box 35.3 and Box 35.4.

Scar Management

A person's skin response to a burn injury can be barely noticeable such as slight color change or lead to cosmetic disfigurement and dysfunction. The goal of scar management is to minimize scarring. It is important to inform the patient that the tissue may not return to the preburn texture or appearance. Hypertrophic scars are red and raised and lack elasticity, and they are painful and itchy. The highest risk

FIG. 35.14 Healed Split-Thickness Skin Graft to Bilateral Feet.

for scar tissue development is associated with deep-dermal partial-thickness and full-thickness burns because of their depth and increased risk of infection. Areas of the skin that required skin grafting also have a visible scar (Fig. 35.14). Scar maturation occurs 6 months to 2 years from the time of the injury. One method to reduce scar formation is timely application of uniform pressure. Custom-made elastic pressure garments are worn for 6 months to 1 year, if needed (Fig. 35.15). These garments reduce scar blood flow and may provide force that helps developing collagen to organize. Although compression therapy is one of the main methods

FIG. 35.15 Compression Garment to Right Leg.

of prophylaxis and treatment of burn scars, its mechanism is not totally understood.

Additional approaches to reduce scarring are scar massage, high-SPF sun protection, silicone gel sheeting, and steroid treatment. Scar massage works by stretching the scar and providing moisture and is most helpful in preventing contractures. Sun protection over the healed burn may decrease the long-term pigment change to the injured area. Silicone gel sheets are used alone over the scar or in conjunction with compression to soften the scar by maintaining scar hydration and tension reduction. Injectable or topical steroids are used for treatment of hypertrophic scars; however, they have some side effects that may make them undesirable. Corticosteroid injections inhibit fibroblast growth and enhance collagen breakdown leading to a flatter and softer scar. Topical steroid treatment poses less risk, but it has been found to be less effective. If less invasive techniques have been unsuccessful for troublesome scars that cause pain or inhibit full range of motion, surgical excision may be recommended.

Itching

Pruritus is common in the maturing burn wound and commonly replaces burn pain. Itching can be extremely uncomfortable for the patient and should be continually assessed.[32] For 6 to 8 weeks, a mild, non–alcohol-based skin cream is applied every 4 hours to healed areas to lubricate the skin until natural lubrication occurs. Patients can be relieved of discomfort by the administration of an antipruritic agent such as diphenhydramine and by the application of moisturizing creams.

Multidisciplinary Care

A multidisciplinary approach to burn treatment is an integral part of providing quality care. This approach involves considering all aspects of the patient's care when treatment decisions are made.[3] The burn team should work together to address all needs of the patient and the family. The team should meet frequently to review patient care and maximize patient and family support. The multidisciplinary team includes, but is not limited to, physicians and nurses and individuals from social work, nutrition, physical and occupational therapy, respiratory therapy, psychology, pain service, child life services, and utilization review.

Outpatient Burn Care

Outpatient burn care can be considered for patients with minor burns. Patients with larger burns can be transitioned to outpatient care when ready. It is cost-effective and removes the potential for a wound infection by endemic, drug-resistant microorganisms within the hospital environment. The hospital environment also changes many self-care routines such as diet, family contact, hygiene, and coping mechanisms. However, patients considered for outpatient burn care must be screened carefully. Nursing evaluation of the patient and the family includes consideration of motivation, willingness to participate in care, ability to understand and perform the necessary procedures, potential aversions to wound care or dressing changes, and reliability of transportation. The transition to outpatient care must also include consideration of physical and occupational therapy needs and involve exercises designed to accelerate return to activities of daily living such as work, school, or both. Home health nurses are helpful in monitoring patients.

Support of the Burn Patient

Burn injuries are physically and psychologically traumatic and life altering for the patient. The family of the burn patient is also affected, and their needs should be remembered during the healing process. Guilt is often associated with burn injuries, especially when the victim is a child. It is important for care providers to support the burn patient physically and psychologically. Health care providers heal and support the patient throughout the hospital stay but often forget that the patient's biggest challenges may still lie ahead after hospitalization.

Many resources are available to help burn patients cope after they are home, and these resources should be provided by the hospital team during the inpatient stay. Research has shown that many patients have difficulty returning to work and desire a coordinator during the rehabilitation process to assess work capacity.[33] Programs are available to help with issues including social and school reentry, support for sexual considerations, and dealing with scars.

STRESSORS OF BURN NURSING

Burn units can be stimulating workplaces in that they offer the fast-paced, high-technology atmosphere of any critical care setting; the complexity of advanced nursing management; and the dynamics of an interdisciplinary, collaborative model of practice. However, all these elements combined contribute to a potentially stressful work environment for the staff. The physical environment can be a difficult one for a variety of reasons. The amount of equipment necessary to maintain the patient can be overwhelming and can limit the workspace dramatically. The temperature of the room usually is kept at approximately 85°F and can become much warmer, depending on the amount of equipment in the room. The various odors in the room may be very unpleasant. Noise levels within a unit also are distressing. Research has shown that although nurses are emotionally supportive to patients and families, the emotional support available to staff is lacking.[34] Self-care and care of other nurses and staff are issues just as important as the care of the patient and the family. The decision to specialize in burn nursing requires careful consideration.

CASE STUDY 35.1 Patient With Burns

Brief Patient History

Ms. J is a 40-year-old victim of a car crash. She was found conscious at the scene and pulled out of a burning car to safety by a passerby. The paramedics at the scene reported her as awake but disoriented and anxious. She is otherwise healthy and is the mother of a 5-year-old child, who was also rescued at the scene with no injuries.

Clinical Assessment

Ms. J is sent from the emergency department to the trauma unit. She is intubated and sedated on arrival. She has partial-thickness burns covering her face, including her nose, lips, and neck. She has areas of partial-thickness and full-thickness burns to both her hands and to her chest and left leg. Her breath sounds are auscultated as present bilaterally, but she is wheezing, and her sputum has a dark carbon appearance. She has a triple-lumen catheter in her right femoral vein with good blood return to all ports.

Diagnostic Procedures

Ms. J has a carboxyhemoglobin level of 3.4% and arterial blood gas values as follows: pH of 7.27, arterial partial pressure of carbon dioxide of 29 mm Hg, arterial partial pressure of oxygen of 313 mm Hg, bicarbonate of 14 mEq/L (mmol/L), and oxygen saturation of 88% on 100% fraction of inspired oxygen. Her serum cyanide level is 45 mmol/L. The chest radiograph obtained on arrival in the emergency department was normal. Blood pressure is 85/50 mm Hg, heart rate is 136 beats/min (sinus tachycardia), respiratory rate is 14 breaths/min, and temperature is 96.3°F.

Medical Diagnosis

Ms. J is diagnosed with burns covering 40% of total body surface area, inhalation injury, and cyanide toxicity.

Questions

1. What major outcomes do you expect to achieve for this patient?
2. What problems or risks must be managed to achieve these outcomes?
3. What interventions must be initiated to monitor, prevent, manage, or eliminate the problems and risks identified?
4. What interventions should be initiated to promote optimal functioning, safety, and well-being of the patient?
5. What possible learning needs do you anticipate for this patient?
6. What cultural and age-related factors may have a bearing on the patient's plan of care?

QSEN BOX 35.5 QSEN: Informatics

Internet Resources

American Burn Association: http://www.ameriburn.org

SUMMARY

- Burn care is highly complex, and decisions regarding appropriate management of burn injuries are best managed by certified burn centers, where the most accurate burn size estimates can be made.
- Burn size, type of injury, location of the burn, and the patient's age and history all are determinants of survival.
- Size and depth of burns are divided into four main categories: (1) superficial (first-degree) burns, which are injuries to epidermis; (2) partial-thickness (second-degree) burns, which involve the epidermis and dermis of the skin; (3) deep-dermal partial-thickness (second-degree) burns, which involve the entire epidermal layer of the skin and part of the dermis; and (4) full-thickness (third-degree) burns, which involve destruction of skin layers from the epidermis down to and including the subcutaneous tissue.
- Accurate fluid resuscitation of a burn patient for more severe burn injuries (greater than 10% of TBSA) is crucial to prevent AKI that may result in acute kidney failure, cardiovascular collapse, and death from burn shock. The Parkland formula is a guide for determining resuscitation fluid (Ringer lactate) volume.
- Careful assessment of intake and output of the burn patient is critical to achieve the optimal patient response to fluid resuscitation.
- After the resuscitative phase of burn patients, the acute care phase of wound healing, wound closure, and prevention of infection begins. This hypermetabolic phase can be complicated by wound infection and sepsis.
- The gold standard of burn wound care includes the application of a topical antimicrobial agent, followed by a gauze dressing to absorb excess drainage, with an outer layer to provide increased absorption, compression, and occlusion. Silver dressings have shown positive results in the prevention of bacterial growth without silver toxicity.
- The rehabilitative phase of care of the burn patient starts from admission of the patient and may last years, depending on future surgical procedures, therapy needs, contracture prevention, and psychological or emotional needs of the patient.
- All the multidisciplinary needs of burn patients must be addressed for these patients to be able to perform in and feel accepted back into society.

ⓔ Visit the Evolve site for additional study materials.

REFERENCES

1. Klein MB, et al. Benchmarking outcomes in the critically injured burn patient. *Ann Surg*. 2014;259(5):833-841.
2. American Burn Association. *Burn Incidence and Treatment in United States Fact Sheet*; 2015. http://www.ameriburn.org. Accessed September 20, 2015.
3. U.S. Department of Health and Human Services Children's Bureau. *Child Maltreatment*. 2012;2013. http://www.acf.hhs.gov/programs/cb/resource/child-maltreatment-2012. Accessed March 26, 2016.
4. Jamshidi R, Sato TT. Initial assessment and management of thermal burn injuries in children. *Pediatr Rev*. 2013;34:395–404.
5. Lloyd E, et al. Outpatient burns: Prevention and care. *Am Fam Physician*. 2012;85(1):25.
6. Haines, et al. Optimizing emergency management to reduce morbidity and mortality in pediatric burn patients. *Pediatr Emerg Med Pract*. 2015;12(5):1-24.
7. Ellison DL. Burns. *Crit Care Nurs Clin North Am*. 2013;25(2):273-285.
8. Jeschke MG, et al. Morbidity and survival probability in burn patients in modern burn care. *Crit Care Med*. 2015;43:808-815.
9. Pape SA, et al. Burn wound healing time assessed by laser Doppler imaging (LDI). Part 1: Derivation of a dedicated colour code for image interpretation. *Burns*. 2012;38:187-194.
10. Kaiser M, et al. Noninvasive assessment of burn wound severity using optical technology: A review of current and future modalities. *Burns*. 2011;37:377-386.
11. Glatstein MM, et al. Pediatric electrical burn injuries: Experience of a large tertiary care hospital and a review of electrical injury. *Pediatr Emerg Care*. 2013;29(6):737-740.

12. D'Cruz R, et al. Chemical burns in children: Aetiology and prevention. *Burns.* 2015;41:764-769.
13. McPhee SJ, et al. *Current Medical Diagnosis and Treatment.* 51st ed. New York: McGraw-Hill; 2012.
14. Toon MH, et al. Children with burn injuries—assessment of trauma, neglect, violence and abuse. *J Inj Violence Res.* 2011;3(2):98.
15. Horner G. Medical evaluation for child physical abuse: What the PNP needs to know. *J Pediatr Health Care.* 2012;26(3):163-170.
16. Williams F, et al. What, how, and how much should patients with burns be fed? *Surg Clin North Am.* 2011;91(3):609.
17. Brunicardi FC, et al. *Schwartz's Principles of Surgery.* 9th ed. New York: McGraw-Hill; 2010.
18. Tintinalli JE, et al. *Tintinalli's Emergency Medicine: A Comprehensive Study Guide.* 7th ed. New York: McGraw-Hill; 2011.
19. Krishnamoorthy V, Ramaiah R, Bhananker SM. Pediatric burn injuries. *Int J Crit Illn Inj Sci.* 2012;2:128-134.
20. Keltz E, Khan FY, Mann G, Rhabdomyolysis. The role of diagnostic and prognostic factors. *Muscles Ligaments Tendons J.* 2013;3(4):303-312.
21. Kraft R, et al. Occurrence of multi-organ dysfunction in pediatric burn patients—incidence and clinical outcome. *Ann Surg.* 2014;259:381-387.
22. Simon PE. Skin Wound Healing. *Medscape.* 2014. http://emedicine.medscape.com/article/884594-overview. Accessed August 15, 2015.
23. Chong SJ, et al. 5 year analysis of bacteriology culture in a tropical burns ICU. *Burns.* 2011;37:1349-1353.
24. Barajas-Nava LA, et al. Antibiotic prophylaxis for preventing burn wound infection. *Cochrane Database Syst Rev.* 2013;(6):CD008738.
25. Davison PG, Loiselle FB, Nickerson D. Survey on current hydrotherapy use among North American burn centers. *J Burn Care Res.* 2010;31(3):393-399.
26. Glasser JS, et al. Activity of topical antimicrobial agents against multidrug-resistant bacteria recovered from burn patients. *Burns.* 2010;36(8):1172-1184.
27. Gunjan K, et al. A comparative study of the effect of different topical agents on burn wound infections. *Indian J Plast Surg.* 2012;45(2):374.
28. Shimizu R, Kazuo K. Skin Graft Plastic Surgery International 2012. http://dx.doi.org/10.1155/2012/563493. Accessed October 16, 2016.
29. Petkar KS, et al. A prospective randomized controlled trial comparing negative pressure dressing and conventional dressing methods on split-thickness skin grafts in burned patients. *Burns.* 2011;37(6):925-929.
30. Nguyen DQ, Potokar TS, Price P. An objective long-term evaluation of Integra (a dermal skin substitute) and split thickness skin grafts, in acute burns and reconstructive surgery. *Burns.* 2010;36(1):23-28.
31. Barr J, et al. Clinical practice guidelines for the management of pain, agitation, and delirium in adult patients in the intensive care unit. *Crit Care Med.* 2013;41(1):263-306.
32. Carrougher GJ, et al. Pruritus in adult burn survivors: Postburn prevalence and risk factors associated with increased intensity. *J Burn Care Res.* 2013;34(1):94-101.
33. Oster C. Return to work after burn injury: Burn-injured individual's perception of barriers and facilitators. *J Burn Care Res.* 2010;31(4):540.
34. Kellogg MB, Barker M, McCune N. The lived experience of pediatric burn nurses following patient death. *Pediatr Nurs.* 2013;40(6):297-301.

36

Organ Donation and Transplantation

Inna Goldvarg-Abud, Christine Hartley, Mary E. Lough, Teresa J. Shafer, and Schawnté Williams-Taylor

Organ transplantation provides the only opportunity for patients with end-stage organ disease to have an enhanced quality of life and an extended survival. Organ transplantation is accepted as the preferred and often only treatment option for end-stage organ disease. Success rates in patients treated—as well as increases in organ donation from the general public—have improved as the field of organ donation and transplantation has evolved. Such evolution came as a result of increased cultural acceptance of brain death, donation, and transplantation; legal and political efforts to facilitate organ donation; improved procurement and allocation processes; advances in organ preservation, organ recovery, surgical techniques in transplantation, immunology, and immunosuppression; and management of infectious diseases.[1]

In the United States, more than 121,139 people are waiting for a lifesaving or life-enhancing organ transplant. In 2015, the Organ Procurement Transplant Network (OPTN) reported 15,067 donors, of which 9080 were deceased donors and 5987 were living donors (Fig. 36.1). The categories of organ donors are described in Table 36.1. In 2014, 31,868 transplants were performed. This number is encouraging, although insufficient, as one patient is added to a transplant waiting list every 10 minutes.[2] Ongoing collaboration between organ procurement organizations; transplant centers; and critical care nurses, physicians, and other health care workers is necessary to have a significant impact in saving lives through organ and tissue donation and transplantation.

ORGAN DONATION

Role of the Critical Care Nurse in Organ Donation

The critical care nurse is an essential member of the team in the donation process, linking the hospital to the *organ procurement organization* (OPO), physicians, and families of potential donors. The Centers for Medicare and Medicaid Services (CMS) guidelines, The Joint Commission standards, and hospital policies require that patients meeting criteria for imminent death and cardiac death be referred to an OPO in a timely manner.[3] Once the notification has been made, nurses must follow the established donation policies for their hospital in accordance with federal guidelines and state laws. Hospitals will already have worked with their federally designated OPO to develop their hospital policy to ensure that it meets these regulations and laws.

Continued hemodynamic support is necessary during the process of declaration of brain death. Patients progressing to brain death undergo many physiologic changes that can compromise the viability of organs for transplantation. Ensuring that oxygenation and perfusion of the organs is maintained along with electrolyte and acid–base balance preserves the opportunity for donation.

Collaboration between the nurse and the OPO staff is necessary to protect the right of the patient, who may already have made the decision to donate by indicating his or her wishes on a donor registry. After declaration of death, the family is informed that the patient has died. OPO staff will already have checked the donor registry to determine if the individual is a donor and, if so, will inform the family of such and what and how the donation will proceed. If the patient has not made the first-person decision to be a donor, the family will be approached by OPO staff and informed of what can be donated. The family can then make the decision about donation.

Because organ donation and transplantation is now mainstream, families often talk about donation well in advance of brain death declaration because they anticipate in what direction the patient's condition is proceeding. Exactly when donation is discussed varies, and the nurse should be flexible and attentive to the family's informational needs, ensuring first and foremost that the experts, the OPO staff, are there to guide the information-giving process.

During the interval after pronouncement of death and until donation authorization is obtained either by checking the donor registry or by receiving authorization from the family, medical management of the potential donor is continued by the medical and nursing staff, as required by state law, the Uniform Anatomical Gift Act. Following authorization for donation, the OPO assumes the care of the donor, providing direction for medical management. The goal of medical management of the patient shifts toward optimal preservation of organ function so that the organs are suitable for transplant.

After death of the patient, nurses advocate for their patient by ensuring the patient's donation decision is honored or—if the patient had not made such a decision during his or her lifetime—upholding the family's right to be offered the opportunity to donate organs and tissues.[4] Once authorization (formerly known as "consent") is obtained, the OPO coordinator and nurse collaborate on management of the donor according to established donor management protocols. Such protocols include managing fluid and electrolyte imbalances secondary to brain death. Patients commonly have a low circulating volume or high serum sodium levels, as hypertonic sodium may have been administered to prevent brain herniation. The donor management phase corrects deficits in the patient's physiologic status to provide optimal organ function before surgical recovery and preservation.

At a Glance

119,916

people need a lifesaving organ transplant (total waiting list candidates). Of those, **77,290** people are <u>active</u> waiting list candidates. Totals as today 2:25pm

24,892

organ transplants performed so far in 2016

Total Transplants January - September 2016 as of 11/04/2016

11,777

donors

Total Donors January - September 2016 as of 11/04/2016

FIG. 36.1 Growth in US Organ Transplant Waiting List Outpaces Growth in Deceased Organ Donors. (From Department of Health and Human Services. Organ Procurement Transplant Network. The need continues to grow. http://optn.transplant.hrsa.gov/.)

TABLE 36.1	**Categories of Organ Donors**
Brain dead donor	Donor declared dead by neurologic criteria for brain death.
Donation after cardiac death	Donor declared dead by circulatory criteria for death.
Living related donor	Living family member related by blood who donates a kidney, portion of the liver, pancreas, intestine, or lung to another family member.
Living, unrelated donor (directed/ nondirected)	Living individual not related to a patient requiring a transplant who donates a kidney, portion of the liver, pancreas, intestine, or lung to another individual. The donor may be anonymous or altruistic.
Living donor, paired donation	Allocated paired kidney exchange or paired exchange involves two pairs of living kidney donors and transplant candidates who do not have matching blood types. The two candidates "trade" donors so that each candidate receives a kidney from a donor with compatible blood type.

From United Network for Organ Sharing website. http://www.unos.org/donation. Accessed October 6, 2015.

Nursing care shifts from cerebral protective strategies to aggressive donor management along with continued support of the family.[5]

The critical care nurse monitors and records vital signs, intake and output, and oxygenation status; obtains specimens for laboratory tests; and assists with central line insertions and multiple diagnostic assessments such as chest radiograph, bronchoscopy, electrocardiogram (ECG), or echocardiogram to evaluate organ function. This donor management phase of the donation process starts after brain death and continues until the patient is taken to the operating room and organs are recovered.

A study of hospital donation practices and their impact on organ donation outcomes revealed gaps in knowledge of organ donation, brain death, and referral criteria and sometimes a poor relationship between the hospital and OPO.[6] It is important that nurses are knowledgeable about the organ donation process. Nurses must assess their own beliefs that pertain to organ donation, as the attitude of the nurse and care given to the family can impact the outcome of the donation.

Organ Procurement Organization as Part of the Health Care Team

Nurses, physicians, respiratory therapists, social workers, and members of other health care disciplines practice in the hospital because that is where the patients are. OPO staff practice in hospitals because that is where the potential donors are. The 2003 Organ Donation Breakthrough Collaborative focused on interprofessional teamwork to increase organ donation.[7-9]

Gone are the days when hospitals and hospitals staff considered donation "nice-to-do" and an "add-on" in terms of care. The federal government has made clear the responsibility placed on hospitals to actively engage and work through the donation process with OPOs, caring for the donor while the OPO is leading and managing the donor assessment, obtaining authorization, and facilitating the recovery process.

Because only OPO staff or trained designated requestors can make the request for donation, they are part of the health care team. In one of the largest donor family studies in the United States, a primary finding was that speaking to an OPO staff member was one of the few variables highly associated with authorization (vs nonauthorization) for donation.[10] A successful donation environment depends on a deep, close, and open

TABLE 36.2   National Organ Donation and Transplantation Laws

Laws	Type	First Enacted
Uniform Anatomical Gift Act (UAGA)	State law	1968; revised in 1987 and 2006
National Organ Transplant Act (NOTA)	Federal law	1984
Uniform Determination of Death Act (UDDA)	State laws	1980
Hospital conditions of participation— organ donation; Centers for Medicare and Medicaid Services (CMS)	Federal regulation	1998
Medical examiner laws restricting ability of medical examiner or coroner to deny organ donation	State laws	Year varies by state
Omnibus Budget Reconciliation Act (OBRA)	Federal law	1986

relationship with a hospital's designated OPO. The OPO should be called before the patient has died when death is imminent. This requirement is established by federal regulation and state law and is practiced by most hospitals and critical care units as policy and best practice.[3]

National Donation and Transplantation Laws

Organ transplantation is the only medical and surgical therapy that is regulated entirely by law. From donation to transplantation, the federal government—and to some extent state governments—monitor the administrative and financial aspects of this process. These regulations ensure that organs are shared on a fair and equitable basis. In addition, the responsibilities and functions of health care professionals are sanctioned and safeguarded by these laws so that their responsibilities may be discharged with assurance and protection medically, legally, and ethically. The major laws are listed in Table 36.2.

Uniform Anatomical Gift Act

The Uniform Anatomical Gift Act of 1968 established the legal framework for organ and tissue donation and donor designation as well as the priority of legal next-of-kin for authorization in the absence of donor designation. It required that the physician pronouncing or certifying death may not in any way participate in the procedures for removing or transplanting anatomic gifts. It also protects health care professionals from liability associated with donation. The act was later amended to require hospitals to establish agreements with an OPO to coordinate recovery. It prohibits the sale or purchase of organs or tissues. This act clarifies who can provide authorization for donation in the absence of known donor wishes.[11]

Uniform Determination of Death Act

The Uniform Determination of Death Act of 1981 states that an individual who has sustained either (1) irreversible cessation of circulatory and respiratory functions or (2) irreversible cessation of all functions of the entire brain including the brainstem is dead. A determination of death must be made in accordance with accepted medical standards. Most states have adopted similarly worded Determination of Death Acts in their state statutes.

National Organ Transplant Act

The National Organ Transplant Act of 1984 mandated the establishment of the national Organ Procurement and Transplantation Network (OPTN). The United Network for Organ Sharing (UNOS) administers the national contract to operate the OPTN and houses the database that contains the list of waiting recipients nationwide and by which all donor and recipient matches are determined. This act also made it illegal to buy or sell organs and tissues.

Omnibus Budget Reconciliation Act

The Omnibus Budget Reconciliation Act requires OPOs to coordinate the recovery and transplantation process at local levels and requires hospitals to be affiliated with a federally mandated OPO. There is only one designated OPO per service area. This act gave families the right to know about organ and tissue donation by mandating that all hospitals participating in the CMS reimbursement program institute a "required request" policy to ensure that families of potential donors are made aware of the option of organ or tissue donation and their option to decline. Hospitals must have a signed agreement with an OPO, tissue bank, and eye bank.[3]

Medical Examiner State Laws

Medical examiner laws encourage or require the release of organs for transplantation. In some states, medical examiners or justices of the peace cannot deny organ donation, under any circumstances. In other states, they cannot deny organ donation unless they are physically present at the donation surgery viewing the organ(s). In situations such as these, the medical examiner or justice of the peace may request a biopsy while in surgery. These state laws were passed to provide protection for recipients waiting at centers so that every possible organ that can be recovered is being recovered to save a life (see Table 36.2).

Overview of Donation Process

The CMS requires hospitals to notify their respective OPOs of all deaths including patients meeting imminent death criteria and cardiac death to increase the potential for organ, tissue, and eye donation. Table 36.3 lists the types of organ donor referrals made to the OPO. All patients meeting imminent death criteria must be referred within the agreed-on time (usually within 1 hour) of meeting criteria. All cardiac deaths must be referred, regardless of age, medical condition, or cause of death.[3] The nurse or hospital designee makes the initial call to the OPO to provide demographic information, admitting diagnosis, and current neurologic status of the patient. Most OPOs have either in-house staff or on-call coordinators who respond to the initial referral call from the hospital. On-site, the OPO coordinator communicates with the bedside nurse and physicians involved in the care of the patient to obtain information about the patient's present hospital course, the past medical history, and the plan of care.

Determining medical suitability is solely the responsibility of the OPO. Speaking to the family about donation is also the responsibility of the OPO, unless designated requestors at the hospital have been trained to do so.[3]

Types of Referrals

Imminent death referrals include patients with severe acute brain injury who (1) require mechanical ventilation; (2) are in a critical care unit or emergency department; and (3) have clinical findings consistent with a low Glasgow Coma Score, typically 5 or less, for whom physicians are evaluating the diagnosis of brain death or have ordered that life-sustaining therapies be

TABLE 36.3   Types of Referrals to the Organ Procurement Organization

	ORGAN REFERRAL		TISSUE REFERRAL
Brain Death	**Donation After Circulatory Determination of Death**		**Cardiac Arrest**
Irreversible, nonsurvivable brain injury	Irreversible, nonsurvivable brain injury		Patient may or may not have sustained a brain injury
Patient currently maintained on a ventilator	Patient currently maintained on a ventilator		Patient not currently on a ventilator
Tests performed to confirm brain death (eg, clinical examination, apnea test)	Any ventilator-dependent patient where plans are to forego life-sustaining treatment		No cardiac or respiratory activity
First person authorization/authorizing agent gives authorization for donation	Patient has not progressed to brain death		First person authorization/authorizing agent gives authorization for donation
Patient in maintained in ICU while donation evaluation and work-up is completed	Family decides to withdraw life-sustaining therapies		May donate tissue and corneas (eg, bone, heart valves, skin)
To operating room for organ recovery	Family authorizes donation		
Organ donors may also donate tissue and corneas	Patient is extubated, circulatory arrest within 60–90 min, rapid recovery of organs in operating room		
	Organ donors may also donate tissue and corneas		

Developed by staff at LifeGift, Houston, TX.

withdrawn, pursuant to the family's decision.[9] Patients meeting the imminent death referral criteria may be or become brain dead (discussed later in chapter), resulting in *donation after brain death* (DBD).

Cardiac Death

Cardiac death referrals provide the opportunity for patients to be tissue and eye donors (discussed later in chapter) after cardiac asystole. Because of the relatively rare occurrence of brain death or withdrawal of treatment, many more deceased patients have the opportunity to donate tissue and eyes. Transplantable tissues include bone, skin, fascia, cartilage, tendons, ligaments, saphenous veins, heart valves, eyes, and corneas.

The decision to withdraw life-sustaining support, whether due to an advance directive or surrogate decision making, must always be separated from the organ donation decision. When a patient from whom treatment is being withdrawn has also executed a legal document or gift (as a document or gift or on a donor registry), that legal document must be honored, regardless of the mode of death (eg, brain death or cardiac circulatory death). To accomplish both compassionate end-of-life care and the patient's goal of donation, the withdrawal of care and family support need to be carefully coordinated.

Donor Evaluation

Once the initial call is made to the OPO, an organ coordinator will contact the critical care nurse and request specific information regarding the patient's age; sex; race; and neurologic, ventilatory, and hemodynamic status as well as the hospital's plan of care. On-site, the OPO coordinator will assess the patient and review the medical records, history of the current hospitalization, and major procedures to obtain information on surgeries, therapies, current medications, past medical history, laboratory values specific to each organ, pulmonary status, systemic infection, diagnostic reports, and hemodynamic status.[12] The time between brain death declaration and organ procurement is often marked by significant instability. During this time, optimal medical management is crucial to ensure posttransplant graft survival.

If the patient is not brain dead or there are no plans to withdraw or decelerate support, the OPO coordinator collaborates with the critical care nurse on a follow-up plan for ongoing evaluation. The OPO continues to follow the patient until the patient meets neurologic criteria for brain death, death is declared, or there is a plan to withdraw life-sustaining support. Many patients referred to the OPO do not become donors because they do not meet brain death criteria or there are no plans to withdraw life-sustaining support, as the patient's status may improve. Patients declared dead by neurologic criteria constitute only 1% of total deaths in the United States.[13]

Brain Death

Brain death is the irreversible cessation of all brain functions including the brainstem. The clinical diagnosis of brain death is based on guidelines established by the American Academy of Neurology. The practice of brain death declaration varies based on hospital policy and state legislation. Neurologists, neurosurgeons, intensivists, and anesthesiologists usually perform the brain death evaluation. Before establishing brain death, certain conditions must be confirmed, including the cause and the irreversibility of coma and confounding factors such as the following:

- Absence of severe hypothermia, defined as a core temperature of 32°C or less
- Absence of hypotension, defined as a systolic blood pressure of 90 mm Hg or less
- Absence of evidence of drug intoxication or poisoning, defined by a careful history, calculation of clearance, and, if needed, a normal drug screen
- Absence of recent or current administration of neuromuscular-blocking medications, defined by the presence of four twitches with maximal ulnar nerve stimulation by a train-of-four peripheral nerve stimulation as shown in Fig. 20.17 in Chapter 20
- Absence of electrolyte, acid–base, or endocrine dysfunction, as defined by severe acidosis and marked deviation from normal values

Clinical Examination for Brain Death

The bedside clinical examination has three components: (1) absence of cerebral motor reflexes, (2) absence of brainstem reflexes, and (3) absence of respiratory drive.

Cerebral motor responses. Cerebral motor responses to pain in all extremities are absent in brain death. These motor responses can be stimulated by the application of pressure to the nail beds or supraorbital ridge. Some motor responses may occur spontaneously during apnea testing because of the presence of hypoxia or hypotension and are considered spinal cord reflexes. These may also be elicited in the presence of respiratory acidosis and can include spontaneous flexion and muscle stretch reflexes in the arms and legs that can resemble grasping movements. It is important to determine whether the patient has been given any neuromuscular blocking medications that may induce pharmacologic motor weakness.

Brainstem reflexes. Brainstem reflexes that are tested include pupillary signs, ocular movements, facial sensory and motor responses, and pharyngeal and tracheal reflexes.

Pupillary reflexes. Pupillary signs are evaluated by absence of the light reflex, which is consistent with brain death. Most often the pupils are round, oval, or irregularly shaped, although dilated pupils may remain even after brain death has occurred. This dilation may exist if the sympathetic cervical pathways to the pupillary dilator muscle are intact. Medications do not normally alter pupil response, although the application of topical medications or severe trauma to the eye may affect pupil reactivity.[14]

Oculocephalic reflex. Ocular movements are lost with brain death. The *oculocephalic reflex,* also described as *doll's eyes,* involves fast turning of the head to both sides. In brain death, this should not generate any eye movements. Neck movements should be avoided in patients with a traumatic brain injury or cervical spine injury.

Oculovestibular reflex. Because the oculovestibular reflex is tested using iced water or normal saline, it is sometimes called *cold calorics.* The head of the bed is elevated 30 degrees, and approximately 50 mL of ice water or normal saline is injected into the ear; no movement of the eye toward the side of the stimulus should be present. It is recommended that the patient be observed for up to 1 minute after each ear irrigation, and 5 minutes should be allowed before testing the opposite ear. Medications that can influence the oculovestibular reflex include sedatives, aminoglycosides, tricyclic antidepressants, anticholinergics, and antiseizure agents.

Corneal and jaw reflexes. Facial sensory and motor responses are elicited by testing for corneal and jaw reflexes. Stroking a cotton-tipped swab gently across the cornea tests the corneal reflexes. Grimacing in response to pain can be elicited by applying deep pressure to the nail beds, the supraorbital ridge, or the temporomandibular joint. Severe trauma within these areas could inhibit interpretation of facial brainstem reflexes.[14]

Gag and cough reflexes. Pharyngeal and tracheal reflexes are absent in patients with brain death. The gag reflex can be evaluated by stimulating the posterior part of the pharynx with a tongue blade. The cough reflex can be tested with bronchial suctioning.[14]

Apnea testing. The loss of brainstem function results in the loss of centrally controlled breathing with resultant apnea. The respiratory neurons are controlled by cerebral chemoreceptors that sense changes in the arterial partial pressure of carbon dioxide ($Paco_2$) and pH of the cerebrospinal fluid that accurately reflect changes in plasma $Paco_2$.

Guidelines for determination of death recommend achieving $Paco_2$ levels greater than 60 mm Hg for maximal stimulation of brainstem respiratory centers. Prerequisites and the procedure for apnea testing are outlined in Box 36.1. The prerequisites

---

BOX 36.1 Apnea Test

Prerequisites
1. Normothermia
2. Systolic blood pressure ≥90 mm Hg
3. Euvolemia
4. Eucapnia
5. Normoxemia

Procedure
- Pulse oximeter is connected to the patient to monitor oxygen saturation.
- Preoxygenate for 10 min with fraction of inspired oxygen of 100%.
- Reduce ventilation frequency to 10 breaths/min and reduce positive end-expiratory pressure to 5 cm H_2O.
- If pulse oximetry oxygen saturation remains >90%, obtain baseline arterial blood gas, including arterial partial pressure of carbon dioxide ($PaCO_2$), pH, bicarbonate, and base excess.
- Disconnect ventilator.
- Place a cannula at the level of the carina and deliver 100% O_2, 6 L/min.
- Observe closely for respiratory movements for 8–10 min. Respiration is defined as abdominal or chest excursions that produce adequate tidal volumes.
- Abort if blood pressure remains <90 mm Hg systolic or declining despite increasing vasopressors.
- Abort if oxygen saturation is <80% for 2 min or drops steadily (consider retry with T-piece and continuous positive airway pressure).
- If no breathing drive is observed, measure arterial partial pressure of oxygen, $PaCO_2$, and pH after approximately 8 min.
- If respiratory movements are absent and $PaCO_2$ is ≥60 mm Hg (or 20 mm Hg increase in $PaCO_2$ over a baseline normal $PaCO_2$), the apnea test result is positive (ie, it supports the clinical diagnosis of brain death).
- If the patient breathes, repeat test a few hours later.

From Wijdicks EFM. The clinical diagnosis of brain death. In: *The Comatose Patient.* New York: Oxford University Press; 2008.

---

that should be addressed before the apnea test are to prevent cardiac dysrhythmias, hypotension, and decreased oxygen saturation. If any of these conditions occur during the apnea test, the test should be aborted, and additional brain death confirmatory testing should be performed (Box 36.2). In cases where a patient is a carbon dioxide retainer or the clinical examination is unreliable because of head trauma, confirmatory testing is necessary. Confirmatory testing is mandatory in children.

Confirmatory Tests

Additional confirmatory testing for the determination of brain death may include cerebral angiography, electroencephalography, transcranial Doppler, and cerebral scintigraphy, although these diagnostic procedures are not required (see Box 36.2).

Donation After Circulatory Determination of Death

Patients not meeting all necessary criteria for brain death but who have an unsurvivable injury when the family and physician make a decision to withdraw life support are potential donors after circulatory death determination. *Donation after circulatory determination of death* (DCDD) is based on the cessation of circulatory and respiratory functions.[15] Previously, DCDD donors were known as non–heart-beating donors, asystolic donors, or donation after cardiac death (DCD) donors. Patients who do not meet brain death criteria but have an unsurvivable condition such as a catastrophic neurologic injury, high spinal cord injury, or a

BOX 36.2   Confirmatory Tests in Brain Death

Cerebral Angiography

- Contrast medium under high pressure in both anterior and posterior circulation injections
- No intracerebral filling at the level of the carotid or vertebral artery entry to the skull
- Patent external carotid circulation
- Possible delayed filling of superior longitudinal sinus

Electroencephalography

- Minimum of eight scalp electrodes
- Electrode dependencies should be between 100 and 10,000
- Integrity of entire recording system should be tested
- Electrode distances should be at least 10 cm
- Sensitivity should be increased to at least 2 microvolts for 30 min with inclusion of appropriate calibrations
- High-frequency filter setting should be at 30 Hz, and low-frequency setting should not be below 1 Hz
- There should be no electroencephalographic reactivity to intense somatosensory or audiovisual stimuli

Transcranial Doppler Ultrasonography

- Bilateral insonation
- The probe is placed at the temporal bone above the zygomatic arch or the vertebrobasilar arteries through the suboccipital transcranial window
- The abnormalities should include a lack of diastolic or reverberating flow, small systolic peaks in early systole, and a lack of flow found by the investigator who previously demonstrated normal velocities

Cerebral Scintigraphy (Technetium Tc 99m Exametazime)

- Injection of isotope within 30 min of reconstitution
- Static image of 500,000 counts at several time intervals: immediately, between 30 and 60 min, and at 2 h
- Correct intravenous injection needs to be confirmed with additional liver images demonstrating uptake (optional)

This information is based on the American Academy of Neurology Guidelines. From Wijdicks EFM. The clinical diagnosis of brain death. In: *The Comatose Patient.* New York: Oxford University Press; 2008.

medical condition requiring mechanical ventilation are candidates for DCDD. Organs are recovered after cardiac asystole and a 3- to 5-minute wait period. Cardiac asystole must occur within 60 to 90 minutes for organ donation to occur. Before the enactment of brain death laws in the 1970s, all organ donors were DCD donors. Interest in DCDD has increased because of (1) family interest in organ donation when neurologic criteria for brain death have not been met and (2) the continued national demand for organs.[16,17]

Controlled Donation After Circulatory Determination of Death

DCDD donors are classified as controlled and uncontrolled DCDD donors. *Controlled DCDD* occurs when the family has made a decision to withdraw life-sustaining support and death is declared at the time of circulatory arrest. In controlled DCDD, families, health care providers, and OPO staff are involved in the timing and planning of the time when support will be withdrawn.[14]

Uncontrolled Donation After Circulatory Determination of Death

Uncontrolled DCDD describes a situation in which cardiac arrest has occurred and resuscitation efforts are determined

to be futile. The uncontrolled DCDD process is rapid, as the patient is undergoing cardiopulmonary resuscitation. After authorization from the family, the patient is taken to the operating room for immediate recovery of organs, primarily kidneys.[18]

DCDD is an opportunity to increase the number of organs available for transplantation. The 5-year organ survival rates in kidney and pancreas recipients from DCDD donors and brain-dead donors are similar.[19] Complications with liver transplant grafts from DCDD donors can occur secondary to *ischemic cholangiopathy* (damage to the bile ducts from an impaired blood supply); consequently, many transplant centers have changed their criteria for acceptance of DCDD donors based on the age of the donor.[20] DCDD lung donor outcomes compare favorably with outcomes of brain-dead lung donors.[21]

Authorization for Donation

"Presumed consent" is the donation law existing in many European countries. This is a system in which one is deemed a donor unless the person has taken action not to be a donor. That is not the law in the United States. The United States retains a voluntary system, often referred to as "opting-in." The architecture of US organ donation law, also termed "Gift Law," is the Uniform Anatomical Gift Act, which is enacted in all 50 states.

The OPO coordinator is an advocate for the donor/donor family and potential recipients. Many factors are important in working with potential donor families. The nurse and OPO coordinator are important in providing a safe, comfortable environment for families in a position to make decisions about donation.[22] Assessing the needs of the family is crucial to the outcome of the donation conversation. Timing of the conversation is also important. Donation does not consist of simply asking the family if they wish to donate.[15] The critical care nurse should inform the family that an expert member of the health care team is available to provide information and answer their questions about donation.[23]

Many myths and misconceptions surround organ donation. Common misconceptions from families surround religious beliefs, cultural milieus, and concerns about possible body disfigurement, concern about the ability to have an open casket funeral, and costs to family.[24] Another common misperception is that hospital staff will not attempt to save the life of their loved one if they believe the patient could be a donor.[24] These misperceptions must be debunked with the family. Finally, research has shown that the manner in which the donation request is made is the main factor in a family's ultimate decision regardless of preexisting attitudes.[25] Many families report that donation has helped their healing in the grieving process and say that donation represents something positive in their loss.[25]

Donor Management

The donor management phase includes ongoing collaboration between the OPO coordinator and OPO medical director, critical care nurse, intensivist, respiratory therapist, and transplant professionals to ensure optimal preservation of organ function for organ recovery and transplantation. Standing orders for the care of an organ donor are provided by the OPO. These encompass required testing and screening of donors as well as parameters for continued medical management of the cadaveric donor, as listed in Box 36.3.

BOX 36.3 Donor Care Protocols

The Organ Procurement Organization (OPO) coordinator should write orders to initiate standard donor care.

1. Transfer care to [Name of OPO].
2. Discontinue all prior orders.
3. Assess blood pressure, heart rate, temperature, urine output, central venous pressure (CVP) (if central venous catheter present), pulmonary artery occlusion pressure (PAOP) (if pulmonary artery [PA] catheter present) every 1 h.
4. Reorder mechanical ventilator parameters as previously set.
5. Maintain head of bed at 30–40 degrees elevation.
6. Continue routine pulmonary suctioning and side-to-side body positioning.
7. Warming blanket to maintain body temperature above 36.5°C.
8. Maintain sequential compression devices.
9. Continue chest tube suction or water seal as previously ordered (if present).
10. Nasogastric (orogastric) tube to low intermittent suction (if present).
11. Intravenous fluid: dextrose 5% in 0.45% saline plus 20 mEq potassium chloride per liter at 75 mL/h.
12. Call OPO coordinator if mean arterial pressure is <70 mm Hg, systolic pressure is >170 mm Hg, heart rate is <60 or >130 beats/min, temperature is <36.5°C or >37.8°C, urine output is <75 or >250 mL/hr, or CVP or PAOP is <8 or >18 mm Hg.
13. Medications:
    Pantoprazole 40 mg intravenously every 24 h, first dose now
    Artificial tears every 1 h and as needed to prevent corneal drying
    Albuterol and Atrovent unit dose per aerosol every 4 h
    Antibiotics previously ordered continued at same dose and frequency
    Vasoactive medication infusions (dopamine, norepinephrine) at previously ordered concentrations and infusion rates
14. Review all medications previously ordered. Most anticonvulsants, pain medications, laxatives, gastrointestinal motility agents, eye drops, antihypertensives, antinausea agents, subcutaneous heparin, osmotic agents (mannitol), and diuretics are unnecessary during donor care and will be discontinued automatically with order number 2 above. Review any other medications in question with the physician.
15. Send electrolytes, magnesium, ionized calcium, complete blood count, platelets, glucose, blood urea nitrogen, creatinine, phosphorus, arterial blood gas, prothrombin time/international normalized ratio, and partial thromboplastin time STAT and repeat every 4 h.
16. Send blood for type and screen with above blood draw (if not previously done).
17. Fingerstick blood glucose every 2 h—call OPO coordinator if blood glucose <90 or >180 mg/dL.
18. Order electrocardiogram STAT.
19. Order radiography STAT with indication "initial donor evaluation."
20. Add other orders for specific organ evaluation as indicated.

The above order set provides a "safety net" of call orders so that the coordinator is alerted to significant changes in donor status. It also prescribes the foundation for ongoing monitoring of physiologic and laboratory variables.

Modified from Powner DJ, O'Connor KJ. Adult clinical donor care. In: LaPointe-Rudow D, Ohler L, Shafer TJ, eds. *A Clinician's Guide to Donation and Transplantation.* Lenexa, KS: Applied Measurement Professionals; 2006.

TABLE 36.4 Donor Management Clinical Parameters

Parameter	Clinical Goal
1. Mean arterial pressure	60–100 mm Hg
2. Central venous pressure	4–10 mm Hg
3. Ejection fraction	>50%
4. Vasopressors	<1 and low dose
5. Arterial blood gas pH	7.3–7.45
6. Pa_{O_2}/Fi_{O_2} ratio	>300
7. Serum sodium	135–155 mEq/L
8. Blood glucose	<150 mg/dL
9. Urine output (averaged over 4 h)	0.5–3.0 mL/kg/h over 4 h

Fi_{O_2}, fraction of inspired oxygen; Pa_{O_2}, arterial partial pressure of oxygen.

Administration has advocated for the implementation of donor management goals by OPOs.[23,26]

Patients with critical neurologic impairment present with many clinical challenges including hypotension (81%), diabetes insipidus (65%), disseminated intravascular coagulation (28%), cardiac arrhythmias (25%), pulmonary edema (18%), and metabolic acidosis (11%). There is increasing evidence that control of these pathophysiologic changes by active clinical management increases the number and quality of organs available for transplantation, which ultimately impacts the potential recipient.[27]

Further assessment of the donor by the OPO coordinator includes screening for any transmissible diseases, including serologic tests for infectious diseases such as human immunodeficiency virus (HIV), hepatitis, syphilis, cytomegalovirus (CMV), and Epstein-Barr virus. The OPO coordinator conducts a medical social history questionnaire with the authorizing person or others who can provide information on the donor's past medical and social history. The questionnaire comprises standard questions about the donor's past behavioral, medical, social, and sexual health. These survey questions are approved by UNOS, by the US Food and Drug Administration, and by other accrediting agencies for organ and tissue donation.

Organ Allocation

The OPTN is responsible for operating the national database, which lists all patients waiting for an organ transplant in the United States. The UNOS manages the national list. The OPO coordinator accesses the UNOS computer to generate a donor-specific list of potential recipients from the national list. Potential recipients are matched with the donor based on blood type, height, weight, human leukocyte antigen (HLA), distance from the donor, waiting time on the list, and severity of illness. The national system in place for organ allocation is fair and equitable for patients requiring a transplant. The list does not reference race, sex, or socioeconomic status. Organs are offered electronically to the transplant team of the first person on the list. If the organ is refused for any reason, the transplant hospital of the next patient on the list is contacted. The process continues until a match is made. Once a patient is selected and contacted and all testing is complete, surgery is scheduled, and the transplant takes place.

Role of Medical Examiners and Coroners in Organ and Tissue Donation

Medical examiners and coroners play a vital role in organ and tissue donation. These individuals are responsible for

The goals of donor management are to maximize oxygenation and provide optimal organ perfusion to maintain the viability of organs for transplantation.

Donor Management Goals

Donor management goals are preset critical care end points used to increase the number of organs transplanted per donor as listed in Table 36.4. The Health Resources and Services investigating and determining the cause and manner of deaths that occur in cases falling within their jurisdiction. Deaths falling within the jurisdiction of medical examiners and coroners include deaths that occur from unexpected and violent circumstances and any death in a child younger than age 6 in many states. These cases account for most potential organ donors. Thus, organ and tissue donation and activities of medical examiners and coroners directly intersect. Medical examiners and coroners must review these cases and release them in a timely manner for donation to occur.

Organ Recovery

Once all recipients have been identified, the OPO coordinator schedules the operating room time and coordinates arrival of the surgical recovery teams for organ retrieval. The OPO coordinator and critical care nurse coordinate the transport, collaborating with operating room and anesthesiology staff. The nurse ensures the donor is connected to a transport monitor; oxygen and emergency medications must be available. In the operating room, hemodynamic support and continued medical management are coordinated between the OPO staff, anesthesiologist, and recovery surgeons.

Organs are first flushed with preservative solution containing electrolytes and nutrients. The organs are then removed from the donor, examined individually in a sterile basin, and packed in sterile containers for transport. For heart, heart and lung, and lungs, transport is immediate. For pancreas and liver, time to transplant ranges from 6 to 20 hours. For kidneys, approximately 24 hours may elapse before transplantation. Tissue typing is primarily carried out between kidney and pancreas donors and recipients and is less frequently done between heart, heart and lung, and single-lung donors and recipients.

Tissue Donation

Families have the opportunity to enhance and save many lives through tissue and eye donation. This donation could impact the lives of 60 to 80 individuals awaiting tissue transplantation. There are approximately 40,000 tissue donors per year, and an estimated 1 million Americans receive tissue transplants each year, from sight-saving corneas to hip replacements, bone repair, and heart valves.[9] Patients with cardiac death are able to donate tissues if deemed medically suitable by the OPO. After the authorization process, if tissue recovery is going to be delayed, it is imperative that the body of the donor is cooled. The American Association of Tissue Banks standards require that tissue be recovered within 24 hours of cardiac death, provided that the body has received sufficient cooling. The recovery of tissue is performed in the operating room using sterile technique. Donors may be both organ and tissue donors with tissue recovery following organ recovery. OPO-trained specialists perform the recovery and bring the necessary supplies required for tissue recovery; hospital operating room staff are not needed for tissue recovery.[12]

Organ Donation Summary

Organ and tissue donation saves lives. Critical care nurses are in a unique position to impact the lives of many patients— patients who are able to give the gift of life and patients awaiting a lifesaving transplant. Nurses collaborate closely with the OPO to honor the wishes of patients and their families. Nursing care does not stop when a patient meets the criteria to become an organ donor. Provision of expert nursing care, compassion, and support of families facing end-of-life decisions is part of daily practice.

IMMUNOLOGY OF TRANSPLANT REJECTION

Organ transplantation has become a widely accepted treatment for end-stage heart, lung, liver, kidney, and pancreatic disease. Major advances have been made in organ procurement and preservation; surgical techniques; and prevention, identification, and treatment of rejection. Ultimately, the long-term success of transplantation depends on the immune system's tolerance for the transplanted organ. Virtually every cell in the human body carries distinctive molecules that enable the immune system to distinguish self from nonself. An intact immune system recognizes and eliminates any foreign biologic material recognized as nonself. Successful organ transplantation requires suppression or downregulation of the immune response. To understand the principles of immunosuppressive therapy, it is important to have some understanding of the cells of the immune system, the immune response, and the process of organ rejection.

Immune Mechanism

Whenever the body is presented with a substance recognized as nonself, a *primary immune response* is elicited. There are three phases of any primary immune response: (1) recognition of the substance as nonself, (2) proliferation of immunocompetent cells, and (3) action against the foreign substance (effector phase). During the primary response, immunologic memory is established so that any subsequent encounter with the same substance induces a more rapid and intense immune response. Subsequent encounters are called *secondary immune responses.*

An *antigen* is a substance that is capable of eliciting an immune response. Every cell has antigens on its surface that are determined by a series of linked genes known as the *major histocompatibility complex* (MHC). If tissue from one person is transplanted into a genetically different person, the antigens on the transplanted tissue cells are immediately recognized as nonself, and rejection occurs. The MHC determines the antigens to which the immune system should respond. The human MHC is called the HLA complex because these markers were first discovered on lymphocytes.

HLAs are divided into two classes. *Class I antigens* consist of HLA-A, HLA-B, HLA-C, and HLA-D loci and are expressed on the plasma membranes of all nucleated cells. *Class II antigens* consist of HLA-DR, HLA-DQ, and HLA-DP loci and are expressed on activated immune cells.[28] Because of the potential for millions of different arrangements of these antigens, the chances of finding a donor organ with the same genes as a recipient are almost nil unless the donor and recipient are identical twins.

Cells of the Immune System

The immune system contains a variety of cells responsible for general defense as well as very specific immune responses. When a particular antigen (foreign protein) appears, the cells of the immune system are stimulated to multiply and mount a response. Immune cells are originally produced in the bone marrow as stem cells; their descendants become lymphocytes or phagocytes (Fig. 36.2).

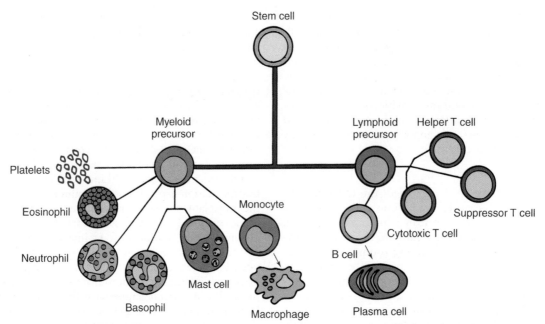

FIG. 36.2 All Cells of Immune System Originate From Stem Cells in Bone Marrow. (From Schindler LW. *Understanding the Immune System.* NIH publication no. 92-529. Bethesda, MD: Department of Health and Human Services; 1991.)

The two major classes of lymphocytes are *B cells* and *T cells*. B cells remain in the bone marrow to complete their maturation. T cells migrate to the thymus gland and mature there. In the thymus, T cells acquire the ability to distinguish self from nonself. After they have matured, some B and T cells are stored in the lymph nodes, whereas others circulate in the blood and lymphatic system.

Humoral Immunity

Humoral immunity is mediated by B cells, which are responsible for the production of antibody or immunoglobulin. When a B cell encounters an antigen to which it is specifically coded to respond, the B cell enlarges, divides, and differentiates into a *plasma cell*. The plasma cell actually produces and secretes *antigen-specific antibody* (Fig. 36.3). B cells function as *antigen presenting cells*.[29] After exposure to an antigen, the immune system retains a memory of that antigen. Subsequent exposure stimulates the B-cell memory cells, resulting in a rapid mobilization of antibody-secreting cells. Antibodies work in several ways, but their primary purpose is to mark an antigen for destruction by the immune system. Other antibodies are capable of neutralizing toxins produced by bacteria, or they can trigger the release of serum proteins known as *complement*.

Cell-Mediated Immunity

T cells provide cell-mediated immunity. Approximately 65% to 80% of all lymphocytes are T cells, of which there are three basic types: *cytotoxic T cells, helper T cells,* and *suppressor T cells.*

Cytotoxic T cells. Cytotoxic T cells are cells responsible for killing invading cells. Their primary role is to rid the body of cells that have become infected, have been transformed by cancer, or are nonself (eg, transplanted tissue). They are also called *T8* or *CD8 lymphocytes,* referring to a marker that distinguishes cytotoxic T cells from other T cells. Cytotoxic T cells are activated by macrophages that present the foreign antigen to immature cytotoxic T cells. With the assistance

of helper T cells and their release of chemical mediators, the cytotoxic T cells mature and kill foreign cells that carry that specific antigen (Fig. 36.4).

Helper T cells. Helper T cells upregulate the immune response by stimulating B cells to differentiate into plasma cells and begin antibody production, by activating cytotoxic T cells, and by stimulating natural killer (NK) cells and macrophages. Helper T cells are identified by surface glycoproteins known as CD4 or T4 markers. Fig. 36.5 illustrates the process responsible for activating helper T cells. *Macrophages* present processed antigen to the immature helper T cells. With the assistance of chemical mediators (interleukins) released by the macrophages, the helper T cells mature and begin to activate other cells of the immune system previously described.

Suppressor T cells. A third type of T cell is the suppressor T cell. These cells suppress, or downregulate, the immune response. They play an important role in keeping the immune response controlled and in turning off the response after the antigenic threat is no longer present.

Other Immune System Defenses

T and B cells work with other parts of the immune system, notably NK cells, phagocytic cells, and complement, to enhance the immune response.

Natural killer cells. NK cells are another type of lymphocyte. They are not targeted for any specific antigen but attack and destroy any cell that is identified as nonself. NK cells contain granules filled with potent chemicals that are released when they bind to the targeted nonself cell. These chemicals are capable of lysing the cell membrane and causing the cell's death. NK cells can also cause tissue inflammation through the release of proinflammatory cytokines.[30]

Phagocytes. Phagocytes are a major category of immune cells capable of destroying foreign cells. Critical phagocytes include monocytes, macrophages, neutrophils, eosinophils, and basophils. Table 36.5 outlines the primary functions of

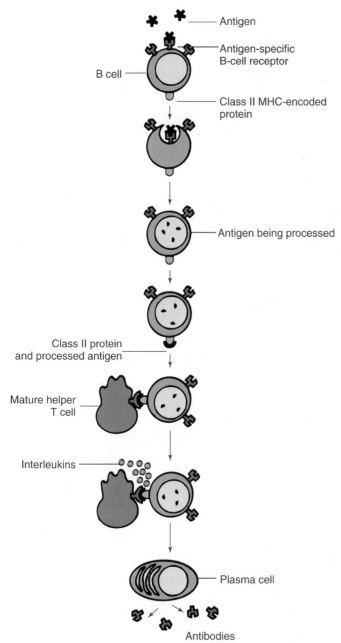

FIG. 36.3 Foreign antigen is processed by the B cell and displayed with its major histocompatibility complex (MHC) class II antigen (protein), which attracts helper T cells. The release of interleukins by the helper T cell stimulates differentiation of the B cell into a plasma cell, which begins to produce antibody. (From Schindler LW. *Understanding the Immune System.* NIH publication no. 92-529. Bethesda, MD: Department of Health and Human Services; 1991.)

these cells. Macrophages are vitally important to the immune response because of their role in "presenting" antigens to the helper and cytotoxic T cells. This presentation alerts T cells to the presence of antigen. Macrophages also produce chemical regulators, or interleukins, that stimulate the maturation of helper and cytotoxic T cells.

Complement. An important system in the immune response is complement. Complement consists of a series of 25 proteins that when activated develop into powerful enzymes capable of lysing alien cell walls. Complement is triggered by the presence of antibody bound to a foreign cell or antigen (antigen–antibody complex). Complement also stimulates basophils, attracts neutrophils, and coats foreign cells to make them more attractive to phagocytes. The latter action is called *opsonization.*

Graft Rejection

Rejection of any transplanted organ occurs when the transplanted tissue is recognized as nonself by the immune system. Cellular-mediated rejection occurs when HLA class I antigens, displayed on cells of the donor organ, activate helper T cells that promote the expansion of cytotoxic T cells and recruit macrophages into the transplanted tissue. NK cells also begin to attack any cell with foreign HLA class I antigens. Left untreated, the transplanted organ becomes infiltrated with these cells leading to the eventual destruction of the foreign graft tissue.

At the same time, antibody-mediated or humoral-mediated rejection occurs as antigen–antibody complexes form. These complexes are present in the transplanted organ and release complement that is capable of cell destruction. Complement plays a role in recruiting basophils and tissue-destroying neutrophils to the site. Antibody also coats the foreign cells, making them more attractive to macrophages.

Graft rejection can occur at different time intervals and has different injury patterns. The three types of rejection patterns are hyperacute rejection, acute rejection, and chronic rejection.

Hyperacute Rejection

Hyperacute rejection is a humoral-mediated response that occurs within hours after transplantation and results in immediate graft failure. The rapid immune response is caused by the presence of preformed reactive antibodies as a consequence of previous exposure to antigens. Presensitization can be the result of previous blood transfusions, multiple pregnancies, or previous organ transplantation.[28] Left ventricular assist devices, which are used as a bridge to eventual heart transplantation, can also sensitize potential recipients because of the physical properties of the device itself, activation of the immune system, and increased production of antibodies.[31] Transplantation of an organ from a donor with an incompatible blood type can have the same effect.[32] Hyperacute rejection is prevented by testing for the presence of preformed antibodies in the recipient and by selecting donors with compatible blood types.

Acute Rejection

Acute rejection tends to occur weeks to months after transplantation but can occur at any time. Class I or II antigens on the cells of the transplanted graft activate a cellular-mediated response.

Chronic Rejection

Chronic rejection occurs at varying times after transplantation and progresses for years until it leads to ultimate failure of the transplanted organ. Chronic rejection is the result of both humoral-mediated and cellular-mediated immune responses. Chronic inflammation results in diffuse scarring of tissue and stenosis of the organ's vasculature, eventually leading to ischemia and necrosis of tissue.

Immunosuppressive Medications

Immunosuppression protocols vary among institutions and according to the type of organ transplanted. The primary goal of immunosuppressive therapies is to suppress the activity of

FIG. 36.4 Macrophage presents the processed antigen from the foreign organism on the major histocompatibility complex (MHC) class I protein to cytotoxic and helper T cells. Aided by the release of interleukins from the helper T cell, the cytotoxic T cell matures and kills the foreign cell. (From Schindler LW. *Understanding the Immune System*. NIH publication no. 92-529. Bethesda, MD: Department of Health and Human Services; 1991.)

FIG. 36.5 Helper T cell is activated by the presence of processed antigen in combination with the major histocompatibility complex (MHC) class II antigen (protein) on the surface of a macrophage. It matures with the stimulus from interleukins. (From Schindler LW. *Understanding the Immune System*. NIH publication no. 92-529. Bethesda, MD: Department of Health and Human Services; 1991.)

helper and cytotoxic T cells. In general, most protocols combine high-dose corticosteroids with a *calcineurin inhibitor* such as cyclosporine or tacrolimus in addition to mycophenolate mofetil, sirolimus, or occasionally azathioprine. These

"triple-drug" regimens are designed to prevent rejection, while reducing the toxicity of the individual medications. In addition to these primary agents, cytolytic therapy is often used in an attempt to induce graft tolerance and prevent early rejection. Cytolytic agents include antilymphocyte globulins and antithymocyte globulins. Table 36.6 summarizes immunosuppressive medications. Absolute care must be taken to monitor the effectiveness of medication therapy and to minimize unnecessarily high doses of these agents, which could predispose patients to greater risks for infection, malignancy, or other toxic effects.

Corticosteroids

Corticosteroids—intravenous methylprednisolone (Solu-Medrol) and oral prednisone—have complex and diverse effects on the immune system. They are used for maintenance therapy and to treat acute rejection. The antiinflammatory actions of steroids provide important protection of the transplanted organ against permanent damage from the body's natural immune response. As maintenance therapy, steroids impair the sensitivity of T cells to antigen, decrease the proliferation of sensitized T cells, and impair the production of interleukins. Steroids also decrease macrophage mobility.

TABLE 36.5 Phagocytes and Their Functions

Phagocyte	Function
Monocytes	Migrate from blood tissues to become macrophages
	Act as scavenger cells in tissues
	Present antigen to T cells
Macrophages	Secrete enzymes, complement proteins, and immune regulatory factors (cytokines)
	Activated by lymphokines
Neutrophils	Contain granules capable of destroying alien organisms
	Key role in inflammatory reactions
Eosinophils	Contain granules capable of destroying alien organisms
	Weaker phagocyte
Basophils	Contain granules capable of destroying alien organisms
	Key role in allergic reaction

TABLE 36.6 Pharmacologic Management
Organ Transplantation

Medication	Dosage[a]	Action	Special Considerations
Azathioprine	Titrate to WBC count of 3000–6000 cells/mm^3	Inhibits purine synthesis	Monitor for bone marrow depression
Cyclosporine gelatin (Neoral),[b] oral solution, and capsules	Therapeutic range: 100–400 ng/mL	Suppresses T lymphocytes	Hold for elevated levels
	Standard dosage ranges for specific organs[c]		Monitor for nephrotoxicity, HTN, hepatotoxicity, tremors, and seizures
	Liver: 14–18 mg/kg/day		Monitor for medications that exhibit nephrotoxic synergy (eg, gentamicin, tobramycin, vancomycin, amphotericin B, ketoconazole, cimetidine, ranitidine)
	Kidney: 10–14 mg/kg/day, tapered to 5–10 mg/kg/day		
	Heart: 4–6 mg/kg/day		
Mycophenolate mofetil (CellCept)	2–3 g/day[c]	Similar to azathioprine but less toxic to bone marrow	Increased blood level concentrations when used with other medications excreted through the kidney tubules
Prednisone	1 mg/kg/day, tapered to 0.3 mg/kg/day or off, if tolerated	Suppresses inflammatory response	Tapered to as low a dosage as tolerated; dosage is increased with rejection
Rabbit antithymocyte globulin (Thymoglobulin)	1.5 mg/kg for 1–7 days; may be given once daily initially then every other day	Suppresses circulating T lymphocytes	Used in lung transplantation for induction therapy
			Used as rescue therapy for other transplantation procedures
			Monitor for reactions
			Pretreatment may be used
Sirolimus (Rapamune)	10 mg/day, tapered to trough level of 12–20 mg/mL (depending on organ and center)	Blocks ability of cytokines to activate T and B lymphocytes	Synergistic effects when used with cyclosporine or tacrolimus
			Monitor for thrombocytopenia
			Used in place of azathioprine or mycophenolate mofetil
Tacrolimus (Prograf)	0.1–0.3 mg/kg/day[c]	Inhibition of interleukin release	Nephrotoxicity with high doses
	Therapeutic range: 5–20 mg/mL		Hyperkalemia

[a]These dosage ranges are general guidelines. Significant variations in dosages occur based on institutional practices, other medications being used in combination, type of transplantation, and patient response to the medications.
[b]Cyclosporine preparations Neoral and Sandimmune are not bioequivalent and cannot be used interchangeably; Gengraf and Neoral are bioequivalent.
[c]Daily dose is divided and administered 12 hours apart.
HTN, hypertension; *WBC*, white blood cell.

Long-term steroid therapy is associated with numerous adverse effects and predisposes the patient to an increased risk of infection (see Table 36.6). A primary goal of corticosteroid therapy is to titrate the medication dose to as low a level as possible. An ideal therapeutic regimen would allow for elimination of the medication altogether. Long-term use of corticosteroids is associated with painful osteoporosis, avascular necrosis of joints, fragile skin that is easily traumatized, poor wound healing, susceptibility to skin cancers, steroid-induced acne, insulin resistance, and obesity.

Cyclosporine

Cyclosporine belongs to a class of immunosuppressants called *calcineurin inhibitors*. The primary mechanism of action is to suppress activation of T lymphocytes, which inhibits the production of interleukin-2 (IL-2).[31] Because cyclosporine is specifically targeted to T cells, the patient's immune system is not completely impaired, and some ability to protect the body from infection is preserved.

Several pharmacologic preparations of cyclosporine are available with varying bioavailability and dose equivalency. Care must be taken when changing brands of cyclosporine with close monitoring of medication levels. The most common side effects of cyclosporine are hypertension, hyperlipidemia, hirsutism, gingival hyperplasia, nephrotoxicity, hepatotoxicity, and seizures.[31] At the present time, cyclosporine is less frequently used than tacrolimus, a newer calcineurin inhibitor.

Tacrolimus

Tacrolimus (Prograf) is a calcineurin inhibitor with similar activity to cyclosporine in that it also impairs T-cell activation by inhibiting the formation of IL-2.[31] Tacrolimus is used in the immunosuppressive regimen of most transplant programs because of its favorable side-effect profile. Tacrolimus is less likely than cyclosporine to cause hyperlipidemia, hypertension, and hirsutism.[31] The most common side effects of tacrolimus are diabetes mellitus, electrolyte imbalances (hyperkalemia, hypophosphatemia, hypomagnesemia), nephrotoxicity, and tremor.[31] Studies comparing cyclosporine with tacrolimus as a primary immunosuppressant in kidney and liver transplant recipients have found tacrolimus to be superior in improving patient survival, improving graft survival, and preventing acute rejection.

Azathioprine

Azathioprine (Imuran) is an antimetabolite that interferes with purine synthesis, which is necessary for the production of antibodies and for the synthesis of nucleic acids in rapidly proliferating cells, such as the cells of the immune system. Azathioprine is used as a maintenance medication to prevent the activation and rapid proliferation of T cells responding to an antigen. A common adverse effect is suppression of other rapidly proliferating cells, resulting in leukopenia, thrombocytopenia, and anemia. The medication dose is adjusted to keep the white blood cell count between 3000 and 5000 cells/mm³ to decrease risk of infection. The actual minimum acceptable white blood cell count varies with institutional preferences and the type of organ transplanted. Most centers have abandoned the use of azathioprine in favor of mycophenolate mofetil.[33]

Mycophenolate Mofetil

Mycophenolate mofetil (CellCept) is a derivative of mycophenolic acid. Mycophenolic acid is a selective inhibitor of the enzyme *inosine monophosphate dehydrogenase,* which is crucial in the pathway for purine synthesis. Because this pathway is responsible for signaling lymphocyte proliferation, mycophenolate mofetil is a potent inhibitor of T- and B-lymphocyte proliferation.[33] This inhibition also disrupts antibody formation and the generation of cytotoxic T cells, effectively suppressing cellular-mediated and humoral-mediated immunity. The mechanism of action is similar to that of azathioprine except that mycophenolate mofetil selectively inhibits T and B cells.

The use of mycophenolate mofetil in transplant recipients was associated with significant reduction in mortality and graft loss as well as a significant reduction in severe rejection requiring treatment.[33] Its use was also associated with delayed progression of coronary artery intimal thickening, a type of proliferative arteriopathy associated with chronic rejection in heart transplant recipients. Side effects consist mainly of gastrointestinal symptoms such as nausea, vomiting, diarrhea, gastritis, and anorexia. Leukopenia is sometimes seen, although not to the same extent as with azathioprine.

The gastrointestinal side effects of mycophenolate mofetil are sometimes difficult to tolerate for patients and can lead to dose interruptions or omissions. A newer and better-tolerated enteric-coated formulation of mycophenolate, mycophenolate sodium, is available; this is helpful for patients who do not tolerate the traditional mycophenolate mofetil formulation. Several studies have shown that mycophenolate sodium is therapeutically similar and has a comparable safety profile. Mycophenolate is typically combined with a calcineurin inhibitor (cyclosporine or tacrolimus).[33]

Sirolimus

Sirolimus (Rapamune), formerly rapamycin, is an immunosuppressive agent that is also a macrolide antibiotic known for its powerful antifungal properties. Cyclosporine and tacrolimus inhibit cytokine production, whereas the mechanism of action of sirolimus is to block the effect of cytokines on the proliferation of lymphoid cells (T and B lymphocytes) by inhibiting a protein (mammalian target of rapamycin [mTOR]) that is essential for cytokine-driven T-cell proliferation. These medications are known as *proliferation signal inhibitors*, or *mTOR inhibitors*.[34,35]

Sirolimus inhibits the proliferation of nonlymphoid cells such as endothelial and smooth muscle cells as well as fibroblasts, which slows the progression of graft vasculopathy in heart transplant recipients. However, the fibroblasts and endothelial cells that are inhibited by sirolimus are also responsible for wound healing leading to an increase in the incidence of impaired wound healing compared with patients who received other immunosuppressants.[35,36] Many centers delay the introduction of sirolimus into the immunosuppressant regimen until the recipient is several months from transplantation and has had the opportunity to heal any surgical wounds. Another immunosuppressant agent is often substituted for sirolimus for several weeks to months before any scheduled surgical procedure to lessen the risk of delayed wound healing. Other primary side effects of this medication include hyperlipidemia and myelosuppression. Most of the myelosuppressive effect is directed at platelets, and severe thrombocytopenias can result, making it necessary to discontinue the medication.

Although dosages vary among institutions, a loading dose is often administered before initiating a maintenance dose to achieve serum levels of 5 to 15 ng/mL. Because of its prolonged half-life, sirolimus is administered once daily. Sirolimus has also been shown to have synergistic effects when combined with cyclosporine and tacrolimus, which can result in a lower dose requirement for these medications. Because cyclosporine and tacrolimus can be nephrotoxic, lower doses of these two medications can be advantageous. Sirolimus also specifically interacts with cyclosporine and must be administered 4 hours after the dose of cyclosporine.

Everolimus

Everolimus is an analogue of sirolimus with a shorter half-life and more rapid time to steady state. Everolimus is also more convenient to administer in that, in contrast to sirolimus, it can be given concomitantly with cyclosporine. Similar to sirolimus, everolimus is a proliferation signal inhibitor and works by blocking IL-2 receptor signal transduction in activated lymphocytes. A synergistic effect of everolimus and calcineurin inhibitors such as cyclosporine and tacrolimus allows for lower doses of those medications to be used. Several trials have been conducted to study the safety and efficacy of everolimus in calcineurin inhibitor-free regimens.

Side effects of sirolimus and everolimus are similar. Both can cause hypertension, hypercholesterolemia, hypertriglyceridemia, thrombocytopenia, diabetes, edema, acne, rash, and mouth sores.[31,35]

Induction Therapy

Induction therapy involves the intraoperative or postoperative use of an immunosuppressive agent for a limited period of time. The purpose of induction therapy is to induce tolerance to the transplanted graft. Induction is used by about half of all transplant centers.[37] There is ongoing debate regarding the need for and effectiveness of induction therapy. According to the 2013 Annual Report from the Scientific Registry of Transplant Recipients, approximately 50% of heart transplant recipients, 58% of lung transplant recipients, 90% of kidney recipients, and 30% of liver recipients receive induction therapy.[38]

Antithymocyte Preparations

Antithymocyte preparations are made by injecting human thymocytes into an animal, usually a horse, rabbit, or goat. The animal produces antibody in response to the foreign human antigen. Antibody to human thymocytes can then be extracted from the serum of the animal. Antithymocyte medications cause depletion of T cells by promoting T-cell clearance from the circulation and modulation of T-cell activation.[31] Depending on the protocol of the institution, antithymocyte preparations may be administered as induction therapy or to treat acute rejection. Patients are subject to reactions caused by the release of pyrogens during the massive T-cell lysis and by the foreign animal protein contained in the preparation.

Antilymphocyte and antithymocyte preparations are *cytolytic* medications. Use of cytolytic medications has been associated with an increased incidence of malignancy, most likely caused by the suppression of cytotoxic T cells, which normally play an important role in identifying and eliminating malignant cells. For that reason, many centers use these medications only to reverse rejections that are unresponsive to conventional treatment with increased corticosteroids.

TABLE 36.7   New York Heart Association Class and Physical Manifestation of Heart Failure

NYHA Class	Physical Manifestation
I	No limitation of physical activity; no dyspnea, fatigue, or palpitations with ordinary activity
II	Slight limitation of physical activity; patients have fatigue, palpitations, and dyspnea with ordinary physical activity but are comfortable at rest
III	Marked limitation of activity; less than ordinary physical activity results in symptoms, but patients are comfortable at rest
IV	Symptoms are present at rest, and any physical exertion exacerbates symptoms

NYHA, New York Heart Association.

Interleukin-2 Receptor Antagonists

Basiliximab is currently the only interleukin-2 receptor antagonist (IL-2Ra) available in the United States. IL-2Ra are antibodies to a receptor found on activated T lymphocytes. As discussed earlier, IL-2 mediates the activation of T lymphocytes; IL-2Ra competitively antagonizes this function. IL-2Ra agents are generally better tolerated than other induction agents, with fewer incidences of fever, leukopenia, thrombocytopenia, and other adverse reactions.

HEART TRANSPLANTATION

The first human heart transplantation was performed at the University of Cape Town, South Africa, in 1967 by Christian Barnard; the patient survived 18 days. In 1968, Shumway and colleagues performed the first successful heart transplant in the United States at Stanford University. The number of heart transplantation procedures grew dramatically for the first few years and then rapidly declined because of poor results. Over time, technologic and surgical advancements in addition to pharmacologic developments have led to significantly increased survival. These advancements included the development of the endomyocardial biopsy to detect allograft rejection, the introduction of T cell–specific agents such as rabbit antithymocyte globulin, the ability of laboratories to measure specific T cells (rosette counts) in the blood, and the introduction of the immunosuppressive medication cyclosporine (previously described). More than 112,000 adult and pediatric heart transplants have been performed in the United States since 1982,[37] with 1-year survival of 82%, 5-year survival of 69%, and a median survival of 11 years.[37]

Indications and Selection

Heart transplantation is indicated for individuals with end-stage cardiac disease if the symptoms of heart failure can no longer be managed with conventional medical therapy, if there are no surgical options offering more favorable long-term outcomes, and if the individual's short-term prognosis is poor without transplantation.[39] The most common conditions necessitating heart transplantation are nonischemic cardiomyopathies of various origins (idiopathic, viral, valvular) and coronary artery disease.[37] Other, less common etiologic factors include severe heart failure resulting from chemotherapy, radiation treatment, myocardial tumor, and complex congenital defects. Many

BOX 36.4   Heart Transplantation Contraindications

Medical Contraindication

Absolute	Relative
Elevated pulmonary artery pressures	Advanced age (>70 y)
Irreversible severe renal, hepatic, or pulmonary disease	Diabetes mellitus with end-organ damage and/or poor glycemic control
Kidney dysfunction	Obesity
Chronic liver dysfunction	Severe cachexia or malnutrition
Recent or unresolved pulmonary infarction	Systemic disease with high probability of recurrence in transplanted heart
Active uncontrolled infection	Severe peripheral vascular disease or cerebrovascular disease
Active malignancy or recent malignancy with high risk of recurrence	History of multiple prior sternotomies
	High level of allosensitization

Psychosocial Contraindications

Absolute	Relative
Inadequate social support system	Inadequate social support system
Illicit substance use	Illicit substance use
Alcohol dependence	Alcohol dependence
Nicotine abuse	Nicotine abuse
Active psychotic symptoms	Active psychotic symptoms
Dementia	Dementia
History of multiple suicide attempts	History of multiple suicide attempts

TABLE 36.8   Classification of Heart Transplant Candidates

Status	Definition
1A	Admitted to listing transplant center hospital and has at least one of the following devices or therapies in place: • Mechanical circulatory support such as left and/or right ventricular assist device (may be listed for 30 days at any point after being implanted) • Total artificial heart • Intraaortic balloon pump • Extracorporeal membrane oxygenator • Mechanical circulatory support with objective medical evidence of significant device-related complications such as thromboembolism, device infection, mechanical failure, or life-threatening ventricular arrhythmias • Continuous mechanical ventilation • Continuous infusion of single high-dose intravenous inotrope or multiple intravenous inotropes, in addition to continuous hemodynamic monitoring of left ventricular filling pressures
1B	At least one of the following devices or therapies in place: • Left and/or right ventricular assist device implanted • Continuous infusion of intravenous inotropes
2	Candidate who does not meet the criteria for status 1A or 1B

Organ Procurement and Transplantation Network Policies. Policy 6: Allocation of Heart and Heart-Lungs. http://optn.transplant.hrsa.gov/media/1200/optn_policies.pdf. Accessed 10-1-2016.

centers grade the severity of heart failure by the classification developed by the New York Heart Association (NYHA) (Table 36.7), which is based on the amount of exertion required to cause symptoms. Most patients who need a heart transplant are categorized as NYHA class III to IV.

In addition to satisfying medical criteria, patients generally are evaluated for the presence of family or social support, absence of chemical dependence, and commitment to adhering to a strict lifelong medical regimen and follow-up. Specific contraindications to heart transplantation are listed in Box 36.4. Heart transplant recipients range from neonates to adults in their 60s and older, with upper age limits varying among transplant institutions. Advanced age was previously considered an absolute contraindication to transplantation, but it is now considered a relative contraindication, based on the findings of several studies that demonstrated excellent survival in carefully selected older recipients.[37]

Preexisting malignancy, once considered an absolute contraindication because of the potential for recurring cancer or development of second cancers resulting from therapeutic immunosuppression, is now considered only a relative contraindication if the potential recipient has been free of malignancy for a specific number of years and if there are no signs of metastasis. Severe liver and kidney dysfunction that is not thought to be reversible by an increase in cardiac output is a contraindication for transplantation. However, combined organ transplants such as heart and kidney or heart and liver transplant can be considered for certain individuals.[40] Diabetes mellitus is not an absolute contraindication if hyperglycemia is adequately treated and there is no sign of end-organ damage such as nephropathy, neuropathy, or retinopathy. If the patient has an active infection, transplantation is delayed until the infection has cleared. Recent pulmonary infarctions increase the risk for postoperative infection and complicate oxygenation and ventilation; a recent history of infarction often precludes transplantation.

Distribution of organs is strictly regulated by a regional, state, and national network organized and managed by the UNOS and contracted by the federal government. Heart transplant candidates are prioritized based on medical urgency, which is determined by the patient's need for inotropic support with invasive hemodynamic monitoring, mechanical ventilation, or mechanical assist devices such as left ventricular assist devices or intraaortic balloon pumps. Patients who require this degree of assistance are listed as status 1A or 1B; all other heart transplantation candidates are listed as status 2 (Table 36.8).

In addition to candidate status, other variables such as blood type impact the length of time a candidate will wait for a transplant. For example, blood type O organs are compatible with recipients with all blood types. Because these organs can be allocated to non–type O recipients, patients who are blood type O generally spend more time on the waiting list before receiving their organ.

There is also some regional variability that can affect median wait times. The region that includes Arizona, California, Nevada, New Mexico, and Utah has a median waiting time of 645 days for blood type O recipients, whereas the region consisting of Alaska, Hawaii, Idaho, Montana, Oregon, and Washington has a median wait time of 196 days.[41] This variability is due to population density of the regions and the number of transplant centers within each region, which can often compete for the same donors. Donor hearts continue to be a limited resource. In 2013, 3817 adult heart transplants were performed worldwide at 252 centers.[37]

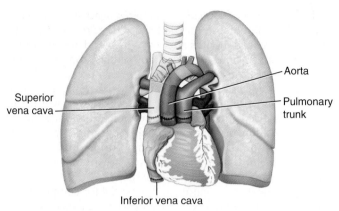

FIG. 36.6 Surgical Procedure for Heart Transplantation.

Transplantation Surgical Procedure

Biatrial Technique

The standard surgical procedure for orthotopic heart transplantation was originally developed by Lower and Shumway in 1960.[42] A standard median sternotomy is used, the great vessels are cannulated, and cardiopulmonary bypass is instituted after anticoagulation and standard hypothermia are achieved. The donor heart is prepared by interconnecting the pulmonary veins to form a single left atrial cuff and by trimming the aorta and pulmonary artery to fit the recipient's anatomy. All of the recipient's heart is removed except the posterior walls of the atria that contain the openings of the pulmonary veins and vena cava. Four major anastomoses are performed between the donor heart and the recipient's native atrial remnant and great vessels: In order, they are anastomoses of the right and left atria, the aorta, and the pulmonary artery (Fig. 36.6). The posterior native atrial remnant remains innervated by the parasympathetic and sympathetic nerve fibers from the autonomic nervous system. However, the donor heart is denervated, resulting in a faster resting heart rate of 90 to 100 beats/min. The rate of the transplanted heart is the normal intrinsic rate generated by the donor sinoatrial node located in the right atrium.

Although it was long regarded as the gold standard for heart transplantation, the standard biatrial technique had disadvantages related to the large atrial cavities. The loss of normal atrial anatomy increased the risk of mitral and tricuspid valve regurgitation, atrial septal aneurysm, atrial thrombus formation, and tachydysrhythmias.

Bicaval Technique

The bicaval technique was originally reported by Sievers et al[43] in 1991 and is now the usual method for orthotopic heart transplant. The anastomotic sites of the bicaval technique include the left atrial cuff, which contains the orifices of pulmonary veins; the superior vena cava and inferior vena cava; and the aorta and the main pulmonary artery (see Fig. 36.6). This technique leaves the recipient with a more anatomically normal atria. Benefits of the bicaval technique include preserved sinoatrial node function with decreased incidence of atrial dysrhythmias and mitral and tricuspid regurgitation.

Postoperative Medical and Nursing Management

Immediate postoperative management of the heart transplant recipient is similar to management of patients undergoing other cardiac surgery procedures. Nursing care of the transplant recipient involves several nursing diagnoses, as listed in Box 36.5. The most frequently used diagnosis is decreased cardiac output. Possible causes for a decrease in cardiac output include right heart dysfunction, dysrhythmias, hypothermia, myocardial depression, tamponade, and rejection.

Variables that influence myocardial performance include prolonged ischemic time (time from excision of the donor heart to removal of the aortic cross-clamp after implantation into the recipient), reperfusion injury, and hypothermia. Dysrhythmias may occur as a result of myocardial irritation, local ischemia, edema around the atrial suture line, and disruption of the sinoatrial nodal blood supply.

An ECG abnormality unique to a transplanted heart is the presence of a second P wave, which is generated by the native sinoatrial node that has been left in the atrial cuff. Because this impulse does not cross the suture line, it is capable of conducting only through the remnant of the native recipient atria. This impulse is not seen in hearts transplanted using the bicaval technique because the native right atrium and its sinoatrial node are removed.

Temporary epicardial pacing or isoproterenol, a powerful beta-adrenergic agonist, are sometimes used in the postoperative period for chronotropic (heart rate) support. The chronotropic and vasodilator properties of isoproterenol effectively sustain the heart rate, increase cardiac output, and decrease pulmonary vascular resistance. Pulmonary vascular resistance may be increased as a result of preexisting left ventricular failure and may be a cause of transient right ventricular dysfunction in the newly transplanted heart. Dopamine and epinephrine are often used for inotropic support in the postoperative period. However, the use of inotropic and chronotropic medications is highly individualized based on institutional preference. Generally, inotropic medications are gradually discontinued over 24 to 48 hours as tolerated by the patient, and the need for isoproterenol decreases as the heart begins to maintain its normal intrinsic rate of approximately 100 beats/min. Temporary pacing is required only occasionally, and less than 10% of transplant recipients require a permanent pacemaker implant.

Cardiac tamponade does not occur with greater frequency in heart transplantation compared with other heart surgeries, but it may be more difficult to detect as a result of an enlarged pericardial sac secondary to long-standing cardiomyopathy.

Signs and Symptoms of Rejection

The occurrence of hyperacute rejection in heart transplants is uniformly fatal unless emergency hemodynamic support

BOX 36.6 Signs and Symptoms of Heart Transplant Rejection

R   Rub (pericardial friction)
E   Electrocardiogram voltage decreased
J   Jugular venous distention
E   Edema (peripheral, sudden onset)
C   Cardiac dysrhythmias (atrial, bradycardia)
T   Tiredness
I   Intolerance of exercise
O   Onset of low-grade fever
N   New S_3 or S_4 heart sound
E   Enlarged cardiac silhouette
P   Pulmonary crackles, wheezes
I   Increased weight
S   Shortness of breath
O   Onset of hypotension
D   Disturbance in mood
E   Echocardiogram findings (systolic function, left ventricular mass/thickness)

From Cupples SA. Heart transplantation. In: Cupples SA, Ohler L, eds. *Transplantation Nursing Secrets*. Philadelphia: Hanley & Belfus; 2003.

TABLE 36.9 Cardiac Biopsy Grading

Grade	Nomenclature
0R	No rejection
1R, mild	Interstitial and/or perivascular infiltrate with up to one focus of myocyte damage
2R, moderate	Two or more foci of infiltrate with associated myocyte damage
3R, severe	Diffuse infiltrate with multifocal myocyte damage, ± edema, ± hemorrhage, ± vasculitis

such as extracorporeal membrane oxygenation is initiated until retransplantation can be performed. Signs and symptoms of hyperacute rejection are not subtle. The donor heart becomes cyanotic, and graft failure and hemodynamic collapse occur within minutes. Careful ABO matching and advances in antibody screening have made occurrence of hyperacute rejection rare.[32] Acute cellular rejection in heart transplant recipients can occur at any time, although it is most likely to occur during the first 3 to 6 months after transplantation. Box 36.6 lists the signs and symptoms of rejection.

Rejection Surveillance

Diagnosis of heart transplant rejection is determined by fluoroscopic- or echocardiography-guided endomyocardial biopsy. A bioptome is percutaneously inserted through the right internal jugular vein and advanced through the right atrium to the right ventricle. The femoral, subclavian, and left internal jugular veins are alternative sites for venous access, although the right internal jugular vein provides the most direct access. Endomyocardial tissue is obtained from the interventricular septum. The samples are microscopically evaluated for interstitial and perivascular infiltration. Heart biopsies are graded according to the severity of the interstitial infiltration of lymphocytes. The standardized cardiac biopsy grading scale ranges from mild to severe (Table 36.9).[44]

The frequency of surveillance biopsies varies from center to center. Generally, biopsies are performed more frequently in the first few weeks and months after transplant and are performed less frequently as time goes on. Many centers stop performing routine biopsies after 2 to 5 years and rely instead on clinical assessment to determine the need for biopsy. A major but rare complication of biopsy is ventricular perforation, which can result in cardiac tamponade. Pneumothorax is another potential complication of endomyocardial biopsy and may result from perforation of the visceral pleura during cannulation of the jugular vein; clinical manifestations are a sudden onset of sharp pain in the affected side and dyspnea.

Despite the invasive nature and potential for complications associated with endomyocardial biopsy, it remains the gold standard of rejection surveillance in heart transplantation. Alternative methods for noninvasive monitoring with comparable sensitivity and specificity remain elusive, although some progress has been made with the development of the AlloMap test. This blood test measures the genes expressed by activated T cells as a marker of possible rejection. Some heart transplant programs use the test as a trigger for performing endomyocardial biopsy. If the AlloMap indicates increased T-cell gene expression, patients undergo a biopsy to rule out rejection.

Treatment of acute rejection episodes may require intravenously administered corticosteroids. Recurrence of acute rejection is managed with various pharmacologic agents, depending on the patient's clinical condition and institutional preference. Strategies include augmenting current maintenance immunosuppression or switching to alternatives such as tacrolimus, mycophenolate mofetil, or sirolimus. Other agents used for recurrent rejection include polyclonal antibodies such as antilymphocyte globulin or antithymocyte globulin. Salvage therapy for persistent rejection that has not responded to conventional immunosuppression includes multiple steroid boluses, anti–T cell antibodies, or total lymphoid irradiation in which low-dose ionizing radiation is used to treat the lymphoid tissue.

Infection Surveillance

Infection surveillance is a high priority for an immunocompromised patient. It is well known that immunosuppression predisposes the patient to infection by a multitude of opportunistic pathogens that cannot easily be prevented with infection control. Development of infection is encountered most often in the early postoperative period, when immunosuppression is maximized. Infection is a leading cause of death during this period (up to 2 years after surgery). Great care must be taken to use aseptic technique for all intravenous line and dressing changes. Centers differ widely in their protective practices regarding the transplant recipient. Some use reverse isolation, whereas others put transplant recipients in rooms with other patients and simply use standard precautions.

Development of fever is aggressively investigated, with systematic blood, wound, and respiratory tract cultures; chest radiographs; and observation. Because steroids are known to suppress the body's inflammatory reaction, an elevated temperature generally is considered significant when it reaches 38°C (100.4°F). Nurses must be suspicious of any new productive cough, dry cough, change in type of secretions, or change in chest radiograph findings.

CMV is a particular threat to transplant recipients. CMV is a herpesvirus that can produce latent infection that persists throughout life. In the United States, 50% to 80% of adults are infected with CMV by age 40 years.[45] CMV can be transmitted

Coronary artery is occluded by focal atherosclerotic plaque.

Coronary artery is narrowed by diffuse thickening of the arterial wall in response to chronic rejection. This is known as allograft vasculopathy.

Typical atherosclerosis

Allograft vasculopathy

(Lipid   ● Macrophages   ● T lymphocytes   ◗ Smooth muscle cells

FIG. 36.7 Allograft Vasculopathy Compared With Typical Atherosclerosis.

through organ and blood product donation. Transplantation from a CMV-seropositive donor to a CMV-seronegative recipient poses the highest risk to the recipient for acquiring a primary infection. The antiviral agent ganciclovir can inhibit viral replication and ameliorate symptoms and is used in the prophylaxis and treatment of CMV infections. CMV immune globulin can be administered for prevention of primary CMV disease and for treatment of CMV disease.

Patient Education

Thorough, effective, and ongoing education of patients and their caregivers is vital to successful long-term outcomes after heart transplantation. The education process begins before the transplant and continues throughout the patient's life. Many members of the health care team provide education about posttransplant care, including nurses, transplant coordinators, pharmacists, dietitians, physical therapists, occupational therapists, and other health professionals. Patients and caregivers are taught about transplant medications, self-monitoring for signs of infection and rejection, and safety precautions and are provided with guidelines for

maintaining a heart-healthy diet and increasing physical activity. Patients may be required to check their blood glucose, blood pressure, temperature, and daily weight at home. At first, frequent clinic visits are needed to monitor progress and adjust medications. A schedule is established for routine laboratory tests and clinic visits to ensure long-term success of the transplant.

Long-Term Considerations

Chronic immunosuppression results in significant morbidity. Steroid administration can result in osteoporosis, avascular necrosis of joints, fragile skin, and obesity. Cyclosporine can cause kidney damage, excessive hair growth, gingival hyperplasia, tremor, and hypertension necessitating pharmacologic control. Azathioprine can be hepatotoxic (see Table 36.7). Concomitant use of these immunosuppressants also leaves patients more susceptible to malignancies and late infections.[37]

Initial causes of death include graft failure, infection, and multiorgan failure.[37] Cause of death 3 to 5 years after transplant is most often due to malignancy, cardiac allograft vasculopathy, and kidney failure.[37]

Cardiac Graft Vasculopathy

Cardiac graft vasculopathy, or coronary artery disease in the transplanted heart, is thought to develop as a result of chronic rejection and is a major cause of late morbidity and mortality. It is a diffuse and rapidly progressive type of coronary disease that causes concentric narrowing of the coronary arteries. Because the lesions are discrete, they are generally not amenable to interventions such as angioplasty or bypass grafting. The pathophysiology is completely different from typical atherosclerotic coronary artery disease as illustrated in Fig. 36.7.

Patients with denervated hearts usually cannot feel anginal pain, although reinnervation of transplanted hearts can occur over time. Cardiac graft vasculopathy can cause ischemic injury, heart failure, or sudden death. Graft vasculopathy is diagnosed initially by angiographic screening and later in the course of the disease by silent infarctions observed on the 12-lead ECG. Patients may have the disease and demonstrate no clinical sequelae. Many transplant programs have initiated baseline and annual angiographic studies to look for the development and progression of graft vasculopathy. Proliferation signal inhibitor medications such as sirolimus and everolimus are sometimes used as prophylaxis against graft vasculopathy or to slow its progression.[46] However, the only definitive treatment for advanced graft vasculopathy is retransplantation.

Compared with end-stage heart disease before transplant, heart transplant recipients report improvement in their functional status and health-related quality of life. The median recipient age is 54 years.[37] At 1 to 3 years after transplant, 90% of recipients report no activity limitations, and 25% are employed.[37]

HEART-LUNG TRANSPLANTATION

Before the first human heart-lung en bloc transplant in 1981, the technique of heart-lung transplantation was perfected in dogs in the 1940s and primates in the 1970s with good success. This success was in part due to improvements in immunosuppressant medications (described earlier in the chapter) that prevented rejection. Reitz and colleagues performed the first heart-lung transplant at Stanford University in 1981 in a 45-year-old woman with end-stage primary pulmonary hypertension, who survived for more than 5 years.[47,48] Heart-lung transplantation is a viable option for patients with end-stage cardiopulmonary failure such as congenital cardiac anomalies with pulmonary hypertension, primary pulmonary hypertension with irreversible right heart failure, and primary parenchymal lung disease with severe right-sided heart failure.

Indications and Selection

Compared with other transplants, relatively few heart-lung transplants are performed each year. In 2013, only 46 heart-lung transplants were performed from 29 centers worldwide.[49] Box 36.7 lists indications for heart-lung, single-lung, and double-lung transplantation. Although there are general standards that all centers adhere to in the candidate selection process, relative contraindications vary case by case in most centers. Box 36.8 lists absolute

---

BOX 36.7   Indications for Heart-Lung and Lung Transplant

Pulmonary Vascular Disease
Primary pulmonary hypertension
Eisenmenger syndrome
Cardiomyopathy with pulmonary hypertension

Restrictive Lung Disease
Idiopathic pulmonary fibrosis
Sarcoidosis
Asbestosis
Histiocytosis X
Bronchiolitis obliterans organizing pneumonia
Desquamative interstitial pneumonitis

Obstructive Lung Disease
Emphysema—idiopathic
Emphysema—alpha-1-antitrypsin deficiency
Cystic fibrosis
Bronchiectasis
Bronchopulmonary dysplasia
Idiopathic and posttransplant obliterative bronchiolitis
Lymphangioleiomyomatosis

BOX 36.8   Contraindications for Heart-Lung and Lung Transplant

Absolute Contraindications
- Malignancy in the last 5 y; lung transplantation for localized bronchoalveolar cell carcinoma is considered on a case-by-case basis
- Ductal carcinoma of the breast is considered on a case-by-case basis
- Untreatable advanced dysfunction of another major organ system
- Coronary artery disease with significant impairment of left ventricular function; heart-lung transplantation may be considered
- *Burkholderia cepacia* genomovar I, III, VI
- Noncurable chronic extrapulmonary infection
- Significant chest wall/spinal deformity
- Mantle radiation
- Documented nonadherence to follow-through with medical therapy or office follow-up, or both
- Untreatable psychologic condition associated with inability to comply with medical therapy
- Absence of consistent or reliable social support system
- Active substance addiction

Relative Contraindications
- Age older than 65 y for single-lung transplant
- Age older than 60 y for bilateral lung transplant
- Corticosteroid >20 mg/day
- Critical or unstable clinical condition
- Severely limited functional status with poor rehabilitation potential
- Colonization with highly resistant or highly virulent bacteria, fungi, or mycobacteria
- Obesity defined as body mass index exceeding 30 kg/m²
- Symptomatic osteoporosis
- Mechanical ventilation
- Coronary artery disease with percutaneous intervention with no cardiac dysfunction

Other medical conditions that have not resulted in end-stage organ damage such as diabetes mellitus, systemic hypertension, peptic ulcer disease, or gastroesophageal reflux should be optimally treated before transplant.

and relative contraindications for heart-lung, single-lung, and double-lung transplantation.

Any patient with end-stage cardiopulmonary or pulmonary disease who has exhausted medical management with the capacity for full rehabilitation may be considered for transplantation. Patients are assessed with regard to the "transplant window." The patient must be terminally ill to require a transplant but also maintain the strength and stamina to survive the long wait, complex surgery, and rigorous rehabilitation after transplantation.

Heart-Lung Transplant Surgical Procedure

Suitable donors are required for the success of a heart-lung transplant. All potential donors are brain dead from an event that leads to donor ventilator dependence to keep potential organs viable. Lungs are at risk for pulmonary edema, embolism, infectious processes, and atelectasis. Besides these risks, underlying donor pathology and chest trauma also determine whether donor organs are suitable for placement.

Donor Criteria and Management for Heart-Lung Transplant

Lung tissue has a relatively short preservation time, generally 4 to 6 hours, leading to procurement distance limits. Donors must first meet brain death criteria, be free of cardiopulmonary pathology, and have preserved lung function with no evidence of infection or malignancy. Donors with a history of smoking may be accepted if they meet the above-mentioned criteria.

To overcome the shortage of donor lungs, marginal donor lungs—lungs that do not meet all criteria—may be accepted. Although most donors are younger than age 55, older donors may be accepted if they meet all other criteria. Lung fields must be clear on radiologic findings with arterial oxygenation greater than 100 mm Hg on 40% inspired oxygen. A 100% oxygen challenge must show an arterial partial pressure of oxygen greater than 300 mm Hg.[50,51]

The donor and potential recipients are matched for ABO compatibility and organ size. Chest circumference, wall dimensions, and height-adjusted and weight-adjusted lung volumes are assessed. A donor with slightly smaller lungs than the recipient helps prevent postoperative compression atelectasis. Finally, inspection of the donor organs during procurement is essential for assessing lesions and trauma, which may impact transplant outcomes.[50,51]

During procurement, a sternotomy is made to inspect the heart and lungs. Once it is determined that the organs are suitable, the heart and lungs are mobilized. Prostaglandins are administered into the pulmonary artery.[52] The donor heart is then flushed with cold cardioplegia solution while the donor lungs are flushed with cold modified Collins solution, Perfadex, or University of Wisconsin solution.[53] Once the heart and lungs are perfused, they are removed and placed in cold electrolyte solution for transport using sterile technique.[54]

Recipient Heart-Lung Transplant Surgery

Cardiopulmonary bypass is used for the recipient operation. The phrenic nerves and bronchial artery circulation are preserved and maintained to prevent bleeding complications in the postoperative period. The heart-lung en bloc is placed with the tracheal anastomosis performed first, followed by the atrial anastomosis and then the aortic anastomosis. The donor trachea is kept short because of limited vascular blood supply in the area (Fig. 36.8).

Postoperative Management of Heart-Lung Transplant Recipient

The heart-lung transplant recipient is admitted to the critical care unit immediately after surgery and monitored for general hemodynamic stability, oxygenation, bleeding, ischemia-reperfusion injury, acute rejection, infection, deep vein thrombosis, pulmonary emboli, and multiorgan function.

Ventilation

Ventilation settings are determined partially by the underlying disease process and patient progression. Regular suctioning of secretions is crucial to maintain airway clearance. Extubation is performed after satisfactory gas exchange and lung mechanics are accomplished, and most patients are extubated within 24 to 48 hours. Evaluation for graft dysfunction, reperfusion injury, gas trapping, and phrenic nerve injury is ongoing. Early mobilization after extubation is essential for improved pulmonary toilet and helps prevent reintubation. Bronchoscopy is used to assess for potential complications such as stenosis, dehiscence, infection, and rejection and to assess the anastomosis.

Fluids

Care must be maintained when managing fluids in the early postoperative period. The lungs are extremely sensitive to volume overload. Pulmonary artery occlusion pressure and daily weight may be used to determine volume status and the need for diuretics. Overdiuresis results in hypotension and prerenal azotemia. Most patients are maintained on low-dose dopamine for the first 24 to 48 hours for inotropic support and kidney vasodilation. Epinephrine may also be used for inotropic support. Prostaglandin E_1 and nitroprusside provide pulmonary and systemic vasodilation. Nitric oxide, a potent vasodilator, is useful in decreasing pulmonary artery pressures and improving oxygenation.[53]

Pleural Drainage

Pleural drainage must be observed and documented, and careful attention should be paid to signs of active bleeding from the mediastinal and pleural chest tubes. Frank blood of more than 100 mL per hour over 3 hours should be a concern in patients with normal coagulation. Exploratory surgery of the chest may be required to find the source of bleeding. When chest tube drainage produces less than 200 mL in 24 hours without a noted air leak, chest tubes can be removed.

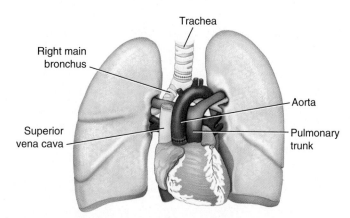

FIG. 36.8 Heart-Lung Transplant En Bloc Surgical Procedure. Incisions in trachea and aorta are shown. The heart is attached to a remnant atrial cuff, which contains the openings of the superior and inferior vena cava and pulmonary veins (not shown).

Ischemia-Reperfusion Injury

Reperfusion injury, also called primary graft dysfunction, usually occurs within the first 72 hours after transplantation and is typified by nonspecific alveolar damage with pulmonary infiltrates on radiography, hypoxemia, lung edema with poor pulmonary compliance, and normal or low left atrial filling pressures. Severe cases require ventilation, moderate levels of positive end-expiratory pressure and fraction of inspired oxygen, pharmacologic therapy, and perhaps nitric oxide or extracorporeal membrane oxygenation.[53]

Rejection Surveillance

Rejection is diagnosed by transbronchial biopsy of the lung or endomyocardial biopsy of the heart. The symptoms of rejection are the same whether the episode of rejection is cellular or antibody mediated. Shortness of breath, cough, fever, fatigue, wheezes, crackles, and decrease in lung function noted on pulmonary function tests all are potential signs of rejection but can also be present with infection. Most centers perform surveillance bronchoscopies at 1 month, 3 months, 6 months, and 1 year after heart-lung or lung transplant for early diagnosis and treatment of a rejection episode.[55]

Rejection of the lung is often followed by rejection of the heart. Heart biopsy is not recommended after 4 to 6 months posttransplant and is performed only with symptoms of heart failure or left ventricular or biventricular dysfunction on echocardiography. Rejection of the lungs can be detected by a decline in lung function on pulmonary function tests with a decrease in forced expiratory volume in 1 second greater than 10% and a decrease in forced vital capacity greater than 10%. Desaturation may also occur in the patient on exercise oximetry.

Spirometry has been shown to have a sensitivity of greater than 60% for detecting infection or rejection grade A2 and higher, but it cannot differentiate between the two. The ability to detect rejection diminishes further in single-lung transplants because of the impact of native lung dysfunction hindering the results.[55] Pulmonary function testing should be used as an adjunct to clinical evaluation and biopsy, not solely to diagnose acute lung rejection.[55] Some centers treat patients empirically with high doses of steroids, normally methylprednisolone 10 mg/kg intravenously daily for 3 consecutive days. Severe grades of rejection may also warrant the use of rabbit antithymocyte globulin. Table 36.10 depicts pulmonary grading of lung rejection.[55]

Humoral rejection is mediated by antibody and complement.[55] It can occur immediately after transplantation (hyperacute) or months later. Antibodies are either preformed antibodies or represent antidonor antibodies that develop after transplantation. Blood testing for donor-specific antibodies provides a method for determining whether a recipient has built antibodies specific to the donor after transplant. Treatment for antibody-mediated rejection warrants high-dose steroids, plasmapheresis, immunoglobulin, and rituximab (Rituxan). Intractable rejection can be treated with monoclonal or polyclonal antibodies, total lymphoid irradiation, or methotrexate.

Infection

Infectious complications are one of the most common causes of morbidity and mortality after heart-lung transplantation. Direct exposure to microbes, denervation of the graft with impaired cough reflex, impaired lymphatic drainage, infections transferred from the donor, infection from the native lung in single-lung transplants, and immunosuppression all contribute to infection risk.[56] Evidence of infection after heart-lung transplantation can be found in blood cultures, sputum, and urine and while performing a bronchoscopy with bronchoalveolar lavage. Bronchoscopies with lavage are done before extubation while assessing anastomotic patency and during routine surveillance. Bronchial lavage washings are sent for cultures to assess for bacteria, fungi, and viruses.

Antimicrobial prophylaxis for *Pneumocystis jiroveci* with sulfamethoxazole and trimethoprim is used in most centers because of successful prevention of this bacterial infection with additional antimicrobial effects against *Toxoplasma gondii* and

TABLE 36.10   Pathologic Grading of Lung Rejection

Category	Grade	Meaning	Appearance
A: Acute rejection	0	None	Normal lung parenchyma
	1	Minimal	Inconspicuous small mononuclear perivascular infiltrates
	2	Mild	More frequent, more obvious perivascular infiltrates; eosinophils may be present
	3	Moderate	Dense perivascular infiltrates; extension into interstitial space; can involve endothelialitis, eosinophils, and neutrophils
	4	Severe	Diffuse perivascular, interstitial, and air-space infiltrates with lung injury; neutrophils may be present
B: Airway inflammation	0	None	No evidence of bronchiolar inflammation
	1R	Low grade	Infrequent, scattered, or single-layer mononuclear cells in bronchiolar submucosa
	2R	High grade	Larger infiltrates of larger and activated lymphocytes in bronchiolar submucosa; can involve eosinophils and plasmacytoid cells
	X	Ungradable	No bronchiolar tissue available
C: Chronic airway rejection—obliterative bronchiolitis	0	Absent	If present describes intraluminal airway obliteration with fibrous connective tissue
	1	Present	
D: Chronic vascular rejection—accelerated graft vascular sclerosis		Not graded	Fibrointimal thickening of arteries and poor cellular hyaline sclerosis of veins; usually requires open lung biopsy for diagnosis

Modified from Martinu T, Chen DF, Palmer SM. Acute rejection and humoral sensitization in lung transplant recipients. *Proc Am Thorac Soc.* 2009;6(1):54.

Nocardia species. There are many other bacterial colonizers and infections seen after heart-lung transplantation and lung transplantation but no widely used prophylaxis.[56]

Candida and *Aspergillus* infections are the most common fungal infections in transplant patients. Prophylactic antifungal medications are used by many centers, but there are no clear data regarding optimal treatment or duration.

CMV is the most common viral infection in transplant recipients (described earlier in chapter). CMV may occur within the first few months after transplantation and may occur later on. Universal prophylaxis and preemptive therapy are the main measures taken to prevent occurrence. CMV infection occurs in 25% to 50% of heart transplant recipients but is highest in lung transplant recipients, with a reported incidence of 54% to 92% in recipients not taking prophylactic antiviral medications.[57] Intravenous ganciclovir followed by oral valganciclovir (Valcyte) are the primary prophylactic antiviral medications to prevent CMV infection.

Other common viruses after transplant include respiratory syncytial virus, influenza, adenovirus, human metapneumovirus, and parainfluenza. These are not treated prophylactically but as they occur. Nevertheless, they still pose a threat to recipient health and may lead to allograft injury over time.

Immunosuppression

Immunosuppressive therapy begins with the induction phase, perioperatively and immediately after transplantation, followed by maintenance therapy that continues for the life of the allograft. As noted earlier in this chapter, induction medication regimens are different from maintenance medications, and their use varies by transplant center. Maintenance immunosuppression is the key to prevention of acute and chronic rejections throughout the life of the graft. Most centers use a three-medication regimen consisting of a calcineurin inhibitor, antimetabolite, and corticosteroid (see previous section on immunosuppressive medications).

Patient Education

Patient education begins during the evaluation process and continues after transplant. Primary caregivers must be part of the learning experience to ensure understanding of the entire process from selection through posttransplantation. Transplant pharmacology, signs and symptoms of infection and rejection, and follow-up requirements all are part of the discussion during pretransplant and posttransplant teaching.

Long-Term Considerations
Bronchiolitis Obliterans Syndrome

Chronic rejection—termed *bronchiolitis obliterans syndrome* (BOS)—is the primary cause of morbidity and mortality after heart-lung transplantation and lung transplantation.[58] BOS is defined as an irreversible decline in forced expiratory volume in 1 second, with measurements taken 3 weeks apart, after excluding other causes of allograft dysfunction.[58] By 5 years after lung transplant, more than 50% of survivors have BOS symptoms.[58]

Factors such as acute cellular rejection and lymphocytic bronchiolitis are known to be associated with BOS. Nonimmune mechanisms such as primary graft dysfunction, infections, airway ischemia, and gastroesophageal reflux may also trigger an inflammatory-immune response leading to BOS.[58] Therefore, the balancing act with immunosuppression dosage to prevent rejection and infection is a careful art. Investigation of patient gastrointestinal complaints should be done promptly to avoid

TABLE 36.11 Bronchiolitis Obliterans Syndrome Classification System

BOS Stage	Description
0[a]	FEV_1 >90% of baseline and $FEF_{25\%-75\%}$ >75% of baseline
0[a]	$pFEV_1$ 81%–90% of baseline and/or $FEF_{25\%-75\%}$ ≤75% of baseline
1	FEV_1 66%–80% of baseline
2	FEV_1 51%–65% of baseline
3	FEV_1 ≤50% of baseline

[a]Potential BOS.

BOS, bronchiolitis obliterans syndrome; $FEF_{25\%-75\%}$, forced expiratory flow, midexpiratory phase; FEV_1, forced expiratory volume in 1 second; $pFEV_1$, potential FEV_1.
Modified from Ahmad S, Shlobin OA, Nathan SD. Pulmonary complications of lung transplantation. *Chest.* 2011;139(2):402.

aspiration risk leading to allograft damage. At the present time, there is no cure for chronic rejection; however, researchers are trying to find interventions to slow the process and eliminate BOS. Table 36.11 depicts the BOS classification system.[58]

Comorbidities

Numerous morbidities develop over time in transplant patients including hypertension and hyperlipidemia from calcineurin inhibitor medications, diabetes mellitus from corticosteroids and calcineurin inhibitors, kidney disease from calcineurin inhibitors, cancers such as skin cancer, and posttransplant lymphoproliferative disease from immunosuppressive agents.

Although the success rate for heart-lung transplantation is not at the level of other organ transplants, heart-lung transplantation remains a viable option for patients with cardiopulmonary end-stage disease. The survival for 3695 adult recipients of heart-lung transplants from January 1982 to June 2013 was reported by the International Society for Heart and Lung Transplantation as follows: 63% 1-year survival, 45% 3-year survival, and 32% 10-year.[49]

SINGLE-LUNG AND DOUBLE-LUNG TRANSPLANTATION

Single-Lung Transplantation Indications

Lung transplantation is a viable option for patients with end-stage pulmonary disease without end-stage cardiac disease. Chronic obstructive pulmonary disease (32%), interstitial lung diseases (24%), cystic fibrosis (16%), and alpha-antitrypsin deficiency (5%) are the main diseases warranting a lung transplant.[49] Lung transplantation is considered when life expectancy is no more than 36 months despite maximum medical management with disease symptoms classified as NYHA class III or IV.

Suitable donor lungs are a scarce resource; consequently single-lung versus double-lung transplant surgery is always a major topic for discussion. Single-lung transplantation benefits two recipients from one donor. Some advantages of a single-lung transplant include shorter extubation time, less need for cardiopulmonary bypass, and a shorter hospitalization. However, improved quality of life and success rates of double-lung transplants have made double-lung transplantation the preferred method of surgery.

Lung hyperinflation is a common complication after single-lung transplantation.[54] Graft compression by the hyperinflated native lung can cause mediastinal shift and respiratory

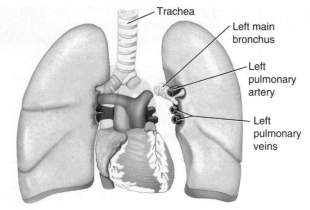

FIG. 36.9 Single-lung transplantation procedure shows where incisions will be for the left main bronchus, left pulmonary artery, and left pulmonary veins.

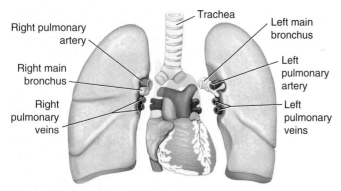

FIG. 36.10 Simultaneous double-lung transplantation procedure in which both lungs are sequentially replaced shows where incisions will occur between the right and left pulmonary veins, right and left pulmonary arteries, and right and left bronchi.

failure. Lobectomy and lung volume reduction surgery (LVRS) are two methods to prevent graft compression leading to decreased ventilation of the allograft. The native lung can also be a source of infections or problematic for a pneumothorax.

Single-Lung Transplant Surgical Procedure

The lung with the worst function is chosen for excision. If both lungs have equal function, the right lung is chosen for explantation with a new donor lung inserted to avoid maneuvering around the heart. A thoracotomy incision is made anteriorly or posteriorly at the fourth or fifth intercostal space. Alternatively, a sternotomy incision can be used. The lung is collapsed while the blood vessels are tied off. The lung is then removed at the bronchus. Next, the donor lung is placed, and the blood vessels are attached. Finally, the implanted lung is inflated, and the incision is closed.[54] Fig. 36.9 shows the surgical procedure for single-lung transplantation.

Double-Lung Transplantation Surgical Procedure

Double-lung transplantation is the preferred surgical procedure for patients with cystic fibrosis or bronchiectasis given the significance of infections in both lungs, which would remain in the native lung if both lungs were not transplanted. A double-lung transplant can also be performed sequentially (Fig. 36.10) or simultaneously, also known as *en bloc* (see Fig. 36.8). Bilateral lung transplant is increasingly selected over single-lung transplant.

Transverse thoracosternotomy, clamshell incision, and median sternotomy are the incisional approaches used in double-lung transplant surgery. The first lung is collapsed, and the blood vessel is tied off and cut at the corresponding bronchi. The new lung is then placed, and the vessels are reattached. The same process is repeated for the second lung to be placed. Patients with pulmonary hypertension may be placed on cardiopulmonary bypass during the surgery to avoid right heart failure.[54] Fig. 36.10 shows the surgical procedure for a double-lung transplant.

Lung Volume Reduction Surgery

LVRS is an option that may be available to patients with end-stage lung disease with comorbidities. LVRS may be indicated in patients with emphysema who have relative or absolute contraindications to transplant. The technique involves reducing the lung volume by wedge resection of the emphysematous tissue.[54] LVRS may decrease the mismatch between the hyperinflated lungs and the chest cavity. This may lead to elastic recoil and improved expiratory flow.

LVRS should be considered for patients with chronic medical conditions such as active hepatitis B, hepatitis C with biopsy-proven liver disease, HIV infection, and organ system dysfunction. Conditions that make patients ineligible for transplant may be acceptable for LVRS, including limited-stage non–small cell cancer with resection, lack of family support, psychiatric conditions, or a history of poor compliance.

Living Donor Lobar Lung Transplantation

Living lobar lung transplant was introduced at the University of Southern California in 1993 for patients who were too ill to wait for cadaveric organs. Two donors are required to donate either a right or left lower lobe of their own lung. The recipient must meet the requirements for cadaveric lung transplant and be on the waiting list. The risk of complication or death is higher than in cadaveric donor transplants because it involves two healthy living donors as well as the recipient.

After surgery, donor lung function has been shown to decline over time. Forced vital capacity has been shown to decrease by 17%, whereas total lung capacity has been shown to decrease by 16% within the first year after donation. Pulmonary function, exercise capacity, and freedom from bronchiolitis obliterans in recipients were equal to recipients of lungs from deceased donors. However, survival rates after 3 months were significantly lower, possibly as a result of more serious illness before transplant in the living lobar transplant group.

Postoperative Management

Postoperative management for lung transplant recipients is similar to management for heart-lung transplant recipients. Ventilation, hemodynamic monitoring, fluid management, drainage, immunosuppression, ischemia-reperfusion injury, rejection, and infection are monitored in the same way. Typically, single-lung transplant recipients have an easier time weaning off the ventilator and have shorter hospitalizations. Ventilation issues may warrant bronchoscopy while the patient is still intubated. Airway complications such as partial anastomotic dehiscence and stenosis are common and are diagnosed by bronchoscopy. Airway dehiscence is treated by reoperation or close observation and supportive care, whereas stenosis may require stent placement in the affected airway.

Aggressive postoperative pulmonary toilet is essential to promote airway clearance because surgical denervation of the lungs diminishes the cough reflex after surgery. Ischemia-reperfusion injury and disrupted pulmonary lymphatics can increase vascular permeability, leading to interstitial edema. Other potential postoperative complications are dysrhythmias, deep vein thrombosis, pulmonary emboli, and pneumothorax, all of which are prevalent in the early postoperative period.

Patient Education

Patient and caregiver education begins before transplant in the evaluation period and continues throughout the life of the patient. Similarly to heart-lung transplantation, information is provided about signs and symptoms of infection and rejection as well as follow-up care.

Long-Term Considerations

BOS is the histopathologic finding of chronic lung rejection, which affects 10%, 27%, and 50% of lung transplant recipients at 1, 3, and 5 years.[59] Acute rejection, infectious episodes, cancer, hypertension, diabetes mellitus, kidney dysfunction, gastrointestinal disturbances, and psychosocial issues all are very common short-term and long-term problems after transplantation and need to be addressed regularly.

LIVER TRANSPLANTATION

Liver transplantation was first attempted in canine models in the 1950s. The outcomes were unsuccessful because of technical complications, infection, and graft failure. Efforts to improve surgical technique continued, and successful liver transplantation in dogs was achieved several years later. In 1963, Starzl and colleagues performed the first human liver transplant, although the patient died intraoperatively. Starzl subsequently performed the first successful human liver transplant in 1967 in a patient with malignant hepatoma.[60]

By 2014, adjusted patient survival rate after liver transplantation was approximately 90% at one year, approximately 85% at 3 years and approximately 70% at 5 years.[61] Survival is affected by the pre-transplant diagnosis, donor liver (deceased or living donation) and age.[61] Liver transplant recipients older than 65 years have lower survival rates.[61]

Indications and Selection

Liver transplantation must be considered for any patient who has irreversible acute or chronic liver disease that is progressive and for which there is no therapy of established efficacy. Diseases of the liver may be categorized as chronic, vascular, fulminant or subfulminant, inborn errors of metabolism, and hepatic malignancies. Box 36.9 lists the most common diseases in patients who undergo liver transplantation. In the United States, the most common indication for liver transplantation in adults is chronic viral hepatitis C. New interferon-free treatment of hepatitis C patients with advanced liver cirrhosis restores liver function and may reduce the need for liver transplantations.[62] Cholestatic disease, biliary atresia, and metabolic disorders are the most common diseases leading to transplantation in pediatric patients.

Candidate selection is an important aspect of transplantation. Given the shortage of available organs, the transplantation team must have reasonable assurance of a successful outcome. The timing of transplantation is of utmost importance. The patient must not be so ill as to be unable to survive the surgery, yet must be experiencing deterioration in the quality of life. Body mass index (BMI) plays a role in posttransplantation

> ### BOX 36.9   End-Stage Liver Diseases Commonly Treated With Liver Transplantation
>
> **Cholestatic Liver Diseases**
> - Biliary atresia
> - Primary sclerosing cholangitis
> - Primary biliary cirrhosis
>
> **Chronic Hepatocellular Diseases**
> - Viral hepatitis (types A, B, C, D, E)
> - Alcoholic liver disease (Laennec disease)
> - Autoimmune hepatitis
> - Cryptogenic cirrhosis
> - Medication-induced liver disease
>
> **Vascular Diseases**
> - Budd-Chiari syndrome
> - Venoocclusive disease
>
> **Acute and Subacute Liver Failure**
> - Viral hepatitis (types A, B, C, D, E)
> - Medication-induced liver failure (acetaminophen, isoniazid overdoses)
> - Fulminant Wilson disease
>
> **Inborn Metabolic Disorders**
> - Wilson disease
> - Alpha-1-antitrypsin deficiency
> - Hemochromatosis
> - Tyrosinemia
> - Glycogen storage disease, types I and II
>
> **Primary Hepatic Malignancies**
> - Hepatocellular carcinoma
> - Hemangioendothelioma
> - Hepatoblastoma

survival. Patients who are underweight (BMI less than 20) or morbidly obese (BMI greater than 40) are at greater risk for death after transplantation. In general, liver transplantation is not to be offered to patients in the following groups:

- Patients who would be unlikely to survive major surgery
- Patients who would not survive the effects of long-term immunosuppression
- Patients who have a disease that is likely to recur quickly and fatally after transplantation
- Patients who are unwilling to comply with long-term and sometimes difficult and demanding medical regimens

The absolute contraindications listed in Box 36.10 fall under these four specific categories. Having one relative contraindication may not rule out transplantation, but having several predicts a poor outcome. Chronologic age is less important than physiologic age. Reports of transplantation in older patients describe favorable results. The UNOS reports that 1054 patients age 65 years or older received a liver transplant in 2014.[61] Certain diseases can recur after transplantation including viral hepatitis, sclerosing cholangitis, and biliary malignancies. In the case of viral hepatitis, serologic indicators of viral replication are monitored closely. Early treatment is indicated. Multicenter protocols are important in evaluating the outcomes of transplantations in patients with diseases that recur. The decision to offer liver transplantation to any patient must be based on evaluation criteria, which vary among institutions and

BOX 36.10   Contraindications to Liver Transplantation

Absolute Contraindications	Relative Contraindications
Brain death	Physiologic age
Metastatic malignancy	Advanced renal disease
Extrahepatic malignancy	Multiple hepatic malignancies
Active drug or alcohol abuse	Moderate cardiopulmonary disease
Advanced cardiopulmonary disease	Peripheral vascular disease
Acquired immunodeficiency syndrome	Psychosocial behaviors indicating non-compliance with medical regimens
Extrahepatic sepsis	Human immunodeficiency virus infection

BOX 36.11   Pretransplantation History for a Patient With End-Stage Liver Disease

- Risk factors for viral hepatitis: transfusions, intravenous drug abuse, tattoos, other parenteral exposure
- Family history of liver disease
- Associated disorders: hypothyroidism, osteoporosis, infertility, arthritis
- Onset, duration, and description of symptoms and complications: jaundice, lethargy, bleeding disorders, pruritus, confusion, ascites, edema, melenic stools, abdominal pain, bone pain or fractures, chronic diarrhea, gynecomastia (in men), amenorrhea (in women)
- Current and past medical history: hospitalizations, surgeries
- Social history: exposure to alcohol, drugs, toxins, tobacco products
- Status of immunizations

BOX 36.12   Sample Evaluation Before Liver Transplantation

Laboratory Tests
- Liver function profile: transaminases (aspartate transaminase, alanine transaminase, gamma-glutamyltransferase), alkaline phosphatase, bilirubin, albumin, prothrombin time, partial thromboplastin time, clotting factors, cholesterol, triglycerides
- Kidney function profile with electrolytes: blood urea nitrogen, creatinine, sodium, potassium, carbon dioxide, chloride
- Hematology: complete blood count, reticulocytes, erythrocyte sedimentation rate
- Thyroid function: serum triiodothyronine (T_3) radioimmunoassay, serum thyroxine (T_4) radioimmunoassay, thyroid-stimulating hormone, T_4 and T_3 uptake
- Serology studies for hepatic viruses and other infectious diseases: viral hepatitis (A, B, C, D, E), cytomegalovirus, Epstein-Barr virus, herpesvirus 1 and 2, parvovirus, human immunodeficiency virus, rapid plasma reagin
- Blood type and antibody screen
- Immunologic profiles: antinuclear antibody, antimitochondrial antibody, anti–smooth muscle antibody, immunoglobulins (IgA, IgG, IgM)
- Nutrition profiles: vitamin levels (A, D, E, B_{12}, folate), iron studies with ferritin
- Tumor markers: alpha-fetoprotein, carcinoembryonic antigen, prostate-specific antigen
- Miscellaneous: ceruloplasmin, alpha-1-antitrypsin level and phenotype

Urine
- 24-h protein and electrolytes, cultures, creatinine clearance, urinalysis, copper

Stool
- Ova, cysts, parasites, occult blood, 48-h fecal fat, cultures

Gastrointestinal Work-Up
- Endoscopy, colonoscopy, endoscopic retrograde cholangiopancreatography, liver biopsy

Pulmonary Profile
- Arterial blood gases, pulmonary function studies

Radiographic and Diagnostic Tests
- Chest radiograph, ultrasound studies of liver including vascular studies

Optional Tests
- Doppler studies, sinus radiography, computed tomography (abdomen, chest, head), electrocardiography, echocardiography, cardiac stress test, cardiac catheterization, mammography, peripheral vascular studies, carotid ultrasonography, abdominal angiography, percutaneous cholangiography, bone mineral density

which are modified as advances in technical ability, immunosuppression, and perioperative management continue.

Recipient Evaluation

A candidate for liver transplantation undergoes a thorough evaluation to determine the cause and severity of the liver disease, to establish the need for transplantation rather than other interventions, and to identify objective indications and contraindications. Evaluation begins with a carefully elicited patient history (Box 36.11). A comprehensive approach includes laboratory, radiographic, and diagnostic testing and multidisciplinary consultations (Box 36.12). Not every patient undergoes every test and consultation. Careful history taking and a good physical examination direct initial diagnostic testing. For example, a patient with a past history of malignancy would undergo extensive testing to rule out metastases, whereas a patient with acute liver failure may have a more abbreviated work-up focused on determining the cause and potential for hepatic recovery.

Initially, the transplant candidate is seen and examined by a hepatologist and transplant surgeon. The patient is evaluated for comorbidities that can potentially decrease a good outcome. Any history of drug and alcohol use is also discussed, and if this is an issue, referral to addictive behavior psychiatry is made for further evaluation. Additionally, the impact of liver disease on the patient's functional level and the availability of social support are reviewed. The transplant candidate should have financial clearance to ensure coverage for liver transplant and immunosuppressive medications. Physical examination not only serves as a confirmation of advanced liver disease but also is an opportunity to document clinical signs that may affect successful liver transplant, including loss of muscle mass and debility. Discussions

regarding recurrent disease after transplantation and possible hepatitis C virus antiviral therapies before or after transplantation are just as important. Surgical evaluation may identify additional factors that may complicate the transplant operation including prior abdominal surgery, obesity, and the candidate's general health and ability to undergo a major surgical procedure. During the evaluation, the surgeon educates the patient and family about the spectrum of donor and graft types, the complexity of the proposed surgery, potential complications, rejection rates, and other aspects of liver transplant including long-term immunosuppression and its side effects.

Other services such as nutrition, cardiology, nephrology, psychiatry, gynecology, anesthesia, infectious disease, endocrinology, hematology, rheumatology, and oral surgery or dentistry also are included in the evaluation. Ideally, all immunizations are brought up to date in an attempt to minimize postoperative infections. The patient and family receive education regarding the evaluation, waiting list, surgery, postoperative management including immunosuppression, and long-term follow-up. At the conclusion of the evaluation, one of several outcomes is possible: (1) The patient is a transplant candidate, (2) the patient is not a candidate, or (3) the patient may be a candidate sometime in the future if certain criteria are met. These criteria may be of a physical nature (eg, it is too early in the disease process to list now, in which case the patient will be reevaluated at set intervals), or they may be of a psychosocial nature (eg, the patient must attend a formal alcohol or drug rehabilitation program or undergo treatment for depression).

After candidacy has been determined and the patient is ready for transplantation, the candidate is entered into the national computer system operated by UNOS. Objective criteria are used to place a patient on the waiting list. These data are used in a formula to determine the patient's liver disease score, which is directly associated with risk of death within 3 months (the higher the score, the higher the risk of death).

Model for end-stage liver disease formula. The Model for End-Stage Liver Disease (MELD) formula is used in all US transplant centers to calculate risk of 3-month mortality in patients 12 years old or older.[63] The MELD objective criteria include serum total bilirubin, serum creatinine, prothrombin time, international normalized ratio, and whether the patient has undergone hemodialysis at least twice in the past 2 weeks.

Pediatric end-stage liver disease formula. The Pediatric End-Stage Liver Disease (PELD) formula is used to calculate risk of 3-month mortality for patients 11 years old or younger.[63] The PELD objective criteria include date of birth, sex, weight, height, serum albumin, serum total bilirubin, prothrombin time, and international normalized ratio.

Waitlist placement. The current liver allocation policy is basically "sickest first." There are many factors that influence access to donor organs such as local organ donation rate, area population, number of transplant centers, blood type, age, and diagnosis. The exceptions to MELD are the categories known as status 1A and 1B that are placed at the top of the list. Status 1A patients have acute liver failure and a life expectancy of hours to a few days without transplant. Status 1B is for very sick pediatric patients (UNOS.org/liver allocation).

The "Share 35" policy was approved and implemented on June 18, 2013, mandating that deceased donor livers are offered to regional candidates with MELD score 35 or greater before local candidates with MELD score less than 35. The policy was implemented to reduce geographic disparities in waitlist mortality.

Additionally, requests may be made to the UNOS regional review board to assign a higher than calculated score for a patient with special problems that are not addressed by the use of only objective criteria, such as children with intractable pruritus. Patients who have hepatocellular carcinoma that meet specific tumor criteria are automatically given a MELD score of 22 because the risk of metastasis outside the liver within 3 months is high. Once metastasis occurs, the patient is no longer deemed a transplant candidate. Other exceptions include disorders such as primary sclerosing cholangitis and polycystic liver disease.

The frequency of recalculation of the MELD score is determined by the score itself. MELD scores greater than 25 are evaluated every 7 days, scores between 19 and 24 are evaluated every 30 days, and scores between 11 and 18 are evaluated every 90 days.[63] A score of less than 10 is recalculated yearly,[63] barring any exacerbation of the liver disease or patient condition.

Next, one of the most difficult phases begins: the waiting period. It is impossible to anticipate when an appropriate organ will become available. The patient may feel that his or her life is being put "on hold." Because of the shortage of donors, it is common for patients in critical care units to die while awaiting transplantation; this is especially true for pediatric recipients. Moreover, knowing that another person must die so that he or she may live can cause feelings of guilt as the patient hopes for a liver to become available. Patients with end-stage liver disease know that the only alternative to transplantation is death. By understanding the basic social processes that patients experience while awaiting transplantation, nurses can facilitate health promotion activities. It is important for the patient and family to receive ongoing psychosocial assessment and to attend pretransplantation support groups, which are available at most transplant centers.

Pretransplantation Phase

A patient with end-stage liver disease who is awaiting a transplant may pose one of the greatest care challenges in the critical care unit. Hepatic encephalopathy, coagulopathies, portal hypertension, severe fluid and electrolyte imbalances, heart failure, pulmonary compromise, and kidney failure are common. Frequent mental status assessments are important in determining the patient's continued candidacy for transplantation. Hepatic encephalopathy may improve with the administration of antibiotics and laxatives, or the patient may proceed to stage IV coma. Later stages of hepatic encephalopathy may be clinically indistinguishable from cerebral hemorrhage. Diagnostic studies may be needed to evaluate the possibility of an intracranial bleed. Some centers use intracranial pressure monitoring catheters with these patients. The head of the patient's bed is maintained at 30 to 45 degrees to avoid even slight increases in intracranial pressure. Protection of the airway is especially important in an encephalopathic patient who is not intubated. In these circumstances, if hematemesis or vomiting occurs, intubation and use of paralytic agents may be necessary to protect the patient's airway.

Patients who have chronic liver disease are malnourished because of poor dietary intake and impaired digestion, absorption, and metabolism of nutrients. They require supplements of the fat-soluble vitamins (A, D, E, and K). Recommended dietary intake for patients with chronic liver disease includes 35 to 40 kcal/kg per day and 1.2 to 1.5 g/kg per day of protein using ideal body weight for patients with ascites and actual body weight for patients without ascites.

Consequences of portal hypertension must be corrected. Gastrointestinal hemorrhage from varices may respond to administration of propranolol or to procedures such as banding and sclerotherapy. Portal hypertension may be reduced by a transjugular intrahepatic portosystemic shunt performed by an interventional radiologist. Rarely, the patient may need to undergo surgical intervention with a vascular shunt created between the portacaval system and the mesangial, splenic, or renal vascular system. However, surgically created vascular shunts are usually not considered in patients who are transplant candidates. Patients with massive ascites usually have total body fluid overload but are intravascularly contracted and require sodium restriction and administration of colloidal fluids (eg, albumin) along with diuretics. Careful documentation of fluid intake and output, daily weight determinations, and frequent measurement of vital signs are needed to monitor fluid status. Ascites can interfere with lung expansion and can compromise oxygenation. Patients with large, distended abdomens also find adequate oral nutrition difficult. Use of diuretics to control ascites is common but can compromise kidney function or worsen hepatorenal syndrome. *Paracentesis* (removal of ascites) may be required for intractable ascites. However, frequent large-volume paracentesis procedures can contribute to kidney and heart compromise related to fluid volume shifts.

Spontaneous bacterial peritonitis can manifest in a patient with end-stage liver disease by an acute decline in liver and kidney function accompanied by fever, abdominal pain, and hepatic encephalopathy. The paracentesis fluid shows increased white blood cells, with or without a positive culture. Patients are treated aggressively with antibiotics and are temporarily deferred from transplantation during treatment for and recovery from bacterial peritonitis.

Determining Donor Suitability

The two criteria necessary for matching a donor liver to a recipient are blood type and body size. HLA tissue typing is not used in the matching of donor livers because it has not been shown to significantly affect patient outcomes. Donors are carefully screened for infectious diseases and metastatic carcinomas because these can be transmitted to the recipient. The transplant center is notified by the regional OPO that a liver is available. If the organ is accepted, a member of the transplant team contacts the patient.

In very urgent situations, the donor blood type (eg, type O) may be incompatible with the recipient blood type (eg, type A). Despite this ABO incompatibility, liver transplants can occur in urgent situations and can be successful. There may be some early postoperative complications, such as mild hemolysis, higher incidence of acute cellular rejection, and increased postoperative hepatic vascular and biliary complications, but innovative use of immunosuppressive regimens and plasmapheresis have improved graft survival of patients with recipient-donor ABO incompatibility.

Extended-criteria donor (ECD) livers, including livers from DCD donors, livers with a cold ischemia time longer than 12 hours, hepatitis C antibody–positive livers, and livers from donors older than 60 years, are expanding the donor pool and shortening waiting times.[64] The use of ECD livers can lead to complications and worsen outcomes. For example, the use of livers from DCD donors leads to biliary complications, livers from donors with advanced age or fatty liver can cause delayed graft function, and livers from Centers for Disease Control high-risk donors can increase the rate of infection in the recipient.[65] Despite the shortcomings of ECD livers, many lives are saved.

After a donor liver becomes available, it is necessary to expedite the preoperative preparation of the recipient. The use of newer preservation solutions has allowed for longer cold ischemia time (ie, the length of time from when the organ is removed from the donor, flushed, and packed in ice for storage until the time when it is transplanted).

Living Donor Liver Transplantation

Since 1985, approximately 23,000 people have died while registered and awaiting a liver from a deceased donor. Many liver transplant centers in the United States now offer *living donor liver transplantation* (LDLT). In 2014, 4.2% of transplanted livers were from living donors.[61] LDLT is more common in pediatric liver transplantation.[61]

LDLT began in 1989 with adult-to-child donations, commonly from a parent to his or her infant. The left lateral hepatic lobe is resected, leaving the donor with the larger mass of liver remaining. LDLT of the lateral segment of the left lobe of the liver has become highly successful in pediatric transplantation. Adult-to-adult LDLT began in the 1990s. Some transplant centers perform adult-to-adult right lobe and, less frequently, left lobe LDLT.

Living donor liver transplantation complications. Complications for the donor after partial hepatectomy are graded by the Clavien severity system I through IV.[66] Grade I complications are not life-threatening and do not result in permanent disability. Grade II complications require medications or transfusion. Grade III complications can be potentially life-threatening and require invasive therapy including a return to the operating room. Grade IV complications lead to disability or death. Most LDLT complications are grade I and II and include urinary tract infection, rash, dysrhythmia, wound infection, pulmonary emboli, pleural effusion, postoperative bleeding, bile leak, or biliary stricture.[66] More serious grade III and IV complications that have been reported for the liver donor include pleural effusions requiring chest tubes, bleeding requiring surgery, biliary complications requiring surgery, wound dehiscence, hepatic artery thrombosis, intraabdominal abscess, splenectomy, perforated gastric ulcer, deep vein thrombosis, and death.[66]

Individuals who donate a part of their liver in the United States have a perioperative risk of mortality of 1.7 per 1000 donors.[67] The risk of a catastrophic donor outcome such as acute liver failure or early death is estimated at 2.9 per 1000 donors.[67] Living donors must undergo a rigorous evaluation to determine eligibility to donate. This evaluation includes both physical health and psychosocial assessments. During this evaluation, the mass of the liver is measured, and the volume that can be safely removed is determined. The volume of liver that can safely be removed must be of sufficient mass so as to be able to support the recipient adequately.[67]

Donor advocate. Each center that performs living donor procedures must have a *donor advocate* who is not a member of the transplant team. The donor advocate is involved in all phases of the procedure to ensure donor safety and well-being.

Postoperative care of the living donor. Postoperative care of the living donor is similar to any patient who has undergone a liver resection. Liver regenerates rapidly after LDLT. Full restoration of liver volume appears to occur more slowly in the donor than in the recipient.[67] Critical care nurses play an important role in caring for donors and must be vigilant in assessing for complications and initiating early interventions.

Liver Transplantation Surgical Procedure

Liver transplantation surgery is lengthy and technically difficult, often lasting 4 to 12 hours. The patient is taken to the operating room for anesthesia induction, insertion of large-bore intravenous catheters that allow high-volume fluid infusion, and insertion of a pulmonary artery catheter for hemodynamic monitoring. Continuous renal replacement therapy may be continued or initiated in the operating room. The patient is positioned on the operating room table in such a way as to minimize pressure that could cause ischemia and chronic injury to tissue and peripheral nerves. Liver transplantation surgery can be divided into three stages: (1) recipient hepatectomy, (2) vascular anastomoses with donor liver, and (3) biliary anastomosis.

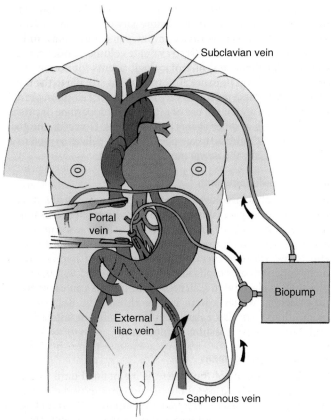

FIG. 36.11 **Venovenous Bypass During Removal of Native Liver.** The portal and iliac veins are cannulated, and blood is circulated by a centrifugal pump to the subclavian vein.

Recipient Hepatectomy

Stage 1 is the longest and most difficult part of the surgery because it involves removal of the native liver. It is further complicated by coagulopathies, adhesions, portal hypertension, and venous collaterals. Before completion of this stage, the patient may be placed on venovenous bypass (Fig. 36.11), although not all patients require this procedure. A centrifugal pump cycles the blood out through iliac and portal vein cannulas and returns it to the central circulation through the axillary or subclavian vein. Advances in surgical techniques, anesthesia, and fluid management have shortened the length of surgery enough to warrant elimination of venovenous bypass in many cases.

Vascular Anastomoses With Donor Liver

Stage 2 comprises the four vascular anastomoses: suprahepatic inferior vena cava, infrahepatic vena cava, hepatic artery, and portal vein. Many variations and adaptations such as vascular patches may be used, depending on the anatomy of the donor and the recipient. If venovenous bypass is used, it is removed after the infrahepatic vena cava anastomosis and before the hepatic artery anastomosis.

Biliary Anastomosis

Stage 3 can be achieved by *choledochojejunostomy* (bile duct to jejunum) or by *choledochocholedochostomy* (bile duct to bile duct). Choledochojejunostomy is performed in patients with diseased bile ducts such as patients with biliary atresia or sclerosing cholangitis (Fig. 36.12). It is also known as a *Roux-en-Y* procedure. Choledochocholedochostomy is performed in patients who have a healthy and intact common bile duct

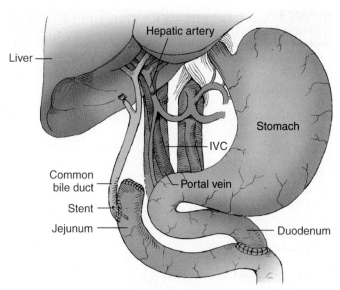

FIG. 36.12 **Roux-en-Y Procedure (Choledochojejunostomy) for liver transplant.** IVC, inferior vena cava.

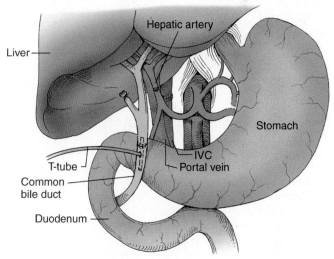

FIG. 36.13 **Choledochocholedochostomy Procedure for liver transplantation.** IVC, inferior vena cava.

(Fig. 36.13). The patient returns from surgery with or without an external stent or T-tube that is connected to a bag into which bile drains. Patients who do not have external biliary tubes may have an internal stent inserted in the bile duct across the biliary anastomosis. The internal stent eventually moves and usually is passed with the stool. Sometimes the internal biliary stent must be removed by an endoscopic procedure.

Bile Drains

Careful attention to any external biliary drain line is important. If the patient has an external biliary drain, the critical care nurse documents color, character, and amount of drainage and reports any changes. Biliary complications can occur after liver transplantation (Box 36.13).

Postoperative Medical and Nursing Management

Nursing diagnoses associated with liver transplantation are listed in Box 36.14. After surgery, some patients are extubated before they arrive in the critical care unit, but most arrive before reversal of anesthesia and remain intubated for 12 to 24 hours. Immediate goals include (1) reestablishment of normal body temperature, (2) hemodynamic stabilization, and (3) maintenance of an effective airway. Postoperative hypothermia is common after orthotopic liver transplantation. The critical care nurse must achieve rewarming safely by the use of methods such as warming blankets, heating lamps, and head covers.

Hemodynamics

Hemodynamic stabilization is a particular challenge because the patient may arrive hypervolemic, euvolemic, or hypovolemic and may be hypertensive or hypotensive. Assessment of total body fluids compared with intravascular fluid status is important. Because of inherent presurgical problems with decreased serum albumin, some centers tend to keep the patient "dry." Hypervolemia often results in third spacing, with resultant ascites and a leaking wound. Accurate measurements of hemodynamic function such as arterial blood pressure, peripheral blood pressure, central venous pressure, pulmonary artery occlusion pressure or wedge pressure, urinary output, patency of drains, and bile totals are assessed frequently to evaluate volume status. Choice of replacement fluids and pharmacologic agents for correction of volume and blood pressure abnormalities is specific to the transplant center. These protocols vary in their use of albumin or fresh frozen plasma and in the use of intravenous dopamine or prostaglandin as well as other agents and solutions. However, the goals are the same: Optimize tissue perfusion and deliver oxygen to all tissues, especially the newly transplanted graft.

Electrolyte Management

Electrolyte abnormalities can occur after liver transplantation. Disturbances in potassium and magnesium levels are common. High serum levels of electrolytes are usually associated with acute kidney injury; low levels can be due to medication side effects (eg, diuretic therapy). The presence of hypernatremia or hyponatremia complicates the correction of volume status and fluid replacement. Calcineurin inhibitors can cause hypomagnesemia, which lowers seizure thresholds. Because these medications can also cause seizures, careful monitoring and replacement of magnesium is important.

Pulmonary Management

Ventilatory support of the patient is maintained until the anesthetic agent has been metabolized and cleared by the new liver and the patient awakens. Frequent measurement of arterial blood gas levels, continuous pulse oximetry, and assessment of breath sounds are needed. The patient may require changes in ventilatory settings, suctioning to remove secretions, or administration of pharmacologic agents to correct acid–base imbalances. Pulmonary complications are common, as listed in Box 36.13. While the patient is on ventilatory support, pneumonia can be avoided by maintaining the head of bed elevated at 30 degrees, turning the patient frequently, providing good oral care, and brushing the patient's teeth. After extubation, patients must be encouraged to perform incentive spirometry exercises and to turn, cough, and deep breathe frequently to help prevent atelectasis and pneumonia. Respiratory treatments with bronchodilators, prophylactic antimicrobials, and chest physiotherapy also may be used. Early mobilization and physical therapy are encouraged.

Coagulopathy Management

Management of coagulopathies is important in the early postoperative phase. Characterization and careful measurement of drain lines and drainage from incisions are needed along with other nursing assessments of blood loss such as identifying signs of hypovolemia, tachypnea, tachycardia, or poor peripheral oxygenation. A sudden increase in abdominal girth, sanguineous drainage or nasogastric output, and black tarry stools are hallmarks of bleeding problems and must be reported immediately. Laboratory monitoring during the first 24 hours after surgery is necessary to assess blood loss and coagulopathies and includes hematocrit, hemoglobin, platelet count, prothrombin time, partial thromboplastin time, fibrinogen, and fibrin split products. Reversal of coagulopathies is done judiciously, with consideration for the potential to thrombose newly anastomosed blood vessels in the liver. Blood products such as platelets, fresh frozen plasma, and specific factors can be given along with pharmacologic agents such as vitamin K.

Neurologic Management

Neurologic assessment of the patient is important in the early postoperative phase to determine mental status and graft function. Patients who were encephalopathic preoperatively are usually slower to clear mentally. Nevertheless, with good liver function, the patient should be alert and oriented within 1 to 2 days; the improved mental status is a reflection of a functional new liver. Certain pharmacologic agents, including immunosuppressants, can cause peripheral and central neurologic side effects that may alter neurologic status. Induction therapy may be used to delay the initiation of immunosuppressant medications associated with neurologic and nephrogenic side effects.

Pain Management

The critical care nurse must always be aware of the potential for intracranial bleeds in a patient who has coagulopathies, serum sodium imbalances, and hemodynamic instability. All these conditions can interfere with pain management because the pharmacologic agents used for pain can mask deterioration in mental status. Medications to relieve pain are administered, but other nonpharmacologic nursing interventions also must be used.

Blood Glucose Management

Blood glucose levels after liver transplant can be altered by steroid administration, graft function, calcineurin inhibitors, and preexisting diabetes. Intensive blood glucose control (less than 150 mg/dL) during liver transplantation surgery has been associated with a lower infection rate and lower mortality. Perioperative hyperglycemia was associated with increased risk of liver allograft rejection in a retrospective study.[68] Low serum glucose in the absence of insulin administration can indicate primary nonfunction of the liver allograft.

Kidney Function

Kidney function can be altered by several mechanisms after liver transplantation, including cyclosporine or tacrolimus administration, acute kidney injury, intrinsic kidney disease, and poor liver function. Patients are managed with attention to fluid and electrolyte imbalances; by avoidance of nephrotoxic medications; and occasionally with ultrafiltration, continuous renal replacement therapy, or intermittent hemodialysis. With good liver function, kidney function usually improves. However, certain immunosuppressive agents and antimicrobials can deleteriously affect the kidney. Adjustments in dose or avoidance of use must be balanced with assessment of kidney and liver function. Daily monitoring of cyclosporine or tacrolimus serum levels is vital to determining adequate immunosuppression, and daily serum creatinine levels are necessary to monitor for acute kidney injury. As the patient's condition continues to improve, the frequency of laboratory testing may decrease.

Infection Prevention

Immunosuppressive therapy places the transplant recipient at an increased risk for infection. Infectious complications are common and continue to be the leading cause of death among orthotopic liver transplant recipients.[68,69] The potential for infection is greatest when patients receive high doses of immunosuppressants. All persons who come into contact with the transplant recipient throughout the hospitalization must practice good handwashing techniques and standard precautions to prevent the transmission of infection. Infections are treated with appropriate antimicrobials specific to the invading organism. Prophylactic therapies are commonly used as well.[68,69] Removal of central lines, arterial lines, urinary catheters, and drains is accomplished as early as is safe for the patient to avoid line-associated infections.

Nutrition Management

The nasogastric tube is removed when its output is minimal, bowel sounds have returned, and the patient is extubated. Patients who undergo a Roux-en-Y biliary anastomosis keep the nasogastric tube longer because postoperative ileus is more common. If oral nutrition is delayed longer than several days, total parenteral nutrition may be started. Consultation with a dietitian should be sought. Prealbumin levels may be measured to assess nutrition status. Otherwise, nutrition may begin orally or through a feeding tube as soon as the patient is extubated. When bowel function returns, the diet is advanced as tolerated.

Liver Function Tests

Graft function is monitored with standard laboratory biomarkers serum aspartate aminotransferase (AST), alanine aminotransferase (ALT), alkaline phosphatase, and gamma-glutamyltransferase; serum bilirubin; and prothrombin time. The serum levels of the biomarkers are measured frequently during the first few postoperative days. These levels may continue to rise for a few days before peaking and subsequently falling. As liver function improves, the frequency of laboratory testing decreases.

Liver Graft Nonfunction

A patient with suspected primary nonfunction of a liver graft demonstrates (1) hemodynamic instability, (2) progressive deterioration of kidney function, (3) coagulopathies and abnormal serum liver function laboratory tests, (4) hypoglycemia, (5) continued ventilatory dependence, and (6) an inability to awaken from anesthesia. Continued nonfunction of the graft necessitates relisting the patient for another donor liver. Early signs of optimal graft function include improving kidney function, mental alertness, a high to normal serum glucose concentration, and early extubation. The serum ALT, AST, gamma-glutamyltransferase, and alkaline phosphatase levels may peak on the third or fourth day but should subsequently decrease. The serum bilirubin concentration may take 1 week before beginning to decrease, and there may be a mild elevation when the external biliary drainage tube is clamped or after a blood transfusion.

Rejection Surveillance

Acute rejection is a cellular-mediated event and should be suspected if the serum liver enzymes, especially AST and ALT, become elevated compared with previous levels. These elevations can be followed by elevations in total bilirubin; such elevations usually precede any other sign of acute rejection of the liver allograft. Sometimes the patient also exhibits fever, a drop in bile output (if a T-tube is still connected to a drainage bag), and a change in the color and viscosity of the bile. At first, the patient may not have any other physical symptoms, but eventually late signs of rejection may occur, including jaundice, malaise, dark urine, and clay-colored stools. Certain infections, such as CMV, can also cause liver function test values to increase.

Rejection is suspected when liver function test values increase, but other reasons for these elevations need to be ruled out. Mechanical and vascular complications are ruled out by Doppler ultrasonography and angiography. Endoscopic retrograde cholangiopancreatography, hepatoiminodiacetic acid scanning, or transhepatic cholangiography may reveal biliary obstruction or leakage. A liver biopsy may be indicated to determine the cause of liver dysfunction if the other tests are inconclusive. Acute rejection can occur at any time after transplantation, but most commonly it occurs during the first few months and sometimes the first week after surgery. Most liver transplant recipients experience at least one acute rejection episode. Treatment of acute rejection requires increasing immunosuppression. Immunosuppressant protocols vary from center to center and are usually successful at reversing acute rejection.

Chronic rejection is both a humoral and a cellular event and is progressive over time and nonreversible. It results in destruction and loss of bile ducts. It is sometimes treated with plasmapheresis to remove circulating antibodies along with pharmacologic immunotherapies that bind B cells. Chronic rejection in a liver transplant recipient usually requires retransplantation if the patient is still a candidate.

Transfer Out of Critical Care

After the patient is stable and the transplanted liver is functional, central venous catheters and arterial lines are removed. The urinary catheter is removed as soon as the patient is awake enough to be continent. Drain lines are removed as drainage outputs become minimal. As the patient begins to participate in self-care, plans are made for transfer out of the critical care unit to the transplant step-down nursing unit.

On the transplant medical-surgical unit, laboratory data and vital signs continue to be routinely monitored. Self-care is promoted. Increasing levels of physical therapy are encouraged, diet is advanced, and much of the nurse's interventions are directed toward teaching the patient and family.

Patient Education

Considerable attention is focused on patient education and discharge planning. Discharge booklets are helpful in the education process. It is important for the patient to learn how to self-administer medications, monitor vital signs, care for the incision and the T-tube (if present), prevent infections, follow safe living practices, and identify problems that must promptly receive medical attention.[70] Because patients are commonly discharged within 2 weeks after orthotopic liver transplant, it is important for discharge instructions to begin as soon as the patient is mentally alert. Patients discharged early may require home health nurse referrals to assist with follow-up of incision care, intravenous therapies, and other procedures. Education must be provided about rejection surveillance, signs and symptoms of infection, lifestyle changes as needed, long-term medication considerations, and the follow-up visit schedule.

Long-Term Follow-Up

Liver transplant recipients who do not live in the same city in which their surgery was performed usually remain in the immediate area of the transplant center after discharge before returning home. During this period, they may be monitored by a home health nurse and be seen in clinic several times a week by the transplant team. Continued serologic testing is performed to monitor graft function, to determine blood levels of certain immunosuppressive agents, and to identify postoperative complications. Although many of these complications can be managed successfully in the outpatient setting, readmissions do occur. Because rejections, readmissions, grieving for the donor, and pharmacologic side effects can create anxiety for the family and the patient, they are encouraged to attend transplantation support groups if offered by the center. After patients return home, they are encouraged to resume a close relationship with their local primary care physician and gastroenterologist.

With the proliferation in the number of liver transplantations being performed, it is not unreasonable for recipients to be admitted to a non–tertiary care hospital for management of some long-term posttransplantation complications. Nurses who work for hospitals that do not perform transplants may have the opportunity to care for these patients. Nurses in these settings must also become knowledgeable about the signs and symptoms of rejection, administration of immunosuppressant medications, monitoring of immunosuppressant levels, and medication-to-medication interactions with the immunosuppressants. Every transplant recipient has a coordinator who follows the patient at the transplant center. The transplant coordinator is also available for consultation with community health care providers who have questions about transplant recipients.

Liver transplant recipients need long-term follow-up surveillance for hypertension, kidney failure, obesity, dyslipidemias, biliary and infectious complications, and malignancies. Early intervention affects the quality and length of life. Behavior modifications and therapeutic lifestyle changes should be frequently reinforced to positively affect long-term health. Financial concerns are a major source of stress in these patients.[71] Many transplant recipients had chronic liver disease before their surgery. They often were disabled for some time and already have experienced financial stressors related to illness. As these patients live longer with liver transplants, issues of insurability, continued disability, and the ability to obtain work will have to be addressed.[71]

Transplantation offers hope for survival but at considerable expense. Many insurance providers, including Medicare, provide partial reimbursement for liver transplant procedures. The costs to patients can be staggering.[71] Transplant centers must find innovative ways to control rising costs because of decreasing reimbursements, complexity of patient care, and increasing patient loads. Close management of posttransplant complications and avoidance of rehospitalization is important in reducing costs. Advanced practice nurses who work in transplant centers offer an effective economic model in the delivery of safe patient care.[72]

Future Considerations

Clinical trials are in process to identify new medications and define improved treatment protocols. With increasing choices of therapies, medications will be selected for patients after other immunosuppressive therapies have failed or severe side effects have occurred. As recipients spend more time on the waiting list, improved methods of medical management of end-stage liver disease and bridges to transplantation become increasingly necessary, including transarterial chemoembolization of hepatocellular cancer and transjugular intrahepatic portosystemic shunt placement.[73]

A limiting factor in liver transplantation continues to be the shortage of organ donors (see Fig. 36.1). Attention is being focused on ways to increase the number and availability of donor organs. This includes reduced-size organs, split-liver technique (in which one liver is divided and transplanted into two recipients), and living liver donors. Expanded criteria for deceased liver donors can include donation after cardiac death, advanced donor age, steatosis, hepatitis C–positive allografts, human T-cell lymphotropic virus–positive allografts, hepatitis B core antibody–positive allografts, donors with active infections, and high-risk donors.[74] Studies are exploring the roles of xenografts and bioartificial liver devices that can support a patient who is awaiting a homograft.[73] Recipient selection criteria also will continue to be redefined for diseases and conditions such as hepatic malignancies, HIV positivity, and alcoholism. As recipients live longer and healthier lives, pregnancy after transplantation will become more common.[75]

The number of liver transplants in the United States has declined in the last 10 years, partially because of worsening donor organ quality. If donor liver utilization practices remain constant, liver transplant will decrease from 78% to 44% by 2030, resulting in greater than 2000 fewer liver transplants. One option is use of marginal donor grafts.[74]

The use of ex vivo perfusion techniques may stabilize liver transplant volume. Otherwise, the number of liver transplants in the United States will decrease substantially over the next 20 years. New strategies for increasing organ donation including use of DCD donors are required to maintain the number of liver transplants at the current level.[74] These and other factors will influence the future of liver transplantation.

KIDNEY TRANSPLANTATION

The first successful kidney transplantation was performed in 1954 in Boston. Today, it is the treatment of choice for patients with end-stage kidney disease. Kidney transplantation allows the recipient to lead a much less restricted lifestyle and provides a more cost-effective treatment method than long-term dialysis. Advances in the study of the immune system and the development of new immunosuppressant medications have allowed for increased graft survival rates for deceased donor and living donor kidney transplants. Transplant centers use a combination of immunosuppressive medications to prevent rejection in an attempt to lower the doses of each agent so that the associated side effects can be minimized.

In 2013, 16,830 kidney transplantations were performed in the United States.[76] However, 96,607 patients were listed with the Scientific Registry of Transplant Recipients awaiting a donor kidney.[76] Discovery of new medications and finding ways to increase the number of donor organs recovered are major challenges faced by the transplantation community.

Indications and Selection

Many disease processes can lead to end-stage kidney disease. For this reason, potential recipients must undergo numerous laboratory tests and some noninvasive physical testing before they can be approved as candidates (Box 36.15). Because after transplantation the patient's immune system will be purposely and controllably compromised, there are several contraindications to kidney transplantation (Box 36.16). If any of these risk factors is present, the patient's risk is determined to be too high for transplantation and the immunosuppressant regimen that follows. The alternative for such a patient is to decrease or eliminate the risk factors that can be controlled and be reevaluated

---

BOX 36.15   Evaluation Before Kidney Transplantation

- Chemistry 24 panel test; human leukocyte antigen tissue typing; prothrombin time; partial thromboplastin time; complete blood count with differential; platelet count; human immunodeficiency virus; hepatitis; cytomegalovirus; Epstein-Barr virus; lipid profile; urine for analysis, culture, and sensitivities; 24-h urine for creatinine clearance and protein (if patient still produces urine); dialysate fluid for culture and sensitivity (if patient is undergoing continuous ambulatory peritoneal dialysis)
- Kidney ultrasonography or spiral computed tomography, chest radiography (posteroanterior and lateral views), electrocardiography, stress test and cardiac catheterization (if indicated), weight management (if indicated), colonoscopy (if age >55 y), mammography (for women age >35 y), venography (for patients with diabetes)
- Consultants: psychologist or psychiatrist, urologist, transplantation surgeon or transplantation nephrologist, social worker, dietitian, chaplain, financial counselor

---

BOX 36.16   Contraindications to Kidney Transplantation

- Malignancy during the past 3 y
- Active infectious process
- Advanced cardiopulmonary disease
- High risk for surgery
- Nonadherence to current medical regimen
- Recreational drug use
- Other serious contributing disease processes

---

at a later date. If the candidate is unwilling to eliminate controllable high-risk behaviors, the only alternative for survival is to remain on dialysis.

Deceased Kidney Donation

Most kidneys transplanted in the United States come from a deceased donor who meets the criteria for brain death or cardiac death (described earlier in the chapter). Donor and recipient are matched by ABO blood type. A simplified description of the current organ allocation criteria is provided.

The first priority for a deceased donor kidney is to candidates who are listed for a kidney and a simultaneous second organ (pancreas, heart, or liver) transplant.[76,77] Second priority is given to candidates who have a perfect HLA match with the donor kidney because this optimizes graft survival. The third priority is by local geographic region.[76,77] Organ allocation is managed through the OPTN/UNOS registry (described in the beginning of the chapter).[76,77] Deceased kidney donors are further classified as (1) standard criteria donor kidneys, delineated by donor age, whether younger than 35 years or older than 35 years; (2) ECD kidneys; and (3) DCD donor kidneys.[76,77]

Living Kidney Donation

The first successful kidney transplant was a living donor transplant between identical twins in 1954. In most cases today, the living donor is related to the recipient.[76]

Living kidney paired donation. An innovative newer option is *kidney paired donation.* A person may want to donate one of his or her kidneys to a family member, but the person's blood type

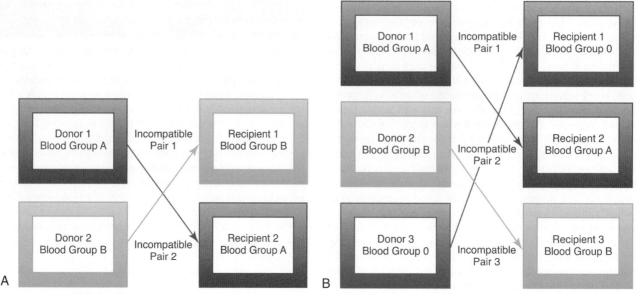

FIG. 36.14 Kidney paired donation is an option for a person who wants to donate a kidney to a family member but does not have a compatible blood type with the intended recipient. With this option, donors can participate in a donation exchange with another living donor-recipient pair (A). There could also be a three-way living donor exchange (B).

is incompatible with the intended recipient. In this situation, they could participate in a donation exchange with another living donor–recipient pair as shown in Fig. 36.14A. This could also be a three-way living donor exchange as shown in Fig. 36.14B. Several other variations have also been used involving a "chain" of donor-to-recipient transplants.[78-80]

Kidney Transplantation Surgical Procedure

When the kidney to be transplanted is procured from the donor—whether living or deceased—the ureter, renal vein, and renal artery are dissected, leaving as much length as possible. When kidneys are retrieved from a deceased donor, an aortic patch is often taken where the renal artery inserts in to the aorta. The minimizes posttransplant renal artery stenosis.[81]

Living Donor Kidney Transplantation

If the donor is living, the procurement is typically by laparoscopic nephrectomy.[81] Open surgical kidney removal is rare today. After the kidney is secured, it is flushed with a cold electrolyte preservative solution until the venous return is clear. This usually requires 100 to 200 mL of solution. The kidney is then transported to the operating room to be transplanted.

Deceased Donor Kidney Transplantation

If the kidney is from a deceased donor, it is flushed with a cold electrolyte preservative solution and simultaneously cooled externally as quickly as possible. It can be transported on a kidney perfusion machine or packed in an iced preservation solution. After the kidney is procured and placed in the hypothermic solution, it can be maintained for 48 to 72 hours before it must be transplanted. Most transplant centers attempt to transplant the organ within 24 hours after procurement to avoid cold ischemic injury and acute kidney injury. At the time of procurement, the kidney is assessed in situ for color, shape, and form. It is palpated to determine firmness, and often a biopsy sample is taken to rule out undiagnosed kidney dysfunction.

Kidney Transplant Recipient Surgery

The patient is anesthetized, and a urinary catheter is placed. A curvilinear incision is made 3 to 4 cm above the symphysis pubis and extended to the iliac crest (Fig. 36.15A). The muscles and fascia are divided and retracted medially to expose the iliac vessels. The kidney is placed in the extraperitoneal space of the right or left iliac fossa. The donor renal artery is anastomosed to the external iliac artery, and the donor renal vein is sutured to the external iliac vein (Fig. 36.15B).[81]

After the revascularization procedures are completed, the ureteral anastomosis is performed. The most common method used is *ureteroneocystostomy*. During this procedure, an incision is made in the dome of the recipient's bladder, and the donor ureter is tunneled through the recipient's mucosal layer and sutured to the mucosal opening. Tunneling of the ureter prevents urinary reflux into the transplanted kidney (Fig. 36.16).[81] A stent is often placed in the ureter to decrease postoperative risk of stenosis of the ureter. The stent is retrieved 2 to 4 weeks after transplant.[81]

During the surgery, a central venous pressure of 8 to 16 mm Hg is maintained, and a systolic blood pressure at least as high as the patient's baseline value should be maintained to ensure adequate perfusion of the transplanted kidney.

Postoperative Medical Management and Nursing Care of the Kidney Transplant Recipient

After the transplantation is completed and the patient is stable and ready for discharge from the recovery room, most transplant centers admit the patient directly to the organ transplantation unit or to the critical care unit. Serious complications can occur in the immediate postoperative period, and a sound knowledge base of medical/surgical nursing, kidney function, anatomy, and immunosuppressive medications is imperative. Relevant nursing diagnoses are listed in Box 36.17.

Fluid Status

If the transplanted kidney is producing urine, the patient's fluid status is monitored closely. Adequate hydration is an absolute

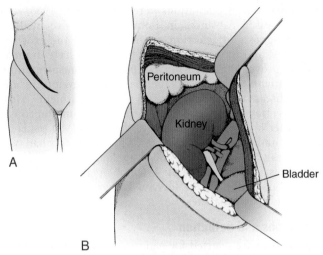

FIG. 36.15 Placement of the kidney graft into the iliac fossa. (A) The incision in the right side of the abdomen is used for graft implantation in the right iliac fossa. (B) The iliac vessels are exposed. (Modified from Smith SL. *AACN Tissue and Organ Transplantation: Implications for Professional Nursing Practice.* St. Louis: Mosby; 1990.)

FIG. 36.16 Ureteroneocystostomy Reconstruction of the Urinary Tract. The donor ureter is passed through a posterior bladder wall tunnel and anastomosed to the bladder mucosa. (From Smith SL. *AACN Tissue and Organ Transplantation: Implications for Professional Nursing Practice.* St. Louis: Mosby; 1990.)

⊚ **BOX 36.17   NURSING DIAGNOSES**

Kidney Transplantation

- Deficient Fluid Volume related to absolute loss, p. 1019
- Risk for Ineffective Renal Perfusion related to decreased blood flow to the kidney, p. 1045
- Risk for Infection: Immunosuppressive medications to prevent rejection of the transplanted kidney, p. 1046
- Disturbed Body Image related to actual change in body structure, function, or appearance, p. 1022
- Anxiety related to threat to biologic, psychologic, and social integrity, p. 1012

---

necessity for continued graft function in the immediate postoperative period. Hypovolemia can lead to compromised blood flow to the kidney, acute kidney injury, and possible graft failure. Urine output volume and color should be monitored at least every 30 minutes. The new kidney will be producing large amounts of urine, and fluid replacement, usually maintained in a 1:1 ratio, must be sustained.

Electrolytes

Electrolyte balance is also of grave concern. Because of the large volumes of urine produced, the potential exists for hypokalemia, hypomagnesemia, and hypocalcemia, leading to possible cardiac compromise. Electrolytes must be monitored at least every 4 to 6 hours and replaced as necessary. Assessment of the blood urea nitrogen and the creatinine concentration also is necessary every 4 to 6 hours to monitor graft function and determine the need for dialysis.

Postoperative Complications

The complete blood count and platelet count should be monitored every 4 to 6 hours. Blood loss during the operation is minimal, usually 500 mL or less. Abrupt decreases or continuously falling counts may indicate hemorrhage at an anastomosis site, which requires a return to the operating room for repair. Even with minimal blood loss during surgery, transfusion of blood products after the surgery is often necessary. Frequent observation and assessment of the surgical incision are needed to evaluate for drainage and swelling. Urine output volume and color should be monitored at least every 30 minutes. The bladder anastomosis is fragile, and clots can commonly occlude the catheter. The bladder must remain decompressed for several days to promote proper healing. If clots occlude the end of the catheter, gentle irrigation or aspiration may be necessary. If the clot cannot be dislodged or aspirated out, it may be necessary to change the catheter. Painful bladder spasms also can occur, and opiates, usually in the form of a belladonna and opium suppository, may be required to relax the bladder.

Immunosuppression

Initiation of induction immunosuppressant therapy begins at the time of transplantation, usually in the form of a polyclonal antithymocyte/antilymphocyte intravenous compound or an intravenous monoclonal antibody compound. These compounds remove the lymphocytes from the patient's system, preventing rejection and suppressing the immune system until oral medications can be safely administered and blood levels are sufficient to allow discontinuation of the intravenous agent. Because the patient is now immunocompromised, strict aseptic technique is required for all procedures to prevent infection.

Infection Risk

Thorough handwashing, aseptic dressing changes, discontinuation of any unnecessary invasive lines, and limiting the number of visitors are necessary protective measures. Because of the patient's immunocompromised status, subtle changes in the temperature, white blood cell count, or wound drainage can signal an active infection. Patients also are susceptible to infection by opportunistic native organisms such as *Candida*, pneumocystis pneumonia, CMV, Epstein-Barr virus, and herpes simplex virus.

Preparation for Discharge Home

The average length of hospital stay after uncomplicated kidney transplantation is 5 to 7 days. During the first few days, the patient must learn the self-care routines essential for graft survival. Medication regimens are complex, and most centers initiate a self-medication program at the patient's bedside as a training tool. Patients are taught the signs and symptoms of infection and graft rejection (Box 36.18), the protocols of the transplant clinic, and new dietary limitations. Frequent transplant clinic visits to check the functioning of the organ and to adjust down the doses of immunosuppressant medications are necessary for the first few months after transplantation.

Long-Term Considerations

Rejection of the transplanted kidney is an ongoing concern for all kidney transplant recipients. The graft function is monitored closely, and if rejection is suspected, a biopsy is performed. If the biopsy reveals acute rejection, rescue therapy is initiated. This therapy can be in the form of high-dose intravenous steroids for mild rejection or intravenous monoclonal antibody for moderate to severe rejection. If the biopsy reveals chronic rejection, the oral immunosuppressant medications are increased or returned to the higher doses used immediately after transplantation. No two patients' immune systems are exactly alike, and the immunosuppressant medication regimen required to prevent rejection must be tailored to each patient individually. The goal is to create a balance among medications that allows the patient to fight off most infections but avoid rejection of the transplanted organ.

Patient adherence to the medical regimen that is required to maintain a transplanted organ is a major concern. Adequate education of the patient and family regarding the importance of taking the medications as instructed is of paramount importance. Patients are reluctant to take the medications appropriately if they are experiencing severe side effects. Decreasing the dosage of the medications can often alleviate these symptoms but may lead to a rejection episode.

Patients often have financial concerns. The federal government helps to pay for the immunosuppressant medications for 36 months after transplantation for recipients younger than 65 years of age. Recipients older than age 65 with Medicare are covered for life.[82] However, the Medicare copayment system is complex, and many transplant recipients have financial concerns about the costs of their immunosuppressive medications.[82]

PANCREAS TRANSPLANTATION

Pancreas transplantation offers the opportunity of normal glucose control without the use of exogenous insulin. The first pancreas transplantations were performed in 1966, with little success.[83] Advances in immunosuppressive medications, diagnosis of rejection, management of the exocrine secretions, and improved surgical techniques have dramatically improved the success rate of pancreas transplantation. Many patients with type 1 diabetes mellitus develop chronic kidney disease requiring long-term dialysis treatments. Most pancreas transplantations are performed simultaneously with other organs, usually kidneys.[84] In 2014, 954 pancreas transplantations were performed.[85] Most recipients had type 1 diabetes (745 recipients), and a smaller number had type 2 diabetes or received multi–visceral organ transplants.[85] There is no difference in survival between recipients with type 1 and type 2 diabetes.[85]

Indications and Selection

Patients who are selected for pancreas transplantation must undergo a thorough evaluation similar to that for other organ transplantation (Box 36.19). The disease processes involved in diabetes mellitus and their effects on all major body systems require that special care be taken to ensure the candidate is in the best possible condition before transplantation. Severe and often life-threatening complications can occur after transplantation if the major body systems have not been properly evaluated beforehand. As with other organ transplants, organ allocation is managed through the OPTN/UNOS registry.[85]

Pancreas Transplantation Surgical Procedure

The surgical techniques for pancreas transplantation are diverse, and different programs use different methods. However, the principles are consistent, and all include the following three precepts:

1. Provide adequate arterial blood flow to the pancreas and duodenal segment.
2. Provide adequate venous outflow from the pancreas.
3. Provide management of the pancreatic exocrine secretions.

The cold-ischemia time of the pancreas before implantation should be minimized because pancreas allografts do not tolerate cold ischemia as well as kidney allografts. Ideally, the pancreas should be revascularized within 24 hours from the time of cross-clamping.

The abdomen is entered through a midline incision. The pancreas graft is transplanted into the right iliac fossa, with the head of the pancreas placed downward into the pelvis.[83] Most transplantation centers place both organs on the right side, although some put the pancreas on the right and the kidney on the left. The native pancreas is not removed.

BOX 36.18   Signs and Symptoms of Kidney Rejection

- Increased tenderness over transplanted kidney site
- Decreased urine output
- Increased serum creatinine levels, greater than patient's baseline level
- Fever
- Rapid weight gain (4–6 lb in a 24-h period)
- Swelling, usually in the hands and feet

BOX 36.19   Evaluation Before Pancreas Transplantation

- Blood chemistries, tissue typing, and viral studies similar to those for kidney transplantation candidates
- Complete cardiovascular work-up, including cardiac catheterization
- Complete vascular studies, particularly of the lower extremities, to ensure proper vascularization of graft
- Nerve conduction studies to evaluate for neuropathy
- Urologic and bladder function studies
- Consultations as required for all transplantation candidates

Arterial and Venous Revascularization

Arterial flow to the pancreas graft is provided from the recipient's iliac artery (Fig. 36.17). Venous outflow from the transplanted graft can be via an anastomosis to the portal vein or to the iliac vein.[83] The iliac vein is more commonly used.[83] Graft outcomes and survival are similar with both venous anastomosis methods.[83]

Exocrine Drainage

The exocrine drainage of the pancreas is one of the most challenging aspects of the transplantation procedure. The head of the pancreas is positioned to drain downward into either the bladder (see Fig. 36.17) or the bowel (Fig. 36.18).

Enteric exocrine drainage. Enteric drainage is the draining of pancreatic exocrine secretions into the bowel. The pancreas and a segment of the donor duodenum are transplanted onto the recipient's small bowel. All the enzymes drain into the bowel and are excreted with the stool. Exocrine drainage into the duodenum most closely approximates normal physiology. However, complications with the side-to-side anastomosis can cause peritonitis. To decrease this risk, a Roux-en-Y duodenojejunostomy is constructed (see Fig. 36.18).[83] One disadvantage of enteric drainage is that it is impossible to monitor pancreatic enzymes as a direct measure of pancreatic function. Nevertheless, enteric drainage is the more commonly used technique.[83]

Bladder exocrine drainage. Bladder drainage is the draining of pancreatic exocrine secretions into the bladder (see Fig. 36.17). A major advantage of this method is that direct monitoring of graft function is possible by measuring urinary amylase. A decrease in urinary amylase precedes irreversible hyperglycemia associated with acute cellular rejection of the transplanted pancreas.[83] The disadvantage of bladder exocrine drainage is that it is associated with genitourinary complications such as recurrent urinary tract infections, prostatitis, urethritis, and hematuria. Other complications include urinary bicarbonate loss and metabolic acidois.[83] Additional surgery to change the drainage method from bladder to enteric drainage is required in 30% of pancreas transplant recipients within 5 years and in 50% of recipients within 15 years.[83]

Postoperative Medical and Nursing Management

After surgery, the patient is taken to the critical care unit. Although these patients now have a functioning pancreas, they are at high risk for surgical complications because of the long-term effects of diabetes. Oxygenation, hemodynamics, and cardiac status must be monitored closely. If simultaneous kidney-pancreas transplantation is performed, fluid and electrolyte management is indicated including intravenous fluid replacement; monitoring of intake and output; and measurements of potassium, blood urea nitrogen, and creatinine levels. A nasogastric tube is usually placed and remains for 24 to 48 hours after surgery. A continuous insulin drip may be used to prevent hyperglycemia until the new pancreas graft is fully functional. Frequent blood glucose monitoring is essential for patient safety while the continuous insulin infusion is in place.

The same aseptic techniques used for kidney transplant recipients are used for pancreas transplant recipients. An increased potential for urinary catheter occlusion exists for pancreas transplant recipients who have undergone a urinary diversion procedure. The exocrine pancreatic enzymes make the urine more viscous and may irritate the anastomosis site on the bladder, causing an increased risk of bleeding. Continuous bladder irrigation may be necessary to keep the urinary drainage catheter patent. Relevant nursing diagnoses are listed in Box 36.20.

Long-Term Considerations

Rejection in this patient population can be very difficult to detect. Serum amylase levels after pancreas-only transplantation are ineffective in monitoring graft function, and blood glucose levels become elevated only in the late stages of rejection. Urine amylase levels in patients with the urinary diversion are an effective means of monitoring for rejection. If kidney transplantation has been performed simultaneously, an increase in

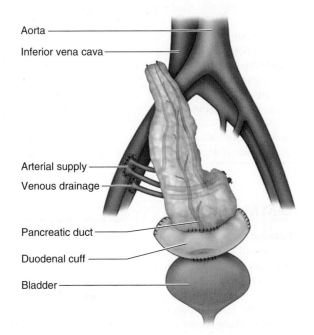

FIG. 36.17 Exocrine Management by Urinary Diversion. (Modified from Smith SL. *AACN Tissue and Organ Transplantation in pancreas transplantation: Implications for Professional Nursing Practice.* St. Louis: Mosby; 1990.)

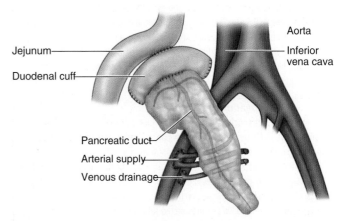

FIG. 36.18 Exocrine Management by Enteric Exocrine Diversion. A segment of the donor duodenum (oversewn duodenal cuff) is transplanted with the pancreas graft.

the serum creatinine level is predictive of rejection. Because of the fragility of pancreas tissue, a pancreas biopsy is rarely performed. However, a kidney biopsy specimen may be obtained to determine rejection and treatment options. Treatment of pancreas rejection is the same as for all other types of organ rejection.

Adherence to the medication regimen is always a concern. It is very important that the patient take the immunosuppressants as prescribed by the physician. Patients with functional pancreas grafts continue to need glucose monitoring at home but often forget to continue this practice after they no longer require insulin. Continued monitoring with frequent clinic visits is required for several months after pancreas transplantation.

◎ **BOX 36.20   NURSING DIAGNOSES**

Pancreas Transplantation

- Risk for Infection: Immunosuppressive medications required to prevent rejection of pancreas, p. 1046
- Imbalanced Nutrition: Less Than Body Requirements related to lack of exogenous nutrients and increased metabolic demand, p. 1029
- Disturbed Body Image related to actual change in body structure, function, or appearance, p. 1022
- Anxiety related to threat to biologic, psychologic, and social integrity, p. 1012
- Activity Intolerance related to prolonged immobility or deconditioning, p. 1006

CASE STUDY 36.1   Patient With a Transplant

Brief Patient History

Mr. V is a 42-year-old man with chronic viral hepatitis C. He has a Model for End-Stage Liver Disease (MELD) score greater than 25. Mr. V is in acute fulminant liver failure and is on the waiting list to receive a liver transplant. Mr. V was hospitalized 2 weeks ago with ascites, hepatorenal syndrome, and hepatic encephalopathy. He has been treated with diuretics, antibiotics, and laxatives. Before transplantation, he remained in the intermediate care unit and was not intubated. He is now undergoing liver transplantation.

Clinical Assessment

Mr. V is admitted to the critical care unit from the operating room after receiving an orthotopic liver transplant. He is intubated and sedated. Mr. V moves all extremities but does not follow commands. He has a nasogastric tube, pulmonary artery catheter, arterial line, urinary catheter, abdominal drain (draining bright red blood), and external biliary drain in place. Continuous renal replacement therapy is in progress.

Diagnostic Procedures

Baseline vital signs include the following: blood pressure of 100/60 mm Hg, heart rate of 118 beats/min (sinus tachycardia), respiratory rate of 20 breaths/min, temperature of 98.3°F, and oxygen saturation of 98%.

Urine output was 75 mL/h and is now 15 mL/h. Central venous pressure is 14 mm Hg, pulmonary artery pressure is 30/16 mm Hg, pulmonary artery occlusion pressure is 18 mm Hg, and intraabdominal pressure is greater than 25 mm Hg.

His current laboratory values include the following:

White blood cell count: 3100 cells/mm³
Hematocrit: 25.3%
Hemoglobin: 8.6 g/dL
Platelet count: 47,000/microliter
Aspartate aminotransferase: 315 units/L
Aminotransferase: 230 units/L
Alkaline phosphatase: 380 units/L
Gamma-glutamyltransferase: 1040 units/L
Total bilirubin: 12.5 mg/dL
Prothrombin time: 21.3 s
International normalized ratio: 2.5
Partial thromboplastin time: 69.9 s
Blood urea nitrogen: 39 mg/dL
Serum creatinine: 1.4 mg/dL
Potassium: 3.8 mEq/L (mmol/L)

Medical Diagnosis

Mr. V is diagnosed with intraabdominal hypertension and abdominal compartment syndrome.

Questions

1. What major outcomes do you expect to achieve for this patient?
2. What problems or risks must be managed to achieve these outcomes?
3. What interventions must be initiated to monitor, prevent, manage, or eliminate the problems and risks identified?
4. What interventions should be initiated to promote optimal functioning, safety, and well-being of the patient?
5. What possible learning needs do you anticipate for this patient?
6. What cultural and age-related factors may have a bearing on the patient's plan of care?

QSEN   BOX 36.21   **QSEN: Informatics**

Internet Resources
Donation

US Government on Organ Donation and Transplantation	http://organdonor.gov
United Network for Organ Sharing (UNOS)	https://www.unos.org

Transplantation

International Society for Heart and Lung Transplantation (ISHLT)	http://www.ishlt.org
International Liver transplantation Society (ILTS)	https://ilts.org
National Kidney Foundation (NKF)	https://www.kidney.org
International Pancreas and Islet Transplant Association	https://www.tts.org/
International Transplant Nurses Society (ITNS)	http://www.itns.org
The Transplantation Society (TTS)	https://www.tts.org

SUMMARY

Organ Donation

- The fields of organ donation and solid-organ transplantation have made dramatic progress in the past 50 years, this trajectory is expected to continue. As transplantation becomes more widespread, more nurses will encounter patients who have undergone solid-organ transplantation. Even more likely is that critical care nurses will assist with the care of a potential organ donor. Knowledge of the rationales for care is essential to delivering safe and high-quality patient care.

- There are 58 OPOs in the United States, Puerto Rico, Guam, and Bermuda. They are nonprofit corporations that provide organ donation services to a designated regional area.
- There are many more individuals listed for transplants than the number of donor organs available.
- The recipient of an organ transplant is required to adhere to a strict regimen of immunosuppressive medications to avoid rejection of the organ by the recipient's own immune system, which recognizes the foreign graft as nonself. The immunosuppressants increase vulnerability to infection. The goal is to create a balance among medications that allows the patient to fight off most infections but avoid rejection of the transplanted organ.

Heart Transplantation

- A transplanted heart must come from a deceased donor. Immediate postoperative management of the heart transplant recipient is similar to that for patients undergoing other heart surgery procedures.

Lung Transplantation

- Transplanted lungs come from a deceased donor. Lungs have a limited ischemic time of approximately 4 hours, which limits the geographic area for donor procurement. Relatively few lungs are available for donation.

Liver Transplantation

- Liver transplants may come from a deceased donor or from a living donor who donates a section of the liver. Before transplantation, the severity of liver disease and level of placement on the transplantation waiting list is determined by the MELD score for patients older than 12 years. The postoperative course is highly variable. Many liver transplant recipients were encephalopathic before transplantation and may have a complicated course afterward. Other patients who have a lower MELD score and receive a functional liver may recover very quickly and should be alert and oriented within 1 to 2 days.

Kidney Transplantation

- Kidney transplants come from a deceased donor or from a living donor who donates one kidney. Postoperative management of fluid status is vital to ensure that the kidney is functional and to avoid volume overload. The bladder must remain decompressed by a urinary catheter for several days to promote effective healing.

Pancreas Transplantation

- Pancreas transplantation is usually performed in tandem with kidney transplantation because most recipients have type 1 diabetes mellitus that has caused their kidneys to fail.

ⓔ Visit the Evolve site for additional study materials.

REFERENCES

1. Linden PK. History of solid organ transplantation and organ donation. *Crit Care Clin.* 2009;1(25):165.
2. Organ Procurement and Transplantation Network. http://optn.transplant.hrsa.govAccessed April 29, 2016.
3. *Federal Register*/Vol. 63, No. 119/Monday, June 22, 1998/Rules and Regulations. 33856–33875; US Department of Health and Human Services; Health Care Financing Administration 42 CFR Part 482 [HCFA-3005 F] RIN: 0938-AI95.
4. Tamburri LM. The role of critical care nurse in the organ donation breakthrough collaborative. *Crit Care Nurse.* 2006;2(26):20.
5. Walton-Tanner K. Maximizing organ donation through aggressive donor management. *Am Nurse Today.* 2011;6:2.
6. Siminoff LA, Traino HM. Improving donation outcomes: hospital development and the rapid assessment of hospital procurement barriers in donation. *Prog Transplant.* 2009;19(2):180.
7. Shafer TJ, et al. U.S. organ donation breakthrough collaborative increases organ donation. *Crit Care Nurse Q.* 2008;51(3):190.
8. Shafer TJ, et al. Organ donation breakthrough collaborative: Increasing organ donation through system redesign. *Crit Care Nurse.* 2006;26(2):44.
9. Shafer TJ, et al. The organ donation breakthrough collaborative. In: LaPointe-Rudow D, Ohler L, Shafer TJ, eds. *A Clinician's Guide to Donation and Transplantation.* Lenexa, KS: Applied Measurement Professionals, Inc; 2006:711.
10. Siminoff LA, et al. Factors influencing families' consent for donation of solid organs for transplantation. *JAMA.* 2001;286(1):71.
11. *Revised Uniform Anatomical Gift Act; 2006.* National Conference of Commissioners on Uniform State Law; July 7-14, 2006.
12. Shafer TJ. The forensic nurse examiner and organ donation: A partnership for life. In: Lynch V, ed. *Forensic Nursing.* St. Louis: Mosby; 2006.
13. Rushton CH. Donation after cardiac death: Ethical implications and implementation strategies. *AACN Adv Crit Care Nurse.* 2006;17(3):345.
14. Wijdicks EFM. The clinical diagnosis of brain death. In: *The Comatose Patient.* New York: Oxford University Press; 2008:102–103.
15. Bernat JL, et al. The circulatory-respiratory determination of death in organ donation. *Crit Care Med.* 2010;38(3):963.
16. Non-Heart Beating Organ Transplantation, Practice and Protocols, Institute of Medicine, Committee on Non-Heart-Beating Transplantation II. *The Scientific and Ethical Basis for Practice and Protocol* Division of Healthcare Services Institute of Medicine. Washington, DC: National Academy of Sciences; 2000:9.
17. Sills P, et al. Donation after cardiac death: Lessons learned. *J Trauma Nurs.* 2007;14(1):47.
18. Edwards J, et al. Maximizing organ donation opportunities through donation after cardiac death. In: LaPointe-Rudow D, Ohler L, Shafer TJ, eds. *A Clinician's Guide to Donation and Transplantation.* Lenexa, KS: Applied Measurement Professionals, Inc; 2006:878.
19. Pine JK, et al. Comparable outcomes in donation after cardiac death and donation after brainstem death: a matched analysis of renal transplants. *Transplant Proc.* 2010;42(10):3947.
20. Reich DJ, Hong JC. Current status of donation after cardiac death liver transplantation. *Curr Opin Organ Transplant.* 2010;15(3):316.
21. De Oliveira NC, et al. Lung transplantation with donation after cardiac death donors: long-term follow-up in a single center. *J Thorac Cardiovasc Surg.* 2010;139(5):1306.
22. Siminoff LA, et al. Requesting organ donation: effective communication. In: LaPointe-Rudow D, Ohler L, Shafer TJ, eds. *A Clinician's Guide to Donation and Transplantation.* Lenexa, KS: Applied Measurement Professionals, Inc; 2006:878.
23. Malinoski DJ, et al. The impact of meeting donor management goals on the development of delayed graft function in kidney transplant recipients. *Am J Transplant.* 2013;13(5):993.
24. Anker AE, Feely TH. Why families decline donation: the perspective of the organ procurement coordinators. *Prog Transplant.* 2010;20(3):239.
25. Strouder DB, et al. Family, faith and friends: how organ donor families heal. *Prog Transplant.* 2009;19(4):358.
26. Malinoski DJ, et al. The impact of meeting donor management goals on the number of organs transplanted per donor: results from the United Network for Organ Sharing Region 5 prospective donor management goals study. *Crit Care Med.* 2012;40(10):2773.
27. McKeown DW, et al. Management of the heartbeating brain-dead organ donor. *Br J Anaesth.* 2012;108(suppl 1):96.
28. Van Gelder FEL, Ohler L. Basics in transplant immunology. In: Ohler L, Cupples S, eds. *Core Curriculum for Transplant Nurses.* Philadelphia: Mosby; 2008.
29. Stolp J, Turka LA, Wood KJ. B cells with immune-regulating function in transplantation. *Nat Rev Nephrol.* 2014;10(7):389.

30. Kroemer A, et al. The innate natural killer cells in transplant rejection and tolerance induction. *Curr Opin Organ Transplant.* 2008;13:339.

31. Costello A, Pearson GJ. Transplant pharmacology. In: Ohler L, Cupples S, eds. *Core Curriculum for Transplant Nurses.* Philadelphia: Mosby; 2008.

32. Becker LE, Morath C, Suesal C. Immune mechanisms of acute and chronic rejection. *Clin Biochem.* 2016;49(4-5):320.

33. Staatz CE, Tett SE. Pharmacology and toxicology of mycophenolate in organ transplant recipients: an update. *Arch Toxicol.* 2014;88(7):1351.

34. Zeiser R, et al. Unlocking the potential of purinergic signaling in transplantation. *Am J Transplant.* 2016;16(10):2781.

35. Ventura-Aguiar P, Campistol JM, Diekmann F. Safety of mTOR inhibitors in adult solid organ transplantation. *Expert Opin Drug Saf.* 2016;15(3):303.

36. Katabathina V, et al. Complications of immunosuppressive therapy in solid organ transplantation. *Radiol Clin North Am.* 2016;54(2):303.

37. Lund LH, et al. The Registry of the International Society for Heart and Lung Transplantation: Thirty-second Official Adult Heart Transplantation Report—2015; Focus Theme: Early Graft Failure. *J Heart Lung Transplant.* 2015;34(10):1244.

38. Colvin-Adams M, et al. OPTN/SRTR 2013 Annual Data Report: heart. *Am J Transplant.* 2015;15(suppl 2):1.

39. Hartley C, et al. Heart transplantation. In: Ohler L, Cupples S, eds. *Core Curriculum for Transplant Nurses.* Philadelphia: Mosby Elsevier; 2008.

40. Cannon RM, et al. A review of the United States experience with combined heart-liver transplantation. *Transplant Int.* 2012;25:1223.

41. Health Resources and Services Administration. Transplants in the US by gender. http://optn.transplant.hrsa.gov/converge/latestData/rptData.asp Accessed November 4, 2015.

42. Lower RR, Shumway NE. Studies on the orthotopic homotransplantations of the canine heart. *Surg Forum.* 1960;11:18.

43. Sievers HH, et al. An alternative technique for orthotopic cardiac transplantation with preservation of the normal anatomy of the right atrium. *Thorac Cardiovasc.* 1991;39:70.

44. Stewart S, et al. Revision of the 1990 working formulation for the standardization of nomenclature in the diagnosis of heart rejection. *J Heart Lung Transplant.* 2005;24:1710.

45. Centers for Disease Control and Prevention. Cytomegalovirus (CMV) and Congenital CMV Infection. http://www.cdc.gov/cmv/index.html Accessed November 4, 2015.

46. Hollis IB, et al. Medication management of cardiac allograft vasculopathy after heart transplantation. *Pharmacotherapy.* 2015;35(5):489–501.

47. Reitz B. The first successful combined heart-lung transplantation. *J Thorac Cardiovasc Surg.* 2011;141(4):867.

48. Deuse T, et al. Review of heart-lung transplantation at Stanford. *Ann Thorac Surg.* 2010;90:329.

49. Yusen RD, et al. The Registry of the International Society for Heart and Lung Transplantation: thirty-second Official Adult Lung and Heart-Lung Transplantation Report—2015; Focus Theme: Early Graft Failure. *J Heart Lung Transplant.* 2015;34(10):1264.

50. Snell GI, Westall GP. Selection and management of the lung donor. *Clin Chest Med.* 2011;32:223.

51. Naik PN, Angel LF. Special issues in the management and selection of the donor for lung transplantation. *Semin Immunopathol.* 2011;33:201.

52. Latchana N, et al. Preservation solutions for cardiac and pulmonary donor grafts: a review of the current literature. *J Thorac Dis.* 2014;6(8):1143.

53. Hayanga JA, et al. Procedural volume and survival after lung transplantation in the United States: the need to look beyond volume in the establishment of quality metrics. *Am J Surg.* 2016;211(4):671.

54. Boasquevisque CHR, et al. Surgical techniques: lung transplant and lung volume reduction. *Proc Am Thorac Soc.* 2009;6:66.

55. Martinu T, et al. Acute allograft rejection: cellular and humoral processes. *Clin Chest Med.* 2011;32:295.

56. Remund KF, et al. Infections relevant to lung transplantation. *Proc Am Thorac Soc.* 2009;6(1):94.

57. Kotton CN. Management of cytomegalovirus infection in solid organ transplantation. *Nat Rev Nephrol.* 2010;6:711.

58. Meyer KC, et al. An international ISHLT/ATS/ERS clinical practice guideline: diagnosis and management of bronchiolitis obliterans syndrome. *Eur Respir J.* 2014;44(6):1479.

59. Knoop C, Estenne M. Chronic allograft dysfunction. *Clin Chest Med.* 2011;32:311.

60. Starzl TE, et al. Orthotopic homotransplantation of the human liver. *Ann Surg.* 1968;168(3):392.

61. Kim WR, et al. OPTN/SRTR 2014 Annual Data Report Liver. *Am J Transplant.* 2016;16(S2):69–98. http://onlinelibrary.wiley.com/doi/10.1111/ajt.13668/full. Accessed September 25, 2016.

62. Deterding K, et al. Improvement of liver function parameters in advanced HCV-associated liver cirrhosis by IFN-free antiviral therapies. *Aliment Pharmacol Ther.* 2015;42(7):889.

63. Organ Procurement and Transplantation MELD Calculator. https://optn.transplant.hrsa.gov/resources/allocation-calculators/meld-calculator/Accessed September 25, 2016.

64. Haring T, O'Mahoney C, Goss J. Extended criteria donors in liver transplantation. *Clin Liver Dis.* 2011;15(4):879.

65. deLemos AS, Vagefi PA. Expanding the donor pool in liver transplantation—expanded criteria donors. *Clin Liver Dis.* 2013;2(4):156.

66. Hall EC, et al. Perioperative complications after live-donor hepatectomy. *JAMA Surg.* 2014;149(3):288.

67. Muzaale AD, et al. Estimates of early death, acute liver failure, and long-term mortality among live liver donors. *Gastroenterology.* 2012;142(2):273–280.

68. Wallia A, et al. Post-transplant hyperglycemia is associated with increased risk of liver allograft rejection. *Transplantation.* 2010;89(2):222.

69. Kumar D, Humar A, eds. *The AST Handbook of Transplant Infections.* Hoboken, NJ: Blackwell Publishing; 2011.

70. Ford E, John E. Patient education for the transplant recipient. In: Ohler L, Cupples S, eds. *Core Curriculum for Transplant Nurses.* St. Louis: Mosby; 2008:51.

71. Kendall K, O'Dell M. Psychosocial issues in transplantation. In: Ohler L, Cupples S, eds. *Core Curriculum for Transplant Nurses.* St. Louis: Mosby; 2008:629.

72. Hoch D, Maynard E, Whiting J. Billing and reimbursement for advanced practice in solid organ transplantation. *Prog Transplant.* 2011;21(4):274.

73. Grogan TA. Liver transplantation: nursing care issues. *Crit Care Nurs Clin North Am.* 2011;23(3):443.

74. Haring T, O'Mahoney C, Goss J. Extended criteria donors in liver transplantation. *Clin Liver Dis.* 2011;15(4):879.

75. Durst JK, Rampersad RM. Pregnancy in women with solid-organ transplants: a review. *Obstet Gynecol Surv.* 2015;70(6):408.

76. Matas AJ, et al. OPTN/SRTR 2013 Annual Data Report: Kidney. *Am J Transplant.* 2015;15(S2):1.

77. Smith JM, et al. Kidney, pancreas and liver allocation and distribution in the United States. *Am J Transplant.* 2012;12:3191.

78. Melcher ML, et al. Chain transplantation: Initial experience of a large multicenter program. *Am J Transplant.* 2012;12:2429.

79. Melcher ML, et al. Dynamic challenges inhibiting optimal adoption of kidney paired donation: findings of a consensus conference. *Am J Transplant.* 2013;13:851.

80. Leeser DB, et al. Living donor kidney paired donation transplantation: experience as a founding member center of the National Kidney Registry. *Clin Transplant.* 2012;26. E213.

81. Lenihan CR, Busque S, Tan JC. Clinical management of the adult kidney transplant recipient. In: Skorecki K, Chertow GM, eds. *Benner & Rector's The Kidney.* 10th ed. St. Louis: Elsevier; 2016:2251.

82. Tanriover B, et al. Future of Medicare immunosuppressive drug coverage for kidney transplant recipients in the United States. *Clin J Am Soc Nephrol.* 2013;8(7):1258.

83. Dhanireddy KK. Pancreas transplantation. *Gastroenterol Clin North Am.* 2012;41(1):133.

84. Redfield RR, et al. Pancreas transplantation in the modern era. *Gastroenterol Clin North Am.* 2016;45(1):145.

85. Kandaswamy R, et al. OPTN/SRTR 2013 Annual Data Report: pancreas. *Am J Transplant.* 2015;15(suppl 2):1.

Hematologic and Oncologic Emergencies

Carol Suarez

Understanding the pathology of a disease, the areas of assessment on which to focus, and the usual medical management allows the critical care nurse to more accurately anticipate and plan nursing interventions. This chapter focuses on hematologic and oncologic disorders commonly seen in the critical care environment.

OVERVIEW OF COAGULATION AND FIBRINOLYSIS

Hemostasis, the ability of the body to control bleeding and clotting, is an intricate balancing act between the coagulation mechanism and fibrinolysis. The following four major actions are involved in achieving hemostasis: (1) local vasoconstriction to reduce blood flow, (2) platelet aggregation at the injury site and formation of a platelet plug, (3) formation of a fibrin mesh to strengthen the plug, and (4) dissolution of the clot after tissue repair is complete.[1] Disruption of the normal hemostatic balance can result in devastating hemorrhagic or thrombotic conditions.

Coagulation Mechanism

The coagulation mechanism consists of 13 factors that work together through a series of feedback loops to achieve hemostasis (Table 37.1 and Fig. 37.1). Depending on the initial triggering event, the extrinsic or intrinsic coagulation pathway is initiated.[1,2] The extrinsic pathway begins when vascular injury occurs, resulting in release of tissue factor and activation of coagulation factor VII. The intrinsic pathway is activated when the damaged subendothelium comes into direct contact with

circulating blood. In this contact phase, proteins activate additional coagulation factors (XII, XI, IX, and VIII).[1] At this point, the two pathways converge into a common pathway, and prothrombin and fibrinogen are converted to their active forms, resulting in clot formation.[3,4]

Clot Formation

Platelets are activated by the arrival of thrombin at the site of injury (Fig. 37.2). Local platelets change shape, become sticky, and begin to aggregate along the vessel wall. Activated platelets undergo degranulation, releasing several factors to assist in clot formation. Serotonin and histamine, two potent vasoconstrictors, help limit blood loss while the clot is forming. The prostaglandin thromboxane A_2 contributes to vasoconstriction and promotes further platelet degranulation. Adenosine diphosphate recruits platelets by increasing adherence and degranulation,[2,3] and the process continues.

At the convergence of the intrinsic and extrinsic pathways, factor X is converted into its active form, enabling the conversion of prothrombin to thrombin. Thrombin then converts fibrinogen to fibrin. Strands of fibrin form and radiate around the newly formed clot, essentially creating a net in which platelets, red blood cells (RBCs), and white blood cells (WBCs) are trapped.[1] The clot is further secured to the site as platelet actomyosin causes the clot to contract and consolidate.[2]

Regulatory Mechanisms

Under normal conditions, feedback systems prevent the coagulation process from spinning out of control. Prostacyclin I_2, a prostaglandin released from damaged endothelial cells, counteracts the effects of thromboxane A_2, serotonin, and histamine through vasodilation and inhibition of platelet degranulation.[1-3] Another means of regulating clot formation is through inhibition of enzymes necessary for activation of coagulation factors along the intrinsic and extrinsic pathways, preventing the conversion of prothrombin to thrombin. The most important of these regulators is antithrombin III; however, protein C and protein S also play a role in thrombin inhibition.[5]

Fibrinolysis

The process of fibrinolysis promotes dissolution and remolding of the clot to promote repair of the vessel wall and maintain flow through the vessel lumen (see Fig. 37.2D). Fibrinolysis begins as soon as the fibrin clot is formed. Circulating plasminogen, a precursor to the powerful enzyme plasmin, binds to fibrin and is trapped within the newly formed clot. The injured epithelial wall releases tissue-type plasminogen activator, which converts

TABLE 37.1	Coagulation Factors
Factor	**Common Name**
I	Fibrinogen
II	Prothrombin
III	Tissue factor
IV	Calcium
V	Proaccelerin
VI	Accelerin
VII	Proconvertin
VIII	Antihemophilic factor
IX	Christmas factor
X	Stuart factor
XI	Plasma thromboplastin antecedent
XII	Hageman factor
XIII	Fibrin-stabilizing factor

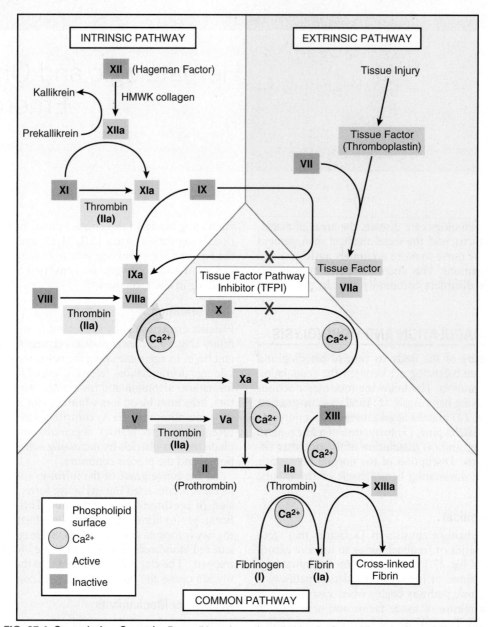

FIG. 37.1 Coagulation Cascade. Factor IX can be activated either by factor XIa or by factor VIIa; in laboratory tests, activation predominantly depends on factor XIa of the intrinsic pathway. Factors in red boxes represent inactive molecules; activated factors are indicated with a lower case "a" and a green box. Note also the multiple points where thrombin (factor IIa; light blue boxes) contributes to coagulation through positive feedback loops. The red "X's" denote points of action of tissue factor pathway inhibitor (TFPI), which inhibits the activation of factors X and IX by factor VIIa. HMWK, high-molecular-weight kininogen; PL, phospholipid. (From Kumar V, Abbas AK, Aster JC. *Robbins and Cotran Pathologic Basis of Disease.* 8th ed. Philadelphia: Saunders; 2010.)

plasminogen to its active state, plasmin. The plasmin begins to digest the fibrin, rapidly breaking down the clot.[2,4] When fibrin is broken down, the fibrin degradation products released act as anticoagulants.

DISSEMINATED INTRAVASCULAR COAGULATION

Description

Disseminated intravascular coagulation (DIC) is a syndrome that arises as a complication of other serious or life-threatening conditions. Although DIC is not seen often, it can seriously hamper diagnostic and treatment efforts for critically ill patients. An understanding of the etiologic and pathophysiologic mechanisms of DIC can assist in anticipating occurrence of the syndrome, recognizing its signs and symptoms, and prompting intervention. Also known as consumptive *coagulopathy*, DIC is characterized by bleeding and thrombosis, both of which result from depletion of clotting factors, platelets, and RBCs. If not treated quickly, DIC will progress to multiple organ failure and death.[6]

A. VASOCONSTRICTION

B. PRIMARY HEMOSTASIS

C. SECONDARY HEMOSTASIS

D. THROMBUS AND ANTITHROMBOTIC EVENTS

FIG. 37.2 Normal Hemostatic Process. Diagrammatic representation of the normal hemostatic process. (A) After vascular injury, local neurohumoral factors induce a transient vasoconstriction. (B) Platelets adhere to exposed extracellular matrix (ECM) by means of von Willebrand factor (vWF) and are activated, undergoing a shape change and granule release. Released adenosine diphosphate (ADP) and thromboxane A_2 (TxA_2) lead to further platelet aggregation to form the primary hemostatic plug. (C) Local activation of the coagulation cascade (involving tissue factor and platelet phospholipids) results in fibrin polymerization, "cementing" the platelets into a definitive secondary hemostatic plug. (D) Counterregulatory mechanisms, such as release of tissue-type plasminogen activator (t-PA) (fibrinolytic) and thrombomodulin (interfering with the coagulation cascade), limit the hemostatic process to the site of injury. (From Kumar V, Abbas AK, Aster JC. *Robbins and Cotran Pathologic Basis of Disease*. 9th ed. Philadelphia: Elsevier; 2015.)

Etiology

Many clinical events can prompt the development of DIC in a critically ill patient, but the exact underlying trigger may not be identifiable (Box 37.1). However, there are some commonly known conditions associated with the development of DIC.

Sepsis, particularly sepsis resulting from gram-negative organisms, can be identified as the cause of DIC in 20% of cases, making it the most common cause of DIC. Endotoxins serve as a trigger for activation of tissue factor and the extrinsic coagulation pathway. Metabolic acidosis and hypoperfusion associated with shock syndromes can result in increased formation of free radicals and damage to tissues. Tissue factor is activated, resulting in DIC. Massive trauma or burns are frequently associated with DIC. Direct tissue damage activates the extrinsic coagulation pathway, and damage to endothelial surfaces activates the intrinsic pathway.[3] Obstetric emergencies, such as abruptio placentae,

BOX 37.1   Causes of Disseminated Intravascular Coagulation

Obstetric Complications
- Abruptio placentae
- Placenta previa
- Retained dead fetus
- Septic abortion
- Amniotic fluid embolism
- Toxemia of pregnancy

Infections
- Gram-negative sepsis
- Gram-positive sepsis
- Meningococcemia
- Rocky Mountain spotted fever
- Histoplasmosis
- Aspergillosis
- Malaria

Neoplasms
- Carcinomas of pancreas, prostate, lung, and stomach
- Acute promyelocytic leukemia
- Tumor lysis syndrome
- Chemotherapy

Massive Tissue Injury
- Traumatic
- Crush injuries
- Burns
- Extensive surgery
- Heat stroke
- Acute transplant rejection

Miscellaneous
- Acute intravascular hemolysis
- Snakebite
- Giant hemangioma
- Shock
- Heat stroke
- Vasculitis
- Aortic aneurysm
- Liver disease
- Cardiac arrest

retained placenta, or incomplete abortion, are also associated with the development of DIC. Tissue factor is concentrated in the placenta, and damage or disruption of this structure can activate coagulation pathways, resulting in coagulopathy.[7]

Pathophysiology

Regardless of the cause, the common thread in the development of DIC is damage to the endothelium that results in activation of the coagulation mechanism (Fig. 37.3).[1] The extrinsic coagulation pathway plays a major role in the development of DIC. Direct damage to the endothelium results in the release of tissue factor and activation of this pathway. The secondary surge of thrombin formation as a result of activation of the intrinsic coagulation pathway leads to the massive disruption of the delicate balance that is hemostasis. Excessive thrombin formation results in rapid consumption of coagulation factors and depletion of regulatory substances—protein C, protein S, and antithrombin.[5] With no checks and balances, thrombi continue to form along damaged epithelial walls, resulting in occlusion of the vessels. As occlusion reaches a critical level, tissue ischemia ensues, leading to further tissue damage and perpetuating the process. Eventually, end-organ function is affected by the ischemia, and failure is evident.[1]

In response to the formation of clots, the fibrinolytic system is activated. As plasmin breaks down the fibrin clots, fibrin split products are released, and they act as anticoagulants.[3,6] Coupled with depletion of circulating clotting factors, activation of fibrinolysis results in excessive bleeding. The end result is shock and further tissue ischemia that aggravate end-organ dysfunction and failure. Death is imminent if this destructive cycle is not interrupted.[7]

Assessment and Diagnosis

Favorable outcomes for patients with DIC depend on accurate and timely diagnosis of the condition. Realization of the role underlying pathology plays, recognition of clinical manifestations, and assessment of appropriate laboratory values are key steps in this process.

Clinical Manifestations

Clinical manifestations are related to the two primary pathophysiologic mechanisms of DIC: the formation of thrombi and bleeding. Thrombi in peripheral capillaries can lead to cyanosis, particularly in the fingers, toes, ears, and nose. In severe, untreated cases, this peripheral ischemia may progress to gangrene.[3,6] As the condition progresses, ischemia worsens, and end organs are affected. The result of this more central ischemia can be respiratory insufficiency and failure, acute kidney injury, bowel infarction, and ischemic stroke. The tissue damage that results perpetuates the anomalies of DIC.[3]

As coagulation factors are depleted, bleeding from intravenous and other puncture sites is observed. Ecchymoses may result from routine interventions such as the use of a manual blood pressure cuff, bathing, or turning. Bloody drainage may also occur from surgical sites, drains, and urinary catheters. With progression of DIC, the patient is at risk for severe gastrointestinal or subarachnoid hemorrhage.[3,6] Table 37.2 lists common signs and symptoms of DIC.

Laboratory Findings

Laboratory tests used to diagnose DIC essentially assess the four basic characteristics of this syndrome: (1) increased coagulant activity, (2) increased fibrinolytic activity, (3) impaired regulatory function, and (4) end-organ failure.[3,6]

Continuous activation of the coagulation pathways results in consumption of coagulation factors. Because of this, prothrombin time, activated partial thromboplastin time, and international normalized ratio values are elevated. Although the platelet count may be within normal ranges, serial examination reveals a declining trend in values. An unexpected drop of at least 50% in the platelet count, particularly in the presence of known contributing factors and associated signs and symptoms, strongly indicates DIC.[1] Fibrinogen levels drop as more and more clots are formed. Thrombus formation in small vessels narrows the vessel lumen, forcing RBCs to squeeze through. The resulting damage and fragmentation of these cells can be seen on microscopic examination of blood samples. Damaged, fragmented RBCs are called *schistocytes.*[3,6]

In response to the excess clotting activity, the fibrinolytic process accelerates, and levels of by-products increase. This is reflected in markedly elevated levels of fibrin degradation products. Another key laboratory test used to evaluate the degree of

clot dissolution—and the severity of the coagulopathy—is the D-dimer level.[1] D-Dimers exclusively indicate clot degradation because, in contrast to fibrin degradation products, which also result from the breakdown of free circulating fibrin, D-dimers result only from dissolution of clots.[3] With progression of the coagulopathy, normal regulatory mechanisms are disrupted, as reflected in decreasing levels of inhibitory factors such as protein C, factor V, and antithrombin III.[3,6,8]

Unchecked DIC resulting in occlusion of vessels and tissue ischemia leads to end-organ dysfunction. Common findings in advanced DIC include respiratory failure, indicated by abnormal arterial blood gas (ABG) levels; liver failure, indicated by increasing liver enzymes; and renal impairment, indicated by increasing blood urea nitrogen (BUN) and creatinine levels.[8]

No single laboratory study can confirm the diagnosis of DIC, but several key results are strong indicators of the condition (Table 37.3). The International Society of Thrombosis and Hemostasis emphasizes early detection of DIC through observation of abnormal trends in laboratory values.[9]

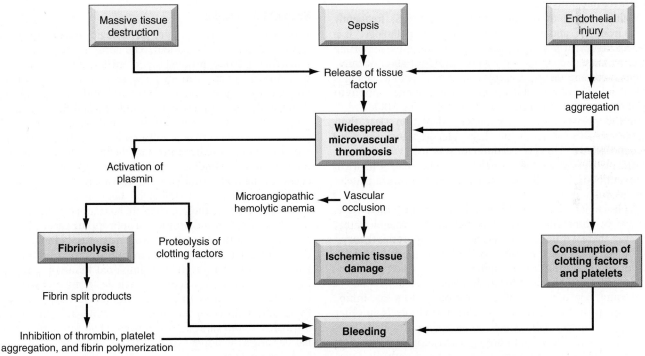

FIG. 37.3 Pathophysiology of Disseminated Intravascular Coagulation. (From Kumar V, Abbas AK, Aster JC. *Robbins and Cotran Pathologic Basis of Disease*. 9th ed. Philadelphia: Elsevier; 2015.)

TABLE 37.2 Signs and Symptoms of Disseminated Intravascular Coagulation

System	Signs Related to Hemorrhage	Signs Related to Thrombi
Integumentary	Bleeding from gums, venipunctures, and old surgical sites; epistaxis; ecchymoses	Peripheral cyanosis, gangrene
Cardiopulmonary	Hemoptysis	Dysrhythmias, chest pain, acute myocardial infarction, pulmonary embolus, respiratory failure
Renal	Hematuria	Oliguria, acute kidney injury
Gastrointestinal	Abdominal distention, hemorrhage	Diarrhea, constipation, bowel infarct
Neurologic	Subarachnoid hemorrhage	Altered level of consciousness, ischemic stroke

TABLE 37.3 Laboratory Studies in Disseminated Intravascular Coagulation

Test	Value
Prothrombin time (PT)	>12.5 s
Platelets	<50,000/mm³, or at least 50% drop from baseline
Activated partial thromboplastin time (aPTT)	>40 s
D-dimer	>250 ng/mL
Fibrin degradation products (FDP)	>40 mg/mL
Fibrinogen	<100 mg/dL

Medical Management

The primary intervention in DIC is prevention. Being aware of the conditions that commonly contribute to the development of DIC and treating them vigorously and without delay provide the best defense against this devastating condition.[3,6,8] After DIC is identified, maintaining organ perfusion and slowing consumption of coagulation factors are paramount to achieving a favorable outcome.[1,3]

Multiple organ dysfunction syndrome (MODS) frequently results from DIC and exacerbates the underlying pathology.[7] It is essential to prevent end-organ ischemia and damage by supporting blood pressure and circulating volume. Administration of intravenous fluids and inotropic agents and, if overt hemorrhaging is evident, infusion of packed RBCs are appropriate interventions to replace blood volume and essential, oxygen-carrying RBCs.

In the presence of severe platelet depletion (less than 50,000/mm³) and severe hemorrhage, platelet transfusions are often indicated.[6,8] However, caution must be used when administering platelets because antiplatelet antibodies may be formed. These antibodies may become activated during future platelet transfusions and elicit DIC.[3]

Replacement of clotting factors in a patient with DIC is thought by some authorities to perpetuate the coagulopathy; however, there is little scientific evidence to support this theory.[1] Fibrinogen levels less than 100 mg/dL indicate the appropriateness of administering cryoprecipitate. A prolonged prothrombin time indicates the need for fresh frozen plasma.[3,6,8]

Slowing consumption of coagulation factors by inhibiting the processes involved in clot formation is another strategy used to treat DIC. The use of heparin, particularly low-molecular-weight heparin, to prevent formation of future clots is controversial.[6] It is contraindicated in patients with DIC associated with recent surgery or with gastrointestinal or central nervous system bleeding. However, heparin has been beneficial in obstetric emergencies such as retained placenta or incomplete abortion, severe arterial occlusions, or MODS caused by microemboli.[3,6] Inhibitors such as aminocaproic acid may be used in conjunction with heparin.[3,6]

Thrombin production in DIC surpasses production of antithrombins and other regulatory factors that would normally be present to inactivate thrombin and its subsequent actions. The use of antithrombin III has been approved in the United States. Ongoing research is yielding mixed results in the treatment of DIC.[3]

Nursing Management

The nursing management plan for a patient with DIC incorporates a variety of nursing diagnoses (Box 37.2). Assessment and monitoring are the primary weapons in the arsenal against DIC. Knowing the diseases and conditions that are most often associated with DIC and understanding the pathophysiologic mechanisms involved enables appropriate monitoring and intervention should the situation arise. Nursing actions are driven by the specific cause of the DIC, although some common interventions are appropriate for all patients with DIC. The nurse has a significant role in supporting the patient's vital functions, initiating bleeding precautions, providing comfort and emotional support, and maintaining surveillance for complications.

Support Vital Functions

Supporting the patient's vital physiologic functions is critical to the outcome of the patient. The administration of intravenous fluids, blood products, and medications is essential to providing adequate hemodynamic support and ensuring adequate tissue oxygenation to combat DIC and prevent end-organ damage. Blood products may include packed RBCs, fresh frozen plasma, platelet concentrations, and cryoprecipitates. The patient should be closely monitored for any adverse reaction to blood products. Medications may include heparin, antibiotics for infection (depending on the underlying cause), vasoactive agents for hemodynamic support, and analgesics for pain.

Close monitoring of vital signs, hemodynamic parameters, intake and output, and appropriate laboratory values assists in the administration and titration of appropriate agents. Frequent assessments of the patient's neurologic status, kidney function, cardiopulmonary function, and integumentary condition facilitate the early identification of impaired tissue or organ perfusion. Particular parameters to include are mental status and level of consciousness; BUN and creatinine levels; prothrombin time, activated partial thromboplastin time, and international normalized ratio values; urine output; vital signs and hemodynamic values including cardiac rhythm and oxygen saturation; and skin integrity.

Initiate Bleeding Precautions

Awareness of the patient's bleeding potential necessitates adjustments to normal nursing interventions (Box 37.3). Unnecessary venipunctures or arterial punctures that may result in bleeding, bruising, or hematomas are avoided. Blood is drawn from existing arterial or venous lines. The use of manual or automatic blood pressure cuffs is avoided whenever possible. If tracheal or oral suctioning is necessary, the use of low-level suction is recommended. Meticulous skin care is advised, keeping the skin moist and using specialty mattresses and beds as appropriate to prevent breakdown. Gentle care is used when bathing or turning the patient to prevent bruising or hematoma formation. The patient is continually assessed for signs of bleeding, petechiae, and ecchymosis.

QSEN BOX 37.3   **QSEN: Patient Safety Alert**

Bleeding Precautions and Injury Prevention

- Handle the patient gently.
  - Use a draw sheet when repositioning the patient in bed.
  - Instruct the patient to notify the nurse immediately if bleeding or bruising is noted.
- Protect the patient from trauma.
  - Avoid rectal temperatures, enemas, and suppositories. If suppositories are prescribed, lubricate liberally and administer with caution.
  - Initiate fall precautions.
  - Instruct the patient to notify the nurse immediately if any trauma occurs.
- Avoid IM injections and venipunctures.
  - If necessary, use a small-gauge needle or IV cannula
- Apply firm pressure to any puncture sites for at least 10 min or until site no longer oozes blood.
- Apply ice to areas of trauma.
- Avoid the use of manual or automatic blood pressure cuff.
  - If necessary, remove cuff immediately after using it.
  - Do not leave cuff on the patient.
- Observe IV sites every few hours for bleeding.
- Shave the patient with an electric shaver only.
- Use a soft-bristled toothbrush when providing mouth care.
- Test urine and stool for occult blood as ordered.

IM, intramuscular; *IV,* intravenous.

QSEN BOX 37.4   **QSEN: Teamwork and Collaboration**

Interprofessional Collaborative Practice: Disseminated Intravascular Coagulation

- Identify and eliminate underlying cause.
- Provide hemodynamic support to prevent end-organ ischemia.
  - Intravenous fluids
  - Positive inotropic agents
- Administer blood and blood components.
  - Fresh frozen plasma
  - Platelets
  - Cryoprecipitate
  - Antithrombin III
- Administer medications.
  - Heparin
  - Aminocaproic acid
  - Antithrombin III
- Initiate bleeding precautions.
- Maintain surveillance for complications.
  - Hypovolemic shock
  - Peripheral ischemia
  - Central ischemia
  - MODS
- Provide comfort and emotional support.

MODS, multiple-organ dysfunction syndrome.

Provide Comfort and Emotional Support

The development of DIC in an already critically ill patient can be stressful for the patient and his or her significant others. It is imperative to provide psychosocial support throughout this crisis. Calm reassurance and uncomplicated explanations of the care the patient is receiving can help to allay much of the anxiety experienced. All treatments and interventions are explained before carrying them out, and questions should be answered at a level understandable to the patient and family. The use of an interpreter when English is not the primary language can enhance understanding and help avoid misconceptions. Providing spiritual support as requested may also be of assistance.

Intraprofessional collaborative management of the patient with DIC is outlined in Box 37.4.

THROMBOCYTOPENIA

Description

Thrombocytopenia is defined as a platelet count less than 150,000/mm^3 or a decrease of greater than 50% from the last measurement.[10,11] This disorder is described as mild when the platelet count is between 70,000/mm^3 and 150,000/mm^3, moderate when the platelet count is between 20,000/mm^3 and 70,000/mm^3, and severe when the platelet count is less 20,000/mm^3.[10] When the platelet count decreases to less than 50,000/mm^3, the patient is at severe risk for bleeding.[10,11] Thrombocytopenia occurs in 20% to 45% of critically ill patients.[11]

Etiology

Onset of thrombocytopenia often follows a viral infection, pregnancy, administration of certain medications (eg, heparin, thiazide diuretics, chemotherapeutic agents), malignancies, splenomegaly, blood transfusions, or alcoholism.[11] Regardless of the precipitating condition, the development of thrombocytopenia occurs via one of the following five mechanisms: (1) decreased platelet production, (2) increased platelet destruction, (3) splenic sequestration of platelets, (4) massive consumption of platelets,[11,12] and (5) hemodilution.[12] One form of thrombocytopenia seen in critically ill patients is immune thrombocytopenic purpura (ITP), which may also be referred to as idiopathic thrombocytopenic purpura.[11,12]

Pathophysiology

In ITP, lymphocytes produce antibodies that begin to destroy existing platelets. The cause of this autoimmune response is unknown.[13] With insufficient platelets available, the normal coagulation pathways are disrupted. Inadequate hemostasis ensues, and bleeding results. Life-threatening gastrointestinal or intracerebral bleeding can occur.[13,14]

Assessment and Diagnosis

ITP is characterized by the gradual onset of signs and symptoms.[13] The diagnosis of ITP is a diagnosis of exclusion and is primarily based on findings in the patient's history and physical examination. ITP is thought to be present when the patient develops a low platelet count and no other cause can be identified.[14]

Clinical Manifestations

Petechial hemorrhages, which manifest as small red spots primarily on legs and oral mucosa, are most indicative of a platelet disorder. In contrast, larger hematomas are most commonly associated with coagulation disorders. Bruising unrelated to trauma is another common sign of ITP.[13] The signs and symptoms of ITP are listed in Table 37.4.

TABLE 37.4 Diagnostic Data for Immune Thrombocytopenic Purpura

System or Study	Signs and Symptoms
Integumentary	Petechial hemorrhage of lower extremities, ecchymoses, gingival bleeding, spontaneous epistaxis
Neurologic	Sudden, severe headache; nausea and vomiting; seizures; focal neurologic deficits; decreased level of consciousness
Renal	Hematuria
Gastrointestinal	Hematemesis, melena, hematochezia
Other	Heavy menses in women, retinal hemorrhage
Laboratory	Decreased platelet count, often <30,000 mm³

Unusual bleeding is a hallmark of ITP. Excessive bleeding from the gums after dental work, spontaneous epistaxis, blood in the urine or stool, and unusually heavy menses in women are typical features of ITP. Rarely, retinal hemorrhage or intracerebral bleeding may be observed.

Laboratory Findings

A complete blood cell count reveals a severely diminished platelet count, often falling below 30,000/mm³, for a patient with ITP.[14] However, the numbers of RBCs and WBCs, the hemoglobin level, results of coagulation studies, and bleeding times are normal.[14]

Medical Management

In most cases, ITP resolves spontaneously, and treatment is unnecessary. In mild cases in which diminished platelet counts result in symptoms, administration of oral corticosteroids is appropriate.[13,14] Platelet counts increase to normal levels within 2 to 6 weeks, and dosages can then be tapered.

In patients exhibiting life-threatening hemorrhage, rapid intervention is necessary. Administration of intravenous immunoglobulin suppresses the platelet-destroying antibody response. This therapy is extremely expensive and is reserved for the most severe manifestations of ITP.[13] High-dose methylprednisolone can be given intravenously and is very effective in treating ITP.[13] Platelet transfusion is recommended after administration of intravenous immunoglobulin or methylprednisolone. When steroid therapy fails to arrest the condition, surgical removal of the spleen is considered.[14]

Nursing Management

The nursing management plan for a patient with ITP incorporates a variety of nursing diagnoses (Box 37.5). The nurse has a significant role in supporting the patient's vital functions, initiating bleeding precautions, providing comfort and emotional support, and maintaining surveillance for complications.

Recognizing potential hazards and providing a safe care environment is of utmost importance (see Box 37.3). For example, padding bed rails can protect the patient from bruising. Substituting sponge-tipped oral care devices for firm-bristled toothbrushes can help minimize mucosal trauma and bleeding. The patient is instructed on how to blow the nose gently to avoid instigating epistaxis. When shaving patients, an electric razor is used to reduce the risk of laceration associated with a blade. Venipuncture and intramuscular injections are avoided. In the event venipuncture is required, prolonged pressure on the site may be necessary to arrest bleeding. Careful administration

BOX 37.5 NURSING DIAGNOSES

Immune Thrombocytopenic Purpura

- Deficient Fluid Volume related to active blood loss, p. 1019
- Powerlessness related to lack of control over current situation and/or disease progression, p. 1038
- Disturbed Body Image related to actual change in body structure, function, or appearance, p. 1022

QSEN BOX 37.6 QSEN: Teamwork and Collaboration

Interprofessional Collaborative Practice: Immune Thrombocytopenic Purpura

- Administer medications.
  - Glucocorticoids
  - Intravenous immunoglobulin
- Prepare patient for splenectomy if unresponsive to medication therapy.
- Administer platelets.
- Initiate bleeding precautions.
- Maintain surveillance for complications.
  - Intracranial or other major hemorrhage
  - Severe blood loss
- Provide comfort and emotional support.

of prescribed medications and monitoring for adverse effects of platelet transfusions and for complicating or contributing factors, such as hemorrhage and infection, are critical to the patient's outcome.

Interprofessional collaborative management of the patient with ITP is outlined in Box 37.6.

HEPARIN-INDUCED THROMBOCYTOPENIA

Description

Another form of thrombocytopenia seen in critical care patients is heparin-induced thrombocytopenia (HIT). There are two distinct types of HIT. The most common form is non–immune-mediated HIT, formally known as type 1 HIT.[15] Seen in 30% of patients receiving heparin therapy, this nonautoimmune condition manifests within a few days of initiation of therapy. Platelet depletion is moderate, counts are usually less than 100,000/mm³, and the condition is transient, often resolving spontaneously. Discontinuation of heparin is not required. The second form is type 2 HIT, or immune-mediated HIT,[15] which is less commonly encountered but is more severe.[15,16] This discussion is limited to immune-mediated HIT.

Etiology

Immune-mediated HIT is a response to the administration of heparin therapy. It has been observed in 0.5% to 5% of patients treated with unfractionated heparin and has occurred after exposure to low-molecular–weight heparin, although to a lesser degree.[15] The disorder is characterized by severe thrombocytopenia during heparin therapy. Diagnostically it is identified by a platelet count less than 50,000/mm³ or at least a 50% decrease from the baseline platelet count from the initiation of therapy. Onset usually occurs 5 to 10 days from the first exposure to heparin, but the onset can occur within hours of a reexposure to

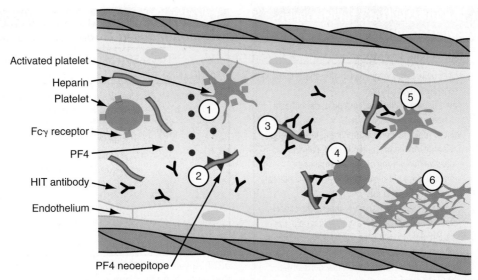

FIG. 37.4 Pathophysiology of Heparin-Induced Thrombocytopenia (HIT). *(1)* Activated platelets release procoagulant proteins from α-granules, including platelet factor 4 (PF4). Administered heparin binds PF4 *(2)*, which undergoes a conformation change and expresses a new antigen (neoepitope). Individuals with HIT produce an immunoglobulin G (IgG) antibody that specifically reacts *(3)* with multiple identical neoepitopes on the heparin-PF4 complex. The reaction forms heparin-PF4-IgG immune complexes. Platelets express FcγRIIa receptors (Fcγ receptor) that react *(4)* with the Fc portion of IgG in immune complexes. Cross-linking of Fc receptors *(5)* results in FcγRIIa-dependent platelet activation. The activated platelets mediate a series of events that lead to further activation of the coagulation cascade, resulting in thrombin generation. Further release of PF4 from newly activated platelets leads to a cycle of continuing platelet activation and *(6)* formation of a primary clot. The reaction can be enhanced by the release of platelet-derived microparticles that are rich in surface phosphatidylserine and increase activation of coagulation and by the binding of heparin-PF4 complexes and HIT-IgG to the vascular endothelium (not shown). (From McCance KL, Huether SE: *Pathophysiology: The Biologic Basis for Disease in Adults and Children.* 7th ed. St. Louis: Elsevier; 2014.)

heparin.[15,16] The risk of developing HIT is higher in women, surgical patients, and patients with major trauma.[15] High-risk surgical procedures include cardiac surgery and orthopedic surgery.[15]

Pathophysiology

The thrombocytopenia that occurs with immune-mediated HIT is related to the formation of heparin-antibody complexes. These complexes release a substance known as platelet factor 4. Platelet factor 4 attracts heparin molecules, forming immunogenic complexes that adhere to platelet and endothelial surfaces (Fig. 37.4). Activation of platelets stimulates the release of thrombin and the subsequent formation of platelet clumps.[15,16]

Patients with immune-mediated HIT are at greater risk for thrombosis than bleeding. Thrombotic complications develop in 20% to 50% of patients and can occur in both the venous and the arterial system.[15] Vessel occlusion can result in the need for limb amputation, stroke, acute myocardial infarction, and death.[15-17] The resultant formation of fibrin- and platelet-rich thrombi is the primary characteristic of HIT that distinguishes it from other forms of thrombocytopenia and gives rise to its more descriptive name: white clot syndrome.[16]

Assessment and Diagnosis

HIT can be associated with severe consequences. Rapid recognition of risk factors and subsequent development of signs and symptoms is essential in treating this condition.

Clinical Manifestations

Common signs and symptoms are listed in Table 37.5. The clinical manifestations of HIT are related to the formation of thrombi and subsequent vessel occlusion.[15] Most thrombotic events are venous, although venous and arterial thrombosis can occur. Thrombotic events typically include deep vein thrombosis, pulmonary embolism, limb ischemia thrombosis, thrombotic stroke, and myocardial infarction.[15,18] The presence of blanching and the loss of peripheral pulses, sensation, or motor function in a limb indicate peripheral vascular thrombi. Neurologic signs and symptoms such as confusion, headache, and impaired speech can signal the onset of cerebral artery occlusion and stroke. Acute myocardial infarction may be heralded by dyspnea, chest pain, pallor, and alterations in blood pressure. Thrombi in the pulmonary vasculature may be evidenced by pleuritic pain, rales, and dyspnea.

Laboratory Findings

The key indicator for identifying HIT is the platelet count. General consensus in the literature considers a platelet count of less than $100,000/mm^3$ or a sudden drop of 50% from the patient's baseline after initiation of heparin therapy to strongly indicate HIT.[15-18]

Two types of assays are available to assist in confirming the diagnosis of HIT: activation assays, based on platelet aggregation or the release of granular contents such as serotonin, and

TABLE 37.5   Diagnostic Data for Heparin-Induced Thrombocytopenia

System or Study	Signs and Symptoms
Cardiac	Chest pain, diaphoresis, pallor, alterations in blood pressure, dysrhythmias
Vascular	Arterial: pain, pallor, pulselessness, paresthesia, paralysis
	Venous: pain, tenderness, unilateral leg swelling, warmth, erythema, palpable cord, pain on passive dorsiflexion of foot, spontaneous maintenance of relaxed foot in abnormal plantar flexion (Homans sign)
Pulmonary	Dyspnea, pleuritic pain, rales, chest pain, chest wall tenderness, back pain, shoulder pain, upper abdominal pain, syncope, hemoptysis, shortness of breath, wheezing
Renal	Thirst, decreased urine output, dizziness, orthostatic hypotension
Gastrointestinal	Abdominal pain, vomiting, bloody diarrhea, abnormal bowel sounds
Neurologic	Confusion, headache, impaired speech patterns, hemiparesis or hemiplegia, vision disturbances, dysarthria, aphasia, ataxia, vertigo, nystagmus, sudden decrease in consciousness
Laboratory	Platelets <50,000/mm^3 or sudden drop of 30%–50% from baseline; positive results for HIPA, SRA, ELISA

ELISA, enzyme-linked immunosorbent assay; *HIPA*, heparin-induced platelet aggregation; *SRA*, serotonin release assay.

TABLE 37.6   Pharmacologic Management

Heparin-Induced Thrombocytopenia

Medication	Dosage	Action	Special Considerations
Argatroban	Loading dose: None	Used to inhibit thrombin	Obtain baseline aPTT 2 h after therapy started
	IV infusion: 2 mcg/kg/min not to exceed 10 mcg/kg/min		Monitor aPTT; maintain INR 1.5–3.0 times initial baseline
			Reduce dosage in patients with known or suspected hepatic impairment

aPTT, Activated partial thromboplastin time; *INR*, international normalized ratio; *IV*, intravenous.

assays that identify the HIT antigen. Activation assays are highly sensitive in detecting the presence of HIT. The most common assay used is heparin-induced platelet aggregation. Serotonin release assay is used by a few institutions. The enzyme-linked immunosorbent assay identifies the presence of the HIT antigen.[16,17]

Medical Management

Early identification is critical to managing the effects of immune-mediated HIT. Current guidelines suggest that platelet count monitoring be performed every 2 or 3 days from day 4 to day 14 for high-risk patients.[19] When a decrease in the platelet count is detected, heparin therapy is discontinued immediately, and the patient is tested for the presence of heparin antibodies.[15-19] If the original indication for heparin still exists or new thromboses occur, an alternative form of anticoagulation is usually necessary.[19]

Direct Thrombin Inhibitors

Direct thrombin inhibitors (DTIs) are being used with increasing frequency to treat HIT. DTIs bind directly to the thrombin molecule, inhibiting its action.[18] Argatroban is the only medication approved for use in the United States at the present time (Table 37.6). Warfarin, although commonly used to treat deep vein thrombosis, is not indicated as a sole agent in treating HIT because of its prolonged onset of action. Studies have shown that the use of warfarin without concomitant use of DTIs can significantly increase the incidence of thrombosis in patients with HIT.[18]

Nursing Management

The nursing management plan for a patient with HIT incorporates a variety of nursing diagnoses (Box 37.7). The nurse has a significant role in decreasing the incidence of heparin exposure, maintaining surveillance for complications, providing comfort and emotional support, and educating the patient and family. Prevention of HIT is a major nursing focus because most critically ill patients receive heparin as part of their plan of care and thus are at risk for this disorder. Initial assessment is crucial to identifying patients at risk for HIT. A medical history that includes previous heparin therapy, deep vein thrombosis, or cardiovascular surgery that involved the use of cardiopulmonary bypass can signal potential problems.

Decrease Incidence of Heparin Exposure

Ensuring that all heparin has been removed from the patient's hemodynamic pressure monitoring system, avoiding the use of heparin-coated catheters, and discontinuing heparin flushes to maintain the patency of other intravenous lines are essential elements of nursing management.

Maintain Surveillance for Complications

Patients with HIT remain at high risk for thrombotic complications for several days or weeks after cessation of heparin. Key nursing actions include vigilant monitoring, early recognition of signs and symptoms, and strategies to prevent deep vein thrombosis. Prompt notification of the physician of any complications that occur is critical to patient outcome.

Educate the Patient and Family

Early in the patient's hospital stay, the patient and family are taught about HIT, its etiologies, and its treatment (Box 37.8). Education of the patient and family is part of prevention of subsequent episodes in patients sensitized to heparin. Closer to discharge, the patient's education plan focuses on the interventions necessary for preventing the reoccurrence of HIT, including measures to avoid future exposure to heparin. The use of medical alert bracelets and listing heparin allergies in the medical record are necessary to avoid this serious complication in the future.

Interprofessional collaborative management of the patient with HIT is outlined in Box 37.9.

BOX 37.7 NURSING DIAGNOSES

Heparin-Induced Thrombocytopenia

- Risk for Decreased Cardiac Tissue Perfusion, p. 1041
- Risk for Ineffective Peripheral Tissue Perfusion, p. 1044
- Risk for Ineffective Renal Perfusion, p. 1045
- Risk for Ineffective Gastrointestinal Perfusion, p. 1043
- Risk for Ineffective Cerebral Tissue Perfusion, p. 1042
- Powerlessness related to lack of control over current situation or disease progression, p. 1038
- Deficient Knowledge related to lack of previous exposure to information, p. 1020 (see Box 37.8, Patient Education Plan for Heparin-Induced Thrombocytopenia)

BOX 37.8 PATIENT EDUCATION PLAN

Heparin-Induced Thrombocytopenia

Before the patient's discharge, the patient should be able to teach back the following topics:

- Pathophysiology of disease
- Purpose of heparin
- Measures to avoid future exposure to heparin
- Identify different types of heparin (unfractionated and low-molecular-weight forms)
- Encourage purchase of medical alert bracelet or similar type of warning device
- Tell any new health care provider about the heparin allergy and previous reaction

  Additional information for the patient can be found at the following websites:

Healthfinder—US Department of Health and Human Services: http://healthfinder.gov

WebMD: http://www.webmd.com

BOX 37.9 QSEN: Teamwork and Collaboration

Interprofessional Collaborative Practice: Heparin-Induced Thrombocytopenia

- Stop all heparin exposure.
  - Unfractionated and low–molecular-weight heparin by any route
  - Heparin flushes
  - Heparin-coated vascular access devices
- Begin therapy with alternative anticoagulant.
  - Argatroban
- Maintain surveillance for complications.
  - Deep vein thrombosis
  - Pulmonary emboli
  - Acute limb ischemia
  - Ischemic stroke
  - Acute myocardial infarction
- Administer antifibrinolytic therapy (as indicated) if thrombosis occurs.
- Prepare patient for surgical embolectomy (as indicated) if thrombosis occurs.
- Provide comfort and emotional support.

SICKLE CELL ANEMIA

Description

Sickle cell anemia (SCA) is a hereditary disease in which RBCs form an abnormal sickle or crescent shape. RBCs carry oxygen to the body and are normally shaped like a disk.[20,21] The sickle-shaped cells have a shortened life span; are unable to carry adequate oxygen to tissues and become trapped in the vasculature because of their shape; and can cause severe pain, increased risk of infection, and life-threatening complications.[20,21]

Etiology

SCA is an autosomal recessive genetic disorder. An individual with normal hemoglobin has two copies of hemoglobin A (HbA) gene. An individual with SCA has two copies of hemoglobin S (HbS) gene. Individuals who have one gene for HbS and one gene for HbA are known as "carriers" of the sickle cell trait (HbAS). When two carriers have a child, there is a 25% chance that the child will have SCA (HbSS), a 50% chance that the child will have sickle cell trait (HbAS), and a 25% chance that the child will have entirely normal hemoglobin (HbAA).[22] This genetic trait is found in people of African, Caribbean, Central American, South American, Saudi Arabian, Indian, and Mediterranean descent.[21] Most patients in the United States are African American.[21] The disease is not prevalent in persons of Asian or Pacific Islander descent.

SCA is usually diagnosed during the first few years of life secondary to manifestation of initial symptoms. Prenatal screening that consists of DNA analysis from fetal cells is now available for at-risk couples.[22] This screening should be offered as part of their prenatal counseling. More than 40 states offer universal neonatal screening for hemoglobinopathies.[22]

Pathophysiology

Sickle cell disease (SCD) is a chronic inflammatory condition that is characterized by hemolysis and vasoocclusion. The cause of SCA is a mutation in the genetic sequence in the beta chain gene of the hemoglobin. This results in a sequence of the replacement of valine with glutamic acid at the N-terminal amino acid position 6 of the protein chain.[20] This substitution leads to the production of HbS.[21]

Normal RBCs contain hemoglobin that are flexible, biconcave disks. When deoxygenated, RBCs containing predominantly HbS distort into a crescent or sickle shape. In this form, the hemoglobin becomes rigid and friable, causing vasoocclusion in the small vessels of the circulatory system.[20] This tends to occur during times of physiologic stress, such as physical overexertion, muscle tissue ischemia, dehydration, infection, or extreme temperatures.[21] Although these conditions have a tendency to exacerbate the condition, most of the sickling events have no identifying cause.[21]

The RBCs become lodged in the vasculature and the microcirculation causing stasis and obstruction of blood flow and damage to the surrounding organs, tissue ischemia, infarction, and, if not corrected, eventually necrosis (Fig. 37.5). In addition, hemolysis of the RBCs occurs, resulting in anemia.[20]

Assessment and Diagnosis

SCA can be associated with severe consequences. Rapid recognition of signs and symptoms is essential in treating this condition.

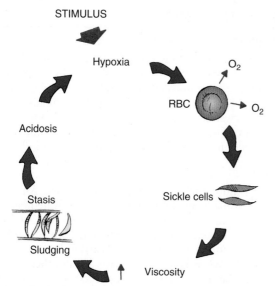

STIMULUS

Hypoxia

O_2

RBC

O_2

Acidosis

Stasis

Sickle cells

Sludging

↑ Viscosity

FIG. 37.5 Cycle Causing Vasoocclusive Episodes in Sickle Cell Anemia. *RBC*, red blood cell. (From Hockenberry M, Coody D. *Pediatric Oncology and Hematology: Perspectives on Care.* St. Louis: Mosby; 1986.)

Clinical Manifestations

Various clinical manifestations are associated with SCA (Fig. 37.6). The patient may present with a low-grade fever, bone or joint pain, pinpoint pupils, inability to follow commands, photophobia, tachycardia, tachypnea, decreased respiratory excursion, hepatomegaly, nonpalpable spleen, and pretibial ulcers.[23]

Laboratory Studies

Initial laboratory studies include a complete blood count, a peripheral blood smear, and a quantitative hemoglobin electrophoresis. Sickle cells constitute 5% to 10% of the blood smear. The elevated reticulocyte count (greater than 10%) is characteristically accompanied by the presence of Howell-Jolly bodies. Howell-Jolly bodies are small remnants of nuclear material from hemolyzed erythrocytes reflective of hyposplenia or autoinfarction and target cells (an erythrocyte with a deeply stained core surrounded by a lighter stained margin that resembles a target with a bull's eye). Typically, an elevated WBC count occurs during and after a crisis. Other tests might include an indirect bilirubin level, which will be elevated following hemolysis. The haptoglobin level will be low or absent because it cannot be replaced quickly enough after severe hemolysis. Haptoglobin, a glycoprotein, exists to bind free hemoglobin that is released from hemolyzed erythrocytes.

Medical Management

SCA is an incurable disease; however, treatment options are available for management of symptoms and complications. Bone marrow transplant offers a cure in a limited number of cases.[20] Medical interventions are aimed at preventing infections, managing pain, transfusing RBCs, and administering hydroxyurea. Patients with chronic disease are more effectively managed through a multidisciplinary approach.[20] It is also important to look at other issues that may exacerbate the patient disease process, such as diet, poor housing, inadequate housing, lack of education, poor access to services, and poor lifestyle choices.

Prevent Infection

Both children and adults with SCA are more prone to infection and have a more difficult time fighting off infection.[23] SCA can result in damage to the spleen from constant sickling of the RBCs, and damage to the spleen can prevent the destruction of bacteria in the blood. Prophylactic administration of oral antibiotics starting at age 2 months can decrease the chances of a pneumococcal infection and early death. Vaccinations against pneumococcal infections, meningitis, hepatitis, and influenza are important to prevent future infections.[23]

Pain Management

Pain associated with SCA can be acute or chronic in nature. The most common type of pain associated with SCA is vasoocclusive pain. It is commonly treated with antiinflammatory and opioid or nonopioid analgesics.[23,24] The pain associated with SCA can vary enormously; therefore, numerous different approaches may be required. The medication of choice is influenced by the patient's history of analgesia use. Some patients may have extremely intricate medication regimens.[23] Paracetamol and nonsteroidal antiinflammatory drugs are used for mild to moderate pain relief. If this approach is ineffective, oral or parenteral opiates may be an alternative.[23,24]

For patients who wish to try nonpharmacologic pain control, approaches include psychologic support, massage, acupuncture, and transcutaneous electrical nerve stimulation. Distraction can be another valuable tool to use. The use of television, video games, repeating inspirational phrases, and mental calculations can also be a form of distraction. Studies suggested that cognitive-behavioral therapy can help teach patients coping strategies for acute and chronic pain.[23]

Transfusion Therapy

RBC transfusion therapy in SCD is an important lifesaving treatment option but should be performed only after careful consideration. Transfusion therapy is primarily used for treatment of patients who are experiencing complications secondary to SCD or as an emergency measure.[24] Transfusion therapy is used with extreme caution because of risks such as iron overload; exposure to hepatitis, human immunodeficiency virus, and other infectious agents; alloimmunization; induction of hyperviscosity; and limitations on resources. The indications for having a blood transfusion or exchange are recurrent painful vasoocclusive crises with long hospital admissions, acute chest syndrome, stroke, priapism, and leg ulcers. Blood transfusions or exchange can also be performed before major operations, such as hip replacement because of avascular necrosis of the hip bone.[23]

Administration of Hydroxyurea

Hydroxyurea is an oral agent that is a safe and effective treatment for children and adults with SCA. It works by increasing the level of fetal hemoglobin in the RBCs, reducing the concentration of sickle hemoglobin and sickling itself.[23] The patient is usually started at a dosage of 15 mg/kg orally once a day. The dosage is increased by 5 mg/kg every 12 weeks until 35 mg/kg is reached, provided that the patient's blood count remains within an acceptable range. Research shows that patients receiving hydroxyurea had fewer episodes of pain and acute chest syndrome and had a decreased need for blood transfusion and hospitalizations compared with patients who received no treatment. Research showed that

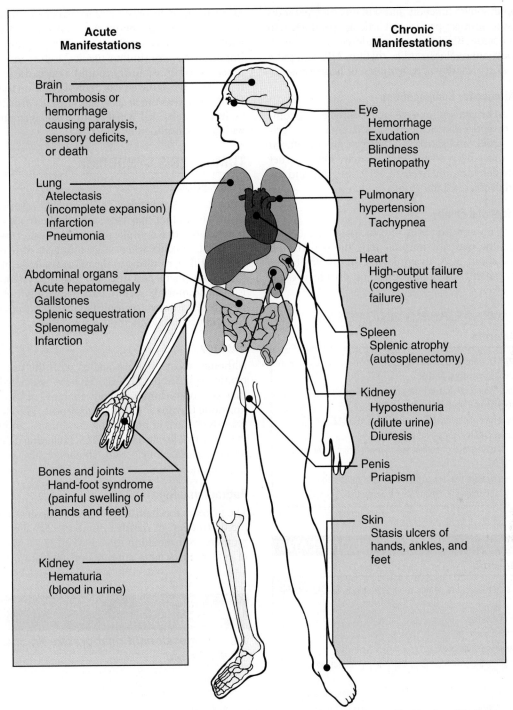

Acute Manifestations

Brain
  Thrombosis or
  hemorrhage
  causing paralysis,
  sensory deficits,
  or death

Lung
  Atelectasis
  (incomplete expansion)
  Infarction
  Pneumonia

Abdominal organs
  Acute hepatomegaly
  Gallstones
  Splenic sequestration
  Splenomegaly
  Infarction

Bones and joints
  Hand-foot syndrome
  (painful swelling of
  hands and feet)

Kidney
  Hematuria
  (blood in urine)

Chronic Manifestations

Eye
  Hemorrhage
  Exudation
  Blindness
  Retinopathy

Pulmonary
hypertension
  Tachypnea

Heart
  High-output failure
  (congestive heart
  failure)

Spleen
  Splenic atrophy
  (autosplenectomy)

Kidney
  Hyposthenuria
  (dilute urine)
  Diuresis

Penis
  Priapism

Skin
  Stasis ulcers of
  hands, ankles, and
  feet

FIG. 37.6 Clinical Manifestations of Sickle Cell Disease. (From McCance KL, Huether SE: *Pathophysiology: The Biologic Basis for Disease in Adults and Children.* 7th ed. St. Louis: Elsevier; 2014.)

hydroxyurea can be used as an alternative to regular blood transfusions.[24]

Nursing Management

The nursing management plan for a patient with SCA incorporates a variety of nursing diagnoses (Box 37.10). The nurse has a significant role in supporting the patient's vital functions, providing comfort and emotional support, maintaining surveillance for complications, and educating the patient and family.

Support Vital Functions

The nurse must recognize and support the patient's vital physiologic functions. Administration of intravenous fluids, blood products, and inotropic agents to provide adequate hemodynamic support and tissue oxygenation is essential in preventing or combating end-organ damage. Close monitoring of vital signs, hemodynamic parameters, intake and output, and appropriate laboratory values assists the critical care nurse in administering and titrating appropriate agents.[24] Frequent assessments include parameters for neurologic status, kidney function, cardiopulmonary function, and skin integrity that indicate impaired tissue or organ perfusion. Particular parameters to include are mental status, BUN and creatinine levels, urine output, vital signs, hemodynamic values, cardiac rhythm, ABG and pulse oximetry values, skin breakdown, ecchymoses, or hematomas.[24]

Maintain Surveillance for Complications

The nurse needs to be vigilant for signs of life-threatening complications such as septicemia, acute myocardial infarction, priapism, ischemic stroke, and shock.[20] If there are any significant concerns, these must be reported immediately. Other issues that may arise are dehydration, hypoxia, infection, skin and tissue viability, and decreased hemoglobin levels.

Educate the Patient and Family

Although there is no cure for SCA, the focus of care is prevention. Early in the patient's hospital stay, the patient and family are taught about SCA, its etiologies, and its treatment (Box 37.11). The patient and family education plan focuses on

BOX 37.10　NURSING DIAGNOSES

Sickle Cell Anemia

- Acute Pain related to transmission and perception of cutaneous, visceral, muscular, or ischemic impulses, p. 1010
- Risk for Ineffective Peripheral Tissue Perfusion, p. 1044
- Risk for Ineffective Renal Tissue Perfusion, p. 1045
- Risk for Ineffective Gastrointestinal Tissue Perfusion, p. 1043
- Risk for Ineffective Cerebral Tissue Perfusion, p. 1042
- Powerlessness related to lack of control over current situation or disease progression, p. 1038
- Deficient Knowledge related to lack of previous exposure to information, p. 1020 (see Box 37.11, Patient Education Plan for Sickle Cell Anemia)

BOX 37.11　PATIENT EDUCATION PLAN

Sickle Cell Anemia

Before the patient's discharge, the patient should be able to teach back the following topics:
- Pathophysiology of disease
- Precipitating factor modification
- Importance of taking medications
- Maintenance of adequate hydration (especially during febrile periods and hot weather)
- Use of pharmacologic and nonpharmacologic methods of pain management
- Avoidance of situations that can precipitate condition such as extreme cold
- Smoking cessation and avoidance of secondhand smoke
- Importance of plenty of rest and relaxation and avoiding exhaustive exercise
- Genetic screening
- Encourage purchase of medical alert bracelet or similar type of warning device

Additional information for the patient can be found at the following websites:
- Sickle Cell Disease Association of America: http://www.sicklecelldisease.org
- Smokefree.gov: http://smokefree.gov
- Healthfinder—US Department of Health and Human Services: http://healthfinder.gov
- WebMD: http://www.webmd.com

measures to help prevent reoccurrence of painful episodes. If the patient smokes, he or she is encouraged to stop smoking and is referred to a smoking cessation program. In addition, the importance of continuous medical follow-up is stressed. While research continues to try to find a cure, nurses must continue to be sensitive to the effects of the disease on the patient and the family as well as the need to be culturally sensitive.[20]

Interprofessional collaborative management of the patient with SCA is outlined in Box 37.12.

TUMOR LYSIS SYNDROME

Description

Tumor lysis syndrome (TLS) refers to a variety of metabolic disturbances that may be seen with the treatment of cancer. A potentially lethal complication of various forms of cancer treatment, TLS occurs when large numbers of neoplastic cells are rapidly killed, resulting in the release of large amounts of potassium, phosphate, and uric acid into the systemic circulation. It is most commonly seen in patients with lymphoma, leukemia, large bulky tumors, or multiple metastatic conditions who are receiving cytotoxic chemotherapy.[25,26]

Etiology

Although most often associated with the use of chemotherapeutic medications, TLS has also been associated with immunotherapy, monoclonal antibody therapy, radiation therapy, and hormone therapy.[25-27] In rare instances, TLS can occur spontaneously.[25] Certain preexisting conditions can place the patient at higher risk for developing TLS, including dehydration, hypotension, elevated uric acid, splenomegaly, and chronic renal insufficiency.[25,27]

Pathophysiology

The primary mechanism involved in the development of TLS is the destruction of massive numbers of malignant cells by chemotherapy or radiation therapy (Fig. 37.7). Massive destruction of cells releases large amounts of potassium, phosphorus, and

BOX 37.12　QSEN: Teamwork and Collaboration

Interprofessional Collaborative Practice: Sickle Cell Anemia

- Prevent infection
  - Prophylactic antibiotics
  - Vaccinations
- Manage pain
  - Pharmacologic management
  - Nonpharmacologic management
- Administration of blood
- Administration of hydroxyurea
- Maintain surveillance for complications
  - Septicemia
  - Acute kidney injury
  - Acute myocardial infarction
  - Acute limb ischemia
  - Ischemic stroke
  - Anemia
- Provide comfort and emotional support

nucleic acids, leading to severe metabolic disturbances such as hyperuricemia, hyperkalemia, hyperphosphatemia, and hypocalcemia (Table 37.7). Vomiting, diarrhea, and other insensible fluid losses from fever or tachypnea also contribute to these electrolyte disturbances.[25] Death of patients with TLS is most often caused by complications of acute kidney injury or cardiac arrest.[25-27]

Hyperuricemia

Hyperuricemia occurs 48 to 72 hours after the initiation of anticancer therapy.[25] Tumor cells undergo rapid growth and development, and large amounts of nucleic acids are present within them. When therapy is initiated, tumor cell destruction releases nucleic acids, which are metabolized into uric acid. Metabolic acidosis ensues, resulting in crystallization of the uric acid in the distal tubules of the kidney and leading to obstruction of urine flow. Glomerular filtration rates decrease as the kidneys are unable to clear the increasing amounts of uric acid. Consequently, acute kidney injury eventually occurs.[28] Acute kidney injury is discussed further in Chapter 26.

Hyperuricemia associated with TLS can be potentiated by several other factors, including elevated uric acid levels before the initiation of therapy. Other causes of increased uric acid production are elevated WBC counts; destruction of WBCs; and enlargement of the lymph nodes, spleen, or liver.[25]

FIG. 37.7 Tumor Lysis Syndrome. Metabolic abnormalities in tumor lysis syndrome and clinical consequences. AKI, acute kidney injury. (From Abu-Alfa AK, Younes A; Tumor lysis syndrome and acute kidney injury: evaluation, prevention and management. *Am J Kidney Dis.* 2010;55[5 suppl 3]:S1–S13.)

TABLE 37.7 Electrolyte Abnormalities in Tumor Lysis Syndrome

Electrolyte	Pathophysiology	Clinical Consequence	Treatment Options
Potassium	Rapid expulsion of intracellular K+ into circulation due to cell lysis	Adverse skeletal and cardiac manifestations (eg, ventricular dysrhythmias, weakness, paresthesias)	Insulin/glucose, sodium bicarbonate, inhaled beta-agonist, K+-binding resins, dialysis, calcium gluconate
Phosphate May be compounded by renal dysfunction	Release of intracellular PO4− due to cell lysis Muscle cramps, tetany, dysrhythmias, seizures	Dialysis, phosphate binders	
Calcium	Precipitation of calcium phosphate complex because of rapid increase in phosphorus concentration	Muscle cramps, tetany, dysrhythmias, seizures, acute kidney injury (acute nephrocalcinosis)	Calcium gluconate (treatment should be reserved for patients with neuromuscular irritability)
Uric acid	Cell lysis leads to increased levels of purine nucleic acids into circulation that are metabolized to uric acid	Renal failure (uric acid nephropathy)	Hydration, dialysis, xanthine oxidase inhibitors, alkalization of urine, urate oxidase

From Davidson MB, et al. Pathophysiology, clinical consequences, and treatment of tumor lysis syndrome. *Am J Med.* 2004;116(8):546–554.

Hyperkalemia

Hyperkalemia occurs within 6 to 72 hours after the initiation of chemotherapy. This is the most deleterious of all the manifestations of TLS.[25] In addition to the release of nucleic acids, tumor cell destruction also results in the release of potassium. Renal insufficiency related to hyperuricemia prevents adequate excretion of potassium, and levels rise. The resultant hyperkalemia may have a profound effect on intracellular and extracellular fluid levels.[29] Left untreated, hyperkalemia can have devastating consequences, including cardiac arrest and death.[25]

Hyperphosphatemia and Hypocalcemia

Hyperphosphatemia and hypocalcemia occur 24 to 48 hours after the initiation of therapy.[25] Phosphorus levels also rise as a consequence of tumor cell destruction. Calcium ions then bind with the excess phosphorus, creating calcium phosphate salts and bringing about hypocalcemia. These salts precipitate in the kidney tubules, worsening renal insufficiency. Hypocalcemia causes tetany and cardiac dysrhythmias, which can result in cardiac arrest and death.[28,29]

Assessment and Diagnosis

Detection and recognition of TLS is accomplished through assessment of clinical manifestations, evaluation of laboratory findings, and other diagnostic tests. Table 37.8 summarizes common findings in TLS.[25,27]

Clinical Manifestations

Clinical manifestations are related to the metabolic disturbances associated with TLS.[27] The patient's history reveals an unexplained weight gain after initiation of chemotherapy or radiation therapy. The weight gain is associated with fluid retention secondary to electrolyte disturbances. Other early signs heralding the onset of TLS include diarrhea, lethargy, muscle cramps, nausea, vomiting, paresthesias, and weakness.[26]

Laboratory Findings

Laboratory findings demonstrate electrolyte disturbances such as elevated potassium and phosphorus levels and a decreased calcium level. Uric acid levels are increased. Elevated levels of BUN and creatinine and decreased creatinine clearance also indicate TLS. Metabolic acidosis is confirmed by the presence of decreased pH, bicarbonate levels, and arterial partial pressure of carbon dioxide ($Paco_2$) on ABG measurements.[26]

TABLE 37.8   Diagnostic Data for Tumor Lysis Syndrome

Diagnostic Parameter	Findings
Clinical	Weight gain, edema, diarrhea, lethargy, muscle cramps, nausea and vomiting, paresthesia, weakness, oliguria, uremia, seizures
Laboratory	↑ Potassium, phosphorus, uric acid, BUN, Cr ↓ Calcium, Cr clearance, pH, bicarbonate, $Paco_2$
Diagnostic	Positive Chvostek and Trousseau signs, hyperactive deep tendon reflexes, dysrhythmias, ECG changes

BUN, blood urea nitrogen; *Cr*, creatinine; *ECG*, electrocardiogram; *Paco₂*, arterial partial pressure of carbon dioxide; ↑, increased; ↓, decreased.

Other Diagnostic Tests

Physical examination reveals positive Chvostek and Trousseau signs related to hypocalcemia. Hyperactive deep tendon reflexes indicate hyperkalemia and hypocalcemia.[27] Potassium and calcium disturbances result in changes that can be seen on the electrocardiogram, such as peaked or inverted T waves, altered Q–T intervals, widened QRS complexes, and dysrhythmias.[25]

Medical Management

Medical interventions are aimed at maintaining adequate hydration, treating metabolic imbalances, and preventing life-threatening complications (see Table 37.7).[26,29]

Adequate Hydration

Administration of intravenous fluids may be necessary early in the course of treatment if inadequate hydration exists. The administration of isotonic saline (0.9% normal saline) reduces serum concentrations of uric acid, phosphate, and potassium.[27] The use of nonthiazide diuretics to maintain adequate urine output may be required. If acute kidney injury occurs, hemodialysis is considered.[27]

Metabolic Imbalances

Electrolytes and ABGs are closely monitored. Dietary restrictions of potassium and phosphorus may be necessary. The goals in treating hyperuricemia are to inhibit uric acid formation and to increase renal clearance.[29] This can be accomplished through the administration of sodium bicarbonate to increase the pH of the urine to greater than 7.0, which increases the solubility of uric acid, preventing subsequent crystallization. Allopurinol administration can also inhibit uric acid formation.[27]

Life-Threatening Complications

If potassium levels rise dangerously, sodium polystyrene sulfonate (Kayexalate) may be given orally, or if the patient is unable to tolerate oral medications because of nausea and vomiting, rectal instillation may be used. If the patient is oliguric, glucose and insulin infusions may be given to facilitate lowering the potassium levels. A 10% solution of calcium gluconate may be administered to stabilize cardiac tissue membranes to prevent life-threatening dysrhythmias.[30] Phosphorus-binding antacids can be used for treating hyperphosphatemia. Stool softeners may be necessary to treat the constipation often associated with the administration of these antacids. Calcium gluconate may be required to replace calcium, but it should be used judiciously.[25]

Nursing Management

The nursing management plan for a patient with TLS incorporates a variety of nursing diagnoses (Box 37.13). The nurse has a significant role in monitoring fluid and electrolytes, providing comfort and emotional support, maintaining surveillance for complications, and education of the patient and family.

BOX 37.13   NURSING DIAGNOSES

Tumor Lysis Syndrome

- Excess Fluid Volume related to renal dysfunction, p. 1025
- Decreased Cardiac Output related to alterations in contractility, p. 1016
- Anxiety related to threat to biologic, psychologic, or social integrity, p. 1012
- Ineffective Coping related to a situational crisis and personal vulnerability, p. 1036

Monitor Fluid and Electrolytes

Assessment and continued monitoring of the patient is an important role of the critical care nurse when caring for a patient with TLS. Recognizing critical laboratory changes or development of symptoms and notifying the physician in a timely manner are essential. Insertion of a urinary catheter and maintenance of the intravenous line site are necessary to ensure adequate intake and output. Vital signs are monitored frequently, and the patient's weight is monitored daily.

Maintain Surveillance for Complications

Nursing interventions are aimed at preventing complications. Seizure precautions are instituted, especially if calcium levels are disrupted. Insertion of a nasogastric tube is appropriate if nausea or vomiting occurs. Dietary adjustments are necessary, such as potassium and phosphorus restrictions in the presence of elevated serum levels and providing additional fiber to combat the constipation associated with the administration of antacids.[30]

Educate the Patient and Family

Early in the patient's hospital stay, the patient and family are taught about TLS, its etiologies, and its treatment. All treatments and interventions are explained before carrying them out, and questions should be answered at a level understandable to the patient and family. Before discharge, potential risk factors and identification of early signs and symptoms are reviewed.

Interprofessional collaborative management of the patient with TLS is outlined in Box 37.14.

ANEMIA OF CRITICAL ILLNESS

Etiology

Anemia of critical illness is a hospital-acquired disorder commonly seen in critically ill patients. It is the result of inflammation, iron deficiency, trauma, surgery, gastrointestinal bleeding, and iatrogenic blood loss from diagnostic testing. Inflammation causes decreased RBC production and increased destruction of RBCs by macrophages. Frequent phlebotomy, coagulopathies, and nutritional deficits are just a few reasons for this increasing problem.[31,32] Studies have shown that 50% of transfusions administered in the critical care unit are related to hospital-acquired anemia.[33] For these reasons, research has been focused on determining ways to minimize iatrogenic blood losses, improve blood salvage techniques, and develop alternatives to traditional blood transfusion therapy.

Blood Conservation Strategies

As more patients and clinicians opt for the limited use of blood products, strategies for conserving blood and preventing unnecessary loss become an important part of the critical care nurse's standard of care. These strategies include minimizing blood loss, managing oxygen delivery and consumption, stimulating production of RBCs, and understanding transfusion safety and alternative agents.[34,35]

Minimizing Blood Loss

Frequent blood draws in a critically ill patient have been associated with the development of anemia. Blood losses correspond to actual volume of samples and discards when drawing from venous access lines. Critical care nurses can be instrumental in significantly decreasing blood loss in this area. The use of pediatric collection tubes and point-of-care testing are techniques that yield valid diagnostic results but require smaller blood samples. Closed-loop vascular devices that retain the sterility of the potential discard and allow its return to the patient are also being used.[36] Noninvasive monitoring devices such as pulse oximetry and capnography can reduce the need for ABG analysis.

The critical care nurse plays a key role in preventing and managing hemorrhagic blood loss in critically ill patients. Control of hypertension, which can contribute to significant hemorrhage, can be accomplished through fluid management and administration of antihypertensive and vasodilatory medications as needed.[37] Blood salvage devices can be employed to collect shed blood and return it to the patient.[35] Several pharmacologic agents can assist in achieving hemostasis and can prevent further blood loss. Desmopressin is a potent vasoconstrictor that also affects clotting factor VIII.[34] Aminocaproic acid (Amicar) inhibits activation of plasminogen.[34] All these agents and devices work to control bleeding.

Managing Oxygen Delivery and Consumption

Illness-related stress, blood loss from surgery, infection, pain, and anxiety contribute to the higher than normal need for oxygen by critically ill patients.[32] Monitoring pulse oximetry is useful in identifying activities and interventions that can contribute to the imbalance between supply and demand. Supplemental oxygen therapy assists in maintaining available oxygen supplies. Promoting a restful environment through modulation of nursing care activities and providing pain and sedation control can assist in decreasing the demand for oxygen. It is important to monitor cardiac output and other hemodynamic parameters to manage interventions that optimize oxygen delivery. Administration of fluids and inotropic agents optimizes blood pressure and cardiac output, and vasodilators are used to decrease afterload and improve efficiency of cardiovascular function.[35]

QSEN BOX 37.14   QSEN: Teamwork and Collaboration

Interprofessional Collaborative Practice: Tumor Lysis Syndrome

- Facilitate adequate kidney function.
  - Volume hydration with 0.9% normal saline
  - Nonthiazide diuretics
- Treat hyperkalemia.
  - Kayexalate
  - Glucose and insulin
- Treat hyperuricemia.
  - Sodium bicarbonate
  - Allopurinol
- Treat hyperphosphatemia.
  - Dietary restrictions
  - Phosphorus-binding antacids
- Treat hypocalcemia.
  - Calcium gluconate
- Maintain surveillance for complications.
  - Acute kidney injury
  - Cardiac dysrhythmias
- Provide comfort and emotional support.

Encouraging Safer Transfusions and Alternative Agents

Finding ways to decrease the risks associated with blood transfusions and make the blood supply safer for patients is a high priority. Better and more sensitive screening tests, irradiation, and removal of leukocytes are a few of the current methods in use. Plasma expanders manufactured from nonhuman sources are also available. Autologous transfusion, in which the patient donates his or her own blood before a surgical procedure or other anticipated need, has also been a common practice for many years. Recombinant DNA technology is being used to develop safe alternatives to blood transfusions. The use of blood from other species is being researched in the quest to provide safe and effective products for use in severe anemia.[34] Current guidelines for the management of anemia and RBC transfusions are presented in Box 37.15.

QSEN **BOX 37.15** **QSEN: Evidence-Based Practice**

Management of Anemia and Red Blood Cell Transfusions Guidelines

Transfusion Triggers in General Critical Care Populations

- A transfusion threshold of 7 g/dL or below, with a target hemoglobin range of 7–9 g/dL, should be the default for all critically ill patients, unless specific comorbidities or acute illness–related factors modify clinical decision making.
- Transfusion triggers should not exceed 9 g/dL in most critically ill patients.

Alternatives to RBC Transfusions

- Erythropoietin should not be used to treat anemia in critically ill patients until further safety and efficacy data are available.
- In the absence of clear evidence of iron deficiency, routine iron supplementation is not recommended during critical illness.

Blood Sampling Techniques to Reduce Iatrogenic Blood Loss

- Introduction of blood conservation sampling devices should be considered to reduce phlebotomy-associated blood loss.
- Pediatric blood sampling tubes should be considered for reducing iatrogenic blood loss.

Adverse Consequences Associated With RBC Transfusion in Critical Care

- Pretransfusion assessment should include observing for conditions that increase risk of TACO (cardiac failure, renal impairment, hypoalbuminemia, fluid overload).
- Attention to the rate of transfusion together with careful fluid balance and appropriate use of diuretic cover (eg, furosemide) can reduce the risk of TACO.
- Patients developing hypoxia and bilateral pulmonary infiltrates during or within 6 h of transfusion should be carefully assessed for the development of TRALI.
- Any adverse events or reactions related to transfusion should be appropriately investigated and reported.

RBC Storage Duration

- There is insufficient evidence to support the administration of "fresher blood" to critically ill patients.

RBC, red blood cell; *TACO*, transfusion-associated circulatory overload; *TRALI*, transfusion-related acute lung injury
Modified from Retter A, et al: Guidelines for the management anaemia and red cell transfusion in adult critically ill patients. *Br J Haematol.* 2013;160(4):445–465.

CASE STUDY 37.1 **Patient With Hematologic Disorders and Oncologic Emergencies**

Brief Patient History

Mr. L, an otherwise healthy, 23-year-old African American man, presents with a week-long history of diarrhea, nausea, and vomiting after attending a barbecue the previous weekend.

Clinical Assessment

Mr. L is admitted to the critical care unit from the emergency department with hypotension, fever, and leukocytosis.

Diagnostic Procedures

Vital signs are as follows: blood pressure of 65/42 mm Hg, heart rate of 145 beats/min (sinus tachycardia), respiratory rate of 35 breaths/min, and temperature of 102.4°F. His white blood cell count is 25,000/mm³ with 15% bands, lactate level is 7 mmol/L, prothrombin time is 25 s, and platelet count is 22,000/mm³. Blood cultures show gram-negative bacilli.

Medical Diagnosis

Mr. L is diagnosed with severe sepsis and disseminated intravascular coagulation.

Questions

1. What major outcomes do you expect to achieve for this patient?
2. What problems or risks must be managed to achieve these outcomes?
3. What interventions must be initiated to monitor, prevent, manage, or eliminate the problems and risks identified?
4. What interventions should be initiated to promote optimal functioning, safety, and well-being of the patient?
5. What possible learning needs do you anticipate for this patient?
6. What cultural and age-related factors may have a bearing on the patient's plan of care?

SUMMARY

Coagulation and Fibrinolysis

- Hemostasis is the ability of the body to control bleeding and clotting.
- Four actions are involved in achieving hemostasis: local vasoconstriction to reduce blood flow, platelet aggregation at the injury site and formation of a platelet plug, formation of a fibrin mesh to strengthen the plug, and dissolution of the clot after tissue repair.

Disseminated Intravascular Coagulation

- DIC is characterized by bleeding and thrombosis, which result from depletion of clotting factors, platelets, and RBCs and, if left untreated, will result in death.
- Medical management focuses on identification of the underlying cause; provision of hemodynamic support to preserve end-organ function; and administration of blood, blood components, and medications to interrupt the process.
- Nursing actions include initiating bleeding precautions, providing comfort and emotional support, and maintaining surveillance for complications (eg, hypovolemic shock, ischemia, multiple-organ dysfunction syndrome).

Idiopathic Thrombocytopenia Purpura

- Idiopathic thrombocytopenia purpura is caused by an autoimmune response that results in the destruction of existing platelets.
- Medical management focuses on administration of glucocorticoids, immunoglobulin, and platelets.
- Nursing actions include initiating bleeding precautions, providing comfort and emotional support, and maintaining surveillance for complications (eg, intracranial hemorrhage, severe blood loss).

Heparin-Induced Thrombocytopenia

- There are two forms of heparin-induced thrombocytopenia: type 1 and type 2. Type 1 is more common, milder, and transient. Type 2 is the result of an autoimmune response to the administration of heparin and is more severe than type 1.
- Medical management focuses on discontinuation of all heparin, initiation of anticoagulation with an alternative anticoagulant, and treatment of thrombosis.
- Nursing actions include providing comfort and emotional support and maintaining surveillance for complications (eg, deep vein thrombosis, pulmonary emboli, limb ischemia, ischemic stroke, acute myocardial infarction).

Sickle Cell Anemia

- SCA is a disease passed down through families in which RBCs form an abnormal sickle or crescent shape.
- Medical management focuses on prevention of infection, management of pain, and administration of RBCs and hydroxyurea.
- Nursing actions include supporting the patient's vital functions, providing comfort and emotional support, maintaining surveillance for complications (eg, ischemic stroke, acute myocardial infarction, acute limb ischemia, acute kidney injury), and educating the patient and family.

Tumor Lysis Syndrome

- Tumor lysis syndrome occurs when a large number of neoplastic cells are rapidly killed, resulting in the release of large amounts of potassium, phosphate, and uric acid in the systemic circulation.
- Medical management focuses on preservation of kidney function and treatment of electrolyte disorders (hyperkalemia, hyperuricemia, hyperphosphatemia, and hypocalcemia).
- Nursing actions include providing comfort and emotional support and maintaining surveillance for complications (eg, acute kidney injury, dysrhythmias).

Hospital-Acquired Anemia

- Anemia of critical illness occurs as a result of inflammation, iron deficiency, trauma, surgery, gastrointestinal bleeding, and iatrogenic blood loss from diagnostic testing.
- Blood conservation strategies include minimizing blood loss, managing oxygen delivery and consumption, and stimulating production of RBCs.

ⓔ Visit the Evolve site for additional study materials.

REFERENCES

1. Rote NS, McCance KL. Structure and function of the hematologic system. In: McCance KL, Huether SE, eds. *Pathophysiology: The Biologic Basis for Disease in Adults and Children*. ed 7. St. Louis: Elsevier; 2014.
2. Furie B, Furie BC. Mechanisms of thrombus formation. *N Engl J Med*. 2008;359(9):938-949.
3. Levi M, van der Poll T. Disseminated intravascular coagulation: a review for the internist. *Intern Emerg Med*. 2013;8(1):23-32.
4. Chapin JC, Hajjar KA. Fibrinolysis and the control of blood coagulation. *Blood Rev*. 2015;29(1):17-24.
5. Mackavey C, Hanks R. Hemostasis, coagulation abnormalities, and liver disease. *Crit Care Nurs Clin North Am*. 2013;25(4):435-446.
6. Levi M. Diagnosis and treatment of disseminated intravascular coagulation. *Int J Lab Hematol*. 2014;36(3):228-236.
7. Gando S. Microvascular thrombosis and multiple organ dysfunction. *Crit Care Med*. 2010;38(2 Suppl):S35-S42.
8. Blaisdell FW. Causes, prevention, and treatment of intravascular coagulation and disseminated intravascular coagulation. *J Trauma Acute Care Surg*. 2012;72(6):1719-1722.
9. Levi M, van der Poll T. A short contemporary history of disseminated intravascular coagulation. *Semin Thromb Hemost*. 2014;40(8):874-880.
10. Greenberg EM, Kaled ES. Thrombocytopenia. *Crit Care Nurs Clin North Am*. 2013;25(4):427-434.
11. Wang HL, et al. Thrombocytopenia in the intensive care unit. *J Intensive Care Med*. 2013;28(5):268-280.
12. Thiele T, et al. Thrombocytopenia in the intensive care unit—diagnostic approach and management. *Semin Hematol*. 2013;50(3):239-250.
13. Neunert CE. Current management of immune thrombocytopenia. *Hematology Am Soc Hematol Educ Program*. 2013;2013:276-282.
14. Winkeljohn D. Diagnosis, treatment, and management of immune thrombocytopenia. *Clin J Oncol Nurs*. 2013;17(6):664-666.
15. Gupta S, et al. Heparin-induced thrombocytopenia in critically ill: diagnostic dilemmas and management conundrums. *World J Crit Care Med*. 2015;4(3):202-212.
16. Greinacher A. Heparin-induced thrombocytopenia. *N Engl J Med*. 2015;373(3):252-261.
17. Sakr Y. What's new about heparin-induced thrombocytopenia type II. *Intensive Care Med*. 2015;41(10):1824-1827.
18. Donavan JL, Tran MT, Kanaan AO. An overview of heparin-induced thrombocytopenia. *J Pharm Pract*. 2010;23(3):226-234.
19. Linkins LA, et al. Treatment and prevention of heparin-induced thrombocytopenia: antithrombotic therapy and prevention of thrombosis, 9th ed: American College of Chest Physicians Evidence-Based Clinical Practice Guidelines. *Chest*. 2012;141(2 Suppl):e495S-e530S.
20. Matthie N, Jenerette C. Sickle cell disease in adults: developing an appropriate care plan. *Clin J Oncol Nurs*. 2015;19(5):562-567.
21. Paradowski K. Pathophysiology and perioperative management of sickle cell disease. *J Perioper Pract*. 2015;25(6):101-104.

22. Jorde LB. Genes and genetic diseases. In: McCance KL, Huether SE, eds. *Pathophysiology: The Biologic Basis for Disease in Adults and Children.* ed 7. St. Louis: Elsevier; 2014.

23. Addis G. Sickle cell disease, part 1: understanding the condition. *Br J Nurs.* 2010;5(5):136-139.

24. Brown M. Managing the acutely ill adult with sickle cell disease. *Br J Nurs.* 2012;21(2):90-96.

25. Wilson FP, Berns JS. Tumor lysis syndrome: new challenges and recent advances. *Chronic Kidney Dis.* 2014;21(1):18-26.

26. Maloney KW. Metabolic emergencies. In: Itano JK, ed. *Core Curriculum for Oncology Nursing.* St. Louis: Elsevier; 2016.

27. Wagner J, Arora S. Oncologic metabolic emergencies. *Emerg Med Clin North Am.* 2014;32(3):509-525.

28. Shelton BK. Tumor lysis syndrome. In: Chernecky CC, Murphy-Ende K, eds. *Acute Care Oncology.* ed 2. St. Louis: Mosby; 2009.

29. Abu-Alfa AK, Younes A. Tumor lysis syndrome and acute kidney injury: evaluation, prevention and management. *Am J Kidney Dis 2010.* 2010;55(5 Suppl 3):S1-S13.

30. Mirrakhimov AE, et al: Tumor lysis syndrome: a clinical review. *World J Crit Care Med* 4(2):130-138.

31. Brophy DF, et al. An epidemiological study of anemia and renal dysfunction in patients admitted to ICUs across the United States. *Anemia.* 2012;2102:938140.

32. Prakash D. Anemia in the ICU: anemia of chronic disease versus anemia of acute illness. *Crit Care Clin.* 2012;28(3):333-343.

33. Collins TA. Packed red blood cell transfusions in critically ill patients. *Crit Care Nurse.* 2011;31(1):25-33.

34. Hayden SJ, et al. Anemia in critical illness: insights into etiology, consequences, and management. *Am J Respir Crit Care Med.* 2012;185(10):1049-1057.

35. Ahmed AH. Prevention and management of hospital-acquired anemia. *Hosp Med Clin.* 2014;3(1):e71-e84.

36. Mukhopadhyay A, et al. The use of blood conservation device to reduce red blood cell transfusion requirements: a before and after study. *Crit Care.* 2010;14(1):R7.

37. Cannon-Diehl MR. Transfusion in the critically ill: does it affect outcome? *Crit Care Nurs Q.* 2010;33(4):324-338.

38

The Obstetric Patient

Susie Hutchins

Innovations in technology and advances in treatment options have placed the worlds of critical care and obstetrics on a pathway of collaboration and sometimes of conflict. Traditionally, the two specialties have been separated, in part because of the typical normalcy and health-oriented approach of obstetrics and the crisis and illness orientation of critical care. Pregnancy alters the function of virtually every organ system, and the baseline state and patient response to physiologic changes are very different in pregnant patients. Fetal considerations often are important in designing and leading the clinical approach to the critically ill pregnant woman. Many common conditions in pregnancy require special medical care with associated complications that have the potential for serious maternal morbidity and mortality.

Critical care obstetrics encompasses two distinct populations: (1) women with preexisting disease who become pregnant and (2) women with normal pregnancies who become compromised by critical illness or injury. The two priorities for a pregnant critically ill woman are (1) supporting fetal growth and development and (2) optimizing maternal and family experiences.

The latest statistics of the growing maternal mortality rates in the United States demonstrate the need to continue diligence and research in providing care to this population. Data from the World Bank showed an increase of 28 maternal deaths per 100,000 live births compared with 12 per 100,000 in 1990. This represents approximately 1200 women who died from maternal causes in 2013.[1] A portion of this increase observed over the past decades may have been caused by changes in the coding and classification of maternal deaths. Although the reason for the increased risk of a woman dying from pregnancy-related causes is unclear, several studies show that an increasing number of pregnant women in the United States have chronic health conditions such as hypertension, diabetes, and chronic heart disease.[2] These conditions may put a pregnant woman at higher risk of pregnancy complications. Cardiovascular disease is the leading cause of death in pregnant women (Box 38.1).[2]

At the global level, the World Health Organization assessed trends in maternal mortality rate from the period 1990–2013 and revealed that the number of women dying of pregnancy and childbirth related complications has almost halved in 23 years.[1] An alarming trend in maternal mortality in the United States is race-specific pregnancy-related mortality rates. Analysis of rates has demonstrated that compared with White women, African American women have 2.7 times the risk of dying as a result of childbirth and that the maternal mortality rate among Hispanic women was approximately 0.8% less than that of White women.[3] High rates of obesity and hypertension and inadequate prenatal care cause death from childbirth more often for African Americans in the United States than for Whites and other ethnic groups.

It is impossible to discuss in one chapter every aspect of management of critically ill obstetric patients. Instead, the focus is to provide a synopsis of the more commonly seen conditions or concerns in the realm of critical care obstetrics and to emphasize the collaborative nature of this emerging field, recognizing that the manifestations and management of many critical illnesses are typically identical in pregnant and nonpregnant patients, although the data value changes associated with pregnancy must be considered. Nursing management, unless unique to the critically ill obstetric patient, is not detailed here.

PHYSIOLOGIC ALTERATIONS IN PREGNANCY

During pregnancy, a woman's body undergoes profound physiologic changes. These changes are necessary to maintain the pregnancy and to allow for fetal growth and development. The changes are so dramatic that they would probably be considered pathologic in a nonpregnant woman. Adaptations occur in nearly every organ system, beginning during the first week of gestation and continuing until up to 6 weeks after delivery. The only system in which no documented characteristic changes occur is the nervous system. Boxes 38.2 and 38.3 and Tables 38.1 to 38.4 summarize the various systems and alterations during pregnancy.[4-7] Understanding the physiologic adaptations is important to the management of a critically ill pregnant woman. More detailed information can be found in textbooks dedicated to obstetric issues.

PHYSIOLOGIC CHANGES DURING LABOR AND DELIVERY

Labor and delivery bring additional stresses to the maternal system, especially as a result of the pain and anxiety associated with labor. The most dramatic requirements are for the cardiopulmonary system. During labor, uterine contractions produce cyclic

BOX 38.1   Pregnancy-Related Deaths

Cardiovascular diseases—15.1%
Noncardiovascular diseases—14.1%
Infection or sepsis—14.0%
Hemorrhage—11.3%
Cardiomyopathy—10.1%
Thrombotic pulmonary embolism—9.8%
Hypertensive disorders of pregnancy—8.4%
Amniotic fluid embolism—5.6%
Cerebrovascular accidents—5.4%
Anesthesia complications—0.3%
Unknown—5.9%

CDC Reproductive Health, Pregnancy Mortality Surveillance System 2014, http://www.cdc.gov/reproductivehealth/maternalinfanthealth/pmss.html. Accessed September 19, 2016.

BOX 38.2   Primary Functions and Implications of Estrogen and Progesterone

Functions and Effects of Estrogen

Promote growth and function of the uterus
Cause uterine musculature hypertrophy and hyperplasia
Increase blood supply to uteroplacental unit
Promote breast (ductal, alveolar, nipple) development
Increase pliability of connective tissue
Relax pelvic joints and ligaments
Allow cervical softening
Promote sodium and water retention
Produce psychologic changes leading to emotional lability
Decrease gastric secretion of hydrochloric acid and pepsin
Increase sensitivity to carbon dioxide (CO_2) levels in blood
Produce integumentary changes
Hyperpigmentation
Striae gravidarum
Affect blood component concentrations
Increase fibrinogen (factor I) concentration
Decrease plasma protein concentration
Cause leukocytosis

Functions and Effects of Progesterone

Decrease maternal smooth muscle contractility
Uterus: Prevent contractility
Gastrointestinal tract: Contribute to nausea, heartburn, and constipation
Renal system: Contribute to urinary dilation leading to urinary stasis
Vascular system: Dilate vessels and contribute to peripheral edema
Produce metabolic effects
Reset hypothalamus up approximately 0.2°C (0.5°F)
Promote fat storage
Stimulate respiratory center to decrease CO_2 retention
Stimulate secretion of sodium in urine, stimulating aldosterone production
Promote breast development and inhibit the action of prolactin

BOX 38.3   Indications for Hemodynamic Monitoring in Pregnancy

Severe pregnancy-induced hypertension with persistent oliguria or pulmonary edema
Massive hemorrhage or volume replacement needs
Acute respiratory distress syndrome
Shock of unknown cause
Sepsis with oliguria or refractory hypotension
Cardiovascular decompression during intrapartum or intraoperative periods
Chronic disease during labor or intraoperatively (New York Heart Association class III or IV cardiac disease)
Pulmonary edema, oliguria, or heart failure refractory to treatment or of unknown cause

TABLE 38.1   Positional Cardiac Output Changes in Pregnancy

Maternal Position	Cardiac Output (L/min)
Knee-chest	6.9 ± 2.1
Right lateral	6.8 ± 1.3
Left lateral	6.6 ± 1.4
Sitting	6.2 ± 0.0
Supine	6.0 ± 0.4
Standing	5.4 ± 2.0

TABLE 38.2   Hemodynamic Changes Associated With Term Pregnancy

Parameter	Pregnancy Normal Value	Change
Mean arterial pressure (mm Hg)	90 ± 6	No significant change
Central venous pressure (mm Hg)	8 ± 2	No significant change
Pulmonary artery occlusion pressure (mm Hg)	4 ± 3	No significant change
Heart rate (beats/min)	83 ± 10	Increase 17%
Cardiac output (L/min)	6.2 ± 1.0	Increase 43%
Systemic vascular resistance (dyn · sec · cm^{-5})	1210 ± 266	Decrease 21%
Pulmonary vascular resistance (dyn · sec · cm^{-5})	78 ± 22	Decrease 34%
Serum colloid oncotic pressure (mm Hg)	18 ± 1.5	Decrease 14%
Left ventricular stroke work index (g-m/m^2)	48 ± 6	No significant change

autotransfusions of approximately 300 to 500 mL. Immediately after birth, cardiac output peaks, with an 80% increase over prelabor values.[4] This increase occurs because of the contracted uterus shunting its blood, the sudden removal of fetal supply demands, and the resolution of vena cava compression. Table 38.5 summarizes the cardiac output changes in labor and delivery.[4,6,7]

Normal blood loss from a vaginal birth is typically 500 mL; blood loss from cesarean deliveries usually is 1000 mL. Clinical estimates tend to underestimate actual blood loss by up to 50%.[8] The cardiopulmonary changes occurring during labor and delivery are of significant concern because they occur over a short period and because maternal decompensation may occur.

In summary, maternal physiology is profoundly and rapidly affected by pregnancy. Adaptations begin early in the pregnancy and continue through the postpartum period, gradually returning to prepregnant states over 6 weeks. Understanding the physiologic stresses uniquely present during pregnancy allows the clinician to provide comprehensive care to the pregnant woman experiencing critical illness or injury.

TABLE 38.3 Physiologic Adaptation of the Gastrointestinal System During Pregnancy

Gastrointestinal Function Change	Presumed Cause
Heartburn	Progesterone and estrogen; size of gravid uterus impeding gastroesophageal junction
Bleeding gums	Hyperemia
Constipation	Progesterone, causing decreased motility and intestinal secretion, enhanced water absorption
Hemorrhoids	Hyperemia, pelvic congestion, obstruction of venous return
"Morning sickness" or nausea	Increased levels of estrogen and human chorionic gonadotropin
Risk for aspiration	Displacement of lower esophageal sphincter and reduced gastric motility
Gallstones	Decreased gallbladder activity, impaired emptying

TABLE 38.4 Renal Physiologic Changes in Pregnancy

Parameter	Percent Change	Normal Levels in Pregnancy (mL/min)
Renal blood flow	Increase 25%–50%	1250–1500
Glomerular filtration rate	Increase 50%	140–170
Renal plasma flow	Increase 35%	700–900

TABLE 38.5 Cardiac Output Changes in Labor and Delivery

Stage of Labor or Delivery	Change in Cardiac Output
Early first stage of labor	↑ 15% plus additional 15% with each contraction
Last first state of labor	↑ 30% plus additional 15% with each contraction
Second stage of labor	↑ 45% plus additional 15% with each contraction
First 5 min postpartum	↑ 80% secondary to autotransfusion
First hour postpartum	↑ 25%

CARDIAC DISORDERS IN PREGNANCY

Cardiac disease ranks fourth after pregnancy-induced hypertension, hemorrhage, and infection as a cause of maternal mortality.[9] Several factors have to be taken into consideration in the care of a pregnant woman with cardiac disease. Cardiac disease during pregnancy may be a result of preexisting conditions such as congenital diseases, or it may be a result of primary cardiac disease arising before or during pregnancy. A pregnant woman with heart disease has decreased cardiac reserve, making it more difficult for her heart to accommodate the higher workload of pregnancy. Thus, prepregnancy counseling is highly recommended for women with known cardiac disease. Counseling would include determining the New York Heart Association functional class, which is especially useful for pregnant women with structural heart disease, and determining the maternal and fetal risks associated with the pregnancy (Box 38.4).[7,10] Major

BOX 38.4 Maternal Mortality Risks

Group 1: Mortality <1%
Atrial septal defect
Ventricular septal defect
Patent ductus arteriosus
Pulmonic tricuspid disease
Tetralogy of Fallot, corrected
Bioprosthetic valve
Mitral stenosis, NYHA classes I and II

Group 2: Mortality 5%–15%
Group 2A
Mitral stenosis, NYHA classes III and IV
Aortic stenosis
Coarctation of aorta, without valvular involvement
Tetralogy of Fallot, uncorrected
Previous myocardial infarction
Marfan syndrome with normal aorta

Group 2B
Mitral stenosis with atrial fibrillation
Artificial valve

Group 3: Mortality 25%–50%
Pulmonary hypertension
Coarctation of aorta, with valvular involvement
Marfan syndrome with aortic involvement

NYHA, New York Heart Association.

fetal risks include fetal development of congenital heart disease, prematurity, intrauterine growth restriction, and intrauterine fetal demise.

The method and timing of delivery are decided primarily by obstetric considerations, taking into account the woman's ability to tolerate the labor process and associated physiologic changes. Selection of anesthesia techniques involves weighing the risks and benefits of the procedures. As a general rule, most patients tolerate epidural anesthesia more favorably than they tolerate general anesthesia (see Chapter 41).

Congenital Cardiac Disorders

Congenital heart defects have become a more common finding in pregnant women as improved surgical techniques have enabled females born with heart defects to live to childbearing age. When surgical repair can be accomplished with no remaining evidence of organic heart disease, pregnancy may be undertaken with confidence. When congenital heart disease is associated with cyanosis, whether the defect was originally uncorrected or the correction failed to relieve the cyanosis, the woman should be counseled about risks to both herself and to her fetus. Of equal concern in pregnant women with congenital heart disease is the risk of fetal congenital cardiac anomalies, which is approximately 5%. During the antepartum period, serial ultrasonography should be performed to access the fetus for appropriate interval growth.[11]

Atrial Septal Defect

Atrial septal defect (ASD) is the most common congenital anomaly seen during pregnancy, and most women with ASD tolerate pregnancy, labor, and delivery without complications. The decrease in systemic vascular resistance lessens the degree of left-to-right shunt, whereas the hypervolemic state may slightly worsen the shunt and increase right ventricular workload. The most common complications seen with ASD are dysrhythmias, heart failure, and thromboembolism.[12]

Ventricular Septal Defect

The outcome for a pregnant woman with ventricular septal defect (VSD) and resultant left-to-right shunt depends on the size of the defect, with larger defects producing a less favorable prognosis. Most VSDs are diagnosed and repaired before women reach childbearing age. In the absence of significant symptoms and pulmonary hypertension, pregnancy is typically well tolerated. Therapy is aimed at early recognition and treatments of signs of heart failure.[13] Common complications include tachycardia, heart failure, and pulmonary hypertension.

Patent Ductus Arteriosus

During pregnancy, patent ductus arteriosus (PDA) is an unusual finding, as it is generally detected and closed during the newborn period. Patients who present with a PDA during pregnancy usually tolerate the hemodynamic stress of labor and delivery without difficulty. Precautions against the risks of infective endocarditis and thromboembolism may be taken. Severe PDA may produce large left-to-right shunts, causing acute heart failure or pulmonary hypertension that is associated with significant maternal mortality.[8]

Tetralogy of Fallot

Tetralogy of Fallot (TOF) is the most common cyanotic heart defect in individuals who survive to adulthood.[14] The four primary lesions associated with TOF are (1) VSD, (2) overriding aorta, (3) right ventricular hypertrophy, and (4) pulmonary stenosis. Women with corrected TOF generally can tolerate pregnancy well. Although rare, if the congenital anomalies are not corrected, maternal mortality rate and fetal complications increase significantly.[14] Cardiopulmonary function must be maximized by measures that include treatment of dysrhythmias and use of prophylaxis for endocarditis. Considerations during labor and delivery include maintenance of adequate preload and blood pressure.

Coarctation of the Aorta

Coarctation of the aorta may occur in isolation or, most often, in combination with valvular or septal anomalies. Patients with uncomplicated coarctation of the aorta who are relatively asymptomatic (New York Heart Association class I or II) have demonstrated good prognosis and minimal risk of complications or death.[4] Assessment of the aortic gradient may also be useful in predicting pregnancy outcome in patients with coarctation of the aorta. In general, aortic gradients across the site of coarctation that are less than 20 mm Hg are associated with good maternal and fetal outcomes.[12] Intrapartum management focuses on the prevention of hypertension to avoid aortic wall stress. Careful management of fluid balance and left ventricular function must occur to prevent congestive heart failure and to promote adequate perfusion.

Eisenmenger Syndrome

Eisenmenger syndrome is not a single congenital defect but a complication that may be the result of other cardiac lesions that cause left-to-right shunting. This syndrome is more likely to occur with VDS or ASD because of the high pressure and high flow associated with these defects. This shunting may result in progressive pulmonary hypertension, leading to shunt reversal or bidirectional shunting.[15] Regardless of the cause, the risk of sudden death because of pulmonary hypertension in pregnancy is 40%, which has remained unchanged for the past 50 years. Avoidance or termination of pregnancy is commonly recommended. If pregnancy is continued, therapeutic management is directed at avoidance of pulmonary vasoconstrictors, thromboembolism, and hypotension; maintenance of adequate preload and oxygenation; fetal surveillance; and reduction of stress at the time of delivery.[15]

Acquired Cardiac Disorders

Special consideration must be given to physical assessment during the antepartum period. Normal physiologic changes such as murmur development or shortness of breath may mask symptoms of cardiac disease or make diagnosis more challenging.

Mitral Stenosis

The presence of a stenotic mitral valve is the most common rheumatic valve disease of pregnancy. The primary concern with mitral stenosis during pregnancy is the impedance to ventricular filling, which produces a relatively fixed cardiac output. Additional risks include thromboembolism, heart failure, and arrhythmias, especially atrial fibrillation. Cardiac output in the face of mitral stenosis is determined by two primary factors: (1) length of diastolic filling and (2) left ventricular preload. The length of diastolic filling may be negatively affected because of the increased pulse rate during a normal pregnancy. Discomfort or anxiety associated with labor may produce a tachycardic state, which may drastically impede ventricular filling, producing an even lower cardiac output, with resultant heart failure and pulmonary edema. Because pregnancy is a hypercoagulable state, thrombi may rapidly form, and fibrillation may dislodge the thrombi and cause arterial embolism. Thus, prophylactic anticoagulation should be considered in this subset of women.[16,17]

Maintenance and management of left ventricular preload is the second important consideration in mitral stenosis. Patients may require high-normal or slightly elevated left ventricular filling pressures to maintain adequate flow across the stenotic mitral valve. It is especially important to assess the patient's fluid status. Caution must be exercised when employing therapies that decrease preload (eg, diuresis or epidural anesthesia).[16] Invasive hemodynamic monitoring may be indicated to carefully tailor therapy.

In the immediate postpartum period, careful monitoring is essential because of the massive fluid shifts and large increases in cardiac output. Authorities recommend that optimal predelivery pulmonary artery occlusion pressures be maintained at 14 mm Hg or less to accommodate the increase in occlusion pressure of up to 16 mm Hg that may occur in the immediate postpartum period.[16]

Aortic Stenosis

Other valvular disease, especially disease affecting the mitral valve, often accompanies aortic stenosis. The hallmark of aortic stenosis is decreased left ventricular ejection.[4] Mild aortic stenosis is usually well tolerated during pregnancy because of the natural hypervolemic state. Significant aortic stenosis can produce left ventricular hypertrophy and dilation. Thromboembolic prophylaxis is recommended. Critical to successful management is maintenance of cardiac output through prevention of hypovolemia, especially at the time of delivery. The maintenance of adequate cardiac output and oxygen transport is vital in the clinical management of pregnant women with aortic stenosis. Any factor that diminishes venous return or produces hypotension worsens the effects of aortic stenosis and significantly reduces cardiac output. Heart failure occurs in less than 10% of patients with severe aortic stenosis, and arrhythmias occur in 3% to 25%.[18] Mortality is rare if careful management is provided.

Marfan Syndrome

Marfan syndrome is an autosomal dominant disorder of connective tissue, in which serious cardiovascular involvement, usually dissection or rupture of the aorta, may occur. Prognosis is based on aortic root and wall involvement, with most authorities citing 40 mm as maximal root diameter, after which significant increases in mortality occur.[17,19] Prevention of tachydysrhythmias and hypertension is recommended, along with endocarditis prophylaxis. Beta-blockade therapy may be initiated for cardiac rate control and to decrease pressure on the weakened aortic wall. Goals of management include maintenance of cardiac output to meet physiologic needs without producing undue stress on the aortic wall, use of regional anesthesia, and avoidance of Valsalva maneuver by shortening the second stage of labor. Careful blood pressure maintenance is essential. Differential diagnosis of chest and back pain is essential, along with recognition of other signs of aortic dissection. Because of its inheritance pattern, there is a 50% risk that the disease will be transmitted to the infant.[19]

Peripartum Cardiomyopathy

Peripartum cardiomyopathy (PPCM) is a type of left ventricular dysfunction of unknown origin that occurs in the last month of pregnancy and up to 5 months after delivery in women with no previous history of heart disease. PPCM is a diagnosis of exclusion. Occurring in 1 in 3000 to 4000 live births, it is a relatively rare but serious condition. Early reports suggested a mortality rate of nearly 50%, but more recent studies indicate a 0% to 5% mortality rate in the United States.[20,21] Controversy regarding exact causes of PPCM continues, as symptoms that are often attributable to viral and immune sources, chronic hypertension, mitral stenosis, obesity, and myocarditis all have been proposed.[21] Definitive diagnosis of PPCM depends on the echocardiographic identification of new-onset heart failure during a limited period toward the end of pregnancy or in the months following delivery.[18,21,22]

Symptoms are identical to those of classic heart failure, but treatment depends on the pregnancy status of the patient. Women who present with PPCM during pregnancy require joint cardiac and obstetric care, but as soon as the baby is born and the patient is hemodynamically stable, standard therapy for heart failure may be applied.[18] This would include treatment with diuretics, digoxin, beta-blockade, and afterload reduction. Angiotensin-converting enzyme inhibitors, angiotensin receptor blockers, and renin inhibitors are contraindicated during pregnancy because of fetotoxicity but may be used after the infant is born.[18,22] Once the bleeding has been stopped after delivery, anticoagulation is commonly employed to prevent thromboembolism and the formation of left ventricular thrombus, which is associated with a worse prognosis.[22] The clinical course of PPCM is quite variable, but 50% to 60% of patients show clinical recovery within the first 6 months after delivery.[23] The prognosis of PPCM is positively related to the recovery of ventricular function. Medical therapy as outlined in the American College of Cardiology Foundation and American Heart Association guidelines should be continued when a woman does not recover function.[22] Subsequent pregnancy is associated with a recurrence risk for PPCM of 30% to 50%.[18]

Ischemic Cardiac Disease
Acute Myocardial Infarction

Although acute myocardial infarction (AMI) during pregnancy is rare; pregnancy has been shown to increase the risk of AMI three to fourfold.[24] With the continuing trend of childbearing at older ages and advances in reproductive technology enabling many older women to conceive, it may be expected that the occurrence of AMI will increase. Mortality rates from AMI during pregnancy range from 37% to 50%, depending on the timing of the myocardial event.[25] However, most occurrences of AMI in pregnancy are not related to atherosclerosis; approximately 50% of ischemic heart disease in pregnancy is linked to idiopathic dissections of the coronary arteries. Other reported conditions that contribute to AMI risk are eclampsia, thrombophilia, postpartum infections, and severe postpartum hemorrhage.[18] Increased mortality is associated with many factors, including occurrence of the event during the third trimester, multigravidas older than 33 years, cesarean section, and delivery occurring within 2 weeks of infarction.[25]

Clinical diagnostics are similar to those for standard AMI detection, although the diagnosis must be made with consideration of the normal physiologic cardiovascular changes. Coronary angiography with the possibility of coronary intervention is preferred to thrombolysis, as it will also diagnose coronary artery dissection.[25]

Treatment of AMI during pregnancy is focused on restoring myocardial blood flow and balancing myocardial oxygen supply and demand.[25] Management may include percutaneous coronary intervention; nitrate therapy, beta-blockade therapy, or both; cardiac monitoring; oxygen therapy; management of pain and anxiety; and afterload reduction. Angiotensin-converting enzyme inhibitors, angiotensin receptor blockers, and renin inhibitors are not indicated during pregnancy.[18] Coronary angiograms, angioplasty, bypass surgery, and intraaortic balloon pumps all have been successfully used during pregnancy. Special consideration is given to the maternal physiologic demands required during the labor and delivery processes. Operative delivery interventions, such as forceps or cesarean section, may be necessary (see "Myocardial Infarction" in Chapter 14).

Prior Myocardial Infarction

The outcome in a pregnant woman with prior myocardial damage depends on many factors. The length of time between the myocardial event and delivery is especially important.[47] Increased myocardial oxygen demands during pregnancy must be considered, and therapy is usually supportive in nature. Careful attention to preload is essential to prevent burdening the heart and producing congestive failure (see "Heart Failure" in Chapter 14).

Cardiac Arrest in Pregnancy

The occurrence of cardiopulmonary arrest during pregnancy is uncommon. Successful management of the pregnant patient in cardiac arrest requires integration of physiologic changes present during pregnancy and adaptations for those from standard resuscitative guidelines. Fetal outcomes are directly related to the mother's condition and well-being. The interrelationship between fetal and maternal well-being may present unique ethical dilemmas for health care providers and family members. Causes of obstetric and nonobstetric cardiopulmonary arrest during pregnancy are summarized in Table 38.6.

Basic cardiac life support. The American Heart Association recommendations include only minor deviations from usual life support procedures.[26] The facilitation of venous return is critically important. This is accomplished by performing chest compressions slightly above the center of the sternum and lateral displacement of the uterus through manual manipulation or through the use of a wedge under the woman's hip, as this improves venous return by decreasing compression of the vena cava by the gravid uterus.[26] Physiologic adaptations in pregnancy place the woman at greater risk for complications from cardiopulmonary resuscitation such as fractured ribs and sternum, hemothorax, hemopericardium, and internal organ damage. Specific organs of concern include the uterus, spleen, and liver.

Advanced cardiac life support. The American Heart Association recommends that the standard resuscitation algorithm be followed for advanced cardiac life support, with a few modifications to compensate for the altered anatomy and physiology of pregnancy.[27] The airway should be secured early with effective preoxygenation, and cricoid pressure should be applied both to aid in intubation and to prevent aspiration. As pregnancy progresses, edema of the oropharynx increases, necessitating the use of a smaller endotracheal tube than in a nonpregnant woman.[27] Careful attention to confirmation of tube placement and oxygenation is important because of the enhanced oxygen demands during pregnancy.

Standard advanced cardiac life support recommendations should be followed for administration of resuscitation medications. Use of lower extremity sites or the femoral vein for venous access should be avoided because of the potential of the gravid uterus to impede venous return.[27] Epinephrine may decrease uteroplacental perfusion because of its vasoconstrictive nature; however, the benefits outweigh the risks of administration. Lidocaine crosses the placenta, but it does not have adverse fetal or uteroplacental effects at therapeutic levels. If maternal toxicity occurs, fetal cardiac and central nervous system depression may occur. No contraindications exist for use of atropine in pregnancy. Administration of sodium bicarbonate

should be undertaken cautiously. Maternal acidosis increases uteroplacental adrenergic reactivity and must be avoided, although maternal alkalosis may impair oxygen exchange to the fetus. Electrical therapies such as defibrillation, cardioversion, and pacing are not contraindicated in pregnancy, but all fetal monitoring devices should be removed because a theoretical risk of the scalp electrode arcing and electrocuting the infant does exist.

Evaluation of fetal tolerance of the mother's condition is essential during cardiopulmonary arrest. Fetal hypoxia may develop because of decreased uteroplacental perfusion. Fetal gestational age is a prime consideration when determining a course of action. Before 24 weeks' gestation, resuscitative efforts are focused primarily on maternal outcome. After the 24th week of gestation, evaluation includes maternal and fetal responses to resuscitative efforts. Emergent cesarean section may be undertaken for fetal distress or to improve maternal status, although consideration also must be given to the stress that cesarean section produces. In late pregnancy, survival of the infant is directly proportional to the time interval between death of the mother and delivery of the infant. Infant viability is best if delivery occurs within 5 minutes of cardiac arrest.[25,27]

HYPERTENSIVE DISEASE

Hypertensive disease is present in 5% of pregnant women.[28] Hypertension is defined as systolic blood pressure of 140 mm Hg or greater or diastolic blood pressure of 90 mm Hg or greater, or both.[28] It is the second leading cause of death in childbearing women, and it contributes to high rates of newborn morbidity and mortality.[4,29,30] Maternal complications include pathologic compromise of the cardiovascular, pulmonary, renal, neurologic, and hepatic systems (Table 38.7).[30-32] Understanding of hypertensive disease in pregnancy is based on (1) a classification according to manifestations and time of onset in relation to gestation, (2) the fact that pregnancy could induce hypertension in women without a history of high blood pressure, and (3) the fact that elevated blood pressure in pregnancy could occur without the presence of generalized edema or proteinuria (transient hypertension).[31] Proper diagnosis of hypertensive complications is critical and requires in-depth knowledge of disease pathophysiology to prevent or decrease the risk of maternal or fetal compromise.

Classification of Hypertension

The National Institutes of Health Working Group on High Blood Pressure has endorsed the classification and terminology of the American Congress of Obstetricians and Gynecologists for hypertensive disease in pregnancy.[28,30] The following

TABLE 38.6 Obstetric and Nonobstetric Causes of Cardiac Arrest in Pregnancy

Obstetric Causes	Nonobstetric Causes
Hemorrhage (17%)	Pulmonary embolism (19%)
Pregnancy-induced hypertension (16%)	Infection or sepsis (13%)
Idiopathic peripartum cardiomyopathy (8%)	Stroke (5%)
Anesthetic complications (2%)	Myocardial infarction
Amniotic fluid embolism	Trauma

From Campbell T, Sanson T. Cardiac arrest and pregnancy. *J Emerg Trauma Shock.* 2009;2(1):34.

TABLE 38.7 Complications of Hypertensive Disease in Pregnancy

Body System	Complication
Cardiovascular	Dysrhythmias, acute heart failure, severe hypertension
Pulmonary	Pulmonary edema, acute airway obstruction
Renal	Oliguria, renal failure, acute kidney injury
Neurologic	Cerebral edema, eclampsia, cerebral hemorrhage, coma
Hepatic	Necrosis, rupture, periportal and subcapsular hemorrhage
Hematologic	DIC, hemolysis thrombocytopenia

DIC, disseminated intravascular coagulation.

definitions have proved useful in establishing consistent guidelines for pregnancy management:[33]

Chronic hypertension is hypertension before conception or diagnosed before 20 weeks' gestation.

Preeclampsia and eclampsia constitute a systemic syndrome of hypertensive disease, with proteinuria diagnosed after 20 weeks' gestation. Eclampsia indicates the additional presence of convulsions.

Preeclampsia superimposed on chronic hypertension may occur before 20 weeks' gestation or have a sudden onset.

Gestational hypertension is hypertension without proteinuria after 20 weeks' gestation.

Preeclampsia and Eclampsia

Preeclampsia is the most common hypertensive disorder of pregnancy. It is estimated that 50,000 women die as a result of preeclampsia each year worldwide. Among women with chronic hypertension, 22% to 25% develop this complication.[34,35] Preeclampsia is a syndrome that affects both the mother and the fetus. It is clinically defined as an increase in blood pressure after 20 weeks' gestation accompanied by proteinuria in a previously normotensive woman.[35,36] Eclampsia is the occurrence of a seizure in a woman with preeclampsia who has no other cause for seizure.

Preeclampsia has been called a "disease of theories" because true mechanisms behind the pathogenesis remain unclear. It is a multisystem disorder unique to humans and difficult to study in laboratory animals, which creates an obstacle to discovering its exact etiology.[36]

One of the key features of preeclampsia involves the failure of uterine spiral arteries to transform from thick-walled muscular vessels to sac-like flaccid vessels, exaggerated inflammatory response, and inappropriate endothelial cell activation.[37] Characteristics of preeclampsia include widespread arteriolar vasospasms resulting in decreased perfusion to virtually all organs including the placenta, a decrease in plasma volume, activation of the coagulation cascade, and alteration in glomerular capillary endothelium. These generalized cyclic vasospasms lead to tissue ischemia and eventually end-organ dysfunction (Fig. 38.1).[32]

A serious problem related to preeclampsia is pulmonary edema caused by increased capillary permeability. Thrombocytopenia complicates severe preeclampsia in approximately 7% to 11% of women.[37,38] Abruptio placentae and the release of procoagulants such as thromboplastin may result in acute disseminated intravascular coagulation (DIC). Women who develop preeclampsia are more sensitive to pressor agents, and this response has been linked to the ratio between prostaglandins, prostacyclin, and thromboxane. Prostacyclin is decreased in preeclampsia, allowing the potent vasoconstrictor and platelet-aggregating effects of thromboxane to dominate. No effective intervention seems to be available, although low-dose aspirin may lead to modest risk reduction of the disease.[37]

New research suggests that pathogenesis related to imbalance between circulating antiangiogenesis-related factors.[39,40] These antiangiogenic factors produce systemic endothelial dysfunction, resulting in hypertension, proteinuria, and other systemic expressions of preeclampsia. The molecular basis for placental misuse

FIG. 38.1 Pathophysiologic Changes of Pregnancy-Induced Hypertension. *AST,* aspartate aminotransferase; *DIC,* disseminated intravascular coagulation; *LDH,* lactate dehydrogenase. (From Gilbert E. *Manual of High Risk Pregnancy and Delivery.* 5th ed. St. Louis: Mosby; 2010.)

of these pathogenic factors remains unknown, and the role of angiogenic proteins in early placental vascular development and trophoblast invasion is just beginning to be explored. Widespread systemic vascular dysfunction and microangiopathy is demonstrated in the mother but not in the fetus.[39,40] With preeclampsia, decreased production of nitric oxide, which is a potent vasodilator and important regulator of maternal blood pressure, also occurs.

Hyperhomocysteinemia may play role in the etiology or pathophysiology of preeclampsia.[41] Mild elevations of homocysteine have been found in women with normal blood pressures who go on to develop preeclampsia. Once preeclampsia is established, homocysteine levels are considerably increased. It is unclear whether the increased levels of homocysteine caused the disease or if they reflect the metabolic alterations resulting from preeclampsia. Deficiencies of vitamin B_6, vitamin B_{12}, or folic acid may cause an increase in homocysteine. In one study in which approximately 4000 women received folic acid supplements, the results demonstrated a decrease in plasma homocysteine and a reduced risk of preeclampsia.[41]

Intracerebral hemorrhage is a rare complication, but it is the most common cause of death in women with severe preeclampsia and eclampsia, being fatal in 50% to 60% of the cases. Infants of women with preeclampsia tend to be small for gestational age because of intrauterine growth restriction. In addition, the maternal condition may warrant early termination of pregnancy, which leads to a severely premature infant. Placental abruption secondary to hypertension may result in fetal hypoxia or death.[35,36]

The treatment goals of severe preeclampsia are to prevent seizures, decrease arterial spasms, and effect prompt delivery of the fetus. Magnesium sulfate ($MgSO_4$) is the standard treatment for the prevention and control of seizures in women with preeclampsia or eclampsia. Serum magnesium levels of 4 to 7 mEq/L are thought to be therapeutic for prevention of seizure activity. A loading dose of 4 to 6 g is given by infusion pump over 15 to 20 minutes, followed by a maintenance infusion of 2 to 3 g/h.[4]

Control of eclamptic seizures is accomplished through administration of 4 to 6 g of intravenous $MgSO_4$ over 5 to 10 minutes. This bolus is followed by a continuous infusion of 2 to 3 g/h. If a patient has a recurrent seizure, another bolus of 2 to 4 g may be given over 3 to 5 minutes. Amobarbital sodium, benzodiazepines, or phenytoin may be used for treating seizures that are not responsive to $MgSO_4$.[29,42] The use of multiple agents to decrease eclamptic seizures should be avoided, unless necessary.

Severe hypertension must be addressed after magnesium infusions. Antihypertensive agents need to be used to keep diastolic blood pressure between 90 and 100 mm Hg. The main drugs used to achieve this are hydralazine hydrochloride or labetalol.[29,42] Diuretics are used only in the setting of pulmonary edema. The placenta plays a central role in the development of the disease, for which the only known cure is delivery of the fetus and removal of the placenta.

Hemolysis, Elevated Liver Enzymes, and Low Platelet Syndrome

Hemolysis, elevated liver enzymes, and low platelet (HELLP) syndrome affects 2% to 20% of patients with severe preeclampsia or eclampsia.[34,43] Maternal mortality ranges from 3.5% to 24%, whereas perinatal mortality is 10% to 60%.[31] Approximately 10% to 15% of pregnant patients with HELLP syndrome do not have elevated proteinuria of hypertensive disease.[36,44,45] The clinical manifestations of HELLP syndrome, which include nausea, vomiting, malaise, flu-like symptoms, and epigastric pain, may

suggest a multitude of other clinical diagnoses. Misdiagnosis is common and may result in a delay of correct treatment. HELLP syndrome may be confused with acute renal disease, gastroenteritis, hepatitis, gallbladder disease, pyelonephritis, or thrombotic thrombocytopenic purpura.[6] Any pregnant woman demonstrating clinical manifestations and showing hemolysis, elevated liver enzymes, and low platelets must be diagnosed with HELLP syndrome. Complications of HELLP syndrome include abruptio placentae, liver hematoma, DIC, pulmonary edema, liver rupture, and acute kidney injury.[4,36]

Collaborative management for patients with severe preeclampsia or eclampsia or with HELLP syndrome is based on stabilization of the mother and the fetus. Continuous assessment of the cardiovascular, renal, central nervous, and pulmonary systems provides early indications of worsening maternal condition. Fetal surveillance may include continuous fetal monitoring, biophysical profile, and fetal lung maturity testing. Delivery of the fetus may be indicated because of the maternal condition or fetal compromise. The goal of the health care team is to accurately monitor ongoing organ system dysfunction and prevent further damage leading to end-organ failure and maternal-fetal mortality.

DISSEMINATED INTRAVASCULAR COAGULATION

DIC is not a separate clinical entity; rather, it is an effect of other disease processes. The obstetric causes of DIC include abruptio placentae, preeclampsia or eclampsia, dead fetus syndrome, septic abortion, and amniotic fluid embolus. In DIC, fibrinogen levels and platelet counts are usually decreased, whereas prothrombin time and partial thromboplastin time are normal to prolonged.[46] The pathophysiologic mechanisms of DIC are summarized in Table 38.8.[4,31] Primary treatment goals include identification of the underlying disorder, removal of the trigger or initiating event, and volume replacement including blood component therapy. Secondary treatment may include anticoagulation therapy. Heparin therapy is controversial.

Abruptio Placentae

Because abruptio placentae is the most common obstetric cause of DIC, evaluating the results of coagulation tests is imperative.

TABLE 38.8 **Conditions Associated With Disseminated Intravascular Coagulation**

Obstetric	Obstetric or Nonobstetric	Nonobstetric
Abruptio placentae	Prolonged shock, any cause	Malignancy
Amniotic fluid embolism	Transfusion-incompatible blood	Extensive surgery
Eclampsia, preeclampsia	Septicemia: bacterial fungal, viral	Collagen vascular disease
Abortion	Septic abortion	Central nervous system trauma
Dead fetus syndrome	Severe chorioamnionitis	Allergic reactions
Hydatidiform mole		Burns
Retained placenta		Vascular malformations
Uterine rupture		Pancreatitis
Maternal hemorrhage		

Of pregnant women experiencing abruption, 20% have a significant clotting defect, with 25% of this group experiencing postpartum hemorrhage.[44] Supportive treatment to decrease risk of DIC includes a type and crossmatching for blood transfusions, clotting mechanism evaluation, and the administration of intravenous fluids.[46] If DIC is established, the basic element of treatment is the removal of blood clots from the uterus, blood component therapy, and fluid volume resuscitation.

Dead Fetus Syndrome

Prolonged retention of a dead fetus may lead to development of DIC, also called *consumption coagulopathy,* in the mother. After the release of thromboplastin from the degenerating fetal tissues into the maternal bloodstream, the extrinsic clotting system is activated, triggering the formation of multiple tiny blood clots. Fibrinogen and factors V and VII are subsequently depleted, and the woman begins to display symptoms of DIC. Fibrinogen levels begin a linear descent 3 to 4 weeks after the death of the fetus and continue to decrease in the absence of appropriate medical intervention.[6] Because of the risk of DIC, the once common practice of waiting for the onset of labor has largely been abandoned.[47]

Septic Abortion

Although septic abortion is a well-documented cause of obstetric DIC, since the legalization of abortion, a large reduction in the number of cases of septic abortion has occurred.[6] Bacterial endotoxins are the most likely initiating mechanism. The clinical findings of gram-negative septic shock are applicable to this condition. The severity of the disease correlates well with the degree of coagulopathy. Aggressive antibiotic therapy and evacuation of the uterus are the frontline therapies for patients who are hemodynamically stable.

SHOCK

Shock is defined as tissue hypoxia resulting from decreased perfusion secondary to decreased intravascular volume. Because pregnancy is a hyperdynamic, low-resistance state with increased oxygen delivery and consumption requirements, the management of shock in a pregnant woman necessitates an approach that is different from the approach for a nonpregnant woman. Normal physiologic adaptations that occur during pregnancy may alter ranges in vital signs and laboratory values, which may mislead the practitioner and complicate timely diagnosis and early treatment. Frequently, the clinician may be obtaining data from and managing two patients—the mother and the fetus.

Causes of hemorrhagic shock unique to pregnancy include abruptio placentae, ectopic pregnancy, placenta previa, and postpartum hemorrhage.[4,6] Postpartum hemorrhage may be attributed to uterine atony, genital tract lacerations, hematoma formation, retained placenta, and uterine prolapse. Unique causes of septic shock in pregnant women include chorioamnionitis, septic abortion, and postpartum pyelonephritis.[4] Cardiogenic shock is most frequently a result of the presence of severe valve disease. Regardless of the cause, whether specific to pregnancy or not, the occurrence of shock requires aggressive intervention with treatment of the underlying cause.

Management of shock in pregnancy focuses on optimizing maternal stability in an effort to provide the most stable uterine environment. Clinical judgments include assessment of the risks and benefits of therapeutic interventions and fetal viability. Consideration must be given to the potential vasoconstrictive nature of some pharmacotherapeutics and the potential for uteroplacental insufficiency.

PULMONARY DYSFUNCTION

Oxygen consumption increases by approximately 15% to 25% throughout pregnancy.[6] To meet these needs for additional oxygen, ventilatory changes (Fig. 38.2) must occur. Pulmonary dysfunction is of clinical significance because of the normally slightly hyperoxygenated condition associated with the physiologic changes in pregnancy. As a result of normal cardiorespiratory changes that occur during pregnancy, a pregnant woman has very limited cardiopulmonary reserve. Therefore, it is relatively easy for the pregnant woman to demonstrate pulmonary decompensation in the presence of any respiratory compromise.

Compromise of respiratory function places the mother and the fetus at risk. Maternal hypoxia may be the end result of several conditions, including pneumonia, asthma, cystic fibrosis (CF), trauma, acute respiratory distress syndrome (ARDS), and pulmonary embolism (PE). Contributing factors (eg, smoking, drug use, preexisting disease states), manifestations, and management differ very little from those seen in a nonpregnant woman. Common to these respiratory disorders is the issue of maternal-fetal hypoxia. Sufficient fetal oxygenation requires a maternal arterial partial pressure of oxygen (Pao_2) greater than 70 mm Hg, which corresponds to an oxygen saturation of 95%.[48] Hyperventilation, shortness of breath, and dyspnea are commonly seen in pregnancy and must be differentiated from the usual maternal complaints.

Asthma

Although asthma is an increasingly common chronic pulmonary complication in women in the reproductive age group, the management strategies do not differ significantly in pregnant women with asthma from women who do not have asthma.[49] Women who may not be compliant with medical regimens while pregnant for fear of fetal harm should be informed that well-controlled asthma does not appear to affect pregnancy adversely, whereas poorly controlled asthma greatly increases pregnancy risk.[50,51] Poorly controlled asthma during pregnancy has been associated with an increased incidence of pneumonia (more than 60% of pneumonias that arise during pregnancy occur in women with asthma), hyperemesis gravidarum, gastroesophageal reflux disease, preeclampsia, chronic hypertension, preterm labor or birth, perinatal mortality, spontaneous abortion, complicated labor, and low birth weight.[52,53] The literature indicates that maternal and fetal outcomes are related to the severity of the disease and the degree of control achieved with medical management.

It is estimated that approximately one-third of patients experience no change in asthma symptoms, one-third experience improvement, and one-third have worsening of symptoms. The peak incidence of asthma exacerbation occurs during the second and early third trimesters; exacerbations during labor are rare because of the naturally occurring increase of endogenous epinephrine and steroids.[51,53] The lessening of asthma symptoms during pregnancy is the result of smooth muscle relaxation caused by progesterone. Decreased cell-mediated immunity and an increased level of corticosteroids may assist in diminishing the inflammatory response. Cyclic adenosine monophosphate levels are increased and aid in maintaining an ongoing energy supply to cells.

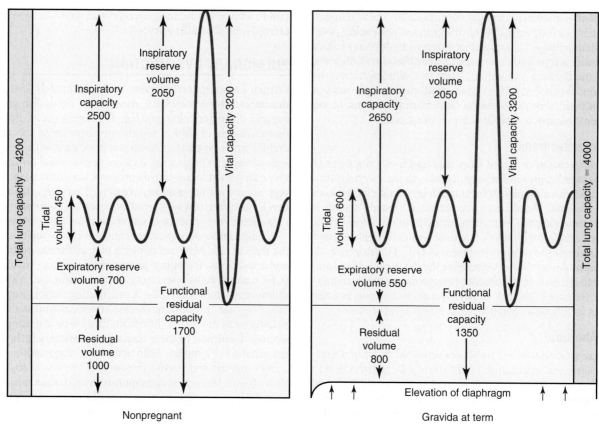

FIG. 38.2 Pulmonary Volumes and Capacities (in milliliters) During Pregnancy, Labor, and the Postpartum Period. (From Bonica JJ, MacDonald J. *Principles and Practice of Obstetric Analgesia and Anesthesia.* 2nd ed. Philadelphia: Williams & Wilkins; 1995.)

Factors that may contribute to exacerbation of asthma symptoms include nasal congestion, decreased functional residual volume, anxiety, noncompliance with medical regimens, stress, exercise, exposure to allergens, environmental irritants, respiratory infections, sinusitis, and smoking.[51-53] The decrease in cell-mediated immunity may predispose the mother to viral infections.

Management recommendations include use of a peak flow meter twice per day to assist in objectively measuring maternal pulmonary function. A decrease in peak expiratory flow rate (PEFR) of more than 20% of the patient's personal best requires a call to the physician; a decrease of greater than 50% of the patient's personal best signals the need for a visit to the emergency department for rapid assessment and intervention.[51,53] Pharmacologic agents used to treat asthma in pregnancy fall into two principal categories: (1) maintenance agents and (2) rescue agents. The most commonly used agents in this category that are safe for use during pregnancy are inhaled steroids, systemic steroids, mast cell stabilizers, methylxanthines, and leukotriene antagonists. Rescue agents, used to provide immediate symptomatic relief, include inhaled beta-agonists and inhaled anticholinergics.[50-52,54]

Cystic Fibrosis

Cystic fibrosis is an autosomal recessive, multisystem disease that affects the exocrine glands and epithelial tissues of the pancreas, sweat glands, and mucous glands of the respiratory, digestive, and reproductive tracts.[52,55] Pulmonary disease is the leading cause of morbidity and mortality in patients with CF. More women with CF are living to reproductive age and becoming pregnant because of improved pulmonary and pharmacologic therapies and because of the opportunity of lung transplantation. The normal pulmonary changes of pregnancy (eg, increased resting minute ventilation; upward displacement of the diaphragm, with resultant decrease in functional residual volume; widened alveolar-arterial oxygen gradient) lead to pulmonary decompensation and increased morbidity and mortality for the mother and the fetus. In advanced lung disease, pulmonary hypertension may be present. Pulmonary hypertension, combined with the normal pregnancy-related increase in blood volume and the consequent inability to increase cardiac output, may lead to uteroplacental insufficiency and cardiovascular collapse, especially during labor and delivery.[52] Management recommendations include ongoing cardiopulmonary assessment (chest radiography, pulmonary function studies, oxygen saturation measured by pulse oximetry [Spo$_2$], arterial blood gas determinations, pulmonary artery pressure monitoring), bronchial drainage and chest physiotherapy, ongoing replacement of pancreatic enzymes and supplementation of nutrition, and antibiotic administration for persistently present organisms such as *Pseudomonas aeruginosa* and *Burkholderia cepacia.*[44,52,53] Historically, women with CF had poor pregnancy outcomes; however, more recent reports suggest that in women with milder disease, pregnancy outcome may be favorable. Additionally, the patient should receive genetic counseling on the risk of her children being affected by CF.[56]

Pneumonia

Pneumonia is a leading cause of infection-related death in the United States and remains a leading cause of maternal and fetal morbidity and mortality.[57,58] Although data suggest that infants born to mothers whose pregnancies have been complicated by pneumonia are more likely to be born preterm and to have a lower birth weight, care must be taken to balance treatment to serve both the mother and the fetus.[59] Exacerbations are more common in the second and third trimesters, and they are often associated with other maternal disease processes. Prior respiratory disease, concurrent illness, human immunodeficiency virus (HIV) infection, drug or tobacco use, aspiration, and anemia have been linked with an increased maternal risk of pneumonia.[57,58]

Pregnancy itself appears to be an independent risk factor for considerable complications of pneumonia. Major complications such as empyema or pneumothorax may occur in 40% of pregnant women with pneumonia. Physiologic changes of pregnancy decrease the mother's ability to clear secretions and place her at increased risk for gastric aspiration. In the fetus, growth restriction, which leads to small-for-gestational-age neonates, occurs in approximately 12% of cases; intrauterine and neonatal death rates of 12% have been reported [57]

Typically, pneumonia is of bacterial origin; however, various organisms may be seen. Some of the more common pathogens identified are *Streptococcus pneumoniae*, responsible for approximately 50% of bacterial pneumonias, and *Haemophilus influenzae*, which is the second most common causative organism. *Mycoplasma pneumoniae* and *Chlamydia pneumoniae* may account for a substantial number of cases and should be considered when selecting empiric treatment.[4,44] Pregnant women may be uniquely susceptible to viral pneumonia secondary to the reduction in cell-mediated immunity that is associated with pregnancy.[59]

Clinicians may be reluctant to obtain chest radiographs; however, the hazard to both the mother and the fetus of delaying the diagnosis is far greater than the small dose (approximately 300 microrads) to the fetus from standard chest radiography. *Pneumocystis jiroveci* (formerly *Pneumocystis carinii*) pneumonia and resistant strains of tuberculosis are a growing concern because many women who are HIV positive or have acquired immunodeficiency syndrome are in their reproductive years.[57,60]

Acute Respiratory Distress Syndrome

ARDS in pregnancy is often the result of a variety of conditions, including aspiration; preeclampsia; abruptio placentae; postpartum hemorrhage; massive blood transfusions; sepsis; amniotic fluid embolism (AFE); and certain drugs such as tocolytics and aspirin, which lead to the development of pulmonary edema (noncardiogenic). An important presenting symptom is dyspnea, especially if it is associated with a degree of anxiety or tachypnea. As dyspnea evolves, pulmonary function rapidly deteriorates over a 24-hour period. Symptoms include coughing, wheezing, diffuse crackles, pulmonary infiltrates or pleural effusion on the chest radiograph, and a deteriorating Pao_2 with increasing fraction of inspired oxygen (Fio_2) demands and declining Pao_2/Fio_2 ratio.[60] Pulmonary compliance may decrease from the normal average of 75 mL/cm H_2O to 20 mL/cm H_2O in severe ARDS.[4] In all suspected cases of ARDS, additional laboratory tests and examinations must be completed to differentiate this syndrome from other conditions such as fluid overload and heart failure that may sometimes be seen in the last trimester.

Management of Respiratory Failure

Management of maternal hypoxia includes restoration and maintenance of the hypervolemic state without inducing fluid overload and further compromising cardiopulmonary function. Because colloidal osmotic pressure is decreased, great care must be taken to prevent the development of pulmonary edema when providing fluid replacement therapy. Oxygen is administered at a high flow rate by mask to achieve an optimal Pao_2 greater than 100 mm Hg and Spo_2 greater than 95%. Noninvasive mechanical ventilation should be used with caution because of the risk of gastric aspiration. If intubation is required, placement of an orotracheal tube is more desirable than a nasotracheal tube because of hyperemic nasal passageways. If nasotracheal intubation is required, the smallest tube possible that still allows adequate ventilation is used. Gastric decompression is instituted with a small-bore nasogastric or orogastric tube.[44,58] Precautions must be taken to maintain the maternal $Paco_2$ of 28 to 32 mm Hg because respiratory alkalosis may lead to decreased uterine blood flow. Pulmonary compliance should be routinely assessed to evaluate the effectiveness of interventions. Pharmacologic therapies must consider maternal-fetal risk and benefits. Table 38.9 summarizes common medications used in pulmonary dysfunction and obstetric concerns regarding their use.[49,52,53]

Pulmonary Embolism

Venous thromboembolism (VTE), including PE, results from a variety of causes, many of which are related to the physiologic changes in pregnancy. Deep vein thrombosis (DVT) during pregnancy is far more common in the left leg than in the right leg. In one study of 60 pregnant women with a first episode of VTE, 58 had isolated left lower extremity DVTs, 2 had bilateral DVTs, and no isolated right lower extremity DVTs occurred.[61] This unusual distribution has been attributed to increased venous stasis in the left leg related to compression of the left iliac vein by the right iliac artery, combined with compression of the inferior vena cava by the gravid uterus itself. Pelvic vein DVT is also more likely in pregnancy, making the diagnosis more difficult. Other factors to be considered include the increasing frequency of long-term bed rest for high-risk multiple pregnancies, preterm labor, maternal age older than 35 years, obesity, smoking, cancer, surgery, and a history of VTE or PE.[62-65]

PE remains a leading cause of maternal mortality and accounts for 20% of pregnancy-related deaths.[61] The greatest risk for developing PE is in the immediate postpartum period, especially if a cesarean section was performed. Two-thirds of the patients who die of PE do so within 30 minutes of the initial event. Physiologic changes associated with pregnancy may obscure the diagnosis of VTE during pregnancy. Assessment, management, and complications associated with PE are essentially no different from those in a nonpregnant woman; however, differential diagnosis of AFE must be considered.[62] If DVT or PE is diagnosed, anticoagulation should be initiated. Either unfractionated heparin or low-molecular-weight heparin is an acceptable treatment for acute VTE. Both have risks and benefits, but both may be used safely during pregnancy. Intravenous heparin is the treatment of choice surrounding delivery because

TABLE 38.9 Common Medications Used in Pulmonary Dysfunction During Pregnancy

Medication	Considerations
Antibiotics	Cephalosporins and erythromycin are generally well tolerated.
	Tetracyclines and quinolones should be avoided.
	Vancomycin and aminoglycosides may lead to fetotoxicity.
	Acyclovir improves maternal morbidity and appears to improve fetal outcomes.
Inhaled corticosteroids	Beclomethasone is generally considered safe.
Systemic corticosteroids	Decreased birth weights and increase in small-for-date infants are documented.
	Most drug is metabolized by placental enzymes before entering the fetal circulation.
	Small amount of steroid may cross into breast milk, but breastfeeding is still considered safe.
Mast cell stabilizers	Cromolyn and nedocromil are generally considered safe.
	They are not associated with increased risks to the fetus.
Beta-adrenergic agonists	Epinephrine and isoproterenol may contribute to maternal-fetal tachycardia.
	Albuterol and terbutaline have fewer side effects and may have additional benefit of tocolytic actions.
Leukotriene receptor antagonists	They appear to be safe for management of chronic, mild to moderate asthma.
Inhaled anticholinergics	Ipratropium is beneficial for acute asthma attack.
	They probably are safe for the fetus because they are poorly absorbed by bronchial mucosa, decreasing the risk of fetal exposure.
Theophylline	It is not commonly used because of maternal side effects.
	It is recommended that serum levels be maintained between 5 and 12 mg/mL to prevent complications of toxicity.
Analgesics	Morphine and meperidine should be avoided in active labor because they can worsen bronchospasm.
	They cross the placenta and should be considered when completing a fetal assessment.
	Fentanyl may be a better agent to use.
	Epidural analgesia is considered safe.
Beta-mimetic tocolytics	These are contraindicated because they may worsen maternal lung damage.
Labor induction	Oxytocin is drug of choice.
	Prostaglandin F_2 should be avoided because it is a bronchoconstrictor.
Neuromuscular blockade	It can be administered safely as long as peripheral nerve testing is conducted to monitor drug dosages.
	These agents cross the placenta, which should be considered when assessing fetal activity.

of its short half-life. Because of the risk of adverse effects on the fetus, warfarin is not generally used until the postpartum period.[66,67] A vena cava filter may be implanted, but a suprarenal position is selected to prevent restriction of venous blood coming from the left ovary and draining into the left renal vein.

Amniotic Fluid Embolism

Amniotic fluid embolism, also known as anaphylactoid syndrome of pregnancy (ASP), is a potentially disastrous complication involving cardiopulmonary collapse in a pregnant woman.[68] AFE is rare. Most studies indicate that the incidence rate is between 1 and 12 cases per 100,000 deliveries.[68,69] The maternal mortality rate from AFE has been reported to range from 10% to 90%, although more recent data from large unselected populations suggest that overall mortality rates may be closer to 20%.[70] Women who survive generally have a poor outcome, with up to 85% sustaining significant neurologic injury from cerebral hypoxia.[68,69] AFE is one of the leading causes of maternal mortality.

The most common precipitating factors associated with the syndrome are a large fetus, multiparity, premature separation of the placenta, induction of labor, tumultuous labor, and small tears in the endocervical veins that may occur during normal labor.[58,68,70,71] An increased risk also was noted in older women from ethnic minority groups.[70] Placental abruption is seen in almost half of the cases, with fetal death having occurred before the event.[71] Fig. 38.3 presents the pathophysiology of AFE.[72]

A patient with AFE may present with sudden onset of agitation and dyspnea, followed by symptomatic hypoxia, hypotension, and later DIC. Signs spend symptoms of shock out of proportion to blood loss and altered mental status may also be observed. Chest pain and bronchospasm are uncommon. In a small percentage of patients, a grand mal seizure may be the initial symptom. More than 25% to 50% of patients die within the first hour, 80% die within the first 9 hours, and 40% of survivors develop DIC.[58,71] The fetal mortality rate is 21%.[71]

No specific diagnostic test exists for AFE, although the presence of fetal squamous cells, lanugo, vernix caseosa, meconium, and mucin in blood aspirated from the pulmonary artery indicates a possibility of its occurrence; however, this debris has been reported in blood samples obtained from normal pregnant women.[58,70] Testing should be done to rule out DIC. Chest radiography may show pulmonary edema, effusions, and cardiac enlargement. Electrocardiogram may show tachycardia, nonspecific ST wave changes, and right ventricular strain. Lung scans may indicate perfusion defects.

Management consists of maintaining oxygenation and supporting cardiac function. Supportive therapy consists of maintenance of blood pressure through aggressive volume replacement and inotropic support, intubation and mechanical ventilation, and blood component therapy for hemorrhage.[58,68] Other therapies such as low-dose heparin, bronchodilators, and steroids may be used.

TRAUMA

Trauma is the leading nonobstetric cause of death among pregnant women; the rate has been estimated to be approximately 6% to 7%, although a precise number is difficult to obtain because injuries may range from minor to life-threatening.[73,74] Motor vehicle accidents are the leading cause of maternal blunt trauma and account for 55% to 82% of maternal trauma.[75]

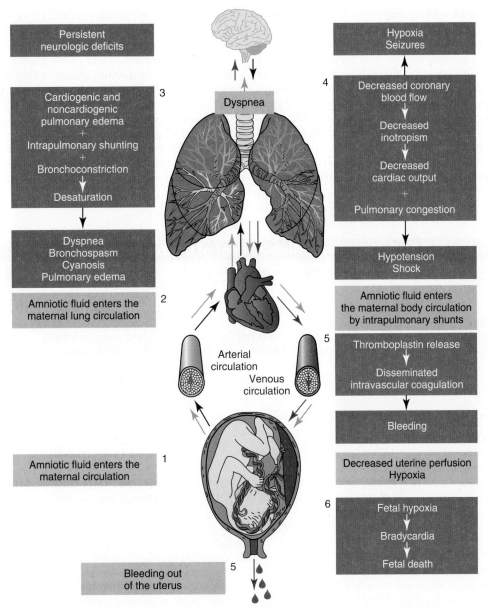

FIG. 38.3 Pathophysiology of Amniotic Fluid Embolism. (From Gei G, Hankins GDV. Amniotic fluid embolism: An update. *Contemp Ob Gyn.* 2000;45:53.)

Blunt abdominal trauma is associated with a 3% to 38% incidence of fetal mortality. Direct fetal injury is not usually seen with blunt trauma because of the absorption of forces by the uterus, placenta, and amniotic fluid. Fetal injury and death are more indirect results of maternal shock and death. When the mother survives, abruption is the next leading cause of fetal mortality, followed by uterine rupture.[75]

Rates of domestic violence or intimate partner violence (IPV) are estimated to be 4% to 17%; exact rates are unknown because of underreporting and differences in methods of data collection. Injuries associated with IPV include defensive wounds; multiple blunt trauma injuries; penetrating injuries; bruises in various stages of healing; injuries to the face, neck, and especially the abdomen; and uterine rupture.[76-79] It may be difficult to differentiate between injury occurring as a result of an accidental fall and injury resulting from being pushed or struck; therefore, the patient should be carefully interviewed. Reports of violence are more likely to be associated with alcohol consumption, drugs, inadequate prenatal care (contributing to low birth weight), and a history of a fetal death and previous induced or spontaneous abortion.[80] The attacks may also become increasingly violent and include knife wounds, gunshot wounds, and homicide.[81] Additionally, if IPV is suspected as the cause of maternal injury, appropriate reporting and referrals should be initiated without delay.

Burn injuries during pregnancy may be caused by exposure to a thermal, chemical, or electrical source. The severity of total body surface area of thermal injury in the mother correlates with deteriorating fetal outcomes related to prolonged hypotension, inadequate volume resuscitation, sepsis, hypernatremia, and carbon monoxide exposure.[73,82,83] The best chance of fetal survival is maternal survival.

Approximately 10% of traumatic injuries occur in the first trimester, 40% occur in the second trimester, and 50% occur in the third trimester.[82] As women continue to work late into their pregnancies and become involved in higher risk activities, the type and severity of injuries may begin to increase. Most mechanisms that produce injuries in pregnant patients are no different from mechanisms that injure nonpregnant women.

Some types of fall injuries may be associated with the stage of pregnancy. In the first trimester, fall injuries may result from fainting from fatigue, hypoglycemia, and normal physiologic changes. At this stage, the fetus is usually well protected from external trauma because the uterus is located within the pelvis and is protected by bony structures. In the second and third trimesters, as the enlarging uterus expands out of the pelvis, maternal abdominal organs are displaced upward and laterally. Some protection is provided to the maternal abdominal organs because the uterus and fetus now occupy much of the abdominal cavity; however, the growing fetus becomes more vulnerable to injury. Hyperventilation and fainting are common as the fetus grows and places greater metabolic demands on the mother. By the third trimester, the fetus has begun to settle into the pelvis in preparation for birth. As relaxin secretion increases, the end effect of relaxed pelvic ligaments may lead to lordosis and pelvic tilt. This produces a change in gait and in the center of gravity and balance, which may increase the risk of falls.[4] Normal physiologic changes associated with pregnancy may mask assessment findings and affect decisions about interventions that are provided (Table 38.10).[80,82]

TABLE 38.10   Initial Assessment and Management of Obstetric Trauma

Assessment	Management, Rationale, or Purpose
Primary Survey	
Airway	
Signs of Obstruction	
Same as for nonpregnant patient	Remove visible debris with caution because of increased hyperemia of nasal or oral area.
	Decrease risk of aspiration (because of enlarged uterus and effects of progesterone) by lateral tilt or by inserting NGT or OGT.
	Emergency cricoidthyrotomy or tracheotomy, if performed, is done above usual site because of upward displacement of thoracic structures.
Breathing	
Signs of Ineffective Respiration	
Same as for nonpregnant patient with exception of the following:	100% oxygen by mask because passages tend to be hyperemic and a tendency for breathing through mouth exists.
SpO_2 <95	Elevate head of bed, if possible, to decrease pressure on thoracic structures caused by elevated diaphragm.
PaO_2 <100 mm Hg	Oral intubation using smaller size (5.5 to 7.0 Fr) endotracheal tubes to reduce risk of bleeding caused by increased vascularity of area.
$PaCO_2$ >30 mm Hg	Gastric decompression with OGT (or small NGT if patient does not tolerate OGT placement) because prone to ileus and gastric reflux.
pH <7.40	Physiologic monitoring (RR, SpO_2, $ETcO_2$).
Tidal volume <800 mL	Obtain ABGs, chest radiograph.
Labored respirations	Emergent needle decompression or chest tube insertion for hemopneumothorax; may need to reassess entry point because of upward or outward displacement of thorax.
RR <20 breaths/min or >24 beats/min	
Circulation	
Signs of Ineffective Circulation	
Same as for nonpregnant patient with exception of the following:	Diagnostic peritoneal lavage may be performed; open technique is usually preferred.
Systolic blood pressure <110 mm Hg	Assess for possible placental abruption.
Mean arterial pressure <80 mm Hg	Normally hypervolemic skin is warm and slightly moist because of progesterone and may mask signs of hypoperfusion.
Central venous pressure <6 mm Hg	Central venous catheter or large-bore IV access to upper extremity sites because of potential for impeded venous return from lower extremities.
Pale, moist, cool skin	Fluid resuscitation.
	LR solution is recommended because it has the potential to metabolize into bicarbonate through intrinsic body pathways; do not administer blood products through same IV line.
	With 0.9 NS, can administer blood products through line; may decrease risk of developing maternal alkalosis (compared with LR solution).
	O-negative blood may be given until type and crossmatching are done.
	Replace 3 mL per 1 mL of blood lost to compensate for hypervolemia associated with pregnancy.
	Use caution because of increased risk of pulmonary edema caused by decreased colloidal osmotic pressure.
	May apply MAST, but *do not* inflate abdominal compartment.
	Tilt the patient to her side, even if on a backboard, to maximize venous return.

TABLE 38.10   Initial Assessment and Management of Obstetric Trauma—cont'd

Assessment	Management, Rationale, or Purpose
Secondary Survey	
Focused Obstetric History	
Gestational age	Keep the mother alive.
Single versus multiple pregnancy	Keep the baby where it is.
Number of pregnancies, live births, abortions	Perform vaginal examination to determine fetal presentation, status of amniotic membrane, and presence of fetal parts or umbilical cord in vagina.
Name of obstetrician	Avoid manipulating cord because of risk of spasms.
Rh factor	Emergent delivery; vaginal versus cesarean; live versus perimortem.
Prenatal complications	
Past vaginal drainage, bleeding, clots	
Past abdominal pain or uterine contractions	
Maternal Studies	
Unexpected Diagnostic Study Results	
CBC:	Insert a urinary Foley catheter with caution because of risk of bleeding caused by increased pelvic vascularity; consider using a smaller size catheter.
WBC >18,000/mm^3	Consider significance of positive toxicity results. Is the fetus at risk for issues such as drug withdrawal or fetal alcohol syndrome?
RBC <6,500,000/mm^3	Hct and Hg values that are below those identified may put the mother and fetus at risk for hypoxia.
Hg <12 g/dL	Use caution when performing a rectal examination to assist in determining fetal position or traumatic damage; pelvic vascular congestion contributes to development of hemorrhoids and predisposes the mother to bleeding from this site.
Hct <32%	Obtain radiologic studies, as needed; however, implement measures to decrease risk to fetus.
Platelets <200,000/mm^3	Left axis deviation may be seen on 12-lead ECG as a normal variant.
Fibrinogen >400 mg/dL	
Chemistries:	
BUN <9 mg/dL	
Creatinine >0.5 mg/dL	
Na$^+$ slightly increased	
Glucose slightly decreased	
Fetal Studies	
Signs of Fetal Distress	
Fetal heart rate <100–110 beats/min	Ultrasound to evaluate fetus.
Nonreassuring patterns on fetal monitor	Assess fundal height, firmness, contractions every 30 min.
Fundal height not appropriate for gestational age	Fetal monitoring (with pocket Doppler, ultrasonography, or fetal monitor) as allowed based on interventions provided to mother.
	Differentiate uterine pain or contractions from other sources of abdominal pain.
Vaginal drainage, bleeding, clots present	Administer tocolytics, as needed.
Abdominal pain, uterine firmness, or contractions present	L/S ratio and presence of PG to determine fetal lung maturity.
Amniocentesis:	Kleihauer-Betke result indicates break in the integrity of placental circulation if fetal cells are present.
Presence of RBCs	
L/S ratio and presence of PG	
Kleihauer-Betke test to detect presence of fetal blood in maternal bloodstream	
Tertiary Survey	
Aspect of Care	
Administer "follow-up meds"	Prophylactic measures:
	Choose broad-spectrum antibiotics, nonteratogenic agents.
	Tetanus toxoid does not cross placenta.
	Rh-negative mothers:
	May become Rh immunized within 72 h.
	Administer Rh immune globulin (300 mcg/15 mL of fetal blood or 30 mL of whole blood) if possibility of mother having received Rh-positive blood.
	Breach in integrity of the placenta of Rh-positive fetus as evidenced by positive Kleihauer-Betke test result.

ABGs, arterial blood gases; *BUN,* blood urea nitrogen; *CBC,* complete blood count; *ECG,* electrocardiogram; *ETco$_2$,* end-tidal carbon dioxide; *Hct,* hematocrit; *Hg,* hemoglobin; *IV,* intravenous; *LR,* lactated Ringer; *L/S,* lecithin-to-sphingomyelin ratio; *MAST,* military antishock trousers; *Na$^+$,* sodium ion; *NGT,* nasogastric tube; *NS,* normal saline; *OGT,* orogastric tube; *Paco$_2$,* arterial partial pressure of carbon dioxide; *Pao$_2$,* arterial partial pressure of oxygen; *PG,* phosphatidylglycerol; *RBC,* red blood cell; *RR,* respiration rate; *Spo$_2$,* oxygen saturation measured by pulse oximetry; *WBC,* white blood cell.

Types of Injuries

Cardiovascular Injuries

Manifestations related to cardiovascular injury may be masked because of normal physiologic changes in pregnancy. The hypervolemic, low systemic resistance state, and increased heart rate that occur during pregnancy may mask shock because significant blood volume may have been lost before the classic manifestations are seen.[4] Therefore, tachycardia and hypotension in a pregnant trauma patient are clinically significant findings that require careful evaluation and should not be solely attributed to pregnancy. Because of venous congestion of the lower extremities, leg wounds may bleed more vigorously than expected.[84]

Pulmonary Injuries

Pregnant patients have diminished oxygen reserves and decreased blood-buffering capacity. This leaves the pregnant trauma patient vulnerable to hypoxemia and less able to compensate when acidemia ensues. During pregnancy, as the uterus grows, the maternal diaphragm is displaced 4 cm above its normal location. This change in location must be considered if placement of a chest tube is necessary to avoid injury to the diaphragm. The insertion point during pregnancy is usually between the third and fourth intercostal spaces.[85]

Neurologic Injuries

Spinal cord injury (SCI) in pregnancy may be acute (result of recent trauma) or may be chronic (from preexisting damage). Initial management of pregnant patients with acute SCI is the same as for nonpregnant patients, including the administration of steroids. Adequate uterine perfusion may be evaluated by observing for a reassuring fetal heart rate tracing and lack of uterine contractions.[86] Patients with SCI, similar to pregnant women, are at high risk for DVT, which necessitates the provision of prophylactic anticoagulation. Disruption of autonomic nervous system activity is not associated with labor dysfunction; vaginal delivery with a SCI is possible. Patients with injuries above T6 are at risk to developing autonomic dysreflexia reaction and may require assisted vaginal delivery or a cesarean section.[86-88] Uterine sensory nerves enter the spinal cord at T11 to L1; women with SCI above T10 are unable to feel uterine contractions.[87] They must rely on fetal monitoring of contractions or uterine palpation and symptoms such as shortness of breath and abdominal spasms to determine labor. Of most importance is that autonomic dysreflexia often occurs with uterine contractions at the time of labor and delivery. Appropriate anesthesia or antihypertensives may treat the problem, but immediate delivery of the infant and placenta is vital.[88]

If SCI is severe, irreversible traumatic brain injury occurs, or maternal brain death occurs, the fetus may remain viable and continue to develop in utero. The issue of pregnancy maintenance in an irreversibly brain-damaged or brain-dead mother is a controversial ethical issue.

Abdominal and Pelvic Injuries

As stated earlier, motor vehicle accidents are the primary cause of blunt trauma during pregnancy. Failure to wear seat belts or the improper use of seat belts increases the likelihood of abdominal injury, causes excessive maternal bleeding, and increases the risk of fetal death. The engorgement of pelvic vasculature increases the risk of retroperitoneal hemorrhage after lower abdominal trauma.[75] Because the uterus displaces maternal abdominal structures, the traditional assessment findings and sites of referred pain may be altered. Peritoneal signs such as tenderness, rigidity, and rebound tenderness are unreliable indicators because of stretching of the abdominal wall. All these factors may contribute to delayed detection of abdominal injuries. Splenic injuries are seen more commonly in the third trimester, and damage with blood loss may be seen after relatively mild trauma from vascular engorgement.

Penetrating abdominal injuries are also seen, with gunshot and stab wounds being the most common causes of a penetrating injury. Mortality rates after gunshot or stab wounds are lower in pregnant women because of the anatomic changes that occur related to the growing uterus. In contrast, the fetal mortality rate ranges from 40% to 70%, and fetal mortality generally results from either direct fetal injury from the object of penetration or preterm delivery following the injury.[81]

Blunt abdominal trauma may also be one of the more common types of injury from IPV during pregnancy. The abuser tends to focus the attacks on the abdomen, breasts, and genitalia (the "swimsuit" area). The effects of this violence may include placental abruption and uterine injury.[81]

Reproductive System Injuries

The uterus is a pelvic organ until 12 weeks' gestation. As the uterus enlarges, it may assist in protecting other organs, but it becomes more vulnerable to injury. Direct trauma to the uterus or placenta reverses protective hemostasis by releasing an increased concentration of placental thromboplastin, a plasminogen activator, from the myometrium. The uteroplacental bed functions as a dilated, passive, low-resistance system that lacks autoregulation and has few or no compensatory mechanisms.[4]

Abruptio placentae, commonly seen with blunt abdominal trauma and pelvic fractures, may occur immediately, within 48 hours, or up to 5 days after injury.[81] Uterine damage or rupture is rare, but if it occurs, it is commonly at the fundus or the site of a previous cesarean section and usually results in fetal death. Even if no identifiable damage is present after trauma, the risk for premature rupture of membranes, premature labor, fetal or maternal hemorrhage, or fetal damage or demise is increased. It is recommended that pregnant patients with trauma be admitted to the hospital for 24 to 48 hours of fetal monitoring because latent injuries or the need for tocolytics may be present.[84,85]

Fetal Injuries

The fetus is usually well cushioned by the amniotic fluid, the gravid uterus, and the abdominal wall, which distribute the force of injury. In most cases of minor trauma, the fetus survives intact. The most common cause of fetal death in maternal trauma is maternal death. The second leading cause of fetal death is placental abruption.[4] Although uncommon, fetal death may occur in the absence of significant maternal injury. During the third trimester, direct fetal injury is more common, as the uterine wall has thinned and the amniotic fluid may have decreased and is unable to absorb the impact. Additionally, the fetal head may be engaged in the pelvis; a resulting pelvic trauma may lead to a skull fracture in the fetus. Potential predictors of fetal demise vary depending on the study. Increased maternal injury severity score, increased maternal hypoxia and acidemia, need for blood replacement, and presence of DIC have been associated with increased fetal mortality rates.[75]

POSTPARTUM HEMORRHAGE

Postpartum hemorrhage (PPH) is the leading cause of maternal mortality. All women beyond 20 weeks' gestation are at risk for PPH and its complications. The direct pregnancy-related maternal mortality rate in the United States is approximately 7 to 10 women per 100,000 live births. The Centers for Disease Control and Prevention states that approximately 11% of these deaths are caused by PPH.[89]

Risk Factors and Causes

PPH is best defined and diagnosed clinically as excessive bleeding that makes the patient symptomatic (pallor, light-headedness, weakness, palpitations, diaphoresis, restlessness, confusion, air hunger, syncope), results in signs of hypovolemia (hypotension, tachycardia, oliguria, low oxygen saturation of less than 95%), or both.[90] Other definitions that have been suggested have been problematic. The most common definition of PPH is estimated blood loss of greater than 500 mL after vaginal birth or greater than 1000 mL after cesarean delivery. The inadequacy of this definition was illustrated in studies that assessed blood loss using various objective methods; also, clinicians were likely to underestimate the volume of blood lost.[91]

Another classic definition of PPH is a 10% decline in post-partum hemoglobin concentration from antepartum levels. However, this is not a clinically useful definition, as rapid blood loss may trigger a medical emergency before observation of a fall in hemoglobin concentration; also, laboratory changes that are not correlated with events that endanger the patient should not be used to define a medical emergency.[91] In a randomized trial, increased risk of PPH was associated with the infant's birth weight, labor induction and augmentation, chorioamnionitis, $MgSO_4$ use, and previous PPH.[90]

PPH has many potential causes. As a way of remembering the causes of PPH, several sources have suggested using the four "T's" as a mnemonic: (1) tone, (2) tissue, (3) trauma, and (4) thrombosis.[92] *Tone* refers to uterine atony, which is the most common cause of PPH. Overdistention of the uterus, fatigue caused by prolonged labor or rapid forceful labor, and inhibition of contractions by drugs constitute major risk factor for atony. *Tissue* includes retained placenta or failure of complete separation of the placenta, which occurs with placenta accreta. Any damage to the genital tract during delivery constitutes *trauma*. Trauma also includes cesarean delivery, uterine rupture, and cervical or vaginal sidewall lacerations. With *thrombosis,* the abnormalities may be preexisting or acquired. Thrombocytopenia may be related to a preexisting disease such as idiopathic thrombocytopenic purpura or acquired secondary to HELLP syndrome, abruptio placentae, DIC, or sepsis.[93]

Prevention

Research suggests that active management of the third stage of labor reduces the incidence and severity of PPH.[94] Active management consists of a uterine-contracting medication (preferably oxytocin) immediately on delivery of the infant, early cord clamping and cutting, and gentle cord traction with uterine countertraction when the uterus is well contracted (Brandt-Andrews maneuver). One research demonstrated that early administration of oxytocin (before placental delivery) did not increase the rate of retained placenta, as initially suspected. Plus, the trial showed trends toward a benefit for early

---

BOX 38.5   FDA Pregnancy and Lactation Labeling Rule (PLLR)

PRESCRIPTION DRUG LABELING SECTIONS 8.1–8.3 USE IN SPECIFIC POPULATIONS

Former Labeling	New Labeling
8.1 Pregnancy	8.1 Pregnancy—includes labor and Delivery
8.2 Labor and Delivery	8.2 Lactation—includes Nursing Mothers
8.3 Nursing Mothers	8.3 Females and Males of Reproductive Potential

From U.S. Federal Drug Administration. Pregnancy and lactation labeling (drugs) final rule. http://www.fda.gov/Drugs/DevelopmentApprovalProcess/DevelopmentResources/Labeling/ucm093307.htm. Accessed September 19, 2016.

---

administration of oxytocin, including a 25% reduction in PPH and a 50% reduction in the need for transfusion.[94]

Rapid recognition and diagnosis of PPH is essential to successful management. Resuscitative measures and the diagnosis and treatment of the underlying cause must occur quickly before complication of severe hypovolemia develops.

RISKS TO FETAL DEVELOPMENT

Medication use in critically ill obstetric patients requires analysis of the risk-benefit ratio. It is important to consider the influence that drug exposure could have on the developing fetus, but often, the benefit may outweigh the potential fetal risk when all factors are considered.[54] Also, fetal and newborn outcomes may be dependent on timely maternal stabilization on potential harmful medication. Critically ill obstetric patients may be reluctant to take medication during pregnancy because of the possibility or perceived possibility of the adverse effects on the fetus. The 2001, the US Food and Drug Administration (FDA) placed medications into risk categories regarding use during pregnancy along with potential effects on the growing fetus.[54,95]

In 2014, the FDA completed major revisions to prescription drug labeling to more thoroughly cover the use of medicines during pregnancy and breastfeeding. They published the *Content and Format of Labeling for Human Prescription Drug and Biological Products: Requirements for Pregnancy and Lactation Labeling,* referred to as the "Pregnancy and Lactation Labeling Rule" (PLLR). This new ruling went into effect June 30, 2015. The PLLR format assists health care providers in rating the risks and benefits of the drugs, which enables providers to provide informed counseling to nursing mothers. The pregnancy letter categories—A, B, C, D, and X—were removed. Box 38.5 is a comparison of the old prescription drug labeling with the new PLLR labeling. The "Females and Males of Reproductive Potential" subsection (8.3) is a new labeling that includes pregnancy testing, contraception recommendations, and information about infertility as it relates to the drug.[96]

Factors that influence embryonic and fetal development may be intrinsic or extrinsic in nature. Intrinsic factors such as chromosomal abnormalities and congenital anomalies account for 25% of all birth defects. Extrinsic factors, also known as *teratogens,* account for the remaining factors.[97] A teratogen is any chemical, substance, or exposure that may cause any form of birth defects in a developing fetus. This would include medicines, radiation, and agents of infection. The effects of teratogens depend on maternal and fetal genotypes, the stage of development when exposure occurs, and the dose and duration of the exposure of the agent.[98] Exposure to ionizing radiation is usually not a concern until more than a cumulative 100 to 200 mGy (10 to 20 rads) has been exceeded, but some experts recommend caution in the first 25 weeks because of fetal organogenesis and central nervous system development.[97,99] At doses less than 0.05 Gy, no evidence of an increased risk of fetal anomalies, intellectual disability, growth restriction, or pregnancy loss from ionizing radiation is present. A small increased risk of childhood cancer, 1 in 2000 versus the 1 in 3000 background rate, may exist.[97]

Prematurity

The condition or illness in a critically ill pregnant patient may justify an early termination of pregnancy to prevent serious complications in or death of the patient. Depending on the duration of gestation, a severely premature infant may result. Technologic advances, improvements in maternal-fetal diagnostics, and aggressive neonatal interventions have improved the survival of extremely-low-birth-weight infants. Research has placed minimal viability parameters between 23 and 24 weeks' gestation and fetal weight between 500 and 1000 g (0.5 and 1 kg).[5] Critical care clinicians may encounter situations in which extrauterine viability, fetal outcomes, and maternal stability are uncertain. Clinical decisions must be made in light of the maternal-fetal risk-benefit ratio. Personal, cultural, spiritual, and social beliefs regarding viability may affect the clinical decision-making process. Parental and family beliefs and desires may conflict with the thoughts and priorities of the health care team. When confronting the dilemma of viability, the parameters of gestational age, fetal weight, parental desires, and maternal-fetal mortality must be considered.

QSEN | CASE STUDY 38.1 | **Patient With Obstetric Issues**

Brief Patient History

Mrs. S is 33 years old, gravida 2, para 1. She delivered a term baby boy by cesarean section this morning. Mrs. S has experienced chills, malaise, and abdominal pain since the operation, and she has been given morphine for pain relief but is still complaining of abdominal pain.

Clinical Assessment

Mrs. S is admitted to the critical care unit with hypotension, tachypnea, and tachycardia. She is lethargic, curled up in bed, and groaning. She does not follow commands or answer questions. No urine output has occurred over the last 4 h, and since placement of a urinary catheter, only 10 mL of dark amber urine has accumulated.

Diagnostic Procedures

Her admission vital signs are as follows: blood pressure of 60/35 mm Hg, heart rate of 145 beats/min (sinus tachycardia), respiratory rate of 30 breaths/min, temperature of 97.5°F, hemoglobin level of 5 g/dL, and platelet level of 30,000/μL. Ultrasound reveals a large fluid collection in the abdomen.

Medical Diagnosis

Mrs. S is diagnosed with an intraabdominal bleed.

Questions

1. What major outcomes do you expect to achieve for this patient?
2. What problems or risks must be managed to achieve these outcomes?
3. What interventions must be initiated to monitor, prevent, manage, or eliminate the problems and risks identified?
4. What interventions should be initiated to promote optimal functioning, safety, and well-being of the patient?
5. What possible learning needs do you anticipate for this patient?
6. What cultural and age-related factors may have a bearing on the patient's plan of care?

▎SUMMARY

- Optimal care for a critically ill obstetric patient or one who has sustained injuries requires persistent application of physiologic changes of pregnancy to normal adult values.
- Symptoms of serious disorders may be altered because of the pregnant state.
- Understanding the intricate maternal-fetal relationship provides practitioners with a focus of maintaining maternal stability to enhance uteroplacental perfusion and an optimal in utero environment.
- All potential therapeutic and pharmacologic interventions must be weighed in light of the risk-benefit ratio to maternal-infant status.
- Critical situations may bring personal, cultural, social, spiritual, and ethical values into conflict.
- Determining the appropriate environment may be challenging. Some institutions have created dedicated obstetric intensive care units, whereas others provide care in the obstetric care unit or critical care unit.
- Decision making must occur in collaboration with family and health care team members, and all options should be considered.
- The key factor is collaboration among specialties to optimize maternal-fetal outcomes and facilitate the family experience. ⓔ Visit the Evolve site for additional study materials.

REFERENCES

1. WHO, UNICEF, UNFPA. *The World Bank, and the United Nations Population Division. Trends in Maternal Mortality: 1990 to 2013.* Geneva: World Health Organization; 2014.
2. *CDC Reproductive Health, Pregnancy Mortality Surveillance System.* ; 2014. http://www.cdc.gov/reproductivehealth/maternalinfanthealth/pmss.html. Accessed September 19, 2016.
3. Xu K, et al. Deaths: Final data for 2007. *National Vital Statistics Report.* 2010;58:19. Hyattsville, MD: National Center for Health Statistics.
4. Cunningham FG, et al. *Williams Obstetrics.* 24th ed. New York: McGraw-Hill; 2014.
5. American Academy of Pediatrics and American College of Obstetricians and Gynecologists. Antepartum care. In: *Guidelines for Perinatal Care.* Elk Grove Village, IL: Author; 2007.
6. Davidson M, London M, Ladewig P. *Old's Maternal-Newborn Nursing and Women's Health Across the Lifespan.* 9th ed. Upper Saddle River, NJ: Pearson Prentice Hall; 2012.
7. Monga M, Creasy R. Cardiovascular and renal adaptation to pregnancy. In: Creasy R, Resnik R, Iams JD, eds. *Creasy and Resnik's Maternal-Fetal Medicine, Principle and Practice.* 7th ed. Philadelphia: Elsevier; 2014.
8. Oyelese Y, Ananth CV. Postpartum hemorrhage. Epidemiology, risk factors and causes. *Clin Obstet Gynecol.* 2010;53(1):147.

9. Curry R, Swan L, Steer PJ. Cardiac disease in pregnancy. *Curr Opin Obstetrics Gynecol.* 2009;21:508.

10. Criteria Committee of the New York Heart Association. *Nomenclature and Criteria for Diagnosis of Disease of the Heart and Great Vessels.* 9th ed. Boston: Little, Brown; 1994.

11. Foley MR. Cardiac disease. In: Dildy GA, et al., ed. *Critical Care Obstetrics.* 5th ed. Malden, MA: Blackwell Publishing; 2010.

12. Hameed AB, Sklansky MS. Pregnancy: Maternal and fetal heart disease. *Curr Probl Cardiol.* 2007;32:419.

13. Shabetai R. Cardiac disease. In: Creasy R, Resnik R, Iams JD, eds. *Creasy and Resnik's Maternal-Fetal Medicine: Principles and Practice.* 7th ed. Philadelphia: Elsevier; 2014.

14. Bashore TG. Adult congenital heart disease: Right ventricular outflow tract lesions. *Circulation.* 2007;115:1933.

15. Makaryus AN, Forouzesh A, Johnson M. Pregnancy in the patient with Eisenmenger's syndrome. *Mt Sinai J Med.* 2006;73(7):1033.

16. Vasu S, Stergiopoulos K. Valvular heart disease in pregnancy. *Hellenic J Cardiol.* 2009;50:498.

17. Rutherford JD, Hands M. Pregnancy with preexisting heart disease. In: Douglas PS, ed. *Cardiovascular Health and Disease in Women.* Philadelphia: Saunders; 2002.

18. Regitz-Zagroske V, et al. ESC guidelines on the management of cardiovascular diseases during pregnancy. The task force on the management of cardiovascular diseases during pregnancy of the European Society of Cardiology (ESC). *Eur Heart J.* 2011;32:3147.

19. Pacini L, et al. Maternal complication of pregnancy in Marfan syndrome. *Int J Cardiol.* 2009;136(2):156.

20. Ramaraj R, Sorrell VL. Peripartum cardiomyopathy: Causes, diagnosis, and treatment. *Cleve Clin J Med.* 2009;76(5):289.

21. Brar S, et al. Incidence, mortality, and racial differences in peripartum cardiomyopathy. *Am J Cardiol.* 2007;100(2):302-304.

22. Johnson-Coyle L, Jensen L, Sobey A. Peripartum cardiomyopathy: Review and practice guidelines. *Am J Crit Care.* 2012;21(2):89.

23. Abboud J, et al. Peripartum cardiomyopathy: a comprehensive review. *Int J Cardiol.* 2007;118(3):295.

24. Roth A, Elkayam U. Acute myocardial infarction associated with pregnancy. *J Am Coll Cardiol.* 2008;52:171.

25. James AH, et al. Acute myocardial infarction in pregnancy: a United States population-based study. *Circulation.* 2006;113(12):1564.

26. American Heart Association. 2015 American Heart Association guidelines for cardiopulmonary resuscitation and emergency cardiovascular care. *Circulation.* 2015;112(suppl IV). IV150.

27. American Heart Association. 2015 American Heart Association guidelines for advanced cardiac life support. *Circulation.* 2015:172.

28. American College of Obstetricians and Gynecologists. Chronic hypertension in pregnancy, ACOG practice bulletin no 125. *Obstet Gynecol.* 2012;119:396.

29. Habli M, Sabai B. Hypertensive disorders of pregnancy. In: Gibbs RS, et al, ed. *Danforth's Obstetrics and Gynecology.* 10th ed. Philadelphia: Lippincott, Williams & Wilkins; 2008.

30. National High Blood Pressure Education Working Group on High Blood Pressure in Pregnancy. Report of the National High Blood Pressure Education Working Group on High Blood Pressure in Pregnancy. *Am J Obstet Gynecol.* 2000;183(1):S1.

31. Belfort M, et al. *Critical Care Obstetrics.* 5th ed. Boston: Blackwell Publishing Co; 2010.

32. Gilbert E. *Manual of High Risk Pregnancy and Delivery.* 5th ed. St Louis: Mosby; 2011.

33. Leeman L, Fontaine P. Hypertensive disorders of pregnancy. *Am Fam Physician.* 2008;78(1):93.

34. American College of Obstetricians and Gynecologists. *Diagnosis and Management of Preeclampsia and Eclampsia.* Washington, DC: ACOG; 2008. ACOG practice bulletin no 33.

35. Chappell LC, et al. Adverse perinatal outcomes and risk factors for preeclampsia in women with chronic hypertension. A prospective study. *Hypertension.* 2008;51(4):354.

36. Martin D. HELLP syndrome A-Z: Facing an obstetric emergency. In: Davidson M, et al, ed. *Old's Maternal-Newborn Nursing and Women's Health Across the Lifespan.* 9th ed. Upper Saddle River, NJ: Pearson Prentice Hall; 2012.

37. Barton JR, Sibai BM. Prediction and prevention of recurrent preeclampsia. *Obstet Gynecol.* 2008;11(2):359.

38. Ghulmiyyah LM, Sibai BM. Managing an eclamptic seizure and its aftermath. *Contemp Ob Gyn.* 2006;51(3):54.

39. Karumanchi SA, Lindheimer MD. Preeclampsia pathogenesis: Triple A rating—autoantibodies and antiangiogenic factors. *Hypertension.* 2008;51(4):991.

40. Wang A, Rana S, Karumanch SA. Preeclampsia: The role of angiogenic factors in its pathogenesis. *Physiology.* 2009;24(3):147.

41. Wen SW, et al. Folic acid supplementation in early second trimester and the risk of preeclampsia. *Am J Obstet Gynecol.* 2008;198(1):45.

42. Ross MG, et al. Eclampsia. http://emedicine.medscape.com/article/253960-overview #a3. Accessed July 20, 2012.

43. Hay JE. Liver disease in pregnancy. *Hepatology.* 2008;47(3):1067.

44. Clark S. Critical care obstetric. In: Gibbs RS, et al, ed. *Danforth's Obstetrics and Gynecology.* 10th ed. Philadelphia: Lippincott, Williams & Wilkins; 2008.

45. Airoldi J, Weinstein L. Clinical significance of proteinuria in pregnancy. In: Davidson M, et al, ed. *Old's Maternal-Newborn Nursing & Women's Health Across the Lifespan.* 9th ed. Upper Saddle River, NJ: Pearson Prentice Hall; 2012.

46. Rodger MA, Silver RM. Coagulation disorders in pregnancy. In: Creasy R, Resnik R, Iams JD, eds. *Creasy and Resnik's Maternal-Fetal Medicine, Principle and Practice.* 7th ed. Philadelphia: Elsevier; 2014.

47. Lindsey JL. *Evaluation of fetal death*; 2010. http://emedicine.medscape.com/article/259165-overview. Accessed April 18, 2012.

48. Cole DE, et al. Acute respiratory distress syndrome in pregnancy. *Crit Care Med.* 2005;33:S269.

49. Powrie R. Respiratory disease. In: James D, et al, ed. *High Risk Pregnancy: Management Options.* 4th ed. Philadelphia: Saunders; 2010.

50. Schatz M, et al. National Heart, Lung and Blood Institute: The relationship of asthma medication use in perinatal outcomes. *J Allergy Clin Immunol.* 2004;113:1040.

51. Montoro M. Pulmonary disorders in pregnancy. In: DeCherney A, et al, ed. *Current Diagnosis and Treatment Obstetrics and Gynecology.* 11th ed. New York: McGraw-Hill; 2012.

52. Schatz M. Asthma. In: Queenan J, ed. *Management of High-Risk Pregnancies.* 6th ed. Malden, MA: Blackwell Publishing; 2012.

53. Whitty J, Dombrowski M. Respiratory diseases in pregnancy. In: Gabbe S, ed. *Obstetrics: Normal and Problem Pregnancies.* 5th ed. Philadelphia: Elsevier; 2007.

54. Briggs G, et al. *Drugs in Pregnancy and Lactation.* 9th ed. Baltimore: Williams & Wilkins; 2011.

55. O'Sullivan BP, Freedman SD. Cystic fibrosis. *Lancet.* 2009;373:1891.

56. Katkin JP. *Cystic fibrosis: Clinical manifestations and diagnosis*; 2015. http://www.uptodate.com/hme/index.html. Accessed February 20, 2016.

57. Smith SE, Osborne K. What are the risks of pneumonia in pregnancy? http://www.wisegeek.com/what-are-the-risks-of-pneumonia-in-pregnncy.htm Accessed July 22, 2012.

58. American Lung Association. *Trends in pneumonia and influenza morbidity and mortality. American Lung Association Research and Program Services Epidemiology and Statistics Unit. Author*; April 2010.

59. Graves C. Pneumonia in pregnancy. *Clin Obstet Gynecol.* 2010;53(2):329.

60. Goldberg J, Smith R. Critical care obstetrics. In: DeCherney A, et al, ed. *Current Diagnosis and Treatment Obstetrics and Gynecology.* 11th ed. New York: McGraw-Hill; 2012.

61. Schwartz DR, Malhotra A, Weinberger SE. *Deep vein thrombosis and pulmonary embolism in pregnancy: Epidemiology, pathogenesis, and diagnosis*; 2014. http://UpToDate.com. Accessed February 20, 2016.

62. Laros R. Thromboembolic disease. In: Creasy R, Resnik R, Iams JD, eds. *Creasy and Resnik's Maternal-Fetal Medicine, Principle and Practice.* 7th ed. Philadelphia: Elsevier; 2014.

63. Pettker C, Lockwood C. Thromboembolic disorders. In: Gabbe S, et al, ed. *Obstetrics: Normal and Problem Pregnancies.* 6th ed. Philadelphia: Elsevier; 2012.

64. Pettker C, Lockwood C. Pathophysiology and diagnosis of thromboembolic disorders in pregnancy. In: Queenan J, et al, ed. *Management of High-Risk Pregnancies.* 6th ed. Malden, MA: Blackwell Publishing; 2012.

65. Shaughnessy K. Massive pulmonary embolism. *Crit Care Nurs.* 2007;27(1):39.

66. Schwartz DR, Malhotra A, Weinberger SE. *Deep vein thrombosis and pulmonary embolism in pregnancy*; 2014. http://www.uptodate.com/hme/index.html. Accessed February 20, 2016.

67. Cooney M. Heparin-induced thrombocytopenia: advances in diagnosis and treatment. *Crit Care Nurs.* 2006;26(6):30.

68. Stafford I, Sheffield J. Amniotic fluid embolism. *Obstet Gynecol Clin North Am.* 2007;34:545.

69. Baldisseri MR. *Amniotic fluid embolism syndrome*; 2016. http://UpToDate.com. Accessed February 20, 2016.

70. Knight M, et al. Incidence and risk factors for amniotic-fluid embolism. *Obstet Gynecol.* 2010;115:910.

71. Dildy GA, Clark SL. Anaphylactoid syndrome of pregnancy (amniotic fluid embolism). In: Dildy GA, ed. *Critical Care Obstetrics.* 5th ed. Malden, MA: Blackwell Scientific; 2010.

72. Gei G, Hankins GDV. Amniotic fluid embolism: an update. *Contemp Ob Gyn.* 2000;45(53):66.

73. El Kady D. Perinatal outcomes of traumatic injuries during pregnancy. *Clin Obstet Gynecol.* 2007;50(3):582.

74. Tweedale C. Trauma during pregnancy. *Crit Care Nurs Q.* 2006;29(1):53-67.

75. El-Kady D, et al. Trauma during pregnancy: an analysis of maternal and fetal outcomes in a large population. *Am J Obstet Gynecol.* 2004;190(6):1661.

76. American College of Obstetricians and Gynecologists (ACOG). *Intimate Partner Violence and Domestic Violence. Committee on Health Care for Underserved Women.* Washington, DC: ACOG; 2012.

77. Weil A. *Intimate partner violence: Diagnosis and screening*; 2016. http://UpToDate.com. Accessed February 21, 2016.

78. Lu M, et al. Domestic violence and sexual assault. In: DeCherney A, et al, ed. *Current Diagnosis and Treatment Obstetrics and Gynecology.* 11th ed. New York: McGraw-Hill; 2012.

79. Gunter J. Intimate partner violence. *Obstet Gynecol Clin North Am.* 2007;34:367.

80. American College of Obstetricians and Gynecologists (ACOG). *Screening Tools: Domestic Violence.* Washington, DC: ACOG; 2008.

81. Chambliss L. Intimate partner violence and its implication for pregnancy. *Clin Obstet Gynecol.* 2008;51(2):385.

82. Muench MV, Canterino JC. Trauma in pregnancy. *Obstet Gynecol Clin North Am.* 2007;34:555.

83. Kennedy BB, Baird SM, Troiano NH. Burn injuries and pregnancy. *J Perinat Neonatal Nurs.* 2008;22(1):21.

84. Bobrowski R. Trauma. In: James D, et al, ed. *High Risk Pregnancy: management Options.* 4th ed. Philadelphia: Elsevier; 2011.

85. Cusick S, Tibbles C. Trauma in pregnancy. *Emerg Med Clin North Am.* 2007;25:861.

86. Ghidini A, et al. Pregnancy and women with spinal cord injuries. *Obstet Gynecol Surv.* 2009;64(3):141.

87. American College of Obstetricians and Gynecologists. *Obstetric management of patients with spinal cord injuries, ACOG committee opinion 275.* Washington, DC: ACOG; reaffirmed; 2014.

88. Carhuapoma F, et al. Neurologic disorders. In: James D, et al, ed. *High Risk Pregnancy: Management Options.* 4th ed. Philadelphia: Saunders; 2011.

89. Centers for Disease Control and Prevention. National Center for Chronic Disease Prevention and Health Promotion. Pregnancy mortality surveillance system. http://www.cdc.gov/reproductivehealth/maternalinfanthealth/pregnancy-relatedmortality.htm. Accessed February 20, 2016.

90. Jacobs AJ, Lockwood CJ. Overview of postpartum hemorrhage. http://UpToDate.com. Accessed July 22, 2012.

91. Prata N, Gerdts C. Measurement of postpartum blood loss. *BMJ.* 2010;340:555.

92. Society of Obstetrics and Gynecology of Canada. Active management of the third stage of labour: prevention and treatment of postpartum hemorrhage. *SOGC Clinical Practice Guidelines.* 2009. No. 235.

93. James AH, et al. Von Willebrand disease and other bleeding disorders in women: Consensus on diagnosis and management from an international expert panel. *Am J Obstet Gynecol.* 2009;6(24):45.

94. Prendiville WJ, Elbourne D, McDonald S. Active versus expectant management in the third stage of labor. *Cochrane Database Syst Rev.* 2009;(3):CD000007.

95. Riordan J, Auerbach K. *Breastfeeding and Human Lactation.* 4th ed. Boston: Jones & Bartlett; 2009.

96. U.S. Federal Drug Administration. Pregnancy and lactation labeling (drugs) final rule. http://www.fda.gov/Drugs/DevelopmentApprovalProcess/DevelopmentResources/Labeling/ucm093307.htm. Accessed September 19, 2016.

97. Austin LM, Frush DP. Compendium of national guidelines for imaging the pregnant patient. *AJR Am J Roentgenol.* 2011;197:737.

98. Niebyl J. Teratology and drugs in pregnancy. In: Scott JR, et al, ed. *Danforth's Obstetrics and Gynecology.* 10th ed. Philadelphia: Lippincott; 2008.

99. McCollough C, et al. Radiation exposure and pregnancy: when should we be concerned? *Radiographics.* 2007;24:909.

39

The Pediatric Patient

Cynthia A. Lewis

Some of the developmental and physiologic differences between adults and children older than 1 month are discussed in this chapter. Although children may experience medical conditions similar to those of adults, they are assessed and managed differently. During periods of stress, children may maintain physiologic stability for a period, but they may then decompensate quickly. Children are *not* small adults. Box 39.1 describes the differences between children and adults. Many of the laboratory values, medications, blood product dosages and methods of administration, and other therapeutic modalities for children are different from those used with adults. Heart rate and blood pressure should be within normal range for age (Tables 39.1 and 39.2). Measurement of blood pressure is the most important diagnostic tool in the detection of hypertension in a child.[1]

Regardless of the anticipated outcome, admission to a critical care unit is stressful for families. Critical care nurses who successfully deal with pediatric patients see the child and the family as an integral unit and are perceptive to the needs of the entire family.[2] Knowledge of normal growth and development and the ability to assess the child's developmental level are important for working with children and their parents. Nurses who take care of pediatric patients can conceptualize using a developmental perspective as the ideal norm.[2] The developmental stages include the different age groups: infancy (0 to 12 months), toddlers (1 to 3 years), preschoolers (3 to 5 years), school-age children (6 to 12 years), and adolescents (12 to 18 years).

Although some critically ill children may be managed in adult critical care units in certain situations, children need the services of various pediatric subspecialists or pediatric intensivists, and they must be transferred to a tertiary care pediatric critical care unit. This also is true for pediatric trauma patients. The risk of death is significantly lower for patients receiving care in a facility with a designated trauma center.[3] Conditions that may require transfer to a hospital with a pediatric critical care unit include the need for high-frequency ventilation, extracorporeal membrane oxygenation, or cardiac surgery and treatment for some neurologic conditions that require intracranial pressure (ICP) monitoring. Transfer is also considered for children who do not respond to treatment.

RESPIRATORY SYSTEM

Anatomy and Physiology

Upper Airway

The upper airway of the infant and child is different from that of the adult. The epiglottis is located at the level of the cervical spine. It is located at C1 in the newborn, at C3 in the older infant, and at C4 to C5 in the adult.

The infant's epiglottis is large and floppy, and because of its high placement, it may press against the pharyngeal soft palate on inspiration. The infant's tongue is large relative to its head size. The tongue fills most of the oral cavity. Because of this anatomy, the infant usually is an obligate nose breather until 4 to 6 months of age, after which the larynx descends with growth.[2] Oral breathing is a very complex process for an infant, and it never occurs alone. Oronasal breathing is possible, but only 30% to 40% of ventilation may be provided orally. During sleep, oronasal breathing may occur spontaneously and last for about 20 seconds.

The larynx of the infant and young child, in contrast to that of the adult, is a funnel-shaped structure, with the narrowest portion at the cricoid ring.[4] The larynx is pliable because the cartilage is less developed, making it easier to collapse on inspiration or expiration. With changes in intrathoracic pressure, collapse may occur even with crying.[4] By age 8 to 10 years, the larynx has grown cylindrical; has assumed the narrowest portion at the glottic opening; and has increased in length, width, and internal diameter. By age 12 years, the diameter has grown to 1.8 cm.

The submucosal layer of the larynx is also looser in the infant and young child, and fluid accumulates more easily in that space. Within the airway's relatively rigid confines, any accumulation of fluid encroaches into the airway space. Along with a shorter and narrower airway, any decrease in airway radius leads to an exponential increase in airflow resistance, which increases the work of breathing. Turbulent airflow, as occurs with crying, doubles the already increased airflow resistance.[5] Fig. 39.1 illustrates the changes in airway diameter and airflow resistance with obstruction from edema in an adult and in an infant. An infant or child with an abnormally small jaw and low-set ears should be considered as having a potentially difficult airway to manage, and a consultation with an anesthesiologist is needed if airway management is required.

Lower Airway

Alveolar collapse is more likely in the infant and young child because of the smaller alveolar size. Infants and young children are at greater risk for ventilation-perfusion mismatch and atelectasis without this collateral ventilation. Infants and children have a higher metabolic rate compared with adults, and oxygen consumption per kilogram is higher. Hypoxemia develops more rapidly in the context of respiratory compromise in young children than in adults.[4]

Chest Mechanics

The respiratory structure and mechanics of infants and young children are very different from those of mature adults. In

TABLE 39.2 Normal Blood Pressures in Children[a]

Age	Systolic Pressure (mm Hg)	Diastolic Pressure (mm Hg)	Mean Arterial Pressure (mm Hg)
Birth (12 h, <1000 g)	39–59	16–36	28–42
Birth (12 h, 3 kg)	60–76	31–45	48–57
Neonate (96 h)	67–84	35–53	45–60
Infant (1–12 mo)	72–104	37–56	50–62
Toddler (1–2 y)	86–106	42–63	49–62
Preschooler (3–5 y)	89–112	46–72	58–69
School-age child (7 y)	97–115	57–76	66–72
Preadolescent (10–12 y)	102–120	61–80	71–79
Adolescent (15 y)	110–131	64–83	73–84

[a]Blood pressure ranges are taken from the following sources. *Neonate:* Versmold H, et al. Aortic blood pressure during the first 12 hours of life in infants with birth weight 610-4220 g. *Pediatrics.* 1981;67:107. Ranges are 10th through 90th percentile. *Others:* Horan MJ, chairman. Task Force on Blood Pressure Control in Children, report of the Second Task Force on Blood Pressure in Children. *Pediatrics.* 1987;79:1. Ranges are 50th through 90th percentile.
Modified from Hazinski MF. *Nursing Care of the Critically Ill Child.* 3rd ed. St. Louis: Elsevier; 2013.

TABLE 39.1 Normal Heart Rates in Children

Age	Awake Heart Rate (per minute)	Sleeping Heart Rate (per minute)
Neonate	100–205	90–160
Infant (6 mo)	100–180	90–160
Toddler	98–140	80–120
Preschooler	80–120	65–100
School-age child	75–118	58–90
Adolescent	60–100	50–90

From Hazinski MF. *Nursing Care of the Critically Ill Child.* 3rd ed. St. Louis: Elsevier; 2013.

FIG. 39.1 Effects of Edema on Airway Resistance. Effects of edema on airway resistance are shown by proportional increases in airflow resistance with 1 mm of circumferential edema in an infant versus an adult. (From Hazinski MF. Children are different. In: Hazinski MF, ed. *Nursing Care of the Critically Ill Child.* 3rd ed. St. Louis: Elsevier; 2013.)

the infant and young child, the chest wall is more compliant because the bones are smaller and more cartilaginous. The ribs are more horizontally placed, providing less of a bellowing action on inspiration. Accessory muscles are less developed, and the external intercostals do not contribute to pulling the ribs up on inspiration. The diaphragm is the principal muscle for inspiration. The diaphragm is more horizontal in the chest of an infant and tends to pull the lower ribs inward on inspiration.[6] Because of these mechanics, infants and toddlers depend almost totally on diaphragmatic contraction for lung expansion. Anything that impedes diaphragmatic contractions may result in respiratory compromise. The intercostal muscles are inadequately developed before school age, and they are unlikely to help with effective ventilation if the diaphragm is impaired.[4] With any decrease in lung compliance, as with lung disease, diaphragmatic contractions, which cause decreased intrathoracic pressure, produce intercostal and substernal retractions rather than inflation of the lungs.[6] The greater the chest wall retractions, the more the diaphragm must contract to offset the changes in intrathoracic pressure to generate an adequate tidal volume for the child. The compliant chest wall of the infant or the young child should expand easily outward with positive-pressure ventilation. If the chest wall does not expand bilaterally during positive-pressure ventilation, either the ventilation effort is inadequate or the airway is obstructed.[4]

Assessment and Oxygen Devices

An infant or child usually experiences respiratory failure more often than primary heart failure. In contrast to older adults, who may have underlying cardiovascular disease, infants and children tend to demonstrate bradycardia and apnea in cardiopulmonary failure and not ventricular dysrhythmias.[5] For an

TABLE 39.3   Clinical Indicators for Infants or Children at Risk for Respiratory Failure

Assessment Area	Physical Findings	Discussion Points
Respiratory rate	Infant: >60 breaths/min	Tachypnea usually first sign of distress in an infant; fatigue is a common contributing factor in respiratory failure
	Child: >40 breaths/min	Late signs: apnea, gasping or agonal respirations
	Slow or irregular	
Mechanics	Retractions (intercostal, supraclavicular, substernal)	
	Paradoxic movements (chest in and abdomen out)	
	Signs of diaphragm fatigue, respiratory alternans	
	Grunting	Closing of glottis to create "auto-PEEP" to keep alveoli open at end-expiration
	Stridor	Sign of upper airway obstruction
	Wheezing	Sign of lower airway obstruction
Air entry	Changes in pitch rather than volume of breath sounds	Chest expansion sometimes is barely perceptible in normal, spontaneously breathing infant. Small, thin chest wall causes breath sounds from any area of the lungs to be easily referred throughout the chest, even over fluid or atelectasis. Listen for bilateral breath sounds high in the axillae because these are the two most separated points
Color or temperature	Central coolness, pallor, or cyanosis	Peripheral changes may be normal in an infant or child
Heart rate	<5 y: <60 or >180 beats/min	Infants and children have limited ability to increase stroke volume; with hypoxemia, the heart rate increases to improve cardiac output. If bradycardia occurs with cardiorespiratory distress, arrest may be imminent
	5–10 y: <60 or >160 beats/min	
	>10 y: <50 or >140 beats/min	
Neurologic status	Infant: hypotonia	Sign of hypoxia for infants
	Child: irritability	Early sign of hypoxia, often manifested as a decreased responsiveness to parents or to pain
	Decreased level of consciousness	

PEEP, positive end-expiratory pressure.
Based on data from Kline-Tilford A, et al. Pulmonary disorders. In: Hazinski MF, ed. *Nursing Care of the Critically Ill Child.* 3rd ed. St. Louis: Elsevier; 2013.

infant or child who is conscious and needs supplemental oxygen, the device of comfort must be selected.[4] Minimizing anxiety and fear in the child is paramount to decrease the work of breathing. Table 39.3 outlines the assessment areas for pediatric patients at risk for respiratory failure.[4]

Airway Positioning

Knowledge of childhood anatomy is necessary to establish a patent airway. An infant or toddler younger than 2 years of age, because of the large occiput, needs to have a small roll or towel placed under the upper shoulders, with the jaw slightly extended into a "sniffing" position.[5] Optimal positioning of the head should assist in maintenance of a patent airway or help when bag-mask ventilation is required.[5] This head positioning displaces the tongue and lines up the posterior pharynx and tracheal opening for a clear airway. For infants younger than 6 months, correct head positioning still may not prevent the large tongue from falling back into the posterior pharynx. Oral airways must not be used unless the infant is unconscious because the airway tip may stimulate laryngospasm as a result of the higher placement of the larynx. Side-lying placement, with the neck in a neutral position, should be attempted.[4] The older child needs to have a folded towel placed under the head, with the neck in an extended position to maintain a patent airway.[4] Fig. 39.2 illustrates proper head positioning for the infant and the child. A child who is conscious must be allowed to assume a position of choice for airway maintenance.

FIG. 39.2 Correct Airway Positioning for Ventilation. Correct airway positioning for ventilation is shown for (A) an infant and (B) a child. Better airflow is provided with straight alignment of the oropharynx *(O)*, pharynx *(P)*, and trachea *(T)*.[46]

Supplemental Oxygen Devices

Many of the oxygen devices used for adults also are used for children. One technique is oxygen "blow-by," which uses oxygen tubing to blow oxygen approximately 2 to 3 inches from the child's face. Because of the unpredictability of the actual oxygen percentage that is delivered, the child should never be left unattended with blow-by as an oxygen delivery method. Oxygen masks may aggravate the child and often are not well tolerated because of the snug fit of the mask to ensure adequate delivery of oxygen.[7] One option in older infants and children is to use a nasal prong or cannula.[6] This method allows the child to talk and eat without a facial obstruction.

The appropriate device for oxygen delivery is determined by the patient's age, size, inspiratory flow rate (tidal volume mL/s), and fraction of inspired oxygen (FIO_2) needed.[8] Oxygen delivery devices may be divided into two different classes: low-flow devices and high-flow devices. Low-flow (variable performance) devices are unable to deliver an oxygen flow rate sufficient to supply the patient's inspiratory flow rate. This allows the child to entrain room air with supplemental oxygen on inspiration. The FIO_2 the child receives depends on his or her respiratory rate and tidal volume. High-flow (fixed performance) devices may deliver an oxygen flow rate that meets or exceeds the child's inspiratory flow rate. This allows a higher FIO_2 to be consistently delivered.[8] Nursing care for a child receiving supplemental oxygen delivery should include monitoring and recording the type of oxygen delivery device, the liter flow (L/min), the FIO_2, and the patient's response to the oxygen therapy.

An adult-sized, self-inflating resuscitation bag may be carefully used on an infant, provided that only the force needed to cause appropriate chest expansion is used.[4] In general, two types of manual resuscitation bags are used: the self-inflating bag and the flow-dependent bag. Self-inflating bags do not require a gas source to provide ventilation, but flow-dependent bags do require a gas flow.[8] Resuscitation bag sizes, along with other supplemental oxygen devices and oxygen administration, are summarized in Table 39.4. Leaf-flap outlet valves should be avoided when a self-inflating bag is used to assist spontaneous ventilation in an infant because the infant cannot generate enough negative inspiratory pressure to open the valve.[4] Resuscitation bags equipped with spring-loaded, positive end-expiratory pressure (PEEP) valves to provide continuous positive airway pressure (CPAP) must not be used with a spontaneously breathing child for the same reason previously discussed.[4] Flow-inflating bags have no flow valves that require opening on inspiration and therefore may be used to provide supplemental oxygen, PEEP, or CPAP to a spontaneously breathing infant or child.[4] Pressure manometers may be attached to these bags to measure peak inspiratory pressure. Ventilatory masks are measured in the child, as in the adult, from the bridge of the nose to the point before the end of the chin. Using a correctly sized mask for an infant or child is critical for adequate oxygenation and ventilation of the patient.

TABLE 39.4 Supplemental Oxygen Devices and Oxygen Administration in Infants and Children

Device	Administration	Discussion Points
Nasal cannula	Infant	Minute volume, inspiratory/expiratory times, and amount of mouth breathing affects infant FIO_2 by nasal cannula differently from an adult given the same gas flow and O_2 percent
	Child	Low-flow O_2 devices are inaccurate for FIO_2 delivery. Titrate to patient's O_2 saturation readings
O_2 hood	10–15 L/min = nearly 100% O_2	Use with infants <1 year old
O_2 blow-by	10–15 L/min	Better tolerated than O_2 masks
		Short-term method of O_2 delivery
		Titrated to child's O_2 saturation
		Allows child or parent to hold tubing
Simple mask	0.4–0.5 FIO_2	Entrains room air. FIO_2 does not correlate with high flow rates
Nonrebreather mask	0.9–0.95 FIO_2	No entrainment of room air. O_2 flow is determined by child's minute ventilation

Self-inflating resuscitation bag	Infant
	  <3 mo: 0.25-L bag
	  3 mo–4 y: 0.5-L bag
	Child
	  5–10 y: 1-L bag
	  >10 y: 1.5-L bag
		Do not use bags with leaf-flap outlet valves or with spring-loaded PEEP valves

Flow-inflating resuscitation bag	Spontaneously breathing Flow rate 3 × minute ventilation Not spontaneously breathing 8–10 L/min flow rate	Set O_2 flow rate at level necessary to achieve desired level of ventilation
Peak inspiratory pressure	≤20–30 cm H_2O	
Ventilatory mask size	<6 mo old: 0 6 mo–3 y: 1 3–6 y: 2 >6 y: 3	Fit and placement on face same as for adult

FIO_2, fraction of inspired oxygen; *O_2*, oxygen; *PEEP*, positive end-expiratory pressure.
Based on data from Kuch B. Respiratory monitoring and support. In: Hazinski MF, ed. *Nursing Care of the Critically Ill Child.* 3rd ed. St. Louis: Elsevier; 2013:1007.

Endotracheal Intubation

Procedure

Endotracheal tube (ETT) placement and management is an important intervention to maintain the airway in a pediatric patient with respiratory failure.[5] Preoxygenation of the child before intubation is very important. Bag-mask ventilation is an effective way to assist the child's ventilation. Attempts for intubation should to be no longer than approximately 30 seconds per attempt to prevent deterioration in heart rate or the child's appearance. Box 39.2 provides formulas as a guideline for ETT measurements in pediatric patients. It is important to ensure that pediatric emergency equipment of the correct size is used. Many facilities use length-based or color-coded resuscitation tapes such as the Broselow system.[5,9] This tape gives an estimate of the child's body weight based on the crown-to-heel length and may be used to determine the appropriate size of resuscitation equipment and medication dosages for the child. Fig. 39.3 provides an illustration of a Broselow tape.

When correctly placed, the tip of the ETT should be 1 to 2 cm above the carina, no higher than the first rib.[4] After the child is intubated, bilateral breath sounds should be assessed high in the axillae along with bilateral chest expansion. The easy transmission of sounds in the chest of the child may be mistaken for breath sounds in the event of accidental esophageal intubation. Initial confirmation of tube placement after assessment of bilateral breath sounds and adequate chest expansion is made with the use of the colorimetric carbon dioxide (CO_2) detector. This device detects the delivery of CO_2 after six breaths. Additional confirmation of the correct placement of the ETT must be obtained by using a capnography waveform.[5] This is a very reliable indicator of exhaled CO_2 and tracheal tube placement because a perfusing cardiac rhythm is needed to deliver CO_2 to the lungs. During a cardiac arrest, CO_2 may not be present, and CO_2 may not be detected even if the ETT is in the correct location. Reexpansion of the bulb of the esophageal detector device indicates ETT placement.[10] A chest radiograph is obtained once the ETT is taped in place to confirm proper tube depth and the position.

ETT dislodgment may occur more easily in an infant or young child and cause acute deterioration of the patient's condition. The tip of the ETT is pulled upward with neck extension or when the head is turned completely to the side. Conversely, the ETT moves downward with neck flexion. With the trachea of the young child being short, an ETT placed higher or lower may become dislodged or intubate the bronchus. ETT obstruction may occur with high placement, neck flexion, or head rotation, which may cause the bevel of the ETT to press against the tracheal wall, occluding the lumen. Secretions and mucous plugs may more easily occlude the lumen of a small-diameter ETT. Assessment of the tube by the bedside nurse is critical in the evaluation of proper functioning of the child's ETT.

The nurse and the respiratory therapist must ensure that the child's ETT remains patent and in correct placement to maintain correct oxygenation and ventilation. Causes of acute deterioration in an intubated pediatric patient may be remembered by using the mnemonic DOPE[4]:

Displacement of the tube
Obstruction of the tube
Pneumothorax (or other air leak)
Equipment failure

Suction equipment and a bag-valve mask need to be readily available for resuscitation if any of the above-mentioned intubation complications occur.

Securing Endotracheal and Nasotracheal Tubes

A small infant or child has less facial area for tape adherence for securing the tubes. A method with a low incidence of accidental extubation uses two pieces of cloth tape, split halfway down the middle, creating a "Y" shape (Fig. 39.4). The skin of a child is more fragile than that of an adult. Cloth tape may be irritating to the child's skin. A soft foam dressing (eg, Mepilex) may be applied to the cheeks, with the securing tape attached on top of the dressing. Breath sounds should be auscultated before and after taping or retaping of the tubing to ensure that the ETT position has not changed.[4] Commercially manufactured devices to secure ETTs are available, but these may be limited in infant and pediatric sizes. No single method of securing a tube has been identified as superior for minimizing ETT dislodgment.[10]

Mechanical Ventilation

Many types of unconventional mechanical ventilation (eg, high-frequency, oscillation, jet ventilation) are used, but for most infants and children, standard means of positive-pressure ventilation support use volume or pressure-controlled ventilators. The type of ventilation chosen depends on the child's size, minute ventilation requirements, and lung compliance. Newer ventilators have flow and pressure triggers that are sensitive enough to ventilate infants and children.[11]

For the older child, non–continuous-flow, volume-limited ventilation in synchronized intermittent mandatory ventilation mode is used most often. Pressure support ventilation is also used in the child in conjunction with other modes to assist with spontaneous breathing, especially during the weaning process. Currently used ventilators have flow triggering designed for infants. Some type of synchronized ventilation mode is used almost exclusively for the ventilation of infants and children. Box 39.3 outlines the characteristics for the ideal pediatric ventilator for the infant and child.[12]

Ventilator-patient asynchrony may have several causes. The Hering-Breuer reflex is a vagal reflex in which the child's sensing of positive lung inflation sets off immediate expiration, and lung deflation stimulates inspiration. Apnea, or active expiration during the ventilator's inspiratory cycle, also may cause asynchrony. The use of adult ventilators not appropriately

---

BOX 39.2   Endotracheal Tube Measurement

Size

- For infants and toddlers: size based on age 1 to 2 y = 3.5 mm
- For children >2 years old: (age in years + 16) ÷ 4
- For any age: compare circumference of the child's little finger with the external diameter size of the ETT
- Cuffed tube: external diameter one-half size smaller than appropriate-sized uncuffed tube

Depth of Insertion

- From teeth to midtrachea: internal diameter of ETT × 3

Cuff Pressure

- Allow for a slight air glottic leak

ETT, endotracheal tube.
Modified from Hazinski MF. *Nursing Care of the Critically Ill Child.* 3rd ed. St. Louis: Elsevier; 2013.

Equipment	GRAY* 3-5 kg	PINK Small Infant 6-7 kg	RED Infant 8-9 kg	PURPLE Toddler 10-11 kg	YELLOW Small Child 12-14 kg	WHITE Child 15-18 kg	BLUE Child 19-23 kg	ORANGE Large Child 24-29 kg	GREEN Adult 30-36 kg
Resuscitation bag		Infant/child	Infant/child	Child	Child	Child	Child	Child	Adult
Oxygen mask (NRB)		Pediatric	Pediatric	Pediatric	Pediatric	Pediatric	Pediatric	Pediatric	Pediatric/adult
Oral airway (mm)		50	50	60	60	60	70	80	80
Laryngoscope blade (size)		1 Straight	1 Straight	1 Straight	2 Straight	2 Straight	2 Straight or curved	2 Straight or curved	3 Straight or curved
ET tube (mm)†		3.5 Uncuffed 3.0 Cuffed	3.5 Uncuffed 3.0 Cuffed	4.0 Uncuffed 3.5 Cuffed	4.5 Uncuffed 4.0 Cuffed	5.0 Uncuffed 4.5 Cuffed	5.5 Uncuffed 5.0 Cuffed	6.0 Cuffed	6.5 Cuffed
ET tube insertion length (cm)	3 kg 9-9.5 4 kg 9.5-10 5 kg 10-10.5	10.5-11	10.5-11	11-12	13.5	14-15	16.5	17-18	18.5-19.5
Suction catheter (F)		8	8	10	10	10	10	10	10-12
BP cuff	Neonatal #5/infant	Infant/child	Infant/child	Child	Child	Child	Child	Child	Small adult
IV catheter (ga)		22-24	22-24	20-24	18-22	18-22	18-20	18-20	16-20
IO (ga)		18/15	18/15	15	15	15	15	15	15
NG tube (F)		5-8	5-8	8-10	10	10	12-14	14-18	16-18
Urinary catheter (F)	5	8	8	8-10	10	10-12	10-12	12	12
Chest tube (F)		10-12	10-12	16-20	20-24	20-24	24-32	28-32	32-38

FIG. 39.3 Broselow Pediatric Color-Coded Resuscitation Tape. BP, blood pressure; ET, endotracheal; F, French; IO, intraosseous; IV, intravenous; NG, nasogastric; NRB, nonrebreathing.*For Gray column, use Pink or Red equipment sizes if no size is listed. †Per 2010 AHA Guidelines, in the hospital, cuffed or uncuffed tubes may be used. (Adapted from Broselow Pediatric Emergency Tap. Distributed by Armstrong Medical Industries, Lincolnshire, IL. Copyright © 2007 Vital Signs, Inc. All rights reserved.)

FIG. 39.4 Securing an Endotracheal Tube With Split Taping. (Modified from Kline-Tilford A, et al. Pulmonary disorders. In: Hazinski MF, ed. *Nursing Care of the Critically Ill Child*. 3rd ed. St. Louis: Elsevier; 2013.)

adapted for an infant or child may cause asynchrony. In a small child, decreased tidal volume and increased respiratory rates occur to cope with respiratory compromise. Adult ventilators may not sense rapidly enough, if at all, any spontaneous respiratory efforts, which leads to increased work of breathing in the child.

Asynchrony may lead to poor oxygenation or volutrauma. Significant asynchrony may require sedation, alone or with neuromuscular blockade. Criteria for weaning and extubation are much more extensive for adults than for children, but some guidelines exist for these procedures. Synchronized intermittent mandatory ventilation with pressure support ventilation is used for weaning from positive-pressure ventilation. Pressure support ventilation allows the child to have greater control over breathing, and asynchrony is not a problem. Box 39.4 outlines the indicators for initiating weaning and extubation.[10,11] Supplemental oxygen may be supplied after extubation by a nasal cannula, ventilation mask, or oxygen hood. Noninvasive ventilation devices such as nasal or facial CPAP may be an option for the patient, but if the child cannot be managed using these options, reintubation may be necessary.

Extubation Complications

Postextubation croup may occur in small children. Manifestations arising from airway edema include hoarseness, stridor, or a crowing cough that begins immediately or up to 3 hours after extubation. Initial treatment consists of keeping the child calm. Procedures must be withheld, if possible, and crying must be prevented to avoid increasing airway resistance. Supplemental humidified oxygen should be administered to the

---

BOX 39.3 Characteristics of a Pediatric Ventilator

Specifications

- Volume, pressure or time cycled, mixed modes of ventilation
- Assist/control, CPAP, PSV, SIMV
- Tidal volume range of 20–450 mL/breath (minute ventilation of 0.4–0.6 L/min)
- Respiratory rate of 1–1000/min (high-frequency ventilation capability is also desirable)
- Variable inspiratory flow of 0.5–40 L/min
- Variable inspiratory/expiratory flow ratios
- Adjustable peak inspiratory pressure of 10–80 cm H_2O
- Adequate humidification
- Provision for PEEP/CPAP

Visual Indicators

- Proximal airway pressure (patent airway)
- Proximal airway temperature (patent airway)
- F_{IO_2} (high and low)
- Inspiratory/expiratory times
- Flow rate (L/min)
- Tidal volume
- Minute ventilation

Alarms

- High and low pressure
- Apnea
- Loss of PEEP
- Power failure/disconnect
- Loss of air/oxygen
- High temperature
- Failure to cycle
- Output jacks to allow ventilator alarms to be connected to a remote alarm in nursing stations

CPAP, continuous positive airway pressure; F_{IO_2}, fraction of inspired oxygen; *PEEP*, positive end-expiratory pressure; *PSV*, pressure support ventilation; *SIMV*, synchronized intermittent mandatory ventilation.
Modified from Kuch B. Respiratory monitoring and support. In: Hazinski MF, ed. *Nursing Care of the Critically Ill Child*. 3rd ed. St. Louis: Elsevier; 2013.

BOX 39.4 Indicators for Initiating Weaning of a Pediatric Patient

- Achievement of baseline mental status
- Presence of cough and gag reflexes
- Absence of fever
- Spontaneous respiratory effort
- Normal acid–base balance
- Oxyhemoglobin saturation ≥90% or Pao_2 ≥60 mm Hg (in the absence of cyanotic heart disease)
- F_{IO_2} <0.5
- PEEP <7 cm H_2O
- $Paco_2$ <50 mm Hg
- Stable hemodynamically
- Stable ventilation support for ≥24 h
- No plans that will require significant sedation or operative procedures in the next 12 h

F$_{IO_2}$, fraction of inspired oxygen; *Paco$_2$*, arterial partial pressure of carbon dioxide; *Pao$_2$*, arterial partial pressure of oxygen; *PEEP*, positive end-expiratory pressure.
From Kline-Tilford A, et al. Pulmonary disorders. In: Hazinski MF, ed. *Nursing Care of the Critically Ill Child*. 3rd ed. St. Louis: Elsevier; 2013:483.

child immediately after extubation, and a cool mist should continue to be provided. More severe symptoms may be treated with racemic epinephrine and with intravenous or inhaled steroid therapy. Intubation equipment and personnel qualified to intubate should be available after extubation, in case the patient requires reintubation.

Tracheostomy

Over the past 3 decades, tracheostomy has become an increasingly common procedure in children. The primary reasons for having a tracheotomy performed include upper airway obstruction caused by anatomic abnormalities, the anticipated need for prolonged ventilation, or the need for effective pulmonary toilet.[13] Most children who require a tracheostomy are younger than 1 year, and a higher incidence is seen among boys.[13] A tracheotomy is recommended if an older child is to remain intubated for longer than 2 to 3 weeks.

Several types of tracheostomy tubes are available for children; the plastic, single-cannula type is the most popular for in-hospital care because it has few complications. Silastic tubes have been recommended for the infant and the child because they are pliable and bend with tracheal movement. Uncuffed tubes usually are preferred for pediatric patients to prevent subglottic stenosis.[14] The diameter of the tracheostomy tube should be carefully selected to avoid any damage to the tracheal wall, to minimize the work of breathing, and to promote translaryngeal airflow, when possible. Table 39.5 describes tracheostomy tube sizes for infants and children.

Bronchiolitis

Bronchiolitis is one of the diseases that primarily affects very young infants and is the most common disease in infants and children younger than 2 years of age.[15] *Bronchiolitis* is a term used to describe a condition that affects the lower respiratory tract and results in obstruction of the small airways. Although this disease has a relatively low mortality rate (200 to 500 deaths per year), it is the most frequent cause of hospitalization in the infant population.[15] Bronchiolitis is one of the most common

diagnoses in children who present in the critical care unit with respiratory failure.[16] The disease is characterized by mucosal edema, inflammation, increased mucus production, and sloughing of epithelial cells. Obstruction of the bronchioles occurs, resulting in hypoxemia and hypercapnia.[15] Widespread fine end-inspiratory crackles and an expiratory wheeze are heard on auscultation. This clinical pattern may be seen during the first year of life, with most hospital admissions occurring within the first 6 months of life.[15] Respiratory syncytial virus (RSV) is the most common cause of viral bronchiolitis, and it infects almost all children by the age of 2 years.[17] The peak incidence for viral bronchiolitis occurs during midwinter and into early spring. RSV is highly contagious and may be spread by close contact through droplets. Meticulous handwashing by clinical staff is the most important step to prevent hospital-acquired infections in other patients or staff members.[18]

Pathophysiology

RSV infection has an overall low mortality rate, but the mortality rate is 37% among infected infants with congenital heart disease. In children younger than 2 years of age, 40% of RSV infections may progress to lower respiratory infections.[15] Patients with cystic fibrosis or bronchopulmonary dysplasia or who are immunocompromised are also at greater risk for more serious disease and for occurrence beyond 1 year of age. The chance of recovery from RSV may be excellent, but residual effects of reactive airways disease may be seen several years after infection.[19] RSV involves inflammation of respiratory epithelium, which leads to necrosis. The epithelium is replaced with nonciliated tissue. Submucosal edema forms with lymphocytic infiltrates and other alveolar debris. Obstruction occurs from mucous secretions and debris not being cleared because of the lack of ciliated epithelium. Pathologic pulmonary dynamics involve lung hyperinflation almost two times normal. Obstruction occurs in a patchy distribution with complete obstruction, leading to atelectasis and partial obstruction, which results in hyperinflation. Inspiratory resistance and expiratory resistance are present, along with ventilation-perfusion

TABLE 39.5	Guidelines for Intubation Equipment and Tracheostomy Tubes for Pediatrics							
	EQUIPMENT CHOICES BASED ON AGE AND WEIGHT							
	3 mo	6 mo	1 y	3 y	6 y	8 y	12 y	16 y
Factors	**6 kg**	**8 kg**	**10 kg**	**15 kg**	**20 kg**	**25 kg**	**40 kg**	**60 kg**
ETT size (mm)	3.0–3.5	3.5–4.0	4.0–4.5	4.5–5.0	5.0–5.5	6.0 c/u	7.0 c	7.0–8.0 c
Laryngoscope blade	0–1 s	0–1 s	1 s	2 s	2 s	2 s/c	3 s/c	3 s/c
Stylet (Fr)	6	6	6	6	14	14	14	14
Suction catheter (Fr)[a]	6–8	8	8	8–10	10	10–12	12–14	12–14
Shiley Tracheostomy								
Shiley size (mm)	0	1	1–12	4	4	4	6	6
Internal diameter (mm ID)	3.4	3.7	3.7–4.1	5	5	5	7	7
Length (cm)	4	4.1	4.1–4.2	4.6	4.6	4.6	6.7	6.7

[a]Catheter size twice the ID size of any tracheal tube.

c/u, cuffed or uncuffed; *ETT*, endotracheal tube; *ID*, internal diameter; *s/c*, straight or curved; *Fr*, French sizing.
Based on data from Kuch B. Respiratory monitoring and support. In: Hazinski MF, ed. *Nursing Care of the Critically Ill Child*. 3rd ed. St. Louis: Elsevier; 2013:1007.

mismatch, which leads to hypoxemia and some degree of CO_2 retention. The probable mechanism in addition to the ventilation-perfusion mismatch is hypoventilation, which results from a marked increase in the work of breathing in the infant.[19]

Clinical Assessment

The first symptoms to appear are symptoms of an upper respiratory tract infection—sneezing and rhinorrhea. In many cases, a family member has had a respiratory illness. After 2 to 3 days, respiratory distress ensues with increased respirations, coughing, nasal flaring, chest retractions, wheezing, irritability, and feeding difficulties. Fever and lung rhonchi may or may not occur. After bronchiolar obstruction has occurred, patients present with increased work of breathing. This may lead to muscle fatigue and respiratory failure if the work of breathing exceeds the capacity of the patient's respiratory muscles. Infants tolerate respiratory loads poorly and are susceptible to fatigue because of the immature pattern of their muscle fibers.[20]

Treatment

The overall treatment for bronchiolitis is supportive. Oxygen continues to be the primary therapy to decrease the work of breathing and oxygen demands. Depending on the severity of illness, the infant may receive supplemental humidified oxygen by mask, nasal CPAP (despite lung hyperinflation), or mechanical ventilation.[6,21] RSV causes airway obstruction, and no therapy has demonstrated an ability to rapidly reduce this obstruction.

Suctioning of the airways will be required to help alleviate the signs and symptoms of airway obstruction from mucous secretions. The mucus will be thick and initially cause the infant to be suctioned frequently. Inhaled beta-2 agonists, anticholinergic agents, and corticosteroids during the acute or recovery phase have been tried with various degrees of success.[15] The use of a clinical pathway for bronchiolitis has been shown to be effective in the literature. A decrease in the use of therapies such as bronchodilators, glucocorticoids, antibiotics, and chest physiotherapy and a decrease in admission rates and length of stay have occurred in association with the use of a bronchiolitis clinical pathway.[15]

The current recommendation from the American Academy of Pediatrics for the prevention of RSV is administration of the monoclonal antibody palivizumab (Synagis; MedImmune). Clinicians may administer palivizumab prophylactically to selected infants and children with chronic lung disease or a history of prematurity (<29 weeks' gestation) or with congenital heart disease.[18] Palivizumab is administered in five monthly doses, 15 mg/kg per dose administered intramuscularly, during the RSV season, usually beginning in November or December.[18]

Status Asthmaticus
Pathophysiology

Asthma is a chronic inflammatory disorder of the airways in which many cells and cellular elements, including mast cells, eosinophils, T lymphocytes, neutrophils, and epithelial cells, play a role.[22] An acute asthma exacerbation is an event of progressive wheezing, cough, chest tightness, shortness of breath, or a combination of all these symptoms. Asthma is identified as the disease with a triad of physiologic processes—airway inflammation, edema, and airway hyperactivity. Inflammation has been recognized as the primary underlying cause in the

pathogenesis of this disease.[22] The treatment for asthma is aimed at decreasing and reducing airway inflammation.

The universal feature of the inflammatory response in asthma includes the activation and infiltration of the airway by cells. The early phase in the inflammation reaction is caused by a trigger, and this may be different with each child. The immediate response to this trigger is bronchospasm and smooth muscle contraction caused by the mediators from the various inflammatory cells in the airway. If this early phase is not responsive to beta-2 agonists, a late phase will occur approximately 6 to 9 hours after the initial exposure to the trigger.[22] This will lead to increased release of the mediator cells in the airway and produce cellular infiltration, airway edema, mucus secretions, bronchospasm, and smooth muscle contraction. Without treatment, atelectasis and mucous plugging may occur in the child.

Clinical Assessment

Assessing severe asthma in an infant is different compared with assessment in an older child because of the anatomic and physiologic differences between them. Physiologic changes may progress rapidly to respiratory failure in the infant. Table 39.6 outlines guidelines for classifying the severity of an asthma exacerbation. A moderate asthma episode requires hospitalization with close monitoring. In a severe event, the child may be able to speak only in short phrases or not at all. The position of comfort or degree of agitation should be noted; sitting upright and unable to lie down indicates severe distress.[23] A severe episode requires critical care, with intubation and ventilation equipment readily available.[6]

Treatment

Standard treatment for a pediatric patient who has asthma includes receiving oxygen, beta-adrenergic therapy, corticosteroids, and anticholinergic medications, as indicated.[6,22] Pharmacologic therapy is based on the concept of reducing airway inflammation. Beta-adrenergic agonists are the first-line agents in the treatment of asthma. Beta-agonist medications that are selective for beta-2 receptors on airway smooth muscle (eg, albuterol, levalbuterol) are preferred to avoid the stimulation of the beta-1 cardiac receptors.[22] These medications are given by nebulization intermittently or continuously. Anticholinergic medications in conjunction with beta agonists improve pulmonary function in children, especially school-age patients.[22] These medications may decrease bronchomotor tone and secretions. The most commonly administered inhaled anticholinergic is ipratropium bromide. This medication works synergistically with beta agonists to improve and prolong bronchodilation. Ipratropium bromide should be administered with albuterol in a nebulizer and not given alone. Corticosteroids are also an important part of the treatment for airway inflammation. Corticosteroids may be administered enterally or parenterally. Both methods are equally efficacious in the treatment of asthma.[22] The peak effect for corticosteroids is virtually the same with either route. Treatment for asthma does not have to be delayed because of a lack of intravenous access in a pediatric patient. The corticosteroid of choice is a glucocorticoid (eg, prednisone, prednisolone, methylprednisolone). Intravenous magnesium sulfate is administered to pediatric patients as an adjunct therapy, as it provides smooth muscle relaxation to patients with severe or life-threatening asthma events.[23] Magnesium is a physiologic calcium

TABLE 39.6   Guidelines for Assessing Severe Asthma in Infants and Children

ASSESSMENT	PHYSICAL FINDINGS		
Area	Infant	Child	Discussion Points
Respiratory rate	Increase of >50% above normal	Can range from normal to >95th percentile for age	Sleeping rates in infants and resting rates in children are good measures of obstruction; awake or activity rates are too variable.
Level of consciousness	Decreased	May be decreased	Assess response to parents and pain.
Accessory muscle use	Retractions in less-than-severe states	Severe intercostal, tracheosternal, and sternocleidomastoid retractions and nasal flaring	In infants, compliant chest wall produces retractions earlier in course. In children, retractions and flaring correlate well with degree of obstruction and with PEF <50% of predicted for age.
Color	Pallor, grayness, or cyanosis	Possible cyanosis	
Dyspnea		Can speak only single words or short phrases; cannot count to 10 in one breath	Infants and children are drowsy or confused.
Quality of cry	Softer and shorter as FEV_1 decreases		
Oxygen saturation	<90% in less-than-severe states	<90% on room air	Infants have greater ventilation-perfusion mismatch. In children, hypoxemia correlates well with degree of obstruction.
Auscultation (breath sounds)	Wheezing; becoming inaudible because of decreased air movement	Same as in infant	Presence and volume of wheezing is the least sensitive predictor of obstruction.
$Paco_2$	If >50 mm Hg or if rising 5–10 mm Hg/h, consider mechanical ventilation	Can range from <40 mm Hg with respiratory distress to >40 mm Hg as air movement significantly decreases	$Paco_2$ is best measure of ventilation in infants. Continually rising $Paco_2$ of >40 mm Hg in a child occurs when PEF is <20% of predicted for age. Hypercapnia develops more readily in young children than adults.
PEF	≥70%		PEF is not needed in cases of severe asthmatic exacerbation. This is used after asthma is under control.
Feeding/sucking ability	Decreased or absent		

FEV₁, forced expiratory volume in 1 second; *Paco₂*, arterial partial pressure of carbon dioxide; *PEF*, peak expiratory flow.
Based on data from Gomez M, Felauer A. Asthma. In: Reuter-Rice K, et al, eds. *Pediatric Acute Care: A Guide for Interprofessional Practice*. Burlington, MA: Jones & Bartlett Learning; 2012; and Marcoux K. Current management of status asthmaticus in the pediatric ICU. *Crit Care Nurs Clin North Am*. 2005;17:463.

antagonist, which has a direct effect on the calcium uptake in the muscle, causing smooth muscle relaxation.[6] Magnesium sulfate (12 to 50 mg/kg) is administered intravenously, usually over 20 minutes.[24]

Critical care management of a child with status asthmaticus involves humidified oxygen to maintain an oxygen saturation of more than 95%, combined with the pharmacologic therapies. Heliox is a mixture of 80% helium and 20% oxygen, which makes this mixture lighter than air. Administration of heliox is effective in decreasing airway resistance and in decreasing the work of breathing. The use of heliox does not appear to have adverse effects, and its administration may improve the status of the child.[22] The use of noninvasive positive-pressure ventilation by means of nasal prongs or a facemask may avoid the need for intubation. Some indications for considering mechanical ventilation are respiratory muscle fatigue, markedly diminished or absent breath sounds, pulsus paradoxus greater than 20 to 40 mm Hg, deterioration in mental status, and arterial partial pressure of oxygen (Pao_2) less than 70 mm Hg on 100% FIO_2.[22] The child and family should be informed of the management approach and plan of care. If properly and effectively treated, pediatric patients who have status asthmaticus may return to their usual state of health, but they will require close follow-up by a pediatrician or pulmonologist.[22]

CARDIOVASCULAR SYSTEM

Anatomy and Physiology

The differences in cardiovascular function between children and adults are related to early physical development and the presence or absence of congenital cardiac disease. Congenital heart defects (CHDs) occur during the embryologic development of the heart, whereas acquired defects occur after birth. Most fetal cardiac development occurs between the fourth and seventh weeks of fetal life. The heart is most susceptible to teratogenic influences at this time.[4] Approximately 90% of CHDs are caused by a genetic predisposition and an adverse response to environmental teratogens during cardiac development. Environmental factors alone account for only approximately 1% of all CHDs. Approximately 5% to 8% of CHDs are associated with genetic anomalies or syndromes.[4] Although more than 35 well-recognized cardiac defects have been documented, the most common is ventricular septal defect.

Congenital Heart Defects

Some CHDs may be diagnosed with ultrasonography before birth, and some parents decide to undergo delivery at a tertiary center affiliated with a pediatric cardiac surgery program. Other newborns with cardiac anomalies are diagnosed after birth and transferred to tertiary care centers for further evaluation and often immediate surgery. Certain defects are completely repaired in the first few days of life, other defects are repaired in stages, and some are repaired when the child is older. Infants with CHDs may develop complications after discharge, after a surgical procedure, or while waiting for surgery, and they may be admitted to an adult critical care unit.

Cardiac Monitoring

In pediatric patients, monitoring of respiratory rate and oxygen saturation is done concurrently with cardiac monitoring. It is important to recognize the manifestations of impending respiratory failure in a pediatric patient because respiratory failure precedes heart failure and potential cardiac arrest. Electrocardiogram monitoring electrodes are placed along the nipple line on the chest to facilitate monitoring of cardiac rate and rhythm and respiratory rate. Dysrhythmias may result from many different causes. Some of these include CHD, surgical correction, hypoxia, electrolyte or acid–base imbalances, drug toxicity, or myocardial injury.[4] Dysrhythmias may be symptomatic or asymptomatic, but they have the potential to deteriorate into a symptomatic condition for the child. The three most common types of clinically significant pediatric dysrhythmias are (1) bradyarrhythmias, (2) tachyarrhythmias, and (3) dysrhythmias that produce cardiac collapse or loss of pulses.[4,5] Hypoxia and heart block are the most common causes of bradyarrhythmias. Supraventricular tachycardia (SVT) is probably the most common form of pediatric tachyarrhythmias. Sinus tachycardia is not considered a dysrhythmia; it is the most efficient method of increasing cardiac output and the chief method of increasing cardiac output in a child. Tachycardia is normally observed in a child who is febrile, scared, or stressed. However, a heart rate that goes to extremely high rates, such as greater than 220 beats/min, may actually reduce the child's cardiac output.[4]

The most common symptomatic tachyarrhythmia in children is SVT. P waves may or may not be seen, and the rate often exceeds 220 beats/min. Wide-QRS SVT is uncommon in children, and any wide-QRS tachycardia must be treated as ventricular in origin until proved otherwise. If the child in SVT is unstable and shows signs of decreased cardiac output and poor perfusion, immediate treatment is indicated.[5] If the child has intravenous access readily available, adenosine (0.1 mg/kg) should be administered up to a maximum of a 6-mg rapid bolus. This dose may be doubled up to a maximum of 12 mg for a second dose. Adenosine should be given as a rapid intravenous bolus because of the drug's short half-life of about 10 seconds. If intravenous access is not readily available, synchronized cardioversion is indicated.[5] The initial energy dose is 0.5 to 1 J/kg. If the SVT persists, the dose of electricity is doubled to 2 J/kg.[5]

Bradycardias

Bradycardia may result from hypoxia, acidosis, or hypothermia. Bradycardia is defined as a cardiac rate less than 100 beats/min for an infant and less than 60 beats/min for a child.[4] Treatment initially includes adequate oxygenation and ventilation for the pediatric patient. If bradycardia continues to cause cardiopulmonary compromise despite oxygenation and ventilation, compressions are started for a heart rate of less than 60 beats/min. If increased vagal tone or a primary atrioventricular block is the cause of the bradycardia, atropine (0.02 mg/kg) may be given to the child.

Shock in Infants and Children

Shock is a critical condition that results from inadequate delivery of oxygen and nutrients to the tissues to meet the metabolic demand.[4] Shock frequently is the end result of severe dehydration, hemorrhage, progressive heart failure, or sepsis. The treatment goal for a child in shock is to prevent end-organ injury and stop the progression from cardiopulmonary failure to cardiac arrest. Shock is typically classified by the etiologic mechanism. These classifications include hypovolemic, distributive or septic, cardiogenic, or obstructive.[5]

Shock may be present in a pediatric patient with normal or abnormal blood pressure. The blood pressure reading may be used to classify the shock further as compensated or hypotensive shock.[5] Compensated shock describes a child with signs of poor perfusion but normal blood pressure. The systolic reading may be normal, but the diastolic pressure may not be normal because of increased systemic vascular resistance with a narrowing pulse pressure.[5] In hypotensive shock, the blood pressure is low, and cardiopulmonary failure may be imminent.[4]

Hypovolemic Shock

Hypovolemic shock is the most common cause of shock in children worldwide.[5] Fluid loss from diarrhea is the leading cause of hypovolemic shock.[5] Causes of volume loss that may lead to hypovolemic shock include diarrhea, hemorrhage, vomiting, inadequate fluid intake, osmotic diuresis, third space losses, and burns.[5] The treatment for hypovolemic shock is fluid resuscitation. Pediatric patients with hypovolemic shock need to receive the appropriate volume of fluid within the first hour of resuscitation to have the best chance of survival and recovery. Fluid resuscitation should start with rapid infusion of isotonic crystalloid in boluses of 20 mL/kg.[5] With severe fluid losses, the child may require two to three fluid boluses initially. If blood replacement is required, packed red cells should be considered, starting with 10 mL/kg. The child must be closely monitored and reassessed after each fluid bolus for effectiveness of the fluid resuscitation on end-organ perfusion.

Cardiogenic Shock

Cardiogenic shock is a condition of inadequate tissue perfusion resulting from myocardial dysfunction. This dysfunction may be the result of pump failure, congenital heart disease, or a rhythm abnormality.[5] Cardiogenic shock is characterized by decreased cardiac output, marked tachycardia, and a high systemic vascular output. The child has decreased urine output (less than 0.5 to 1 mL/kg/h) and changes in mental status as end-organ perfusion is affected. Crackles may be heard on lung auscultation, and frothy sputum may be present. Increased respiratory effort often distinguishes cardiogenic shock from hypovolemic shock.[5]

The main treatment objectives are to improve the effectiveness of cardiac function and overall cardiac output by increasing the efficiency of ventricular emptying.[5,25] Many children with cardiogenic shock have a high preload and do not require additional fluids. However, if the child's history is consistent with fluid loss, a fluid bolus of 5 to 10 mL/kg may be cautiously given. Frequent assessments of the child's respiratory function should be performed in anticipation of respiratory failure. Supplemental oxygen should be given, but the nurse should be prepared to assist with ventilation with intubation and helping to establish a central venous access in the child.[5] This approach allows for the measurement of the central venous pressure and provides access for fluid and medication infusion.

Typical pharmacologic support of a child with cardiogenic shock includes the use of diuretics and vasodilators. Diuretics are indicated when the child has evidence of pulmonary edema. The vasodilators are given as a continuous infusion. Milrinone is the preferred medication for cardiogenic shock (loading dose 50 mcg/kg, followed by an infusion at 0.25 to 0.75 mcg/kg/min).[5]

Distributive Shock, Sepsis, and Septic Shock

Septic shock is the most common form of distributive shock. This condition is caused by infectious agents or their endotoxins, which stimulate the child's immune system and trigger release or activation of inflammatory mediators. Septic shock in children typically evolves along a continuum from a systemic inflammatory response in the early stages to septic shock later on.[5] The child exhibits manifestations of systemic inflammatory response syndrome with severe sepsis or septic shock. The infant or child may have a temperature elevation, a low temperature, or temperature instability. Along with changes in level of consciousness, the child may be irritable, restless, or lethargic. Urine output is decreased, the skin may be warm or mottled, and peripheral pulses may be strong and bounding. The child does not feed well, and decreased fluid intake may precipitate dehydration. Blood pressure is maintained within normal limits from activation of the body's compensatory mechanisms. Parents may remark that the child "does not seem right" or "something is different" with the child. It is important to listen to the parents' assessment of the child's status.

Severe sepsis or septic shock is diagnosed when perfusion decreases and the child becomes hypotensive. If the child is receiving inotropic agents, the blood pressure may be normal, but a change occurs in perfusion. The patient exhibits metabolic acidosis and hypoxemia. This may require intubation, mechanical ventilation, sedation, fluids, and vasopressor medications. Complications of septic shock include acute respiratory distress syndrome, acute kidney injury, disseminated intravascular coagulation, and multiple-organ dysfunction syndrome. Fig. 34.6 in Chapter 34 presents a concept map of septic shock that depicts the process from etiology through treatment.

Obstructive Shock

Obstructive shock is a condition of impaired cardiac output caused by some physical obstruction of blood flow. The physiology of the clinical symptoms varies according to the cause of the obstruction.[5] Four types of obstructive shock occur in children.

One type of obstructive shock is caused by a *cardiac tamponade*.[5] This occurs when fluid, blood, or air accumulates in the pericardial space around the heart. This condition is seen after cardiac surgery or a penetrating cardiac injury. Symptoms of a cardiac tamponade include muffled or distant heart sounds, distended neck veins, or pulsus paradoxus (ie, decrease in systolic blood pressure by more than 10 mm Hg during inspiration). The treatment is supportive and includes fluids, adequate

oxygenation and ventilation, vasopressors, and a possible pericardiocentesis.[5]

A second type of obstructive shock is caused by a *tension pneumothorax*,[5] which is caused by entry of air into the pleural space. This is most often seen in a pediatric patient when chest trauma has occurred or when an intubated child on positive-pressure ventilation deteriorates suddenly. The signs and symptoms include diminished breath sounds on the affected side; distended neck veins; tracheal deviation; and a rapidly deteriorating clinical condition of the child that may result in bradycardia, hypotension, and hypoxemia. The treatment is immediate needle decompression over the third rib at the midclavicular line. The decompression should lead to an escaping of air. The decompression should be followed by an insertion of a chest tube.

A third but rare cause of obstructive shock is caused by a *massive pulmonary embolism*,[5] which results from partial or total obstruction of the pulmonary artery. The symptoms include signs of cyanosis, hypotension, and right heart failure. Treatment includes adequate oxygenation and ventilation, and fluid therapy is administered if the patient is poorly perfused. Additional diagnostic tests and medications such as fibrinolytic agents may be required.

A fourth type of obstructive shock is caused by a *ductal-dependent congenital heart lesion*.[5] Because systemic circulation is supported by the right side of the heart through the ductus arteriosus, these lesions are called *ductal-dependent lesions*. The affected infant shows signs of severe shock, congestive heart failure, hypotension, poor perfusion, lethargy, and acidosis. The infant is treated with prostaglandin E_1 to maintain the patency of the ductus arteriosus.

Cardiopulmonary Arrest

The pediatric patient must be assessed for manifestations of respiratory failure and shock, as failure to recognize these problems may result in the development of cardiopulmonary failure and respiratory or cardiac arrest. In pediatric patients, respiratory arrest usually precedes cardiac arrest. In an arrest situation, oxygen is administered, and an airway is established and maintained (see "Assessment and Oxygen Devices"). In the event of a cardiac arrest, compressions are started, and an intravenous or intraosseous line is established. Intraosseous placement is recommended as an alternative means to deliver intravenous fluids and medications in children of all ages when vascular access is not obtained within 90 seconds or after three attempts. Intraosseous access often is achieved in 30 to 60 seconds and is the preferred route over the endotracheal route for medications. Any medication or fluid that is administered by a peripheral intravenous line may be given by the intraosseous route.[5] The preferred site is the broad, flat portion of the anteromedial surface of the tibia approximately 1 to 2 cm below the tibial tuberosity. Other interventions are based on the cardiac rhythm and the cause of the arrest.

Pulseless arrest includes the following dysrhythmias: asystole, ventricular fibrillation (VF), pulseless ventricular tachycardia (VT), and pulseless electrical activity (PEA).[5] Treatment of asystole starts with cardiopulmonary resuscitation (CPR; rate of 15 compressions to two breaths with two rescuers), airway maintenance with oxygenation, attachment to a monitor or defibrillator, and obtaining intravenous or intraosseous access. After an advanced airway is in place, chest compressions may continue without pauses for breaths. A child requires 8 to 10 breaths per minute. The next step in the treatment algorithm depends on whether the rhythm is shockable.[5] The rhythms of VF or VT are shockable. On a manual defibrillator, the initial dose of electricity is 2 J/kg. Immediately after the shock, compressions are resumed for 2 minutes (five cycles). The compressions support the heart while it is in a recovery state, even if a perfusion rhythm has returned.[5] If VT or VF persists, another shock is administered at 4 J/kg, compressions are resumed, and epinephrine is given. The first dose of epinephrine is 0.01 mg/kg (1:10,000 at 0.1 mL/kg) given intravenously or intraosseously; if given endotracheally, the dose is 0.1 mg/kg (1:1000 at 0.1 mL/kg). Subsequent doses may be given every 3 to 5 minutes. Maximum dosage is 1 mg (1 mL). After 2 minutes of CPR, the patient's rhythm should be checked. If the VT or VF rhythm continues, the patient is defibrillated again at 4 J/kg, compressions are resumed immediately, and an antiarrhythmic medication such as amiodarone (5 mg/kg) is given intravenously or intraosseously.

If the rhythm is not shockable, as in asystole or PEA, the first action after starting CPR is to give epinephrine at the same dose listed previously. After five cycles or 2 minutes of CPR, the patient's rhythm is checked, and if asystole or PEA persists, CPR and dosing with epinephrine every 3 to 5 minutes are continued. The treatment needs to include reversible causes, which include hypovolemia, hypoxia, hydrogen ion (acidosis), hypoglycemia, hypokalemia or hyperkalemia, hypothermia, tension pneumothorax, tamponade, toxins, and thrombosis (pulmonary or coronary).

The primary goals of postresuscitation management of a pediatric patient include the following:[5]
1. Optimization of cardiopulmonary function to restore and maintain vital organ perfusion and function, especially the brain
2. Prevention of any secondary organ injury
3. Identification and treatment of the cause of any acute illnesses
4. Initiation of measures to help improve long-term, neurologically intact survival of the child

The nurse should assess the patient using a systematic approach. In addition to primary assessments, the approach should include review of the patient's history, a thorough physical examination, the use of invasive and noninvasive monitoring techniques, and use of appropriate laboratory testing.[5]

NERVOUS SYSTEM

Anatomy

The nervous system grows rapidly before birth, and growth continues during infancy and childhood. Compared with an adult, an infant or toddler's head size is proportionally larger than the rest of the body. When infants fall, the head usually leads, and a significant head injury may occur.[4] The skull is more flexible because the skull bones are not fused and are separated by spaces called *fontanels*. The anterior fontanel is the junction of the coronal, sagittal, and frontal sutures, whereas the posterior fontanel is the junction of the parietal and occipital bones. By age 3 months, the posterior fontanel is usually closed, and the anterior fontanel is closed by age 20 months.

The brain of a young child has a high water content and contains less myelin compared with the brain of an adult. This makes the child's brain more homogeneous and less compartmentalized.[4] Shear hemorrhages and diffuse brain injuries are more common in children than in adults.

Spinal cord injuries are less common in children than in adults because the spine of the child is elastic, and the vertebrae are less likely to fracture. However, in children with head injuries or multisystem trauma, spinal cord injuries should always be suspected until ruled out.[4]

Physiology

Cerebral blood flow and oxygen consumption are increased in childhood in relation to increased metabolic needs. Hyperemia, tissue hypoxia, and acidosis result in cerebral arterial dilation and increased cerebral blood flow. Hyperventilation decreases cerebral blood flow, but severe hypercarbia may result in decreased oxygen consumption and use. Normal cerebral perfusion pressure (CPP) values in children are unknown. It is thought that CPP should be in the range of 40 to 60 mm Hg, but this figure may vary because perfusion is determined by blood flow and not by blood pressure.[4] CPP must be maintained at a level to maintain blood flow. A patient with a normal CPP does not necessarily have effective cerebral perfusion.

Assessment

Cognitive function cannot be evaluated until the preschool and early childhood years, but level of consciousness, movement, and pupils can be evaluated in pediatric patients. The Glasgow Coma Scale (GCS) is used for older children and has been modified for use in infants and younger children (Table 39.7). Survival and recovery of a patient with a GCS score of 5 to 8 are better for children than for adults.[4] Evaluation of reflexes in children is similar to that in adults, with a couple of exceptions. Although a positive Babinski reflex is an abnormal response in adults, this response is normal in children until age 1 year.[7] In the first few months of life, grasp is reflexive in an infant. With severe neurologic disease or injury, grasp may revert to a reflex as opposed to a purposeful response, and the grasp response may not indicate improvement of the child's neurologic status.

Responsiveness in a pediatric patient should be evaluated in relation to the child's age, clinical condition, and changes in responsiveness over time. Infants and children should always respond to their parents or caregivers and to a painful stimulus. A decrease in responsiveness is abnormal and should be investigated.[4] If the child is older than 2 years, the ability to follow commands may be assessed by asking him or her to hold up two fingers or wiggle the toes. This action is not accomplished by a reflex action.

When a child is unconscious, the most important component of the GCS to assess is the motor function.[4] The patient's central and peripheral responses to a painful stimulus need to be assessed. A central stimulus is applied to the head and trunk, above the nipple line. The peripheral stimulus may be assessed at the medial aspect of each extremity. The patient's best response is the one that is recorded for the GCS score.

Signs of increased ICP in pediatric patients include a change in responsiveness, a deterioration in the ability to follow commands, a change in the response to pain, and pupil dilation with light stimulation.[4] The Cushing triad sign of an increased ICP may be observed only during cerebral herniation and should not be used as an early indicator or ICP. If any neurologic deterioration is detected in a pediatric patient, a complete neurologic assessment is required, including the child's vital signs and consultation with the patient's physician.

TABLE 39.7 Modified Glasgow Coma Scale for Infants and Children[a]

	Child	Infant	Score
Eye opening	Spontaneous	Spontaneous	4
	To verbal stimuli	To verbal stimuli	3
	To pain only	To pain only	2
	No response	No response	1
Verbal response	Oriented, appropriate	Coos and babbles	5
	Confused	Irritable cries	4
	Inappropriate words	Cries to pain	3
	Incomprehensible words or nonspecific sounds	Moans to pain	2
	No response	No response	1
Motor response	Obeys command (eg, child holds up two fingers, wiggles toes, or sticks out tongue)	Moves spontaneously and purposefully	6
	Localizes painful stimulus (eg, child reaches for hand that is rubbing sternum or pinching trapezius)	Withdraws to touch	5
	Withdraws in response to pain (eg, child adducts each extremity when medial aspect is pinched)	Withdraws in response to pain	4
	Flexion in response to pain (eg, decorticate posturing when sternum is rubbed or trapezius muscle pinched)	Decorticate posturing (abnormal flexion) in response to pain	3
	Extension in response to pain (eg, decerebrate posturing when sternum rubbed or trapezius pinched)	Decerebrate posturing (abnormal extension) in response to pain	2
	No response (flaccid)	No response (flaccid)	1

[a]Modifications in parentheses from Milonovich L, Eichler V. Neurological disorders. In: Hazinski MF, ed. *Nursing Care of the Critically Ill Child*. 3rd ed. St. Louis: Elsevier; 2013:587.

Data from Tasker RC. Head and spinal cord trauma. In Nichols DG, ed. *Rodgers Textbook of Pediatric Intensive Care*. 4th ed. Philadelphia: Lippincott Williams & Wilkins, 2008; originally proposed in Morray JP, et al. Coma scale for use in brain-injured children. *Crit Care Med*. 1984;12:1018.

Seizures

Seizures are brief manifestations of the brain's electrical system that result from cortical neuronal discharge. Regardless of the etiology, the basic mechanism of a seizure is the same. Abnormal electrical discharge may arise from central areas of the brain that may affect consciousness. This activity may be restricted to one area of the cerebral cortex or spread to other portions of the brain. Seizures are the most commonly observed neurologic deficit in children and may occur with various central nervous system conditions. The symptoms depend on the origin of the electrical location in the brain (Box 39.5). At least 8% of the general population will experience one or more seizures in their lifetime, and approximately 1% will develop epilepsy, involving recurring seizures.[26] The incidence of causative factors that are associated with seizures in children is related to the child's age. In infants, the most common factors are related to birth traumas (ie, anoxia, congenital defects, intracranial bleeds).[26] Acute infections are a common cause in late infancy and early childhood but uncommon in a child who is in middle childhood. In children who are older than 3 years, the most common cause of seizures is idiopathic epilepsy.[26] As children enter adolescence, hormonal and metabolic changes may alter the seizure threshold. A child who is in an unconscious state must be evaluated for a history of seizures because unconsciousness may be the result of a postictal state.

Nursing management of seizures includes providing a safe environment for the child, monitoring respiratory status and perfusion, assessing for the cause of the seizure, determining methods to prevent additional seizures, and documenting the seizure activity. Children admitted to the critical care unit may require intubation for respiratory complications of seizures, for the sedative effects of anticonvulsants, or for status epilepticus. Anticonvulsant therapy may be indicated for prolonged or recurrent seizures. The primary therapy for seizure disorders is

BOX 39.5 Causes of Seizures in Children

Nonrecurrent (Acute)

- Febrile episodes
- Intracranial infection
- Intracranial hemorrhage
- Space-occupying lesions (cyst, tumor)
- Acute cerebral edema
- Anoxia
- Toxins
  - Drugs
  - Tetanus
  - Lead (encephalopathy)
  - *Shigella, Salmonella*
- Metabolic alterations
  - Hypocalcemia
  - Hypoglycemia
  - Hyponatremia or hypernatremia
  - Hypomagnesemia
  - Alkalosis
  - Disorders of amino acid metabolism
  - Deficiency states
  - Hyperbilirubinemia

Recurrent (Chronic)

- Idiopathic epilepsy
- Epilepsy resulting from
  - Trauma
  - Hemorrhage
  - Anoxia
  - Infections
  - Toxins
  - Degenerative phenomena
  - Congenital defects
  - Parasitic brain disease
  - Hypoglycemic injury
- Epilepsy—sensory stimulus
- Epilepsy—stimulating states
  - Narcolepsy and catalepsy
  - Psychogenic causes
  - Tetany from hypocalcemia, alkalosis
- Hypoglycemic states
  - Hyperinsulinism
  - Hypopituitarism
  - Adrenocortical insufficiency
  - Hepatic disorders
- Uremia
- Allergy
- Cardiovascular dysfunction or syncopal episodes
- Migraine

Modified from Schultz R, Hockenberry M. The child with cerebral dysfunction. In: Hockenberry MJ, Wilson D, eds. *Wong's Nursing Care of Infants and Children*. 9th ed. St. Louis: Mosby; 2011.

administration of the appropriate antiepileptic medication or a combination of medications to provide the desired effort without causing undesirable side efforts. Medications that may be used for a child with seizures include phenobarbital, phenytoin (Dilantin), levetiracetam (Keppra), fosphenytoin, and benzodiazepines (lorazepam, diazepam).[26]

Status Epilepticus

Status epilepticus is a medical emergency that requires immediate intervention to prevent possible brain injury or death.[26] This condition is characterized by two or more unprovoked seizures that may be caused by a variety of pathologic processes in the brain.[26] Causes may include high fever, meningitis, encephalitis, metabolic disorders, and abrupt cessation of anticonvulsant medications. Cerebral blood flow, metabolic requirements, and oxygen needs all increase when a seizure occurs. A video electroencephalogram is required to confirm status epilepticus in patients in a deep coma or with pharmacologic paralysis. Magnetic resonance imaging may be performed to evaluate the brain for any anatomic abnormalities. The goal of treatment is to control the seizures or reduce their frequency and severity, to discover the correct cause of the seizures, or to evaluate the child for possible epilepsy surgery.[27] This will allow the child live as normal a life as possible. Treatment includes short-term administration of anticonvulsant medications such as diazepam, lorazepam, or midazolam. The critical care nurse should assess and evaluate the child to ensure that the patient has a patent airway, adequate ventilation effort, and adequate oxygenation and systemic perfusion. Clinical documentation should contain the patient's neurologic assessment, including the seizure manifestation and duration. With rapid treatment of the seizures, it may be possible to prevent neuronal damage, systemic complications, and even death from status epilepticus.[28]

Bacterial Meningitis

Meningitis is an acute inflammation of the meninges, the outer covering of the brain and spinal cord, and cerebrospinal fluid. The pathogens usually come from a distant site and colonize. They enter the bloodstream, producing sepsis, and they invade the meninges.[29] The highest incidence is found among infants younger than age 1 year. Meningococcal meningitis is readily transmitted by droplet infection from nasopharyngeal secretions. The risk of transmission increases with the number of contacts. This may occur most frequently in school-age children or adolescents.[26]

The clinical manifestations of bacterial meningitis include fever, chills, headache, vomiting, irritability or lethargy, photophobia, nuchal rigidity, and a positive Kernig (pain with extension of the legs) or Brudzinski sign (flexion of the neck stimulates flexion at the knees and hips). One of the most dramatic and serious complications usually associated with meningococcal infection is meningococcal sepsis or meningococcemia. When the onset is severe and sudden, it is known as *Waterhouse-Friderichsen syndrome*. This syndrome is characterized by overwhelming septic shock, disseminated intravascular coagulation, massive bilateral adrenal hemorrhage, and purpura.[26] Meningococcemia requires emergency treatment and critical care because of the high mortality rate.[26] The late stages of this disease may produce increased ICP and cardiovascular collapse. Symptoms in infants are less specific and may include lethargy, vomiting, bulging fontanels, hypothermia or hyperthermia, diarrhea, and poor feeding.

Nursing management must include early recognition and immediate start of therapies to prevent possible disabilities. Initial management includes use of isolation precautions, initiation of antibiotic therapy, maintenance of ventilation and hydration, reduction of increased ICP, management of systemic shock, control of seizures and temperature, and provision of family education and support.[26] Because of the sudden nature of the illness, emotional support of the child and parents is extremely important. Parents frequently feel guilty for not having suspected the seriousness of this disease. They should be kept informed about their child's progress and all procedures and results.[26] The complications of bacterial meningitis may include the development of hearing loss, hydrocephalus, loss of digits or parts of extremities, and possible death. The long-term effect on infants manifests as communicating hydrocephalus; in the older child, the effects are related to the inflammatory process or vasculitis associated with the disease. Hearing impairment is the most common sequela of this disease.[26] Evaluation of the child's hearing for possible hearing loss is needed for at least 6 months after the infection.

Head Trauma

Unintentional injury is the leading cause of death in children between ages 1 and 17 years. The number of children in this age range dying of their injuries is higher compared with the total number of pediatric patients dying of the next nine leading causes.[3] Current evidence suggests that most injured children are not being treated in pediatric trauma centers. Approximately 47% of pediatric trauma care occurs in nontrauma centers.[30] The best outcome after pediatric trauma occurs when the clinical team is prepared and knowledgeable about the unique aspects of the injured child.[9] Much of the anxiety of taking care of injured pediatric patients is eliminated by having instruments, equipment, and medication dosages carefully precalculated. One effective practice in many centers is the use of the Broselow tape that is color coded for specific weight groups of infants and children (see Fig. 39.3).

Head trauma in pediatric patients is due to closed head injuries resulting from motor vehicle accidents, bicycle crashes, falls, or child abuse.[31] During infancy and childhood, the head is proportionally larger compared with the rest of the body. As a result, a child may be propelled head first in unrestrained crashes, causing acceleration-deceleration injuries when their heads hit objects. Child abuse resulting from blunt trauma to the head or from shaking is the leading cause of head injury among infants and young children.[31]

Traumatic brain injury (TBI) is the leading cause of childhood death and disability in developing nations. In the United States, 435,000 children visit the emergency department each year because of head trauma; of these patients, 37,000 require hospitalization.[32] Morbidity and mortality associated with head trauma are attributed to injury suffered in two distinct phases: the *primary* phase and the *secondary* phase. The primary phase of injury occurs at the moment of impact, when the mechanical forces cause direct disruption of the brain parenchyma. Primary injuries may be focal or diffuse in nature. Examples of focal brain injuries include intracranial contusion and extraaxial hemorrhage (epidural, subdural, or subarachnoid hemorrhage). Diffuse brain injury is typically produced by acceleration or deceleration forces that result in shear trauma at the interface of the white and gray matter.[32]

The secondary phase of injury comprises sequelae of local and systemic events triggered by the primary injury. The three basic mechanisms leading to secondary brain injury are ischemia, energy failure, and excitotoxicity resulting in cell death.[32] Other factors that may contribute to secondary brain injury include axonal injury and death, cerebral edema, and ICP abnormalities.[32]

Head injuries are classified on the basis of the GCS score for the patient: mild injuries with a GCS score of 13 to 15, which may be associated with brief loss of consciousness, disorientation, headache, or vomiting; moderate TBI with a GCS score of 9 to 12; and severe TBI with a GCS score of less than 8. Patients with moderate or severe TBI typically have more significant symptoms compared with symptoms seen with mild TBI as well as abnormal brain imaging. Children with severe TBI need to be admitted to a critical care unit for aggressive management and treatment of increased ICP.[31] Several studies on children with severe TBI have reported that an ICP greater than 20 mm Hg is associated with a poor outcome.[32] Thus therapy should be directed to maintain ICP below this level. Treatment goals include measures to ensure adequate cerebral oxygenation and prevention of secondary brain injury. The child's plan of care includes providing optimal ventilation and oxygenation, maintenance of a normal arterial partial pressure of carbon dioxide (Pco_2), maintenance of a normal ICP with monitoring and interventions, and maintenance of adequate systemic and cerebral perfusion pressures.[31]

Complications of head injuries include hemorrhage, infections, cerebral bleeding, cerebral edema, seizures, and brain herniation. Treatment is based on the clinical signs in the patient. Treatment for epidural hematoma is surgical intervention. Subdural hematomas are more common in children; treatment of a subdural hematoma may also be surgical intervention for large hematomas associated with increased ICP.[4]

Children, especially infants, are at risk for seizures after severe head injury. A child admitted to the critical care unit with a TBI must be constantly monitored for cerebral edema and signs of increased ICP. Two other potential complications of head injury—diabetes insipidus and syndrome of inappropriate antidiuretic hormone—are discussed in Chapter 32.

Nursing interventions include precise neurologic assessment, which includes use of GCS scores and monitoring for signs of increased ICP. The psychologic impact of injury on a child cannot be underestimated. Studies have shown that 60% of injured children have posttraumatic stress disorder symptoms immediately after the injury. Symptoms continue to be experienced 18 months after injury in 38% of children.[9] Children who survive severe head injuries often require extended rehabilitation services to improve long-term outcomes. The pediatric rehabilitation team should be involved in the care of the child while the child is in the critical care unit.

Working with the family of a child with a head injury is challenging. Information given to the parents must be accurate and consistent. The parents may be guilt-ridden, especially if they feel they could have prevented the injury. Parents are encouraged to interact with the child soothingly and gently, even if the child cannot respond. Reading books, making a tape of home activities, and bringing familiar toys or stuffed animals to the child are ways to involve the family in the care of the child.

If the child is not expected to survive, the parents should be informed. The child should be evaluated for brain death and possible organ donation. Before the tests begin, the parents are offered the opportunity to spend time with the child. If brain death has been determined, the parents are informed of the test results. Parents may be asked to participate in deciding when, not if, to discontinue support. If the decision has been made to discontinue the critical care treatment, the priorities for the critical care nurse include providing comfort and dignity for the child and the family.[33] The most important aspects of care for the families at this time are to show a genuinely caring attitude, to extend kindness and understanding, and to be present with them.[33] Parents must always be approached in a sensitive and compassionate manner. The critical care nurse is typically the member of the team who is closest to the family and the best person to help the family members prepare for the death of the child. Special circumstances such as the impending arrival of additional family members may influence the timing of the decision. Parents must be allowed to spend as much time as they desire with the child to see that everything possible has been done for their child.

GASTROINTESTINAL SYSTEM, FLUIDS, AND NUTRITION

Anatomy and Physiology

After birth, growth and maintenance of the small intestine require nutritional components and the stimulation that comes from having food in the gut lumen. The intestinal tracts of infants and young children are larger in relation to body weight compared with intestinal tracts of adults. Sodium and water conservation, which occurs in the large intestine, is an immature process in the infant. For the first 2 years of life, gut immunity is lower, and mucosal binding for bacterial toxins is greater. With these differences in immunity, sensitivity, and greater potential for fluid loss, infants and toddlers have greater morbidity and mortality rates associated with enteric infections compared with adults.[4]

Assessment and Treatment

The child's fluid requirements involve replacing output and insensible losses and extra fluid for the production of new intracellular and extracellular fluid during growth. Fluid maintenance for a child with normal renal and cardiac status may be calculated using several formulas, but these account only for basal metabolic needs and growth. The amount of fluid given to a pediatric patient must be determined by the child's clinical condition, fluid balance, and insensible water losses.[4] Table 39.8 provides guidelines for normal fluid and electrolyte maintenance for infants and children. Box 39.6 provides adjustments to fluid maintenance based on level of activity or increased metabolic rate associated with disease.

Fluid and electrolyte requirements are based on the patient's history, degree of dehydration, and presenting symptoms. Infants and children need more calories per body weight compared with adults for energy expenditure because of growth. Critical illness has a major impact on the nutritional status of a child. If a child is in a critical care unit for longer than 5 to 7 days, the chances of developing a serious nutritional deficiency increase significantly.[34] Suboptimal nutritional intake may result in malnutrition as well as poor recovery and outcomes. Nutritional support after the initial nutritional assessment is an essential aspect of care for the

TABLE 39.8 Normal Fluid and Electrolyte Maintenance for Infants and Children[4]

Component	Weight of Infant or Child	Total Amount
Fluids	1–10 kg	100 mL/kg/d (may be increased to 150 mL/kg for caloric requirements)
	11–20 kg	1000 mL + 50 mL/each kg over 10 kg
	>20 kg	1500 mL + 25 mL/each kg over 20 kg or 100 mL/100 kcal/d can be used for children of any weight or 1500 mL/m²/d can be used for children >10 g
Sodium		2–4 mEq/kg/d
Potassium		1–2 mEq/kg/d
Hourly fluid maintenance	1–10 kg	4 mL/kg/hr
	11–20 kg	40 mL + 2 mL/kg over 10 kg
	>20 kg	60 mL + 1 mL/kg over 20 kg

BOX 39.6 Adjustments to Fluid Maintenance

- Fever or hypothermia: increases or decreases 0.42 mL/kg for each 1°C > or < 37°C.
- Tachypnea: increases 25%–30%
- Humidified mechanical ventilation: decreases 12%
- Activity of non–critically ill, resting child: increases 10%
- Restless or active child: increases 30%
- Diaphoresis: increases 10%–25%
- High-humidity environment: decreases 25%–40%

Modified from Hazinski MF. *Nursing Care of the Critically Ill Child.* 3rd ed. St. Louis: Elsevier; 2013.

child. Malnutrition is a chronic problem among chronically ill hospitalized pediatric patients, and children younger than 5 years old are at an increased risk of death. Critical care nurses play an important role in the feeding of critically ill children. Many procedures such as placing feeding tubes, checking gastric retentions, performing mouth care, and administering enteral or parenteral nutrition are within the nursing domain.[34]

Parenteral Nutrition

Providing needed calories in the face of fluid restrictions is a significant problem for an infant or child who is critically ill if the intestinal tract is nonfunctional. One method that may provide the necessary nutrition is parenteral nutrition. This form of nutrition is given by the intravascular route, and although it does not provide greater nutrition compared with enteral feedings, it may give sufficient support until enteral feeding is possible.[4] Table 39.9 outlines daily dextrose, lipid, and amino acid amounts; administration rates; and intravenous line concentration limits for an infant or child receiving total parenteral nutrition. The total parenteral nutrition solution should be tailored to account for the unique needs of each patient. Determination of the child's individual nutrient requirements

may vary, depending on such factors as age, weight, organ dysfunction, disease state, metabolic condition, body composition, and current medications.[35]

Enteral Nutrition

The enteral route is important for providing nutrition to a child.[34] Its advantages are convenience, safety, and low cost. The enteral route also is important in maintaining gastrointestinal mucosal integrity and immunologic function.[34]

Many different formulas based on age, host factors, and nutritional requirements are available for the infant or child. Amounts for formula feeds are based on needed kilocalories per kilogram per day and tolerance for each child and the clinical condition. For a full-term infant younger than 1 year, cow's milk–based formulas (Enfamil, Similac) or soy-based formulas (Isomil, ProSobee) are most commonly given. Standard dilution for infant formulas is 20 kcal/ounce.[36] Human breast milk is highly recommended for feedings for infants. Feedings designed specifically for children between 1 and 6 years old include infant formulas, pediatric follow-up formulas, pediatric enteral formulas, various homemade and pureed feedings, and commercial adult formulas.[36] Adult formulas may be given to children older than 6 years. Osmolite and Isocal are preferred for their isotonicity and caloric and protein content.

Continuous gavage feedings have advantages over bolus feedings. The risk for aspiration is less, particularly for an infant with reflux. In practice, the individual child's tolerance ultimately dictates the method on how the formula is delivered. Feeding pumps are typically used to control the rate of continuous-drip feeding. The important features of the enteral pump for use with children is the ability to provide low delivery rates (less than 5 mL/h) and to advance in small increments (1 to 5 mL/h).[36]

Gastric and duodenal or jejunal feeding tubes are used to administer enteral feeds in a critically ill child.[34] Gastric feeding tubes can be placed easily at the bedside by the nurse. Determining the insertion length of a nasogastric tube in a child has traditionally been the same as that in an adult—naris to ear to xyphoid process. However, this measurement may not always allow for all the side holes of a feeding tube to be in the stomach. Measuring to a point between the xyphoid and the umbilicus is a safer method. Table 39.10 provides guidelines for gavage feeding tube sizes and feeding rates for infants and children. Nasoduodenal or transpyloric tubes are recommended to reduce the risk of aspiration in the presence of delayed gastric emptying or reflux. These tubes also ensure the delivery of enteral feeds to the main sites of nutrient absorption. Gastric retention, diarrhea, and abdominal distention may limit the use of enteral nutrition. Parenteral nutrition should be considered when it is impossible to obtain enteral access or when enteral nutrition cannot meet the child's nutritional requirements.[34]

PAIN MANAGEMENT

The past 20 years of research has witnessed remarkable growth in pediatric pain management. Research has proven that infants and children do feel pain; when they are not treated, morbidity and mortality rates and hyperalgesia are increased. A negative impact on development of the infant or child may occur. Children experience pain not only from life-threatening

TABLE 39.9   Total Parenteral Nutrition Administration for Term Infants and Children

Per 24 Hours	INFANTS AND CHILDREN			
	10 kg	10–20 kg	20 kg	Adolescents
Fluids (mL/kg)	100–125	1000 mL: add 50 mL/kg for each extra kg >10 kg		1500 mL: add 20–25 mL for each extra kg >20 kg
Calories (kcal/kg)	75–90	75–90	>40	30–60
Protein (g/kg) Maximum peripheral: 2 g/kg/d Maximum central: 3.5 g/kg/d	2–2.5	1.5–2.5	1.5–2.5	1–2
Dextrose (%) Maximum peripheral: 10%–12.5% Maximum central: 30%	5–30	5–30	5–30	5–30
Fat (g/kg/d)	1–3	1–3	1–3	1–3
	Infants and Children (>2.5 kg and <11 y)		Children and Adults (>11 y)	
Vitamins (mL/d) MVI-peds (vitamin K = 0.2 mg/5 mL) MVI-13 (vitamin K = 0.15 mg/10 mL)	5 mL/d		10 mL/d	
Heparin[a]	0–0.5 U/mL		0–0.5 U/mL	
Levocarnitine[b]	>30 days = 5 mg/kg/d		>30 days = 1–5 mg/kg/d	

MVI, multiple vitamins for infusion; *PN,* parenteral nutrition; *TPN,* total parenteral nutrition.
[a]Recommended for slow infusion rates.
[b]Prematurity or TPN dependent.
Based on the guidelines from American Society for Parenteral and Enteral Nutrition.[45]

TABLE 39.10   Guidelines for Gavage Feeding in Infants and Children[35]

Parameters	Age and Size Determinations				
Age	3 mo	6 mo	2 y	5 y	10 y
Tube size	6 Fr	8 Fr	10 Fr	12 Fr	14 Fr

Method	Initial Volume and Rate	Advancement Volume and Rate
Bolus	2–5 mL/kg every 3–4 h over 20 min	2–5 mL/kg every other feeding
Continuous	1–2 mL/kg/h; initial volume not to exceed 55 mL/h regardless of child's weight	1–2 mL/kg every 8–12 h

Fr, French sizing.

diseases but also from injuries, surgeries, burns, and infections. Children also experience pain from many of the procedures and investigations used by physicians and nurses to investigate and treat disease.[37]

Physiology and Pharmacokinetics

Neurotransmitters and peripheral and central neural pathways for pain transmission are developed and are functional before birth, and they continue to mature during the first 2 years of life. After age 2 years, the perception of pain is the same for adults and children, but the psychosocial and behavioral expressions of the responses to pain change with the child's growth and developmental stage.[4] The nerve tracts to the brain are myelinated by 30 weeks of gestation, and the thalamocortical tracts are myelinated by 37 weeks of gestation, indicating that neonates are able to perceive all forms of pain. No perfect guide exists for providing analgesia to a pediatric patient. Children may demonstrate wide variations in the medications needed, the duration and dosing requirements, and the responses to the medications.[4] Each child must be monitored for his or her response to the pain therapy.

The physiologic effects of untreated pain in a child may result in the following:
- Hyperglycemia from decreased insulin secretion with breakdown of carbohydrate and fat stores
- Metabolic acidosis from increased use of fat
- Increased corticosteroids, growth hormone, and catecholamines
- Increased pulmonary vascular resistance
- Hypoxemia

Assessment

Pain assessment is the key to effective pain management. Many of the factors that influence pain in an adult also influence pain in a child. One difference is the influence of parental anxiety and behavior regarding their child's overall experience of pain. Although most pain research has involved procedural pain, it is important to be cognizant of the acute and chronic pain and distress associated with the critical care unit and its repetitive procedures.

The child may not spontaneously express his or her need for pain treatment. Staff members must be vigilant and actively explore a child's level of pain whenever the potential for pain exists. A child's verbal statement of pain is the most reliable indicator in acute pain management. However, this approach may not be possible with a preverbal child, a child who cannot comprehend the request to symbolically identify pain, or a child who has a significantly altered level of consciousness. For children up to age 3 years, behavioral scales are used as the primary source for pain assessment, and physiologic parameters are used as secondary sources. One such tool is the Face, Legs, Activity, Crying, and Consolability (FLACC) postoperative pain scale.

For children at least 6 years old, self-reports are the primary assessment tool, with behavioral scales used as secondary sources. For children 3 to 6 years old, self-reports may be used, but with a caveat. Many self-report scales have been tested as effective with this age group, but younger children 3 to 4 years old may have difficulty using them. Cognitive ability may not be advanced enough, or the child might have regressed in cognitive ability because of the illness. The child's rating may indicate a mood state rather than pain. Within this age group, self-reports and behavioral scales may need to be used together to get a true picture of the child's pain. One of the most valuable clues to pain relief is a change in behavior and vital signs after the administration of pain medication.

Parents often are the primary source of information about how their child exhibits pain. Parents are sensitive to changes in the child's behavior and often want to be involved in efforts for the child's pain relief. Encouraging parents to be involved gives them a sense of control and helping. Parents usually know what comfort measures to take with their children when they are in pain. For most children, having the supportive presence of their parents provides the most comfort. (See Chapter 8 for a discussion of pain-rating scales.)

Treatment of Pain

Some general principles are applied to the management of pain in children, as follows:

- *Prevention of pain:* If pain can be anticipated, pain should be treated prophylactically.
- *Adequate assessment:* Developmentally appropriate assessment tools are available.
- *Multimodal approach:* Analgesics; physical strategies such as massage, acupuncture, and hot or cold therapies; and behavioral, cognitive, and psychological approaches are available.
- *Parental involvement:* Parents are the best source of information about their child. They should be taught different strategies to help their child cope with the pain.
- *Nonnoxious routes:* The route of administration of analgesia should be as painless as possible.
- *Pain control during procedures:* Inadequate pain control during procedures may create an atmosphere of anxiety and increased pain during subsequent procedures.

Nonsteroidal Antiinflammatory Drugs

Nonsteroidal antiinflammatory drugs (NSAIDs) are effective for the management of mild to moderate pain, and they may be used in combination with opioids. They have superior antiinflammatory properties compared with aspirin or acetaminophen.[4] The drawbacks to NSAIDs is that a ceiling effect exists, and they affect the gastric mucosa, decrease platelet aggregation, and cause peptic ulcer formation and hepatic dysfunction. It is recommended that a histamine-2 receptor blocker be given concurrently for prolonged use of these medications.[24] The use of NSAIDs should be avoided in children with a history of severe renal disease, dehydration, or heart failure.[24] Examples of NSAIDs commonly used are ibuprofen and ketorolac. Ketorolac is the only NSAID that is approved for parenteral use by the US Food and Drug Administration.[38]

Opioid Analgesics

Narcotic analgesics are the most important class of medications for the relief of moderate to severe pain. Administration of narcotics requires decisions about the route of administration of the medication, the choice of narcotic, and the method of administration. The most commonly used narcotics for children are morphine, fentanyl, and hydromorphone. Methadone is an extremely long-acting narcotic, but it is not used as commonly for acute pain control. This medication is used for weaning from iatrogenic narcotic dependency or for control of chronic pain.[4] Meperidine is not a medication of choice because it decreases cardiac output and causes tachycardia. The medication's metabolite lowers the child's seizure threshold, causing hyperexcitability with multiple dosing. Opioids are given by intravenous push, continuous infusion, patient-controlled analgesia, or epidural injection. Table 39.11 outlines standard dosages of morphine, fentanyl, and hydromorphone for infants and children. Ketorolac in combination with morphine patient-controlled analgesia has provided a very effective combination of analgesia in children.[38]

Naloxone is an opioid antagonist that is required if the child becomes unresponsive after receiving narcotics, the respirations become shallow and less than 8 per minute, and the pupils become pinpoint. The initial dose is 1 to 2 mcg/kg/dose given intravenously over 2 minutes. The patient will need to be observed for the response to the medication. If patient is not responsive, the medication is continued until a total dose of 10 mcg/kg/dose has been given.[24]

Topical Anesthetics

The use of topical analgesic ointments reduces the local pain of procedures such as suturing or venipuncture and reduces the child's anticipated pain and anxiety over the upcoming procedure. The use of these agents has been expanded to include pain reduction for lumbar punctures or bone marrow aspiration. Some ointments take approximately 10 to 60 minutes to be effective. Ela-Max is a topical formulation of 4% lidocaine that is encapsulated by liposomes, which create lipid solubility and allow transdermal medication delivery. Ela-Max provides anesthesia in approximately 30 minutes.[24] A transdermal patch, Synera, containing lidocaine and tetracaine, may also be used on children older than age 3 years.[24] Lidocaine iontophoresis allows active transdermal delivery of lidocaine under the influence of a low-level electric current. It is available as Numby Stuff. Numby Stuff provides topical anesthesia to a child in 10 minutes.

Nonpharmacologic Management of Pain

Nonpharmacologic techniques should be used to supplement, not replace, the use of pain medications. Some nonpharmacologic interventions that may be used in children include distraction, relaxation, guided imagery, and cutaneous stimulation. The use of these techniques may decrease the perceived threat of pain, provide a sense of control, enhance the child's comfort, and promote rest or sleep. These nonpharmacologic techniques

TABLE 39.11	Opioid Dosages for Infants and Children	
Agent	**Age**	**Dosage**
Morphine		
IVP	<6 mo	0.025–0.03 mg/kg/dose. Lower dosage recommended for infants ≤3 months old.
	>6 mo	0.1 mg/kg/dose
Continuous infusion		Titrate to 0.01–0.14 mg/kg/h; maximum 10 mcg/kg/h
PCA		For children ≥5 years old and weighing ≤50 kg
		Usual concentration: 1 mg/mL
		Demand dose: 0.01–0.003 mg/kg/dose
		Usual basal rate: 0–0.03 mg/kg/h
Epidural		0.001–0.005 mg/kg/h for continuous infusions
Fentanyl		
Intravenous (short procedure), intermittent		1–2 mcg/kg/dose (if sedation used: 1–2 mcg/kg/dose)
Continuous infusion		1–3 mcg/kg/h
Epidural		0.2–2 mcg/kg/h, possibly with bupivacaine
Hydromorphone		
Intravenous		0.015 mg/kg/dose every 3–6 h
PCA		For children ≥5 years weighing ≤50 kg
		Usual concentration: 0.2 mg/mL
		Demand dose: 0.003–0.004 mg/kg/dose
		Usual basal rate: 0–0.004 mg/kg/h

IVP, intravenous push; *PCA*, patient-controlled analgesia.
From *Lexi-Comp Online Formulary*. http://www.crlonline.com/crlsql/servlet/crlonline. Accessed September 2015.

are safe, noninvasive, and usually inexpensive, and most are independent nursing functions.

Oral sucrose is a valuable analgesic option for neonates undergoing a brief painful procedure. It has a rapid onset of effect and short-lived action thought to be mediated by the release of endogenous brain opioids. Use of sugar has a low risk, and it is simple to administer to the neonate.[39]

PSYCHOSOCIAL ISSUES OF THE CHILD AND FAMILY

An unplanned admission of a child to a critical care unit, including children with illnesses or injuries, is a traumatic event for parents and for the child. In a crisis situation, parents may feel overwhelmed and become focused solely on the physiologic well-being of their child. If the child is conscious, he or she desperately needs the continual physical presence and emotional support of the parents; however, this is a time when it may be very difficult for the parents to help their child emotionally. Critical care nurses encounter the child and family at a very emotionally vulnerable time. Parents may view the nurses and physicians as their lifeline, controlling the needs and the life of their child.[4] A common complaint of families and patients is the lack of accuracy, clarity, and consistency of the information that is presented to them. Family members indicate a willingness and desire that bad news be empathetically communicated.[40] The critical care nurse needs to be knowledgeable about childhood cognitive and emotional development and about family dynamics to assist the child and the family through this health crisis. The following sections address some common issues that hospitalized children and their families face during hospitalization.

The Ill Child's Experience of Critical Illness

The term *family-centered care* defines the focus of care for a child because the nursing care of a child involves not only the child but also the family as a whole. Family-centered care supports the child's family by prioritizing the family members' needs and values and empowering the family unit.[41] Two basic concepts in family-centered care are *enabling* and *empowering*. The critical care staff enable families by creating opportunities and means for family members to be present during examinations and procedures.[32] Empowerment describes the interaction of the staff members with the families in a way that allows the families to maintain control or acquire a sense of control over their lives.

The emotional reactions of the child to hospitalization depend on the type and quantity of stress produced by the illness itself, the hospitalization experience, and the notions that the child has about the situation. The final outcome is influenced by the child's age and level of development. A child in the critical care unit experiences significant stress, and the important question is whether the child's capacity to cope physically or emotionally in an age-appropriate fashion is exceeded.

Three elements help a child cope successfully with a crisis: (1) a resilient personality, (2) a supportive family, and (3) an outside support system.[4] The critical care health team members serve as the outside support system, applying the family-centered concept as they reinforce and strengthen the coping efforts of the child and family. Nurses must take every opportunity to reassure the parents that they are an integral part of their child's care and recovery. When children were asked who or what helped the most while they were in the pediatric critical care unit, 43% stated their nurses were the most helpful, and 29% said that it was their families.[42] This is not a surprising finding considering that the critical care nurse has the most contact with the child in the critical care unit and provides most of the care to the child.[42]

A child who is critically ill needs the physical presence of the parents (or primary caretaker) at the bedside. Young children are most frightened by the separation from their parents. Unrestricted visitation (ie, 24 h/day) for parents is imperative. The parents are the most reassuring persons in the child's eyes and are needed psychologically by the child to believe that he or she will not be abandoned, left to be unsafe, or left in pain and distress. Anxiety and fear are easily heightened when the child recognizes scary words or fills in ambiguities heard with his or her own distorted interpretations. For a child who is very ill and prostrate, anxieties may fester within, unknown to staff members. Every member of the health care team should have an understanding of the five phases of development of logical thought—infancy, toddlerhood, preschool age, school age, and adolescence—to communicate effectively with a child and should understand the basis of a child's perceptions, fears, and misunderstandings.[4]

Parents' Experience of a Child's Critical Illness

When their child is admitted to the critical care unit, parents may experience a staged response similar to the grief process.[4] With a sudden illness or injury, the initial emotions may be shock, disbelief, and denial. These feelings may last for a few hours or a few days. Parents may question the diagnosis or want to prove the physician wrong. The situation may feel unreal, as if it were not happening to them. It may be difficult to grasp the totality of what has happened to their child. They may feel paralyzed and not know what they should do next. The parents may find it difficult to remember and process explanations given to them about what is happening with their child. This is usually a defense against pain. Forgetting may result in some parents feeling that staff members do not explain much to them. Other parents may feel that this is a sign of their own inadequacy. Explanations about their child's condition may have to be given in small increments of information with compassion and repetition. Some parents may appear to be competent and composed during the height of the crisis, but this should not be interpreted as their being less stressed or anxious.

Parents need to be reunited with their child, if this is their wish, as soon as they have been prepared about what to expect. However, parents may be afraid to see their child. Changes in their child's appearance and in the child's emotional reactions will be very upsetting to parents. If the child is conscious and relatively alert, the parents need to be informed that their child may show some form of regressive behavior such as withdrawal or anger, which is to be expected given the stress of the situation and the degree of illness or injury. Parents also may feel frightened about touching or talking to their child, believing that this may harm the child. They must be reassured that they can do this and that if they have any concerns, staff members will be present in the room to help them.

Intense anxiety may make parents question whether their reactions are normal. They wonder how other parents feel or behave. They may be extremely frightened by the intensity of their feelings and may wonder whether they are going to have a breakdown. These feelings are common in a crisis, and parents need to hear that their feelings are understandable. Some parents may behave with hostility toward staff or family members. Some may behave quite rigidly, visiting only briefly or not asking questions in an attempt to maintain composure.

Anger is an emotion that usually takes its toll after the crisis period, usually with longer critical care unit stays. Destructive anger occurs when parents seek justification for their anger by blaming others for their child's condition. They are unreasonably critical of the health care team and may make complaints about the child's care as a manifestation of the anger. Parents may become depressed as they realize the severity of their child's condition. At this time, parents should be given an opportunity to express their feelings and participate in activities such as bathing the child.

The critical care nurse can assist the parents by clarifying information and by helping them support their child.[44] During crises, communication with the parents must be frequent and clear. Key elements to effective communication include communication at frequent, predictable intervals; use of consistent, understandable terminology; provision of opportunities for

parents to ask questions and express opinions; and assistance of support personnel.[4] The primary focus in decision making should be the interests of the child.[40]

Critical care nurses who provide direct care to the child and parents have the greatest degree of contact with the family. In addition to the nurse's role in psychological assessment and intervention, other support staff members should be available to assist the family. The creation of an ethical working environment in the critical care unit is a necessary precondition for addressing ethical issues raised by specific parent situations.[40] Clinical nurse specialists assess parental worries and concerns and, based on the assessment, help the parents to make plans to address their concerns.[43] Social workers provide the family with support and advocacy during their time of crisis. Many critical care units also have access to child life specialists, chaplains, discharge planners, and ethicists to assist in providing psychosocial support to the families. Concern for the psychosocial and developmental well-being of pediatric patients and their families is the primary focus of the child life specialist.[41] An important role of the critical care nurse is to mobilize and introduce the families to the support staff available in their institutions for their support. The following case study discusses some of these concepts.

CASE STUDY 39.1 Pediatric Patient

Brief Patient History

A 2-month-old infant is admitted directly to the critical care unit with a history of vomiting and diarrhea over the past 24 hours. The mother reports that the infant was irritable yesterday but is more lethargic today. The infant has had three wet diapers over the past 24 hours, and the urine appears dark. She does not tolerate any formula or Pedialyte.

Clinical Assessment

Physical assessment reveals the following: weight, 6.84 kg (weight 1 week prior, 7.6 kg); temperature, 38.5°C; pulse, 180 beats/min; respiratory rate, 46–50 breaths/min; blood pressure, 60/43 mm Hg; and pulse oximetry, 93%. The infant's lips and mucous membranes are dry and tacky. Her fontanel is sunken. Extremities are cool and mottled, nail beds are dusky, and capillary refill is 4 seconds. Pulses are rapid and weak centrally and peripherally. The infant is lethargic.

Diagnostic Procedures

The infant is placed on oxygen, and intravenous access is attained. A point-of-care glucose test reveals blood sugar of 60 mg/dL.

Medical Diagnosis

The infant is diagnosed with hypovolemic, hypotensive shock.

Questions

1. For the bedside nurse, what is the priority in caring for this infant?
2. What category of shock applies to this situation?
3. Describe the pathophysiology of hypovolemic shock in a pediatric patient.
4. What are the two goals of therapy?
5. What level of dehydration does this infant appear to have?
6. Describe how and when to treat hypoglycemia in infants.
7. What is the fluid of choice to treat the volume deficit?
8. After the infant has received the initial volume replacement of two normal saline boluses, she is arousable. Vital signs are as follows: pulse of 160 beats/min, blood pressure of 70/40 mm Hg, capillary refill of 3 seconds, and blood glucose of 80 mg/dL. What is the next step in the treatment of the infant's hypovolemic shock?

SUMMARY

- Children are physically, physiologically, and emotionally immature, and they are different from adults.
- Complete respiratory failure may develop rapidly in a child when respiratory distress is present.
- In infants and children, most cardiac arrests result from progressive respiratory failure, shock, or both.
- Bradycardia is an ominous sign in a seriously ill or injured child.
- Hypotension is typically only a late sign of hypotensive shock in children.
- Head injury is a primary insult to a child. Patient outcomes are compromised if secondary insults such as hypotension or hypoxemia occur.
- Most children in the critical care unit experience pain and anxiety, and they should be treated accordingly.
- The concept of family-centered care recognizes that the family is the one constant in a child's life.

ⓔ Visit the Evolve Site for additional study materials.

REFERENCES

1. Park M: *Pediatric Cardiology for Practioners*, ed 5, Phildadelphia, 2008, Mosby.
2. Mullen J, Frances M: Caring for critically ill children and their families. In Slota M, editor: *Core Curriculum for Pediatric Critical Care Nursing*, ed 2, St. Louis, 2006, Mosby.
3. Guice K, et al.: Traumatic injury and children: a national assessment, *J Trauma* 36:S68, 2007.
4. Hazinski MF: Children are different. In Hazinski MF, editor: *Nursing Care of the Critically Ill Child*, ed 3, St. Louis, 2013, Elsevier, p 1.
5. American Heart Association: Pediatric Advanced Life Support, *Dallas*, 2011. ISBN 978-0-87493-527-1.
6. Grant M, Webster H: Pulmonary system. In Slota M, editor: *Core Curriculum for Pediatric Critical Care Nursing*, ed 2, St. Louis, 2006, Mosby.
7. Wilson D: The child with disturbance of oxygen and carbon dioxide. In Hockenberry M, et al, editors: *Wong's Nursing Care of Infants and Children*, ed 9, St. Louis, 2011, Mosby.
8. Slota M: Bioinstrumentation: principles and techniques. In Hazinski MF, editor: *Nursing Care of the Critically Ill Child*, ed 3, St. Louis, 2013, Elsevier, p 961.
9. Knudson M, McGrath J: Improving outcomes in pediatric trauma care: essential characteristics of the trauma center, *J Trauma* 63:S140, 2007.
10. Kline-Tilford A, et al.: Pulmonary disorders. In Hazinski MF, editor: *Nursing Care of the Critically Ill Child*, ed 3, St. Louis, 2013, Elsevier, p 483.
11. Kacmarek R, et al.: *The Essentials of Respiratory Care*, ed 4, St. Louis, 2005, Mosby.
12. Kuch B: Respiratory monitoring and support. In Hazinski MF, editor: *Nursing Care of the Critically Ill Child*, ed 3, St. Louis, 2013, Elsevier, p 1007.
13. Amin R: Chronic respiratory failure. In Chernick V, et al, editors: *Kendig's Disorders of the Respiratory Tract in Children*, ed 7, Philadelphia, 2006, Saunders.
14. Frankel L, Kache S: Mechanical ventilation. In Kliegman R, et al, editors: *Nelson's Textbook of Pediatrics*, ed 18, Philadelphia, 2007, Saunders.
15. Zentz S: Care of infants and children with bronchiolitis: a systematic review, *J Pediatr Nurs* 26:519, 2011.
16. Langley J, Bradley J: Defining pneumonia in critically ill infants and children, *Pediatr Crit Care Med* 6:S9, 2005.
17. Mansbach J, et al.: US outpatient office visits for bronchiolitis, 1993-2004, *Ambul Pediatr* 7:304, 2007.
18. American Academy of Pediatrics: AAP Updates Recommendations for Use of Palivizumub Against RSV. Released July 28th, 2014. Accessed on September 7th, 2015. https://www.aap.org/en-us/about-the-aap/aap-press-room/Pages/AAP-Updates-Recommendations-for-Use-of-Palivizumab-Against-RSV.aspx.
19. Wohl M: Bronchiolitis. In Chernick V, et al, editors: *Kendig's Disorders of the Respiratory Tract in Children*, ed 7, Philadelphia, 2006, Saunders.
20. Cambonie G, et al.: Clinical effects of Heliox administration for acute bronchiolitis in young infants, *Chest* 129:676, 2006.
21. Buckmaster A, et al.: Continuous positive airway pressure therapy for infants with respiratory distress in nontertiary care centers: a randomized controlled trial, *Pediatrics* 120:509, 2007.
22. Marcoux K: Current management of status asthmaticus in the pediatric ICU, *Crit Care Nurs Clin North Am* 17:463, 2005.
23. Gomez M, Felauer A: Asthma. In Reuter-Rice K, et al, editors: *Pediatric Acute Care: A Guide for Interprofessional Practice*, Burlington, MA, 2012, Jones & Bartlett Learning.
24. Lexi-Comp Online Formulary. Accessed on September 7th, 2015. http://www.crlonline.com/crlsql/servlet/crlonline.
25. Callow L, Suddaby E: Cardiovascular system. In Slota M, editor: *Core Curriculum for Pediatric Critical Care Nursing*, ed 2, St. Louis, 2006, Saunders.
26. Schultz R, Hockenberry M: The child with cerebral dysfunction. In Hockenberry MJ, et al, editors: *Wong's Nursing Care of Infants and Children*, ed 9, St. Louis, 2011, Mosby.
27. Schultz R, et al.: The child with cerebral dysfunction. In Hockenbery MJ, Wilson D, editors: *Wong's Nursing Care of Infants and Children*, ed 9, St. Louis, 2011, Mosby.
28. Smith G, et al.: Epilepsy update, part I: reining our understanding of a complex disease, *Am J Nurs* 115:40–56, 2015.
29. Vernon-Levett P: Neurologic system. In Slota M, editor: *Core Curriculum for Pediatric Critical Care Nursing*, ed 2, St. Louis, 2006, Saunders.
30. Ochoa C, et al.: Prior studies comparing outcomes from trauma care at children's hospitals versus adult hospitals, *J Trauma* 63:S87, 2007.
31. Pasek TA, Etzel KA: Multisystem issues. In Slota M, editor: *Core Curriculum for Pediatric Critical Care Nursing*, ed 2, St. Louis, 2006, Saunders.
32. O'Brien N: Traumatic brain injury. In Reuter-Rice K, et al, editors: *Pediatric Acute Care: A Guide for Interprofessional Practice*, Burlington, MA, 2012, Jones & Bartlett Learning.
33. Smith J, Martin S: Caring practice: providing developmentally supportive care. In Curley M, Maloney-Harmon P, editors: *Critical Care Nursing of Infants and Children*, ed 2, Philadelphia, 2001, Saunders.
34. Ista E, Joosten K: Nutritional assessment and enteral support of critically ill children, *Crit Care Nurs Clin North Am* 17:385, 2005.
35. Ratz N: Parental Nutrition. In Reuter-Rice K, et al, editors: *Pediatric Acute Care: A Guide for Interprofessional Practice*, Burlington, MA, 2012, Jones & Bartlett Learning.
36. Nevin-Filino N, Miller M: Enteral nutrition. In Samour P, King K, editors: *Handbook of Pediatric Nutrition*, ed 3, Sudbury, MA, 2003, Jones & Bartlett.
37. The International Association for the Study of Pain (IASP): Children's Pain Matters! Priority on Pain in Infants, Children and Adolescents. Accessed on September 7th, 2015. http://iasp.files.cms-plus.com/Content/Content Folders/GlobalYearAgainstPain2/20052006PaininChildren/8x5.pdf.
38. Drain C: *Perianesthesia Nursing: A Critical Care Approach*, ed 4, St. Louis, 2003, Saunders.
39. Paske T, et al.: Hospitalized infants who hurt: a sweet solution with oral sucrose, *Crit Care Nurse* 32(1):61, 2012.
40. Perkin R: Ethical issues in pediatric critical care. In Hazinski MF, editor: *Nursing Care of the Critically Ill Child*, ed 3, St. Louis, 2013, Elsevier, p 1071.
41. Pike M, Enright K: Child life: developmental considerations. In Reuter-Rice K, et al, editors: *Pediatric Acute Care: A Guide for Interprofessional Practice*, Burlington, MA, 2012, Jones & Bartlett Learning.
42. Board R: School-age children's perceptions of their PICU hospitalization, *Pediatr Nurse* 31:166, 2005.
43. McNelis A, et al.: Concerns with needs of children with epilepsy and their parents, *Clin Nurse Spec* 21:195, 2007.
44. Pietsch J, Chung D: Care of the child with burns. In Hazinski MF, editor: *Nursing Care of the Critically Ill Child*, ed 3, St. Louis, 2013, Elsevier, p 921.
45. Ayers P, et al.: A.S.P.E.N. parenteral nutrition safety consensus recommendations, *JPEN J Parenter Enteral Nutr* 38:296–333, 2014.
46. Cote CJ, Todres ID: The Pediatric airway. In Cote CJ, et al, editors: *A Practice of Anesthesia for Infants and Children*, ed 2, Philadelphia, 1993, WB Saunders CO, p 55.

40

The Older Adult Patient

Fiona Winterbottom and Misty Jenkins

The population of older adults in the United States is increasing as improvements in health care technology and therapies have led to an extended life expectancy.[1] This chapter provides an overview of the information a critical care nurse needs to know to properly care for an older adult patient.

In 2030, approximately 20% of the US population will be composed of older adults compared with 13% in 2010, and the average life expectancy will be approximately 79 years.[1,2] The societal implications of the aging population are far reaching, especially in health care. Scientific advances in medical therapies enhance the ability to resuscitate older adults, but the health care industry must be mindful and responsible in resource allocation and provision of services. Healthy People 2020 is a nationwide program created by the US Department Health and Human Services to address some of these issues with specific targets, which were developed in consultation with experts using the most current scientific knowledge.[1] These objectives help guide states, communities, and professional organizations to identify, develop, and evaluate programs and policies that promote healthy aging as well as measure the impact of prevention activities by encouraging collaboration across communities and empowering individuals to make informed health decisions.[1]

CHRONIC DISEASE IN OLDER ADULTS

Approximately 80% of older Americans are living with at least one chronic condition, and almost two-thirds have multiple chronic conditions including cardiovascular disease, cancer, chronic respiratory diseases, accidents, stroke, Alzheimer disease, diabetes, frailty, and significant physical and cognitive disabilities.[3] Chronic diseases pose significant individual and societal burden in terms of symptoms, functional ability, disability, and diminished quality of life (QOL). Of health care costs for older Americans, 95% are for chronic diseases; the cost of treating chronic illness in adults older than 65 is nearly three to five times higher compared with younger patients with chronic illness. Medicare health care spending is projected to increase from $555 billion in 2011 to $903 billion in 2020.[1,3,4]

The Society of Critical Care Medicine estimates that 45% of annual intensive care unit (ICU) admissions are patients older than age 65; 10% of ICU admissions are for patients 85 years old or older. Additionally, increasing numbers of elderly patients are admitted to medical ICUs compared with surgical ICUs with higher inpatient and 90-day mortality.[4] Older adults are frequently admitted for congestive heart failure, pneumonia, irregular heartbeat, septicemia, osteoarthritis, chronic obstructive pulmonary disease, urinary tract infections, and hip fractures. Common procedures performed for elderly patients include blood transfusion, diagnostic cardiac procedures, echocardiogram, upper gastrointestinal endoscopy, intubation/mechanical ventilation, and hemodialysis.[4] See Table 40.1 for leading causes of death in elderly adults.

HEART DISEASE AND AGE-RELATED CHANGES OF THE CARDIOVASCULAR SYSTEM

Age-related structural and cellular changes in the myocardium and peripheral vasculature have a significant impact on critically ill older adults.[5] The largest risk factor for cardiovascular disease in older adults is age. Cardiac and arterial system changes result in reduced cardiovascular function and reserve, leaving an older adult at increased risk for cardiac decompensation.

Myocardial Changes

The aging heart undergoes a modest degree of hypertrophy and thickening of the left ventricular (LV) wall without significant changes in LV cavity size.[6] Increase in LV wall thickness is primarily due to growth in muscle cell size, which can lead to reduced early diastolic filling and increased cardiac pressures.[7] Diastolic filling occurs in two cycles: passive (early diastolic phase) and active (late diastolic phase).[6] As early diastolic filling is reduced, most ventricular filling shifts to the active phase of late diastole relying on the atrial contraction.[6] Atrial contractions can contribute 70% of LV end-diastolic volume.[8] These alterations explain the relative intolerance of atrial fibrillation in some older adults.[8] Several other factors contribute to the changes in the myocardium including a decrease in the number of cardiomyocytes, increase in collagen accumulation, fibrosis, increased inflammatory cells and proteins, and changes in calcium signaling of cardiomyocytes.[8] Myocardial contraction is dependent on intracellular levels of free calcium and the sensitivity of the contractile proteins for calcium. The changes in calcium signaling lead to a prolonged duration of contraction (systole), which is caused in part by a slowed or delayed rate of myocardial relaxation.[6] Presence of an S_4 heart sound may be evident with reduced LV compliance.[9]

Vascular Changes

Vascular changes include endothelial dysfunction and arterial stiffness. The endothelium regulates vascular homeostasis by balancing vasodilators and vasoconstrictors.[8] A decrease in vasodilating substances such as nitric oxide has been well documented with aging.[8] Endothelial dysfunction results in arterial stiffening, which reduces blood flow and promotes atherosclerosis and thrombosis.[8] Atherosclerosis is the accumulation of

TABLE 40.1 Leading Causes of Death in Adults Older than 65 Years of Age

Cause of Death	Number of Deaths (per 100,000 Standard Population)
Heart disease	611,105
Cancer	584,881
Chronic lower respiratory diseases	149,205
Accidents (unintentional injuries)	130,557
Stroke (cerebrovascular diseases)	128,978
Alzheimer disease	84,767
Diabetes	75,578
Influenza and pneumonia	56,979
Nephritis, nephrotic syndrome, and nephrosis	47,112
Intentional self-harm (suicide)	41,149

Adapted from Murphy SL, et al. *Mortality in the United States, 2014.* NCHS data brief, no 229. Hyattsville, MD: National Center for Health Statistics; 2015.

lipoproteins and fibrinous products such as platelets, macrophages, and leukocytes within a vessel.[7] Arteriosclerosis is a gradual decrease in arterial compliance, or "stiffening of the arteries," that occurs as a result of the thickening of the intimal layer of the large and distal arteries secondary to an increase in smooth muscle cells and connective tissue.[7] Atherosclerotic and arteriosclerotic processes in older adults cause arteries to become progressively less distensible and alter the vascular pressure-volume relationship, leading to increases in afterload and development of concentric (pressure-induced) ventricular hypertrophy.[7] Increased arterial stiffness occurs from alterations in the arterial wall resulting in an increase in systolic blood pressure (BP), decrease in diastolic BP, and widening of pulse pressure. The effects of these changes can complicate treatment for systolic hypertension because of excessive lowering of diastolic BP and the risk for postural hypotension.[7]

Conduction and Beta-Adrenergic Changes

Heart rate modulation and adrenergic responsiveness are important changes in the aging cardiovascular system.[7] Heart rate decreases in both variability and maximal heart rate by loss of cells in the sinoatrial node, fibrosis, and hypertrophy, resulting in a slower conduction of electrical impulses throughout the heart.[7] Beta-adrenoceptors are located on cardiac and smooth muscle tissues. The cardiovascular system is affected by two types of beta-adrenoceptors: beta-1-adrenoceptors, primarily located in the heart, and beta-2-adrenoceptors, which are found within the smooth muscle of blood vessels. Beta-adrenoceptors bind to catecholamines, epinephrine, and norepinephrine, resulting in elevated heart rate, contractility, conduction velocity, relaxation, and systemic vasodilation. Normally during exercise or acute stress, there is an increase in heart rate, augmentation of myocardial contractility and relaxation, and reduced LV afterload.[6] With aging, these responses are diminished from a reduction in beta-adrenergic stimulation and an increase in parasympathetic vagal tone (slowing heart rate).[8] Decreased cyclic adenosine monophosphate generation, reduced beta-receptors, and increased inhibitory G protein activity are thought to be responsible for these alterations.[8] These deficits in sympathetic modulation occur in the presence of an increased production and release of circulating

catecholamines as a compensatory response to fewer cardiac muscarinic beta-receptors.[6,8] The changes consequently blunt the stress response and may cause orthostatic hypotension, syncope, and cardiac decompensation from lack of cardiac reserve.[8]

Electrocardiogram Changes

Changes in the electrocardiogram (ECG) include decreased R wave and S wave amplitude, increased P–R interval, and increased Q–T interval duration reflective of prolonged rate of relaxation.[6] The QRS axis shifts leftward with age, perhaps as a result of increased LV wall thickness or hypertrophy.[6] The senescent myocardium may have a lower threshold for atrial and ventricular arrhythmias because of changes in gene expression of proteins that regulate calcium.[6] Cardiac dysrhythmias include atrial fibrillation and paroxysmal supraventricular tachycardia; the most common dysrhythmia is premature ventricular contraction.[6] Reports show that 3% to 4% of patients older than 60 years experience atrial fibrillation, and the incidence may be 10% in patients 80 to 89 years old.[6,9] A study of healthy older patients with 24-hour ambulatory ECG recordings showed that 13% to 50% experienced short runs of paroxysmal supraventricular tachycardia (3-5 beats) in healthy adults.[6] Older individuals also have a high prevalence of LV hypertrophy, which predisposes them to ventricular arrhythmias and sudden death. Atrial fibrillation is thought to be related to increased arterial stiffness, reduced LV compliance, and reduced rate control, and anticoagulation is recommended for most patients.[10] Age-associated cardiac conduction changes (even if asymptomatic) are predictive of future cardiac morbidity and mortality in older adults.[6]

Left Ventricular Changes

Aging is associated with a decline in exercise performance secondary to many physiologic variables. Cardiac performance is dependent on the heart's ability to increase and maintain cardiac output (CO), allowing oxygen delivery to the peripheral tissues. During exercise, CO is increased by several mechanisms, the most important of which are increased heart rate, increased inotropic state of the myocardium, and decreased aortic impedance.[6] The Baltimore Longitudinal Study of Aging reported that older adults' diminished ability to exercise was not related to a difference in CO response.[6] Maximal heart rate achieved during exercise is attenuated in older adults; however, decreased heart rate response is accompanied by increased LV end-diastolic volume. As adults age, there is a progressive decline in maximum oxygen consumption, which begins in the second decade of life and decreases by approximately 10% per decade. As a result, an older individual's ability to exercise may be limited by reduction in cardiac reserve, increased vascular afterload, arterial-ventricular load mismatching, pulmonary function, reduced intrinsic myocardial contractility, impaired autonomic regulation, and physical deconditioning.[6]

Baroreceptor Changes

Baroreceptors are mechanoreceptors that respond to stretch and other changes in the blood vessel wall. They are located at the bifurcation of the common carotid artery and the aortic arch.[11] Impulses arising in the baroreceptor region project to the vasomotor center (nucleus of tractus solitarius) in the medulla. Abrupt changes in BP caused by changes in peripheral resistance, CO, or blood volume are sensed by baroreceptors, resulting in an increase in impulse frequency to the vasomotor center within the medulla. This increase inhibits vasoconstrictor impulses arising from the vasoconstrictor region within the medulla, resulting in a decrease in heart rate and peripheral vasodilation returning BP to within normal limits.[11] The baroreflex can be tested by measuring heart rate response (ie, increase or decrease in heart rate) after administration of a pressor or a depressor agent and by changing the patient's position from lying to standing. Baroreflex-mediated tachycardia response to depressor agents is also attenuated in older adults. There are several reports of attenuation in heart rate response of older adults after changes in position.[11] When an individual changes position from supine to standing, distribution of blood volume changes, resulting in a reduction in CO and BP. A simultaneous response by baroreceptors increases heart rate and maintains BP by increasing CO.[11] This is known as orthostatic hypotension.[12] The baroreceptor reflex response also mediates changes in peripheral resistance and force of myocardial contraction, which offsets the decrease in BP. Prevalence of orthostatic hypotension is greater in older patients, especially older patients in critical care, and judicious use of antihypertensive medications is recommended.[11]

Heart Failure and Myocardial Infarction

Chronic heart failure affects approximately 5.7 million people in the United States and may be a contributing cause of death in 282,000 individuals per year, at a predicted cost of $39 billion annually.[13] Approximately 50% of heart failure cases are found within the 6% of the US population older than age 75.[6] Chronic heart failure is the leading cause of hospitalizations for adults older than 65 years with an average 1-year mortality of 33% to 35%.[13] Incidence of myocardial infarction (MI) in the Framingham Heart Study demonstrated that the rate of MI doubles for older men and increases more than fivefold in older women.[13] Similar results were seen in the Atherosclerosis Risk in Communities surveillance study.[13] Critical care nurses should recognize that older adult patients not only are more likely than young patients to experience an MI, but also are more likely to die of MI.

MI is one of the most common causes of chronic heart failure leading to heart failure via an intricate process known as LV remodeling.[13] Age-associated changes in arterial structure and function cause large vessels to become less distensible, leading to prolonged systolic contraction, lengthened diastolic relaxation, increased myocardial oxygen demand, and diminished organ perfusion.[6] Additionally, atherosclerotic coronary arteries may limit blood flow to the myocardium, creating a higher risk of developing myocardial ischemia or MI. MI in older adults is often associated with ST segment depression rather than ST segment elevation. Sensation of chest pain may be altered and may be less intense and of shorter duration.[5] Other atypical symptoms may include dyspnea, confusion, and failure to thrive, which results in unrecognized signs and symptoms of cardiac problems and delays in diagnosis and treatment.[5]

Hypertension

The population is aging, and hypertension affects most individuals older than 65 years of age.[10] Pathophysiology of hypertension in older adults results from changes in arterial structure and function that decrease distensibility of large vessels, reduce forward circulation flow, increase pulse wave velocity, cause late systolic BP augmentation, and increase myocardial oxygen demand, all of which limit organ perfusion.[10] Older adults

with poor BP control have an increased risk of cerebrovascular disease, coronary artery disease (CAD), disorders of LV structure and function, aortic and peripheral arterial disease, chronic kidney disease (CKD), ophthalmologic disorders, and QOL issues.[10] Secondary issues related to hypertension include renal artery stenosis, obstructive sleep apnea, primary aldosteronism, and thyroid disorders. Older adult patients with higher baseline systolic BP or longer duration of hypertension often experience autonomic dysfunction, microvascular damage, and CKD related to reduced renal tubular mass, fewer transport pathways for potassium excretion, and hyperkalemia.[10] Glomerulosclerosis and interstitial fibrosis lead to progressive renal dysfunction and reduction in glomerular filtration rate, increased intracellular sodium, reduced sodium-calcium exchange, and volume expansion.[10] Older adults generally have contracted intravascular volumes and impaired baroreflexes, which may be exacerbated by diuretics, sodium, and water depletion, causing orthostatic hypotension. Volume overload is commonly due to excessive salt intake, inadequate kidney function, or insufficient diuretic therapy. An age-related decline in plasma renin activity, tubular function, and glomerular filtration rate affects overall sodium and water homeostasis.[5]

Hyperlipidemia and Metabolic Syndrome

Improved cardiovascular care has led to delay of cardiovascular disease; however, monitoring of cardiovascular risk factors such as cholesterol, BP, and obesity is now needed in the older adult population.[14] Lipoprotein levels increase with advancing age, adding to risk factors for development and progression of atherosclerosis. Serum lipoproteins are particles that contain various amounts of cholesterol, triglycerides, phospholipids, and apoproteins. The classification of lipoproteins is based on their size and relative concentration of cholesterol, triglycerides, and apoproteins. The five principal serum lipoproteins are chylomicrons, low-density lipoproteins (LDLs), very-low-density lipoproteins, intermediate-density lipoproteins, and high-density lipoproteins. Lp(a) lipoprotein is composed of an LDL-like particle that in elevated levels has been implicated as a strong risk factor for coronary heart disease and stroke.[15] Timely identification of high-risk individuals with high Lp(a) lipoprotein may allow for therapy such as statins to reduce LDL cholesterol to recommended levels.[15]

Another condition that may warrant attention in patients older than 65 years is metabolic syndrome. Metabolic syndrome is characterized by a group of risk factors including abdominal obesity; high triglycerides; low high-density lipoproteins; small LDL particles; elevated BP; proinflammatory, prothrombotic states; and high plasma insulin (insulin resistance).[14] Metabolic syndrome has been reported to increase cardiovascular and mortality risk in middle-aged adults secondary to glucose metabolism and insulin resistance that is linked to cholesterol metabolism.[14] Reduction of risk associated with diabetes and metabolic syndrome may be modulated by manipulation of cholesterol absorption, leading to fewer events and improved survival in older adult cardiovascular patients.[14]

Heart Disease Management

Risk stratification tools such as the Framingham Risk Score can be used to predict MI, stroke, or cerebrovascular disease.[10] Evaluation of older adult patients with known or suspected hypertension should include identification of reversible or treatable causes, evaluation of organ damage, assessment for other risk factors, and identification of treatment barriers. Recommended laboratory testing for hypertensive patients includes urinalysis, serum chemistries, lipid profile, blood glucose testing (including hemoglobin A_{1c}), ECG and echocardiography.[10]

Treatment of cardiovascular risk factors in older adults includes aggressive treatment of dyslipidemia with lipid-lowering medication, control of blood glucose, and lifestyle modification. There should be consideration that QOL issues such as cognitive function, physical activity, and sexual function are reduced by aging and disease.[10] Drug treatment is recommended for older adult hypertensive patients with attention to alterations in medication distribution and disposal, changes in homeostatic cardiovascular control, and QOL factors. Lifestyle modification may be the only treatment necessary for milder forms of hypertension in older adults. Smoking cessation, weight reduction, increased physical activity, and sodium restriction result in greater benefit in older individuals than in younger adults.[10]

Pharmacologic Management of Hypertension

The Eighth Joint National Committee Guidelines set BP goals based on age, diabetes, and CKD.[12] In adults older than 60 years without diabetes or CKD, BP goals are systolic BP less than 150 mm Hg and diastolic BP less than 90 mm Hg.[12] If diabetes is present without CKD or CKD is present with or without diabetes, BP goals are systolic BP less than 140 mm Hg and diastolic BP less than 90 mm Hg.[12] Pharmacologic recommendations vary based on age, underlying comorbidities, and race.[12] For African Americans of any age with diabetes without CKD and African Americans older than 60 years, initial treatment consists of a thiazide-type diuretic or calcium channel blocker alone or in combination.[12] An angiotensin-converting enzyme inhibitor or angiotensin receptor blocker may be used alone or in combination with a thiazide-type diuretic and calcium channel blocker as an initial treatment for adults of all other races who are older than 60 years old or adults of any age with diabetes without CKD.[12] If CKD is present, an angiotensin-converting enzyme inhibitor or angiotensin receptor blocker alone or in combination with other drug classes is recommended.[12] Beta-blockers are no longer used as first-line antihypertensive agents.[12]

Cardiac Medication Considerations in Older Adults

Treatment with medication should be considered when nonpharmacologic interventions are unsuccessful (Table 40.2). Heart rate control can be managed with beta-blockers and calcium channel blockers. Amiodarone can be used for conversion and maintenance of sinus rhythm with atrial fibrillation.[10] Aging increases the risk of major hemorrhage in patients with atrial fibrillation, with or without warfarin therapy.[10] Anticoagulation therapy can be complicated by polypharmacy, simultaneous use of antiplatelet medications, uncontrolled hypertension, and poorly controlled anticoagulation therapy.[16] Ventricular dysrhythmias are best managed with pharmacologic therapy and cardiac resynchronization therapy (CRT) in patients with advanced heart failure.[17] CRT involves a type of pacemaker or pacemaker/defibrillator that resynchronizes the contractions of the heart's ventricles by sending electrical impulses to the heart muscle, assisting blood flow and vascular remodeling. CRT has become an established therapy for advanced heart failure LV reverse remodeling, with significant reduction in LV

volumes and improvement in LV ejection fraction.[17] CRT has been shown to improve QOL in patients with advanced heart failure.[18] Cardiac defibrillators implanted after MI may be considered in patients with New York Heart Association class II or III chronic heart failure and LV ejection fraction of 35% or less to prevent sudden cardiac death.[18] Implantable cardioverter defibrillators deliver an electrical shock when an abnormal rhythm is detected. This therapy has been shown to reduce overall mortality by 23%; however, there is no improvement in symptoms or QOL; therefore careful consideration of the risk and benefits of this therapy should be discussed with patients, families, and the health care team.[18]

Combination pharmacologic therapy in older adult patients provides opportunity for enhanced efficacy, avoidance of adverse effects, enhanced convenience, and compliance.[16] Table 40.3 lists potentially inappropriate symptom management medications for older adults. Older adult patients often discontinue medications or take medications inappropriately, resulting in failure to reach recommended targets and outcomes and may result in hospital admission.[16] The average older adult patient takes six prescription medications daily; therefore, polypharmacy, nonadherence, and potential medication interactions are important concerns in this group.[16] Nonadherence to medication regimens may be due to competing health problems, socioeconomic status, treatment complexity, side effects, and cost of medications.[19] Clinical and fiscal consequences of medication nonadherence can lead to increased hospital readmissions and adverse medical events.[19] Assessing factors that affect medication adherence such as literacy, eyesight, understanding of directions, education level, severity of disease, and comorbid conditions may assist in understanding barriers to compliance.[16] Patient management is most effective when intraprofessional health care teams collaborate to achieve and maintain goals. Novel opportunities for therapeutic management and compliance include smartphones, telemedicine, and computerized technologies. Other collaborative efforts include effective communication with local pharmacies, medication reconciliation at discharge, follow-up discharge phone calls, and timely provider handoff.

ONCOLOGIC ISSUES IN CRITICALLY ILL OLDER ADULTS

Cancer diagnoses in older adults are increasing with improving cancer survival rates.[20] In addition to various solid tumors, there has been an increase in the number of hematologic diseases seen in older adults.[20] Limited evidence exists for treatment of older adults with cancer because clinical trials have excluded this patient population.[21] Older patients with cancer respond differently to cancer therapies than younger patients because of age-related physiologic changes and comorbid chronic conditions; therefore, functional age may be more important than chronologic age when considering the health status of older adults.[21] The comprehensive geriatric assessment is a complex but standardized instrument that is used to assess frailty and identify older adults at risk for treatment-related complications.[22] The comprehensive geriatric assessment has shown predictive value in older adults in surgical oncology in regard to 30-day postoperative complications, mortality, and discharge to a nonhome institution.[22]

Older hematology/oncology patients are often admitted to the ICU for diagnoses such as respiratory failure, renal failure,

TABLE 40.2 Cardiac Medication Considerations in Older Adults

Medication	Clinical Considerations

Thiazide Diuretics
Hydrochlorothiazide
Chlorthalidone
Bendrofluazide
	Recommended for initial hypertensive therapy
	  ↓ Peripheral vascular resistance
	  ↓ Intravascular volume
	  ↓ BP
	  Generally well tolerated in older adults
	  ↓ Cardiovascular, cerebrovascular, renal adverse outcomes
	  May exacerbate arrhythmias, hyperuricemia, glucose intolerance, dyslipidemia

Nonthiazide Diuretics Indapamide—sulfonamide diuretic Furosemide—loop diuretic	Increase blood glucose Do not increase uric acid Can cause potassium-independent prolongation of Q–T interval Increase glucose May cause headaches, fever, anemia May cause electrolyte disturbances

Mineralocorticoid Antagonists
Spironolactone/eplerenone
	Useful in hypertension when combined with other agents
	  Cause potassium retention
	  Not associated with adverse metabolic effects

Beta-Blockers
Metoprolol
	Indicated for older adult patients with:
	  Hypertension, CAD, HF
	  Certain arrhythmias
	  Migraine headaches
	  Senile tremor

Calcium antagonists
Phenylalkylamines—verapamil
 	
Benzothiazepines—diltiazem
 	
Dihydropyridines—nicardipine
	Variable effects on heart muscle, sinus node function, atrioventricular conduction,
	  peripheral arteries, coronary circulation
	Effective in older adult patients with hypertension due to increasing arterial stiffness,
	  decreased vascular angina and supraventricular arrhythmias, compliance, diastolic dysfunction

ACEIs Captopril (Capoten) Enalapril (Vasotec) Lisinopril (Prinivil, Zestril)	Block conversion of angiotensin I to angiotensin II in tissue and plasma Lower peripheral vascular resistance and BP without reflex stimulation of heart rate and contractility Reduce morbidity and mortality in patients with HF, reduced systolic function, post-MI Retard progression of diabetic renal disease and hypertensive nephrosclerosis

Angiotensin Receptor Blockers
Losartan (Cozaar)
Valsartan (Diovan)
	Selectively block AT1 receptor subtype to:
	  Reduce BP
	  Protect kidneys
	  Reduce mortality and morbidity in HF patients
	Considered first line and as an alternative to ACEIs in older adult hypertensive
	  patients with diabetes mellitus, hypertension, and HF who cannot tolerate ACEIs

Direct Renin Inhibitors Aliskiren	Effective for BP lowering without dose-related increases in adverse events in older adult patients May be used in combination therapy
Nonspecific Vasodilators Hydralazine	Fourth-line antihypertensive because of unfavorable side effects

Continued

TABLE 40.2   Cardiac Medication Considerations in Older Adults—cont'd

Medication	Clinical Considerations
Minoxidil	Tachycardia Fluid accumulation and atrial arrhythmias (minoxidil) when used as part of combination regimens Centrally acting agents (eg, clonidine) are not first-line treatments in older adults because of sedation and/or bradycardia Abrupt discontinuation leads to increased BP and heart rate, which may aggravate ischemia and/or HF These agents should not be considered in noncompliant patients but may be used as part of a combination regimen if needed after several other agents are deployed
Centrally Acting Agents	
Clonidine	Not first-line treatments in older adults because of sedation and/or bradycardia Abrupt discontinuation leads to increased BP and HR

ACEIs, angiotensin-converting enzyme inhibitors; *BP,* blood pressure; *CAD,* coronary artery disease; *HF,* heart failure; *MI,* myocardial infarction.
Adapted from Aronow WS, et al. ACCF/AHA 2011 expert consensus document on hypertension in the elderly: A report of the American College of Cardiology Foundation Task Force on Clinical Expert Consensus Documents. *J Am Coll Cardiol.* 2011;57:2037.

TABLE 40.3   Potentially Inappropriate Symptom Management Medications for Older Adults

Medication	Possible Side Effect
NSAIDs[a]	
Indomethacin	CNS effects (highest of all NSAIDs)[b]
Ketorolac	Asymptomatic gastrointestinal conditions (ulcers[b])
Aspirin (>325 mg)	Asymptomatic gastrointestinal conditions (ulcers[b])
Naproxen	Gastrointestinal bleeding,[b] renal failure,[b] high blood pressure,[b] heart failure[b]
Opioids	
Meperidine	Intense side-effect profile for adverse effects, especially CNS effects (seizures) Most critical in individuals with renal compromise[b]
Morphine, hydromorphone, fentanyl	Intense side-effect profile at higher doses, especially CNS effects (eg, somnolence, respiratory depression, delirium)[b]
Adjuvant Medications	
Muscle relaxants (methocarbamol, carisoprodol, chlorzoxazone, metaxalone, cyclobenzaprine, baclofen)	Anticholinergic effects,[b,c] sedation,[b] weakness,[b] cognitive impairment[b]
Tricyclic antidepressants (amitriptyline and amitriptyline compounds)	Strong anticholinergic effects[b,c]; may lead to ataxia, impaired psychomotor function, syncope, falls; cardiac arrhythmias (Q–T interval changes)[b]; may produce polyuria or lead to urinary incontinence[b]; may exacerbate chronic constipation
Doxepin	Cardiac arrhythmias,[b] may produce polyuria or lead to urinary incontinence,[b] may exacerbate chronic constipation
Antihistamines (diphenhydramine, hydroxyzine, promethazine)	Potent anticholinergic properties[b,c] May lead to confusion and sedation
Benzodiazepines	Increased sensitivity at higher doses with prolonged sedation and increased risk for falls
Short acting (lorazepam ≥3 mg, oxazepam ≥60 mg, alprazolam ≥2 mg)	May produce or exacerbate depression; smaller doses may be both effective and safer
Long acting (diazepam)	CNS effects,[b] may cause or exacerbate respiratory depression in chronic obstructive pulmonary disease,[b] may produce polyuria or lead to urinary incontinence[b]
Selective serotonin reuptake inhibitor antidepressants (fluoxetine, citalopram, paroxetine, sertraline)	May produce CNS stimulation, sleep disturbances, and increasing agitation[b]; may exacerbate or cause syndrome of inappropriate secretion of antidiuretic hormone or hyponatremia
Decongestants	High level of CNS stimulation, which may lead to insomnia[b]
CNS stimulants (methylphenidate)	Altered CNS function, leading to cognitive impairment[b]; appetite-suppressing effect[b]

[a]May cause or exacerbate gastric or duodenal ulcers, prolonged clotting time and international normalized ratio, and decreased platelet function.
[b]High-severity rating.
[c]Anticholinergic effects include some of the following symptoms: blurred vision, constipation, drowsiness, sedation, dry mouth, tachycardia, urinary retention, confusion, disorientation, memory impairment, dizziness, nausea, nervousness, agitation, anxiety, facial flushing, weakness, and delirium.
Based on data from Fick DM, et al. Updating the Beers criteria for potentially inappropriate medication use in older adults: Results of a U.S. consensus panel of experts. *Arch Intern Med.* 2003;163(22):2716; and Laroche ML, Charmes JP, Merle L. Potentially inappropriate medications in the elderly: A French consensus panel. *Eur J Clin Pharmacol.* 2007;63(8):725.
CNS, central nervous system; *NSAIDs,* nonsteroidal antiinflammatory drugs.

and septic shock related to antineoplastic therapies or postsurgical complications.[21,23] Other reasons for ICU admission include prevention and management of oncologic emergencies such as tumor lysis syndrome, superior vena cava syndrome, spinal cord compression, increased intracranial pressure, cardiac tamponade, febrile neutropenia, disseminated intravascular coagulation, syndrome of inappropriate secretion of antidiuretic hormone, hyperammonemia, hypoglycemia/hyperglycemia, and hypercalcemia of malignancy.[20,23] Treatment of oncologic emergencies is the same in older patients as in younger patients; however, older adults may be less able to withstand the treatments.

Patients with cancer may be medically or surgically managed with preferential surgical removal of solid tumors.[24] Care of an elderly patient in the surgical ICU can be challenging particularly if surgical intervention is emergent and functional status has not been optimized before surgery.[24] In the immediate postoperative period, volume resuscitation in elderly critically ill patients with cardiac or renal issues can predispose them to complications related to volume overload, pulmonary edema, acute respiratory distress syndrome, electrolyte abnormalities, and cardiac failure. Early use of advanced monitoring to evaluate response to resuscitative efforts is particularly important in older adult patients. Preoperative status and ability to compensate direct the duration of monitoring and depend on the patient's response to resuscitation as well as clinical status. Hemodynamics and blood urea nitrogen, creatinine, and serum osmolality should be monitored during diuretic use. Transfusion is not without risk, and red blood cell transfusion is generally recommended for a hemoglobin level of less than 7.0 g/dL in all critically ill patients. For patients with active bleeding or coronary ischemia, a higher hemoglobin level between 7.0 and 9.0 g/dL may be targeted.[24]

Common postoperative complications in elderly patients include respiratory failure, atrial fibrillation, myocardial ischemia, and coagulopathies.[24] Pulmonary complications occur in 2% to 10% of older adults with the chance of mechanical ventilation increasing between the ages of 55 and 85 years. Extubation may be challenging for some elderly patients, which may lead to the need for tracheostomy to assist with weaning. Atrial fibrillation occurs in 3.7% to 6.7% of elderly patients within 3 days of surgery.[24] Age older than 70 years is an independent risk factor for the development of postoperative atrial fibrillation. Cardiac complications pose the greatest risk of mortality in older adults undergoing surgery with MI being the leading cause of postoperative death in patients older than 80 years. Although risk is higher in older adults, treatment modalities are the same as in younger adults. Treatment options for some medical conditions including cardiovascular conditions include anticoagulants and antiplatelet medications, which can result in life-threatening coagulopathies.

AGE-RELATED CHANGES OF THE RESPIRATORY SYSTEM AND PULMONARY DISEASE

Significant age-related changes affect the pulmonary system including alterations in compliance of the chest wall, strength of respiratory muscles, and static elastic recoil of the lung.[25] As a result, older adult patients have less pulmonary reserve along with increased susceptibility to infections. Given the prevalence of lung disease in the growing older adult population, it is important to understand the effects of these changes to provide optimal care (Fig. 40.1).[26]

Thoracic Wall and Respiratory Muscles

The thoracic cavity, which houses and protects the lungs, becomes progressively smaller with aging as a result of a loss of height of the intervertebral disk leading to narrowing of the rib spaces.[26] This narrowing or kyphosis increases after 40 years of age.[26] Thoracic stiffening occurs from a decline in rib mobility secondary to contractures of intercostal muscles and calcification of costal cartilage. Additionally, prevalence of vertebral fractures increases with age, particularly in women, as a result of osteoporosis.[25] Progressive decreases in chest wall compliance and changes in the shape of the thorax alter chest wall mechanics leading to a deterioration in respiratory function.[25] A decrease in forced expiratory volume and forced vital capacity is seen with significant kyphosis of greater than 55 degrees.[27]

Strength of the diaphragm and intercostal muscles decreases with age with a 2% annual decline in muscle function.[26] The diaphragm is the most important inspiratory muscle because its movement accounts for 75% of change in intrathoracic volume during quiet respiration. Other factors such as an increase in abdominal girth and change in posture also decrease thoracic excursion. Respiratory muscle function is affected by skeletal muscle and peripheral muscle strength.[20] During aging, skeletal muscle progressively atrophies, and its energy metabolism decreases, which may partially explain the declining strength of the respiratory muscles.[20] Handgrip strength testing can be a simple and useful measurement in assessment of muscle function.[20] Age-related reductions in maximal inspiratory pressure and maximal expiratory pressure are likely a consequence of impaired respiratory mechanics and sarcopenia (age-related atrophy of muscle fibers).[21,26] Sarcopenia describes reduced muscle mass and function, which may be related to decreased muscle protein synthesis, increased muscle proteolysis, motor neuron loss, and increased muscle fat content.[28] Respiratory muscle strength is additionally affected by nutritional status, which is often deficient in older adults.[25] At a cellular level, respiratory muscle strength relies on available energy.[25] Adenosine triphosphate reserves are decreased in older adults.[26] Chronic heart failure, Parkinson disease, sequelae of cerebrovascular disease, and myasthenia gravis can produce diminished respiratory muscle function.[25] Accessory inspiratory muscles (sternocleidomastoid, scalene, and trapezius) facilitate inspiration during exercise or increased respiratory demands. Use of accessory muscles is an important factor for critical care nurses to recognize as a precursor to respiratory failure.

The aging pulmonary system has a reduced ability to clear mucus from the airways. As respiratory muscle declines, the ability to generate the necessary high forced expiratory flow for an effective cough is reduced.[26] This is accompanied by alterations in mucociliary cells located in the upper and lower airways where they function to remove large and small particles.[26] The cilia beat in synchrony to trap and clear mucus from the airways.[26] A decrease in beat frequency may be responsible for these age-related changes in mucociliary clearance.[26] This leads to an increased risk of aspiration and hospital-acquired infections in older adults.[5] These changes emphasize the importance of dysphagia screening, deep breathing, and coughing for older patients in the critical care unit.

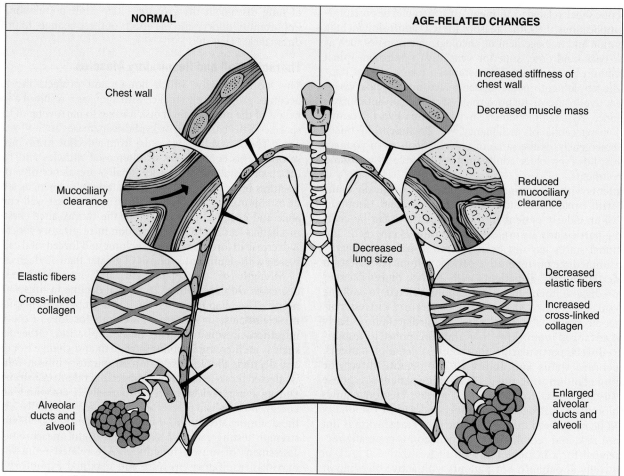

NORMAL	AGE-RELATED CHANGES
Chest wall	Increased stiffness of chest wall
	Decreased muscle mass
Mucociliary clearance	Reduced mucociliary clearance
	Decreased lung size
Elastic fibers	Decreased elastic fibers
Cross-linked collagen	Increased cross-linked collagen
Alveolar ducts and alveoli	Enlarged alveolar ducts and alveoli

FIG. 40.1 Age-Related Changes in the Respiratory System. With advancing age, the compliance of the chest wall and lung tissue changes. There is also a reduced clearance of mucus by the cilia that line the pulmonary tree and an enlargement of the alveolar ducts and alveoli.

Lung Parenchyma and Volumes

Diminished recoil of the lung occurs with aging, causing increased lung volume and distention of the alveolar spaces.[25] The residual volume results in an increase in air trapping by approximately 50% between ages 20 and 70 years.[25] Reduced lung elasticity results from changes in the ratio of elastic to support tissue that occur with advancing age.[29] To maintain a consistent total lung capacity, the elastic load from the chest wall increases secondary to augmented thoracic wall stiffness and counteracts the reduced lung elasticity.[25]

Pulmonary function studies may be the best way to assess respiratory impairment in older adults.[28] Dynamic lung volumes and flow rates depend on resistance of airways and chest wall compliance and are limited by collapse of small airways during forced expiration. Age-related changes in respiratory mechanics lead to airflow restrictions, which are reflected in decreased 1-second forced expiratory volume.[28] Maximal expiratory flow rate and maximal midexpiratory flow rate are also decreased.[28] Age-related decrease in dynamic lung volume is probably caused by decreased chest wall compliance, small airways closure during forced expiration, and decreased strength of expiratory muscles. Breathing exercises generate lung volumes of forced vital capacity, which is an untimed lung volume, and 1-second forced expiratory volume, which is a timed lung volume. These spirometry tests can assist in assessing restrictive respiratory patterns.[21] Reduced timed lung volume is exhibited in chronic obstructive pulmonary disease (COPD), asthma, bronchiectasis, and cystic fibrosis.[28] Other conditions that display reductions in timed and untimed lung volumes include kyphosis, scoliosis, myasthenia gravis, diaphragmatic paralysis, pleural effusions or fibrosis, and pulmonary hypertension.[21] These anatomic changes are reflected by an increase in residual volume and decrease in vital capacity. The application of conventional quality control standards to objective assessment of pulmonary function in older patients may prove difficult because of mood alterations, fatigability, lack of cooperation, or cognitive impairment.[28]

Pulmonary Gas Exchange

Ventilation and diffusion depend on numerous factors including lung surface area. Displacement of inhaled air volume away from the alveoli limits the surface area available for gas exchange. This may partly explain the progressive and linear decrease in pulmonary diffusion capacity, which depends on surface area and capillary blood volume.[29] Capillary blood volume and surface area have also been reported to decrease with advancing age. Changes in pulmonary circulation result in a ventilation-perfusion mismatch.[28] Ventilation-perfusion mismatch leads to a decline in arterial partial pressure of oxygen (Pao_2) of approximately 0.3 mm Hg per year from the age of 30 years.[5] The typical Pao_2 for healthy adults older than 65 years is approximately 89 mm Hg compared with 100 mm Hg for adults 18 to 24 years old.[28] Age-related changes in ventilation and arterial partial pressure of carbon dioxide ($Paco_2$) occur across the adult life span. Total minute ventilation must increase with advancing age to maintain $Paco_2$. $Paco_2$ is largely dependent on the minute ventilation, which is the sum of alveolar ventilation and dead space ventilation. Ventilation-perfusion inequality may exist with decreased diffusion capacity of the lung for carbon monoxide and the transfer capacity of oxygen across the alveolar–capillary interface.[28]

Control of respiratory responses to hypoxia and hypercapnia decreases by 50% and 40%, respectively, in older adults, which may be due to declining chemoreceptor function.[5] Decreases in Pao_2 may be the result of an increase in closing volume in dependent lung zones during resting tidal breathing in older patients.[30,31] Consequently, dependent lung zones may be ventilated intermittently, leading to regional differences. Alterations in blood volume and vascular resistance within the pulmonary circulation may also contribute to ventilation-perfusion mismatching. Important considerations for critical care nurses with regard to older adult patients includes recognition of decreased respiratory reserve and more rapid decompensation than in younger patients.[5] Other factors such as exposure to environmental pollutants and COPD have an impact on the ability to compensate for respiratory conditions or wean from mechanical ventilation.[5]

Pulmonary Diseases

Older adults are more susceptible to respiratory infections as a result of changes in pulmonary immunity.[26] The complex changes of the immune system include a phenomenon known as *inflamm-aging,* in which there is an increase in circulating proinflammatory cytokines.[26] The chronic inflammatory state may contribute to the destruction of the lung parenchyma and loss of elasticity.[26] This process is coupled with a blunted immune response often called *immunosenescence* and subsequently leads to a decrease in both innate and adaptive immune responses. As a result, the aging immune system contributes to the increase in morbidity and mortality in this population.[26]

Older individuals are less able to protect against environmental injury and infection of the respiratory system. Decreases in T-cell function, decline in mucociliary clearance, and a decrease swallowing ability (dysphagia) with loss of cough reflex can increase the frequency and severity of pneumonia in older adults. Poor dentition, nutrition, and oral hygiene also play a role in the incidence of oropharyngeal colonization with gram-negative bacteria and aspiration pneumonia.[5]

Lung diseases are more common in older adults and have significant consequences given the many age-related changes that occur.[27] Incidence of COPD is two to three times higher in people older than age 60 and is the third leading cause of death in the United States.[26] It also accounts for 20% of hospital admissions for adults 65 to 75 years old.[26,27] The greatest risk factor for developing COPD in genetically susceptible individuals is cigarette smoking.[26] Acute exacerbations of COPD are due to viral or bacterial infections in 70% of cases.[27] The clinical presentation of pneumonia in older adults may be atypical and include a nonproductive cough, delirium, anorexia, falls, and dizziness.[27] Noninvasive ventilation is highly effective for respiratory support during COPD exacerbations.[27] Absolute contraindications for noninvasive ventilation include respiratory arrest, inability to maintain one's own airway, loss of airway reflexes, upper airway obstruction, copious secretions, emesis, and patient refusal.[27] The occurrence of pulmonary embolism is higher in older adults as a result of predisposing conditions such as malignancy, postoperative states, and immobility.[27] Treatment with systemic anticoagulation places an older adult at a greater risk for adverse events.[27] Other pulmonary processes potentially resulting in respiratory emergencies include acute decompensated heart failure, influenza, and pneumonia.[27] Respiratory emergencies can progress to acute respiratory failure and require mechanical ventilation; however, controversy exists as to whether age is an independent predictor of outcome.[32] A study by Barnato et al[33] showed larger increases in disability after discharge from the hospital in patients with mechanical ventilation compared with patients after hospitalizations without mechanical ventilation. Additionally, 90-day survival after mechanical ventilation has not improved despite a decrease in hospital mortality from mechanical ventilation, as death rate trends are increasing in the postacute setting.[33,34] Prolonged mechanical ventilation has a 1-year survival rate of 49% to 77%.[34] Postoperative respiratory complications often occur in elderly patients with a dramatic increase in respiratory failure requiring mechanical ventilation for patients older than 65 years old.[24,35] Elective surgeries for this population require careful consideration in light of the increased risks for complications and mortality.[36] Use of mechanical ventilation has shown an increase in recent years when measured from 1993 to 2009 with a substantial increase because of pneumonia compared with COPD exacerbations and heart failure.[37] There was a decline in mortality rates in patients with pneumonia and COPD exacerbations despite increasing comorbidities .[37] These trends in outcomes could be related to intensive care bundles, including sedation interruptions, ventilator-associated pneumonia interventions, and lung protective strategies.[37]

ACCIDENTS AND TRAUMA IN OLDER ADULTS

As the elderly population increases and older adults have more independent and active lifestyles, there is an increased risk for traumatic events, delayed recovery from trauma, and severe disability. At the present time, 23% of all trauma admissions occur in adults older than 65 years with accidents representing the fourth leading cause of death in this population.[38]

Several factors place older adults at particular risk. Conditions such as weakness, deconditioning, cognitive impairments, gait instability, loss of sensory perception, delayed reaction times, and chronic illnesses can lead to an increase in accidents and traumatic events in older adults. Trauma often occurs before risk factors are identified. Elderly patients who have sustained trauma in the past are three times more likely to have a future traumatic event.[38] The mechanism of trauma in elderly patients is usually blunt trauma rather than penetrating trauma. Approximately three-quarters of all traumas in older adults are related to simple falls, such as falls from standing.[38] Fall injury is often underrecognized leading to delay in treatment and poorer outcomes. Falls related to blunt cerebral injury and long bone fractures combined with comorbid conditions result in the greatest mortality. Underlying conditions such as cardiovascular disease (including hypertension and arrhythmias), previous stroke, COPD, dementia, endocrine disorders, cancers, hepatic disease, and chronic renal failure increase risk of poor outcomes after trauma.[38] Treatments for these conditions such as beta-blockers, pacemakers, steroids, anticoagulants, and antiplatelet medications may mask abnormal vital signs and confound evaluation of older adults experiencing accidents or trauma. Referral to a trauma center is recommended if the patient meets trauma activation criteria on initial evaluation. Despite improvements in access to trauma care and medical advances, elderly patients who experience traumatic injury still remain at high risk for poor outcomes, ranging from loss of independence to death.[38,39]

Cognitive Functioning and Neuromuscular Aging

Cognitive functioning has become one of the greatest threats of old age, with more than 50% of adults older than age 85 years affected by Alzheimer disease.[40] Structural and neurophysiologic changes occur in the brain with aging; however, it is unclear which changes are a normal process of aging or pathology of neurogenic disorders.[40] Cognitive function involves transforming, synthesizing, storing, and retrieving sensory input in addition to perception, attention, thinking, memory, and problem solving. Neuropsychological assessment of older adults can be achieved with psychometric and clinical neuropsychological assessment and standardized testing. Cognitive profile information can be helpful in differentiating between normal aging, mild cognitive impairment, early dementia, depression, mental health issues, and progressive neurologic disease. An assessment may also be useful after a stroke or in conditions such as Parkinson disease to assist in decision making about ability to drive or about the extent to which the individual has capacity to make specific decisions (eg, medical treatment, financial affairs, or self-care).[41] The rate at which complex tasks are completed may diminish; however, this is not synonymous with cognitive impairment, as deterioration of cognitive functioning is not a normal expectation of the aging process. Some slight memory dysfunction is common with increasing age, but significant decline may be a result of acute or chronic conditions. Acute mental status changes resulting from infection, metabolic imbalances, or medications are usually reversible after identification and treatment.

Delirium is a frequent complication in critical care but is often unrecognized in hospitalized critically ill older adults.[42] Delirium is been reported in up to 80% of all mechanically ventilated patients.[43] A critically ill older adult is especially susceptible to delirium when age-related changes are coupled with the acute stress of critical illness.[43] In the aging brain, a decline in hormonal and immunologic feedback mechanisms can lead to a cycle of excessive inflammatory response to an acute stress such as sepsis resulting in neurodegeneration and further inflammation.[43] Although the exact mechanism of delirium is unclear, it is associated with neuroinflammation and neurodegeneration leading to brain atrophy and cognitive impairment.[43,44] Delirium is characterized by acute changes in mental status from baseline, inattention, and disorganized thinking or changes in level of consciousness. Cost estimates for care associated with delirium including postcare range from $38 billion to $152 billion annually.[42] Risk factors for delirium include alterations in sleep-wake cycle, sepsis, hypoxemia, electrolyte imbalances, metabolic alterations, and medications that induce delirium.[36] Critical care nurses play a vital role in implementing interventions to prevent the occurrence of delirium through promoting orientation, encouraging mobility, minimizing noise and sleep disturbances, and reducing use of restraints and devices such as Foley catheters.[36]

Postoperative cognitive dysfunction (POCD) is an acute and short-term disorder of cognition, memory, and attention that may be seen in critical care patients. Distinction should be made between etiologic factors and this syndrome. A study of long-term postoperative cognitive dysfunction in the elderly found that POCD was present in 26% of patients 1 week after surgery and in 9.9% 3 months after surgery compared with 3.4% and 2.8% of control subjects.[5] Increasing age, duration of anesthesia, postoperative infections, and respiratory complications were risk factors for early POCD. Only age was a risk factor for prolonged POCD after cardiac surgery in older adults, with an incidence of up to 80% at discharge and 50% at 6 weeks. In some cases, neurocognitive decline lasted 5 years following some cardiac surgeries. Cardiopulmonary bypass appears to be a factor in short-term and long-term POCD.[5]

Delusions and hallucinations may be present in delirium but are also evident in other psychiatric disorders. Chronic impairment develops from more organic causes, such as changes associated with neurodegenerative dementias (eg, Alzheimer disease) or nonneurodegenerative types (eg, multiinfarct dementia, traumatic brain injury). Although dementia is pathology-based, there is an increased incidence associated with advanced age, especially in adults older than 85 years.[40] Alzheimer disease is identified by amyloid-containing neuritic plaques and intraneuronal neurofibrillary tangles in various areas of the cortex.[40] Alzheimer disease is characterized initially by progressive short-term memory loss and later by long-term memory loss. Marked decline in memory leaves individuals functionally impaired and physically dependent. In contrast, nonneurodegenerative dementias, such as multiinfarct types, manifest as fixed deficits associated with the area of brain injury. In contrast to Alzheimer type of dementia, cognitive impairment may be associated with significant impairment after stroke rather than over time.[41]

Baseline dementia, stress of surgery or acute illness, and hospitalization can cause cognitive decline and significantly increase risk for delirium in older adults. Sensory perception decreases with age, resulting in difficulties for older patients in unfamiliar surroundings such as hospitals. Immobility and deprivation of vision and hearing increase the likelihood of dehydration, anorexia, confusion, depression, and disorientation.[5]

Structure and Morphology

The brain decreases approximately 20% in size between 25 and 95 years of age (Fig. 40.2).[46] Reduction in brain weight may be related to the overall decrease in the number of neurons that occurs with advancing age. Neurons are lost from the hippocampus; amygdala; cerebellum; and areas of the brainstem such as the locus caeruleus, dorsal motor nucleus of the vagus, and substantia nigra. Conversely, very few neurons disappear from the hypothalamus with advancing age.[40] Portions of the cerebral cortex atrophy, predominantly the frontal and temporal cortical association areas (superior frontal gyrus and superior temporal gyrus, respectively).[40] Cerebral blood flow and brain weight decrease with advancing age, most likely as a result of reduction in neuron number and metabolic needs of cerebral tissue.[46] Cerebral blood flow is also influenced by age-related changes in BP, barometric response to positional change, and severity of cerebrovascular disease. Accompanying the loss of neurons

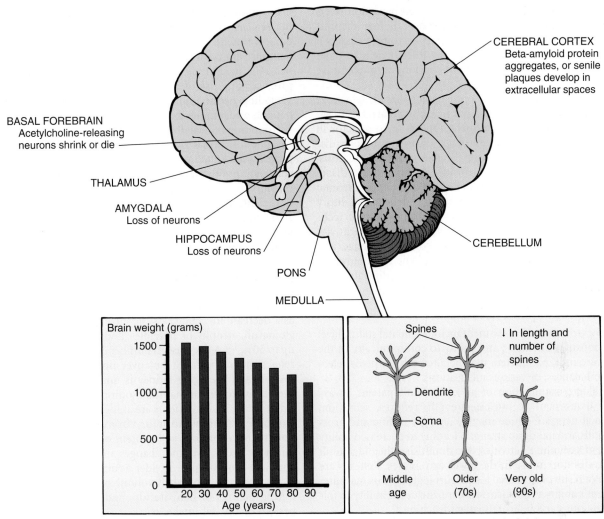

FIG. 40.2 Age-Related Changes in the Brain. (From Selkoe DJ. Aging brain, aging mind. *Sci Am.* 1992;267:134.)

are changes in ultrastructure and intracellular structures of the neuron. The neuron is composed of a cell body, dendrite, and axon. Dendrites are long, spiny processes that extend out from the cell body. Dendrite spines decrease in number with age; the length of dendritic spines increases in middle and late old age and then decreases after late old age (older than 90 years).[46] Shrinking of large neurons and degenerative changes occurring in cell bodies and axons of some acetylcholine-secreting neurons have been reported. These changes may explain alterations in processing and receiving of information.[46]

Lipofuscins, neuritic plaques, and neurofibrillary bodies appear within the cytoplasm of the neuron.[47] Lipofuscins, or age pigments, are granules containing a dark, fluorescent pigment and derive from lipid-rich membranes that have been partially disintegrated and oxidized. It is unclear whether lipofuscin accumulation is harmful to the brain.[47] Neuritic, or senile, plaques are aggregates of beta-amyloid protein that accumulate in the brain of normal senescent individuals. Neuritic plaques are found in the hippocampus, cerebral cortex, and other brain regions.[47] Neurofibrillary tangles, which are bundles of helically wound protein filaments, occur in the hippocampus with advancing age in healthy persons. They are present in larger numbers in persons with neuropathologic disorders

such as Alzheimer disease and may affect neuronal signaling.[47] Synaptogenesis or synaptic regeneration still occurs after partial nerve degeneration but at a slower rate in the older brain. After a nerve fiber is damaged, neighboring undamaged neurons often sprout new fibers and form new connections.[48]

Cognitive Function

Cognitive and brain reserve are well studied in the context of age-associated cognitive impairment and dementia. However, there is a paucity of research that examines the role of cognitive or brain reserve in delirium.[49] Brain and cognitive reserve concepts developed from observations that some individuals demonstrate less cognitive impairment than others with comparable brain injury or neuropathology. Most research on reserve is based on studies in chronic progressive disorders such as Alzheimer disease. Brain and cognitive reserve describes variability across persons in the relationship of pathologic changes with clinical expression of disease. *Brain reserve* refers to structural aspects of the brain, and *cognitive reserve* relates to how cognitive tasks are initiated and coordinated. Cognitive reserve comprises neural reserve and neural compensation. Neural reserve describes the efficiency, capacity, or flexibility of brain networks or cognitive paradigms that underlie task performance in the healthy brain. Neural compensation refers to the ability to function optimally when pathology disrupts standard processing networks. Studies are ongoing to assess if these processes are modifiable and may offer benefit to older adults for the prevention of delirium and long-term cognitive decline.[49]

Cognitive impairment is a core element shared by a large number of different neurologic and neuropsychiatric diseases. Some form of cognitive impairment appears to be a factor in many neuropsychiatric and neurologic disorders (bipolar disease, stroke, epilepsy, Parkinson disease, multiple sclerosis, Alzheimer disease, and other neurodegenerative brain disorders).[50] Cognitive decline seems to be linked to temporofrontal functional deficiency, which is expressed as deficient auditory discrimination and orienting.[50] New electrophysiologic technology is known as mismatch negativity. Mismatch negativity abnormality is closely associated with cognitive change and decline occurring in many different neurologic and neuropsychiatric illnesses as well as in normal aging, providing ability to measure cognitive decline.[50]

Central Nervous System Assessment

Central nervous system assessment includes mental status, level of consciousness, memory, and ability to communicate. In the critical care unit, parameters may be altered by hypoxia, electrolyte imbalances, or various medications.

Neurologic examination of an older adult patient always includes assessment of muscle strength, reflexes, sensation, and cranial nerves.[40] There may be changes in fine and gross motor skills and handgrip strength, leading to decreased ability to perform fine motor activities. Age diminishes the older adult patient's vibratory sense in the lower extremities. Reflexes are slowed as a result of neuronal loss. Neurologic deficits may alter the patient's ability to perform self-care, including ability to follow instructions and interpret patient teaching.[40]

Several standardized neurologic assessments are available for use in critical care.[51] Most of these assessments can be used for all critical care patients to define patient status accurately and consistently. Examples of scales that should be used routinely in critical care—particularly in care of older adult patients—include the Glasgow Coma Scale, National Institutes of Health Stroke Scale, International Standards for Neurological Classification of Spinal Cord Injury, Mini-Cog Assessment Instrument for Dementia, and the Confusion Assessment Method for the ICU. Assessment of older adults in critical care should also include consideration of age-related changes such as vision impairment, hearing deficits (particularly low-pitched and high-pitched sounds), slight loss of taste/dentition, and diminished sense of smell.

Studies have identified a relationship between critical illness and long-term cognitive impairment, including dementia and accelerated cognitive decline.[44,45,51] Executive function, attention, and memory appear to be affected for up to 6 years after a critical illness. One of the strongest independent predictors of cognitive decline for critical illness is length of delirium.[44] Delirium and immobility are the two most common and modifiable risk factors for disability.[43] An ICU-focused multidisciplinary approach known as the "ABCEDF bundle" is being implemented in many hospitals and specifically addresses delirium and early mobilization. The evidenced based ABCDEF bundle includes *A*ssessing, preventing, and managing pain; *B*oth spontaneous awakening and spontaneous breathing trial;

*C*hoosing lighter sedation and only when necessary; screening for *D*elirium; *E*arly mobility; and *F*amily engagement and empowerment.[45] Because most studies have been unable to demonstrate cognitive function objectively before critical illness, the magnitude of the problem is unclear. The ability to prognosticate risk of cognitive impairment would be useful in providing better information about long-term outcomes for patients and families and allow them to make difficult decisions surrounding critical illness.[52] Several tools are available to assess baseline functional and cognitive status, as this contributes to posthospital outcomes; however, incorporating these tools is challenging with many critically ill older adults as a result of the inability to communicate because of endotracheal tubes, sedation, delirium, and busy ICU work flow.[43] Brummel et al[43] created a modified pragmatic functional and cognitive assessment for older adults with critical illnesses to assess activities of daily living, mobility, and cognition.

RENAL SYSTEM IN OLDER ADULTS

Aging produces changes in renal structure and function such as a decrease in renal mass, nephron hypertrophy, sclerosis of glomeruli, atrophy of arterioles, and reduced renal blood flow up to 50%.[5,53] A decrease in number of nephrons does not affect renal function initially, but over time older adults lose renal reserve, and the aging kidney is unable to concentrate urine, excrete hydrogen, or maintain sodium/potassium balance.[5,53,54] Additionally, older patients are at high risk for dehydration and are more vulnerable to injury from decreases in renal blood flow such as episodes of hypotension leading to acute kidney injury or from extreme changes in body fluid composition and acid–base balance.[5] Older adults have reduced capability to excrete free water when volume overloaded, conserve water during periods of dehydration, and conserve sodium during periods of low salt intake.[5]

Demographic changes are leading to increased numbers of people with CKD and end-stage renal disease requiring dialysis.[54] In the United States, 40% of patients with end-stage renal disease are older than 65 years of age.[55] CKD is defined as a glomerular filtration rate less than 60 mL/min/1.73 m² or by the presence of kidney damage for 3 or more months.[54] Acute kidney injury and CKD are often seen in critically ill patients. Recognition by critical care nurses by trending patient's normal renal function can assist with prompt interventions to prevent progressive and irreversible renal injury.

GASTROINTESTINAL SYSTEM IN OLDER ADULTS

Age-related gastrointestinal changes include poor dentition, salivary dysfunction, dysphagia, *presbyesophagus* (reduced esophageal motility), and diminished peristalsis. Gastric mucosa weakens and atrophies with age resulting in hyposecretion of pepsin and acid, achlorhydria (decreased acid secretion), mucin secretion from mucus cells altering the protective function of the gastric mucosa and leading to esophageal reflux, esophagitis, and gastric ulcerations.[56] Gastric and duodenal ulcers often occur in the presence of *Helicobacter pylori* with the combination of nonsteroidal antiinflammatory drugs and *H. pylori* posing a significant risk for gastrointestinal bleeding in critically ill older adults.[56]

Sensory alterations of taste, smell, gastric motility, and motor function occur with aging. Gag reflex may be absent in 40%

of healthy elderly adults resulting in dysphagia as a particular hazard for silent aspiration and aspiration pneumonia.[57] Other age-related issues of the gastrointestinal tract include weakening of intestinal and colonic muscles, altered rectal sensation, and decreased mucus production that may lead to constipation, fecal impaction, fecal incontinence, and diverticulosis.[57,58]

Nutritional support may be challenging in hospitalized critically ill elderly patients depending on whether the patient is ventilated or able to take enteral nutrition. Dietary consultation and dysphagia screening during the critical care admission may identify preexisting problems and determine specific nutritional needs.[57]

Age-Related Changes in the Liver

Age-related changes in the liver include a decrease in hepatocytes, liver weight, hepatic volume, and perfusion with a loss of smooth-surfaced endoplasmic reticulum, diminished bile acid secretion, increased biliary cholesterol, and increased hepatocyte polyploidy.[59,60] Functions of the liver include detoxification of toxins and medications, carbohydrate storage, ketone body formation, reduction and conjugation of adrenal and gonadal steroid hormones, synthesis of plasma proteins, deamination of amino acids, urea formation, and synthesis and storage of cholesterol.[59,60] Age-related changes in hepatic function include a reduction in synthesis of cholesterol, total bile acid pool, and bile acid from cholesterol. There is also a reduced capacity of the liver for regeneration in response to injury compared with younger patients. Despite these age-related changes, liver function is not appreciably affected.[60]

Tests of liver function such as serum bilirubin, alkaline phosphatase, and aspartate aminotransferase levels are unaltered with advancing age. First-pass clearance of medications may be reduced because of decreases in total liver blood flow. The most important age-related change in liver function decreases the capacity of the liver to metabolize medications.[60] Although clinical tests of liver function do not reflect this change in metabolism, it is well recognized that medication side effects and toxic effects occur more frequently in older adults than in younger adults. Polypharmacy is cited as a common cause of adverse medication reactions in older adults.[60] Reduced medication-metabolizing capacity is caused by a decline in activity of the medication-metabolizing enzyme system and microsomal ethanol oxidizing system and decrease in total liver blood flow.[60] Medications that depend on the cytochrome P450 group of liver enzymes are most affected because age-associated changes can cause a 50% decline in enzymatic function.[60]

A clinically significant age-related change is decline in the rate of hepatic regeneration after partial liver resection (hepatectomy) or injury.[61] The rate of liver regeneration (hepatocyte proliferation) after injury is decreased in older adults, which may enhance the progress of hepatic diseases and compromise liver transplantation in older adults.[60] Liver transplantation is a complex issue, as some evidence reports that livers from older donors may be less viable than livers from young donors. Recipient age should also be a consideration, as posttransplant mortality increases by 15% between 55 and 75 years of age. The impact of age is modest with respect to recipient and graft survival, at least during the first few posttransplantation years, as recipient and graft survival rates decline in older adult patients receiving livers from older donors by only 10% to 15% in the initial years after transplant.[61]

Age, Disease, and the Liver

Aging alters hepatic function and structure by a decrease in hepatocytes, liver weight, hepatic volume, and perfusion with an ensuing fourfold increase in mortality of adults 45 to 85 years old.[59,60] Nonalcoholic fatty liver disease (NAFLD) is the most common chronic liver pathology in the United States affecting approximately one-third of the overall population.[59] NAFLD is most frequently seen in obese individuals and may be a hepatic manifestation of metabolic syndrome.[59] The hallmark of NAFLD is the intrahepatic accumulation of lipids that may develop into nonalcoholic steatohepatitis, a risk factor for liver diseases such as cirrhosis and hepatocellular carcinoma (HCC) seen in elderly patients.[59] Variation in inflammatory markers such as cytokines, chemokines, reactive oxygen species, and antioxidant enzymes may support the theory of inflamm-aging. Redistribution of adipose tissue from subcutaneous to visceral sites can result in ectopic lipid accumulation in nonadipose tissues including heart, skeletal muscle, and liver, increasing risk of disorders such as hypertension, atherosclerosis, hyperlipidemia, insulin resistance, and diabetes. Inflamm-aging may be counteracted through lifestyle changes—regular physical activity and reduced caloric intake may be key factors for healthy aging.[59]

HCC is one of the most common causes of cancer-related mortality worldwide and is predisposed by nonalcoholic steatohepatitis progress to cirrhosis in 8% to 26% of patients.[59] Treatment options include percutaneous ablation or radiofrequency ablation, surgical resection, and transplantation. In most cases, HCC arises in the setting of cirrhosis, but hepatitis B virus (HBV) and hepatitis C virus (HCV) are the most common underlying etiologies; HCC can also develop in a background of "pure" steatohepatitis.[59] HCC is very rare before age 40; it increases progressively with older age and peaks in incidence at approximately age 75 years.[59] Older adults with HBV may develop subclinical hepatitis with a low rate of HBV clearance but are highly infective chronic HBV surface antigen carriers.[62] HCV prevalence increases with advancing age with estimates of infected elderly adults ranging from 5.2% to 42.1%.[62] Alcohol consumption and liver disease are common in older adults with some reports indicating that 5% to 15% of older adults have alcohol-related problems.[62] Individuals with alcoholic hepatitis and underlying alcoholic cirrhosis have a higher chance of developing HCC and a higher mortality.[62]

DIABETES IN OLDER ADULTS

Diabetes affects approximately 25% of elderly adults, and this prevalence is expected to increase in the next 20 years.[63] In addition, diabetes is undiagnosed in one-third of older adults.[63] Elderly African Americans and Hispanics have a greater rate of type 2 diabetes.[63] The effects of diabetes can be significant resulting in higher mortality, reduced functional status, and increased risk for institutionalization along with higher risk for acute and chronic microvascular and cardiovascular complications.[63]

Of the two types of diabetes, type 2 diabetes is considerably more common in older adults; this has been linked to the increasing incidence of overweight and obesity. Furthermore, age-related changes such as insulin resistance and diminished pancreatic islet function add to the risk for developing type 2 diabetes in older adults. Recommendations for diabetic management reflect the three major classes of older adults: relatively healthy older adults, older adults with complex medical conditions, and older adults with a very significant comorbid illness and functional impairment.[63] Older adults with limited life expectancy are unlikely to benefit from intensive glucose control.

Older adults, particularly adults with diabetes, are more likely to require hospitalization than younger adults. Recommendations from the American Diabetes Association for critically ill hospitalized patients suggest starting insulin treatment for persistent hyperglycemia greater than 180 mg/dL with glucose targets of 140 to 180 mg/dL after insulin therapy is started.[64] As older adults recover from critical illness, insulin regimens may need to be adjusted. Less strict targets may be appropriate for patients with multiple comorbidities and reduced life expectancy.[63]

Geriatric syndrome refers to conditions that are more likely to occur in older adults with diabetes. Cognitive dysfunction is more frequent in elderly patients with diabetes and varies from subtle dysfunction to dementia and memory loss.[63] Additionally, diabetes increases the risk for functional impairment and falls. This increased risk is likely due to peripheral neuropathy, vision and hearing difficulty, and gait and balance problems.[63] Peripheral neuropathy occurs in 50% to 70% of older adults with diabetes and can cause significant pain. The risk for falls and fractures also rises.[63] Depression is also common in these patients, and periodic screening should be performed.[63,64] For elderly patients who require insulin, it is important to remember that insulin therapy requires good visual and motor coordination, which may be challenging for some older adults.[64] Strategies essential to patient safety and prevention of readmission include medication reconciliation, patient and caregiver education, and close communication between inpatient and outpatient care teams.[63] Critical care nurses need to be conscious of the prevalence of diabetes and issues surrounding its management in the older population.[63]

IMMUNE SYSTEM IN OLDER ADULTS

Infections in older adults are generally more complicated, serious, and lethal than infections in younger individuals.[65] Adults older than 65 years are the fastest growing segment of the population, and they are hospitalized at more than three times the rate of people of all ages.[65] Older adults are often more frail than younger adults and have comorbidities that make them more susceptible to infections such as pneumonia, urinary tract infections, and bacteremia.[65]

Elderly patients with infections often present with nonspecific symptoms including altered mental status, anorexia, and generalized weakness and can often deteriorate quickly to severe sepsis and septic shock.[66] The cornerstones of treatment for severe sepsis and septic shock include early recognition, early resuscitation, early antibiotics, and early source control.[67] Early and aggressive treatment can save lives and prevent further deterioration in condition.

INTEGUMENTARY AND MUSCULOSKELETAL SYSTEMS IN OLDER ADULTS

Skin disorders common in older adults include seborrheic keratosis, xerosis, Campbell de Morgan spots, and other dermatologic disorders caused by degenerative and metabolic changes.[67] Overall skin elasticity decreases as a result of collagen depletion affecting the skin's protective capability.[67] Protective layers of subcutaneous tissue decrease as capillary fragility increases leading to acute and chronic wounds. Annual prevalence of chronic wounds in older adults is approximately 10% to 35%.[68] Wound healing is diminished because of decreased cytokine and growth factor production, diminished inflammatory response, and reduction of cell proliferation.[68] Diminished wound healing is particularly important in the critical care environment where increased opportunity to develop pressure ulcers and infections exists.

Decreased lean body mass, increased body fat, and decline in muscle strength occur in aging adults. Energy expenditure is reduced by 15% in older adults.[5]

Bone demineralization and decreased bone mass occurs with aging as a result of an increase in osteoblast and osteoclast activity, which decreases calcium absorption into bone, causing osteoporosis.[68] Osteoporosis is more common in women and results in bones that are delicate and at risk for fractures. Fractures often increase mortality and decrease QOL in older adults. Critical care nurses should consider the complications of critical illness and should promote early mobility and participation in activities of daily living to reduce post-ICU impairment.[69] Approximately 50% of patients discharged from the critical care unit, especially patients who were mechanically ventilated, develop a new or worsening disability in the first year after hospitalization.[69] Many older adults do not regain preillness functional ability and are unable to return home or provide self-care.[69,70]

PHARMACOLOGIC THERAPY IN OLDER ADULTS

Approximately 40% of older adults are prescribed more than five medications per day, and older adults are particularly vulnerable to adverse medication interactions.[71,73] The Critical Care Safety Study found that approximately 61% of adverse events in critical care units were linked with medications.[74] Medication-related adverse events account for costs of approximately $76.6 billion in the ambulatory care setting, $20 billion in hospitals, and $4 billion in nursing homes.[71] Medications most often associated with adverse events include cardiovascular medications (24%), anticoagulants (20%), antiinfective agents (13%), and hypoglycemic agents.[71] The Beers Criteria list contains medications that are potentially inappropriate for use in older adults.[72] Alterations in absorption, distribution, metabolism, and excretion are responsible for many adverse events. Alterations in gastric acid secretion, solubility of medications, and hepatic and renal function result in changes to absorption rates.[75] Distribution of medication is affected by changes in lean body mass and total body water.[68] See Table 40.4 for more details.

LONG-TERM COMPLICATIONS OF CRITICAL CARE FOR OLDER ADULTS

Improved critical care outcomes have led to an increase in survivors of critical illness and additional challenges related to long-term complications of critical care.[70,73] Adults older than 65 account for approximately 50% of ICU admissions in the United States.[73] Nurses Improving Care for Health-system Elders (NICHE) is a program that promotes evidence-based practices for patient-centered care of older adults.[73] Because older adults are a vulnerable population, they have unique needs during hospitalization such as prevention of functional decline, avoidance of post-ICU syndrome, and reduction of polypharmacy.[73] Functional decline can occur 1 day after

TABLE 40.4 Age-Related Changes in Pharmacokinetics

Pharmacokinetic Parameter	Definition	Age-Related Changes
Absorption	Medication moves from site of administration to bloodstream; affected by mode of administration	Decreased absorptive surface area of small intestine and gastrointestinal motility Decreased splanchnic blood flow Increased gastric acid pH Changes in body skin/fat
Distribution	Medication is delivered from bloodstream to target tissues; affected by blood flow	Decreased lean body mass and total body water Increased total body fat Decreased serum albumin/plasma proteins Decreased red blood cells
Metabolism	Metabolic breakdown of a medication that renders it active or inactive; affected by mode of administration	Decreased liver mass Decreased medication metabolism Decreased total liver blood flow
Excretion	Removal of medication through an eliminating organ, often the kidney; some medications are excreted in bile or feces, in saliva, or through the lungs	Decreased renal blood flow/glomerular filtration rate Decreased distal renal tubular secretory function

Data from Gilman AG, et al, eds. *Goodman and Gilman's the Pharmacological Basis of Therapeutics*. 8th ed. London: Pergamon Press; 1990; Vestal RE, Cusack BJ. Pharmacology and aging. In: Schneider EL, Rowe JW, eds. *Handbook of the Biology of Aging*, San Diego: Academic Press; 1990; and Kaplow R. Oncologic issues in the older adult in critical care. *Crit Care Nurs Clin North Am.* 2014;26(1):147.

admission, leading to decreasing muscle strength and increasing risk of complications each day of the ICU stay.[73] Complications of immobility include aspiration pneumonia, falls, deep vein thrombosis, loss of independence, pulmonary emboli, deconditioning, pressure ulcers, bowel paralysis, and increased length of stay. Table 40.5 presents details of functional decline. Pain is a particular problem in elderly patients—80% of older adults potentially experience and are undertreated for pain.[73]

Approximately 50% of patients who are discharged from the ICU require caregiving assistance for 1 year after discharge. Most family caregivers receive little advice or education on medication management or clinical care before discharge. Several instruments exist to assist with family caregiving assessment such as the Family Preferences Index tool. This tool can be used to assess if families wish to participate in patient care and for teaching opportunities.[73]

Functional status before illness appears to be a strong predictor of disability after critical illness with studies showing that many elderly patients who are discharged from the ICU die within 12 months of hospital discharge.[69] Elderly patients who require mechanical ventilation for extended periods experience chronic critical illness and have the highest rate of mortality.[76]

Assessments such as the Katz Index of Activities of Daily Living, Barthel Index, and frailty index are useful and validated instruments to assess functional status in elderly adults.[43] The most modifiable factors to reduce disability after critical illness include prevention of immobility and recognition of delirium (previously discussed in this chapter).[43] Delirium can be reduced by noise reduction, medication review, avoidance of restraints, and early mobility.[77] Understanding prehospital function, effect of critical care treatments, and post-ICU follow-up can decrease negative physical, functional, and cognitive long-term outcomes associated with critical illness.[78] Critical care nurses must recognize the need to prevent and manage long-term complications of critical care.[78] Critical care nurses have an essential role to advocate for multidisciplinary collaboration in the care of older adults to promote decreased sedation, prompt extubation, and early progressive mobility.[79]

TABLE 40.5 Decline in Functional Status

Hospital Day	Characteristics
1	Early initiation of contractions Muscle atrophy Pressure ulcers
2	Continued decrease in muscle strength
3	Decreased plasma volume Decreased stroke volume and cardiac output Increased heart rate and cardiovascular workload Orthostatic hypotension
5	Insulin resistance Microvascular dysfunction
7	Visible muscle weakness Postural muscle strength is decreased
8	Bone degradation begins

Adapted from Giambattista L, et al. NICHE recommended care of the critically ill older adult. *Crit Care Nurs Q.* 2015;38(3):223.

Palliative and End-of-Life Care

Palliative care is frequently misconstrued as synonymous with withdrawal of life support or hospice care. Palliative care is focused on the relief of suffering, in all its dimensions, throughout the course of a patient's illness. Palliative care specialists provide medical care for patients with serious illnesses with emphasis on relief from undesirable symptoms such as pain, shortness of breath, fatigue, anorexia, and nausea and vomiting. The goal of palliative care is to improve QOL for both the patient and the family; therefore, holistic assessment includes social, spiritual, and patient-centered goals of care.[80] Compassionate end-of-life care in accordance with patient wishes is an essential component of critical care. The Institute of Medicine[3] report described the need for improvement in end-of-life care through enhanced communication, professional education, person-centered care, and advanced care planning. Financial concerns about the cost of health care and the increasing elderly population have also led to questions about supply, demand, and sustainability of

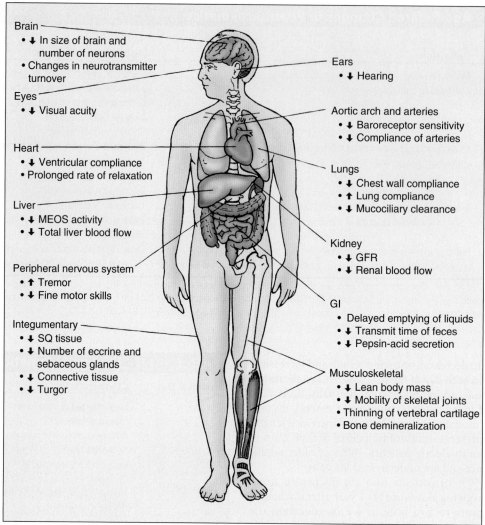

FIG. 40.3 Physiologic Changes That Occur in All Systems and That the Critical Care Nurse Must Consider in Caring for an Older Adult Patient in the Critical Care Unit. GFR, glomerular filtration rate; GI, gastrointestinal; MEOS, microsomal enzyme oxidative system; SQ, subcutaneous.

high-cost therapies.[81] A systematic review found that palliative care consultation resulted in decreased costs between 9% and 25%.[82] The Study to Understand Prognoses and Preferences for Outcomes and Risks of Treatments (SUPPORT) indicated that hospitalized patients often received care they did not want at the end of life.[83] Palliative care provides a mechanism for patients and families to continue therapeutic treatment options at the same time as declining interventions that may be harmful or painful such as cardiopulmonary resuscitation. A "Do Not Resuscitate" order does not equate to "Do Not Treat" and should never be a reason to deny a patient treatment that has potential benefit. The responsibility of the critical care nurse is to advocate for holistic and appropriate treatment for all patient without judgment or prejudice.

CONCLUSION

Older adults, especially individuals without family or friends, are particularly vulnerable during hospital stays and transitions of care. Fragmented communication and inadequate assessment can pose significant risk for iatrogenic complications of

critical illness. Critical care nurses must consider all factors that affect the care of older adult patients in the intensive care unit. Fig. 40.3 summarizes changes that occur in elderly adults.

CASE STUDY 40.1   The Older Patient

Brief Patient History

Mr. S is a 70-year-old man with a history of atrial fibrillation for which he takes warfarin, hypertension, and chronic obstructive pulmonary disease who presented to the emergency department at 3 am after tripping and falling while walking to the bathroom. He reported no loss of consciousness.

Clinical Assessment

Mr. S is admitted to the critical care unit from the emergency department. Nursing assessment findings include drowsiness, confusion, and mild left hemiparesis. He also has a raised area of ecchymosis on his right forehead and complains of a headache.

Diagnostic Procedures

The patient's admission laboratory test results are unremarkable except for an international normalized ratio of 4. Computed tomography scan of the head without contrast shows a right-sided subdural hematoma. Baseline vital signs are as follows: blood pressure of 170/65 mm Hg, heart rate of 80 beats/min (atrial fibrillation), respiratory rate of 20 breaths/min, and temperature of 98.4°F.

Medical Diagnosis
Mr. S is diagnosed with acute traumatic subdural hematoma.

Questions
1. What major outcomes do you expect to achieve for this patient?
2. What problems or risks must be managed to achieve these outcomes?
3. What interventions must be initiated to monitor, prevent, manage, or eliminate the problems and risks identified?
5. What possible learning needs do you anticipate for this patient?
6. What cultural and age-related factors may have a bearing on the patient's plan of care?

SUMMARY

REFERENCES

1. Centers for Disease Control and Prevention. *The State of Aging and Health in America 2013*. Atlanta, GA: Centers for Disease Control and Prevention, US Dept of Health and Human Services; 2013.
2. Murphy SL, et al. *Mortality in the United States, 2014. NCHS data brief, no 229*. Hyattsville, MD: National Center for Health Statistics; 2015. Retrieved on March 30th 2016 from http://www.cdc.gov/nchs/data/data-briefs/db178.htm.
3. IOM (Institute of Medicine). *Dying in America: Improving quality and honoring individual preferences near the end of life*. Washington, DC: The National Academies Press; 2015. Retrieved on March 30th 2016 from http://www.cdc.gov/nchs/fastats/deaths.htm.
4. Bell L. The epidemiology of acute and critical illness in older adults. *Crit Care Nurs Clin North Am*. 2014;26(1):1.
5. Marik P. Management of the critically ill geriatric patient. In: O'Donnell JM, Nacul FE, eds. *Surgical Intensive Care Medicine*. 2nd ed. New York: Springer Science; 2010.
6. Strait J, et al. Aging-associated cardiovascular changes and their relationship to heart failure. *Heart Fail Clin*. 2012;8(1):143.
7. North BJ. The intersection between aging and cardiovascular disease. *Circ Res*. 2012;110(8):1097.
8. Dai X, et al. Cardiovascular physiology in the older adults. *J Geriatr Cardiol*. 2015;12(3):196.
9. Francis GS, et al. Pathophysiology of heart failure. In: Fuster V, et al., ed. *Hurst's the Heart*. 12th ed. New York: McGraw-Hill; 2008.
10. Aronow WS, et al. ACCF/AHA 2011 Expert Consensus Document on Hypertension in the Elderly: A report of the American College of Cardiology Foundation Task Force on Clinical Expert Consensus Documents. *J Am Coll Cardiol*. 2011;57(20):2037.
11. Hajjar I. Postural blood pressure changes and orthostatic hypotension in elderly patients: Impact of antihypertensive medications. *Drugs Aging*. 2005;22(1):55.
12. James PA, et al. 2014 evidence-based guideline for the management of high blood pressure in adults: Report from the panel members appointed to the Eighth Joint National Committee (JNC 8). *JAMA*. 2014;311(5):507.
13. Shih H, et al. The aging heart and post-infarction left ventricular remodeling. *J Am Coll Cardiol*. 2010;57(1):9.
14. Strandberg TE, et al. Cholesterol and glucose metabolism and recurrent cardiovascular events among the elderly: A prospective study. *J Am Coll Cardiol*. 2006;48(4):708.
15. Nenseter MS. Lipoprotein(a) levels in coronary heart disease-susceptible and -resistant patients with familial hypercholesterolemia. *Atherosclerosis*. 2011;216(2):426.
16. Cooney D, Pascuzzi K. Polypharmacy in the elderly: Focus on drug interactions and adherence in hypertension. *Clin Geriatr Med*. 2009;25:221.
17. Moss AJ, et al. Cardiac resynchronization therapy for the prevention of heart failure events. *N Engl J Med*. 2009;361:1.
18. Azad N, Lemay G. Management of chronic heart failure in the older population. *J Geriatr Cardiol*. 2014;11(4):329.
19. Resnick B, Pacala JT. 2012 Beers criteria. *J Am Geriatr Soc*. 2012;60(4):612.
20. Carella AM, et al. Metabolic disorders in elderly patients with hematologic malignancies. A review. *World*. 2015;2:29.
21. Hurria A, et al. Improving the evidence base for treating older adults with cancer: American Society of Clinical Oncology statement. *J Clin Oncol*. 2015;33(32):3826.
22. Korc-Grodzicki B, et al. Surgical considerations in older adults with cancer. *J Clin Oncol*. 2014;32(24):2647.
23. Kaplow R. Oncologic issues in the older adult in critical care. *Crit Care Nurs Clin North Am*. 2014;26(1):147.
24. Menaker J, Scalea TM. Geriatric care in the surgical intensive care unit. *Crit Care Med*. 2010;38(9):S452.
25. Janssens JP. Aging of the respiratory system: Impact on pulmonary function tests and adaptation to exertion. *Clin Chest Med*. 2005;26:469.
26. Lowery EM, et al. The aging lung. *Clin Interv Aging*. 2013;8:1489.
27. Tyler K, Stevenson D. Respiratory emergencies in geriatric patients. *Emerg Med Clin North Am*. 2016;34(1):39.
28. Fragoso CAV, Gill TM. Respiratory impairment and the aging lung: A novel paradigm for assessing pulmonary function. *J Gerontol A Biol Sci Med Sci*. 2011;67A(3):264.
29. Bonomo L, et al. Aging and the respiratory system. *Radiol Clin North Am*. 2008;46:685.
30. LeBlanc P, et al. Effects of age and body position on "airway closure" in man. *J Appl Physiol*. 1970;28:448.
31. Holland J, et al. Regional distribution of pulmonary ventilation and perfusion in elderly subjects. *J Clin Invest*. 1968;47:81.
32. Rosenthal RA, Kavic SM. Assessment and management of the geriatric patient. *Crit Care Med*. 2004;32(4):S92.
33. Barnato AE, et al. Disability among elderly survivors of mechanical ventilation. *Am J Respir Crit Care Med*. 2011;183(8):1037.
34. Kahn JM, et al. Long-term acute care hospital utilization after critical illness. *JAMA*. 2010;303(22):2253.
35. Behrendt CE. Acute respiratory failure in the United States: Incidence and 31-day survival. *Chest J*. 2000;18(4):1100.
36. Marik PE. Management of the critically ill geriatric patient. *Crit Care Med*. 2006;34(9):S176.
37. Mehta AB, et al. Epidemiological trends in invasive mechanical ventilation in the United States: A population-based study. *J Crit Care*. 2015;30(6):1217.
38. Bonne S, Schuerer DJE. Trauma in the older adult: Epidemiology and evolving geriatric trauma principles. *Clin Geriatr Med*. 2013;29(1):137.
39. Stevens CL, Torke AM. Geriatric trauma: A clinical and ethical review. *J Trauma Nurs*. 2016;23(1):36.
40. Bishop NA, Lu T, Yankner BA. Neural mechanisms of ageing and cognitive decline. *Nature*. 2010;464:529.
41. Clare L. Neuropsychological assessment. In: Abou-Saleh MT, Katona C, Kumar A, eds. *Principles and Practice of Geriatric Psychiatry*. 3rd ed. London: John Wiley & Sons; 2011.
42. Rice KL, et al. Nurses' recognition of delirium in the hospitalized older adult. *Clin Nurse Specialist*. 2011;25(6):299.
43. Brummel NE, et al. Understanding and reducing disability in older adults following critical illness. *Crit Care Med*. 2015;43(6):1265.
44. Pandharipande PP, et al. Long-term cognitive impairment after critical illness. *N Engl J Med*. 2013;369(14):1306.
45. Balas Michele C, et al. Effectiveness and safety of the awakening and breathing coordination, delirium monitoring/management, and early exercise/mobility (ABCDE) bundle. *Critical care medicine*. 2014;42.5:1024. Retrieved on May 30th 2016 from http://www.icudelirium.org/medicalprofessionals.html.
46. Quinn J, Kaye J. The neurology of aging. *Neurologist*. 2001;7:98.
47. Selkoe DJ. Aging brain, aging mind. *Sci Am*. 1992;267:134.
48. Gottstein U, Held K. Effects of aging on cerebral circulation and metabolism in man. *Acta Neurol Scand Suppl*. 1979;72:54.

49. Jones RN, et al. Aging, brain disease, and reserve: Implications for delirium. *Am J Geriatr Psychiatry*. 2010;18(2):117.

50. Naatanen R, et al. The mismatch negativity: An index of cognitive decline in neuropsychiatric and neurological diseases and in ageing. *Brain*. 2011;134:3435.

51. Mink J. The neurologic assessment toolbox: Key assessments at critical times. *Nurs Crit Care*. 2012;7(3):12.

52. Ehlenbach WJ, et al. Association between acute care and critical illness hospitalization and cognitive function in older adults. *JAMA*. 2010;303(8):763.

53. Walker M, Spivak M, Sebastian M. The impact of aging physiology in critical care. *Crit Care Nurs Clin North Am*. 2014;26(1):7.

54. Garasto S, et al. Estimating glomerular filtration rate in older people. *Biomed Res Int*. 2014;2014.

55. Fassett RG. Current and emerging treatment options for the elderly patient with chronic kidney disease. *Clin Interv Aging*. 2014;9:191.

56. Clark JA, Coopersmith CM. Intestinal crosstalk: A new paradigm for understanding the gut as the "motor" of critical illness. *Shock*. 2007;28:384.

57. Bitar K, et al. Aging and gastrointestinal neuromuscular function: Insights from within and outside the gut. *Neurogastroenterol Motil*. 2011;23:490.

58. Lacasse C. Polypharmacy and symptom management in older adults. *Clin J Oncol Nurs*. 2010;15(1):27.

59. Sheedfar F, et al. Liver diseases and aging: friends or foes? *Aging Cell*. 2013;12(6):950.

60. Schmucker DL. Age-related changes in liver structure and function: Implications for disease? *Exp Gerontol*. 2005;40:650.

61. Schmucker DL, Sanchez H. Liver regeneration and aging: A current perspective. *Curr Gerontol Geriatr Res*. 2011.

62. Floreani A. Liver disorders in the elderly. *Best Pract Res Clin Gastroenterol*. 2009;23:909.

63. Kirkman MS, et al. Diabetes in older adults. *Diabetes Care*. 2012;35(12):2650.

64. Grant RW, Kirkman MS. Trends in the evidence level for the American Diabetes Association's "Standards of Medical Care in Diabetes" from 2005 to 2014. *Diabetes Care*. 2015;38(1):6.

65. Htwe TH, et al. Infection in the elderly. *Infect Dis Clin North Am*. 2007;21(3):711.

66. Dellinger R Phillip, et al. Surviving Sepsis Campaign: international guidelines for management of severe sepsis and septic shock, 2012. *Intensive care medicine*. 2013;39.2:165-228. Retrieved March 20th 2016 from http://www.survivingsepsis.org.

67. Smith DR, Leggat PA. Prevalence of skin disease among the elderly in different clinical environments. *Austral J Ageing*. 2005;24(2):71.

68. Pittman J. Effect of aging on wound healing current concepts. *J Wound Ostomy Continence Nurs*. 2007;34:412.

69. Black DM, Rosen CJ. Following the bone density trail: A clinical perspective. *J Clin Endocrinol Metabol*. 2012;97(4):1176.

70. Desai SV, Law TJ, Needham DM. Long-term complications of critical care. *Crit Care Med*. 2011;39(2):371.

71. Fick DM, et al. Updating the Beers criteria for potentially inappropriate medication use in older adults: Results of a US consensus panel of experts. *Arch Intern Med*. 2003;163:2716.

72. Campanelli Christine M. American Geriatrics Society updated beers criteria for potentially inappropriate medication use in older adults: the American Geriatrics Society 2012 Beers Criteria Update Expert Panel. *Journal of the American Geriatrics Society*. 2012;60.4:616. Retrieved September 26, 2016 from http://www.americangeriatrics.org/files/documents/beers/2012AGSBeersCriteriaCitations.pdf.

73. Giambattista L, et al. NICHE recommended care of the critically ill older adult. *Crit Care Nurs Q*. 2015;38(3):223.

74. Rothschild JM, et al. The critical care safety study: The incidence and nature of adverse events and serious errors in intensive care. *Crit Care Med*. 2005;33:1694.

75. Yuen GJ. Altered pharmacokinetics in the elderly. *Clin Geriatr Med*. 1990;6:257.

76. Baldwin MR. Measuring and predicting long-term outcomes in older survivors of critical illness. *Minerva Anestesiol*. 2014.

77. Balas M, et al. Critical care nurses' role in implementing the "ABCDE bundle" into practice. *Crit Care Nurse*. 2012;32(2):35.

78. Covinsky KE, Pierluissi E, Johnston CB. Hospitalization-associated disability. *JAMA*. 2011;306(16):1783.

79. Pandharipande P, et al. Liberation and animation for ventilated ICU patients: The ABCDE bundle for the back-end of critical care. *Crit Care*. 2010;14(3):157.

80. Frost DW, Cook DJ, Heyland DK. Patient and healthcare professional factors influencing end-of-life decision-making during critical illness: A systematic review. *Crit Care Med*. 2011;39(5):1134.

81. Newman R, Thomas K. Failing to plan is planning to fail: Advance care planning for people nearing the end of life. *Aging Health*. 2011;7(5):677.

82. May P, Normand C, Morrison RS. Economic impact of hospital inpatient palliative care consultation: Review of current evidence and directions for future research. *J Palliat Med*. 2014;17:1054.

83. Connors AF, et al. A controlled trial to improve care for seriously ill hospitalized patients: The study to understand prognoses and preferences for outcomes and risks of treatments (SUPPORT). *JAMA*. 1995;274(20):1591.

41

The Perianesthesia Patient

Denise O'Brien

Advances in anesthetic agents and monitoring have resulted in more precise and safer delivery of anesthetic agents. Caring for a critically ill patient who is emerging from anesthesia requires diligent monitoring of the patient's physical and psychological status to prevent potential complications that may occur as a result of the anesthetic agents or techniques. To provide safe and competent patient care, the critical care nurse needs to have knowledge of anesthetic agents and techniques and the physiologic and psychological responses of patients who receive anesthesia.[1,2]

SELECTION OF ANESTHESIA

The complex structure of anesthetic agents, combined with potential medication interactions and the patient's physical condition, can make it difficult to predict the patient's response when emerging from anesthesia. Knowledge of the general principles of anesthesia prepares the nurse for the most commonly expected outcomes.[2,3] The American Society of Anesthesiologists (ASA) physical status classification is widely accepted as a method of preoperative patient evaluation.[4] It guides communication of clinical conditions and predicts risks for anesthesia (Box 41.1). Preoperative evaluation allows the anesthesia care provider to individualize and modify care for patients at high risk for surgery.[4]

The type of anesthesia used for surgery may be local, regional, or general. Local and regional anesthetics eliminate the sensation of pain to a specific part of the body without loss of protective reflexes or consciousness. Many patients also receive intravenous sedation with benzodiazepines to relieve anxiety, provide amnesia, and promote relaxation. Local anesthesia with sedation may be defined as moderate or *procedural* sedation. Another term used is *monitored anesthesia care*. Depending on the sedation given and the patient's response, the level of consciousness can range from light to deep. Further information on sedation is provided in Chapter 9. Regional anesthesia includes peripheral and central neuraxial (spinal, epidural, caudal) blocks. Blocks include single injection and continuous infusion techniques, typically used for postoperative or postprocedural analgesia. Spinal anesthesia involves injecting local anesthetic into cerebrospinal fluid contained within the subarachnoid space, below L1 in an adult and L3 in a child.[5] Epidural anesthesia involves injecting the epidural space, which lies within the vertebral canal but outside the dural sac, with local anesthetics. Epidurals may be performed at all levels of the neuraxis. Spinal and epidural anesthesia cause sensory and motor anesthesia. The advantages of epidural over spinal anesthesia are decreased incidence of spinal headache, less incidence of systemic hypotension, ability to provide a segmental sensory block, and increased ability to provide postoperative pain management.[6]

General anesthesia is a controlled, reversible state of unconsciousness: The patient is not arousable, there is partial or complete loss of protective reflexes, and the airway and ventilation needs to be continuously monitored and maintained. An endotracheal tube is commonly used for airway maintenance for general anesthesia, although a laryngeal mask airway may also be used.[7]

Several factors influence the choice of anesthetic agent and the mode of delivery. These factors include age, coexisting diseases, site of surgery, position of the patient during surgery, type of surgery (ie, elective, emergent), duration of the procedure, the skills of the anesthesia care provider and the surgeon, and patient preference.[8]

GENERAL ANESTHESIA

The goals of general anesthesia are analgesia, amnesia/hypnosis, suppression of autonomic and sensory reflexes, and skeletal muscle relaxation.[9] Stages of anesthesia, defined by Guedel around the time of World War I, were initially used to identify the patient's physiologic state and monitor anesthetic depth. These stages are less relevant today because of technologic advances in monitoring and anesthetic agents with faster onset and elimination, limiting the usefulness of the classic signs and symptoms associated with the stages to assessment and care of the patient after surgery.[10]

Stage I, commonly called the *stage of analgesia*, begins with the initiation of an anesthetic agent and ends with the loss of consciousness. This stage has been described as the lightest level of anesthesia and represents mild sensory and mental depression. Patients can open their eyes on command, breathe normally, and maintain protective reflexes. The patient's pain threshold is not appreciably lowered during this stage.

Stage II, also called the *stage of delirium*, begins with the loss of consciousness and ends with the onset of a regular pattern of breathing and the disappearance of the eyelid reflex. It is characterized by excitement, which can include uncontrolled movement and potentially dangerous responses to noxious stimuli. Other responses include vomiting, laryngospasm, tachycardia, and cardiac arrest. If vomiting occurs, the patient is at risk for aspiration because of the loss of protective reflexes that is associated with this stage of anesthesia. With the use of newer and faster acting anesthetic agents, this stage is passed through rapidly, decreasing the risk of complications. The use of propofol, etomidate, or short-acting barbiturates during the induction of anesthesia also facilitates rapid transition through stage II.

Stage III is the *stage of surgical anesthesia*. It lasts from the onset of a regular pattern of breathing to the cessation of breathing. This is the goal for anesthesia because the response

983

- Category 1: Normal, healthy patient
- Category 2: Patient with mild systemic disease
- Category 3: Patient with severe systemic disease (eg, hypertension, diabetes)
- Category 4: Patient with severe systemic disease that is life-threatening
- Category 5: Patient with high morbidity
- Category 6: Patient with brain death

to surgical incision is absent. Patients experience a depression in all elements of nervous system function (e.g., sensory depression, loss of recall, reflex depression, and some skeletal muscle relaxation). Each anesthetic agent affects the patient's clinical signs differently, and monitoring the effects of anesthesia depends on the specific properties of each agent.

Stage IV is considered the *stage of overdose* and occurs when the patient receives too much anesthesia. In this stage, the patient shows signs of circulatory failure, and full cardiovascular and pulmonary support must be provided.

During general anesthesia, the goal is to keep the patient insensate, immobile, and safe. Recall or awareness during surgery can occur when the depth of anesthesia is inadequate (Box 41.2).

QSEN BOX 41.2   QSEN: Patient Safety Alert

Preventing and Managing the Impact of Anesthesia Awareness

Anesthesia awareness, also called *unintended intraoperative awareness*, occurs under general anesthesia when a patient becomes cognizant of some or all events during a procedure and has direct recall of those events. Because of the routine use of neuromuscular blocking agents (paralytics) during general anesthesia, the patient is often unable to communicate with the surgical team when this occurs.

The frequency of anesthesia awareness has been found in multiple studies to be between 0.1% and 0.2% of all patients undergoing general anesthesia.[1-3] General anesthesia is administered to 21 million patients annually in the United States, so 20,000 to 40,000 cases of anesthesia awareness occur each year. Patients experiencing awareness report auditory recollections (48%), sensations of not being able to breathe (48%), and pain (28%).[1] More than 50% experience mental distress after surgery, including an indeterminate number with posttraumatic stress syndrome.[2,3] Some patients describe these occurrences as their "worst hospital experience," and some determine to never again undergo surgery.

The incidence of awareness is reported to be greater in patients for whom the dose of general anesthetic must be smaller and carefully titrated to decrease significant side effects, such as a patient who is hemodynamically unstable. Procedures typically identified as falling into this category are some cardiac, obstetric, and major trauma cases.[4] Factors contributing to the risk of anesthesia awareness include the increasing use of intravenous delivery of anesthesia, as opposed to inhalation, and the premature lightening of anesthesia at the end of procedures to facilitate operating room turnover.

Monitoring of patients under general anesthesia to prevent anesthesia awareness can be challenging. Despite a variety of available monitoring methods, awareness is difficult to recognize while it is occurring. Typical indicators of physiologic and motor response, such as high blood pressure, fast heart rate, movement, and hemodynamic changes, are often masked by the use of paralytic agents to achieve necessary muscle relaxation during the procedure, as well as the concurrent administration of other medications necessary to the patient's management such as beta-blockers or calcium channel blockers.

To overcome the limitations of current methods to detect anesthesia awareness, new methods are being developed that are less affected by the medications typically used during general anesthesia. These devices measure brain activity rather than physiologic responses. These electroencephalography devices (also called level-of-consciousness, sedation-level, or anesthesia-depth monitors) include bispectral index (BIS), spectral edge frequency, and median frequency monitors. These devices may have a role in preventing and detecting anesthesia awareness in patients with the highest risk, ameliorating the impact of anesthesia awareness. A body of evidence has not yet accumulated to define precisely the role of these devices in detecting and

preventing anesthesia awareness; The Joint Commission expects additional studies on these subjects to emerge. In its review of the BIS monitor, the US Food and Drug Administration determined that "Use of BIS monitoring to help guide anesthetic administration may be associated with the reduction of the incidence of awareness with recall in adults during general anesthesia and sedation."

The anesthesia professional must often balance the psychological risks of anesthesia awareness against the physiologic risks of excessive anesthesia for many critical medical conditions. The Joint Commission has asked the American Society of Anesthesiologists (ASA) and the American Association of Nurse Anesthetists (AANA) to address the adequacy of current monitoring practices regarding anesthesia levels, including practices that involve little or no technologic support. In its 2006 practice advisory, the ASA recommended that intraoperative monitoring include clinical monitoring (eg, noting purposeful or reflex movement), conventional monitors (eg, end-tidal anesthetic analyzer, heart rate, blood pressure), and brain function monitoring on a case-by-case basis.[5] Multimodal monitoring is suggested rather than reliance on any single monitor.

Reducing the Risk of Anesthesia Awareness

The ASA and the AANA provide guidelines for administering and monitoring anesthesia. Specific recommendations for the prevention of awareness were addressed in the February 2000 issue of *Anesthesiology*[4]:

- Consider premedication with amnesic medications (eg, benzodiazepines, scopolamine), particularly when light anesthesia is anticipated.
- Administer more than a "sleep dose" of induction agents if they will be followed immediately by tracheal intubation. Avoid muscle paralysis unless absolutely necessary and, even then, avoid total paralysis (by using only the amount clinically required).
- Conduct periodic maintenance of the anesthesia machine and its vaporizers, and meticulously check the machine and its ventilator before administering anesthesia.
- Be alert to patients taking beta-blockers, calcium channel blockers, or other medications that can mask physiologic responses to inadequate anesthesia.

Managing the Impact of Anesthesia Awareness

Anesthesia awareness cannot always be prevented. Health care practitioners must be prepared to acknowledge and manage the occurrence of anesthesia awareness with compassion and diligence. The following practices are suggested when patients report awareness[4]:

- Interview the patient after the procedure, taking a detailed account of his or her experience and including it in the patient's chart.
- Apologize to the patient if anesthesia awareness occurred.

Preventing and Managing the Impact of Anesthesia Awareness

- Assure the patient of the credibility of his or her account, and sympathize with the patient's suffering.
- Explain what happened and its reasons (eg, the necessity to administer light anesthesia in the presence of significant cardiovascular instability).
- Offer the patient psychological or psychiatric support including referral to a psychologist or psychiatrist.
- Notify the patient's surgeon, nurse, and other key personnel about the incident and the subsequent interview with the patient.
  Surgical team members should also be educated about anesthesia awareness and its management.

The Joint Commission Recommendations

Anesthesia awareness is underrecognized and undertreated in health care organizations. The Joint Commission recommends that health care organizations performing procedures under general anesthesia take the following steps to help prevent and manage anesthesia awareness:

1. Develop and implement an anesthesia awareness policy that addresses the following:
   - Education of clinical staff about anesthesia awareness and how to manage patients who have experienced awareness
   - Identification of patients at proportionately higher risk for an awareness experience and discussion with such patients before surgery of the potential for anesthesia awareness
   - The effective application of available anesthesia monitoring techniques including timely maintenance of anesthesia equipment
   - Appropriate postoperative follow-up of all patients who have undergone general anesthesia including children
   - The identification, management, and, if appropriate, referral of patients who have experienced awareness
2. Ensure access to necessary counseling or other support for patients who experience posttraumatic stress syndrome or other mental distress.

References

1. Sebel PS, et al. The incidence of awareness during anesthesia: a multicenter United States study. *Anesth Analg.* 2004;99(3):833.
2. Lennmarken C, Sandin R. Neuromonitoring for awareness during surgery. *Lancet.* 2004;363(9423):1747.
3. Osterman JE, et al. Awareness under anesthesia and the development of posttraumatic stress disorder. *Gen Hosp Psychiatry.* 2001;23(4):198.
4. Ghoneim MM. Awareness during anesthesia. *Anesthesiology.* 2000;92(2):597.
5. Practice advisory for intraoperative awareness and brain function monitoring. A report by the American Society of Anesthesiologists Task Force on Intraoperative Awareness. *Anesthesiology.* 2006;104:847.

Bibliography

Ekman A, et al. Reduction in the incidence of awareness using BIS monitoring. *Acta Anaesthesiol Scand.* 2004;48(1):20.
Liska JM. *Silenced Screams: Surviving Anesthetic Awareness During Surgery—a True-Life Account.* Park Ridge, IL: AANA Publishing, Council for Public Interest in Anesthesia; 2002.
Myles PS, et al. Bispectral index monitoring to prevent awareness during anaesthesia: the B-Aware randomised controlled trial. *Lancet.* 2004;363(9423):1757.

Modified from The Joint Commission: Sentinel Event Alert. http://www.jointcommission.org/SentinelEvents/SentinelEventAlert/sea_32.htm Accessed January 11, 2016.

Excessive anesthesia may stress the patient and increase emergence and recovery time. The level of anesthesia is monitored by continual assessment of the patient's clinical presentation. Basic anesthetic monitoring standards adopted by the ASA mandate the use of pulse oximetry, capnography, an oxygen analyzer, disconnect alarms, body temperature measurements, arterial blood pressure and heart rate every 5 minutes, and a visual display of an electrocardiogram (ECG) during the intraoperative period in all patients undergoing anesthesia.[11] The standard may be exceeded and additional monitors used as warranted by the patient's condition. External monitoring devices used to assess levels of anesthesia include lower esophageal contractility, heart rate variability, surface electromyogram, spontaneous electroencephalographic activity monitors, and evoked potentials.

ANESTHETIC AGENTS

Typically two or more anesthetic agents are used in combination to achieve the desired level of anesthesia. To anticipate the patient's response, it is important for the nurse to have knowledge of the anesthetic agents that are used and their usual physiologic effects.[2] The characteristics of ideal anesthetic agents and adjuncts are listed in Box 41.3.

Inhalation Agents

Inhalation agents are used for induction and maintenance of anesthesia or, in combination with other anesthetic agents, to maintain surgical anesthesia. They can be classified as volatile

BOX 41.3   Characteristics of Ideal Anesthetic Agents and Adjuncts

- Rapid onset of action
- Controllable duration of action
- Identifiable levels of depth
- Technically easy to administer
- No untoward effects on hemodynamic status
- No toxic metabolites
- Predictable elimination
- High specificity of action
- High margin of safety
- Useful with all ages
- Cost-effective
- Rapid emergence

or gaseous. Volatile agents are further classified as halogenated hydrocarbons or ethers, are liquid at room temperature, and have a boiling point of 20°C. Gaseous agents are gases at room temperature. Inhaled anesthetics are delivered through the respiratory tract and are absorbed into the circulation through the alveoli. The effects of inhalation agents depend on alveolar ventilation, the ventilation-perfusion ratio, coadministered gases, gas flow, and the physicochemical properties of the gas. Their exact mechanism of action is unknown, but all cause central nervous system (CNS) depression and a state of unconsciousness that is deep enough to allow surgery. Table 41.1 lists

TABLE 41.1   Inhalation Anesthetics

Medication	Characteristics	Effects	Considerations
Nitrous oxide	Light anesthetic; inorganic gas; nontoxic, nonirritating; carrier for other inhalation agents; always given with oxygen	Anesthetic and analgesic; minimal pulmonary, cardiac, or CNS effects; increases intracranial pressure; amnesia	Eliminated by ventilation; PONV; diffusion hypoxia; mild myocardial depression
Isoflurane (Forane)	Pungent, ether-like odor; low potential for toxicity; volatile agent	Higher cardiovascular stability; potentiates muscle relaxants	Mild depression of spontaneous ventilation; may trigger malignant hypothermia; postoperative shivering; fewer dysrhythmias noted
Desflurane (Suprane)	Strong, pungent odor; rapid onset; volatile agent; requires warmed vaporizer for administration	Minimal metabolism; respiratory depression; cardiovascular depression; no lingering analgesia	Observe for breath holding; coughing and laryngospasm; may trigger malignant hypothermia; needs immediate postoperative analgesia
Sevoflurane (Ultane)	Nonirritating to airway; volatile agent; choice for pediatric anesthetic	Minimal airway irritation; rapid elimination; great precision and control over anesthetic depth; decreases SVR	May trigger malignant hypothermia; observe for breath holding; needs immediate postoperative analgesia

CNS, central nervous system; *PONV,* postoperative nausea and vomiting; *SVR,* systemic vascular resistance.

inhalation anesthetics used at the present time and their chief characteristics, effects, and nursing implications.[10]

Intravenous Anesthetics

Because inhalation anesthetics can produce adverse effects such as vasodilation, hypotension, dysrhythmias, and myocardial depression, other medications and methods of delivery have been sought to provide general anesthesia. Intravenous anesthetics are commonly used in the perioperative period. Intravenous anesthetics are grouped by their primary pharmacologic action as nonopioid or opioid intravenous agents.[12-14] Nonopioid agents are further divided into barbiturates, nonbarbiturates, and sedatives. These medications can be administered by intermittent intravenous push dosing to induce anesthesia or by continuous intravenous drip to maintain anesthesia.

Nonopioid Intravenous Anesthetics

Gamma-aminobutyric acid (GABA) is an inhibitory neurotransmitter. Nonopioid medications appear to interact with GABA in the brain. Activation of the GABA receptors inhibits the postsynaptic neurons and results in a loss of consciousness. Barbiturates bind to GABA postsynaptic receptors, inhibiting neuronal activity and causing a loss of consciousness. Sedatives such as benzodiazepines potentiate the action of GABA, leading to inhibition of neuronal activity. Nonbarbiturate induction agents, such as etomidate, antagonize the muscarinic receptors in the CNS and work as opioid agonists, resulting in a hypnotic state and loss of consciousness. Table 41.2 lists the nonopioid intravenous anesthetics and their effects and nursing considerations.[12]

Benzodiazepine Antagonists

Flumazenil (Romazicon) reverses the sedative, amnesic, respiratory depressant, and muscle-relaxant effects of benzodiazepines.[14] This medication is specific for the benzodiazepine receptors and does not reverse the effects of barbiturates or opiates. It should be used with caution in patients who have a history of seizures or long-term benzodiazepine use, as it can precipitate seizures. Because flumazenil has a shorter duration of action than most of the benzodiazepines, the risk of resedation can occur after the initial dose starts to wear off, especially when high doses of benzodiazepines are administered. The patient must be monitored for resedation and other residual effects. If the patient develops signs of resedation, flumazenil is repeated at 20-minute intervals. Flumazenil has proved to be valuable in the care of the patient who has received an excessive dose of a benzodiazepine such as midazolam or lorazepam. Consequently, flumazenil is very useful intraoperatively, postoperatively, and in the critical care unit.

Opioid Intravenous Analgesics

Intravenous opioid analgesics play an important role in clinical anesthesia care. These medications enhance the effectiveness of inhalation agents by providing the analgesic portion of the anesthetic process. Intravenous opioids blunt the sympathetic response to painful stimuli during anesthesia. The use of opioids allows for reduction in the concentration of the inhalation agent to be administered, increasing safety. Opioids bind to specific receptors and produce a morphine-like or opioid agonist effect. Opioids are used to manage acute and chronic pain and are administered for general anesthesia, sedation, and pain relief during regional anesthesia; they are important in all phases of the perioperative experience. Table 41.3 lists clinical uses and nursing implications for the most frequently used opioids.[13]

Opioid Antagonists

Opioid antagonists are used to reverse the effects of opioids, particularly respiratory depression, restoring spontaneous ventilation in patients who are breathing inadequately. The medication of choice in perianesthesia care is naloxone (Narcan). Naloxone competes with and displaces the opioid on the receptor site; it reverses respiratory depressant and analgesic effects of opioids. Naloxone is diluted and then titrated to the patient's response, minimizing the risk of rapid reversal and subsequent adverse effects. The onset of action is 1 to 2 minutes, and the duration of action is 1 to 4 hours. If adequate reversal has not been achieved after 3 to 5 minutes, naloxone administration is repeated until reversal is complete.[15]

If long-acting opioids are used, the patient must be monitored for respiratory insufficiency because the depressant effects of the opioids may return. Often, a low-dose, continuous intravenous drip of naloxone proves effective. Close monitoring of vital signs is critical. The patient should be monitored for increased blood pressure, which may occur in response to pain after large doses

TABLE 41.2   Nonopioid Intravenous Anesthetics

Medication	Characteristics	Effects	Considerations
Barbiturates			
Methohexital (Brevital)	Good patient acceptance; no analgesia; hepatic metabolism; ultra-fast onset of action, brief duration	CNS depression, spontaneous ventilation arrested; loss of laryngeal reflexes; causes histamine release (vasodilation, hypotension, flushing); lowers seizure threshold (epileptiform)	IV administration painful, may cause myoclonus, coughing, and hiccoughs; increased risk of aspiration
Nonbarbiturates			
Etomidate (Amidate)	Agent of choice in patients with cardiovascular dysfunction	Heart rate and cardiac output remain constant; minimal negative inotropic effects; suppression of adrenal function up to 5–8 hours after a single dose	May cause nausea and vomiting; burns when given IV; may cause myoclonus, laryngospasm, cough, and hiccoughs; no analgesic effects
Propofol (Diprivan)	No analgesic effect; avoid in patients with coronary stenosis, ischemia, or hypovolemia; antiemetic properties; hepatic metabolism	Minimal residual CNS effects; myocardial depressant; may decrease blood pressure 20%–25%	Rapid emergence may hasten pain awareness; low incidence of postoperative side effects; pain on administration; dose reduction in older adults, patients with cardiac disease, and patients with hypovolemia; long-term or high-dose infusions can result in hypertriglyceridemia; contraindicated in patients allergic to soybean oil, egg lecithin, or glycerol
Dissociative Anesthetic			
Ketamine (Ketalar)	Profound analgesia and unconsciousness; provides amnesia; may be used alone; may be given IV, IM, or PO	Produces cardiovascular and respiratory stimulation; may increase blood pressure and heart rate 10%–50%; increases intracranial pressure	Monitor for and prevent emergent reactions; minimize stimulation of patient during emergence; titrate pain medications; benzodiazepines or dexmedetomidine may help reduce agitation during emergence; may be used in subanesthetic doses for opioid-sparing effects for pain management
Butyrophenones			
Haloperidol (Haldol)	Limited use in anesthesia because of long duration; antipsychotic; antiemetic, prevents and treats nausea and vomiting in low doses (recommended adult dose 1 mg); dopamine antagonist	—	In tranquilizing doses, high incidence of extrapyramidal reactions; potential for torsades de pointes because of prolongation of Q–T interval
Benzodiazepines			
Diazepam (Valium)	Rapid onset; long half-life; anterograde amnesic; effective anxiolysis; renal excretion	—	Titrate opioid medications and monitor for respiratory depression; used orally as premedicant
Midazolam (Versed)	Rapid onset; short duration; potent amnesic; effective anxiolysis; hepatic metabolism	—	Reduce dose in older adults and debilitated patients; use cautiously in patients with myocardial ischemia, COPD, and hepatic disease; titrate opioid medications; monitor for respiratory depression
Lorazepam (Ativan)	Slow onset of action; long duration; anticonvulsant action; hepatic metabolism; renal excretion; no active metabolites	Pronounced sedation; minimal cardiovascular effects	Poor IV compatibility; titrate opioid medications and monitor for respiratory depression; watch for orthostatic hypotension

CNS, central nervous system; *COPD,* chronic obstructive pulmonary disease; *IM,* intramuscularly; *IV,* intravenous/intravenously; *PO,* per os (orally).

TABLE 41.3   Opioid Adjunctive Agents[a]

Clinical Uses	Implications	Considerations
Preoperative sedation	Monitor for hypotension	Keep naloxone (Narcan) available
Induction of anesthesia	Monitor for bradycardia	Keep resuscitation equipment available
Maintenance of anesthesia	Monitor for respiratory depression	Respiratory depressant effect may outlast analgesia
Postoperative pain management	May cause nausea and vomiting	Monitor for respiratory depression, sedation

[a]Agents include alfentanil (Alfenta), fentanyl (Sublimaze), ketorolac (Toradol), morphine, sufentanil (Sufenta), remifentanil (Ultiva), and hydromorphone (Dilaudid).

of naloxone. In addition, tachycardia, nausea, vomiting, or dia-phoresis may occur if the reversal is too rapid. Naloxone must be used with caution in patients with cardiac irritability and in patients who are physically dependent on opioids because reversal may precipitate an acute withdrawal syndrome.

Neuromuscular Blocking Agents

Neuromuscular blocking agents (NMBAs), or muscle relaxants, interrupt the transmission of impulses from the nerve to the muscle, causing a decrease in muscle activity. Decreasing muscle activity allows the surgeon to operate in a quiet field and decreases the need for deep anesthesia. These medications have contributed greatly to clinical anesthesia care. Use of NMBAs is not limited to the operating room; they are used to facilitate endotracheal intubation, to terminate laryngospasm, to eliminate chest wall rigidity that may occur after the rapid injection of potent opioids, and to facilitate mechanical ventilation by producing total paralysis of the respiratory muscles.[15]

NMBAs cause paralysis of the respiratory muscles, and the patient receiving these agents requires ventilatory support with a handheld bag-valve-mask device or a mechanical ventilator. NMBAs do not have analgesic, amnesic, anxiolytic, or sedative effects. The paralyzed patient is unable to communicate his or her needs; NMBAs must be used in combination with other medications to prevent pain and provide sedation.

Skeletal muscle contraction occurs when acetylcholine is released from the motor neuron and binds to receptor sites on the muscle fiber (ie, neuromuscular junction), resulting in depolarization. Skeletal muscle relaxation occurs when the release of acetylcholine ceases and any residual acetylcholine is destroyed by the enzyme acetylcholinesterase, resulting in repolarization. NMBAs interfere with the relationship between acetylcholine and the receptor. There are two general categories of skeletal muscle relaxants: nondepolarizing and depolarizing.

Depolarizing agents compete with acetylcholine at the neuromuscular junction, causing the muscle to depolarize and inhibiting repolarization. The muscle stays in a prolonged depolarized state, and movement is inhibited. The principal depolarizing skeletal muscle agent is succinylcholine (Anectine). After succinylcholine attaches to the receptor, a brief period of depolarization occurs, which is manifested by transient muscular fasciculations. Succinylcholine has a rapid onset of 60 to 90 seconds and a short duration of action of 5 to 10 minutes. It is frequently used to facilitate intubation. Succinylcholine cannot be pharmacologically reversed.

Nondepolarizing NMBAs are typically longer acting agents than depolarizing agents. Nondepolarizing agents do not cause initial muscle contraction or depolarization. They compete with and block the uptake of acetylcholine at the muscle receptor site and prevent repolarization. Sustained muscle relaxation occurs, and voluntary control of skeletal muscle contraction is weakened or lost.

Table 41.4 presents a pharmacologic overview of the commonly used skeletal muscle relaxants.[16] Many factors can potentiate or antagonize the effects of nondepolarizing NMBAs; these factors are listed in Box 41.4.[17]

Neuromuscular Blocking Agent Antagonists

The pharmacologic actions of nondepolarizing NMBAs can be reversed by anticholinesterase medications such as neostigmine (Prostigmin). These medications increase the amount of acetylcholine available at the receptor sites by preventing its destruction by acetylcholinesterase. This promotes more effective competition of acetylcholine with the nondepolarizing skeletal muscle relaxant that is occupying the receptor sites. Because of the increased availability and mobilization of the acetylcholine, the concentration gradient favors acetylcholine and the removal of the nondepolarizing agent from the receptors, resulting in the return of normal skeletal muscle depolarization and contraction.[18] These medications also produce undesirable side effects by increasing the level of acetylcholine at receptor sites in the heart, lungs, eyes, and gastrointestinal tract, which can lead to bradycardia, bronchospasm, miosis, and increased peristalsis and secretion. To prevent or minimize these effects,

TABLE 41.4   Neuromuscular Blocking Agents[a]

Characteristics	IMPLICATIONS	
	Depolarizing	Nondepolarizing
Compete with acetylcholine at myoneural junction	Nonreversible	Reversible with time and anticholinesterases
	Use cautiously in patients with neuromuscular disease such as myasthenia gravis or muscular dystrophy; contraindicated for pediatric use except in emergencies	Use cautiously in patients with hepatic or renal disease, obesity, asthma, or COPD
Shorter acting agents are most appropriate for anesthesia	Adverse effects include bradycardia, tachycardia, ventricular dysrhythmias, asystole, hypertension, and hyperkalemia	Adverse effects include tachycardia, hypertension, hypotension, bronchospasm, and flushing
Provide surgical relaxation Facilitate intubation	Increases intraocular, intracranial, and intragastric pressure	
Assist in ventilatory support	Precipitates muscle fasciculations and pain	
	Prolongs respiratory depression	
	Histamine release causes hypotension	
	Use cautiously in patients with head injury, cerebral edema, trauma, burns, electrolyte imbalances, and renal or hepatic disease	
	Monitor for clinical signs of malignant hyperthermia	

[a]Long-acting agents include pancuronium (Pavulon); intermediate-acting agents include atracurium (Tracrium), vecuronium (Norcuron), rocuronium (Zemuron), and cisatracurium (Nimbex); and short-acting agents include succinylcholine (Anectine), which is a depolarizing agent.
COPD, chronic obstructive pulmonary disease.

anticholinergic agents such as atropine or glycopyrrolate (Robinul) are given with the anticholinesterase agent.

In 2015, sugammadex (Bridion) was approved for use in the United States by the Food and Drug Administration for the reversal of neuromuscular blockade associated with rocuronium and vecuronium. This new reversal agent, the first selective relaxant binding agent, encapsulates the NMBA, terminating the neuromuscular blockade without the need for anticholinergic drugs because sugammadex has no effect on acetylcholinesterases or any other receptor system in the body.[18] Table 41.5 lists the common NMBA reversal agents used in anesthesia and their nursing implications.[19]

BOX 41.4   Factors Influencing Neuromuscular Blockade

Potentiating Factors
- Hypocalcemia
- Hypokalemia
- Hyponatremia
- Hypermagnesemia
- Acidosis
- Hypothermia
- Antibiotics
  - Gentamicin
  - Tobramycin
  - Amikacin
  - Kanamycin
  - Neomycin
  - Polymyxin B
  - Clindamycin
  - Tetracyclines
  - Piperacillin
  - Streptomycin
- Antidysrhythmics
  - Procainamide
  - Lidocaine
  - Quinidine
- Beta-adrenergic blockers
- Calcium channel blockers
- Diuretics
  - Furosemide
  - Thiazides
- Inhalation agents
- Local anesthetics
- Cyclosporine
- Lithium
- Dantrolene
- Etomidate
- Hepatobiliary disease
- Renal failure
- Neuromuscular diseases

Antagonizing Factors
- Phenytoin
- Carbamazepine
- Aminophylline
- Theophylline
- Sympathomimetic agents
- Corticosteroids
- Azathioprine

PERIANESTHESIA ASSESSMENT AND CARE

The goal of management in the immediate postoperative period is the recognition and immediate treatment of any problems to eliminate or lessen complications that may occur. This requires the collaborative effort of the nurse, the anesthesiologist, and the surgeon. Physical assessment of the postanesthesia patient begins immediately on admission to the unit. This initial assessment focuses on airway, ventilation, and circulation (heart rate, rhythm, and blood pressure). After the brief initial assessment, the nurse admitting the patient receives a verbal report from the anesthesia care provider and surgeon. The report includes information about the patient's general condition, the patient's significant past history or comorbidities, the operation performed, the type of anesthesia administered, the estimated blood loss, the total intake and output during surgery, and any problems or complications encountered in the operating room.[20]

Assessment of the cardiopulmonary system is the immediate priority. The patient's airway is assessed to ensure that it is patent, with or without adjuncts, and the patient's breathing pattern is evaluated to ensure that it is unlabored. The patient's blood pressure, pulse, rate of respiration, oxygen saturation level, and temperature are measured and recorded. All dressings and drains are quickly inspected for integrity and gross bleeding. After these initial observations have been made, it is essential to systematically assess the patient's total condition.

Respiratory Function

Because patients have experienced some interference with their respiratory system, postanesthesia maintenance of adequate gas exchange is a crucial aspect of care in the immediate postoperative period. Supplemental oxygen administration may be used in the immediate postoperative phase. Any change in respiratory function must be detected early so that appropriate measures can be taken to ensure adequate oxygenation and ventilation. Respiratory function is evaluated by using physical assessment skills: inspection, palpation, percussion, and auscultation. Several preexisting conditions can increase the probability that ventilatory support will be needed in the postoperative period. These include preexisting pulmonary disease, thoracic or upper abdominal surgery, history of smoking, recent significant opioid administration, and low oxygen saturation before surgery.

Pulse oximetry, a noninvasive technique, indirectly measures oxygen saturation of functional hemoglobin. Pulse oximetry can be used to identify hypoxemia, and its use should be standard on all postoperative patients. If the patient is intubated and mechanically ventilated, capnography can be used to assess for adequate ventilation. Arterial blood gas measurements are appropriate to confirm abnormal pulse oximetry or capnography values. Normal pulse oximetry values are 97% to 99%; however, preanesthetic baseline values must be noted. Some patients normally have lower saturation values on room air for various reasons, and attempting to maintain higher oxygen saturation levels may result in prolonged oxygen therapy.[21]

For spontaneously breathing patients, supplemental oxygen may be needed, typically using nasal cannula (prongs) or simple facemask. Surgery and anesthesia often interrupt the normal functioning of the nose, so humidification or nebulization with oxygen delivery may be needed. Humidifiers convert water from the liquid to the gaseous state, whereas nebulizers produce tiny water particles. This is especially helpful at higher flow rates.[21]

TABLE 41.5   Neuromuscular Blocking Agent Reversal Agents

Medication	Characteristics	Effects	Considerations
Anticholinesterase			
Neostigmine (Prostigmin)	Binds with cholinesterase and inactivates it	Antidote for nondepolarizing NMBAs	Does not cross blood–brain barrier
	Preserves endogenous anticholinesterase	Prevents postoperative distention and urinary retention	Lasts 30–90 min
	More effective in antagonizing intense blocks than pyridostigmine or edrophonium	Muscarinic effects cause bradycardia, bronchoconstriction, peripheral vasodilation, and coronary vasoconstriction	May be given with atropine and glycopyrrolate to decrease muscarinic effects; most commonly given with glycopyrrolate
			Use cautiously in patients with asthma or coronary artery disease
Edrophonium (Tensilon)	Cholinergic	Parasympathetic effects:	Must be given with atropine
	Short-acting anticholinesterase	GI: salivation, dysphasia, nausea, vomiting, increased peristalsis	Very rapid onset but brief duration of action
		CV: bradycardia, cardiac dysrhythmias, hypotension	Use cautiously in presence of asthma, peptic ulcer, or bradycardia
		RESP: increased pharyngeal and tracheobronchial secretions	
		EENT: lacrimation, miosis, diplopia	
Anticholinergic			
Atropine	Anticholinergic	Preanesthetic medication to prevent or reduce respiratory tract secretions	Crosses blood–brain barrier
	Antimuscarinic	Restoration of cardiac rate during anesthesia	Ensures adequate hydration
	Chronotropic stimulator in event of bradycardia	Antidote for cholinesterase inhibitors	Provides temperature control to prevent hyperpyrexia
		Causes decreased sweating and predisposition to heat prostration	
Glycopyrrolate (Robinul)	Similar to atropine	Less incidence of dysrhythmias	Does not cross blood–brain barrier
	Longer duration	Slow increase in heart rate	Contraindicated in presence of glaucoma, peptic ulcer, or COPD
		Protection against peripheral muscarinic effects of neostigmine and pyridostigmine	
Selective Relaxant Binding Agent			
Sugammadex (Bridion)	First selective relaxant binding agent for steroidal agents, only for reversal of rocuronium and vecuronium	No effects on acetylcholinesterases—no anticholinergic agent needed	Approximately 75% of dose eliminated through the urine; avoid in patients with creatinine clearance of <30 mL/min
			Patients on oral contraceptives need an additional dose (interacts with oral contraceptives reducing effectiveness similar to one missed dose); patients on nonoral hormonal contraceptives need to use additional nonhormonal contraceptive for 7 days after dose of sugammadex

COPD, chronic obstructive pulmonary disease; *CV,* cardiovascular; *EENT,* eyes, ears, nose, and throat; *GI,* gastrointestinal; *NMBA,* neuromuscular blocking agent; *RESP,* respiratory.

Patients may require mechanical ventilation after anesthesia. Various modes, such as positive end-expiratory pressure (PEEP), continuous positive airway pressure (CPAP), assist control ventilation, and synchronized intermittent mandatory ventilation, are used to improve the respiratory status of the patient.[22]

Stir-Up Regimen

A significant aspect of perianesthesia nursing management is the stir-up regimen,[23] which is aimed at the prevention of complications, primarily atelectasis and venous stasis. The stir-up regimen consists of five major activities—deep-breathing exercises, coughing, positioning, mobilization, and pain management.

Deep-breathing exercises. The major factor contributing to postoperative pulmonary complications is low lung volumes resulting from a shallow, monotonous, sighless breathing pattern caused by general anesthesia, opioids, and pain. The patient must be stimulated to take three or four deep breaths every 5 to 10 minutes. Full lung expansion is important, and every effort must be made to enhance the patient's ability to accomplish it.

The sustained maximal inspiration (SMI) maneuver is a method to enhance the lung volumes of postoperative patients.[23] The SMI maneuver consists of having the patient inhale as close to lung capacity as possible and, at the peak of inspiration, hold that volume for 3 to 5 seconds before exhaling it. This maneuver is more effective than simple deep breathing in preventing reduced lung volumes in the immediate postanesthesia period. If the patient's vital capacity is inadequate or if anesthesia respiratory depression is prolonged, deep breathing and the SMI maneuver may be augmented with a manual resuscitation bag connected to an oxygen source or with an intermittent positive-pressure breathing apparatus.

Incentive spirometry is used to assist with preventing and treating atelectasis, promoting normal lung expansion, and improving oxygenation. Incentive spirometry devices provide visual feedback to patients and observation of inspiratory volume. Instruction and practice before surgery provide patients with the opportunity to master the device and establish their baseline levels before anesthetic and surgical interventions.

Coughing. A purposeful cough is the most effective method to clear the air passages of obstructive secretions.[23] For a patient recovering from anesthesia, the cascade cough is the most effective coughing maneuver. Instruct the patient to take a rapid, deep inhalation. This will increase the volume of air in the lungs and dilate the airways, allowing air to pass behind the retained secretions. On exhalation, have the patient perform multiple coughs. With each cough, the length of the airways increases, enhancing the effectiveness of the cough.

Coughing is most effective with the patient sitting upright. Splinting of incisions and adequate analgesia facilitate coughing. If the patient is unable to sit upright, place the patient in a side-lying position with hips and knees flexed, or in a semi-Fowler position with the head and arms supported with pillows and the knees flexed. This positioning decreases abdominal tension and allows maximal movement of the diaphragm, improving the effectiveness of the cough.

Between cascade cough maneuvers, the patient is encouraged to inhale and close the glottis. This dilates the airways, increases intrathoracic pressure, and compresses the smaller airways, pushing the secretions toward the larger airways where they can be expectorated in succeeding cough maneuvers.

When a large amount of secretions accumulates in the patient's lungs and cannot be handled effectively by coughing, suctioning must be instituted. Suctioning is associated with complications and should be done only when necessary and not routinely.

Positioning. Ideally, patients recovering from anesthesia are positioned in a semiprone, side-lying position if possible. The semiprone position promotes maintenance of a patent airway, prevents aspiration, and permits optimal ventilation of the lower lung lobes. Frequent repositioning of patients (at least every hour) from side to side is essential for the prevention of atelectasis and venous stasis. Patients are encouraged to turn and change positions as soon as possible. Positioning changes may be limited by the operative procedure or special needs of the patient.

Mobilization. To prevent venous stasis, patients must be encouraged to move their legs and arms rhythmically, flexing and extending their extremities. Mobilization and flexion of the muscles aids venous return, improves cardiac output (CO), and prevents venous stasis and the formation of deep vein thrombosis.

Pain management. Adequate analgesia is a major consideration in the recovering patient. Without adequate pain management, it is difficult to implement the first four interventions of the stir-up regimen. Poorly controlled pain can have serious consequences in terms of hemodynamic responses to catecholamines and physical limitations on respiratory function. However, the medications used to control pain may have deleterious effects on hemodynamic and respiratory function. Opioids depress the cough reflex, ciliary activity, and respiratory center in the brain and should not be used indiscriminately. However, if the patient refuses to deep breathe, cough, or move because of pain, he or she is at risk for postoperative respiratory and embolic complications.

Pain accelerates the cardiovascular system by activating the sympathetic nervous system and the adrenal system. Normally, this causes an increase in heart rate and blood pressure. However, anesthesia and some cardiac medications can blunt the sympathetic response; asking the patient his or her pain level is the most valid method of assessing pain levels (see Chapter 8). It has been suggested that pain, especially at upper abdominal and thoracic sites, decreases or eliminates the normal sighing (yawning) mechanism. The absence of an appropriate sigh leads to reduced lung volumes and ultimately to atelectasis and pneumonia. Appropriate pain relief in these patients reduces the postoperative incidence of atelectasis and pneumonia.[24]

After the assessment has been completed and it has been determined that the patient is experiencing acute postoperative pain, certain interventions are suggested. If the patient has received an inhalation anesthetic, such as isoflurane, and demonstrates manifestations of acute pain, relief is instituted early in the postanesthetic period. Similarly, patients undergoing a nitrous oxide–opioid technique are medicated early in the immediate postoperative period, particularly if the intraoperative opioids (eg, fentanyl, remifentanil) were of short duration. If medications such as sufentanil and morphine were used intraoperatively, opioids must be administered with caution to avoid respiratory depression as a result of the synergistic action of the intraoperative and postoperative opioid agonists. Because of the synergistic effects of the medications, it may be necessary to decrease the amount of opioids administered during the first 24 hours after administration of anesthesia, but this decision must always be based on the patient's report of pain and his or her clinical status.[25-27]

Cardiovascular Function

Evaluation of the cardiovascular system involves assessment of the heart, circulating blood, and arteriovenous system. These three basic components control CO. Because tissue perfusion depends on a satisfactory CO, most of the assessment is aimed at evaluating this component.[28]

In most patients, the nurse uses physical assessment skills to evaluate cardiovascular function.[29] The patient's overall condition is observed, especially skin color and turgor. Peripheral cyanosis, edema, jugular venous distention, shortness of breath, and many other findings may be indicative of cardiovascular problems. All operative and access sites are checked for bleeding, and the amount of blood lost during surgery and the patient's most recent hemoglobin level are noted.

The patient's blood pressure must be assessed and correlated to the preoperative assessment, intraoperative course, and anesthetic course. The major component of systolic pressure is stroke volume, and the major component of diastolic pressure is systemic vascular resistance (SVR). Changes in the patient's systolic or diastolic pressure or narrowing of the pulse pressure may indicate cardiovascular compromise.[29] Peripheral pulses are assessed bilaterally. The rate, character, and any irregularities are documented and reported to the physician if clinically indicated.[29] ECG monitoring is also essential in the immediate postoperative recovery period. During the postoperative period, dysrhythmias of any type may occur at any time and in any patient.[29,30]

Two components of CO are heart rate and stroke volume. If CO is compromised, one of the first compensatory responses is an increase in heart rate, followed by peripheral vasoconstriction. Medications such as beta-blockers and angiotensin-converting enzyme inhibitors as well as anesthetic agents can impair the patient's ability to initiate that response. The nurse must be aware of the patient's preoperative medications and the impact they may have in the initial phase of recovery. Hemodynamic monitoring is commonly used with higher acuity patients in the postanesthesia recovery period. A pulmonary artery catheter and arterial blood pressure monitoring are used for hemodynamic monitoring.

Central Nervous System Function

Assessment of the CNS in the immediate postanesthesia period typically involves gross evaluation of behavior, level of consciousness, intellectual performance, and emotional status. Anesthetic agents are typically stopped before the patient leaves the operating room; timing depends on the agent, its duration, and the type of the procedure. The nurse should anticipate that the patient will be responsive on arriving in the postanesthesia setting. However, even if anesthesia is not stopped until just before the procedure ends, most patients can respond within 60 to 90 minutes from time of admission to the unit.[31]

In patients undergoing general anesthesia, perioperative stroke can occur in 7% of patients after noncardiac and non-neurosurgical procedures.[32] Because of this risk, the nurse caring for a postanesthesia patient following general anesthesia should complete a neurologic assessment that includes stroke assessment (facial symmetry, vocalization to assess for slurred speech, strength, and movement of extremities) and pupillary check. In addition, Glasgow Coma Scale assessment may be completed. For patients who have undergone neurosurgical procedures, a more detailed assessment of the CNS is necessary.

Occasionally, a patient becomes agitated and thrashes about; when extreme, this behavior is referred to as *emergence delirium*. It occurs more often in children and younger adults (younger than 40 years), older adults (older than 64 years), and patients with a history of drug dependency or psychiatric disorder.[30] Emergence delirium also tends to occur more commonly in patients who were induced with etomidate, received benzodiazepines, and underwent musculoskeletal procedures.[33]

Thermal Balance

Measurement of the patient's body temperature in the immediate postanesthesia recovery period is particularly important. Factors influencing the body temperature include type of anesthesia, preoperative medication, age of the patient, site and temperature of intravenous fluids, body surface exposure, temperature of irrigation solutions, temperature of the ambient air, and vasoconstriction (from blood loss or anesthetic agents). Hypothermia (temperature less than 36°C) and hyperthermia (temperature greater than 38°C) are associated with physiologic alterations that may interfere with recovery.[34]

The body maintains its temperature in a narrow range of 36°C to 38°C. This is accomplished by a balance of heat production and heat loss that is controlled by the thermoregulation mechanisms in the CNS. These mechanisms receive input from various thermoreceptors located in the skin, nose, oral cavity, thoracic viscera, and spinal cord. They then send sensory information in hierarchic order to the spinal cord, the reticular formation, and the primary control center in the hypothalamic region of the brain.[35]

The central temperature controls maintain body temperature through physiologic and behavioral responses. Physiologic thermoregulatory responses consist of sweating, shivering, and alterations in peripheral vasomotor tone. These responses fine-tune the regulatory process of body temperature; heat is conserved by vasoconstriction and lost by vasodilation and sweating. The physiologic responses also can lower the metabolic rate to decrease heat production or increase muscle tone and shivering to increase heat production. Behavioral thermoregulation is accomplished by subjective feelings of discomfort or comfort. For example, in a hot environment, a person seeks air conditioning, and a person seeks heat in a cold environment. Behavioral thermoregulation is a stronger response mechanism, but it cannot fine-tune body temperature as the physiologic responses can.[35]

Fluid and Electrolyte Balance

Evaluation of a patient's fluid and electrolyte status involves total body assessment. Imbalances readily occur in postoperative patients secondary to many factors, including restriction of food and fluids preoperatively, fluid loss during surgery, and stress. The normal body response to stress, surgery, trauma, and anesthesia is to release the antidiuretic hormone responsible for the retention of water and sodium. Postanesthesia patients often have abnormal avenues of fluid loss after surgery.

Each patient must be evaluated to determine his or her baseline requirements and the fluid needed to replace abnormal losses. Most patients in the immediate postanesthesia recovery period receive intravenous fluids. It is important to know what fluids, if any, are to follow and whether the infusion is to be discontinued. All intravenous sites are checked regularly for signs of extravasation, phlebitis, and infection.

Oral intake is prohibited after anesthesia until the patient regains laryngeal and pharyngeal reflexes. These reflexes are demonstrated by the patient's ability to gag and swallow effectively. The management of postoperative nausea and vomiting (PONV) is critical.

Normal output in an average adult results from urinary output and insensible losses, including evaporation of water from the skin and exhalation during respiration.[36] A lower-than-normal urinary output can be expected in the immediate postanesthesia recovery period as a result of the body's normal reaction to stress and anesthetics. External losses from vomiting, nasogastric tubes, drain tubes, and wound drainage are assessed and monitored. Accurate measurement and recording of all intake and output is vital in the assessment of the patient's fluid and electrolyte status.[36]

In a surgical patient, intravenous access to the circulatory system is necessary for the administration of anesthesia, resuscitation medications, blood and blood products, and fluid and electrolyte solutions. Postoperative parenteral fluid requirements vary with the patient's preoperative status and with the surgical procedure. Disease processes, tissue injuries, and operative procedures greatly influence the physiology of fluids and electrolytes in the body.

In deciding the type of fluid to use in the postanesthesia recovery period, the clinician can differentiate between crystalloids and colloids, between maintenance and replacement fluids, and among fluids of differing tonicity. Because of the large variety of fluid solutions, some general guidelines are recommended in clinical practice.[36] Crystalloids are typically used as maintenance fluids to compensate for insensible fluid losses and as replacement fluids to correct body fluid deficits (ie, treatment of specific fluid and electrolyte disturbances). Maintenance fluid requirements are calculated according to body weight and are used to replace insensible losses from the lungs, skin, urine, and feces. Adults typically require 1.5 to 2 mL/kg per hour. When crystalloids are used to replace blood loss, the replacement factor is 3 mL of crystalloid for each 1 mL of blood loss.[37] Isotonic solution, 0.9% normal saline, or lactated Ringer solution is usually administered in the immediate postoperative period. Colloids typically are used for fluid replacement associated with severe hypotension or shock resuscitation. In general, colloids do not leave the intravascular space and require lower infusion volumes to achieve volume replacement.

The goal of fluid therapy in the immediate postanesthesia recovery period is the restoration of blood volume and tissue perfusion. Recovery after surgery is a dynamic process, and fluid reassessment is conducted periodically. Fluid challenges may be necessary in hypovolemic patients or in patients with clinical manifestations of hypoperfusion. The decision whether to use crystalloids or colloids for fluid resuscitation is complex, controversial, and often determined by physician preference. Either can meet the replacement needs of the patient and achieve the desired outcome when administered appropriately. As with any therapeutic intervention, complications can occur with fluid administration, and the patient should be monitored closely.

Blood and blood components are reserved for specific patient situations.[37] Red blood cells are indicated to increase oxygen-carrying capacity in patients with anemia.

Platelets are used to treat bleeding associated with deficiencies in platelet number or function. Fresh-frozen plasma is transfused to increase clotting factor levels in patients with demonstrated deficiencies. A good understanding of the fluid types available, a systematic approach to evaluating fluid depletion, and awareness of the indications for blood component therapy allow the nurse to make appropriate decisions when implementing fluid therapy in the immediate postanesthesia period.

Psychosocial Status

Assessment of the patient's psychosocial status and emotional well-being is an important component of perianesthesia care. As with any other assessment, this must be made in the context of the whole patient. Almost all patients experience a degree of anxiety about anesthesia and the surgical procedure and a fear of postoperative pain.[38] Physical manifestations include increased heart rate and blood pressure; pale, cool skin; increased respiratory rate; increased muscle tone; restlessness; agitation; and dilated pupils.

Other Nursing Considerations

In the postanesthesia care unit (PACU), assessment and nursing care are based on the complexity and acuity of the patient's condition.[39] Concerns exist regarding the use of the PACU as an overflow unit for critically ill patients.[40] Issues surrounding these concerns are competencies of staff; adequacy of equipment, medications, supplies, and technology; and appropriate nurse staffing. Box 41.5 provides guidelines for the overflow of critical care patients into the PACU.[40]

General Comfort Management

Postanesthesia care includes general comfort and safety measures.[22] Whenever patients are recovering, at least two nurses (one of whom is an RN competent in Phase I perianesthesia nursing) must always be present in the same room or unit for safety.[41] Patients should not be left alone, especially when unconscious and emerging from anesthesia. Side rails should be

---

QSEN BOX 41.5   QSEN: Patient Safety Alert

A Joint Position Statement on ICU Overflow Patients

Issue

A Phase I postanesthesia care unit (PACU) is a critical care area providing postanesthesia nursing care for patients immediately after operative and invasive procedures prior to discharge to the Phase II ambulatory setting, the inpatient surgical unit, or the intensive care unit (ICU).

Perianesthesia nurses have identified concerns regarding the increasing use of the Phase I PACU for the care of the surgical and nonsurgical ICU patients when ICU beds are not available in the facility.

Purpose

As professional societies involved in the provision of care for operative and invasive procedures and critically ill patients, the American Society of PeriAnesthesia Nurses (ASPAN), the American Association of Critical-Care Nurses (AACN), and the American Society of Anesthesiologists (ASA) collaborated to develop criteria for the purposes of maintaining quality care in the PACU, ensuring quality care for the ICU patient, and promoting the safe practice of perianesthesia and critical care nursing.

ASPAN exists to promote quality and cost-effective care for patients, their families, and the community through public and professional education,

research, and standards of practice. ASPAN has the responsibility for defining the scope of practice for perianesthesia nursing. An integral part of this responsibility involves identifying the educational requirements and competencies essential to perianesthesia practice as well as recommending acceptable staffing requirements for the perianesthesia environment.

AACN was established to provide the highest quality resources to maximize nurses' contributions to care for critically ill patients and their families. AACN provides and inspires leadership to develop standards and guidelines that establish work and care environments that are respectful, healing, and humane.

ASA was established to raise and maintain the standard of the medical practice of anesthesiology and improve the care of the patient during anesthesia and recovery and is involved in the provision of critical care medicine in the ICU.

Background

In response to concerns expressed by perianesthesia nurses around the country, the ASPAN Standards and Guidelines Committee conducted a review of current literature and perianesthesia nursing practice to identify issues related to the care of critically ill surgical and nonsurgical patients in Phase I PACUs during times when all other ICU beds are full. The review identified the following trends:

continued

QSEN BOX 41.5   **QSEN: Patient Safety Alert—cont'd**

A Joint Position Statement on ICU Overflow Patients

1. Staffing requirements identified for Phase I PACUs may be exceeded during times when PACUs are being utilized for ICU overflow patients.[1-4]
2. The Phase I PACU nurse may be required to provide care to a surgical or nonsurgical ICU patient he/she has not been properly trained to care for or for which he/she has not had the required care competencies validated.[1,2]
3. Phase I PACUs may be unable to receive patients normally admitted from the operating room when staff is being utilized to care for ICU overflow patients.[1,3]
4. Because the need to send ICU overflow patients to the Phase I PACU might not regularly occur, both the PACU and hospital management may not be properly prepared to deal with the care and management of both PACU and ICU patients.[1,5]

Statement

Therefore, when it is necessary to admit ICU overflow patients or prolong the stay of the surgical ICU patient in the Phase I PACU, ASPAN, AACN, and ASA recommend that the following criteria be met:

1. It must be recognized that the primary responsibility for Phase I PACU is to provide the optimal standard of care to the postanesthesia patient and to effectively maintain the flow of the surgery schedule.[4]
2. Appropriate staffing requirements should be met to maintain safe, competent nursing care of the postanesthesia patient as well as the ICU patient.[4] Staffing criteria for the ICU patient should be consistent with institution specific ICU guidelines and based on individual patient acuity and needs.[6]
3. Phase I PACUs are by their nature critical care units, and as such staff should meet the competencies required for the care of the critically ill patient. These competencies should include, but are not limited to, ventilator management, hemodynamic monitoring, and medication administration, as appropriate to their patient population.[4,7]
4. The primary goal when determining the postoperative setting for the critically ill surgical patient is to ensure the best environment for the patient, aligning both nurse and physician characteristics and competencies.[8]
5. Critical care nurses providing Phase I recovery should also meet the competencies necessary to provide postanesthesia care to patients.[8,9]
6. Management should develop and implement a comprehensive resource utilization plan with ongoing assessment that supports the staffing needs for both the PACU and ICU patients when the need for overflow admission arises.[4]
7. Management should have a multidisciplinary plan to address appropriate utilization of ICU beds. Admission and discharge criteria should be utilized to evaluate the necessity for critical care and to determine the priority for admissions.[10]
8. Medical management of the patient must be established.[9,10]

Expected Actions

ASPAN, AACN, and the ASA Committee on Surgical Anesthesia recognize the complexity of caring for patients in a dynamic health care environment where reduced availability of resources and expanding roles for the RN have an impact on patient care. Thus, we encourage all members to actively pursue the education and development of competencies required for the care of the critically ill patient in the perianesthesia environment. We encourage organizations to set policies that identify the medical management of the extended care of surgical patients in this population. We also encourage members to actively identify strategies for collaboration and problem solving to address complex staffing issues. This information and position is to be shared with all individuals, organizations, and institutions involved in the care of the critically ill patient in the perianesthesia environment.

Approval Statement

This statement was recommended by a vote of the ASPAN Board of Directors on April 14, 2000, in Kansas City, Missouri, and approved by a vote of the ASPAN Representative Assembly on April 16, 2000, in Kansas City, Missouri. This position statement was updated and revised at the October 2013 meeting of the Standards and Guidelines Strategic Work Team in Batesville, Indiana.

References

1. Mamaril M, Sullivan E: Safe staffing for the postanesthesia care unit: weighing the evidence and identifying the gaps, *J PeriAnesth Nurs* 22(6):393, 2007.
2. Clifford T: The ICU patient, *J PeriAnesth Nurs* 25(2):114, 2010.
3. Lalani SB, Kanji K, Ali F: Experiences of nurses related to prolonged-stay patients in a postanesthesia care unit in Karachi, Pakistan, *J PeriAnesth Nurs* 27(1):26, 2012.
4. American Society of PeriAnesthesia Nurses. Practice recommendation 1: patient classification/recommended staffing guidelines. In *2012-2014 Perianesthesia Nursing Standards, Practice Recommendations and Interpretive Statements*, Cherry Hill, NJ, 2012, ASPAN, pp 30-33.
5. Lanai SB, Ali F, Kanji Z: Prolonged stay patients in the PACU: a review of the literature, *J PeriAnesth Nurs* 28(3):151, 2013.
6. Hardin S, Kaplow R: *Synergy for Clinical Excellence: The AACN Synergy Model for Patient Care*, Sudbury, MD, 2005, Jones & Bartlett.
7. Odom-Forren J: The PACU as a critical care unit, *J PeriAnesth Nurs* 18(6):431, 2003.
8. Mamaril M: Standards of perianesthesia nursing practice: advocating for patient safety, *J PeriAnesth Nurs* 18(3):168, 2003.
9. Barone CP, Pablo CS, Barone GW: Postanesthesia care in the critical care unit, *Crit Care Nurse* 24(1):38, 2004.
10. Hegedus MB: Taking the fear out of postanesthesia care in the intensive care unit, *Dimens Crit Care Nurs* 22(6):237, 2003.

Bibliography

AACN standards for establishing and sustaining healthy work environments: a journey to excellence, *Am J Crit Care* 3(14):187, 2005.

Kiekkas P, et al: Workload of postanesthesia care unit nurses and intensive care overflow, *Br J Nurs* 8(14):434, 2005.

Schweizer A, et al: Opening of a new postanesthesia care unit: impact on critical care utilization and complications following major vascular and thoracic surgery, *J Clin Anesth* 14:486, 2002.

Sullivan E: Teamwork and collaboration, *J PeriAnesth Nurs* 17:334, 2002.

Weissman C: The enhanced postoperative care system, *J Clin Anesth* (17)314, 2005.

From American Society of Perianesthesia Nurses: Position Statement 4: A joint position statement on ICU overflow patients developed by ASPAN, AACN, and ASA's Committee on Surgical Anesthesia. http://www.aspan.org/Portals/6/docs/ClinicalPractice/PositionStatement/Current/PS4_2015.pdf. Accessed January 11, 2016.

in the up position and locked when care is not being provided. Wheel locks prevent sliding off the bed.

General physical measures such as cleaning and comfort measures are important to the total well-being of postanesthesia patients and are often overlooked. After the initial assessment and when safe, the skin should be cleansed of preparation solutions, and electrodes or sensors that are not in use should be removed. Repositioning in a position different from the operative position may prevent future complaints of discomfort and skin alterations for patients who have undergone lengthy operative procedures. While repositioning, patient movement and deep breathing may help prevent atelectasis, promote circulation, and prevent pressure ulcers from developing on skin surfaces.

Oral care is comforting to the patient who has had no oral intake and has received drying medications. Ice chips and small

- Intraoperative complications
- Type of anesthetic technique
- Patient comorbidities and preexisting diseases
- Preoperative condition of patient
- Length and type of surgery
- Urgency of surgery
- Poorly controlled pain
- Other medications administered intraoperatively
- Changes in fluid status and electrolyte balance
- Alterations in body temperature

sips of water or juice may be offered to patients who can tolerate fluids. A non–petroleum-based ointment is applied to the lips after oral care to prevent drying and cracking.

Patients often complain of being cold when returning from the operating room. This is a result of the effects of anesthesia and premedications and the cool atmosphere of the operating room. A normothermic patient may shiver or complain of feeling cold, so warm blankets may provide psychological comfort. However, blankets of any type must not obscure the intravenous lines, arterial lines, or other monitoring apparatus from the direct view of the attending nurse. The patient's temperature must be monitored closely to avoid overheating.

In addition to physical comfort measures, psychological comfort should be provided. Reorientation, especially to time and place, is important to the postanesthesia patient, as is constant reassurance that the procedure has been completed and the patient is now recovering. The nurse's presence at the bedside or gentle touch may also be comforting to the patient.

MANAGEMENT OF POSTANESTHESIA PROBLEMS AND EMERGENCIES

In the immediate postoperative period, significant physiologic changes occur as the patient emerges from the effects of anesthesia. Factors that influence the development of problems are listed in Box 41.6.[42]

Respiratory Complications and Emergencies

Respiratory complications are common in the postanesthesia period. All general anesthetic agents and opioid analgesic medications have respiratory depressant effects. Acute pain also impairs the ability to breathe deeply. Most respiratory complications are related to upper airway obstruction, although other problems can occur, including acute respiratory failure, aspiration, pulmonary edema, and respiratory arrest.[30]

Airway Obstruction

Relaxed nasal or oropharyngeal muscles, rigid neck muscles, or secretions in the upper respiratory tract can cause obstruction of the airway. Soft tissue obstruction occurs when the pharynx is blocked and air cannot flow in and out. The most common cause of soft tissue obstruction is the tongue. Clinical manifestations of an airway obstruction include snoring, stridor, flaring of the nostrils, retractions at the intercostal spaces and the suprasternal notch, abnormal use of accessory muscles, asynchronous movements of the chest and abdomen, increased

pulse rate, decreased oxygen saturation level, and decreased breath sounds.[43]

Management of an airway obstruction begins with immediate recognition. Stimulation may be all that is necessary to relieve the obstruction and obtain a patent airway. With a nonreactive patient, the head tilt–chin lift maneuver or elevation of the mandible at its angles (jaw thrust) can be used to displace the tongue and open the airway. If patency of the airway cannot be achieved by either of these methods, an oropharyngeal or nasopharyngeal airway is inserted. A nasopharyngeal airway is usually better tolerated, although it can occasionally cause nasal bleeding. Oropharyngeal airways should be used only for unconscious patients because they can cause gagging, vomiting, and laryngospasm in awake patients. The patient can also be turned on his or her side to a lateral position, which facilitates displacement of the tongue and drainage of secretions. If the obstruction is still unrelieved, positive-pressure mask ventilation, intubation, tracheotomy, or cricothyrotomy may be required.[4,30,43]

Laryngeal Edema

Laryngeal edema is defined as swelling of the laryngeal tissue. This edema can cause various degrees of airway obstruction. Manifestations include stridor, retraction, hoarseness, and a croup-like cough. Apprehension and restlessness may be present in an awake patient.

Management consists of placing the patient in the upright position; using cool, humidified oxygen; and administering nebulized racemic epinephrine. If laryngeal edema is a result of an allergic reaction, the reaction must be managed with epinephrine, bronchodilators, and antihistamines. Reintubation is performed only if the patient's symptoms cannot be controlled by an inhalation treatment within 30 minutes, if hypercarbia persists, or if the patient appears to be in respiratory distress. If reintubation is done, the endotracheal tube must be at least one size smaller than the previous tube used, and an air leak must be present around the cuff.[30,43]

Laryngospasm

Laryngospasm is caused by reflex contractions of the pharyngeal muscles, which results in spasms of the vocal cords and the inability of the patient to take a breath. The spasms may result in partial or complete airway obstruction. Involvement of the intrinsic laryngeal muscles causes a reflex closure of the glottis, which results in an incomplete obstruction. Involvement of the extrinsic muscles causes a reflex closure of the larynx, which results in a complete airway obstruction. Signs and symptoms of laryngospasm include dyspnea, hypoxia, hypoventilation, absence of breath sounds, and hypercarbia. Crowing sounds may be heard if the spasm is incomplete. The chest does not expand normally, and a rocking motion of the chest wall that stimulates abdominal breathing may be present. The patient panics if awake.

Several factors can help identify a patient at risk for a laryngospasm. Preoperatively, risks include a history of asthma, chronic obstructive pulmonary disease (COPD), or smoking. Intraoperatively, risks include the use of an endotracheal tube, anesthetic agents, "light" anesthesia, multiple attempts at intubation, and surgical airway manipulation. After surgery, risks include coughing, "bucking" on the endotracheal tube, repeated suctioning, and excessive secretions in the nasopharyngeal area. Laryngospasm may also be precipitated by irritants and foreign bodies.

Laryngospasm is an emergency that requires an immediate response; otherwise, the patient may rapidly deteriorate. Management is initiated by removing the stimulus, along with any irritants such as secretions, blood, or an artificial airway that is too long. The patient's head must be hyperextended (unless contraindicated), and positive-pressure mask ventilation is instituted on 100% oxygen. The anesthesiologist is notified immediately. If complete obstruction is unrelieved by positive-pressure ventilations, a small dose of succinylcholine (10 to 20 mg) may be needed to relax the vocal cords to allow for ventilation. Positive-pressure mask ventilation is continued until full muscle function has resumed. Although it may cause further irritation of the airways, endotracheal intubation is required if the laryngospasm persists or if refractory hypoxemia develops. Lidocaine, steroids, and atropine are medications that may be used in the treatment of laryngospasm.

After the spasm, the patient continues to receive supplemental oxygen until he or she is stable. It is also important at that time for the nurse to reassure the patient that the spasm has resolved. The patient's feelings of being unable to breathe during laryngospasm are intense, and emotional support from the nurse is imperative.[30,44]

Bronchospasm

Bronchospasm is a lower airway obstruction that is characterized by spasmodic contractions of the bronchial tubes. Bronchial airway constriction is a result of an increase in smooth muscle tone in the airways, and bronchospasms develop when the smooth muscles constrict and obstruct the airway. Inflammation has also been recognized as a fundamental component of bronchospasms.

Bronchiolar constriction may be centrally generated, as in asthma, or it may be a local response to airway irritation. Manifestations include wheezing; noisy, shallow respirations; chest retractions; and use of accessory muscles. The patient can exhibit shortness of breath, coughing, and a prolonged expiratory phase of respiration. Hypertension and tachycardia may be present. The patient's level of consciousness may range from lethargy to extreme anxiety.

Patients who smoke and patients with chronic bronchitis have irritable airways that react to stimulation. A preoperative history of asthma, a recent upper respiratory infection, severe emphysema, pulmonary fibrosis, and radiation pneumonitis are indicators of a greater risk of bronchospasm. Stimuli that may produce a bronchospasm postoperatively include secretions, vomitus, and blood. Patients who have had laryngoscopy, bronchoscopy, or other surgical stimulation are also at increased risk of bronchospasm. Some medications are also thought to predispose the patient to bronchoconstriction resulting from cholinomimetic stimulation; these medications include physostigmine, neostigmine, edrophonium, and barbiturates. Other histamine-releasing medications, such as morphine and atracurium, may potentially foster bronchospasm.

Bronchospasm is treated initially by removal of any possible irritants or medications. First-line therapy consists of inhaled bronchodilators. These inhalants cause fewer cardiovascular side effects than systemically administered medications. Common inhalant medications used are albuterol and metaproterenol. Systemic bronchodilators and antiinflammatory agents may sometimes be required. Epinephrine is occasionally needed as a continuous infusion. Intravenous methylprednisolone manages the inflammatory aspect of bronchospasm. Cholinergics have been given by nebulizer to decrease secretions.[30,44]

Noncardiogenic Pulmonary Edema

Pulmonary edema may be defined simply as increased total lung water. Fluid can accumulate in the interstitial spaces or in the alveoli as a result of cardiogenic or pulmonary capillary processes. Noncardiogenic pulmonary edema, also known as postobstructive pulmonary edema, in the postanesthesia recovery period can result from pulmonary aspiration, blood transfusion reaction, allergic medication reaction, upper airway obstruction, or sepsis.[45] The most common causative factor seems to be an upper airway obstruction, usually laryngospasm. Often, a short episode of airway obstruction occurred in the operating room. Noncardiogenic pulmonary edema has also been reported after administration of naloxone to patients who have received general anesthesia. Abrupt reversal of analgesics causes an increase in the level of adrenal catecholamines, which can lead to pulmonary hypertension and probably increased pulmonary vascular permeability.

During laryngospasm, the patient is inhaling against a closed glottis. This generates an increase in negative intrathoracic pressure. A tremendous subatmospheric transpulmonary pressure gradient is created that causes transudation, or leakage of fluid, from the pulmonary capillaries into the interstitium.

Management consists of maintenance of an unobstructed airway and supplemental oxygen to correct hypoxemia. Patients who cannot maintain adequate oxygenation with a mask may require the use of CPAP or mechanical ventilation with PEEP. The use of PEEP or CPAP improves hypoxemia by restoring the functional residual capacity (FRC). Vigorous pulmonary toilet and the use of hemodynamic monitoring may be required if the patient's blood pressure is labile and fluid balance is difficult to maintain. Morphine can be titrated to relieve anxiety. Corticosteroid therapy can be used to decrease laryngeal edema and stabilize the pulmonary membrane. Noncardiogenic pulmonary edema occurs rapidly and requires early assessment and immediate intervention.

Aspiration

Aspiration can be defined as the passage of regurgitated gastric contents or other foreign materials into the trachea and down to the smaller air units. It can occur during the period of reduced protective airway reflexes. The most common and most severe form of aspiration is the aspiration of gastric contents. The gastric acid in gastric contents damages the alveolar and capillary endothelial cells. Fluid rich with protein leaks into the interstitium and alveoli; this results in atelectasis and consolidation. Pulmonary compliance and FRC are decreased, and airway resistance and intrapulmonary shunting are increased, with hypoxemia resulting.

If aspiration is suspected, management begins with lowering the patient's head, if possible. The patient is positioned to the side or the head is turned to the side to permit gravity to pull secretions from the trachea. Management centers on promoting tissue oxygenation by maintaining arterial oxygenation by means of CPAP and supplemental oxygen. Positive-pressure ventilation by mask can be applied if the patient is awake and can protect his or her airway or by an endotracheal tube if the patient cannot tolerate the mask or requires higher levels of airway pressure.[30,44]

Hypoxemia

Administration of oxygen by facemask or nasal cannula may be needed to prevent hypoxemia in postoperative patients, based on oxygen saturation levels that may be assessed noninvasively by pulse oximetry. Respiratory depressant effects of residual agents may result in a shallow breathing pattern with an increased ratio of dead space to tidal volume. This is even more evident in patients after upper abdominal surgery, and the reduction in effective ventilation can have serious effects on oxygenation.[42]

The most common cause of hypoxemia is ventilation-perfusion mismatching. Atelectasis often occurs as a result of bronchial obstruction by secretions or blood. Reduction in FRC is caused by the effects of anesthesia and, in the case of upper abdominal surgery, by the surgical procedure. When FRC falls below closing capacity, dependent alveoli occlude, leading to increased mismatching. Impairment of hypoxic pulmonary vasoconstriction by inhalation agents and some vasoactive medications potentiates this effect.[30]

Hypoventilation

Central respiratory depression is caused by all anesthetic agents and may lead to significant hypoventilation and hypercarbia. Impaired respiratory muscle function, particularly after upper abdominal surgery, may contribute to the problem of carbon dioxide elimination. Incomplete reversal of neuromuscular blockade must also be considered. Other contributory factors may include tight dressings and body casts, obesity, and gastric dilation. Increased carbon dioxide production may occur as a result of shivering or sepsis. This leads to hypercarbia in patients who are unable to increase ventilation enough to compensate.

Hypercarbia resulting from postoperative hypoventilation may cause hypertension and tachycardia, increasing the risk of myocardial ischemia in susceptible individuals. Hypoventilation, by itself or in combination with the other factors previously discussed, can cause hypoxemia. Very high levels of carbon dioxide may have sedative effects. Evaluation of suspected hypoventilation requires measurement of arterial blood gases. Capnographic monitoring may be especially useful in patients at high risk for hypoxemia.[30]

Careful titration of opioid antagonists, such as naloxone, may be effective in improving ventilation without compromising pain relief. Planning ahead to provide adequate postoperative analgesia is essential for maintaining ventilation, particularly in patients undergoing abdominal or thoracic procedures. Placing obese patients in a semi-Fowler position and relieving the effects of tight dressings and casts can also be important. Hypoventilation that cannot be improved sufficiently by noninvasive means requires intubation and mechanical ventilation until the patient can maintain adequate ventilation.[44]

Cardiovascular Problems and Emergencies

In the immediate postoperative period, cardiovascular complications causing an alteration in CO can occur. These include anesthetic effects on cardiac function, myocardial dysfunction, dysrhythmias, hypertension, and hypotension. These conditions may occur individually or in combination.[30,46]

Effects of Anesthesia on Cardiac Function

In the immediate postoperative period, the residual effects of anesthetic agents and their adjuncts must be considered in the evaluation of a patient who has cardiac dysfunction. Volatile anesthetic agents such as sevoflurane and isoflurane can cause a dose-related reduction in myocardial function. The actions of these agents may be observed for several hours after the conclusion of surgery.[4] Nitrous oxide is an inhalation agent that demonstrates insignificant cardiac depression. However, the combined action of opioids given during emergence from nitrous oxide can result in marked cardiovascular depression.[3]

Therapy directed toward mitigating the myocardial depressant effects of inhalation anesthetic agents primarily focuses on increasing preload. Elevation of the legs and a crystalloid fluid bolus are commonly sufficient treatment, but ephedrine or other positive inotropic agents may be needed.[24]

Individually, most opioids and benzodiazepines result in only moderate depression of cardiac function. Opioids reduce the sympathetic response and enhance vagal and parasympathetic tone. This results in vasodilation and a decrease in SVR. Benzodiazepines also cause vasodilation and a decrease in the SVR. Used in combination, these medications can have a significant effect on the cardiovascular system. Specifically, the overall reaction may include lowered SVR, heart rate, ventricular contractility, catecholamine level, baroreceptor reflex, CO, and blood pressure. Aggressive administration of crystalloid solutions may be required to counteract these effects. High-dose opioids combined with vecuronium produce a negative inotropic and chronotropic effect. Patients may require short-term vascular support until these medications dissipate.[30,47]

Barbiturates depress the activity of the vasomotor center, causing peripheral vasodilation and hypotension. These actions are dose related and are more marked in the presence of underlying cardiovascular disease. Ketamine, in an anesthetic dose, has a direct myocardial depressant effect that is usually counterbalanced by its indirect effect on the autonomic nervous system to increase heart rate and blood pressure. In patients who are unable to mount a sympathetic response to stress, ketamine causes a net decrease in CO. Propofol causes a dose-dependent decrease in blood pressure primarily because of a decrease in SVR. This must be considered when caring for patients who are hypovolemic or have minimal cardiac reserves.[44,48]

Local anesthetic agents can cause cardiovascular toxicity if inadvertently injected into the systemic circulation or if an excessive dosage of the agent is used. Decreased myocardial contractility, reduced SVR, and diminished CO have resulted from these agents. Cardiovascular compromise appears to occur in a dose-related fashion. Management of cardiovascular complications associated with local anesthetic agents includes measures to increase preload—elevation of legs and fluid administration. In refractory cases, ephedrine may also be needed.[4,30]

Myocardial Dysfunction

During the immediate postoperative period, the causes of myocardial depression include pathologic processes and aberrant physiologic states, in addition to anesthetic side effects. These processes may occur alone or in combination and may be particularly hazardous in the presence of underlying cardiac disease.

Myocardial ischemia results from an imbalance of oxygen supply and demand. Commonly, ischemia results from a decrease in myocardial blood flow caused by atherosclerosis, vasospasm, or hypotension. In the postoperative period, the stress of surgery and the actions of certain anesthetic agents can increase myocardial ischemia.[30,46]

Dysrhythmias

In the immediate postanesthetic period, patients are predisposed to various cardiac dysrhythmias. The most common dysrhythmias are sinus tachycardia, sinus bradycardia, premature ventricular contractions, supraventricular tachydysrhythmias, and ventricular tachycardia. A variety of causes can result in dysrhythmias, including circulatory instability, preexisting heart disease, an increase in vagal tone, medications, pain, electrolyte disturbances, and hypoxemia.[49]

Accurate interpretation and identification of the dysrhythmia are essential because therapeutic intervention is based on diagnosis. Appropriate skin preparation and lead placement are extremely important to ensure a clear, readable tracing that is free from artifact. Additional 12-lead ECG capabilities should be used if an interpretation cannot be made from tracings obtained with bedside monitoring.

The hemodynamic effects of the dysrhythmia also should be thoroughly assessed. The clinical presentation of the dysrhythmia determines the severity of underlying cardiac disease and the type of treatment. Tachydysrhythmias shorten diastolic filling time and interfere with coronary artery perfusion. These two effects, coupled with an increase in myocardial oxygen consumption, may produce cardiac decompensation. Bradycardia can produce a clinically significant decrease in CO if stroke volume is limited by underlying cardiac disease or if the venous return is reduced. The cause of the rhythm disturbance should be considered.[48]

General anesthesia lowers the dysrhythmia threshold of the myocardium. Inhalation agents sensitize the myocardium to catecholamines and depress sinoatrial and atrioventricular nodal function. Junctional rhythms and premature ventricular contractions are the most common dysrhythmias. Ketamine produces sympathetic stimulation, resulting in tachycardia and hypertension. Succinylcholine stimulates the cholinergic receptors, enhancing vagal tone, and it can produce sinus bradycardia or junctional escape rhythms. Opioids may cause bradycardia because of direct stimulation of the vagus nerve.

Endogenous catecholamine levels in postoperative patients are elevated because of the pain and stress of surgery. Increased catecholamine levels increase sinus and atrioventricular node rates, as well as atrial and ventricular irritability. The direct result is tachydysrhythmias and atrial or ventricular premature contractions.[30,46,48]

Postoperative Hypertension

Hypertension is not an unusual occurrence in the immediate postoperative period. The diagnosis of hypertension must be considered in the context of an elevated blood pressure in relation to the patient's preoperative and intraoperative blood pressure range. Most commonly, postoperative hypertension is related to fluid overload, heightened sympathetic nervous system activity, or preexisting hypertension. Postoperative hypertension, even as a transient episode, can have significant cardiovascular and intracranial consequences, so aggressive diagnosis and treatment are indicated.

Increased sympathetic tone in the immediate postoperative period may result from the stress of surgery, postoperative pain, anxiety or restlessness during emergence from anesthesia, bladder or bowel distention, or hypothermia. Stimulation of the autonomic nervous system can occur because of hypoxia or hypercarbia. These factors can occur alone or in combination.

Pain is one of the most common sources of increased sympathetic tone. Administering adequate amounts of analgesics, repositioning the patient for comfort, providing reassurance, and limiting environmental stimuli can contribute to alleviating postoperative pain and to lowering blood pressure. Hypothermia and shivering also contribute to postoperative hypertension and are easily treated with warm blankets, active warming devices, and warm intravenous fluids. Bladder distention contributes to postoperative hypertension and must be alleviated. Placement of a urinary catheter may be needed. Hypoxia and hypercarbia must also be treated.

Pharmacologic treatment of postoperative hypertension includes the use of vasodilators, beta-adrenergic blockers, and calcium channel blockers. The use of these agents is necessary when hypertension persists despite conservative measures previously mentioned.[30,46]

Postoperative Hypotension

Maintenance of blood pressure depends on adequate preload, myocardial contractility, and afterload. The most common cause of hypotension is intravascular volume depletion caused by inadequate replacement of blood loss, third space fluid loss, insensible loss, and urinary output. Pulmonary embolism may also reduce preload by blocking flow of blood to the left side of the heart. Reduced myocardial contractility may be a result of the effects of anesthetic medications, myocardial ischemia, or dysrhythmias. Reduced afterload in the form of low SVR may occur as a result of sepsis, hyperthermia, sympathectomy, or large arteriovenous shunts, as seen in chronic liver failure.

Prolonged hypotension can lead to serious ischemic organ damage. Prompt treatment is essential. If the underlying cause is not immediately apparent, the first treatment is an attempt to increase preload by elevating the patient's legs and infusing fluids. Examination of the ECG monitor for dysrhythmias or evidence of ischemia may help guide therapy. The lungs are examined for evidence of pulmonary edema or tension pneumothorax. Vasopressors may be administered to maintain perfusion while additional monitoring modalities are evaluated and established. Insertion of a central venous catheter allows measurement of right ventricular filling pressure and may be used to guide fluid administration in patients with normal myocardial function. In the presence of left ventricular dysfunction or when the cause remains unclear, a pulmonary artery catheter may be inserted to guide therapy through evaluation of left-sided filling pressure, CO, and SVR. The use of additional fluids, inotropic agents, or vasoconstrictor or vasodilator medications is determined by these measurements.[49]

Thermoregulatory Problems and Emergencies

Patients recovering from anesthesia usually experience some form of thermoregulatory imbalance (ie, a core body temperature that is outside the normothermic range of 36°C to 38°C). Hypothermia and hyperthermia can occur in the postoperative patient. Management of these alterations is important because they are associated with other physiologic alterations that may interfere with recovery.

Hypothermia

Hypothermia is a common occurrence intraoperatively and postoperatively because the conditions associated with surgery and anesthesia typically inhibit the body's heat-generating mechanisms and favor its heat-loss mechanisms.[50] Hypothermia occurs when systemic heat loss lowers core body temperature below 36°C. Causes include wound and skin exposure, respiratory gas exchange, fluid and blood administration, use of mechanical warming or cooling devices, chemical reactions, alterations in body temperature regulation, and disease states. Clinical manifestations of hypothermia include bluish tint to the skin (peripheral cyanosis); shivering and an increase in metabolic rate (early sign); dysrhythmias; and a decrease in metabolic rate (late sign), oxygen consumption, muscle tone, heart rate, and level of consciousness.[35]

Hypothermia has several adverse effects, including discomfort, vasoconstriction, and shivering. It depresses the myocardium and increases susceptibility to ventricular dysrhythmias. Significant hypothermia slows metabolic processes, leading to reduced medication biotransformation and impaired renal transport. This may prolong medication effects and delay emergence.[35,50]

Shivering

Shivering may be a result of the compensatory response to hypothermia or the effects of anesthetic agents, and it can produce an increase in the metabolic rate. Under these conditions, increased oxygen consumption and greater carbon dioxide production can increase the ventilatory requirements. If these requirements are not met, the arterial partial pressure of carbon dioxide ($Paco_2$) increases, and the arterial partial pressure of oxygen (Pao_2) can decrease, especially if any significant intrapulmonary shunting coexists. The demand for blood flow by the diaphragm can increase sharply, requiring CO and myocardial workload to increase and causing an increase in myocardial oxygen consumption. Myocardial ischemia can result, particularly in older patients and patients with coronary artery disease.[35,50]

Vasoconstriction, a particularly deleterious consequence of postoperative hypothermia, may be responsible for unexplained hypertension in the postanesthesia period. Because vasoconstriction can increase SVR and myocardial workload, the potential for myocardial ischemia exists. Vasoconstriction can mask hypovolemia, and sudden reductions in blood pressure can occur as the patient warms and vasodilates.[51] Delayed medication clearance as a consequence of hypothermia is particularly significant in older patients who may already have impaired medication-clearing mechanisms and a decreased metabolic rate. For example, the maximal rate of renal excretion of a medication can decline by 10% for every 0.6°C drop in body temperature. Older patients with hypothermia are more likely to have residual paralysis because of muscle relaxants that are difficult to reverse pharmacologically.[52]

Management of hypothermic patients is directed toward the restoration of normothermia. Rewarming prevents the thermoregulatory responses to cold, such as shivering. Management depends on the degree of temperature loss. If the patient's body temperature is between 36°C and 37°C, the patient can simply be covered with warmed blankets, and overhead heat lamps can be used to keep the patient adequately warm. If the patient's body temperature is less than 36°C, rapid rewarming is required to decrease the possible complications of hypothermia and the postanesthesia recovery time. Convective warming devices provide a safe and effective means of rewarming the patient.[34] In patients with a normal metabolic rate, a setting of "low" or "medium" increases the mean body temperature by about 1°C per hour. A "high" setting increases the mean body temperature by about 1.5°C per hour.[4] Other methods of rewarming are thermal mattresses, fluid and blood warming, and environmental warming. Supplemental oxygen may be needed to meet the increased metabolic demand in shivering patients. Patients who are shivering may respond to a small dose of meperidine (Demerol).[51]

Hyperthermia

By definition, hyperthermia occurs at any core body temperature above normal. Severe, clinically significant hyperthermia results when core temperature exceeds 40°C. Although it is not as common perioperatively as hypothermia, hyperthermia is nevertheless a serious complication of surgery. Postoperative temperature elevations may be caused by accidental overwarming of the patient during surgery, infection, sepsis, or transfusion reactions. Because an elevated temperature increases oxygen demand and, subsequently, the ventilatory and cardiac workload, a hyperthermic patient with poor cardiac reserve experiences serious consequences.[53]

Postoperative fever must be distinguished from other hyperthermic syndromes. A fundamental difference exists between fever and specific hyperthermic states. In non–fever-related hyperthermic states, body temperature rises above normal despite the body's heat-dissipating mechanisms (eg, vasodilation, sweating). Excessive heat gain from internal or external factors exceeds the body's cooling capabilities, with a consequent increase in body temperature.[2,4]

In contrast, fever results from a resetting to a higher temperature from the normal set-point. Until the body reaches its new set-point temperature, heat-generating mechanisms (ie, vasoconstriction and shivering) are activated. After the new set-point temperature is reached, there is an equilibrium between heat generation and heat loss. In contrast to hyperthermia, with fever there is no physiologic activity to bring body temperature back to normal. Factors that can contribute to raising core body temperature and fever during the perioperative period are listed in Box 41.7.[50]

Primary therapy for hyperthermia includes cooling and decreasing thermogenesis. Cooling by evaporative or direct external methods is effective. This includes ice packs, a cool environment, and cooling blankets. Gastric and bladder lavage have also proved effective. Although physical cooling is an appropriate therapy for other hyperthermias, attempts to cool a febrile patient may be resisted by the thermoregulatory system. Consequently, the first course of action is to restore normothermia with the use of antipyretic medications. Antipyretics are useful because they have the ability to prevent prostaglandin synthesis in the hypothalamus. Measures to manage febrile patients include using antipyretics (as indicated), providing a sponge bath with tepid water, keeping the environment cool, using a cooling blanket for sustained fever, and monitoring fluid and electrolyte balance as fluid needs increase during fever. The possibility of malignant hyperthermia (MH) must always be considered.[53]

Malignant Hyperthermia

MH is a genetically determined condition. MH is precipitated by certain general inhalation anesthetics, depolarizing skeletal muscle relaxants, local anesthetics, and stress in susceptible patients. The incidence of MH ranges from 1 in 15,000 in children to 1 in 50,000 in adults. The onset of MH usually occurs during induction of anesthesia but may occur within the first few hours of recovery from anesthesia.[3] Because successful management of MH depends on early assessment and prompt intervention, the nurse must be knowledgeable about the pathophysiology and treatment of this syndrome.

Identification before anesthesia of patients who may be susceptible to MH is of major therapeutic importance.[54] Patient history or genealogy going back two generations may be

BOX 41.7   Factors Influencing Temperature and Fever

Causes of Elevated Core Temperature	Causes of Postoperative Fever
Blood transfusion	Atelectasis
Medication-induced fever	Wound infection
Overuse of techniques to prevent hypothermia	Abscess formation
Hypothalamic injury	Fat emboli after bone trauma
Malignant hyperthermia	Medication reactions
Warm environment	Malignancy
Use of anticholinergics	Silent aspiration
Endocrine disorders	Dehydration
Neurogenic hyperthermia	Blood transfusion reaction
	Central nervous system damage
	Urinary tract infections
	Phlebitis, deep vein thrombosis
	Pulmonary emboli

BOX 41.8   Signs and Symptoms of Malignant Hyperthermia

- Muscle rigidity
- Increased carbon dioxide production (hypercapnia)
- Rhabdomyolysis
- Marked temperature elevation (hyperthermia)
- Tachycardia
- Tachypnea
- Metabolic acidosis
- Respiratory acidosis
- Hyperkalemia
- Myoglobinuria
- Elevated creatine phosphokinase
- Ventricular dysrhythmias
- Cyanosis
- Skin mottling
- Hot, flushed skin
- Rigidity
- Profuse sweating
- Unstable blood pressure

Modified from Odom-Forren J. *Drain's Perianesthesia Nursing: A Critical Care Approach.* 6th ed. St. Louis: Elsevier; 2013.

BOX 41.9   Environmental and Pharmacologic Triggers of Malignant Hyperthermia

Environmental Stimuli
- Extremely hot and humid weather
- Strenuous and prolonged exercise

Pharmacologic Agents
- Isoflurane
- Sevoflurane
- Desflurane
- Succinylcholine

Modified from Odom-Forren J. *Drain's Perianesthesia Nursing: A Critical Care Approach.* 6th ed. St. Louis: Elsevier; 2013.

positive. Physical examination may reveal myopathies such as cryptorchidism, pectus carinatum, kyphosis, lordosis, ptosis, or hypoplastic mandible. Electromyographic changes are seen in less than half of MH-susceptible patients.

The most definitive test for detecting MH susceptibility is a biopsy of skeletal muscle.[54] Samples are obtained from the quadriceps muscles and are subjected to isometric contractor testing. The skeletal muscle of a patient susceptible to MH has an increased isometric tension when exposed to caffeine or halothane. Genetic testing for the presence of a ryanodine mutation that predicts MH susceptibility may ultimately replace the invasive diagnostic tests.[3]

When a susceptible patient is exposed to a triggering agent for MH, such as isoflurane, the clinical features are produced by an excess of calcium ions in the myoplasm. With an elevated calcium ion concentration in the myoplasm, skeletal muscle contraction is intense and prolonged, leading to a hypermetabolic state of acid and heat production. More specifically, heat is produced by the accelerated and continued synthesis and use of adenosine triphosphate during glycolysis. The metabolic by-product of glycolysis, lactic acid, is transported to the liver and then back to the metabolically active muscle, where the cycle repeats. Respiratory acidosis and metabolic acidosis develop because of this hypermetabolic state, and symptoms such as tachycardia, tachypnea, ventricular dysrhythmias, and unstable blood pressure appear. Because of intense vasoconstriction, the skin is mottled and cyanotic.[55] Box 41.8 lists the clinical manifestations of MH.

Elevated body temperature can be a late sign of MH. For this reason, the nurse must not prolong the assessment of the patient on the assumption that the patient's temperature must be significantly elevated before intervention is attempted. After the patient's temperature begins to rise, it may increase at a rate of 1°C every 3 to 5 minutes and may approach 46°C.[30]

Muscle rigidity occurs in about 75% of patients who experience MH. This is especially true in MH-susceptible patients after the administration of succinylcholine. Muscle rigidity may be so severe that the nurse cannot open the patient's mouth to insert an airway. The onset of skeletal muscle rigidity after the administration of succinylcholine could be a sign of impending development of MH.[53,55]

Various environmental and pharmacologic agents can stimulate an acute episode of MH (Box 41.9).[54] Fatigue, emotional upset, or very hot and humid weather can trigger a waking febrile episode. The anesthetic agents that may trigger MH seem to affect the sarcoplasmic reticulum. Because of their widespread use, volatile anesthetic agents (eg, isoflurane) and succinylcholine are the most common triggering agents. In MH-susceptible patients and in patients who have had an episode of MH in the operating room, all possible triggering agents must be stringently avoided. As another precaution, because emotional upsets trigger MH, nurses must provide a stress-free environment for a patient susceptible to MH.

The cornerstone of successful management of MH is early detection. If the patient develops acute MH, all inhalation anesthetics are stopped, the patient is hyperventilated with 100% oxygen, and dantrolene is given. To be administered, dantrolene must be diluted with sterile water. Cooling measures, such as administering cold intravenous fluids, packing the patient in ice, and irrigating body cavities (eg, stomach, bladder) with cold fluids, are initiated as needed based on the patient's temperature. Accurate intake and output records are essential because large amounts of fluids and diuretics are given. Laboratory tests such as complete blood cell count and coagulation studies are closely scrutinized for signs of bleeding or onset of disseminated intravascular clotting. Ongoing ECG and temperature monitoring are also essential. It is recommended that all emergency medications be available on a special cart in the operating room or in the PACU.

Neurologic Problems and Emergencies

Almost all patients exhibit some level of arousal within 15 minutes after anesthesia is completed.[3] Although many factors are known to prolong anesthetic effects, most reports of delayed emergence and emergence delirium are anecdotal.

Delayed Emergence

Delayed awakening after general anesthesia occurs occasionally; this is defined as a failure to regain consciousness within 20 to 30 minutes after the anesthetic ends.[56] It can usually be attributed to prolonged action of anesthetic medications, metabolic causes, or neurologic injury.[30] In most cases, prolonged sedation is the result of residual general anesthetic. Hypoventilation resulting from a high concentration of inhaled anesthetic limits exhalation of the agent and prolongs its retention. Opioids used as adjunct therapy may contribute to hypercarbia and sedation as well. Hypothermia, advanced age, hepatic dysfunction, and renal disease may contribute to prolonged recovery from anesthetics by heightening sensitivity or delaying elimination, or both. The use of premedication may also prolong recovery, especially if opioids or benzodiazepines, particularly lorazepam, are used.[57]

In addition to experiencing a slowing elimination of potent inhalation anesthetic, a hypoventilating patient may develop hypoxia and hypercapnia. The hypercapnia may cause significant narcosis and may potentiate the depressive effects of the anesthetics. In diabetic patients, fasting or excessive insulin may cause electrolyte abnormalities, leading to unconsciousness or coma.[56]

Severe electrolyte disturbances are most commonly seen after excessive water absorption during hysteroscopy or transurethral prostate surgery. The subsequent dilution hyponatremia may manifest as sedation, coma, or hemiparesis. Dilution hyponatremia may also be seen after the inappropriate release of antidiuretic hormone. Hypocalcemia after parathyroid surgery may result in delayed awakening. High magnesium levels after prolonged administration of magnesium sulfate to a patient with eclampsia or preeclampsia may also result in prolonged postoperative sedation and in muscle weakness after cesarean section under general anesthesia.[36]

Neurologic injury and subsequent unconsciousness may be the result of an unsuspected cerebrovascular accident. Intracranial hemorrhage may result from hypertensive responses to anesthetic agents or surgical manipulations, especially in patients receiving anticoagulant therapy. Paradoxic air emboli may cross a patent foramen ovale in the presence of a right-to-left shunt. Direct emboli from cardiac valves, intracardiac thrombi, and atherosclerotic vessels may also be a threat. Fat emboli can occur after massive long-bone or tissue damage and may not appear until during or after surgical manipulation

or reduction of the fracture. Deliberate, induced hypotension in healthy patients is not usually associated with neurologic damage. However, uncontrolled intraoperative hypotension may result in ischemia, especially in a patient with hypertension or carotid occlusive disease.[57]

The successful management of delayed arousal depends on careful consideration of the differential diagnosis. A thorough review of the patient's preoperative medical condition and the intraoperative course (surgical and anesthetic) usually points to a cause. If the cause of the sedation is not immediately obvious, the first consideration must be assessing the patient's oxygenation and ensuring adequate gas exchange. Pulse oximetry, end-tidal carbon dioxide measurement (capnography), and arterial blood gas analysis can give an estimate of any ventilatory depression and rule out ongoing hypoxia and hypercarbia factors.[57,58]

If the cause is thought to be residual inhalation anesthetic, maintenance of adequate ventilation should be sufficient treatment. Residual opioids can be reversed by naloxone, and anticholinergic CNS depression can be reversed by physostigmine. The benzodiazepine antagonist flumazenil has been shown to directly antagonize the CNS sedative and amnesic effects of benzodiazepines.[4]

Body temperature is measured, and warming is instituted if hypothermia exists. Serum electrolytes and magnesium and calcium levels are checked if ion disturbance is suspected. Blood for a serum glucose assay may also be drawn, but the simple fingerstick glucose determination is faster and accurate enough to exclude hypoglycemia from consideration if the result is normal. Other laboratory tests may be useful if hepatic or renal disease is being considered. Unless perioperative events point specifically to it, neurologic injury is usually a diagnosis of exclusion. If other causes of prolonged arousal have been excluded, a thorough neurologic consultation is obtained.[57]

Emergence Delirium

Most patients emerge from general anesthesia in a calm, tranquil manner. However, some patients emerge in a state of excitement, a condition characterized by restlessness, disorientation, crying, moaning, or irrational talking. In the extreme form of excitement, which is referred to as *emergence delirium*, the patient screams, shouts, and thrashes about wildly. This condition is seen most frequently after tonsillectomy, thyroid surgery, circumcision, hysterectomy, and perineal and abdominal wall procedures.[30,58]

Hypoxia with resulting air hunger and hypercarbia may appear as restlessness, disorientation, slurred speech, and agitation. Hyponatremia, hypochloremia, and acid–base changes all can be seen during the immediate postoperative period and can be the cause of mental confusion. Pain is a common cause of restlessness and is frequently seen postoperatively. Urinary bladder and gastric distention, which can cause considerable discomfort, are easily overlooked.[30,58]

Medication reactions are commonly implicated as the cause of postoperative agitation. Such reactions are less common than they were previously because the use of offending medications is less prevalent. The most frequently implicated medications are the anticholinergics, most notably scopolamine and atropine. They have been shown to have toxic CNS effects that can include psychotic behavior, delirium, and motor disturbance. Ketamine in anesthetic doses is also associated with a high incidence of unpleasant agitation. Neuroleptic medications such as haloperidol, especially in rarely used high doses for PONV, may be associated with development of dyskinesia and involuntary muscle activity and with postoperative confusion.[57]

The patient's state of apprehension or anxiety can have a marked effect on emergence agitation; it is especially notable in apprehensive patients and, conversely, in patients who are seemingly unconcerned about forthcoming major surgery. Factors such as fear of disfigurement (eg, caused by cancer surgery) and feelings of suffocation also increase the likelihood of emergence excitement. Young patients tend to have an increased incidence of postoperative excitation, as do patients undergoing emergency procedures. Several psychiatric factors have been shown to increase the incidence of postoperative delirium, including a history of alcoholism, insomnia, depression, or debility.[30,58]

If emergence delirium occurs, the patient's status is thoroughly evaluated. Management includes determining a cause, initiating specific therapy, and protecting patients from injuring themselves. When the nurse encounters a restless, confused postoperative patient, the first measure is to ensure that the agitation is not the result of hypoxia. Presuming pain to be the cause of agitation in a hypoxic patient and treating the excitement with opioids or sedatives can have disastrous consequences. Hypoxia must be quickly excluded from the differential diagnosis by pulse oximetry, arterial blood gas determination, or both.[2,59]

Hyponatremia may be suspected in a confused patient after hysteroscopy or prostate surgery, especially if the surgery was prolonged. A serum electrolyte determination can confirm the diagnosis. Treatment usually consists of fluid restriction and, rarely, hypertonic saline administration. Severe acid–base disturbances can be diagnosed, and therapy is directed by arterial blood gas determination. If pain appears to be the diagnosis after exclusion of hypoxia, intravenous opioids may be administered in small increments. The CNS effects of the anticholinergics are usually dramatically reversed by the administration of physostigmine. The incidence of hallucinations with ketamine may be decreased by benzodiazepine administration. Gastric distention may be relieved by nasogastric aspiration, and urinary bladder distention is easily treated with catheterization.[4]

When dealing with perioperative anxiety, the best treatment is prevention. Some patients need reassurance that they will not experience intraoperative awareness and will receive pain medication, if needed, on awakening.

Occasionally, the nurse is faced with a restless postoperative patient who does not seem to be getting relief from opioid administration. Small intravenous doses of a short-acting benzodiazepine such as midazolam may be warranted. Anxiolytics are administered in reduced doses because their respiratory depressant effects are cumulative with those of existing opioids, sedatives, and residual general anesthetics. If overt psychotic behavior is apparent despite adequate treatment, psychiatric consultation should be obtained.[58]

The patient's respiratory function and airway patency are checked first because restlessness is a well-known manifestation of hypoxia. Other causes of emergence delirium include a full bladder, cramped or sore muscles and joints from prolonged abnormal positioning on the operating table, pain, incomplete reversal of NMBAs, withdrawal from alcohol and medications, acid–base disturbances, and electrolyte abnormalities. A restless patient requires constant, careful observation. Gentle physical restraint may be required to prevent injury. Several nurses or other personnel may be needed. If hypoxia, pain, and a full bladder are ruled out, a change in positioning may have a quieting effect.[2]

Nausea and Vomiting

Nausea and vomiting, although usually not life-threatening, are probably the most unpleasant and lasting memories many patients have of their anesthesia.[60] Although the incidence has decreased in recent years, nausea and vomiting still result in significant postoperative morbidity and patient discomfort. Nausea is described as a subjective, unpleasant mental experience that usually leads to vomiting. Retching is the rhythmic muscular activity that usually precedes vomiting. Vomiting is defined as the forceful expulsion of gastrointestinal contents through the mouth.[61]

Vomiting can be significant.[62] The physical exertion may increase postoperative bleeding and disrupt delicate suture lines. Tearing or rupture of the esophagus is probably rare but must be a concern in patients with a history of esophageal pathology. Aspiration of emesis is a life-threatening complication in a patient whose airway-protective reflexes are blunted by residual anesthetic or sedative medications or damaged by surgical activity. If vomiting is protracted, dangerous hypokalemia, hypochloremia, hyponatremia, and dehydration may develop. Nausea and vomiting are also the leading causes of unexpected hospitalization after surgery.[61,63]

Risk factors most strongly associated with PONV include female sex, history of PONV, history of motion sickness (subjective as reported by patient), nonsmoker, postoperative use/administration of opioids, use of volatile anesthetics, and use of nitrous oxide.[64] Weak or conflicting evidence shows age, duration of surgery, and type of surgery as risk factors.

The most effective treatment of PONV is prevention.[62] Several maneuvers warrant mention as being simple to perform and effective. Avoidance of gastric insufflation is paramount. Swallowing of blood should be prevented during oral, pharyngeal, or nasal surgery. If distention is suspected, it should be decompressed intraoperatively.[4,52] A nasogastric tube is placed to empty fluid and gases from the stomach, but its presence may trigger gagging and subsequent vomiting. An oral airway may elicit the same response in a partially conscious patient and is removed at the first signs of gagging to prevent vomiting and subsequent aspiration.[65]

Many medications have been shown to possess antiemetic qualities, and prophylactic antiemetics and combination medications have been shown to be effective in decreasing or preventing PONV. Available antiemetics include anticholinergics, phenothiazines, antihistamines, butyrophenones, and antidopaminergics. Complementary therapies, including acupressure, ginger gum, and aromatherapy with peppermint oil, have also been shown to be effective in relieving symptoms.[66] It is important to remember the supportive care of a patient with nausea and vomiting. If vomiting is severe, electrolyte replacement must be considered. Prolonged vomiting may result in hypovolemia. Intravenous fluids may need to be increased to compensate for fluid losses. Decreased opioid doses may be needed to reduce the risk of nausea and vomiting; adding nonopioids, such as nonsteroidal antiinflammatory drugs or acetaminophen, may allow for adequate analgesia with less risk of nausea.[67]

CASE STUDY 41.1 Patient With Complex Perianesthesia Management

Brief Patient History

Ms. C is a 60-year-old, bilingual Hispanic woman. She has a history of colon cancer with metastasis, and she has been taking the equivalent of 400 mg of morphine each day for the past 2 weeks to manage her pain. Ms. C is a recovering alcoholic and opioid addict but has been "clean" for 6 years. Other significant medical history includes hypertension, which has been controlled for the past 2 years with lisinopril 10 mg daily. She has undergone a colon resection with general anesthesia (combination of inhalation and intravenous opioid and nonopioid agents), which took several hours to complete. Her vital signs were stable throughout the surgical procedure. Ms. C received 20 mg of morphine during the 4 hours she was in the postanesthesia care unit (PACU).

Clinical Assessment

Ms. C is admitted to the surgical critical care unit from the PACU because of difficulty in controlling her hypertension. She is somnolent but arousable to painful stimuli; however, she states in Spanish that she is having abdominal pain. Her skin is warm and dry; her breaths are being taken through her nose, but respirations are slow and shallow.

Diagnostic Procedures

Her baseline vital signs are blood pressure, 190/92 mm Hg; heart rate, 120 beats/min (sinus tachycardia); respiratory rate, 14 breaths/min; temperature, 36.5°C; chest x-ray, right lower lobe atelectasis; hemoglobin, 9 g/dL; hematocrit, 27; pulse oximetry oxygen saturation, 80% on 100% oxygen via nonrebreather mask; end-tidal carbon dioxide, 70 mm Hg. Ms. C reports that her pain is an 8 out of 10. Riker Sedation-Agitation Scale score is 2.

Medical Diagnosis

Ms. C is diagnosed with respiratory depression and hypoxemia secondary to opioid analgesia.

Questions

1. What major outcomes do you expect to achieve for this patient?
2. What problems or risks must be managed to achieve these outcomes?
3. What interventions must be initiated to monitor, prevent, manage, or eliminate the problems and risks identified?
4. What interventions should be initiated to promote optimal functioning, safety, and well-being of the patient?
5. What possible learning needs would you anticipate for this patient?
6. What cultural and age-related factors might have a bearing on the patient's plan of care?

QSEN BOX 41.10 QSEN: Informatics

Internet Resources

American Association of Critical-Care Nurses: http://www.aacn.org
American Association of Nurse Anesthetists: http://www.aana.com
American College of Surgeons: http://www.facs.org
American Society for Pain Management Nursing: http://www.aspmn.org
American Society of Anesthesiologists: http://www.asahq.org
American Society of PeriAnesthesia Nurses: http://www.aspan.org
British Anaesthetic and Recovery Nurses Association: http://www.barna.co.uk
Malignant Hyperthermia Association of the United States: http://www.mhaus.org
National Association of PeriAnesthesia Nurses of Canada: http://www.napanc.org
National Institutes for Health: http://www.nih.gov
PubMed Health: http://www.ncbi.nlm.nih.gov/pubmedhealth
Society for Critical Care Medicine: http://www.sccm.org

SUMMARY

Selection of Anesthesia

- The type of anesthesia used for surgery may be local, regional, or general.
- Local and regional anesthetics eliminate the sensation of pain to a specific part of the body without loss of protective reflexes or consciousness.
- General anesthesia is a controlled state of unconsciousness; the patient is not arousable, there is partial or complete loss of protective reflexes, and the airway needs to be continuously monitored and maintained.

Perianesthesia Assessment and Care

- Caring for a critically ill patient who is emerging from anesthesia requires monitoring of the patient's physical and psychological status to prevent potential complications that may occur as a result of anesthesia or surgical procedures.
- Knowledge of the preoperative history is important in evaluating and managing postoperative care.
- Communication and hand-off among the anesthesia care provider, the perioperative nurse, and the RN caring for the patient in the immediate postoperative period is important for continuity and safe patient care.
- The goal of patient management in the immediate postoperative period is recognition and immediate treatment of any problems to eliminate or lessen complications.
- Assessment of the cardiopulmonary system is the immediate priority.
- The stir-up regimen is probably the most important aspect of perianesthesia nursing management and consists of five major activities: deep-breathing exercises, coughing, positioning, mobilization, and pain management.

Management of Postanesthesia Problems and Emergencies

- The most frequent complications include respiratory compromise, hypovolemia, hypothermia, and cardiac dysrhythmias.
- The most common adverse reaction is PONV.
- The most lethal complication is malignant hyperthermia.
- Respiratory issues include upper airway obstruction, laryngeal edema, laryngospasm, bronchospasm, acute respiratory failure, aspiration, pulmonary edema, and respiratory arrest.
- Pain management is a priority; inadequate analgesia can interfere with respiratory function and adequate ventilation, affect hemodynamic status, and have a prolonged psychological impact.

ⓔ Visit the Evolve site for additional study materials.

REFERENCES

1. Krenzischek DA, et al. Patient safety: perianesthesia nursing's essential role in safe practice. *J Perianesth Nurs.* 2007;22:385–392.
2. Cartwright SMI, Andrews SM. Perianesthesia nursing as a specialty. In: Odom-Forren J, ed. *Drain's Perianesthesia Nursing: A Critical Care Approach.* ed 6. St. Louis: Elsevier; 2013.
3. Barash PG, Cullen BF, Stoelting RK. *Handbook of Clinical Anesthesia.* ed 5. Philadelphia: Lippincott Williams & Wilkins; 2006.
4. Neuman MD, Fleisher LA. Risk of anesthesia. In: Miller RD, ed. *Miller's Anesthesia.* ed 8. Philadelphia: Elsevier; 2015.
5. Duke J. *Anesthesia Secrets.* ed 5. Philadelphia: Elsevier; 2015.
6. Drasner K, Larson MD. Spinal and epidural anesthesia. In: Miller RD, Pardo Jr MC, eds. *Basics of Anesthesia.* ed 6. St. Louis: Elsevier; 2011.

7. Hagberg CA, Artime CA. Airway management in the adult. In: Miller RD, ed. *Miller's Anesthesia*. ed 8. Philadelphia: Elsevier; 2015.

8. Miller RD. Choice of anesthetic technique. In: Miller RD, Pardo Jr MC, eds. *Basics of Anesthesia*. ed 6. St. Louis: Elsevier; 2011.

9. Pazdernik TL, Kerecsen L. Anesthetics. In: Paxdernik TL, Kercsen L, eds. *Rapid Review of Pharmacology*. ed 3. St. Louis: Elsevier; 2010.

10. Drain CB. Inhalation anesthesia. In: Odom-Forren J, ed. *Drain's Perianesthesia Nursing: A Critical Care Approach*. ed 6. St. Louis: Elsevier; 2013.

11. American Society of Anesthesiologists. *Standards for Basic Monitoring, Reaffirmed*; October 28, 2015. http://www.asahq.org/~/media/Sites/ASAHQ/Files/Public/Resources/standards-guidelines/standards-for-basic-anesthetic-monitoring.pdf. Accessed January 10, 2016.

12. Drain CB. Nonopioid intravenous anesthetics. In: Odom-Forren J, ed. *Drain's Perianesthesia Nursing: A Critical Care Approach*. ed 6. St. Louis: Elsevier; 2013.

13. Drain CB. Opioid intravenous anesthetics. In: Odom-Forren J, ed. *Drain's Perianesthesia Nursing: A Critical Care Approach*. ed 6. St. Louis: Elsevier; 2013.

14. Vuyk J, Sitsen E, Reekers M. Intravenous anesthetics. In: Miller RD, ed. *Miller's Anesthesia*. ed 8. Philadelphia: Elsevier; 2015.

15. Gahart BL, Nazareno AR, Ortega MQ. *Intravenous Medications: A Handbook for Nurses and Health Professionals*. ed 32. St. Louis: Elsevier; 2016.

16. Drain CB. Neuromuscular blocking agents. In: Odom-Forren J, ed. *Drain's Perianesthesia Nursing: A Critical Care Approach*. ed 6. St. Louis: Elsevier; 2013.

17. Wilson J, Collins AS, Rowan BO. Residual neuromuscular blockade in critical care. *Crit Care Nurse*. 2012;32(3):e1–e9.

18. Naguib M, Brull SJ. Sugammadex: a novel selective relaxant binding agent. *Expert Rev Clin Pharmacol*. 2009;2:37–53.

19. Murphy GS, et al. Reversal (antagonism) of neuromuscular blockade. In: Miller RD, ed. *Miller's anesthesia*. ed 8. Philadelphia: Elsevier; 2015.

20. American Society of PeriAnesthesia Nurses. Practice recommendation 6: safe transfer of care: handoff and transportation. In: *2015-2017 Perianesthesia Nursing Standards, Practice Recommendations and Interpretive Statements*. Cherry Hill, NJ: American Society of PeriAnesthesia Nurses; 2015.

21. Schutz SL. Oxygen saturation monitoring by pulse oximetry. In: Wiegand DLM, ed. *AACN Procedure Manual for Critical Care*. ed 6. Philadelphia: Elsevier; 2011.

22. International Anesthesia Research Society. Open Anesthesia Encyclopedia: Critical Care and Perioperative Medicine. Modes of Mechanical Ventilation. http://www.openanesthesia.org/modes_of_mechanical_ventilation/. Accessed January 10, 2016.

23. O'Brien D. Patient education and care of the perianesthesia patient. In: Odom-Forren J, ed. *Drain's Perianesthesia Nursing: A Critical Care Approach*. ed 6. St. Louis: Elsevier; 2013.

24. Dunwoody CJ, et al. Assessment, physiological monitoring, and consequences of inadequately treated acute pain. *J PeriAnesth Nurs*. 2008;23(suppl):S15–S27.

25. Cohen SP, Raja SN. Pain. In: Goldman L, Schafer AI, eds. *Goldman's Cecil Medicine*. ed 24. St. Louis: Elsevier; 2011.

26. Aubrun F, et al. Relationships between measurement of pain using visual analog score and morphine requirements during postoperative intravenous morphine titration. *Anesthesiology*. 2003;98:1415.

27. Polomano RC, et al. Perspective on pain management in the 21st century. *Pain Manag Nurs*. 2008;9(suppl 1):S3–S10.

28. Sun LS, Schwarzenberger JC. Cardiac physiology. In: Miller RD, ed. *Miller's Anesthesia*. ed 8. Philadelphia: Elsevier; 2015.

29. Schick L, Windle PE. *Perianesthesia Nursing Core Curriculum*. ed 3. St. Louis: Elsevier; 2016.

30. O'Brien D. Postanesthesia care complications. In: Odom-Forren J, ed. *Drain's Perianesthesia Nursing: A Critical Care Approach*. ed 6. St. Louis: Elsevier; 2013.

31. Brown EN, Lydic R, Schiff ND. General anesthesia, sleep, and coma. *N Engl J Med*. 2010;363:2638–2650.

32. Ng JLW, Chan MT, Gelb AW. Perioperative stroke in noncardiac, non-neurosurgical surgery. *Anesthesiology*. 2011;115:879–890.

33. Radtke FMF. Risk factors for inadequate emergence after anesthesia: emergence delirium and hypoactive emergence. *Minerva Anestesiol*. 2010;76:394–403.

34. Hooper VD, et al. ASPAN's evidence-based clinical practice guideline for the promotion of perioperative normothermia: second edition. *J PeriAnesth Nurs*. 2010;25:346–365.

35. AORN Recommended Practice Committee. Recommended practices for the prevention of unplanned perioperative hypothermia. *AORN J*. 2007;85(85):972–974, 976-984, 986-988.

36. Edwards MR, Grocutt MPW. Perioperative fluid and electrolyte therapy. In: Miller RD, ed. *Miller's Anesthesia*. ed 8. Philadelphia: Elsevier; 2015.

37. Malina DP. Fluid and electrolytes. In: Odom-Forren J, ed. *Drain's Perianesthesia Nursing: A Critical Care Approach*. ed 6. St. Louis: Elsevier; 2013.

38. Rosén S, Svensson M, Nilsson U. Calm or not calm: the question of anxiety in the perianesthesia patient. *J PeriAnesth Nurs*. 2008;23:237–246.

39. Kiekkas P, et al. Nursing activities and use of time in the postanesthesia care unit. *J PeriAnesth Nurs*. 2005;20:311–322.

40. American Society of PeriAnesthesia Nurses. Position statement 4: A joint position statement on ICU overflow patients developed by ASPAN, AACN, and ASA's Committee on Surgical Anesthesia. http://www.aspan.org/Portals/6/docs/ClinicalPractice/PositionStatement/Current/PS4_2015.pdf. Accessed January 10, 2016.

41. American Society of PeriAnesthesia Nurses. Practice recommendation 1: patient classification/staffing recommendations. In: *2015-2017 Perianesthesia Nursing Standards, Practice Recommendations and Interpretive Statements*. Cherry Hill, NJ: American Society of PeriAnesthesia Nurses; 2015.

42. Litwack K. *Post Anesthesia Care Nursing*. ed 2. St. Louis: Mosby; 1995.

43. Wright SM. Assessment and management of the airway. In: Odom-Forren J, ed. *Drain's Perianesthesia Nursing: A Critical Care Approach*. ed 6. St. Louis: Elsevier; 2013.

44. Odom JL. Airway emergencies in the post anesthesia care unit. *Nurs Clin North Am*. 1993;28:483–491.

45. Udeshi A, Cantie SM, Pierre E. Postobstructive pulmonary edema. *J Crit Care*. 2010;25:508.e1–508.e5.

46. Weitz HH. Perioperative cardiac complications. *Med Clin North Am*. 2001;85:1151–1169.

47. Mokhlesi B, Corbridge T. Toxicology in the critically ill patient. *Clin Chest Med*. 2003;24:689–711.

48. Sloan SB, Weitz HH. Postoperative arrhythmias and conduction disorders. *Med Clin North Am*. 2001;85:1171–1189.

49. Nicholau D. Postanesthesia recovery. In: Miller RD, Pardo Jr MC, eds. *Basics of Anesthesia*. ed 6. St. Louis: Elsevier; 2011.

50. Kurz A. Thermal care in the perioperative period. *Best Pract Res Clin Anaesthesiol*. 2008;22:39–62.

51. De Witte J, Sessler DI. Perioperative shivering: physiology and pharmacology. *Anesthesiology*. 2002;96:467–484.

52. Warttig SS. Interventions for treating inadvertent postoperative hypothermia. *Cochrane Database Syst Rev*. 2014;11:CD009892.

53. Sessler DI. Temperature regulation and monitoring. In: Miller RD, ed. *Miller's Anesthesia*. ed 8. Philadelphia: Elsevier; 2015.

54. Rosenberg H, et al. Malignant hyperthermia. *Orphanet J Rare Dis*. 2007;2:21.

55. Hommertzheim R, Steinke EE. Malignant hyperthermia: the perioperative nurse's role. *AORN J*. 2006;83:149–156, 159–160.

56. McClain DA. Delayed emergence. In: Atlee JL, ed. *Complications in Anesthesia*. ed 2. St. Louis: Saunders; 2007.

57. Mecca RS. Coma and delayed emergence. In: Lobato EB, Gravenstein N, Kirby RR, eds. *Complications in Anesthesiology*. ed 4. Philadelphia: Lippincott Williams & Wilkins; 2008.

58. O'Brien D. Acute postoperative delirium: definitions, incidence, recognition, and interventions. *J Perianesth Nurs*. 2002;17:384–392.

59. Hagberg CA. *Benumof's and Hagberg's Airway Management*. ed 3. Philadelphia: Mosby; 2013.

60. Chandrakantan A, Glass PS. Multimodal therapies for postoperative nausea and vomiting, and pain. *Br J Anaesth*. 2011;107(suppl 1):i27–i40.

61. Ho K-Y, Gan TJ. Postoperative nausea and vomiting. In: Lobato EB, Gravenstein N, Kirby RR, eds. *Complications in Anesthesiology*. ed 4. Philadelphia: Lippincott Williams & Wilkins; 2008.

62. Kranke P, Eberhart LH. Possibilities and limitations in the pharmacological management of postoperative nausea and vomiting. *Eur J Anaesthesiol*. 2011;28:758–765.

63. Gan TJ, et al. Consensus guidelines for the management of postoperative nausea and vomiting. *Anesth Analg*. 2014;118:85–113.

64. American Society of PeriAnesthesia Nurses PONV/PDNV Strategic Work Team. ASPAN'S evidence-based clinical practice guideline for the prevention and/or management of PONV/PDNV. *J PeriAnesth Nurs*. 2006;21:230–250.

65. Odom-Forren J, Fetzer SJ, Moser DK. Evidence-based interventions for post discharge nausea and vomiting: a review of the literature. *J Perianesth Nurs*. 2006;21:411–430.

66. Mamaril ME, Windle PE, Burkard JF. Prevention and management of postoperative nausea and vomiting: a look at complementary techniques. *J Perianesth Nurs*. 2006;21:404–410.

67. Pasero C, McCaffery M. *Pain Assessment and Pharmacologic Management*. St. Louis: Elsevier; 2011.

Nursing Management Plans of Care

◎ **NURSING MANAGEMENT PLAN**

Activity Intolerance

Definition: Insufficient physiologic or psychologic energy to endure or complete required or desired daily activities.

Activity Intolerance Related to Cardiopulmonary Dysfunction

Defining Characteristics

- Chest pain with activity
- Electrocardiogram (ECG) changes with activity
- Heart rate is >15 beats/min above baseline with activity for patients on beta-blockers or calcium channel blockers
- Heart rate remains elevated above baseline 5 min after activity
- Breathlessness with activity
- SpO_2 <92% with activity
- Postural hypotension when moving from supine to upright position
- Patient reports fatigue with activity

Outcome Criteria

- Heart rate is <20 beats/min above baseline with activity and is <10 beats/min above baseline with activity for patients on beta-blockers or calcium channel blockers.
- Heart rate returns to baseline 5 min after activity.
- Chest pain with activity is absent.
- Patient reports tolerance to activity.

Nursing Interventions and Rationale

1. Encourage active or passive range-of-motion exercises while the patient is in bed *to keep joints flexible and muscles stretched.*
2. Teach the patient to refrain from holding breath while performing exercises and *to avoid Valsalva maneuver.*
3. Encourage performance of muscle-toning exercises at least three times daily *because a toned muscle uses less oxygen when performing work than an untoned muscle.*
4. Progress ambulation *to increase tolerance to activity.*
5. Teach the patient to take pulse *to determine activity tolerance:* Take pulse for a full minute before exercise and then for 10 s and multiply by 6 at exercise peak.
6. Collaborate with the practitioner regarding administration of fluids to ensure that the patient is hydrated to 24-h fluid requirements per body surface area *to increase preload and increase stroke volume and cardiac output.*

Activity Intolerance Related to Prolonged Immobility or Deconditioning

Defining Characteristics

- Decrease in systolic blood pressure is >20 mm Hg
- Increase in heart rate is >20 beats/min with postural change
- Syncope with postural change
- Patient reports lightheadedness with postural change

Outcome Criteria

- Decrease in systolic blood pressure is <10 mm Hg.
- Increase in heart rate is <10 beats/min with postural change.
- Syncope or lightheadedness is absent with postural change.
- Hypoxemia is absent.
- Patient reports tolerance to activity.

Nursing Interventions and Rationale

1. Collaborate with the practitioner regarding the patient's activity level and the need for physical therapy *to ensure the patient's safety.*
2. Collaborate with the physical therapist to develop progressive activity plan for the patient *to return to prior level of function.*

For Patient on Bed Rest

1. Instruct the patient how to perform straight-leg raises, dorsiflexion or plantar flexion, and quadriceps-setting and gluteal-setting exercises *to increase muscular and vascular tone.*
2. Reposition the patient incrementally *to avoid syncope:*
   a. Head of bed to 45 degrees and hold until symptom-free
   b. Head of bed to 90 degrees and hold until symptom-free
   c. Dangle until symptom-free
   d. Stand until symptom-free and ambulate

For Patient on Ventilator

1. Collaborate with the practitioner, respiratory care practitioner, and physical therapist regarding the patient's eligibility for early progressive mobility *to ensure patient is ready and able to participate.*
2. Initiate early progressive mobility program when the patient is ready *to limit the effects of prolonged immobility.*
   a. Elevation of the head of the bed
   b. Turn patient every 2 h
   c. Perform passive range of motion at least three times a day
   d. Progress patient to active range of motion when ready
   e. Place bed in chair position to position patient in upright/leg-down position
   f. Initiate bed mobility activities such as sitting on the edge of the bed (dangling)
   g. Initiate transfer training
   h. Implement pregait activities such as standing at the side of the bed and marching in place
   i. Progress patient to ambulation
3. Monitor the patient's response to activity and discontinue activity if patient shows signs of intolerance *to ensure patient safety:*
   a. Hypoxemia
   b. Hypotension
   c. Dysrhythmias or ECG changes

NURSING MANAGEMENT PLAN

Acute Confusion

Definition: Abrupt onset of reversible disturbances of consciousness, attention, cognition, and perception that develop over a short period of time.

Acute Confusion Related to Sensory Overload, Sensory Deprivation, and Sleep Pattern Disturbance

Defining Characteristics

Early Symptoms

- Sudden onset of global cognitive function impairment (hours to days)
- Restlessness, agitation, and combative behavior
- Drowsiness (can lead to loss of consciousness)
- Slurring of speech, inappropriate statements or "word salad," mumbling, or inappropriate gestures
- Short attention span (needs questions repeated); inability to learn new material
- Disordered sleep/wake cycle
- Disorientation to person, time, place, and situation
- Difficulty in separating dreams from reality (may experience bizarre dreams or nightmares)
- Anger at staff for continued questions about his or her orientation

Later Symptoms

- Symptoms that tend to fluctuate throughout the day and night
- Continuations of early symptoms, which may be more frequent or of longer duration
- Illusions
- Hallucinations
- Extreme agitation (eg, attempts to climb out of bed, pull out catheters, rip off dressings)
- Calling out in loud voice, swearing, or attempting to bite or hit people who approach patient

Nursing Interventions and Rationale

1. Determine and document the patient's dominant spoken language, his or her literacy, and the languages in which he or she is literate. *Sometimes people are not literate in their spoken language, or, less commonly, they are literate only in their second language.*
2. Determine and document the patient's premorbid degree of orientation, cognitive capabilities, and any sensory/perceptual deficits.

For Sensory Overload

1. Initiate each nurse-patient encounter by calling the patient by name and identifying yourself by name. *This fosters reality orientation and assists the patient in filtering irrelevant or impersonal conversation.*
2. Assess the patient's immediate physical environment from his or her viewpoint, and explain equipment, its sounds, and its therapeutic purpose. Demonstrate audible and visual alarms, and explain possible alarm conditions. *This decreases alienation of the patient from the technologic environment and reduces the inherent sense of fear and urgency accompanying alarm conditions.*
3. Provide preparatory sensory information by explaining procedures in relation to the sensations the patient will experience including duration of sensations. *Preparatory sensory information enhances learning and lessens anticipatory anxiety.*
4. Limit noise levels. *Audible alarms cannot and must not be silenced, and many critical but noisy activities must take place in the critical care unit. However, it has been shown that noise levels produced by clinical personnel exceed levels designated as acceptable and are often greater than levels generated by technologic devices.*

   a. Keep staff conversations soft enough that they are inaudible to the patient whenever possible.
   b. Assume that everything said at or around a patient's bedside is intended for that patient's awareness and that it will be interpreted as pertaining to him or her. *As in the discussion that follows, conversations about the patient but not to him or her foster depersonalization and delusions of reference.*
   c. Enforce nighttime noise limits.
5. Readjust alarm limits on physiologic monitoring devices as the patient's condition changes (improves or deteriorates) *to lessen unnecessary alarm states.*
6. Consider use of headphones and digital music player with the patient's favorite music and/or subliminal or classical music. *This can effectively filter out assaultive noise of the critical care environment and supplant it with familiar, soothing sounds and rhythms.*
7. Modify lighting. *Day and night cycles need to be simulated with environmental lighting.*

   a. Never turn on overhead fluorescent lights abruptly without warning the patient, assisting him or her out of the supine position, and shielding his or her eyes with gauze or a face cloth. *Continuous bright lighting sustains anxiety and promotes circadian rhythm desynchronization.*
8. Shield patients from viewing urgent and emergent events in the critical care unit. *Resuscitation efforts, albeit difficult to conceal, engender fear in the patient and a sense of instability and vulnerability (eg, "I'm next").*

   a. When such an event occurs, elicit the patient's cognitive and emotional reaction; *thoughts, impressions, and feelings need to be shared, and misconceptions need to be clarified.*
9. Ensure patients' privacy, modesty, and dignity. *Physical exposure and nudity, although they seemingly pale in importance compared with priorities such as physiologic assessment and stabilization, are primal indignities for all individuals.*

   a. Keep the patient minimally exposed. When it becomes necessary to expose the patient, verbally apologize for this necessity. *To be naked is to feel vulnerable; to be vulnerable is to feel fearful.*

For Sensory Deprivation

1. Provide reality orientation in four spheres (personal, place, time, and situation) at more frequent intervals than when testing.

   a. Convey this information in the context of routine conversation. *Sample statements:* "Mr. Clark, this is Tuesday morning and you're in University Hospital. Your heart surgery was yesterday morning, and you're doing well. My name is Joe, and I'm your nurse today." *The patient is made to feel patronized by repetitions such as, "Do you know where you are?" Given the effects of general anesthesia, opioid analgesics, sedatives, and sleep, it is expected that some degree of disorientation will exist normally.*
2. Ensure the patient's visual access to a calendar.
3. Apprise the patient of daily news events and the weather.
4. Touch patients for the express purpose of communicating caring. Hold their hands, stroke their brows, and rub the skin on an aspect of the arms. *Touch is the universal language of caring. In the setting of critical care, in which there is considerable physical body manipulation, it is useful and important to contrast assaultive touch with comforting touch. Touch can be used as a technique for distraction from painful stimuli when used in conjunction with uncomfortable procedures. (See later discussion of the use of touch in management of the patient experiencing hallucinations.)*

Continued

NURSING MANAGEMENT PLAN

Acute Confusion—cont'd

5. Foster liberal visitation by family members and significant others. Encourage significant others to touch the patient as consistent with their individual comfort level and cultural norms.

6. Structure and identify opportunities for the patient to exercise decision-making skills, however small. *Although not so designated, patients with sensory alterations also experience a type of cognitive deprivation.*

7. Assist patients to find meaning in their experiences. *Patients need to find meaning and to identify their roles in the experience of critical illness and critical care.*
   a. Explain the therapeutic purpose of all they are asked to do for themselves and all that is done with them and for them.
   b. Avoid statements such as, "Will you turn to that side for me?" or "I need you to swallow this medication." *These statements implicitly convey that the maneuver has some value for the nurses instead of the patients.*
   c. Similarly, use "thank you" judiciously. *This simple salutation, when used indiscriminately, suggests something was done to benefit the nurses, not the patients.*

For Hallucinations

1. Approach the patient with a calm, matter-of-fact demeanor. *The goal of this interaction is for the nurse to demonstrate external control. This helps decrease the anxiety and fear that generally accompany hallucinations and allows the patient to feel safe. Anxiety is transferable.*

2. Address the patient by name. *This is a useful presentation of reality because self-identity is the last sphere of orientation to vanish.*

3. In responding to the patient's description of the hallucination, do not deny, argue, or attempt to disprove the existence of the perceived event. Statements such as, "There are no voices coming from that air vent" or "Look, I'm brushing my hand across the wall, and there are no bugs" confuse the patient further *because the hallucination, although frightening, is his or her perceived reality.*

4. Express to the patient that your experiences are dissimilar, and acknowledge how frightening his or hers must be. *Sample statements:* "I don't hear (or see) what you do, but I know how frightening such an experience must be to you. I'm Joe, your nurse, and I'm going to stay with you until the voices (or visions) go away." *Validating the patient's feelings demonstrates acceptance and sensitivity to the experience and promotes trust.*

5. Remain with any patient who is experiencing a hallucination. *Feelings of fear and anxiety often accelerate when a patient is left alone. He or she needs someone to represent a nonthreatening reality.*

6. Do not explore the content of the hallucination with the patient by asking about its nature or character. *The nurse is the patient's link with reality. Pursuit of a detailed description of a hallucination may signify to the patient that the nurse accepts his or her sensory distortion as factual. This may further confuse the patient and distance him or her more from reality.*
   a. Ascertain that the voices are not telling the patient to harm himself or herself by asking simply and concretely, "What are the voices saying?" *The nurse can help bridge the gap between the patient's misperception and reality by addressing the feelings (eg, fear, anxiety) and/or meanings (eg, danger, death) engendered by the hallucination.*
   b. Determine how the misperception affects the patient emotionally; acknowledge those feelings; and use a calm, controlled, matter-of-fact approach to provide the trust and comfort the patient needs to tolerate this frightening experience. *In other words, the nurse should deal*

with the intent more than the content of the hallucination. The resultant decrease in anxiety will enable the patient to focus more accurately on his or her immediate environment.

7. Talk concretely with the patient about things that are really happening. *Sample statements:* "How does your chest incision feel this afternoon, Mr. Clark?" "Your sister Kate was here to see you, but you were sleeping. She went down to the cafeteria and will be back." "Your secretions are a little easier for you to cough up today." *Interpretation of reality-based stimuli by the nurse encourages the patient to focus on actual circumstances and discourages a preoccupation with sensory misperceptions.*

8. Distract the patient by changing the topic. *This tactic is useful in situations of escalating anxiety and confusion or when all else fails. Topics need to consist of basic themes that are universally understood and culturally congruent such as music, food, or weather or topics of special interest to the patient such as hobbies, crafts, or sports.*
   a. Avoid topics that evoke strong emotions such as politics, religion, or sexuality. *This is especially true in regard to a patient with reality distortions; sometimes hallucinations and delusions are expressions of repressed conflicts associated with religious, sexual, or aggressive issues. Pursuit of such subjects could increase confusion and anxiety.*

9. Avoid the use of touch as an intervention strategy for any patient who demonstrates escalating anxiety or paranoid, suspicious, or mistrustful thoughts. *Although touch can be useful in the management of patients with sensory alterations, for patients experiencing hallucinations (as well as delusions and illusions), touch can be readily misinterpreted as aggression or pain, and it can provide the basis for a tactile illusion.*

10. For auditory hallucinations:
    a. *Patient behaviors:* Head cocked as if listening to an unseen presence; lips moving.
    b. *Therapeutic nurse responses:* "Mr. Clark, you appear to be listening to something." If the patient acknowledges voices: "I don't hear any voices, but I know this is troubling you. The voices will go away. Nothing is going to harm you. I'm Joe, your nurse, and I'll be here with you."
    c. *Nontherapeutic nurse responses:* "Tell me about your conversations with these voices." "To whom do these voices belong—anyone you know?"

11. For visual hallucinations:
    a. *Patient behaviors:* Staring into space as if focused on an unseen object; startled movements and anxious facial expression.
    b. *Therapeutic nurse responses:* "Mr. Clark, something seems to be troubling you. Tell me what it is." If patient states he visualizes people, images, or the devil in his environment and implies a sense of danger, respond, "There are only nurses and doctors here, Mr. Clark. I know this must be upsetting, but these images will go away. We're here with you in the hospital. Nothing will happen to you."
    c. *Nontherapeutic nurse responses:* "Describe the people you see. What are they wearing?" "What does the devil mean in your life? What about God?"

For Delusions

1. Explain all unseen noises, voices, and activity simply and clearly. *They readily feed a delusional system. Sample statements:* "That is Dr. Smith. He's come to see you and other patients here in the hospital." "The voices and activity you hear are from the bedside of the patient behind this curtain. He's being helped by one of the nurses."

NURSING MANAGEMENT PLAN

Acute Confusion—cont'd

2. Avoid the "negative challenge" of the patient's delusions (eg, "Nobody here stole your belongings" or "Doctors and nurses do not harm people"). Similarly, avoid defending the referents of the patient's belief: "Nurses are good" and "Doctors mean well." *A delusion is a belief, albeit false, that cannot be changed with logic. To attempt this change is to challenge the patient's belief system and escalate his or her anxiety, further blurring the boundaries between reality and the patient's internally based "logic."*

3. For the patient with persecutory delusions who refuses food, fluids, or medications because of a belief that he or she has been poisoned or the medications are tainted, permit the refusal unless it is a life-threatening event. Try again in 20 minutes; allow the patient to choose an alternative selection of food or to read the label on the unit's medication. *Coercion, show of force, or engagement in complicated, logical justifications will heighten the patient's suspiciousness and possibly reinforce the delusional belief. When the patient feels more in control, he or she need not rely on the "paradoxical" quality of the delusion to equip him or her with a false sense of power. His or her power instead is derived from making reality-based decisions.*

4. Staff members should be particularly careful not to engage in unnecessary laughter or whispering within view of a delusional patient. *The delusional patient is hypervigilant, scanning the environment for evidence to corroborate or confirm his or her belief that staff members are colluding against him or her; laughter and whispers easily suggest this belief, this delusion of reference. This rationale also pertains to the patient experiencing hallucinations and/or illusions.*

5. Observe the principles detailed in the third intervention in the "For Hallucinations" section.

For Illusions

1. Interpret a reality-based stimulus for the patient in a calm, matter-of-fact manner. *Seen and unseen noises, voices, activity, and people can provide the stimulus for a sensory misinterpretation, an illusion.*

2. Minimize stimulation in the patient's immediate environment. *Nursing interventions detailed previously under "Sensory Overload" are especially relevant here.*

3. Address the feeling and meaning associated with the experience, not the content of the sensory misinterpretation.
   a. *Patient behaviors:* Eyes darting, startled movements, frightened facial expression. "I know who you are. You're the devil come to take me to hell."
   b. *Therapeutic nurse responses:* "I'm Joe, your nurse. I know this experience is troubling for you. You're in the hospital, and no one here will harm you."
   c. Nontherapeutic nurse responses: "There are no such things as devils and angels." "Do you think the devil would be dressed in white?" *The first nontherapeutic nurse response carries a parental tone (ie, "You know better than that."), infantilizing the patient and adding to his or her feelings of powerlessness over the environment. The second nontherapeutic response reflects obvious logic, which is not in the patient's sensory domain; it cannot be processed and only adds to his or her confused state.*

4. Observe the principles detailed in the fifth intervention of the "For Hallucinations" section.

NURSING MANAGEMENT PLAN

Acute Pain

Definition: Unpleasant sensory and emotional experience arising from actual or potential tissue damage or described in terms of such damage (International Association for the Study of Pain); sudden or slow onset of any intensity from mild to severe with an anticipated or predictable end and a duration of less than 6 months.

Acute Pain Related to Transmission and Perception of Cutaneous, Visceral, Muscular, or Ischemic Impulses
Defining Characteristics
Subjective

- Patient verbalizes presence of pain
- Patient rates pain on a scale of 1 to 10 using a visual analog scale

Objective

- Increase in blood pressure, heart rate, and respiratory rate
- Pupillary dilation
- Diaphoresis, pallor
- Skeletal muscle reactions (eg, grimacing, clenching fists, writhing, pacing, guarding or splinting of affected part)
- Apprehension, fearful appearance
- May not exhibit any physiologic change

Outcome Criteria

- Patient verbalizes that pain is reduced to a tolerable level or is totally relieved.
- Patient's pain rating is lower on a scale of 1 to 10.
- Blood pressure, heart rate, and respiratory rate return to baseline 5 min after intravenous (IV) administration of an opioid analgesic or 20 min after intramuscular administration of an opioid analgesic.

Nursing Interventions and Rationale

1. Modify variables that heighten the patient's experience of pain.
   a. Explain to the patient that frequent, detailed, and seemingly repetitive assessments will be conducted to allow the nurse to better understand the patient's pain experience, not because the existence of pain is in question.
   b. Explain the factors responsible for pain production in the individual. Estimate the expected duration of the pain if possible.
   c. Explain diagnostic and therapeutic procedures to the patient in relation to sensations the patient should expect to feel.
   d. Reduce the patient's fear of addiction by explaining the difference between drug tolerance and drug dependence. *Drug tolerance is a physiologic phenomenon in which a medication begins to lose effectiveness after repeated doses; drug dependence is a psychologic phenomenon in which opioids are used regularly for emotional, not medical, reasons.*
   e. Instruct the patient to ask for pain medication when pain is beginning and not to wait until it is intolerable.
   f. Explain that the practitioner will be consulted if pain relief is inadequate with the present medication.
   g. Instruct the patient in the importance of adequate rest, especially when it reduces pain *to maintain strength and coping abilities and to reduce stress.*
2. Collaborate with the practitioner regarding pharmacologic interventions.
   - **For postoperative or posttraumatic cutaneous, muscular, or visceral pain,** perform the following:
   a. Medicate with an opioid analgesic to break the pain cycles as long as level of consciousness and vital signs are stable.
   b. Check the patient's previous response to similar dosage and opioids.

c. Establish optimal analgesic dose that brings optimal pain relief.
d. Offer pain medication at prescribed regular intervals rather than making the patient ask for it *to maintain more steady blood levels.*
e. Consider waking the patient to avoid loss of opiate blood levels during sleep.
f. If administering medication on as-needed (PRN) basis, give it when the patient's pain is just beginning, rather than at its peak.
   (1) Advise the patient to intercept pain, not endure it, or several hours and higher doses of opioid analgesics may be necessary to relieve pain, leading to a cycle of undermedication and pain alternating with overmedication and drug toxicity.
g. Perform rehabilitation exercises (turn, deep breathe, leg exercises, ambulate) shortly before peak of drug effect *because this will be the optimal time for the patient to increase activity with the least risk of increasing pain.*
h. When making the transition from one drug to another or from intramuscular or IV to oral medication, use an equianalgesic chart. *Equianalgesic means approximately the same pain relief. The patient's response should be closely monitored to determine if the right analgesic choice was made.*
i. To assess effectiveness of pain medication, do the following:
   (1) Reevaluate pain 15 to 30 min after IV and 30 to 60 min after oral medication administration; observe the patient's behavior, and ask the patient to rate pain on a scale of 1 to 10.
   (2) Collaborate with the practitioner to add or delete other medications that potentiate the action of analgesics, such as antiemetics, hypnotics, sedatives, or muscle relaxants.
   (3) Observe for indicators of undertreatment: report of pain not relieved; observed restlessness, sleeplessness, irritability, and anorexia; decreased activity level.
   (4) Observe for indicators of overtreatment: hypotension or bradycardia; respiratory rate <10/min; excessive sedation.
j. Evaluate the patient's level of sedation and respiratory rate at regular intervals *to avoid oversedation.*
   (1) Respirations should be counted for a full minute and qualified according to rhythm and depth of chest excursion.
   (2) Consider the use of capnography (end-tidal carbon dioxide monitoring) as an early indicator of hypoventilation and oversedation.
k. If patient-controlled analgesia (PCA) is used, perform the following:
   (1) Instruct the patient on what the drug is, the dose, and how often it can be self-administered by pushing the button to activate the PCA machine. For example, "When you have pain, instead of asking the nurse to bring medication, push the button that activates the machine and a small dose of the pain medicine will be injected into your IV line. You can keep your pain under control by administering additional medicine as soon as your pain begins to return or increases. Push the button before undertaking a painful activity, such as ambulation. Try to balance your pain relief against sleepiness, and don't activate the machine if you start to feel sleepy. If your pain medicine seems to stop working despite pushing the button several times, call the nurse to check your IV. If you are not receiving adequate pain relief, the nurse will call your doctor."
   (2) Monitor vital signs, especially blood pressure and respiratory rate, every hour for the first 4 h, and assess postural heart rate and blood pressure before initial ambulation.
   (3) Monitor respiratory rate every 2 h while the patient is on PCA.
   (4) If the patient's respiratory rate decreases to <10 breaths/min or if patient is overly sedated, anticipate administration of naloxone.

NURSING MANAGEMENT PLAN

Acute Pain—cont'd

l. If epidural opioid analgesia is used, do the following:
   (1) Keep the patient's head elevated 30 to 45 degrees after injection *to prevent respiratory depressant effects.*
   (2) Observe closely for respiratory depression for 24 h after injection. Monitor respiratory rate every 15 min for 1 h, every 30 min for 7 h, and every hour for the remaining 16 h.
   (3) Assess for adequate cough reflex.
   (4) Avoid use of other central nervous system depressants, such as sedatives.
   (5) Observe for reports of pruritus, nausea, and vomiting.
   (6) Anticipate administration of naloxone for respiratory depression (and smaller doses of naloxone for pruritus).
   (7) Assess for and treat urinary retention.
   (8) Assess epidural catheter site for local infection. Keep the catheter taped securely *to prevent catheter migration.*

- For peripheral vascular ischemic pain (hypothetic vascular occlusion of leg), do the following:

a. Correctly identify and differentiate ischemic pain from other types of pain. *(NOTE: Ischemic pain is usually a burning, aching pain made worse by exercise and lessened or relieved by rest. Eventually, the pain occurs at rest. Coldness and pallor of extremity may be noted, especially if the limb is elevated above the heart level. Rubor and mottling of the skin may be evident from prolonged tissue anoxia and inability of damaged vessels to constrict. Eventually, cyanosis and gangrenous tissue will be evident. Chronic ischemia leads to visible changes in the limb, such as flaking skin, brittle nails and hair, leg ulcers, and cellulitis.)*

b. Administer pain medications, and evaluate their effectiveness as previously described. *The pain of ischemia is chronic and continuous and can make the patient irritable and depressed.*

c. Treat the cause of the ischemic pain, and institute measures *to increase circulation to the affected part.*

3. Initiate nonpharmacologic interventions.
   a. Treat contributing factors.
   b. Apply comfort measures.
      (1) Use relaxation techniques, such as back rubs, massage, warm baths, music, and aromatherapy.
         (a) Use blankets and pillows to support the painful part and reduce muscle tension.
         (b) Encourage slow, rhythmic breathing.
      (2) Encourage progressive muscle relaxation techniques.
         (a) Instruct the patient to inhale and tense (tighten) specific muscle groups and then relax the muscles as exhalation occurs.
         (b) Suggest an order for performing the tension and relaxation cycle (eg, start with facial muscles and move down body, ending with toes).
      (3) Encourage guided imagery.
         (a) Ask the patient to recall an experienced image that is very pleasurable and relaxing and involves at least two senses.
         (b) Have the patient begin with rhythmic breathing and progressive relaxation and then travel mentally to the scene.
         (c) Have the patient slowly experience the scene (eg, how it looks, sounds, smells, feels).
         (d) Ask the patient to practice this imagery in private.
         (e) Instruct the patient to end the imagery by counting to three and saying, "Now I'm relaxed." If the person does not end the imagery and falls asleep, the purpose of the technique is defeated.

NURSING MANAGEMENT PLAN

Anxiety

Definition: Vague uneasy feeling of discomfort or dread accompanied by an autonomic response (the source often nonspecific or unknown to the individual); a feeling of apprehension caused by anticipation of danger. It is an alerting signal that warns of impending danger and enables the individual to take measures to deal with threat.

Anxiety Related to Threat to Biologic, Psychologic, or Social Integrity
Defining Characteristics
Subjective

- Verbalizes increased muscle tension
- Expresses frequent sensation of tingling in hands and feet
- Relates continuous feeling of apprehension
- Expresses preoccupation with a sense of impending doom
- Reports difficulty falling asleep
- Repeatedly expresses concerns about changes in health status and outcome of illness

Objective

- Psychomotor agitation (fidgeting, jitteriness, restlessness)
- Tightened, wrinkled brow
- Strained (worried) facial expression
- Hypervigilance (scans environment)
- Startles easily
- Distractibility
- Sweaty palms
- Fragmented sleep patterns
- Tachycardia
- Tachypnea

Outcome Criteria

- Patient effectively uses learned relaxation strategies.
- Patient demonstrates significant decrease in psychomotor agitation.
- Patient verbalizes reduction in tingling sensations in hands and feet.
- Patient is able to focus on the tasks at hand.
- Patient expresses positive, future-based plans to family and staff.
- Patient's heart rate and rhythm remain within limits commensurate with physiologic status.

Nursing Interventions and Rationale

1. Instruct the patient in the following simple, effective relaxation strategies:
   a. If not contraindicated for cardiovascular reasons, tense and relax all muscles progressively from toes to head. *Progressive toe-to-head relaxation releases the muscular tension that may be a stress-related effect resulting from the threat or change in the patient's health status and outcome of illness.*
   b. Perform slow deep-breathing exercises. *Deep-breathing exercises provide slow, rhythmic, controlled breathing patterns that relax the patient and distract him or her from the effects of his or her illness and hospitalization.*
   c. Focus on a single object or person in the environment. *Focusing on a single object or person helps the patient dismiss myriad disorienting stimuli from his or her visual-perceptual field, which can have a dizzying, distorted effect. A clear sensorium allows him or her to feel more in control of his or her environment.*
   d. Listen to soothing music or relaxation tapes with eyes closed. *Music or words expressed in soft, low tones tend to produce soothing, relaxing effects that counteract or inhibit escalating anxiety and provide respites from the patient's situational crisis. Closed eyes eliminate distracting visual stimuli and promote a more restful environment.*
2. Actively listen to and accept the patient's concerns regarding the threats from his or her illness, outcome, and hospitalization. *Active listening and unconditional acceptance validate the patient as a worthwhile individual and assure him or her that his or her concerns, no matter how great, will be addressed. Knowledge that he or she has an avenue for ventilation will assuage anxiety.*
3. Help the patient distinguish between realistic concerns and exaggerated fears through clear, simple explanations. *Sample statements:* "Your lab results show that you're doing okay right now." "The shortness of breath you're experiencing is not unusual." "The pain you described is expected, and this medication will relieve it." *A patient who is informed about his or her progress and is reassured about expected symptoms and management of care will be better equipped to maintain a more realistic perspective of his or her illness and its outcome. Anxiety emanating from imagined or exaggerated fears will likely be assuaged or averted.*
4. Provide simple clarification of environmental events and stimuli that are not related to the patient's illness and care. *Sample statements:* "That loud noise is coming from a machine that is helping another patient." "The visitor behind the curtain is crying because she's had an upsetting day." "That gurney is here to take another patient to x-ray." *Clarification of events and stimuli that are unrelated to the patient helps to disengage him or her from the extant anxiety-provoking situations surrounding him or her, avoiding further anxiety and apprehension.*
5. Assist the patient in focusing on building on prior coping strategies to deal with the effects of his or her illness and care. *Sample statements:* "What methods have helped you get through difficult times in the past?" "How can we help you use those methods now?" (See the nursing management plan for Ineffective Coping for interventions that assist patients to use coping strategies effectively.) *Use of previously successful coping strategies in conjunction with newly learned techniques arms the patient with an arsenal of weapons against anxiety, providing him or her with greater control over the situational crisis and decreased feelings of doom and despair.*
6. Give the patient permission to deny or suppress the effects of his or her illness and hospitalization with which he or she cannot cope or control. *Sample statements:* "It's perfectly okay to ignore things you can't handle right now." "How can we help ease your mind during this time?" "What are some things or tasks that may help distract you?" *Adaptive denial can be helpful in reducing feelings of anxiety in patients with life-threatening illness.*

NURSING MANAGEMENT PLAN

Autonomic Dysreflexia

Definition: Life-threatening, uninhibited sympathetic response of the nervous system to a noxious stimulus after a spinal cord injury at the seventh thoracic vertebra (T7) or above.

Autonomic Dysreflexia Related to Excessive Autonomic Response to Noxious Stimuli

Defining Characteristics

- Paroxysmal hypertension (sudden increase in both systolic and diastolic blood pressure [BP] >20 mm Hg above patient's normal BP); for many patients with spinal cord injury, normal BP may be 90/60 mm Hg
- Pounding headache
- Bradycardia (may be a relative slowing, so the heart rate may still appear within the normal range)
- Profuse sweating (above the level of the injury) especially in the face, neck, and shoulders
- Pilomotor erection (goose bumps) above the level of the injury
- Cardiac dysrhythmias (atrial fibrillation, premature ventricular contractions, and atrioventricular conduction abnormalities)
- Flushing of the skin (above the level of the injury) especially in the face, neck, and shoulders
- Blurred vision
- Appearance of spots in the visual fields
- Nasal congestion
- Feelings of apprehension or anxiety

Outcome Criteria

- BP returns to patient's baseline level.
- Heart rate and rhythm returns to patient's baseline level.
- Headache is absent.
- Sweating, flushing, and piloerection above level of injury are absent.
- Visual disturbances and nasal congestion are absent.
- Feelings of apprehension or anxiety are absent.

Nursing Interventions and Rationale

1. Place the patient on cardiac monitor, and assess for bradycardia or other dysrhythmias. *Disturbances of cardiac rate and rhythm can occur because of autonomic dysfunction associated with dysreflexia.*
2. Check the patient's BP every 3 to 5 min, *as BP may fluctuate very quickly.*
3. Sit the patient upright and lower his or her legs if possible *to decrease venous return and BP.*
4. Loosen any clothing or constrictive devices *to decrease venous return and BP.*
5. Investigate for and remove instigating cause of dysreflexia:

a. Bladder
   (1) If indwelling catheter not in place, catheterize the patient immediately.
      (a) Before inserting the catheter, instill 2% lidocaine jelly into the urethra and wait 2 min, if possible.
      (b) Drain 500 mL of urine, and recheck BP.
      (c) If BP is still elevated, drain another 500 mL of urine.
      (d) If BP declines after the bladder is empty, serial BP must be monitored closely because the bladder can go into severe contractions causing hypertension to recur.
   (2) If indwelling catheter is in place, check the catheter and tubing for kinks, folds, constrictions, or obstructions and for correct placement. If problem is found, correct it immediately.
   (3) If catheter is plugged, irrigate it gently with no more than 10 to 15 mL of sterile normal saline solution at body temperature.
   (4) If unable to irrigate catheter, remove it and prepare to reinsert a new catheter: Proceed with its lubrication, drainage, and observation as outlined above.
   (5) Avoid manually compressing or tapping on the bladder.
b. Bowel: If systolic BP is >150 mm Hg, proceed to no. 6 before checking for a fecal impaction.
   (1) With a gloved hand, instill a topical anesthetic agent (2% lidocaine jelly) generously into the rectum *to decrease flow of impulses from bowel.*
   (2) Wait 2 min if possible *for sensation in area to decrease.*
   (3) With a gloved hand, insert a lubricated finger into the rectum and check for the presence of stool.
   (4) If stool is felt, gently remove, if possible.
c. Skin
   (1) Loosen clothing or bed linens as indicated.
   (2) Inspect skin for pimples, boils, pressure ulcers, and ingrown toenails, and treat as indicated.
6. If symptoms of dysreflexia do not subside, collaborate with the practitioner regarding the administration of antihypertensive medications (eg, nifedipine [immediate-release form], nitrates [sodium nitroprusside, isosorbide dinitrate, or nitroglycerin ointment], hydralazine, mecamylamine, diazoxide, phenoxybenzamine, captopril, prazosin).
   a. Administer medications, and monitor their effectiveness.
   b. Assess BP and heart rate.
7. Instruct the patient about causes, symptoms, treatment, and prevention of dysreflexia.
8. Encourage the patient to carry a medical bracelet or informational card to present to medical personnel in the event dysreflexia may be developing.

⊚ NURSING MANAGEMENT PLAN

Compromised Family Coping

Definition: A usually supportive primary person (family member, significant other, or close friend) provides insufficient, ineffective, or compromised support, comfort, assistance, or encouragement that may be needed by the patient to manage or master adaptive tasks related to his or her health challenge.

Compromised Family Coping Related to Critically Ill Family Member

Defining Characteristics

- Disruption of usual family functions and roles
- Inability to accept or deal with crisis situation; use of defense mechanisms (eg, denial, anger); unrealistic expectations of patient's outcome and care provided; judgmental toward health care providers
- Nonrecognition that family is in state of crisis
- Inappropriate emotional outbursts; arguments among family and with others; inability to respond to each other's feelings or support each other
- Misinterpretation of information; short attention span with repeated questions about information already provided; members not sharing information with each other
- Inability to make decisions regarding changes in family structure or about course of care for ill member; noncooperation among family members
- Expressions of grief, hopelessness, powerlessness, and isolation; do not seek or respond to support services
- Hesitancy to spend time with ill person in the critical care unit or inappropriate behavior when visiting (may upset patient)
- Neglect of own personal health; fatigue, apathy; refusal of offers for respite time

Outcome Criteria

- The family will express an understanding of course and prognosis of illness, therapies, and alternative measures.
- The family will diminish or resolve conflicts and cooperate in decision making.
- The family will develop trust and mutual support for each member and form a cohesive unit.
- The family will support ill person in making decisions (if capable) or respect prior wishes regarding provision of health care.
- Family efforts will be directed toward a purpose and readjust to changes in life patterns and role function. Members will accept responsibility for changes.
- The family will identify and use effective coping strategies.
- The family will identify and use available resources as needed to facilitate resolution of the crisis.
- The family will have a sense of control and confidence in meeting personal and collective needs.

Nursing Interventions and Rationale

1. Identify family's perception of the crisis situation. *All initial nursing interventions should be directed toward resolving the crisis situation. Understanding and using family theory principles will facilitate this process and individualize care.*
   a. Determine family structure; developmental phase of roles; and ethnic, cultural, and belief factors that may affect communication with family and the plan of care.
   b. Identify strengths of the family.

2. Provide honest and accurate information in language persons can understand. Give updated information as appropriate. Listen. *This facilitates open communication among family and health care providers, projects a caring attitude and concern for them and the patient, and assists the family in making decisions and being involved with the plan and goals of care.*

3. Encourage liberal visitation with the patient.
   a. Before the visit, prepare family members for what they will observe in a technical environment. *This prevents a strong emotional reaction to an unfamiliar and frightening situation.*
      (1) Inform them about the patient's appearance and behaviors that may be distressing to them.
      (2) Explain the cause of the patient's responses to stimuli (eg, pain, trauma, surgery, medication), and explain that these behaviors are being monitored and are usually temporary.
   b. Encourage them to touch the patient and let the patient know of their presence.

4. Identify and support effective coping behaviors. *This aids in the family's sense of control and resolution of helplessness/powerlessness.*

5. Observe for signs of fatigue and the need for emotional/spiritual support and respite from hospital waiting routine. *This provides support and comfort, facilitates hope, resolves sense of isolation, gives sense of security, and diminishes guilt feeling for attending to personal needs.*
   a. Encourage family to verbalize feelings.
   b. Provide information on available resources.
   c. Alert interdisciplinary team members (social, psychologic, spiritual) to family needs.
   d. Provide pager device (if available) or obtain phone numbers when family leaves the hospital premises.

6. Instruct family in simple caregiving techniques, and encourage participation in the patient's care. *This facilitates giving a sense of normalcy to the experience, self-confidence, and assurance that good care is being provided.*

7. Serve as advocate for the patient and family. Teach family how to negotiate with the health care delivery system, and include them in health care team conferences when appropriate. *This facilitates informed decision making, promotes control and satisfaction, and permits mutual goal setting.*

8. Consider nonbiologic or nonlegal family relationships. Encourage contact with the patient and participation in care. *This facilitates holistic care and support of emotional ties and demonstrates respect for the family unit and relationships.*

9. Provide emotional support and compassion when the patient's condition worsens or deteriorates. *The use of touch and expression of concern for the patient and family convey comfort and trust in the health care provider and respect and assurance that the family's loved one will receive appropriate care and attention.*

◎ NURSING MANAGEMENT PLAN

Decreased Cardiac Output

Definition: Inadequate blood pumped by the heart to meet the metabolic demands of the body.

Decreased Cardiac Output Related to Alterations in Preload
Defining Characteristics
- Cardiac output is <4.0 L/min
- Cardiac index is <2.5 L/min/m^2
- Heart rate is >100 beats/min
- Urine output is <30 mL/h or 0.5 mL/kg/h
- Decreased mentation, restlessness, agitation, confusion
- Diminished peripheral pulses
- Blue, gray, or dark purple tint to tongue and sublingual area
- Systolic blood pressure is <90 mm Hg
- Subjective complaints of fatigue

Reduced Preload
- Right atrial pressure is <2 mm Hg
- Pulmonary artery occlusion pressure is <6 mm Hg

Excessive Preload
- Right atrial pressure is >8 mm Hg
- Pulmonary artery occlusion pressure is >12 mm Hg

Outcome Criteria
- Cardiac output is 4–8 L/min.
- Cardiac index is 2.5–4 L/min/m^2.
- Right atrial pressure is 2–8 mm Hg.
- Pulmonary artery occlusion pressure is 6–12 mm Hg.

Nursing Interventions and Rationale
1. Collaborate with the practitioner regarding administration of oxygen to maintain oxygen saturation measured by pulse oximetry (Spo$_2$) >92% *to prevent tissue hypoxia.*
2. Maintain surveillance for signs of decreased tissue perfusion and acidosis *to facilitate early identification and treatment of complications.*
3. Monitor fluid balance and daily weights *to facilitate regulation of the patient's fluid balance.*

For Reduced Preload Resulting From Volume Loss
1. Collaborate with the practitioner regarding administration of crystalloids, colloids, blood, and blood products *to increase circulating volume.*
2. Limit blood sampling, observe intravenous lines for accidental disconnection, apply direct pressure to bleeding sites, and maintain normal body temperature *to minimize fluid loss.*
3. Position the patient with legs elevated, trunk flat, and head and shoulders above the chest *to enhance venous return.*
4. Encourage oral fluids (as appropriate), administer free water with tube feedings, and replace fluids that are lost through wound or tube drainage *to promote adequate fluid intake.*
5. Maintain surveillance for signs of fluid volume excess and adverse effects of blood and blood product administration *to facilitate early identification and treatment of complications.*

For Reduced Preload Resulting From Venous Dilation
1. Collaborate with the practitioner regarding administration of vasoconstrictors *to increase venous return.*
2. Maintain surveillance for adverse effects of vasoconstrictor therapy *to facilitate early identification and treatment of complications.*

3. If the patient is hyperthermic, administer tepid bath, hypothermia blanket, or ice bags to axilla and groin *to decrease temperature and promote vasoconstriction.*

For Excessive Preload Resulting From Volume Overload
1. Collaborate with the practitioner regarding administration of the following:
   a. Diuretics to remove excessive fluid
   b. Vasodilators to decrease venous return
   c. Inotropes to increase myocardial contractility
2. Restrict fluid intake and double-concentrate intravenous drips *to minimize fluid intake.*
3. Position the patient in semi-Fowler or high-Fowler position *to reduce venous return.*
4. Maintain surveillance for signs of fluid volume deficit and adverse effects of diuretic, vasodilator, and inotropic therapies *to facilitate early identification and treatment of complications.*

For Excessive Preload Resulting From Venous Constriction
1. Collaborate with the practitioner regarding administration of vasodilators *to promote venous dilation.*
2. Maintain surveillance for adverse effects of vasodilator therapy *to facilitate early identification and treatment of complications.*
3. If the patient is hypothermic, wrap him or her in warm blankets or administer hyperthermia blanket *to increase temperature and promote vasodilation.*

Decreased Cardiac Output Related to Alterations in Afterload
Defining Characteristics
- Cardiac output is <4 L/min
- Cardiac index is <2.5 L/min/m^2
- Heart rate is >100 beats/min
- Urine output is <30 mL/h
- Decreased mentation, restlessness, agitation, confusion
- Diminished peripheral pulses
- Blue, gray, or dark purple tint to tongue and sublingual area
- Systolic blood pressure is <90 mm Hg
- Subjective complaints of fatigue

Reduced Afterload
- Pulmonary vascular resistance is <100 dyn • s • cm^{-5}
- Systemic vascular resistance is <800 dyn • s • cm^{-5}

Excessive Afterload
- Pulmonary vascular resistance is >250 dyn • s • cm^{-5}
- Systemic vascular resistance is >1200 dyn • s • cm^{-5}

Outcome Criteria
- Cardiac output is 4–8 L/min.
- Cardiac index is 2.5–4 L/min/m^2.
- Pulmonary vascular resistance is 80–250 dyn • s • cm^{-5}.
- Systemic vascular resistance is 800–1200 dyn • s • cm^{-5}.

Nursing Interventions and Rationale
1. Collaborate with the practitioner regarding administration of oxygen to maintain Spo$_2$ >92% *to prevent tissue hypoxia.*
2. Maintain surveillance for signs of decreased tissue perfusion and acidosis *to facilitate early identification and treatment of complications.*

Continued

◎ NURSING MANAGEMENT PLAN

Decreased Cardiac Output—cont'd

For Reduced Afterload

1. Collaborate with the practitioner regarding administration of vasoconstrictors *to promote arterial vasoconstriction and prevent relative hypovolemia.* If decreased preload is present, implement nursing management plan for Decreased Cardiac Output Related to Alterations in Preload.
2. Maintain surveillance for adverse effects of vasoconstrictor therapy *to facilitate early identification and treatment of complications.*
3. If the patient is hyperthermic, administer tepid bath, hypothermia blanket, or ice bags to axilla and groin *to decrease temperature and promote vasoconstriction.*

For Excessive Afterload

1. Collaborate with the practitioner regarding administration of vasodilators *to promote arterial vasodilation.*
2. Collaborate with the practitioner regarding initiation of intraaortic balloon pump *to facilitate afterload reduction.*
3. Promote rest and relaxation and decrease environmental stimulation *to minimize sympathetic stimulation.*
4. Maintain surveillance for adverse effects of vasodilator therapy *to facilitate early identification and treatment of complications.*
5. If the patient is hypothermic, wrap the patient in warm blankets or administer hyperthermia blanket *to increase temperature and promote vasodilation.*
6. If the patient is in pain, treat pain *to reduce sympathetic stimulation.* Implement nursing management plan for Acute Pain Related to Transmission and Perception of Cutaneous, Visceral, Muscular, or Ischemic Impulses.

Decreased Cardiac Output Related to Alterations in Contractility
Defining Characteristics

* Cardiac output is <4 L/min
* Cardiac index is <2.5 L/min/m^2
* Heart rate is >100 beats/min
* Urine output is <30 mL/h
* Decreased mentation, restlessness, agitation, confusion
* Diminished peripheral pulses
* Blue, gray, or dark purple tint to tongue and sublingual area
* Systolic blood pressure is <90 mm Hg
* Subjective complaints of fatigue
* Right ventricular stroke work index is <7 g/m^2/beat
* Left ventricular stroke work index is <35 g/m^2/beat

Outcome Criteria

* Cardiac output is 4–8 L/min.
* Cardiac index is 2.5–4 L/min/m^2.
* Right ventricular stroke work index is 7–12 g/m^2/beat.
* Left ventricular stroke work index is 35–85 g/m^2/beat.

Nursing Interventions and Rationale

1. Collaborate with the practitioner regarding administration of oxygen to maintain Spo$_2$ >92% *to prevent tissue hypoxia.*
2. Maintain surveillance for signs of decreased tissue perfusion and acidosis *to facilitate early identification and treatment of complications.*
3. Ensure preload is optimized. If preload is reduced or excessive, implement nursing management plan for Decreased Cardiac Output Related to Alterations in Preload.
4. Ensure afterload is optimized. If afterload is reduced or excessive, implement nursing management plan for Decreased Cardiac Output Related to Alterations in Afterload.

5. Ensure electrolytes are optimized. Collaborate with the practitioner regarding administration of electrolyte replacement therapy *to enhance cellular ionic environment.*
6. Collaborate with the practitioner regarding administration of inotropes *to enhance myocardial contractility.*
7. Monitor ST segment continuously *to determine changes in myocardial tissue perfusion.* If myocardial ischemia is present, implement nursing management plan for Ineffective Cardiopulmonary Tissue Perfusion.

Decreased Cardiac Output Related to Alterations in Heart Rate or Rhythm
Defining Characteristics

* Cardiac output is <4 L/min
* Cardiac index is <2.5 L/min/m^2
* Heart rate is >100 beats/min or <60 beats/min
* Urine output is <30 mL/h or 0.5 mL/kg/h
* Decreased mentation, restlessness, agitation, confusion
* Diminished peripheral pulses
* Blue, gray, or dark purple tint to tongue and sublingual area
* Systolic blood pressure is <90 mm Hg
* Subjective complaints of fatigue
* Dysrhythmias

Outcome Criteria

* Cardiac output is 4–8 L/min.
* Cardiac index is 2.5–4 L/min/m^2.
* Dysrhythmias are absent or return to baseline.
* Heart rate is >60 beats/min or <100 beats/min.

Nursing Interventions and Rationale

1. Collaborate with the practitioner regarding administration of oxygen to maintain Spo$_2$ >92% *to prevent tissue hypoxia.*
2. Ensure electrolytes are optimized. Collaborate with the practitioner regarding administration of electrolyte therapy *to enhance cellular ionic environment and avoid precipitation of dysrhythmias.*
3. Collaborate with the practitioner and pharmacist regarding the patient's current medications and their effect on heart rate and rhythm *to identify any prodysrhythmic or bradycardic side effects.*
4. Maintain surveillance for signs of decreased tissue perfusion and acidosis *to facilitate early identification and treatment of complications.*
5. Monitor ST segment continuously *to determine changes in myocardial tissue perfusion.* If myocardial ischemia is present, implement nursing management plan for Altered Cardiopulmonary Tissue Perfusion.

For Lethal Dysrhythmias or Asystole

1. Initiate advanced cardiac life support interventions, and notify the practitioner immediately.

For Nonlethal Dysrhythmias

1. Collaborate with the practitioner regarding administration of antidysrhythmic therapy, synchronized cardioversion, or overdrive pacing *to control dysrhythmias.*
2. Maintain surveillance for adverse effects of antidysrhythmic therapy *to facilitate early identification and treatment of complications.*

For Heart Rate <60 Beats/Min

1. Collaborate with the practitioner regarding initiation of temporary pacing *to increase heart rate.*

⊚ NURSING MANAGEMENT PLAN

Decreased Cardiac Output—cont'd

Decreased Cardiac Output Related to Sympathetic Blockade

Defining Characteristics

- Decreased cardiac output and cardiac index
- Systolic blood pressure is <90 mm Hg or below patient's baseline
- Decreased right atrial pressure and pulmonary artery occlusion pressure
- Decreased systemic vascular resistance
- Bradycardia
- Cardiac dysrhythmias
- Postural hypotension

Outcome Criteria

- Cardiac output and cardiac index are within normal limits.
- Systolic blood pressure is >90 mm Hg or returns to baseline.
- Right atrial pressure and pulmonary artery occlusion pressure are within normal limits.
- Systemic vascular resistance is within normal limits.
- Sinus rhythm is present.
- Dysrhythmias are absent.
- Fainting or dizziness with position change is absent.

Nursing Interventions and Rationale

1. Implement measures to prevent episodes of postural hypertension:
   a. Change the patient's position slowly *to allow the cardiovascular system time to compensate.*
   b. Apply pneumatic compression stockings *to promote venous return.*
   c. Perform range-of-motion exercises every 2 h *to prevent venous pooling.*
   d. Collaborate with the practitioner and physical therapist regarding the use of a tilt table *to progress the patient from supine to upright position.*
2. Collaborate with the practitioner regarding administration of the following:
   a. Crystalloids and/or colloids to increase the patient's circulating volume, *which increases stroke volume and subsequently cardiac output.*
   b. Vasopressors if fluids are ineffective to constrict the patient's vascular system, *which increases resistance and subsequently blood pressure.*
3. Monitor cardiac rhythm for bradycardia and/or dysrhythmias, *which can further decrease cardiac output.*
4. Avoid any activity that can stimulate the vagal response *because bradycardia can result.*
5. Treat symptomatic bradycardia and symptomatic dysrhythmias according to unit's emergency protocol or advanced cardiac life support guidelines.

NURSING MANAGEMENT PLAN

Decreased Intracranial Adaptive Capacity

Definition: Intracranial fluid dynamic mechanisms that normally compensate for increases in intracranial volumes are compromised, resulting in repeated disproportionate increases in intracranial pressure (ICP) in response to various noxious and nonnoxious stimuli.

Decreased Intracranial Adaptive Capacity Related to Failure of Normal Intracranial Compensatory Mechanisms

Defining Characteristics

- ICP is >15 mm Hg, sustained for 15 to 30 min
- Headache
- Vomiting, with or without nausea
- Seizures
- Decrease in Glasgow Coma Scale score of 2 or more points from baseline
- Alteration in level of consciousness, ranging from restlessness to coma
- Change in orientation: disoriented to time, place, or person or all three
- Difficulty or inability to follow simple commands
- Increasing systolic blood pressure of more than 20 mm Hg with widening pulse pressure
- Bradycardia
- Irregular respiratory pattern (eg, Cheyne-Stokes, central neurogenic hyperventilation, ataxic, apneustic)
- Change in response to painful stimuli (eg, purposeful to inappropriate or absent response)
- Signs of impending brain herniation:
  - Hemiparesis or hemiplegia
  - Hemisensory changes
  - Unequal pupil size (1 mm or more difference)
  - Failure of pupil to react to light
  - Disconjugate gaze and inability to move one eye beyond midline if third, fourth, or sixth cranial nerves involved
  - Loss of oculocephalic or oculovestibular reflexes
  - Possible decorticate or decerebrate posturing

Outcome Criteria

- ICP is <15 mm Hg.
- Cerebral perfusion pressure is >60 mm Hg.
- Clinical signs of increased ICP are absent.

Nursing Interventions and Rationale

1. Maintain adequate cerebral perfusion pressure.
   a. Collaborate with the practitioner regarding administration of volume expanders, vasopressors, or antihypertensives *to maintain the patient's blood pressure within normal range.*
   b. Implement measures to reduce ICP.
   (1) Elevate head of bed 30 to 45 degrees *to facilitate venous return.*
   (2) Maintain head and neck in neutral (avoid flexion, extension, or lateral rotation) *to enhance venous drainage from the head.*
   (3) Avoid extreme hip flexion.
   (4) Collaborate with the practitioner regarding administration of steroids, osmotic agents, and diuretics and need for drainage of cerebrospinal fluid if a ventriculostomy is in place.
   (5) Assist the patient to turn and move self in bed (instruct the patient to exhale while turning or pushing up in bed) *to avoid isometric contractions and Valsalva maneuver.*
2. Maintain patent airway and adequate ventilation, and supply oxygen *to prevent hypoxemia and hypercarbia.*
3. Monitor arterial blood gas values and maintain arterial partial pressure of oxygen (PaO$_2$) >80 mm Hg, arterial partial pressure of carbon dioxide (PaCO$_2$) >35 mm Hg, and pH at 7.35–7.45 *to prevent cerebral vasodilation.*
4. Avoid suctioning beyond 10 s at a time; hyperoxygenate and hyperventilate before and after suctioning *to avoid hypoxemia.*
5. Plan patient care activities and nursing interventions around the patient's ICP response. Avoid unnecessary additional disturbances, and allow the patient up to 1 h of rest between activities as frequently as possible. *Studies have shown the direct correlation between nursing care activities and increases in ICP.*
6. Maintain normothermia with external cooling or heating measures as necessary. Wrap hands, feet, and male genitalia in soft towels before cooling measures *to prevent shivering and frostbite.*
7. Collaborate with the practitioner to control seizures with prophylactic and as-needed (PRN) anticonvulsants. *Seizures can greatly increase the cerebral metabolic rate.*
8. Collaborate with the practitioner regarding administration of sedatives, barbiturates, or paralyzing agents *to reduce cerebral metabolic rate.*
9. Counsel family members to maintain calm atmosphere and avoid disturbing topics of conversation (eg, patient condition, pain, prognosis, family crisis, financial difficulties).
10. If signs of impending brain herniation are present, implement the following:
    a. Notify the practitioner at once.
    b. Ensure that head of bed is elevated 45 degrees and that the patient's head is in neutral plane.
    c. Administer mainline intravenous infusion slowly to keep-open rate.
    d. Drain cerebrospinal fluid as ordered if a ventriculostomy is in place.
    e. Prepare to administer osmotic agents and/or diuretics.
    f. Prepare the patient for emergency computed tomography head scan and/or emergency surgery.

◎ NURSING MANAGEMENT PLAN

Deficient Fluid Volume

Definition: Decreased intravascular, interstitial, or intracellular fluid. This refers to dehydration, water loss alone without a change in sodium concentration.

Deficient Fluid Volume Related to Absolute Loss
Defining Characteristics
- Cardiac output is <4 L/min
- Cardiac index is <2.2 L/min
- Pulmonary artery occlusion pressure is <6 mm Hg
- Right atrial pressure is <2 mm Hg
- Tachycardia
- Narrowed pulse pressure
- Systolic blood pressure is <100 mm Hg
- Urinary output is <30 mL/h
- Pale, cool, moist skin
- Apprehensiveness

Outcome Criteria
- Cardiac output is >4 L/min, and cardiac index is >2.2 L/min.
- Pulmonary artery occlusion pressure is >6 mm Hg or returns to baseline level.
- Right atrial pressure is >2 mm Hg or returns to baseline level.
- Heart rate is normal or returns to baseline level.
- Systolic blood pressure is >90 mm Hg.
- Urinary output is >30 mL/h.

Nursing Interventions and Rationale
1. Secure airway and administer oxygen to maintain oxygen saturation >92%.
2. Place the patient in supine position with legs elevated *to increase pre-load.* For the patient with head injury, consider using low-Fowler position with legs elevated.
3. For fluid repletion, use the 3:1 rule, replacing 3 parts of fluid for every unit of blood lost.
4. Administer crystalloid solutions using the fluid challenge technique: Infuse precise boluses of fluid (usually 5–20 mL/min) over 10-min periods; monitor hemodynamic pressures serially *to determine successful challenging.* If the pulmonary artery occlusion pressure elevates >7 mm Hg above beginning level, the infusion should be stopped. If the pulmonary artery occlusion pressure rises only to 3 mm Hg above baseline or falls, another fluid challenge should be administered.
5. Replete fluids first before considering use of vasopressors *because vaso-pressors increase myocardial oxygen consumption out of proportion to the reestablishment of coronary perfusion in the early phases of treatment.*
6. When blood replacement is indicated, replace it with fresh packed red blood cells and fresh frozen plasma *to keep clotting factors intact.*
7. Move or reposition the patient minimally *to decrease or limit tissue oxygen demands.*
8. Evaluate the patient's anxiety level, and intervene through patient education or sedation *to decrease tissue oxygen demands.*
9. Maintain surveillance for signs and symptoms of fluid overload.

Deficient Fluid Volume Related to Decreased Secretion of Antidiuretic Hormone (ADH)
Defining Characteristics
- Confusion and lethargy
- Decreased skin turgor
- Thirst
- Weight loss over short period
- Decreased pulmonary artery occlusion pressure
- Decreased right atrial pressure
- Urinary output is >6 L/day
- Serum sodium is >148 mEq/L
- Serum osmolality is >295 mOsm/kg

- Urine osmolality is <100 mOsm/kg
- Urine specific gravity is <1.005

Outcome Criteria
- Weight returns to baseline.
- Urinary output is >30 mL/h and <200 mL/h.
- Serum osmolality is 280–295 mOsm/kg.
- Urine specific gravity is 1.010–1.030.

Nursing Interventions and Rationale
1. Record intake and output every hour, noting color and clarity of urine *because color and clarity are an indication of urine concentration.*
2. Monitor cardiac rhythm continuously for dysrhythmias *caused by electrolyte imbalance.*
3. Collaborate with the practitioner regarding administration of vasopressin or desmopressin *to replace ADH.*
   a. Monitor the patient for adverse effects of medications (eg, headache, chest pain, abdominal pain) *caused by vasoconstriction.*
   b. Report adverse effects to the practitioner immediately.
4. Collaborate with the practitioner regarding intravenous fluid and electrolyte replacement therapy *to restore fluid balance, correct dehydration, and maintain electrolyte balance.*
   a. Administer hypotonic saline *to replace free water deficit.*
5. Provide oral fluids low in sodium such as water, coffee, tea, or orange juice *to decrease sodium intake.*
6. Weigh the patient daily at same time, in same amount of clothing, and preferably with same scale *to ensure accuracy of readings.*
7. Reposition the patient every 2 h *to prevent skin integrity issues caused by dehydration.*
8. Provide mouth care every 4 h *to prevent breakdown of oral mucous membranes.*
9. Collaborate with the practitioner regarding administration of medications to prevent constipation *caused by dehydration.*
10. Maintain surveillance for symptoms of hypernatremia (muscle twitching, irritability, seizures), hypovolemic shock (hypotension, tachycardia, decreased central venous pressure and pulmonary artery occlusion pressure), and deep vein thrombosis (calf pain, tenderness, swelling).

Deficient Fluid Volume Related to Relative Loss
Defining Characteristics
- Pulmonary artery occlusion pressure is <6 mm Hg
- Right atrial pressure is <2 mm Hg
- Tachycardia
- Narrowed pulse pressure
- Systolic blood pressure is <100 mm Hg
- Urinary output is <30 mL/h
- Increased hematocrit level

Outcome Criteria
- Pulmonary artery occlusion pressure is >6 mm Hg or returns to baseline level.
- Right atrial pressure is >2 mm Hg or returns to baseline level.
- Systolic blood pressure is >90 mm Hg.
- Urinary output is >30 mL/h.
- Hematocrit level is normal.

Nursing Interventions and Rationale
1. Collaborate with the practitioner regarding administration of intravenous fluid replacements (usually normal saline solution or lactated Ringer solution) at a rate sufficient to maintain urinary output >30 mL/h. Colloid solutions are avoided in the initial phases (but can be used later) because of the possibility of increased edema formation *as a result of increased capillary permeability.*

NURSING MANAGEMENT PLAN

Deficient Knowledge

Definition: Absence or deficiency of cognitive information related to a specific topic.

Deficient Knowledge Related to Cognitive or Perceptual Learning Limitations

Defining Characteristics

- Verbalized statement of inadequate knowledge of skills
- Verbalization of inadequate recall of information
- Verbalization of inadequate understanding of information
- Evidence of inaccurate follow-through of instructions
- Inadequate demonstration of a skill
- Lack of compliance with prescribed behavior

Outcome Criteria

- Patient participates actively in necessary and prescribed health behaviors.
- Patient verbalizes adequate knowledge or demonstrates adequate skills.

Nursing Interventions and Rationale

1. Determine specific cause of the patient's cognitive or perceptual limitation.
2. Provide uninterrupted rest period before teaching session to decrease fatigue and encourage optimal state for learning and retention.
3. Manipulate environment as much as possible to provide quiet and uninterrupted learning sessions.
   a. Ensure that lights are bright enough to see teaching aids but not too bright.
   b. Schedule care and medications to allow uninterrupted teaching periods.
   c. Move the patient to a quiet, private room for teaching if possible.
4. Adapt teaching sessions and materials to level of education and ability to understand of the patient and family.
   a. Provide printed material appropriate to reading level.
   b. Use terminology understood by the patient.
   c. Provide printed materials in the patient's primary language if possible.
   d. Use interpreters during teaching sessions *when necessary.*
5. Teach only present-tense focus during periods of sensory overload.
6. Determine potential effects of medications on ability to retain or recall information. Avoid teaching critical content while the patient is taking sedatives, analgesics, or other medications that affect memory.
7. Reinforce new skills and information in several teaching sessions. Use several senses when possible in teaching session (eg, see a film, hear a discussion, read printed information, demonstrate skills related to self-injection of insulin).
8. Reduce the patient's anxiety.
   a. Listen attentively, and encourage verbalization of feelings.
   b. Answer questions as they arise in a clear and succinct manner.
   c. Elicit the patient's concerns, and address those issues first.
   d. Give only correct and relevant information.
   e. Continually assess response to teaching session, and discontinue if anxiety increases or physical condition becomes unstable.
   f. Provide nonthreatening information before more anxiety-producing information is presented.
   g. Plan for several teaching sessions so that information can be divided into small, manageable packages.

Deficient Knowledge Related to Lack of Previous Exposure to Information

Defining Characteristics

- Verbalized statement of inadequate knowledge or skills
- New diagnosis or health problem requiring self-management or care

- Lack of prior formal or informal education about the specific health problem
- Demonstration of inappropriate behaviors related to management of health problem

Outcome Criteria

- Patient verbalizes adequate knowledge about or performs skills related to disease process, its causes, factors related to onset of symptoms, and self-management of disease or health problem.
- Patient actively participates in health behaviors required for performance of a procedure or in behaviors enhancing recovery from illness and preventing recurrence or complications.

Nursing Interventions and Rationale

1. Determine existing level of knowledge or skill.
2. Assess factors that affect the knowledge deficit:
   a. Learning needs, including patient's priorities and the necessary knowledge and skills for safety
   b. Learning ability of the patient, including language skills, level of education, ability to read, and preferred learning style
   c. Physical ability to perform prescribed skills or procedures; consider effect of limitations imposed by treatment such as bed rest, restriction of movement by intravenous or other equipment, or effect of sedatives or analgesics
   d. Psychologic effect of stage of adaptation to disease
   e. Activity tolerance and ability to concentrate
   f. Motivation to learn new skills or gain new knowledge
3. Reduce or limit barriers to learning:
   a. Provide consistent nurse-patient contact to encourage development of trusting and therapeutic relationship.
   b. Structure environment to enhance learning and control unnecessary noise or interruptions.
   c. Individualize teaching plan to fit the patient's current physical and psychologic status.
   d. Delay teaching until the patient is ready to learn.
   e. Conduct teaching sessions during time of day when the patient is most alert and receptive.
   f. Meet the patient's immediate learning needs as they arise (eg, give brief explanation of procedures when they are performed).
4. Promote active participation in the teaching plan by the patient and family:
   a. Solicit input during development of plan.
   b. Develop mutually acceptable goals and outcomes.
   c. Solicit expression of feelings and emotions related to new responsibilities.
   d. Encourage questions.
5. Conduct teaching sessions, using the most appropriate teaching methods.
6. Use the "teach-back" method *to confirm that you have explained to the patient what they need to know in a manner that the patient understands.*
   a. Use simple lay language, explain the concept, or demonstrate the process to the patient/caregiver.
      (1) Avoid technical terms to avoid misunderstandings.
      (2) If the patient/caregiver has limited English proficiency, use a professional translator to reduce miscommunication.
   b. Ask the patient/caregiver to repeat in his or her own words how he or she understands the concept explained. If a process was demonstrated to the patient, ask the patient/caregiver to demonstrate it independent of assistance.
   c. Identify and correct misunderstandings of or incorrect procedures by the patient/caregiver.

NURSING MANAGEMENT PLAN

Deficient Knowledge—cont'd

d. Ask the patient/caregiver to demonstrate his or her understanding or procedural ability again *to ensure the above-noted misunderstandings are now corrected.*

e. Repeat steps until convinced the patient/caregiver comprehends the concept or possesses the ability to perform the procedure accurately and safely.

7. Provide written materials that enhance health literacy:

a. Limit content to one or two key objectives. Do not provide too much information or try to cover everything at once.

b. Limit content to what patients really need to know. Avoid information overload.

c. Use only words that are well known to individuals without medical training.

d. Ensure that content is appropriate for age and culture of the target audience.

e. Write at or below the sixth-grade level.

f. Use words of one or two syllables.

g. Use short paragraphs.

h. Use active voice.

i. Avoid all but the simplest tables and graphs. Clear explanations (legends) should be placed adjacent to the table or graph as well as in the text.

j. Use large font (minimum 12 point) with serifs. (Serif text has the little horizontal lines that you see at the bottoms of letters such as "f," "x," "n," and others.)

k. Do not use more than two or three font styles on a page. *Consistency in appearance is important.*

l. Use uppercase and lowercase text. ALL UPPERCASE TEXT IS HARD TO READ.

m. Ensure a good amount of empty space on the page. Do not clutter the page with text or pictures.

n. Use headings and subheadings to separate blocks of text.

o. Bulleted lists are preferable to blocks of text in paragraphs.

p. Illustrations are useful if they depict common, easy-to-recognize objects. Images of people, places, and things should be age and culturally appropriate to the target audience. Avoid complex anatomic diagrams.

8. Initiate referrals for follow-up if necessary:

a. Health educators

b. Home health care

c. Rehabilitation programs

d. Social services

9. Evaluate effectiveness of teaching plan, based on the patient's ability to meet preset goals and objectives *to determine need for further teaching.*

NURSING MANAGEMENT PLAN

Disturbed Body Image

Definition: Confusion in mental picture of one's physical self.

Disturbed Body Image Related to Actual Change in Body Structure, Function, or Appearance

Defining Characteristics

- Actual change in appearance, structure, or function
- Avoidance of looking at body part
- Avoidance of touching body part
- Hiding or overexposing body part (intentional or unintentional)
- Trauma to nonfunctioning part
- Change in ability to estimate spatial relationship of body to environment
- Verbalization of the following:
  - Fear of rejection or reaction by others
  - Negative feeling about body
  - Preoccupation with change or loss
  - Refusal to participate in or to accept responsibility for self-care of altered body part
- Personalization of part or loss with a name
- Depersonalization of part or loss by use of impersonal pronouns
- Refusal to verify actual change

Outcome Criteria

- Patient verbalizes the specific meaning of the change to him or her.
- Patient requests appropriate information about self-care.
- Patient completes personal hygiene and grooming daily with or without help.
- Patient interacts freely with family or other visitors.
- Patient participates in the discussions and conferences related to planning his or her medical and nursing management in the critical care unit and transfer from the unit.
- Patient talks with trained visitors (support group representatives) at least twice about his or her loss.

Nursing Interventions and Rationale

1. Evaluate the patient's mental, physical, and emotional state; recognize assets, strengths, response to illness, coping mechanisms, past experience with stress, and support system.
2. Appraise the response of the family and significant others. *Body image is derived from the "reflected appraisals" of family and significant others.*
3. Determine the patient's goals and readiness for learning.
4. Provide the necessary information to help the patient and family adapt to the change. Clarify misconceptions about future limitations.
5. Permit and encourage the patient to express the significance of the loss or change; note nonverbal behavior responses.
6. Allow and encourage the patient's expression of anxiety. *Anxiety is the most predominant emotional response to a body image disturbance.*
7. Recognize and accept the use of denial as an adaptive defense mechanism when used early and temporarily.
8. Recognize maladaptive denial as that which interferes with the patient's progress and/or alienates support systems. Use confrontation.
9. Provide an opportunity for the patient to discuss sexual concerns.
10. Touch the affected body part *to provide the patient with sensory information about altered body structure and/or function.*
11. Encourage and provide movement of altered body part *to establish kinesthetic feedback. This enables the patient to know his or her body as it now exists.*
12. Prepare the patient to look at the body part. Call the body part by its anatomic name (eg, stump, stoma, limb) as opposed to "it." *The use of impersonal pronouns increases a sense of fantasy and depersonalization of the body part.*

13. Allow the patient to experience excellence in some aspect of physical functioning—walking, turning, deep breathing, healing, self-care—and point out progress and accomplishment. *This helps to balance the patient's sense of dysfunction with function.*
14. Avoid false reassurance. Acknowledge the difficulty of incorporating the altered body part or function into one's body image. *This evidences the nurse's sensitivity and promotes trust.*
15. Talk with the patient about his or her life, generativity, and accomplishments. *Patients with disturbances in body image frequently see themselves in a distortedly "narrow" sense. Encouraging a wider focus of themselves and their life reduces this distortion.*
16. Help the patient explore realistic alternatives.
17. Recognize that incorporating a body change into one's body image takes time. Avoid setting unrealistic expectations and *inadvertently reinforcing a low self-esteem.*
18. Suggest the use of additional resources such as trained visitors who have mastered situations similar to those of the patient.
    a. Refer the patient to a psychiatric nurse, psychologist, or psychiatrist if needed.

Disturbed Body Image Related to Functional Dependence on Life-Sustaining Technology

Defining Characteristics

- Actual change in function requiring permanent or temporary replacement
- Refusal to verify actual loss
- Verbalization of the following: feelings of helplessness, hopelessness, powerlessness, fear of failure to wean from technology

Outcome Criteria

- Patient verifies actual change in function.
- Patient does not refuse or fight technologic intervention.
- Patient verbalizes acceptance of expected change in lifestyle.

Nursing Interventions and Rationale

1. Evaluate the patient's response to the technologic intervention.
2. Assess responses of the family and significant others. *Body image is derived from the "reflected appraisals" of family and significant others.*
3. Provide information needed by the patient and family.
4. Promote trust, security, comfort, and privacy.
5. Recognize anxiety. Allow and encourage its expression. *Anxiety is the most predominant emotion accompanying body image alterations.* Implement nursing management plan for Anxiety Related to Threat to Biologic, Psychologic, or Social Integrity.
6. Assist the patient to recognize his or her own functioning and performance in the face of technology. For example, assist the patient to distinguish spontaneous breaths from mechanically delivered breaths. *The activity will assist in weaning the patient from the ventilator when feasible. To establish realistic, accurate body boundaries, a patient needs help to separate himself or herself from the technology that is supporting his or her functioning. Any participation or function on the part of the patient during periods of dependency is helpful in preventing and/or resolving an alteration in body image.*
7. Plan for discontinuation of the treatment (eg, weaning from ventilator). Explain the procedure that will be followed and be present during its initiation.
8. Plan for transfer from the critical care environment.
9. Document care, ensuring an up-to-date management plan is available to all involved caregivers.

NURSING MANAGEMENT PLAN

Disturbed Sleep Pattern

Definition: Time-limited interruptions of sleep amount and quality as a result of external factors.

Disturbed Sleep Pattern Related to Fragmented Sleep
Defining Characteristics
- Decreased sleep during one block of sleep time
- Daytime sleepiness
- Decreased sleep
- Less than one-half of normal total sleep time
- Decreased slow-wave or rapid-eye-movement (REM) sleep
- Anxiety
- Fatigue
- Restlessness
- Disorientation and hallucinations
- Combativeness
- Frequent awakenings

Outcome Criteria
- Patient's total sleep time approximates patient's normal sleep time.
- Patient can complete sleep cycles of 90 min without interruption.
- Patient has no delusions or hallucinations.
- Patient has reality-based thought content.

Nursing Interventions and Rationale
1. Assess normal sleep pattern on admission and any history of sleep disturbance or chronic illness that may affect sleep or sedative/hypnotic use.
   a. Promote normal sleep activity while the patient is in the critical care unit.
   b. Assess sleep effectiveness by asking the patient how his or her sleep in the hospital compares with sleep at home.
2. Promote comfort, relaxation, and a sense of well-being.
   a. Treat pain; change, smooth, or refresh bed linens at bedtime; and provide oral hygiene.
   b. Eliminate stressful situations before bedtime.
   c. Use relaxation techniques, imagery, music, massage, or warm blankets.
   d. Have a close family member sit beside the bed and provide the patient with his or her own garments or coverings.
   e. Provide quiet or background noise of the television or music (patient preference) *to best promote sleep.*
   f. Provide a comfortable room temperature.
3. Minimize noise, particularly noise generated by the staff and equipment.
   a. Reduce the level of environmental stimuli.
   b. Dim the lights at night.
4. Foods containing tryptophan (eg, milk, turkey) may be appropriate *because these promote sleep.*
5. Plan nap times to assist in approximating the patient's normal 24-h sleep time.
6. Minimize awakenings *to allow for at least 90-min sleep cycles.*
   a. Continually assess the need to awaken the patient, particularly at night. Distinguish between essential and nonessential nursing tasks.
   b. Organize nursing management to allow for maximal amount of uninterrupted sleep, while ensuring close monitoring of the patient's condition. Whenever possible, monitor physiologic parameters without waking the patient.
   c. Coordinate awakenings with other departments, such as laboratory and radiography, *to minimize sleep interruptions.*
7. Be aware of the effects of commonly used medications on sleep. *Many sedative/hypnotic medications decrease REM sleep.*
   a. Use sedative and analgesic medications that minimally disrupt sleep to complement comfort measures, with dosages reduced gradually as the medication is no longer necessary.
   b. Do not abruptly withdraw REM-suppressing medications *because this can result in REM rebound.*
8. Document amount of uninterrupted sleep per shift, especially sleep episodes lasting longer than 2 h. *Sleep pattern disturbance is diagnosed, treated, and resolved more efficiently when formally documented in this manner.*

◎ NURSING MANAGEMENT PLAN

Dysfunctional Ventilatory Weaning Response

Definition: Inability to adjust to lowered levels of mechanical ventilator support that interrupts and prolongs the weaning process.

Dysfunctional Ventilatory Weaning Response (DVWR) Related to Physical, Psychosocial, or Situational Factors

Defining Characteristics

Mild DVWR

- Responds to lowered levels of mechanical ventilator support with:
  - Restlessness
  - Slightly increased respiratory rate from baseline
  - Expressed feelings of increased need for oxygen, breathing discomfort, fatigue, warmth
  - Queries about possible machine malfunction
  - Increased concentration on breathing

Moderate DVWR

- Responds to lowered levels of mechanical ventilator support with:
  - Slight baseline increase in blood pressure <20 mm Hg
  - Slight baseline increase in heart rate <20 beats/min
  - Baseline increase in respiratory rate <5 breaths/min
  - Hypervigilance to activities
  - Inability to respond to coaching
  - Inability to cooperate
  - Apprehension
  - Diaphoresis
  - Eye widening ("wide-eyed look")
  - Decreased air entry on auscultation
  - Color changes: pale, slight cyanosis
  - Slight respiratory accessory muscle use

Severe DVWR

- Responds to lowered levels of mechanical ventilator support with:
  - Agitation
  - Deterioration in arterial blood gases from current baseline
  - Baseline increase in blood pressure >20 mm Hg
  - Baseline increase in heart rate >20 beats/min
  - Respiratory rate increases significantly from baseline
  - Profuse diaphoresis
  - Full respiratory accessory muscle use
  - Shallow, gasping breaths
  - Paradoxic abdominal breathing
  - Discoordinated breathing with the ventilator
  - Decreased level of consciousness
  - Adventitious breath sounds, audible airway secretions
  - Cyanosis

Outcome Criteria

- Airway is clear.
- Underlying disorder is resolving.
- Patient is rested, and pain is controlled.
- Nutrition status is adequate.
- Patient has feelings of perceived control, situational security, and trust in the nurses.
- Patient is able to adapt to selected levels of ventilator support without undue fatigue.

Nursing Interventions and Rationale

1. Communicate interest and concern for the patient's well-being, and demonstrate confidence in ability to manage weaning process *to instill trust in the patient.*
2. Use normalizing strategies (eg, grooming, dressing, mobilizing, social conversation) *to reinforce the patient's self-esteem and feeling of identity.*
3. Identify parameters of the patient's usual functioning before the weaning process begins *to facilitate early identification of problems.*
4. Identify the patient's strengths and resources that can be mobilized *to enhance the patient's coping and maximize weaning effort.*
5. Note concerns that adversely affect the patient's comfort and confidence, and manage them discreetly *to facilitate the patient's ease.*
6. Praise successful activities, encourage a positive outlook, and review the patient's positive progress *to increase the patient's perceived self-efficacy.*
7. Inform the patient of his or her situation and weaning progress *to permit the patient as much control as possible.*
8. Teach the patient about the weaning process and how he or she can participate in the process.
9. Negotiate daily weaning goals with the patient *to gain cooperation.*
10. Position the patient with the head of the bed elevated *to optimize respiratory efforts.*
11. Coach the patient in breath control by regular demonstrations of slow, deep, rhythmic patterns of breathing *to assist with dyspnea.*
12. Remain visible in the room and reassure the patient that help is immediately available if needed *to reduce the patient's anxiety and fearfulness.*
13. Encourage the patient to view weaning trials as a form of training, regardless of whether the weaning goal is achieved, *to avoid discouragement.*
14. Encourage the patient to maintain emotional calmness by reassuring, being present, comforting, talking down if emotionally aroused, and reinforcing the idea that he or she can and will succeed.
15. Monitor the patient's status frequently *to avoid undue fatigue and anxiety.*
16. Provide regular periods of rest by reducing activities, maintaining or increasing ventilator support, and providing oxygen as needed before fatigue advances.
17. Provide distraction (eg, visitors, radio, television, conversation) when the patient's concentration starts to create tension and increases anxiety.
18. Ensure adequate nutrition support, sufficient rest and sleep time, and sedation or pain control *to promote the patient's optimal physical and emotional comfort.*
19. Start weaning early in the day *when the patient is most rested.*
20. Restrict unnecessary activities and visitors who do not cooperate with weaning strategies *to minimize energy demands on the patient during the weaning process.*
21. Coordinate necessary activities to promote adequate time for rest and relaxation. Implement the nursing management plan for Activity Intolerance Related to Prolonged Immobility or Deconditioning.
22. Monitor the patient's underlying disease process *to ensure it is stabilized and under control.*
23. Advocate for additional resources (eg, sedation, analgesia, rest) needed by the patient *to maximize comfort status.*
24. Develop and adhere to an individualized plan of care *to promote the patient's feelings of control.*

NURSING MANAGEMENT PLAN

Excess Fluid Volume

Definition: Increased isotonic fluid retention.

Excess Fluid Volume Related to Increased Secretion of Antidiuretic Hormone (ADH)
Defining Characteristics
- Headache
- Decreased sensorium
- Weight gain over short period
- Intake greater than output
- Increased pulmonary artery occlusion pressure
- Increased right atrial pressure
- Urine output is <30 mL/h
- Serum sodium is <120 mEq/L
- Serum osmolality is <275 mOsm/kg
- Urine osmolality greater than serum osmolality
- Urine sodium is >200 mEq/L
- Urine specific gravity is >1.03

Outcome Criteria
- Weight returns to baseline.
- Urine output is >30 mL/h.
- Serum sodium is 135–145 mEq/L.
- Urine specific gravity is 1.005–1030.

Nursing Interventions and Rationale
1. Monitor cardiac rhythm continuously for dysrhythmias *caused by electrolyte imbalance.*
2. Restrict the patient's fluids to 500 mL less than output per day *to decrease fluid retention.*
3. Provide the patient chilled beverages high in sodium content such as tomato juice or broth *to increase sodium intake.*
4. Collaborate with the practitioner regarding administration of demeclocycline, lithium, or opioid agonists *to inhibit renal response to ADH.*
5. Collaborate with the practitioner regarding administration of hypertonic saline and furosemide *for rapid correction of severe sodium deficit and diuresis of free water.*
   a. Administer hypertonic saline at a rate of 1–2 mL/kg/h until the patient's serum sodium is increased no greater than 1–2 mEq/L/h.
6. Weigh the patient daily (at same time, in same amount of clothing, and preferably with same scale) *to ensure accuracy of readings.*
7. Provide frequent mouth care to prevent breakdown of oral mucous membranes.
8. Initiate seizure precautions because the patient is at high risk as a result of hyponatremia.
   a. Pad side rails of bed to protect the patient from injury.
   b. Remove any objects from immediate environment that could injure the patient in the event of a seizure.

   c. Keep appropriate-size oral airway at bedside to assist with airway management after the seizure.
9. Collaborate with the practitioner regarding administration of medications to prevent constipation *caused by decreased fluid intake and immobility.*
10. Maintain surveillance for symptoms of hyponatremia (eg, headache, abdominal cramps, weakness) and congestive heart failure (eg, dyspnea, rales, increased central venous pressure, and pulmonary artery occlusion pressure).

Excess Fluid Volume Related to Renal Dysfunction
Defining Characteristics
- Weight gain that occurs during a 24- to 48-h period
- Dependent pitting edema
- Ascites in severe cases
- Fluid crackles on lung auscultation
- Exertional dyspnea
- Oliguria or anuria
- Hypertension
- Engorged neck veins
- Decrease in urinary osmolality as renal failure progresses
- Right atrial pressure is >8 mm Hg
- Pulmonary artery occlusion pressure is >12 mm Hg

Outcome Criteria
- Weight returns to baseline.
- Edema or ascites is absent or reduced to baseline.
- Lungs are clear to auscultation.
- Exertional dyspnea is absent.
- Blood pressure returns to baseline.
- Heart rate returns to baseline.
- Neck veins are flat.
- Mucous membranes are moist.

Nursing Interventions and Rationale
1. Promote skin integrity of edematous areas by frequent repositioning and elevation of areas where possible. Avoid massaging pressure points or reddened areas of skin *because this results in further tissue trauma.*
2. Plan patient care to provide rest periods *so as not to heighten exertional dyspnea.*
3. Weigh the patient daily at same time, in same amount of clothing, and preferably with same scale.
4. Instruct the patient about the correlation between fluid intake and weight gain, using commonly understood fluid measurements; for example, ingesting 4 cups (1000 mL) of fluid results in an approximate 2-lb weight gain in the anuric patient.

NURSING MANAGEMENT PLAN

Hyperthermia

Definition: Core body temperature above the normal diurnal range due to failure of thermoregulation.

Hyperthermia Related to Increased Metabolic Rate
Defining Characteristics
- Increased body temperature above normal range
- Seizures
- Flushed skin
- Increased respiratory rate
- Tachycardia
- Skin warm to touch
- Diaphoresis

Outcome Criteria
- Temperature is within normal range.
- Respiratory rate and heart rate are within patient's baseline range.
- Skin is warm and dry.

Nursing Interventions and Rationale
1. Monitor temperature every 15 min to 1 h until within normal range and stable, then every 4 h *to maintain close surveillance for temperature fluctuations and evaluate effectiveness of interventions.*
   a. Use temperature taken from the pulmonary artery catheter or bladder catheter if available *because these methods closely reflect core body temperature.*
   b. Use tympanic membrane temperature if core body temperature devices are unavailable.
   c. Use rectal temperature if none of the above-listed methods are available.
2. Collaborate with the practitioner regarding administration of antithyroid medications *to block the synthesis and release of thyroid hormone.*
3. Collaborate with the practitioner regarding the use of a cooling blanket *to facilitate heat loss by conduction.*
   a. Wrap hands, feet, and male genitalia *to protect them from maceration during cooling and decrease chance of shivering.*
   b. Avoid rapidly cooling the patient and overcooling the patient *because this initiates the heat-conserving response (ie, shivering).*
4. Place ice packs in patient's groin and axilla *to facilitate heat loss by conduction.*
5. Maintain the patient on bed rest *to decrease the effects of activity on the patient's metabolic rate.*
6. Provide tepid sponge baths *to facilitate heat loss by evaporation.*
7. Decrease the patient's room temperature *to facilitate radiant heat loss.*
8. Place fan near patient to circulate cool air *to facilitate heat loss by convection.*
9. Provide the patient with a nonrestrictive gown and lightweight bed coverings *to allow heat to escape from the patient's trunk.*
10. Collaborate with the practitioner and the respiratory care practitioner regarding administration of oxygen to maintain oxygen saturation >90% *because patient has increased oxygen consumption resulting from an increased metabolic rate.*
11. Collaborate with the practitioner regarding use of antipyretic medications *to facilitate patient comfort.*
12. Collaborate with the practitioner regarding use of intravenous (IV) and oral fluids *to maintain adequate hydration of the patient.*

Hyperthermia Related to Pharmaceutical Agent (Malignant Hyperthermia)
Defining Characteristics
Early Signs
- Blood pressure is >140/90 mm Hg
- Profuse diaphoresis
- Heart rate is >100 beats/min
- Masseter and general skeletal muscle rigidity and fasciculations
- Tachypnea
- Decreased level of consciousness
- Increased end-tidal carbon dioxide pressure (P_{ETCO_2})

Late Signs
- Increasing core body temperature up to 42°C to 43°C (107.6°F to 109.4°F)
- Hot skin
- Systolic blood pressure is <90 mm Hg
- Heart rate is >100 beats/min and ventricular dysrhythmias
- Cardiac index is >4.0 L/min/m²
- Pulmonary artery occlusion pressure is >12 mm Hg
- Continued skeletal muscle rigidity and fasciculations
- PaO_2 is <80 mm Hg
- Respiratory and metabolic acidosis
- Fixed, dilated pupils
- Seizures, coma, or decerebrate posturing
- Urinary output is <30 mL/h; urine color reddish brown (myoglobinuria)
- Prolonged bleeding (disseminated intravascular coagulation [DIC])

Outcome Criteria
- Core body temperature is <38.3°C (101°F).
- Muscle rigidity and fasciculations are absent.
- Patient is alert and oriented.
- Pupils are normoreactive.

Nursing Interventions and Rationale
1. Obtain the emergency kit for malignant hyperthermia. *It is recommended that health care institutions have an emergency malignant hyperthermia kit available that contains the items mentioned in the following plan.* Call the malignant hyperthermia hotline for more information (1-800-644-9737).
2. Collaborate with the practitioner to implement measures to rapidly decrease metabolism:
   a. Administer dantrolene (Dantrium) at a dose of 2.5 mg/kg rapidly through a large-bore IV line, *which relaxes skeletal muscles by reducing the release of calcium from the sarcoplasmic reticulum.*
   b. Observe for infiltration of dantrolene into surrounding tissues. *Dantrolene is very alkaline and irritating to tissues.*
3. Collaborate with the practitioner to initiate cooling measures:
   a. Administer cold IV solutions (IV bag has been submerged in ice bath before solution is administered).
   b. Provide cool-water sponge bath.
   c. Apply cooling blanket until temperature is within 1°F to 3°F of desired level *to avoid "overshoot," in which excessive cooling lowers the body temperature below the desired range.*
   d. Institute iced saline lavages of stomach, rectum, and bladder.
   e. Monitor core temperature continuously *to avoid overcooling.*

◎ NURSING MANAGEMENT PLAN

Hyperthermia—cont'd

4. Collaborate with the practitioner to implement interventions to reverse metabolic and respiratory acidosis:
   a. Administer intravenous sodium bicarbonate at a dose of 1–2 mEq/kg as necessary *to treat metabolic acidosis and hyperkalemia.*
   b. Hyperventilate the patient with 100% oxygen; then ventilate with 15–20 mL/kg tidal volume at 15–20 breaths/min.
   c. Assess arterial blood gas values frequently, and make ventilatory adjustments as necessary *to remedy hypoxemia and hypercarbia.*
5. Collaborate with the practitioner to provide adequate nutrients to the tissues, and correct electrolyte imbalances:
   a. Administer 50% dextrose and regular insulin to *increase glucose uptake into the liver to meet hypermetabolic needs of the body and enhance the movement of potassium from extracellular fluid back into the cells.*
   b. Administer intravenous calcium chloride at a dose of 10 mg/kg or calcium gluconate at a dose of 10–50 mg/kg *for life-threatening hyperkalemia.*
   c. Monitor serum electrolytes *to assess efficacy of previously mentioned action.*
   d. Monitor blood urea nitrogen and creatinine levels *to evaluate for renal failure.*
   e. Monitor serum enzyme levels, particularly creatine phosphokinase elevations, *for indication of degree of muscle hyperactivity.*
6. Collaborate with the practitioner to correct cardiovascular instability and dysrhythmias:
   a. Titrate vasoactive and inotropic drips *per protocol* to desired systemic blood pressure, pulmonary artery occlusion pressure, or pulmonary artery diastolic pressure.
   b. Follow critical care emergency standing orders about administration of antidysrhythmic agents.
   c. Do not administer calcium channel blockers, *as they may cause hyperkalemia and cardiac arrest in the presence of dantrolene.*
7. Collaborate with the practitioner to maintain a high urinary output (>50 mL/h):
   a. Administer osmotic agents (mannitol) *for excretion of excess fluid load and to increase urinary output to prevent renal failure.*
   b. Administer diuretics (furosemide) *to enhance secretion of myoglobin, potassium, sodium, and magnesium.*
   c. Administer supplemental potassium chloride as indicated by serum potassium levels.
   d. Administer steroids (eg, Solu-Cortef) *for mineralocorticoid effect of potassium excretion, to increase glomerular filtration rate, and to reduce cerebral edema.*
8. Maintain surveillance for hematologic abnormalities:
   a. Monitor coagulation studies *for indications of DIC and for efficacy of heparin therapy.*
   b. Assess stool, urinary, and nasogastric drainage for occult blood.
9. Weigh the patient daily at same time, in same amount of clothing, and preferably with same scale *to assist in assessment of hydration status.*

◎ NURSING MANAGEMENT PLAN

Hypothermia

Definition: Core body temperature below normal diurnal range failure of thermoregulation.

Hypothermia Related to Decreased Metabolic Rate
Defining Characteristics
- Reduction in body temperature below normal range
- Shivering
- Pallor
- Piloerection
- Hypertension
- Skin cool to touch
- Tachycardia
- Decreased capillary refill

Outcome Criteria
- Temperature is within normal range.
- Heart rate is within patient's baseline range.
- Skin is warm and dry.
- Capillary refill is normal.

Nursing Interventions and Rationale
1. Monitor temperature every 15 min to 1 h until within normal range and stable and then every 4 h *to maintain close surveillance for temperature fluctuations and to evaluate effectiveness of interventions.*
   a. Use temperature taken from pulmonary artery catheter or bladder catheter if available *because these methods closely reflect core body temperature.*
   b. Use tympanic membrane temperature *if core body temperature devices are unavailable.*
   c. Use rectal temperature if none of the above-listed methods are available.
2. Collaborate with the practitioner regarding administration of thyroid medications *to replace lacking thyroid hormone.*
3. Collaborate with the practitioner regarding the use of a fluid-filled heating blanket *to facilitate rewarming by conduction.*
4. Initiate forced air-warming therapy *to facilitate convective heat gain.*
5. Provide the patient with warm blankets *to facilitate heat transfer to the patient.*
6. Increase the patient's room temperature *to decrease radiant heat loss.*
7. Replace wet patient gown and bed linen promptly *to decrease evaporative heat loss.*
8. Warm intravenous fluids and blood products *to facilitate rewarming by conduction.*

Hypothermia Related to Exposure to Cold Environment, Trauma, or Damage to the Hypothalamus
Defining Characteristics
- Core body temperature <35°C (95°F)
- Skin cold to touch
- Slurred speech, incoordination
- At temperature <33°C (91.4°F):
  - Cardiac dysrhythmias (atrial fibrillation, bradycardia)
  - Cyanosis
  - Respiratory alkalosis
- At temperatures <32°C (89.6°F):
  - Shivering replaced by muscle rigidity
  - Hypotension

- Dilated pupils
- At temperatures <28°C to 29°C (82.4°F to 84.2°F):
  - Absent deep tendon reflexes
  - Three to four breaths/min to apnea
  - Ventricular fibrillation possible
- At temperatures <26°C to 27°C (78.8°F to 80.6°F):
  - Coma
  - Flaccid muscles
  - Fixed, dilated pupils
  - Ventricular fibrillation to cardiac standstill
  - Apnea

Outcome Criteria
- Core body temperature is >35°C (95°F).
- Patient is alert and oriented.
- Cardiac dysrhythmias are absent.
- Acid–base balance is normal.
- Pupils are normoreactive.

Nursing Interventions and Rationale
1. Monitor the patient's core body temperature continuously.
2. Collaborate with the practitioner regarding the need for intubation and mechanical ventilation.
   a. Heated air or oxygen can be added *to help rewarm the body core.*
   b. Do not hyperventilate a patient with hypothermia *because carbon dioxide production is low, and this action may induce severe alkalosis and precipitate ventricular fibrillation.*
3. Maintain cardiopulmonary resuscitation and advanced cardiac life support until core body temperature is at least 29.5°C (85.1°F) before determining that patient cannot be resuscitated. *Electrical defibrillation is usually successful in terminating ventricular fibrillation if the temperature is >28°C (82.4°F).*
4. Administer cardiac resuscitation drugs sparingly *because as the body warms, peripheral vasodilation occurs. Drugs that remain in the periphery are suddenly released, leading to a bolus effect that may cause fatal dysrhythmias.*
5. Monitor arterial blood gas values *to direct further therapy, and ensure that pH, arterial partial pressure of oxygen (PaO$_2$), and arterial partial pressure of carbon dioxide (PaCO$_2$) are corrected for temperature.*
6. Rewarm the patient rapidly *because the pathophysiologic changes associated with chronic hypothermia have not had time to evolve.*
   a. Institute rapid, active rewarming by immersion in warm water (38°C to 43°C) (100.4°F to 109.4°F).
   b. Apply thermal blanket at 36.6°C to 37.7°C (97.9°F to 99.9°F). Some researchers suggest rewarming only the torso or trunk first, leaving the extremities exposed to room temperature. *This is done to prevent early peripheral vasodilation with abrupt redistribution of intravascular volume. This also prevents colder blood trapped in the extremities from returning to the body core before the heart is rewarmed.*
   c. Perform rapid core rewarming with heated (37° to 43°C [98.6° to 109.4°F]) intravenous infusion, hemodialysis, peritoneal dialysis, and colonic or gastric irrigation fluids.
7. Monitor peripheral circulation *because gangrene of the fingers and toes is a common complication of accidental hypothermia.*

NURSING MANAGEMENT PLAN

Imbalanced Nutrition: Less than Body Requirements

Definition: Intake of nutrients insufficient to meet metabolic needs.

Imbalanced Nutrition: Less Than Body Requirements Related to Lack of Exogenous Nutrients and Increased Metabolic Demand

Defining Characteristics

- Unplanned weight loss of 20% of body weight within past 6 months
- Serum albumin is <3.5 g/dL
- Total lymphocytes are <1500/mm^3
- Anergy
- Negative nitrogen balance
- Fatigue; lack of energy and endurance
- Nonhealing wounds
- Daily caloric intake less than estimated nutrition requirements
- Presence of factors known to increase nutrition requirements (eg, sepsis, trauma, multiple-organ dysfunction syndrome)
- Maintenance of nothing by mouth (NPO) status for >10 days
- Long-term use of intravenous 5% dextrose
- Documentation of suboptimal calorie counts
- Drug or nutrient interaction that might decrease oral intake (eg, chronic use of bronchodilators, laxatives, anticonvulsives, diuretics, antacids, opioids)
- Physical problems with chewing, swallowing, choking, and salivation and presence of altered taste, anorexia, nausea, vomiting, diarrhea, or constipation

Outcome Criteria

- Patient exhibits stabilization of weight loss or weight gain of 0.5 lb daily.

- Serum albumin is >3.5 g/dL.
- Total lymphocytes are <1500/mm^3.
- Patient has positive response to cutaneous skin antigen testing.
- Patient is in positive nitrogen balance.
- Wound healing is evident.
- Daily caloric intake equals estimated nutrition requirements.
- Increased ambulation and endurance are evident.

Nursing Interventions and Rationale

1. Inquire if the patient has any food allergies and food preferences *to ensure the food provided to the patient is not contraindicated.*
2. Monitor the patient's caloric intake and weight daily *to ensure adequacy of nutrition interventions.*
3. Collaborate with the dietitian regarding the patient's nutrition and caloric needs *to determine the appropriateness of the patient's diet to meet those needs.*
4. Monitor the patient for signs of nutrition deficiencies *to facilitate evaluation of extent of nutrition deficient.*
5. Provide the patient with oral care before eating *to ensure optimal consumption of diet.*
6. Assist the patient to eat as appropriate *to ensure optimal consumption of diet.*
7. Collaborate with the practitioner and dietitian regarding administration of parenteral and enteral nutrition as needed.

◎ NURSING MANAGEMENT PLAN

Impaired Gas Exchange

Definition: Excess or deficit in oxygenation and/or carbon dioxide elimination at the alveolar-capillary membrane.

Impaired Gas Exchange Related to Alveolar Hypoventilation
Defining Characteristics

- Abnormal arterial blood gas (ABG) values (decreased arterial partial pressure of oxygen [PaO$_2$], increased arterial partial pressure of carbon dioxide [PaCO$_2$], decreased pH, decreased arterial oxygen saturation [Sao$_2$])
- Somnolence
- Neurobehavioral changes (eg, restlessness, irritability, confusion)
- Tachycardia or dysrhythmias
- Central cyanosis

Outcome Criteria

- ABG values are within patient's baseline.
- Central cyanosis is absent.

Nursing Interventions and Rationale

1. Initiate continuous pulse oximetry or monitor oxygen saturation measured by pulse oximetry [Spo$_2$] every hour.
2. Collaborate with the practitioner and respiratory care practitioner regarding administration of oxygen to maintain Spo$_2$ >90%.
   a. Administer supplemental oxygen by an appropriate oxygen delivery device *to increase driving pressure of oxygen in the alveoli.*
   b. If supplemental oxygen alone is ineffective, administer high-flow oxygen via high-flow nasal cannula, bilevel positive airway pressure (BiPAP) via noninvasive ventilation (NIV), or positive end-expiratory pressure (PEEP) via invasive mechanical ventilation *to open collapsed alveoli and increase the surface area for gas exchange.*
3. Prevent hypoventilation.
   a. Position the patient in high-Fowler or semi-Fowler position *to promote diaphragmatic descent and maximal inhalation.*
   b. Assist with deep-breathing exercises and/or incentive spirometry with sustained maximal inspiration 5 to 10 times/h *to help reinflate collapsed portions of the lung.* See the nursing management plan for Ineffective Breathing Pattern Related to Decreased Lung Expansion for further instructions.
   c. Treat pain, if present, *to prevent hypoventilation and atelectasis.* Implement the nursing management plan for Acute Pain Related to Transmission and Perception of Cutaneous, Visceral, Muscular, or Ischemic Impulses.
4. Assist the practitioner with intubation and initiation of mechanical ventilation as indicated.

Impaired Gas Exchange Related to Ventilation-Perfusion Mismatching or Intrapulmonary Shunting
Defining Characteristics

- Abnormal ABG values (decreased PaO$_2$, decreased Sao$_2$)
- Somnolence

- Neurobehavioral changes (restlessness, irritability, confusion)
- Central cyanosis

Outcome Criteria

- ABG values are within patient's baseline.
- Central cyanosis is absent.

Nursing Interventions and Rationale

1. Initiate continuous pulse oximetry, or monitor Spo$_2$ every hour.
2. Collaborate with the practitioner and respiratory care practitioner regarding administration of oxygen to maintain an Spo$_2$ >90%.
   a. Administer supplemental oxygen by an appropriate oxygen delivery device *to increase driving pressure of oxygen in the alveoli.*
   b. If supplemental oxygen alone is ineffective, administer high-flow oxygen via high-flow nasal cannula, BiPAP via NIV, or positive end-expiratory pressure (PEEP) via invasive mechanical ventilation *to open collapsed alveoli and increase the surface area for gas exchange.*
3. Position the patient to optimize ventilation-perfusion matching.
   a. For a patient with unilateral lung disease, position with the good lung down *because gravity will improve perfusion to this area, and this will best match ventilation with perfusion.*
   b. For a patient with bilateral lung disease, position with the right lung down *because this lung is larger than the left and affords a greater area for ventilation and perfusion, or change position every 2 h, favoring positions that improve oxygenation.*
   c. For a patient with diffuse bilateral disease, collaborate with the practitioner regarding the use of prone positioning *to encourage perfusion to the anterior region of the lungs, which are usually less damaged than the posterior region.*
   d. Avoid any position that seriously compromises oxygenation status.
4. Perform procedures only as needed, and provide adequate rest and recovery time in between *to prevent desaturation.*
5. Collaborate with the practitioner regarding administration of the following:
   a. Sedatives *to decrease ventilator asynchrony and facilitate the patient's sense of control.*
   b. Neuromuscular blocking agents *to prevent ventilator asynchrony and decrease oxygen demand.*
   c. Analgesics *to treat pain if present.* Implement the nursing management plan for Acute Pain Related to Transmission and Perception of Cutaneous, Visceral, Muscular, or Ischemic Impulses.
6. Evaluate the patient for the presence of secretions. If secretions are present, implement the nursing management plan for Ineffective Airway Clearance Related to Excessive Secretions or Abnormal Viscosity of Mucus.

◉ NURSING MANAGEMENT PLAN

Impaired Spontaneous Ventilation

Definition: Decreased energy reserves result in an inability to maintain independent breathing that is adequate to support life.

Impaired Spontaneous Ventilation Related to Respiratory Muscle Fatigue or Metabolic Factors

Defining Characteristics

- Dyspnea and apprehension
- Increased metabolic rate
- Increased restlessness
- Increased use of accessory muscles
- Decreased tidal volume
- Increased heart rate
- Abnormal arterial blood gas (ABG) values (decreased arterial partial pressure of oxygen [PaO_2], increased arterial partial pressure of carbon dioxide [$PaCO_2$], decreased pH, decreased arterial oxygen saturation [SaO_2])
- Decreased cooperation

Outcome Criteria

- Metabolic rate and heart rate are within patient's baseline.
- Patient experiences eupnea.
- ABG values are within patient's baseline.

Nursing Interventions and Rationale

1. Collaborate with the practitioner regarding application of pressure support to the ventilator *to assist the patient in overcoming the work of breathing imposed by the ventilator and endotracheal tube.*
2. Carefully snip excess length from the proximal end of the endotracheal tube *to decrease dead space and decrease the work of breathing.*
3. Collaborate with the practitioner and dietitian to ensure that at least 50% of the diet's nonprotein caloric source is in the form of fat rather than carbohydrates *to prevent excess carbon dioxide production.*
4. Collaborate with the practitioner and respiratory care practitioner regarding the best method of weaning for individual patients *because each situation is different, and various weaning options are available.*

   a. Consider initiating a daily spontaneous awakening trial ("sedation vacation") and spontaneous breathing trial.

   b. Monitor the patient for signs of weaning intolerance.
5. Collaborate with the practitioner and physical therapist regarding a progressive ambulation and conditioning plan *to promote overall muscle conditioning and respiratory muscle functioning.* Implement the nursing management plan for Activity Intolerance Related to Prolonged Immobility or Deconditioning.
6. Determine the most effective means of communication for the patient *to promote independence and reduce anxiety.*
7. Develop a daily schedule and post it in the patient's room *to coordinate care and facilitate the patient's involvement in the plan.*
8. Treat pain, if present, *to prevent respiratory splinting and hypoventilation.* Implement the nursing management plan for Acute Pain Related to Transmission and Perception of Cutaneous, Visceral, Muscular, or Ischemic Impulses.
9. Ensure that the patient receives at least 2- to 4-h intervals of uninterrupted sleep in a quiet, dark room. Collaborate with the practitioner and respiratory care practitioner regarding use of full ventilatory support at night *to provide respiratory muscle rest.*
10. Place the patient in semi-Fowler position or in a chair at the bedside *for best use of ventilatory muscles and to facilitate diaphragmatic descent.*
11. Explain the weaning procedure to the patient before the trial *so that the patient will understand what to expect and how to participate.*
12. Monitor the patient during the weaning trial for evidence of respiratory muscle fatigue *to avoid overtiring the patient.*
13. Collaborate with the practitioner and occupational therapist to provide diversional activities during the weaning trial *to reduce the patient's anxiety.*
14. Collaborate with the practitioner and respiratory care practitioner regarding removal of the ventilator and artificial airway *after the patient has been successfully weaned.*

NURSING MANAGEMENT PLAN

Impaired Swallowing

Definition: Abnormal functioning of the swallowing mechanism associated with deficits in oral, pharyngeal, or esophageal structure or function.

Impaired Swallowing Related to Neuromuscular Impairment, Fatigue, and Limited Awareness

Defining Characteristics
- Evidence of difficulty swallowing:
  - Drooling
  - Difficulty handling oral secretions
  - Absence of gag, cough, or swallow reflex
  - Moist, wet, gurgling voice quality
  - Decreased tongue and mouth movements
  - Presence of dysarthria
- Difficulty handling solid foods:
  - Uncoordinated chewing or swallowing
  - Stasis of food in oral cavity
  - Wet-sounding voice or change in voice quality
  - Sneezing, coughing, or choking with eating
  - Delay in swallowing of more than 5 s
  - Change in respiratory patterns
- Difficulty handling liquids:
  - Momentary loss of voice or change in voice quality
  - Nasal regurgitation of liquids
  - Coughing with drinking
- Evidence of aspiration:
  - Hypoxemia
  - Productive cough
  - Frothy sputum
  - Wheezing, crackles, or rhonchi
  - Temperature elevation

Outcome Criteria
- Evidence of swallowing difficulties is absent.
- Evidence of aspiration is absent.

Nursing Interventions and Rationale
1. Collaborate with the practitioner and speech therapist regarding swallowing evaluation and rehabilitation program *to decrease the incidence of aspiration.*
2. Collaborate with the practitioner and dietitian regarding a nutrition assessment and nutrition plan *to ensure that the patient is receiving adequate nutrition.*
3. Place the patient in an upright position with the head midline and the chin slightly down *to keep food in the anterior portion of the mouth and to prevent it from falling over the base of the tongue into the open airway.*
4. Provide the patient with single-textured soft foods (eg, cream cereals) that maintain their shape *because these foods require minimal oral manipulation.*
5. Avoid particulate foods (eg, hamburger) and foods containing more than one texture (eg, stew) *because these foods require more chewing and oral manipulation.*
6. Avoid dry foods (eg, popcorn, rice, crackers) and sticky foods (eg, peanut butter, bananas) *because these foods are difficult to manipulate orally.*
7. Provide the patient with thick liquids (eg, fruit nectar, yogurt) *because thick liquids are more easily controlled in the mouth.*
8. Thicken thin liquids (eg, water, juice) with a thickening preparation or avoid them *because thin liquids are easily aspirated.*
9. Place foods in the uninvolved side of the mouth *because oral sensitivity and function are greatest in this area.*
10. Avoid the use of straws *because they can deposit the liquid too far back in the mouth for the patient to handle.*
11. Serve foods and liquids at room temperature *because the patient may be overly sensitive to heat or cold.*
12. Offer solids and liquids at different times *to avoid swallowing solids before being properly chewed.*
13. Provide oral hygiene after meals *to clear food particles from the mouth that could be aspirated.*
14. Collaborate with the practitioner and pharmacist regarding oral medication administration *to adjust medication regimen to prevent aspiration and choking and to ensure all prescribed medications are swallowed.*
15. Crush tablets (if appropriate) and mix with food that is easily formed into a bolus, use thickened liquid medications (if available), or embed small capsules into food *to facilitate oral medication administration.*
16. Inspect mouth for residue after all medication administration *to ensure medication has been swallowed.*
17. Educate the patient and family on the swallowing problem, rehabilitation program, and emergency measures for choking.

NURSING MANAGEMENT PLAN

Impaired Verbal Communication

Definition: Decreased, delayed, or absent ability to receive, process, transmit, or use a system of symbols.

Impaired Verbal Communication Related to Cerebral Speech Center Injury

Defining Characteristics

* Inappropriate or absent speech or responses to questions
* Inability to speak spontaneously
* Inability to understand spoken words
* Inability to follow commands appropriately through gestures
* Difficulty or inability to understand written language
* Difficulty or inability to express ideas in writing
* Difficulty or inability to name objects

Outcome Criterion

* Patient is able to make basic needs known.

Nursing Interventions and Rationale

1. Collaborate with the practitioner and speech pathologist *to determine the extent of the patient's communication deficit (eg, whether fluent, nonfluent, or global aphasia is involved).*
2. Have the speech therapist post a list of appropriate ways to communicate with the patient in the patient's room *so that all nursing personnel can be consistent in their efforts.*
3. Assess the patient's ability to comprehend, speak, read, and write.
   a. Ask questions that can be answered with "yes" or "no." If a patient answers "yes" to a question, ask the opposite (eg, "Are you hot?" "Yes." "Are you cold?" "Yes."). *This may help determine whether the patient understands what is being said.*
   b. Ask simple, short questions, and use gestures, pantomime, and facial expressions to give the patient additional clues.
   c. Stand in the patient's line of vision, giving a good view of your face and hands.
   d. Have the patient try to write with a pad and pencil. Offer pictures and alphabet letters at which to point.
   e. Make flash cards with pictures or words depicting frequently used phrases (eg, glass of water, bedpan).
4. Maintain an uncluttered environment, and decrease external distractions *to enhance communication.*
5. Maintain a relaxed and calm manner, and explain all diagnostic, therapeutic, and comfort measures before initiating them.
6. Do not shout or speak in a loud voice. *Hearing loss is not a factor in aphasia, and shouting will not help.*
7. Have only one person talk at a time. *It is more difficult for the patient to follow a multisided conversation.*
8. Use direct eye contact, and speak directly to the patient in unhurried, short phrases.
9. Give one-step commands and directions, and provide cues through pictures and gestures.

10. Try to ask questions that can be answered with a "yes" or a "no," and avoid topics that are controversial, emotional, abstract, or lengthy.
11. Listen to the patient in an unhurried manner, and wait for his or her attempt to communicate.
    a. Expect a time lag from when you ask the patient something until the patient responds.
    b. Accept the patient's statement of essential words without expecting complete sentences.
    c. Avoid finishing the sentence for the patient if possible.
    d. Wait approximately 30 s before providing the word the patient may be attempting to find (except when the patient is very frustrated and needs something quickly, such as a bedpan).
    e. Rephrase the patient's message aloud *to validate it.*
    f. Do not pretend to understand the patient's message if you do not.
12. Encourage the patient to speak slowly in short phrases and to say each word clearly.
13. Ask the patient to write the message, if able, or draw pictures if only verbal communication is affected.
14. Observe the patient's nonverbal clues for validation (eg, answers "yes" but shakes head "no").
15. When handing an object to the patient, state what it is *because hearing language spoken is necessary to stimulate language development.*
16. Explain what has happened to the patient, and offer reassurance about the plan of care.
17. Verbally address the problem of frustration over the inability to communicate, and explain that both the nurse and the patient need patience.
18. Maintain a calm, positive manner, and offer reassurance (eg, "I know this is very hard for you, but it will get better if we work on it together").
19. Talk to the patient as an adult. Be respectful, and avoid talking down to the patient.
20. Do not discuss the patient's condition or hold conversations in the patient's presence without including him or her in the discussion. *This may be the reason some aphasic patients develop paranoid thoughts.*
21. Do not exhibit disapproval of emotional utterances or spontaneous use of profanity; instead, offer calm, quiet reassurance.
22. If the patient makes an error in speech, do not reprimand or scold, but try to compliment the patient by saying, "That was a good try."
23. Delay conversation if the patient is tired. *The symptoms of aphasia worsen if the patient is fatigued, anxious, or upset.*
24. Be prepared for emotional outbursts and tears from patients who have more difficulty in expressing themselves than with understanding. *The patient may become depressed, refuse treatment and food, ignore relatives, and push objects away.* Comfort the patient with statements such as, "I know it's frustrating and you feel sad, but you are not alone. Other people who have had strokes have felt the way you do. We will be here to help you get through this."

NURSING MANAGEMENT PLAN

Ineffective Airway Clearance

Definition: Inability to clear secretions or obstructions from the respiratory tract to maintain a clear airway.

Ineffective Airway Clearance Related to Excessive Secretions or Abnormal Viscosity of Mucus
Defining Characteristics

- Abnormal breath sounds (displaced normal sounds, adventitious sounds, diminished or absent sounds)
- Ineffective cough with or without sputum
- Tachypnea, dyspnea
- Verbal reports of inability to clear airway

Outcome Criteria

- Cough produces thin mucus.
- Lungs are clear to auscultation.
- Respiratory rate, depth, and rhythm return to baseline.

Nursing Interventions and Rationale

1. Assess sputum for color, consistency, and amount.
2. Assess for clinical manifestations of pneumonia.
3. Provide for maximal thoracic expansion by repositioning, deep breathing, splinting, and pain management *to avoid hypoventilation and atelectasis.* If hypoventilation is present, implement the nursing management plan for Ineffective Breathing Pattern Related to Decreased Lung Expansion.
4. Maintain adequate hydration by administering oral and intravenous fluids (as ordered) *to thin secretions and facilitate airway clearance.*
5. Provide humidification to airways by an oxygen delivery device or artificial airway *to thin secretions and facilitate airway clearance.*
6. Administer bland aerosol every 4 h *to facilitate expectoration of sputum.*
7. Collaborate with the practitioner regarding administration of the following:
   a. Bronchodilators *to treat or prevent bronchospasms and facilitate expectoration of mucus.*
   b. Mucolytics and expectorants *to enhance mobilization and removal of secretions.*
   c. Antibiotics *to treat infection.*
8. Assist with directed coughing exercises *to facilitate expectoration of secretions.* If the patient is unable to perform cascade cough, consider using huff cough (patients with hyperactive airways), end-expiratory cough

(patient with secretions in distal airway), or augmented cough (patient with weakened abdominal muscle).
   a. Cascade cough—instruct the patient to do the following:
      (1) Take a deep breath, and hold it for 1 to 3 s.
      (2) Cough out forcefully several times until all air is exhaled.
      (3) Inhale slowly through the nose.
      (4) Repeat once.
      (5) Rest, and then repeat as necessary.
   b. Huff cough—instruct the patient to do the following:
      (1) Take a deep breath, and hold it for 1 to 3 s.
      (2) Say the word "huff" while coughing out several times until air is exhaled.
      (3) Inhale slowly through the nose.
      (4) Repeat as necessary.
   c. End-expiratory cough—instruct the patient to do the following:
      (1) Take a deep breath, and hold it for 1 to 3 s.
      (2) Exhale slowly.
      (3) At the end of exhalation, cough once.
      (4) Inhale slowly through the nose.
      (5) Repeat as necessary, or follow with cascade cough.
   d. Augmented cough—instruct the patient to do the following:
      (1) Take a deep breath, and hold it for 1 to 3 s.
      (2) Perform one or more of the following maneuvers to increase intraabdominal pressure:
         (a) Tighten knees and buttocks.
         (b) Bend forward at the waist.
         (c) Place a hand flat on the upper abdomen just under the xiphoid process and press in and up abruptly during coughing.
         (d) Keep hands on the chest wall and press inward with each cough.
      (3) Inhale slowly through the nose.
      (4) Rest and repeat as necessary.
9. Suction nasotracheally or endotracheally as necessary *to assist with secretion removal.*
10. Reposition the patient at least every 2 h or use kinetic therapy *to mobilize and prevent stasis of secretions.*
11. Allow rest periods between coughing sessions, suctioning, or any other demanding activities *to promote energy conservation.*

NURSING MANAGEMENT PLAN

Ineffective Breathing Pattern

Definition: Inspiration and/or expiration that does not provide adequate ventilation.

Ineffective Breathing Pattern Related to Decreased Lung Expansion

Defining Characteristics
- Abnormal respiratory patterns (hypoventilation, hyperventilation, tachypnea, bradypnea, obstructive breathing)
- Abnormal arterial blood gas (ABG) values (increased arterial partial pressure of carbon dioxide [$PaCO_2$], decreased pH)
- Unequal chest movement
- Shortness of breath, dyspnea

Outcome Criteria
- Respiratory rate, rhythm, and depth return to baseline.
- Minimal or absent use of accessory muscles.
- Chest expands symmetrically.
- ABG values return to baseline.

Nursing Interventions and Rationale
1. Treat pain, if present, *to prevent hypoventilation and atelectasis.* Implement the nursing management plan for Acute Pain Related to Transmission and Perception of Cutaneous, Visceral, Muscular, or Ischemic Impulses.
2. Position the patient in high-Fowler or semi-Fowler position *to promote diaphragmatic descent and maximal inhalation.*
3. Assist with deep-breathing exercises and incentive spirometry with sustained maximal inspiration 5 to 10 times/h *to help reinflate collapsed portions of the lung.*
   a. Deep breathing—instruct the patient to do the following:
      (1) Sit up straight or lean forward slightly while sitting on edge of bed or chair (if possible).
      (2) Take in a slow, deep breath.
      (3) Pause slightly, or hold breath for at least 3 s.
      (4) Exhale slowly.
      (5) Rest, and repeat.
   b. Incentive spirometry—instruct the patient to do the following:
      (1) Exhale normally.
      (2) Place lips around the mouthpiece, and close mouth tightly around it.
      (3) Inhale slowly and as deeply as possible, noting the maximal volume of air inspired.
      (4) Hold maximal inhalation for 3 s.
      (5) Take the mouthpiece out of mouth, and slowly exhale.
      (6) Rest, and repeat.
4. Assist the practitioner with intubation and initiation of mechanical ventilation as indicated.

Ineffective Breathing Pattern Related to Musculoskeletal Fatigue or Neuromuscular Impairment

Defining Characteristics
- Unequal chest movement
- Shortness of breath, dyspnea
- Use of accessory muscles
- Tachypnea
- Thoracoabdominal asynchrony
- Abnormal ABG values (increased $PaCO_2$, decreased pH)
- Nasal flaring
- Assumption of three-point position

Outcome Criteria
- Respiratory rate, rhythm, and depth return to baseline.
- Use of accessory muscles is minimal or absent.
- Chest expands symmetrically.
- ABG values return to baseline.

Nursing Interventions and Rationale
1. Prevent unnecessary exertion *to limit drain on the patient's ventilatory reserve.*
2. Instruct the patient in energy-saving techniques *to conserve the patient's ventilatory reserve.*
3. Assist with pursed-lip and diaphragmatic breathing techniques *to facilitate diaphragmatic descent and improved ventilation.*
   a. Diaphragmatic breathing—instruct the patient to do the following:
      (1) Sit in the upright position.
      (2) Place one hand on the abdomen just above the waist and the other on the upper chest.
      (3) Breathe in through the nose, and feel the lower hand push out; the upper hand should not move.
      (4) Breathe out through pursed lips, and feel the lower hand move in.
4. Position the patient in high-Fowler or semi-Fowler position *to promote diaphragmatic descent and maximal inhalation.*
5. Assist the practitioner with intubation and initiation of mechanical ventilation as indicated.

◎ NURSING MANAGEMENT PLAN

Ineffective Coping

Definition: Inability to form a valid appraisal of the stressors, inadequate choices of practiced responses, or inability to use available resources.

Ineffective Coping Related to Situational Crisis and Personal Vulnerability

Defining Characteristics

- Verbalization of inability to cope. *Sample statements:* "I can't take this anymore." "I don't know how to deal with this."
- Ineffective problem solving (problem lumping). *Sample statements:* "I have to eliminate salt from my diet. They tell me I can no longer mow the lawn. This hospitalization is costing a mint. What about my kids' future? Who's going to change the oil in the car? This is an incredible amount of time away from work."
- Ineffective use of coping mechanisms
- Projection: blames others for illness or pain
- Displacement: directs anger and/or aggression toward family
- *Sample statements:* "Get out of here. Leave me alone."
- Cursing, shouting, or demanding attention; striking out or throwing objects
- Denial: of severity of illness and need for treatment
- Noncompliance. *Examples:* activity restriction; refusal to allow treatment or to take medications
- Suicidal thoughts (verbalizes desire to end life)
- Self-directed aggression. *Examples:* disconnects or attempts to disconnect life-sustaining equipment; deliberately tries to harm self
- Failure to progress from dependent to more independent state (refusal or resistance to care for self)

Outcome Criteria

- Patient verbalizes beginning ability to cope with illness, pain, and hospitalization. *Sample statements:* "I'm trying to do the best I can." "I want to help myself get better."
- Patient demonstrates effective problem solving (lists and prioritizes problems from most to least urgent).
- Patient uses effective behavioral strategies to manage the stress of illness and care.
- Patient demonstrates interest or involvement in illness or environment. *Examples:* Patient does the following:
  - Requests medications when anticipating pain
  - Questions course of treatment, progress, and prognosis
  - Asks for clarification of environmental stimuli and events
  - Seeks out supportive individuals in his or her environment
  - Uses coping mechanisms and strategies more effectively to manage situational crisis
  - Demonstrates significant reduction in impulsive, angry, or aggressive outbursts (projection, shouting, cursing) directed toward family
  - Verbalizes future-based plans, with cessation of self-directed aggressive acts and suicidal thoughts
  - Willingly complies with treatment regimen
  - Begins to participate in self-care

Nursing Interventions and Rationale

1. Actively listen and respond to the patient's verbal and behavioral expressions. *Active listening signifies unconditional respect and acceptance for the patient as a worthwhile individual. It builds trust and rapport, guides the nurse toward problem areas, encourages the patient to express concerns, and promotes compliance.*

2. Offer effective coping strategies to help the patient better tolerate the stressors related to his or her illness and care. Give permission to vent feelings in a safe setting. *Sample statements:* "I don't blame you for feeling angry or frustrated." "Others who are ill like you have expressed similar feelings." "I will listen to anything you want to share with me." "We don't have to talk; I'd like to sit here with you." "It's perfectly okay to cry." *Individuals who are provided with opportunities to express their feelings will be better able to release pent-up emotions and derive a greater sense of relief and comfort. They are less likely to resort to overly impulsive, aggressive acts, which may harm self or others.*

3. Inform the family of the patient's need to displace anger occasionally but that you will be working with the patient to help him or her release his or her feelings in a more constructive, effective way. *Family members who are well informed are better equipped to cope with their loved one's emotional anguish and outbursts. They are less likely to waste energy on feelings of guilt, fear, anger, or despair and can use their strength to help the patient in more constructive ways. The knowledge that their loved one is being cared for emotionally as well as physically provides family members with a greater sense of comfort and understanding. They will feel nurtured and respected by the nurse's attempt to include them in the process.*

4. With the patient, list and number problems from the most to least urgent. Assist the patient in finding immediate solutions for the most urgent problems, postpone finding solutions for problems that can wait, delegate some problems to family members, and help the patient to acknowledge problems that are beyond his or her control. *Listing and numbering problems in an organized fashion helps to break them down into more manageable "pieces" so that the patient is better able to identify solutions for problems that are solvable and to suppress problems that are less relevant or not amenable to interventions.*

5. Identify individuals in the patient's environment who best help him or her to cope, and identify those who do not. Validate your observations with the patient. *Sample statements:* "I notice you seemed more relaxed during your daughter's visit." "After the chaplain left, you were able to sleep a bit longer than usual; would you like to see him more often?" "Your grandson was a bit upset today; I'll be glad to talk to him if you like." *Supportive persons can invoke a calming effect on the patient's physiologic and psychologic states. Conversely, well-meaning but nonsupportive individuals can have a deleterious effect on the patient's ability to cope and must be carefully screened and counseled by the nurse.*

6. Teach the patient effective cognitive strategies to help him or her better manage the stress of critical illness and care. Help the patient construct pleasant thoughts, situations, or images that can simultaneously inhibit unpleasant realities. Examples: a day at the beach, a walk in the park, drinking a glass of wine, or being with a loved one. *Pleasant thoughts and images constructed during critical illness and care tend to inhibit or reduce the intensity of the unpleasant, stressful effects of the experience.*

7. Assist the patient in using coping mechanisms more effectively so that the patient can better manage his or her situational crisis.
   a. Suppression of problems beyond his or her control
   b. Compensation for illness and its effects; focusing on his or her strengths, interests, family, and spiritual beliefs

⊚ NURSING MANAGEMENT PLAN

Ineffective Coping—cont'd

c. Adaptive displacement of anger, fear, or frustration through healthy, verbal expressions to staff. *Effective use of coping mechanisms helps to assuage the patient's painful feelings in a safe setting. The patient is strengthened and need not resort to the use of more ineffective defenses to eliminate anxiety.*

8. Initiate a suicidal assessment if the patient verbalizes the desire to die, states that life is not worth living, or exhibits self-directed aggression. *Sample statement:* "We know that this is a bad time for you. You're saying repeatedly that you want to die. Are you planning to harm yourself?" If the response is "yes," remain with the patient, alert staff members, and provide for psychiatric consultation as soon as possible. Continue to express concern to the patient and protect him or her from harm. *Suicidal thoughts as a result of ineffective coping or exhaustion of coping devices are a common occurrence in critically ill patients. If the mood state is distressing enough, a patient may seek relief by attempting a self-destructive act. Although the patient may not imminently have the energy to succeed in his or her attempt, voicing a specific plan signifies a depressed mood state and depletion of coping strategies. Immediate intervention is needed because the attempt may be successful when the patient's energy is restored.*

9. Encourage the patient to participate in self-care activities and treatment regimen in accordance with his or her level of progress. Offer praise for his or her efforts toward self-care. *Patients who take an active role in their own treatment and progress are less apt to feel like helpless or powerless victims. This greater sense of control over their illness and environment will guide them more swiftly toward becoming as independent as possible.*

◎ NURSING MANAGEMENT PLAN

Powerlessness

Definition: The lived experience of lack of control over a situation, including a perception that one's actions do not significantly affect an outcome.

Powerlessness Related to Lack of Control Over Current Situation or Disease Progression

Defining Characteristics

Severe
- Verbal expressions of having no control or influence over situation
- Verbal expressions of having no control or influence over outcome
- Verbal expressions of having no control over self-care
- Depression over physical deterioration that occurs despite patient's compliance with regimens
- Apathy

Moderate
- Nonparticipation in care or decision making when opportunities are provided
- Expressions of dissatisfaction and frustration about inability to perform previous tasks and/or activities
- Lack of progress monitoring
- Expressions of doubt about role performance
- Reluctance to express true feelings, fearing alienation from caregivers
- Passivity
- Inability to seek information about care
- Dependence on others that may result in irritability, resentment, anger, and guilt
- No defense of self-care practices when challenged

Low
- Passivity

Outcome Criteria
- Patient verbalizes increased control over situation by wanting to do things his or her way.
- Patient actively participates in planning care.
- Patient requests needed information.
- Patient chooses to participate in self-care activities.
- Patient monitors progress.

Nursing Interventions and Rationale

1. Evaluate the patient's feelings and perception of the reasons for lack of power and sense of helplessness.
2. Determine as far as possible the patient's usual response to limited control situations. Determine through ongoing assessment the patient's usual locus of control (ie, believes that influence over his or her life is exerted by luck, fate, powerful persons [external locus of control] or that influence is exerted through personal choices, self-effort, self-determination [internal locus of control]).
3. Support the patient's physical control of the environment by involving him or her in care activities; knock before entering room if appropriate; ask permission before moving personal belongings. Inform the patient that, although an activity may not be to his or her liking, it is necessary. *This gives the patient permission to express dissatisfaction with the environment and the regimen.*
4. Personalize the patient's care using his or her preferred name. *This supports the patient's psychologic control.*
5. Provide therapeutic rationale for all the patient is asked to do for himself or herself and for all that is being done for and with him or her. Reinforce the practitioner's explanations; clarify misconceptions about the illness situation and treatment plans. *This supports the patient's cognitive control.*
6. Include the patient in care planning by encouraging participation and allowing choices wherever possible (eg, timing of personal care activities; deciding when pain medicines are needed). Point out situations in which no choices exist.
7. Provide opportunities for the patient to exert influence over himself or herself and his or her body, affecting an outcome. For example, share with the patient the nurse's assessment of his or her breath sounds and explain that they can be improved by self-initiated deep-breathing exercises. *Feedback that the patient has been successful in helping clear his or her lungs reinforces the influence he or she does retain.*
8. Encourage the family to permit the patient to do as much independently as possible *to foster perception of personal power.*
9. Assist the patient to establish realistic short-term and long-term goals. *Setting unrealistic or unattainable goals inadvertently reinforces the patient's perception of powerlessness.*
10. Document care to provide for continuity *so that the patient can maintain appropriate control over the environment.*
11. Assist the patient to regain strength and activity tolerance as appropriate, *increasing a sense of control and self-reliance.*
12. Increase the sensitivity of the health team members and significant others to the patient's sense of powerlessness. Use power over the patient carefully. Use the words *must, should,* and *have to* with caution *because they communicate coercive powers and imply that the objects of "musts" and "shoulds" are of benefit to the nurse instead of the patient.*
13. Plan with the patient for transfer from the critical care unit to the intermediate unit and eventually to home.

◎ NURSING MANAGEMENT PLAN

Relocation Stress Syndrome

Definition: Physiologic and/or psychosocial disturbance following transfer from one environment to another.

Relocation Stress Syndrome Related to Transfer Out of the Critical Care Unit

Defining Characteristics

- Alienation
- Aloneness
- Anger
- Anxiety
- Concern over relocation
- Dependency
- Depression
- Fear of an unknown environment
- Frustration
- Increased illness
- Increased physical symptoms
- Increased verbalization of needs
- Insecurity
- Loneliness
- Loss of identify
- Loss of self-esteem
- Loss of self-worth
- Move from critical care unit to another environment
- Pessimism
- Sleep disturbance
- Unwillingness to move
- Withdrawal
- Worry

Outcome Criteria

- Patient will express willingness to move to new environment.
- Anxiety will be absent.

Nursing Interventions and Rationale

1. Initiate pretransfer teaching as soon as appropriate during the patient's stay in the critical care unit *to ease the transition from the critical care unit to the next environment.* Teaching should focus on the differences in the environment and the care the patient would receive.
2. Provide the patient and family written information regarding the transfer (if available) *to enhance effectiveness of teaching.*
3. Help the patient see that progress is being made *in preparation for transfer.* Each time a tube is removed or a treatment frequency is decreased, reinforce with the patient and family that the patient is progressing.
4. Remove monitoring and supportive equipment from the patient's room when no longer needed *to allow the patient to experience the loss of technology while still in the critical care unit.*
5. Encourage the patient and family to discuss concerns regarding relocation.
6. Assist the patient and family members to develop and maintain a positive perception of the transfer.
7. Arrange for the patient's family to have a tour of the new unit *as a means of familiarizing them with the unit before the patient's transfer.*

◎ NURSING MANAGEMENT PLAN

Risk for Aspiration

Definition: Vulnerable to entry of gastrointestinal secretions, oropharyngeal secretions, solids, or fluids into tracheobronchial passages, which may compromise health.

Risk Factors
- Impaired laryngeal sensation or reflex
  - Reduced level of consciousness
  - Extubation
- Impaired pharyngeal peristalsis or tongue function
  - Neuromuscular dysfunction
  - Central nervous system dysfunction
  - Head or neck injury
- Impaired laryngeal closure or elevation
  - Laryngeal nerve dysfunction
  - Artificial airways
  - Gastrointestinal tubes
- Increased gastric volume
  - Delayed gastric emptying
  - Enteral feedings
  - Medication administration
- Increased intragastric pressure
  - Upper abdominal surgery
  - Obesity
  - Pregnancy
  - Ascites
- Decreased lower esophageal sphincter pressure
  - Increased gastric acidity
  - Gastrointestinal tubes
- Decreased antegrade esophageal propulsion
  - Trendelenburg or supine position
  - Esophageal dysmotility
  - Esophageal structural defects or lesions

Outcome Criteria
- Breath sounds are normal, or there is no change in patient's baseline breath sounds.
- Arterial blood gas values remain within patient's baseline.
- There is no evidence of gastric contents in lung secretions.

Nursing Interventions and Rationale
1. Assess gastrointestinal function *to rule out hypoactive peristalsis and abdominal distention.*
2. Position the patient with the head of the bed elevated 30 degrees *to prevent gastric reflux through gravity.* If head elevation is contraindicated, position the patient in the right lateral decubitus position *to facilitate passage of gastric contents across the pylorus.*
3. Maintain patency and functioning of nasogastric suction apparatus *to prevent accumulation of gastric contents.*
4. Provide frequent and scrupulous mouth care *to prevent colonization of the oropharynx with bacteria and inoculation of the lower airways.*
5. Ensure that the endotracheal or tracheostomy cuff is properly inflated *to limit aspiration of oropharyngeal secretions.*
6. Treat nausea promptly; collaborate with the practitioner on an order for an antiemetic *to prevent vomiting and resultant aspiration.*

Additional Interventions for Patient Receiving Continuous or Intermittent Enteral Tube Feedings
1. Position the patient with the head of the bed elevated 45 degrees *to prevent gastric reflux.* If a head-down position becomes necessary at any time, interrupt the feeding 30 min before the position change.
2. Check placement of feeding tube by auscultation or radiographically at regular intervals (eg, before administering intermittent feedings and after position changes, suctioning, coughing episodes, or vomiting) *to ensure proper placement of the tube.*
3. Monitor the patient for signs of delayed gastric emptying *to decrease potential for vomiting and aspiration.*
   a. For large-bore tubes, check residuals of tube feedings before intermittent feedings and every 4 h during continuous feedings. Consider withholding feedings for residuals >150% of the hourly rate (continuous feeding) or >50% of the previous feeding (intermittent feeding).
   b. For small-bore tubes, observe abdomen for distention, palpate abdomen for hardness or tautness, and auscultate abdomen for bowel sounds.

◎ NURSING MANAGEMENT PLAN

Risk for Decreased Cardiac Tissue Perfusion

Definition: Vulnerable to a decrease in cardiac (coronary) circulation, which may compromise health.

Risk Factors
- Hypovolemia
- Hypoxemia
- Hypertension
- Hypotension
- Vasoconstriction
- Vasodilation
- Embolism
- Stenosis
- Coronary artery disease
- Trauma
- Cardiac tamponade

Outcome Criteria
- Systolic blood pressure is >90 mm Hg.
- Mean arterial pressure is >60 mm Hg.
- Heart rate is <100 beats/min.
- Pulmonary artery pressures are within normal limits or back to baseline.
- Cardiac index is >2.2 L/min/m^2.
- Urine output is >0.5 mL/kg/h or >30 mL/h.
- The 12-lead electrocardiogram is normalized without new Q waves.
- Chest pain is absent.
- CK-MB enzymes, troponin I, and myoglobin levels are within normal range.

Nursing Interventions and Rationale
1. Collaborate with the practitioner regarding administration of fibrinolytic therapy or the preparation of the patient for percutaneous coronary intervention *to restore myocardial blood flow.*
2. Collaborate with the practitioner regarding administration of oxygen at 2 L/min to achieve oxygen saturation measured >90% *to maximize myocardial oxygen supply.*
3. Collaborate with the practitioner regarding administration of sublingual nitroglycerin and/or intravenous nitroglycerin infusion *to augment coronary blood flow and reduce cardiac work by decreasing preload and afterload.*

   a. Do not administer nitrates to patients who have taken phosphodiesterase inhibitors for erectile dysfunction within the last 24 or 48 h (depending on the medication), *as severe hypotension may occur.*

4. Collaborate with the practitioner regarding administration of morphine *to control pain.*
5. Collaborate with the practitioner regarding administration of aspirin, antiplatelet therapy, and heparin *to prevent recurrent thrombosis and inhibit platelet function.*
6. Collaborate with the practitioner regarding administration of beta-blockers *to decrease myocardial oxygen demand and prevent recurrent ischemia.*
7. Collaborate with the practitioner regarding administration of angiotensin-converting enzyme inhibitors *to block the conversion of angiotensin I to angiotensin II, a potent vasoconstrictor.*
8. Maintain the patient on bed rest with bedside commode privileges *to minimize myocardial oxygen demand.*
9. Monitor the patient's hemodynamic and cardiac rhythm status:
   a. Select cardiac monitoring leads based on infarct location and rhythm to obtain the best rhythm for monitoring.
   b. Evaluate cardiac rhythm for the presence of dysrhythmias, which are common complications of myocardial ischemia.
   c. Collaborate with the practitioner regarding administration of antidysrhythmic medications.
   d. Assess serum electrolytes (potassium and magnesium) and arterial blood gases.
   e. Collaborate with the practitioner regarding administration of electrolytes to correct any imbalances.
   f. Monitor ST segment continuously to determine changes in myocardial tissue perfusion.
   g. Monitor the patient's blood pressure at least every hour, as many conditions (eg, drugs, dysrhythmias, myocardial ischemia) may cause hypotension (systolic blood pressure <90 mm Hg).
   h. Treat symptomatic dysrhythmias according to unit's emergency protocol or advanced cardiac life support guidelines.
10. Instruct the patient to avoid Valsalva maneuver, as forced expiration against a closed glottis causes sudden and intense changes in systolic blood pressure and heart rate.

◎ NURSING MANAGEMENT PLAN

Risk for Ineffective Cerebral Tissue Perfusion

Definition: Vulnerable to a decrease in cerebral tissue circulation, which may compromise health.

Risk Factors

- Hypovolemia
- Hypoxemia
- Hypertension
- Hypotension
- Vasoconstriction
- Vasodilation
- Embolism
- Stenosis
- Hemorrhage
- Vascular disease
- Trauma

Outcome Criteria

- Patient is oriented to time, place, person, and situation.
- Pupils are equal and normoreactive.
- Blood pressure is within baseline or ordered parameters.
- Motor function is bilaterally equal.
- Headache, nausea, and vomiting are absent.
- Patient verbalizes importance of and displays compliance with reduced activity.
- Neurologic deficits are absent.

Nursing Interventions and Rationale

For Ischemia

1. Collaborate with the practitioner regarding administration of fibrinolytic therapy *to facilitate lysis of the clot and restoration of blood flow to affected area.*
2. Monitor the patient for alterations in blood pressure, oxygenation, temperature, rhythm, and glucose levels.
3. Collaborate with the practitioner regarding administration of vasodilators for hypertension *to maintain the patient's blood pressure within desired range.* Use caution in lowering blood pressure, *as hypotension decreases cerebral blood flow.*
   a. Patients receiving fibrinolytic therapy—keep systolic blood pressure <185 mm Hg and diastolic blood pressure <110 mm Hg.
   b. Patients not receiving fibrinolytic therapy—keep systolic blood pressure <220 mm Hg and diastolic blood pressure <120 mm Hg.
4. Collaborate with the practitioner regarding administration of intravenous fluids and vasoconstrictors for hypotension, *as hypotension decreases cerebral blood flow.*
5. Collaborate with the practitioner regarding administration of oxygen to maintain oxygen saturation measured >95% *to prevent hypoxemia and potential worsening of the neurologic injury.*
6. Collaborate with the practitioner regarding administration of acetaminophen for elevated temperature *because hyperthermia is associated with increased morbidity in patients with stroke.*
7. Collaborate with the practitioner regarding the treatment of dysrhythmias *resulting from increased sympathetic nervous system stimulation.*
8. Collaborate with the practitioner regarding administration of insulin for hyperglycemia, *as elevated blood glucose has been linked to an increase in the area of infarct.*

9. Collaborate with the speech therapist regarding the patient's ability to swallow before initiating oral feedings *to ensure the patient is not at risk for aspiration.*
10. Collaborate with the physical therapist to assess the patient's ability to ambulate safely *to ensure the patient is not at risk for falling* and ability to perform activities of daily living *to facilitate discharge home.*
11. Maintain surveillance for complications such as increased intracranial pressure, seizures, and acute lung failure.
12. Collaborate with the practitioner and rehabilitation specialist regarding the patient's need for rehabilitation *to maximize the patient's independence.*

For Hemorrhage

1. Assess for indicators of increased intracranial pressure and brain herniation (see the nursing management plan for Decreased Intracranial Adaptive Capacity Related to Failure of Normal Intracranial Compensatory Mechanism).
2. Collaborate with the practitioner regarding administration of anticonvulsant medications *to prevent the onset of seizures or to control seizures.*
3. Collaborate with the practitioner regarding administration of vasodilators for hypertension *to avoid further bleeding.* Use caution in lowering blood pressure, *as hypotension decreases cerebral blood flow.*
   a. If systolic blood pressure is >200 mm Hg or mean arterial pressure is >150 mm Hg, aggressive reduction in blood pressure is indicated.
   b. If systolic blood pressure is >180 mm Hg or mean arterial pressure is >130 mm Hg in the presence of increased intracranial pressure, cautious reduction in pressure is indicated maintaining cerebral perfusion pressure >60–80 mm Hg.
   c. If systolic blood pressure is >180 mm Hg or mean arterial pressure is >130 mm Hg in the absence of elevated intracranial pressure, reduction in blood pressure is indicated with a target of 160/90 mm Hg.
4. Collaborate with the practitioner regarding administration of insulin for hyperglycemia, *as elevated blood glucose has been linked to an increase in the area of infarct.*
5. Collaborate with the practitioner regarding administration of acetaminophen for elevated temperature *because hyperthermia is associated with increased morbidity in patients with stroke.*
6. Initiate precautions *to prevent rebleeding.*
   a. Ensure bed rest in a quiet environment *to lessen external stimuli.*
   b. Maintain a darkened room to lessen symptoms of photophobia.
   c. Restrict visitors, and instruct them to keep conversation as nonstressful as possible.
   d. Administer sedatives as prescribed *to reduce anxiety to promote rest.*
   e. Administer analgesics as prescribed *to relieve or lessen headache.*
   f. Provide a soft, high-fiber diet and stool softeners to prevent constipation, which can lead to straining and increased risk of rebleeding.
   g. Assist with activities of daily living (feeding, bathing, dressing, toileting).
   h. Avoid any activity that could lead to increased intracranial pressure; ensure that the patient does not flex hips beyond 90 degrees and avoids neck hyperflexion, hyperextension, or lateral hyperrotation *that could impede jugular venous return.*
7. Collaborate with the physical therapist to assess the patient's ability to ambulate safely *to ensure the patient is not at risk for falling* and ability to perform activities of daily living *to facilitate discharge home.*
8. Collaborate with the practitioner and rehabilitation specialist regarding the patient's need for rehabilitation *to maximize the patient's independence.*

◎ NURSING MANAGEMENT PLAN

Risk for Ineffective Gastrointestinal Perfusion

Definition: Vulnerable to decrease in gastrointestinal circulation, which may compromise health.

Risk Factors
- Hypovolemia
- Hypoxemia
- Hypertension
- Hypotension
- Vasoconstriction
- Vasodilation
- Embolism
- Stenosis
- Vascular disease
- Trauma

Outcome Criteria
- Normal bowel sounds are present.
- Abdominal pain, distention, and guarding are absent.
- Vital signs are at baseline.

Nursing Interventions and Rationales

1. Collaborate with the practitioner regarding administration of crystalloids, colloids, blood, and blood products *to maintain adequate circulating volume.* Implement the nursing management plan for Deficient Fluid Volume Related to Absolute Loss.
2. Collaborate with the practitioner regarding pain management. Implement the nursing management plan for Acute Pain Related to Transmission and Perception of Cutaneous, Visceral, Muscular, or Ischemic Impulses.
3. Collaborate with the practitioner regarding administration of oxygen to maintain oxygen saturation >92% *to prevent hypoxemia and potential worsening of the gastrointestinal injury.*
4. Collaborate with the practitioner regarding administration of electrolyte replacement therapy *to maintain adequate electrolyte balance.*
5. Collaborate with the dietitian regarding administration of nutrition *because the patient will be unable to eat.* Implement the nursing management plan for Imbalanced Nutrition: Less Than Body Requirements.
6. Maintain surveillance for complications such as gastrointestinal hemorrhage, hypovolemic shock, and septic shock.
7. Collaborate with the practitioner regarding preparation for surgery *to remove infarcted bowel.*

◎ NURSING MANAGEMENT PLAN

Risk for Ineffective Peripheral Tissue Perfusion

Definition: Vulnerable to a decrease in blood circulation to the periphery, which may compromise health.

Risk Factors
- Hypovolemia
- Hypoxemia
- Hypertension
- Hypotension
- Vasoconstriction
- Vasodilation
- Embolism
- Stenosis
- Iatrogenic (arterial catheters, intraaortic balloon pump catheters)
- Vascular disease
- Trauma

Outcome Criteria
- Peripheral pulses are full and equal bilaterally.
- Capillary refill is equal bilaterally.
- Ischemic pain is absent.
- Skin temperature is equal in both extremities.
- Skin is pink and warm in both extremities.
- Paresthesias are absent.

Nursing Interventions and Rationale
1. Collaborate with the practitioner regarding administration of antiplatelet, anticoagulant, or fibrinolytic therapy.
2. Collaborate with the practitioner regarding pain management. Implement the nursing management plan for Acute Pain Related to Transmission and Perception of Cutaneous, Visceral, Muscular, or Ischemic Impulses.
3. Ensure the patient is adequately hydrated *to decrease blood viscosity.*
4. Maintain the affected extremity in dependent position if possible *to enhance blood flow.*
5. Keep the affected extremity warm, and protect it from injury. *Do not apply heat directly to the affected extremity because this can result in injury.*
6. Maintain surveillance for pain, pallor, pulselessness, paresthesia, paralysis, and poikilothermia *as indicators of abrupt change in blood flow.*
7. Maintain surveillance for tissue breakdown and arterial ulcers *as indicators of injury.*
8. Prepare the patient for possible surgery or interventional procedure to restore blood flow.

◉ NURSING MANAGEMENT PLAN

Risk for Ineffective Renal Perfusion

Definition: Vulnerable to a decrease in blood circulation to the kidney, which may compromise health.

Risk Factors
- Hypovolemia
- Hypoxemia
- Hypertension
- Hypotension
- Vasoconstriction
- Vasodilation
- Embolism
- Stenosis
- Nephrotoxic medications
- Vascular disease
- Trauma

Outcome Criteria
- Electrolytes are within normal range.
- Serum creatinine and blood urea nitrogen are within normal range.
- Normal acid–base balance is present.
- Urinary output is within normal limits, or patient is stable on dialysis.
- Hemoglobin and hematocrit values are stable.

Nursing Interventions and Rationale
1. Monitor intake and output, urine output, and the patient's weight.
2. Collaborate with the practitioner regarding administration of crystalloids, colloids, blood, and blood products *to increase circulating volume and maintain mean arterial pressure >70 mm Hg.*
3. Collaborate with the practitioner regarding administration of inotropes *to enhance myocardial contractility and increase cardiac index to >2.5 L/min.*
4. Collaborate with the practitioner regarding administration of diuretics to oliguric patient *to flush out cellular debris and increase urine output.*
5. Minimize the patient's exposure to nephrotoxic medications *to decrease damage to kidneys.*
6. Monitor blood levels of drugs cleared by kidneys *to avoid accumulation.*
7. Monitor the patient for signs of electrolyte imbalance *as a result of impaired electrolyte regulation.*
8. Maintain surveillance for signs and symptoms of fluid overload.
9. Monitor the patient's clinical status and response to dialysis therapy *to ensure the patient is receiving safe and effective dialytic therapy.*

◎ NURSING MANAGEMENT PLAN

Risk for Infection

Definition: Vulnerable to invasion and multiplication of pathogenic organisms, which may compromise health.

Risk Factors

- Inadequate primary defenses (eg, broken skin, traumatized tissue, decreased ciliary action, stasis of body fluids, change in pH secretions, altered peristalsis)
- Inadequate secondary defenses (eg, decreased hemoglobin, leukopenia, suppressed inflammatory or immune response)
- Immunocompromised state
- Inadequate acquired immunity
- Tissue destruction and increased environmental exposure
- Chronic disease
- Invasive procedures
- Malnutrition
- Pharmacologic agents (eg, antibiotics, steroids)

Outcome Criteria

- Total lymphocyte count is >1000/mm³.
- White blood cell count is within normal limits.
- Temperature is within normal limits.
- Blood, urine, wound, and sputum culture results are negative.

Nursing Interventions and Rationale

1. Perform proper hand hygiene before and after patient care *to reduce the transmission of microorganisms.*
2. Use appropriate personal protective equipment in accordance with US Centers for Disease Control and Prevention guidelines.
   a. Ensure the practitioner uses maximum barrier precautions when inserting lines.
      (1) Ensure sterile gloves, gown, and mask are worn.
      (2) Drape the patient completely with a sterile sheet.
3. Use aseptic technique for insertion and manipulation of invasive monitoring devices, intravenous lines, and urinary drainage catheters *to maintain sterility of environment.*
   a. Ensure the practitioner uses maximum barrier precautions when inserting lines.
      (1) Ensure sterile gloves, gown, and mask are worn.
      (2) Drape the patient completely with a sterile sheet.
4. Stabilize all invasive lines and catheters *to avoid unintentional manipulation and contamination.*
5. Use aseptic technique for dressing changes *to prevent contamination of wounds or insertion sites.*
6. Change any line placed under emergent conditions within 24 h *because aseptic technique is usually breached during an emergency.*
7. Collaborate with the practitioner to change any dressing that is saturated with blood or drainage *because these are media for microorganism growth.*
8. Minimize use of stopcocks and maintain caps on all stopcock ports *to reduce the ports of entry for microorganisms.*
9. Avoid the use of nasogastric tubes, nasotracheal tubes, and nasopharyngeal suctioning in the patient with a suspected cerebrospinal fluid leak *to decrease the incidence of central nervous system infection.*
10. Change ventilator circuits with humidifiers when visibly soiled or mechanically malfunctioning *to avoid introducing microorganisms into the system.* Do not change routinely.
11. Provide the patient with a clean manual resuscitation bag *to avoid cross-contamination between patients.*

12. Provide oral care to a patient with an artificial airway or an unresponsive patient every 2–4 h and as needed (PRN) *to decrease the incidence of hospital-acquired pulmonary infections.*
    a. Swab mouth and moisten lips every 4 h.
    b. Brush teeth with in-line suction toothbrush every 12 h. Rinse or swab the patient's mouth with chlorhexidine after brushing.
    c. Suction subglottic secretions (secretions pooling above the cuff of the endotracheal tube or tracheostomy tube) every 12 h and before repositioning the tube or deflation of the cuff.
    d. Provide lip balm to keep the patient's lips moistened PRN.
    e. Provide mouth moisturizer to keep the patient's mouth moistened PRN.
13. Cleanse in-line suction catheters with sterile saline according to the manufacturer's instructions *to avoid accumulation of secretions within the catheter.*
14. Maintain the head of the bed elevated at 30 to 45 degrees in patients with an artificial airway *to decrease the incidence of aspiration.*
15. Use disposable sterile scissors, forceps, and hemostats *to reduce transmission of microorganisms.*
16. Maintain a closed urinary drainage system *to decrease incidence of urinary infections.*
17. Keep the urinary drainage tubing and bag below the level of the patient's bladder *to prevent the backflow of urine.*
18. Assess the urinary drainage tubing for kinks *to prevent stasis of urine.*
19. Protect all access device sites from potential sources of contamination (nasogastric reflux, draining wounds, ostomies, sputum).
20. Refrigerate parenteral nutrition solutions and opened enteral nutrition formulas *to inhibit bacterial growth.*
21. Maintain daily surveillance of invasive devices for signs and symptoms of infection.
22. Notify the practitioner of elevated temperature or if any signs or symptoms of infection are present.

Additional Interventions for Patient Receiving Immunosuppressive Drugs

1. Obtain blood, urine, and sputum cultures for temperature elevations >38°C (100.4°F), *as elevation likely is caused by bacteremia or bladder or pulmonary infection.*
2. Auscultate breath sounds at least every 6 h. *Pulmonary infection is the most common type of infection, and changes in breath sounds might be an early indication.*
3. Inspect wounds at least every 8 h for redness, swelling, or drainage, *which may indicate infection.*
4. Inspect overall skin integrity and oral mucosa for signs of breakdown, *which place the patient at risk for infection.*
5. Notify the practitioner of new-onset cough. *Even a nonproductive cough may indicate pulmonary infection.*
6. Monitor white blood cell count daily, and report leukocytosis or sudden development of leukopenia, *which may indicate an infectious process.*
7. Protect the patient from exposure to any staff or family member with a contagious lesion (eg, herpes simplex) or respiratory infections.
8. Collaborate with the dietitian regarding the patient's nutrition status and need for augmentation of nutrition intake as necessary *to prevent debilitation and increased susceptibility to infection.*
9. Collaborate with the practitioner to remove invasive lines and catheters as soon as possible *to decrease potential portals of entry.*
10. Teach the patient the clinical manifestations of infection. *A knowledgeable patient will seek medical attention promptly, which will result in earlier treatment and a decreased risk that infection will become life-threatening.*

NURSING MANAGEMENT PLAN

Situational Low Self-Esteem

Definition: Development of a negative perception of self-worth in response to a current situation.

Situational Low Self-Esteem Related to Feelings of Guilt About Physical Deterioration
Defining Characteristics
- Inability to accept positive reinforcement
- Lack of follow-through
- Nonparticipation in therapy
- Not taking responsibility for self-care (ie, self-neglect)
- Self-destructive behavior
- Lack of eye contact

Outcome Criteria
- Patient verbalizes feelings of self-worth.
- Patient maintains positive relationships with significant others.
- Patient manifests active interest in appearance by completing personal grooming daily.

Nursing Interventions and Rationale
1. Evaluate the meaning of health-related situation. How does the patient feel about himself or herself, the diagnosis, and the treatment? How does the present situation fit into the larger context of his or her life?
2. Assess the patient's emotional level, interpersonal relationships, and feeling about himself or herself. Recognize the patient's uniqueness (eg, how the hair is worn, preference for name used).
3. Help the patient discover and verbalize feelings and understand the crisis by listening and providing information.
4. Assist the patient to identify strengths and positive qualities that increase the sense of self-worth. Focus on past experiences of accomplishment and competency. Help the patient with positive self-reinforcement. Reinforce the love and affection of family and significant others.
5. Assess coping techniques that have been helpful in the past. Help the patient decide how to handle negative or incongruent feedback about the situation.
6. Encourage visits from family and significant others. Facilitate interactions, and ensure privacy. Help family members entering the critical care unit by explaining what they will see. Increase visitors' comfort with equipment; offer chairs and other courtesies.
7. Encourage the patient to pursue interest in individual or social activities, even though difficult in the critical care unit.
8. Reflect caring, concern, empathy, respect, and unconditional acceptance in nurse-patient relationships.
9. The nurse is a significant other for the patient who provides important appraisals of the patient and who can facilitate the change process.
10. Help the family support the patient's self-esteem.
11. Provide for continuity of nurse assignment to ensure consistent contacts that can *facilitate support of the patient's self-esteem.*

◎ NURSING MANAGEMENT PLAN

Unilateral Neglect

Definition: Impairment in sensory and motor response, mental representation, and spatial attention of the body and the corresponding environment characterized by inattention to one side and overattention to the opposite side. Left-side neglect is more severe and persistent than right-side neglect.

Unilateral Neglect Related to Perceptual Disruption
Defining Characteristics

- Neglect of involved body parts and/or extrapersonal space
- Denial of existence of the affected limb or side of body
- Denial of hemiplegia or other motor and sensory deficits
- Left homonymous hemianopia
- Difficulty with spatial-perceptual tasks
- Left hemiplegia

Outcome Criteria

- Patient is safe and free from injury.
- Patient is able to identify safety hazards in the environment.
- Patient recognizes disability and describes physical deficits present (eg, paralysis, weakness, numbness).
- Patient demonstrates ability to scan the visual field to compensate for loss of function or sensation in affected limbs.

Nursing Interventions and Rationale

1. Adapt environment to the patient's deficits *to maintain patient safety.*
   a. Position the patient's bed with the unaffected side facing the door.
   b. Approach and speak to the patient from the unaffected side. If the patient must be approached from the affected side, announce your presence as soon as entering the room *to avoid startling the patient.*
   c. Position the call light, bedside stand, and personal items on the patient's unaffected side.
   d. If the patient will be assisted out of bed, simplify the environment *to eliminate hazards* by removing unnecessary furniture and equipment.
   e. Provide frequent reorientation of the patient to the environment.
   f. Observe the patient closely, and anticipate his or her needs. *Despite repeated explanations, the patient may have difficulty retaining information about the deficits.*
   g. When the patient is in bed, elevate his or her affected arm on a pillow *to prevent dependent edema and support the hand in a position of function.*
2. Assist the patient to recognize the perceptual defect.
   a. Encourage the patient to wear any prescriptive corrective glasses or hearing aids *to facilitate communication.*
   b. Instruct the patient to turn the head past midline *to view the environment on the affected side.*
   c. Encourage patient to look at the affected side and to stroke the limbs with the unaffected hand. Encourage handling of the affected limbs *to reinforce awareness of the affected side.*
   d. Instruct the patient to look for the affected extremity when performing simple tasks *to know where it is at all times.*
   e. After pointing to them, have the patient name the affected parts.
   f. Encourage the patient to use self-exercises (eg, lifting the affected arm with the unaffected hand).
   g. If the patient is unable to discriminate between the concepts of *right* and *left*, use descriptive adjectives such as "the weak arm," "the affected leg," or "the good arm" to refer to the body. Use gestures, not just words, to indicate right and left.

3. Collaborate with the patient, practitioner, and rehabilitation team *to design and implement a beginning rehabilitation program for use during the critical care unit stay.*
   a. Use adaptive equipment (braces, splints, slings) as appropriate.
   b. Teach the patient the individual components of any activity separately, and then proceed to integrate the component parts into a completed activity.
   c. Instruct the patient to attend to the affected side, if able, and to assist with bathing or other tasks.
   d. Use tactile stimulation to reintroduce the arm or leg to the patient. Rub the affected parts with different textured materials to stimulate sensations (eg, warm, cold, rough, soft).
   e. Encourage activities that require the patient to turn the head toward the affected side, and retrain the patient to scan the affected side and environment visually.
   f. If the patient is allowed out of bed, cue him or her with reminders to scan visually when ambulating. Assist and remain in constant attendance *because the patient may have difficulty maintaining correct posture, balance, and locomotion.* There may be vertical-horizontal perceptual problems, with the patient leaning to the affected side to align with the perceived vertical. Provide sitting, standing, and balancing exercises before getting the patient out of bed.
4. Assist the patient with oral feedings.
   a. Avoid giving the patient any very hot food items that could cause injury.
   b. Place the patient in an upright sitting position if possible.
   c. Encourage the patient to feed himself or herself; if necessary, guide the patient's hand to the mouth.
   d. If the patient is able to feed himself or herself, place one dish at a time in front of the patient. When the patient is finished with the first, add another dish. Tell the patient what he or she is eating.
   e. Initially, place food in the patient's visual field; then gradually move the food out of the field of vision and teach the patient to scan the entire visual field.
   f. When the patient has learned to visually scan the environment, offer a tray of food with various dishes.
   g. Instruct the patient to take small bites of food and to place the food in the unaffected side of the mouth.
   h. Teach the patient to sweep out pockets of food with the tongue after every bite *to eliminate retained food in the affected side of the mouth.*
   i. After meals or oral medications, check the patient's oral cavity for pockets of retained material.
5. Initiate patient and family health teaching.
   a. Assess to ensure that the patient and the family understand the nature of the neurologic deficits and the purpose of the rehabilitation plan.
   b. Teach the proper application and use of any adaptive equipment.
   c. Teach the importance of maintaining a safe environment, and point out potential environmental hazards.
   d. Instruct family members how to facilitate relearning techniques (eg, cueing, scanning visual fields).

Physiologic Formulas for Critical Care

HEMODYNAMIC EQUATIONS

Mean (Systemic) Arterial Pressure (MAP)

$$MAP = \frac{(Diastolic \times 2) + (Systolic \times 1)}{3}$$

Systemic Vascular Resistance (SVR)

$$\frac{MAP - RAP}{CO} = SVR \text{ in Wood units}$$

Normal range is 10–18 Wood units.

$$\frac{MAP - RAP}{CO} \times 80 = SVR \text{ in dyn·sec·cm}^{-5}$$

Normal range is 800–1400 dyn·s·cm^{-5}.

Systemic Vascular Resistance Index (SVRI)

$$\frac{MAP - RAP}{CI} \times 80 = SVR \text{ in dyn·sec·cm}^{-5}/m^2$$

Normal range is 2000–2400 dyn·s·cm^{-5}/m^2.

Pulmonary Vascular Resistance (PVR)

$$\frac{PAP \text{ mean} - RAP}{CO} = PVR \text{ in units}$$

Normal range is 1.2–3 units.

$$\frac{PAP \text{ mean} - RAP}{CO} \times 80 = PVR \text{ in dyn·sec·cm}^{-5}$$

Normal range is 100–250 dyn·s·cm^{-5}.

Pulmonary Vascular Resistance Index (PVRI)

$$\frac{PAP \text{ mean} - PAOP}{CI} \times 80 = PVR \text{ in dyn·sec·cm}^{-5}/m^2$$

Normal range is 225–315 dyn·s·cm^{-5}/m^2.

CI, cardiac index; CO, cardiac output; PAOP, pulmonary arterial occlusion pressure (wedge pressure); PAP, pulmonary arterial pressure; RAP, right atrial pressure.

Left Cardiac Work Index (LCWI)

Step 1. $MAP \times CO \times 0.0136 = LCW$

Step 2. $\dfrac{LCW}{BSA} = LCWI$

Normal range is 3.4–4.2 kg-m/m^2.

Left Ventricular Stroke Work Index (LVSWI)

Step 1. $MAP \times SV \times 0.0136 = LVSW$

Step 2. $\dfrac{LVSW}{BSA} = LVSWI$

Normal range is 50–62 g-m/m^2.

Right Cardiac Work Index (RCWI)

Step 1. $PAP \text{ mean} \times CO \times 0.0136 = RCW$

Step 2. $\dfrac{RCW}{BSA} = RCWI$

Normal range is 0.54–0.66 kg-m/m^2.

Right Ventricular Stroke Work Index (RVSWI)

Step 1. $PAP \text{ mean} \times SV \times 0.0136 = RVSW$

Step 2. $\dfrac{RVSW}{BSA} = RVSWI$

Normal range is 7.9–9.7 g-m/m^2.

Corrected Q–T Interval (Q–Tc)

$$\frac{QT}{\sqrt{(RR \text{ interval})}} = QTc$$

Body Surface Area (BSA)

Many hemodynamic formulas can be indexed or adjusted to body size by use of a BSA nomogram (Fig. B.1). To calculate BSA:
1. Obtain height and weight.
2. Mark height on the left scale and weight on the right scale.
3. Draw a straight line between the two points marked on the nomogram.

The number where the line crosses the middle scale is the BSA value.

FIG. B.1 Body surface area (BSA) nomogram.

PULMONARY FORMULAS

Shunt Equation (Qs/Qt)

$$\frac{Qs}{Qt} = \frac{Cc_{O_2} - Ca_{O_2}}{Cc_{O_2} - Cv_{O_2}}$$

Cc_{O_2} = Pulmonary capillary oxygen content (calculated value)
Ca_{O_2} = Arterial oxygen content (calculated value)
Cv_{O_2} = Venous oxygen content (calculated value)
Normal range is less than 5%.

Pulmonary Capillary Oxygen Content (Cc_{O_2})

$$Cc_{O_2} = (Hgb \times 1.34 \times Sc_{O_2}) + (Pc_{O_2} \times 0.003)$$

Hgb = Hemoglobin (measured via laboratory sample or arterial blood gas)
Sc_{O_2} = Pulmonary capillary oxygen saturation
Pc_{O_2} = Partial pressure of oxygen in capillary blood
Normal range is greater than 19 mL/dL.

Arterial Oxygen Content (Ca_{O_2})

$$Ca_{O_2} = (Hgb \times 1.34 \times Sa_{O_2}) + (0.003 \times Pa_{O_2})$$

Hgb = Hemoglobin (measured via laboratory sample or arterial blood gas)
Sa_{O_2} = Arterial oxygen saturation (measured via arterial blood gas)
Pa_{O_2} = Partial pressure of oxygen in arterial blood (measured via arterial blood gas)
Normal range is 17–20 mL/dL.

Venous Oxygen Content (Cv_{O_2})

$$Cv_{O_2} = (Hgb \times 1.34 \times Sv_{O_2}) + (0.003 \times Pv_{O_2})$$

Hgb = Hemoglobin (measured via laboratory sample or arterial blood gas)
Sv_{O_2} = Mixed venous oxygen saturation (measured via mixed venous blood gas)
Pv_{O_2} = Partial pressure of oxygen in mixed venous blood (measured via mixed venous blood gas)
Normal range is 12–15 mL/dL.

Alveolar Pressure of Oxygen (Pa_{O_2})

$$Pa_{O_2} = Fi_{O_2} \times (Pb - Ph_2O) - Pac_{O_2}/RQ$$

Fi_{O_2} = Fraction of inspired oxygen (obtained from oxygen settings)
Pb = Barometric pressure (assumed to be 760 mm Hg at sea level)
Ph_2O = Water pressure in the lungs (assumed to be 47 mm Hg)
Pac_{O_2} = Partial pressure of carbon dioxide in arterial blood (measured via arterial blood gas)
RQ = Respiratory quotient (assumed to be 0.8)
Normal range is 60–100 mm Hg.

Arterial/Inspired Oxygen Ratio

$$Pa_{O_2}/Fi_{O_2} \text{ ratio} = \frac{Pa_{O_2}}{Fi_{O_2}}$$

Pa_{O_2} = Partial pressure of oxygen in arterial blood (measured via arterial blood gas)

FIO_2 = Fraction of inspired oxygen (obtained from oxygen settings)
Normal range is greater than 300.

Arterial/Alveolar Oxygen Ratio

$$PaO_2/PAO_2 = \frac{PaO_2}{PAO_2}$$

PaO_2 = Partial pressure of oxygen in arterial blood (measured via arterial blood gas)
PAO_2 = Partial pressure of oxygen in alveoli (calculated value)
Normal range is greater than 0.75 (75%).

Alveolar-Arterial Gradient

$$P(A-a)O_2 = PAO_2 - PaO_2$$

PAO_2 = Partial pressure of oxygen in alveoli (calculated value)
PaO_2 = Partial pressure of oxygen in arterial blood (measured via arterial blood gas)
Normal range is 25–65 mm Hg.

Dead Space Equation (Vd/VT)

$$Vd/Vt = \frac{PaCO_2 - PETCO_2}{VtPaCO_2}$$

$PaCO_2$ = Partial pressure of carbon dioxide in arterial blood (measured via arterial blood gas)
$PETCO_2$ = Partial pressure of carbon dioxide in exhaled gas (measured via end-tidal CO_2 monitor)
Normal range is 0.2–0.4 (20%–40%).

Static Compliance (C_ST)

This value is calculated for mechanically ventilated patients.

$$C_{ST} = \frac{VT}{PP} - PEEP$$

VT = Tidal volume (obtained from ventilator)
PP = Plateau pressure (measured via ventilator)
$PEEP$ = Positive end-expiratory pressure (obtained from ventilator)
Normal range is 60–100 mL/cm H_2O.

Dynamic Compliance (C_DY)

Also called *characteristic*, this value is calculated for mechanically ventilated patients.

$$C_{DY} = \frac{VT}{PIP} - PEEP$$

VT = Tidal volume (obtained from ventilator)
PIP = Peak inspiratory pressure (obtained from ventilator)
$PEEP$ = Positive end-expiratory pressure (obtained from ventilator)
Normal range is 40–80 mL/cm H_2O.

NEUROLOGIC FORMULAS

Cerebral Perfusion Pressure (CPP)

$$CCP = MAP - ICP$$

MAP = Mean arterial pressure (measured via arterial line or blood pressure cuff)

ICP = Intracranial pressure (measured via ICP monitoring device)
Normal range is 60–150 mm Hg.

Arteriojugular Oxygen Difference (AjDO_2)

$$AjDO_2 = (SaO_2 - SjvO_2) \times 1.34 \times Hgb$$

SaO_2 = Arterial oxygen saturation (measured via arterial blood gas)
$SjvO_2$ = Jugular venous oxygen saturation (measured via jugular blood gas or jugular venous catheter)
Hgb = Hemoglobin (measured via laboratory sample or arterial blood gas)
Normal range is 5–7.5 mL/dL.

ENDOCRINE FORMULAS

Serum Osmolality

$$Serum\ osmolality = 2(Na^+ + K^+) + \frac{Glucose}{18} + \frac{BUN}{2.8}$$

Na^+ = Sodium
K^+ = Potassium
BUN = Blood urea nitrogen
Normal range is 275–295 mOsm/kg of water.

Fluid Volume Deficit in Liters

$$Fluid\ volume\ deficit = \frac{0.6(kg/weight) \times (Na^+ - 140)}{140}$$

Na^+ = Sodium

KIDNEY FORMULAS

Anion Gap

$$[Na^+] - ([Cl^-] + [HCO_3^-])$$

Normal range is 8–16 mEq.

Clearance

$$Clearance = U \times \frac{(V)}{(P)}$$

U = Concentration of substance in urine
V = Time
P = Concentration of substance in plasma
Normal range depends on substance measured.

NUTRITIONAL FORMULAS

Caloric and Protein Needs[1]

Estimating Caloric Needs

Indirect calorimetry is the most accurate way to estimate energy needs. When indirect calorimetry is unavailable, there are many predictive equations, some are derived from testing hospitalized patients (e.g. Penn State, Ireton-Jones, and Swinamer equations) and some are derived from testing healthy volunteers (e.g. Harris-Benedict, Mifflin St Jeor equations). For critically ill patients, currently guidelines recommend using indirect calorimetry if available. In the absence of indirect calorimetry, guidelines recommend using a simple weight-based equation of 25 – 30 kcal/kg/day to estimate energy requirements. The weight used for this calculation should be dry weight or usual body weight if patients are following aggressive volume resuscitation or have edema or anasarca. Note that predictive equations in general are less accurate in underweight and obese patients.

For obese critically ill patients, if indirect calorimetry is unavailable, current guidelines recommend using the weight-based equation of 11 – 14 kcal/kg of *actual* body weight per day for patients with BMI in the range of 30 – 50 kg/m², and 22 – 25 kcal/kg *ideal* body weight per day for patients with BMI >50 kg/m².

Estimating Protein Needs

Protein needs vary with the degree of malnutrition and stress. In the critical care setting, adequate protein provision is key in ensuring healing, immune function, and maintaining lean body mass. Nitrogen balance studies are the most accurate way to assess protein needs. When nitrogen balance studies are unavailable, weight-based equations of 1.2 – 2.0 g/kg *actual* body weight/day are recommended. Patients with burns and/ or have multi-trauma may require protein provision on the higher end of recommendations or may be in the range of 1.5 – 2.0 g/kg/day.

For obese critically ill patients, protein should be provided in a range from 2.0 g/kg *ideal* body weight per day for patients with BMI of 30 – 40 kg/m² up to 2.5 g/kg *ideal* body weight per day for patients with BMI >40 kg/m². Protein recommendations should be re-evaluated based on nitrogen balance studies with the goal of achieving nitrogen equilibrium.

REFERENCE

1. Mclave, Stephen A, et al. Guidelines for the Provision and Assessment of Nutrition Support Therapy in the Adult Critically Ill Patient: Society of Critical Care Medicine (SCCM) and American Society for Parenteral and Enteral Nutrition (ASPEN). *Journal of Parenteral & Enteral Nutrition.* 2016;40.2:159.

Note: Page numbers followed by *f* indicate figure, by *t* table, and by *b* box.

1053

SPECIAL FEATURES